KEEP THIS BOOK!

WHEN YOU **PURCHASED**

Physical Rehabilitation, you didn't just buy a required text for your course, you invested in a curriculum-spanning resource that will guide you from your first class to preparing for the NPTE.

WHEN YOU
START YOUR CAREER

Physical Rehabilitation will be your most trusted reference for client/patient care in whichever setting you work.

WHEN YOU
THINK ABOUT SELLING

Physical Rehabilitation at the end of the semester for a few dollars, don't. Use it as you grow from a rookie to a seasoned clinician.

A Classic and a must in your shelf of PT books. "I have had this book ever since I was in college and it has proven to be valuable to me now that I am in my 11th year of practice as it was when I was still in my budding internship."

Five Stars. "This book is very comprehensive and contains almost everything you need to know for the NPTE exam."

This book is every Physical Therapy Students Bible. "...if you purchase this book during your first semester of PT school, it will help you immensely! Don't wait until Neuro PT to purchase this book. Use this book as a guide for every PT class from Integumentary to Pediatrics to Neuroanatomy!"

—Online Reviewers

O'Sullivan & Schmitz's
PHYSICAL REHABILITATION

EIGHTH EDITION

KEEP THIS BOOK!

WHEN YOU **PURCHASED**

Physical Rehabilitation, you didn't just buy a required text for your course, you invested in a curriculum-spanning resource that will guide you from your first class to preparing for the NPTE.

WHEN YOU **START YOUR CAREER**

Physical Rehabilitation will be your most trusted reference for client/patient care in whichever setting you work.

WHEN YOU **THINK ABOUT SELLING**

Physical Rehabilitation at the end of the semester for a few dollars, don't. Use it as you grow from a rookie to a seasoned clinician.

A Classic and a must in your shelf of PT books. "I have had this book ever since I was in college and it has proven to be valuable to me now that I am in my 11th year of practice as it was when I was still in my budding internship."

Five Stars. "This book is very comprehensive and contains almost everything you need to know for the NPTE exam."

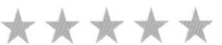

This book is every Physical Therapy Students Bible. "...if you purchase this book during your first semester of PT school, it will help you immensely! Don't wait until Neuro PT to purchase this book. Use this book as a guide for every PT class from Integumentary to Pediatrics to Neuroanatomy!"

—Online Reviewers

O'Sullivan & Schmitz's
PHYSICAL REHABILITATION
EIGHTH EDITION

George D. Fulk, PT, PhD, FAPTA
Professor and Director of the Center for Physical Therapy and Movement Science
Director of the Division of Physical Therapy
Department of Rehabilitation Medicine
School of Medicine
Emory University
Atlanta, Georgia

Kevin K. Chui, PT, DPT, PhD, GCS, OCS, CEEAA, FAAOMPT
Endowed Chair and Professor
Department of Physical Therapy
Waldron College of Health and Human Services
Radford University
Roanoke, Virginia

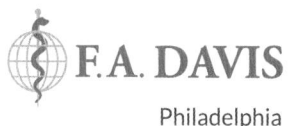
F.A. DAVIS
Philadelphia

F. A. Davis Company
1915 Arch Street
Philadelphia, PA 19103
www.fadavis.com

Printed in the United States of America

Last digit indicates print number: 10 9 8 7 6 5 4 3 2 1

Acquisitions Editor: Jennifer A. Pine
Director of Content Development: George W. Lang
Developmental Editor: Laura S. Horowitz
Content Project Manager: Julie Chase
Art and Design Manager: Carolyn O'Brien

As new scientific information becomes available through basic and clinical research, recommended treatments and drug therapies undergo changes. The author(s) and publisher have done everything possible to make this book accurate, up to date, and in accord with accepted standards at the time of publication. The author(s), editors, and publisher are not responsible for errors or omissions or for consequences from application of the book, and make no warranty, expressed or implied, in regard to the contents of the book. Any practice described in this book should be applied by the reader in accordance with professional standards of care used in regard to the unique circumstances that may apply in each situation. The reader is advised always to check product information (package inserts) for changes and new information regarding dose and contraindications before administering any drug. Caution is especially urged when using new or infrequently ordered drugs.

Library of Congress Cataloging-in-Publication Data

Names: Fulk, George D., editor. | Chui, Kevin K., editor.
Title: O'Sullivan and Schmitz's physical rehabilitation / [edited by]
  George D. Fulk, Kevin K. Chui.
Other titles: Physical rehabilitation | Physical rehabilitation
Description: Eighth edition. | Philadelphia : F. A. Davis Company, [2024] |
  Preceded by Physical rehabilitation / [edited by] Susan B. O'Sullivan,
  Thomas J. Schmitz, George Fulk. Seventh edition. 2019. | Includes
  bibliographical references and index.
Identifiers: LCCN 2023042727 (print) | LCCN 2023042728 (ebook) | ISBN
  9781719646918 (hardback) | ISBN 9781719651479 (epub) | ISBN
  9781719651486 (Adobe PDF)
Subjects: MESH: Physical Therapy Modalities | Physical Examination--methods
  | Disability Evaluation | Orthopedic Equipment
Classification: LCC RM700 (print) | LCC RM700 (ebook) | NLM WB 460 | DDC
  615.8/2--dc23/eng/20231117
LC record available at https://lccn.loc.gov/2023042727
LC ebook record available at https://lccn.loc.gov/2023042728

The eighth edition of *O'Sullivan and Schmitz's Physical Rehabilitation* is dedicated to Dr. Susan O'Sullivan and Dr. Tom Schmitz. As faculty members at Boston University in the mid-1970s, Susan and Tom saw a need for a textbook that covered the breadth of adult rehabilitation. At the time, there were no textbooks dedicated to physical therapy. First published in 1980, *Physical Rehabilitation* was one of the first, if not the first, textbook that was written by and for physical therapists. Through their continued efforts, in concert with the outstanding authors who have contributed to the book, *Physical Rehabilitation* has facilitated physical therapy student and physical therapist assistant student learning for over 40 years. Susan and Tom's excellence is supported by the fact that *Physical Rehabilitation* is consistently among the most widely used textbooks in physical therapy and physical therapist assistant education. The impact Susan and Tom have had on physical therapy education and practice through this book is immeasurable. The profession of physical therapy is indebted to Susan and Tom.

With the eighth edition of *O'Sullivan and Schmitz's Physical Rehabilitation,* we continue a tradition of striving for excellence that was started by Dr. O'Sullivan and Dr. Schmitz more than 40 years ago. They had a vision to create a comprehensive textbook that was written by and for physical therapists. The addition of "O'Sullivan and Schmitz" to the title of the textbook honors the amazing work and broad influence on physical therapy education and practice that Susan and Tom have had over the life span of the textbook. We are humbled and appreciative of the trust that they have placed in us to continue their legacy as the editors of the *O'Sullivan and Schmitz's Physical Rehabilitation.* We will continue to strive for excellence.

The text is designed to provide a comprehensive approach to the rehabilitation management of adult patients and clients. As such, it is intended to serve as a primary textbook for physical therapy students and as an important resource for practicing therapists as well as for other rehabilitation professionals. The eighth edition recognizes the continuing evolution of the profession and integrates basic and applied research to guide and inform evidence-based practice. It also integrates principles of patient/client management (examination, evaluation, diagnosis, prognosis, intervention, and outcomes) presented in the American Physical Therapy Association's *Guide to Physical Therapist Practice* and terminology from the World Health Organization's International Classification of Functioning, Disability, and Health.

O'Sullivan and Schmitz's Physical Rehabilitation is organized into three sections. Section One (Chapters 1 to 9) includes chapters on clinical decision-making and examination of basic systems as well as examination of function and the environment. Section Two (Chapters 10 to 29) addresses many of the diseases, disorders, and health conditions commonly seen in the rehabilitation setting. Appropriate examination and intervention strategies are discussed for related body structure/function impairments, activity limitations, participation restrictions in societal interactions, and quality of life. Health promotion and wellness strategies are also considered. Emphasis is placed on parameters of learning critical to ensuring the patient/client can achieve identified goals and expected outcomes. The final section, Section Three (Chapters 30 to 32), includes orthotics, prosthetics, and seating and wheeled mobility.

A central element of the text is a strong pedagogical format designed to facilitate and reinforce the learning of key concepts. Each chapter of *O'Sullivan and Schmitz's Physical Rehabilitation* includes an initial content outline, learning objectives, an introduction and summary, questions for review (self-assessment), and extensive references. Web-based resources for clinicians and patients/families are also provided. Application of important concepts is promoted through end-of-chapter case studies, which include guiding questions designed to enhance clinical decision-making skills. Many health condition–focused chapters contain *Tables of Outcome Measures* emphasizing tests and measures commonly used in clinical practice, and *tables* that summarize and critically appraise research relevant to the chapter content. Our hope is that these tables may provide a model for readers to continue to critically examine clinical practice using high-quality research findings. We also hope it will inspire enthusiasm about the importance of lifelong and self-directed learning.

The visuals have been enhanced with the addition of new illustrations and photographs. Design changes and a full-color format provide a reader-friendly environment and augment understanding of content. Valuable resources for the eighth edition include seven immersive online case studies with accompanying video segments and guiding questions. These video cases illustrate important components of the history taking, initial examination, and interventions for patients undergoing rehabilitation. Importantly, these video cases provide students with opportunities for critical thinking and clinical decision-making and to receive feedback from expert clinicians on why certain tests and interventions were performed. The cases were authored by practicing therapists from various parts of the country who were directly involved in the care of the case study patient participant. The clinical decision-making skills and clinical skills of these dedicated case study contributors are well represented in the online materials. The case studies include the following:

Immersive Case A: A Patient With Long COVID/
Post-Acute Sequelae of COVID-19

Immersive Case B: A Patient With Acute COVID-19

Immersive Case C: A Patient With Stroke

Immersive Case D: A Patient With Multiple Sclerosis

Immersive Case E: A Patient With Mild Parkinson
Disease (**mini-case**)

Immersive Case F: A Patient With Freezing of Gait
Due to Parkinson Disease

Immersive Case G: A Patient With a Lower Extremity
Limb Loss Following Amputation

Questions are posed that address key elements in developing the plan of care for each patient. All case study materials (patient history, examination data, video segments, answers to guiding questions for student feedback) are available online at www.FADavis.com. Suggested answers to the end-of-chapter case study *Guiding Questions* and *Questions for Review* (self-assessment) are also available online. In separate files, also available at www.FADavis.com, answers to the questions are provided for student feedback.

As we have gratefully noted with previous editions, our greatest asset and inspiration in preparing the eighth edition of *O'Sullivan and Schmitz's Physical Rehabilitation* has been an extraordinary group of contributing authors. We are most fortunate to have this group of talented individuals whose breadth and scope of professional knowledge and experience seem unparalleled. These individuals are recognized experts from a variety of specialty areas who have graciously shared their knowledge and clinical practice expertise by providing relevant, up-to-date, and practical information within their respective content areas.

The eighth edition has also benefited from the input of numerous individuals engaged in both academic and clinical practice settings who have used and reviewed the content. We are grateful for their constructive feedback and have instituted many of their suggestions and changes. As always, we welcome suggestions for improvements from our colleagues and students.

As physical therapists continue to take on more and greater professional responsibilities and challenges, the very nature of this text makes it a perpetual "work in progress." We are grateful for the opportunity to contribute to the academic literature in physical therapy, as well as to the professional development of those preparing to enter a career devoted to improving the quality of life of those we serve.

We acknowledge the very important contributions that physical therapists make in the lives of their patients. This book is dedicated to those therapists—past, present, and future—who guide and challenge their patients to lead a successful and independent life and who work toward building a community to improve the health of society.

—GEORGE D. FULK
KEVIN K. CHUI

Edward W. Bezkor, PT, DPT, OCS, MTC, CAFS
Assistant Program Director
Department of Physical Therapy, University of St. Augustine
for Health Sciences
San Marcos, California

Janet R. Bezner, PT, DPT, PhD, NBC-HWC, FAPTA
Professor and Chair
Department of Physical Therapy
Associate Dean, College of Health Professions
Texas State University
Round Rock, Texas

Beth Black, PT, DSc
Professor Emerita
Physical Therapy Program
School of Health Sciences
Oakland University
Rochester, Michigan

Mark Bowden, PT, PhD
*Professor and Director, MUSC Division of Physical
Therapy*
Research Health Scientist, Ralph H. Johnson VA Medical
Center
Charleston, South Carolina

Judith M. Burnfield, PT, PhD
Vice President Research
Director Movement and Neurosciences Center
Clifton Chair in Physical Therapy and Movement Science
Madonna Rehabilitation Hospitals
Lincoln, Nebraska

Guilherme M. Cesar, PT, PhD
Department of Physical Therapy
Brooks College of Health
University of North Florida
Jacksonville, Florida

Heidi Cheerman, PT, MS, DPT, NCS
Assistant Clinical Professor
Department of Physical Therapy, Movement and
Rehabilitation Sciences
Bouvé College of Health Sciences
Northeastern University
Boston, Massachusetts

Tzurei Chen, PT, PhD, GCS
Associate Professor
School of Physical Therapy and Athletic Training
College of Health Professions
Pacific University
Hillsboro, Oregon

Kevin K. Chui, PT, DPT, PhD, GCS, OCS, CEEAA,
FAAOMPT
Endowed Chair and Professor
Department of Physical Therapy
Waldron College of Health and Human Services
Radford University
Roanoke, Virginia

Laura J. Cohen, PhD, PT, ATP/SMS, RESNA
Fellow
Founder and Principal
Rehabilitation and Technology Consultants, LLC
Arlington, Virginia

Shala Cunningham, PT, DPT, PhD, OCS,
FAAOMPT
Associate Professor
Department of Physical Therapy
Waldron College of Health and Human Services
Radford University
Roanoke, Virginia

Vanina Dal Bello-Haas, PT, PhD
Professor
School of Rehabilitation Science
McMaster University
Hamilton, Ontario, Canada

Amy DeBlois, PT, DPT, NCS
Department of Physical Therapy Education
SUNY Upstate Medical University
Syracuse, New York

Judith E. Deutsch, PT, PhD, FAPTA
Professor and Director Rivers Lab
Department of Rehabilitation and Movement Sciences
Rutgers Biomedical and Health Science
School of Health Professions
Rutgers University
Newark, New Jersey

Konrad J. Dias, PT, DPT, PhD, CCS
Professor
Department of Physical Therapy
College of Health and Human Services
California State University, Sacramento
Sacramento, CA

Lee Dibble, PT, PhD, ATC, FAPTA
Professor, Department Chair
Department of Physical Therapy and Athletic Training
University of Utah
Salt Lake City, Utah

Nora E. Fritz, PT, DPT, PhD, NCS
Associate Professor
Departments of Physical Therapy and Neurology
Wayne State University
Detroit, Michigan

George D. Fulk, PT, PhD, FAPTA
Professor and Director
Division of Physical Therapy
Department of Rehabilitation Medicine
Emory University School of Medicine
Atlanta, Georgia

Jessica Galgano, PhD, CCC-SLP
NYU Grossman School of Medicine
Open Lines Speech and Communication PLLC
LSVT Global, Inc.
New York, New York

Tamara N. Gravano, PT, DPT, MSPT, EdD
Board-Certified Specialist in Geriatric Physical Therapy
Certified Exercise Expert for Aging Adults

Eric J. Hegedus, PT, DPT, PhD, MHSc, OCS
Program Director
Doctor of Physical Therapy Program
Department of Public Health and Community Medicine
School of Medicine
Tufts University
Phoenix, Arizona

Maura Daly Iversen, PT, DPT, SD, MPH, FNAP, FAPTA
Dean, College of Health Professions
Professor of Physical Therapy and Public Health
Sacred Heart University
Fairfield, Connecticut
Epidemiologist, Division of Rheumatology, Immunology and Immunity
Brigham and Women's Hospital
Boston, Massachusetts

Deborah G. Kelly, PT, MSEd, DPT, CLT-LANA
Associate Professor
Department of Physical Therapy
College of Health Sciences
University of Kentucky
Lexington, Kentucky

Dennis W. Klima, PT, MS, PhD, DPT, GCS, NCS
Professor
Department of Physical Therapy
University of Maryland Eastern Shore
Princess Anne, Maryland

Daniel J. Lee, PT, DPT, PhD, GCS, OCS, COMT
Chair and Clinical Associate Professor
Department of Physical Therapy
School of Health Professions
Stony Brook University
Stony Brook, NY

Margery A. Lockard, PT, PhD
Clinical Professor (retired)
Health Sciences Department
Physical Therapy and Rehabilitation Sciences Department
College of Nursing and Health Professions
Drexel University
Philadelphia, Pennsylvania

Kimberly L. Malin, PT, MS, DHSc, NCS
Associate Professor
School of Physical Therapy and Athletic Training
College of Health Professions
Pacific University
Hillsboro, Oregon

Jessica Maxwell, PT, DPT, PhD
Professor and Program Director
School of Physical Therapy
South College
Nashville, Tennessee

Tara L. McIsaac, PT, PhD
Professor
Department of Physical Therapy
School of Pharmacy and Health Professions
Creighton University – Phoenix
Phoenix, Arizona

Richard J. McKibben, PT, DSc, ECS
Faculty, Doctor of Science in Health Science
Rocky Mountain University of Health Professions
Provo, Utah
Owner/Electromyographer
Integrity Rehab Management, LLC
Hamilton, Georgia

Coby D. Nirider, PT, DPT
Chief Clinical Officer/Administrator
Brookhaven Hospital, LLC
Tulsa, Oklahoma

Susan B. O'Sullivan, PT, EdD
Professor Emerita
Department of Physical Therapy and Kinesiology
Zuckerberg College of Health Sciences
University of Massachusetts Lowell
Lowell, Massachusetts

Evangelos Pappas, PT, MSc, PhD
Professor and Associate Dean (intoHEALTH)
University of Wollongong
Wollongong, Australia
Honorary Professor, Discipline of Physiotherapy,
The University of Sydney

Kevin M. Parcetich Jr., PT, DPT, NCS
Assistant Professor
Department of Physical Therapy
Waldron College of Health and Human Services
Radford University
Roanoke, Virginia

Ingrid S. Parry, MS, PT, BT-C
Shriners Hospitals for Children, Northern California
University of California, Davis
Sacramento, California

Pat Precin, PhD, PsyaD, NCPsyA, LP, OTR/L, FAOTA
Assistant Professor of Rehabilitation and Regenerative Medicine
Programs in Occupational Therapy
Columbia University
New York, New York

Leslie N. Russek, PT, DPT, PhD, OCS
Professor Emeritus
Physical Therapy Department
Lewis School of Health Sciences
Clarkson University
Potsdam, New York

Martha Taylor Sarno CCC-SLP; MA, Fellow ASHA; Honors of the Association, MD *(hon)*
Research Professor
Department of Rehabilitation Medicine
NYU School of Medicine
New York, New York

Faith Saftler Savage, PT, ATP
Seating Specialist
The Boston Home
Boston, Massachusetts

David A. Scalzitti, PT, PhD
Associate Professor
Department of Health, Human Function, & Rehabilitation Sciences
George Washington University
Washington, District of Columbia

Thomas J. Schmitz, PT, PhD
Professor Emeritus
Department of Physical Therapy
School of Health Professions
Long Island University
Brooklyn, New York

Michael C. Schubert, PT, PhD, FAPTA
Professor
Laboratory of Vestibular NeuroAdaptation
Department of Otolaryngology—Head and Neck Surgery
Department of Physical Medicine and Rehabilitation
Johns Hopkins University School of Medicine
Baltimore, Maryland

Scott W. Shaffer, PT, PhD, ECS
Associate Dean/Professor
School of Physical Therapy
University of the Incarnate Word
San Antonio, Texas

Wagner H. Souza, PT, PhD
Postdoctoral Fellow
Laboratory of Vestibular NeuroAdaptation
Department of Otolaryngology—Head and Neck Surgery
Department of Biomedical Engineering
Johns Hopkins University School of Medicine
Baltimore, Maryland

Julie Ann Starr, PT, DPT, CCS, FAPTA
Clinical Associate Professor Emerita
Department of Physical Therapy
College of Health and Rehabilitation Sciences: Sargent College
Boston University
Boston, Massachusetts

Tina M Stoeckmann, PT, DSc
Clinical Professor
Residency Program Academic Coordinator
Department of Physical Therapy
Marquette University
Milwaukee, Wisconsin

Carolyn A. Unsworth, PhD, BAppSci(OccTher), GCTE, OTR, MRCOT, FOTARA
Discipline Lead Occupational Therapy
Institute of Health and Wellbeing
Federation University Australia
Adjunct Professor, Monash University, Australia
Adjunct Professor, Jönköping University, Sweden
Adjunct Professor, James Cook University, Australia
Melbourne, Victoria, Australia

R. Scott Ward, PT, PhD, FAPTA, BT-C, Certified Burn Therapist
Professor
Department of Physical Therapy and Athletic Training
University of Utah
Salt Lake City, Utah

Brian J. Wilkinson, PT, DPT, CHT, CLT
Associate Professor
School of Physical Therapy and Athletic Training
College of Health Professions
Pacific University
Hillsboro, Oregon

Gavin Williams, PT, PhD, FACP
Professor of Physiotherapy Rehabilitation
Epworth Healthcare and The University of Melbourne
Melbourne, Victoria, Australia

Christopher Kevin Wong, PT, PhD, OCS
Professor
Programs in Physical Therapy
Vagelos College of Physicians and Surgeons
Columbia University
New York, New York

2222

Michelle Wormley, PT, MPT, PhD, CLT
Associate Professor
Department of Physical Therapy and Human Movement
   Science
College of Health Professions
Sacred Heart University
Fairfield, Connecticut

Pei-Tzu Wu, PT, PhD, CCS
Assistant Professor
School of Physical Therapy and Athletic Training
College of Health Professions
Pacific University
Hillsboro, Oregon

Sheng-Che Yen, PT, PhD
Clinical Professor
Department of Physical Therapy, Movement and
   Rehabilitation Sciences
Bouvé College of Health Sciences
Northeastern University
Boston, Massachusetts

ACKNOWLEDGMENTS

The ongoing development of *O'Sullivan and Schmitz's Physical Rehabilitation* has been in all aspects a collaborative venture. Its fruition has been made possible only through the expertise and gracious contributions of many talented individuals. Our appreciation is considerable.

Heartfelt thanks are extended to our contributing authors. Each has brought a unique body of knowledge, as well as distinct clinical practice expertise, to their respective chapters. Their commitment to physical therapist education is collectively displayed in content presentations that carefully reflect the scope of knowledge and skills required of a dynamic, evolving physical therapy practice environment. We are extremely grateful to each of our contributors and heartened by the excellence they bring to the eighth edition.

Heartfelt thanks are also extended to the practicing clinicians who prepared the case studies and video segments. Their contributions expertly move text content to clinical practice and significantly add to the development of the clinical reasoning skills of our readers.

Our appreciation goes to the dedicated professionals at F.A. Davis Company: Margaret Biblis, Editor-in-Chief; Jennifer Pine, Acquisitions Editor; Julie Chase, Content Project Manager; George Lang, Content Director; Paul Marino, and Amy Gibbons, former and current Senior Developmental Editors of Digital Products; Michael Kern, Editorial Department Associate; and Kate Margeson, Illustration Coordinator. These individuals are recognized for their continued support, encouragement, and unwavering commitment to excellence. Thanks also are extended to Cassie Carey, Senior Production Editor, and Rose Boul, Senior Art Coordinator, at Graphic World Publishing Services.

Importantly, we cannot thank Laura Horowitz, from York Content Development, enough for her assistance with editing. Her skills and knowledge have greatly enhanced the textbook, and the final product would not have been as good without her.

We wish to thank the numerous students, faculty, and clinicians who over the years have used *O'Sullivan and Schmitz's Physical Rehabilitation* and provided us with meaningful and constructive comments that have greatly enhanced this edition. It is our sincere hope that this feedback will continue.

Finally, we are grateful to Drs. O'Sullivan and Schmitz for providing us with this opportunity. We hope to continue to build on their work with the goal of continually improving the text to meet the evolving needs of physical therapy students, educators, clinicians, and other health-care professionals.

—George D. Fulk
Kevin K. Chui

Physical Rehabilitation was first published in 1981, and through its seven editions since, has become one of the most used and beloved texts in physical therapy education. Even as leadership of the eighth edition transfers into the capable hands of Dr. George Fulk and Dr. Kevin Chui, the contributions and impact of Dr. O'Sullivan and Dr. Schmitz's work endures. F. A. Davis Company is proud to have been a partner in this title's success and henceforth recognizes the original author's work with the permanent addition of their names to the title.

CONTENTS

SECTION ONE: ## Clinical Decision-Making and Examination

Chapter 1: **Clinical Decision-Making** *1*
Judith E. Deutsch • Susan B. O'Sullivan

Chapter 2: **Examination of Vital Signs** *31*
Shala Cunningham • Thomas J. Schmitz

Chapter 3: **Examination of Sensory Function** *67*
Kimberly L. Malin • Heidi Cheerman • Kevin K. Chui • Sheng-Che Yen

Chapter 4: **Musculoskeletal Examination** *103*
Evangelos Pappas • Eric J. Hegedus

Chapter 5: **Examination of Motor Function: Motor Control and Motor Learning** *125*
Susan B. O'Sullivan • Scott W. Shaffer • Richard J. McKibben

Chapter 6: **Examination of Coordination and Balance** *181*
Dennis W. Klima • Thomas J. Schmitz • Susan B. O'Sullivan

Chapter 7: **Examination of Gait** *216*
Judith M. Burnfield • Guilherme M. Cesar

Chapter 8: **Examination of Function** *271*
David A. Scalzitti

Chapter 9: **Examination and Modification of the Environment** *293*
Kevin M. Parcetich Jr. • Thomas J. Schmitz

SECTION TWO: ## Intervention Strategies for Rehabilitation

Chapter 10: **Strategies to Improve Motor Function** *333*
Tina M. Stoeckmann • Susan B. O'Sullivan

Chapter 11: **Strategies to Improve Locomotor Function** *368*
George D. Fulk • Lee Dibble

Chapter 12: **Chronic Pulmonary Dysfunction** *382*
Pei-Tzu Wu • Julie Ann Starr

Chapter 13: **Heart Disease** *415*
Konrad J. Dias

Chapter 14: **Vascular, Lymphatic, and Integumentary Disorders** *469*
Tamara N. Gravano • Brian J. Wilkinson • Deborah G. Kelly

Chapter 15: **Stroke** *523*
Judith E. Deutsch

Chapter 16: **Multiple Sclerosis** *588*
Nora E. Fritz • Tara L. McIsaac

Chapter 17: **Amyotrophic Lateral Sclerosis** *635*
Vanina Dal Bello-Haas

Chapter 18: **Parkinson Disease** *679*
Tara L. McIsaac • Edward W. Bezkor

Chapter 19: **Traumatic Brain Injury** *726*
George D. Fulk • Coby Nirider • Gavin Williams • Amy DeBlois

Chapter 20: **Traumatic Spinal Cord Injury** *759*
Amy DeBlois • Mark Bowden • George D. Fulk

Chapter 21:   **Vestibular Disorders** *815*
Wagner H. Souza • Michael C. Schubert

Chapter 22:   **Amputation** *849*
Tzurei Chen • Kevin K. Chui • Sheng-Che Yen • Kevin M. Parcetich • Margery A. Lockard

Chapter 23:   **Arthritis** *889*
Maura Daly Iversen • Michelle Wormley

Chapter 24:   **Burns** *939*
R. Scott Ward • Ingrid S. Parry

Chapter 25:   **Chronic Pain** *966*
Leslie N. Russek

Chapter 26:   **Psychosocial Issues in Physical Rehabilitation** *1012*
Pat Precin

Chapter 27:   **Cognitive and Perceptual Dysfunction** *1054*
Carolyn A. Unsworth

Chapter 28:   **Neurogenic Disorders of Speech and Language** *1098*
Martha Taylor Sarno • Jessica Galgano

Chapter 29:   **Promoting Health and Wellness** *1119*
Janet R. Bezner • Jessica Maxwell • Beth Black

SECTION THREE: # Orthotics, Prosthetics, and Seating and Wheeled Mobility

Chapter 30:   **Orthotics** *1149*
Christopher Kevin Wong • Daniel J. Lee

Chapter 31:   **Prosthetics** *1180*
Christopher Kevin Wong • Daniel J. Lee

Chapter 32:   **Seating and Wheeled Mobility** *1223*
Laura J. Cohen • Faith Saftler Savage

Index *1285*

The immersive case series adheres to a standardized format allowing clinical experts to skillfully lead students through the clinical decision-making process of evaluation and treatment of seven distinct patients experiencing one of six unique health conditions. Rooted in the International Classification of Functioning, Disability, and Health (ICF) framework, the cases are thoughtfully divided into eight segments, with the exception of Case E, which is presented as a condensed mini-case. The segment composition varies from case to case with each segment incorporating an activity designed to refine students' clinical decision-making skills. Throughout the case, subject matter experts remain a constant presence, providing invaluable guidance at every step. They draw attention to key points, ensuring students not only observe but also comprehend the nuances of each case.

Immersive Case Coordinator

Rebecca Martin, PT, DPT, PhD
Board Certified Clinical Specialist in Neurologic Physical Therapy
Co-Chair ANPT CSM Program Committee
Lead Consultant
Wildfire Global Consulting
Potsdam, NY

IMMERSIVE CASE A — A Patient With Long COVID/Post-Acute Sequelae of COVID-19

Jenna L. Tucker, PT, DPT, NCS, CBIS
Clinical Assistant Professor
Kean University
Union, NJ

Lauren Ziaks, PT, DPT, ATC, NCS
Certificate in Vestibular Rehabilitation, 2021
Board Certified Clinical Specialist in Neurologic Physical Therapy
Concussion Specialist, Advanced Rehabilitation Clinician—Intermountain Healthcare, Park City Hospital
Independent Contractor, Washington Orthopedic Spine & Injury Center
Co-founder - Phoenixconcussionrecovery.com
Board of Directors - CONNECT Summit County
Park City, UT

IMMERSIVE CASE B — A Patient With Acute COVID-19

Daniel G. Miner, PT, DPT, NCS
Assistant Professor
Department of Physical Therapy
Radford University Carilion
Roanoke, VA

IMMERSIVE CASE C — A Patient With Stroke

Christina Garrity, PT, DPT, NCS
Founder and Physical Therapist
Labyrinth Physical Therapy & Wellness
Dayton, OH

IMMERSIVE CASE D   # A Patient With Multiple Sclerosis

Rebecca Martin, PT, DPT, PhD
Board Certified Clinical Specialist in Neurologic Physical Therapy
Co-Chair ANPT CSM Program Committee
Lead Consultant
Wildfire Global Consulting
Potsdam, NY

IMMERSIVE CASE E   # A Patient With Mild Parkinson Disease (mini-case)

IMMERSIVE CASE F   # A Patient With Freezing of Gait Due to Parkinson Disease

Tara L. McIsaac, PT, PhD
Professor
Department of Physical Therapy
School of Pharmacy and Health Professions
Creighton University—Phoenix
Phoenix, AZ

Jamie Nesbit, PT, DPT
Board Certified Neurologic Clinical Specialist (ABPTS)
Board Certified Geriatric Clinical Specialist (ABPTS)
Department of Physical Therapy
School of Pharmacy and Health Professions
Assistant Professor
Creighton University—Phoenix
Phoenix, AZ

IMMERSIVE CASE G   # A Patient With a Lower Extremity Limb Loss Following Amputation

William Riddick, PT, DPT, GCS
Board Certified Clinical Specialist in Geriatric Physical Therapy
Outpatient PT Clinical Leader—Sheltering Arms Institute
Clinical Adjunct Faculty
Old Dominion University
Co-Chair Amputation Care Special Interest Group (APTA Federal)

Luke Utley, PT, D.P.T.
Physical Therapist
Department of Physical Medicine and Rehabilitation
Mayo Clinic
Rochester, MN

Fourteen video case studies continued from the seventh edition are available online at https://www.fadavis.com/product/physical-rehabilitation-fulk-8. Each includes a narrative presentation and three accompanying video segments (examination, intervention, and outcomes) together with guiding questions designed to challenge clinical decision-making skills. Student feedback is provided via suggested answers to the guiding questions posted in a separate online file.

CASE STUDY 1: ## Critical Care Patient in the Intensive Care Unit

(applicable to Chapters 1, 2, 12, and 13)

James Tompkins, PT, DPT
Department of Physical Medicine and Rehabilitation
Mayo Clinic Hospital
Phoenix, Arizona

Joseph L. Verheijde, PhD, MBA, PT
Department of Physical Medicine and Rehabilitation
Mayo Clinic Hospital
Scottsdale, Arizona

Bhavesh M. Patel, MD, FRCPC
Departments of Critical Care and Respiratory Care
Mayo Clinic Hospital
Phoenix, Arizona

CASE STUDY 2: ## Patient With Burns

(applicable to Chapter 24)

Jill Quarles, PT, MS • Sophie Manning, PT, BSc
Michigan Medicine
Ann Arbor, Michigan

CASE STUDY 3: ## Patient With a Below Knee Amputation

(applicable to Chapter 22)

Kim Stover Rosso, PT, MSPT • Laura Pink-Baker, PT, DPT
Michigan Medicine
Ann Arbor, Michigan

CASE STUDY 4: ## Patient With Spinal Cord Injury

(applicable to Chapter 20)

Alex Eubank, PT, DPT
Dodd Hall Rehabilitation Services
Ohio State University Wexner Medical Center
Columbus Ohio

CASE STUDY 5: # Patient With Spinal Cord Injury

(applicable to Chapter 20)

Sally Taylor, PT
Shirley Ryan AbilityLab
(Formerly the Rehabilitation Institute of Chicago)
Chicago, Illinois
Assistant Professor
Department of Physical Therapy and Human Movement Sciences
Northwestern University, Feinberg School of Medicine
Chicago, Illinois

CASE STUDY 6: # Patient With Parkinson Disease

(applicable to Chapter 18)

Edward W. Bezkor, PT, DPT, OCS, MTC, CAFS
Assistant Professor
University of St. Augustine for Health Sciences
Doctor of Physical Therapy Program
San Marcos, California

Michelle Farella-Accurso, PT, DPT
New York College of Osteopathic Medicine of New York Institute of Technology
Adele Smithers Parkinson's Disease Research and Treatment Center
Department of Physical Therapy
Old Westbury, New York

CASE STUDY 7: # Patient With Traumatic Brain Injury and Shoulder Amputation

(applicable to Chapters 19 and 22)

Faye Bronstein PT, DPT, NCS
New York University Langone Medical Center
Rusk Institute of Rehabilitation Medicine
New York, New York

CASE STUDY 8: # Patient With Traumatic Brain Injury

(applicable to Chapter 19)

Victoria Stevens, PT, NCS • Kate Rough, PT, DPT, NCS
University of Washington Medical Center
Rehabilitation Medicine
Seattle, Washington

CASE STUDY 9: # Patient With Right Hemorrhagic CVA

(applicable to Chapter 15)

Alicia Esposito O'Hara, PT, DPT, NCS
New York University Langone Medical Center
Rusk Institute of Rehabilitation Medicine
New York, New York

CASE STUDY 10:   # Patient With Left Ischemic CVA

(applicable to Chapter 15)

Greg Hartley, PT, DPT, GCS • Gemma Longfellow, PT, MSPT, GCS • Karen J. Lagares, PT, DPT, GCS
St. Catherine's Rehabilitation Hospital
North Miami, Florida

CASE STUDY 11:   # Patient With Right Thalamic Ischemic Infarct and Left Lateral Medullary Ischemia

(applicable to Chapter 15)

Hendrika Lietz, PT, DPT, NCS
University of Michigan Hospital
Ann Arbor, Michigan

CASE STUDY 12:   # Patient With Right Basal Ganglia Intraparenchymal Hemorrhage

(applicable to Chapter 15)

Patricia Laverty, PT, DPT • Maria Julia Vila, PT, MPT
New York University Langone Medical Center
Rusk Institute of Rehabilitation Medicine
New York, New York

CASE STUDY 13:   # Patient With Vestibular Disorder

(applicable to Chapter 21)

Bryan Hujsak, PT, DPT, NCS
The New York Eye and Ear Infirmary
Vestibular Rehabilitation
New York, New York

CASE STUDY 14:   # Patient With Multiple Sclerosis

(applicable to Chapter 16)

Maria Rundell, PT, DPT, NCS, MSCS
Outpatient Lead Therapist
HealthSouth Rehabilitation Hospital of Colorado Springs
Colorado Springs, Colorado

Clinical Decision-Making and Examination

Clinical Decision-Making

Judith E. Deutsch, PT, PhD, FAPTA
Susan B. O'Sullivan, PT, EdD

Chapter 1

LEARNING OBJECTIVES

1. Describe an integrated framework for making clinical decisions and identify factors that affect clinical decision-making.
2. Describe the International Classification of Function (ICF) and its relationship to physical therapy.
3. Describe the key steps in the *Guide to Physical Therapist Practice* of the patient/client management process.
4. Map a participation goal into its relevant activities (ICF) and tasks (movement science).
5. Explain the role of movement observation of tasks in physical therapist examination.
6. Discuss strategies to promote shared decision-making to develop goals and the plan of care (POC).
7. Identify potential problems that could adversely affect the physical therapist's clinical decision-making.
8. Identify key elements of physical therapy documentation.
9. Discuss the importance of evidence-based practice in examination and developing the POC.
10. Analyze and interpret patient/client data, formulate realistic goals and outcomes, and develop a POC when presented with a clinical case.

CHAPTER OUTLINE

CLINICAL REASONING AND CLINICAL DECISION-MAKING *2*
INTEGRATED FRAMEWORK: ELEMENTS OF CLINICAL REASONING *5*
  Shared Decision-Making *5*
  Hypothesis-Oriented Algorithm for Clinicians (HOAC) *5*
  International Classification of Functioning, Disability, and Health (ICF) *5*
  Movement Science and Movement System *8*
INTEGRATED FRAMEWORK: PATIENT/CLIENT MANAGEMENT *8*
  History and Interview *8*
  Systems Review *9*
  Examination *12*

Evaluation *14*
Diagnosis *15*
Prognosis *16*
Plan of Care *17*
Discharge Planning *22*
Implementation of the Plan of Care *23*
Reexamination of the Patient and Evaluation of Expected Outcomes *23*
DOCUMENTATION *23*
EVIDENCE-BASED PRACTICE *24*
  Using Evidence to Guide Clinical Decisions *24*
SUMMARY *27*

CLINICAL REASONING AND CLINICAL DECISION-MAKING

Clinical reasoning refers to the thinking and decision-making processes that are used in clinical practice.[1] Reasoning is a context-dependent way of thinking and making decisions in professional practice to guide practice actions.[2] It is a multidimensional, nonlinear cognitive process that involves synthesis of information and collaboration with the patient, caregivers, and health-care team. The clinician integrates information about the patient, the task, and the setting to reach decisions and determine actions in accordance with best available evidence. Clinical decisions are the outcomes of the iterative clinical reasoning process and form the basis of patient/client management. Numerous factors influence a clinician's decision-making, including their goals, knowledge base and expertise, psychosocial skills, problem-solving strategies, and procedural skills.

Decision-making is a shared process between the clinician and patient. Each of them brings their characteristics including their beliefs and biases, preferences, and values. The agreed upon goals between the therapist and the patient will be influenced by physical, psychosocial, educational, and cultural factors and overall resources, time, and level of financial and social support.

Frameworks and models may be used to organize the clinical reasoning process. Those frameworks may change over time based on the evolution of the field of physical therapy or the conceptualization of health. For example, the World Health Organization (WHO) used a disablement model (the International Classification of Impairments, Disabilities, and Handicaps [ICIDH]) that evolved into an enablement model called the International Classification of Functioning and Health (ICF).[3] This resulted in changes in vocabulary and perspectives on how to view health (e.g., the term *disease* was replaced with *health condition*). Frameworks can be specific to the profession. In physical therapist practice, the American Physical Therapy Association's (APTA) *Guide to Physical Therapist Practice* is organized using the patient management system. In its third edition,[4] the APTA changed from using the Nagi disablement model[5] to using the enablement model of the ICF.[6] Algorithms are also used to guide decision-making. Physical therapy–specific algorithms include the Hypothesis-Oriented Algorithm for Clinicians (HOAC) I and II.[7] Clinical reasoning is also derived from the knowledge base or science that underpins the profession. Movement science and exercise science are two important bodies of knowledge that inform how we make clinical decisions.

Physical therapists practice in a variety of clinical environments including acute, rehabilitation, and chronic care facilities, as well as schools and community-based settings. They also provide physical therapy remotely (e.g., teleconsultation and telerehabilitation). Therapists have many different roles in these settings, including direct patient care and case management as a member of a collaborative team, with referral to and consultation with other providers and supervision of personnel (e.g., physical therapist assistants, other support staff). Making clinical decisions is influenced by interaction and involvement of other providers, as depicted in Figure 1.1. Decision-making is also influenced by the clinical practice environment.

Primary care is generally the first level of care. Typically, patients are seen by a primary care physician or by a wide range of health-care professionals, including the physical therapist. Therapists provide integrated, accessible health-care services that address a large majority of personal health-care needs; develop a sustained partnership with the physician, other team members, and patient; and practice within the context of family and community. Primary care is provided in a wide variety of settings, including hospitals; rehabilitation centers; clinical practice settings; and school, industrial, or workplace settings.

Secondary care is more specialized and is provided to patients who are initially treated by other practitioners and then referred for specialist treatment and support. Examples of patients who may require secondary care include those with significant spinal cord injury (SCI), traumatic brain injury (TBI), or respiratory or cardiac disease.

Tertiary care is provided to patients in highly specialized, complex, and technology-based settings and in response to requests from other primary or secondary health-care practitioners for consultation and specialized services. Examples include specialized burn units, cancer units, or advanced neonatology services. Across the spectrum of settings, therapists have active roles in prevention and health promotion, wellness, and fitness with a wide variety of populations. Box 1.1 provides a summary of the terminology used to define clinical practice environments.[4]

Physical therapists today practice as primary care providers in complex environments and are called upon to reach increasingly complex decisions under significant practice constraints. For example, a therapist may be required to complete the examination and determine a plan of care (POC) for the patient with complex needs and multiple comorbidities within 24 to 48 hrs of admission to a rehabilitation facility. Limited insurance coverage with high co-pays and limited allocation of physical therapy treatment sessions also complicates the decision-making process.

This chapter presents an integrated framework for clinical decision-making with shared decision-making between the patient and the therapist depicted at the center.[8] It is anchored by the *Guide to Physical Therapist Practice*, uses the language and concepts of the

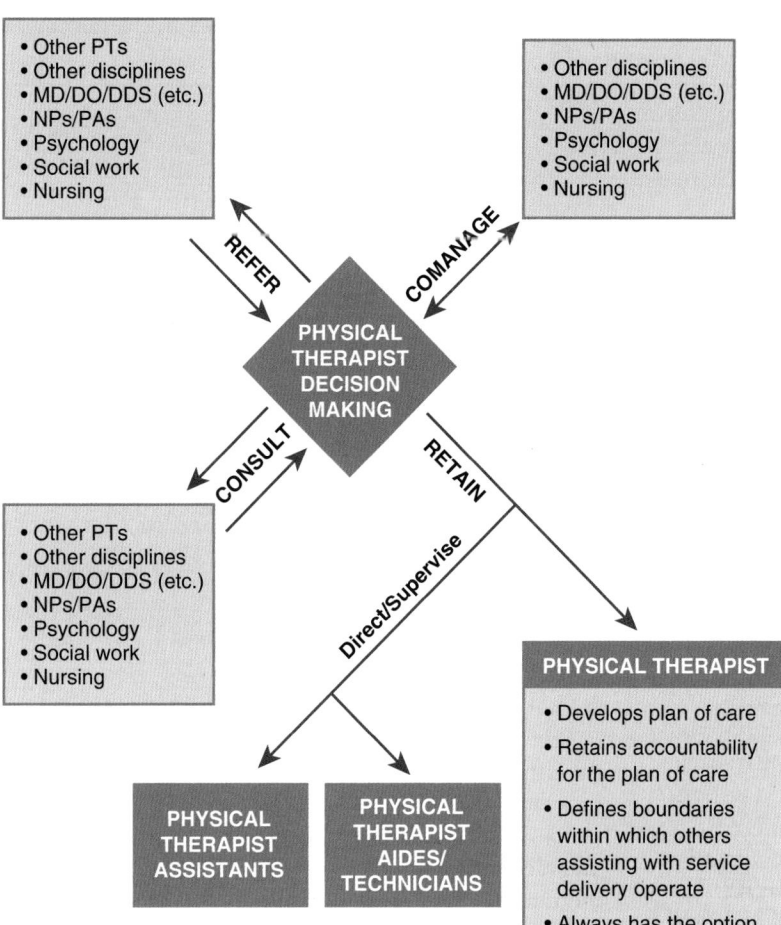

Figure 1.1 Physical therapist decision-making related to the involvement of other providers. *Introduction to the Guide to Physical Therapist Practice.* Guide to Physical Therapist Practice 3.0. *American Physical Therapy Association; 2014. http://guidetopt practice.apta.org/content/1/SEC1.body.*

Box 1.1   Clinical Practice Terminology[4]

Primary care is defined as the provision of integrated, accessible health-care services by clinicians who are accountable for addressing a large majority of personal health-care needs, developing a sustained partnership with patients, and practicing within the context of family and community.

Secondary care is the care provided to patients who are initially treated by other practitioners and then referred to specialists/physical therapists.

Tertiary care is the care provided to patients in highly specialized, complex, and technology-based settings (e.g., burn units) or in response to requests of other health-care practitioners for consultation and specialized services.

Acute care involves the care of individuals with severe symptoms, illnesses, or life- or limb-threatening health conditions, regardless of their cause. It generally serves as an entry point to health care, is short term, and encompasses preventive and primary care.

Rehabilitation includes health-care services that help an individual keep, restore, or improve skills and functioning for daily living that have been lost or impaired because a person was sick, hurt, or disabled. These services may include physical therapy, occupational therapy, speech-language pathology, and psychiatric rehabilitation services in a variety of inpatient and outpatient settings.

Chronic care addresses preexisting or long-term illness and involves a continuum of integrated care over time and delivered in a variety of settings. It addresses loss of functional abilities and assists in helping individuals maintain independence and a high level of functioning. Chronic care encompasses medical care, rehabilitative care, and supportive services.

Telehealth is the delivery of services (consultation-direct care) remotely. May use telecommunications or digital technology.

(Continued)

Box 1.1   Clinical Practice Terminology⁴—cont'd

Prevention is the avoidance, minimization, or delay of the onset of impairment, activity limitation, and/or participation restrictions. Includes primary, secondary, and tertiary prevention initiatives for individuals as well as selective intervention initiatives for subsets of the population at risk for impairments, activity limitations, and/or participation restrictions.

• **Primary prevention** prevents a target condition in a susceptible or potentially susceptible population through specific measures such as general health efforts.
• **Secondary prevention** decreases the duration of illness, severity of disease, and number of sequelae through early diagnosis and prompt intervention.
• **Tertiary prevention** limits the degree of disability and promotes rehabilitation and restoration of function in patients with chronic and irreversible diseases.

Health promotion is any effort taken to allow an individual, group, or community to achieve awareness of—and empowerment to pursue—prevention and wellness. Services include identifying risk factors and implementing services to reduce risk factors, preventing or slowing the functional decline and disability, and enhancing activity, participation, wellness, and fitness.
Wellness is a state of being that incorporates all facets and dimensions of human existence, including physical health, emotional health, spirituality, and social connectivity.
Clinical practice environments include hospitals, rehabilitation centers, outpatient clinical settings, home-based, school-based, sports settings and through telehealth.

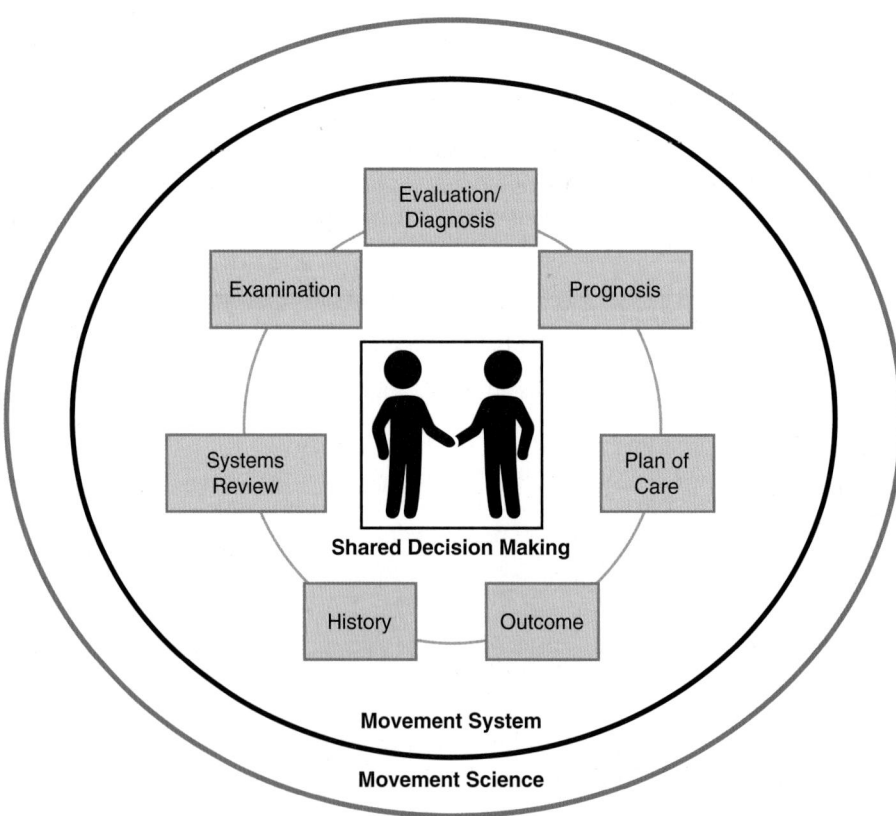

Figure 1.2 Integrated Framework: Illustrates the centrality of the shared decision-making and the influence of both movement science and the movement system in the reasoning process. The patient/client management organizes the steps of the reasoning process. Hypothesis generation occurs at each step. While an episode of care may follow the steps sequentially, a prescribed order is not required.

ICF and Movement Science, as well the Movement System,⁹ and is driven by hypothesis generation and testing consistent with the HOAC. The integration of these frameworks and processes guides patient/client management that can assist in organizing and prioritizing data and in planning effective treatments compatible with the needs and goals of the patient/client and members of the health-care team (see Fig. 1.2). Each of the main elements will be explained further.

■ INTEGRATED FRAMEWORK: ELEMENTS OF CLINICAL REASONING

Shared Decision-Making

The physical therapist and the patient work together to make clinical decisions. Patients are encouraged to consider the benefits and harms of available treatment or management options, communicate their preferences, and collaborate with the clinician to choose the course of action that best fits their preference.[10,11] An integrative model of shared decision-making includes essential elements such as explaining the problem, presenting options, discussing pros and cons of various options, checking patient understanding, deferring a decision about what action to take, and follow-up after the decision is made. Also taken into consideration are individual preferences, abilities, self-efficacy, patient readiness to change, and clinicians' knowledge.[12] A three-phase model of shared decision-making in physical therapy consists of:

1. Preparing for collaboration.
2. Exchanging information on options.
3. Affirming and implementing a decision.[13]

The authors of this model also provided specific evidence-based strategies and resources for implementing shared decision-making including the following:

• Health literacy universal precautions: making sure the clinician's language is simplified.
• Teach back: confirming that the patient understood the communication.
• Motivational interviewing: using techniques to engage the patient by eliciting, understanding, and addressing their ambivalence to adhere to therapy.
• Decision aids: using tools to increase patient knowledge of options and their relative value (for example the Ottawa personal decision guide worksheet to be used across multiple health conditions, https://decisionaid.ohri.ca/decguide.html).[14] These tools have been shown to increase patient confidence, active involvement, and selection of more conservative treatments.[15]

Hypothesis-Oriented Algorithm for Clinicians

Physical therapists may use algorithms to guide their decision-making. An algorithm specific to physical therapy is the hypothesis-oriented algorithm for clinicians (original version, HOAC I, and revised version, HOAC II). The HOAC II[7,16] provides a graphical step-by-step process for clinicians to gather information and tests their hypothesis on how to proceed with the examination and intervention. The HOAC acknowledges that there are both patient-identified problems (PIP) and nonpatient-identified problems (NPIPs). The NPIPs are identified by the clinician, often based on knowledge of

a health condition as well as observation of the patient. Once the problems are identified, there are decision steps and possible choices for evaluation and treatment planning. Hypotheses are generated about why the patient's problems exist, and criteria are generated to test the hypotheses. A series of questions are posed, typically in a branching program of yes/no choices, addressing whether the measurements met testing criteria, the hypotheses generated were viable, goals were met, strategies were appropriate, and tactics were implemented correctly. A "no" response to any of the questions posed in an algorithm is an indication for reevaluation of the viability of the hypotheses generated and reconsideration of the decisions made. In using HOAC as a framework for clinical decision-making, the therapist also distinguishes between existing problems and anticipated problems (including NPIPs), defined as deficits that are likely to occur if an intervention is not used for prevention. The value of an algorithm is that it guides the therapist's decisions and provides an outline of the decisions made. See Chapter 17, Amyotrophic Lateral Sclerosis, for examples of hypothesis-oriented algorithms.

International Classification of Functioning, Disability, and Health

WHO's International Classification of Functioning, Disability, and Health (ICF) provides a model and common language by which to describe health conditions and organize information to classify patient's problems by clearly defining the complex interaction among health condition, body function/structure impairment, activity limitation, participation restriction, and contextual factors.[3] The APTA has joined WHO, World Physical Therapy, and other international professional organizations in endorsing the ICF classification. Figure 1.3 presents the structure of the ICF model.[4]

The ICF provides descriptions of health, health conditions, functioning, and disabilities that are associated with a health condition and contextual factors that can influence outcomes.[17] Health is defined as a state of complete physical, mental, and social well-being and not merely the absence of disease or infirmity. Health condition is an umbrella term for disease, disorder, injury, or trauma and may include other circumstances such as aging, stress, congenital anomaly, or genetic predisposition. It may also include information about pathogeneses and etiology. Health and health condition may be viewed on a continuum from wellness to illness. Body functions are physiological functions of body systems (including psychological functions). Body structures are anatomical parts of the body such as organs, limbs, and their components.

Impairments are the problems an individual may have in body function (physiological functions of body systems) or structure (anatomical parts of the body). The resulting significant deviation or loss is the direct result of the health condition. For example, a patient with

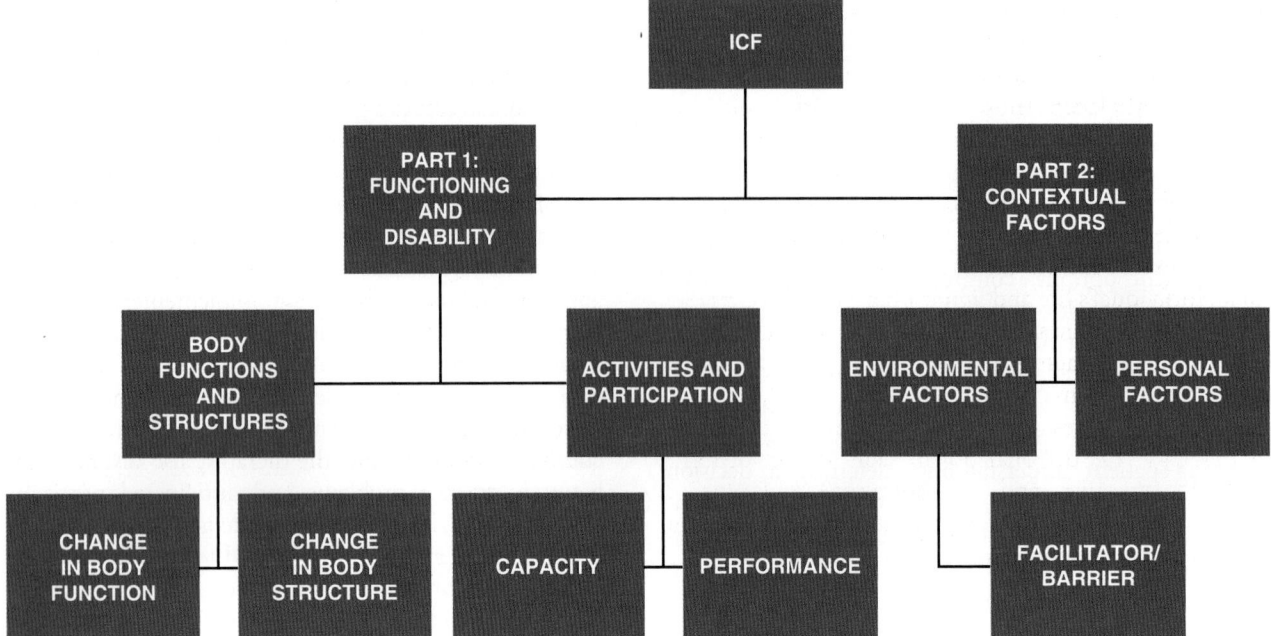

Figure 1.3 Structure of the International Classification of Functioning, Disability, and Health (ICF) model of functioning and disability. *Introduction to the Guide to Physical Therapist Practice.* Guide to Physical Therapist Practice 3.0. *American Physical Therapy Association; 2014. http://guidetoptpractice.apta .org/content/1/SEC1.body.*

stroke may present with sensory loss, paresis, dyspraxia, and hemianopsia (direct impairments). Impairments may be mild, moderate, severe, or complete and may be permanent (e.g., a complete spinal cord injury), resolve as recovery progresses (e.g., normal breathing after pneumonia), or become progressively worse (e.g., for a patient with a neurodegenerative disease such as Parkinson disease). Impairments may also be indirect (secondary), the sequelae or complications that originate from other systems. They can result from preexisting impairments or the expanding multisystem dysfunction that occurs with prolonged bedrest and inactivity, an ineffective POC, or lack of rehabilitation intervention. Examples of indirect impairments for a person with a stroke may include decreased vital capacity and cardiovascular endurance, disuse atrophy and weakness, contractures, pressure injuries, deep vein thrombosis, renal calculi, urinary tract infections, pneumonia, and depression.

Activity is the execution of a task or action by an individual. Activity limitations are difficulties an individual may have in executing tasks or actions. These can include limitations in the performance of cognitive and learning skills; communication skills; functional mobility skills such as transfers, walking, lifting, or carrying objects; and activities of daily living (ADLs). Basic activities of daily living (BADL) include self-care activities of toileting, maintaining hygiene, bathing, dressing, eating, drinking, and having social (interpersonal) interactions. The person with stroke may demonstrate difficulties in all these areas and be unable to perform the actions, tasks, and activities that constitute the "usual activities" for this individual.

Participation is an individual's involvement in a life situation, the societal perspective of functioning. Participation restrictions are problems an individual may experience with involvement in daily life situations and societal interactions. Categories of life roles include home management, work (job/school/play), and community/ leisure. These include instrumental activities of daily living (IADL) such as housecleaning, preparing meals, shopping, telephoning, or other modes of communication, and managing finances, as well as work and leisure activities (e.g., sports, recreation, travel). Thus, the individual with stroke is unable to resume societal roles and activities such as working, parenting, attending church, or playing golf. In the section on examination, the relationships among participation, activity, and body function/structure are further described.

Performance describes what an individual does in their current environment, which includes use of assistive devices or personal assistance, whenever the individual uses them to perform actions or tasks. Performance qualifiers indicate the extent of participation restriction (difficulty) in performing tasks or actions in an individual's current real-life environment. All aspects of the physical, social, and attitudinal world constitute the environment. Difficulty can range from mild to moderate to severe.

Capacity describes an individual's ability to execute a task or an action (highest probable level of functioning in a given domain at a given moment). Capacity qualifiers indicate the extent of activity limitation and are used to describe an individual's highest probable level of functioning (ability to do the task or action). Qualifiers can range from the assistance of a device (e.g., adaptive equipment) or another person (minimal to moderate to maximal assistance) or environmental modification (home, workplace). Thus, the patient with stroke may demonstrate moderate difficulty in locomotion in the home environment (performance qualifiers) and require the use of an ankle-foot orthosis, small-based quad cane, and moderate assistance of one (capacity qualifiers).

Contextual factors represent the entire background of an individual's life and living situation. These include both environmental factors and personal factors. Environmental factors make up the physical, social, and attitudinal environment in which people live and conduct their lives. Factors range from products and technology (for personal use in daily living, communication, mobility, and transportation) and physical factors (home environment, terrain, climate) to social support and relationships (family, friends, personal care

providers), attitudes (individual and societal), and institutions and laws (housing, communication, transportation, legal, financial services, and policies).

Personal factors are the background of an individual's life, including gender, age, coping styles, social background, education, profession, past and current experience, overall behaviors, character, and other factors that influence how disability is experienced by an individual. Qualifiers include factors that serve as barriers or facilitators. Barriers (disablement risk factors) are factors within an individual's environment that, through their absence or presence, limit functioning and create disability. Facilitators (assets) are factors in an individual's environment that, through their absence or presence, improve functioning and disability. Both can range from mild to moderate to strong in their influence on functioning. Box 1.2 summarizes ICF terminology on functioning, disability, and health.[17]

Box 1.2   International Classification of Functioning, Disability, and Health (ICF) Terminology[3,17]

Body functions are physiological functions of body systems (including psychological functions).

Body structures are anatomical parts of the body such as organs, limbs, and their components.

Health is a state of complete physical, mental, and social well-being and not merely the absence of disease or infirmity.

Health condition is an umbrella term for disease, disorder, injury, or trauma and may also include other circumstances, such as aging, stress, congenital anomaly, or genetic predisposition. It may also include information about pathogeneses and etiology.

Impairments are problems in body function or structure such as a significant deviation or loss.

Activity is the execution of a task or action by an individual.

Activity limitations are difficulties an individual may have in executing activities.

Capacity describes an individual's ability to execute a task or an action (probable level of functioning in a given domain at a given moment).

Contextual factors represent the entire background of an individual's life and living situation.

• **Personal factors** are the particular background of an individual's life, including gender, age, coping styles, social background, education, profession, past and current experience, overall behavior pattern, character, and other factors that influence how disability is experienced by an individual.

• **Environmental factors** make up the physical, social, and attitudinal environment in which people live and conduct their lives, including social attitudes, architectural characteristics, and legal and social structures.

• **Barriers** are factors within an individual's environment that, through their absence or presence, limit functioning and create disability.

• **Facilitators** are factors in an individual's environment that, through their absence or presence, improve functioning and disability.

Disability is an umbrella term for impairments, activity limitations, and participation restrictions. It denotes the negative aspects of the interaction between an individual (with a health condition) and that individual's contextual factors (environmental and personal factors).

Functioning encompasses all body functions and structures, activities, and participation.

Participation is an individual's involvement in a life situation; societal perspective of functioning.

Participation restrictions are problems an individual may experience in involvement in life situations. Participation restriction is determined by comparing an individual's participation to that which is expected from an individual without a disability in a particular culture or society.

Performance describes what an individual does in his or her current environment. The current environment includes assistive devices or personal assistance, whenever the individual uses them to perform actions or tasks.

Performance qualifiers indicate the extent of participation restriction (difficulty) in performing tasks or actions in an individual's current real-life environment.

The ICF Checklist is a practical tool to elicit and record information on functioning and disability of an individual.[18] WHO also has Core Sets, which provide a list of body structure/functions, activities, and participation that are commonly seen with certain health conditions. The Core Set is organized into categories such as neurological and musculoskeletal. These can be helpful for novice therapists when first learning the ICF and about a certain health condition (www.icf-research-branch.org/icf-core-sets-projects2).[19]

Movement Science and Movement System

Movement science informs clinical reasoning. Movement science is foundational for physical therapist practice.[20] It includes biomechanics, kinesiology, psychology, and neuroscience.[21] Motor control and motor learning are distinct areas of study within the field of movement science. Many motor control theories guide the examination of movement. One of these is the "systems theory," which frames motor control by examining the relationship between internal attributes of the person (specifically, cognition, perception, and action) and how these interact with the environment and the attributes of the specific movement or task.[22] Movement science terminology provides useful language and tools for the physical therapy examination that are not provided by the ICF.[23] See Chapter 5, Examination of Motor Function, and Chapter 10, Strategies to Improve Motor Function, for further discussion.

The movement system is defined in APTA's vision statement as "a collection of systems (cardiovascular, pulmonary, endocrine, integumentary, nervous, and musculoskeletal) that interact to move the body or its component parts" (www.apta.org/MovementSystem/).[24] In this chapter, it is used as a tool for screening and movement observation. Incorporating the movement system into physical therapy assessment may result in the creation of movement system diagnoses and a guide to interventions. How the movement system is integrated with physical therapist clinical reasoning is an ongoing area of study in the profession.

■ INTEGRATED FRAMEWORK: PATIENT/CLIENT MANAGEMENT

While the ICF offers a high-level model to organize information about a patient's health conditions and many relevant factors to consider when examining and developing a POC for a patient, it is not specific to physical therapy. *The Guide to Physical Therapist Practice*, specifically in the patient/client management section, guides clinical reasoning for physical therapists.

Patient/client management involves identifying and defining the patient's restrictions in participation and activities and impairments of body function and structure as well as the resources available to determine appropriate intervention. It begins with patient referral or initial entry (direct access) and continues as an ongoing process throughout the episode of care. Ongoing reexamination allows the therapist to evaluate progress and modify interventions as appropriate.

The steps in patient/client management include (1) history and interview, (2) systems review, (3) examination, (4) evaluation of the data and identification of problems, (5) determination of the physical therapy diagnosis and prognosis, (6) POC with goals and intervention, and (7) reexamination and evaluation of treatment outcomes (see Fig. 1.2).

History and Interview

Information about the patient's history and current health status is obtained from review of the medical record and interviews with the patient, family, and caregivers. The medical record provides detailed reports from members of the health-care team; processing these reports requires an understanding of the health condition, medical terminology, differential diagnosis, laboratory and other diagnostic tests, and medical management. The use of resource materials or professional consultation can assist the novice clinician.

The initial interview sets the stage for shared decision making. It is an important method used to obtain information from the patient, including learning patient goals, establishing rapport and mutual trust, ensuring open communication lines, and enhancing motivation. Communication skills and questioning techniques (e.g., motivational interviewing) are used to focus on the current health condition, past medical history, personal context, and emotional context. Several strategies are key to ensuring effective patient involvement, including active listening, empathy, building rapport, asking appropriate questions, summarizing and validating patient responses, and effectively using nonverbal communication cues. During the interview, the therapist should listen carefully to what the patient says and ask key questions that allow the patient to express feelings (e.g., What are you most concerned about?) and ideas (e.g., What are your thoughts or ideas about what may have caused this?). What do you expect or hope for? What would be important for us to include in your POC? Empathy is best relayed to the patient by recognizing the patient's feelings and demonstrating understanding of the patient's unique individual experiences (e.g., Can you help me understand how you see or experience your health condition?). Building good rapport allows the patient to feel comfortable and opens the lines of communication. The therapist's communication (e.g., tone of voice, choice of language) and nonverbal communication (e.g., facial expressions, gestures, eye contact) influences the patient's level of comfort with the interviewer and the overall outcome.

Conversely, the therapist should observe the patient for any physical manifestations that reveal emotional context, such as slumped body posture, grimacing, and poor eye contact. The therapist should be sensitive to differences in culture and ethnicity that can influence how the patient or family member responds during the interview or examination process. Biases, prejudices, preconceptions, and judgments on the part of the therapist can interfere with active listening and in processing what the patient is saying. Ensuring effective communication with the patient promotes cooperation and serves to make the therapist's observations more valid, which is crucial to the success of the POC.[25,26]

During the interview, the therapist asks the patient a series of questions, using both open-ended and closed-ended questions. Open-ended questions require more than a simple yes/no response (e.g., What symptoms are you currently experiencing?), while closed-ended questions limit the patient's responses to a yes/no answer or a nod (e.g., Do you have any pain today?).

Questions are posed regarding the history of the present health condition. Specifically, the patient is asked to describe current problems and their reason for seeking physical therapy, and to give a chronological account leading up to the episode of care. Questions then explore location, quality, and severity of the symptoms or problems as well as timing (occurrence), factors that aggravate or relieve them, and associated manifestations (other symptoms or problems) that may be occurring. Questions are posed regarding participation and activity (e.g., How has your health condition affected your daily life? What have you had to give up because of your health condition?). The patient will often describe their difficulties in terms of activity limitations or participation restrictions (what they can or cannot do). General questions about activities and participation should be directed toward delineating the difference between capacity and performance. For example, "Since your stroke, how much difficulty do you have walking long distances?" "How does this compare to before you had the stroke?" (capacity). Questions directed toward examining performance can include "What problem(s) do you have when walking?" "Is this problem with walking made worse or better with the use of an assistive device?" Questions are also posed regarding the patient's past medical history, health habits (e.g., smoking history, alcohol use), family history, and personal and social history. Information about physical environment; vocation; recreational interests; exercise likes and dislikes; and type, frequency, and intensity of regular activity should be obtained.[25–27] The types of data that may be generated from a patient history are presented in Figure 1.4.[4] Sample representative interview questions are included in Box 1.3.

Pertinent information can also be obtained from the patient's family or caregiver. For example, patients with central nervous system involvement and cognitive and/or communication impairments and younger pediatric patients may be unable to accurately communicate their existing problems. The family member/caregiver then assumes the primary role of assisting the therapist in identifying problems and providing relevant aspects of the history. The perceived needs of the family member or caregiver can also be determined during the interview. Some of the information obtained in the history and interview is relevant for the systems review.

Systems Review

The use of a screening examination (brief systems review) allows the therapist to quickly scan the patient's body systems and determine areas of intact function and dysfunction. Known health conditions are an important component of the screen. This information can be obtained by reviewing the medical record, using a medical screening questionnaire, and using the history and interview or specific tests and measures. It is recommended that clinicians collect the minimal data set (MDS) consisting of heart rate, blood pressure, orientation, communication, and learning style. While included in the MDS, it is important to highlight that screening cognitive and communication ability first guides how the examination and management are conducted.

A cognition and communication screening should include the following:

- Communication ability, affect, and language: assessment of the ability to produce and understand speech, and communicate thoughts and feelings
- Cognitive ability: assessment of consciousness, orientation (person, place, and time), expected emotional/behavioral responses, and learning preferences (e.g., learning barriers, education needs)

Then the clinician may conduct a systems screen based on movement system's six systems with information obtained first through interview and then through screening tests and measures. The systems, which are adapted from Deutsch et al.,[23] are presented below:

1. Cardiovascular: assessment (through interview) of shortness of breath, chest pain or pressure, irregular heartbeat, leg cramps with ambulation; and screening tests and measures of heart rate, blood pressure, temperature, pedal pulses, 2- or 6-minute Walk Tests (2MWT; 6MWT).
2. Pulmonary: assessment (through interview or observation) of shortness of breath, difficulty breathing, cough, wheezing; and screening tests and measures of breathing pattern respiratory rate, oxygen saturation, and 2- or 6MWT.
3. Integumentary: assessment and measurement of skin color, temperature, integrity, pliability (texture), presence of scar formation.
4. Musculoskeletal: assessment (through interview or observation) of joint pain, swelling or stiffness, weakness; and screening tests and measures of gross range of motion (ROM), gross strength, posture and symmetry, joint temperature and alignment, Five Times Sit to Stand Test.

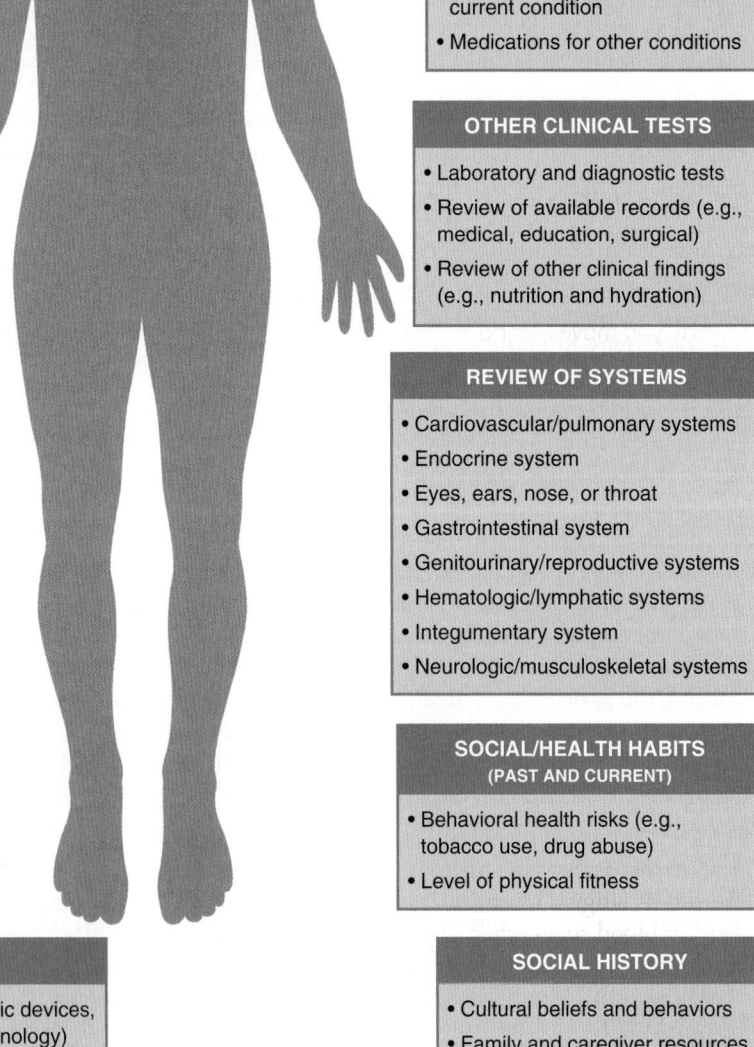

ACTIVITIES AND PARTICIPATION

- Current and prior role functions (e.g., self-care and domestic, education, work, community, social, and civic life)

CURRENT CONDITION(S)

- Concerns that led the patient or client to seek the services of a physical therapist
- Concerns or needs of the patient or client who requires the services of a physical therapist
- Current therapeutic interventions
- Mechanisms of injury or disease, including date of onset and course of events
- Onset and pattern of symptoms
- Patient or client, family, significant other, and caregiver expectations and goals for the therapeutic intervention
- Patient or client, family, significant other, and caregiver perceptions of patient's or client's emotional response to the current clinical situation
- Previous occurrence of current condition(s)
- Prior therapeutic interventions

GENERAL DEMOGRAPHICS

- Age
- Education
- Primary language
- Race/ethnicity
- Sex

FAMILY HISTORY

- Familial health risks

GENERAL HEALTH STATUS
(SELF-REPORT, FAMILY REPORT, CAREGIVER REPORT)

- General health perceptions
- Mental functions (e.g., memory, reasoning ability, depression, anxiety)
- Physical function (e.g., mobility, sleep patterns, restricted bed days)

GROWTH AND DEVELOPMENT

- Developmental history
- Hand dominance

LIVING ENVIRONMENT

- Assistive technology (e.g., aids for locomotion, orthotic devices, prosthetic requirements, seating and positioning technology)
- Living environment and community characteristics
- Projected destination at conclusion of care

MEDICAL/SURGICAL HISTORY

- Cardiovascular
- Endocrine/metabolic
- Gastrointestinal
- Genitourinary
- Gynecological
- Integumentary
- Musculoskeletal
- Neuromuscular
- Obstetrical
- Psychological
- Pulmonary
- Prior hospitalizations, surgeries, and pre+existing medical and other health-related conditions

MEDICATIONS

- Medications for current condition
- Medications previously taken for current condition
- Medications for other conditions

OTHER CLINICAL TESTS

- Laboratory and diagnostic tests
- Review of available records (e.g., medical, education, surgical)
- Review of other clinical findings (e.g., nutrition and hydration)

REVIEW OF SYSTEMS

- Cardiovascular/pulmonary systems
- Endocrine system
- Eyes, ears, nose, or throat
- Gastrointestinal system
- Genitourinary/reproductive systems
- Hematologic/lymphatic systems
- Integumentary system
- Neurologic/musculoskeletal systems

SOCIAL/HEALTH HABITS
(PAST AND CURRENT)

- Behavioral health risks (e.g., tobacco use, drug abuse)
- Level of physical fitness

SOCIAL HISTORY

- Cultural beliefs and behaviors
- Family and caregiver resources
- Social interactions, social activities, and support systems

Figure 1.4 Types of data that may be generated from a patient or client history. *Principles of Physical Therapist Patient and Client Management. Guide to Physical Therapist Practice 3.0. American Physical Therapy Association; 2014. http://guidetoptpractice.apta.org/content/1/SEC2.body.*

Box 1.3 Representative Interview Questions[23,26,27]

Patient's Reasons for Seeking Care

- Why are you seeking care?
- What would you like to do? What activities and experiences are important to you? When was the last time you were able to do the activities you desire? What are you able to do? What are you unable to do?
- How limiting is the problem for which you are seeking care?
- How long have you had this problem?
- What do you think is contributing to this problem? What makes it worse? Better?
- Are there other factors or health conditions that you think I should know about?

Patient's Goals	• What do you hope to achieve with therapy? • What would you consider as benchmarks (examples) of progress toward your goals?
Patient's Role in Society	• What roles do you play (e.g., at home, at work)? • How do the identified problem(s) interfere with your important home, work, and social activities?
Patient's Resources and Constraints (including available social supports)	• What is your prior physical therapy experience, knowledge of your health condition, and recent physical activity? • What kind of assistance do you get daily from family and friends? • What additional assistance do you (or your family members, significant others) think you need from family or others? • How feasible is access to health care—both financially and in terms of accessibility (e.g., distance, transportation, schedule, insurance coverage)?

Environmental Conditions in Which Patient Activities Typically Occur

- Describe your home/school/work environment.
- How do you move around/access areas in the home (i.e., bathroom, bedroom, entering and exiting the home)? How safe do you feel?
- How do you move around/access areas in the community (i.e., workplace, school, grocery store, shopping center, community center, stairs, curbs, ramps)? How safe do you feel?

Patient's Preferences for Solutions	• How do you prefer to learn and remember (e.g., verbal, written)? • How safe do you feel in your home environment? Community environment? • What specific concerns or fears do you have? What is your greatest concern? • What barriers might make it difficult for you to do what you need to do to participate in therapy or reach your goals? • What do you consider as facilitators to reach your goals? • How ready are you to assume an active role in managing your care? • How comfortable are you in changing a particular behavior that needs to change to optimize your outcome from this episode of care? • What problems might be anticipated in the future? What can you do to eliminate or reduce the likelihood of that happening?

5. Endocrine: assessment (through interview or observation) of fatigue, recent weight loss or gain, usual level of blood sugar when checked (diabetes); and screening tests and measures of the Functional Assessment of Chronic Illness Therapy-Fatigue scale, 2- or 6MWT.
6. Neuromuscular: assessment (through interview or observation) of numbness or pins and needles, weakness, dizziness, problem with balance/falls, headaches, loss of consciousness, visual changes; and screening tests and measures of gross sensory screen, gross reflex screen, Romberg test, Single Leg Stance, myotome/dermatome tests, gait observation or the Timed Up and Go Test, Five Times Sit to Stand Test, Tandem Walking Test, 2MWT, 6MWT, 10-meter Walk Test, balance confidence (with the Activities-specific Balance Confidence scale).

It is worth noting that some assessments (e.g., shortness of breath for cardiovascular and pulmonary assessments) or specific measurements (2MWT and 6MWT for cardiovascular, pulmonary, neuromuscular assessment) may be used to assess several systems at the same time. Information is also obtained about other major body systems (e.g., gastrointestinal, genitourinary) to determine if referral for additional medical evaluation is needed. Understanding areas of deficit along with having accurate knowledge of the main health condition allow the clinician to (1) confirm the need for further or more detailed examination; (2) rule out or differentiate specific system involvement; (3) determine if referral to another health-care professional is warranted; and (4) focus the search of the origin of symptoms to a specific location or body part. An important starting point for identification of areas to be examined is consideration of all potential (possible) factors contributing to an observed activity limitation or participation restriction. Consultation is appropriate if the needs of the patient/client are outside the scope of the expertise of the therapist assigned to the case. For example, a patient recovering from stroke is referred to a dysphagia clinic for a detailed examination of swallowing function conducted by a dysphagia specialist (speech-language pathologist).

Screening is also used for healthy populations. For example, the physical therapist can screen individuals to identify risk factors for disease such as decreased activity levels, stress, and obesity. Screening is also conducted for specific populations such as pediatric clients (e.g., for scoliosis), geriatric clients (e.g., to identify fall risk factors),

athletes (e.g., preperformance examinations), and working adults to identify the risk of musculoskeletal injuries in the workplace (e.g., ergonomic examinations). These screens may involve observation, oral history, and a brief examination. Additional screening examinations may be mandated by institutional settings. For example, in a long-term care facility, the therapist may be asked to review the chart or briefly examine a patient for indications of changes in functional status. The therapist then determines the need for physical therapy services based on completing a screening examination.

Examination

The purposes of the examination are to collect baseline data on participation and activity that will be used to determine clinical outcomes of the episode of care. Data from movement observations-analyses and tests/measures of participation, activity, and body function/structure are used to inform the evaluation, diagnosis, and prognosis. Examination consists of:

1. Mapping the patient's participation goals into relevant activities, followed by movement observation and analysis of the relevant activities the patient needs to achieve the participation goals with concurrent hypothesizing about what interferes (body function/structure limitations, the environment, or personal factors) in achieving the goals (see Fig. 1.5, left side).
2. Performance of specific tests and measures that quantify and rule in or out hypotheses related to the movement observation and analysis reasoning (see Fig. 1.5, right side).

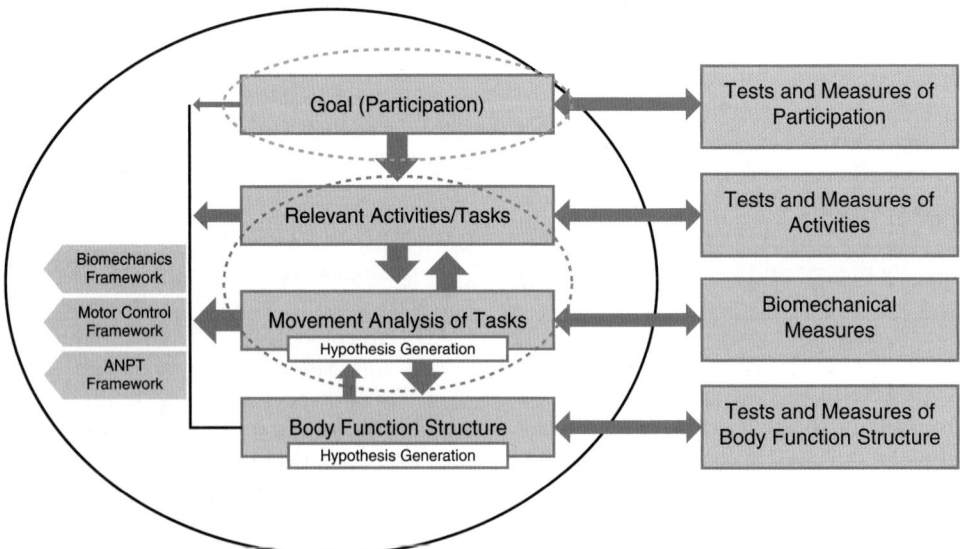

Figure 1.5 Examination consists of complementary processes of dissection of the participation goal into relevant activities, movement observation, and analysis of tasks (using three frameworks: biomechanics, Motor Control Framework, and Academy of Neurologic Physical Therapy (ANPT) Framework), hypothesis generation related to body function structure (left side) and administration of tests and measures (right side). The influences of ICF with personal factors (orange) and the environment (gray) are represented with dotted circles.

Participation Goal Mapping, Movement Observation, and Analysis of Relevant Tasks

First the clinician maps the client's participation goal into relevant component activities ICF or tasks (movement science) in the context of their personal factors identifying what the client is both able and unable to do. Activities that the clinician identifies as resources (able to do) need no further examination; those that are not performed successfully or efficiently require movement observation and are interpreted through a movement analysis of tasks.

The case study at the end of the chapter illustrates the process of mapping participation goals to relevant activities or tasks. One of client's participation goals is to return to gardening in her community garden. This participation goal requires that she walk on uneven surfaces (activity) and carry gardening tools while walking (activity), squat or bend down to the ground (task), sit on the ground (task), get up from the ground (task), shovel mulch into a wheelbarrow (task), transport mulch in the wheelbarrow (task), and manipulate tools and plants (task). These tasks may take place in various environmental conditions (e.g., weather, quality of the ground, and other people in the garden). Consideration will need to be given regarding which tasks she may need to delegate or have adapted to observe her hip precautions (e.g., transporting materials in the wheelbarrow or getting up from the floor).

Next, the clinician performs a movement observation and analysis of the relevant tasks that have been identified as important by the patient and the clinician. The term *tasks* is used here from movement science to be consistent with "task analysis" and "task-specific training." Movement analysis of tasks begins with movement observation, is followed by interpretation/analysis of how the task was performed, and leads to the generation of hypotheses of underlying body structure-function impairments. This information about the patient's movement is then analyzed and compared to what is known about typical performance of the relevant tasks under various environmental and contextual conditions to identify the specific aspects of movement that are problematic for the patient.

It is important that the clinician consider all aspects of the environment (physical, social, and attitudinal) included in the ICF. The environment has also been described from a movement science perspective using Gentile's taxonomy.[28] The taxonomy organizes movement into three factors:

1. Is the person stationary or moving?
2. Is the environment stationary or moving?
3. Is upper extremity manipulation required?

For the client in the case study with a participation goal of gardening, she needs to move and function in a stationary environment (garden) as a moving person with upper extremity (UE) manipulation tasks.

When feasible, movement analysis of activities-tasks should be examined in the environmental context in which the person executes them. For example, in the case study of the widow, the clinician may simulate an uneven surface and have the patient carry a bag with gardening tools while walking. The clinician then generates hypotheses about what may interfere with typical movement performance. Movement analysis of the tasks can be performed using biomechanical analyses of normal movement (e.g., gait, sit-stand, and running)[29–31] compared to movement changes as a result of disease, normal development, and aging.[32–34] There are tools for movement observation and analysis (e.g., Motor Control Framework and the Academy of Neurological Physical Therapy Task Analysis) that can be applied regardless of health condition.[35,36] The Academy of Neurological Physical Therapy Task Analysis framework has "observable constructs of movement" that can be observed across tasks. These would include description of, for example, movement symmetry and speed.[36]

Based on the movement analysis of tasks, the clinician hypothesizes about potential body function/structure impairments that may interfere with optimal movement and activity-task performance. These hypotheses may be tested by combining movement observations with modification to the environment, as well as conducting relevant tests/measures (Fig. 1.5, right side). For example, the clinician may change the height of the chair during sit-stand to differentiate between a force-generation deficit or ROM limitation. Or, the clinician may measure lower extremity force generation using a Five Times Sit to Stand Test (activity) or manual muscle test and range of motion measurements of the hip (body structure/function). Where possible, the therapist should consult the literature for known relationships between body function/structure limitations and activity-task performance.

■ TESTS AND MEASURES

The use of tests and measures (Fig. 1.5, right side) complements the participation goal dissection and movement analysis of tasks (Fig. 1.5, left side). The selection of the tests and measures can occur at any level of the ICF categories (Fig. 1.5, right side) and should align with the patient's goals and as well as confirm the clinician's hypotheses that results from their movement observation. Tests and measures also provide performance-based and patient-reported measures to quantify the baseline participation, activity, and body function/structure impairment status. They are used to support the therapist's clinical judgments about the diagnosis, prognosis, and POC.[4]

Tests and measures may be performed in any order. The decision as to which approach to use is based on the results of the screening examination and the therapist's knowledge of the health condition. Key information to obtain during an examination of participation and activity is the level of independence or dependence, as well as the need for physical assistance, external devices, or environmental modifications.

Selection of specific tests and measures and depth of the examination depends on several factors, including the patient's health condition (severity and complexity of the problem), stage of recovery (acute, subacute, chronic), phase of rehabilitation (early, middle, or late), cognition and behavior (level of arousal, communication ability, ability to participate in the examination), and setting (hospital, home, community, work). Adequate training and skill in performing specific tests and measures are crucial in ensuring both validity and reliability of the tests. Failure to correctly perform an examination procedure can lead to the gathering of inaccurate data and the formation of an inappropriate POC. The use of health condition–specific standardized instruments (e.g., the Fugl-Meyer Assessment of Physical Performance used for individuals with stroke) can facilitate the examination process but may not always be appropriate for every patient. The therapist needs to carefully review the unique problems of the patient to determine the appropriateness and sensitivity of an instrument. The remaining chapters in Section 1 focus on examination and on specific tests and measures.

Several websites also provide rich resources for information on tests and measures. For example, readers can access the Rehabilitation Measures Database developed at the Shirley Ryan Ability Lab at www.rehabmeasures@sralab.org. This site provides a comprehensive description and review of literature on a large number of tests and measures with online links to access the instrument directly (e.g., the Berg Balance Scale). The APTA has an evidence-based resources page (https://www.apta.org/patient-care/evidence-based-practice-resources) that can be accessed to search for tests and measures as well as clinical practice guidelines (CPGs) developed by the professional association. The Academy of Orthopedics of the APTA has produced guidelines for 12 topics which may be found in the *Journal of Orthopedic and Sports Physical Therapy* site, or by searching in The Physiotherapy Evidence Database (PEDro).

Through the Evidence Database to Guide Effectiveness process many APTA academies have identified outcome measures at all levels of the ICF care. Furthermore, they have suggested what might be taught in entry level physical therapist practice. The Academy of Neurological Physical Therapy, for example, has recommended which measures should be used for persons poststroke in acute, inpatient, and outpatient care.[37,38] It is important that tests be selected that are valid and reliable for the patient's health condition. For example, see Chapter 15, Stroke, for an in-depth discussion on outcome measures for people with stroke.

Novice therapists should resist the tendency to gather excessive and extraneous data in the mistaken belief that more information is better. Unnecessary data will only confuse the picture, rendering clinical decision-making more difficult and unnecessarily raising the cost of care. If problems arise that are not initially identified in the history or systems review, or if the data obtained are inconsistent, additional tests and measures may be indicated. Consultation with an experienced clinician can provide an important means of clarifying inconsistencies and determining the appropriateness of specific tests and measures.

Evaluation

As part of the evaluation, the therapist synthesizes and interprets the results of the movement analysis and tests and measures, along with other history/examination data, to arrive at working hypotheses underlying the patient's limitations and restrictions in activity and participation. Relevant personal or environmental factors that impact, in a positive or negative manner, the patient's ability to achieve their stated goals are summarized. The steps to follow in formulating the evaluation may be summarized in this way:

1. What does the patient wish to achieve? What is the patient's (participation level) goal?
2. Are there any NPIPs identified by the clinician and/or caregiver that also need to be addressed? (HOAC)
3. What are the contextual (personal and environmental) factors that need to be considered? (ICF and movement science)?
4. What are the primary movement problems, or key movement-related elements, underlying the patient's inability to perform the desired task and roles? Examples of some key movement-related elements include postural control, verticality, alignment, movement symmetry, movement speed, movement amplitude, motor control, muscle performance, and symptom provocation (movement science and movement system).[36]
5. Is the patient's ability to perform the desired task different or consistent across various environmental conditions (moving vs. stationary environment)?[28]

The therapist identifies and prioritizes the patient's participation restrictions, activity limitations, and body function/structure impairments and develops a problem list. Table 1.1 presents a sample problem list. Organization of the information allows the hypothesis generation of how the participation and activity limitations may be related to body function/structure impairments. For example, a person with Parkinson disease may be able to walk independently in their home but have difficulty walking in a crowded store. The therapists may assess dual task ability as a possible explanation for the walking challenges in a more complex environment. The body function/structure impairment of cognition may be revealed by increasing the complexity of the task or the environment. Identifying the causative factors is a difficult yet critical step in determining appropriate

Table 1.1 Sample Prioritized Problem List for a Patient with Stroke

Participation Restrictions	Activity Limitations	Direct Body Function/ Structure Impairments	Indirect Body Function/ Structure Impairments
Patient-Identified Problems (PIPs)			
Housekeeping (modA for cooking and maxA for cleaning)	Bed mobility–minA BADL–min–modA Transfers–modA	Dec. selective capacity, force generation of upper and lower limbs, motor planning, balance	Shoulder subluxation Dec. shoulder ROM Dec. endurance
Gardening–max A	Walking on even surfaces–modA Carrying gardening bag–maxA Stand-floor transfer–unable	Dec. selective capacity, force generation of upper and lower limbs; motor planning ability balance	Dec. endurance Dec. ankle ROM
Attending church–modA	Transfers modA Limited Community ambulation Dec. expressive communication Dec. problem solving	Same as above Dysarthria	
Non–Patient-Identified Problems (NPIPs)			
Mild diabetic neuropathy Cataracts		Dec. sensation–inc risk for ulcer Dec. balance–inc risk for falls	
Contextual Factors			

Personal Factors	Social Factors	Environmental Factors
Wife, gardener, church member, highly motivated	Spouse is primary caregiver; has two involved sons living within 30-mile radius. Highly educated, former high school chemistry teacher	Lives in one-level ranch house; entry with two steps, no handrails; church has a parking lot and stairs to enter, long hallway to reach the pews.

BADL = basic activities of daily living; Dec = decreased; Inc = increased; MinA = minimal assistance; ModA = moderate assistance; MaxA = maximal assistance; ROM = range of motion

treatment interventions and guiding the patient to achieve their goal. The skilled clinician is also able to identify the impact of barriers and facilitators in the patient's environment to incorporate strategies to minimize or maximize these factors within the POC. A POC that emphasizes and reinforces facilitators enhances function and the patient's ability to experience success. Improved motivation and engagement are the natural outcomes of reinforcement of facilitators.

Accurate collection and interpretation of data allow the therapist to determine a diagnosis and prognosis and to develop a POC. Examination and evaluation are ongoing processes that continue throughout the episode of care and are essential in formulating a diagnosis and prognosis and determining success reaching stated goals

and outcomes and responses to selected interventions.[4] It is important to share the results of the evaluation with the patient. This provides valuable information to the patient, promotes continued exchange of information between the patient and clinician, and reinforces shared decision-making.

Diagnosis

The physical therapy diagnostic process (differential diagnosis) requires the clinician to collect, evaluate, and categorize data according to a classification scheme relevant to the clinician and to determine whether the patient's presenting problems are amenable to physical therapy intervention. It guides the prognosis and selection of interventions during the development of the POC. Physical therapy diagnosis refers to the cluster of signs and symptoms, syndromes, or categories that best characterize the patient's primary problem. *The Guide to Physical Therapist Practice* describes the process as using "labels that identify the impact of a condition or function at the level of the system (especially the movement system) and at the level of the whole person."[4] *The Guide* indicates that diagnosis is typically made at the impairment, activity, and participation levels. In contrast, the medical diagnosis refers to the identification of a disease, disorder, or condition (pathology/pathophysiology) primarily at the cellular, tissue, or organ level. Thus, the diagnosis reflects the professional body of knowledge, the expertise and clinical reasoning of the physical therapist, and the boundaries placed on the profession by the law and health-care agencies.[4] Examples include the following:

- Physical therapy diagnosis: Dependent mobility and ADL with impaired motor function and sensory integrity affecting the left nondominant side.
- Medical diagnosis: Cerebrovascular accident.
- Physical therapy diagnosis: Dependent mobility and ADL with impaired motor function, peripheral nerve integrity, and sensory integrity.
- Medical diagnosis: SCI.
- Physical therapy diagnosis: Dependent mobility and ADL with impaired balance and motor control involving upper and lower extremities, as well as the trunk
- Medical diagnosis: Cerebral palsy.

Physical therapy diagnoses are an area of exploration and refinement. Recently, the Movement System Task Force within the APTA's Academy of Neurology has proposed that each movement system diagnosis should be "associated with a clear description of a unique cluster of movement observations and associated examination findings" that are health-condition neutral and emphasize the role of movement analysis of tasks.[36] They have offered diagnoses for balance that are based on understanding the motor control and the movement problem.[39] The balance diagnoses are intended to guide specific treatment. For example, balance can be classified as reactive, which would require using perturbations for training.

The use of diagnostic categories specific to physical therapy allows for successful communication with colleagues and patients/caregivers about the conditions that require the physical therapist's expertise, provides an appropriate classification for establishing standards of examination and treatment, and directs examination of treatment effectiveness, thereby enhancing evidence-based practice (EBP). Physical therapy diagnostic categories also facilitate successful reimbursement when linked to functional outcomes and enhance direct access of physical therapy services.[40]

Prognosis

Prognosis represents a synthesis that is based on an understanding of the examination findings, health condition, foundational knowledge, theory, evidence, and experience. Prognosis may be related to the health condition, body structure/function, activity, and participation. The patient's resources and constraints, based on personal factors (e.g., their social, emotional, and motivational status), environmental factors, and social factors will affect the prognosis.

Knowledge of the health condition may guide the expected level and rate of recovery. Issues to consider include the nature of the pathology as well as stage, acuity, and tissue irritability. The evidence regarding plasticity, healing, and natural recovery of a variety of health conditions informs the prognosis. It may be adversely affected when there are several health conditions or comorbidities.

Prognosis should be specific to different aspects of activity and participation. For example, a patient may have an excellent prognosis for return to independent ambulation and an excellent prognosis for returning to independent living, but also have a guarded prognosis for independent community ambulation. This degree of specificity for prognosis will facilitate the process of a realistic ongoing negotiation (shared decision-making) between the patient and the clinician.

For example, a patient sustained a lower limb amputation due to dysvascularity. The patient's goal is to return to work, which requires walking, and to do so within 4 months. Regarding the health condition, the clinician draws from information related to expected outcomes following dysvascular amputation. For example, 10% to 15% of people with a lower limb amputation will have wound-healing complications within the first year of the amputation,[41,42] nearly 50% of similar patients with amputations due to dysvascularity have a second amputation within 3 years of the initial amputation,[43] and over half will fall within a year.[44] This knowledge is consistent with the HOAC in which the clinician, based on the knowledge of the health condition, may anticipate problems (NPIPs) and factor the information into prognosis.

With regard to activity and participation, only 33% of patients achieve independent ambulation within 1 year post-amputation;[45] following a first amputation individuals take an average of 1,721 steps/day, compared to 7,817 steps/day for healthy adults of similar age.[46] Furthermore, only 40% to 50% of individuals are able to ambulate in the community, and these individuals report more disability than 95% of the population.[46–48] The clinician keeps these types of data in mind but tempers expectations for this particular patient with respect to important modifiers that may be facilitators or barriers to recovery. Examples that should be considered specific to amputation include the patient's activity and endurance prior to surgery, previous engagement, and success with physical therapy, other health conditions, emotional status, motivation, access to rehabilitation services, and social and emotional support.

An accurate prognosis may be determined at the onset of treatment for some patients. For other patients with more complicated conditions, such as severe TBI accompanied by extensive disability and multisystem involvement, a prognosis or prediction of level of improvement can be determined only at various increments during rehabilitation.

Therapists also need to compare levels of habitual performance (what a person currently does) to highest level an individual is capable of (what a person could potentially do) to arrive at realistic outcomes. The amount of time needed to reach optimal recovery is an important determination, one that is required by Medicare and many other insurance providers. Predicting optimal levels of recovery and time frames can be a challenging process for the novice therapist. Use of experienced clinicians as resources and mentors as well as referring to the literature can facilitate this step in the decision-making process. In rehabilitation settings, the POC may also include a more general statement regarding the patient's overall rehabilitation potential. This is typically expressed in one word: excellent, good, fair, or poor.

Plan of Care

The POC outlines anticipated patient management. The therapist evaluates and integrates data obtained from the patient/client history, the systems review, tests, measures, evaluation, diagnosis, and prognosis. The therapist must consider multiple factors when determining the POC, such as the patient's current condition (stability, chronicity, or severity of the condition; level of impairment and physical function), comorbidities (premorbid conditions, complications, secondary impairments), age, overall health status, resources (psychosocial, economic), living environment, and potential discharge placement (e.g., home or another health-care facility).

Multisystem involvement, severe impairment and functional loss, extended time of involvement (chronicity), and multiple comorbid conditions are parameters that significantly increase the complexity of the decision-making process. Professional consultation with expert clinicians and mentors is an effective means of helping the novice sort through the complex issues involved in decision-making, especially when complicating factors intervene.[49] There is an accumulating body of evidence on expertise in physical therapy practice, spearheaded by the pivotal work of Jensen and colleagues.[49-51] These researchers have shown that the knowledge, skills, and decision-making abilities used by expert clinicians can be identified, nurtured, and taught. The novice therapist may benefit from a period of active mentoring by expert clinicians early in clinical practice (e.g., clinical residency program).

Respecting patient values and incorporating patient preferences and needs into the POC are key elements in successful outcomes. Patient-centered care is defined by the Institute of Medicine as "providing care that is respectful of and responsive to individual patient preferences, needs, values and ensuring that patient values guide all clinical decisions."[52] The patient is viewed as an active participant and collaborative partner who participates in the goal-setting process, makes informed choices, and assumes responsibility for their health care. Therapists who place strong emphasis on communicating effectively; educating their patients, families, and caregivers; and teaching self-management skills can successfully empower patients. The natural outcomes of this approach are improved satisfaction with care, improved therapy outcomes, and improved adherence to suggested lifestyle changes.

Some rehabilitation plans fail simply because the therapist did not fully involve the patient in the planning process, producing goals or outcomes that were not meaningful to the patient (e.g., independent wheelchair mobility for the patient with incomplete SCI). That same patient may have established a very different set of personal goals and expectations (e.g., return to walking). For many patients for whom complete recovery is not expected, the overall "goal of any rehabilitation program must be to increase the ability of individuals to manage their lives in the context of ongoing disability, to the greatest extent possible."[26(p11)] This cannot be effectively done if the therapist assumes the role of expert and sole planner, establishing the rules, regulations, and instructions for rehabilitation. Rather, it is critical to engage the patient in problem-solving and promoting lifelong skills in their own health management.

The patient's ability and motivation to participate in planning or share in the decision-making can vary. Sometimes severe illness may interfere with shared decision-making. As the illness resolves and the patient begins to improve, they may be more able to engage in planning the treatment. Also, the more difficult the problems encountered, the more likely patients are to put their trust in "the experts" and the less likely they are to trust their own abilities to reach effective decisions. The therapist needs to guard against promoting dependence on the expert (the "my therapist syndrome") to the exclusion of the patient listening to their own thoughts and feelings and participating in problem-solving. In this instance, the patient's feelings of perceived helplessness are increased while the patient's ability to utilize their own decision-making abilities is delayed or restricted.[26,53] Refer to Box 1.3 for sample questions to promote shared decision-making.

A major focus of the POC is producing meaningful changes in participation and activity such as achieving independence in locomotion or in ADL, returning to work, or participating in recreational activities that are important to the patient/client in terms of improving quality of life (QOL). QOL is defined as the sense of total well-being that encompasses both physical and psychosocial aspects of the patient's life. Finally, not all participation and activity restrictions and body function/structure impairments can be remedied by physical therapy. Some restrictions and impairments are permanent or progressive, the direct result of an unrelenting health condition such as amyotrophic lateral sclerosis. In this example, a primary emphasis on reducing the number and severity of indirect impairments and activity limitations is appropriate.

Essential components of the POC include goals and expected outcomes and a general statement of the interventions to be used, including proposed duration and frequency required to reach the goals, as well as anticipated discharge plans.

Goals and Outcomes

An important first step in the development of the POC is determining goals (the intended impact on functioning) and outcomes (the predicted level of optimal functioning at the conclusion of the episode of care). Goals are the interim steps necessary to achieve expected outcomes. They address PIPs, NPIPs, and predicted changes in impairments, activity limitations, and participation restrictions. They also address predicted changes in overall health, risk reduction and prevention, wellness and fitness, and optimization of patient/client satisfaction.

Goal statements should be measurable, functionally driven, and time limited. They also involve a negotiated process of reconciling goals related to PIPs and NPIPs. Decision aids may be a useful tool in aiding the patient to contribute to their goals. There are four essential elements to each goal:

- Individual: Who will perform the specific behavior, activity required, or aspect of care? Goals and outcomes are focused on the patient/client. This includes individuals who receive direct-care physical therapy services and/or individuals who benefit from consultation and advice, or services focused on promoting, health, wellness, and fitness. Goals can also be focused on family members or caregivers, for example, the parent of a child with a developmental disability.
- Behavior/activity: What is the specific behavior or activity the patient/client will demonstrate? This includes changes in activity limitations (e.g., transfers, ambulation), ADL changes in participation restrictions (e.g., community mobility, return to school or work), and changes in body function and structure (e.g., ROM, strength, balance). Changes should be measurable, attainable, and relevant.
- Condition: What are the conditions under which the patient/client's behavior is measured? The statement specifies the specific conditions or measures required for successful achievement; for example,

amount of assistance required, distance achieved, required time to perform the activity, the specific number of successful attempts out of a specific number of trials. Statements focused on functional changes should include a description of the conditions required for acceptable performance. For example, the Functional Independence Measure (FIM) describes the amount of physical assistance a person requires to perform various functional tasks such as transfers and ambulation. This instrument grades levels from No Helper/Independence (grade 7) to No Helper/Modified Independence (grade 6; device), to Helper/Modified Dependence (grades 5, 4, and 3; supervision, minimal, moderate, assistance), to Helper/Complete Dependence (grades 2 and 1; maximal, total assistance) (see Chapter 8, Examination of Function for a complete description of this instrument).[54] The type of environment required for a successful outcome of the behavior should also be specified: clinic environment (e.g., quiet room, level floor surface, physical therapy gym), home (e.g., one flight of eight stairs, carpeted surfaces), and community (e.g., uneven grassy surfaces, curbs, ramps).

- Time: How long will it take to achieve the stated goal? Goals can be short term (generally considered to be 2 to 3 weeks) and long term (longer than 3 weeks).

Outcomes describe the predicted level of optimal improvement attained. In instances of severe disability and incomplete recovery (e.g., TBI), the patient, therapist, and team members may have difficulty determining the expected outcomes at the beginning of rehabilitation. Long-term and short-term goals can be used that focus on the expectations for a specific time period, stage of recovery (e.g., in TBI, minimally conscious states, confusional states), or setting/episode of care. Goals should be measurable, functionally driven, time limited, and with the same four essential elements.

Each POC has multiple goals and outcomes. Goals may be linked to the successful attainment of more than one outcome. For example, attaining a short-term goal of ROM in dorsiflexion may be important to the long-term goal of independence in transfers and locomotion and outcome of reducing activity limitations. The successful attainment of an outcome is also dependent on achieving many different goals. For instance, the ability to perform physical actions, tasks, or activities is dependent on independent locomotion with an assistive device in home and community environments (long-term goal) that is dependent on increasing strength, ROM, and balance skills (short-term goals). In formulating a POC, the therapist accurately identifies the relationship between and among goals and then sequences them appropriately. Goals and outcomes are modified following a significant change in patient status. Box 1.4 presents examples of outcome and goal statements.

Box 1.4 Examples of Outcome and Goal Statements

Outcomes

The following are examples of expected outcomes:

• Impact of impairments is reduced.
• Ability to perform physical actions, tasks, or activities is improved.
• Health status and QOL are improved.
• Patient/client satisfaction is enhanced.

Goals

The following are examples of anticipated goals with variable time frames:

Short-Term Goals

• The patient will increase strength in shoulder depressor muscles and elbow extensor muscles in both upper extremities from good to normal within 3 weeks.
• The patient will increase ROM 10 degrees in knee extension bilaterally to within normal limits within 3 weeks.
• The patient will be independent in the application of lower-extremity orthoses within 1 week.
• The patient and family will recognize personal and environmental factors associated with falls during ambulation within 2 weeks.
• The patient will attend to task for 5 minutes out of a 30-minute treatment session within 3 weeks.

Long-Term Goals

• The patient will independently perform transfers from wheelchair to car within 4 weeks.
• The patient will be independent in ambulation using an ankle-foot orthosis and a quad cane on level surfaces for unlimited community distances and for all daily activities within 8 weeks.
• Patient will increase their score on the DGI from 20–22 to reduce risk for falls.
• The patient will demonstrate supervision with BADL with minimal setup and equipment (use of a reacher) within 6 weeks.

BADL = basic activities of daily living; DGI = Dynamic Gait Index; QOL = quality of life; ROM = range of motion.

Interventions

The next step is to determine the intervention, defined as the purposeful interaction of the physical therapist with the patient/client and, when appropriate, other individuals involved in their care. The intervention focuses on the patient's participation goals and related activities and body function/structure requirements. The Guide to Physical Therapist Practice identifies interventions that can be delivered three ways: through consultation, direct intervention, and education (see Fig. 1.6).

Coordination and Communication

Case management requires therapists to be able to communicate effectively with all members of the rehabilitation team, directly or indirectly. For example, the therapist communicates directly with other professionals at case conferences, team meetings, or rounds or indirectly through documentation in the medical record. Effective communication enhances collaboration and understanding. Therapists are also responsible for coordinating care at many different levels. The therapist delegates appropriate aspects of treatment to physical therapy assistants and oversees the responsibilities of physical therapy aides. The therapist coordinates care

with other professionals, family, or caregivers regarding specific interventions and times. For example, for early transfer training to be effective, consistency in how everyone transfers the patient is important. The therapist also coordinates discharge planning with the patient and family and other team members. Therapists may be involved in providing POC recommendations to other facilities such as long-term care facilities.

Direct Intervention

Skilled physical therapy includes a wide variety of direct interventions, which can be broadly classified into three main groups: recovery, compensatory, and preventive. Recovery interventions are directed toward restoring the patient's premorbid status across the ICF. This approach is based on knowledge and evidence for existing potential for change (e.g., neural plasticity; potential for muscle strengthening or improving aerobic endurance). For example, the patient poststroke undergoes high-intensity stepping training to restore locomotion.

Compensatory interventions promote optimal function across the ICF without full recovery. These can result from the adaptation of remaining motor elements (using involved segments) or substitution. In substitution,

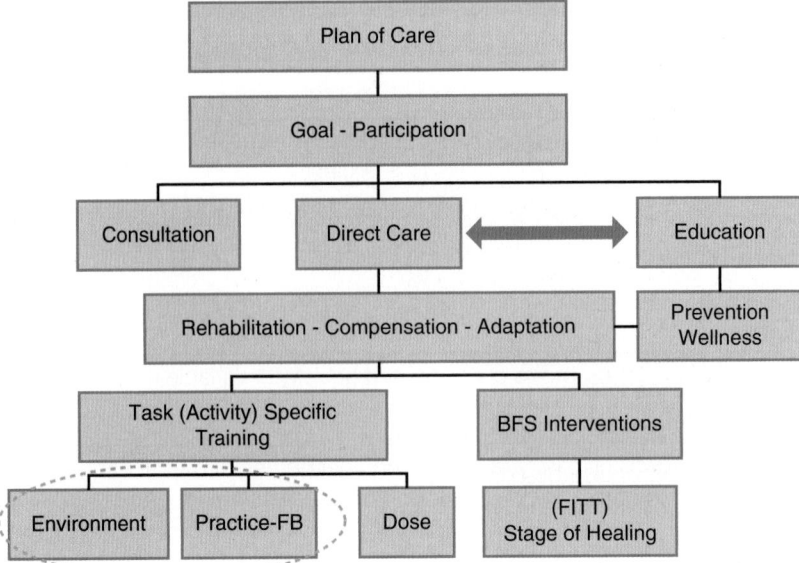

Figure 1.6 Plan of care organized at a high level using the *Guide to Physical Therapist Practice*. It incorporates the language of the ICF. Interventions are based on movement science and physiology principles. The process uses shared decision-making.

functions are taken over or replaced by different body segments using different motor patterns. The activity (task) can be adapted (changed) to achieve function. In substitution, the uninvolved or less-involved extremities are targeted for intervention. For example, the patient with left hemiplegia learns to eat or dress using the less-involved right UE; the patient with complete T1 paraplegia learns to roll using UEs and momentum. Environmental adaptations are also used to facilitate relearning of functional skills and optimal performance. For example, the patient with TBI can dress by selecting clothing from color-coded drawers. Compensatory/substitution interventions can be used in conjunction with restorative interventions to maximize function or when restorative interventions are unrealistic or unsuccessful (e.g., the patient with severe impairment, declining health condition, and multiple co-morbidities).

Preventive interventions are directed toward minimizing potential problems (e.g., anticipated indirect impairments, activity limitations, and participation restrictions) and maintaining health. For example, early resumption of upright standing using a tilt table minimizes the risk of pneumonia, bone loss, and renal calculi in the patient with SCI. A successful educational program for frequent skin inspection can prevent the development of pressure injuries in that same patient. Preventive interventions also encompass promoting health and wellness. They are often delivered through education and are guide by NPIPs. See Chapter 29, Promoting Health and Wellness, for a complete discussion of the role of physical therapists in health promotion.

Interventions are chosen based on the examination and evaluation of the patient, the physical therapy diagnosis, the prognosis, and the goals and expected outcomes. The therapist relies on knowledge of foundational science and interventions (e.g., principles of motor learning, motor control, muscle performance,

task-specific training, and cardiovascular endurance) to determine those interventions that are likely to achieve successful outcomes. In particular, task-specific training incorporating elements of motor learning form the basis for many interventions. It is important to identify all possible interventions early in the process, to carefully weigh those alternatives, and then to decide on the interventions that have the best probability of success. This is an opportunity to used shared decision-making to give the patient choices of activities. This will promote autonomy and engagement. Narrowly adhering to one treatment approach reduces the available options and may limit or preclude successful outcomes. Use of a protocol (e.g., predetermined exercises for the patient with hip fracture) standardizes aspects of care but may not meet the individual needs of the patient. Protocols can foster a separation of examination/evaluation findings from the selection of interventions.

A POC is ideally organized based on the patient's participation goals and relevant activities. Thus, treatments occur at the level of the relevant activities using task-specific training. To do this the clinician identifies the correct environment in which to train, how they will structure practice and offer feedback. It is important that they have a treatment dose that will, based on evidence, achieve the treatment goals. An outline for ensuring that all the elements of the intervention are delivered is presented in Box 1.5. Special attention is placed on how to dose the intervention organized by using the FITT (frequency, intensity, time, type) equation, presented in Box 1.6.

The therapist and patient should choose interventions that accomplish more than one goal and are linked to the expected outcomes. The interventions should be effectively sequenced to address key activities and impairments first and to achieve optimum motivational effect, interspacing the more difficult or

Box 1.5 Elements of Task-Specific Training

Environment

Will training occur in a stationary or moving environment?
  Will it be closed and stable or open and variable?
  What is the physical setup (height and texture) or support surface?
  What is the lighting? (stable, variable, low, high)
  What is the sound level? (quiet, noisy)
  Is it possible to simulate the conditions of the environment required for the participation goal and activities to be practiced?

Practice Schedule

How will practice be structured?

• Type: Massed, or distributed?
• Practice schedule: Random: blocked serial, or faded?

Feedback

How will feedback be provided?

• Knowledge of performance: information on movement kinematics
• Knowledge of results: information on movement outcome
• Augmented feedback: given in the form of manual cueing or guidance
• Faded feedback: given in decreasing frequency
• Bandwidth feedback: given when performance deviates from boundaries of correct performance

Dose

Dose the intervention by using the FITT (see Box 1.6).

See Chapter 10, Strategies to Improve Motor Function, for a complete description of these elements.
FITT = frequency, intensity, time, type.

Box 1.6 The FITT Equation for Exercise Intervention

Frequency: How Often Will the Patient Exercise?

This is typically defined in terms of the number of times per week exercise or activity training is performed (e.g., daily or three times per week) or the number of visits before a specific date. Rest days may be specified.

Intensity: What Is the Prescribed Intensity of Exercises or Activity Training?

Intensity refers to how hard the person will work. For example, the POC includes sit-to-stand repetitions, three sets of five reps each, progressing from high seat to low. Intensity is usually monitored by heart rate, perceived exertion, talk test, and fatigue levels.

Time (duration): How Long Will the Patient Exercise?

This is typically defined in terms of days or weeks (e.g., three times per week for 6 weeks). The duration (how long the person exercises during an anticipated session) should also be defined (e.g., 30- or 60-minute sessions).

Type: What Are the Specific Exercises or Activities?

What is the specific exercise intervention performed? Examples include:

• **Cardiovascular training:** walking, running, cycling, dancing, swimming, aerobics routines
• **Strength training:** use of resistance (bands, dumbbells, machines), functional/body weight training
• **Neuromuscular training:** locomotor and balance training, UE training

POC = plan of care; UE = upper extremity.

uncomfortable procedures with easier ones. The therapist should include tasks that motivate the patient and ensure success during the treatment session. Whenever possible, the therapist should end each treatment session on a positive note. This helps the patient retain a positive feeling of success and look forward to the next treatment.

Patient/Client Education

Educational interventions are directed toward ensuring an understanding of the patient's health condition, results of the examination and evaluation, and explanation of the interventions. There is a large role for education as it relates to prevention and wellness. Here the clinician's knowledge of health condition is very important.

In addition, educational interventions are directed toward ensuring a successful transition to the home environment (instruction in home exercise programs [HEP]), returning to work (ergonomic instruction), or resuming social activities in the community (environmental access). It is important to document what was taught, who participated, when the instruction occurred, and overall effectiveness. The need for repetition and reinforcement of educational content should also be documented in the medical record.

Communication strategies are developed within the context of the patient/client's age, cultural background, language skills, and educational level, and the presence of specific communication or cognition impairments. Therapists may provide direct one-on-one instruction to a variety of individuals, including patients/clients, families, caregivers, and other interested persons. Additional strategies can include group discussions or classes, or instruction through printed or audiovisual materials. There is mounting evidence that shared decision-making has a positive impact when coupled with patient education.[55]

Discharge Planning

Discharge planning is initiated early in the rehabilitation process during the data collection phase and intensifies as goals and expected outcomes are close to being reached. Discharge planning may also be initiated if the patient refuses further treatment or becomes medically or psychologically unstable. If the patient is discharged before outcomes are reached, the reasons for discontinuation of services must be carefully documented.

In the discharge summary, the therapist should include current physical/functional status, degree of goals/outcomes achieved, reasons for goals/outcomes not being achieved, and the discharge prognosis. This is typically a one-word response such as excellent, good, fair, or poor. It reflects the therapist's judgment of the patient's ability to maintain the level of function achieved at the end of rehabilitation without continued skilled intervention. Elements of an effective discharge plan are included in Box 1.7.

Box 1.7   Elements of the Discharge Plan

Patient, family, or caregiver education—instruction includes information regarding the following:

- Current health condition (pathology), impairments, activity limitations, and participation restrictions
- Ways to reduce risk factors for recurrence of condition and developing complications, indirect impairments, activity limitations, and participation restrictions
- Ways to maintain/enhance performance and functional independence
- Ways to foster healthy habits, wellness, and prevention
- Ways to assist in transition to a new setting (e.g., home, skilled nursing facility)
- Ways to assist in transition to new roles

Plans for follow-up care or referral to another agency: patient and caregiver are provided with the following:

- Information regarding follow-up physical therapy care or referral for additional services to another agency (e.g., home care agency, outpatient facility) as needed
- Information regarding community support group and community fitness center as appropriate

Instruction in a home exercise plan: patient/caregiver instruction regarding the following:

- HEP, activity training, ADL training
- Use of assistive technology (e.g., assistive devices, orthoses, prosthetics, wheelchairs) provided

Evaluation/modification of the home environment:

- Planning regarding the home environment and modifications needed to assist the patient in the home (e.g., installation of ramps and rails, bathroom equipment such as tub seats, raised toilet seats, bathroom rails, furniture rearrangement or removal to ease functional mobility). See Chapter 9, Examination and Modification of the Environment.
- All essential equipment and renovations should be in place before discharge.

ADL = activities of daily living; HEP = home exercise program.

Implementation of the Plan of Care

The therapist must consider many factors in structuring an effective treatment session. The patient's involvement, comfort, motivation, and optimal performance should be a priority along with safety and privacy during the treatment session. The environment should be structured appropriately to reduce distractions and improve motor learning. See Chapter 10, Strategies to Improve Motor Control, for more information on interventions to enhance motor function.

The patient's immediate pretreatment level of function or initial state should be carefully examined. A wide range of influences, from emotional to cognitive to organic, may affect how a patient reacts to a particular treatment. Some patients who are overly stressed may demonstrate altered homeostatic responses. For example, the patient with TBI who presents with high arousal and agitated behaviors can be expected to react to treatment in unpredictable ways, frequently demonstrating "fight or flight" responses. Similarly, patients with TBI who are lethargic may be difficult to arouse and demonstrate limited ability to participate in therapy sessions. Changes in patient/client status and responses to individual treatment sessions should be carefully monitored and documented.

Expert clinicians develop the "art of clinical practice" by learning to adjust their input (e.g., verbal commands and manual contacts) based on patient response. Treatment thus becomes a dynamic and interactive process between patient and therapist. Shaping of behavior can be further enhanced by careful orientation to the purpose of the tasks and how they meet the patient's needs and the plan for subsequent sessions. This helps to engage the patient and ensure optimal cooperation and motivation.

Reexamination of the Patient and Evaluation of Expected Outcomes

This step is ongoing and involves continuous reexamination of the patient and a determination of the effectiveness of treatment. Data are evaluated within the context of the patient's progress toward goals and expected outcomes set forth in the POC. A determination is made whether the goals and outcomes are reasonable given the patient's diagnosis and progress. If the patient attains the desired level of competence for the stated goals, revisions in the POC are indicated. If the patient attains the desired level of competence for the expected outcomes, discharge is considered. If the patient fails to achieve the stated goals or outcomes, the therapist must determine why. Were the goals and outcomes realistic given the clinical problems and database? Were the interventions selected at an appropriate level to challenge the patient, or were they too easy or too difficult? Were facilitators appropriately identified and

the patient sufficiently motivated? Were intervening and constraining factors (barriers) identified? If the interventions were not appropriate, additional information is sought, goals modified, and different treatment interventions selected. Revision in the POC is also indicated if the patient progresses more rapidly or slowly than expected. Each modification must be evaluated in terms of its overall impact on the POC. Thus, the plan becomes a fluid statement of how the patient is progressing and what goals and outcomes are achievable. Its overall success depends on the therapist's ongoing clinical decision-making skills and on engaging the patient's cooperation and motivation.

■ DOCUMENTATION

Documentation is an essential requirement that serves as a record of patient/client care, including patient/client status, physical therapy management, and outcome of physical therapy intervention. Importantly, it demonstrates appropriate utilization of services for timely reimbursement from third-party payers. It also provides a mechanism for communication among the rehabilitation team members and may be used for policy or research purposes and outcomes analysis.[1] Written documentation is formally done at the time of admission and discharge, and at periodic intervals during rehabilitation (interim or progress notes). Many clinical settings require documentation for every treatment session. The format and timing of notes will vary according to the regulatory requirements specified by institutional policy, Medicare and third-party payers, state law, and specific accreditation organization (i.e., The Joint Commission, Commission on the Accreditation of Rehabilitation Facilities [CARF], and so forth). Data included in the medical record should be meaningful (important, not just nice to have), complete and accurate (valid and reliable), timely (recorded promptly), and systematic (regularly recorded). Patient involvement in the development and monitoring of the POC should be carefully documented. A description of specific interventions, any modifications needed, and communication/collaboration with other providers/patients/family/caregivers should also be included. Defensible Documentation for Patient/Client Management is a comprehensive series of documents available from APTA that includes Documentation Elements, General Guidelines, Current Concerns, Improving Your Clinical Documentation, and a Documentation Review Sample Checklist. These documents can be accessed at www.practice-dept@apta.org.[56]

In the United States, all health-care facilities must comply with Medicare coding and billing using the ICD-10-CM Official Guidelines for Coding and Reporting. These codes are developed by the Centers for Medicare and Medicaid Services (CMS) and the National Center for Health Statistics (NCHS). Adherence to these guidelines is required under the Health

Insurance Portability and Accountability Act. Thus, therapists need to be informed about current coding and include pertinent information consisting of the medical diagnosis code (e.g., G460 Middle cerebral artery syndrome) and the reason the patient/client is being seen (e.g., G8194 Hemiplegia, unspecified affecting left nondominant side). For current ICD-10 coding resources, visit the Provider Resources section of the CMS.org website.[57] APTA provides guidelines and information on how to identify the correct codes for ICD-10.[58]

Electronic documentation systems have expanded use in physical therapy and provide a fully integrated and completely paperless workflow for managing patient care. This includes managing referrals, initial intake data, progress and discharge notes, scheduling, and billing. Advantages of electronic documentation include standardization of data entry, increased speed of access to data, and integration of data that can be used for a wide variety of applications (e.g., clinical management of patients, quality control, clinical research). Information about the patient and his or her medical history is readily available from any computer or electronic device with Internet access. Therapists also can receive notification of when the patient arrives or checks in, as well as notice of scheduled evaluations and required POC updates. Software programs typically do not allow notes to be filed unless all the required elements are completed. Thus, overall efficiency of practice management is increased with decreased errors in documentation and improved accuracy of reimbursements. Many different companies provide software programs for physical therapy that focus on specific practice settings (e.g., outpatient rehabilitation, home care, private practice). Therapists using documentation software for electronic entry of patient data should ensure that programs comply with appropriate provisions for security and confidentiality.

■ EVIDENCE-BASED PRACTICE

Improved patient outcomes can be achieved by EBP, defined as "the integration of best research evidence with our clinical expertise and our patient's unique values and circumstances."[59] Therapists should utilize tests and measures and interventions that have undergone rigorous scientific examination while resisting use of interventions simply because they are in widespread clinical use. Numerous resources are available to assist the therapist in this process. The APTA has published a Clinical Research Agenda designed to support, explain, and enhance physical therapy clinical practice.[60] EBP tools are available on the APTA's evidence-based webpage. This site allows easy access to journals, clinical summaries, tests and measures, CPGs, Cochrane Reviews, and the Rehabilitation

Reference Center (see Table 1.2) Several texts are available that summarize valuable information regarding principles of EBP.[61–63] Components of EBP are summarized in Figure 1.7. Commonly used electronic databases are listed in Table 1.2.

The essential steps of EBP[59] are as follows:

Step 1: A clinical problem is identified, and an answerable question is formulated.
Step 2: A systematic literature review is conducted, and evidence collected.
Step 3: The research evidence is critically appraised for its validity (closeness to the truth), impact (size of the effect), and applicability (usefulness in clinical practice).
Step 4: The critical appraisal is synthesized and integrated with the clinician's expertise and the patient's unique values and circumstances.
Step 5: The effectiveness and efficiency of the steps in the evidence-based process are evaluated.

A well-constructed clinical question contains four elements: (1) the patient/client or population and clinical characteristics, (2) the specific intervention to be studied, (3) the comparison to an alternative intervention, and (4) the outcome achieved. This is represented by the acronym PICO—patient, intervention, comparison, outcome. For example, one study examined patients with low back pain (P) and compared specific interventions (I, C) (therapeutic exercise, transcutaneous electrical nerve stimulation, thermotherapy, ultrasound, massage, E-stim system, and traction). Outcomes (O) identified as being important to the patient (pain, function, patient global assessment, QOL, and return to work) were examined.[62]

Using Evidence to Guide Clinical Decisions

A hierarchy of evidence should be considered. At the top of the hierarchy are CPGs and systematic reviews (e.g., Cochrane Database of Systematic Reviews, Physiotherapy Evidence Database). Next is a consideration of individual randomized controlled trials (RCTs) followed by other less rigorous research designs (e.g., cohort design, case-control designs, single-subject design, qualitative design).

CPGs are defined as systematically developed statements to guide clinicians in using the best available evidence in patient care. They are developed through a combination of (1) expert consensus; (2) systematic reviews and meta-analysis; and (3) analysis of patient preferences combined with outcome-based guidelines. CPGs include an evaluation of the quality of relevant scientific literature and recommendations for treatment likely to be effective and beneficial as well as those likely to be ineffective or harmful. APTA has endorsed

Table 1.2	Commonly Used Electronic Databases for Evidence-Based Resources in Physical Therapy
Database or Search Engine	**Website**
MEDLINE and PubMed—U.S. National Library of Medicine: search service to Medline and Pre-Medline (database of medical and biomedical research), free public access	www.ncbi.nlm.nih.gov https://pubmed.ncbi.nlm.nih.gov/
PEDro, Physiotherapy Evidence Database: Includes abstracts, systematic reviews, and clinical practice guidelines in physiotherapy. PEDro is produced by the Centre for Evidence-Based Physiotherapy at the George Institute for Global Health, University of Sydney. They have initiatives to increase evidence in practice. Consider following them on X, formerly known as Twitter.	www.pedro.org.au @PEDro_database (twitter)
Cochrane Library: UK funded evidence-based–resource portal: You can access it as an app.	https://www.cochranelibrary.com/
Cochrane Database of Systematic Reviews: Gold standard for systematic reviews	https://www.cochranelibrary.com/cdsr/reviews
Cochrane Central Register of Controlled Trials (CCTR): A bibliographic database of definitive clinical trials	
Cochrane rehabilitation: special collection of rehabilitation-related articles. Consider signing up for their alerts.	https://rehabilitation.cochrane.org/
ECRI Guidelines Trust Repository for Clinical Practice Guidelines. They are rated for quality. You may wish to create your own account (it is free).	https://guidelines.ecri.org/
Guidelines International Network (GIN) Global network that supports guideline development and aggregates high-quality guidelines.	https://g-i-n.net/
National Institute for Health and Care Excellence (NICE) UK National Health Service Repository	https://www.nice.org.uk/guidance/published?ngt=NICE%20guidelines
American Physical Therapy Association (APTA) Evidence-Based Resources A landing page for APTA-sponsored resources such as clinical practice guidelines, tests and measures, clinical summaries, and the rehabilitation reference center. This is one of many member benefits.	https://www.apta.org/patient-care/evidence-based-practice-resources
National Rehabilitation Information Center (NARIC) citations and abstracts of research articles and books on all aspects of rehabilitation	www.naric.com
Clinical Trials Registry, National Institutes of Health (NIH): Provides information about ongoing clinical trials	www.clinicaltrials.gov
Database of Abstracts of Reviews of Effects (DARE): Reviews of evidence-based medicine including abstracts of systematic reviews	www.york.ac.uk/inst/crd
Cumulative Index to Nursing and Allied Health Literature (CINAHL): Includes abstracts and bibliographies	https://www.ebsco.com/products/research-databases/cinahl-database
Health Information Research Unit, McMaster University: Evidence-Based Health Informatics: Includes the Canadian Cochrane database	http://hiru.mcmaster.ca
Center for International Rehabilitation Research Information and Exchange: Maintains a database of rehabilitation research	https://publichealth.buffalo.edu/rehabilitation-science/research-and-facilities/funded-research/center-for-international-rehab-research-info-exchange.html
Rehabilitation Measures Database, Shirley Ryan Ability Lab, was developed by the Rehabilitation Institute of Chicago: Maintains a comprehensive database of rehabilitation tests and measures	www.rehabmeasures@.sralab.org

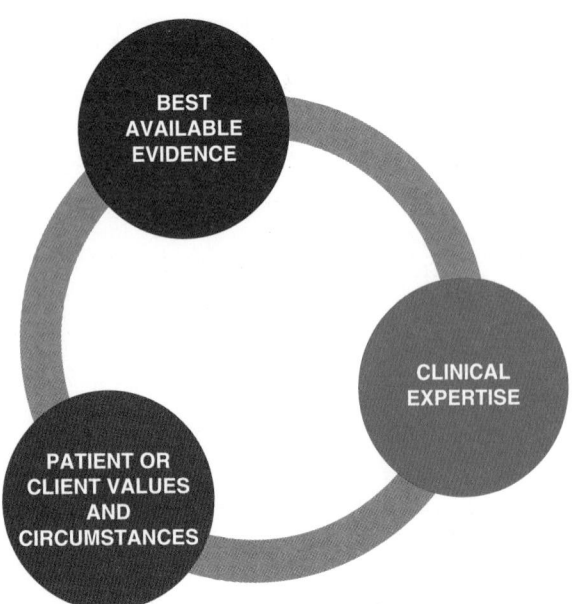

Figure 1.7 Components of EBP. *Introduction to the Guide to Physical Therapist Practice.* Guide to Physical Therapist Practice. *American Physical Therapy Association; 2014.* http://guidetoptpractice.apta.org/content/1/SEC1.body.

a process for establishing CPGs and has published a number of CPGs in conjunction with APTA sections. Selected examples include:

- Academy of Orthopedic Physical Therapy: published CPGs for the rehabilitation of patients with low back pain,[64] hip pain and mobility impairments,[65,66] knee pain and mobility impairments,[67,68] ankle stability and movement coordination impairments,[69,70] heel pain,[71] neck pain,[72] and shoulder impairments.[73]
- Academy of Cardiovascular and Pulmonary Physical Therapy and the Academy of Acute Care: published CPG on the management of individuals at risk for or diagnosed with venous thromboembolism.[74]
- Academy of Geriatric Physical Therapy: published CPG on the management of falls in community-dwelling older adults.[75]
- Academy of Neurologic Physical Therapy: published multiple CPGs. A couple of examples are vestibular rehabilitation for peripheral vestibular hypofunction[76] measurement of outcomes,[77] use of ankle-foot orthoses and electrical stimulation for persons poststroke.[78]

It important to consider the overall quality of the CPG document and to consider the methodology used. The Appraisal of Guidelines for Research and Evaluation Enterprise (AGREE) was developed to contribute to the science and advancement of practice guidelines through various programs of research and international collaborations. CPGs can be evaluated using the AGREE II Instrument.[79] This is used by the APTA for its resources, including *Physical Therapy* (journal of the APTA). This process helps to ensure that published guidelines are trustworthy. CPGs provide a summation of the best possible evidence for use in clinical practice. They should be viewed as general recommendations and do not provide detail regarding specific recommendations (e.g., aerobic exercise is recommended but the specifics of frequency, intensity, and time are not).

A systematic review (SR) is a comprehensive examination and analysis of the literature using critical appraisal skills. The researcher determines key resources to provide the evidence. These include peer-reviewed and evidence-based journals, electronic medical databases, and online search engines (e.g., PubMed). Table 1.2 includes commonly used electronic databases in physical therapy. Specific criteria are developed for the inclusion and exclusion of the research studies selected for review. Studies employing different designs may be analyzed individually or compared qualitatively; studies of similar design may be combined quantitatively (e.g., meta-analysis).

Critical analysis of research findings involves detailed examination of methodology, results, and conclusions. The clinician should be able to answer the following questions: (1) What is the level of evidence? (2) Is the evidence valid? and (3) Are the results important and clinically relevant? The PEDro scale was developed by physiotherapists at the University of Sydney to assist clinicians in evaluating the quality of rehabilitation literature (see Table 1.2). Interpretation and synthesis of the evidence must be considered within the context of the specific patient/client problem. Examination begins with the purpose of the study, which should be clearly stated, and the review of literature, which should be relevant in terms of the specific question asked. The methods/design should be closely examined. Research design varies and can be evaluated in terms of levels of evidence and grades of recommendation in order of most to least rigorous (Table 1.3). Although an RCT provides the most rigorous design, there are times when other designs are indicated. For example, there may be ethical issues involving control groups that receive no treatment when treatment is clearly beneficial. In addition, when outcomes are not clearly understood or defined (e.g., QOL issues), designs such as single-case studies may be indicated. See Chapter 8, Examination of Function, for additional discussion.

Table 1.3	Levels of Evidence and Grades of Recommendation	
Level	Intervention	Grade of Recommendation
1	a. SR[a] of RCT[b] b. Individual RCT with narrow confidence interval	A: Strong evidence
2	a. SR of cohort studies[c] b. Individual cohort study or individual low-quality RCT	B: Moderate evidence
3	a. SR of case-control studies[d] b. Individual case-control study	B: Moderate evidence
4	Case-series,[e] cohort or poor-quality cohort and case-control studies	C: Weak evidence
5	Expert opinion or bench research	D: Theoretical/foundational None or conflicting evidence

[a]SR, systematic review: A review in which the primary studies are summarized, critically appraised, and statistically combined; usually quantitative in nature with specific inclusion/exclusion criteria.

[b]RCT, randomized controlled trial: An experimental study in which participants are randomly assigned to either an experimental or control group to receive different interventions or a placebo; the most rigorous study design.

[c]Cohort study: A prospective (forward-in-time) study; a group of participants (cohort) with a similar condition receives an intervention and is followed over time and outcome evaluated; comparison is made to a matched group who do receive the intervention (quasi-experimental with no randomization).

[d]Case-control study: A retrospective study in which a group of subjects with a condition of interest are identified for research after outcomes are achieved (e.g., studying the impact of an intervention on level of participation); a comparison group is used.

[e]Case series: Clinical outcomes are evaluated of a single group of patients with a similar condition.

Adapted from Oxford Centre for Evidence-Based Medicine: Levels of Evidence. May 2001. Retrieved September 10, 2016, from www.cebm.net

SUMMARY

An organized process of clinical decision-making allows the therapist to systematically manage patients. Clinical decision-making is a shared process between the therapist and the patient. It is influenced by the clinician's foundation knowledge of movement science, and WHO's International Classification of Function, the Hypothesis-Oriented Algorithm for Clinical Decision-Making. It can be organized in steps of the *Guide to Physical Therapist Practice* for the patient/client management process, which are (1) history and interview; (2) systems review; (3) examination; including mapping participation goals to activities, movement observation and analysis, and tests and measures; (4) evaluation of the data and identify problems; (5) determine the diagnosis and prognosis; (6) determine the POC; (7) implement the POC; and (8) reexamine the patient and evaluating treatment outcomes. Patient participation through shared decision-making throughout the episode of care is essential in ensuring successful outcomes. Evidence-based practice allows the therapist to select interventions that have been shown to provide meaningful change in patients' lives. Inherent to the therapist's success in this process are an appropriate knowledge base and experience, critical-thinking and decision-making skills, and communication and teaching skills. Documentation is an essential requirement for effective communication among the rehabilitation team members and for timely reimbursement of services.

Note: The authors gratefully acknowledge the contributions to this chapter by Kathleen Gill Body PT, DPT, NCS, FAPTA; Margaret Schenkman PT, PhD, FAPTA; and George D. Fulk, PT, PhD, FAPTA.

Questions for Review

1. What is shared decision-making and where in the patient/client management would you use it?

2. What are the key steps in patient/client management?

3. Differentiate between participation restrictions, activity limitations, and body function/structure impairments. Define and give an example of each.

4. What are the essential elements of goal statements? Write two examples of each.

5. Differentiate between recovery and compensatory interventions. Give an example of each.

6. What is the FITT equation? Give an example of how each is used in formulating interventions for a POC.

7. What are the essential steps in EBP?

8. In EBP, what are the elements of a well-constructed clinical question? Give an example.

CASE STUDY

The patient is a 78-year-old woman who is a retired schoolteacher who was recently widowed after 48 years of marriage. She has two sons, one daughter, and four grandchildren; all live within an hour's driving distance. One of her children visits every weekend. She has a rambunctious black Labrador puppy that is 8 months old and was given to her "for company" at the time her husband died. She was walking the dog at the time of the accident. She is an active participant in a garden club, which meets twice a month, and in weekly events at the local senior center. Previously she was driving her car for all community activities and would like to return to driving.

She lives alone in a large old New England farmhouse. Her home has an entry with four stairs and no rail. Inside there are 14 rooms on two floors. The downstairs living area has a step down into the family room with no rail. There are 14 stairs to the second floor, with rails on either side. The upstairs sleeping area is cluttered with large, heavy furniture. The second-floor bathroom is small, with a high claw-foot tub with pedestal feet and a lip. There is no added equipment.

HISTORY INTERVIEW AND GOALS

The patient tripped and fell at home ascending the stairs outside the front door. She was admitted to the hospital after sustaining a transcervical, intracapsular fracture of the right femur. The patient had an open reduction and internal fixation procedure of the right lower extremity (RLE) to reduce and pin the fracture. After 2 weeks of acute hospital admission, the patient is at home and referred for home care physical therapy.

Patient states "I want to get my life back together, get my dog home again so I can take care of him. I want to be independent in my home and return to gardening."

PAST MEDICAL HISTORY–COMORBIDITIES

Patient has a long-standing problem with osteoporosis (on medication for 5 years). She has a history of falls, three in the last year alone. Approximately 3 years ago she had a myocardial infarction and presented with third-degree heart block, requiring implantation of a permanent pacemaker. She underwent cataract surgery with lens implantation in the right eye 2 years ago; the left eye is scheduled for similar surgery within the next few months.

OTHER HEALTH CONDITIONS (MEDICAL DIAGNOSES)

Coronary artery disease, hypertension (HTN), mitral valve prolapse, s/p permanent heart pacer, s/p right cataract with implant, osteoporosis (moderate to severe in the spine, hips, and pelvis), osteoarthritis with mild pain in right knee, s/p left elbow fracture (1 year ago), left ankle fracture (2 years ago), urinary stress incontinence.

MEDICATIONS

Fosamax 70 mg weekly
Atenolol 24 mg PO daily
MVI (multivitamin concentrate) with Fe tab PO daily
Metamucil 1 tb prn PO daily, Colace 100 mg PO bid
Tylenol No. 3 tab prn/mild pain

SYSTEMS REVIEW
Minimal Data Set—Including Cognition and Communication

Alert and oriented ×3; height 5 feet, weight 98 pounds
Pleasant, cooperative, articulate
No apparent memory deficits
Good problem-solving and safety awareness about hip precautions

CASE STUDY—cont'd

Cardiovascular
Pulse 74; BP 110/75

Pulmonary
RR 12 BPM

Neuro
Vision: wears glasses; cloudy vision L eye; impaired depth perception
Hearing: WFL
Sensation: BLEs intact
Sits unsupported and maintains balance

Integumentary
Incision healed and well approximated
Wears bilateral TEDs q a.m. × 6 wks

Musculoskeletal ROM LLE, BUEs: WFL

Posture
Flexed, stooped posture: moderate kyphosis, flexed hips and knees
Mild resting head tremor

Strength (MMT)
LLE, BUEs: WFL

EXAMINATION

Participation:
Gardening: unable
Walking dog–max assistance
Driving–unable

Activities—Functional Status (patient was completely independent [I] before her fall)
I bed mobility
Modified I in sit-to-stand and stand-to-sit transfers
Uses 2-in. foam cushions to elevate seat of kitchen chair and living room chair to assist in standing up.
Unable to do tub transfers at present
I dressing—upper
Modified I dressing—lower, uses reacher device
Bathing, minimal assist (MinA) of home health aide for sponge baths
IADL: requires moderate assistance (ModA) of home health aide for homemaker activities.

Berg Balance Test: Total Score: 42/56
Item 2 Standing, unsupported, EO: 4—able to stand safely for 2 minutes.
Item 6 Standing unsupported EC: 3—able to stand for 10 seconds with supervision.
Item 7 Standing unsupported feet together: 1—needs help, can stand for 15 seconds.
Item 8 Forward reach: 3—can safely reach 5 in. (12 cm)
Item 13 (tandem stance) and Item 14 (stand on one leg): 0—unable

Gait
Ambulates with standard walker and supervision approximately 200 feet on level surfaces, partial weight-bearing
Stairs: modified dependence—one flight of stairs with rail, small base quad cane and supervision
Gait speed and endurance: not tested at this time

Body Structure/Function
Range of Motion
Right hip:
Flex: 0° to 85°
Ext: NT (not tested)
Abd: 0° to 20°
Add: NT
IR, ER: NT

Right knee and ankle: WFL

(Continued)

CASE STUDY—cont'd

Strength (MMT)
RLE:
Hip flex NT
Hip ext NT
Hip abd NT
Knee ext: 4/5
Ankle: DF 4/5, PF 4/5

PRIMARY INSURANCE
Medicare with supplemental policy

Guiding Questions
1. Dissect the patient's participation goals into the relevant activities required to achieve them.
2. What are the patient's primary participation and activity limitations? Identify the body function/structure impairments that will need to be addressed to reduce the activity and participation limitations.
3. What are the facilitators for recovery, and what are the barriers?
4. What information is available about her functional status within the home in terms of performance versus capacity qualifiers?
5. What is her rehabilitation prognosis?
6. Write two long-term and two short-term goal statements to direct her POC.
7. Identify two direct treatment interventions and one patient education for her POC.
8. What interventions can be done for prevention and wellness?
9. What tests and measures can be used to determine successful attainment of outcomes?

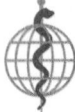

For additional resources, including answers to the questions for review, new immersive cases, case study guiding questions, references, and more, please visit **https://www.fadavis.com/product/physical -rehabilitation-fulk-8**. You may also quickly find the resources by entering this title's four-digit ISBN, 4691, in the search field at **http://fadavis.com** and logging in at the prompt.

Examination of Vital Signs

Shala Cunningham, PT, DPT, PhD, OCS, FAAOMPT
Thomas J. Schmitz, PT, PhD

Chapter 2

LEARNING OBJECTIVES

1. Discuss the rationale for including vital sign and pulse oximetry measures in the patient examination.
2. Explain the relevance of vital signs data when developing a diagnosis, determining the prognosis, and establishing a plan of care.
3. Recognize the importance of vital signs data in determining physiological response to treatment and evaluating patient progress.
4. Describe the procedure for monitoring temperature, pulse, respiration, blood pressure, and oxygenation saturation (pulse oximetry).
5. Differentiate between normal and abnormal values or ranges for each vital sign.
6. Identify the normative variations in vital signs and the factors that influence these changes.
7. Describe the recommended elements for documentation of vital signs data.

CHAPTER OUTLINE

NORMATIVE VITAL SIGN DATA *32*
ALTERATIONS IN VITAL SIGN VALUES: OVERVIEW OF INFLUENTIAL VARIABLES *33*
  Lifestyle Patterns and Patient Characteristics *33*
  Culture *33*
PATIENT OBSERVATION *34*
TEMPERATURE *35*
  Thermoregulatory System *36*
  Abnormalities in Body Temperature *38*
  Factors Influencing Body Temperature *39*
  Types of Thermometers *40*
  Hand Hygiene *42*
  Measuring Body Temperature *42*
PULSE *43*
  Rate *43*
  Rhythm *43*
  Quality *44*
  Factors Influencing Heart Rate *44*
  Pulse Sites *46*
  Monitoring Pulse *46*
  Automated Heart Rate Monitoring *49*
  Doppler Ultrasound *50*
RESPIRATION *50*
  Respiratory System *50*
  Regulatory Mechanisms *51*
  Factors Influencing Respiration *52*
  Parameters of Respiration *53*
  Patterns of Respiration *54*
  Respiratory Examination *55*
BLOOD PRESSURE *55*
  Blood Pressure Regulation *56*
  Factors Influencing Blood Pressure *56*
  Equipment Requirements *58*
  Korotkoff Sounds *59*
  Measuring Brachial Blood Pressure *61*
  Measuring Popliteal (Thigh) Blood Pressure *62*
PULSE OXIMETRY *63*
  Measuring Pulse Oximetry *63*
  Sources of Error *63*
RECORDING RESULTS *64*
RESOURCES *65*
SUMMARY *65*

Examination of body temperature, heart rate (HR), respiratory rate (RR), and blood pressure (BP) provides the physical therapist with important data about the status of the cardiovascular/pulmonary system. Owing to their importance as indicators of the body's physiological status and response to physical activity, environmental conditions, and emotional stressors, they are collectively referred to as vital signs. For many patients, measurement of vital signs is a crucial component of the clinical examination. Because many important clinical decisions are based in part on these measures, accuracy is essential.

The *American Physical Therapy Association (APTA) Guide to Physical Therapist Practice* includes examination of vital signs (HR, RR, and BP) in the cardiovascular/pulmonary systems review and among the tests and measures used to characterize or quantify aerobic capacity/endurance, circulation (arterial, venous, lymphatic), and ventilation and respiration. Pulse oximetry is included among the tests and measures used for examination of ventilation and respiration and aerobic capacity/endurance.[1] Although not considered a primary vital sign, pulse oximetry is an important related measure that provides information on arterial blood (hemoglobin) oxygen saturation levels (amount of oxygen available for tissues).[2] Data obtained allow the therapist to screen and monitor for *hypoxemia*—decreased oxygen concentrations of arterial blood. Hypoxemia is often associated with pulmonary disorders that impair ventilation of the lungs (e.g., pneumonia, chronic obstructive pulmonary disease [COPD], anemia, respiratory muscle weakness, and circulatory impairments).

Also referred to as *cardinal signs*, vital signs data represent quantitative measures of the body's essential physiological functions. Variations in vital signs are a clear indicator that some change in the patient's physiological status has occurred. Taken at rest and during and after exercise, these measures also provide important data on aerobic capacity and endurance. Taken together with other examination data, vital sign measures assist the physical therapist in making clinical judgments to do the following:[1]

1. Determine the patient's baseline status.
2. Identify potential risk factors, suspected pathology, and impairments of body functions and structures.
3. Develop the diagnosis, prognosis, and plan of care (POC).
4. Reexamine the patient periodically throughout the episode of care to determine if outcome expectations are being met.
5. Evaluate the effectiveness of interventions in achieving goals (intended impact on functioning) and outcomes (results of implementing POC that indicate the impact on functioning).
6. Determine whether a referral or consultation with another practitioner is indicated.

The physical therapist's clinical decision-making will determine which vital signs should be measured and the frequency of measurement for an individual patient within a specific context (e.g., self-paced ambulation on level surfaces vs. stair climbing). Although taking vital sign measures may be delegated to a physical therapist assistant, the physical therapist evaluates and determines the significance of the data.

■ NORMATIVE VITAL SIGN DATA

Many resources provide vital signs values across age groups. Normative data are typically presented as averages or as a range of values for the age group from which they were derived; using a range reflects the variability of values designated as normal. Table 2.1 provides examples of normative vital signs data presented by age ranges.[3-5]

Clinical Note. Normative vital sign data provide the physical therapist with a *general reference* for comparison during evaluation of clinical findings. Values included in normative tables should be considered cautiously because discrepancies and inconsistencies exist among sources. As discussed later in this chapter, another consideration in using these data is that vital sign values are specific to the individual (may typically run slightly higher or lower) and are influenced by multiple factors, such as normal diurnal patterns, environmental temperature, physical activity, medications, and emotions. Accurate interpretation requires knowledge of an individual's baseline measures as well as existing influencing factors at the time measures are taken.

"Normal" resting vital sign measures are specific to the individual and are referred to as *baseline values*. Some people typically display baseline values in a way that is different from values represented by normative data. For example, aerobically trained individuals often have resting HRs of less than 60 beats per minute (bpm), with some reports of values in the low 30s.[6] Such variation underscores the importance of knowing baseline measures and of monitoring vital signs as a sequential process for each individual. Vital sign measurements yield the most useful information when performed and recorded at *periodic intervals over time* as opposed to a single measurement taken at a given point in time. Serial recording allows changes in patient status or response to treatment to be monitored over time and can indicate an acute change in physiological status at a specific point in time (e.g., response to an exercise test).

On examination, initial vital sign measures may be well within normal ranges. In these circumstances, Wilkinson et al. suggest that one should "not become complacent when a client's vital signs are within normal limits. Although stable vital signs *indicate* physiological

Table 2.1	Comparison of Normal Vital Signs for Various Ages 35				
Age	Temperature F° (C°)	Blood Pressure (mm Hg) 50th to 90th Percentile Systolic	Diastolic	Respiratory Rate	Pulse Rate
Newborn	97.9–100.3	72–104	37–56	30–60	100–170
1–2 yrs	97.9–100.3	85–106	41–62	24–20	80–150
3–5 yrs	97.9–100.3	90–110	47–73	20–34	70–130
6–12 yrs	97.9–100.3	90–121	59–78	15–30	65–120
Adolescent	98.0–100.3	102–124	64–80	12–20	55–90
Adult	98.0–100.3	<120	<80	12–18	60–100
Older Adult	97.8–100.3	<120	<80	12–20	60–100

well-being, they do not *guarantee* it. Vital signs alone are limited in detecting some important physiological changes; for example, vital signs may sometimes remain stable in the presence of moderately large blood loss. Evaluate the vital signs in the context of your overall assessment of the client."[7]

At times, an abnormally high or low value for a vital sign may be obtained. In such situations, it is important to maintain a calm, professional demeanor and not react adversely to the information. As discussed later in this chapter, multiple factors can alter vital sign values, including those that are patient related (e.g., emotions, stress, excessive caffeine ingestion, medication intake) and/or practitioner related (e.g., faulty positioning and measurement, incorrect BP cuff size). Any abnormal values should be investigated and, if deemed appropriate, repeated to confirm accuracy. A comparison should be made of subjective and objective data to determine if what the patient states is consistent with data obtained.[8] It is also important to ensure that vital sign data is consistent with key patient information such as symptoms, comorbidities, medications, and laboratory values.

Clinical Note. As with all physical therapy examinations, before a vital sign measure is taken, the procedure and its rationale should be explained in terms appropriate to the patient's understanding and confirmation made of the patient's safety, privacy, modesty, comfort, and understanding.

■ ALTERATIONS IN VITAL SIGN VALUES: OVERVIEW OF INFLUENTIAL VARIABLES

Lifestyle Patterns and Patient Characteristics

Several lifestyle patterns (modifiable) and patient characteristics (nonmodifiable) influence vital sign measures. Lifestyle patterns include, but are not limited to, caffeine intake, tobacco use, diet, alcohol consumption, response to stress, obesity, physical activity level, medications, and use of illegal drugs. Patient characteristics include hormonal status, age, sex, and family history. Other variables that affect vital sign measures include time of day, general health status, emotional distress, and pain. Information about lifestyle patterns and patient characteristics is gathered from the patient history, the systems review, and tests and measures. Factors identified as modifiable become the focus of patient-related instruction (e.g., current condition, risk factor reduction) and/or health promotion and wellness strategies. Specific factors influencing each vital sign are addressed in greater detail later in the chapter.

Culture

As with any physical therapy test or measure, the influence of culture on vital sign measures can vary from subtle to marked. *Culture* refers to an integration of learned behaviors (not biologically inherited), norms, and symbols characteristic of a society that are passed from generation to generation.[9] It is a set of shared behavioral standards that include fundamental values, beliefs, attitudes, and customs, including those related to health care and illness.[10,11] *Cultural competence* in health care refers to the ability to effectively provide care consistent with the patient's cultural needs. The Centers for Disease Control and Prevention (CDC) broadly defines cultural competence as "a set of congruent behaviors, attitudes, and policies that come together in a system, agency, or among professionals that enable effective work in cross-cultural situations."[12] The APTA supports this holistic definition of cultural competence.[13] Emphasizing the overarching importance of cultural competence, Leavitt proposes that "for physical therapy practitioners, cultural competence is an essential element in making effective and efficient examination, evaluation, diagnosis, prognosis, and intervention possible. Developing rapport, collecting and synthesizing patient data, recognizing personal functional concerns, and developing the plan of care for a particular patient requires cultural competence."[9] Recent demographic changes in the United States have created greater societal diversity and have heightened the need for culturally competent physical therapists. Data from the 2020 Census (conducted every 10 years) demonstrate the evolving diversity of cultures and ethnicities that comprise the U.S. population.[14]

Reflective of the importance of cultural competence in understanding and responding effectively to the cultural needs of patients in health-care settings, the U.S. Department of Health and Human Service's Office of Minority Health published *National Standards for Culturally and Linguistically Appropriate Services in Health Care* with input from a national advisory committee. The 15 standards are offered as guidelines for providers, policymakers, accreditation and credentialing agencies, purchasers of health benefits (including labor unions), patients, and advocates (e.g., local and national ethnic-, immigrant-, and other community-focused organizations), as well as educators and other members of the health-care community.[15] The principal standard is to "Provide effective, equitable, understandable, and respectful quality care and services that are responsive to diverse cultural health beliefs and practices, preferred languages, health literacy, and other communication needs."[10] Physical therapists should be knowledgeable of the diversity within and among the patient populations they serve. Examination strategies and plans of care should be developed that carefully consider and incorporate the patient's beliefs and attitudes related to both health care and illness.[10,11,16]

■ PATIENT OBSERVATION

Observation refers to the deliberate use of the senses (vision, hearing, smell) to gather information about the patient.[7,8] Observation alone will not provide definitive diagnostic information, nor will it allow one to draw conclusions or inferences; however, observation may provide clues to underlying problems, guide selection of screening examinations, and assist with prioritizing tests and measurements, especially those related to the medical stability of the patient.[17–19] Using a logical, consistent sequence will create a systematic approach to observation (e.g., first facial expression and overall appearance, signs of pain or distress, skin condition). This will improve efficiency, conserve time, and help ensure that no areas are overlooked. The following are examples of the types of information and clues to underlying problems that may be gathered via observation:

- Signs of immediate patient distress or discomfort (e.g., pain, grimacing, difficulty breathing) are typically evident by observation of facial expressions, use of accessory muscles for breathing, an irregular or labored breathing pattern, and frequent positional changes. Use of accessory muscles of breathing may be indicative of cardiac or pulmonary impairments.
- *Diaphoresis* (profuse perspiration) may indicate that the body is working to compensate for a reduced cardiac output. It is associated with a variety of potential causes, including myocardial infarct, hypotension, and shock; it may also be associated with hyperthermia (e.g., faulty thermoregulation), thyroid hyperactivity, anxiety, and overactive sweat glands. Excessive sweating may also be related to environmental conditions or patient participation in strenuous physical activity prior to visit. The term *hyperhidrosis* also refers to abnormally increased perspiration. In addition, the timing of sweating can be suggestive of underlying problems. For example, nocturnal sweating may suggest malignancy and intermittent sweating may be associated with infection.[20]
- A disagreeable body odor may suggest poor hygiene (e.g., impaired self-care abilities or lack of resources) or the presence of a wound (e.g., infected drainage) or underlying disease; a fruity breath smell may be suggestive of high blood glucose or diabetic ketoacidosis.[7,19]
- Various sounds of respiration may be heard, such as wheezing, crackles, or sighs (discussed later in this chapter and in Chapter 12, Chronic Pulmonary Dysfunction). Potential considerations include a narrowed airway, COPD, presence of foreign object, or secretions partially blocking an airway.
- The presence of a cough may be caused by a relatively benign airway irritant (e.g., dust particles) or may indicate the presence of a disease such as asthma, bronchitis, COPD, lung cancer, or pneumonia. An acute cough typically resolves within 3 weeks or less (e.g., upper respiratory tract infection). A chronic or persistent cough is typically defined as lasting more than 8 weeks.
- The skin is the largest organ of the body; observation of skin color provides important preliminary data about the efficiency of the cardiovascular/pulmonary system and may be an indicator of disease, inflammation, and infection.[17,19] Common skin color changes with associated causes are presented in Box 2.1.
- The skin should also be observed for changes in texture and hair growth. Patients with diabetes mellitus or atherosclerosis typically lack hair growth on the legs and display thickening of the nails of the fingers and toes. Skin texture also varies with age and poor nutritional status. Skin lesions may be indicative of pathological changes or trauma.
- The color and appearance of fingernails should be noted. With normal circulation and oxygen supply, they should be pink (or light brown in dark-skinned individuals) and free of irregularities. Examples of pathological changes in nails include the following:
  - *Beau lines* are deep grooved (indented) transverse lines across the nail resulting from disruption of nail growth caused by trauma or disorders such as Raynaud disease (decreased blood flow to fingers), psoriasis, or infection around the nail plate.
  - *Clubbing* is a bulbous swelling of fingertips secondary to proliferation of connective tissue between the nail matrix and distal phalanx, accompanied by a loss of the normal angle between the nailbed and the skin; nails appear bluish gray (cyanotic) and become soft and boggy (spongy).[21] Clubbing develops gradually over time and is associated with diagnoses that involve long-standing hypoxia, such as congenital heart defects and cardiopulmonary diseases (Fig. 2.1).
  - *Half-and-half nails* (also called *Lindsay nails*) are seen with renal failure; the distal portion of the nail turns red, pink, or brown; there is a distinct line of demarcation between the two halves.
  - *Onycholysis* is detachment of the nail from the nailbed; associated with trauma, fungal infections, psoriasis, and overactive thyroid gland.
  - *Mee lines* are transverse white lines across the breadth of the nail associated with systemic diseases such as renal failure, Hodgkin disease, malaria, and sickle cell disease; classically associated with arsenic poisoning.
  - *Pitting* is characterized by tiny punctate depressions in the nail caused by systemic diseases such as reactive arthritis, psoriasis, and eczema.
  - *Splinter hemorrhages* are tiny hemorrhages creating reddish lines of blood under the nail (appears as if a "splinter" is lodged under the nail) and is associated with bacterial endocarditis and trauma.

Box 2.1 Common Skin Color Changes

- **Cyanosis:** In patients with light skin tones, may present as a bluish-gray discoloration of the skin and mucous membranes. In patients with dark skin tones, cyanosis may present as gray or whitish discoloration. In patients with yellow-toned skin, cyanosis may be grayish-greenish in appearance.
- **Central cyanosis:** Caused by hypoxia and results in color changes in central aspects of body and mucous membranes; associated with diseases of the cardiovascular and pulmonary system and CNS disorders that impair respiration.
- **Peripheral cyanosis:** Caused by hypoxia with color changes in the nailbeds and lips; associated with decreased cardiac output, exposure to cold (extreme vasoconstriction), and arterial (peripheral vascular disease) or venous obstruction (deep vein thrombosis).
- **Acute cyanosis:** Caused by hypoxia from a blocked airway (asphyxiation or choking), with rapid onset of skin color changes initially in the face, lips, and nailbeds.
- **Ecchymosis:** Caused by bruising (bleeding under the skin) and may be seen anywhere on the body; new bruises appear bluish purple whereas older bruises are greenish yellow; often caused by trauma (e.g., falls, sports injury, physical abuse); patients on blood thinning agents (e.g., Coumadin) tend to bruise more easily. In patients with dark skin tones, new bruises may be purple, dark brown, or black.
- **Erythema:** Reddened area of skin caused by increased blood flow (hyperemia); associated with skin irritation or injury, infection, and inflammation; redness over a bony prominence warns of the potential development of a decubitus ulcer. In patients with dark skin tones, erythema may appear as hyperpigmentation.
- **Flushing:** Diffuse redness of face; may involve other body areas; related to emotions (embarrassment, anger), physical exertion, fever, and increased temperature of environment.
- **Jaundice:** Caused by impaired liver function (e.g., hepatitis, liver cancer), the skin takes on a yellow-orange hue; it is best observed in the sclera, mucous membranes, and palm of hands and sole of the feet.
- **Pallor (pale):** The skin takes on a lighter tone (whiter, with decreased pink hue) than normal for the individual (a normally "fair" skin color should be ruled out); for darker skin, pallor is apparent by loss of red tones; associated with anemia (low hemoglobin) and impaired circulation; observed in the face, palms, mucous membranes, and nailbeds.
- **Petechiae:** Tiny red or purple hemorrhagic spots caused by capillary bleeding with subsequent leakage of blood into the skin; tend to appear in clusters and are often seen on the ankles and feet, but can occur anywhere on body; may be a sign of thrombocytopenia (low platelet count); as platelets play a critical role in clotting, reduced counts impair clotting and increase the risk of bleeding; low platelet counts are associated with a variety of medications (e.g., anticoagulants, aspirin, steroids, and chemotherapy drugs) and disorders (e.g., acute and chronic infections, leukemia, systemic lupus erythematosus, and scleroderma).

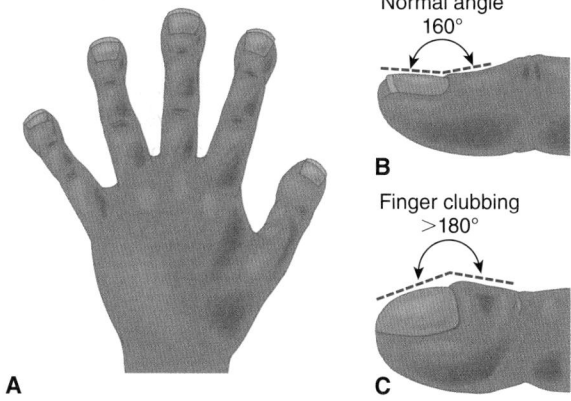

Figure 2.1 (A) Clubbing of fingertips is associated with long-term hypoxic states; (B) normal nail plate angle of 160°; (C) a nail plate angle of 180° or more occurs with clubbing.

- Abnormal posture may be suggestive of pain or structural abnormalities of the pelvis (pelvic obliquity), pectoral, or vertebral regions that may also interfere with respiratory patterns.

- Edema may be associated with congestive heart failure (CHF), liver failure, lymphedema, venous insufficiency, or severe hypothyroidism triggering myxedema; localized edema may result from varicose veins, thrombophlebitis, or trauma.

■ TEMPERATURE

Body temperature represents a balance between the heat produced or acquired by the body and the amount of heat lost. Because humans are warm-blooded, or *homoiothermic*, body temperature remains relatively constant despite changes in the external environment. This is in contrast to cold-blooded, or *poikilothermic*, animals (such as reptiles), in which body temperature varies with that of their environment.

Figure 2.2 presents a comparison of Fahrenheit and centigrade temperature values with ranges of normal and altered body temperature. Oral temperatures will be affected by oral intake, including smoking. Patients should refrain from smoking or eating for at least 15 minutes prior to an oral temperature reading.

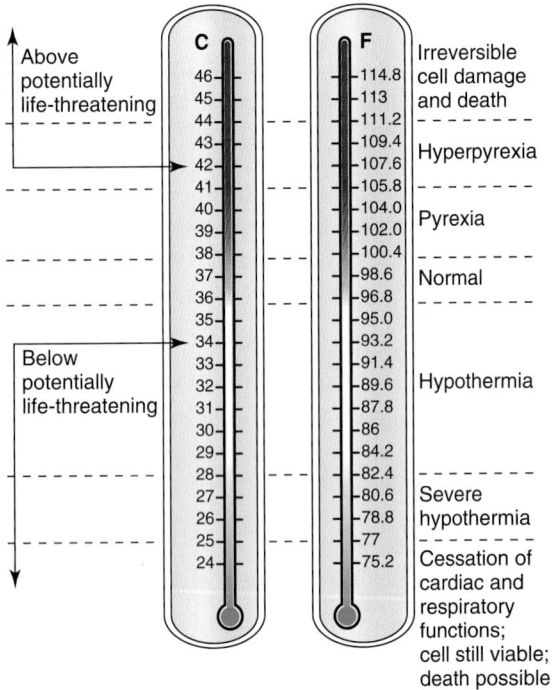

Figure 2.2 Comparison of Fahrenheit and centigrade scales indicating ranges of normal and altered body temperature. *(Adapted from Wilkinson, et al., 8, p. 423 with permission.)*

Clinical Note. If a situation occurs that requires changing a temperature reading from one scale to the other, a conversion formula can be used. To convert centigrade into Fahrenheit, multiply the centigrade value by 9/5 and add 32 (F = [9/5 × C°] + 32°). To change from Fahrenheit into centigrade, subtract 32 from the Fahrenheit value and multiply by 5/9 (C = [F − 32°] × 5/9).

Thermoregulatory System

The purpose of the thermoregulatory system is to maintain a relatively constant internal body temperature. This system monitors and acts to maintain temperatures that are optimal for normal cellular and vital organ function. The thermoregulatory system consists of three primary components: the thermoreceptors, the regulating center, and the effector organs.[22,23]

Thermoreceptors

The thermoreceptors provide input to the temperature-regulating center located in the hypothalamus. The regulating center depends on information from thermoreceptors to achieve constant temperatures. Once this information reaches the regulatory center, it is compared with a "set point" standard or optimal temperature value. Depending on the contrast between the "set" value and incoming information, mechanisms may be activated to either conserve or dissipate heat.[24]

Peripheral and central thermoreceptors provide afferent temperature input to the regulating center. The peripheral receptors (skin temperature), composed primarily of free nerve endings, have a high distribution in the skin. Central thermoreceptors (core temperature) are located in the deep tissues (e.g., abdominal organs), nervous system, and the hypothalamus.[24,25] The thermoreceptors located in the hypothalamus are sensitive to temperature changes in blood perfusing the hypothalamus. These cells also can initiate responses to either conserve or dissipate heat. They are particularly sensitive to core temperature changes and monitoring body warmth.[22] The thermoreceptors permit *feedforward* responses to expected changes in core temperature (e.g., change in environmental temperature).

The cutaneous peripheral thermoreceptors demonstrate a larger distribution of cold receptors than warmth receptors and are sensitive to rapid changes in temperature.[22] Signals from these receptors enter the spinal cord through afferent nerves and travel to the hypothalamus via the lateral spinothalamic tract.

Regulating Center

The temperature-regulating center of the body is located in the hypothalamus. The hypothalamus coordinates the heat production and loss processes, much like a thermostat, ensuring an essentially constant, stable body temperature. By influencing the effector organs, the hypothalamus achieves a relatively precise balance between heat production and heat loss. In a healthy individual, the hypothalamic thermostat is set and carefully maintained at 98.6° ± 1.8°F (37° ± 1°C).[22] In situations in which input from thermoreceptors indicates a drop in temperature below the "set" value, mechanisms are activated to conserve heat. Conversely, a rise in temperature will activate mechanisms to dissipate heat. Mechanisms to dissipate heat are particularly important during strenuous exercise. Figure 2.3 summarizes the primary physiological adjustments to exercise or increases in environmental temperature that occur during heat acclimation (physiological adaptations to dissipate and improve tolerance to heat). These responses are activated through hypothalamic control of the effector organs. Input to the effector organs is transmitted through pathways of both the somatic and autonomic nervous systems.[22,23,26,27]

Clinical Note. It is important to note that the normal human body temperature ranges have been expanded to range from 97° to 100.3°F.[28,29]

Effector Organs

The effector organs respond to both increases and decreases in temperature. The primary effector systems include vascular, metabolic, skeletal muscle (shivering),

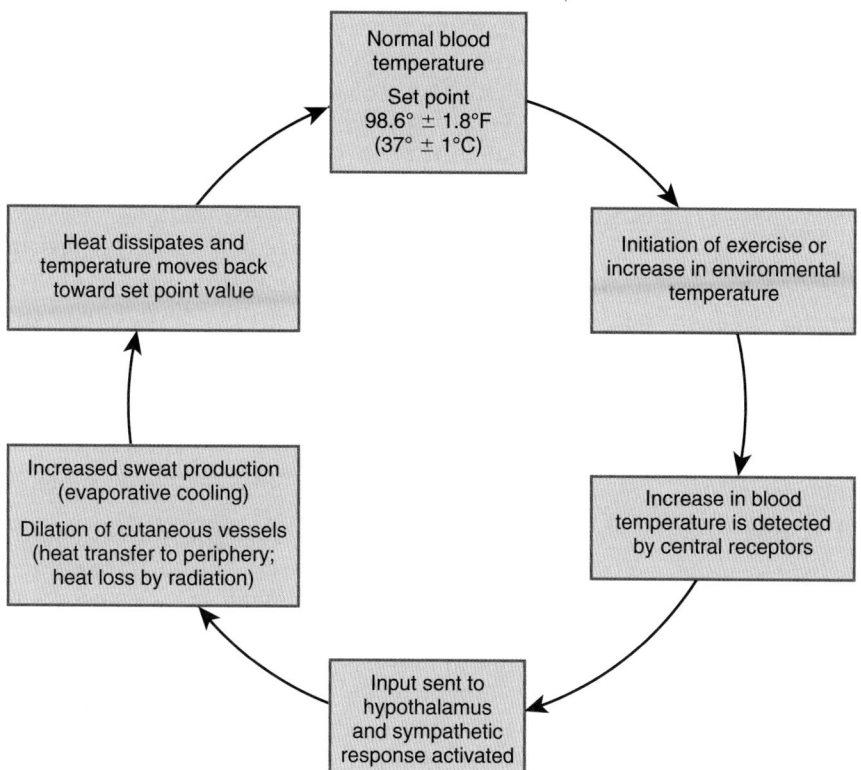

Figure 2.3 Thermoregulatory response during heat acclimation. Increased body temperature activates heat (loss) dissipation to maintain normal body temperature.

and sweating. These effector systems function either to increase or to dissipate body heat.

Conservation and Production of Body Heat

When body temperature is lowered, mechanisms are activated to conserve heat and increase heat production. The following are descriptions of heat conservation and production mechanisms:

- *Vasoconstriction of blood vessels:* The hypothalamus activates sympathetic nerves, an action that results in vasoconstriction of cutaneous vessels throughout the body. This significantly reduces the lumen of the vessels and decreases blood flow near the surface of the skin, where the blood would normally be cooled. Thus, the amount of heat lost to the environment is decreased.
- *Decrease (or absence) of sweat gland activity:* To reduce or to prevent heat loss by evaporation, sweat gland activity is diminished. Sweating is totally abolished with cooling of the hypothalamic thermostat below approximately 98.6°F (37°C).[22]
- *Cutis anserina or piloerection*: Also a response to cooling of the hypothalamus, this heat conservation mechanism is commonly described as "gooseflesh." The term *piloerection* means "hairs standing on end." Although of less significance in humans, this mechanism functions to trap a layer of insulating air near the skin and decrease heat loss in lower mammals with greater hair covering.

The body also responds to decreased temperature with several mechanisms, including shivering and hormonal regulation, designed to produce heat. These mechanisms are activated when body temperature falls below a critical temperature level.[23] The primary motor center for shivering is located in the posterior hypothalamus. This area is activated by cold signals from the skin and spinal cord. In response to cold, impulses from the hypothalamus activate the efferent somatic nervous system, causing increased tone of skeletal muscles. As the tone gradually increases to a certain threshold level, *shivering* (involuntary muscle contraction) is initiated, and heat is produced. This shivering reflex can be at least partially suppressed through conscious cortical control and voluntary muscle activity.[30]

The function of hormonal influence in thermal regulation is to increase cellular metabolism, which subsequently increases body heat. Increased metabolism occurs through circulation of two hormones from the adrenal medulla: *norepinephrine* and *epinephrine*. This is called *chemical thermogenesis*. Circulating levels of these hormones, however, are of greater significance in maintaining body temperature in infants than in adults. Heat production by these hormones can be increased in an infant by as much as 100%, as opposed to 10% to 15% in an adult.[23]

A second form of hormonal regulation involves increased output of *thyroxine* by the thyroid gland. Thyroxine increases the rate of cellular metabolism throughout the body. This response, however, occurs only as a result of prolonged cooling, and heat production is not immediate.[22] The thyroid gland requires several weeks to hypertrophy before increased demands for thyroxine can be achieved.

Loss of Body Heat

Excess heat is dissipated from the body through four primary methods: radiation, conduction, convection, and evaporation.

- *Radiation:* The transfer of heat by electromagnetic waves from one object to another is accomplished by radiation. This heat transfer occurs through the air between objects that are not in direct contact. Heat is lost to surrounding objects that are colder than the body (e.g., a wall or surrounding objects in the room).
- *Conduction:* The transfer of heat from one object to another through a liquid, solid, or gas takes place by conduction. This type of heat transfer requires direct molecular contact between two objects, as when a person is sitting on a cold surface or when heat is lost in a cool swimming pool. Heat is also lost by conduction to air.
- *Convection:* The transfer of heat by movement of air or liquid (water) is achieved by convection. This form of heat loss is accomplished secondary to conduction. Once the heat is conducted to the air, the air is then moved away from the body by convection currents. Use of a fan or a cool breeze provides convection currents. Heat loss by convection is most effective when the air or liquid surrounding the body is continually moved away and replaced.
- *Evaporation:* Dissipation of body heat by the conversion of a liquid to a vapor occurs by evaporation. This form of heat loss occurs on a continual basis through the respiratory tract and through perspiration from the skin. Evaporation provides the major mechanism of heat loss during heavy exercise. Profuse sweating provides a significant cooling effect on the skin as it evaporates. In addition, this cooling of the skin functions to further cool the blood as it is shunted from internal structures to cutaneous areas.

Abnormalities in Body Temperature
Increased Body Temperature

Pyrexia is the elevation of normal body temperature, more commonly referred to as fever.[26,27] Fever is part of the body's natural defense against infectious disease (invading pathogens). Increasing internal temperatures creates an environment less favorable for viruses and bacteria to replicate. Fever occurs when the "set" value of the hypothalamic thermostat is triggered to rise by circulating pyrogens (fever-producing substances) secreted primarily from toxic bacteria, viruses, or injured body tissue. The effects of these pyrogens result in fever during illness. As a result of the new, higher thermostat value, the body responds by activating its heat conservation and production mechanisms. These mechanisms

raise body temperature to a new, higher value over a period of several hours. Thus a fever, or febrile state, is produced.

The clinical signs and symptoms of a fever vary with the level of disturbance of the thermoregulatory center and with the phase of the fever. These signs and symptoms may include general malaise, headache, increased pulse and RR, chills, piloerection, shivering, loss of appetite (anorexia), pale skin that later becomes flushed and hot to the touch, nausea, irritability, restlessness, constipation, sweating, thirst, coated tongue, decreased urinary output, weakness, and insomnia.[17,31]

Several types of fevers present unique characteristics that are named based on their distinguishing clinical feature: *continuous, intermittent, relapsing,* or *remittent* (Box 2.2).

An unusually high fever above 106.7°F (41.5°C) is called *hyperpyrexia.* Hyperthermia is an uncontrolled increase in body temperature with an unchanged setting of the thermoregulatory center. Excessively high body temperatures are caused by an inability of the thermoregulatory system to lose heat fast enough to balance excessive heat production or high environmental temperatures. Examples of hyperthermia include heat exhaustion and heat stroke. *Heat exhaustion* is associated with exercise and physical exertion in high environmental temperatures where the cardiovascular system cannot meet the demands of blood flow to the skin (thermoregulation) and to the muscles (metabolic exercise requirements). Symptoms include profuse sweating, fatigue,

---

Box 2.2   Common Types of Fever

Continuous (also known as constant or sustained): Body temperature is constantly elevated above normal throughout day but does not fluctuate by more than 1.8°F (1°C) in 24 hrs; seen in uncomplicated minor infection, urinary tract infection, lobar pneumonia, typhoid (foodborne illness), infective endocarditis, and typhus (flea-borne disease).

Intermittent: Body temperature alternates between periods of fever for some hours of the day with return to normal temperatures for the remaining hours; seen in malaria and septicemia.

Relapsing (also known as recurrent or periodic): Periods of fever are interspersed with normal temperatures; each lasts at least one day; seen in noninfectious inflammatory diseases such as rheumatoid arthritis and Crohn's disease, recurrent infections, malignancy (neoplastic fever), and infections caused by certain species of *Borrelia* spirochetes (ticks and lice).

Remittent: Elevated body temperature throughout day that fluctuates more than 3.6°F (2°C) within a 24-hr period but never returns to normal; seen in infective endocarditis and typhoid infection.

faintness, dizziness, weak and rapid pulse, nausea, headache, and vomiting. Treatment typically includes stopping physical activity, moving to a cooler environment, drinking fluid, removing tight clothing, assuming a supine position with legs elevated, and applying available cooling methods such as fans or ice packs or towels. *Heat stroke* is a more severe form of hyperthermia in which the thermoregulatory system essentially fails. It can be life-threatening and requires immediate emergency medical attention to rapidly reduce body temperature (ice water immersion, ice packs). Symptoms include rapid and shallow breathing; mental status changes (confusion, delirium); strong, rapid pulse; lack of sweating; faintness; throbbing headache; and eventually loss of consciousness or death.[7,23,32–35]

Decreased Body Temperature

Exposure to extreme cold produces a lowered body temperature called *hypothermia*. With prolonged exposure to cold, there is a decrease in metabolic rate, and body temperature gradually falls. As cooling of the brain occurs, there is a depression of the thermoregulatory center. The function of the thermoregulatory center becomes seriously impaired when body temperature falls below approximately 94°F (34.4°C) and is completely lost with temperatures below 85°F (29.4°C).[36] Therefore, the body's heat regulatory and protection mechanism is lost. Symptoms of hypothermia include decreased HR and RR, cold and pale skin, cyanosis, decreased cutaneous sensation, depression of mental and muscular responses, and drowsiness, which may eventually lead to coma. If hypothermia is left untreated, the progression of these symptoms may lead to death.

Factors Influencing Body Temperature

A statistical average or normal temperature of 98.6°F (37°C) taken orally has been established for body temperature in an adult population. However, a range of values is more representative of normal body temperature because certain everyday circumstances (e.g., time of day) or activities (e.g., exercise) influence the body's temperature. In addition, some individuals typically run a *slightly higher* or *lower* body temperature than the statistical average. Therefore, deviations from the average will be apparent from individual to individual, as well as between measures taken from the same person under varying circumstances.

Time of Day

The term *circadian rhythm* describes a 24-hr cycle of normal variations in body temperature. Certain predictable and regular changes in temperature occur on a daily basis. Body temperature tends to be lowest between 4:00 and 6:00 a.m. and highest between 4:00 and 8:00 p.m. Digestive processes and the level of skeletal muscle activity significantly influence these regular changes in body temperature. For individuals who work at night, this pattern is usually inverted.[22,24]

Age

Compared with adults, infants demonstrate a higher normal temperature owing to the immaturity of the thermoregulatory system. Infants are particularly susceptible to environmental temperature changes, and their body temperature will fluctuate accordingly. Young children also average higher normal temperatures because of the heat production associated with increased metabolic rate and high physical activity levels. Older adults tend to demonstrate lower than average body temperatures owing to a variety of factors, including lower metabolic rates, decreased subcutaneous tissue mass (which normally insulates the body against heat loss), decreased physical activity levels, and inadequate diet.

Emotions/Stress

Stimulation of the sympathetic nervous system causes increased production of epinephrine and norepinephrine with a subsequent increase in metabolic rate.

Exercise

The effects of exercise on body temperature are an important consideration for physical therapists. Strenuous exercise significantly increases body temperature because of an increase in metabolic rate. Active muscle contractions are an important and potent source of heat production. During exercise, body temperature increases are proportional to the relative intensity of the workload. The magnitude of temperature change appears to be influenced by fitness level.[37] Vigorous exercise can increase the metabolic rate by as much as 20 to 25 times that of the basal level.[22]

External Environment

Generally, warm weather tends to increase body temperature, and cold weather decreases body temperature. Environmental conditions influence the body's ability to maintain constant temperatures. For example, in hot, humid environments, the effectiveness of evaporative cooling is severely diminished because the air is already heavily moisture laden. Other forms of heat dissipation are also dependent on environmental factors such as movement of air currents (convection). Clothing also can be an important external consideration because it can function either to conserve or to facilitate release of body heat. The amount and type of clothing are important. To dissipate heat, absorbent, loose-fitting, light-colored clothing is most effective. To conserve heat, several layers of lightweight clothing to trap air and to insulate the body are recommended.

Medications

Several medications may cause an increase in body temperature. For example, neuroleptic malignant syndrome is a relatively rare but serious reaction to the use of

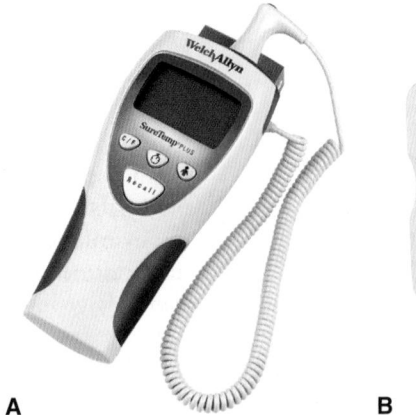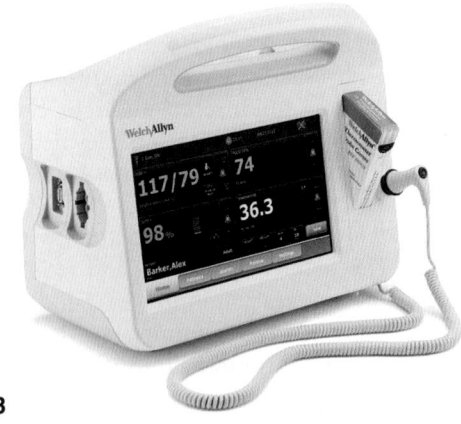

Figure 2.4 (A) Handheld electronic thermometer with disposable probe covers reduces the risk of cross-contamination. (B) This device interfaces with the electronic health record. The unit measures temperature, BP, and oxygen saturation levels (pulse oximetry). *(Courtesy of Welch Allyn, Skaneateles Falls, NY 13153-0220.)*

A   **B**

antipsychotic drugs and includes fever as a symptom.[38] Antibiotics normally will resolve fever when treating infection. However, antibiotics can paradoxically cause a fever. (A paradoxical drug reaction refers to an outcome opposite from the known action of a medication.) Late state serotonin syndrome, caused by an accumulation of high levels of serotonin in the body, may lead to a fever.[39] This can result from initiation of a selective serotonin reuptake inhibitor (SSRI) drug, or from a new medication added to an existing SSRI. Appendix 2.A (online) provides a list of common medications by drug classification, indications, side/adverse effects, as well as potential impact on vital signs.

Measurement Site

Body temperatures vary among body parts. Rectal and tympanic (ear) membrane temperatures are from 0.5°F to 0.9°F (0.3° to 0.5°C) higher than oral temperatures; axillary temperatures are approximately 1.1°F (0.6°C) lower than oral temperatures. Oral temperature in a healthy adult population is generally considered to be 98.6°F (37°C), and for rectal and tympanic membrane temperatures the value is 99.5°F (37.5°C). Being an external measure, the axillary value is somewhat lower at 97.6°F (36.5°C).[40]

Types of Thermometers
Glass Mercury Thermometers

For many years, temperatures had been taken using a glass thermometer, which consists of a glass tube with a bulbous tip filled with mercury. Owing to the highly poisonous nature of mercury and breakability of glass, automated thermometers have largely replaced their use in patient care settings. The U.S. Environmental Protection Agency warns against using mercury thermometers and encourages replacement with non-mercury-containing devices whenever possible.[41]

Automated Thermometers

Automated thermometers are widely used in patient care and community settings. They provide a rapid (several seconds), highly accurate measure of body temperature,

displayed digitally. Standard clinical automated thermometers consist of a portable battery-operated unit, an attached probe, and plastic disposable probe covers (Fig. 2.4). An important advantage of these thermometers is the low chance of cross-infection.

> **Clinical Note.** Depending on the manufacturer, a variety of features may be available on automated thermometers such as memory recall of previous recording(s), the ability to toggle between Fahrenheit and Celsius values, timers (e.g., pulse measures), and auto shutoff.

Oral Thermometers

Handheld automated oral (digital "stick") thermometers are readily available commercially. These units are typically about 5 in. in length with a tapered design (Fig. 2.5). One end of the device has a narrow tip and serves as the probe; in some models the tip is flexible. The opposite end is broad and houses the battery. These thermometers also provide a flashed, digital display of body temperature; most models have memory capabilities. Typically, these devices are used for a single patient; however, they can also be used with disposable probe covers.

Temporal Artery Thermometer

Noninvasive temporal artery thermometers measure body temperature by sliding a probe, held flat against the skin, in a straight line from the center of the forehead, across the temporal artery area to the hairline. The probe is then lifted from the forehead, centered on the mastoid process behind the ear, and slid down to the soft depression behind the earlobe (this helps eliminate the possibility of a false low temperature caused by evaporative cooling in the presence of forehead perspiration). The thermometer detects heat emitting from the skin surface over the temporal artery. The probe can be cleaned with an alcohol swab or used with disposable probe caps. For patients in isolation, tubular sheaths that cover the entire unit are available

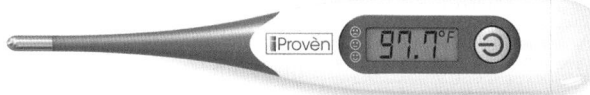

Figure 2.5 Handheld automated oral thermometers are self-contained with an internal battery; the proximal end houses the digital display and battery, and the distal end serves as the temperature probe. *(Courtesy of iProvèn, Netherlands.)*

for optimum infection control. As a measurement site, the temporal artery is easily accessible and poses low risk of injury as there is no contact with mucous membranes.

Tympanic Thermometer

Tympanic (ear) infrared thermometers measure body temperature through a sensor probe placed in the ear that detects infrared (thermal) radiation from the tympanic membrane. This location provides an important reflection of core temperature because the tympanic membrane receives its blood supply from a tributary of the internal carotid artery, which supplies the hypothalamus (temperature-regulating center). These handheld portable thermometers include an ear probe (used with a single-use disposable cover) and provide a digital display of body temperature within several seconds (Fig. 2.6A). They are particularly useful when oral monitoring is contraindicated, for patients not capable of cooperating or following directions, in emergency situations where rapid temperature values are required, and for children who may have difficulty remaining still during other types of monitoring.

Noncontact Infrared Thermometers

Noncontact infrared thermometers (NCIT) measure temperature using the surface area of the forehead

(Fig. 2.6B). Because these thermometers do not touch the patient, there is no risk of contamination. Based on manufacturer's specifications, the thermometers are held a specified distance from the center of the forehead. If the forehead is perspiring, temperature can be measured over other surface areas (e.g., neck, axilla). As they are noncontact, they are practical for large-scale screenings (e.g., emergency department entry, community centers, epidemic infectious disease control).

Clinical Note. A large clinical study found that some NCIT devices may not be consistently accurate compared to oral thermometers to determine if an individual's temperature exceeds a specific threshold for large-scale screenings.[36]

Disposable Skin Surface Thermometers

Skin surface thermometers consist of heat-sensitive strips (tape, patches, or disks) that provide a general measure of body surface temperature. They also respond to body temperature by changing color and are more frequently used with children. They must be applied to dry skin. The forehead and abdomen are common placement sites. The temperature readings are non-specific and are usually confirmed with a more precise measuring instrument.

Clinical Note. A variety of devices are available to measure temperature. However, only two noninvasive measurements have been found to accurately represent core body temperature: oral and tympanic thermometers.[42,43] Neither of these devices is recommended for critical care patients. Bladder temperature, through the use of temperature-sensing indwelling urinary catheters, is often considered ideal in this environment.[44]

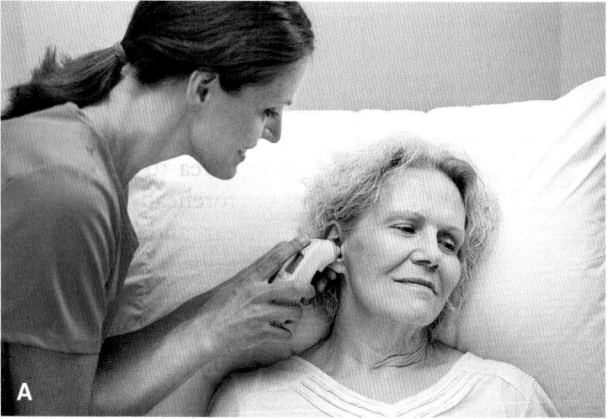
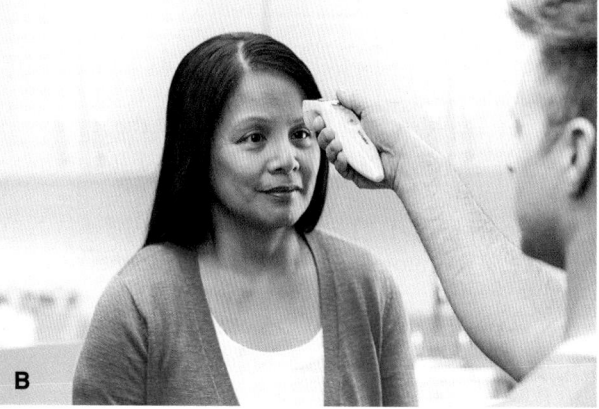

Figure 2.6 (A) Tympanic (ear) thermometer. (B) Noncontact forehead thermometer. *(Courtesy of Welch Allyn, Skaneateles Falls, NY 13153-0220.)*

Hand Hygiene

Although addressed here as a precursor to examining vital signs, hand hygiene is a paramount consideration with all aspects of patient care, as it plays a critical role in preventing transmission of pathogens in health-care settings.[45] Hand hygiene is accomplished by washing hands with soap and water or by rubbing hands with an alcohol-based formula. Alcohol-based hand rubs are an efficient and effective way to inactivate a broad spectrum of microorganisms from the hands.[46]

When using soap and water, enough product should be used to cover all hand surfaces. Clean running water assists with removing microorganisms, and a warm temperature removes less protective oil from the hands than does hot water. The force of the water should not cause splashing, which can promote the transfer of microorganisms. Care should be taken not to lean against the sink to avoid contact with a potentially contaminated area.

Measuring Body Temperature

Oral temperatures are contraindicated for patients with *dyspnea* or who are mouth breathers, have had oral surgery, or have a history of epilepsy or are prone to seizures. They also should not be used with infants or small children or patients who are irrational, unconscious, or uncooperative. In situations in which oral temperatures may be contraindicated, an automated unit with a tympanic sensor may be substituted.

Measuring Oral Temperature: Automated Thermometer

A. Assemble equipment: An automated thermometer with disposable probe covers or sheaths.
B. Wash hands.
C. Procedure:
　1. Turn on the power.
　2. Grasp the proximal aspect of the thermometer with the thumb and forefinger and attach the disposable cover over the distal probe tip until it snaps or locks in place. (Some units have a proximal button that releases the probe cover after temperature reading is complete.) For a small handheld automated unit, the probe covers are designed as a plastic sheath.
　3. Ask the patient to open their mouth and place the covered probe at the posterior base of the tongue to the right or left of the frenulum in the sublingual pocket. This placement positions the tip of the thermometer over superficial blood vessels that reflect core body temperature. Instruct the patient to close the lips (not teeth) around the thermometer. Continue to hold the probe in place, because the weight of the probe may displace it from the sublingual pocket.

4. Hold the probe in the sublingual pocket until an audible beep is heard (several seconds). The beep indicates maximum temperature has been reached. Remove the probe from the patient's mouth and note the temperature reading on the digital display for recording.
5. Remove the probe cover over a waste receptacle for disposal. If available on the unit, use the probe release mechanism; if a plastic sheath cover is used, use a clean paper towel for removal. (Cover sheath with paper towel, place thumb and forefinger proximally on probe over paper towel, and slide fingers distally.)
6. Return thermometer to appropriate storage cradle.
7. Wash hands.

Clinical Note. Generally, a temperature reading is assumed to be an oral measure unless otherwise noted. Documentation software typically includes entry labels for temperature source (e.g., oral, rectal, tympanic).

Measuring Temporal Artery Temperature

A. Assemble equipment: temporal artery thermometer and disposable probe cover.
B. Wash hands.
C. Procedure:
　1. Attach the disposable cover to the probe, holding the edges with the thumb and forefinger. (Ensure that the firm circular collar of the cover engages with the base by gently pushing it down to snap it into place; do not touch the plastic film of the probe cover.)
　2. Place the probe in the center of the forehead.
　3. Press the on button. Depending on manufacturer, the ON button may need to be held throughout the procedure.
　4. Slowly slide the probe across the forehead along the hairline. A rapid clicking or beeping indicates an increase in temperature.
　5. If required based on manufacturer directions, the probe is lifted from the forehead and placed on the neck below the ear in the depression just behind the mastoid.
　6. Remove the probe cover over a waste receptacle for disposal. If a plastic sheath cover is used, use a clean paper towel for removal. (Cover sheath with paper towel, place thumb and forefinger proximally on probe over paper towel, and slide fingers distally.)
　7. Return thermometer to appropriate storage cradle.
　8. Wash hands.

Clinical Note. Midline on the forehead the temporal artery is less than 2 mm below the skin surface, making this an ideal location for temperature measurement.

Measuring Tympanic Membrane Temperature: Automated Tympanic Thermometer

A. Assemble equipment: Tympanic (infrared) thermometer and disposable probe covers.
B. Wash hands.
C. Procedure:
  1. Attach the disposable cover to the probe, holding the edges with the thumb and forefinger. (Ensure that the firm circular collar of the cover engages with the base by gently pushing it down to snap it into place; do not touch the plastic film of the probe cover.)
  2. Turn the patient's head to one side. Follow the manufacturer's recommendation for positioning of the ear and insertion. Some tympanic thermometers require straightening of the ear canal before insertion by pulling the ear up and back for adults and pulling down and back for a child.
  3. Insert the probe snugly into the ear canal. Use a firm, gentle pressure; avoid forcing the probe too deeply. The probe should seal the opening of the ear canal. To ensure accurate reading, the probe should be angled anteriorly toward the jawline, as if approaching the patient from behind.
  4. Press the button that activates the thermometer. The temperature is displayed within several seconds. An audible beep or flashing light will signal when the maximum temperature is reached.
  5. Gently remove the probe from the ear. Eject or remove the probe cover over a waste receptacle for disposal. For manual removal of the probe cover, use a clean paper towel or tissue.
  6. Return tympanic thermometer to protective case or storage base. Most units include a protective cap that fits over the probe tip.
  7. Wash hands.

■ PULSE

The *pulse* is the wave of blood in the artery created by contraction of the left ventricle during a cardiac cycle (one complete cycle of cardiac muscle contraction and relaxation). With each contraction, blood is pumped into an already full aorta. The inherent elasticity of the aortic walls allows expansion and acceptance of the new supply. The blood is then forced out and surges through the systemic arteries. It is this wave or surge of blood that is felt as the pulse. The strength or amplitude of the pulse reflects the amount of blood ejected with each myocardial contraction, or *stroke volume* (SV). The *apical pulse* is located at the apex of the heart and is monitored using a stethoscope.

Peripheral pulses are those located in the periphery of the body that can be felt by palpating an artery over a bony prominence or other firm surface. Examples of peripheral pulses include the radial, carotid, and popliteal pulses. Of the peripheral pulses, examination of the carotid pulse provides the most accurate representation of the central aortic pulse.

Pressure changes in the large arteries during the cardiac cycle are reflected in the relatively smooth and rounded appearance of the normal arterial waveform. The lowest point of pressure occurs during ventricular diastole, while the highest point occurs during ventricular systole (peak ejection). The notch on the descending slope of the pulse wave represents closure of the aortic valve and is not palpable. A healthy adult heart beats an average of 70 times per minute, a rate that provides continuous circulation of approximately 5 to 6 liters of blood through the body. The pulse can be palpated wherever a superficial artery can be stabilized over an underlying surface. In monitoring the pulse, specific attention is directed toward determining three parameters: *rate*, *rhythm*, and *quality*.

Rate

The HR is the number of pulsations (peripheral pulse waves) or frequency per minute. Bradycardia is an abnormally slow HR, less than 60 bpm. Tachycardia is an excessively high HR, greater than 100 bpm. *Palpitation* refers to the sensation of a rapid or irregular HR perceived by the patient without actually palpating a peripheral pulse. Multiple factors influence the HR, including age, sex, emotional status, stress, and physical activity level. Body size and stature also influence HR. Tall, thin individuals generally have a slower HR than those who are obese or have stout frames.

Rhythm

The pulse *rhythm* is the pattern of pulsations and the intervals between them. In a healthy individual, the rhythm is regular and indicates that the time intervals between pulse beats are essentially equal. *Dysrhythmia* refers to an irregular rhythm in which pulses are not evenly spaced. An irregular rhythm may present as premature, late, or missed pulse beats, or random, irregular beats in either a predictable or an unpredictable pattern.[46] Irregular rhythms are often associated with conduction abnormalities or an impulse originating from a site other than the sinoatrial node.

Quality

The *quality* (force, volume) of the pulse refers to the amount of force created by the ejected blood volume against the arterial wall during each ventricular contraction. In examining the quality of the pulse, the therapist is determining the feel of the blood as it passes through a vessel. The quantity (volume) of blood within the vessel produces the force of the pulse. Normally, the pulse volume of each beat is the same. The force of the pulse is greater with a higher blood volume and weaker with a lower blood volume. The volume is examined by noting how easily the pulse can be obliterated. A normal pulse is described as full or strong and can be palpated using moderate pressure of the fingers over a bony landmark. With lower volumes, the pulse is small, is easily obliterated, and is termed *weak* or *thready*. With increased volume, the pulse is large, is difficult to obliterate, and is termed a *bounding* (or *full*) pulse; a feeling of high tension is noted. A numerical scale is often used to document the quality (strength) of the pulse (see Table 2.2).

In addition to rate, rhythm, and quality, the feel of the arterial wall under the examiner's fingertips should be determined. Normally, a vessel will feel smooth, elastic, soft, flexible, and relatively straight. With advancing age, vessels may demonstrate sclerotic changes. These changes frequently cause the vessels to feel twisted, hard, or cordlike, with decreased elasticity and smoothness.

Several other important terms are used to describe variations in pulse. The term *bigeminal* is used to describe an abnormality in pulse rhythm where two beats occur in rapid succession (double systolic peak). *Pulsus alternans* (alternating pulse) is marked by a fluctuation in amplitude between beats (a strong and a weak), with minimal change in overall rhythm. A normal pulse beat is followed by a premature beat of diminished amplitude. A *paradoxical* pulse (pulsus paradoxus) is decreased amplitude of the pressure wave detected during quiet inspiration with a return to full amplitude on expiration; it is often associated with obstructive lung disease. See Fig. 2.7 for a schematic illustration of normal and common alterations in arterial pulse waveforms. See Chapter 13, Heart Disease, for a thorough discussion of cardiac pathologies and the cardiac examination.

Factors Influencing Heart Rate

Essentially, any factor that alters the metabolic rate will also influence HR. Several factors are of particular importance when considering HR.

Age

The adult HR range is generally considered to be between 60 and 100 bpm; however, in highly trained athletes, the resting value may be considerably lower. This lowered resting value occurs because the effectiveness of each cardiac contraction is 40% to 50% greater in the trained versus untrained individual.[23]

Sex

Men and boys typically have slightly lower HR than women and girls.

Emotions/Stress

Responses to a variety of emotions (grief, fear, anger, excitement, anxiety) activate the sympathetic nervous system, with a resultant increase in HR. The stress-inducing effects of moderate to severe pain will also elevate HR.

Exercise

Oxygen demands of skeletal muscles are significantly increased during physical activity. At rest, only 20% to 25% of the available muscle capillaries are open.[22,24] During vigorous exercise, extensive vasodilation causes all capillaries to open. The HR increases to provide additional blood flow to muscles and to meet the increased oxygen requirement. For physical therapists, monitoring a patient's HR is an important method of evaluating response to exercise. Typically, HR will increase as a function of the activity's intensity (termed *chronotropic competence*).

A linear relationship exists between HR and intensity of workload. To use the HR effectively to prescribe exercise, both the patient's resting and predicted maximal HRs must be determined. Maximum HR values can be

Table 2.2	Numerical Scale for Grading Pulse Quality (Strength)	
Grade	Pulse	Description
0	Absent	No perceptible pulse even with maximum pressure
1+	Thready	Barely perceptible; easily obliterated with slight pressure; fades in and out
2+	Weak	Difficult to palpate; slightly stronger than thready; can be obliterated with light pressure
3+	Normal	Easy to palpate; requires moderate pressure to obliterate
4+	Bounding	Very strong; hyperactive; is not obliterated with moderate pressure

Description   **Possible Cause**

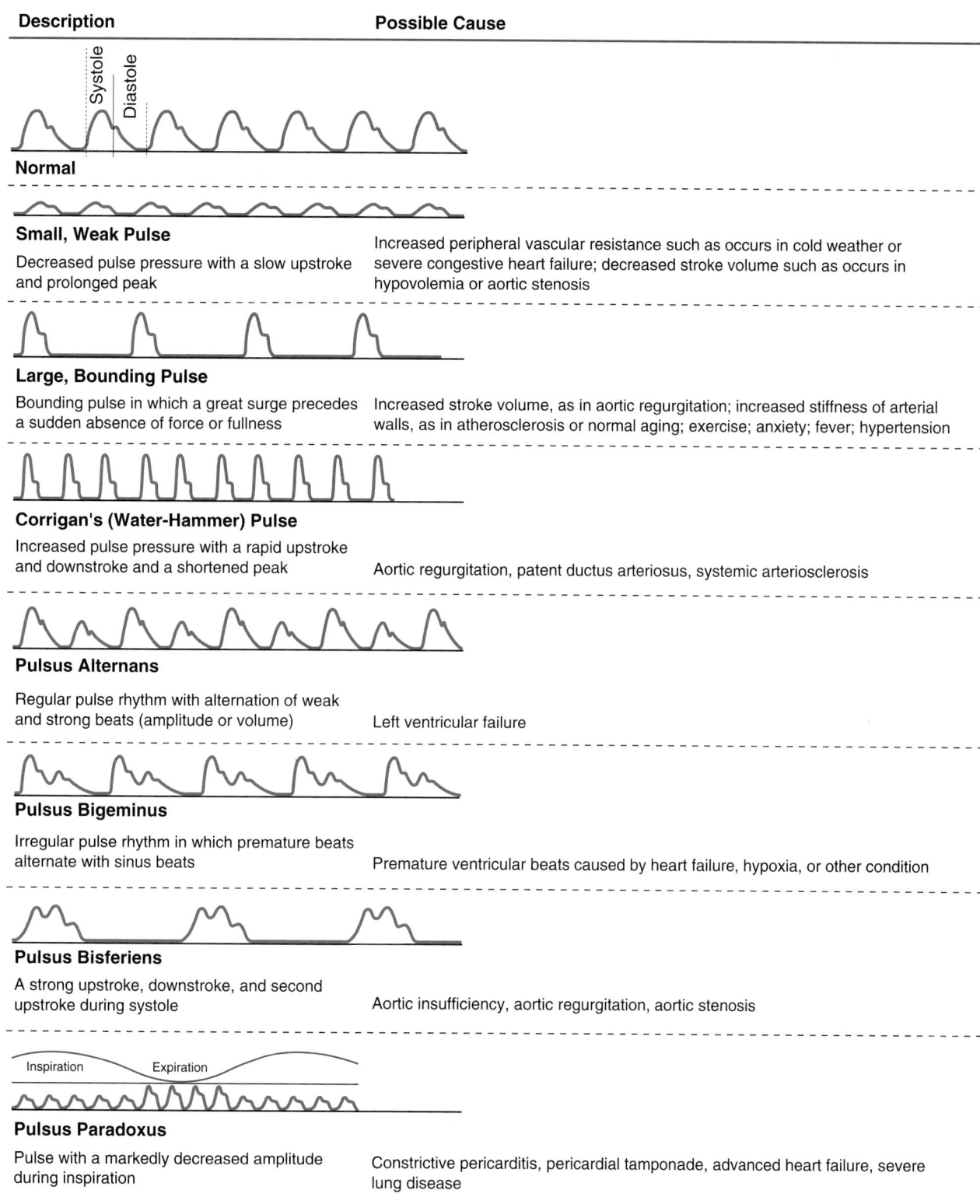

Normal

Small, Weak Pulse

Decreased pulse pressure with a slow upstroke
and prolonged peak

Increased peripheral vascular resistance such as occurs in cold weather or
severe congestive heart failure; decreased stroke volume such as occurs in
hypovolemia or aortic stenosis

Large, Bounding Pulse

Bounding pulse in which a great surge precedes
a sudden absence of force or fullness

Increased stroke volume, as in aortic regurgitation; increased stiffness of arterial
walls, as in atherosclerosis or normal aging; exercise; anxiety; fever; hypertension

Corrigan's (Water-Hammer) Pulse

Increased pulse pressure with a rapid upstroke
and downstroke and a shortened peak

Aortic regurgitation, patent ductus arteriosus, systemic arteriosclerosis

Pulsus Alternans

Regular pulse rhythm with alternation of weak
and strong beats (amplitude or volume)

Left ventricular failure

Pulsus Bigeminus

Irregular pulse rhythm in which premature beats
alternate with sinus beats

Premature ventricular beats caused by heart failure, hypoxia, or other condition

Pulsus Bisferiens

A strong upstroke, downstroke, and second
upstroke during systole

Aortic insufficiency, aortic regurgitation, aortic stenosis

Pulsus Paradoxus

Pulse with a markedly decreased amplitude
during inspiration

Constrictive pericarditis, pericardial tamponade, advanced heart failure, severe
lung disease

Figure 2.7 Normal and abnormal pulses, as reflected in arterial waveforms. *(From Dillon, 2, p. 477
with permission.)*

determined by a maximal graded exercise test, whenever
possible, or by using various published formulas. Common formulas include:

- Age-adjusted HR formula: maximum HR [HR_{max}] =
  220 minus age

- Karvonen formula: target HR = [(HR_{max} − HR_{rest}) ×
  % intensity] + HR_{rest}

For moderate-intensity exercise, the CDC recommends that the target HR be 50% to 70% of predicted
HR maximum, and for vigorous-intensity exercise, it

should be 70% to 85%.[47] Lower exercise intensities are indicated for individuals with low fitness levels.

In examining HR response to exercise, level of aerobic fitness also must be considered. Both resting HR and submaximal exercise HR are typically lower in trained individuals. In response to identical exercise intensity, a sedentary person's HR will demonstrate greater acceleration when compared with a trained individual. Although the metabolic requirements of an activity are the same, the lower HR response in a trained individual occurs as a result of a more efficient (increased) SV owing to greater cardiac strength and efficiency. The linear relationship between HR and workload exists for both trained and untrained individuals. However, the rate of rise will differ. When compared with a sedentary person, the trained individual will achieve a higher work output and greater oxygen consumption before reaching a specified submaximal HR.

Medications

The impact of medications on HR is particularly important for patients with cardiac disease or hypertension. Beta blockers (beta-adrenergic blocking agents) are a category of drugs that block the sympathetic beta receptors and decrease both resting HR and HR response to exercise.[22] They are commonly used in the treatment of angina pectoris, arrhythmias, hypertension, and the acute phase of myocardial infarction. Examples of prescribed beta blockers include acebutolol, atenolol, bisoprolol, carvedilol, labetalol, metoprolol, nadolol, nebivolol, and propranolol. Patients taking beta blockers typically experience early fatigue with exercise; an alternative to HR monitoring, such as Ratings of Perceived Exertion scale, should be considered to monitor exercise intensity.[48] See additional discussion in Chapter 13, Heart Disease.

Systemic or Local Heat

During periods of fever, HR will increase. The body will attempt to dissipate heat by vasodilation of peripheral vessels. HR will increase to shunt blood flow to cutaneous areas for cooling. Local applications of thermal modalities (such as a hot pack) may also elevate HR to increase blood flow to cutaneous areas secondary to arteriolar and capillary dilation.

Pulse Sites

A peripheral pulse can be monitored at a variety of sites on the body (Fig. 2.8). A superficial artery located over a bone or underlying firm surface is easiest to palpate. Box 2.3 identifies the peripheral pulse locations, provides example indications for their use, and shows palpation sites.[7,39,43]

The apical (central) pulse is considered the most accurate because it measures the actual sounds of the heart values opening and closing (Fig. 2.9). It is monitored by auscultation (listening), using a stethoscope

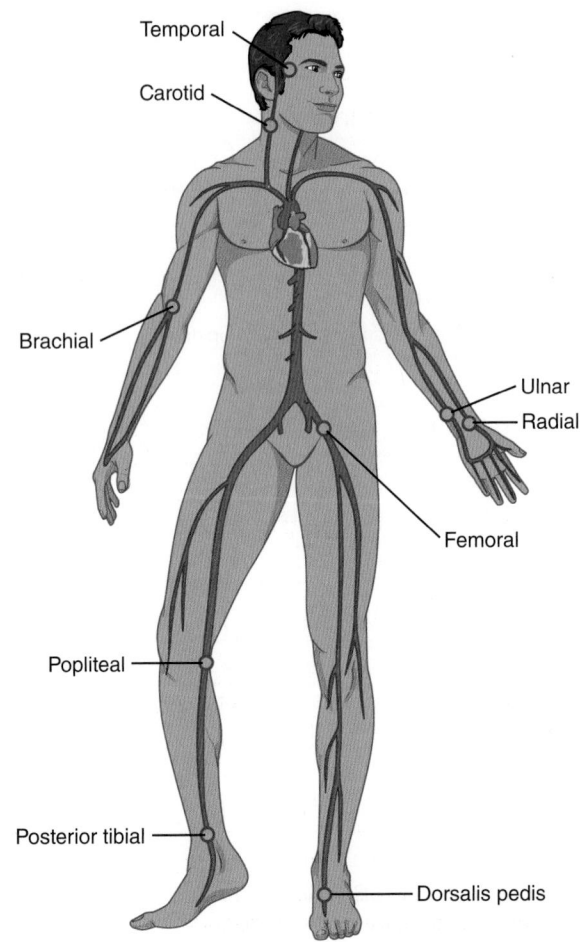

Figure 2.8 Common sites for monitoring peripheral pulses.

directly over the apex (lower portion pointing to the left) of the heart. Apical pulses are used when peripheral pulses are weak or imperceptible, when other sites are either inaccessible (e.g., surgery) or difficult to palpate (e.g., infants), and when the effects of cardiac medications designed to alter HR and rhythm need to be monitored.

Monitoring Pulse

Peripheral pulses are monitored by palpation using the index and third finger of one hand. The thumb should not be used because it has its own pulse, which will interfere with monitoring. Generally, a light pressure is used initially to locate the pulse, and then more firm pressure is used when determining the rate, rhythm, and quality. The fingertips should be moved gently over the selected site until the strongest pulsation is found. To monitor resting values, the patient should be resting quietly for at least 5 minutes prior to the pulse measurement.

The radial artery is the most common site for measuring the pulse. With few modifications, the same procedure can be followed for monitoring at other pulse sites.

Box 2.3   Pulse Location, Indications for Use, and Palpation Sites

Pulse Location and Indications for Use	Palpation Sites
Temporal: Over temporal bone; superior and lateral to the eye. Used with infants, when radial pulse inaccessible, and by anesthesiologists for monitoring during surgery.	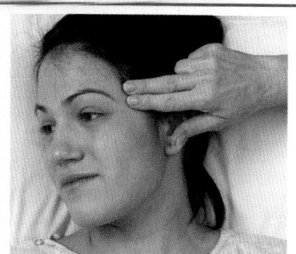
Carotid: On either side of the lower neck, below the jaw, fingers over thyroid cartilage between the trachea and medial border of sternocleidomastoid. Used with infants, during shock or cardiac arrest, to monitor cranial circulation; easily accessible if other peripheral pulses difficult or too weak to locate.[a]	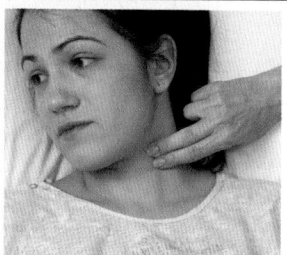
Brachial: Medial aspect of antecubital fossa, elbow should be slightly flexed and supported to avoid contraction of biceps. Used to monitor blood pressure and during cardiac arrest.	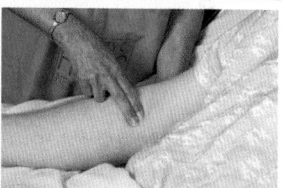
Radial: Distal radius at base of the thumb, lateral to tendon of the flexor carpi radialis. Most common site for peripheral pulse monitoring; easy to locate and easily accessible.	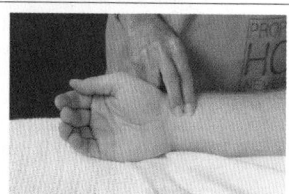
Femoral: Inferior to the inguinal ligament, midway between the anterior superior iliac spine and the symphysis pubis; typically monitored in supine. Used to LE circulation and during cardiac arrest.	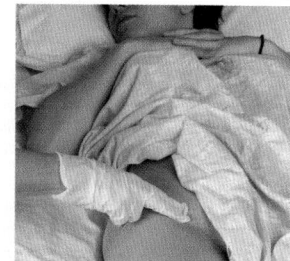
Popliteal: Inferior aspect of popliteal fossa; popliteal artery is deep and at times may be difficult to palpate; typically monitored in prone position with knee flexed to relax hamstrings and popliteal fascia; can also be accomplished in supine position. Used to monitor thigh BP and LE circulation; weak or absent popliteal pulse may indicate impaired flow or blockage in femoral artery.	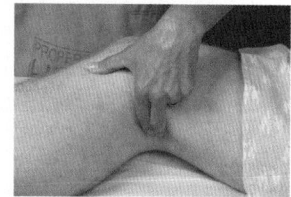

(Continued)

Box 2.3   Pulse Location, Indications for Use, and Palpation Sites—cont'd

Pulse Location and Indications for Use	Palpation Sites
Pedal (dorsalis pedis): Dorsal, medial aspect of foot, lateral to the tendon of the extensor hallucis longus; ankle should be slightly dorsiflexed; some individuals have congenitally nonpalpable pedal pulses. Used to monitor circulation to feet.	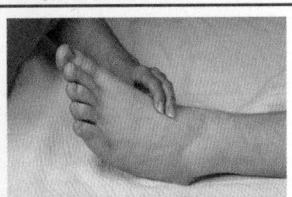
Posterior tibial: Posterior and inferior to the medial malleolus. Used to monitor circulation to feet; weak or absent pulse may be indicative of arterial disease (e.g., atherosclerosis) or occlusion.	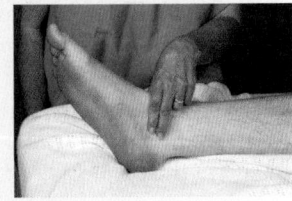

Images from Wilkinson, JM, et al., 47, pp. 191–194 with permission.
ªPrecaution: Pressure should never be applied bilaterally over carotid arteries or high on the neck to avoid stimulation of the
     carotid sinus and a subsequent reflex drop in pulse rate and blood pressure.
BP = blood pressure; LE = lower extremity.

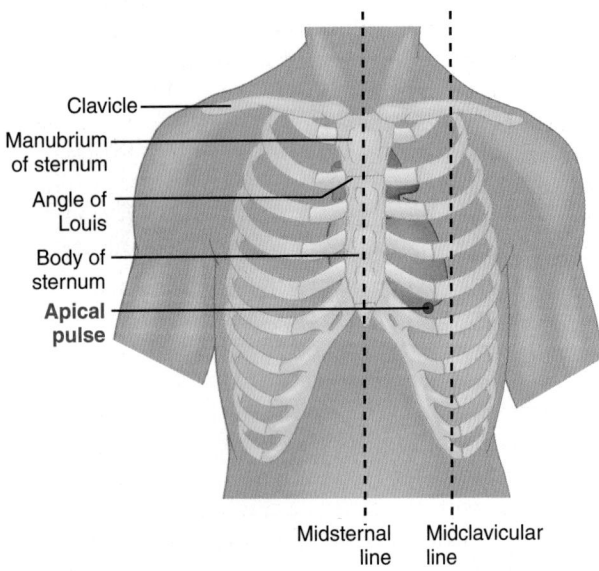

Figure 2.9 The apical pulse is located approximately 3.5 in. to the left of the midsternum, in the fifth intercostal space.

Measuring Radial Pulse

A. Assemble equipment: Watch with a second hand.
B. Wash hands.
C. Procedure:
  1. Explain procedure and rationale in terms appropriate to the patient's understanding.
  2. Ensure patient understanding, modesty, safety, and comfort.
  3. Place the patient's wrist in a neutral position relative to flexion and extension and support the forearm. If measuring from supine, the forearm can be supported across the patient's chest or at

their side with partial flexion of the elbow. From a sitting position, the forearm can rest across the patient's thigh, supported by a pillow or the therapist's arm. This relaxed positioning of the upper extremity (UE) generally facilitates artery palpation.
  4. Place the fingers squarely and firmly over the radial pulse; use only enough pressure to feel the pulse accurately. If the pressure is too great, it will occlude the artery.
  5. Once the strongest pulsation is located, note the position of the second hand on the watch. The first pulsation should be counted as zero to avoid overestimating. Determine the *rate* (number of beats per minute) by counting the pulse for 30 seconds and multiplying by 2; if any irregularities are noted, a full 60-second count should be taken to improve accuracy. Note the *rhythm* (time intervals between pulse beats) and the *quality* (force) of the pulse.
  6. Wash hands.

Measuring Apical Pulse

A. Assemble equipment: Watch with a second hand, stethoscope, and antiseptic wipes for cleaning earpieces and diaphragm of stethoscope before and after use.
B. Wash hands.
C. Procedure:
  1. Explain the procedure and rationale in terms appropriate to the patient's level of understanding. Indicate that there will be a request to remain quiet during monitoring to avoid interference with auscultation.

2. Ensure patient's understanding, modesty, safety, and comfort. Apical pulses are typically monitored with the patient either supine or sitting.

3. Use an antiseptic wipe to clean the earpieces and diaphragm of the stethoscope.

4. Expose the sternum and chest.

5. Locate the site where pulse will be monitored; the apical pulse is located approximately 3.5 in. (8.9 cm) to the left of the midsternum, in the fifth intercostal space, within an inch of the midclavicular line drawn parallel to the sternum (see Fig. 2.9). These landmarks are guides to locating the apical pulse. In some individuals, a stronger pulse may be noted by altering the placement of the stethoscope (e.g., placement in the fourth or sixth intercostal space).

6. Place the earpieces of the stethoscope (tilting slightly forward) into the ears. The tubes of the stethoscope should not be crossed and should hang freely.

7. Place the flat disk diaphragm of the stethoscope over the apex of the heart and locate the point where the apical pulse is heard most clearly. This is called the *point of maximal impulse.* If the rhythm is regular, count the pulse for 30 seconds and multiply by 2. If any irregularities are noted, take a full 60-second count. The pulse will be heard as a *lub-dub.* The first heart sound (S1 ["lub"]) is caused by closure of the atrioventricular (tricuspid and mitral) valves at the beginning of systole. The second heart sound (S2 ["dub"]) is caused by closure of the semilunar (aortic and pulmonic) valves at the end of systole.

8. Wash hands and clean the stethoscope. If the same examiner is using the stethoscope again, it is not necessary to clean the earpieces; the diaphragm should always be cleaned.

Measuring Apical–Radial Pulse

Monitoring the apical–radial pulse involves two examiners simultaneously measuring the pulse at two separate locations: (1) the apical pulse at the apex of the heart; and (2) the radial pulse at the wrist. The values from the two different sites are then compared. Typically, the apical and radial pulse values are the same. However, in some situations (e.g., variations in SV or vascular occlusion), blood pumped from the heart may not be reaching the distal site, causing a weak or imperceptible radial pulse. For example, if the heart contracts prematurely, the ventricles have insufficient time to fill, resulting in a diminished SV and creating an imperceptible pulse in the radial artery.[23] On the other hand, SV may be normal with a weak or imperceptible radial pulse, suggesting a more peripheral problem such as impaired flow or blockage within a vessel. In either situation, there is a deficit in the number of radial pulses when compared with the number of apical pulses.[23] This is called a *pulse deficit,* defined as the difference between the rate of radial and apical pulses. The value of this measure is that it provides important information about the cardiovascular system's ability to perfuse the body.

Automated Heart Rate Monitoring

Advances are continual in the design, features, accuracy, waterproofing, information storage capacity, and Bluetooth capabilities of heart rate monitors (HRMs). In addition to monitoring HR, some HRMs provide data on HR variability (calculation of the time between pulses), real-time display of percentage of maximum HR, and estimates of maximal oxygen uptake (V_2max). Many HRMs allow data to be downloaded wirelessly to a computer (e.g., tablet, smartphone, watch) for analysis and storage using software programs and apps. This provides a permanent record and sequential data on exercise performance. Most models allow programming of a prescribed exercise HR range with an audible and/or visible warning when the HR is outside the predetermined range. Some models include a talking feature that "speaks" HR information. Memory capabilities allow storage of exercise information over a variable number of exercise sessions.

HRMs consist of two basic elements: (1) a sensor that transmits data and (2) a monitor that incorporates a receiver, microprocessor, and display. Wireless HRMs employ technology (Bluetooth, Bluetooth SMART, or ANT+) to allow information transfer between electronic devices, while others include a lead wire with a distal sensor (e.g., earlobe clip, fingertip cover, or finger sleeve). Some monitors integrate sensors into a chest strap that provides wireless transmission of signals to a monitor worn as a wristwatch. Another style replaces the chest strap with fingertip sensors directly on the wristwatch. HR data are recorded when a fingertip is placed in contact with the sensor. Some HRMs are equipped with more than one type of sensor. This feature allows selection of the sensor that is most appropriate for the activity and the user. HRMs are frequently used in prescribed exercise and training programs because they provide a practical, accurate method of pulse monitoring and are lightweight, comfortable, and easy to use. Many types of exercise training devices (e.g., treadmills, stair climbers, stationary bicycles, elliptical machines) incorporate HRMs directly into the unit by means of a metal handgrip sensor device.

Holter monitors are worn for 24 or 48 hrs. A continuous recording is made and later read by a trained provider.[49] Event monitors are worn generally for 30 days. They will detect an abnormal rhythm and transmit the rhythm to a device that is capable of directly contacting an interpreting provider in real time.[49] An implantable loop recorder is invasively inserted (typically under the skin of the chest) and functions as an event monitor for extended periods of time. An implantable loop recorder

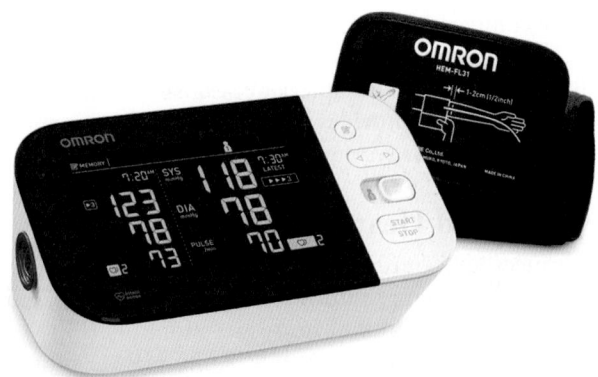

Figure 2.10 Personal HR monitor with waveform *(Courtesy of Withings, Cambridge, MA 02142.)*

may be indicated for individuals experiencing fainting spells or who are at high risk for stroke.[49] They are also used to capture brief episodes of atrial fibrillation to potentially explain the cause of a cryptogenic stroke.

Other HRM features are available and differ with the model and manufacturer (Fig. 2.10). Among the more common features are multifunction wrist monitors (consisting of a watch, stopwatch, alarm clock, lap timer, calendar, and data storage), illuminated and large-number LCD displays (some with a zoom feature that doubles the size of information on the screen), visual graphics (e.g., "time in zone graph"), memory displays of previous training sessions, estimates of calories burned and energy expended during exercise, and HR statistics (average, minimum, maximum). Some units combine the ability to monitor HR with measures of blood oxygenation (oximetry).

Doppler Ultrasound

Doppler ultrasound (DUS) is a noninvasive instrument used to examine pulses that are extremely weak or faint or that are obliterated by even slight pressure or when arterial flow is severely compromised (e.g., superficial thrombophlebitis, arteriosclerosis, thromboangiitis obliterans, vascular tumors of the extremities). DUS is based on the principle that high-frequency ultrasound waves directed at a moving interface (i.e., blood flowing through a vessel) will cause a change in the wave frequency reflective of the velocity of the moving interface (called the *Doppler effect*). In essence, the DUS measures how sound waves are reflected off moving blood cells. The resultant frequency change caused by the movement alters the pitch of the sound waves as they are reflected back to the examiner; the pulse is heard as a swooshing sound.[50] The change in pitch heard by the examiner provides important information about the blood flow through a vessel.

The essential elements of a DUS device include the ultrasound unit, a handheld probe (piezoelectric crystal) that transmits and receives sound waves, and earpieces that look similar to those on a stethoscope or a

small speaker to amplify the sound. Passed gently over the skin surface above an artery using ample coupling gel, the probe transmits high-frequency sound waves to an artery. The waves are disturbed by movement of the red blood cells, reflected back to the probe, and transformed into an amplified audible sound.[51]

The audible sound represents the difference in frequency between the waves directed at the vessel and those reflected back by motion of blood cells; the frequency is proportional to the velocity of the moving red blood cells. The absence of an audible sound indicates no detection of movement and, subsequently, no perfusion.[50] Using a computer interface, the flow measures can be graphically displayed and stored. It should be noted that although the specific characteristics of the reflected sounds are not diagnostic, they can assist in identifying abnormal flow.[52]

■ RESPIRATION

The primary function of respiration (movement of air into and out of the lungs) is to supply the body with oxygen for metabolic activity and to remove carbon dioxide. The respiratory system consists of a series of branching tubes and brings atmospheric oxygen into contact with the gas exchange membrane of the lungs in the alveoli. Oxygen is then transported throughout the body via the cardiovascular system. *External respiration* is the exchange of oxygen and carbon dioxide between the lungs and the environment. *Internal respiration* is the exchange of oxygen and carbon dioxide between the circulating blood and body tissues.

Respiratory System

The entire pathway that transports air from the environment extends from the mouth and nose down to the alveolar sacs. Figure 2.11 illustrates the structures of the respiratory system. The upper respiratory airways include the nose, mouth, pharynx, and larynx. Air enters the body by way of the nose and mouth and is then moved to the pharynx, where it is warmed, filtered, and humidified. The pharynx serves as a common pathway for both air and food. Inspired air is then moved to the larynx, which contains the epiglottis, vocal cords, and cartilaginous structures. The anatomical arrangement of the larynx and pharyngeal muscles provides the critical function of protecting the lungs from foreign particles, as well as assisting with phonation (production of vocal sounds) and coughing, which is the primary physiological mechanism for clearing the airways. The *laryngopharynx* is the area where solid and liquid food intake is separated from inspired air. It is also the site of bifurcation into the larynx and esophagus. The pharyngeal muscles close the glottis during swallowing to protect the lungs from aspiration. If a foreign body passes the glottis and enters the tracheobronchial tree, the cough reflex is initiated to clear the air passage. Immediately below the thyroid cartilage of the larynx (i.e., the Adam's

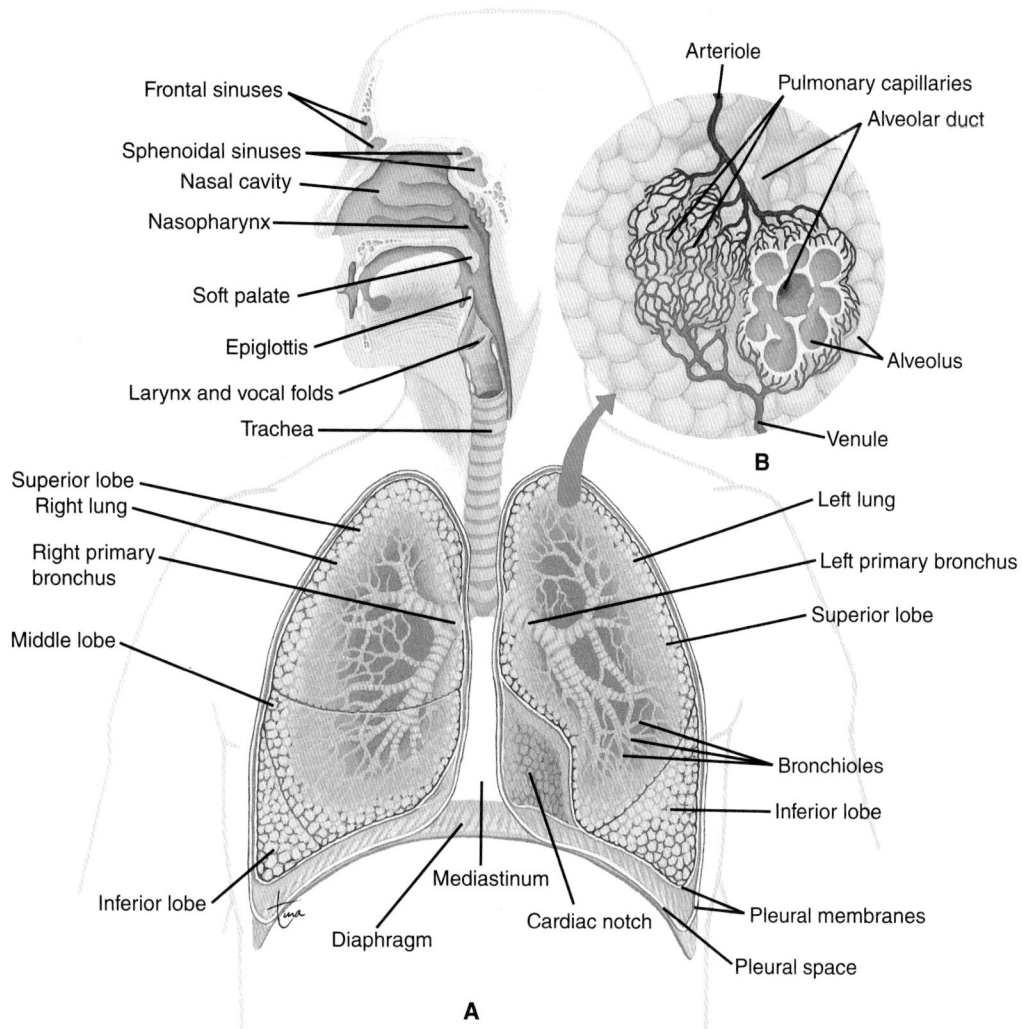

Figure 2.11 Structures of the respiratory system. (A) Anterior view of the upper and lower respiratory tracts. (B) Microscopic view of alveoli and pulmonary capillaries. (The colors represent the vessels, not the oxygen content of the blood within the vessels.) *(From Scanlon and Sanders with permission.)*

apple) is the site for making an emergency opening to the tracheal air pathway (*tracheostomy*).[24,53,54]

The trachea is approximately 4 to 5 in. (11 to 13 cm) long and continues from the cartilaginous structures of the neck into the thorax. At the level of the carina, the trachea divides into two mainstem bronchi. The carina contains the majority of cough receptors and is located approximately between the sternum and manubrium at the second intercostal space. The right and left mainstem bronchi are asymmetrical in size and shape and continue into the lower respiratory tract, further subdividing into the respiratory bronchioles, where gas exchange begins. However, gas exchange primarily occurs in the alveolar ducts and the large surface area provided by the alveoli. The respiratory bronchioles, alveolar ducts, and alveoli (alveolar sacs) comprise the *respiratory zone* for gas exchange (Fig. 2.12). The *conducting zone* (trachea, bronchi, and terminal bronchioles) provides for continuous movement of air into and

out of the lungs; these areas do not contribute to gas exchange.[21,50–53]

Inspiration is initiated by contraction of the diaphragm and intercostal muscles. During contraction of these muscles, the diaphragm moves downward and the intercostals lift the ribs and sternum up and outward. The size of the thoracic cavity is thus increased, allowing for lung expansion. Normal inspiration lasts 1 to 1.5 seconds. During relaxed breathing, expiration is essentially a passive process. Once the respiratory muscles relax, the thorax returns to its resting position, and the lungs recoil. This ability to recoil occurs because of the inherent elastic properties of the lungs. Normal expiration lasts 2 to 3 seconds.[46]

Regulatory Mechanisms

Regulation of respiratory function involves multiple components of both neural and chemical control and is closely integrated with the cardiovascular system.

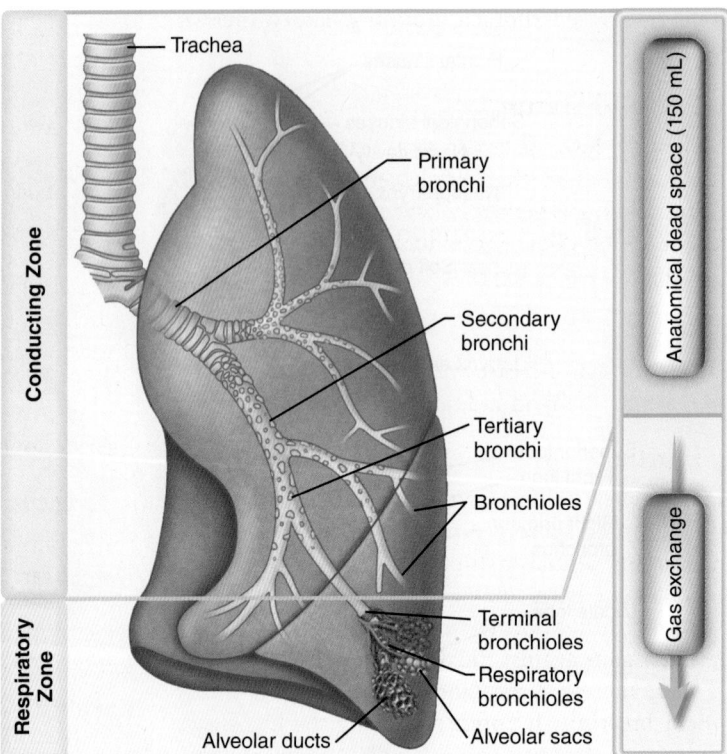

Airway Characteristics

Figure 2.12 Primary components of the conducting and respiratory zones. The conducting zone transports inhaled air to and from the respiratory zone where air exchange takes place. The air exchange occurs in progressively increasing increments in the respiratory bronchioles, alveolar ducts, and alveolar sacs. *(Adapted from Van Guilder and Janot with permission.)*

Breathing is controlled by the respiratory center, which lies bilaterally in the pons and medulla. Motor nerves whose cell bodies are located in this area control the respiratory muscles. The respiratory center provides control of both the *rate* and the *depth* of breathing in response to the metabolic needs of the body.[55]

Both *central* and *peripheral* chemoreceptors influence respiration. *Central* chemoreceptors are located in the respiratory center and are sensitive to changes in either carbon dioxide or hydrogen ion levels of arterial blood. An increase in either carbon dioxide levels or hydrogen ions will stimulate breathing.[23] *Peripheral* chemoreceptors are located at the bifurcation of the carotid arteries (carotid bodies) and in the arch of the aorta (aortic bodies). These receptors are sensitive to the partial pressure of oxygen (Pao_2) in the arterial blood. When Pao_2 levels in arterial blood drop, afferent impulses carry this information to the respiratory center. Motor neurons to the respiratory muscles are stimulated to increase tidal volume (amount of air exchanged with each breath) or, with very low oxygen levels, to increase the RR as well. These peripheral chemoreceptors cause an increase in respiration only when Pao_2 levels fall to approximately 53 mm Hg (from a normal level of about 90 to 100 mm Hg). This is because the receptors are sensitive only to Pao_2 levels in plasma and not to the total oxygen in blood.[23,55]

Respiration also is influenced by a protective stretch mechanism called the *Hering-Breuer reflex*. Pulmonary stretch receptors throughout the walls of the lungs detect the amount of stretch imposed by entering air. When overstretched, these receptors send impulses to the respiratory center to inhibit further inspiration and increase the duration of expiration. Impulses stop at the end of expiration so that another inspiration can be initiated. In adults, this reflex is rarely demonstrated and would likely not be activated until tidal volume reached higher than 1.5 liters.[56] Respiration is also stimulated by vigorous movements of joints and muscle (exercise) and is strongly influenced by voluntary cortical control.

Factors Influencing Respiration

Multiple factors can alter normal, relaxed, effortless respiration. As with temperature and pulse, any influence that increases the metabolic rate also will increase RR. Increased metabolism and subsequent demand for oxygen will stimulate increased respiration. Conversely, as metabolic demands diminish, respirations also will decrease. Several influencing factors are of particular importance when examining respiration. These include age, body size, stature, exercise, and body position.

Age

The RR of an infant is between 30 and 60 breaths per minute.[3] The rate gradually slows until adulthood, when it ranges between 12 and 18 breaths per minute.[3] In older individuals, the RR may increase owing to decreased elasticity of the lungs and decreased efficiency of gas exchange. Other factors associated with normal aging that affect respiratory function include weakening of respiratory muscles, deterioration of alveolar walls, decreased thoracic mobility, and decreased lung volumes.[56,57]

Body Size and Stature

Men generally have a larger vital capacity than do women, adults larger than adolescents, and children. Tall, thin individuals generally have a larger vital capacity than stout or obese individuals. With larger lung capacity, there is also a lower RR.

Exercise

RR and depth will increase with exercise as a result of increased oxygen demand and carbon dioxide production.

Body Position

The recumbent position can significantly affect respiration and predispose the patient to stasis of fluids. Among the influential factors that limit normal lung expansion when lying down are compression of the chest against the supporting surface and pressure from abdominal organs against the diaphragm. Both of these factors cause increased resistance to breathing. Difficult recumbent breathing is common during the late stages of pregnancy as the fetus shifts the diaphragm upward. When lying flat, patients with CHF also experience labored breathing, which improves when standing or sitting up.

Spinal Cord Integrity

The diaphragmatic nerve has its origin from C3, C4, and C5. Spinal cord injuries above this level will cause cessation of respiration. In the presence of exiting nerve impingement, ipsilateral hemidiaphragm elevation may occur; however, the contralateral side maintains respiration.

Environment

Exposure to pollutants such as gas and particle emissions, asbestos, chemical waste products, or coal dust can diminish the ability to transport oxygen. Other common offending pollutants include high ozone concentrations, sulfur dioxide, and carbon monoxide.[27] These respiratory irritants typically increase mucus production. High altitudes also affect the respiratory system owing to reduced air mass (i.e., the partial pressure of oxygen in inspired air is low). This means fewer oxygen molecules per liter of air, reducing arterial blood oxygen levels and triggering shortness of breath (*dyspnea*) and reduced tolerance to activity. Hyperventilation, tachycardia, and pulmonary edema (accumulation of fluid in alveolar walls) can also occur at high altitudes.[58,59]

Emotions/Stress

Stress and emotions can cause an increased rate and depth of respirations owing to stimulation of the sympathetic nervous system.

Pharmacological Agents

Essentially any drug that depresses central nervous system (CNS) function will result in respiratory depression. Narcotic agents (e.g., opioids, meperidine hydrochloride) will decrease the rate and depth of respirations. Other categories of CNS depressant agents include barbiturates (e.g., phenobarbital, secobarbital), benzodiazepines (e.g., lorazepam, midazolam, alprazolam, diazepam), neuroleptics (e.g., chlorpromazine, haloperidol, clozapine), muscle relaxants, tricyclic antidepressants, and antiseizure agents. Conversely, bronchodilators decrease airway resistance and residual volume with a resultant increase in vital capacity and airflow. Common bronchodilator medications include albuterol, bitolterol, epinephrine, formoterol, isoproterenol, metaproterenol, and terbutaline.[60,61]

Parameters of Respiration

In examining respiration, four parameters are considered: rate, depth, rhythm, and sound. The *rate* is the number of breaths per minute. Either inspirations or expirations are counted, but not both. The normal adult RR is 12 to 20 breaths per minute. The rate should be counted for 30 seconds and multiplied by 2. If any irregularities are noted, a full 60-second count is indicated.

The *depth* of respiration refers to the amount (volume) of air exchanged with each breath. Normally, the depth of respirations is consistent, producing a relatively even, uniform movement of the chest. The normal adult tidal volume is approximately 500 mL of air. The depth of respiration is determined by observing chest movements and is usually described as *deep* or *shallow*, depending on whether the amount of air exchanged is greater or less than normal. With deep breaths, a large volume of air is exchanged; with shallow respirations, a small amount of air is exchanged, typically with minimal lung expansion or chest wall movement.

The *rhythm* refers to the regularity of inspirations and expirations. Normally, there is an even time interval between respirations. The respiratory rhythm is described as *regular* (normal) or *irregular* (abnormal).

The *sound* of respirations refers to deviations from normal, quiet, effortless breathing. Although some respiratory sounds are audible, accurate identification requires auscultation (listening with a stethoscope placed directly against the chest wall). Normal (*vesicular*) breath sounds are heard primarily during inspiration and sound relatively smooth and soft.[56] Common abnormal (*adventitious*) sounds of breathing include the following:

- **Wheeze (Wheezing):** A continuous whistling sound produced by air passing through a narrowed airway such as a bronchi or bronchiole. This is often compared to the whistling produced when stretching the neck of a balloon and allowing air to escape slowly through the narrowed passageway. It may be heard on both inspiration and expiration but is more prominent on expiration. Wheezing is a common symptom of asthma and is also seen in CHF. It can also result from an airway obstruction.

- **Stridor:** A harsh, high-pitched crowing sound that occurs with upper airway obstructions resulting in narrowing of the glottis or trachea. It is apparent in patients with tracheal stenosis or presence of a foreign object.
- **Crackles (rales):** Rattling or bubbling sounds caused by secretions in the air passages of the respiratory tract. The sound is often compared to that of rustling a cellophane bag. Crackles may be heard with the ear but are most accurately determined using a stethoscope. Inspiratory crackles often suggest pulmonary fibrosis and expiratory crackles are apparent in patients with CHF or pneumonia.
- **Sigh:** A deep inspiration followed by a prolonged, audible expiration. Occasional sighs are normal and function to expand alveoli; frequent sighs are abnormal and may be indicative of emotional stress.
- **Stertor:** A snoring sound owing to partial obstruction (e.g., secretions) in the upper airway (e.g., trachea, large bronchi).

Patterns of Respiration

Examination of the rate, rhythm, and depth allows the therapist to determine the pattern of respiration. Not all patients will present with a distinct pattern of respiration. However, several patterns occur with sufficient frequency that uniform terminology has been developed for their identification. Common respiratory patterns are presented in Figure 2.13.

Eupnea is the term used to describe a normal breathing pattern of 12 to 20 times per minute in an adult. Hyperventilation is an abnormally fast rate and depth of respiration often associated with anxiety, emotional stress, and panic disorders. A common response to an acute episode is to have the patient rebreathe into a paper bag, which replaces some of the lost carbon dioxide (hypocapnia). CNS or pulmonary disorders may cause prolonged hyperventilation. Hypoventilation is a reduction in the rate and depth of respirations. This decrease in the amount of air entering the lungs causes an increase in arterial carbon dioxide levels.

Difficult or labored breathing is called *dyspnea*. Patients with dyspnea require increased, noticeable effort to breathe and often appear as if struggling to get air into the lungs. In an effort to increase effectiveness of respiration, accessory muscles such as the intercostals and abdominals are often active. The intercostals assist in raising the ribs to expand the thoracic cavity; the abdominals assist the function of the diaphragm. Additional muscles that may provide accessory functions in respiration are the sternocleidomastoid, pectoralis major

TYPE	DESCRIPTION	ILLUSTRATION
Eupnea	Normal respirations, with equal rate and depth, 12–20 breaths/min	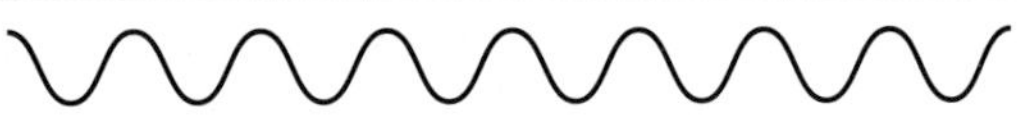
Bradypnea	Slow respirations, < 10 breaths/min	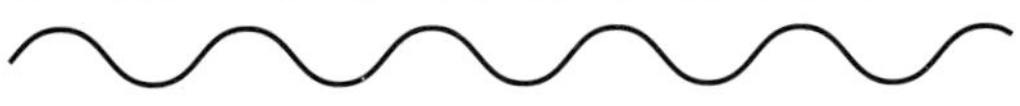
Tachypnea	Fast respirations, > 24 breaths/min, usually shallow	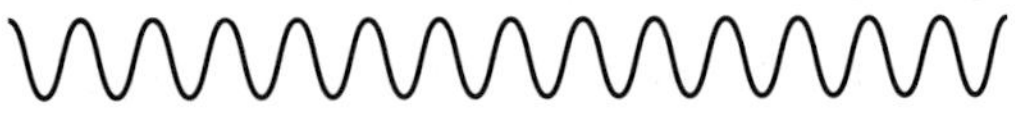
Kussmaul's Respirations	Respirations that are regular but abnormally deep and increased in rate	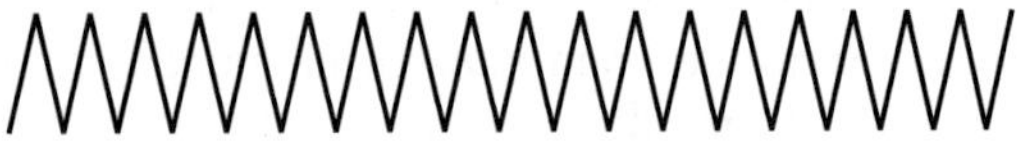
Biot's Respirations	Irregular respirations of variable depth (usually shallow), alternating with periods of apnea (absence of breathing)	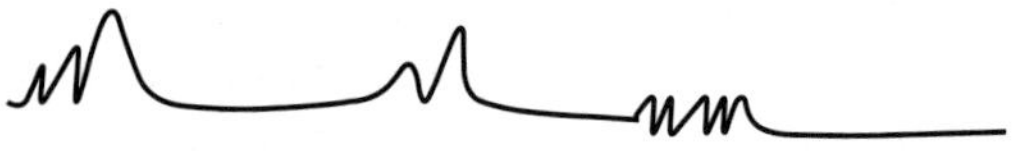
Cheyne-Stokes Respirations	Gradual increase in depth of respirations, followed by gradual decrease and then a period of apnea	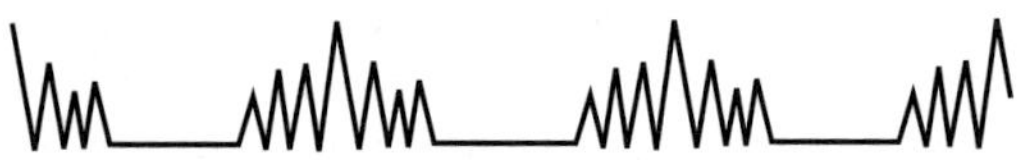
Apnea	Absence of breathing	

Figure 2.13 Normal (eupnea) and abnormal respiratory patterns. *(From Wilkinson, et al. with permission.)*

and minor, scalenes, and subclavius. Use of accessory muscles to breathe is referred to as costal or thoracic breathing. Pain and nasal flaring sometimes accompany dyspnea (to bring in more oxygen). Acute episodes may be brought on by blockage of an air passage, infection of the respiratory tract, or trauma to the thorax. Long-standing dyspnea is a hallmark of COPD, such as asthma or bronchitis.

Orthopnea is difficult or labored breathing (dyspnea) when the patient is lying down that is relieved by sitting or standing. The change in positioning causes gravity to lower the abdominal organs, allowing increased room for chest expansion. Orthopnea is a characteristic symptom of CHF and also may be seen with asthma, advanced emphysema, and pulmonary edema. *Tachypnea* is an abnormally fast RR, usually greater than 24 breaths per minute. This pattern is seen with respiratory insufficiency and fever as the body attempts to rid itself of excess heat. *Bradypnea* is an abnormally slow RR, usually 10 breaths or fewer per minute. Bradypnea is associated with impairment of the respiratory control center, as may occur with increased intracranial pressure (tumor), drug intake (narcotics), or metabolic disorder. *Apnea* is the absence of respirations and is usually transient. If sustained for longer than several minutes, brain damage and death may occur. Cheyne-Stokes respiration is characterized by a period of apnea lasting 10 to 60 seconds, followed by gradually increasing depth and frequency of respirations (hyperventilation). It occurs with depression of the cerebral hemispheres (e.g., coma), in basal ganglia disease, and occasionally in CHF. Among the hallmarks of obstructive sleep apnea is not only loud snoring, but also when bed partner observes 20 to 30 seconds of apnea while asleep (witnessed apnea).[62]

Respiratory Examination

Because respiration is under both voluntary (cortical) and involuntary control, it is important that the patient is unaware that respiration is being examined. Once aware of the examination, characteristics of the breathing pattern will likely be altered. This is a normal reaction to being observed. It is often recommended that respirations be observed immediately after taking the pulse. After monitoring the pulse, the fingers can remain in place at the pulse site, and respirations can be monitored without drawing the patient's conscious attention to their breathing pattern. Ideally, respiration should be examined with the chest exposed. If this is not possible, or if respirations cannot be easily observed through clothing, maintain fingers on the radial pulse site and place the patient's forearm across the chest. This will allow limited palpation without drawing conscious input from the patient. Chapter 12, Chronic Pulmonary Dysfunction, provides a more thorough discussion of the respiratory examination.

Monitoring Respiration

A. Assemble equipment: Watch with a second hand.
B. Wash hands.
C. Procedure:
  1. Ensure patient understanding, safety, modesty, and comfort. Respirations are typically monitored with the patient either supine or sitting. *Note:* The patient should be in a quiet resting position for at least 5 minutes prior to monitoring respirations.
  2. Expose chest area; if area cannot be exposed and respirations are not readily observable, place patient's forearm across chest and keep fingers positioned as if continuing to monitor the radial pulse.
  3. As the patient breathes, observe the rise and fall of the chest; note the amount of effort required or audible sounds produced during breathing. (Normally, respiration is effortless and silent.)
  4. Using the second hand of a watch, determine the rate by counting respirations (either inspirations or expirations, but not both) for 30 seconds and multiply by 2.
  5. Identify the rhythm (regularity of inspirations and expirations); note deviations from normal uninterrupted, even spacing. If any irregularities are noted, count for a full 60 seconds to accommodate the fluctuations and ensure an accurate count.
  6. Observe the depth of respiration; determine if a small, large, or approximately normal volume of air is inspired. Observe involvement of accessory muscles, which suggests weakness in the primary muscles of breathing (diaphragm and external intercostal muscles); if difficult to observe, palpation of chest wall excursion can be used to identify depth of respiration. Record as shallow, deep, or normal.
    Note: Chest wall excursion can also be determined by circumferential chest measures using a tape measure at three specific bony landmarks: (1) the sternal angle of Louis; (2) the xiphoid process; and (3) midway between the xiphoid process and the umbilicus.
  7. If indicated, determine the sound of breathing using a stethoscope.
  8. Return clothing if chest has been exposed.
  9. Wash hands.

■ BLOOD PRESSURE

BP refers to the force the blood exerts against a vessel wall. It is measured in millimeters of mercury (mm Hg) and recorded in the form of a fraction (e.g., 119/79). The top number indicates systolic pressure, and the bottom indicates diastolic pressure. Because liquid flows only from a higher to a lower pressure, the pressure is highest in the arteries, lower in the capillaries, and lowest in veins.[22,24]

The heart is an intermittent pulsatile pump, pressure is measured at both the highest and lowest points of the pulse. These points represent the systolic (ventricular contraction) and diastolic (ventricular relaxation) pressures. The systolic pressure is the highest pressure exerted by the blood against the arterial walls. The diastolic pressure (which is constantly present) is the lowest pressure. The elastic properties of the arterial walls allow for expansion and recoil in response to the changing volume of circulating blood during the cardiac cycle. The mathematical difference between the systolic and diastolic pressures is called the *pulse pressure*. For example, a systolic pressure of 119 mm Hg and a diastolic pressure of 79 mm Hg result in a pulse pressure of 40 mm Hg.

BP is a function of two primary elements: (1) cardiac output (amount of blood flow, CO); and (2) peripheral resistance (impediment to blood flow within a vessel, R) that the heart must overcome. The relationship between BP, CO, and R is expressed in the equation: $BP = CO \times R$. Additional factors that contribute to this relationship include the diameter and elasticity of vessel walls, blood volume, and blood viscosity.

Blood Pressure Regulation

The *vasomotor center* is located bilaterally in the lower pons and upper medulla. It transmits impulses through sympathetic nerves to all vessels of the body. The vasomotor center is tonically active, producing a slow, continual firing in all vasoconstrictor nerve fibers. It is this slow, continual firing that maintains a partial state of contraction of the blood vessels and provides normal *vasomotor tone*.[63] The vasomotor center assists in providing the stable arterial pressure required to maintain blood flow to body tissue and organs. This occurs because of its close connection to the cardiac controlling center in the medulla (because changes in cardiac output will influence BP). In addition, the vasomotor and cardiac controlling centers require input from afferent receptors.

Afferent input regarding BP is provided primarily by *baroreceptors* and *chemoreceptors*. The *baroreceptors* (pressoreceptors) are stimulated by the stretch of the vessel wall from alterations in pressure. These receptors have a high concentration in the walls of the internal carotid arteries above the carotid bifurcation and in the walls of the aortic arch. Baroreceptors located in the *carotid sinuses* of the carotid arteries monitor BP to the brain. Baroreceptors in the *aortic sinuses* of the aortic arch are responsible for monitoring BP throughout the body.

In response to an increase in BP, the baroreceptor input to the vasomotor center results in an inhibition of the vasoconstrictor center of the medulla and excitation of the vagal center.[24] This results in a decreased HR, decreased force of cardiac contraction, and vasodilation, with a subsequent drop in BP. The baroreceptor input during a lowering of BP would produce the opposite effects.

The *chemoreceptors* are stimulated by reduced arterial oxygen concentrations, increases in carbon dioxide tension, and increased hydrogen ion concentrations. These receptors lie close to the baroreceptors. Those located in the carotid artery are called *carotid bodies,* and on the aortic arch they are termed *aortic bodies*. Impulses from these receptors travel to the brain (cardioregulatory and vasomotor centers) via afferent pathways in the vagus and glossopharyngeal nerves. Efferent impulses from these centers, in response to alterations in BP, will alter HR, strength of cardiac contractions, and size of blood vessels.[23]

Factors Influencing Blood Pressure

Many factors influence pressure. As with all vital signs, BP is represented by a range of normal values and will yield the most useful data when monitored over a period of time. Important influences to be considered when examining BP include blood volume, diameter and elasticity of arteries, cardiac output, age, exercise, and arm position.

Blood Volume

The amount of circulating blood in the body directly affects pressure. Blood loss (e.g., hemorrhage) will cause pressure to drop and can result in hypovolemic shock from inadequate tissue perfusion. Conversely, an increase in the amount of circulating blood (e.g., blood transfusion) will cause the pressure to rise. Reduced fluid volume, as may occur with diarrhea or inadequate oral intake (dehydration), will also lower BP; excess fluid, as occurs with CHF, will increase pressure. Essentially, any situation causing a shift (increase or decrease) in body fluids (intravascular, interstitial, or intracellular) will alter BP. Bladder distention can also contribute to BP elevation.

Diameter and Elasticity of Arteries

The diameter (size) of the vessel lumen will provide either *increased peripheral resistance* (vasoconstriction) or *decreased resistance* (vasodilation) to cardiac output. The elasticity of the vessel wall also influences resistance. Normally, the expansion and recoil properties of the arterial walls provide a continuous, smooth flow of blood into the capillaries and veins between heartbeats. With age, these properties are diminished; arterial stiffness decreases vessel wall compliance. Thus, there is a higher resistance to blood flow with resultant *increase* in BP.

A characteristic feature of arteriosclerosis is reduced vessel wall compliance in response to fluctuations in pressure. For older adults, elevated BP is often associated with the degenerative effects of arteriosclerosis. As the disease progresses, small arteries and arterioles lose elasticity, the walls become thick and hard and unable to yield to pressure exerted by blood flow, and the lumen gradually narrows and may eventually become blocked. Multiple factors can contribute to hypertension in elders (e.g., smoking, activity level, obesity, diet, comorbidities such as cardiac or vascular disease). In her extensive literature review, Pinto suggests that "the increase in BP with age is most likely due to complex and varied factors moulded [molded] and influenced by the individual environment and lifestyle."[64]

Cardiac Output

When increased amounts of blood are pumped into the arteries, the walls of the vessels distend, resulting in a higher BP. With lower cardiac output, less blood is pushed into the vessel, and there is a subsequent drop in pressure.

Age

BP varies with age. It normally rises gradually after birth and reaches a peak during puberty. By late adolescence (18 to 19 years), adult BP is reached. For many years, the normal adult BP was considered 120/80 mm Hg. A BP value of 119/79 mm Hg or below is now the normal adult standard.[65,66] Table 2.3 presents new categories of BP from a recent report by the American College of Cardiology (ACC) and the American Heart Association (AHA) titled *Guideline for the Prevention, Detection, Evaluation, and Management of High Blood Pressure in Adults.*[65]

The ACC/AHA guideline recognizes the high prevalence of hypertension that affects millions of individuals in the United States and worldwide and provides comprehensive information addressing its prevention and treatment. Hypertension is an important risk factor for many disorders, including myocardial infarct, heart failure, stroke, and kidney disease. The new ACC/AHA guideline classifies normal adult BP as below 120/80 mm Hg, elevated BP as 120–129/80 mm Hg, hypertension stage 1 as 130–139/80–89 mm Hg, and

hypertension stage 2 as 140/90 mm Hg or higher (see Table 2.3).[65] The ACC/AHA "guideline is intended to be a resource for the clinical and public health practice communities. It is designed to be comprehensive but succinct and practical in providing guidance for prevention, detection, evaluation, and management of high BP."[65] New published recommendations for the guidelines suggest lifestyle modifications for adults with stage 1 hypertension and a low cardiovascular risk. If target BP is not met within 6 months, antihypertensive medications are indicated.[67]

Clinical Note. *White coat hypertension* or *nonsustained hypertension* is seen more frequently in older adults. This occurs in individuals whose BP is higher in a clinical setting than outside the clinic; it is believed to be associated with the stress and anxiety of seeing a health care professional (the "white coat").

Exercise

Physical activity increases cardiac output. In response to the intensity of the workload, there is a progressive increase in systolic BP, no change or a slight increase in diastolic BP, and a widening of pulse pressure. Greater increases are noted in systolic pressure owing to proportional changes in the pressure gradient of peripheral vessels. This means that although cardiac output during exercise is high, vasodilation reduces peripheral resistance to maintain a relatively lower diastolic pressure. A drop in systolic BP of 10 mm Hg or more with increasing exercise intensity or failure of systolic BP to increase with heightened workload is considered an abnormal response and is indication for stopping exercise.[35]

Valsalva Maneuver

The Valsalva maneuver is an attempt to exhale forcibly with the glottis, nose, and mouth closed. It causes an increase in intrathoracic pressure with an accompanying collapse of the veins of the chest wall. There is a subsequent decrease in blood flow to the heart, a decreased venous return, and a drop in BP. This maneuver serves to internally stabilize the abdominal and chest wall during periods of rapid and maximum exertion such as lifting a heavy object. When the breath is released, the intrathoracic pressure decreases, and venous return is suddenly reestablished as an "overshoot" mechanism to compensate for the drop in BP. In turn, there is a marked increase in HR and BP. This rapid rise in arterial pressure causes vagal slowing of the HR (bradycardia). Although the Valsalva maneuver can temporarily enhance muscle function via internal stabilization, it has an indirect undesirable effect of increasing BP and should be avoided by individuals with cardiac impairment and hypertension.[22,26]

Table 2.3	Adult Blood Pressure Categories[62]	
Category	Systolic Blood Pressure (mm Hg)	Diastolic Blood Pressure (mm Hg)
Normal	<120	<80
Elevated	120–129	<80
Hypertension		
Stage 1	130–139	80–89
Stage 2	≥140	≥90
Hypertensive Crisis	>180	>120

Clinical Note. A common misconception concerning the Valsalva maneuver is that it directly increases HR and BP. As described earlier, it is the body's recovery mechanism of suddenly increasing venous return that causes this increase. The subsequent drop in BP due to the Valsalva maneuver may result in seeing "black dots" and the feeling of dizziness that often accompanies straining while lifting a heavy object.

Orthostatic Hypotension

Associated with prolonged immobility and periods of bedrest, orthostatic or postural hypotension is a sudden drop in BP that occurs when movement to upright postures (sitting or standing) is initiated. The positional change causes gravitational blood pooling in the lower extremity (LE) veins. Venous return and cardiac outputs are reduced, with resultant cerebral hypoperfusion. This can trigger an episode of light-headedness, dizziness, or even loss of consciousness (syncope). In response to positional changes under normal circumstances, BP is maintained by reflex vasoconstriction (via baroreceptors), which increases HR. After a period of inactivity, postural hypotension should be anticipated; it requires a gradual acclimation to the upright position until normal reflex control returns.

Other predisposing factors for postural hypotension include exercise, drugs such as antihypertensives and vasodilators, reduction in baroreceptor response with aging, the Valsalva maneuver, and hypovolemia (abnormally low volume of circulating blood).[68,69] Patients with CNS involvement of the autonomic nervous system (e.g., patients with acute cervical spinal cord injury or Parkinson disease) typically exhibit episodes of orthostatic hypotension with position changes. As a useful precaution, any patient restricted to a recumbent position for even short periods should be considered at risk for postural hypotension. These events can be minimized by use of external pressure supports such as abdominal binders and support or full-length elastic stockings (elastic bandages can also be used effectively) and a very gradual acclimation to upright postures. Should postural hypotension occur during the examination, the patient should be moved to a sitting position from standing or a reclined position from sitting with the legs elevated.

Orthostatic hypotension is examined by first taking initial HR and BP with the patient in supine position at rest for 5 minutes. The patient is then moved directly to the standing position; HR and BP are repeated immediately and again after 3 minutes. A patient is orthostatic if systolic BP drops more than 20 mm Hg, if diastolic BP drops more than 10 mm Hg, or if the patient is experiencing light-headedness or dizziness.[70]

Arm Position

BP may vary as much as 20 mm Hg by altering the arm position. For consistency of measurements, the patient should be positioned with the arm in a horizontal, supported position at heart level. If the patient's condition or the type of activity precludes these positions, alterations should be carefully documented. As with other vital signs, factors such as fear, anxiety, or emotional stress also will cause an increase in BP. In addition, some medications can either increase BP or interfere with antihypertensive drugs. These drugs include steroids, NSAIDs, diet pills, cyclosporine, erythropoietin, tricyclic antidepressants, monoamine oxidase inhibitors, and some oral contraceptives.

Note: Ambulatory Blood Pressure Monitoring (ABPM) has been considered to be the reference standard for the diagnosis of hypertension. The 2015 statement from the U.S. Preventive Services Task Force and the 2017 ACC/AHA hypertension guidelines recommend obtaining measurements outside of the clinical setting for diagnostic confirmation of hypertension.[65,71] Compared with ABPM, the sensitivity and specificity of office-based BP measurements are poor.[72–75] However, randomized trials upon which hypertension diagnosis and treatment recommendations are based used office-based BP measurements.[76]

Equipment Requirements

A noninvasive or *indirect* measure of BP is used by physical therapists. In critical care settings, invasive or *direct* measures of BP are obtained by placing a thin catheter directly into an artery. The equipment required for taking BP using the more common noninvasive auscultatory (listening) method includes a *sphygmomanometer* and a *stethoscope*. The sphygmomanometer (frequently referred to as a *blood pressure cuff*) consists of a flat, airtight, inflatable latex bladder. The bladder is covered with a cotton or nylon sleeve that extends beyond the length of the bladder. There are two tubes that extend from the cuff. One is attached to a rubber bulb that has a valve to maintain or to release air from the cuff. The second tube is attached to a pressure manometer (portion of sphygmomanometer that registers the pressure reading). In patient care settings, sphygmomanometers may be wall mounted or placed on a mobile stand with a wheeled base.

BP cuffs are typically secured on the patient's extremity by a hook and loop closure. They come in a variety of sizes. In adults, the width of the bladder should be approximately 40% of the arm circumference, and bladder length should be enough to encircle at least 80% of the arm circumference. Obtaining a cuff of appropriate size is important. Cuffs that are too narrow will show inaccurately high readings; cuffs that are too wide will show inaccurately low readings.[75] The AHA provides the following guidelines for the appropriate cuff size based on arm circumference.[77]

- Arm circumference 22 to 26 cm (7 to 10 in.): Small adult cuff, 12 × 22 cm (5 × 9 in.)
- Arm circumference 27 to 34 cm (11 to 13 in.): Adult cuff, 16 × 30 cm (6 × 12 in.)
- Arm circumference 35 to 44 cm (14 to 17 in.): Large adult cuff, 16 × 36 cm (6 × 14 in.)
- Arm circumference 45 to 52 cm (18 to 20 in.): Adult thigh cuff, 16 × 42 cm (6 × 17 in.)

The manometer registers the BP reading. Manometers are either *aneroid* or *mercury*, with a 300 mm Hg scale marked in 2-mm increments. The aneroid manometer registers BP by way of a circular calibrated dial and needle (see Box 2.4, image A); automated BP units provide a digital LCD or use an app to connect wirelessly to an electronic device (see Box 2.4, images B, C, D). Owing to health and environmental concerns, aneroid manometers and automated displays have largely replaced mercury manometers in patient care settings.

Automated sphygmomanometers are self-inflating battery (rechargeable) or electrically powered units; many battery-powered models are also equipped with an AC adapter. Some include the "average mode" feature that performs two or three readings and then averages the total. Devices designed for clinical use often include several cuff sizes (e.g., small, medium, large, and extra-large). In hospital settings, BP is often included in units designed to measure multiple vital signs. Automated sphygmomanometers designed for home use are described in Box 2.4 (B, C, D).

To monitor BP with an aneroid sphygmomanometer, an acoustic stethoscope is used to listen to the sounds over the artery as pressure is released from the cuff. By a combination of listening through the stethoscope and watching the manometer, the BP reading is obtained. A stethoscope amplifies and carries body sounds to the examiner's ears. Proximally, it consists of two rubber or plastic earpieces attached to narrow metal tubing that projects laterally from the earpieces about 1 in. (2.5 cm) and then downward about 6 in. (15 cm). The tubes are connected by a flexible, semicircular metal spring mechanism that is often rubber-coated. These metal tubes are referred to as *binaurals* (designed for use in both ears). The semicircular spring provides tension to maintain the position of the earpieces in the examiner's ears during use. The metal tubes then insert into fork-shaped rubber or plastic tubing that joins to form a single lumen and attach to the head distally. Some stethoscopes (e.g., Sprague Rappaport–type stethoscope) are designed with two separate tubes that do not join and lead individually directly to the head of the stethoscope (the two tubes are held together with small metal clasps).

There are two types of distal sensing microphones on stethoscopes: a *bell shape* and a *flat-disk diaphragm*. Stethoscopes may have only one type of head; others have a combination design with one side bell shaped and the other a flat disk (see Fig. 2.14). The bell shape amplifies low-frequency sounds such as those produced in blood vessels; this type is generally recommended for determining BP. The flat-disk diaphragm is more useful for high-frequency sounds such as heart and lung sounds.

Another type of sensor incorporates both high- and low-frequency capabilities of the two shapes into a single-sided unit that eliminates the need to turn the head over. To hear low-frequency sound (bell shape), lighter pressure of the examiner's fingers is used; firmer pressure allows high-frequency sounds to be heard.

Battery-powered stethoscopes provide higher levels of amplification with volume control and dual-frequency sound filtering; some are available with interchangeable removable heads. A design variation for emergency medical service personnel provides higher amplification levels by replacing the earpieces with a headset designed to block out noise in a moving ambulance. Disposable stethoscopes are also available for use in high-risk settings where minimizing the risk of cross-infection is essential.

Korotkoff Sounds

When measuring BP, a series of sounds called Korotkoff sounds are heard through the stethoscope. The bell side of the stethoscope is generally recommended for auscultation because Korotkoff sounds are low frequency. Initially when pressure is applied through the cuff around the patient's arm, the blood flow is occluded, and no sound is heard through the stethoscope. As the pressure is gradually released, a series of five phases of sounds can be identified.

The therapist should be alert for the presence of an auscultatory gap, especially in patients with BP above normal values (hypertension). An auscultatory gap is the temporary disappearance of sound normally heard over the brachial artery between phases 1 and 2 and may cover a range of as much as 40 mm Hg. Not identifying this gap may lead to an underestimation of systolic pressure and overestimation of diastolic pressure.

Phase I: The first clear, faint, rhythmic tapping sound, which gradually increases in intensity, is heard. The period when blood initially flows through the artery is recorded as *systolic pressure*. This represents the highest pressure in the arterial system during ventricular contraction. *Be alert for an auscultatory gap.*

Phase II: A murmur or swishing sound is heard as the artery widens and more blood flows through it.

Phase III: Sounds become crisp, more intense, and louder; blood is now flowing relatively unobstructed.

Box 2.4 Examples of Sphygmomanometers

Illustration

Manual

Manual sphygmomanometers have traditionally been used to monitor BP. Air is manually pumped into the inflatable cuff. As pressure is slowly released, heart sounds are monitored using a stethoscope. (A) Courtesy of OMRON, Inc., Lake Forest, IL 60045

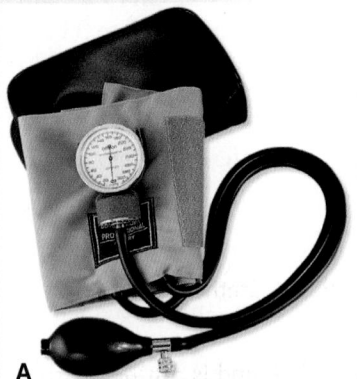

A

Automated

Automated sphygmomanometers, designed for home use, are convenient and practical for patients requiring frequent self-monitoring. They provide a rapid digital display, monitor pulse (in most cases), allow data storage, and are easy to use (place cuff and activate start button). Automated sphygmomanometers do not require a stethoscope; during automated inflation and deflation, the diastolic and systolic pressures are recorded. These devices monitor BP at the traditional arm location (B) or at the wrist (C). Some units provide wireless connectivity. For both arm and wrist cuffs, patients should be instructed that the UE should be relaxed and supported at heart level.

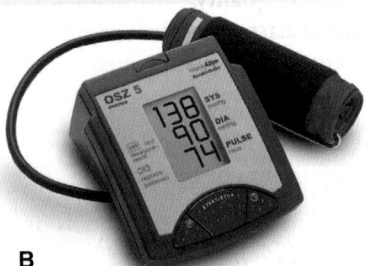

B

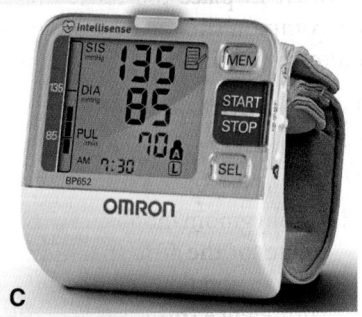

C

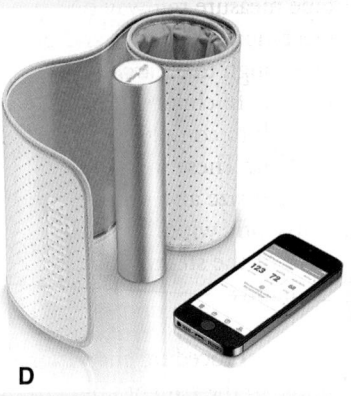

D

Courtesy of OMRON Healthcare, Hoffman Estates, IL 60169.
(B and C courtesy of Welch Allyn, Skaneateles Falls, NY 13153-0220; D courtesy of Withings, Cambridge, MA 02142)

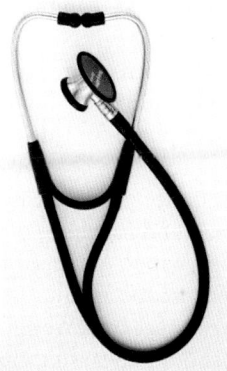

Figure 2.14 Stethoscope with dual head.

Phase IV: Sound is distinct, with abrupt muffling; soft blowing quality.

Phase V: Last sound is heard; recorded as *diastolic pressure* in adults.

A BP reading with a systolic pressure of 117 and a second diastolic reading of 76 would be recorded as 117/76. An important consideration in determining BP is that it should be done in a minimal amount of time. The BP cuff acts as a tourniquet. As such, venous pooling and considerable discomfort to the patient will occur if the cuff is left in place too long. The brachial artery is the most common site for BP monitoring. A description for monitoring BP in the LE is also presented.

Measuring Brachial Blood Pressure

A. Assemble equipment:
   1. A stethoscope.
   2. A sphygmomanometer with a bladder size appropriate for the arm. In adults, the width of the bladder should be about 40% of the arm circumference (measurement can be made using a tape measure midway between the acromion and olecranon processes), and bladder length should be enough to encircle at least 80% of arm circumference. In children, the bladder should be long enough to completely encircle the entire arm.

      Note: These measurements refer to the internal bladder size and not the external encasing cuff.
   3. Antiseptic wipes for cleaning earpieces and the head of the stethoscope before and after use.

B. Wash hands.

C. Procedure:
   1. Explain procedure and rationale in terms appropriate to the patient's understanding. Indicate that there will be a request to remain quiet during monitoring to avoid interference with auscultation.

      Note: As with other vital sign measures, BP is monitored after the patient has been in a relaxed quiet setting for a period of time because activity or physical exertion will cause an elevation in measurements.
   2. Guide the patient to the desired position. The sitting position is recommended with the back supported, the legs uncrossed, and feet flat on floor. The diastolic pressure may be raised by 6 mm Hg if the back is unsupported, and the systolic pressure may be increased by 5 to 8 mm Hg if the legs are crossed.[77] The arm should be supported at the level of the heart.[78] If the arm is allowed to rest unsupported, the measured BP will be increased by 10 to 12 mm Hg owing to the added hydrostatic pressure induced by gravity.[77]

      Placing the chair next to a treatment table will facilitate UE positioning. The UE should be free of clothing. (Rolling up a garment sleeve is not acceptable owing to the tourniquet effect produced and interference with cuff positioning.)

      Note: If a supine position is used, the arm should be at the patient's side and slightly elevated to the middle of the trunk. If measuring BP in a standing position (e.g., monitoring postural hypotension), ensure that the arm is supported at heart level.
   3. Ensure patient understanding, safety, modesty, and comfort.
   4. Use antiseptic wipes to clean the earpieces and head of stethoscope.
   5. Wrap the deflated cuff snugly and evenly around the patient's bare arm approximately 1 in. (2.5 cm) above the antecubital fossa; the center of the cuff should be in line with the brachial artery (Fig. 2.15). Some cuffs have markers to guide positioning over the artery.
   6. Ensure that the aneroid gauge is easily visible. (A mercury manometer must be on a level surface at eye level.) Check that the sphygmomanometer registers zero.

      Note: The first time a patient's BP is measured, an estimation of the systolic pressure should be made. This will ensure that during the actual measure, an adequate level of cuff inflation is used. The procedure is as follows:
      a. Locate and palpate the radial artery on the distal forearm of the cuffed arm.
      b. Close the valve of the BP cuff (turn clockwise).
      c. While continuing to monitor the pulse, rapidly inflate the BP cuff to 30 mm Hg above the level at which the radial pulse is extinguished.
      d. Note the pressure value on the gauge. (This is the estimate of maximum pressure required to measure systolic pressure for the individual patient.)
      e. Allow air to release quickly.

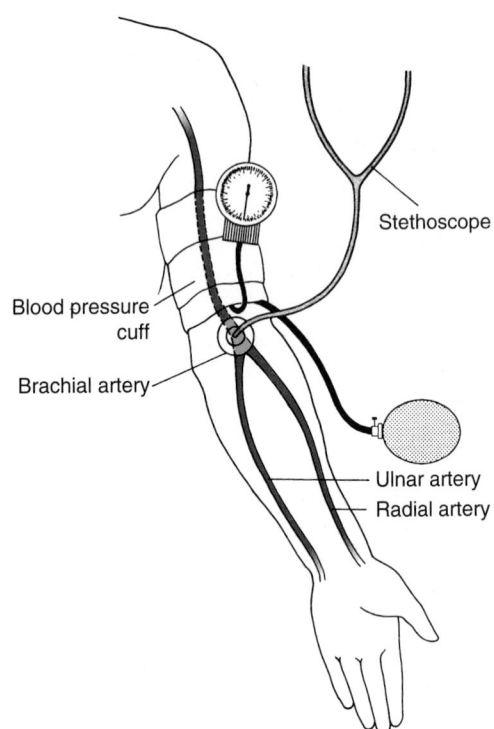

Figure 2.15 Placement of the BP cuff and stethoscope for monitoring brachial artery blood pressure.

Stethoscope

Blood pressure cuff

Brachial artery

Ulnar artery
Radial artery

7. Place the earpieces of the stethoscope (tilting slightly forward) into the ear canals; the tubes of the stethoscope should not be crossed or in contact with each other and should hang freely.

8. Locate and palpate the brachial artery slightly above and medial to the antecubital fossa. Place the head of the stethoscope firmly over the brachial pulse point at the lower border of the BP cuff. Sufficient pressure should be used to avoid gapping between the circumference of the stethoscope head and the skin.

9. Close the valve of the BP cuff (turn clockwise), and rapidly and steadily inflate the cuff to approximately 30 mm Hg above the estimated systolic pressure.

10. Release the thumb valve carefully, allowing air out slowly; air should be released at a rate of 2 mm Hg per heartbeat. Listen for the appearance of Korotkoff sounds.

11. Watch the manometer closely and note the point at which the first rhythmic tapping sound is heard (a mercury manometer must be viewed at eye level); this is the point when blood first begins to flow through the artery and represents the systolic pressure (Korotkoff phase 1). Deflections in the dial or column of mercury will now be noted.

12. Continue to release air carefully at a rate of 2 mm Hg per heartbeat. Note when the sound first becomes muffled (Korotkoff phase 4) because quickly thereafter the sound will disappear (Korotkoff phase 5); this is recorded as the diastolic pressure.

13. Allow remainder of air to release quickly.

14. Clean the head and earpieces of the stethoscope with antiseptic wipes. If the same examiner is using the stethoscope again, it is not necessary to clean the earpieces. However, the head of the stethoscope should always be cleaned between patients.

15. Wash hands.

Note: It is generally recommended that at least two BP measurements be taken and the values averaged.[77] At least a 1-minute interval should elapse between repeated measures. In its examination of hypertension, the ACC/AHA guideline recommends use of BP averages of at least 2 readings obtained on at least 2 occasions.[65] If a 24-hr ABPM is being performed at home, the nondominant arm should be utilized and the patient instructed to keep the arm still during readings.[77,78]

Measuring Popliteal (Thigh) Blood Pressure

Measurement of popliteal BP is indicated in situations in which comparisons between the UE and LE are warranted, such as peripheral vascular disease. They also are used when UE pressures are contraindicated, such as after trauma or surgery. In comparison to the brachial artery, the popliteal artery normally yields a higher systolic pressure; diastolic values are approximately the same. In a systematic review of 44 studies comparing arm and leg BP readings performed in the supine position, mean systolic BP was higher in both the calf (by 10 mm Hg) and the ankle (17 mm Hg) than in the arm.[79] Essentially, the procedure is the same as that for determining pressure at the brachial artery, with the following variations:

1. The patient is in a prone position; alternatively, the supine position may be used. Expose the LE using appropriate draping procedures.

2. Locate the pulse by palpation in the popliteal fossa. Flexing the knee slightly facilitates pulse location, as the artery is deep within the posterior knee. Knee flexion also facilitates stethoscope placement. Because the popliteal pulse is deep, it is often useful to initially palpate it using the first two or three fingers of each hand on either side of the posterior knee. Once a pulse is perceived, attention is then directed to locating the strongest pulse point.

3. Wrap the deflated cuff snugly and evenly around the patient's midthigh. (A wide cuff is used; use guidelines for cuff size described for brachial BP.)

The center of the bladder should be directly over the popliteal artery.

Note: As described for brachial BP, an estimate of maximum pressure required to measure systolic pressure can be made using the popliteal or dorsalis pedis artery.

4. Proceed with auscultating the pressure as for the brachial artery.

■ PULSE OXIMETRY

Pulse oximetry provides a measure of peripheral arterial blood saturation that is updated with each pulse wave. It has become the standard for noninvasive examination of oxygenation.[80] Oxygen is carried in the blood in two forms: (1) dissolved in arterial plasma and (2) combined with hemoglobin.[22] Arterial plasma transports only about 3% of the oxygen in blood and is measured as PaO_2 (partial pressure of oxygen). The greater amount of oxygen (approximately 97%) is carried by hemoglobin and measured as SaO_2 (arterial hemoglobin oxygen saturation). Pulse oximetry measures arterial blood oxygen saturation as a noninvasive intervention.[81] Oxygen saturation via pulse oximetry is reported as SpO_2 and can be measured at any adequately perfused peripheral pulse.[82]

The level of arterial oxygenation measured indirectly by pulse oximetry is documented as SpO_2. A pulse oximeter measures SpO_2 based on the absorption of light by pulsating arterial blood at two specific wavelengths that correspond to the absorption of oxygenated and deoxygenated hemoglobin.[2] Simply stated, it is a measure of the amount of oxygen-carrying hemoglobin in the blood relative to the amount of hemoglobin not carrying oxygen.[37]

Pulse oximetry can alert the therapist to a decline in patient status much sooner than observation alone. Cyanosis may not develop until arterial oxygen saturation drops to approximately 67%.[82] In addition, the threshold at which cyanosis becomes apparent is affected by skin pigmentation, peripheral perfusion, and hemoglobin concentration.[83] Oximetry also provides continuous information to allow administration of supplemental oxygen to be adjusted to a target level. However, it should be noted that the accuracy of pulse oximetry decreases when oxygen saturation is below 90%, and especially below 80%.[84–86] SpO_2 may not be a reliable measure with patients who are critically ill.[84,87]

Normal oxygen saturation levels are between 96% and 100%. A resting SpO_2 less than 93% and a greater than 3% to 5% decrease in SpO_2 with 1 minute of ambulation has been described as hypoxemia.[88] *Hypoxemia* is a term used to describe deficient oxygenation of the blood. *Hypoxia* is a diminished supply of oxygen available to body tissues, and *anoxia* is the complete lack of oxygen,[36] a condition that can be sustained only for a very brief period. In general, saturation levels below 90% are considered significant and warrant additional testing beyond the data provided by pulse oximetry (e.g., arterial blood gas analysis), as well as marking the potential need for administration of supplemental oxygen.[89]

Alterations in heart function (e.g., heart attack, heart failure, arrhythmias) typically reduce cardiac output and the amount of oxygen delivered to tissues. Lung conditions also affect oxygen saturation levels and impair ability of the lungs to oxygenate blood. These include anemia (reduction in number of hemoglobin molecules available to carry oxygen), hypoventilation (e.g., COPD, bronchitis, emphysema, pneumonia, asthma), and diffusion impairments that affect blood–gas exchange (e.g., alveolar fibrosis, interstitial fluid).

Pulse oximetry contributes to (1) early identification of hypoxemia; (2) monitoring patient tolerance to activity; and (3) evaluating patient response to treatment. Pulse oximetry measures may be done continuously, intermittently to generate a series of values over time, or as a single measure at a given point in time (e.g., as an initial screening tool). The measurement pattern will be determined within the context of the patient history and examination findings. Telemetry oximetry monitoring allows continuous communication of SpO_2 data from remote locations.[90]

Measuring Pulse Oximetry

The pulse oximeter provides data on the percentage of oxygen that is combined with hemoglobin. In hospital settings, pulse oximeters are typically included in units designed to gather multiple measures such as pulse, temperature, and BP. Portable units are relatively small (Fig. 2.16), are easy to use and transport, and provide the therapist with immediate information about the patient's saturation levels. The display provides a digital percentage of the amount of hemoglobin saturated with oxygen and a pulsatile waveform and pulse rate, with an audible signal indicating each pulsation. The patient interface is provided by a lead wire and sensor that attaches to the unit. The sensor is placed over a pulsating arteriolar vascular bed.[90] Several types of sensors are available, including fingertip sleeves, adhesive designs for use on fingertips and forehead (temporal artery), as well as nasal, earlobe, and foot styles. Others are self-contained and clip over the distal finger.

Sources of Error

Pulse oximetry is subject to artifactual and patient-related sources of error. If a saturation reading is in doubt, the examiner can place the probe on their own

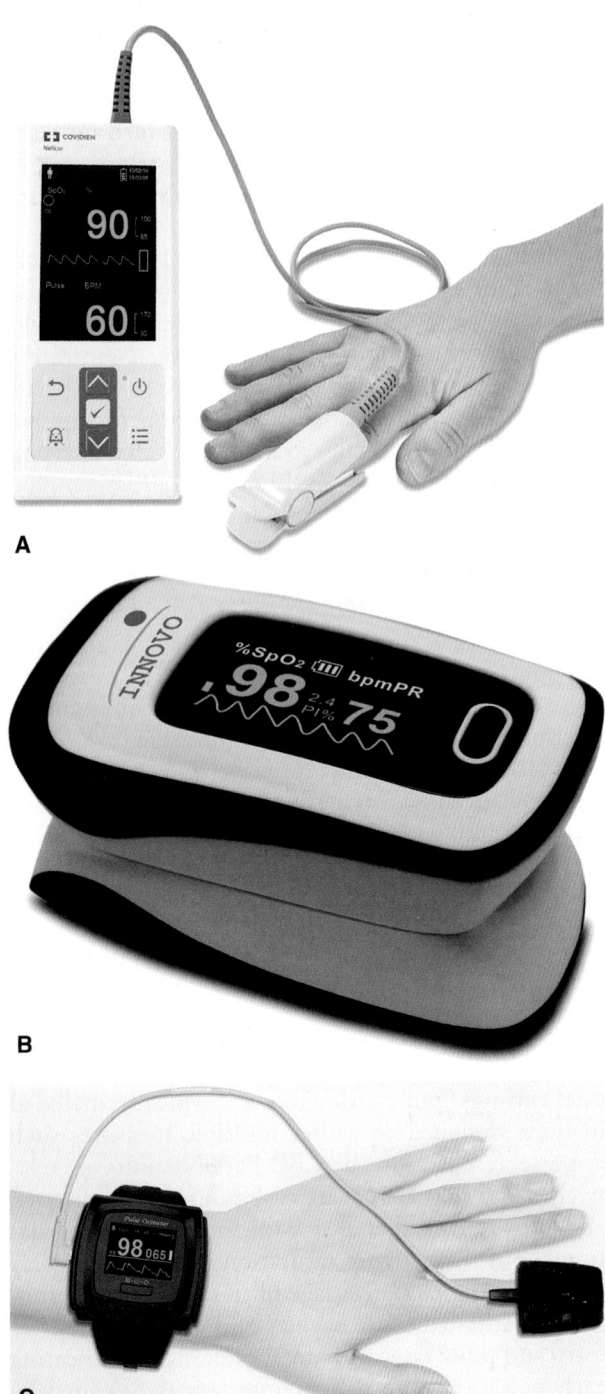

Figure 2.16 Pulse oximeters provide data on arterial blood oxygen saturation as well as pulse rate. (A) Handheld unit with fingertip sensor. *(A, Courtesy of Medtronic, Boulder, CO 80301.)* (B) Fingertip clip design. (C) Wrist unit with finger sleeve. *(B, C, Courtesy of Innovo Medical, Stafford, TX, 77477.)*

Falsely normal or high readings may be present due to interference from high levels of carboxyhemoglobin that may be present with carbon monoxide (CO) poisoning, or from chronic, heavy smoking.[91–93] Glycohemoglobin A1c levels greater than 7% in patients with type 2 diabetes have been shown to result in overestimation of arterial oxygen saturation by pulse oximetry.[87] Nail polish and vital dyes such as methylene blue and indocyanine green may also result in abnormal results.[93–95]

> **Clinical Note.** Caution should be used in interpretation of results as pulse oximeters have been shown to not capture blood oxygenation readings uniformly across different skin colors.[96–98] There is an increased incidence of hidden hypoxemia (Sao_2 < 88% despite Spo_2 > 88%) in individuals with darker pigmented skin.[96–99] In a large multi-institutional study, occult hypoxemia (an Sao_2 < 88% with an Spo_2 of 92% to 96%) was found in up to 17% of Black patients.[100] This highlights the need to use additional signs and symptoms of hypoxemia when examining patients. Signs and symptoms of hypoxemia include tachypnea, dyspnea, use of accessory muscles, flaring of nostrils, ability of patient to speak in full sentences without need to catch breath, irregular or periodic breathing, anxiety, and bluish or grayish color of skin.[101]

■ RECORDING RESULTS

The nursing section of the electronic health record is an important source of vital sign data and should be checked regularly. Here, data are typically provided in numeric and/or graph form, with time represented on the horizontal axis and the measured values on the vertical axis. Many software programs automatically create graphs from numerical data entries. The visual record allows easy identification of data trends reflective of normal variations or a response to disease or therapeutic intervention. For the therapist practicing in facilities where such forms are used, familiarity with the specific recording system is important. For manual documentation, several methods are used to differentiate vital sign entry; they generally include both numeric entries and graphs using some variation of open and closed circles, connecting lines, color codes, or other symbols to discriminate among temperature, HR, RR, BP, and oximetry data.

For purposes of physical therapy documentation, vital signs data entry points are often included in documentation software. Alternatively, vital sign data may be included directly within the narrative portion of the note. An important element in recording this information is that it allows easy comparison from one entry to the next. The date, time of day, patient position, examiner's name, and equipment used should all be clearly

finger.[80] This ensures that abnormal readings are not due to equipment error. Other sources of error include motion or noise artifact, hypothermia, and hypoperfusion. Pulse oximetry readings can be falsely low owing to hemodynamic instability or poor limb perfusion.

indicated. Any deviations from standard measurement protocol should be documented.

■ RESOURCES

Multiple Internet resources are available to enhance patient understanding of the implications of altered vital sign values and the importance of maintaining values within normal ranges, in addition to presenting strategies to prevent, detect, and obtain treatment for the precipitating causes. Many organizations provide a rich source of online information and education for patients and families as well as clinical guidelines and resource materials for health professionals. Examples are provided in Appendix 2.B (online).

SUMMARY

Examination of vital signs is an important component of the review of systems. Vital sign measures provide information about the patient's physiological status, may identify potential risk factors, and can serve as a screening tool for undiagnosed problems. Establishing and maintaining a database of values for an individual patient informs clinical decisions for determining the diagnosis and prognosis, designing the POC, and monitoring response to treatment.

The procedure for measuring each vital sign has been presented. Because multiple factors influence vital signs, the most useful data are obtained when measures are taken at periodic intervals rather than as a single measure in time. Sequential measures allow changes in patient status or response to treatment (e.g., exercise prescription) to be monitored over time, as well as indicating an acute change in status at a specific point in time.

Questions for Review

1. In monitoring a patient's BP, you obtain values that are markedly higher than those documented by another therapist yesterday. How would you respond to this situation?

2. Prior to a vital signs examination, what preliminary data can be obtained by a careful, systematic observation of the patient?

3. Together with other examination data, vital sign measures assist the physical therapist in making clinical decisions about what aspects of patient care?

4. Provide examples of lifestyle patterns (modifiable) and patient characteristics (nonmodifiable) that may influence vital sign measures.

5. What are the mechanisms by which the body conserves and produces heat?

6. What methods are used to dissipate excess heat from the body? Provide a description of each.

7. What is the procedure for measuring oral temperature using a handheld battery-powered thermometer?

8. What three pulse parameters (characteristics) are considered during monitoring? Describe each.

9. What parameters (characteristics) are considered in examining respiration? Describe each.

10. What is the procedure for measuring brachial BP using a stethoscope and aneroid sphygmomanometer?

11. What medical conditions would alert the therapist to the potential need for monitoring oxygen saturation levels using pulse oximetry?

CASE STUDY

An 82-year-old woman has been admitted to the medical surgical floor following a fall in her home. Her left femur was fractured, and an open reduction external fixation was performed.

PAST MEDICAL HISTORY

The patient has a past medical history of hypertension, high cholesterol, type 2 diabetes, and osteoporosis. Her medications include metformin 1000 mg by mouth (PO) twice daily, glipizide 10 mg PO once daily, lisinopril/HCT 20/25 1 tablet PO daily, amlodipine 5 mg PO (by mouth) daily, atorvastatin 10 mg PO at bedtime, Prolia (denosumab) 60 mg subcutaneous injection every 6 months.

(Continued)

CASE STUDY—cont'd

ADMITTING DIAGNOSIS

Left femur fracture.

- **Blood Pressure:** 105/50 mm Hg
- **Pulse:** 60 bpm
- **Respiratory Rate:** 18 breaths per minute
- **Oximetry:** 92% on room air at rest
- **Temperature:** 100.8 F (38.2 C)
- **Cognition:** Able to describe fall and transfer to hospital. Unable to report time and date.
- **Deep tendon reflexes:** Intact right LE. Left LE not tested.
- **Motor function:** Good upper body strength. Unable to contract left quadriceps or actively lift left leg off of bed.
- **Cutaneous sensation:** Decreased sensation of feet bilaterally with known past medical history of neuropathy.
- **Integument:** Incision left hip. Dressing dry and intact.

PHYSICAL THERAPY

The patient is now 12 hrs postoperative and physical therapy has received referral to evaluate and treat.

GUIDING QUESTIONS

1. What potential vital sign precautions may be anticipated based on the patient's medication history?

2. How and when would you monitor vital signs to ensure the patient is sufficiently medically stable to participate in physical therapy and respond appropriately to treatment?

3. What changes in the patient's vital signs would indicate therapy should be modified or discontinued?

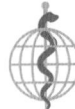

For additional resources, including answers to the questions for review, new immersive cases, case study guiding questions, references, and more, please visit **https://www.fadavis.com/product/physical -rehabilitation-fulk-8**. You may also quickly find the resources by entering this title's four-digit ISBN, 4691, in the search field at **http://fadavis.com** and logging in at the prompt.

Examination of Sensory Function

Kimberly L. Malin, PT, MS, DHSc, NCS
Heidi Cheerman, PT, MS, DPT, NCS
Kevin K. Chui, PT, DPT, PhD, GCS, OCS, CEEAA, FAAOMPT
Sheng-Che Yen, PT, PhD

Chapter 3

LEARNING OBJECTIVES

1. Understand the purpose(s) of performing a sensory examination.
2. Understand the relationship between preliminary mental status screening and tests for sensory function.
3. Describe the classification and function of the receptor mechanisms involved in the perception of sensation.
4. Identify the spinal pathways that mediate sensation.
5. Understand the guidelines for administering an examination of sensory function.
6. Describe the testing protocol for each sensory modality.
7. Apply clinical decision-making skills to application of sensory examination data using the case study example.

CHAPTER OUTLINE

SENSORY INTEGRATION *67*
SENSATION AND MOVEMENT *68*
SENSORY INTEGRITY *68*
CLINICAL INDICATIONS *69*
   Pattern (Distribution) of Sensory Impairment *70*
   Spinal Cord Tracts *72*
AGE-RELATED SENSORY CHANGES *72*
PRELIMINARY CONSIDERATIONS *73*
   Arousal, Attention, Orientation, and Cognition *75*
   Memory, Hearing, and Visual Acuity *76*
CLASSIFICATION OF THE SENSORY SYSTEM *77*
   Sensory Receptors *77*
   Spinal Pathways *78*
TYPES OF SENSORY RECEPTORS *78*
   Cutaneous Receptors *78*
   Deep Sensory Receptors *80*
   Muscle Receptors *80*
   Joint Receptors *80*
PATHWAYS FOR TRANSMISSION OF SOMATIC SENSORY SIGNALS *81*
   Anterolateral Spinothalamic Pathway *81*
   Dorsal Column–Medial Lemniscal Pathway *81*
SOMATOSENSORY CORTEX *82*
PREPARATION FOR ADMINISTERING THE SENSORY EXAMINATION *84*
   Testing Environment *84*

Equipment *84*
Patient Preparation *86*
THE SENSORY EXAMINATION *86*
   Superficial Sensations *87*
   Deep Sensations *90*
   Combined Cortical Sensations *91*
RELIABILITY *93*
QUANTITATIVE SENSORY TESTING AND SPECIALIZED TESTING INSTRUMENTS *94*
   TSA-II NeuroSensory Analyzer + VSA 3000 Vibratory Sensory Analyzer *94*
   Von Frey Aesthesiometer II *95*
   Touch Test Sensory Evaluator *95*
   Rydel-Seiffer 64/128 Hz Graduated Tuning Fork *96*
   Rolltemp II *96*
   Bio-Thesiometer *96*
   MSA (Modular Sensory Analyzer) Thermotest *96*
CRANIAL NERVE FUNCTION *97*
SENSORY INTEGRITY WITHIN THE CONTEXT OF TREATMENT *97*
EDUCATION FOR PATIENTS WITH IMPAIRED SENSORY FUNCTION *97*
GOALS AND OUTCOMES *100*
SUMMARY *100*

■ SENSORY INTEGRATION

"If all of the sensory stimuli which enter the central nervous system were allowed to bombard the higher centers of the brain, the individual would be rendered utterly ineffective. It is the brain's task to filter, organize, and integrate a mass of sensory information so that it can be used for the development and execution of the brain's functions."—A. Jean Ayers, PhD[1(p25)]

The human system is continually inundated with sensory information from a variety of environmental inputs as well as from movement, touch, awareness of the body in space, sight, sound, and smell. "In all higher order motor behaviors, the brain must correlate sensory inputs with motor outputs to accurately assess and control the body's interaction with the environment."[2(p32)]

Sensory integration is the ability of the brain to organize, interpret, and use sensory information. This integration provides an internal representation of the environment that informs and guides motor responses.[2] These sensory representations provide the foundation on which motor programs for purposeful movements are planned, coordinated, and implemented.[3] Ayers defined *sensory integration* as "the neurological process that organizes sensation from one's own body and from the environment and makes it possible to use the body effectively within the environment."[4(p11)] In an intact system, sensory integration occurs automatically without conscious effort.

Sensory integration is a theory developed by A. Jean Ayers (1920–1989), an occupational therapist whose work focused on examining the manner in which sensory integration develops, identifying patterns of dysfunction in children with learning disorders, and developing intervention strategies to improve the processing of sensory information. Mailloux and Miller-Kuhaneck summarized the evidenced-based approach that Ayers used to develop this theory for clinical application.[5] The theory purports that disordered sensory integration directly affects both motor and cognitive learning and that interventions designed to enhance sensory integration will improve learning.[1] Bundy and Murray[6] suggest the value of the theory lies in its usefulness in (1) explaining behaviors of individuals with impaired sensory integration functions, (2) establishing a plan of care (POC) to address specific impairments, and (3) predicting expected outcomes of the selected interventions. A review article by Schaaf and colleagues[7] summarized sensory integration research on children with autism spectrum disorder and to guide future research proposed a three-pillar road map consisting of practice, advocacy, and education. In 2020, Camarata et al. adapted this conceptual theory for sensory integration and processing, highlighting that sensory function is the substratum for motor and social skills impacting behaviors. Any disruption in the modulation of sensory input, sensory discrimination, or sensory integration can impact a person's ability to participate in their roles at home, school/work, and within the community.[8]

■ SENSATION AND MOVEMENT

Motor learning and motor performance are inextricably linked to sensation. As a motor task is practiced, the individual learns to anticipate and correct or modify movements based on sensory input organized and integrated by the central nervous system (CNS). The CNS uses this information to influence movement by both feedback and feedforward control. *Feedback control* uses sensory information received *during the movement* to monitor and adjust output. *Feedforward control* is a proactive strategy that uses sensory information obtained from experience. Signals are sent in *advance of movement,* allowing for anticipatory adjustments in postural control or movement.[3,9] The primary role of sensation in movement is to (1) guide selection of motor responses for effective interaction with the environment and, (2) through feedback, adapt movements and shape motor programs for corrective action. Sensation also provides the important function of protecting the organism from injury. See Chapter 5, Examination of Motor Function: Motor Control and Motor Learning, for a more detailed discussion of CNS control of motor function.

■ SENSORY INTEGRITY

The term *somatosensation* (somatosensory) refers to sensation received from the skin and musculoskeletal system, as opposed to that from specialized senses such as sight or hearing. Examination of sensory function involves testing *sensory integrity* by determining the patient's ability to interpret and discriminate among incoming sensory information. The sensory examination is based on the premise that within the intact human system, sensory information is taken in from the body and the environment; the CNS then processes and integrates the information for use in planning and organizing behavior. This premise is more aptly termed a *theoretical construct* (a concept that represents an *unobservable* event). We cannot *directly* observe CNS processing, integration of sensory information, or the motor planning process. However, our current knowledge of CNS function and motor behavior provides evidence that these unobservable events occur. We *can* observe impairments in motor behavior but can only *hypothesize* that they truly result from faulty sensory integration mechanisms.[6] By performing an accurate examination of body systems, the therapist can determine if more extensive sensory testing is warranted for proper differential diagnosis.

The *Guide to Physical Therapist Practice* defines *sensory integrity* as "the soundness of cortical sensory processing, including proprioception, vibration sense, stereognosis, and cutaneous sensation."[10] Sensory integrity is included among the list of 26 categories of tests and measures that may be used by physical therapists during a patient initial examination or during subsequent visits as part of a reexamination.

This chapter focuses primarily on examination of somatosensory integrity of the face, trunk, and extremities as well as screening for cranial nerve integrity; testing approaches for examining *cranial nerve integrity* and reflex testing are addressed in Chapter 5, Examination of Motor Function: Motor Control and Motor Learning. As the CNS analyzes and uses all sensory input to identify movement errors and initiate corrective responses, examination of sensory function typically precedes examination of motor function. This sequence assists the physical therapist in differentiating the impact of sensory impairments on motor function.

■ CLINICAL INDICATIONS

Indications for examination of sensory function are based on the history and systems review. Data from the history and systems review include family, social, medical, and surgical history; demographics; general health status; activities and participation; current condition(s); growth and development; living environment; social/health habits; medications; and status of body systems (e.g., cardiovascular, pulmonary, integumentary).[10] These data may indicate the existence of pathology or a health condition resulting in sensory function changes. Box 3.1 describes the elements of the examination of sensory function.

Sensory dysfunction may be associated with any pathology or injury affecting either the peripheral nervous system (PNS), the CNS, or both. Deficits may occur at any point within the system, including at the sensory receptors, peripheral nerves, spinal nerves, spinal cord nuclei and tracts, brain stem, thalamus, and sensory cortex.[11] Examples of conditions that generally demonstrate some level of sensory impairment include pathology, disease, or injury to the peripheral nerves, such as trauma (e.g., fracture) that can sever, crush, or damage a nerve; metabolic disturbances (e.g., diabetes, hypothyroidism, alcoholism); infections (e.g., Lyme disease, leprosy, HIV); impingement or compression (e.g., arthritis, carpal tunnel syndrome); burns; toxins (e.g., lead, mercury, chemotherapy); and nutritional deficits (e.g., vitamin B_{12}). Sensory impairments are

---

Box 3.1   Elements of the Examination of Sensory Function

Elements of the examination of sensory function include the Patient/Client History, a Systems Review, and Tests and Measures/Impairments. The physical therapist uses the results of tests and measures to determine the integrity of an individual's sensory, perceptual, and somatosensory processes. Responses monitored at rest, during activity, and after activity may indicate the presence or severity of a body function or structure impairment, activity limitation, or participation restriction.

Patient/Client History

Review for risk factors for impaired sensory integrity
- Lack of safety awareness in all environments
- Risk-prone behaviors (e.g., working without protective gloves)
- Substance abuse

Review for health, wellness, and fitness needs
- Fitness, including physical performance (e.g., inadequate balance, limited perception of arms and legs in space)
- Health and wellness (e.g., inadequate understanding of role of proprioception in balance)

Systems Review

Review history and assess for pathology or health condition
- Cardiovascular (e.g., lymphedema, peripheral vascular disease)
- Integumentary (e.g., burn, frostbite)
- Musculoskeletal (e.g., derangement of joint; disorders of bursa, synovia, and tendon)
- Neuromuscular (e.g., cerebral palsy, stroke, developmental delay, spinal cord injury, traumatic brain injury)
- Pulmonary (e.g., ventilatory pump failure)
- Multisystem (e.g., AIDS, Guillain-Barré syndrome, trauma)

Tests and Measures/Impairments

Select tests and measures that will objectively quantify impairments of body functions and structures
- Circulation (e.g., numb feet)
- Integumentary integrity (e.g., redness under orthosis)
- Muscle performance (e.g., decreased grip strength)
- Posture (e.g., asymmetrical alignment)

Objectively describe activity limitations and participation restrictions
- Self-care (e.g., inability to put on trousers while standing due to foot numbness)
- Domestic life (e.g., difficulty with sorting laundry due to hand numbness)
- Education (e.g., inability to sit for full classes due to sensory loss in trunk and lower extremities)
- Work life (e.g., inability to operate cash register due to clumsiness)
- Community, social, and civic life (e.g., inability to drive car due to loss of spatial awareness, inability to play guitar due to hyperesthesia)

Adapted from *Guide to Physical Therapist Practice*,[9] with permission of the American Physical Therapy Association.® 2014
American Physical Therapy Association. APTA is not responsible for the translation from English.

also associated with injury to nerve roots or spinal cord, cerebral vascular accident (CVA), transient ischemic attack, tumors, multiple sclerosis (MS), and brain injury or disease. These examples, which are not all-inclusive, indicate the wide spectrum of injuries, diseases, and pathologies that may present with some element of sensory deficit. Therefore, when any new-onset change in sensory integrity is noted during a physical therapy examination or treatment, it is important to refer the patient to the appropriate physician for further evaluation. A new medical diagnosis with a change in treatment plan may be necessary.

Pattern (Distribution) of Sensory Impairment

Examination of sensory function contributes critical information to establishing a physical therapy diagnosis and prognosis, identifying goals and expected outcomes, and developing a POC. A seminal feature of the examination involves determining the *pattern* (specific boundaries) of sensory involvement. Pattern identification is accomplished using knowledge of skin segment innervation by the dorsal roots and peripheral nerves (Figs. 3.1 and 3.2). The term *dermatome* (or *skin*

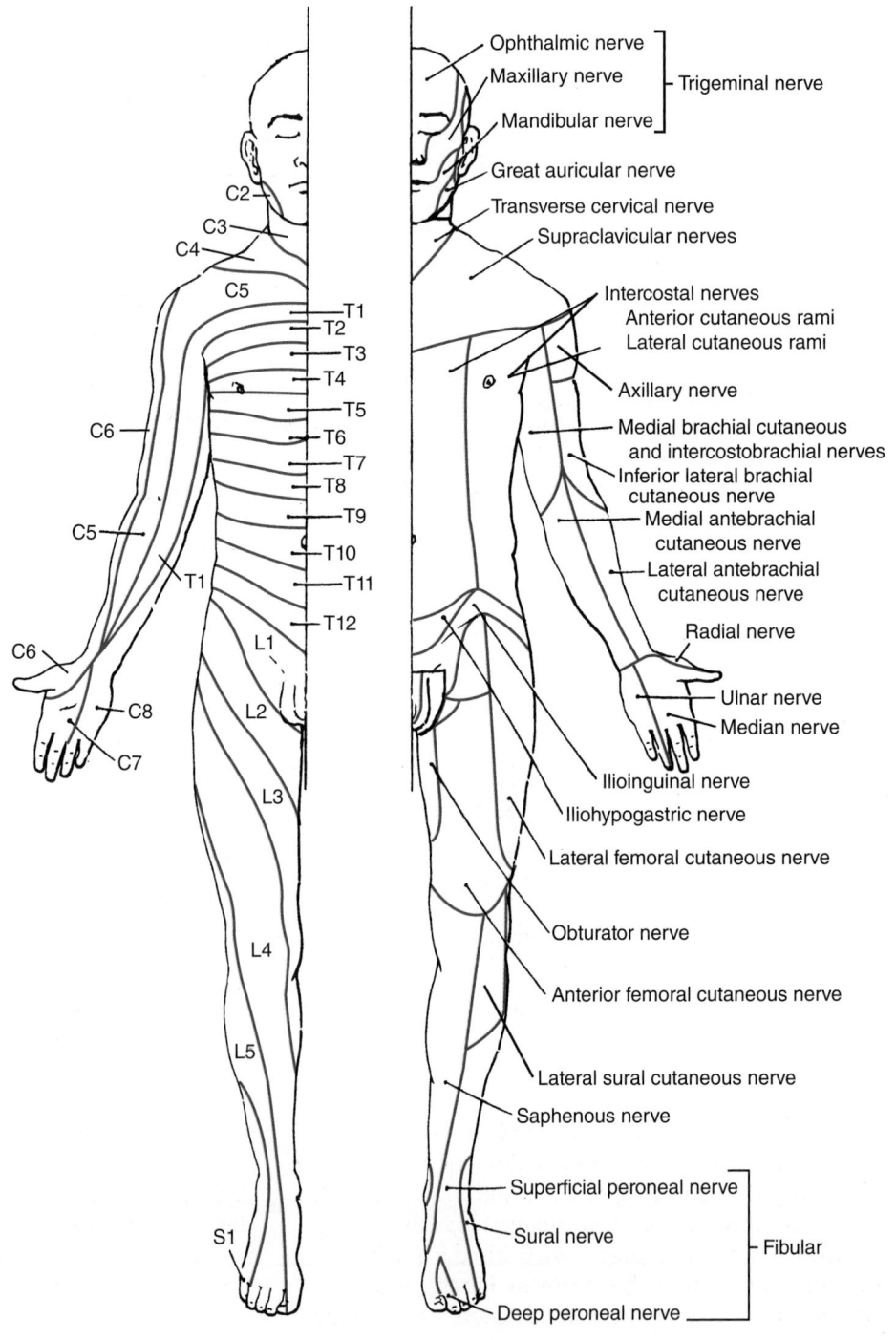

Figure 3.1 Anterior view of skin segment innervation by dorsal roots (left) and peripheral nerves (right). *(From Gilman and Newman,[11(p43)] with permission.)*

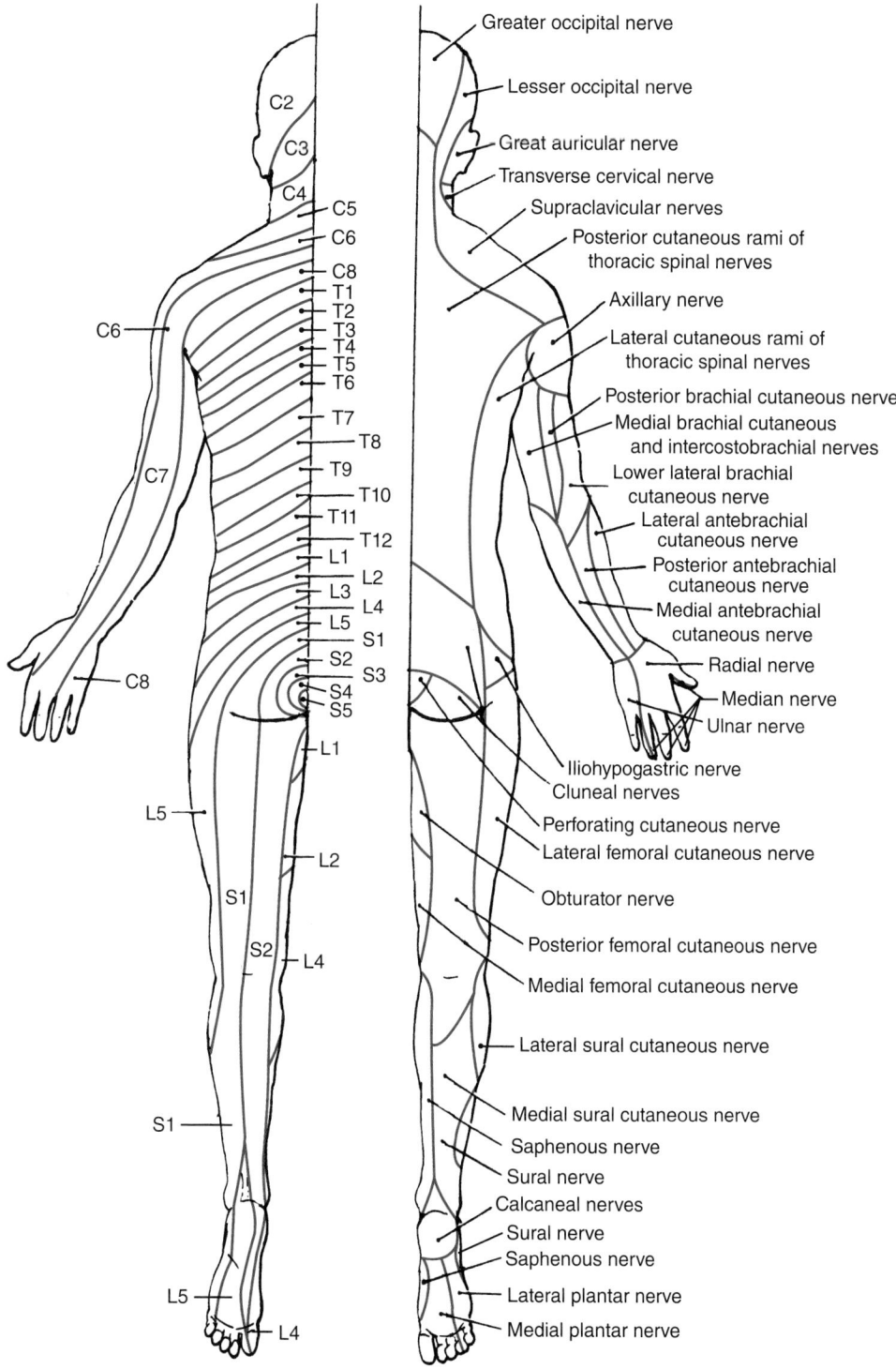

Figure 3.2 Posterior view of skin segment innervation by dorsal roots (left) and peripheral nerves (right). *(From Gilman and Newman,[11](p44) with permission.)*

segment) refers to the skin area supplied by one dorsal root.[12] The graphic illustration of skin segment innervation as presented in Figures 3.1 and 3.2 is referred to as a *dermatome map*. There are discrepancies among published dermatome maps based on the methodologies used to identify skin segment innervation. In a clinical commentary, Downs and Laporte[13] discuss the

history of dermatome mapping, including variations in methodologies employed and inconsistencies in the dermatome maps used in education and practice. In a similar review article by Apok and colleagues, inconsistencies in dermatome pattern distribution and overlap are discussed.[14] A 2014 study by Ladak and colleagues presented preliminary findings, based on a synthesis of literature, of a refined dermatome map that incorporates physical neural connections.[15] In 2020 Weber et al. published a study indicating the possibility of using functional MRI and spatial normalization to develop normative quantitative measures of sensory function that may be more clinically precise, accounting for left/right asymmetry and variability among individuals.[16] As new technology allows for more precise identification of nerve distribution, cutaneous spinal nerve distribution will likely continue to be reevaluated.

Clinical Note. Considerable variation exists in the clinical presentation of sensory impairments. This variability is typically associated with the nervous system involved (CNS vs. PNS); the type of injury, pathology, or disease; as well as the severity, extent, and duration of involvement.

During the review of systems, asking the patient to carefully describe the pattern or distribution of sensory symptoms (e.g., tingling, numbness, diminished, or absent sensation) provides the therapist with preliminary information to help guide the examination and to assist in identifying the dermatome(s) and nerve(s) involved. Peripheral nerve injuries generally present sensory impairments that parallel the distribution of the involved nerve and correspond to its pattern of innervation. For example, if a patient presents with complaints of numbness on the ulnar half of the ring finger, the little finger, and the ulnar side of the hand, the therapist would be alerted to carefully address ulnar nerve (C8 and T1) integrity during the sensory examination.[17] Complaints of sensory disturbances on the palmar surface of the thumb and the palmar and distal dorsal aspects of the index, middle, and the radial half of the ring finger would be indicative of median nerve (C6–C8 and T1) involvement.

Other patterns of sensory loss may be associated with specific pathology. For example, with peripheral neuropathy (e.g., diabetes), sensory loss is often an early symptom and presents in a *glove and stocking* distribution (referring to the typical involvement of the hands and feet that spreads proximally).[18] In contrast, MS frequently presents with an unpredictable or scattered pattern of sensory or motor involvement.[19]

Spinal cord injury (SCI) often presents with a more diffuse pattern of sensory involvement below the lesion level that is typically bilateral, although not necessarily symmetrical.[20] Examination of sensory function following SCI provides critical data that reflect the degree of neurological impairment. Together with other tests and measures, sensory data contribute to determining the relative completeness of the injury, the existence of *zones of partial preservation* (areas distal to a complete or incomplete lesion that retain partial innervation), symmetry or asymmetry of the lesion, and the presence of sacral sensation at S4-S5

below the neurological level of the lesion (a defining feature of an incomplete lesion).[21]

Spinal Cord Tracts

Examination of sensory function also provides data that reflect the integrity of the spinal cord tracts that carry somatosensory information.[20] For example, contralateral loss or impairment of pain and temperature perception is suggestive of lesions in the anterolateral tracts. Deficits in discriminative sensations such as vibration and two-point discrimination suggest lesions of the dorsal column.

Evidence of both sensory and motor loss that correlate with a specific myotome and dermatome is usually indicative of nerve root involvement (recall that the dorsal and ventral roots converge to form the spinal nerves). CNS lesions (e.g., CVA, brain injury) may produce significant sensory impairments characterized by a diffuse pattern of involvement (e.g., head, trunk, and limbs) and can result in significant motor dysfunction (sensory ataxia) and impairment of fine motor control and motor learning. Sensory ataxia is often mistaken for cerebellar ataxia, leading to a misdiagnosis impacting clinical decision-making for a patient's plan of care, prolonging functional recovery.[22] This highlights the importance of performing an accurate examination of systems for proper differential diagnosis. Sensory impairments can also present a significant threat of injury to anesthetic limbs (e.g., an inability to determine the temperature of bathwater).

■ AGE-RELATED SENSORY CHANGES

Alterations in sensory function occur with normal aging and should be clearly differentiated from those associated with specific illness, disease, or pathology. In recent years, there has been an expanding body of literature devoted to the neuroscience of aging and its impact on function and quality of life of older adults.[23–36] The topics addressed are specific age-related changes in vision, hearing, and the somatosensory system; treatment, prevalence, and risk factor information; as well as the role of public policy and public health in addressing age-related sensory loss. *Healthy People 2030*,[37] published by the U.S. Department of Health and Human Services, presents a comprehensive health and well-being agenda for the third decade of the 21st century. The overarching goals of *Healthy People 2030* are to (1) attain healthy, thriving lives and well-being free of preventable disease, disability, injury, and premature death; (2) eliminate health disparities, achieve health equity, and attain health literacy to improve the health and well-being for all; (3) create social, physical, and economic environments that promote attaining the full potential for health and well-being for all; (4) promote healthy development, healthy behaviors, and well-being across all life stages; and (5) engage leadership, key constituents, and the public across multiple sectors to take action and design policies that improve the health and well-being of all. The fourth goal draws national attention to an expanding population of older adults and the impact of age (including changes in sensation such as vision and hearing) on well-being across the life span. Decreased acuity of many sensations is considered a characteristic finding with aging.[38] The exact morphology of diminished sensation with age has not been completely established; however, several neurological changes have been identified and suggest potential explanations.

Over the life span, neurons are replaced at a declining rate, and this may account for the decline of the brain's average weight with aging. Although a feature of Alzheimer disease, normal aging does not produce a significant loss in the number of cortical neurons.[39] Other changes in the brain include degeneration of neurons with the presence of replacement gliosis, lipid accumulation in the neurons, loss of myelin, and development of neurofibrils (masses of small, tangled fibrils) and plaques on the cells.[39,40] There is also a decrease in the number of enzymes responsible for synthesis of dopamine, norepinephrine, and to a lesser degree acetylcholine, as well as depletion of the neuronal dendrites in the aging brain.[41,42]

Electrophysiological studies have identified a gradual reduction in conduction velocity of sensory nerves with advancing age, and this may reflect degenerative changes in myelin sheaths or loss or reduction in size of sensory axons.[43-46] Evoked potentials provide a quantitative measure of sensory function and have been found to decrease in amplitude with age.[47] A reduction in the number of Meissner corpuscles[48] has also been identified. These corpuscles, responsible for touch detection, are limited to hairless areas and become sparse, take on an irregular distribution, and vary in size and shape with age. Age-related changes in morphology and decreased concentrations of pacinian corpuscles, responsive to rapid tissue movement (e.g., vibration), have also been reported.[49]

Degenerative changes in myelin have been documented in both the CNS and PNS.[50] In a review of the literature on the effects of normal aging on myelin and nerve fibers, Peters[51] suggests that (1) age-associated cognitive decline is more likely due to widespread damage to myelin sheaths of cortical neuron axons than to actual loss of these neurons, and (2) the resulting changes in conduction velocity alter the normal timing of neuronal circuits. In a study published in 2020, Bouhrara et al. provide further evidence that myelin content in the human brain follows an inverted U-shaped trajectory with normal aging, suggesting that myelination continues into middle age and then declines. The investigators used an advanced magnetic resonance mapping technique in their study to build on previous studies that had used less-specific technology.[52]

In their review, Mosher and Wyss-Coray suggest that microglial aging is another area of study that may reveal causes of age-related cognitive decline and symptoms related to Alzheimer disease.[53] Microglia are considered the immune cells of the CNS. Age-related changes to microglia, including senescence, dystrophy, impaired motility and signaling, and impaired phagocytosis and proteostasis may contribute to a harmful immune-mediated response resulting in neuroinflammation and a decline in cellular function and signal transmission. In the PNS, a decrease in the distance between the nodes of Ranvier has been associated with advancing age.[54] This finding may be related to a slowing of saltatory conduction as identified by some authors.[39,43] Destruction of myelin sheaths has been linked to a reduced expression of primary myelin proteins and axonal atrophy and to a reduced expression and axonal transport of cytoskeletal proteins.[55] As compared to younger subjects, lower sensory nerve conduction velocities have been documented in older adults.[45,46]

Although not an exhaustive list, other documented, age-related sensory changes include altered postural stability and control,[56-58] diminished response to tactile stimuli,[59-60] reduced vibratory[61,62] and proprioceptive acuity,[63,64] decreased cutaneous temperature thresholds,[65-68] and diminished two-point discrimination.[69,70] These changes frequently appear in the presence of age-related visual or hearing losses that impair compensatory capabilities. In addition, some medications may further influence the distortion of sensory input. This combination of sensory impairments may result in postural instability, exaggerated body sway, balance problems, wide-based gait, diminished fine motor coordination, tendency to drop items held in the hand, and difficulty in recognizing body positions in space. Table 3.1 (Evidence Summary) provides an overview of research exploring age-related sensory changes.

Clinical Note. Activity limitations secondary to impairments associated with age-related somatosensory changes can impact a person's quality of life, limiting their ability to participate in roles outside of the home, leading to feelings of isolation and potential mental health concerns.

PRELIMINARY CONSIDERATIONS

Accuracy of data from examination of sensory function relies on the patient's ability to respond to the application of multiple somatosensory stimuli. Use of several easily administered preliminary tests will provide sufficient data to determine the patient's ability to concentrate on and respond to the battery of sensory test items. The two general categories of preliminary tests

Table 3.1	Evidence Summary: Research Exploring Age-Related Changes in Sensory Function

Senthilkumari et al. (2015)[46]

Methods	Examined age-related differences in nerve conduction velocity of the median nerve. Median motor and sensory conduction velocity was measured.
Subjects/Design	Included 103 individuals without a history of neurological illness, subdivided into three groups: group I (ages 15–30 years, $n = 40$); group II (ages 31–45 years, $n = 31$); and group III (ages 46–60 years, $n = 32$). Groups were not significantly different for gender or body mass index.
Results	Significant differences found in median motor/sensory conduction velocity between groups: group I = 59.5 ± 3.3/64.4 ± 6.8; group II = 56.7 ± 1.1/60.2 ± 5.7; group III = 52.8 ± 4.3/54.5 ± 7.5. The correlation between age and median motor (–0.41) and sensory (–0.54) was significant and negative.
Conclusions/ Comments	There was a significant decrease in median motor and sensory nerve conduction velocity with age. Furthermore, there was a significant inverse relationship between median nerve conduction velocity and age. Age can affect the conduction velocity of the median nerve. This study is limited by its cross-sectional design.

Alanazy et al. (2017)[61]

Methods	Vibration threshold was tested at the distal interphalangeal joint (index finger) and interphalangeal joint (great toe) using a conventional tuning fork (CTF) and a Rydel-Seiffer tuning fork (RSTF).
Subjects/Design	The vibration threshold of normal healthy adults ($n = 281$) was examined using a CTF and RSTF.
Results	Associations between the CTF and RSTF were moderate for finger and toe measures (Spearman correlation coefficient = 0.59 and 0.64, respectively). As a covariate, only age had a significant negative effect on vibration threshold. Reference values for vibration thresholds are also provided.
Conclusions/ Comments	The CTF and RSTF provided comparable results. Among the possible covariates, only age had an effect (negative) on vibration thresholds. Reference values stratified by age are also provided for each instrument and each body part.

Ko et al. (2015)[63]

Methods	Examined ankle proprioception in aging men and women using passive motion detection (threshold) and movement tracking.
Subjects/Design	Examined 289 aging adults (ages 51–95 years) without severe lower limb pain or limited ankle mobility (i.e., <10° of plantarflexion or dorsiflexion). Women ($n = 131$) were significantly younger, shorter, and weighed less when compared to males ($n = 158$).
Results	When adjusting for height and weight, there were several significant findings suggesting an age-associated reduction in proprioception. Age-associated differences in proprioception were also found between genders: men at slower speeds and women at faster speeds.
Conclusions/ Comments	Proprioception of men and women, as measured by threshold and tracking, decreased with increasing age. The paradigm used in this study should be replicated using a longitudinal design.

Bouhrara et al. (2020)[52]

Methods	Investigated differences in myelin water fraction (MWF) related to aging in many brain regions of healthy adults.
Subjects/Design	Used the BMC-mcDESPOT analysis to directly measure MWF in several brain areas of 106 individuals aged 22–94 years without cognitive impairment.

Table 3.1	Evidence Summary: Research Exploring Age-Related Changes in Sensory Function—cont'd

Bouhrara et al. (2020) [52]

Results	A quadratic, inverted U-shaped relationship between MWF and age across brain regions indicates that myelination in the brain continues until middle age and then decreases with further aging.
Conclusions/ Comments	The results of this study support previous, nonspecific MRI studies indicating maturation of brain myelination until middle age and a decrease in myelination with further, normal aging in the absence of disease.

Palve and Palve (2018)[48]

Methods	Investigated electrophysiological data with specific study groups divided into three categories based on age: group I (18–30 years), group II (31–45 years), and group III (46–60 years), to identify when changes in nerve conduction velocity (NCV) occurs.
Subjects/Design	The NCVs were determined for the median, common peroneal (motor and sensory components), along with late responses in the form of H-reflex and F-waves of 150 individuals, of which 93 were male and 57 were female.
Results	Individuals with older age had longer latencies, smaller amplitudes, and slower conduction velocities compared with the younger age group. Of note, the change with age was more significant in sensory nerve conduction and late responses in all the peripheral nerves.
Conclusions/ Comments	The results of this study support that aging has a definitive correlation with NCV and late responses of different peripheral nerves and should be considered in clinical practice.

include the patient's (1) arousal level, attention span, orientation, and cognition;[71] and (2) memory, hearing, and visual acuity. These preliminary tests are typically considered with sensory involvement associated with CNS lesions.

Arousal, Attention, Orientation, and Cognition

A necessary first step is to determine the patient's arousal level for participation in the test protocol. *Arousal* is the state of responsiveness of the human system to sensory stimulation. It is described by using traditionally accepted key terms and definitions to identify the patient's level of consciousness. These terms include *alert, lethargic, obtunded, stupor,* and *coma* and represent a continuum of physiological readiness for activity. They are defined as follows:[71]

- *Alert.* The patient is awake and attentive to normal levels of stimulation. Interactions with the therapist are normal and appropriate.
- *Lethargic.* The patient appears drowsy and may fall asleep if not stimulated in some way. Interactions with the therapist may get diverted. The patient may have difficulty focusing or maintaining attention on a question or task.
- *Obtunded.* The patient is difficult to arouse from a somnolent state and is frequently confused when awake. Repeated stimulation is required to maintain consciousness. Interactions with the therapist may be largely unproductive.

- *Stupor* (semicoma). The patient responds only to strong, generally noxious stimuli and returns to the unconscious state when stimulation is stopped. When aroused, the patient is unable to interact with the therapist.
- *Coma* (deep coma). The patient cannot be aroused by any type of stimulation. Reflex motor responses may or may not be seen.

Reliable information about the integrity of the somatosensory system can be obtained from patients who are alert. Reliability is proportionally reduced in patients with lethargy and nonexistent in patients who are obtunded, stuporous, or comatose.

Clinical Note. While the previous terms (alert, lethargic, obtunded, stupor, coma) are widely used in general practice, it is important to note that those who work with individuals experiencing disorders of consciousness use classifications derived from the JFK Coma Recovery Scale Revised (CRS-R): Consciousness, Minimally Conscious State (MCS), Vegetative State, Coma. The revised scale further breaks down the category of MCS to MCS–, MCS+, and Emergence from MCS (MCSe), as the scale is intended to monitor progress and obtain prognosis for emergence of full consciousness.[72–74] Refer to Chapter 19 for further details related to the use of the CRS-R in rehabilitation for those with traumatic brain injury.

Attention is selective awareness of the environment or responsiveness to a stimulus or task without being distracted by other stimuli.[8,11,75] Attention can be examined by asking the patient to repeat items on a progressively more challenging list. These repetition tasks can begin with two or three items and gradually progress to longer lists. For example, the patient might be asked to count by fives or sevens or to spell words backward.[75] Spelling words backward can be made more challenging by using progressively longer words (e.g., book, fork, telephone, automobile). Individuals with a high attention span will be able to perform the task. In contrast, attention deficits will be apparent when the order of letters is confused.

Orientation refers to the patient's awareness of time, person, and place (or space). In medical record documentation, the results of this mental status screening are often abbreviated "oriented × 3," referring to the three parameters of time, person, and place. If a patient is not fully oriented to one or more domains, the notation would read "oriented × 2 (time)" or "oriented × 1 (time, place)." With partial orientation entries, it is customary to include the *domains of disorientation* within parentheses. Box 3.2 presents sample questions for examining orientation.[11,71,75]

> ### Box 3.2 Sample Questions for Examining Orientation
>
> A series of simple questions is posed to the patient. The questions are designed to determine the patient's understanding of recognition of who the patient is; the location, including the present facility (the name of hospital or clinic); the present time; and the passage of time.
>
> #### Person
> - What is your name?
> - Do you have a middle name?
> - How old are you?
> - When were you born?
>
> #### Place
> - Do you know where you are right now?
> - What kind of a place is this?
> - Do you know what city and state we are in?
> - What city or town do you live in?
> - What is your address at home?
>
> #### Time
> - What is today's date?
> - What day of the week is it?
> - What time is it?
> - Is it morning or afternoon?
> - What season is it?
> - What year is it?
> - How long have you been here?
>
> From Nolan,[64(p26)] with permission.

Cognition is defined as the process of knowing and includes both awareness and judgment.[8] Nolan[71] suggests three areas for testing cognition-dependent functions: (1) fund of knowledge, (2) calculation ability, and (3) proverb interpretation. *Fund of knowledge* is defined as the sum of an individual's learning and experience in life, which will be highly variable and different for each patient. Detailed information about premorbid knowledge base is often not available. However, a number of general categories of information can be used to test this cognitive function. Sample questions might include the following:[71]

- Who was the next Democratic candidate for president after Barack Obama?
- Who is the current vice president of the United States?
- Which is more—a gallon or a liter?
- In what country is the Great Pyramid?
- What would you add to your food to make it sweeter?
- In what state would you find the city of Boston?
- What are the elements that make up water and salt?
- Can you name a car made by General Motors?
- Who is Charles Dickens?

Calculation ability examines foundational mathematical abilities.[71,75] Two associated terms are *acalculia* (inability to calculate) and *dyscalculia* (difficulty in accomplishing calculations).[71] This cognitive screening can be administered either verbally or in written format. The patient is asked to mentally perform a series of calculations when provided with mathematical problems. The test should be initiated with simple problems and progress to the more difficult. Adding and subtracting are generally easier than multiplication and division. An alternative approach is to provide written mathematical problems and ask the patient to fill in the answer: $4 + 4 =$ ____; $10 + 22 =$ ____; $46 \times 8 =$ ____; $13 \times 7 =$ ____; $4 \times 3 =$ ____; $6 \times 6 =$ ____; and so forth.

Proverb interpretation examines the patient's ability to interpret use of words outside of their usual context or meaning. This is a sophisticated cognitive function. During the screening, the patient should be asked to describe the meaning of the proverb. Sample proverbs include the following:[71,75]

- People who live in glass houses should not throw stones.
- A rolling stone gathers no moss.
- A stitch in time saves nine.
- The early bird catches the worm.
- The dog that trots about finds the bone.
- The empty wagon makes the most noise.
- Every cloud has a silver lining.

Memory, Hearing, and Visual Acuity

Also related to the ability to respond during sensory testing is the status of the patient's memory and hearing function as well as visual acuity.

Memory

Both long- and short-term memory should be examined. Impairments of short-term memory will be the most disruptive to collecting sensory information owing to patient difficulties in remembering and following directions. *Long-term (remote) memory* can be examined by requesting information on date and place of birth, parents' names, number of siblings, date of marriage, schools attended, or other historical facts, such as "Where were you on September 11, 2001?"[76] *Short-term memory* can be addressed by verbally providing the patient with a series of words or numbers. For example, ask the patient to repeat a series of three words (e.g., car, book, cup) immediately and again in 5 minutes. Individuals with normal memory function should be able to recall the list 5 minutes later and at least two of the items from the list after 30 minutes.[71] Use of numbers could include a seven-digit list; a short sentence could also be used to test short-term memory. To ensure understanding of the task, the patient should repeat the sequence immediately.

Hearing

Observing the patient's response to conversation can provide a gross assessment of hearing. If a patient at baseline utilizes auditory assistive devices (i.e., amplifier, hearing aids), be sure that these are in place and working properly during observation and testing. Note should be made of how alterations in voice volume and tone influence patient response. Whispering 40 in. (1 meter) from each ear can be used to compare hearing on both sides.

A vibratory tuning fork can be used to examine and compare air conduction hearing with bone conduction hearing. *Air conduction hearing* involves signals transmitted through air to the inner ear and is examined by placing a vibrating tuning fork near the pinna. *Bone conduction hearing* refers to sounds transmitted through bone and is tested by placing a vibrating tuning fork on the mastoid process.[77,78]

Clinical Note. If a patient's hearing is impaired and they are unable to respond to testing with verbal directions, assess their ability to respond with visual directions (i.e., writing down on paper/whiteboard, typing on an electronic device) for accuracy of data.

Visual Acuity

A basic visual examination[78] can be made using a standard Snellen chart mounted on the wall or visual acuity cards for use at bedside. A Snellen chart (standard eye chart) includes a series of uppercase letters that gradually decrease in size as the viewer moves down the chart. If the patient uses corrective lenses, they should be worn during testing and should be clean. Visual acuity is typically recorded at 20 feet (6 m) from the Snellen chart. This distance is then placed over the size of the printed letter the individual is able to read comfortably. For example, on a continuum of visual acuity, 20/20 is considered excellent, and 20/200 is considered poor acuity.[11]

Clinical Note. Some diagnoses or comorbidities directly affect vision such as MS, hypertension, and diabetes. Examining the cranial nerves (CNs) will provide additional information about vision. For example, the oculomotor nerve (CN III) is often affected by diabetes (oculomotor nerve palsy).

Peripheral field vision can be examined by sitting directly in front of the patient with outstretched arms. The index fingers should be extended and gradually brought toward the midline of the patient's face. The patient is asked to identify when the therapist's approaching finger is first seen. Differences between right and left visual field should be noted carefully. Depth perception may be grossly checked by holding two pencils or fingers (one behind the other) directly in front of the patient. The patient is asked to touch or grasp the foreground object.

Because tests of sensory integrity require a verbal response to the stimulus, patients with arousal, attention, orientation, cognitive, or short-term memory impairments generally cannot be accurately tested. However, impairments in vision, hearing, or speech will not adversely affect test results if appropriate adaptations are made in providing instructions and indicating responses (e.g., signaling with either one or two fingers during tests for two-point discrimination, pointing to an area of stimulus contact, mimicking joint position sense or awareness of movement with the contralateral extremity, or identifying an object by selecting from a group of items during tests for stereognosis).

■ CLASSIFICATION OF THE SENSORY SYSTEM

Several different schemes have been proposed for categorizing the sensory system. Among the more common is classification by the type (or location) of *receptors* and the *spinal pathway* mediating information to higher centers.

Sensory Receptors

Sensory receptors (sensory nerve endings) are located at the distal end of an afferent nerve fiber. Once stimulated, they give rise to perception of a specific sensation. Sensory receptors are highly sensitive to the type of stimulus for which they were designed (termed *receptor specificity*). This specificity of nerve fiber sensitivity to a single modality of sensation is called the *labeled line principle*.[79] This means that individual tactile sensations are perceived when specific types of receptors are stimulated. For example, in response to touch, selective activation of Merkel disks and Ruffini endings generates the sensation of steady pressure in the cutaneous area above the active receptors.[80]

It should be noted that the term *modality* has a specific meaning within the context of sensation. Modality "defines a general class of stimulus, determined by the type of energy transmitted by the stimulus and the receptors specialized to sense that energy."[80(p413)] Each type of sensation perceived (e.g., vision, hearing, taste, touch, smell, pain, temperature, proprioception) is referred to as a *modality of sensation.*

The three divisions of sensory receptors include those that mediate the (1) superficial, (2) deep, and (3) combined (cortical) sensations.[11]

Superficial Sensation

Exteroceptors are responsible for the superficial sensations.[81] They receive stimuli from the external environment via the skin and subcutaneous tissue. Exteroceptors are responsible for the perception of pain, temperature, light touch, and pressure.[11,81]

Deep Sensation

Proprioceptors are responsible for the deep sensations. These receptors receive stimuli from muscles, tendons, ligaments, joints, and fascia[75] and are responsible for position sense[82] and awareness of joints at rest, movement awareness (kinesthesia), and vibration.

Combined Cortical Sensations

The combination of both the superficial and deep sensory mechanisms makes up the third category of combined sensations. These sensations require information from both exteroceptive and proprioceptive receptors, as well as intact function of cortical sensory association areas. The combined cortical sensations include stereognosis, two-point discrimination, barognosis, graphesthesia, tactile localization, recognition of texture, and double simultaneous stimulation.

Spinal Pathways

Sensations also have been classified according to the system by which they are mediated to higher centers. Sensations are mediated by either the *anterolateral spinothalamic system* or the *dorsal column–medial lemniscal system*.[39,81,83]

Anterolateral Spinothalamic System

This system initiates self-protective reactions and responds to stimuli that are potentially harmful in nature. It contains slow-conducting fibers of small diameter, some of which are unmyelinated. The system is concerned with transmission of thermal and nociceptive information and mediates pain, temperature, crudely localized touch, tickle, itch, and sexual sensations.

Dorsal Column–Medial Lemniscal System

The dorsal column is the system involved with responses to more discriminative sensations. It contains fast-conducting fibers of large diameter with greater myelination. This system mediates the sensations of discriminative touch and pressure sensations, vibration, movement, position sense, and awareness of joints at rest. The two systems are interdependent and integrated so as to function together.

■ TYPES OF SENSORY RECEPTORS

The sensory receptors frequently are divided according to their structural design and the type of stimulus to which they preferentially respond. These divisions include (1) *mechanoreceptors,* which respond to mechanical deformation of the receptor or surrounding area; (2) deep sensory receptors, which respond to changes and stimuli within muscle, tendon, fascia, ligaments, and joint capsules; (3) *thermoreceptors,* which respond to changes in temperature; (4) *nociceptors,* which respond to noxious stimuli and result in the perception of pain; (5) photic (electromagnetic) receptors, which respond to light within the visible spectrum; and (6) *chemoreceptors,* which respond to chemical substances and are responsible for taste, smell, oxygen levels in arterial blood, carbon dioxide concentration, and osmolality (concentration gradient) of body fluids.[10,11,81,84]

The perception of pain is not limited to stimuli received from nociceptors, because other types of receptors and nerve fibers contribute to this sensation. High intensities of stimuli to any type of receptor may be perceived as pain (e.g., extreme heat or cold and high-intensity mechanical deformation). Refer to Chapter 25 (Table 25.1) for subjective and objective characteristics associated with different types of pain. The management of chronic pain and a description of psychosocial factors contributing to the pain experience are detailed in Chapter 25.

The general classification of sensory receptors is presented in Box 3.3.[65,69,85] Following is a more in-depth description of mechanoreceptors (cutaneous sensory receptors) and deep sensory receptors (muscle and joints receptors). Refer to these receptors for anatomical-clinical correlates to the battery of sensory test items described in this chapter.

Cutaneous Receptors

Cutaneous sensory receptors are located at the terminal portion of the afferent fiber. These include free nerve endings, hair follicle endings, Merkel disks, Ruffini

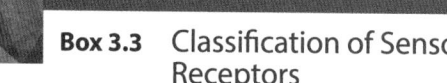

Box 3.3   Classification of Sensory Receptors

I. Mechanoreceptors
   A. Cutaneous sensory receptors
      1. Free nerve endings
      2. Hair follicle endings
      3. Merkel disks
      4. Ruffini endings
      5. Krause end bulbs
      6. Meissner corpuscles
      7. Pacinian corpuscles
II. Deep Sensory Receptors
   A. Muscle receptors
      1. Muscle spindles
      2. Golgi tendon organs
      3. Free nerve endings
      4. Pacinian corpuscles
   B. Joint receptors
      1. Golgi-type endings
      2. Free nerve endings
      3. Ruffini endings
      4. Paciniform endings
III. Thermoreceptors
   A. Cold
      1. Cold receptors
   B. Warmth
      1. Warmth receptors
IV. Nociceptors
   A. Pain
      1. Free nerve endings
      2. Extremes of stimuli*
V. Electromagnetic Receptors
   A. Vision
      1. Rods
      2. Cones
VI. Chemoreceptors
   A. Taste
      1. Receptors of taste buds
   B. Smell
      1. Receptors of olfactory nerves in olfactory epithelium
   C. Arterial oxygen
      1. Receptors of aortic and carotid bodies
   D. Osmolality
      1. Probably neurons of supraoptic nuclei
   E. Blood CO_2
      1. Receptors in or on surface of medulla and in aortic and carotid bodies
   F. Blood glucose, amino acids, fatty acids
      1. Receptors in hypothalamus

*Extremes of stimuli to other sensory receptors will be perceived as pain.
Adapted from Waxman,[65] Hall,[69] and Mtui et al.[75]

endings, Krause end bulbs, Meissner corpuscles, and pacinian corpuscles. The density of these sensory receptors varies for different areas of the body. For example, there are many more tactile receptors in the fingertips than in the back. These areas of higher receptor density correspondingly display a higher cortical representation in somatic sensory area I. Receptor density is a particularly important consideration in interpreting the results of a sensory examination for a given body surface. Figure 3.3 illustrates the cutaneous sensory receptors and their respective locations within the various layers of skin.

Free Nerve Endings

These receptors are found throughout the body. Stimulation of free nerve endings results in the perception of pain, temperature, touch, pressure, tickle, and itch sensations.[10,75]

Hair Follicle Endings (Hair End Organs)

At the base of each hair follicle, a free nerve ending is entwined. The combination of the hair follicle and its nerve provides a sensitive receptor. These receptors are sensitive to mechanical movement and touch.[86,87]

Merkel Disks

These touch receptors are located below the epidermis in hairless, smooth (glabrous) skin with a high density in the fingertips. They are sensitive to low-intensity touch, as well as to the velocity of touch, and respond to constant indentation of the skin (pressure). They provide for the ability to perceive continuous contact of objects against the skin and are believed to play an important role in both two-point discrimination and localization of touch.[81,87] Merkel disks are also believed to contribute to the recognition of texture.

Ruffini Endings

Located in the deeper layers of the dermis, these encapsulated endings are involved with the perception of touch and pressure. They are slowly adapting and particularly important in signaling continuous skin deformation such as tension or stretch; they are also found in joint capsules and assist with joint position sense.[79,87]

Krause End Bulb

The function of these bulbous encapsulated nerve endings is not clearly understood. They are located in the dermis and conjunctiva of the eye. They are believed to be low-threshold mechanical receptors that may play a contributing role in the perception of touch and pressure.

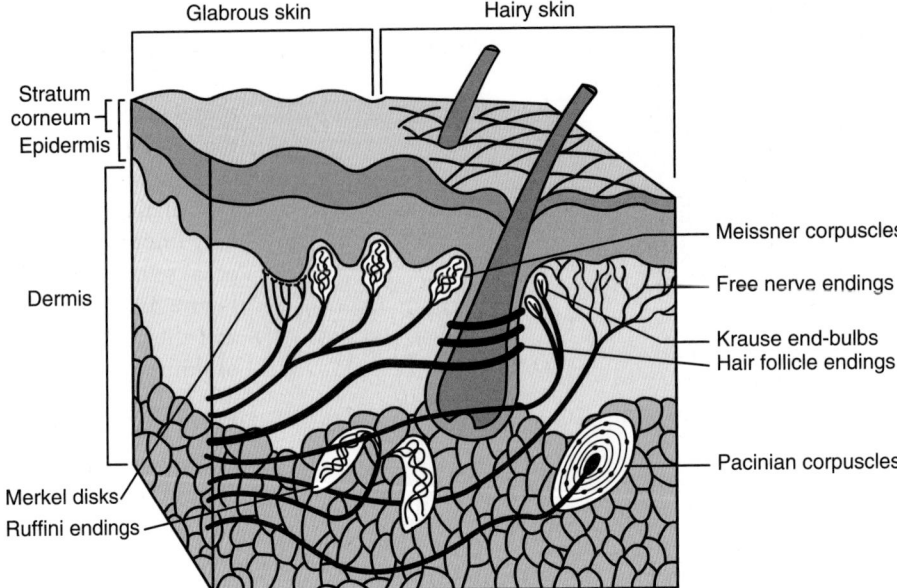

Figure 3.3 The cutaneous sensory receptors and their respective locations within the various layers of skin (epidermis, dermis, and the subcutaneous layer).

Meissner Corpuscles

Located in the dermis, these encapsulated nerve endings contain many branching nerve filaments within the capsule. They are low threshold, rapidly adapting, and in high concentration in the fingertips, lips, and toes, areas that require high levels of discrimination. These receptors play an important role in discriminative touch (e.g., recognition of texture) and movement of objects over skin.[39,79,87]

Pacinian Corpuscles

These receptors are located in the subcutaneous tissue layer of the skin and in deep tissues of the body (including tendons and soft tissues around joints). They are stimulated by rapid movement of tissue and are quickly adapting. They play a significant role in the perception of deep touch and vibration.[87,88]

Deep Sensory Receptors

The deep sensory receptors are located in muscles, tendons, and joints[75,79,83] and include both muscle and joint receptors. They are concerned primarily with posture, position sense, proprioception, muscle tone, and speed and direction of movement. The deep sensory receptors include the muscle spindle, Golgi tendon organs, free nerve endings, pacinian corpuscles, and joint receptors.

Muscle Receptors
Muscle Spindles

The muscle spindle fibers (intrafusal fibers) lie in a parallel arrangement to the muscle fibers (extrafusal fibers). They monitor changes in muscle length (Ia and II spindle afferent endings) as well as velocity (Ia ending) of these changes. The muscle spindle plays a vital role in position and movement sense and in motor learning.

Golgi Tendon Organs

These receptors are located in a series at both the proximal and distal tendinous insertions of the muscle. The Golgi tendon organs function to monitor tension within the muscle (Figure 3.4). They also provide a protective mechanism by preventing structural damage to the muscle in situations of extreme tension. This is accomplished by inhibition of the contracting muscle and facilitation of the antagonist.

Free Nerve Endings

These receptors are within the fascia of the muscle. They are believed to respond to pain and pressure.

Pacinian Corpuscles

Located within the fascia of the muscle, these receptors respond to vibratory stimuli and deep pressure.

Joint Receptors
Golgi-Type Endings

These receptors are located in the ligaments and function to detect the rate of joint movement.

Free Nerve Endings

Found in the joint capsule and ligaments, these receptors are believed to respond to pain and crude awareness of joint motion.

Ruffini Endings

Located in the joint capsule and ligaments, Ruffini endings are responsible for the direction and velocity of joint movement.

Paciniform Endings

These receptors are found in the joint capsule and primarily monitor rapid joint movements.

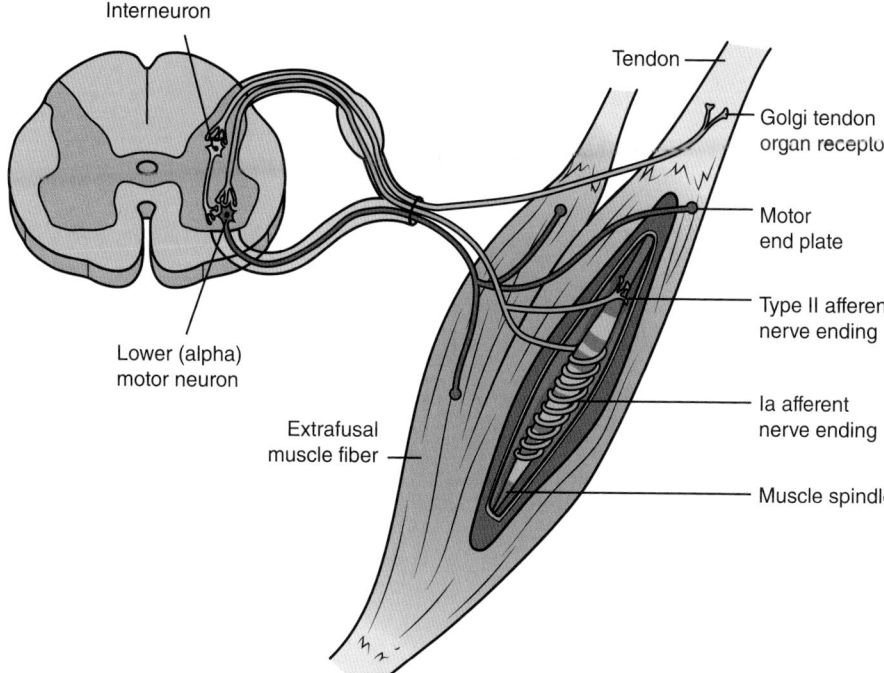

Figure 3.4 Golgi tendon organ monitors tension within the muscle. Type Ia and type II afferent nerve endings within the muscle spindle monitor changes in muscle length (Ia and II) and velocity of change (Ia).

■ PATHWAYS FOR TRANSMISSION OF SOMATIC SENSORY SIGNALS

Somatic sensory information enters the spinal cord through the dorsal roots. Sensory signals are then carried to higher centers via ascending pathways from one of two systems: the *anterolateral spinothalamic system* or the *dorsal column–medial lemniscal system.*[89,90]

Anterolateral Spinothalamic Pathway

The spinothalamic tracts are diffuse pathways concerned with nondiscriminative sensations such as pain, temperature, tickle, itch, and sexual sensations.[75,89,90] This system is activated primarily by mechanoreceptors, thermoreceptors, and nociceptors and is composed of afferent fibers that are small diameter and slowly conducting. Sensory signals transmitted by this system do not require discrete localization of signal source or precise gradations in intensity.

After originating in the dorsal roots, the fibers of the spinothalamic pathway immediately cross and ascend the spinal cord through the medulla, pons, and midbrain to the ventroposterolateral (VPL) nucleus of the thalamus (Fig. 3.5). Axons of the VPL neurons project to the somatosensory cortex via the internal capsule.[39,88]

Compared with the dorsal column–medial lemniscal system, the anterolateral spinothalamic pathways make up a cruder, more primitive system. The spinothalamic tracts are capable of transmitting a wide variety of sensory modalities. However, their diffuse pattern of termination results in only crude abilities to localize the source of a stimulus on the body surface and in poor intensity discrimination.[75] The three major tracts of the spinothalamic system are the (1) *anterior (ventral) spinothalamic tract,* which carries the sensations of crudely localized, light touch and pressure; (2) the *lateral spinothalamic tract,* which carries pain and temperature; and (3) the *spinoreticular tract,* which is involved with pain sensations, especially diffuse, deep, and chronic pain.[75,89,90]

Dorsal Column–Medial Lemniscal Pathway

This system is responsible for the transmission of discriminative sensations received from specialized mechanoreceptors.[75,89,90] Sensory modalities that require fine gradations of intensity and precise localization on the body surface are mediated by this system. Sensations transmitted by the dorsal column–medial lemniscal pathway include discriminative touch, stereognosis, tactile pressure, barognosis, graphesthesia, recognition of texture, kinesthesia, two-point discrimination, proprioception, and vibration.

This system is composed of large, myelinated, rapidly conducting fibers. After entering the dorsal column, the fibers ascend to the medulla and synapse with the dorsal column nuclei (nuclei gracilis and cuneatus). From here they cross to the opposite side and pass up to the thalamus through bilateral pathways called the *medial lemnisci.* Each medial lemniscus terminates in the ventral posterolateral thalamus. From the thalamus, third-order neurons project to the somatosensory cortex. Projection to sensory association areas in the cortex allows for the perception and interpretation of the combined cortical sensations (Fig. 3.6).[75,79,81,88] Table 3.2 presents a comparison of the most salient features of each ascending pathway.

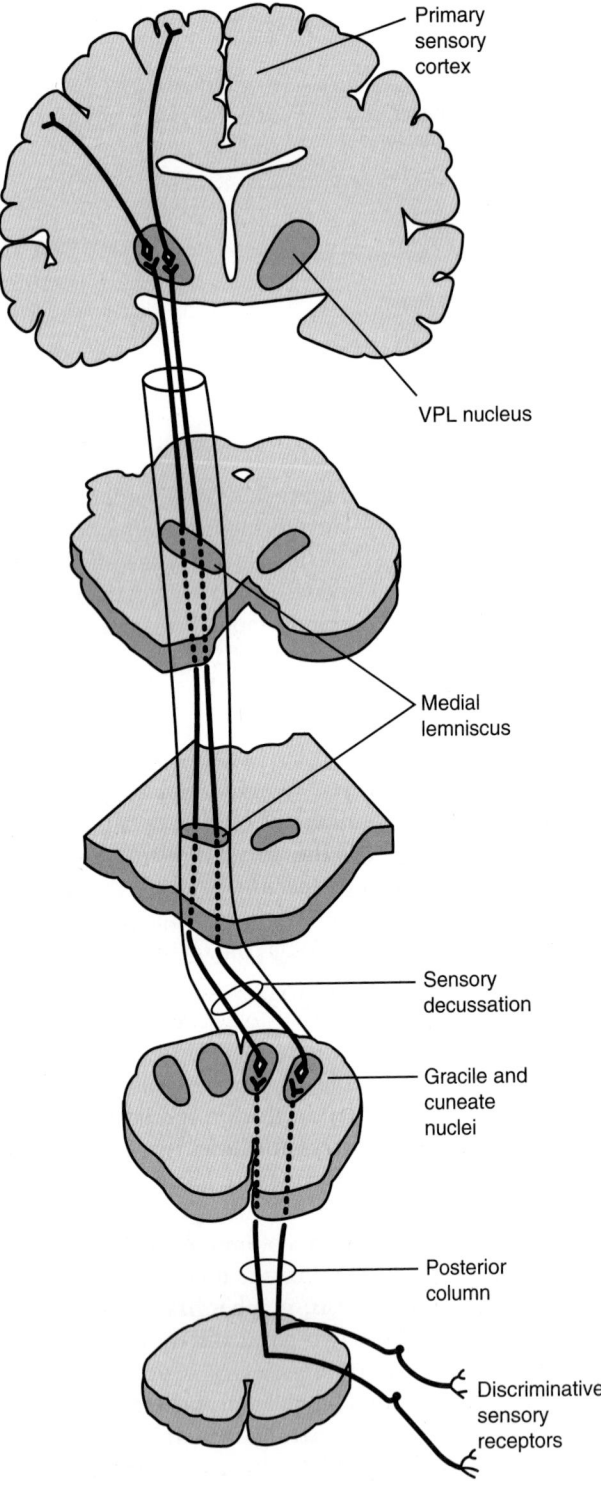

Figure 3.5 Anterolateral spinothalamic tract carrying pain and temperature.

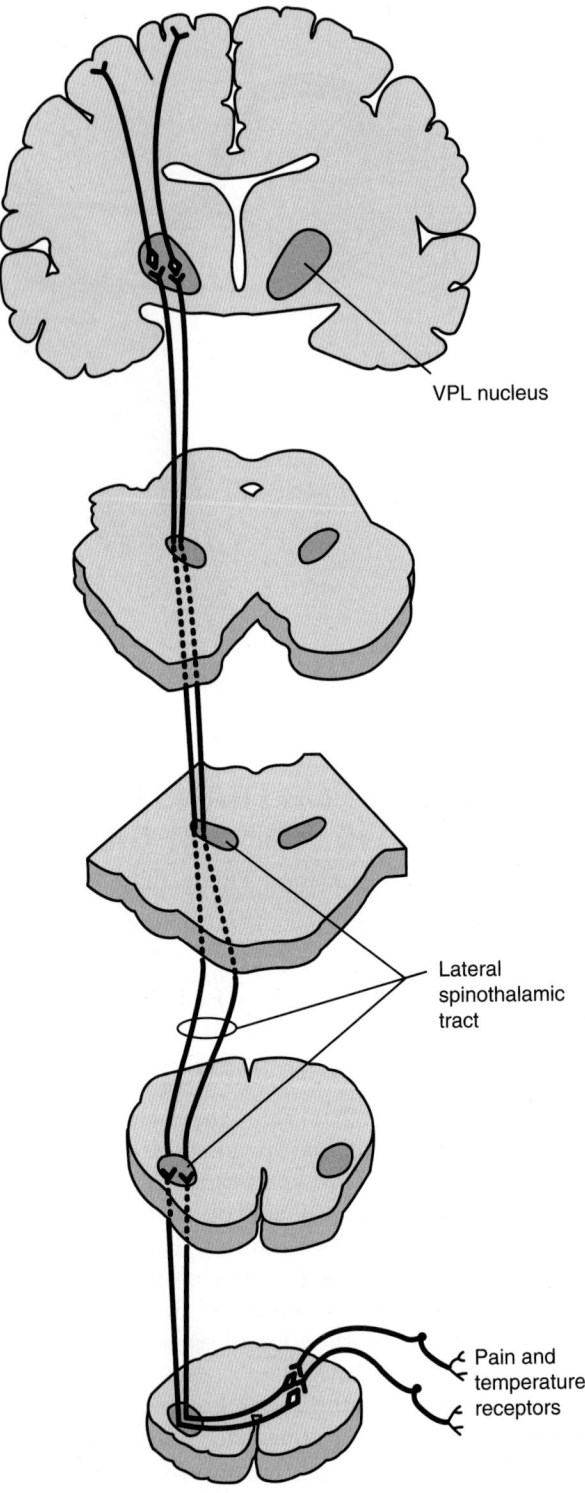

Figure 3.6 Dorsal column–medial lemniscal tract carrying discriminative sensations such as kinesthesia and touch.

■ SOMATOSENSORY CORTEX

The most complex processing of sensory information occurs in the somatosensory cortex, which is divided into three main divisions: primary somatosensory cortex (S-I), secondary somatosensory cortex (S-II), and posterior parietal cortex (Fig. 3.7A). The primary

somatosensory (S-I) area occupies a lateral strip called the *postcentral gyrus* (posterior to the central sulcus) and includes four distinct areas: Brodmann areas 3a, 3b, 1, and 2. S-I neurons identify the location of stimuli as well as discern the size, shape, and texture of objects. At the superior aspect of the lateral sulcus is the secondary somatosensory cortex (S-II), which is innervated by

Table 3.2	Features of Pathways for Transmission of Somatic Sensory Signals			
Pathway	Type of Sensation	Afferent Fibers	Origin	Projection
Anterolateral spinothalamic	Nondiscriminative (e.g., pain, temperature); broad spectrum of sensory modalities; crude localization; poor intensity discrimination; poor spatial orientation relative to origin of stimulus	Small diameter, slowly conducting	Skin: mechanoreceptors, thermoreceptors, nociceptors	From dorsal roots of spinal nerves, synapse at dorsal horns; fibers cross and move up spinal cord, through medulla, pons, and midbrain to the ventroposterolateral nucleus of thalamus
Dorsal column–medial lemniscal	Discriminative (e.g., stereognosis, two-point discrimination); precise localization; fine intensity gradations; high degree of spatial orientation relative to origin of stimulus	Large, rapidly conducting	Skin, joints, tendons: specialized mechanoreceptors	From dorsal roots of spinal nerves, ascend to medulla, synapse with dorsal column nuclei, cross to contralateral side and ascend to thalamus; then project to sensory cortex

neurons from S-I. S-II projects to the insular cortex, which innervates the temporal lobe, believed important in tactile memory. The posterior parietal lobe is behind S-I and consists of areas 5 and 7. Area 5 integrates tactile input from mechanoreceptors of the skin with proprioceptive input from muscles and joints. Area 7 integrates stereognostic and visual information from visual, tactile, and proprioceptive input.[83,88,91,92] These processing areas analyze and integrate somatosensory information and contribute to motor performance by (1) determining the initial position required before a movement occurs, (2) detecting error as movement occurs, and (3) identifying movement outcomes, which helps to shape learning.

Animal models have provided considerable insight into the function of the cortical association areas. Complete removal of area S-I of the somatosensory system produces deficits in position sense and the ability to determine the size, texture, and shape of objects. Temperature and pain perception are diminished but not abolished. Owing to reliance on input from S-I, removal of S-II results in severe impairment of the perception of both shape and texture of objects. Animal models have also shown reduced ability to learn new discriminative tasks, which are based on the shape of an object. Insult to the posterior parietal cortex presents profound impairments in attending to sensory input from the contralateral side of the body.[91]

The sensory homunculus (somatotopic map) represents a cross-sectional view through the postcentral gyrus and identifies the relative size of the cortex devoted to specific body parts (Fig. 3.7B). Note that certain areas of the body are exaggerated, such as the hand, face, and mouth, owing to greater innervation density of the skin. The relative size of body parts represents both the *density* of sensory input from the body region as well as the *importance* of sensory information from the area as it relates to function.[88,91] For example, the relative size of the foot is reflective of its importance in locomotion; the relative size of the index finger reflects its role in fine motor skills. In contrast, cortical areas for the trunk and back are small, implying a lower receptor density and reduced role in sensory perception related to function.

Using two-point discrimination as an example, Bear et al.[93] provide an extraordinary illustration of how our ability to perceive a stimulus varies remarkably across the body:

Two-point discrimination varies at least twentyfold across the body. Fingertips have the highest resolution. The dots of Braille are 1 mm high and 2.5 mm apart; up to six dots make a letter. An experienced Braille reader can scan an index finger across a page of raised dots and read about 600 letters per minute, which is roughly as fast as someone reading aloud. Several reasons explain why the fingertip is so much better than, say, the elbow for Braille reading: (1) There is a much higher density of mechanoreceptors in the skin of the fingertip than on other parts of the body; (2) the fingertips are enriched in receptor types that have small receptive fields; (3) there is more brain tissue (and thus more raw computing power) devoted to the sensory information of each square millimeter of fingertip than elsewhere; and (4) there may be special neural mechanisms devoted to high-resolution discriminations.[93(p392)]

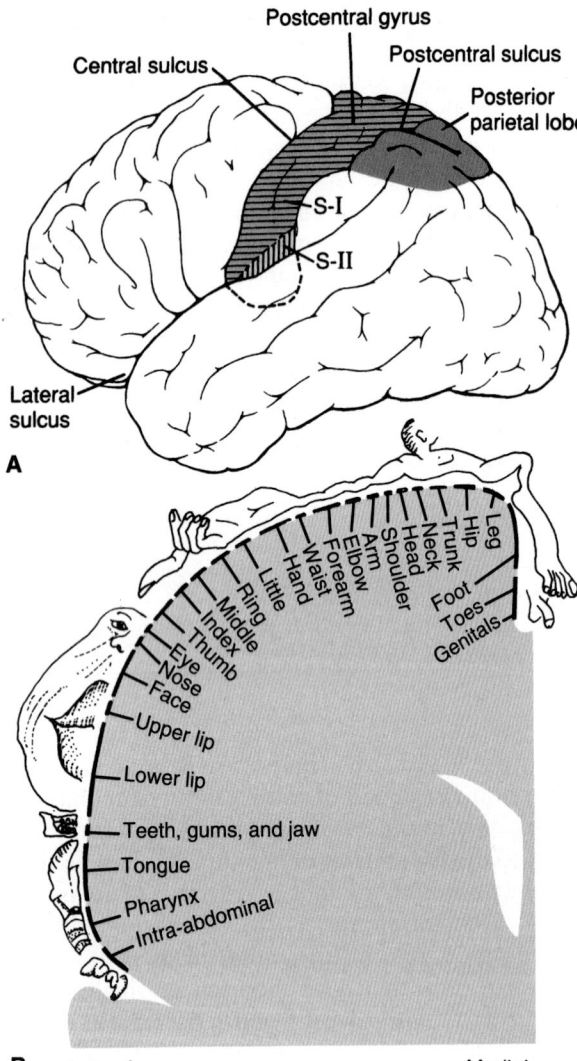

Figure 3.7 (A) The somatosensory cortex has three main divisions: the primary (S-I) and secondary (S-II) areas and the posterior parietal lobe. (B) The sensory homunculus. Areas of the body used for tactile discrimination (e.g., lips, tongue, and fingers) are represented by large areas of cortical tissue. Areas with reduced cortical representation, such as the trunk, are reflective of body parts with lesser roles in sensory perception. *(From Kandel ER, Jessell TM. Touch. In: Kandel ER, Schwartz JH, Jessel TM, eds.* Principles of Neural Science. *3rd ed. Appleton and Lange; 1991:368 [A], 372[B], with permission.)*

■ PREPARATION FOR ADMINISTERING THE SENSORY EXAMINATION

Before initiating the examination of sensory function, the testing environment should be identified and prepared, needed equipment gathered, and consideration given to patient preparation (i.e., what information and instruction will be provided).[77,78,94,95]

Testing Environment

The sensory examination should be administered in a quiet, well-lit area. Depending on the number of body areas to be tested, either a sitting or recumbent position may be used. If full-body testing is indicated, both prone and supine positions will be required, and use of a treatment table is recommended to allow examination of each side of the body.

Equipment

To perform a sensory examination, the following equipment and materials are used:

1. *Pain.* A large-headed safety pin or a large paper clip that has one segment bent open (providing one *sharp* and one *dull* end). The sharp end of the instrument should not be sharp enough to risk puncturing the skin. If a large-headed safety pin is used, the sharp end may be further blunted by light sanding. Commercially available, single-use, protected neurological pins are recommended (Fig. 3.8).

> **Clinical Note.** The Tip-therm is an early detection tool for identification of changes in thermal perception designed for monitoring polyneuropathy associated with diabetes (Fig. 3.9).[96] It provides a method for patients to test temperature sensitivity of their feet independently. It provides only a gross estimate of temperature perception; however, its convenience, low cost, and patients' ability to use it are important characteristics. The tool can be used many times, requires no energy, and uses the special characteristics of synthetic material and metal. One end is metal, and the opposite side is synthetic material. Both materials are essentially at room temperature; however, the metal end takes more heat from the body (metal has a higher conductivity than the synthetic end). As a result, the metal end is perceived as warmer and the synthetic end as cooler.

2. *Temperature.* Two standard laboratory test tubes with stoppers.
3. *Light touch.* A camel-hair brush, a piece of cotton, or a tissue.
4. *Vibration.* Tuning fork and earphones (if available, to reduce auditory clues). Tuning forks are made of steel or magnesium alloy and grossly resemble a two-pronged fork. When the tines are stuck against a surface (usually the palm of the examiner's hand), the fork resonates at a specific pitch (e.g., 128, 256, or 512 Hz), determined by the length of the two U-shaped prongs (tines).
5. *Stereognosis (object recognition).* A variety of small, commonly used articles such as a comb, fork, paper clip, key, marble, coin, pencil, and so forth.

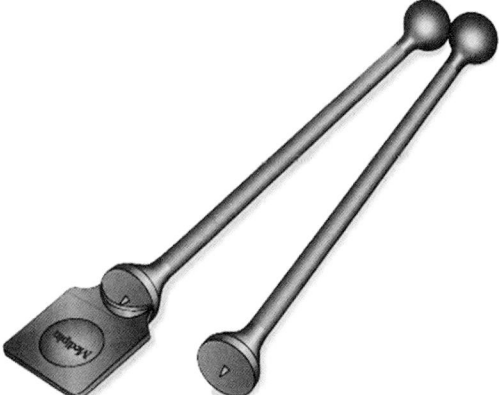

Figure 3.8 Single-use, protected neurological pin. The image on the left shows the pin prior to use with the protective cap intact (although schematically presented to allow visualization of pin location). On the right, the protective cap is removed and the pin exposed. On the opposite end of the pin is a smooth, rounded surface used to randomly intersperse application of a dull stimulus. After use, the point is destroyed by compressing it against a hard surface and disposing in a biohazard receptacle. *(Courtesy of US Neurologicals, Kirkland, WA 98033.)*

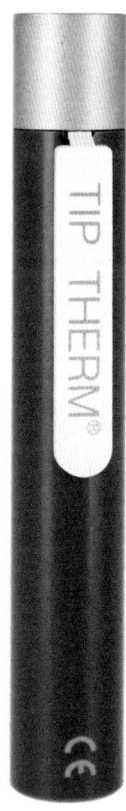

Figure 3.9 The Tip Therm is a thermal instrument designed for patient monitoring of gross temperature perception of the feet. The instrument is 4 in. (100 mm) long with a 0.59-in. (15 mm) diameter. *(Courtesy of Tip Therm GmbH, Düsseldorf, Germany.)*

6. *Two-point discrimination.* Several instruments are available to measure two-point discrimination. A two-point discrimination aesthesiometer (Fig. 3.10) is a small handheld instrument designed to measure the shortest distance that two points of contact on the skin can be distinguished. It consists of a small ruler with one stationary and one moveable (sliding) tip coated with vinyl. The vinyl coverings help to minimize the impact of temperature on perception of contact. Some instruments also have a third tip, allowing ease of alternating from two points to a single point of contact during testing. If used on an uneven body surface, care should be taken not to allow the "ruler" portion of the instrument to make contact with the skin. *Note:* The term *aesthesiometer* is not specific to this instrument; it is used to describe any number of instruments designed to examine touch perception. For finer gradations in measurement (e.g., fingertips), small circular disks can be used to measure two-point discrimination (Fig. 3.11). These instruments typically allow quantification of two-point discrimination from 1 to 25 mm.

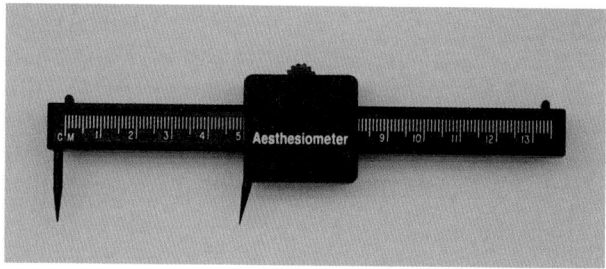

Figure 3.10 A handheld aesthesiometer provides a quantitative measure of two-point discrimination. The two-point threshold is determined by gradually bringing the tips closer together as it is sequentially applied to the patient's skin. The scale is calibrated to the nearest 0.1 cm and measures up to 14 cm.

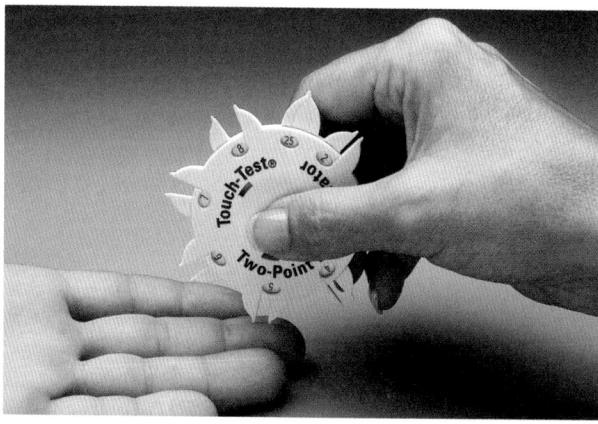

Figure 3.11 This circular two-point discrimination instrument consists of two joined plastic rotating disks with rounded tips placed at standard testing intervals. *(Courtesy of North Coast Medical, Inc., Morgan Hill, CA 95037.)*

7. *Recognition of texture.* Samples of fabrics of various textures such as cotton, wool, burlap, or silk (approximately 4 × 4 in. [10 × 10 cm]).

Patient Preparation

A full explanation of the purpose of the testing should be provided. Sensory testing often involves close contact and touching of multiple body areas. Each individual will have a different level of comfort with this contact, and it is important to have the individual's informed consent before proceeding. Details of the examination along with risks and benefits should be explained in a manner that is understandable to the patient and in accordance with their learning style. In order to obtain informed consent, a narrative approach is recommended. A narrative approach[97] includes ongoing conversation with the individual about their comfort level with the examination and their willingness to continue. These conversations should be documented. Informed consent should be an ongoing process that is reestablished throughout a treatment session and upon subsequent visits. Provider respect for and attentiveness to an individual's change of mind related to informed consent is very important in maintaining a positive patient-provider partnership. During the examination, the patient also should be informed that cooperation is necessary to obtain accurate test results. It is of considerable importance that the patient be requested not to guess if uncertain of the correct response to testing. The patient should be in a comfortable, relaxed position. Preferably, the tests should be performed when the patient is well rested. Considering the high level of concentration required, it is not surprising that fatigue has been noted to adversely affect results of some sensory tests.[98]

> **Clinical Note.** A "trial run" or demonstration of each test should be performed just prior to actual administration. This will orient the patient to the sensation being tested, what to anticipate, and what type of response is required. The importance of this initial trial should not be underestimated. If a practice trial is inadequately or not performed, what appears to be a sensory impairment may in reality only be a reflection of the patient's lack of understanding of the testing protocol or how to respond to a stimulus.

Some method of occluding the patient's vision during the testing should be used (vision should not be occluded during the explanation and demonstration). Visual input is prevented because it may allow for compensation of a sensory deficit and thus decrease the accuracy of test results. The traditional methods of occluding vision include a fabric blindfold (such as those worn by travelers to sleep on an airplane), a small folded towel, or by asking the patient to keep the eyes closed. These methods are practical in most instances. However, in situations of CNS dysfunction, a patient may become anxious or disoriented if vision is occluded for a long period of time. In these situations, a small screen or folder may be preferable as a visual barrier. Whatever method is used, it should be removed between the tests while directions and demonstrations are provided.

■ THE SENSORY EXAMINATION

The superficial (exteroceptive) sensations are usually examined first, as they consist of more primitive responses, followed by the deep (proprioceptive) and then the combined cortical sensations. If a test indicates impairment of the superficial responses, some impairment of the more discriminative (deep and combined) sensations also will be noted and is a contraindication to further testing (e.g., lack of touch sensation would be a contraindication for testing stereognosis). That is, the primary modality of sensation (touch) must be sufficiently intact to permit meaningful testing of cortical sensory function (ability to identify objects placed in the hand).

For each sensory test, the following data will be generated:

- The modality tested
- The quantity of involvement or body surface areas affected (pattern identification)
- The degree or severity of involvement (e.g., absent, impaired, or delayed responses)
- Localization of the exact boundaries of the sensory impairment
- The patient's subjective feelings about changes in sensation
- The potential impact of sensory loss on function (i.e., activity limitation, participation restriction)

Knowledge of skin segment (dermatome) innervation by the dorsal roots and peripheral nerve innervation (see Figs. 3.1 and 3.2) is required for making sound, accurate diagnostic, and prognostic judgments. They serve as critical references during testing as well as provide a framework for documenting results.

Sensory tests are typically performed in a distal-to-proximal direction. This progression will conserve time, particularly when dealing with localized lesions involving a single extremity, where deficits tend to be more severe distally. It is generally not necessary to test every segment of each dermatome; testing general body areas is sufficient. However, once a deficit area is noted, testing must become more discrete, and the exact boundaries of the impairment should be identified. A skin pencil may be useful to mark the boundaries of sensory change directly. This information should be transferred later to a sensory examination form, graphically presented on a dermatome chart, and peripheral nerve involvement identified. Figure 3.12 presents a sample Sensory Examination Form.

A single documentation form applicable to the variety of patients seen in different practice settings does not exist. Specialized centers or organizations have developed specific forms to examine sensory function (e.g., the International Standards for Neurological Classification of Spinal Cord Injury, described in Chapter 20, Traumatic Spinal Cord Injury). However, the following are common elements of sensory examination forms: (1) a dermatome chart to graphically display findings; (2) a grading scale (e.g., 0 = absent, 1 = impaired, 2 = normal, NT = not testable, etc.) to score patient perception of individual modalities; and (3) a section for narrative comments.

Most often the dermatome charts are completed using a color code (i.e., each color represents a different sensory modality). The colors used to plot each sensation are then coded by the examiner directly on the form (see Fig. 3.12). In many instances, hatch marks of varying density are used to represent gradations in sensory impairment (i.e., the closer together, the greater is the sensory impairment). With this method, a completely colored-in area indicates no response to a given sensation. With varied or "spotty" sensory loss, more than one dermatome chart may be required to completely depict all test findings. With use of several dermatome charts, the sensation(s) represented should appear in bold print at the top of each page.

The form presented in Figure 3.12 provides the foundational elements of documentation typically included for sensory examinations. It should be modified or expanded to meet the needs of a given population or facility. Therapists may find it necessary to include sensory testing data within the body of a narrative or progress report.

Clinical Note. Physical therapy electronic documentation software for the sensory examination typically includes some variation of the elements presented in Figure 3.12. If greater detail is warranted, additional dermatome charts may be scanned into the system.

During testing, the application of stimuli should be applied in a random, unpredictable manner with variation in timing. This will improve accuracy of the test results by avoiding a consistent pattern of application, which might provide the patient with "clues" to the correct response. During application of stimuli, consideration must also be given to skin condition. Scar tissue or calloused areas are generally less sensitive and will

demonstrate a diminished response to sensory stimuli. Recall that a trial test is performed to instruct the patient in what to expect and how to respond to application of the specific stimuli. Remember, too, that patient vision is occluded during testing.

The following sections present the individual sensory tests. The tests are subdivided for superficial, deep, and combined cortical sensations. Table 3.3 presents terminology used to describe common sensory impairments.

Clinical Note. Hands should always be washed prior to and after patient contact. "Hand hygiene is a major component of standard precautions and one of the most effective methods to prevent transmission of pathogens associated with health care."[99(p1)] The World Health Organization (WHO) recommends hand washing with soap and water for 40 to 60 seconds and hand rubbing using an alcohol-based hand rub for 20 to 30 seconds.[100] See "Hand Hygiene" in Chapter 2, Examination of Vital Signs, for a more detailed discussion and figures illustrating hand hygiene techniques using soap and water and an alcohol-based hand rub.

Superficial Sensations
Pain Perception

This test is also referred to as *sharp/dull discrimination* and indicates the function of protective sensation. To test pain awareness, the sharp and dull ends of a large-headed safety pin, a reshaped paper clip (the segment pulled away from the body of the paper clip provides a sharp end), or a single-use, protected neurological pin (see Fig. 3.8) are used. The instrument should be carefully cleaned before administering the test and disposed of immediately afterward (owing to the protective cap on the neurological pin, cleaning is not required). The sharp and dull ends of the instrument are randomly applied perpendicularly to the skin. To avoid summation of impulses, the stimuli should not be applied too close to each other or in too rapid a succession. To maintain a uniform pressure with each successive application of stimuli, the safety pin, reshaped paper clip, or protected neurological pin should be held firmly and the fingers allowed to "slide" down the instrument once in contact with the skin. This will avoid the chance of gradually increasing pressure during application. The instrument used to test pain perception should be sharp enough to deflect the skin but not puncture it.

Response

The patient is asked to verbally indicate *sharp* or *dull* when a stimulus is felt. All areas of the body may be tested.

This form provides a record of the type, severity, and location of sensory impairments. It should be used in conjunction with additional dermatome sheets, if needed, to graphically outline the exact boundaries of the impairment. The designations P and D may be added to the grading key to indicate either a proximal (P) or a distal (D) location of the impairment on a limb or body part. The dermatome chart should be color coded and filled in using varying density hatch marks (higher density for more severe areas of impairment). Indicate the color used for documentation in the box titled Color Code (a different color should be used for each sensation). Separate notation should be made for examination of the face and identification of peripheral nerve involvement. Abnormal responses should be briefly described in the comments section.

Patient Name: _____   Date: _____

Examiner: _____

ANTERIOR

POSTERIOR

Sensations	Upper Extremity		Lower Extremity		Trunk		Comments
	Right	Left	Right	Left	Right	Left	
Pain							
Temperature							
Touch							
Vibration							
Two-Point Disk							
Kinesthesia							
Proprioception							
Stereognosis							

Note: Areas shaded indicate sensation not typically tested for corresponding body part.

Key to Grading
0 = Absent, no response
1 = Decreased, delayed response
2 = Increased, exaggerated response
3 = Inconsistent response
4 = Intact, normal response
NT = Unable to test
P = Proximal; D = distal

Indicate Peripheral Nerve Involvement:

Color Code

Color	Sensation

Figure 3.12 Sample Sensory Examination Form.

Table 3.3	Terminology Describing Common Sensory Impairments
Abarognosis	Inability to recognize weight
Allesthesia	Sensation experienced at a site remote from point of stimulation
Allodynia	Pain produced by a non-noxious stimulus
Analgesia	Complete loss of pain sensitivity
Astereognosis	Inability to recognize the form and shape of objects by touch (synonym: *tactile agnosia*)
Atopognosia	Inability to localize a sensation
Causalgia	Painful, burning sensations, usually along the distribution of a nerve
Dysesthesia	Touch sensation experienced as pain
Hypalgesia	Decreased sensitivity to pain
Hyperalgesia	Increased sensitivity to pain
Hyperesthesia	Increased sensitivity to sensory stimuli
Hypoesthesia	Decreased sensitivity to sensory stimuli
Pallanesthesia	Loss or absence of sensibility to vibration
Paresthesia	Abnormal sensation such as numbness, prickling, or tingling, without apparent cause
Thalamic syndrome	Vascular lesion of the thalamus resulting in sensory disturbances and partial or complete paralysis of one side of the body, associated with severe, boring-type pain; sensory stimuli may produce an exaggerated, prolonged, or painful response
Thermanalgesia	Inability to perceive heat
Thermanesthesia	Inability to perceive sensations of heat and cold
Thermhyperesthesia	Increased sensitivity to temperature
Thermhypoesthesia	Decreased temperature sensibility
Thigmanesthesia	Loss of light touch sensibility

Clinical Note. When clinicians are testing individuals for the purpose of determining level of consciousness after a severe traumatic brain injury, the ability of the individual to localize to noxious stimulation (indicate where on the body the painful stimulus is being applied) is a motor function sign denoting emergence from coma to a minimally conscious state.[72–74]

Temperature Awareness

This test determines the ability to distinguish between warm and cool stimuli. One method of examination involves the use of two test tubes with stoppers; one should be filled with warm water and the other with crushed ice. Ideal temperatures for cold are between 5°C (41°F) and 10°C (50°F) and for warmth, between 40°C (104°F) and 45°C (113°F). Caution should be exercised to remain within these ranges, because exceeding these temperatures may elicit a pain response and, consequently, inaccurate test results. The side of the test tube should be placed in contact with the skin (as opposed to only the distal end). This technique provides sufficient surface area contact to determine the temperature. The test tubes are randomly placed in contact with the skin area to be tested. All skin surfaces should be tested.

Response

The patient is asked to reply *hot* or *cold* after each stimulus application.

Clinical Note. The clinical usefulness of thermal testing may be problematic. Nolan[98] points out that the tests are extremely difficult to duplicate on a day-to-day basis, owing to rapid changes in temperature once the test tubes are exposed to room air. Although it is a simple test to perform, determining changes over time is not practical unless a method of monitoring the temperature of the test tubes is used.[98] Monitoring of changes over time may be achieved through an alternate method using two temperature testing paddles (Fig 3.13); each paddle is placed in either warm or cold water, and a thermal strip indicates the temperature of the paddle.

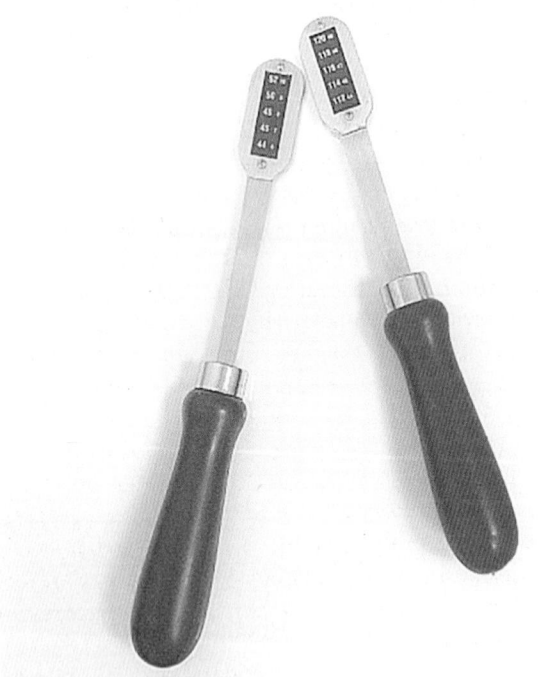

Figure 3.13 Thermal testing strip on temperature testing paddles indicate paddle temperature after being immersed in warm or cold water. *(Courtesy of US Neurologicals, Poulsbo, WA 98370.)*

Touch Awareness

This test determines perception of tactile light touch input. A camel-hair brush, piece of cotton (ball or swab), or tissue is used. The area to be tested is lightly touched or stroked. Examination of finer gradations of light touch can be quantified using monofilaments (see the "Quantitative Sensory Testing and Specialized Testing Instruments" section).

Response

The patient is asked to indicate when they recognize that a stimulus has been applied by responding "yes" or "now."

Note: A quantitative score for pain perception, temperature, and light touch awareness can be obtained by dividing the number of *correct responses* by the *number of stimuli* applied (normal response would be 100%).[101] Also, inability to verbally communicate does not necessarily preclude obtaining accurate data. For example, having the patient hold up one or two fingers might be used for dichotomous responses (yes/no; hot/cold). Other options might include nodding, pointing to index cards containing printed responses, or using hand gestures to indicate recognition of a stimulus.

Pressure Perception

The therapist's fingertip or a double-tipped cotton swab is used to apply a firm pressure on the skin surface. This pressure should be firm enough to indent the skin and to stimulate the deep receptors. This test can also be administered using the thumb and fingers to squeeze the Achilles tendon.[98]

Response

The patient indicates when an applied stimulus is recognized by responding "yes" or "now."

Deep Sensations

The deep sensations include *kinesthesia, proprioception,* and *vibration.* Kinesthesia is the awareness of movement. Proprioception includes position sense and the awareness of joints at rest. *Vibration* refers to the ability to perceive rapidly oscillating or vibratory stimuli. Although these sensations are closely related, they are examined individually.

Kinesthesia Awareness

This test examines *awareness of movement.* The extremity or joint(s) is moved passively through a relatively small range of motion (ROM). Small increments in ROM are used as joint receptors fire at specific points throughout the range. The therapist should identify the range of movement being examined (e.g., initial, mid-, or terminal range). As discussed, a trial run or demonstration of the procedure should be performed prior to actual testing. This will ensure that the patient and the therapist agree on terms to describe the direction of movements.

Response

The patient is asked to describe verbally the direction (up, down, in, out, etc.) and range of movement in terms previously discussed with the therapist while the extremity is *in motion.* The patient may also respond by simultaneously duplicating the movement with the contralateral extremity. This second approach, however, is impractical with proximal lower extremity joints, because of potential stress on the low back. During testing, movement of larger joints is usually discerned more quickly than that of smaller joints. The therapist's grip should remain constant and minimal (fingertip grip over bony prominences) to reduce tactile stimulation.

Proprioceptive Awareness

This test examines *joint position sense* and the *awareness of joints at rest.* The extremity or joint(s) is moved through a ROM and held in a static position. Again, small increments of range are used. The words selected to identify the range of movement examined should be identified to the patient during the practice trial (e.g., initial, mid-, or terminal range). As with kinesthesia, caution should be used with hand placements to avoid excessive tactile stimulation.

Response

While the extremity or joint(s) is held in a static position by the therapist, the patient is asked to describe the position verbally or to duplicate the position of the extremity or joint(s) with the contralateral extremity (position matching). This test may also be performed unilaterally using the same extremity or joint(s); first held in position by the examiner, then returned to resting position, followed by active duplication of position by the patient using the same limb.

Clinical Note. Based on a series of position matching studies conducted in the Motor Control Laboratory at the University of Michigan, Goble[102] presents several important factors to assist clinicians in making informed decisions about proprioceptive matching test outcomes:

- For position matching tests, there are different memory influences and different interhemispheric communication requirements between use of the ipsilateral extremity (same arm positioned by examiner is used to actively replicate the joint angle[s]) versus contralateral limb (patient moves opposite extremity from that used by examiner).
- Likely owing to the enhanced role of the right hemisphere in proprioceptive feedback processing, the left arm appears to have an advantage in matching tasks.
- The magnitude of the reference joint angle (larger magnitudes associated with greater error) and how reference positions are established (fewer errors noted when active movement used to establish position versus passive movement by examiner) will influence performance.
- Proprioceptive acuity must be considered within the context of anticipated changes occurring over the life span or that are diagnosis specific (e.g., stroke).
- Task workspace (area in which activities of daily living are typically performed) appears to influence joint position matching performance. During position matching experiments, greater performance occurred to the left of the body midline with the fewest errors in the far left of the workspace.

Vibration Perception

This test requires a tuning fork that vibrates at 128 Hz.[98] The ability to perceive a vibratory stimulus is tested by placing the base of a vibrating tuning fork on a bony prominence (such as the sternum, elbow, or ankle). The tuning fork base (the "handle" of the fork) is held between the examiner's thumb and index finger without making contact with the tines. The tines are then briskly hit against the open palm of the examiner's opposite hand to initiate the vibration. Care must be taken not to touch the tines, as this will stop the vibration. The base of the fork is then placed over a bony prominence. If vibration sensation is intact, the patient will perceive the vibration. If there is impairment, the patient will be unable to distinguish between a vibrating and nonvibrating tuning fork. Therefore, there should be a random application of vibrating and nonvibrating stimuli.

Auditory clues can pose a challenge in obtaining accurate test results. Typically, it is easy to hear the sound of the tines making vigorous contact with the examiner's hand to initiate the vibration. If the sound is not heard, it provides an easy indicator to the patient that the next application will be nonvibrating. To minimize this effect, the vibration can be initiated for *every* stimulus application; however, when a nonvibrating stimulus is desired, brief contact of the therapist's fingers on the tines will stop the vibration prior to placement on the skin. This, though, does not solve the problem of the auditory cues generated during application of a vibrating stimulus. The best solution is use of sound-occlusive earphones (the type worn by airport ground workers). Unfortunately, such earphones are seldom available in a clinic setting.

Response

The patient is asked to respond by verbally identifying or otherwise indicating if the stimulus is vibrating or nonvibrating each time the fork makes contact.

Combined Cortical Sensations

Stereognosis Perception

This test determines the ability to recognize the form of objects by touch (stereognosis). A variety of small, easily obtainable, and culturally familiar objects of differing size and shape are required (e.g., keys, button, ring, coins,[103] etc.). A single object is placed in the hand, the patient manipulates the object, and then the patient identifies the item verbally. The patient should be allowed to handle several sample test items during the explanation and demonstration of the procedure.

Response

The patient is asked to name the object verbally. For patients with speech impairments, sensory testing shields can be used (Fig. 3.14). Alternatively, the item manipulated can be identified from a group of images presented after each test.

Tactile Localization

This test determines the ability to localize touch sensation on the skin (topognosis). The patient is asked to identify the specific point of application of a touch stimulus (e.g., tip of ring finger, lateral malleolus, and so forth) and not simply the perception of being touched. Tactile localization is typically not tested in isolation and frequently examined in combination with similar tests such as pressure perception or touch awareness.

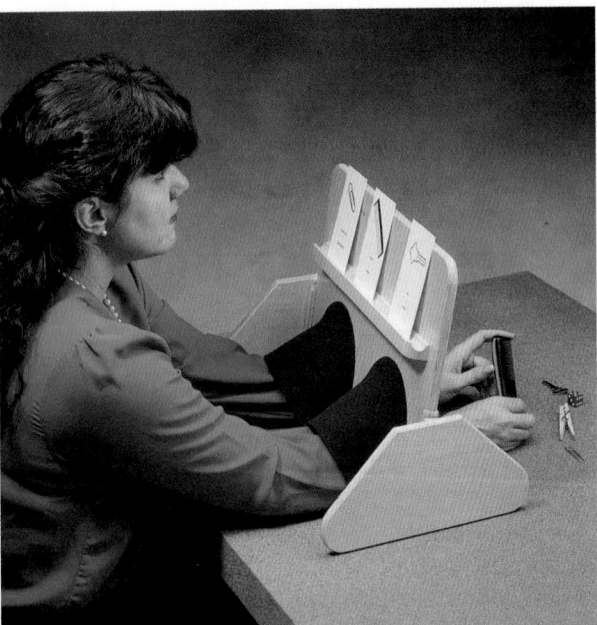

Figure 3.14 A sensory testing shield can be used for examining stereognosis in the presence of speech or language impairments. In this simulation, the subject manipulates the object without the use of visual input. Following manipulation, the subject points to the matching object pictured on the ledge of the testing shield. *(Courtesy of North Coast Medical, Inc., Morgan Hill, CA 95037.)*

Using a cotton swab or fingertip, the therapist touches different skin surfaces. After each application of a stimulus, the patient is given time to respond.

Response

The patient is asked to identify the location of the stimuli by pointing to the area or by verbal description. The patient's eyes may be open during the response component of this test. The distance between the application of the stimulus and the site indicated by the patient can be measured and recorded. Accuracy of localization over various parts of the body may be compared to determine the relative sensitivity of different areas.

Two-Point Discrimination

This test determines the ability to perceive two points applied to the skin simultaneously. It is a measure of the smallest distance between two stimuli (applied simultaneously and with equal pressure) that can still be perceived as two distinct stimuli. Two-point discrimination values vary for different individuals and by gender and body parts and may be negatively influenced by fatigue.[104] As this sensory function is most refined in the distal upper extremities, this is the typical site for testing. It is believed to contribute to precision grip movements and instrumental activities of daily living.[105]

Two-point discrimination is among the most practical and easily duplicated tests for cutaneous sensation. Some years ago, a series of classic two-point discrimination studies were conducted by Nolan.[106–108] The purpose of his research was to establish normative data on two-point discrimination for young adults. His sample consisted of 43 college students ranging in age from 20 to 24 years. Values from Nolan's studies for the upper and lower extremities as well as the face and trunk are presented in Appendix 3.A (online). The results from these studies should be used cautiously because they relate to a specific population. They should not be generalized for interpreting data from older or younger patients. Normative data for two-point discrimination have been documented by several authors, including van Nes et al.,[109] Kaneko et al.,[110] Vriens and van der Glas,[111] and Koo et al.[112]

As mentioned earlier, the aesthesiometer (see Fig. 3.10) and the circular two-point discriminator (see Fig. 3.11) are among the most common devices used for measurement. Two reshaped paper clips can also be used; however, this requires the assistance of a second examiner to measure the distance between the two points using a small ruler. During the test procedure, the two tips of the instrument are applied to the skin simultaneously with tips spread apart. To increase the validity of the test, it is appropriate to alternate the application of two stimuli with the random application of only a single stimulus (the purpose of the third tip on some aesthesiometers). With each successive application, the two tips are gradually brought closer together until the stimuli are perceived as one. The smallest distance between the stimuli that is still perceived as two distinct points is measured.

Response

The patient is asked to identify the perception of "one" or "two" stimuli.

Double Simultaneous Stimulation

This test determines the ability to perceive simultaneous touch stimuli (double simultaneous stimulation). The therapist simultaneously (and with equal pressure) touches (1) identical locations on opposite sides of the body, (2) proximal and distal locations on opposite sides of the body, and/or (3) proximal and distal locations on the same side of the body. The term *extinction phenomenon* is used to describe a situation in which only the proximal stimulus is perceived, with "extinction" of the distal.

Response

The patient verbally states when a touch stimulus is perceived and the number of stimuli felt.

Described next are several additional tests for the combined (cortical) sensations including graphesthesia (traced finger identification), recognition of texture, and barognosis (recognition of weight). However, these tests are usually not performed if stereognosis and two-point discrimination are found to be intact.

Graphesthesia (Traced Figure Identification)

This test determines the ability to recognize letters, numbers, or designs "written" on the skin. Using a fingertip or the eraser end of a pencil, a series of letters, numbers, or shapes is traced on the palm of the patient's hand. During the practice trial, agreement should be reached about the orientation of the tracings (e.g., the bottom of the traced figures will always be oriented toward the base of the patient's hand [wrist]). Between each separate drawing, the palm should be gently wiped with a soft cloth to clearly indicate a change in figures to the patient. This test is a useful substitute for stereognosis when paralysis prevents grasping an object. Talmasov and Ropper[113] described an interesting case report of a patient with a right parietal lesion resulting in isolated agraphesthesia for numbers and letters.

Response

The patient is asked to verbally identify the figures drawn on the skin. For patients with speech or language impairments, the figures can be selected (pointed to) from a series of line drawings.

Recognition of Texture

This test determines the ability to differentiate among various textures. Suitable textures may include cotton, wool, burlap, or silk. The items are placed individually in the patient's hand, and the patient is allowed to manipulate the sample texture.

Response

The patient is asked to identify the individual textures as they are placed in the hand. They may be identified by name (e.g., silk, cotton) or by texture (e.g., rough, smooth).

Barognosis (Recognition of Weight)

This test determines the ability to recognize different weights. A set of discrimination weights consisting of small objects of the same size and shape but of graduated weight is used (Fig. 3.15). The therapist may choose to place a series of different weights in the same hand one at a time, place a different weight in each hand simultaneously, or ask the patient to use a fingertip grip to pick up each weight.

Response

The patient is asked to identify the comparative weight of objects in a series (i.e., to compare the relative weight of the object with the previous one), or when the objects are placed (or picked up) in both hands simultaneously, the patient is asked to compare the weight of the two objects. The patient responds by indicating that the object is "heavier" or "lighter."

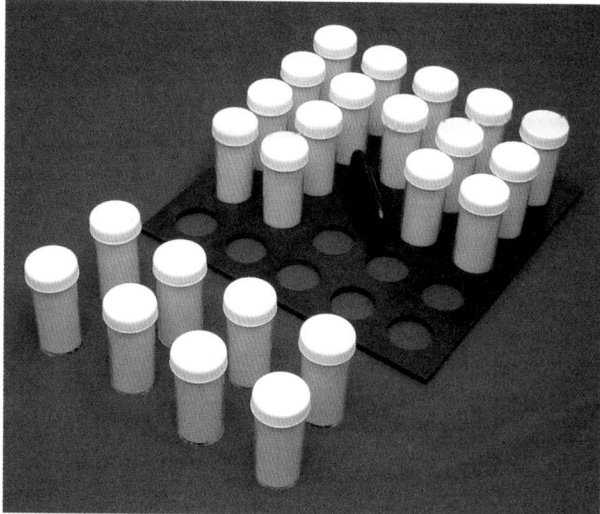

Figure 3.15 Discrimination weights are identical in size, shape, and texture. The only distinguishing feature is their variation in weight. *(Courtesy of Lafayette Instruments, Lafayette, IN 47903.)*

Clinical Note. Impaired sensation is a contraindication to or precaution for use of some physical agents because the end range of intensity or duration is frequently associated with the patient's subjective report of how the intervention feels (i.e., patient tolerance).

■ RELIABILITY

Reliability is an important parameter of any test or measure. However, few systematic reports addressing the reliability of traditional sensory tests appear in the literature. This is likely due to the inability to accurately quantify test results. In an important early reliability study by Kent,[114] the upper limbs of 50 adult patients with hemiplegia were tested for sensory and motor deficits. Three sensory tests were administered and then repeated by the same examiner within 1 to 7 days. Results revealed a high reliability for both stereognosis ($r = 0.97$) and position sense ($r = 0.90$). A lower reliability was reported for two-point discrimination, with correlation coefficients ranging from 0.59 to 0.82, depending on the body area tested.

More recently, Suda et al. examined the reliability and validity of the Semmes-Weinstein monofilament and thumb localization testing for light touch and proprioception in the upper extremities of patients with chronic stroke.[115] The authors found that both the Semmes-Weinstein monofilament and thumb localization tests are reliable and valid for sensory examinations of the upper extremity in people with chronic stroke; however, the Semmes-Weinstein monofilament was found to be more reliable as a screening tool. Moloney et al.[116] examined the interrater reliability of thermal quantitative sensory testing in young healthy adults. The interrater reliability for cold detection threshold (ICC = 0.27–0.55), warm detection threshold (ICC = 0.38–0.69), cold pain threshold (ICC = 0.88–0.94), and heat pain threshold (ICC = 0.52–0.86) ranged from poor to high. Wu and Li[117] examined proprioception using an arm position-matching paradigm. Without visual or auditory cues, healthy older adults were tested in three different joints and positions. Moderate interrater reliability was reported for each position: shoulder flexion at 60° (ICC = 0.49), elbow flexion at 40° (ICC = 0.47), and wrist extension at 50° (ICC = 0.64). Tyros et al.[118] examined vibration disappearance thresholds of the median nerve, using a 128-Hz tuning fork, on patients with chronic whiplash associated disorder. Both intra- (ICC = 0.955) and interrater (0.983) reliability were excellent. Meirte et al.[119] examined the reliability of touch pressure threshold within burn scars and healthy controls using the Semmes-Weinstein monofilament test. Interrater reliability was excellent for burn scars (ICC = 0.908) and fair for the control group (ICC = 0.731). Intrarater reliability was high for burn scars (ICC = 0.822) as well as for the control group (ICC = 0.807). Reidy et al.[103] examined stereognosis in younger and older adults using a house key, button, ring, and coin. When using their dominant hand, there was no significant difference between younger (95%–100% correct) and older adults (87.5%–100% correct) in accurately discriminating individual objects. However, when using the nondominant hand, there was a significant difference between the ability of younger (97.5% correct) and older (75% correct) adults to identify the button.

Although limited published data are available related to reliability measures, several approaches can be used to improve this aspect of the tests, including (1) use of consistent guidelines for completing the tests; (2) administration of the tests by trained, skillful examiners; and (3) subsequent retests performed by the same individual. It also should be noted that the patient's understanding of the test procedure and the patient's ability to communicate results further influence the reliability of sensory tests. As developing advances in technology (see discussion later) provide tools for quantitative sensory testing, greater emphasis on reliability will follow. Additional research related to standardization of testing protocols and identification of normative data for various age groups will improve the overall reliability and interpretation of test results.

■ QUANTITATIVE SENSORY TESTING AND SPECIALIZED TESTING INSTRUMENTS

With the expanding availability of specialized testing systems and instruments, quantitative sensory testing (QST) has gained considerable clinical and research interest. This is clearly evident from the expanding body of literature on this topic.[120–129] QST allows quantification of the level of stimuli required for perception of a sensory modality. Although sufficient data are not available to predict the ultimate integration of QST instrumentation into clinical practice, preliminary information suggests its potential usefulness. This section provides a brief overview of selected QST devices and is certainly not all-inclusive. The Internet provides a rich source of information on this developing technology and instrumentation.

TSA-II NeuroSensory Analyzer + VSA 3000 Vibratory Sensory Analyzer (Medoc, Ltd., Durham, NC)

This computer-controlled system (Fig. 3.16) is capable of generating and recording a response to repeatable vibratory and thermal stimuli (i.e., warmth, cold, heat- or cold-induced pain). For testing thermal sensation, a "thermode" capable of heating or cooling is placed on the patient's skin (Fig. 3.17). The patient is asked to respond to the stimulus by pushing a response button. A sensory threshold is recorded, and a computer comparison to age-matched normative data is generated. The system includes hand and foot (Fig. 3.18) support vibratory stimulators as well as a handheld vibrating device (see Fig 3.16, far left). A variety of report formats can be generated; a sample is presented in Figure 3.19. Several examples of

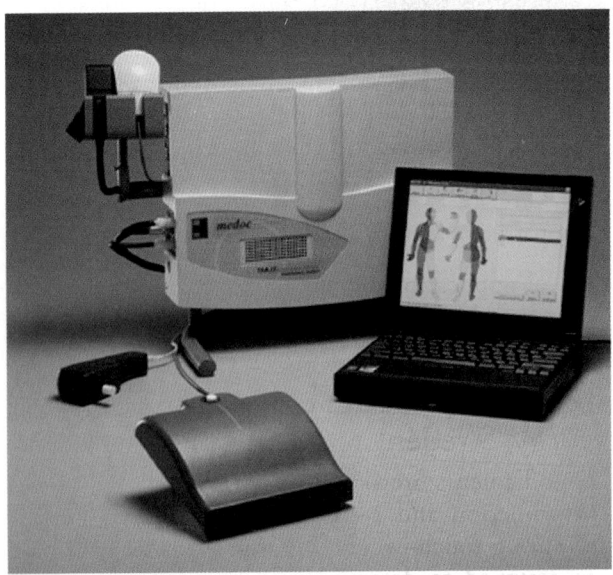

Figure 3.16 TSA-II NeuroSensory Analyzer + VSA 3000 Vibratory Sensory Analyzer. This system provides quantitative measures of both thermal and vibratory stimuli using a variety of patient interfaces. Note the small handheld vibratory device on the far left. *(Courtesy of Medoc, Ltd., Durham, NC 27707.)*

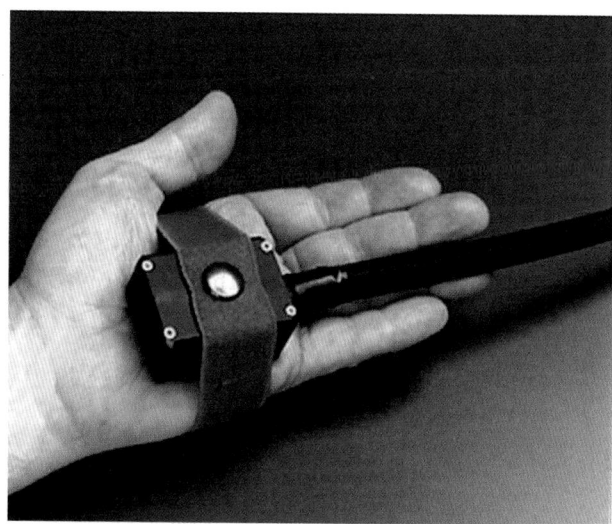

Figure 3.17 Thermode placed in hand for measuring perception of thermal stimuli. *(Courtesy of Medoc, Ltd., Durham, NC 27707.)*

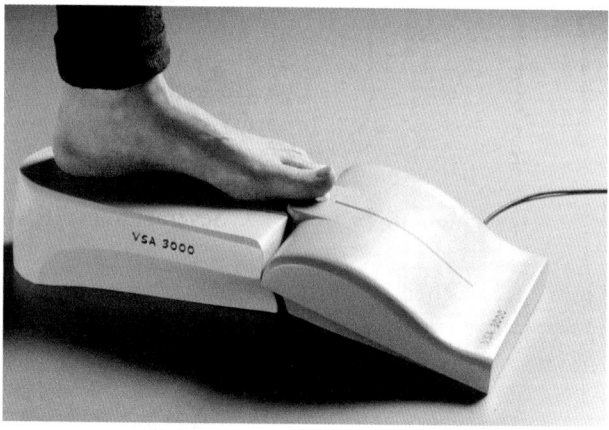

Figure 3.18 Foot support vibratory stimulator. *(Courtesy of Medoc, Ltd., Durham, NC 27707.)*

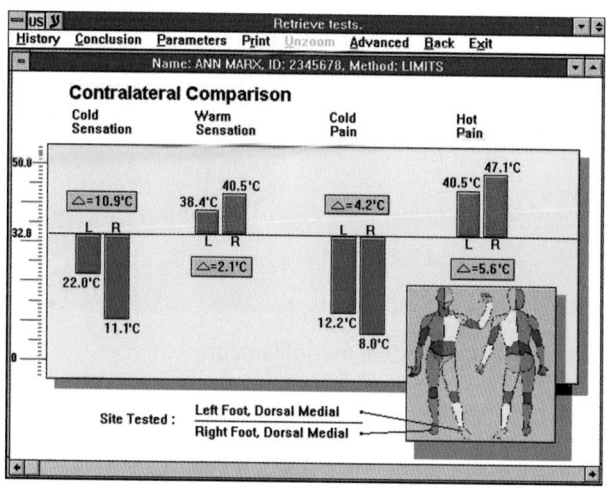

Figure 3.19 Computer-generated data from thermal testing that presents a comparison between the two sides of the body. Note the data for the right foot presents consistently higher threshold values than that of the left. Values are generated for each foot as well as the total difference between the feet. All values are in Celsius. Conversions for the temperature scale on the left border are 32°C = 89.6°F and 50°C = 122°F. *(Courtesy of Medoc, Ltd., Durham, NC 27707.)*

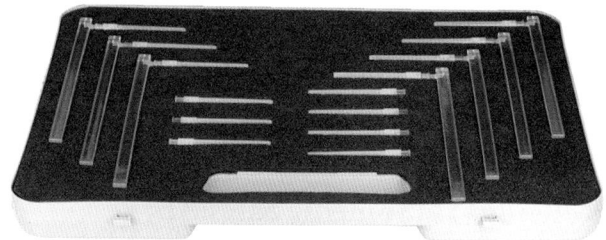

Figure 3.20 von Frey aesthesiometer. This set contains a series of monofilaments mounted on Plexiglas handles. *(Courtesy of Somedic SenseLab AB, Sösdala, Sweden.)*

clinical applications include neuropathies (e.g., diabetic, metabolic, cancer), compression injuries, and pharmacological trials.

von Frey Aesthesiometer II (Somedic AB, Hörby, Sweden)

Monofilaments are not new to examination of sensory function and are considered a classic tool for measuring touch-evoked potentials (Fig. 3.20). They are designed to detect very small changes in touch threshold. The filaments are available as sets, in various sizes (i.e., thicknesses from 0.128 to 0.508 mm), with each mounted on a handle. The nominal force required for bending the monofilament increases from 0.026 g for the first handle to 100 g for the last (pressure range of between 5 and 178 g/mm²).

The filaments are applied individually to the patient's skin until it bends; each filament provides a specific amount of force (thicker filaments are used if the thinner are not perceived). With vision occluded, the patient responds "yes" when a stimulus is felt. The filaments are held perpendicular to the skin, and application is usually repeated three times at each testing site.[101] Monofilaments are frequently used in hand-rehabilitation clinics; other examples of clinical applications include neuropathies (e.g., diabetic) and peripheral nerve injuries.

Touch Test Sensory Evaluator (North Coast Medical, Inc., Morgan Hill, CA)

Individual monofilaments are also available in increments ranging from 0.008 to 300 g (Fig. 3.21). These instruments are convenient and can be carried in a pocket. The

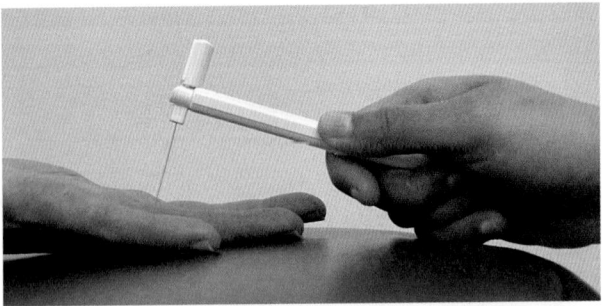

Figure 3.21 Individual monofilament.

handle opens to a 90° angle for testing; when folded, it protects the monofilament when not in use.

Rydel-Seiffer 64/128 Hz Graduated Tuning Fork (US Neurologicals, Kirkland, WA)

This quantitative tuning fork contains small scaled weights on the distal ends of the two prongs, converting it from 128 to 64 Hz (Fig. 3.22). The two triangles move closer together, and their intersection moves upward as the intensity of vibration decreases. The intensity where the patient no longer perceives the vibration is recorded as the number adjacent to the intersection of the triangles. This instrument allows more sensitive and specific testing for detecting sensory changes as compared to qualitative tuning forks and has demonstrated high intertester and intratester reliability.[130]

Rolltemp II (Somedic Sales AB, Hörby, Sweden)

This instrument is used as a screening tool for determining changes in perception of thermal sensation (Fig. 3.23). The rollers are housed in a storage unit to maintain temperature. The individual rollers are placed in contact with the skin to provide a gross estimate of temperature perception.

Bio-Thesiometer (Bio-Medical Instrument Co, Newbury, OH)

This instrument is designed to quantitatively measure threshold perception of a vibratory stimulus (Fig. 3.24). The stimulus is applied using a handheld device applied to the skin. Intensity of stimulation can be preset or gradually increased until the threshold is reached (or gradually lowered until no longer felt).

MSA (Modular Sensory Analyzer) Thermotest (Somedic Sales AB, Hörby, Sweden)

The MSA Thermotest (Fig. 3.25) measures response to thermal (warm and cold) stimuli. Thermodes of

different sizes allow testing of various anatomical locations. A computer interface using SenseLab software sets up and runs the Thermotest and allows for analysis and storage of data. Temperatures range from 5°C to 52°C (41°F–125.6°F).

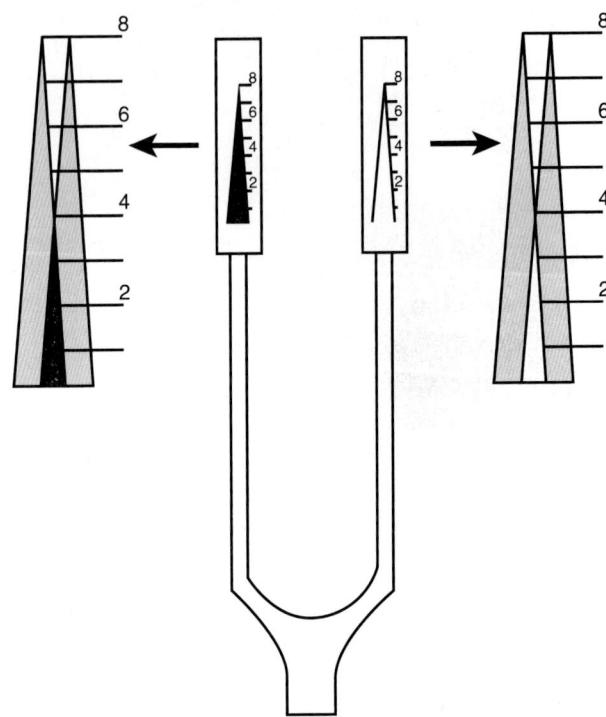

Figure 3.22 Schematic illustration of the Rydel-Seiffer tuning fork. *(Courtesy of US Neurologicals, Kirkland, WA, 98033.)*

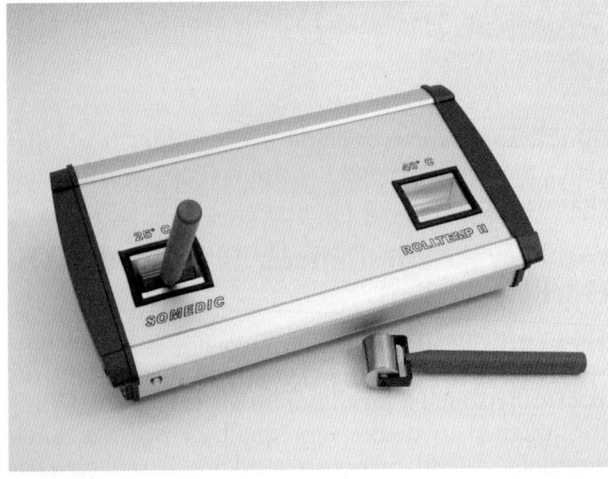

Figure 3.23 The Rolltemp II provides a quick screening tool for thermal sensation. One roller is maintained at 40°C (104°F) and the other at 25°C (77°F). *(Courtesy of Somedic Sales AB, Hörby, Sweden.)*

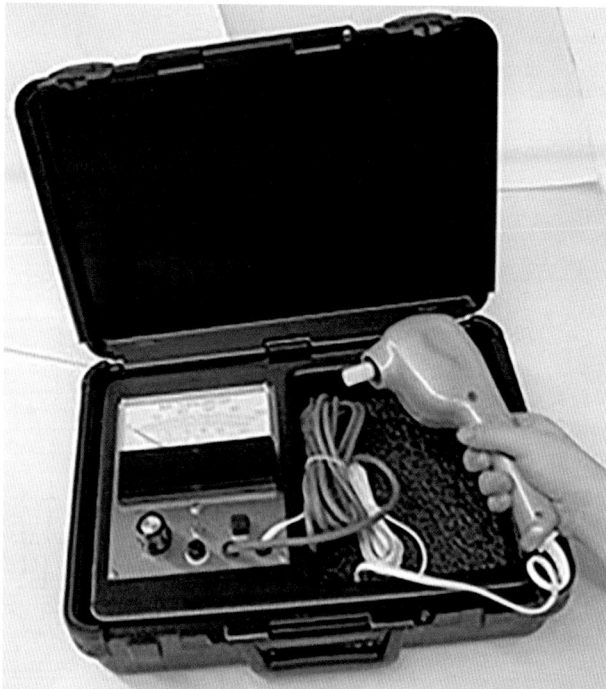

Figure 3.24 Bio-Thesiometer for measuring perception of vibratory stimulus. *(Courtesy of Bio-Thesiometer USA, Newbury, OH 44065.)*

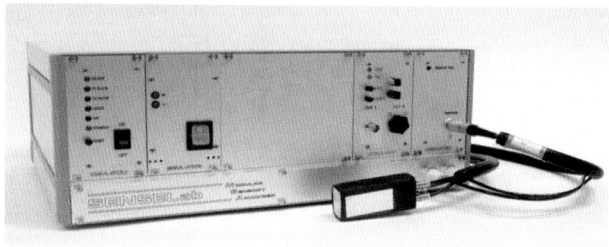

Figure 3.25 MSA Thermotest. In the right foreground is a 1 × 2 in. (25 × 50 mm) standard thermode for application of thermal stimuli.

■ CRANIAL NERVE FUNCTION

An examination of cranial nerves provides information about their individual function as well as insight into the location of intracranial lesions.[132,133] Data generated may include function of muscles innervated by the cranial nerves; visual, auditory, sensory, and gag reflex integrity; perception of taste; swallowing characteristics; eye movements; and constriction and dilation patterns of the pupils.

Table 3.4 provides a summary of the functional components of the cranial nerves. Box 3.4 presents examples of tests appropriate for each cranial nerve. Impairments noted during initial testing may indicate that a more comprehensive examination is warranted. See Chapter 5, Examination of Motor Function: Motor Control and Motor Learning, for additional information on cranial nerve examination.

■ SENSORY INTEGRITY WITHIN THE CONTEXT OF TREATMENT

Learning a motor behavior is dependent on the patient's ability to take in sensory information from the body and the environment (sensory intake), process it (sensory integration), and use it to plan and organize behavior (output). When patients experience impairment in processing sensory intake, deficits typically occur in planning and organizing behavior. This produces behaviors that may interfere with successful motor learning and motor function.

The POC designed for a patient with impaired sensation is typically guided by one of two approaches, the *Sensory Integration Approach* and the *Compensatory Approach*. The selection of a treatment model is based on a complete dataset of information from all examinations together with the established prognosis and diagnosis. The treatment approach depicted in Figure 3.26 is based largely on the Sensory Integration Model developed by Ayers.[1,134–138] The basic premise of this approach is that specific treatment techniques can enhance sensory integration (CNS processing) with a resultant change in motor performance.

Using the Sensory Integration Approach, data obtained from the examination of sensory function inform development of a POC to enhance opportunities for *controlled* sensory intake within a framework of meaningful functional skills. During treatment, the patient is provided guided practice in planning and organizing motor behaviors using both *intrinsic* feedback (from the movement) and *augmented* feedback (cues planned by the therapist). This approach is designed to improve the ability of the CNS to process and integrate information and promote motor learning. The reader is referred to the work of Ayers[1,134–138] and Bundy and Murray[6] for a detailed presentation of both the theory and practice of the Sensory Integration Model.

The compensatory approach is a more traditional intervention that focuses on patient education to accommodate the limitations imposed by the sensory deficit. The therapist's role is to assist the patient in achieving optimum functional capacity, minimizing activity and participation limitations, protecting anesthetic limbs, and creating appropriate environmental adaptations to enhance safety and function.

■ EDUCATION FOR PATIENTS WITH IMPAIRED SENSORY FUNCTION

Frequently, the treatment of individuals with impaired sensory function involves safety concerns that require a compensatory approach focused on patient and caregiver

Table 3.4   Functional Components of the Cranial Nerves

Number	Name	Components	Function
I	Olfactory	Afferent	Olfaction (smell)
II	Optic	Afferent	Vision
III	Oculomotor	Efferent Somatic Visceral	Elevates eyelid Turns eye up, down, in Constricts pupil Accommodates lens
IV	Trochlear	Efferent (somatic)	Turns the adducted eye down and causes intorsion (inward rotation) of eye
V	Trigeminal	Mixed Afferent Efferent	Sensation from face Sensation from cornea Sensation from anterior tongue Muscles of mastication Dampens sound (tensor tympani)
VI	Abducens	Efferent (somatic)	Turns eye out
VII	Facial	Mixed Afferent Efferent (somatic) Efferent (visceral)	Taste from anterior tongue Muscles of facial expression Dampens sound (stapedius) Tearing (lacrimal gland) Salivation (submandibular and sublingual glands)
VIII	Vestibulocochlear	Afferent	Balance (semicircular canals, utricle, saccule) Hearing (organ of Corti)
IX	Glossopharyngeal	Mixed Afferent Efferent	Taste from posterior tongue Sensation from posterior tongue Sensation from oropharynx Salivation (parotid gland)
X	Vagus	Mixed Afferent Efferent	Thoracic and abdominal viscera Muscles of larynx and pharynx Decreases heart rate Increases gastrointestinal motility
XI	Spinal accessory	Efferent	Head movements (sternocleidomastoid and trapezius)
XII	Hypoglossal	Efferent	Tongue movements and shape

From Nolan,[64(p44)] with permission.

education. The therapist instructs the patient and/or caregiver in practical strategies intended to prevent injury and optimize functional mobility. Results of previous cognitive testing preferred learning styles, health literacy, communication impairments, and potential language barriers should be considered before choosing the mode of education delivery. The Foundation for Peripheral Neuropathy (www.foundationforpn.org) provides patient resources and research initiatives to improve the lives of individuals with peripheral neuropathy. Additional web-based resources are provided in Appendix 3.B (online). Examples of areas of focus for patient and family education related to safety include modification of the environment. Insensitivity to temperature presents multiple safety concerns; instruction may be given to wear heat-resistant gloves

Box 3.4 Tests for Cranial Nerve Function[11,64]

Cranial nerve I: Examine olfactory acuity using non-noxious odors such as lemon oil, coffee, cloves, or tobacco.

Cranial nerve II: Examine visual acuity using a Snellen chart; both central and peripheral vision is tested.

Cranial nerves III, IV, and VI: Determine equality and size of pupils, reaction to light, presence of strabismus (loss of ocular alignment), ability of eyes to follow a moving target without head movement, presence of ptosis of eyelid.

Cranial nerve V: Sensory tests of face (sharp/dull discrimination, light touch); open and close jaw against resistance; jaw jerk reflex.

Cranial nerve VII: Examine any asymmetry of face at rest and during voluntary contraction.

Cranial nerve VIII: Test auditory acuity using a vibrating tuning fork (Weber test) placed on vertex of skull or forehead; patient indicates on which side the tone is louder. Rub fingers together at a distance and gradually bring toward patient; note distance when first heard. Alter volume of conversation. Rinne test (conductive hearing loss), vibrating tuning fork placed on mastoid process, then near external ear canal; note hearing acuity.

Cranial nerve IX: Examine taste on posterior one-third of tongue; examine gag reflex.

Cranial nerve X: Examine swallowing; observe uvula and soft palate for any asymmetry (tongue depressor).

Cranial nerve XI: Examine strength of the sternocleidomastoid and trapezius muscles.

Cranial nerve XII: With tongue protruded, examine ability to move tongue rapidly from side to side.

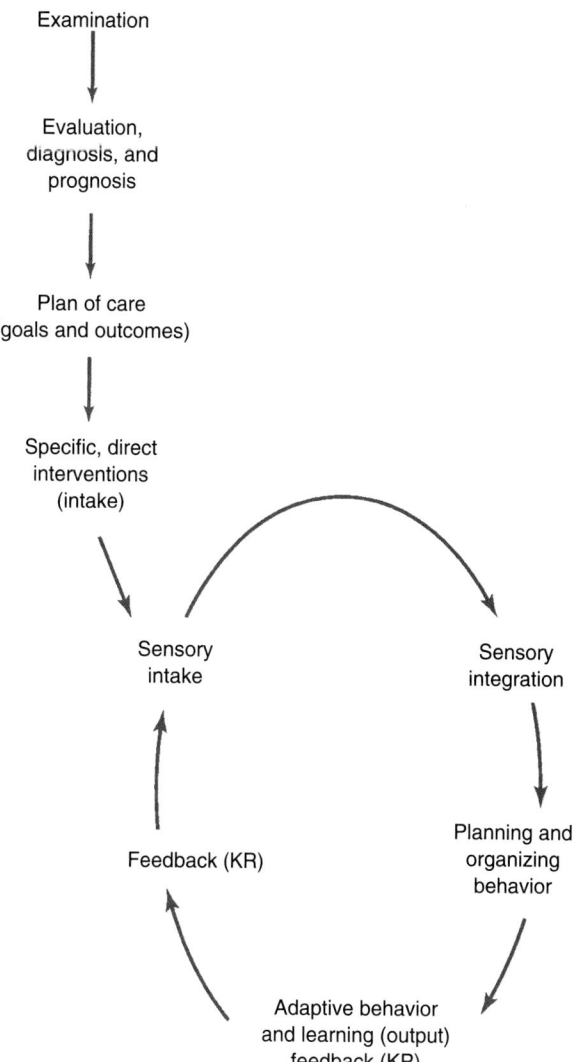

Figure 3.26 Elements of patient management for sensory impairment. KP refers to knowledge of performance (feedback about the quality of movement produced); KR refers to knowledge of result (feedback about the end result or outcome of the movement). *(Adapted from Bundy and Murray.[6(p5)])*

when working in the kitchen and to arrange kitchen supplies to eliminate the need for accessing storage directly over the stove. Visual impairments may require enhanced lighting and contrasting colors denoting steps or changes in ambulatory surface.

- *Use of Augmentative Sensory Devices.* When hearing is impaired, it may be necessary to educate patients about the availability of assistive listening devices (ALDs) or alerting devices. ALDs are used to amplify sound transmission, and alerting devices produce a loud sound or blinking light to alert a person of events such as ringing doorbells, telephones, or alarms.[139] An audiologist and/or speech-language pathologist referral will be warranted for persons with newly discovered or worsening hearing

loss. Similarly, when vision is impaired or worsening, a referral to an optometrist or ophthalmologist should be generated.

- *Self-Monitoring.* Individuals who are insensitive to temperature may be educated to measure the temperature of bathwater before entering or to test the water with a body part with intact sensation. Further, when areas of insensitive skin are detected, patients may be taught not to go barefoot and to perform daily skin checks for cuts, bruises, or development of infection (e.g., due to development of ingrown toenail). This is especially applicable for individuals with diabetic peripheral neuropathy.

Box 3.5   Examples of General Goals and Outcomes for Patients With Sensory Dysfunction

1. **Impact of pathology/pathophysiology is reduced.**
   Decrease: Risk of secondary impairments such as pain, integumentary, range of motion, etc.
   Improve: Patient/client, family and caregiver knowledge of disease, current functional status, prognosis and plan of care; symptom management.

2. **Impact of impairments is reduced.**
   Decrease: Integumentary consequences such as skin breakdown/wounds, pain, joint range of motion limitations, etc.
   Improve: Patient/client, family, and caregiver knowledge of sensory awareness, performing thorough daily skin checks, management of proper skin care, and performing pressure relief and weight shifts as needed to protect skin at bony prominences.

3. **Ability to perform physical activities, tasks, or activities is improved.**
   Decrease: Barriers to performing functional tasks and activities; fall risk.
   Improve: Independence with functional mobility and ADL with proper use of assisted devices as needed to tolerate positions and activities safely using problem-solving and decision-making skills to mitigate fall risk.

4. **Disability associated with chronic illness is reduced.**
   Decrease: Immobility and sedentary lifestyle due to chronic sensory dysfunction.
   Improve: Ability to assume/resume self-care and home management; ability to assume work (job/school/play), community, and leisure roles; patient/client and family knowledge and awareness of personal and environmental factors associated with condition worsening; awareness and use of community resources.

5. **Health status and quality of life are improved.**
   Decrease: Mental health stressors and feelings of isolation.
   Improve: Holistic health-care approach to provide a sense of well-being and independence; equitable provision of support systems and resources based on patient/client-centered needs; self-confidence and self-management skills; health, wellness, and fitness.

6. **Patient/client satisfaction is enhanced.**
   Decrease: Barriers to health accessibility impacted by social determinants of health.
   Improve: Health outcomes with equitable accessibility and quality of health-care services including rehabilitation services to patient/client and family through effective coordination of care with patient/client, family caregivers, and other professionals.

- *Strategies to Promote Safe Balance.* Sensory impairments often lead to difficulties with balance and postural control. Patients will need to be educated in both remediation and compensation strategies for safety. The reader is referred to Box 10.5 in Chapter 10 of this text for strategies to promote safe balance.

■ GOALS AND OUTCOMES

The general goals for patients with sensory dysfunction will depend on the impact this has on activity limitations and participation restrictions. Examples of general goals and outcomes for individuals with sensory dysfunction are presented in Box 3.5.

SUMMARY

Examination of sensory function provides important information about the integrity of the somatosensory system. Findings from the examination assist in making clinical judgments about diagnosis, prognosis, goals, and expected outcomes, as well as establishing the POC. Periodic reexamination provides critical data on changes in patient status and in determining progress toward goals and outcomes. Individual tests for each sensory modality have been presented. Reliability of these test procedures can be improved by careful adherence to consistent guidelines, administration of tests by trained individuals, and subsequent retests performed by the same examiner. Documentation of test results should address the type(s) of sensation affected, the quantity, the degree of involvement, and the localization of the exact boundaries of the sensory deficits. Finally, it should be emphasized that additional research related to sensory testing is warranted. Further development of QST techniques, standardized protocols, validity and reliability measures, and additional normative data will significantly improve the clinical applications of data obtained from the examination of sensory function.

Questions for Review

1. Define sensory integration, and describe the relationship to motor performance.

2. Define a dermatome, and describe a precaution with using published dermatome maps.

3. Identify six pathologies or health conditions that would warrant (or indicate the need for) examination of sensory function.

4. Describe the five terms commonly used to document a patient's level of consciousness.

5. Which type of sensory receptor is responsible for position sense and awareness of joints at rest, during movement, and vibration? How would you comprehensively examine this sensory receptor?

6. Which type of muscle receptor senses tension, and how does it affect the muscle when under extreme tension?

7. For a suspected localized lesion, in which direction would you conduct your examination of sensory function? Why?

8. Describe four purposes of screening the sensory system related to safety.

9. Describe how the data from the examination of sensory function are used by the physical therapist.

10. Describe equipment (items) that can be used to assess stereognosis.

11. Explain why impaired sensation is a contraindication to or precaution for use of some physical agents.

12. What information would you provide to the patient prior to administration of sensory tests to obtain informed consent?

13. Which muscles would you test to assess the spinal accessory cranial nerve?

14. List the six data items that should be generated for each sensory test.

CASE STUDY

HISTORY

A 56-year-old Lebanese landscaper who immigrated to the United States 22 years ago sustained a spinal injury after falling off a ladder while cleaning home gutters. He landed on his back onto equipment, with extreme extension forces placed on his thoracic spine.

Computed tomography (CT) imaging revealed no brain injury and extensive damage at T9 and T10 vertebral bodies with burst fractures and posterior spinal cord injury.

Four weeks post-injury he presents for outpatient physical therapy, and you are the evaluating therapist. His major complaints are numbness and tingling radiating down his lower extremities (left greater than right), low back pain, proximal lower extremity pain, and "having trouble knowing where my legs are."

Past Medical/Surgical History: Long-standing history of hypertension (15 years), hypercholesterolemia (10 years), poorly controlled type 2 diabetes (15 years), anxiety, and one pack per day × 25-year smoker.

Medications: Tylenol, Oxycodone, Lovenox, Lisinopril, Amitriptyline, Metformin, Dulcolax

Social History: Patient lives with his wife and two children ages 20 and 17 years. He lives in a single-level, second-floor, walk-up apartment with one rail on the stairway. His wife is very supportive; however, she works full time and has limited time off available. Per conversation with the patient, his wife has questioned much of his medical management and prefers to consult with close family members and spiritual leaders. Although the patient was high functioning and independent at baseline, he has a history of two mechanical falls within the past year "tripping over things" outside. He is anxious to return to his job in order to provide for his family, expressing much concern about his privately paid health insurance coverage.

GUIDING QUESTIONS: PART 1

1. Considering the visual, somatosensory, and vestibular systems, which is most often affected by the patient's preexisting medical conditions, and how would you assess it?

2. Given his history of falls, which modality(ies) should you examine? Why? Which standardized tests and measures will you administer for data collection?

(Continued)

CASE STUDY—cont'd

3. How would you examine pain sensation, and what findings would you expect given the long-standing history of diabetes along with spine injury? Why is it important to examine pain sensation?

4. How would you quantitatively measure touch awareness (touch-evoked potentials) in this patient?

CASE STUDY PHYSICAL THERAPY EXAMINATION FINDINGS

Arousal, Attention, Communication, and Cognition: Alert, oriented. Able to follow multi-step commands. Lacks insight into the seriousness of his condition and current functional limitations.

Pain: At rest: 2/10 mid to lower back radiating to bilateral lower extremities; achy. With mobility: increases to 4/10; sharp, shooting.

Cardiopulmonary: HR: 78 bpm; BP: 118/76 mm Hg sitting; 128/82 post ambulation

Integument: Bilateral calluses base of hallux metatarsal heads.

Tone: Mild flexor spasticity (1 on the Modified Ashworth Scale) in bilateral hip flexors. Three to four beats bilateral ankle clonus noted with dorsiflexion quick stretch.

Sensory Integrity: Paresthesia in bilateral lower extremities with mild loss of proprioception and vibration (distal more than proximal). Intact sharp/dull discrimination and light touch bilaterally C2-T8; impaired and spotty below T8.

Passive ROM: Screened in supine. All within normal limits except 0° to 5° bilateral ankle dorsiflexion.

Muscle Performance: Screened in supine. Mild weakness in bilateral lower extremities; able to move against gravity, with the greatest weakness noted with hip flexion, extension, and abduction.

Functional Mobility: Bed mobility and supine to/from sitting: Independent rolling to right and left. *Transfers and Ambulation:* Supervision with use of cane; unsteady without loss of balance. *Stairs:* Supervision step-to-step pattern ascending and descending with one railing with increased time needed to complete without loss of balance.

Balance: *Observation of functional activities:* Loss of balance with dynamic gait with body/head turns and starting/stopping with ability to self-correct. *Timed Up and Go Test:* 14.8 seconds.

Gait: Slow, self-selected walking speed; steppage gait with inconsistent base of support; and overall increased step variability. Patient looks down and walks as if throwing his feet, which tend to slap on the ground; worsens with balance and/or terrain challenges.

GUIDING QUESTIONS: PART 2

1. Based on the sensory integrity test findings, what receptors are responsible for these sensory modalities? Where are the receptors located? Identify the ascending pathway that mediates these sensory modalities.

2. Based on the history of this patient's case and the physical therapy examinations findings, what education and resources would you provide to this patient and family? Are there any needed referrals to other health-care providers?

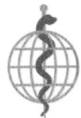

For additional resources, including answers to the questions for review, new immersive cases, case study guiding questions, references, and more, please visit **https://www.fadavis.com/product/physical-rehabilitation-fulk-8**. You may also quickly find the resources by entering this title's four-digit ISBN, 4691, in the search field at **http://fadavis.com** and logging in at the prompt.

Musculoskeletal Examination

Evangelos Pappas, PT, MSc, PhD
Eric J. Hegedus, PT, DPT, PhD, MHSc, OCS

Chapter 4

LEARNING OBJECTIVES

1. Identify the purposes of performing a musculoskeletal examination.
2. Discuss the components of a musculoskeletal examination.
3. Identify questions that should be included in a patient interview.
4. Describe the procedures used to selectively test specific tissue types in a musculoskeletal examination.
5. Identify additional procedures that often complement a musculoskeletal examination.
6. Using the case study examples, apply clinical decision-making skills in evaluating musculoskeletal examination data.

CHAPTER OUTLINE

PURPOSES OF THE MUSCULOSKELETAL EXAMINATION *103*
EXAMINATION PROCEDURES *104*
  Patient History *104*
  Observation/Inspection *110*
  Screening Examination *111*
  Palpation *113*
  Motion *113*

Muscle Performance *118*
Tissue-Specific Tests *120*
Functional Movement Analysis *121*
Additional Tests and Measurements *121*
EVALUATION OF EXAMINATION FINDINGS *122*
SUMMARY *123*

The musculoskeletal system includes bones; muscles with their related tendons and synovial sheaths; bursa; and joint structures such as cartilage, menisci, capsules, and ligaments. The musculoskeletal system works in concert with the nervous system to produce purposeful movement. Injury and disease can greatly affect function by causing impairments such as pain, inflammation, limited movement, instability, and weakness. Examples of diagnoses that result in direct impairment of the musculoskeletal system include fracture, rheumatoid arthritis, and other systemic diseases, osteoarthritis, joint dislocation, tendinosis, bursitis, muscle strain/rupture, and ligament sprain/rupture. Of note is that musculoskeletal disorders are the second most common cause of disability worldwide, measured by years lived with disability, with low back pain being the most frequent condition.[1] In addition to primary musculoskeletal impairments, many pathological conditions that initially affect other body systems, such as the neurological, cardiovascular, or pulmonary systems, can result in secondary or indirect impairment of the musculoskeletal system. Both direct and indirect musculoskeletal impairments can contribute to activity limitations and participation restrictions that affect a patient's ability to perform certain tasks and roles

in society. Thus, performing a systematic, evidence-based, and thorough evaluation is an important skill for health-care professionals who encounter patients with musculoskeletal disorders, as it will form the foundation of an effective treatment plan. In addition to an understanding of the musculoskeletal system and the pathologies that affect it, the clinician must understand psychosocial aspects of care that affect outcome.

This chapter discusses the purposes of, and provides a general framework for, conducting a musculoskeletal examination. Other resources are available that provide detailed musculoskeletal testing procedures of specific body regions.[2]

■ PURPOSES OF THE MUSCULOSKELETAL EXAMINATION

Evaluation of data from the musculoskeletal examination contributes to establishing a diagnosis and prognosis, setting anticipated goals and expected outcomes, and developing and implementing a plan of care (POC). A musculoskeletal examination is also an important component of evaluating treatment effectiveness throughout an episode of care. The purposes of performing a musculoskeletal examination include the following:

1. To determine the presence and extent of impairments, activity limitations, and disability
2. To identify the specific tissues and pathology causing/contributing to the impairment, activity limitation, or disability when possible
3. To establish objective baseline status against which progress will be measured
4. To formulate appropriate goals, expected outcomes, and a POC in consultation with the patient
5. To determine the presence of red flags and yellow flags and determine if consultation with other health-care providers is required
6. To identify risk factors associated with the development or worsening of impairments, activity limitations, or disabilities
7. To determine the need for orthotic and adaptive equipment necessary for functional performance of activities of daily living (ADL) and occupational and/or recreational activities
8. To assess and address psychosocial issues including social determinants of health that may interfere with recovery and motivate the patient
9. To establish a therapeutic alliance with the patient
10. To gather data on prognostic factors that may predict outcome

■ EXAMINATION PROCEDURES

Patient History

Before beginning the physical examination, it is important to gain as much information as possible about the patient's current condition and past medical history. This information will help to direct and focus the physical examination to an area and system of the body. Information on symptoms and functional ability will help to establish a baseline against which treatment effectiveness can be judged. It will also help ensure that the examination and subsequent treatment are conducted safely and efficiently.

In an outpatient setting, most of this information is obtained through intake forms, outcome measures, and while interviewing the patient. However, utilizing other information sources can be efficient and provide objectivity and details to supplement interview data. If the patient is hospitalized in an acute care or rehabilitation setting, the medical records—including admission reports, progress notes, medication sheets, surgical summaries, imaging reports, and laboratory test results—should be available and sought out. Referral summaries from previous medical care settings that review prior treatment approaches and discuss functional status may also be included. Other members of the health-care team can be consulted for their input.

Medications

The type, frequency, dose, and effect of medications the patient is taking should be noted. The use of analgesic or anti-inflammatory medications may reduce the intensity of symptoms at the time of the examination. Changes in the use of these medications may make it difficult to determine the effects of physical therapy treatment. The secondary effects of some medications may necessitate the modification of examination and treatment techniques. For example, prolonged use of corticosteroids is associated with *osteopenia* (reduced bone mass) and reduced tensile strength of ligaments. The therapist should consider these side effects when applying manual force in the course of the examination. The use of anticoagulants may make the patient susceptible to contusions and *hemarthrosis* and require close monitoring for bruising and joint swelling. The amount of force used in exercise and manual therapies may need to be reduced. Medications that affect balance and motor coordination may make the prescription of certain exercises risky. Therapists should investigate the potential side effects of medications that patients are using and make appropriate modifications to the POC. Finally, patients frequently ask therapists about whether they should use certain medications. Therapists are encouraged to obtain a thorough understanding of the physical therapy practice act within their state and ensure that they stay within its limits when they answer questions regarding medications.

Imaging

Due to direct access and changes in tertiary education programs, physical therapists are increasingly becoming the primary care musculoskeletal specialists of choice. As part of this evolving role, they are frequently provided with the opportunity to incorporate the findings of imaging and other medical information into the musculoskeletal assessment. Many physical therapy programs have either dedicated courses or large aspects of courses focusing on imaging. Similarly, dedicated textbooks provide therapists with the necessary expertise to incorporate the findings of imaging studies in the diagnostic process.[3] Incidental findings in imaging studies are common,[4] and so it is important to correlate the findings of the physical examination with imaging findings. Imaging, like other steps of the examination process, is not the definitive diagnostic standard, and it needs to be viewed in the context of the physical examination findings.

Medical History and Systems Review

Outpatient clients often arrive with only a general diagnosis from a referring physician, or they may be self-referred. In such cases, it will be helpful to ask the patient to complete a medical history questionnaire before the examination begins. This questionnaire should include space for the patient to note the chief problem and date of onset; diagnostic tests performed for the problem; name and date of all surgeries; all medications currently being taken; past or current treatment for the problem (including those initiated by patient); a checklist of common medical conditions the patient may have experienced; brief family medical history; and questions regarding patient's age, occupation, and lifestyle, such as smoking, alcohol use, and exercise. Figure 4.1 provides an example of a medical history questionnaire. The *APTA Guide to Physical Therapist Practice* also includes a detailed template for a patient self-administered health questionnaire.[5] The location, intensity, and quality of pain are frequently assessed with a body diagram that is completed by the patient (Fig. 4.2). The McGill Pain Questionnaire[6] can clarify symptoms further (Fig. 4.3).

A thorough understanding of the patient's medical history is critical for selection and safe application of examination and treatment procedures. This history may also indicate a need for further systems review. Conditions involving the cardiac, respiratory, neurological, vascular, metabolic, endocrine, gastrointestinal, genital urinary, visual, and dermatological systems should be noted. It is likely impractical and inefficient to perform a thorough review of all systems on every patient; however, including blood pressure screening or other relevant vital signs (see Chapter 2, Examination of Vital Signs) as part of the physical examination in the outpatient setting has the potential to improve hypertension detection rates and inform rehabilitation programs.[7] Additionally, the systems identified as potential issues on intake forms or in medical records should be further screened. For example, a family history of heart disease or risk factors such as obesity and smoking should prompt the therapist to further investigate symptoms that may indicate cardiovascular system involvement and make appropriate referral. A history of diabetes mellitus should prompt the therapist to suspect and test for potentially compromised peripheral vascular and peripheral nervous systems, and to possibly avoid the use of heat modalities during treatment.

In addition to vital signs, blood and urine laboratory tests may be available, particularly in the inpatient setting, and provide important information that can assist the clinician in the diagnosis and in formulating a POC. For example, laboratory values can provide information about the safety and intensity of exercise interventions. Normal laboratory values vary based on age, sex, and race. Normative values on cholesterol and glucose can be found in Chapter 15, Stroke. The Academy of Acute Care Physical Therapy has a task force on laboratory values that has published a comprehensive resource on this topic (https://www.aptaacutecare.org/page/ResourceGuides). Normal laboratory values can be easily accessed online (https://www.physio-pedia.com/Lab_Value_Interpretation) or as an application on smartphones.

Physical therapists are embracing an increasingly important role in the promotion of health and wellness for their patients, particularly in states with direct access. Thus, it is important that they are competent in the assessment of lifestyle factors and their association with musculoskeletal pathology (see Chapter 29, Promoting Health and Wellness). Therapists need to be especially aware of pathologies that mimic signs and symptoms of the musculoskeletal system. For example, inflammation of the gallbladder (cholecystitis) may result in right shoulder pain. However, shoulder pain related to cholecystitis typically is not mechanical—that is, it will not increase with shoulder movements or testing of shoulder musculature, as would typically occur in the presence of musculoskeletal conditions. Patients with cholecystitis would likely have additional symptoms such as upper abdominal discomfort, bloating, belching, nausea, and intolerance of fried foods. Knowledge of systemic human pathology, part of what are called "red flags," allows the therapist to recognize conditions requiring additional physician evaluation and intervention. For example, a previous history of malignancy increases the likelihood of spinal malignancy, while older age, prolonged corticosteroid use, severe trauma, and the presence of a contusion or abrasion increase the likelihood of spinal fracture.[8] "Yellow flags" are discussed in the patient interview section and refer to psychological factors that are related to outcomes. Physical therapists, especially those with orthopedic board certification, demonstrate very high levels of competence in making correct decisions for medical referral.[9] Clinical practice guidelines frequently recommend red flag screening as an appropriate part of the examination process.[10] Coordinated efforts in recent years to create more evidence-based red flag screening tools are promising and may result in more accurate identification of patients with serious pathology.[11] Having a patient complete a medical history questionnaire before the examination is an efficient means of obtaining this information, but the information should be verified during the interview with targeted questions that aim to elicit information about answers that are not clear in the questionnaire.

Patient-Reported Outcome Measures

A good practice that allows the therapist to establish the impact of injury or pathology at baseline is the use of validated generic, condition- or body region–specific patient-reported outcome measures. These questionnaires are a precursor of the patient interview and are time-efficient, as they can be completed by the patient and reviewed by the therapist, improving the patient interview. They also provide valuable information regarding patient progress when reissued at regular intervals throughout treatment. Clinicians should consider the psychometric properties (e.g., content validity, minimal detectable change, responsiveness) of these patient-reported outcome measures in the population

The purpose of this questionnaire is to assist us in providing you with quality care by obtaining a better understanding of your total health status. This questionnaire is part of your confidential medical record.

NAME: _____ DATE: _____

CHIEF PROBLEM OR COMPLAINT: _____

REFERRING MD: _____ DATE OF NEXT MD VISIT: _____

MEDICATIONS: Please list *all* medications currently being taken, along with the dosage, if known, and frequency.

1. _____   4. _____

2. _____   5. _____

3. _____   6. _____

SURGERY: Please list *all* surgeries and approximate date.

1. _____   DATE: _____

2. _____   DATE: _____

3. _____   DATE: _____

4. _____   DATE: _____

DIAGNOSTIC TESTS: Please check tests for current problem only.

X-rays: _____   CT Scan: _____   MRI: _____   Bone Scan: _____

EMG: _____   Blood Test: _____   Myelogram: _____   Others: _____

OCCUPATION: _____

LIFE STYLE: Non-Smoker: _____ Smoke _____/day

No Alcohol: _____ Alcohol _____/day or _____/week

No Exercise: _____ Exercise _____/day or _____/week

FAMILY HISTORY: Mother, Father, siblings: Alive and healthy: _____

If deceased, cause of death: _____

Figure 4.1 An example of a medical history recording form. *(Courtesy of North Andover Physical Therapy Associates, North Andover, MA.)*

DO YOU HAVE, OR HAVE YOU HAD, ANY OF THE FOLLOWING: Please check *all* that apply.

___ High blood pressure
___ Heart problems
___ Heart palpitations, murmur
___ Chest pain

___ Shortness of breath
___ Coughing

___ Difficulty sleeping lying flat
___ Lung problems
___ Asthma
___ Allergies

___ Ulcers
___ Recent weight gain or loss
___ Nausea, vomiting
___ Bowel or bladder changes
___ Loss of appetite

___ Sexual dysfunction
___ Abnormal or painful menstruation
___ Pelvic inflammatory disease
___ Currently pregnant
___ Date of last mammogram:_____

___ Blood in urine
___ Incontinence

___ Seizures
___ Head trauma
___ Paralysis
___ Loss of consciousness
___ Headaches

___ Numbness or tingling
___ Dizziness
___ Balance problems

___ Arthritis

___ Hot or cold intolerance
___ Diabetes
___ Low blood sugar
___ Thyroid problems

___ Tumors ___ Cancer
___ Bleeding or bruising
___ Dialysis
___ Blood transfusion

___ Rashes
___ Scars
___ Changes in hair or nails

___ Wear eyeglasses, contacts
___ Changes in vision
___ Blurred or double vision

___ Difficulty swallowing
___ Ear pain
___ Vocal changes
___ Ringing in ears

___ Dentures
___ Major dental work
___ Difficulty eating

___ Varicose veins
___ Muscle cramps
___ Joint or muscle pain

___ Psychiatric or psychological care

___ Fractures (broken bones)
      Where?_____
___ Problem requiring orthopedic shoes
___ Hip or ankle problem
___ Unusual illness as child

Please check if you have ever been in a motor vehicle accident _____

Figure 4.1—cont'd

of interest. Examples of such questionnaires include the following:

- Patient-Specific Functional Scale (PSFS) for multiple patient populations[12]
- Western Ontario and McMaster Universities Osteoarthritis Index (WOMAC) for knee and hip osteoarthritis (www.physio-pedia.com/WOMAC_Osteoarthritis_Index)
- Neck Disability Index (NDI) for neck pain (www.physio-pedia.com/Neck_Disability_Index)
- Oswestry Disability Index for low back pain (https://en.wikipedia.org/wiki/Oswestry_Disability_Index)
- Disabilities of the Arm, Shoulder and Hand questionnaire (DASH) for upper extremity disorders (www.physio-pedia.com/DASH_Outcome_Measure)
- Knee injury and Osteoarthritis Outcome Score (www.koos.nu/)
- Fear-Avoidance Beliefs Questionnaire (FABQ) (www.physio-pedia.com/Fear%E2%80%90Avoidance_Belief_Questionnaire)
- Tampa Scale of Kinesiophobia (TSK) (https://www.physio-pedia.com/Tampa_Scale_of_Kinesiophobia)

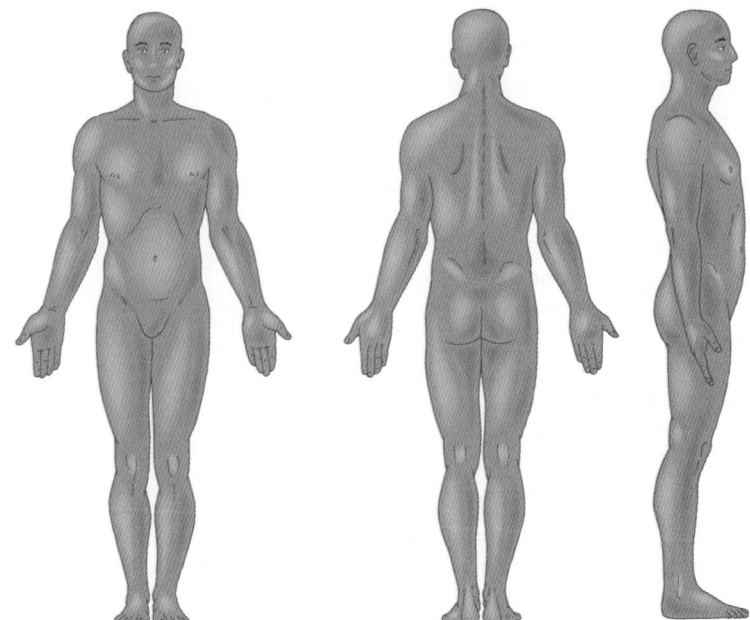

Figure 4.2 This body chart can supplement the patient's verbal description of the location of the pain.

Look carefully at the twenty groups of words. If any word in any group applies to *your* pain, please circle that word — but do not circle more than *one word in any one group* — so you must choose the *most suitable word* in that group.

In groups that do not apply to your pain, there is no need to circle *any* word — just leave them as they are.

Group 1	*Group 2*	*Group 3*	*Group 4*	*Group 5*
Flickering	Jumping	Pricking	Sharp	Pinching
Quivering	Flashing	Boring	Gritting	Pressing
Pulsing	Shooting	Drilling	Lacerating	Gnawing
Throbbing		Stabbing		Cramping
Beating		Lancinating		Crushing
Pounding				
Group 6	*Group 7*	*Group 8*	*Group 9*	*Group 10*
Tugging	Hot	Tingling	Dull	Tender
Pulling	Burning	Itching	Sore	Taut
Wrenching	Scalding	Smarting	Hurting	Rasping
	Searing	Stinging	Aching	Splitting
			Heavy	
Group 11	*Group 12*	*Group 13*	*Group 14*	*Group 15*
Tiring	Sickening	Fearful	Punishing	Wretched
Exhausting	Suffocating	Frightful	Gruelling	Blinding
		Terrifying	Cruel	
			Vicious	
			Killing	
Group 16	*Group 17*	*Group 18*	*Group 19*	*Group 20*
Annoying	Spreading	Tight	Cool	Nagging
Troublesome	Radiating	Numb	Cold	Nauseating
Miserable	Penetrating	Drawing	Freezing	Agonizing
Intense	Piercing	Squeezing		Dreadful
Unbearable		Tearing		Torturing

Figure 4.3 The McGill Pain Questionnaire. The first 10 groups of words are somatic (describing what the pain feels like), 11 to 15 are affective, 16 is evaluative, and 17 to 20 are miscellaneous. *(From Melzack.)*[10]

Clinicians are strongly encouraged to identify appropriate patient-reported outcome measures for their patient population and routinely use them at the initial examination and during reexamination sessions.

Patient Interview

After reviewing the information gained from medical history, imaging, laboratory values, medications, and patient-reported outcome measures, the therapist is ready to begin the patient interview. The interview has many critical functions: (1) establishing rapport, comfort, trust; (2) establishing a partnership or therapeutic alliance; (3) allowing the physical therapist to have a greater understanding of how pain and injury are affecting the patient's life; (4) determining the patient's readiness for behavioral change; (5) gaining insight into any social barriers to care and recovery; (6) understanding the patient's cognitive ability and ability to communicate; (7) discovering any red or yellow flags that require referral or co-treatment by a professional outside of physical therapy; and (8) enhancing the diagnostic process by further ruling in some diagnoses while ruling out others.

The value of this first encounter is so great that many experienced clinicians spend more time in the patient interview than they do in the physical examination. Establishing rapport, comfort, and trust as well as understanding barriers to care and the impact of pain and injury in the patient's life form the foundation for a therapeutic alliance or partnership. Having a strong therapeutic alliance seems to improve outcomes in many patient populations,[13] especially in those with chronic musculoskeletal pain.[14] Many outcomes are reliant on behavioral change by the patient. For example, a patient who has sequelae from obesity-related diabetes will likely need to embrace both dietary changes and activity changes to manage the symptoms effectively. To discover the patient's readiness for change, motivational interviewing is often employed to facilitate discovering the source of the patient's ambivalence for and barriers to change in a way that guides them to finding their own solutions. Motivational interviewing is based on the transtheoretical model of behavior change that includes stages of change: precontemplation, contemplation, preparation, action, and maintenance.[15] Determining the stage of change will assist the clinician to focus interventions, goals, and use of resources. For more information on this topic see Chapter 29, Promoting Health and Wellness.

Gaining insight into any social barriers to care allows the clinician to address some of the social determinants of health, which include access to quality (or any) health care, economic stability, access to education, and neighborhood environment. These social determinants of health have an important relationship to outcome.[16,17]

Communication and cognitive ability such as orientation to person, place, and time, as well as general arousal state are also assessed during the interview. If deficits in these areas are present, the examination may need to be modified to gain accurate information. The use of simple words, concise instructions, and task demonstrations may be helpful. Distractions in the environment should be kept to a minimum. Communication difficulties may be overcome through the use of foreign language interpreters or software applications, gestures, drawings, and language boards. Changes in medications, upright positioning, and access to natural light via windows and skylights may improve patient arousal and orientation to time. Depending on the type of deficit, the patient may benefit from an evaluation by a neurologist, neuropsychologist, speech-language pathologist, and/or occupational therapist.

The therapist should keep in mind that one of the goals of the assessment is to decide whether the pathology falls within the scope of physical therapy practice. In this respect, the therapist should carefully explore the possibility of red (discussed earlier in this chapter) and yellow flags that may require consultation with or referral to a different health-care practitioner. Red flags, signs of more serious pathology, and yellow flags, psychological factors, can be addressed in the patient interview. These psychological factors/yellow flags like kinesiophobia, depression, and anxiety have a relationship with pain and outcomes.[18] Common tools used to screen for yellow flags are the Patient Health Questionnaire for Depression and Anxiety (PHQ-4)[19] and the Optimal Screening for Prediction of Referral and Outcome Yellow Flag (OSPRO-YF).[20]

Finally, information from the patient interview can help increase suspicion of some pathologies while helping to lessen suspicion of some others. A salient example is with rotator cuff tear diagnosis. If the patient answers "no" to either query about pain with overhead activity and pain at night while sleeping on their shoulder, the likelihood is less that the patient's shoulder pain is a torn rotator cuff.[21] On the other hand, if the patient is aged 65 years or older, has pain at night, and presents with weakness in shoulder external rotation during the physical exam, there is a moderate likelihood that the patient has a rotator cuff tear.[22]

The following sequence is suggested as a way of organizing the interview. Similar information on general patient interviewing can be found in other texts.[23,24] The interview should begin with an open-ended question

such as, "I have read the information you filled out, but please tell me more about this issue." It is important to listen actively and reflectively in order to understand all relevant details. All questions should use conversational language rather than medical terminology so the patient easily understands the questions. The therapist should ask one question at a time and obtain a response before proceeding to other questions. Follow-up inquiries may be needed to clarify initial answers. Ideally, the patient interview should be conducted in a quiet, well-lit room that offers a measure of privacy. To encourage good communication, the therapist and patient should be at a similar eye level, facing each other, with a comfortable space between them of about 3 feet (1 meter). The patient should have the therapist's undivided attention; telephone calls and other interruptions should be avoided. The therapist may wish to have paper and pen or an electronic device available to take notes, but the interview should flow as an active conversation, not a dictation session. If the therapist uses an electronic device to document the interview, this should be explained to the patient in advance to avoid misunderstandings.

The patient should be given the opportunity to present their story and what this injury means to them. The therapist should ask follow-up questions to differentiate between pain and loss of function or disability, identify the first occurrence of the symptoms (even if it was several years ago), get a detailed account of the mechanism of injury (if relevant), understand the change in symptoms over time and their behavior during the day, understand the irritability of the condition, identify factors that alleviate or aggravate the symptoms, and establish the type and effectiveness of previous treatments. In the conclusion of this phase of the interview, it is important to understand the goals that your patient has for physical therapy. The patient's goals will provide information that should be used at the end of the physical examination to formulate a mutually agreed upon treatment plan. The therapist should not presume to know what issues are important to the patient. Answers to these questions help the therapist to determine the patient's expectations for their recovery. For example, an older patient who is hospitalized after a fractured hip may expect to remain in the acute care hospital for 2 weeks before being able to independently ambulate and resume self-care. Given current health insurance practices, more realistic goals may need to be discussed, such as discharge from the hospital in 3 or 4 days to a rehabilitation or extended care facility for further nursing care and physical and occupational therapy, or discharge home with home health aides, visiting nurses, and home care physical and occupational therapists.

Finally, it is a good habit for the therapist to conclude the interview by asking the patient if there is anything else to add and allow enough time for a response. The information elicited with the questions discussed earlier may be supplemented with additional questions based on the specific region of the body being examined and suspected etiologies. The physical therapist's knowledge of anatomy, kinesiology, pathokinesiology, physiology, and pathophysiology, as well as the physical presentation and progression of musculoskeletal conditions, provides the appropriate background on which to base and develop patient interview questions.

Observation/Inspection

Observation begins with the therapist's first contact with the patient, whether at bedside or in the examination room. Observation of the patient provides a great deal of information and, after patient interview and systems review, is the next step of the diagnostic process. Observation should be performed with maximum exposure of the patient according to what is clinically appropriate and respecting the patient's privacy. Maximum exposure allows inspection of the integumentary system, a potential window to underlying pathology. A complete guide to integumentary inspection is beyond the scope of this chapter. Briefly, a conscientious clinician will look for the "4 Cs": color or pigmentation, contour, coldness (temperature), and capillary refill. Changes in color or pigmentation may help discern skin diseases that require referral, like tinea versicolor or vitiligo or underlying inflammatory disease in the case of erythema. *Cyanosis* (a blue discoloration of the skin and lips in white people or gray discoloration in people of color) in the hands and feet may indicate serious pathology of the cardiopulmonary system. Contour may reveal edema and lesions of the skin, ranging from malignant (melanoma) to communicable (scabies) to benign (lipoma). *Clubbing,* in which the distal finger and nail become rounded (bulbous), may be caused by chronic hypoxemia and is typically associated with cardiovascular and respiratory diseases or neurovascular abnormalities (see Fig. 2.1 in Chapter 2).[11] Skin tissue thickenings such as *calluses* can indicate areas of repeated stress. Coldness, a reminder to check temperature with palpation, can indicate lack of blood flow to an area or in the case of excessive warmth, an active inflammatory process. Capillary refill is an indication of blood flow to a region and may be limited, for example, in diabetes and atherosclerosis.

Beyond integumentary observation, an astute clinician can determine the patient's desire to move, affect, level of orientation, functional ability, and general health, especially when combined with the detailed history that has already taken place. These vital pieces of information help to guide the individualized physical examination and create greater suspicion of some pathologies while decreasing suspicion of others. For example, imagine two patients with a knee issue, one is overweight, using oxygen, arrives in a wheelchair, and reports a chronic issue, while the other limps in independently and reports a traumatic onset. The therapist can make assumptions about the vitality of these patients and the knee pathologies that might be a greater

possibility in a chronic situation compared to an acute onset. Further, the therapist might want to think about clarifying questions to ask, examination techniques that will be tolerated, and what screening examinations to perform to differentially diagnose, for example, osteoarthritis versus a possible fracture.

As the physical therapist moves from global observation to a more detailed inspection of a region and joint, symmetry takes on heightened importance. The therapist should view the body region/joint anteriorly, posteriorly, and from the sides. Often, detailed palpation, which is discussed later, is combined with observation. Bone shafts and joints are compared against the opposite side of the body for symmetry. Contour and alignment should be considered. Common causes of changes in bone contour include acute fractures, callus formation or bone angulation owing to healed fractures, congenital variations, bone hyperplasia at tendon insertions, and arthritis. Alignment differences can be due to the above conditions as well as muscle and soft tissue tightness, muscle weakness, ligament laxity, and joint dislocation.

For patients with musculoskeletal involvement, an examination for postural alignment is often performed. From an *anterior* view, both eyes, shoulders (acromion processes), iliac crests, anterior superior iliac spines, greater trochanters of the femur, patellae, and ankle medial malleoli should be horizontally level. Waist angles should be symmetrical. Patellae and feet should face anteriorly. *Laterally,* the line of gravity should bisect the external auditory meatus, acromion process, and greater trochanter, and lie just posterior to the patella and anterior to the lateral malleolus (Fig. 4.4).[25]

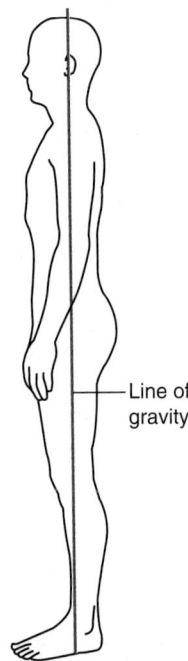

Figure 4.4 The location of the line of gravity from the lateral view. *(From Levangie and Norkin,[25] with permission.)*

The cervical and lumbar spine should exhibit normal lordotic curves and the thoracic spine a normal kyphotic curve. From a *posterior* view, the earlobes, shoulders, inferior angles of the scapula, iliac crests, posterior superior iliac spines, greater trochanters, buttock and knee creases, and malleoli should be level. The spine should be straight, with the medial borders of the scapulae equidistant from the spine. Varus, valgus, and hyperextension knee deformities and pes planus/cavus should be noted.

The therapist should be aware of the mixed evidence regarding the association between posture and pain/pathology and avoid the temptation to make a diagnosis or to attempt to correct small postural deviations that cannot be reasonably linked to patients' impairments. For example, even though increased thoracic kyphosis can restrict shoulder range of motion (ROM), there is currently no evidence that it predisposes people to shoulder pain.[26] On the other hand, there is more evidence that a pronated foot posture is linked to the development of lower extremity (LE) overuse injuries.[27] Postural assessment remains an important aspect of physical therapy examination and should be measured with objective tools when possible as one of the factors that may contribute to the development of pain.[28] Clinicians should critically assess the relationship between the patient's posture and symptoms or pathology and avoid generic advice against sitting or standing "incorrectly," as the evidence between common postures and pain prevention is rather tenuous.[29]

Abnormalities noted during observation may be further documented with objective anthropometric measurements. Using a flexible plastic tape measure, limb lengths are measured between bony landmarks and compared bilaterally. For example, leg length is commonly measured from the anterior superior iliac spine to the lateral malleolus. Circumferential measurements help substantiate joint effusion, edema, and muscle hypertrophy and atrophy. Typically, these measurements are taken at specified distances above or below a bony landmark so they can be reliably reproduced during subsequent measurements. For example, circumference measurements of the upper arm should be taken at noted distances distal to the acromion process or proximal to the olecranon process. If measurements are needed of the hands or feet, volumetric measurements can be taken by submerging the distal extremity in a container of water and noting the volume of water that is displaced.

Screening Examination

The musculoskeletal physical therapist will frequently encounter patients who report symptoms in one area that could be arising from body regions away from that area. For example, patients who report neck and upper extremity (UE) symptoms may have pathology in the neck, in the UE, or in both regions. Screening examinations like the upper quarter and lower quarter screens assess gross ROM, strength, sensation, and reflexes for the purposes of reproducing the concordant sign (usually pain or weakness), determining where best to focus a more detailed examination, and continuing to differentially diagnose. For example, in the case of upper quarter pain (neck and arm), if cervical ROM is full, symmetrical, and painless, it is unlikely that the neck is the source of the symptoms, and the examination should be focused elsewhere in the extremity. If, on the other hand, cervical motion causes change in peripheral symptoms, a more thorough cervical examination is required. The upper and lower quarter screens should not take more than a few minutes to perform, and their findings frequently allow the therapist to have greater suspicion of the pathology (e.g., radiculopathy, peripheral neuropathy, contractile tissue pathology). A detailed knowledge of myotomes, dermatomes, and reflexes based on nerve root level is required to identify the spinal level that causes the symptoms (Fig. 4.5). Dermatomes (sensation), myotomes (strength), and reflex testing all have their limitations. Dermatomal distribution varies and is debatable,[30] and myotomes and reflexes are most reliable when compared to the opposite side of the body. Despite these limitations, upper and lower quarter screening examinations are important as the clinician narrows down the clinical examination to a small number of potential diagnoses while ruling other diagnoses out as a possibility.

In addition to these screens, there are other tools that have been created to assist practitioners, most notably, the Ottawa Knee Rules[31] and the Ottawa Ankle Rules.[32] These tools have high sensitivity so that a negative finding would rule out pathology (and the need for imaging). The Ottawa Knee Rules, for example, are used in the case of acute (7 days or less) traumatic knee pain and state that if the patient has any one of the following—at least 55 years old, inability to bear weight immediately after trauma and in the clinic for four steps regardless of limp, or isolated patellar tenderness, fibular head tenderness, or an inability to flex the knee to at least 90°—then an x-ray must be ordered due to suspicion of fracture. If the patient has none of these signs or symptoms, then a fracture can be ruled out, and x-rays are not necessary. The pooled sensitivity from multiple studies on adults is 99%,[33] and even children as young as 5 years of age may benefit from the Ottawa Knee Rules.[34] The Ottawa Ankle Rules apply to the ankle and midfoot and have similarly high sensitivity.[35] The Ottawa Ankle Rules are also for acute traumatic injuries and state that an x-ray is required if there is pain in the malleolar or midfoot region and any one of the following: pain with palpation at the posterior tip of the medial malleolus, at the posterior tip of the lateral malleolus, base of the fifth metatarsal, over the navicular; or an inability to bear weight regardless of limp immediately and in the clinic. If none of these are present, then a fracture can

SPINAL NERVE AND MUSCLE CHART

NECK, DIAPHRAGM AND UPPER EXTREMITY

Name

Date

PERIPHERAL NERVES

KEY ⟶ D. = Dorsal Prim. Ramus
V. = Vent. Prim. Ramus
P.R. = Plexus Root
S.T. = Superior Trunk
P. = Posterior Cord
L. = Lateral Cord
M. = Medial Cord

Group	Muscle Strength Grade	Muscle	Cervical (D. 1-8, T. 1)	Cervical (V. 1-8, T. 1)	Cervical (V. 1-4)	Phrenic (V. 3, 4, 5)	Long Thor. (P.R. 5, 6, 7, (8))	Dor. Scap (P.R. 4, 5)	N. to Subcl. (S.T. 5, 6)	Suprascap (S.T. 4, 5, 6)	U. Subscap. (P. (4), 5, 6, (7))	Thoracodor (P. (5), 6, 7, 8)	L. Subscap. (P. 5, 6, (7))	Lat. Pect. (L. 5, 6, 7)	Med. Pect. (M. (6), 7, 8, T. 1)	Axillary (P. 5, 6)	Musculocu. (L. (4), 5, 6, 7)	Radial (P. 5, 6, 7, 8, T. 1)	Median (L.M. 5, 6, 7, 8, T. 1)	Ulnar (M. 7, 8, T. 1)	C1	C2	C3	C4	C5	C6	C7	C8	T1
		HEAD & NECK EXTENSORS	•																		1	2	3	4	5	6	7	8	1
Cervical nerves		INFRAHYOID MUSCLES			•																1	2	3						
Cervical nerves		RECTUS CAP ANT. & LAT.			•																1	2							
Cervical nerves		LONGUS CAPITIS			•																1	2	3	(4)					
Cervical nerves		LONGUS COLLI		•																		2	3	4	5	6	(7)		
Cervical nerves		LEVATOR SCAPULAE			•			•															3	4	5				
Cervical nerves		SCALENI (A. M. P.)		•																			3	4	5	6	7	8	
Cervical nerves		STERNOCLEIDOMASTOID			•																(1)	2	3						
Cervical nerves		TRAPEZIUS (U. M. L.)			•																	2	3	4					
Cervical nerves		DIAPHRAGM				•																	3	4	5				
Brachial Plexus – Root		SERRATUS ANTERIOR					•																		5	6	7	8	
Brachial Plexus – Root		RHOMBOIDS MAJ & MIN						•																4	5				
Brachial Plexus – Trunk		SUBCLAVIUS							•																5	6			
Brachial Plexus – Trunk		SUPRASPINATUS								•														4	5	6			
Brachial Plexus – Trunk		INFRASPINATUS								•														(4)	5	6			
Brachial Plexus – P Cord		SUBSCAPULARIS									•		•												5	6	7		
Brachial Plexus – P Cord		LATISSIMUS DORSI										•														6	7	8	
Brachial Plexus – P Cord		TERES MAJOR											•												5	6	7		
Brachial Plexus – L		PECTORALIS MAJ (UPPER)												•											5	6	7		
Brachial Plexus – M&L		PECTORALIS MAJ (LOWER)												•	•											6	7	8	1
Brachial Plexus – M&L		PECTORALIS MINOR													•											(6)	7	8	1
Axil.		TERES MINOR														•									5	6			
Axil.		DELTOID														•									5	6			
Musculo-cutan		CORACOBRACHIALIS															•									6	7		
Musculo-cutan		BICEPS															•								5	6			
Musculo-cutan		BRACHIALIS															•								5	6			
Radial		TRICEPS																•								6	7	8	1
Radial		ANCONEUS																•									7	8	
Radial – Lat.M		BRACHIALIS (SMALL PART)																•							5	6			
Radial – Lat.M		BRACHIORADIALIS																•							5	6			
Radial – Lat.M		EXT CARPI RAD L																•							5	6	7	8	
Radial – Post Inter		EXT CARPI RAD B																•								6	7	(8)	
Radial – Post Inter		SUPINATOR																•							5	6	(7)		
Radial – Post Inter		EXT DIGITORUM																•								6	7	8	
Radial – Post Inter		EXT DIGITI MINIMI																•								6	7	8	
Radial – Post Inter		EXT CARPI ULNARIS																•								6	7	8	
Radial – Post Inter		ABD POLLICIS LONGUS																•								6	7	8	
Radial – Post Inter		EXT POLLICIS BREVIS																•								6	7	8	
Radial – Post Inter		EXT POLLICIS LONGUS																•								6	7	8	
Radial – Post Inter		EXT INDICIS																•								6	7	8	
Median		PRONATOR TERES																	•							6	7		
Median		FLEX CARPI RADIALIS																	•							6	7	8	
Median		PALMARIS LONGUS																	•							(6)	7	8	1
Median		FLEX DIGIT SUPERFICIALIS																	•								7	8	1
Median – A Inter		FLEX DIGIT PROF I & II																	•								7	8	1
Median – A Inter		FLEX POLLICIS LONGUS																	•							(6)	7	8	1
Median – A Inter		PRONATOR QUADRATUS																	•								7	8	1
Median		ABD POLLICIS BREVIS																	•							6	7	8	1
Median		OPPONENS POLLICIS																	•							6	7	8	1
Median		FLEX POLL BREV (SUP. H)																	•							6	7	8	1
Median		LUMBRICALES I & II																	•							(6)	7	8	1
Ulnar		FLEX CARPI ULNARIS																		•							7	8	1
Ulnar		FLEX DIGIT. PROF. III & IV																		•							7	8	1
Ulnar		PALMARIS BREVIS																		•							(7)	8	1
Ulnar		ABD DIGITI MINIMI																		•							(7)	8	1
Ulnar		OPPONENS DIGITI MINIMI																		•							(7)	8	1
Ulnar		FLEX DIGITI MINIMI																		•							(7)	8	1
Ulnar		PALMAR INTEROSSEI																		•								8	1
Ulnar		DORSAL INTEROSSEI																		•								8	1
Ulnar		LUMBRICALES III & IV																		•							(7)	8	1
Ulnar		ADDUCTOR POLLICIS																		•								8	1
Ulnar		FLEX POLL BREV. (DEEP H.)																		•								8	1

SENSORY

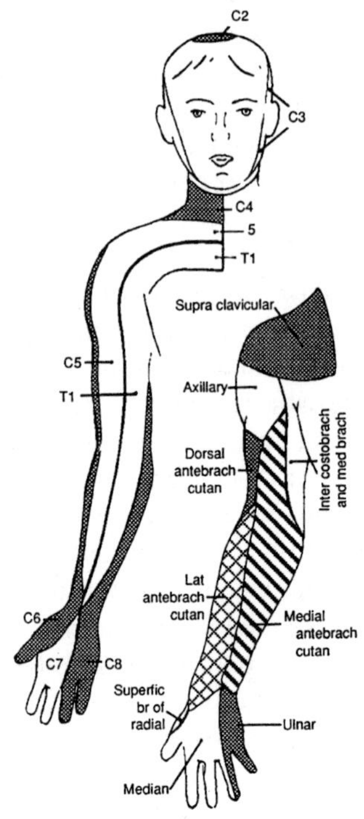

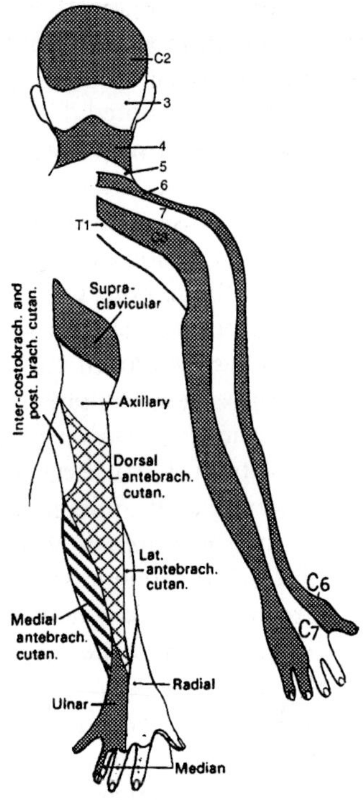

Dermatomes redrawn from Keegan and Garrett Anat Rec 102. 409. 437. 1948
Cutaneous Distribution of peripheral nerves redrawn from Gray's *Anatomy of the Human Body*. 28th ed

Figure 4.5 Manual muscle testing recording forms that aid in determining the site or level of a nerve lesion. *(From Kendall et al.,[59] with permission.)*

be ruled out, and no x-rays are necessary. In general, the tests that have a high negative likelihood ratio are most useful for ruling out diagnoses and should be included in the screening examination, while tests with a high positive likelihood ratio are more useful for ruling in diagnoses and should be included in the tissue-specific test section of the examination to differentiate between the most likely diagnoses at the end stage of the examination (see Appendix 1.C [online]).

Palpation

Palpation is an important physical therapy skill that can provide valuable information. It can be done after observation or later in the examination (especially if there is a risk that palpation can produce high levels of pain, which may then affect proper baseline measures for ROM or strength). Palpation requires detailed knowledge of anatomy and a systematic approach. All structures on one body surface should be systematically palpated before proceeding to another surface. For example, all structures on the patient's anterior surface should be palpated before beginning to palpate structures on the posterior surface. The uninvolved side is palpated first to acquaint the patient with the procedure and, in some cases, to serve as a normative model for comparison. The therapist should develop a system of moving from superior to inferior structures, medial to lateral, or superior and then inferior from a joint line. Which direction the therapist moves is not important, but the palpation process should be consistent and thorough.

Palpation of bone, soft tissue structures, and the skin is performed by varying the therapist's tactile pressure and using various parts of the hands. Light tactile pressure allows palpation of superficial tissues like the skin, whereas more pressure is needed to palpate deeper structures such as bone. Usually, the fingertips are used for palpation, but large, deeper structures such as the greater trochanter of the femur or borders of the scapula are easier to locate using the entire surface of the hand. Changes in skin temperature may be easier to detect using the posterior surface of the therapist's hand. When moving from one area to another, the therapist's hand should stay in firm contact with the skin whenever possible to prevent a tickling sensation. The fingers should not "crawl" or "walk" across the skin.

During palpation, the therapist seeks feedback from the patient to help localize painful structures, especially those that reproduce the concordant sign/symptom. Some lesions in deep or proximal structures will refer symptoms to other body areas, but localized tenderness often helps to implicate particular structures. As mentioned previously, localized skin temperature should be noted: cool temperatures can suggest reduced circulation, whereas warmth can indicate increased circulation and often inflammation. Skin and soft tissue density

and extensibility should be considered. Often, muscle spasms and adhesions in skin and connective tissue can be found with palpation. The quality (amplitude) of peripheral pulses will provide gross information on arterial blood supply. Bilateral edema in the ankles and legs that forms pits with tactile pressure (termed *pitting edema*) can indicate cardiac failure or liver or renal conditions. Unilateral pitting edema is typically associated with obstruction of venous return.

Motion

Joints and their related structures are examined by performing active, passive, and accessory joint motions. Joint motion is a necessary component of functional tasks. Numerous studies have identified the ROM needed in the LE during gait[36] and when climbing stairs,[37] rising from a chair,[38] and squatting, kneeling, and sitting cross-legged.[39,40] The ROM needed in the upper extremity to eat with a spoon[41] and perform many UE activities[42] has been examined. Careful examination of joint movement for ROM restrictions helps identify and quantify impairments causing activity limitations and may assist in the diagnosis.

Active Range of Motion

The examination of joint motion begins by testing *active range of motion* (AROM). The patient is asked to move a body part through the osteokinematic motions at the involved and other biomechanically related joints. *Osteokinematics* refers to the gross angular motions of the shafts of bones. These motions are described as occurring in the three cardinal planes of the body: flexion and extension in the sagittal plane, abduction and adduction in the frontal plane, and medial and lateral rotation in the transverse plane. For example, in the examination of the hip, the patient would be asked to move the hip into flexion, extension, abduction, adduction, and medial and lateral rotation. Often, flexion and extension of the knee, as well as flexion, extension, rotation, and lateral flexion of the lumbar spine, are tested, because knee and spine motions can affect hip function. Some therapists prefer to have the patient move in functional, combined motions rather than in straight plane motions. For example, a patient would be asked to reach a hand behind the head to test shoulder abduction and medial rotation simultaneously rather than perform isolated, individual motions.

Active motion is a good musculoskeletal screening procedure to further focus the physical examination. The amount, quality, and pattern of motion, as well as the occurrence of pain and crepitus, should be noted. For purposes of musculoskeletal screening, AROM can be visually estimated to determine if motion is within functional limits; however, objective and accurate measurements are needed to establish a pathological baseline and to evaluate treatment response. In addition to goniometers and inclinometers, smartphone applications can be used in this regard, as they have excellent psychometric properties.[43,44] Normal ROM varies among individuals and is influenced by factors such as age and sex,[45] as well as measurement methods.[46] Restricted movement can be determined by comparing to the opposite, uninvolved extremity, if possible, or to normative values by age and sex.[47] Complete and painless AROM frequently suggests that further passive testing of that motion is unnecessary unless the therapist needs to assess the end-feel. If, however, the amount of active motion is less than normal, the therapist will not be able to isolate the cause without further testing. Capsule, ligament, muscle, and soft tissue tightness; joint surface abnormalities; and muscle weakness are all capable of causing limitations in AROM. Variations in the quality and pattern of active motion can result from central and peripheral nervous system disorders and metabolic conditions, in addition to disorders involving musculoskeletal structures. So, although active motion is an effective screening procedure, positive findings require further tests to identify the underlying etiology and thus enable effective treatment.

Passive Range of Motion

Passive motions are movements performed by the therapist without the assistance of the patient. The term *passive range of motion* (PROM) typically refers to the amount of osteokinematic motion available when the patient's joint is moved without the patient's assistance. Normally, PROM is slightly greater than AROM because joints have a small amount of motion at the end of the range that is not under voluntary control. PROM is examined not only for amount of motion but also for the motion's effect on symptoms, the type of tissue resistance felt by the therapist at the end of the motion (end-feel), and the pattern of limitation.

Passive range of osteokinematic motion depends on the integrity of joint surfaces and the extensibility of the joint capsule, ligaments, muscles, tendons, and soft tissue. Limitations in PROM may be due to bone or joint abnormalities or shortening of soft tissue structures. Because the therapist, rather than the patient, provides the muscle force needed to perform PROM, it does not depend on the patient's muscle strength and coordination.

Pain during PROM is often due to moving, lengthening, or pinching of noncontractile structures. Pain occurring at the end of PROM may be due to lengthening contractile structures and noncontractile structures. Pain during PROM is not due to the active shortening (contracting) of muscle and the resulting pull on tendon and bone attachments. By comparing active and passive motions that cause pain, and noting the location of the pain, the therapist gains important information about which injured tissues are involved.

For example, on examination, a patient is found to have limited and painful active knee flexion. This pain and limitation may be coming from the contraction of the hamstring muscles, the lengthening of the quadriceps muscle, or the approximation of the tibiofemoral and patellofemoral joint surfaces, menisci, joint capsule, ligaments, or bursae. If the symptoms are eliminated during PROM, the hamstring muscles are likely the source of the symptoms (as they do not contract during PROM). The performance of resisted isometric knee flexion would be used to confirm the presence of a lesion in the hamstring muscles.

Both the beginning and the end of the motion are measured to identify the "range" of movement and are recorded using both the start and end values (e.g., 0°–110°). Using the most common notation system, the 0° to 180° system, all motions except rotation begin in anatomical position at 0° and progress toward 180°. For example, a motion that begins at 0° and ends at 135° would be recorded as 0°–135°. A ROM that does not start with 0° or ends prematurely indicates joint *hypomobility*. Joint *hypermobility* at the beginning of the range is noted by the inclusion of a zero (the normal starting position) between the starting and ending measurements. For example, if the elbow joint has 5° of hypermobility in extension and 140° of flexion, it would be recorded as 5°–0°–140°. Hypermobility at the end of the ROM is denoted by an ending value higher than normal. Measurement results are incorporated into narrative reports or recorded on specialized forms. Specialized ROM recording forms typically have joints and motions listed centrally, with multiple columns on the left and right sides to record the date, examiner's initials, and ROM values of serial measurements (Fig. 4.6). These forms readily allow comparison of serial measurements to assess patient progress.

A systematic review of the reliability of PROM of the UE found 22 relevant studies of usually poor methodological quality. Using an instrument (goniometer or inclinometer) to measure PROM demonstrated higher reliability than visually estimating. Most studies reported acceptable reliability when an inclinometer or a goniometer was used.[48] Lower reliability was found for the LE; however, knee flexion demonstrated acceptable reliability more consistently than other directions of motion.[49] In an often-cited study, Boone et al. found the average standard deviation between measurements made on the same subjects by different testers to be 4.2° for UE motions and 5.2° for LE motions.[50] These issues with reliability have been attributed to difficulties in measuring complex versus simple hinged joints, in palpating bony landmarks, and in moving heavy body parts.[50] The use of standardized positions, stabilization of the body part proximal to the joint being tested, use of bony landmarks to align the goniometer, and repeated testing conducted by the same therapist (rather than multiple therapists) all help to improve the validity and reliability of goniometric measurements.[51]

Range of Motion—Lower Extremity

Patient's Name _____ Date of Birth _____

Left				Right		
			Date			
			Examiner's Initials			
			Hip			
			Flexion			
			Extension			
			Abduction			
			Medial Rotation			
			Lateral Rotation			
			Knee			
			Flexion			
			Ankle			
			Dorsiflexion			
			Plantarflexion			
			Inversion—Tarsal			
			Eversion—Tarsal			
			Inversion—Subtalar			
			Eversion—Subtalar			
			Inversion—Midtarsal			
			Eversion—Midtarsal			
			Great Toe			
			MTP Flexion			
			MTP Extension			
			MTP Abduction			
			IP Flexion			
			Toe			
			MTP Flexion			
			MTP Extension			
			MTP Abduction			
			PIP Flexion			
			DIP Flexion			
			DIP Extension			
			Comments:			

Figure 4.6 Range of motion recording form for the lower extremity. The multiple columns on either side of the centrally listed joints and motions are used to record the date, examiner's initials, and ROM values from serial measurements. *(From Norkin and White,[47] with permission.)*

The end of each motion at each joint is limited from further movement by particular anatomical structures. The type of structure that limits a joint motion has a characteristic feel, which may be detected by the therapist performing the PROM. This feeling, which is experienced by the therapist as resistance, or a barrier to further motion, is called the *end-feel*. A variety of normal (physiological) and abnormal (pathological) end-feels have been described.[52] Normal end-feels are generally described as *hard* (bony), *soft* (soft tissue approximation), *elastic* (elongation of musculotendinous structures), or *capsular* (elongation of capsule or ligaments). Elbow extension that is limited by the contact between the olecranon and the olecranon fossa is an example of a bony end-feel; elbow flexion that is limited by the contact between the biceps and anterior forearm soft tissues is an example of a soft end-feel; hip flexion with the knee straight that is limited by the elongation of the hamstrings is an example of an elastic end-feel; and wrist flexion that is limited by the elongation of the dorsal capsule and ligaments is an example of a capsular end-feel. Even though the assessment of end-feels is frequently taught in physical therapy education and included as part of the typical physical examination, end-feels largely have unacceptable interrater reliability,[49] while intrarater reliability is better.[53]

Cyriax and Cyriax[52] initially described characteristic patterns of restricted joint ROM due to diffuse, intra-articular inflammation involving the entire joint capsule. These patterns of restricted motion, which usually involve multiple motions at a joint, are called *capsular patterns* and are typically associated with osteoarthritis. The restrictions do not involve the loss of a fixed number of degrees but rather the loss of a proportion of one motion relative to another. Capsular patterns vary from joint to joint. Table 4.1 presents common capsular patterns. Although therapists have been using capsular patterns in clinical decision-making for many years, research demonstrates that the patterns of ROM restriction in the presence of osteoarthritis are complex and difficult to summarize.[54] The sole recognition of a capsular or noncapsular pattern is not enough to direct appropriate treatment. Information gained from the patient history, observation, palpation, AROM and PROM, muscle tests, joint mobility tests, and tissue-specific tests must be integrated to determine the most likely cause of the symptoms.

Accessory Joint Motions

If PROM is found to be limited or painful, an examination of arthrokinematic motions is indicated. *Arthrokinematics* refers to the motion of joint surfaces. These motions, often called *accessory* or *joint play motions,* are used to determine joint mobility and integrity. Accessory joint motions are typically described as glides (or slides), spins, and rolls. A *glide* (*slide*) is a linear motion of one surface sliding over another (Fig. 4.7). A *roll* is a rotary motion similar to the bottom of a rocking chair rolling over the floor or a tire rolling over a road

Table 4.1	Capsular Patterns of Extremity Joints
Shoulder (Glenohumeral Joint)	Maximum loss of external rotation Moderate loss of abduction Minimum loss of internal rotation
Elbow Complex	Flexion loss is greater than extension loss
Forearm	Equally restricted in pronation and supination
Wrist	Equally restricted in flexion and extension
Carpometacarpal Joint I Carpometacarpal Joints II–V	Abduction and extension restriction Equally restricted in all directions
Finger Interphalangeal	Flexion loss is greater than extension loss
Hip	Maximum loss of internal rotation, flexion, abduction Minimal loss of extension
Knee (Tibiofemoral Joint)	Flexion loss is greater than extension loss
Ankle (Talocrural Joint)	Plantarflexion loss is greater than extension loss
Subtalar Joint	Restricted varus motion
Midtarsal Joint	Restricted dorsiflexion, plantarflexion, abduction, and medial rotation
Metatarsophalangeal Joint I Metatarsophalangeal Joints II–V Interphalangeal Joints	Extension loss is greater than flexion Variable, tend toward flexion restriction Tend toward extension restriction

Capsular patterns are from Cyriax and Cyriax[52] and Kaltenborn.[55]

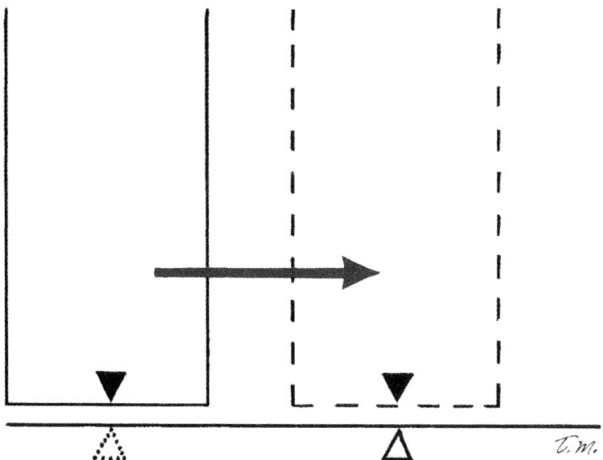

Figure 4.7 A glide (slide) is a type of linear accessory joint motion in which points on a moving joint surface come in contact with new points on the opposing joint surface. *(From Norkin and White,[47] with permission.)*

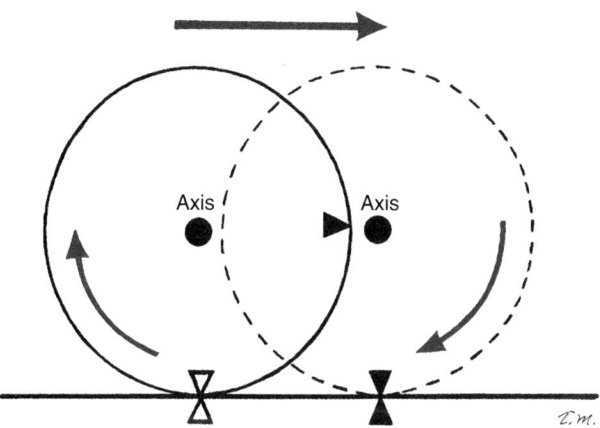

Figure 4.8 During a roll, new points on the moving joint surface come in contact with new points on the opposing surface. The axis of rotation also moves, in this case to the right. *(From Norkin and White,[47] with permission.)*

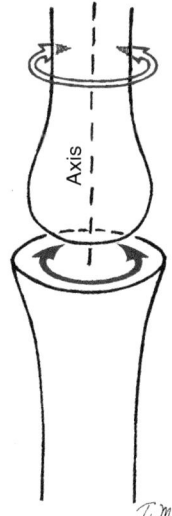

Figure 4.9 A spin is an accessory joint motion in which all the points on the moving surface rotate around a fixed axis. *(From Norkin and White,[47] with permission.)*

(Fig. 4.8). A *spin* is a rotary motion around a fixed point or axis (Fig. 4.9).

Accessory motions usually occur in combination with each other and result in angular movement of the bone shaft, or osteokinematic motion. The combination of a roll and glide allows for increased ROM by re-centering the moving surface on the stable surface. The direction of the rolling and gliding components of roll-gliding depends on whether a concave or convex joint surface is moving. If a concave joint surface is moving, the gliding component occurs in the same direction as the rolling or angular movement of the bone's shaft (Fig. 4.10). For example, during flexion of the knee with the femur fixed, the shaft of the tibia rolls posteriorly while the tibia's joint surface (concave) also glides posteriorly. If

a convex joint surface is moving, the gliding component occurs in the direction opposite to the rolling or angular movement of the bone's shaft. For example, during abduction of the glenohumeral joint, the shaft and humeral head (convex) roll cranially, while the contacting articular surface of the humeral head glides caudally. In the human body, roll-gliding is by far the most frequently occurring arthrokinematic motion, although there are several instances of pure spin motions. An example of a spin joint motion would be supination and pronation of the radius at the humeroradial joint.

The accessory motions most commonly tested are translatory: glides that are parallel to the joint surfaces and *distractions* and *compressions* that are perpendicular to the joint surfaces. Kaltenborn[55] and Hertling and Kessler[24] describe specific testing and treatment techniques that focus on accessory motions—usually under the topic of *joint mobilization*. Careful attention must be given to general patient positioning, specific joint positioning, relaxation of surrounding muscles, stabilization of one joint surface, and mobilization of the other joint surface. As with other manual assessment techniques, the clinician is cautioned against overreliance on accessory motion findings due to questionable reliability.[56]

While it is important for the clinician to understand the principles of accessory motions and, subsequently, joint mobilization, it is important to note that the principles are largely theoretical constructs that can assist with the mental imaging of joint motion[57] but in reality are complicated by the interaction with forces from periarticular structures. The fact that the humeral head remains largely stationary during shoulder abduction, as it has been experimentally verified, provides some evidence that an effective superior roll is combined with

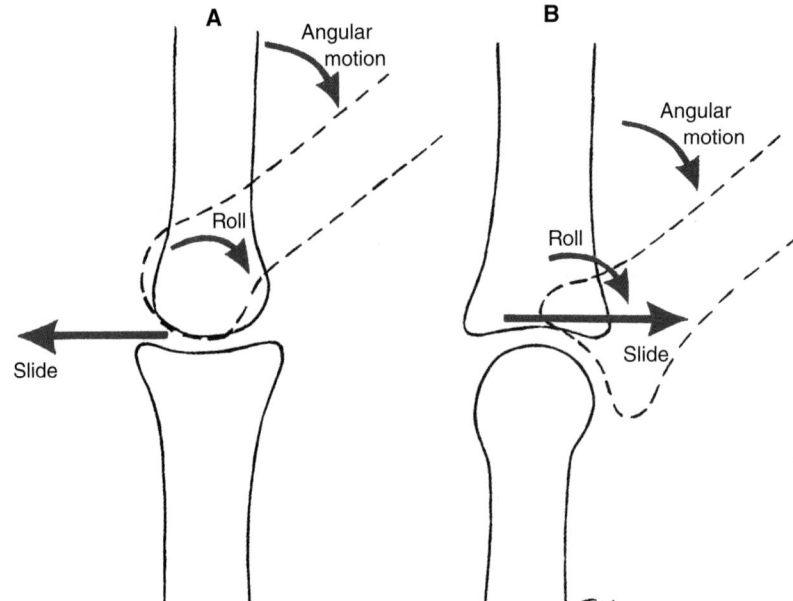

Figure 4.10 The concave-convex rule. (A) If the joint surface of the moving bone is convex, gliding is in the opposite direction of the angular movement of the bone. (B) If the joint surface of the moving bone is concave, gliding is in the same direction as the angular movement of the bone. *(From Norkin and White,[47] with permission.)*

an inferior slide.[57] This, however, does not necessarily mean that joint mobilizations according to the convex-concave rule are effective.

Muscle Performance

Muscle performance is the ability of a muscle to perform work. Strength, power, endurance, and motor control are all components of muscle performance that can be tested and varied throughout a POC as well as the type of muscle contraction: isometric, concentric, eccentric, or plyometric. *Muscle strength* is the force exerted by a muscle or group of muscles to overcome a resistance in one maximal effort. Clinical methods of determining muscle strength include manual muscle testing (MMT), handheld dynamometry, and isokinetic dynamometry. Depending on the patient, other characteristics related to muscle performance may also be tested. *Muscle power* is work produced per unit of time, or the product of strength and speed. *Muscle endurance* is the ability of the muscle to contract repeatedly over time. *Motor control* is the coordinated movement of many muscle groups, and it has been defined as the production of purposeful, coordinated movements by the central nervous system in its interaction with the rest of the body and with the environment.[58] Motor control is addressed later under the section on motion analysis. The purposes of muscle performance testing can include investigation of muscle/tendon contribution to the concordant sign or symptom, to determine the activity level of a muscle/tendon (e.g., postoperative quadriceps inhibition), to establish a baseline of coordinated movement, and to determine progress toward return to activity. The concordant sign or symptom is frequently the reason for the patient seeking care and is often recorded as the chief complaint.

When a lesion presents in the contractile tissues such as muscle or tendons, MMT can be used to elicit pain from muscle contraction or to identify muscle weakness. A painful contraction is often associated with a muscle/tendon issue while a painless but weak contraction is often associated with a neurological issue. For example, bicipital tendinopathy would be painful during resisted isometric testing of elbow flexion and shoulder flexion, while a C5-6 nerve root issue may be painless but weaker when testing the biceps. Muscle weakness may be due to many causes, including pathologies involving upper motor neurons, peripheral nerves, neuromuscular junctions, disuse atrophy, and muscle inhibition, which is why it is critical to continue to build preponderance of evidence for a diagnosis by corroborating muscle testing with patient history, screening, motion testing, and palpation.

MMT can be performed as a "make test" or a "break test." In the make test, the examiner exerts just enough force to prevent joint movement—a true isometric test. In a break test, the examiner provides enough force to overcome the patient's resistance, causing joint movement. The break test is performed at the end of the ROM when testing one-joint muscles and at mid-range when testing two-joint muscles.[59] Table 4.2 presents a commonly used method for interpreting the results of the MMT.

A grading system is used with categories of Normal (grade 5), Good (grade 4), Fair (grade 3), Poor (grade 2), Trace (grade 1), and Zero (Table 4.3).[60] It is important to note that this numerical scale indicates ordinal data, because the intervals between the numbers do not represent equal units of measure. The MMT grades of *Good* and *Normal* typically encompass a large range of muscle strength, whereas the grades of *Fair, Poor,* and *Trace* include a much narrower range. Sharrard,[61] counting alpha motor neurons in spinal cords of individuals with poliomyelitis at the time of autopsy, found that muscles

Table 4.2	Results of Resisted Isometric Testing
Findings	**Possible Pathologies**
Strong and painless	There is no lesion or neurological deficit involving the tested muscle and tendon.
Strong and painful	There is a minor lesion of the tested muscle or tendon.
Weak and painless	There is a disorder of the nervous system, neuromuscular junction, a complete rupture of the tested muscle or tendon, or disuse atrophy.
Weak and painful	There is a serious, painful pathology such as a fracture or neoplasm. Other possibilities include an acute inflammatory process that inhibits muscle contraction, exercise-induced muscle damage, or a partial rupture of the tested muscle or tendon.

Table 4.3	Manual Muscle Testing Grades			
Grade	**Grade Abbreviation**	**0–5 Scale**	**0–10 Scale**	**Criteria**
Normal	N	5	10	Full available ROM, against gravity, strong manual resistance
Good plus	G+	4+	9	Full available ROM, against gravity, nearly strong manual resistance
Good	G	4	8	Full available ROM, against gravity, moderate manual resistance
Good minus	G–	4–	7	Full available ROM, against gravity, nearly moderate manual resistance
Fair plus	F+	3+	6	Full available ROM, against gravity, slight manual resistance
Fair	F	3	5	Full available ROM, against gravity, no resistance
Fair minus	F–	3–	4	At least 50% but not full ROM, against gravity, no resistance
Poor plus	P+	2+	3	Full available ROM, gravity minimized, slight manual resistance
Poor	P	2	2	Full available ROM, gravity minimized, no resistance
Poor minus	P–	2–	1	At least 50% but not full ROM, gravity minimized, no resistance
Trace plus	T+	1+		Minimal observable motion (less than 50% ROM), gravity minimized, no resistance
Trace	T	1	T	No observable motion, palpable muscle contraction, no resistance
Zero	0	0	0	No observable or palpable muscle contraction

ROM = range of motion.

previously receiving a grade of *Good* had 50% of their innervated motor neurons, whereas muscles graded as *Fair* had only 15% of their motor neurons. Beasley[62] noted that patients with poliomyelitis were graded as having *Good, Fair,* and *Poor* knee extension when they had on average only 43%, 9%, and 3% of the knee extension force of normal subjects, respectively. Andres et al.,[63] in a study of four muscle groups in patients with amyotrophic lateral sclerosis, found that the muscles were often graded as *Normal* until up to 50% of strength was lost. Overall, the reliability and validity of MMT are within acceptable limits.[64] However, a wide range of strength values within an MMT grade and an overlap in strength values between adjacent MMT grades has been observed.[65] Global strength scores that average MMT results from multiple muscle groups also resulted in higher reliability.[66]

Although more costly and time-consuming than MMT, handheld dynamometry can be used to improve objectivity and sensitivity of testing. *Handheld dynamometers* (HHDs) are portable devices, placed between the therapist's hand and the patient's body, that measure mechanical force at the point of application (Fig. 4.11). The force measured by the dynamometer

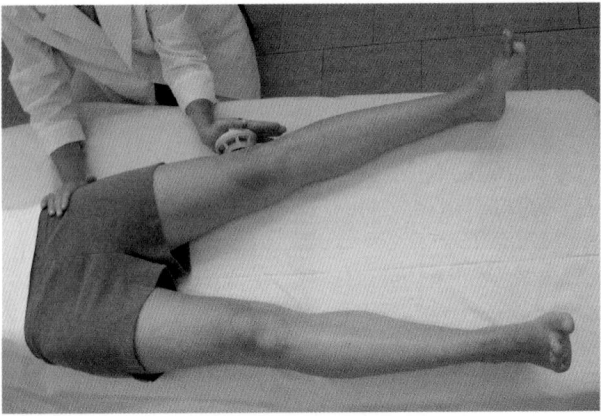

Figure 4.11 Measurement of the strength of the left hip abductors with a handheld dynamometer. The handheld dynamometer measures force at the point of application, which should be converted to torque by multiplying the force by the distance from the joint axis.

will vary depending on the method of applying the resistance (make or break test), the patient's body position in relation to gravity, the joint angle, the dynamometer placement on the patient (lever arm), the stabilization to prevent muscle substitution, and the therapist's strength.[67] Although force values determined with make and break tests are highly correlated, break tests usually result in greater force values than make tests,[68] so they should not be used interchangeably.

The body part proximal to the joint being tested must be well stabilized by the therapist to minimize extraneous muscle substitutions. To reduce the effect of moving a body segment's weight on force measurements, it is recommended that muscle groups be tested in gravity-minimized positions. For example, to test the strength of the hip abductors, the patient would be positioned supine so that the muscle action would pull in a horizontal plane relative to the ground (see Fig. 4.11). The joint should also be positioned at an easily reproducible angle so that muscle length remains constant. The dynamometer is applied perpendicular to the body segment at an established location on the patient's body. When muscles contract, they produce *torque* that creates angular joint motion. The therapist must apply sufficient resistance to oppose the patient's torque to ensure an isometric (make test) or an eccentric contraction (break test). To provide greater resistance than what can be achieved manually, the dynamometer can be attached to a fixed surface, or an isokinetic dynamometer can be used in the isometric setting.

Normative force values for particular muscle groups by age and sex have been reported;[69] however, attention must be directed to replicating methods used in the normative studies to ensure appropriate comparisons. Some authors have also included regression equations to take into account body weight and height.[69] For patients with unilateral conditions, it may be helpful to compare results to that of the uninvolved extremity. In general, it is expected that side-to-side differences are less than 11%.[69,70]

In addition to HHD, there are more complex and expensive devices that can be used to assess muscle strength. *Isokinetic dynamometers* are stationary, electromechanical devices that control the velocity of a moving body segment by resisting and measuring the patient's effort so that the body segment cannot accelerate beyond the predefined angular velocity. Isokinetic dynamometers can be used to measure the torque produced during isometric, concentric, and eccentric contractions. Muscle forces measured with HHD have been compared to forces measured with isokinetic dynamometers to evaluate concurrent validity with good results.[71–73] Reliability seems to be better when testing the UEs than when testing the LEs and trunk.[74–76] Agre et al.[77] found the standard deviation of the repeated measurements expressed as a percentage of the mean force measurements (coefficient of variation of replication) to be 5.1% to 8.3% for the UE muscle groups and 11.3% to 17.8% for the LE muscle groups. Some of the error in using HHDs is due to off-center loading of the dynamometer, difficulties in positioning and stabilization, and limitations in the strength and experience of the examiners.

Tissue-Specific Tests

After completing the patient interview, observation, palpation, examination of motion, and muscle performance, the therapist should have a preponderance of evidence for the most likely one or two diagnoses. Tissue-specific tests (TSTs), also known as "special tests," are designed to focus on specific conditions in a particular region of the body. As such, these tests are best used to confirm a diagnosis. A therapist would ordinarily choose to perform only those tests indicated by previous findings that are relevant to the area of the body being examined and the pathology or pathologies that is/are part of the working hypotheses. A perfectly accurate TST would have either a true positive or a true negative finding 100% of the time. However, no TST has perfect accuracy, so their imperfection is captured through false positives and negatives. False-positive TSTs are those where the test is positive for a pathology that is not present, and false-negative TSTs are negative for a pathology that is present. Despite this imperfection, a positive test finding with a highly specific (high positive likelihood ratio) test or tests in conjunction with other aspects of the examination would be highly suggestive of pathology. A detailed presentation of the many TSTs that are used in orthopedic assessment is beyond the scope of this chapter and can be found elsewhere.[2]

Prior to performing a TST or cluster of TSTs, the clinician should have a good sense of the pretest probability of the pathology that the TSTs are designed to assess, and this comes from a good understanding of incidence and prevalence of the common pathologies in the patient population with whom the therapist works. For example, hip dysplasia is more frequently seen in the pediatric than in the geriatric population. Therefore, a pediatric physical therapist treating a patient with hip pain and gait dysfunction has a greater baseline suspicion of hip dysplasia than of osteoarthritis. Based on the outcome of the TSTs, the clinician should calculate the post-test probability of the pathology (pretest probability × likelihood ratio = post-test probability). For TSTs to be helpful, they need to have good diagnostic properties; tests with strong positive likelihood ratios are useful for ruling in diagnoses. Because there are few TSTs with strong stand-alone diagnostic properties, researchers have used clusters of tests that frequently provide more clinically relevant information and assistance in the diagnostic process.[78] The reader is referred to specialized textbooks that discuss these important concepts in further detail.[79]

Functional Movement Analysis

Physical therapists are experts in the evaluation of motion founded on motor control. The conclusion of the physical examination represents an excellent opportunity to assess the quantity and quality of functional motion, focusing on the motions that are painful, difficult, or relevant to the patient's occupation or recreational activities. For the patients whose job involves the use of a computer and their symptoms exacerbate later in the day, an office *ergonomic evaluation* may provide unique insight into the source of the symptoms and the implementation of simple yet effective solutions. In the musculoskeletal setting, ADL such as gait (see Chapter 7, Examination of Gait) or standing from a chair, athletic activities (e.g., squatting, jumping, throwing a ball), or occupational activities (e.g., lifting boxes) are frequently assessed. The motion should be viewed or recorded from different angles and assessed systematically. While motion analysis with digital equipment used to be available only to few clinicians who had access to a biomechanical laboratory, recent technological advances allow the recording of functional activities with smartphones, tablets, or digital cameras and the careful analysis of angles at different parts of the task. Motions can be slowed down, and relevant frames can be analyzed in detail and compared longitudinally to assess progress. Applications are available that are either free or low cost, and when the process of video data collection is standardized, they have the potential to provide accurate motion analysis that is practical in the clinical setting.[80]

Additional Tests and Measurements

Depending on findings, other tests and measurements may be indicated. Many of these additional examination procedures are discussed in detail in other chapters of this book. For example, patient complaints of paresthesia or difficulty in muscle performance often indicate neurological involvement that calls for testing of superficial, deep, and proprioceptive sensations (see Chapter 3, Examination of Sensory Function), reflexes and motor tone (see Chapter 5, Examination of Motor Function: Motor Control and Motor Learning), and coordination and balance (see Chapter 6, Examination of Coordination and Balance). Data from these tests together with muscle performance results help to identify conditions affecting peripheral nerves, spinal nerve roots, and the central nervous system. Therapists must distinguish peripheral nerve versus nerve root patterns of sensory and motor innervation. Figure 4.5 presents muscle testing recording forms that are helpful in recognizing impaired innervation patterns. Myotomes that are often included as parts of a musculoskeletal examination are shown in Table 4.4, and deep tendon reflexes are presented in Chapter 5. Upper motor neuron lesions usually result in hyperreflexia, whereas lower motor neuron lesions involving the spinal nerve root

Table 4.4	Myotomes[2]	
Level	**Upper Quarter Myotomes**	
	Action to Be Tested	*Muscle*
C5	Shoulder abduction, shoulder flexion	Deltoid
C5, C6	Elbow flexion	Biceps
	Wrist extension	Extensor carpi radialis longus Extensor carpi radialis brevis
C7	Elbow extension	Triceps
	Wrist flexion	Flexor carpi radialis Flexor carpi ulnaris
C8	Ulnar deviation	Flexor carpi ulnaris Extensor carpi ulnaris
T1	Digit abduction/ adduction	Interossei
Level	**Lower Quarter Myotomes**	
	Action to Be Tested	*Muscle*
L2, L3, L4	Knee extension	Quadriceps
L4	Ankle dorsiflexion	Anterior tibialis
L5	Extension of great toe	Extensor hallucis longus
S1	Plantarflexion	Gastrocnemius
	Ankle eversion	Peroneus longus Peroneus brevis

or peripheral nerves usually cause hyporeflexia of deep tendon reflexes. When pain sensitization is suspected, the therapist should utilize appropriate tests that assess relevant properties (e.g., pressure hyperalgesia, thermal hyperalgesia, and temporal summation).[66] For more details on the assessment of pain, see Chapter 25, Chronic Pain.

Impairments in ROM, accessory joint motions, and motor performance may affect ADL and occupational and recreational activities. In such cases, the examination of functional abilities (see Chapter 8, Examination of Function) and environmental surroundings (see Chapter 9, Examination and Modification of the Environment) is often appropriate. Sometimes findings indicate the need for additional testing by other health professionals, such as physician specialists, psychologists, speech-language pathologists, and occupational therapists.

■ EVALUATION OF EXAMINATION FINDINGS

At the conclusion of the musculoskeletal examination, all pertinent historical, patient interview, and physical examination findings are evaluated to establish a physical therapy diagnosis on which treatment is based. A *diagnosis* has been defined as a label encompassing a cluster of signs and symptoms, syndromes, or categories.[5] The specific tissues causing the impairments should be identified when possible so that treatment can be focused and effective. The therapist should be aware that identifying the exact tissue pathology is frequently not possible, particularly for certain categories such as low back pain or in cases of chronic musculoskeletal pain.[4] The therapist must have a thorough understanding of the pathologies commonly affecting the body segment under consideration. The symptoms and clinical manifestations of these pathologies are compared to the current examination findings to establish a diagnosis. The American Physical Therapy Association's revised and adapted *Musculoskeletal Preferred Practice Patterns* can assist students and novice physical therapists in categorizing diagnoses into common clusters. Information is provided on risk factors, examination, evaluation/diagnosis/prognosis, interventions, and outcomes (https://guide.apta.org/).

Sometimes the evaluation process does not yield a clearly identifiable diagnosis. In such cases, a provisional diagnosis and the alleviation of symptoms and impairments become the basis for treatment. In other instances, the evaluation may indicate the presence of two or more conditions. The therapist should then prioritize and focus initially on the condition causing the most serious impairments, activity limitations, and disability.

The evaluation should clearly determine the baseline for the patient's symptoms, impairments, activity limitations, and participation restrictions. This information becomes the basis of the clinical problem list and guides development of anticipated goals and expected outcomes. The results of future examinations can be compared to this baseline to evaluate the effectiveness of treatment.

In addition to establishing a diagnosis and baseline data, the evaluation of findings should ascertain etiological factors. Unless the underlying causes of the condition are recognized and treated, chronic problems can be expected. The therapist must not only direct attention to the specifically involved tissues but also must think more broadly of physiological units of function and biomechanics. For example, a patient with "shin splints" may initially respond well to modality-based treatment and reduced activity. However, since the condition is frequently due to LE mechanics, the resumption of normal weight-bearing activities may cause reinjury unless the biomechanical issues are addressed. Similarly, a patient with supraspinatus tendinopathy may react well to rest and gentle glenohumeral ROM exercises but often also requires eventual strengthening of the rotator cuff and scapulothoracic musculature and restoration of normal scapulohumeral rhythm.

Finally, an analysis of the examination findings should establish the stage of the patient's condition. The stage, whether acute, subacute, or chronic, can indicate how well the patient will tolerate mechanical loads such as those imposed by daily activities or by a therapist during treatment. The *acute stage* is usually defined as occurring up to the first 48 to 72 hrs after onset. The *subacute stage* may continue up to 2 weeks to several months after onset. Typically, conditions are considered in the *chronic stage* after 3 to 6 months. Another way of defining the stages, which is probably more relevant to treatment planning, focuses on tissue inflammation and the repair process. Conditions in an *acute inflammation stage* will show signs and symptoms of inflammation associated with hyperemia, increased capillary permeability with protein and plasma leakage, and an influx of granulocytes and other defensive cells. These signs and symptoms include swelling, elevated skin temperature at the lesion site, and pain at rest that worsens with ROM and resisted isometric contractions that even minimally stress the involved tissues. The *chronic inflammation stage* produces signs and symptoms associated with attempts at tissue repair, including an increase in the number of fibrocytes and the presence of granulation tissue; the patient will now have minimal or no swelling and elevated temperature at the lesion site. Pain tends to occur only at the extremes of ROM when the end-feel is reached, or with a moderate to maximal amount of isometric resistance. Tissues in an acute stage will often not tolerate mechanical loading from daily, recreational, occupational, or therapeutic activities. The force, frequency, and duration of treatment procedures must be monitored closely so as not to increase inflammation and worsen the condition. In contrast, tissues in the chronic stage will usually tolerate and require treatment procedures involving more mechanical loading, frequency, and duration to effect positive changes in the tissues. The stage of the condition also adds prognostic information. Typically, an acute condition will show more spontaneous improvement over a shorter period of time than a chronic condition. A chronic condition usually requires a longer period of treatment to promote a smaller improvement in status.

SUMMARY

The musculoskeletal examination provides important information for diagnosis and treatment. The examination process begins with a review of the patient's medical records and a detailed interview. Careful screening, observation, palpation, motion testing, and muscle performance testing are typically performed. Depending on the findings, TSTs particular to the body region under examination may need to be included. Examination of the peripheral and central nervous systems, gait, functional ability, and the environment is often required. At the conclusion of this process, all findings must be evaluated to determine the diagnosis, baseline status, etiological factors, mode of onset, and stage (acute, subacute, or chronic) of the condition. In addition, the therapist will better understand the patient's goals, time frames, and readiness to begin rehabilitation. At this point, the prognosis, mutual goals, expected outcomes, and POC can be developed.

Questions for Review

1. What are the purposes of a musculoskeletal examination?
2. What information about the patient's symptoms should be obtained during a patient interview?
3. What psychometric property would make a tissue-specific test useful for ruling in a diagnosis?
4. Describe at least three attributes of the physical examination that would help establish good patient rapport.
5. Give at least three examples of osteokinematic and arthrokinematic motions. How do arthrokinematic motions combine to produce osteokinematic motion in a typical synovial joint in which the moving joint surface is concave? Convex?
6. Distinguish between muscle strength, endurance, and power.
7. Discuss the implications of a weak and painful finding during the performance of resisted isometric testing.
8. What factors are important in determining MMT grades? What would be the criteria for MMT grades of *Good, Fair*, and *Poor*?
9. What are the advantages and disadvantages of using MMT, handheld dynamometers, and isokinetic dynamometers to determine muscle strength?
10. What would a positive finding on a glenohumeral apprehension test indicate?

CASE STUDY 1

A 45-year-old man enters the outpatient physical therapy department with a complaint of right shoulder pain of 1 week's duration. The pain began Monday morning following a weekend of scraping and painting his house. The patient describes his pain as aching and troublesome; his pain is a 6 on a pain scale of 0 to 10. He reports that he is married and is having difficulty in home maintenance activities such as lawn mowing. His score on the *Quick*DASH is 50%.

While palpating the shoulder region during the musculoskeletal physical examination, increased tenderness in the region of the bicipital groove of the right anterior shoulder is noted. AROM of the right shoulder reveals increased pain and some limitations during shoulder flexion, abduction, and extension; all other active motions are pain free and within normal ROM limits. Passive shoulder motions are pain free with normal ROM, except for shoulder extension, which is limited and causes an increase in pain toward the end of motion.

(Continued)

CASE STUDY 1—cont'd

GUIDING QUESTIONS

1. What additional information should be gathered during the interview?

2. How do you interpret the 50% score on the *QuickDASH*?

3. The therapist suspects the presence of bicipital tendinopathy. Do the findings during testing of AROM and PROM support this diagnosis? Explain.

4. What additional tests should be performed to selectively examine contractile tissue and help to support or repudiate the diagnosis of bicipital tendinopathy? Provide a rationale for your selection.

5. Create your own case study, and explain to someone why the findings you created would produce the diagnosis you decided on.

CASE STUDY 2

A 14-year-old girl is referred for outpatient physical therapy 12 weeks after sustaining midshaft fractures of her left tibia and fibula from a bicycle accident. Her long leg cast was removed yesterday. The fracture is well healed. The patient reports her left knee and ankle are stiff and painful when she tries to move them. She also describes her left leg as weak. At this time, she is ambulating with two crutches, weight-bearing as tolerated, with hopes of progressing off the crutches as soon as possible.

GUIDING QUESTIONS

1. On observation, the patient's left thigh and calf appear to be thinner than the right. How can this observation be objectively measured and documented? Why might the patient's left leg be thinner than the right?

2. What accessory joint motion should be examined considering the limitation in passive knee flexion ROM? Apply the concave-convex rules for determining the direction of the glide given the shape of the joint surfaces.

3. In addition to observing, palpating, and testing AROM, PROM, accessory joint motions, and muscle performance, what other testing procedures would be important to include in the examination of this patient?

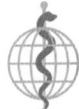 For additional resources, including answers to the questions for review, new immersive cases, case study guiding questions, references, and more, please visit **https://www.fadavis.com/product/physical -rehabilitation-fulk-8**. You may also quickly find the resources by entering this title's four-digit ISBN, 4691, in the search field at **http://fadavis.com** and logging in at the prompt.

Examination of Motor Function: Motor Control and Motor Learning

Susan B. O'Sullivan, PT, EdD
Scott W. Shaffer, PT, PhD, ECS
Richard J. McKibben, PT, DSc, ECS

Chapter **5**

LEARNING OBJECTIVES

1. Identify the purposes and components of the examination of motor structure and function: motor control and motor learning.

2. Discuss potential constraining factors that can affect an examination of motor function, including sensory, perceptual, cognitive, and communication deficits.

3. Describe the examination of activities and participation.

4. Describe the examination of the movement system.

5. Describe the examination of impairments of body structure and function of the movement system and the implication of common deficits for function.

6. Describe the measures used in the assessment of motor learning.

7. Discuss the importance of examining and promoting patient involvement in decision-making and assessment of problem-solving skills.

8. Compare and contrast the advantages, disadvantages, and utilization of imaging tests, including radiography, computed tomography (CT) scan, magnetic resonance imaging (MRI), diffusion tensor imaging (DTI), functional magnetic resonance imaging (fMRI), spectrum photon emission computed tomography (SPECT), and positron emission tomography (PET).

9. Compare and contrast the advantages, disadvantages, and utilization of electrophysiologic neuromuscular assessments to include nerve conduction studies (NCS), electromyography (EMG), electroencephalography (EEG), and transmagnetic stimulation (TMS).

10. Discuss factors that influence determination of the physical therapy diagnosis with disorders of motor function.

11. Analyze and interpret patient data, formulate realistic goals and expected outcomes, and identify appropriate interventions when presented with a clinical case study.

12. Compare and contrast the clinical examination findings associated with various central nervous health conditions (see Table 5.14).

13. Compare and contrast the clinical examination findings associated with various neuromuscular diseases (see Table 5.15).

CHAPTER OUTLINE

OVERVIEW OF MOTOR FUNCTION *126*
  Motor Control and Learning *126*
  Systems Theory *126*
  Motor Structure and Function *127*
  Recovery and Neuroplasticity *129*
COMPONENTS OF THE EXAMINATION *132*
  Patient History *132*
  Systems Review *133*
  Tests and Measures *133*
CONSTRAINTS ON THE MOTOR FUNCTION EXAMINATION *133*
  Sensory Impairments *134*
  Perceptual Impairments *134*
  Altered Consciousness and Arousal *134*
  Cognitive Impairments *135*
  Communication Impairments *135*
MOTOR CONTROL EXAMINATION *136*
  Examination of Functional Activities and Movements *136*
  Movement Observation and Analysis *136*
  Motor Skills *137*
  Motor Coordination *138*

EXAMINATION OF BODY STRUCTURE AND FUNCTION *140*
  Musculoskeletal Impairments *140*
  Neuromuscular Impairments *143*
MEASURES OF MOTOR LEARNING *155*
  Stages of Motor Learning *155*
  Performance Measures *156*
  Retention Tests *156*
  Transfer Tests *158*
  Adaptation *158*
  Documentation *158*
DECISION-MAKING/PROBLEM-SOLVING SKILLS *159*
INSTRUMENTATION AND TECHNOLOGY TO ASSESS MOTOR FUNCTION *160*
  Structural Imaging Techniques *160*
  Functional Imaging Techniques *162*
  Molecular Imaging Techniques *163*
  Electrophysiologic Neuromuscular Assessment *163*
EVALUATION AND DIAGNOSIS *174*
SUMMARY *177*

■ OVERVIEW OF MOTOR STRUCTURE AND FUNCTION

Motor Control and Motor Learning

Motor control evolves from a complex set of neural, physical, and behavioral processes that govern posture and movement. Some movements have a genetic basis and emerge through processes of normal growth and development. Examples of these include the largely reactive reflex patterns that predominate during much of early life and in some patients with brain damage. Other movements, termed *motor skills,* are learned through practice and interaction with the environment. Practice and feedback are important variables in defining motor learning and motor skill development. A *motor program* is defined as "a prestructured set of movement commands that defines the essential details of skilled action, with minimal or no involvement of sensory feedback." An example is the complex neural circuitry in the spinal cord known as *central pattern generators* that control locomotion and gait.

Generalized motor programs (GMPs) are higher level motor programs, defined as "a motor program whose output can vary along certain dimensions to produce novelty and generalizability in movement."[1] GMPs contain information about the order of events, the timing of events (temporal structure), the overall force of contractions, and the muscle(s) or limb(s) used in the movements. *Motor memory* (*procedural memory*) involves the recall of motor programs or subroutines and includes information on (1) initial movement conditions; (2) sensory parameters (how the movement felt, looked, and sounded); (3) specific movement performance parameters (*knowledge of performance*); and (4) outcome of the movement (*knowledge of results*).

Sensory information (see Chapter 3, Examination of Sensory Function, for additional information) is an important component of motor control. Sensory information (feedback) is transmitted in ascending pathways to higher centers. *Feedback* is defined as response-produced information received during or after the movement that allows for appreciation (awareness) of stimuli, modulation of movement, and corrective actions. It is used to assess movement outcomes and shape further movement and learning. Sensory inputs also provide the stimuli for reflexive movement control organized at the spinal cord level. A *closed-loop system* is defined as "a type [of] system control involving feedback, error detection, and error correction that is applicable to maintaining a system goal."[1(p435)] The primary role of closed-loop systems in motor control appears to be in the monitoring of constant states such as posture and balance and the control of slow movements, or those requiring a high degree of precision or accuracy. Feedback is also critically important in motor learning. In contrast, an *open loop system* "is a type of system control in which instructions for the effector system are determined in advance and run off without feedback."[1(p439)] Rapid and skilled movement sequences or well-learned movements can thus be completed without the benefit of sensory feedback (e.g., the skilled piano player). In fact, most movements have elements of both closed- and open-loop control processes (hybrid control system).[2] *Feedforward* is "the anticipated sensory consequences of movement that should occur if the movement is correct."[1(p437)] The sending of signals in advance of movement readies the sensorimotor systems and allows for *proactive (anticipatory)* adjustments in postural activity.

Motor skills are acquired and modified by actions of the central nervous system (CNS) through processes of motor learning. *Motor learning* is defined as "a set of internal processes associated with practice or experience leading to relatively permanent changes in the capability for skilled behavior."[1(p438)]

Processing of sensory information by the CNS is both serial and parallel, leading to the production of coordinated movement. *Coordination* (see Chapter 6 for additional information) is the ability to execute smooth, accurate, and controlled motor responses while moving toward achieving a goal. *Coordinative structures* (synergies) are the functionally linked muscles that are constrained by the nervous system to act cooperatively to produce an intended movement.[2] Box 5.1 summarizes terminology related to motor control.

Systems Theory

The cooperative actions of multiple systems allow for accommodation of movement to match the specific demands of the task and the environment. This is defined by *systems theory,* a distributed model of motor control. The central concept is that many systems interact to produce coordinated movement, not just the nervous system. For example, mechanical factors of the musculoskeletal system (body mass, inertia, and gravity) contribute to the overall quality of the movement produced. Cognition (attention, memory, learning, judgment, and decision-making) and perception (interpretation of sensation) are also critical. Impairments in any of these interacting systems can significantly alter the quality of the movement produced and the level of function achieved. Another concept is that units of the CNS are organized around specific task demands (termed *task systems*). The entire CNS may be necessary for complex tasks, whereas only small portions may be needed for simple tasks. Command levels vary depending on the specific task executed. Thus, the highest level of command (i.e., primary and association motor and sensory cortices) may not be required in the execution of rhythmic (e.g., walking, chewing) and reflexive movements that are typically associated with the brain stem and spinal cord, respectively.[3,4]

Box 5.1   Motor Control Terms

Ability: A genetically predetermined characteristic or trait of a person that underlies performance of certain motor skills.

Coordination: The ability to execute smooth, accurate, and controlled motor responses while moving toward achieving a goal.[1(p436)]

Coordinative structures (synergies): Functionally linked muscles that are constrained by the CNS to act cooperatively to produce an intended movement.[1(p436)]

Degrees of freedom: The collection of separate movements of a system that need to be controlled.[1(p436)]

Feedback: Response-produced information received during or after the movement that allows for appreciation (awareness) of stimuli, modulation of movement, and corrective actions.

Feedforward: The anticipated sensory consequences of movement that should occur if the movement is correct.[1(p437)]

Motor ability: A genetically predetermined characteristic or trait that underlies performance of certain motor skills.

Motor control: The underlying substrates of neural, physical, and behavioral processes that govern posture and movement.

- **Reactive motor control:** Movements are adapted in response to ongoing feedback (e.g., muscle stretch causes an increase in muscle contraction in response to a forward weight shift).
- **Proactive (anticipatory) motor control:** Movements are adapted in advance of ongoing movements via feedforward mechanisms (e.g., the postural adjustments made in preparation for catching a heavy, large ball).

Motor learning: A set of internal processes associated with practice or experience leading to relatively permanent changes in the capability for skilled behavior.[1(p438)]

Motor memory (*procedural memory*): The recall of motor programs or subroutines and the retention (memory) of motor information and movements.

Motor planning (motor praxis): The ability to plan and execute coordinated movement.

Motor program: A prestructured set of movement commands that defines the essential details of skilled action, with minimal or no involvement of sensory feedback.[1(p438)]

Generalized motor program (GMP): A higher level motor program, defined as a motor program whose output can vary along certain dimensions to produce novelty and generalizability in movement (e.g., walking versus running).[1(p437)]

Schema: A learned rule, concept, or generalization relating the outcomes of a class of actions using parameters that were used to produce those outcomes; schema serve to provide a basis for movement decisions and are stored in memory for the reproduction of movement (e.g., recall of past movement initial conditions and past outcomes).[1(p440)]

Motor skill: A goal-directed action or task; acquisition of skill is dependent on practice and experience and is not genetically defined.

Motor Structure and Function

The primary motor cortex and lateral spinal pathways (i.e., lateral corticospinal and rubrospinal tracts) are involved in voluntary movements of distal musculature (see Figs. 5.1 and 5.2). Similar to the somatosensory cortex, the motor cortex has a somatotopic organization (homunculus) with greater cortical representation in areas of increased motor control and dexterity (see Fig. 5.3). Ventromedial pathways (i.e., medial corticospinal, vestibulospinal, tectospinal, and pontine and medullary reticulospinal tracts) are involved in control of posture and locomotion and, with the exception of the medial corticospinal tract, are located at the brain stem (Fig. 5.4). The neurons of the ventral horn (alpha and gamma motor neurons) of the spinal cord and motor unit serve as the *final common pathway* to not only engage the peripheral muscles (extrafusal fibers) but also to regulate muscle spindle alignment (intrafusal fibers) to optimize proprioceptive feedback (see Fig. 5.5).[5]

Optimal neuromuscular transmission requires a healthy motor cortex, brain stem motor nuclei, descending CNS motor tracts, and motor units. A motor unit is

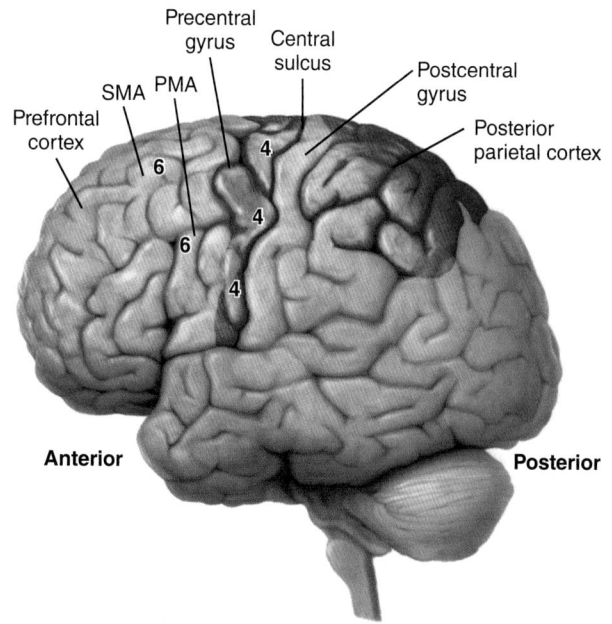

Figure 5.1 Primary areas of the cortex involved in coordinated movement.

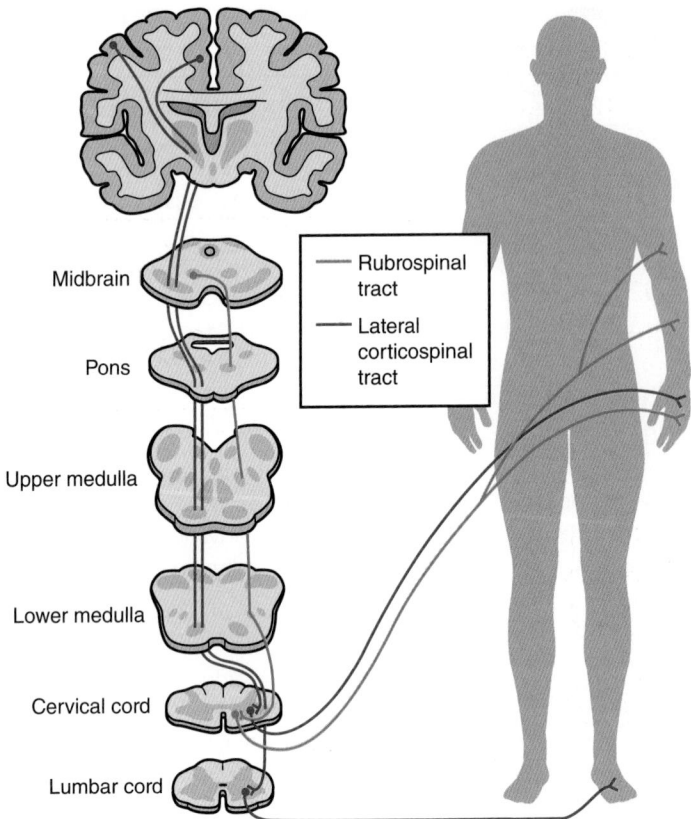

Figure 5.2 Lateral spinal pathways.

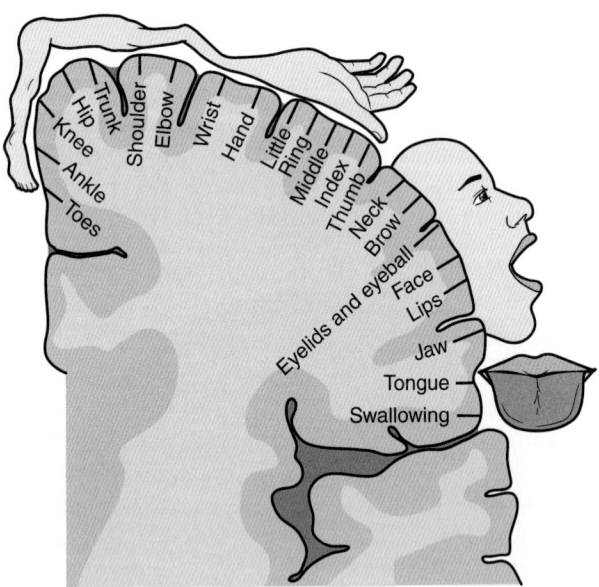

Figure 5.3 The motor homunculus.

composed of one anterior horn cell, one axon, its neuromuscular junction (see Fig. 5.6), and all the muscle fibers innervated by that axon. The health of the anterior horn cell determines cell life or death, and its impact is reflected by the significant motor atrophy and weakness that is demonstrated in patients with motor neuron disease (e.g., amyotrophic lateral sclerosis [ALS], polio; see Chapter 17, Amyotrophic Lateral Sclerosis).[4,5]

Peripheral axons are typically surrounded by some degree of myelin (produced by the Schwann cell) with gaps (nodes of Ranvier) that in combination increase nerve conduction velocity. Peripheral nerve injuries, entrapments, and disease may predominately impact myelin (e.g., early carpal tunnel, Guillain-Barré syndrome), axons (e.g., traumatic injuries), or both (e.g., diabetic polyneuropathy). Peripheral neural connective tissue structures assist in the organization and protection of axons and are known as the endoneurium, perineurium, and epineurium (see Fig. 5.7). The endoneurium surrounds individual axons and provides a conduit for nerves to grow and travel. Perineurium envelopes the fascicles, and the epineurium surrounds the entire nerve trunk.[5] Damage to an axon results in Wallerian degeneration with loss of one to two nodes of Ranvier proximally and complete loss of the axon distal to the site of damage. This process typically requires 5 to 7 days to complete in motor neurons and 7 to 10 days in sensory neurons. If the remaining axon has a healthy environment with connective tissue support, axonal regeneration can occur at approximately 1 mm a day or an inch a month.[6] Nerve classifications by Seddon and Sunderland (see Fig. 5.8) highlight the progression of peripheral nerve injury according to involvement of myelin (i.e., neuropraxia

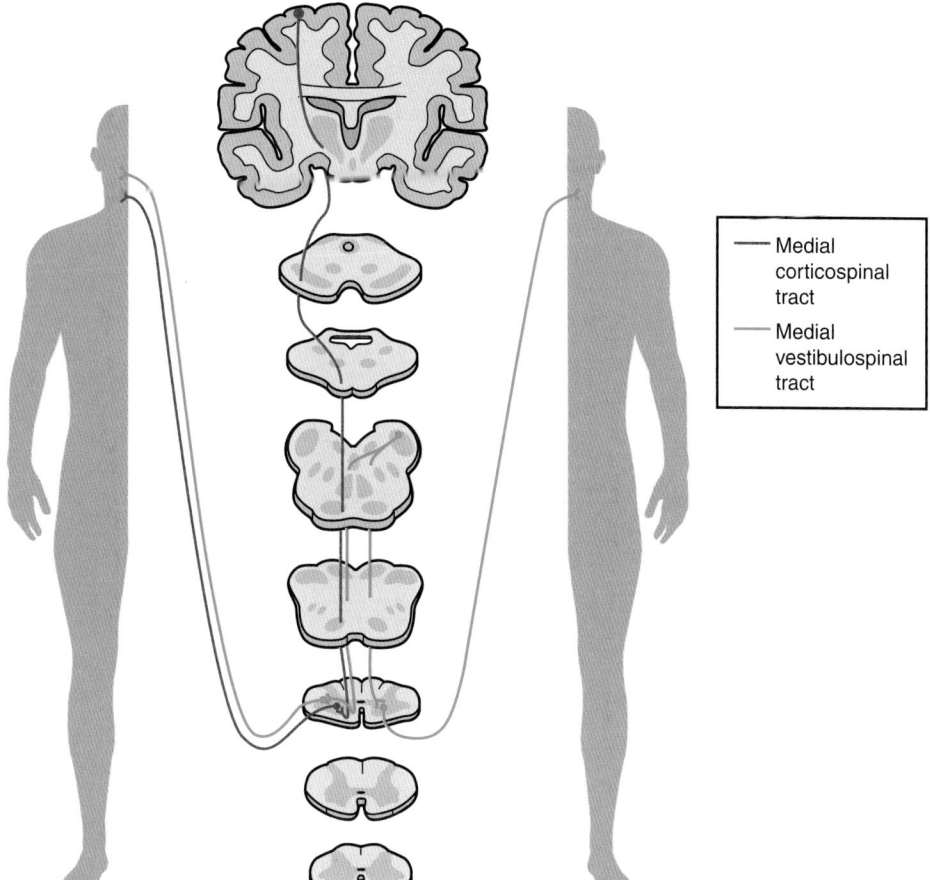

Figure 5.4 Ventromedial pathways.

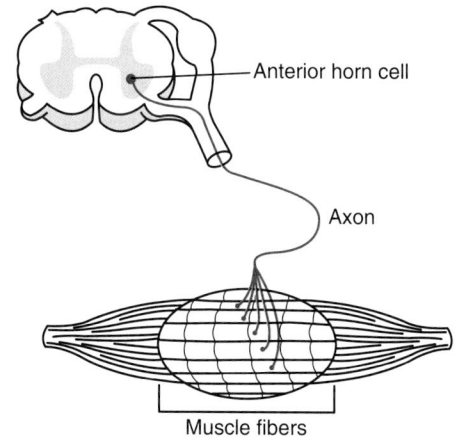

Figure 5.5 The motor unit.

or grade 1) and varying involvement of axons and connective tissue structures (axonotmesis/neurotmesis, grades 2 to 5).[7,8]

Neuromuscular transmission also requires an optimal balance of neurotransmitters, receptors, and ions that assist in the generation of an action potential both within the central motor pathways, anterior horn cells, and neuromuscular junction. For example, neuromuscular junction disease may be presynaptic with antibodies blocking calcium channels, resulting in impaired release of acetylcholine (e.g., Lambert Eaton myasthenia syndrome) or postsynaptic with antibodies blocking or ultimately destroying nicotinic acetylcholine receptors (e.g., myasthenia gravis).[5,9]

Recovery and Neuroplasticity

Recovery is the reacquisition of the ability to perform movement in the same manner as it was performed prior to injury (i.e., using the same body segments). Function is restored in neuromuscular tissue that was initially lost after injury. Task performance is similar to that used by nondisabled individuals. *Compensation* refers to the performance of movement in a new manner. Alternative movements can result from (1) *adaptation* of remaining motor elements or (2) *substitution* of movements using different motor elements or body segments. Neural tissue acquires a new function, and tasks are accomplished using alternate muscles or limbs. For example, the patient with stroke dresses by using the less-involved upper extremity (UE). A determination needs to be made as to whether the movements demonstrate recovery or compensation. If compensatory movements are present, are they of sufficient quality and efficiency to permit return of function?[10,11]

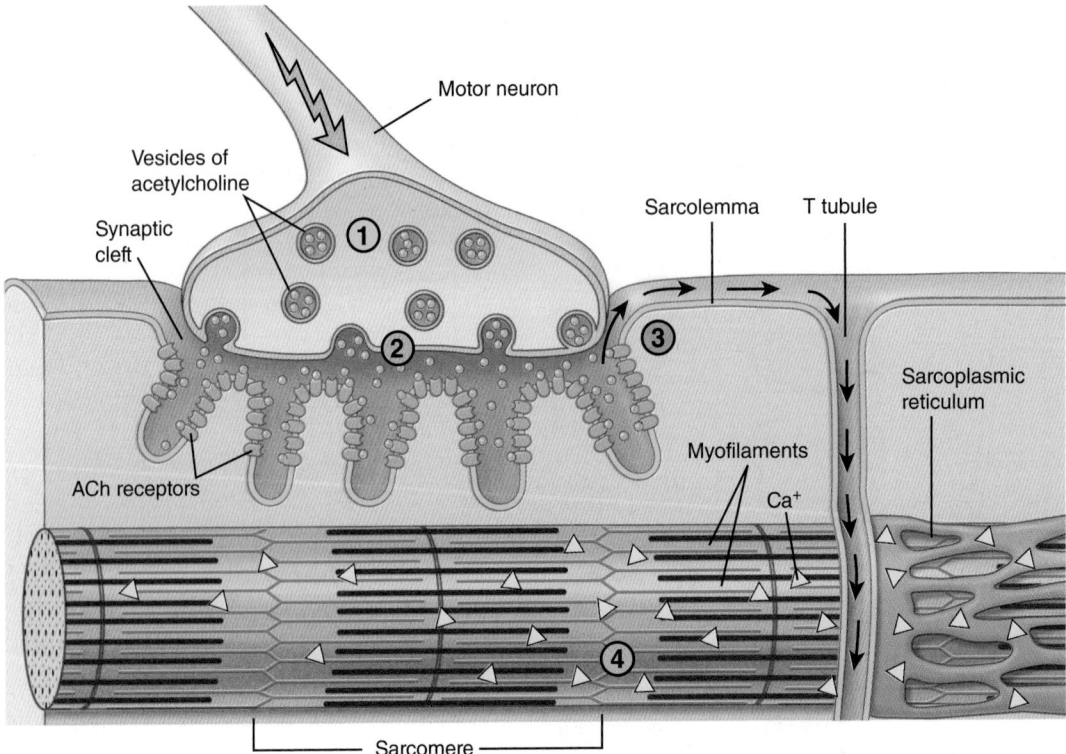

Figure 5.6 Neuromuscular junction activation: 1) Action potential in motor axon results in activation of calcium channels of vesicles of acetylcholine toward the synaptic cleft; 2) Acetylcholine is released into the synaptic cleft; 3) Acetylcholine binds with nicotinic receptors resulting in opening of voltage-gated sodium channels and an action potential that travels from the muscle membrane to T tubules; 4) Sarcoplasmic reticulum releases calcium into the sarcoplasm creating a cascade of events (calcium binds to troponin, tropomyosin moves to expose binding sites on actin, and myosin crossbridges bind to sites on actin) that results in muscle contraction.

Neural plasticity refers to the adaptive capacity of the peripheral nervous system and CNS to change and/or repair itself. Following peripheral nerve injury, the PNS demonstrates neuroplastic recovery via remyelination, axonal regeneration, or collateral sprouting (see Fig. 5.9) Although the human CNS has very limited ability to effectively regrow axons following injury or disease, the brain and spinal cord change in both structure and function via synaptic and neural network plasticity. The CNS has the unique and innate capacity to encode experiences and learn new behaviors (i.e., experience-dependent neural plasticity).[10] Learning involves both short-term changes (e.g., increases in the strength of synaptic connections via modulation of neurotransmitters and receptors) and long-term changes (e.g., modification in genes, neurons, and neuronal networks within specific CNS regions). As learning progresses, there is a shift from short-term to long-term processes. Motor (procedural) memory allows for continued access of this information for repeat performance or modification of existing patterns of movement. Thus, the patient with brain damage (e.g., traumatic brain injury [TBI], stroke) may progress and improve in motor function with an effective rehabilitation plan of care (POC).

Unfortunately, neuroplastic mechanisms may also result in impairments such as chronic pain (e.g., central sensitization), spasticity, and impaired motor control following neural injury.[4] This balance reinforces that the therapist needs to ensure the examination accurately identifies all elements of the patient's motor function. Box 5.2 summarizes terminology related to neuroplasticity and recovery. See additional discussion in Chapter 10, Strategies to Improve Motor Function.

Damage to the nervous and muscular systems interferes with motor function processes. Lesions affecting areas of the PNS, CNS, and muscle can produce specific, recognizable deficits that are relatively consistent among patients (e.g., patients with lower or upper motor neuron syndrome, neuromuscular junction disorders, or myopathy). Individual differences in neural plasticity, recovery, and functional outcomes can also be expected. In conditions with widespread damage to the CNS (e.g., multiple sclerosis [MS] or TBI) the resultant impairments in motor function are numerous, complex, and difficult to delineate. An accurate picture of the scope of deficits may not be readily apparent on initial examination. A process of reexamination over time will generally yield an understanding of

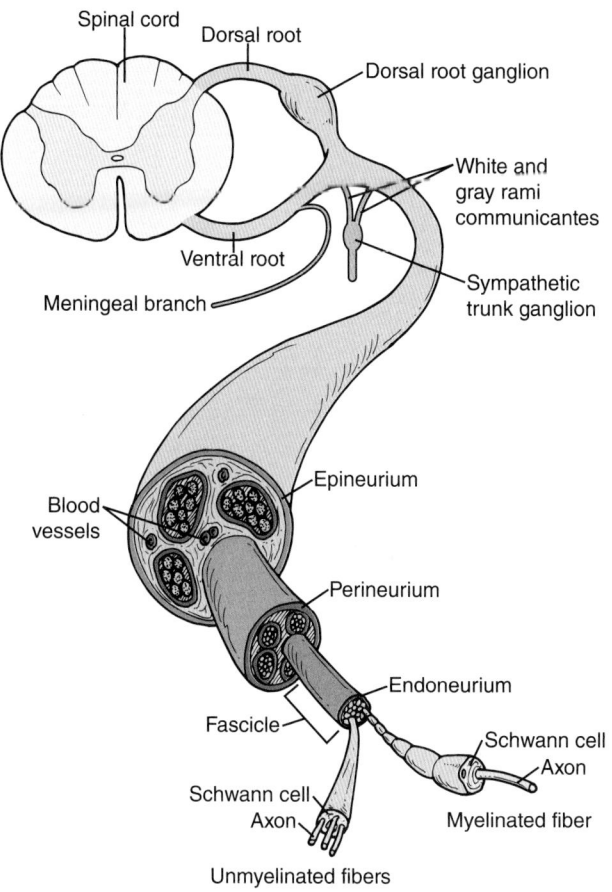

Figure 5.7 The peripheral nerve.

the patient's performance capabilities, deficits, and prognosis. The comprehensive examination focuses on functional activities and participation, movement observations, and impairments of body structure and function that directly affect neuromuscular function. Goals, expected outcomes, and a POC can then be effectively developed.

This chapter reviews the essential components of the neuromuscular examination including functional activities and participation, the movement system and available strategies, system impairments and their impact on movement, and factors that may constrain the motor examination. Excluded is the examination of coordination and balance that is discussed fully in Chapter 6, Examination of Coordination and Balance. Additionally, the chapter provides a discussion of the instrumentation and technology used to assess neuromuscular structure and function including imaging: radiography, CT scan, magnetic resonance imaging (MRI), functional MRI (fMRI), and positron emission tomography (PET)/single photon emission computed tomography (SPECT), as well as electrophysiologic neuromuscular assessments such as electromyography (EMG), nerve conduction velocity (NCV), electroencephalography (EEG), and transmagnetic stimulation (TMS). The chapter concludes with a comparison of clinical findings and differential diagnosis of common peripheral and CNS disorders.

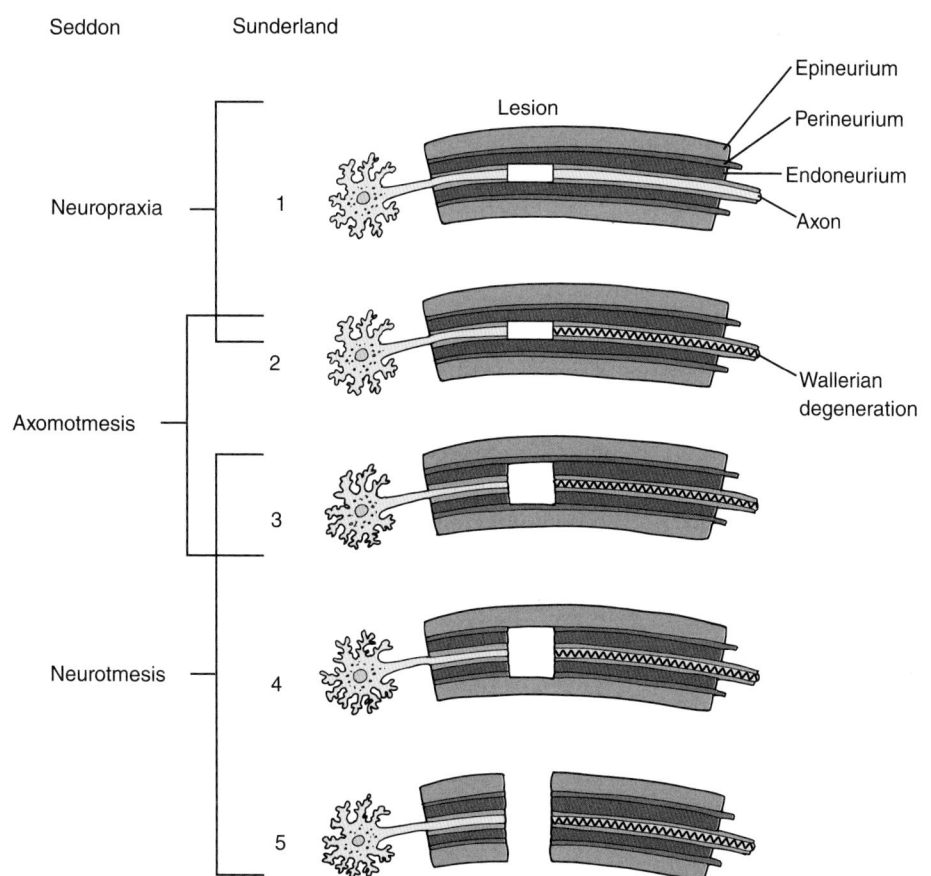

Figure 5.8 Seddon and Sunderland classification of nerve injury.

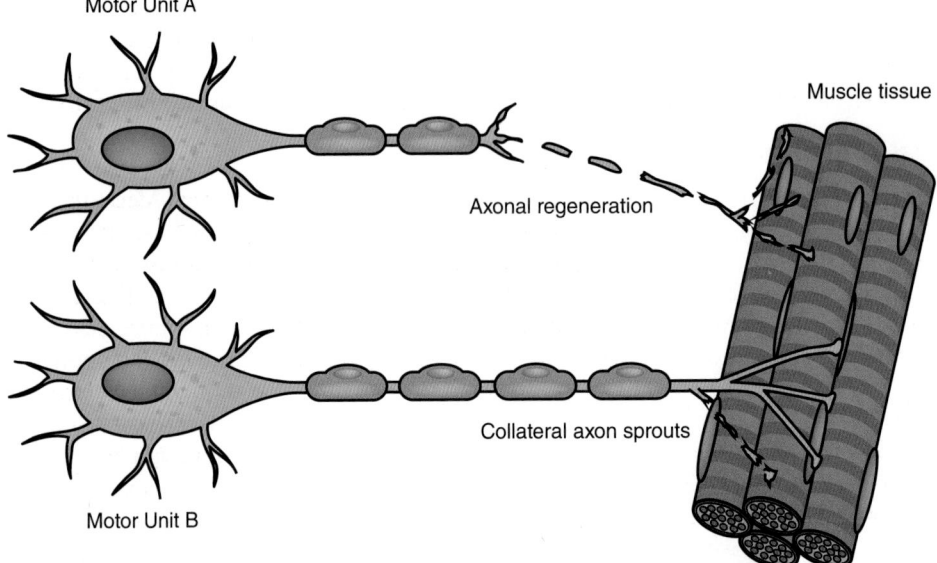

Figure 5.9 Remyelination, axonal regeneration, and collateral sprouting.

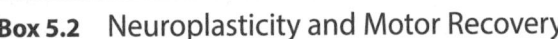

Box 5.2   Neuroplasticity and Motor Recovery

Neuroplasticity: lifelong capacity of the nervous system to continuously change in structure and function. Includes intercellular changes (changes at the synaptic level) and network changes (cortical reorganization).[2(p91)]

Motor recovery: restoration of the ability to perform a movement in the same manner as it was performed prior to injury; tasks are accomplished using limbs or end effectors typically used by nondisabled individuals.

• **Function-induced recovery:** restoration of function resulting from use-dependent cortical reorganization occurring in response to movement of the affected limbs and changes in activity and the environment.

• **Spontaneous recovery:** restoration of function in neural tissue initially lost after injury resulting from naturally occurring repair processes within the CNS.

• **Learned nonuse:** a behavioral learned response to sensory loss or paresis; limbs are capable of movement but are weak and/or clumsy, resulting in preferential use of unaffected limbs; nonuse of the affected extremities interferes with recovery (the *use it or lose it principle*).

Motor compensation: performance of an old movement in a new manner.

• **Adaptation:** appearance of alternative motor patterns using remaining motor elements of the involved limbs or body segments (tasks are accomplished using alternative movement patterns).

• **Substitution:** tasks are accomplished using movements produced by alternate limbs or body segments.

■ COMPONENTS OF THE EXAMINATION

The examination of motor function involves three components: (1) patient history, (2) a review of relevant systems, and (3) specific tests and measures that allow formulation of the diagnosis, prognosis, and POC.[12]

Patient History

During the patient/client history, information is gathered on (1) general demographics, (2) social history, (3) employment/work (job/school/play), (4) living environment, (5) general health status, (6) social/health habits, (7) family history, (8) medical/surgical history, (9) current condition(s)/chief complaint(s), (10) functional status and activity level, (11) medications, and (12) other clinical tests. Information is obtained from the patient and other interested persons (e.g., family members, significant others, and caregivers). If the patient is unable to communicate accurate and meaningful information, as is frequently the case with injury to the brain, data must be gathered from other sources (e.g., family members, caregivers). A review of the medical record can be used to verify and triangulate data obtained from personal communications. Often, the medical record of a patient with pronounced deficits in motor function (e.g., the patient with TBI) contains a large amount of data that can be unwieldy and difficult to sort through. The therapist can benefit from the application of a framework to identify and classify problems. The International Classification of Functioning, Disability and Health (ICF) model[13] focuses on impairments, activity limitations, and participation restrictions, and provides a useful framework. It is discussed fully in Chapter 1, Clinical Decision-Making.

Systems Review

A systems review serves the purpose of a screening examination, that is, a brief or limited examination of body systems. The physical therapist can then use this information to identify potential problems that will require more extensive examination. For example, screening examinations for posture and tone may reveal significant impairments. More detailed tests and measures are then required to delineate the exact nature of the problems uncovered. Sometimes screening examinations reveal problems in communication and/or cognition that preclude further testing. For example, a patient with stroke and severe communication and cognitive impairments will be unable to follow directions and cooperate with many individual tests of physical function. The therapist will document this in the medical record as *unable to test at the present time due to severe communication/cognitive deficits.*

Tests and Measures

Therapists should select standardized tests and outcome measures with established validity and reliability whenever possible, consistent with the American Physical Therapy Association's (APTA) goal of *evidence-based practice.*[12] Examination of motor function is a multifaceted process that typically requires several different tests and measures. Information should be obtained about movement and function (i.e., activity limitations and participation restrictions) and specific impairments (i.e., body functions and structure). Instruments can be general (providing an overall measure of health) or specific (providing condition-specific, body-region specific, or individual-specific data). Instruments can be self-report or performance based with a focus on qualitative or quantitative aspects of movement or both. Many different instruments focusing on the examination of motor function are discussed in later chapters in this text.

The Rehabilitation Measures Database (RMD)-Shirley Ryan Ability Lab contains more than 500 tests and measures and provides a valuable source of information on specific tests and measures (http://www.sralab.org).[14] The RMD is supported by the continuing efforts of numerous contributors (physicians, clinicians, therapists, researchers) and numerous funding sources, including the National Institute of Disability. The RMD collaborates closely with members of the APTA using a framework developed by the APTA Research Section titled EDGE (*Evaluation Database to Guide Effectiveness*). Consensus-based working groups, EDGE task forces, have released several EDGE documents that provide recommendations for outcome measures used in neurologic physical therapy. These include recommendations for the examination of patients with stroke (StrokEDGE),

multiple sclerosis (MSEDGE), spinal cord injury (SCIEDGE), traumatic brain injury (TBIEDGE), vestibular dysfunction (VestibularEDGE), and Parkinson disease (PDEDGE). These can be found on the Academy of Neurologic Physical Therapy (ANPT) website (http://www.neuropt.org) entitled EDGE Taskforce Outcome Measures.[15] ANPT also supported the publication of a clinical practice guideline that recommends a core set of outcome measures to use with people with neurological health conditions.

Qualitative assessment of motor function requires insights and understanding of patterns of movement and functional activities. The therapist uses inductive reasoning processes (formulating generalizations from specific observations). An experienced therapist or expert clinician is far more efficient in reaching decisions about qualitative performance than is the novice therapist. Quantitative instruments use objective measurement as a way of examining performance. Documentation requirements imposed by the health-care system and third-party payers increasingly emphasize objective instruments as evidence of the need for as well as the effectiveness of services. However, many aspects of motor function are not easily measured, especially in the patient with neurological injury. For example, motor learning is not directly measurable but rather is inferred from measures of performance, retention, generalizability, and adaptability. Thus, these constructs are used to infer changes in the CNS that occur with learning. The therapist must be sensitive to the nature of the variables being examined and identify appropriate measures that provide a meaningful analysis of patient function. It is not likely that any one measure will provide all the data needed for the examination of motor function.

Reexamination is performed to determine if goals and outcomes are being met and if the patient is benefiting from the POC. If goals and expected outcomes are not being met, modifications in the POC are needed. The patient who has reached a plateau and does not show continued progress over time is considered for discharge. Many patients with deficits in motor function typically undergo multiple episodes of rehabilitation as recovery occurs (e.g., TBI or stroke). Patients with chronic progressive conditions, such as Parkinson disease (PD) and MS, also typically experience multiple episodes of rehabilitation when deterioration with loss of function occurs.

■ CONSTRAINTS ON THE MOTOR FUNCTION EXAMINATION

Patients who sustain brain damage either through trauma or disease may present with a number of sensory, perceptual, cognitive, communication, and motor system impairments that can significantly affect how they move, experience the environment, and interact with others. It is important to understand how the examination of motor function can be constrained by these impairments.

Sensory Impairments

Sensory system impairments include deficits in somatosensation (e.g., loss of position and movement sense, loss of touch and pressure sensations, pain), vision (e.g., poor eyesight, visual field deficits, homonymous hemianopsia), and vestibular function (e.g., loss of gaze stabilization, dizziness, impaired posture, and balance control). These deficits can have a significant impact on the examination of motor function. Sensory testing involves investigating the ability to detect stimuli, discriminate or distinguish between stimuli, and the ability to organize and utilize sensory inputs appropriately (see Chapter 3, Examination of Sensory Function). The evaluation process seeks to link the identified sensory deficits to loss of function and movement deficiencies. Thus, a thorough sensory examination is an important *first step* in the examination of motor function and ruling out specific health conditions that typically impair both motor and somatosensory function (e.g., radiculopathy, most entrapment mononeuropathies, chronic polyneuropathy, cortical strokes).

Patients who have deficits in any movement-monitoring sensory system may be able to compensate using other sensory systems. For example, the patient with major distal lower extremity (LE) cutaneous and proprioceptive losses with ataxia looking straight ahead can use vision (i.e., looking down) as an error-correcting system to maintain a stable posture and improve gait. When vision is also impaired (e.g., the patient with diabetic neuropathy and retinopathy), however, postural instability becomes readily apparent. Significant sensory losses and inadequate compensatory shifts to other sensory systems may result in severely disordered movement responses. The patient with proprioceptive losses (demyelination in the dorsal columns of the cervical spinal cord) and severe visual disturbances (demyelination in the optic chiasm), such as diplopia (commonly seen in the patient with MS), may be unable to maintain a stable posture. An accurate examination, therefore, requires that the therapist not only look at each individual sensory system but also at the overall sensory interaction and integration and the adequacy of compensatory adjustments.

Perceptual Impairments

Perception is the integration of sensory information that enables an individual to interpret the sensation accurately, and therefore respond appropriately. Accurate perception is a critical component of moving successfully through complex and diverse environments and in motor learning. There are several perceptual impairments that can contribute to difficulties in the examination of motor control that may only become fully apparent over time. Body scheme/body image impairments include unilateral neglect, anosognosia, somatoagnosia, and right-left discrimination. Spatial relation impairments include figure-ground discrimination, form discrimination, position in space, topographical disorientation, depth and distance perception, and vertical disorientation. Agnosia impairments include visual object agnosia, auditory agnosia, and tactile agnosia. Deficits in apraxia include ideomotor apraxia, ideational apraxia, and buccofacial apraxia. The physical therapist should be able to screen for perceptual deficits and initiate appropriate referrals. Consultation with an occupational therapist, optometrist, or audiologist may assist in the examination, evaluation, and holistic treatment of patients with perceptual deficits. See Chapter 27, Cognitive and Perceptual Dysfunction, for discussion of these impairments and their role in impairing function.

Altered Consciousness and Arousal

Examination of consciousness and arousal is important in determining the degree to which an individual is able to respond. The *ascending reticular activating system* includes core neurons in the brain stem, the locus coeruleus, and raphe nuclei that synapse directly on the thalamus, cortex, and other brain regions. It functions to arouse and awaken the brain and control sleep–wake cycles. High levels of activity are associated with extreme excitement (high arousal), whereas lesions in the brain stem are associated with low arousal, sleep, and coma (e.g., the patient with profound brain injury). Additional information on the levels of consciousness and arousal are in Chapter 19, Traumatic Brain Injury.

The *Glasgow Coma Scale* (GCS) is a gold standard instrument used to document level of consciousness in acute brain injury. Three areas of function are examined: eye opening, best motor response, and verbal response. Total GCS scores range from a low of 3 to a high of 15. A total score of 8 or less is indicative of severe brain injury and coma, a score between 9 and 12 is indicative of moderate brain injury, and a score between 13 and 15 is indicative of mild brain injury.[16] The Rancho Los Amigos Levels of Cognitive Function is widely used in rehabilitation facilities to examine the return of the person with brain injury from coma (Level I, no response) to generalized and localized states (Levels II-III) to confused states (Levels IV-VI) to automatic–appropriate state (Level VII), and finally to purposeful–appropriate state (Level VIII).[17] See Chapter 19, Traumatic Brain Injury, for additional discussion.

Examination of the pupillary size and reaction can also reveal important information about the unconscious patient. Pupils that are bilaterally small may be indicative of damage to the sympathetic pathways in the hypothalamus or metabolic encephalopathy. Pinpoint pupils are suggestive of a hemorrhagic pontine lesion or narcotic overdose (e.g., morphine, heroin). Pupils that are fixed in mid-position and slightly dilated are suggestive of midbrain damage, whereas large bilaterally fixed and dilated pupils suggest severe anoxia or drug toxicity (e.g., tricyclic antidepressants). If only one pupil is fixed and dilated, temporal lobe herniation with compression of the oculomotor nerve and midbrain is likely.[18]

Whereas an appropriate level of arousal allows for optimal motor performance, very low or high levels of arousal can cause deterioration in motor performance. This is referred to as the *inverted-U principle* (Yerkes–Dodson law).[19] Patients at either end of the arousal continuum (either very high or very low) may not respond at all or may respond in an unpredictable manner. This phenomenon may explain the reactions of patients with brain damage who are labile and lack homeostatic controls for normal function. Under conditions of severe stress, performance can become severely disrupted.

Cognitive Impairments

Cognitive abilities include orientation, attention, memory, and executive or higher order cognition (e.g., calculating abilities, abstract thinking, constructional ability). Deficits in cognitive function occur with neurological disease (e.g., frontal lobe disease, TBI) or psychiatric illness (e.g., panic attacks, depression following stroke). Impaired function can range from orientation and memory deficits to poor judgment; distractibility; and difficulties in information processing, abstract reasoning, and learning, to name just a few. Patients with deficits across many or all areas of cognitive function demonstrate diffuse or multifocal pathology (e.g., Alzheimer disease [AD], chronic brain syndrome). Patients with deficits in only one or a few areas of testing typically demonstrate focal deficits (e.g., stroke).[20] The physical therapist may be one of the first professionals to interact with the patient and should be able to screen for cognitive deficits and initiate appropriate referrals. Consultation with an occupational therapist or neuropsychologist is necessary to obtain an accurate picture of these deficits and to help structure the examination of motor function (see Chapter 27, Cognitive and Perceptual Dysfunction). Additionally, as outlined in Chapter 3, it is important to assess if a patient with cortical dysfunction has adequate attention, orientation, and memory to complete a reliable motor examination and assess the impact this may have on motor function.

Executive Functions

Executive functions (higher cognitive functions) include abstract thinking, problem-solving, judgment, reasoning, and so forth. They represent advanced cognitive function and are dependent on the presence and interaction of basic cognitive functions (i.e., attention, memory, language). The patient with brain injury may demonstrate an inability to manipulate information, initiate and terminate activities, recognize errors, problem-solve, and think abstractly. Insight (the ability to understand either oneself or an external situation) and judgment (the ability to form an opinion, reach a decision, or plan an action after analyzing a problem and comparing choices) can also be affected by brain injury.[20] The presence of any of these deficits can significantly impact the examination of motor function, as well as learning and performance. Referral to an occupational therapist and/or neuropsychologist is indicated for comprehensive examination and evaluation (see Chapter 27, Cognitive and Perceptual Dysfunction). Recognition and understanding of these deficits can improve the validity of the motor function examination and the effectiveness of the rehabilitation POC. Collaboration and consistency of team members is paramount in order to reduce potential frustrations and inappropriate expectations.

Communication Impairments

The patient's grasp of information and ability to communicate should be ascertained. The physical therapist should listen carefully to spontaneous speech during the initial examination sessions. The patient's understanding of spoken language can be determined using simple tests. Word comprehension can be determined by varying the difficulty of commands, from one- to two- or three-stage commands (e.g., point to your nose; point to your right hand and lift your left hand). Repetition and naming can be tested (repeat after me; name the parts of a watch). Problems with articulation (*dysarthria*) are evidenced by speech errors, such as difficulties with timing, vocal quality, pitch, volume, and breath control. Problems of *fluency*, word flow without pauses or breaks, should be noted. Speech that flows smoothly but contains errors, neologisms (nonsense words), misuse of words, and circumlocutions (word substitution) is indicative of *fluent aphasia* (e.g., Wernicke aphasia, sensory or receptive aphasia). The patient typically demonstrates deficits in auditory comprehension with well-articulated speech marked by word substitutions. Speech that is slow and hesitant with limited vocabulary and impaired syntax is indicative of *nonfluent aphasia* (e.g., Broca or motor aphasia). Articulation is labored and word-finding difficulties are apparent. In some settings, especially the acute hospital setting, the physical therapist may be the first to become aware of communication deficits. Referral to a speech-language pathologist is indicated for comprehensive examination and evaluation (see Chapter 28, Neurogenic Disorders of Speech and Language).

Recognition and understanding of these deficits can improve the validity of the motor function examination and the effectiveness of the POC. This may include simplifying instructions, using written instructions, or using alternative forms of communication such as gestures, pantomime, or communication boards. A common error is to assume that patients understand the task at hand when they really have no idea what is expected. To ensure accuracy of testing, frequent checks for comprehension should be performed throughout the examination. For example, the use of message discrepancies (saying one thing and gesturing another) can be used to test the patient's level of understanding.

■ MOTOR CONTROL EXAMINATION

Examination of Functional Activities and Movements

Examination of functional activities and movements should focus on those key functional activities important to the patient's daily life that were identified in the earlier interview or questionnaire. Functional activities or tasks are commonly grouped into functional categories. *Activities of daily living* (ADL) refer to those daily living skills necessary for an adult to manage life. *Basic ADL* (BADL) includes grooming skills (e.g., oral hygiene, showering or bathing, dressing), toilet hygiene, feeding, and personal device care. Instrumental ADL (IADL) includes money management, functional communication and socialization, functional and community mobility, and health maintenance. *Functional mobility skills* refer to those skills that allow a person to move around in and interact with their environment. Examples include rolling over and sitting up in bed, sit-to-stand transfers, walking, stair climbing, and wheelchair skills.

During an initial examination and periodically throughout the course of rehabilitation, the therapist typically administers performance-based measures in which the patient is examined in the clinical environment. The Functional Independence Measure (FIM)[21] was a widely used 18-item test of physical, psychological, and social function that is part of the Uniform Data System for Medical Rehabilitation (UDSMR).[22] It defines various levels of assistance ranging from dependent to levels of assistance (maximal, moderate, or minimal assist) to contact guard or stand-by assist, to independent. However, in efforts to standardize data across post-acute care settings including inpatient rehabilitation, skilled nursing, home health and long-term care, the Centers for Medicare and Medicaid Services (CMS) has implemented the collection of GG codes in place of the FIM. These codes are the self-care and mobility items from the Continuity Assessment Record and Evaluation (CARE) item set. Each item is scored on a six-point scale from 01 (dependent) to 07 (independent).

Self-report (subjective) measures can be used to provide information about prior functional abilities and participation and can be used when the patient is unable to perform the test items. For example, the Functional Mobility Assessment is a reliable and stable self-report measure that examines wheeled mobility function.[23] Level of participation refers to the patient's ability to perform tasks within the context of his/her environment and life and is a measure of disability. It is measured objectively by quantifying the frequency of participation or level of independence (e.g., FIM, The Continuity Assessment Record and Evaluation [CARE]). Subjective measures focus on the patient's opinions and feelings about their actual level of participation compared to their desired level of participation. Frequency of participation may or may not directly relate to perceived satisfaction.[24] See Chapter 8, Examination of Function, for a complete discussion.

Movement Observation and Analysis

Movement observation and analysis is foundational to the practice of physical therapists as movement system experts. It requires an understanding of normal human movement. By providing a basis for comparison, this information informs the analysis and evaluation of a patient's performance. Analysis focuses on the interaction between the task, the environment, and patient performance. Key movement constructs the clinician must consider include postural control (verticality and stability) and coordination (speed, smoothness, sequencing, timing, and accuracy).[25] See discussion in Chapter 6, Examination of Coordination and Balance.

Movement analysis is best organized according to stages of movement, including movement preparation and initiation, movement execution, movement termination, and movement outcome. Box 5.3 presents suggested questions that can be used to inform analysis during each stage of movement. Critical skills include accurate observation, recognition, and interpretation of movement deficiencies; determination of how underlying impairments relate to the movement deficiencies observed; and determination of what needs be altered and how. For example, the patient who is unable to transfer from bed to wheelchair may lack postural trunk support (stability), adequate LE extensor control (strength), and ability to maintain control while moving from one surface to the other (dynamic control). Or the patient with acute stroke sits up from supine using the less affected UE for support and propulsion. The more affected extremities lag and are not well integrated into the movement pattern. The final sitting position is asymmetrical with most of the weight borne on the less affected side and the more affected UE held in an abnormally flexed and adducted position.

Initial movement conditions should be standardized (conducted in a structured and controlled environment using key instructions). As performance improves, environmental demands can be modified. For example, visual and auditory inputs are altered, assistance or external support is reduced, verbal cueing is reduced. A determination must be made of how these changes affect performance. For example, the patient with TBI can be easily distracted and thus pays poor attention in the busy clinic environment, resulting in an inability to complete a transfer task. However, the patient is able to perform the transfer in a closed, quiet environment. The term *environmental demands* refers to the physical characteristics of the environment or features required for successful performance of movement (regulatory conditions).

Box 5.3   Suggested Questions to Inform Analysis of Stages of Movement

Initial Conditions, Preparation, and Initiation

A.

1. What are the components of the overall movement sequence (motor plan)?
2. What is the initial posture and starting position?
3. What are the requirements for stimulus identification and response programming?
4. How and where is the movement initiated?
5. What are the requirements of the movement being attempted? Consider factors related to timing, direction, and coordination of the movement.
6. What are the initial environmental conditions and interactions required?

B. Movement Execution

1. How well was the movement performed?
2. Were the musculoskeletal and biomechanical components successful? Consider factors related to amplitude of movements, timing, force, and direction of the movements.
3. Were the requirements for postural control and balance met?
4. Were the requirements for cognitive and sensory/perceptual components met?
5. Were the motor control requirements of the activity met (*mobility, stability, dynamic stability,* or *skill*)?

C. Movement Termination

1. Was the movement successfully terminated?
2. Were the requirements for postural control, timing, stability, and accuracy met?

D. Movement Outcome

1. Was the overall movement sequence successfully completed?
2. If unsuccessful, what components of the patient's movements were abnormal, missing, or delayed?
3. What underlying impairments constrain or impair the movements?
4. Do the movement errors increase over time? Is fatigue a constraining factor?
5. Is patient safety maintained throughout the activity?
6. Can the patient effectively analyze their own movements?
7. Can the patient successfully adapt to changing activity or task demands?
8. What difficulties do you expect this patient may have with other functional activities?
9. What compensatory strategies are evident? Are they functional or nonfunctional?
10. What, if any, adaptive equipment is required? What is the level of success in using the adaptive equipment?
11. What environmental factors constrain or impair movements?
12. Can the patient adapt to changing environmental demands?
13. What difficulties do you expect this patient may have in other environments?
14. Are there any sociocultural factors that may influence performance?

Adapted from the Academy of Neurologic Physical Therapy (ANPT) Movement System Task Force (https://www.neuropt.org).

As performance improves, the task or activity can be modified. For example, the base of support (BOS) can be narrowed, the speed increased, perturbation added, and cognitive demands increased (e.g., dual tasks added). It must be determined how these changes affect performance. The term *activity demands* refers to the requirements imbedded in each step of the activity. It is important to document these findings, as they provide valuable information necessary for developing an effective POC to improve motor function.

The Movement System Task Force from the ANPT recommends using six core tasks for analysis: sitting, sit-to-stand, standing, walking, stepping up and down, and reach/grasp/manipulate. This allows a range of task requirements for analysis: ability to maintain position (sitting and standing), ability to move between positions (sit to stand), ability to move through the environment (step up and down, walk, turn), and ability to complete UE functional skills (reach, grasp, manipulate). The reader is referred to the task force paper for additional discussion and recommendations.[25]

Motor Skills

Motor skills can be categorized by different classification schemes.[26] One widely used classification scheme in physical therapy categorizes motor skills according to movement function and postural control. Categories include *stability* (*static postural control*), *dynamic postural control*, and *transitional mobility*. During stability, the individual is required to maintain a posture in a stable, unchanging position with the center of mass (COM) over the BOS. During dynamic postural control, stability is adjusted and maintained (COM over the BOS) while parts of the body (UE or LE) are moving. During transitional mobility, the individual is able to move from one posture to another with the BOS and/or COM changing. Table 5.1 presents postural and movement characteristics, examples, and indicators of impaired function.

Motor skills can be also classified by discrete/continuous/serial dimensions, gross/fine motor dimensions, and simple versus complex dimensions.[1] These terms are defined in Box 5.4, Categories of Motor Skills. Motor skills are shaped to the specific environments in which they occur. These include open versus closed skills, self-paced versus externally paced skills, and anticipation timing, and are they defined in Box 5.5, Motor Skills and the Environment. Analysis using these dimensions allows for a more complete description of available motor behaviors and improved documentation and communication.

Motor Coordination

Coordination is defined as the ability to execute smooth, efficient, accurate, and controlled movement. *Synergies* are functionally linked muscles that are constrained by the CNS to act cooperatively to produce an intended motor action. They are used to simplify control, reduce, or constrain the degrees of freedom, and initiate coordinated patterns of movement. *Degrees of freedom* refers to "the collection of separate movements that need to be controlled"[1(p436)] by engaging these cooperative units of muscle action. Coordinated movements are defined by precise spatial and temporal organization involving control of speed, distance, direction, rhythm, and levels of muscle tension. In individuals with normal motor control, voluntary movement patterns are functional, task specific, and highly variable, depending on the task purpose and environment. The CNS controls patterns of (1) single-limb and multiple-limb movements, (2) bilateral (bimanual) symmetrical and asymmetrical movements, (3) reciprocal movements, and (4) patterns of proximal stabilization and postural support. Examples include eye-head-hand coordination, reaching and grasping, discrete bimanual tasks, and gait transitions. Examination is discussed fully in Chapter 6, Examination of Coordination and Balance.

Documentation

During an analysis of movements, key elements the therapist should observe and document include the following:

1. the type of skill being demonstrated
2. the ability to organize and control movements
3. the overall quality, efficiency, and economy of movement
4. the success in attaining the action-goal (outcome)

Table 5.1	Classification of Motor Skills According to Movement/Postural Control		
Category	Postural and Movement Characteristics	Postural and Movement Examples	Indicators of Impaired Function
Static postural control (stability)	Ability to maintain postural stability and orientation with the COM over the BOS with the body not in motion; BOS is fixed	Holding in antigravity postures: prone on elbows, quadruped, sitting, kneeling, half-kneeling, plantigrade, or standing	Failure to maintain a steady posture; excessive postural sway; wide BOS; high guard arm position or UE handhold; loss of balance; COM exceeds BOS
Dynamic postural control	Ability to maintain postural stability and orientation with the COM over the BOS while parts of the body are in motion; BOS is fixed	Weight shifting; limb movements (UE reaching, LE stepping in plantigrade or standing)	Failure to maintain or control posture during weight shifting or dynamic trunk or extremity movements; loss of balance
Transitional mobility	Ability to move from one posture to another; BOS and/or COM are changing	Rolling; supine to sit; sit-to-stand; transfers	Failure to initiate or sustain movements through the range; poorly controlled movements
Skill	Ability to consistently perform coordinated movement sequences for the purposes of investigation and interaction with the physical and social environment	UE skills: grasp and manipulation; LE skills. Locomotion, stair climbing: body (COM) is in motion and BOS is changing	Poorly coordinated movements (dyssynergia, dysmetria, dysdiadochokinesia); lack of precision, control, consistency, and economy of effort; inability to achieve a task goal

COM = center of mass; BOS = base of support; UE = upper extremity; LE = lower extremity.

Box 5.4   Categories of Motor Skills

Gross motor skill: a motor skill that involves the large musculature of the body and a task goal in which precision of movement is not important to the successful execution of the skill (e.g., running or jumping)

Fine motor skill: a motor skill that requires coordination of small muscles and the eyes to produce small, precise hand movements (e.g., writing, cutting with scissors, buttoning a shirt)

Discrete motor skill: a skill that has a recognizable beginning and end defined by the task (e.g., coming to stand, locking the brake on a wheelchair)

Serial motor skill: a skill composed of several discrete actions strung together, often with the order of actions being critical for success (e.g., transferring from a bed to a wheelchair)

Continuous motor skill: a rhythmic, cyclical motor skill that is performed without any recognizable beginning or end; behavior continues until arbitrarily stopped by the performer or some external agent (e.g., walking, running, swimming, propelling a wheelchair)

Simple motor skill: a skill that involves a single motor program that produces an individual movement response (e.g., kicking a ball)

Complex motor skill: a skill that involves multiple actions and motor programs combined to produce a coordinated movement response (e.g., running and kicking a soccer ball during a game)

Dual-task skills: motor skills that involve simultaneously performing a secondary motor or cognitive task, requiring divided attention; secondary tasks can be (1) motor (e.g., walks while carrying a tray, walks while catching or bouncing a ball) or (2) cognitive (e.g., walks while talking, walks while counting backward)

Box 5.5   Motor Skills and the Environment

Skilled movements are shaped to the specific environments in which they occur.

Anticipation timing (time to contact): the ability to time movements to a target or an event in the environment, requiring precise control of movements (e.g., avoiding an obstacle, stepping onto an escalator or moving walkway)

Regulatory conditions: those features of the environment to which movement must be molded to be successful (e.g., stepping on a moving walkway or into a revolving door)

- **Closed skills:** skills performed in a stable, predictable environment (e.g., activities practiced in a quiet room, walking in a quiet hall)
- **Open skills:** skills performed in a changing or unpredictable environment (e.g., activities practiced in a busy gym, crossing a busy street)
- **Self-paced skills:** movements that are initiated at will and whose timing is controlled or modified by the person (e.g., walking)
- **Externally paced skills:** movements that are initiated and paced by dictates of the external environment (e.g., walking in time with a metronome, crossing at a streetlight)

5. the ability to adapt easily and successfully to changing task demands
6. the ability to adapt easily and successfully to changing environmental demands
7. verbal cues and assistance, if any, required
8. the results of specific tests and measures administered

The qualitative analysis of movements can be enhanced by video-recording the patient's movements (motion capture). Sequential recordings over the course of rehabilitation provide visual documentation of patient progress and can be an important motivational and educational tool for use with the patient and family.[27] Computer-based video analysis of the movements can be used to assist both the therapist and the patient in understanding movement deficits.[28] Movement recordings can be viewed repeatedly at different speeds to determine control during different tasks and at different body segments. For example, a patient's performance in a task such as sitting up from supine can be observed first at regular speeds, then at slow-motion speeds. Stop-action or freezing a frame can be used to isolate a problematic point in the movement sequence. This may be helpful, particularly for the inexperienced therapist, in improving both the quality and reliability of observations. Examples of video-recorded case studies accompanying this text can be viewed online at https://www.fadavis.com/product/physical-rehabilitation-fulk-8.

■ EXAMINATION OF BODY STRUCTURE AND FUNCTION

Pathology of the motor system affecting the motor cortex and subcortical areas (e.g., cerebellum, basal ganglia, spinal cord) produces a wide range of primary musculoskeletal and neuromuscular impairments that directly influence motor function. Secondary impairments develop as a result of inactivity (e.g., muscle atrophy, contracture, decreased endurance) and not because of the original CNS pathology. *Upper motor neuron syndrome (UMN)* occurs after injury to brain (motor cortex or descending motor pathways) or spinal cord. Signs and symptoms include decreased muscle control, weakness, easy fatigability, increased muscle tone, spasticity, exaggerated deep tendon reflexes, hyporeflexia of superficial reflexes, and Babinski sign. See Table 5.2, Positive and Negative Features of Upper Motor Syndrome. Motor impairments associated with subcortical pathology (e.g., cerebellum, basal ganglia) are discussed in Chapter 6. Lower motor neuron syndrome (LMN) arises from pathology affecting the distal motor nerve up to the level of the anterior horn cell in the spinal cord. It can occur as a result of hereditary conditions (e.g., spinal muscle atrophy, familial motor neuron disease) or from injury to the motor neuron. Symptoms include muscle atrophy, weakness, and hyporeflexia with an absence of sensory involvement. An accurate examination depends on the therapist's knowledge and understanding of the pathophysiology and the impact on motor function, discussed in the next sections.

Table 5.2	Positive and Negative Features of Upper Motor Neuron Syndrome
Negative Features	**Positive Features**
Paresis and paralysis	Spasticity
Loss of dexterity	Stereotyped movement synergies; spastic dystonia
Fatigue	Spasms (flexor, extensor/adductor)
	Spastic co-contraction
	Extensor plantar response (Babinski sign)
	Clonus
	Exaggerated deep tendon reflexes
	Associated reactions
	Disturbances in movement efficiency and speed; mass movements

Musculoskeletal Impairments

Examination of the musculoskeletal system is essential. Important elements include joint integrity and mobility, and muscle performance (e.g., strength, power, endurance, and length). This is discussed fully in Chapter 4, Musculoskeletal Examination. This next section will focus on impairments seen in patients with neurological conditions that may impact motor control.

Limitations in Range of Motion and Alignment

Limitations in joint range of motion (ROM) restrict the normal coordinated action of muscles and alter the biomechanical alignment of body segments and posture. Long-standing immobilization or inactivity result in contracture (a fixed resistance resulting from fibrosis of tissues surrounding a joint) and restricted movement. The resultant compensatory movement patterns are frequently dysfunctional, producing additional stresses and strains on the musculoskeletal system. They are also more energy costly and can significantly affect functional performance. For example, shortening of the gastrocnemius muscles results in a toe-walking gait pattern; tightness of the hip adductors results in a scissoring gait pattern. Changes in alignment secondary to muscle tightness alter postural control. For example, in standing, anterior pelvic tilting and flexion of the hips and knees are typically the result of hip flexor tightness. In sitting, posterior pelvic tilting is associated with kyphosis and forward head position and is typically the result of hamstring tightness. Abnormalities in alignment that alter the COM within the BOS place increased demands on the postural control system. For example, the patient with chronic stroke will demonstrate altered postural alignment in standing with more weight distributed over the less affected limb and away from the more affected limb. This patient also typically demonstrates a more forward leaning posture with greater anterior pelvic tilt, resulting in limitations in balance and postural control.[29]

Motor Weakness and Muscle Atrophy

Muscle performance is the capacity of muscle(s) to generate forces whereas *muscle strength* is the force exerted by muscle(s) to overcome a resistance.[12] Isotonic contractions involve active shortening of muscles, and eccentric contractions involve active lengthening of muscles. Isometric contractions produce high levels of tension for holding contractions without overt movement. *Muscle power* is defined as the work produced per unit of time or the product of strength and speed.[12] Muscle performance depends on a number of interrelated factors, including length–tension characteristics, viscoelasticity, velocity, and metabolic adequacy (i.e., fuel storage and delivery). Of equal importance are the integrated actions of the CNS (neuromuscular control factors) acting on motor units, including (1) the number of motor units recruited, (2) the type of motor units recruited, and (3) the discharge rate and continuing modulation of motor units. The CNS controls the recruitment order and timing of muscles. Synergistic movements and postural adjustments also depend on the integrity of the peripheral nerves and on the muscle fibers.

Patients with impairments in motor function and neurological injury pose unique challenges for the examination of muscle strength. *Weakness* is the inability to generate sufficient levels of force and can vary from *paresis* (partial weakness) to *plegia* (absence of muscle strength). Weakness is seen in patients with UMN syndrome. Patients may present with *hemiplegia* (one-sided paralysis), *paraplegia* (LE paralysis), or *tetraplegia* (quadriplegia). Weakness also appears in patients with LMN lesions. Prolonged weakness from neuromuscular impairment can lead to secondary musculoskeletal weakness (peripheral changes in muscle).

Patients with stroke demonstrate significant changes in muscle performance, including altered recruitment patterns, abnormal times to achieve force, and decreased motor unit firing rates.[30] Within 2 months after insult, they also demonstrate up to a 50% decrease in motor units of affected extremities with greater losses of type II (fast twitch) fibers.[31] Muscle performance in patients with stroke is influenced by the presence of other UMN impairments, including spasticity, disordered synergistic activity/mass patterns of movements, abnormal muscle cocontraction, and/or profound sensory deficit.[32-34] Strength losses are typically greater in the distal extremity than the proximal. Strength losses have also been found on the "supposedly normal" extremities.[35,36] The bilateral effects of an ipsilateral cortical lesion are evidence of the small percentage (estimated 10%) of corticospinal tract fibers that remain uncrossed. Possible other unidentified factors may also exist. This information has prompted use of terms such as *less involved* or *less affected* in place of more traditional terms such as *unaffected, uninvolved, sound, normal,* or *good* side. This also casts doubt as to the validity of using the contralateral uninvolved side as a reference for normal muscle strength in patients with hemiplegia.

In patients with chronic symmetrical peripheral sensorimotor neuropathy (e.g., diabetic neuropathy) or acute motor neuropathy (e.g., Guillain-Barré), strength losses are typically greater in distal segments (i.e., foot and ankle) than proximal, with involvement of more proximal segments as the disease progresses. In chronic symmetrical neuropathy, the progression is slow (months or years), whereas in Guillain-Barré the progression is rapid (days or weeks) and more complete (i.e., demyelination of peripheral nerves and nerve roots), involving not just the proximal LEs but also the trunk, UEs, and in some cases the lower CN nerves. Patients with primary muscle disease (e.g., myopathies) typically experience proximal weakness, whereas patients with myasthenia gravis

experience decremental strength losses with greatest initial involvement in the orofacial and proximal extremity muscles. Thus, the first contraction of a muscle may start out strong, and each succeeding contraction gets weaker and weaker.

The clinical examination of muscle strength utilizes standardized methods and protocols (e.g., manual muscle testing [MMT], handheld dynamometers, instrumented isokinetic systems). There are validity issues when MMT is used in the clinical examination of patients with UMN lesions.[37,38] Appropriate criteria are therefore critical in determining whether the standards of validity and reliability of MMT are met. First and foremost, the therapist must consider the patient's movement capabilities. Individual isolated joint movements, mandated by standardized MMT procedures and isokinetic protocols, may not be possible in the presence of an UMN lesion where abnormal obligatory synergies are present. The presence of abnormal coactivation, spasticity, and abnormal posturing may preclude the patient's ability to perform isolated joint movements. These barriers to normal movement are termed *active restraint.* The prescribed test positions may also be precluded by the presence of abnormal reflex activity (e.g., supine testing influenced by presence of the tonic labyrinthine reflex). Muscle and soft tissue changes in viscoelasticity (e.g., contracture) offer a form of *passive restraint* and may also preclude the use of standardized testing. In these instances, the decision should be made *not* to use standardized MMT procedures. An estimation of strength can be made from observations of active movements during performance of functional activities. For example, shallow knee bends or sit-to-stand transfers can be used to examine the strength of hip extensors and knee extensors. Standing heel-rises or toe-rises can be used to examine the strength of foot–ankle muscles (dorsiflexors, plantarflexors). Documentation should clearly indicate that UMN involvement precluded use of standardized MMT procedures. Estimates of strength can be made based on observations during active functional movements. Inability to move or support the body against gravity should receive a poor grade. The ability to move the body against gravity should receive a fair grade, while the ability to move the body against gravity and resistance should receive a good grade. When using functional tasks, it is important to remember that muscle performance is graded using the synergistic actions of muscles acting together and not the isolated actions of individual muscles as required in the MMT.

If MMT is used, therapists should utilize standardized positions whenever possible. If a modified position is required (e.g., the patient lacks full ROM or adequate stabilization), it should be carefully documented. *Substitutions* (muscle actions that compensate for specific muscle weakness) should be identified, eliminated whenever possible, and carefully documented. For example, the patient with spinal cord injury (SCI) typically presents with common muscle substitutions (e.g., wrist extensors are used to close the fingers using tenodesis grasp). Knowledge of common substitutions is very helpful when working with this patient group.

Isokinetic testing may be part of a comprehensive clinical examination or research tool for patients with disorders of motor function. It allows the therapist to quantitatively monitor many important parameters of motor function, including a muscle's ability to generate force throughout the range, peak torques, and ability to generate torques at changing velocities (velocity-spectrum testing). Rate of tension development (time to peak torque) and shape of the torque curve can also be determined. Concentric, isometric, and eccentric contractions and reciprocal agonist/antagonist relationships can be analyzed. Testing results yield important information for understanding functional performance.[39–41] Validity and reliability of isokinetic testing is well established.[42–47]

Patients with stroke typically demonstrate a variety of deficits when tested with an isokinetic dynamometer, including (1) decreased torque overall in the more affected limb when compared to the less affected limb; (2) decreased torque with increasing movement speeds; (3) decreased limb excursion; (4) extended times to peak torque development and the duration time peak torque is held; and (5) increased time intervals between reciprocal contractions. For example, many patients with stroke are unable to develop tension above 70° to 80° per second. When this value is compared to the speed needed for normal walking (100° per second), reasons for gait difficulties become readily apparent. Normative data, when available, can provide an appropriate reference for evaluating and interpreting patient data.[48,49]

Atrophy, the loss of muscle bulk (wasting), occurs when functional mobility is lost (disuse atrophy) and from LMN disease (neurogenic atrophy) or protein–calorie malnutrition. *Disuse atrophy* is evident after periods of inactivity, developing in weeks or months. It is generally widespread and affects antigravity muscles to a greater extent. Strength can be negatively influenced by disuse atrophy. The lack of resistive load on muscle reduces the overall number of sarcomeres and results in diminished capacity of muscle for developing torque (contractile strength). It also results in reduced passive tension of muscle with loss of joint stability and increased risk for postural abnormality. *Neurogenic atrophy* accompanies LMN injury (e.g., peripheral nerve injury, spinal root injury) and occurs rapidly, generally within 2 to 3 weeks. Atrophy is also accompanied by other signs of LMN injury (e.g., decreased or absent tone, decreased or absent deep tendon reflexes [DTRs], fasciculations, weak or absent voluntary movements). Distribution is limited to a segmental or focal pattern (nerve root).

During the examination of muscle atrophy, the therapist should visually inspect the muscle symmetry and

shapes, comparing their size and contour. Muscles that look flat or concave are indicative of atrophy. Comparisons should be made between and within limbs. Is the atrophy unilateral (e.g., radiculopathy, mononeuropathy, cortical stroke) or bilateral (e.g., polyneuropathy, thoracic, or lumbar spinal cord)? Are multiple limbs and/or trunk involved (e.g., cervical myelopathy/SCI, brain stem stroke)? Is the atrophy more proximal (e.g., myopathy), distal (e.g., polyneuropathy), sporadic (e.g., lumbar stenosis with multiple nerve root levels; initial motor neuron disease, ALS; initial MS), or global (e.g., later stages of neurodegenerative diseases)? Limb girth measurements can be used to compare a limb undergoing neurogenic atrophy with the corresponding normal limb. Palpation at rest and during muscle contraction is used to determine muscle tension. Girth measurements or volumetric displacement measures (e.g., hands or feet) can be used to confirm visual inspection findings.

Documentation

Documentation of muscle performance should include:

1. a description of the effects of muscle weakness and contracture on active movements, posture, and function.
2. the specific tests administered and findings.
3. the type and degree of changes present (e.g., paresis, paralysis).
4. whether the changes are symmetrical or asymmetrical, distal or proximal.
5. presence of associated signs and symptoms (e.g., UMN, LMN syndromes).
6. factors that influence muscle performance (e.g., nonfractionated movement, tone).
7. the patient's perceived loss of function and impact on daily life.

When examining functional performance, it is important to remember that strength estimates taken in one position do not necessarily generalize to other positions (e.g., ability to move while supporting full body weight in upright standing).

Motor Endurance and Fatigue

Muscle endurance allows the muscle to sustain forces or to generate forces repeatedly over time.[12] An examination of muscle endurance is important in determining functional capacity. *Fatigue* is an overwhelming sustained sense of exhaustion and decreased capacity for physical and mental work at the usual level. Fatigue can be the result of excessive activity caused by an accumulation of metabolic waste products (e.g., lactic acid); malnutrition (i.e., deficiency of nutrients); cardiorespiratory disturbances (i.e., inadequate oxygen and nutrients to the tissues); emotional stress; and other factors. Although fatigue is protective and serves a useful function in guarding against overwork and injury, it is a serious problem for some individuals. For example, patients with chronic fatigue syndrome (CFS, myalgic encephalomyelitis) experience extreme fatigue that worsens with physical or mental activity and is not relieved by rest. They may experience difficulties with memory, focus, and concentration along with dizziness that worsens with transitional movements (e.g., sit-to-stand). Other groups of individuals who may also experience significant limitations because of fatigue include those with neuromuscular junction disease (myasthenia gravis, Lambert-Eaton syndrome), MS, PD, amyotrophic lateral sclerosis (ALS), myopathy (e.g., Duchenne muscular dystrophy), and Guillain-Barré syndrome. Additional factors that can influence fatigue include health status, environmental context (e.g., stressful environment), and temperature (e.g., heat stress in the patient with MS).[50]

Exhaustion is defined as the limit of endurance, beyond which no further performance is possible. Most patients can report with great accuracy the point at which exhaustion is reached. Of concern with some patients is *overwork weakness (injury),* defined as "a prolonged decrease in absolute strength and endurance due to excessive activity of partially denervated muscle."[46(p22,51)] For example, patients with CFS who report weakness following strenuous activity may have to spend the entire next day in bed. It is therefore important to document the type, length, and effectiveness of rest attempts. *Delayed onset muscle soreness* is prolonged in patients with overwork weakness, peaking between 1 and 5 days after activity.

An examination of fatigue begins with the initial interview. The patient is asked to identify those activities that are fatiguing, the frequency and severity of fatigue episodes, and the circumstances surrounding the onset of fatigue. It is important to identify the *fatigue threshold*, which is that level of exercise that cannot be sustained.[52] In most cases, the onset of fatigue is gradual, not abrupt, and dependent on the intensity and duration of the activity attempted. Precipitating activities should be identified within the context of habitual daily activity. The patient is asked to identify any solutions used to overcome debilitating fatigue and how successful they are.

Self-assessment questionnaires are particularly useful for the patient with significant fatigue. The *Modified Fatigue Impact Scale* is an instrument initially developed to assess quality-of-life problems related to fatigue in patients with MS. The scale has 21 items that focus on three areas of function. It uses a 5-point Likert scale, with 0 = never to 4 = almost always. The total score is 0 to 84, with subscales for physical (0–36), cognitive (0–40), and psychosocial (0–8) functioning.[53,54] It has excellent test-retest reliability (intraclass correlation coefficient = 0.85) when used with patients with MS.[55] The *Fatigue Severity Scale* is a nine-item questionnaire with questions that focus on the severity of fatigue and how it interferes with activity levels and

lifestyle. The items are scored on a 7-point scale, from 1 = strongly disagree to 7 = strongly agree. It has been used with multiple populations, including those with MS, PD, and post-polio syndrome, and has been shown to be a good screening tool in PD.[56–60]

During performance testing, perceived level of fatigue can also be documented using the *Borg Scale for Rating of Perceived Exertion*.[61] To better determine the level of muscle fatigue, the therapist should ask the patient to identify two separate scores, one for the level of muscular fatigue and one for the level of central fatigue (breathlessness). Timed performance on functional tasks (e.g., timed self-care tasks, Time to Walk, 6-minute Walk Test) also provides objective and reproducible measures of levels of fatigue.

Documentation

Documentation of muscle endurance and fatigue should include:

1. a description of the effects of fatigue on activities, active movements, and function, including onset, duration, and recovery
2. the specific questionnaires and tests administered and their findings
3. level of assistance or assistive devices required
4. the time on task
5. the frequency and effectiveness of rest attempts
6. compensatory strategies adopted and their effectiveness
7. the patient's perceived loss of function and impact on daily life.

Social and environmental stressors should also be described along with the patient's emotional/psychological responses (e.g., degree of depression or anxiety).

Neuromuscular Impairments
Abnormal Autonomic Function

Therapists need to examine *autonomic nervous system* (ANS) responses. The actions of the ANS are typically widespread with multiple systems engaged. The ANS has two main divisions: the sympathetic nervous system (SNS) and the parasympathetic nervous system (PNS). See Table 5.3, Effects of Autonomic Nervous System Stimulation. The SNS allows actions to be initiated to protect the individual during conditions of stress (*the alarm system*). Motor systems become engaged in carrying out defensive commands, producing *fight or flight responses* (e.g., the aroused patient with TBI may hit or bite). In one study examining patients with TBI during acute hospitalization, elevated autonomic parameters (heart rate, blood pressure, respiratory rate) were almost universal, seen in 92% of patients 7 days postinjury.[62] The PNS is activated continuously to maintain *homeostasis*. It shuts down when the SNS is activated and works to restore homeostasis afterward.

Table 5.3   Effects of Autonomic Nervous System Stimulation

SNS Stimulation	PNS Stimulation
Fight or flight response	Maintains homeostasis
Hypervigilance; increased awareness of environment	Decreased awareness of environment
Pupils dilate	Pupils constrict
Heart rate increases	Heart rate slows
Blood pressure increases	Blood pressure slows
Respiration increases and quickens	Respiration slows, becomes shallow
Blood flow to muscles increases; blood flow to skin and gastrointestinal track decreases	Blood flow returns to viscera/gastrointestinal tract
Digestion slows; release of insulin and digestive enzymes slows	Digestion returns
Glucose production and release increases	
Activation of mass muscles	Relaxation of most muscle groups
Sweating increases	Sweating ceases

PNS = parasympathetic nervous system; SNS = sympathetic nervous system.

Critical components for baseline examination include (1) a representative sampling of ANS responses, including heart rate, blood pressure, respiratory rate, pupil dilation, and sweating; (2) a determination of patient reactivity, including the degree and rate of response to stimulation; and (3) a determination of physiological stressors (e.g., environmental factors). Careful monitoring during a motor performance examination assists in defining homeostatic stability. Guidelines for the examination of vital functions can be found in Chapter 2, Examination of Vital Signs.

Dysautonomia refers to a medical condition caused by impairments of the ANS. It occurs in certain diseases and conditions that affect the nervous system and can be seen in patients with brain injury, PD, MS, Guillain-Barré syndrome, and SCI (particularly injury above T5). For example, the rate of dysautonomia was 8% on day 14 post TBI.[62] It can also occur with other diseases including diabetes, rheumatoid arthritis, lupus, Crohn disease, Lyme disease, and others. Symptoms of dysautonomia affecting the motor control examination can include fainting or loss of consciousness, dizziness and balance problems, noise/light sensitivity, weakness and ongoing fatigue, visual disturbances (blurred vision), brain fog (lack of focus, forgetfulness), shortness of breath, large swings in heart rate and blood pressure, and swings in body and skin temperature. Different types of dysautonomia include *neurocardiogenic syncope* (vasovagal syncope or situational syncope), caused by a sudden drop in blood pressure often in reaction to an intense emotional stress, dehydration, or hyperventilation and resulting in fainting. Additional symptoms include altered heart rate, palpitations, paleness, sweating, and nausea. *Postural syncope (postural hypotension)* is caused by a sudden drop in blood pressure due to a quick change of position leading to symptoms of fainting upon standing, chest pain, and shortness of breath. *Postural orthostatic tachycardia syndrome* is caused by a very fast heart rate (tachycardia) that happens when a person stands after sitting or lying down. Examination of baseline ANS parameters should, therefore, precede other elements of the motor examination in the patient suspected of autonomic instability. Ongoing monitoring is also critical to ensuring that accurate data are collected and to safeguard the patient.[18]

Abnormal Synergies

Abnormal, obligatory synergies can predominate in patients who lose independent control of select muscle groups and emerge after disruption of the motor system, predominately the corticospinal tracts (e.g., stroke, brain injury). *Abnormal synergies* are defined as stereotyped patterns of muscle coactivation and movement that reflect loss of independent joint control and limit a person's ability to coordinate joints in flexible and adaptable patterns. The performance of many functional activities is disrupted or precluded. Voluntary movements are limited with loss of ability to adapt movements to changing demands. Selective movement control (individuation or fractionation of movement) is the ability to selectively activate a muscle or limited set of muscles and is severely disordered in patients with abnormal synergies.[2] Abnormal synergies following stroke are described as either a flexion or extension synergy and affects both the UE and LE (see Chapter 15, Stroke).[63,64]

The examination of abnormal synergies is both qualitative and quantitative. Obligatory synergy patterns are observed when a patient attempts a voluntary movement. The therapist observes whether voluntary movement can be initiated, whether it can be completed, and how the movement is carried out. If movement is stereotypic and obligatory, what muscle groups are linked together? How strong are the linkages between muscle groups? Are there linkages between upper and lower limbs or one side to another (associated reactions)? Are the movements influenced by other components of UMN syndrome, such as primitive reflexes, spasticity, paresis, or position? (See Table 5.2.) For example, does elbow, wrist, and finger flexion always occur when shoulder flexion is initiated? Is head turning used to initiate or reinforce UE flexion (asymmetric tonic neck reflex [ATNR])? Therapists also need to identify when these patterns occur, under what circumstances, and what variations are possible. In patients with stroke, lessening of abnormal synergy dominance and emergence of selective movement control are evidence of recovery. Disability-specific measures, such as the *Fugl-Meyer Post-Stroke Assessment of Physical Performance*, have been developed to provide an objective and quantifiable measure of obligatory synergies and recovery after stroke (see Chapter 15, Stroke).[65,66] Many of the available standardized tests and measures to assess abnormal movement patterns and function are discussed in later chapters. For example, tests and measures used to assess stroke patients include Rivermead Mobility Index,[67] Wolf Motor Function Test,[68] Action Research Arm Test,[69] and the Stroke Impact Scale.[70] Expert panel recommendations for chronic stroke outcome measures for motor function are presented by Bushnell and colleagues.[71]

Abnormal Postural Control

Postural patterns and control of the trunk are also typically disturbed in patients with brain lesions. Primary impairments seen in patients with stroke or TBI (i.e., changes in strength, tone, muscle activation and timing, and sensation) all contribute to disordered postural control. The therapist needs to closely examine the patient's postural patterns and movement control during changes in position that require greater and greater levels of control. For example, the patient is asked to move from supine to side-lying to sitting and finally to standing. Disordered postural control and loss of balance typically becomes evident as the patient moves into the higher postures characterized by a reduced BOS and higher center of gravity (COG) (e.g., moving from sitting to standing). Examples of the standardized tests and measures include the *Function in Sitting Test*[72] and the *Postural Assessment Scale for Stroke Patients*.[73] Sorrentino et al.[74] provide a systematic review of clinical measurement tools to assess trunk performance after stroke. See discussion in Chapter 6, Coordination and Balance.

Documentation

Documentation of abnormal movements should include:

1. a description of the effects of abnormal tone, movements, and posture on function.
2. the results of individual tests administered and findings.
3. the nature and composition of the abnormal movement patterns observed (e.g., obligatory synergies).
4. factors that influence abnormal movements (e.g., spasticity, hyperreflexia).
5. the patient's perceived loss of function and impact on daily life.

Abnormal Muscle Tone

Tone is defined as the resistance of muscle to passive elongation or stretch. It represents a state of slight residual contraction in normally innervated, resting muscle, or steady-state contraction. Tone is influenced by several factors, including (1) physical inertia, (2) intrinsic mechanical-elastic stiffness of muscle and connective tissues, and (3) spinal reflex muscle contraction (tonic stretch reflexes). It excludes resistance to passive stretch from fixed soft tissue contracture. Because muscles rarely work in isolation, the term *postural tone* may be a more accurate term to describe a pattern of muscular tension that exists throughout the body and affects groups of muscles. Tonal abnormalities exist along a continuum from flaccidity, hypotonia, normal, spasticity, and rigidity. *Dystonia* is impaired or disordered tonicity.

Spasticity

Spasticity is a motor disorder characterized by a velocity-dependent increase in muscle tone with increased resistance to stretching. The larger and quicker the stretch, the stronger the resistance of the spastic muscle. During rapid movement, initial high resistance (spastic catch) may be followed by a sudden inhibition or letting go of the limb (relaxation) in response to a stretch stimulus, termed *clasp-knife response*. Chronic spasticity is associated with contracture, abnormal posturing and deformity, functional limitations, and disability.

Spasticity arises from injury to descending motor pathways from the cortex (pyramidal tracts) or brain stem (medial and lateral vestibulospinal tracts, dorsal reticulospinal tract), producing disinhibition of spinal reflexes with hyperactive tonic stretch reflexes or a failure of reciprocal inhibition. The result is hyperexcitability of the alpha motor neuron pool. It occurs as part of UMN syndrome (see Table 5.2). Typical patterns of spasticity that influence both the resting posture and movement seen in UMN syndrome are outlined in Table 5.4. In addition, the patient with UMN syndrome will also typically present with spasms, spastic cocontraction, associated reactions, clonus, and the Babinski sign. *Associated reactions* are defined as involuntary movements resulting from activity occurring in other parts of the body (e.g., sneezing, yawning, squeezing the hand). The *Babinski sign* is dorsiflexion of the great toe with fanning of the other toes on stimulation of the lateral sole of the foot.[75–77]

Rigidity

Rigidity is a hypertonic state characterized by stiffness and resistance to movement that is independent of the velocity of movement. It is associated with lesions of the basal ganglia and is seen in PD. Rigidity is the result of excessive supraspinal drive (UMN facilitation) acting on alpha motor neurons; spinal reflex mechanisms are typically normal. *Lead-pipe rigidity* refers to a constant

Table 5.4	Typical Patterns of Spasticity in Upper Motor Neuron Syndrome	
Body Part	**Actions**	**Muscles Affected**
	Upper Limbs	
Scapula	Retraction, downward rotation	Rhomboids
Shoulder	Adduction and internal rotation, depression	Pectoralis major, latissimus dorsi, teres major, subscapularis
Elbow	Flexion	Biceps, brachialis, brachioradialis
Forearm	Pronation	Pronator teres, pronator quadratus
Wrist	Flexion, adduction	Flexor carpi radialis
Hand	Finger flexion, clenched fist thumb, adducted in palm	Flexor digitorum profundus/sublimis, adductor pollicis brevis, flexor pollicis brevis
	Lower Limbs	
Pelvis	Retraction (hip hiking)	Quadratus lumborum
Hip	Adduction (scissoring) Internal rotation Extension	Adductor longus/brevis Adductor magnus, gracilis Gluteus maximus
Knee	Extension	Quadriceps
Foot and ankle	Plantarflexion Inversion Equinovarus Toes claw (tarsometatarsal extension, metatarsophalangeal flexion) Toes curl (tarso- and metatarsophalangeal flexion)	Gastrocnemius/soleus Tibialis posterior Long toe flexors Extensor hallucis longus Peroneus longus
Hip and knee (prolonged sitting posture)	Flexion Sacral sitting	Iliopsoas Rectus femoris, pectineus Hamstrings
Trunk	Lateral flexion with concavity Rotation	Rotators Internal/external obliques
Posture forward (prolonged sitting posture)	Excessive forward flexion Forward head	Rectus abdominis, external obliques Psoas minor

The form and intensity of spasticity may vary greatly, depending on the CNS lesion site and extent of damage. The degree of spasticity can fluctuate within each individual (i.e., due to body position, level of excitation, sensory stimulation, and voluntary effort). Spasticity predominates in antigravity muscles (i.e., the flexors of the UE and the extensors of the LE). If left untreated, spasticity can result in movement deficiencies, subsequent contractures, degenerative joint changes, and deformity.

CNS = central nervous system; LE = lower extremity; MP = meta; UE = upper extremity.
Adapted from Mayer.[19]

increase in muscular tone and stiffness of affected muscles. *Cogwheel rigidity* refers to the coexistence of rigidity with tremor, producing stiffness and a ratchet-like jerkiness when a body part is manipulated. It is commonly seen in UE movements (e.g., wrist or elbow flexion and extension). Tremor, bradykinesia, and loss of postural stability are also associated motor deficits in patients with PD.

Decorticate and Decerebrate Rigidity

Severe brain injury can result in coma with decorticate or decerebrate rigidity. *Decorticate rigidity* refers to sustained contraction and posturing of the upper limbs in flexion and the lower limbs in extension. The elbows, wrists, and fingers are held in flexion with shoulders adducted tightly to the sides while the LEs are held in extension, internal rotation, and plantarflexion. *Decerebrate rigidity* (abnormal extensor response) refers to sustained contraction and posturing of the trunk and limbs in a position of full extension. The elbows are extended with shoulders adducted, forearms pronated, and wrists and fingers flexed. The LEs are held in stiff extension with plantarflexion. Decorticate rigidity is indicative of a corticospinal tract lesion at the level of the diencephalon (above the superior colliculus), whereas decerebrate rigidity indicates a corticospinal lesion in the brain stem between the superior colliculus and vestibular nucleus. *Opisthotonus* is characterized by strong and sustained contraction of the extensor muscles of the neck and trunk, resulting in a rigid, hyperextended posture. Extensor muscles of the proximal limbs may also be involved. These postures are considered exaggerated and severe forms of spasticity.

Dystonia

Dystonia is a prolonged involuntary movement disorder characterized by twisting or writhing repetitive movements and increased muscular tone. *Dystonic posturing* refers to sustained abnormal postures caused by co-contraction of muscles that may last for several minutes or hours or may be permanent. Dystonia results from a CNS lesion commonly in the basal ganglia and can be inherited (primary idiopathic dystonia), associated with neurodegenerative disorders (Wilson disease, PD on excessive L-dopa therapy), or metabolic disorders (amino acid or lipid disorders). Dystonia can affect only one part of the body (*focal dystonia*) as seen in spasmodic torticollis (wry neck) or isolated writer's cramp. *Segmental dystonia* affects two or more adjacent areas (e.g., torticollis and dystonic posturing of the UE).[77]

Hypotonia

Hypotonia and *flaccidity* are terms used to define abnormally low tone or absent muscular tone. Resistance to passive movement is diminished, stretch reflexes are dampened or absent, and limbs are easily moved (floppy). Hyperextensibility of joints is common. LMN syndrome produces symptoms of decreased or absent tone, decreased or absent reflexes, paresis, muscle fasciculations and fibrillations with denervation, and neurogenic atrophy. Mild decreases in tone along with asthenia (weakness) can be seen in cerebellar lesions. Acute UMN lesions (e.g., hemiplegia, tetraplegia, paraplegia) can produce temporary hypotonia, termed *spinal shock* or *cerebral shock*, depending on the location of the lesion. The duration of CNS depression and hypotonia that occurs with shock is highly variable, lasting days or weeks. It is typically followed by the development of spasticity and UMN signs.

Examination of Tone

An examination of tone consists of (1) initial observation of resting posture, (2) passive motion testing, and (3) active motion testing. Variability of tone is common. For example, spasticity can vary in presentation from morning to afternoon, day to day, or even hour to hour, depending on several factors, including (1) volitional effort and movement; (2) stress, anxiety, and pain; (3) position and interaction of tonic reflexes; (4) medications; (5) general health; (6) ambient temperature; and (7) state of CNS arousal or alertness. In addition, urinary bladder status (full or empty), fever and infection, and metabolic and/or electrolyte imbalance can also influence spasticity. The therapist should therefore consider the impact of each of these factors in determining tone. Repeat (serial) testing and a consistent approach to examination is necessary to improve the accuracy and reliability of test results.[76]

Initial observation of the patient can reveal abnormal posturing of the limbs or body. Careful inspection should be made regarding the position of the limbs, trunk, and head. With spasticity, posturing in fixed, antigravity positions is common; for example, a spastic UE is typically held fixed against the body with the shoulder adducted, elbow flexed, and forearm supinated with wrist/fingers flexed. In the supine position, the LEs are typically held in extension, with adduction with plantarflexion, and inversion (see Table 5.4).[77] Limbs that appear floppy and lifeless (e.g., LE rolled out to the side in external rotation) may indicate hypotonicity. *Palpation* of the muscle belly may yield additional information about the resting state of muscle. Consistency, firmness, and turgor should all be examined. Hypotonic muscles will feel soft and flabby, whereas hypertonic muscles will feel taut and harder than normal.

Passive motion testing reveals information about the responsiveness of muscles to stretch. Because these responses should be examined in the absence of voluntary control, the patient is instructed to relax, letting the therapist support and move the limb. During a passive motion test, the therapist should maintain firm and constant manual contact, moving the limb in all motions. When tone is normal, the limb moves easily, and the therapist can alter direction and speed without feeling abnormal resistance. The limb is responsive and feels light. Hypertonic limbs generally feel stiff and resistant to movement, whereas flaccid limbs feel heavy and unresponsive. Many older individuals may find it difficult to relax during passive movements (termed *paratonia*); their stiffness should not be mistaken for hypertonicity. Varying the speed of movement is an important determinant of spasticity. In a spastic limb, resistance may be near normal when the limb is moved at a slow velocity. Faster movements intensify the resistance to passive motion. It is also important to remember that muscle stiffness with spasticity will offer the greatest resistance during the first stretch and that with each successive stretch resistance can be reduced by as much as 20% to 60%.[76] In the patient with rigidity, resistance is constant and not responsive to increasing the velocity of passive motion.

Clonus, spasmodic alteration of antagonistic muscle contractions, is examined using a quick stretch stimulus that is then maintained. For example, ankle clonus is tested by sudden dorsiflexion of the foot and maintaining the foot in dorsiflexion. Clasp-knife phenomenon, increased muscle resistance to passive movement followed by a sudden release of the muscle, is examined by passive motion testing. All limbs and body segments are examined, with particular attention given to those identified as problematic in the initial observation. Comparisons should be made between UEs and LEs and right and left extremities. Asymmetrical tonal abnormalities are typically indicative of neurological dysfunction.

MODIFIED ASHWORTH SCALE

The *Modified Ashworth Scale* (MAS) is the most widely used to measure an increase in muscle tone in patients with lesions of the CNS (Table 5.5). The original *Ashworth Scale* (AS), a 5-point ordinal scale, was modified by Bohannon and Smith by adding an additional 1+ grade to increase the sensitivity of the instrument, making it a 6-point scale.[78] The examiner uses passive motion to assess resistance to passive motion due to spasticity. Inter- and intrarater agreement for the MAS scores is satisfactory. Better reliability is exhibited when measuring UEs than when measuring LEs.[79] There is a lack of operational definitions as to how fast to move the limb. Thus, the MAS measures muscle tone at one unspecified velocity, which can result in variation in overall reliability. For example, the MAS has been shown to have moderate to good intrarater reliability but only poor to moderate interrater reliability. Reliability has also been shown to vary with the muscles being tested.[80] Limitations with use of the scale include (1) inability to detect small changes, (2) inability to distinguish between soft tissue viscoelastic and neural changes, and (3) problems with psychometric properties (unequal distances of scores). The lower MAS ratings of 1, 1+, and 2 are most problematic. Training is suggested to improve interrater reliability between examiners.[81–83]

TARDIEU/MODIFIED TARDIEU SCALE

The Tardieu Scale for assessing spasticity is a performance-based test of the quality of muscle tone during three different velocities: slow-velocity stretch (V1, as slow as possible), the speed of the limb falling under gravity (V2), and fast-velocity stretch (V3, moving as fast as possible).[84,85] The quality of muscle reaction is measured using an ordinal scale (0–5), where 0 is no spasticity, 4 is severe spasticity, and 5 is joint immobility. The *Modified Tardieu Scale* uses an additional measurement of joint angles. One goniometric measurement (R1) is taken at the onset of resistance (catch or clonus) to quick stretch (V3). The second measurement (R2) is taken at the full passive ROM and is taken at very slow speed (V1). The difference between the two measures, R2–R1, represents the velocity-dependent tone component of the muscle. Intrarater reliability is adequate to excellent and varies with muscles tested and training. Interrater reliabilities are lower and also vary with training.[86,87]

Documentation

Documentation of tone abnormalities should include

1. a description of the effects of abnormal tone on active movements, posture, and function,
2. the individual tests administered and findings, including the type and degree of abnormality observed (e.g., spasticity, rigidity, dystonia),
3. a determination of the specific body segments affected,
4. whether the changes are symmetrical or asymmetrical,
5. resting postures and associated signs and symptoms (e.g., UMN, LMN syndrome),
6. factors that modify (increase or diminish) tone,
7. the patient's perceived loss of function and impact on daily life.

It is important to remember that measurement of tone in one position does not mean that tone will be the same in other positions or during functional activities. A change in position such as sitting up or standing up can substantially alter the requirements for postural tone. Of great importance is a description of the effects of tone on active movements, posture, and function.

Table 5.5	Modified Ashworth Scale for Grading Spasticity
Grade	**Description**
0	No increase in muscle tone.
1	Slight increase in muscle tone, manifested by a catch and release or by minimal resistance at the end of the ROM when the affected part(s) is moved in flexion or extension.
1+	Slight increase in muscle tone, manifested by a catch, followed by minimal resistance throughout the remainder (less than half) of the ROM.
2	More marked increase in muscle tone through most of the ROM but affected part(s) easily moved.
3	Considerable increase in muscle tone, passive movement difficult.
4	Affected part(s) rigid in flexion or extension.

ROM = range of motion.
From Bohannon and Smith,[21p.207] with permission.

Abnormal Reflex Function

Reflexes are involuntary, predictable, and specific responses to a stimulus that are dependent on an intact reflex arc (afferent or sensory neurons, synaptic connections, efferent or motor neurons, and descending motor pathways). In many neurological conditions, reflexes are altered, and responses are used to provide evidence of CNS disruption and pathology.

Deep Tendon Reflexes

DTRs, also referred to as a muscle stretch reflexes, can be used to assess the state of the CNS. An increased or hyperactive DTR is an indication of disinhibition of the stretch reflex mechanism and is typically seen in patients with UMN syndrome and spasticity. Hyperactive responses are characterized by observable movement of the joint (brisk or strong responses) along with an increased amplitude and decreased threshold of response. *Clonus* is a self-sustained, oscillating stretch reflex consisting of involuntary and rhythmic muscle contractions and caused by a permanent lesion in descending motor

neurons. It is also seen in conditions with muscle spasticity and spasms (UMN syndrome). Clonus may be found at the ankle, wrist, jaw, or other muscles.

A decreased or hypoactive DTR can occur with interruption of the monosynaptic reflex arc or in conditions of shock (e.g., spinal shock after a SCI). They are also decreased in LMN syndrome (e.g., peripheral neuropathy, nerve root compression), cerebellar syndrome, and muscle disease. Because each DTR arises from specific spinal segments, an absent reflex can be used to identify the level of a spinal lesion (e.g., radiculopathy).

DTRs are tested by tapping sharply over the muscle tendon with a standard reflex hammer and observing the response. To ensure adequate response, the muscle is positioned in midrange and the patient is instructed to relax. The quality and magnitude of responses should be carefully documented. The therapist should compare the strength of reflex response elicited with a similar test in the opposite extremity and with other DTR responses within the same extremity. Table 5.6 presents an overview of the examination of DTRs.

Table 5.6 Examination of Deep Tendon Reflexes		
Myostatic Reflexes (Stretch)	**Stimulus**	**Response**
Jaw (Cranial nerve V)	Patient is sitting, with jaw relaxed and slightly open. Place finger on top of chin; tap downward on top of finger in a direction that causes the jaw to open.	Jaw rebounds and closes
Biceps *Musculocutaneous nerve* *(C5, C6)*	Patient is sitting with arm flexed and supported. Place thumb over the biceps tendon in the cubital fossa, stretching it slightly. Tap thumb or directly on tendon.	Slight contraction of elbow flexors
Brachioradialis (supinator) *Radial nerve (C5, C6)*	Patient is sitting with arm flexed onto the abdomen. Place finger on the radial tuberosity and tap finger with hammer.	Slight contraction of elbow flexors, slight wrist extension or radial deviation
Triceps *Radial nerve (C6, C7)*	Patient is sitting with arm supported in abduction, elbow flexed. Palpate triceps tendon just above olecranon. Tap directly on tendon.	Slight contraction of elbow extensors
Finger flexors *Median nerve (C6–T1)*	Hold hand in neutral position. Place finger across palmar surface of distal phalanges of four fingers and tap.	Slight contraction of finger flexors
Hamstrings *Tibial branch, sciatic nerve* *(L5, S1, S2)*	Patient is prone with knee semiflexed and supported. Palpate tendon at the knee. Tap on finger or directly on tendon.	Slight contraction of knee flexors
Quadriceps (patellar, knee jerk) *Femoral nerve (L2, L3, L4)*	Patient is sitting with knee flexed, foot unsupported. Tap tendon of quadriceps muscle between the patella and tibial tuberosity.	Slight contraction of knee extensors
Achilles (ankle jerk) *Tibial (S1–S2)*	Patient is prone with foot over the end of the plinth or sitting with knee flexed and foot held in slight dorsiflexion. Tap tendon just above its insertion on the calcaneus. Maintaining slight tension on the gastrocnemius-soleus group improves the response.	Slight contraction of plantarflexors

If DTRs are difficult to elicit, responses can be enhanced by specific reinforcement maneuvers. In the *Jendrassik maneuver,* the patient hooks the fingers of both hands together and strongly pulls them apart while LE DTRs are tested. During UE testing, the patient can squeeze their knees together, clench their teeth, or make a fist with the contralateral extremity. The use of any reinforcing maneuvers to elicit responses in patients with hyporeflexia should be carefully documented.

Clonus is easily tested at the ankle (ankle clonus). The patient is positioned in sitting or supine with the knee slightly flexed. The therapist gently moves the foot into dorsiflexion and plantarflexion a few times and then rapidly dorsiflexes the foot and holds the ankle in this position. A positive sign is recorded if the therapist feels and sees oscillations of the foot. A grade of 4+ or 5+ is given depending upon whether the clonus is *sustained* (greater than 10 beats) or *nonsustained.*

Reflexes are subjectively graded on a 0 to 5 scale:[88]

0 = No response, always abnormal
1+ = slight but definitely present response; may or may not be normal
2+ = normal
3+ = brisk response, more reflexive than normal
4+ = very brisk, hyperreflexive, with nonsustained clonus
5+ = sustained clonus

Superficial Reflexes

Superficial cutaneous reflexes are elicited by sensory afferents from skin (e.g., a light stroke applied to the skin). They are mediated by UMN pathways that are typically polysynaptic. The expected response is brief contraction of muscles innervated by the same spinal segments receiving the afferent inputs from the cutaneous receptors. A stimulus that is strong in a patient with significant UMN pathology may produce irradiation of cutaneous signals with activation of *protective withdrawal reflexes.* Cutaneous reflexes include the plantar reflex, abdominal reflex, cremaster reflex, and corneal reflex.

The *plantar reflex* (S1, S2) is tested by applying a stroking stimulus on the sole of the foot along the lateral border and up across the ball of the foot. A normal response consists of flexion of the big toe; sometimes the other toes will demonstrate a down going (flexion) response or no response at all. An abnormal response (*positive or upgoing Babinski sign*) consists of extension (upgoing) of the big toe, with fanning of the lateral four toes. It is indicative of an abnormality in the corticospinal system. The *Chaddock sign* is elicited by stroking around the lateral ankle and up the lateral dorsal aspect of the foot. It also produces extension of the big toe and is considered a confirmatory toe sign. The *abdominal reflex* is elicited with brisk, light strokes over the abdomen. A localized contraction under the stimulus is produced, with a resultant deviation of the umbilicus toward the area stimulated. Each of the four quadrants should be tested in a diagonal direction. Umbilical deviation in a superior/lateral direction indicates integrity of spinal segments T8 to T9. Umbilical deviation in an inferior/lateral direction indicates integrity of spinal segments T10 to T12. Loss of response is abnormal and indicative of pathology (e.g., thoracic SCI). Asymmetry from side to side is highly significant in neurological disease. Abdominal reflexes may be absent in patients with obesity or abdominal surgeries. An abnormal corneal reflex is evidence of peripheral nerve damage to the trigeminal nerve (V) or the facial nerve (VII). An abnormal cremasteric reflex may be evidence of testicular torsion. Neither are typically tested by the physical therapist. Table 5.7, Examination of Superficial Reflexes, presents an overview of these examinations.

Table 5.7	Examination of Superficial Reflexes	
Superficial Reflexes (Cutaneous)	**Stimulus**	**Response**
Plantar (S1, S2)	With blunt object (key or wooden end of applicator stick), stroke the lateral aspect of the sole, moving from the heel to the ball of the foot, curving medially across the ball of the foot. Alternate stimuli for plantar (for sensitive feet): • Chaddock: stroke lateral ankle and lateral aspect of foot. • Oppenheim: stroke down tibial crest	Normal response is flexion (plantarflexion) of the great toe and sometimes the other toes (negative Babinski sign). Abnormal response, termed a *positive Babinski sign,* is extension (dorsiflexion) of the great toe with fanning of the four other toes (indicates UMN lesions). Same as for plantar.
Abdominal reflexes Above umbilicus = T8–T10 Below umbilicus = T10–T12	Position patient in supine, relaxed. Make brisk, light strokes over each quadrant of the abdominals from the periphery to the umbilicus.	Localized contraction under the stimulus, causing the umbilicus to move toward the stimulus. Note: can be masked by obesity.

UMN = upper motor neuron.

Primitive and Tonic Reflexes

Primitive and *tonic reflexes* are present during infancy as a stage in normal development and typically become integrated by the CNS at an early age (e.g., 4 to 6 months of age). Once integrated, these reflexes are not generally recognizable in their pure form in older children or adults. They may continue, however, as adaptive fragments of behavior underlying normal motor control. Persistent reflexes (sometimes termed *obligatory reflexes*) beyond the expected age of development or appearing in adult patients following brain injury are always indicative of neurological involvement. Patients who exhibit these reflexes typically present with extensive brain damage (e.g., stroke, TBI) and other UMN signs.

Reflexes examined in the patient with UMN signs and suspected of abnormal reflex activity include flexor withdrawal, traction, grasp, tonic neck, tonic labyrinthine, positive support, and associated reactions. *Flexor withdrawal reflex* is generally the simplest to observe and is judged by the appearance of an overt movement response. *Tonic neck reflexes,* on the other hand, bias the musculature and may not be visible through overt movement responses. In fact, movement is rarely produced, but rather posture is typically influenced through tonal adjustments. Thus, the term *tuning reflexes* is an appropriate description of their function. Abnormal postures should be examined for their reflex dependence (e.g., the patient with brain injury exhibits excessive extensor tone in supine but not in side-lying position). To obtain an accurate examination, the therapist must be concerned with several factors. The patient must be positioned appropriately to allow for the expected response. An adequate test stimulus is essential, including both an adequate magnitude and duration of stimulation. Keen observation skills are needed to detect what may be subtle movement changes and abnormal responses. Palpation skills can assist in identifying tonal changes not readily apparent to the eye. Primitive and tonic reflexes are graded using a 0 to 4+ scale:[88]

0+ Absent
1+ Tone change: slight, transient with no movement of the extremities
2+ Visible movement of extremities
3+ Exaggerated, full movement of extremities
4+ Obligatory and sustained movement, lasting for more than 30 seconds

Table 5.8 presents an overview of the examination of primitive and tonic reflexes.

Documentation

Documentation of reflex abnormalities should include:

1. a description of the effects of abnormal reflexes on active movements, posture, and function.
2. the specific tests administered and their findings.
3. a determination of the specific reflexes affected.

4. the presence of associated signs and symptoms (e.g., UMN syndrome).
5. factors that influence or modify reflexes.
6. the patient's perceived loss of function and impact on daily life.

Abnormal Cranial Nerve Function

There are 12 pairs of CNs, all distributed to the head and neck, with the exception of CN X (vagus), which is distributed to the thorax and abdomen. CNs I, II, and VIII are purely sensory and carry the special senses of smell, vision, hearing, and equilibrium. Cranial nerves III, IV, and VI are purely motor and control pupillary constriction and eye movements. CNs XI and XII are also purely motor, innervating the sternocleidomastoid, trapezius, and tongue muscles. CNs V, VII, IX, and X are mixed, containing both motor and sensory fibers. Motor functions include chewing (V), facial expression (VII), swallowing (IX, X), and vocal sounds (X). Sensations are carried from the face and head (V, VII, IX); alimentary tract, heart, vessels, lungs (IX, X); and tongue, mouth, and palate (VII, IX, X). Parasympathetic secretomotor fibers (ANS) are carried by CN III for control of smooth muscles in the eyeball, VII for control of salivary and lacrimal glands, IX to the parotid salivary gland, and X to the heart, lungs, and most of the digestive system.[89]

An examination of CN function should be performed with suspected lesions of the brain, brain stem, and cervical spine. Deficits in olfactory function (CN I) should be suspected with lesions of the nasal cavity and anterior/inferior cerebrum. Lesions of the optic pathways (optic nerve [CN II], optic chiasma, optic tract, lateral geniculate body, superior colliculus) and visual cortex may produce visual deficits. Midbrain (mesencephalic) lesions may result in deficits of CNs III and IV (oculomotor, trochlear). Pontine lesions may involve several CNs, including V (ophthalmic, maxillary, and mandibular branches) and VI (abducens). Nuclei of CNs VII (facial) and VIII (vestibular and cochlear branches) are located at the junction of the pons and medulla. Lesions affecting the medulla may involve CNs IX (glossopharyngeal), X (vagus), XI (spinal accessory), and XII (hypoglossal). The spinal root of XI is found in the upper five cervical segments. The CNs, their function, clinical tests, and possible abnormal findings are presented in Table 5.9, Examination of Cranial Nerve Integrity.

Documentation

Documentation of an examination of CN integrity should include:

1. a description of the effects of abnormal reflexes on active movements, posture, and function.
2. the specific tests administered and findings, including specific deficits.
3. the patient's perceived loss of function.

Table 5.8   Examination of Primitive and Tonic Reflexes

Reflexes	Stimulus	Response
Primitive Reflexes		
Flexor withdrawal	Noxious stimulus (pinprick) to sole of foot. Tested in supine or sitting position.	Toes extend, foot dorsiflexes, entire LE flexes uncontrollably. Onset: 28 weeks of gestation. Integrated: 1–2 months.
Crossed extension	Noxious stimulus to ball of foot of LE fixed in extension; tested in supine position.	Opposite LE flexes, then adducts and extends. Onset: 28 weeks' gestation. Integrated: 1–2 months.
Traction	Grasp forearm and pull up from supine into sitting position.	Grasp and total flexion of the UE. Onset: 28 weeks' gestation. Integrated: 2–5 months.
Moro	Sudden change in position of head in relation to trunk; drop patient backward from sitting position.	Extension, abduction of UEs, hand opening, and crying followed by flexion, adduction of arms across chest. Onset: 28 weeks' gestation. Integrated: 5–6 months.
Startle	Sudden loud or harsh noise.	Sudden extension or abduction of UEs, crying. Onset: birth. Integrated: persists.
Grasp	Maintained pressure to palm of hand (palmar grasp) or to ball of foot under toes (plantar grasp).	Maintained flexion of fingers or toes. Onset: palmar, birth; plantar, 28 weeks' gestation. Integrated: palmer, 4–6 months; plantar, 9 months.
Tonic Reflexes		
Asymmetrical tonic neck (ATNR)	Rotation of the head to one side.	Flexion of skull limbs, extension of the jaw limbs, "bow and arrow" or "fencing" posture. Onset: birth. Integrated: 4–6 months.
Symmetrical tonic neck (STNR)	Flexion or extension of the head.	With head flexion: flexion of UEs, extension of LEs; with head extension: extension of UEs, flexion of LEs. Onset: 4–6 months. Integrated: 8–12 months.
Symmetrical tonic labyrinthine (TLR or STLR)	Prone or supine position.	With prone position: increased flexor tone/flexion of all limbs; with supine: increased extensor tone/extension of all limbs. Onset: birth. Integrated: 6 months.
Positive supporting	Contact to the ball of the foot in upright standing position.	Rigid extension (co-contraction) of the LEs. Onset: birth. Integrated: 6 months.
Associated reactions	Resisted voluntary movement in any part of the body.	Involuntary movement in a resting extremity. Onset: birth–3 months. Integrated: 8–9 years.

LE = lower extremity; UE = upper extremity.

Table 5.9	Examination of Cranial Nerve Integrity		
Cranial Nerve	**Function**	**Test**	**Possible Abnormal Findings**
I *Olfactory*	Olfaction (smell)	Test sense of smell on each side (close off other nostril): use common, nonirritating odors.	Anosmia (inability to detect smells), seen with frontal lobe lesions
II *Optic*	Vision	Visual acuity test: uses Snellen eye chart; test each eye separately (covering other eye); test at distance of 20 ft. Visual field test: test temporal and vertical peripheral vision (visual fields) by confrontation.	Blindness, myopia (impaired far vision), presbyopia (impaired near vision) Field defects: homonymous hemianopsia
III *Oculomotor*	Pupillary reflex Accommodation Convergence	Shine light in eye: pupil constricts. Eye accommodates to light. Pupils move medially when viewing object at close range.	Absence of pupillary constriction Lateral strabismus (exotropia) Anisocoria (unequal pupils) Horner syndrome, CN III paralysis
III, IV, VI *Oculomotor, trochlear, and abducens (tested simultaneously)*	Extraocular movements CN III: turns eye up, down, in; elevates eyelid CN IV: turns eye down when adducted CN VI: turns eye out	Test saccadic movements: ask patient to look up, down, medial, and lateral. Test pursuit eye movements: ask patient to follow moving finger. Test one eye at a time; other eye occluded.	Lateral strabismus: eyeball turns lateral; can cause diplopia or nystagmus Impaired eye movements Ptosis Medial strabismus: eyeball turns inward; can cause diplopia or nystagmus
V *Trigeminal: ophthalmic, maxillary, mandibular divisions*	Sensory function: face Sensory: cornea Motor function: muscles of mastication	Test pain, light touch sensations: forehead, cheeks, inner oral cavity (occlude vision). Test corneal reflex: touch lightly with wisp of cotton. Palpate temporal and masseter muscles. Observe spontaneous movements. Have patient open mouth, move jaw side to side. Bite down on tongue depressor and hold against resistance.	Loss of facial sensations, numbness with CN V lesion Trigger area with trigeminal neuralgia Loss of corneal reflex ipsilaterally (blinking in response to corneal touch) Weakness, wasting of muscles When opened, deviation of jaw to ipsilateral side Asymmetry of jaw movement Asymmetry of jaw strength
VII *Facial*	Motor function: facial muscles Sensory function: taste to anterior two-thirds of tongue	Test strength and symmetry of facial muscles: have patient elevate eyebrows and forehead; wrinkle forehead, smile, frown, and pucker lips, close eyes tightly, puff out both cheeks. Apply sweet, salty, and sour solutions to outer and lateral portions of anterior tongue using a cotton swab (occlude vision).	Paralysis: Inability to close eye, drooping corner of mouth, difficulty with speech articulation Unilateral LMN: Bell palsy Bilateral LMN: Guillain-Barré Unilateral UMN: stroke Incorrectly identifies solution Decreased taste

(Continued)

Table 5.9   Examination of Cranial Nerve Integrity—cont'd

Cranial Nerve	Function	Test	Possible Abnormal Findings
VIII Vestibulocochlear	Vestibular function	Test balance and protective functions: vestibulospinal function.	Vertigo, decreased balance, decreased protective responses (disequilibrium)
		Test eye–head coordination: vestibular ocular reflex.	Gaze instability with head rotations, nystagmus (constant, involuntary cyclical movement of the eyeball)
	Cochlear function	Test auditory acuity Weber test for lateralization: place vibrating tuning fork on top of head, midposition; check if sound heard in one ear, or equally in both. Rinne test: Compares air and bone conduction. Place vibrating tuning fork on mastoid bone, then close to ear canal; sound heard longer through air than bone.	Deafness, impaired hearing, tinnitus Unilateral conductive loss: sound lateralized to impaired ear Sensorineural loss: sound heard in good ear Conductive loss: sound heard through bone is equal to or longer than air Sensorineural loss: sound heard longer through air
IX Glossopharyngeal	Sensory function: posterior one-third of tongue, pharynx, middle ear	Apply sweet, salty, and sour solutions to posterior tongue.	Incorrectly identifies solution, loss of taste on posterior tongue
IX, X Glossopharyngeal and vagus (tested simultaneously)	Phonation	Listen to voice quality.	Dysphonia: hoarse voice; denotes vocal cord weakness; nasal quality denotes palatal weakness
	Swallowing	Examine for difficulty in swallowing: glass of water, different consistencies of food.	Dysphagia: difficulty swallowing; loss of swallowing reflexes
	Palatal, pharynx control	Have patient say "ah," then observe motion of soft palate (elevates) and position of uvula (remains midline).	Dysarthria: difficulty articulating words clearly, slurs words Palate fails to elevate (lesion of CN X); asymmetrical elevation with unilateral paralysis
	Gag reflex	Stimulate back of throat lightly on each side.	Loss of gag reflex: lesion of CN IX; possibly CN X
XI Accessory	Motor function Spinal nerve root Trapezius muscle	Examine bulk, strength. In sitting, ask patient to elevate the shoulder upward against resistance applied in the direction of depression.	LMN: atrophy, fasciculations, weakness Weakness, inability to approximate the acromion and the occiput
	Sternocleidomastoid	In supine, ask patient to flex head anterolaterally and rotate head to opposite side; resistance is applied in an obliquely posterior direction.	Weakness, inability to flex head laterally and forward, rotate head to contralateral side
	Cranial nerve root	Examine laryngeal elevation by placing index and middle fingers over patient's Adam's apple (laryngeal muscles); ask patient to swallow.	Dysphagia due to decreased laryngeal elevation

Table 5.9	Examination of Cranial Nerve Integrity—cont'd		
Cranial Nerve	**Function**	**Test**	**Possible Abnormal Findings**
XII *Hypoglossal*	Motor function: tongue movements	Listen to patient's articulation.	Dysarthria (seen with lesions of CN X or CN XII, also V, VII)
		Examine resting position of tongue.	Atrophy or fasciculations of tongue (LMN, ALS)
		Ask patient to protrude tongue, move tongue side to side.	Impaired movements with deviation of tongue to weak side UMN lesion: tongue deviates away from side of cortical lesion Check for tongue tremors or involuntary tongue movements

ALS = amyotrophic lateral sclerosis; CN = cranial nerve; LMN = Lower motor neuron; UMN = Upper motor neuron.

■ MEASURES OF MOTOR LEARNING

Motor learning is "a set of internal processes associated with practice or experience leading to relatively permanent gains in the capability for skilled performance."[1(p438)] As mentioned earlier, changes in the CNS are not directly observable, but rather they are inferred from improvement in performance as a result of practice or experience. Individual differences in learning are expected and influence both the rate and degree of learning possible. Motor learning abilities among individuals vary across three main foundational categories of abilities: cognitive abilities, perceptual speed ability, and psychomotor ability. Differences are a result of both genetics and experience. The therapist should be sensitive to such factors as alertness, anxiety, memory, speed of processing information, speed and accuracy of movements, and uniqueness of the setting. In addition, recovering patients may vary in their learning potential according to the pathology present, the number and type of impairments, recovery potential and general health status, and comorbidities. Although most skills can be learned through practice or experience, the therapist should be sensitive to the patient's underlying capabilities (abilities) that support certain skills. For example, some patients with SCI may not be able to learn to manage curbs using "wheelies" because of the difficulty of the task, their residual abilities, and their general health status.

Stages of Motor Learning

Fitts and Posner described three main stages in learning a motor skill: (1) the cognitive stage, (2) the associative stage, and (3) the autonomous stage of learning.[90] Their model provides a useful framework for examining and developing strategies to improve motor learning. A three-stage process was also supported by the work of Anderson.[91,92] It is important to remember that these stages are not fixed or discrete but rather have overlapping borders.

In the early *cognitive stage,* the learner develops an understanding of the task. During practice, *cognitive mapping* allows the learner to assess abilities and task demands, identify relevant and important stimuli, and develop an initial movement strategy (motor program) based on explicit memory of prior movement experiences. The learner performs initial practice of the task, retaining some strategies while discarding others to develop an initial movement strategy. During successive practice trials, the learner modifies and refines the movements. During this stage, there is considerable cognitive activity, and each movement requires a high degree of conscious attention and thought. Most learners are highly dependent on the use of visual feedback to shape movements. Performance is initially inconsistent, with large gains occurring as the patient progresses toward the next stage. The basic "What to do?" decision is answered.

The second and middle stage is the *associative stage* of motor learning (fixation). During this stage, the learner selects the best strategy and focuses on refining the pattern. Spatial and temporal organization increases while errors and extraneous movements decrease. Performance becomes more consistent, and cognitive activity decreases. The learner is less dependent on visual feedback while use of proprioceptive feedback increases. Thus, the learner begins to learn the "feel" of the movement. This stage can persist, depending on the learner and the level of practice. The "How to do?" decision is answered.

The third and final stage is the *autonomous phase* of motor learning. The learner continues to practice and refine motor patterns. The spatial and temporal components of movement become highly organized over time with extensive periods of practice (e.g., weeks, months, or years). Performance is at a very high level (e.g., skilled gymnast). At this stage of learning, movements are largely error-free and automatic, with only a minimal level of cognitive monitoring and attention. The learner is now free to concentrate on other things such as a secondary task (dual-task performance) or on other aspects of the environment (e.g., sports competition). The "How to succeed?" decision has been answered.

Patients with brain injury admitted to active rehabilitation often must relearn basic motor skills using entirely different motor control mechanisms and strategies. Activities and movements that were easily done previously now become unfamiliar and challenging. These patients can persist in the cognitive learning stage for some time before they develop the idea of a movement. Impairments in motor control can influence performance and learning during the associated stage, which can also be prolonged. Many times, patients are discharged from rehabilitation before the skills become refined and learning completed. Many patients fail to reach the third autonomous stage of learning evidenced by a low degree of attention given to performance. See Chapter 10, Strategies to Improve Motor Control, for additional discussion on motor learning.

Performance Measures

Traditionally, changes in performance resulting from practice have been used to assess motor learning. However, it is possible to improve performance during the initial practice session (acquisition phase) while not retaining the skill. For example, the patient with stroke demonstrates improved sitting posture and balance at the end of a therapy session, but on return the next day they continue to demonstrate prior poor sitting posture and loss of balance. This is indicative of temporary changes associated with practice versus true motor learning (retained motor skills), which may only become evident with repeat practice sessions. In addition, factors such as fatigue, anxiety, poor motivation, boredom, or drugs can cause performance to deteriorate during practice while learning may still be occurring. For example, the patient with MS who is fatigued and stressed performs very poorly during scheduled treatment but returns after the weekend rested and calm and is able to perform the task with ease.

Performance is best used as a measure of motor learning during a retention test or a transfer test (discussed later in this section). Table 5.10 presents some possible measures of motor performance. For example, an individual recovering from stroke can demonstrate functional independence in transfers after a series of training sessions. Improvement in functional scores (e.g., FIM scores) documents changes in the level of assistance needed. Qualitative changes in performance compared to the criterion skill can also be used to document motor learning. Thus, the movement is performed with improved motor control, indicative of changes in spatial and temporal organization. Error scores can be used to document accuracy of movement. Therefore, therapists can report the number and type of errors (constant, variable) that occur within a given practice session and across practice attempts. A decrease in the frequency of error provides indirect evidence of improvements in learning. One common measurement problem in skill learning is the *speed–accuracy trade-off.* Typically, initial practice sessions are characterized by slowed performance in order to improve movement accuracy. As learning progresses, performance speed is increased once accuracy demands are satisfied. The therapist documents the time it takes to complete the activity along with the number of errors. Reduced effort and concentration are indicative of improved performance and should be documented. A high degree of cognitive monitoring is necessary in early learning (cognitive stage). In contrast, performance across the associative and autonomous stages of motor learning is characterized by a reduced level of cognitive monitoring and increased automaticity. As learning progresses, performance is increasingly characterized by consistency and accuracy. Thus, the acquired skills are observed for variability within and across practice sessions, which can be expected to decrease.[93]

Performance plateaus, defined as the leveling off of performance after a period of steady improvement, characterize normal practice and can be expected. During plateaus, learning may still be going on, whereas performance is not changing. Problems can also occur with the measurement instruments selected. Failure to demonstrate improved performance can be the result of *ceiling effects,* defined as a high level of performance in which further improvement cannot be detected owing to limitations in the performance measure. Conversely, *floor effects* are a low level of performance in which further decreases cannot be detected by limitations in the performance measure. They can affect a determination of negative learning.

Retention Tests

Reliable inferences about motor learning can be made by using retention tests, sometimes called a transfer test. *Retention* refers to the ability of the learner to demonstrate the skill over time and after a period of no practice (*retention interval*). A *retention test* is defined as "a performance test on a given task provided after a retention interval without practice."[1(p440)] Retention intervals can be of varying lengths. For example, a patient who is seen only once a week in an outpatient clinic is asked to demonstrate a skill practiced the previous week. Performance after the retention interval is compared to performance on the initial practice session. A *difference score* can be determined and documented—that is, the difference in performance scores from the end of the original acquisition phase and the beginning of the retention phase. Performance may show a slight initial decrease but should return to original performance levels within relatively few practice trials after the retention interval if learning has occurred (termed *warm-up decrement*). It is important not to provide any verbal cueing or knowledge of results during the retention test. This same patient may have been given a home exercise program (HEP)

Table 5.10   Measures of Motor Performance

Examples of Measures	Performance Examples
Outcome Measures	
Movement Time: The time interval between the initiation of a movement and completion of a movement, in seconds or minutes	10MWT Time to complete a functional task (e.g., transfer wheelchair to mat) Minnesota Rate of Manipulation Test
Reaction Time: The time interval between the presentation of a stimulus and the initiation of a response, in seconds or minutes	Time to initiate a functional task after cueing is provided (e.g., supine-to-sit or sit-to-stand transfers)
Distance: The total distance completed, in meters or feet	6MWT or 12MWT
Observational Performance Changes: Observation of deviations of performance with respect to target behaviors	Observational gait analysis: Systematic examination of movement patterns of body segments at each point in the gait cycle
Changes in Performance Scores using a standardized outcome measure	Changes in scores on the Functional Independence Measure, Barthel Index, Berg Balance Scale, or Purdue Pegboard Test
Errors in Performance using a criterion task	*Error in program selection*: Patient with stroke incorrectly transfers to the less affected side when asked to transfer to the more affected side. *Error in program execution*: Patient with TBI becomes distracted and is unable to complete a transfer.
Constant Error: The average error of a set of scores from a target value; a measure of average bias	Patient exhibits an average distance on a Functional Reach Test of 6 in. on 3 trials; mean for age (72 years, women; ≥13.8 in.).
Variable Error: The SD of a set of scores about the subject's own average score; a measure of movement consistency	Patient exhibits an average SD on a Functional Reach Test of 3 in. on three trials.
Number of Successful Attempts: During practice of an activity compared to total number of attempts **Percentage of Successful Attempts**	Patient performs an independent sit-to-stand transfer 4 out of 10 attempts. Patient performs an independent sit-to-stand transfer 40% of attempts.
Time on Target, compared to total time of the activity, in seconds or minutes	Patient is able to maintain independent stability in sitting (or standing) for 2 minutes during a 5-minute trial.
Time in Balance	Number of seconds patient is able to maintain BOS within COM while standing on foam
Trials to Completion: Number of trials required until correct response obtained	Ten practice trials required for patient to be independent in wheelchair-to-mat transfers
Instrumental Response Measures	
Limb displacement, trajectory	Distance limb(s) traveled to produce response during instrumental motion analysis, kinematic gait analysis
Velocity	Speed limb(s) moved while performing response during instrumental motion analysis or isokinetic dynamometry
Acceleration/deceleration	Acceleration/deceleration pattern while moving during instrumental motion analysis or isokinetic dynamometry
Joint angle	Angle of each joint during instrumental motion analysis, or using electrogoniometry

BOS = base of support; COM = center of mass; 6MWT = 6-minute Walk Test; SD = standard deviation; 10MWT = 10-meter Walk Test; TBI = traumatic brain injury; 12MWT = 12-minute Walk Test.

that includes daily practice of the desired skill. If, on return to the clinic some weeks later, performance of the desired skill has not been maintained or has deteriorated, the therapist might reasonably conclude that the patient has not been diligent with the HEP and learning has not been retained.

Transfer Tests

Transfer of learning refers to "the gain (or loss) in the capability for performance in one task as a result of practice or experience on another task. A transfer test is a performance test in which the task or task conditions have changed; often provided after a retention interval without practice."[1(p441)] Learning obtained from the criterion task can result in *positive transfer* or learning or it can detract from the criterion task, termed *negative transfer*. For example, the patient with stroke practices feeding skills using the less affected UE. The feeding task is then practiced using the more affected UE. During a transfer test, the therapist observes and documents the effectiveness of task performance on the second task and compares it with the performance on the first criterion task. *Generalizability* is "the ability of applying what is learned in the practice of one task to one or more other unpracticed tasks."[1(p437)] For example, the patient practices wheelchair transfers in the clinic, followed by practice of transfers to a toilet and to a car. When the tasks have a high degree of similarity, the success rate is improved.

Adaptation

Adaptation refers to the process of adjusting a movement (adapting) to changing task and environmental demands. This can include changing one or more parameters of the movement (e.g., force or direction) while maintaining the skill (e.g., walking). Adaptation also refers to the ability of the individual to apply a learned motor skill to the learning of other similar or related skills. For example, individuals who learn to transfer from wheelchair to platform mat can apply that learning to other variations of transfers (e.g., wheelchair to car, wheelchair to bathtub). The therapist observes and documents how successful the patient was in learning the variation of the skill (i.e., number of practice trials, time, and effort required to perform these new types of transfers). These parameters are typically reduced from that required to learn the initial skill.

Observing performance under conditions of changing environmental demands is also an important measure of adaptation. Thus, an individual who has learned a skill (e.g., walking with a cane in the physical therapy clinic) should be able to apply that learning to new and variable environments (e.g., walking at home, outdoors, or on a busy street). The therapist observes and documents how successful the patient is in performing the skill in new and varied environments. The patient who is able to perform the skill in only one type of environment—for example, the patient with TBI who is only able to function within a tightly controlled, clinic environment (*closed environment*) demonstrates limited and largely nonfunctional skills in more *open environments*. This patient is not likely to return home and be independent in the community environment and will likely require placement in a more structured, assisted living setting. Terminology related to motor learning is summarized in Box 5.6.

Documentation

Documentation of motor learning should include:

1. a description of the changes in performance (skill development) associated with practice, including the amount and type of practice, number and frequency of practice trials, time, and effort.
2. a description of the type and amount feedback used (see Box 5.6 for types of feedback).
3. a level of cognitive-verbal-visual monitoring required during early stage 1 (cognitive) learning.

Box 5.6   Motor Learning Terms

Motor learning: "a set of internal processes associated with practice or experience leading to relatively permanent gains in the capability for skilled performance."[1(p438)]

Procedural or implicit learning: the learning and execution of motor skills and nondeclarative cognitive skills, especially those involving sequences of movement. It occurs through trial-and-error practice and involves actions occurring in a normal setting. Tasks can be performed automatically without attention or conscious thought.[2(p85)]

Stages of motor learning (Fitts and Posner 3-stage model)[86]

• **Cognitive stage:** the learner develops an initial understanding of the task with practice that involves high levels of cognitive processes (attention and concentration) and dependence on visual inputs; performance is inconsistent with multiple errors.

• **Associative stage:** the learner selects, practices, and refines a motor pattern resulting in spatial and temporal organization of movements; learner becomes less dependent on visual feedback while use of proprioceptive feedback increases; performance is more consistent with a decrease in errors and extraneous movements.

• **Autonomous stage:** the learner continues to practice and refine a motor pattern; skills are acquired, movements are highly coordinated, largely error free, the shift to automaticity with only minimal cognitive monitoring evident.

Box 5.6 Motor Learning Terms—cont'd

Measures of motor learning

- **Performance measures:** assess changes in performance of a task as a result of practice, with attention to the quality of movements and the success of movement outcome.
- **Retention test:** defined as a performance test on a given task provided after a retention interval and without practice.[1(p440)]
- **Transfer of learning** refers to the gain (or loss) in the capability for performance in one task as a result of practice or experience on another task.[1(p440)]
- **Transfer test:** refers a performance test in which the task or task conditions have changed; often provided after a retention interval without practice."[1(p440)]
- **Adaptation:** refers to the process of adjusting a movement (adapting) to changing task and environmental demands.

Knowledge of Performance: augmented feedback about the movement pattern the learner has just made; sometimes referred to kinematic feedback.[1(p438)]

Knowledge of Results: augmented verbal feedback given back to the learner about the success of an action with respect to an environmental goal.[1(p438)]

---

4. a level of cognitive-verbal-proprioceptive monitoring required during stage 2 (associative) learning.
5. a level of decreased monitoring and automaticity of movements during stage 3 (autonomous) learning.
6. the retention of skills after a period of no practice.
7. the generalizability of a skill to other related tasks.
8. the ability to adapt a skill to changing task and environmental demands.

■ DECISION-MAKING/PROBLEM-SOLVING SKILLS

The patient who is able to engage in active introspection and self-evaluation of performance and reach decisions independently about how to improve performance demonstrates an important element of learning. In contrast, physical therapists who overemphasize guided or assisted movements and errorless practice may be limiting the patient's learning. Although this may be important for safety reasons, lack of exposure to performance errors may preclude the patient from developing capabilities for self-evaluation. In an era of fiscal responsibility and limitations on the amount of physical therapy sessions allowed, many patients are able to learn only the very basic skills while in active rehabilitation. Much of the necessary learning of functional skills occurs after discharge and during outpatient episodes of care. The therapist cannot possibly structure practice sessions to meet all of the functional challenges the patient may face. The acquisition of independent problem-solving/decision-making skills ensures that the final goal of rehabilitation—independent function—can be achieved. The therapist needs to observe and document this very important function, including the patient's self-perceptions of the effectiveness of the decisions reached. See Box 5.7, Questions to Examine of the Patient's Ability to Actively Problem Solve, and additional discussion in Chapter 10.

Motivational factors include personal sense of self-determination (i.e., choice and collaboration), self-efficacy

Box 5.7 Questions Examining the Patient's Ability to Actively Problem Solve

1. Does the patient understand the goal of the intended movement?
2. Is the patient able to recognize/describe the intended outcome of the movement? Determine if it was successful or not successful?
3. Is the patient able to recognize/describe any problems encountered during the movement? Suggest solutions to correct the problems?
4. Is the patient able to identify/sequence component steps of a complex task?
5. Is the patient able to recognize aspects of the environment that can lead to success or failure in reaching the intended goal?
6. Is the patient motivated and confident in the performance of the skill?
7. Is the patient motivated and confident to return home and be safe in the home environment?

(i.e., confidence in one's capabilities), and focused attention. They are important factors to assess in order to ensure active participation, learning, and retention of motor skills.[92] Highly motivated individuals devote greater effort to learning a task and are willing to devote more focused time to practice. Individuals who are not motivated to learn are not engaged and limit their effort and practice. Therapists need to explore with the patient their perceptions about their disability or injury, their personal goals, their feelings about competence, and perceptions for success in achieving their goals. Equally important is an assessment of the patient's understanding of the relevance of the learning activity or skill to their daily life. A rehabilitation POC that focuses on involved decision-making, active participation, and self-direction is critical in ensuring that the patient will be able to continue practice once discharged and to retain learned motor skills. Self-determination and self-management are key elements in ensuring success in real-world environments. Assessment of these factors should be an ongoing process throughout the rehabilitation episode of care. It is important to remember that the patient will experience a number of motivational "ups and downs." The therapist who accurately identifies and reacts to these changes can provide effective intervention, including encouragement and positive reinforcement. Continuing documentation of the patient's motivational and emotional status is necessary.

Learning styles differ according to several factors, including personality characteristics, reasoning styles (inductive or deductive), and initiative (active or passive). Some individuals utilize an *analytical/objective* learning style. They process information in a step-by-step order and learn best with factual information and structure. Other individuals are more *intuitive/global* learners. They tend to process information all at once and learn best when information is personalized and presented within the context of practical, real-life examples. They may have difficulty in ordering steps and comprehending details. Hemispheric differences between right and left hemisphere lesions seen after stroke are examples of these behavioral differences (see Chapter 15, Stroke). Some individuals rely heavily on visual processing and demonstration to learn a task. Others depend more on auditory processing, talking themselves through a task. Individual characteristics and preferences are best determined by talking with the patient and family, using careful listening and observation skills. The medical record may also provide information concerning relevant premorbid history (e.g., educational level, occupation, interests). A thorough understanding of each of these factors allows the therapist to appropriately structure the examination, learning environment, and therapist–patient interactions.

■ INSTRUMENTATION AND TECHNOLOGY TO ASSESS MOTOR FUNCTION

Imaging and electrophysiological testing have vastly expanded the diagnosis, prognosis, and treatment of patients with movement disorders.[94,95] They also provide a means for assessing neural plastic mechanisms, motor control, and motor learning in both healthy individuals and those facing diverse neuromusculoskeletal health conditions.[96,97] In combination, imaging and electrophysiological testing provide structural and functional information on the spatial (i.e., location and area) and temporal (i.e., timing) characteristics of the neuromuscular system. This section will discuss the basic mechanisms and relevance of various imaging and electrophysiology (NCS, EMG, EEG, and TMS) techniques used in the assessment of neuromusculoskeletal health conditions and motor function.

Imaging has fundamentally shaped how health-care providers evaluate, diagnosis, and treat patients with neuromuscular and skeletal dysfunction. With direct access to physical therapy services approved in all states and the District of Columbia, physical therapists have the responsibility to understand the indications and limitations of various imaging modalities. Rehabilitation providers, regardless of practice setting, must recognize the indications for imaging and how their results impact patient prognosis and management.[98] Additionally, modern neuroimaging provides capabilities beyond *structural imaging* of pathology (i.e., radiograph, CT scan, standard MRI, DTI) and now allows for the molecular *(PET)* and *functional* (fMRI) *imaging* of the brain during resting and task specific activities.[99,100]

Structural Imaging
Radiography (X-Ray)
Radiographic images (i.e., x-rays) are foundational to the assessment of motor function. A radiographic image is the result of electromagnetic radiation that is projected through the body and captured by a radiographic detector (e.g., plate/plain film). The x-ray is absorbed differently based on tissue density with structures like metal and bone appearing radiopaque (i.e., white and light gray) and air or fat appearing radiolucent (i.e., black or dark gray). Radiographic images provide visualization of significant fractures (see Figure 5.10), dislocations, compromised joint space or erosion (e.g., osteoarthritis, degenerative disc disease), or shifts in bone density (e.g., osteopenia, some osseous tumors). Since x-ray images typically only provide a two-dimensional view in one plane, examination of multiple views for a specific area or joint is warranted. Despite the low cost and relatively small degree of radiation, radiographs have limited capability to detect soft tissue (e.g., muscle, tendon) or nervous system involvement.[98,101]

Computed Tomography
CT also uses x-rays but incorporates computerized reconstruction of specifically target cross-sections at multiple angles to allow circumferential analysis of an anatomical area, to include specific plane or 3-D analysis.[101] Noncontrast CT provides rapid (minutes) and enhanced imaging of cortical bone, soft-tissue, and vascular structures following trauma. It is also seen as the initial imaging technique for the differential diagnosis of TBI (e.g., subdural, epidural, and intraventricular hematomas) and hemorrhagic versus ischemic cerebral strokes (see Fig. 5.11).[101] CT scans combined with contrast agents also increase sensitivity to detecting emerging hemorrhagic strokes and cerebral vasospasms following TBI. Although recent advancements in CT imaging have resulted in reduced radiation dosage and enhanced imaging quality, limitations still exist with regards to detection of ischemic cortical lesions

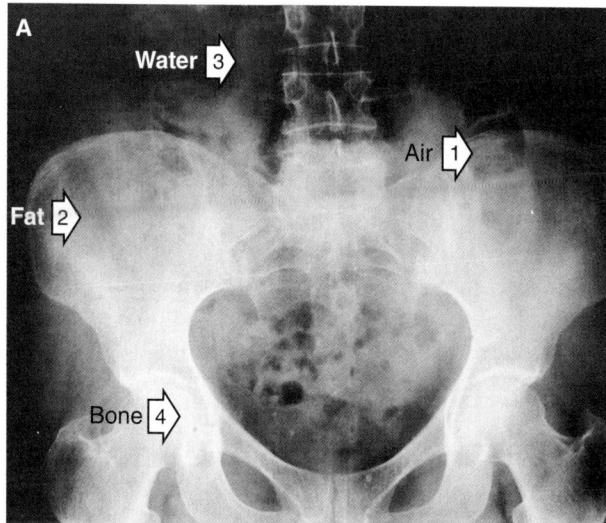

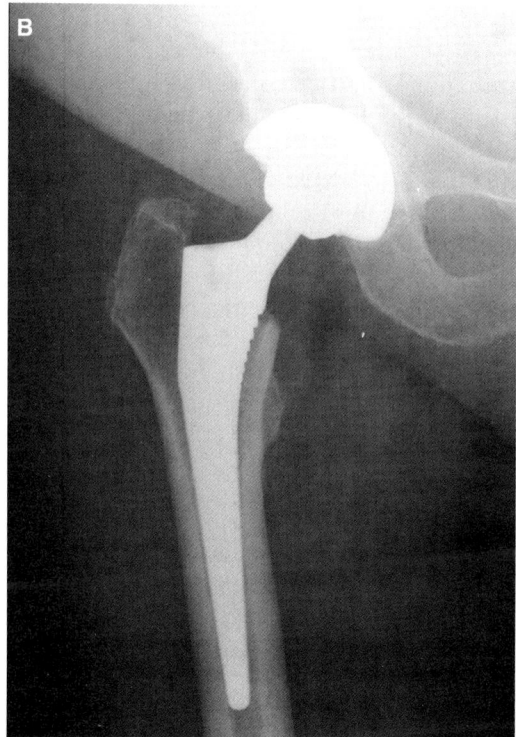

Figure 5.10 (A and B) Standard radiographs.

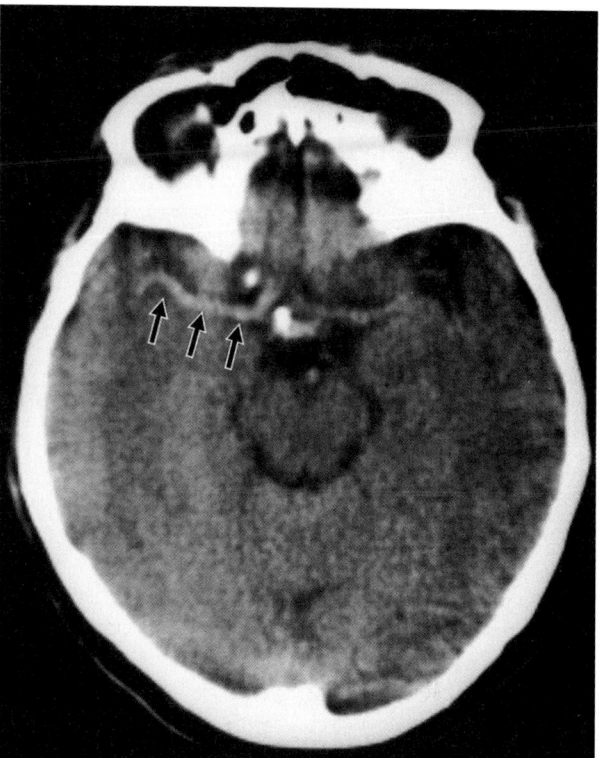

Figure 5.11 Computed tomography (CT) scan of acute stroke.

and ability to predict recovery following brain injury or stroke.[94]

Magnetic Resonance Imaging

Magnetic resonance imaging (MRI) has the clear advantages of no radiation exposure and superior visualization of soft tissue, cartilage, bone marrow, and the nervous system, thus placing it as the reference standard for various neuromusculoskeletal health conditions.[98,101] MRI images are the result of the body in the presence of a strong magnetic field, introduction of radiofrequency pulses, and subsequent image capture (relaxation) times (T1 and T2). T1 and T2 weighted sequences are standard with T1 showing bright or high signal intensity for fat (e.g., myelinated structures) and T2 demonstrating bright signal for structures with increased water content (e.g., cerebrospinal fluid).[101] Although MRI takes longer to complete, it is often the initial choice or conducted in addition to a CT scan secondary to optimize imaging of cortical lesions (see Figure 5.12).[94] MRI also serves as the preferred imaging technique for the diagnosis and medical management of various PNS and CNS conditions.[101–103] Despite various advantages, standard sequence MRI is costly and contraindications and suboptimal imaging exist related to metal and movement artifact and the magnetic field.[101,104] Clinical limitations of standard T1-T2 MRI also include the inability to detect axonal injuries that occur after mild brain injuries.[94]

Diffusion Tensor Imaging

Diffusion tensor imaging (DTI) expands on the standard capabilities of MRI by providing microscopic-level assessment of water diffusion rate and orientation along white matter tracts. In effect, DTI produces 3-D images (see Fig. 5.13) that provide visualization and anisotropic diffusion measurement of myelinated axons and corresponding tracts (e.g., lateral corticospinal tracts, corpus callosum).[94] The initial clinical utility and research on DTI involved patients with mild TBI and normal standard sequence MRI. This research and subsequent studies have assisted in identifying areas of axonal injury

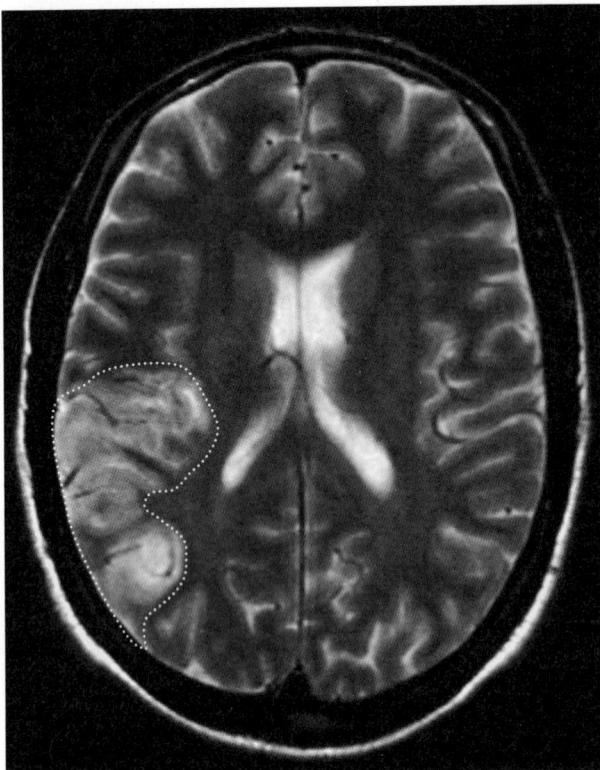

Figure 5.12 Magnetic resonance image (MRI) of T2 sequence.

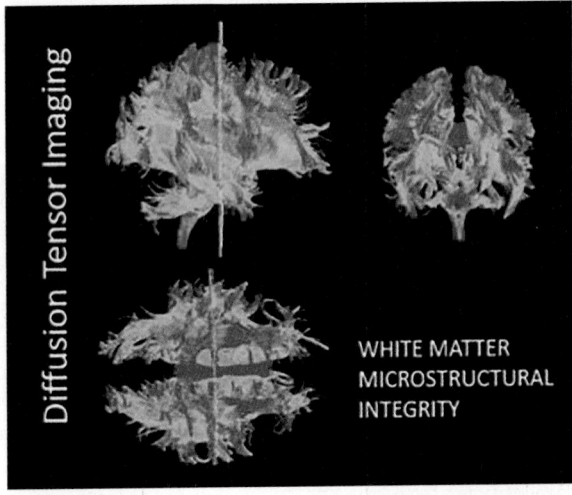

Figure 5.13 Diffusion tensor imaging (DTI).

that correlate to clinic findings in patients with mild TBI.[105] DTI changes in white matter tracts are also seen in patients following acute stroke, with specific changes in the corticospinal tracts demonstrating some association with motor outcomes at 3 months.[100] DTI investigation over the past decade has vastly expanded to include patients with SCI, neurodegenerative disease (e.g., PD, ALS, and MS), and peripheral nervous system pathology (e.g., carpal tunnel syndrome and lumbar radiculopathy).[105–107] Although DTI provides a sensitive response to axonal injury, it lacks specificity, and future

research is needed to clearly assess its prognostic capability and responsiveness to therapeutic techniques.[94,100]

Functional Imaging Techniques

Functional MRI

Functional imaging techniques, such as fMRI, have vastly enhanced the ability to indirectly assess neural activity and functional connectivity between various areas of the brain. In comparison to standard CT and MRI, fMRI moves beyond analysis of local neural lesions and allows for the investigation of functional connectivity both within and outside the areas of pathology. Specifically, fMRI has been invaluable for identifying brain neuroplastic reorganization following central and peripheral nervous system dysfunction.[99,108,109] Consistent patterns of ipsilateral reorganization after stroke include upregulation of communication between the frontoparietal and motor cortex regions, suggesting greater dependence on cognitive level motor control.[99] Functional MRI cortical reorganization is also demonstrated in various regions in patients with phantom limb pain and early diabetic polyneuropathy.[108,109]

fMRI indirectly measures neural activity by assessing changes in blood flow, volume, and local rate of metabolism of oxygen. The blood oxygen level dependent (BOLD) signal captured on MRI represents the amount of deoxyhemoglobin in the examined tissue. As neural activity increases in a region of the brain, oxygen use and deoxyhemoglobin levels correspondingly increase over a 2 to 5 second duration creating the BOLD signal seen on MRI (see Fig. 5.14). The BOLD signal, also referred to as the hemodynamic response, provides an opportunity to study the brain at rest (resting-state fMRI) and during performance of cognitive or sensorimotor tasks (task-based fMRI).[99,110] Evidence supports that resting-state fMRI is useful in identifying disrupted functional connections within 1 hour of acute cortical strokes. Additionally, resting-state fMRI has shown restoration of cortical-level functional networks in patients who exhibited rapid (within 1 week) recovery of hand function following stroke. Secondary to the 2- to 5-second time lag seen with the hemodynamic response, tasked-based fMRI protocols typically employ a block design to allow for appropriate periods of rest (i.e., control) and stimulus (e.g., sensory stimulus, motor task) for accurate signal capture. Tasked-based fMRI informs the capacity of both short- and long-term neuroplastic recovery and specifically in relationship to motor function and learning. For example, previous research utilizing task specific practice in patients with chronic stroke showed improved autonomous movement and a supporting reduction of contralateral cortical activity (i.e., less reliance on the injured cortex) with use of the paretic UE.[99] Task-specific fMRI has also provided integral information on commonly used interventions (e.g. constraint induced movement therapy, bilateral training, sensory and proprioceptive training) and corresponding neural structures and networks activated

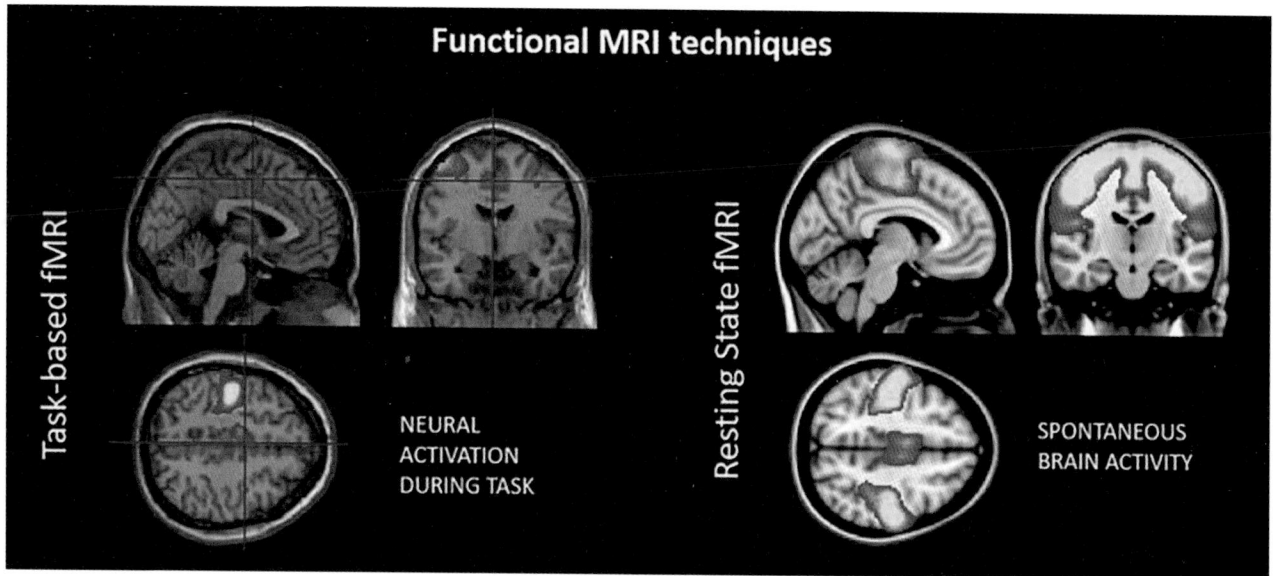

Figure 5.14 Functional MRI (fMRI).

in both healthy individuals and patients with central nervous dysfunction.[96,99] Despite the advantages fMRI provides over structural imaging for examining neuroplasticity, recovery and motor learning, some limitations do exist. Primary areas of consideration and limitations include poor temporal resolution, extraneous head and eye movement creating image artifacts, patient's emotional status and focus, and standard MRI precautions.

Molecular Imaging Techniques

PET/Single Photon Emission Computed Tomography

PET and SPECT provide noninvasive means to identify the molecular processes associated with cancer, heart conditions, and neurodegenerative diseases. PET/SPECT creates images by measuring high energy gamma rays created by the decay of various radioisotopes (fluorine-18 and carbon-11). Radioisotopes are combined with a specific metabolic radiotracer (e.g., ^{18}F = 2 fluro-2deoxy-D-glucose = FDG) or imaging agent such as dopamine (flourine-18 combined with dopamine = F-FDOPA) and injected intravenously into the area of interest. The combination of metabolic tracers and specific imaging agents enhances PET/SPECT ability to investigate metabolic pathways such as glucose utilization (i.e., increased with cancer and neurodegenerative disorders like AD) or specific ion, neurotransmitter, or receptor deficits (e.g., PD). Additionally, this level of molecular imaging makes it possible to detect pathologies prior to clinical impairments, allowing for diagnosis and therapeutic trials of various CNS disorders.[111,112] Dopaminergic PET/SPECT images have been shown to improve the diagnosis of PD and are recognized as valuable biomarkers for the status and disease progression of patients with early to middle stage PD (see Fig. 5.15).[112,113] PET has also assisted in identifying amyloid-beta (A-beta) and tau pathology that is common in patients with AD. In fact,

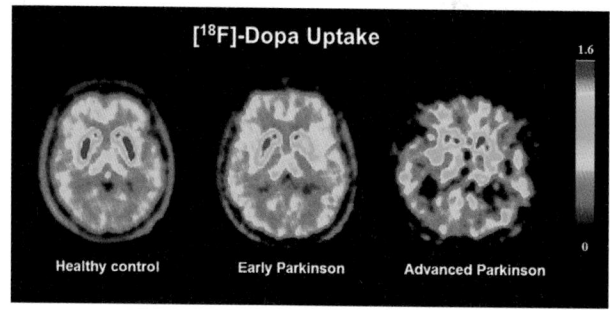

Figure 5.15 Positron emission tomography (PET).

PET guidelines are now approved in several countries to assist in the diagnosis of AD and A-beta PET scans have shown promise as an adjunct measure for the early management and longitudinal assessment of patients with mild cognitive impairment.[114] PET is costly secondary to the requirements for a cyclotron to produced radiotracers and both PET and SPECT have radiation risk. Although SPECT is less costly, it lacks the specificity of PET and future research into the cost-benefit of PET versus SPECT and responsiveness of both imaging techniques to rehabilitation is needed.[111] See Table 5.11 for a summary of physical principles, advantages, disadvantages, and typical use of different types of imaging.

Electrophysiologic Neuromuscular Assessment

Similar to imaging, electrophysiological assessment serves an extension of a detailed and evidence-based historical and physical examination. Electrophysiological techniques result in useful information for assessing peripheral and CNS function that is inaccessible to standard structural imaging techniques. Specifically, in contrast to structural (i.e., minutes to days) and functional neuroimaging techniques (e.g., fMRI = seconds), electrophysiologic

Table 5.11   Characteristics of Imaging Modalities

Imaging Modality	Physical Principles	Advantages	Disadvantages	Typical Use
Structural Imaging				
Radiography	X-ray Two-dimensional image	Fast; Visualization of various densities (e.g., bone, gas, fat) and basic bony anatomy (e.g., joint alignment, fractures)	Limited for complex anatomy and soft-tissue visualization; Radiation exposure*	Initial assessment of musculoskeletal conditions
Noncontrast CT Scan	X-ray; computer image reconstruction of cross-section and 3-D images	Fast (minutes); High spatial resolution (50–200 μm); detailed visualization of cortical bone lesions or fluid contrast (e.g., bleeding)	Insensitive to some soft tissue and neural lesions secondary to low image contrast; Increased radiation exposure	Initial assessment of polytrauma and some neurologic injuries (e.g., head injuries and vascular strokes); assists acute surgical and medical (TPA) management
Contrast CT, to include angiography	Addition of oral, intravenous, or intrathecal induced contrast agent	Enhanced visualization of vascular structures or scar tissue	Reaction to contrast agent	Vascular injury or breakdown of the blood-brain barrier; CT myelogram-dura and nerve root compromise
MRI (T1–T2 sequence)	Radio waves and use of magnetic fields to produce multiplanar and 3-D images	High spatial resolution (25–100 μm); detailed views of soft tissue, bone marrow, vascular and neurologic tissue; no radiation	Longer scanning time; higher cost Lower sensitivity to cortical bone injuries, axonal injuries, and early infarction	Reference standard for various neuromusculoskeletal conditions; detection of small neurovascular changes (hematoma, edema) related to head injuries and stroke
Diffusion-Tensor MRI	Modified MRI sequence; assesses water diffusion rate and orientation in white matter	Sensitive to axonal injury and moderate to large changes in white matter	Limited specificity	Clinical research; assessment of white tracts following injury and response to therapeutic interventions
Molecular Imaging				
PET/SPECT	Measures high (PET) and low (SPECT) energy gamma rays created by decay of various radioisotopes and imaging agents	High sensitivity for detection of normal and impaired metabolic pathways or neural transmission	Higher cost to produce isotopes/radiotracers; Radiation exposure	Detection of certain cancers; assists in diagnosis of PD; potential biomarker for neurodegenerative disease (e.g., AD and PD) progression and responsiveness to therapies
Functional Imaging				
Resting-state functional MRI	BOLD signal assessed while the patient is at rest	High spatial resolution; localization of cortical/subcortical activity throughout the brain	Sensitive to patient movement; poor temporal resolution (2- to 5-second lag)	Clinical research; identification and recovery of brain activity and connectivity following CNS/PNS lesions
Tasked-based functional MRI	BOLD signal assessed prior to and soon after a during a specific task	High spatial resolution following specific stimulus; ability to assess recovery and motor control/learning	Similar to resting state; limited to individuals who can complete task	Clinic and motor control/learning research: healthy individuals and patients following CNS/PNS lesions

* = radiation exposure varies by body region; BOLD = blood oxygen level dependent; CT = computed tomography; TPA = tissue plasminogen activator; MRI = magnetic resonance imaging; PET = positron emission tomography; SPECT = single photon emission computed tomography; PD = Parkinson disease; AD = Alzheimer disease; CNS = central nervous system; PNS = peripheral nervous system.

assessment provides quantitative temporal information with millisecond precision. Electrophysiologic techniques also directly assess neural activation (i.e., anterior horn cell, motor units, pyramidal cells activity) that is not reliant on indirect (fMRI) vascular changes.

Nerve Conduction Studies

Electrodiagnostic testing in the form of *NCS* is most often used to the assess the functional integrity of the peripheral nervous and muscular systems. Peripheral NCS assess sensory axons, motor axons, the neuromuscular junction, and the muscle fibers activated. Nerve conduction studies in the form of somatosensory evoked potentials also allow for the evaluation of sensory nerve conduction from the peripheral to CNS (see additional information on CNS-evoked potentials in the EEG section later in this chapter). Typical nerve conduction studies are divided according to the anatomy investigated and include motor nerve conduction, sensory nerve conduction, late responses (F-wave and H-reflex), and repetitive nerve stimulation.

Typical NCS involve direct stimulation to initiate an impulse in a motor or sensory nerve. The impulse that results from the stimulation creates a waveform or evoked potential that is referred to as *compound motor action potential* (CMAP) or *sensory nerve action potential* (SNAP). Figures 5.16 and 5.17 provide examples of a normal SNAP and CMAP. The SNAP and CMAP provide key information on the *evoked potential's* conduction time (i.e., distal latency), amplitude, duration, and overall appearance (i.e., morphology). NCV can also be calculated and represents the speed of a nerve over a specific distance (NCV = Conduction distance/Proximal latency – Distal latency). Although NCV can be used in sensory nerves, it is most often employed to assess motor NCV between two stimulation sites (e.g., see Fig. 5.17; elbow-wrist median motor NCV = 61 meters/second). Normal NCS values for latency, NCV, and amplitude exist for various peripheral nerves and provide a reliable and valid means for determining nerve pathology.[115]

Distal motor and sensory latencies (measured in milliseconds) and respective nerve conduction velocities (measured in meter/seconds) reflect the fastest axons of the nerve and are used to assess myelin health. Figure 5.18A demonstrates slowing of the median distal motor latency and wrist-to-palm NCV, consistent with mild to moderate median nerve demyelination (i.e., motor fiber myelinopathy). In comparison, the amplitude of the CMAP is normal, suggesting overall healthy physiological functioning of motor axons. Sensory or motor amplitudes require further analysis and maybe reduced secondary to the following: (1) varying degrees of myelin loss across axons resulting in *temporal dispersion* of the waveform; (2) *partial neuropraxia (myelinopathy) and conduction block* stopping axonal transmission despite the axon remaining intact; or (3) *axonal degeneration* (i.e., Wallerian degeneration). Critical evaluation of sensory and motor amplitudes provides important

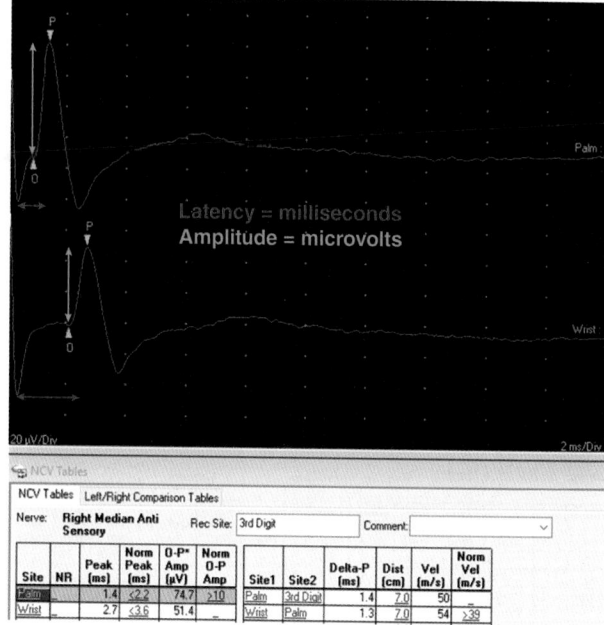

Figure 5.16 Normal median sensory nerve conduction study.

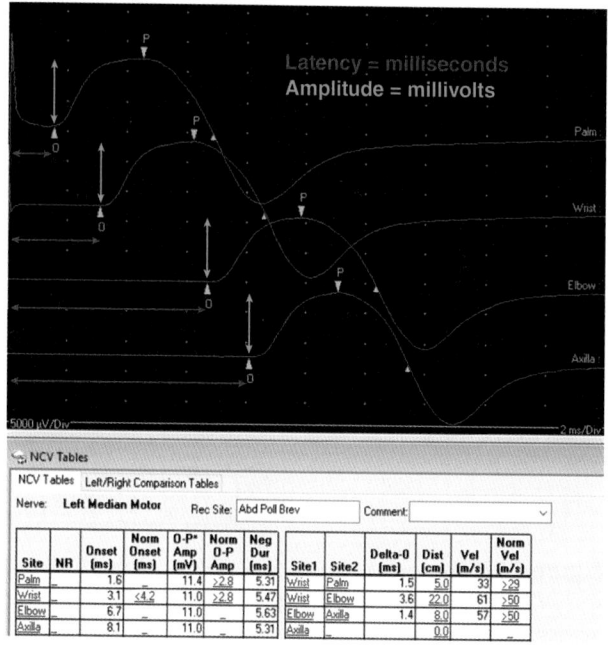

Figure 5.17 Normal median motor nerve conduction.

diagnostic and prognostic information for patient management. In general, temporal dispersion and conduction block represent myelin pathology, and in the case of conduction block, the potential for a timelier recovery. Figure 5.18B shows NCV slowing with partial conduction block of ulnar motor axons (≈30%) occurring at or just distal to the medial epicondyle of a patient with cubital tunnel syndrome. Despite the drop in amplitude near the elbow, the duration of the overall wave forms are minimally changed, suggesting this patient has a positive prognosis.[116] Collectively, the findings of a normal

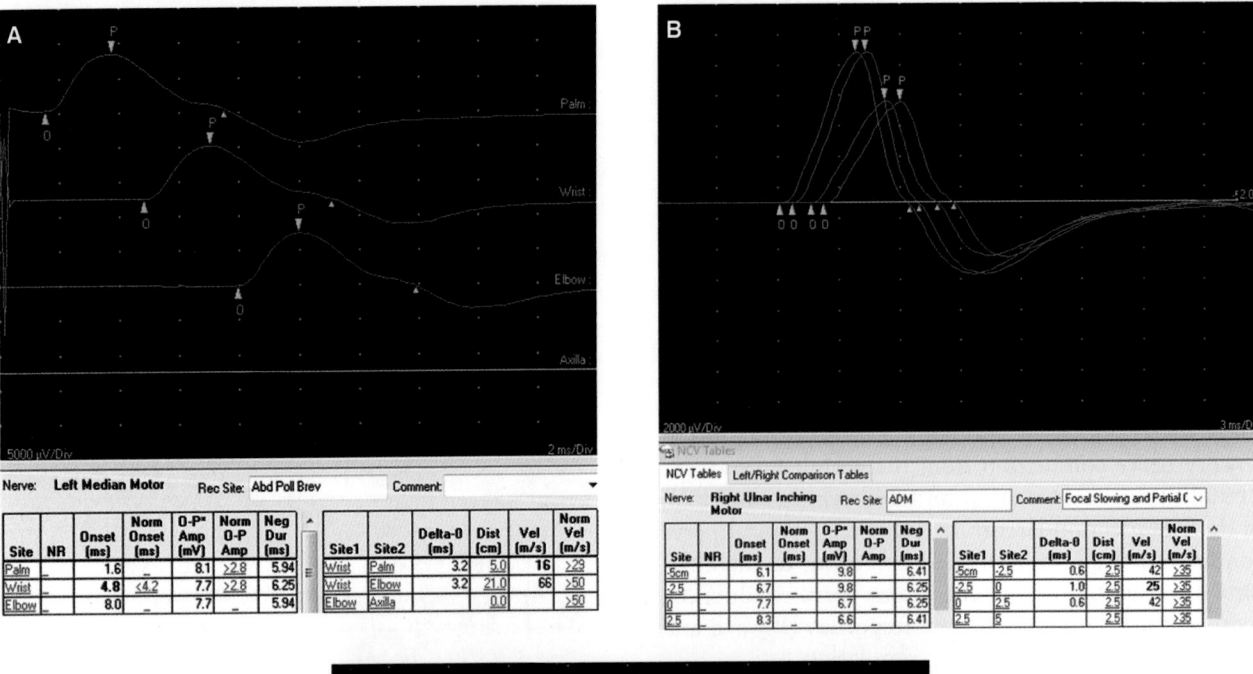

Nerve: **Left Median Motor**   Rec Site: Abd Poll Brev   Comment:

Site	NR	Onset (ms)	Norm Onset (ms)	O-P* Amp (mV)	Norm O-P Amp	Neg Dur (ms)
Palm		1.6	—	8.1	≥2.8	5.94
Wrist		4.8	≤4.2	7.7	≥2.8	6.25
Elbow		8.0	—	7.7	—	5.94

Site1	Site2	Delta-O (ms)	Dist (cm)	Vel (m/s)	Norm Vel (m/s)
Wrist	Palm	3.2	5.0	16	≥29
Wrist	Elbow	3.2	21.0	66	≥50
Elbow	Axilla		0.0		≥50

NCV Tables   Left/Right Comparison Tables

Nerve: **Right Ulnar Inching Motor**   Rec Site: ADM   Comment: Focal Slowing and Partial C ∨

Site	NR	Onset (ms)	Norm Onset (ms)	O-P* Amp (mV)	Norm O-P Amp	Neg Dur (ms)
-5cm		6.1		9.8		6.41
-2.5		6.7		9.8		6.25
0		7.7		6.7		6.25
2.5		8.3		6.6		6.41

Site1	Site2	Delta-O (ms)	Dist (cm)	Vel (m/s)	Norm Vel (m/s)
-5cm	-2.5	0.6	2.5	42	≥35
-2.5	0	1.0	2.5	25	≥35
0	2.5	0.6	2.5	42	≥35
2.5	5		2.5		≥35

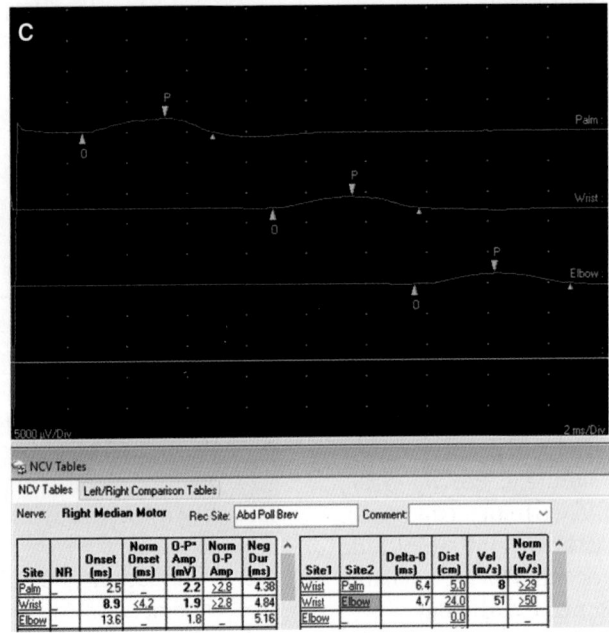

NCV Tables   Left/Right Comparison Tables

Nerve: **Right Median Motor**   Rec Site: Abd Poll Brev   Comment: ∨

Site	NR	Onset (ms)	Norm Onset (ms)	O-P* Amp (mV)	Norm O-P Amp	Neg Dur (ms)
Palm		2.5	—	2.2	≥2.8	4.38
Wrist		8.9	≤4.2	1.9	≥2.8	4.84
Elbow		13.6	—	1.8	—	5.16

Site1	Site2	Delta-O (ms)	Dist (cm)	Vel (m/s)	Norm Vel (m/s)
Wrist	Palm	6.4	5.0	8	≥29
Wrist	Elbow	4.7	24.0	51	≥50
Elbow			0.0		—

Figure 5.18 Abnormal motor nerve conduction studies. (A) Mild median slowing focally across the wrist. (B) Partial motor conduction block of ulnar nerve at elbow. (C) Severe median slowing across the wrist with partial axon loss.

distal (wrist) CMAP with only partial conduction block of the ulnar nerve at the elbow reflect a lesser degree of nerve injury (neuropraxia) without the need for an extended recovery for axonal regeneration. In contrast, Figure 5.18C shows a patient with severe carpal tunnel that includes axonal motor loss. In addition, to median nerve myelinopathy (significantly prolonged wrist distal motor latency), the patient exhibits axonal degeneration as supported by a lower than normal CMAP amplitude distal to the lesion. This finding can be confirmed by needle EMG of the abductor pollicis brevis. Taken together, these findings reinforce that a more significant axonal

injury (i.e., axonotmesis, see Fig. 5.5) has occurred. Overall, the benefits of motor and sensory nerve conduction testing include enhanced diagnostic accuracy of peripheral nerve entrapments and polyneuropathy, detailed physiological assessment of sensorimotor myelin and collective axonal involvement, and prognostic (mild vs. moderate vs. severe) information for patient management. Despite the benefits, NCS are not able to diagnosis small neural fiber dysfunction (pain, impaired temperature, or crude touch), are reliant on needle EMG to confirm motor axonopathy and recovery, and may result in transient discomfort during testing.[117,118]

Late-evoked or long-latency responses, such as F-waves and H-reflexes, are appropriately named because they occur after the CMAP. Both F-waves and H-reflexes allow for the assessment of longer and more proximal nerve segments that would otherwise be inaccessible to routine nerve conduction studies. The F wave is elicited by the supramaximal stimulus of a peripheral nerve at a distal site (e.g., median nerve at the wrist), leading to propagation of impulses both toward the nearby recording muscle (e.g., abductor pollicis brevis) and returning back to the muscle from the anterior horn cell. Since no synapse is involved, the F-wave is not considered a reflex but rather a measure of motor neuron conduction. The F-wave assists in the diagnosis of conditions where the entire length (Guillain-Barré syndrome) or most proximal portion of the myelin and/or collective axon health is involved (e.g., brachial plexus injuries, multilevel radiculopathies).[119,120]

The *H reflex* is also a useful long-latency electrodiagnostic measure, and like a monosynaptic reflex, will demonstrate impairments (a prolonged latency or absent response) in cases of radiculopathy, polyneuropathy, or respective peripheral nerve involvement. Its most common application is in testing the monosynaptic pathways of S1 nerve roots via the tibial nerve and to a lesser extent at C6–C7 and L3–L4 via the median or femoral nerves. The H-reflex is the result of an action potential's travel along the IA afferent sensory axon toward the dorsal horn and synapsing directly and/or through interneurons on the alpha motor neurons (e.g., S1 level), leading to an impulse traveling peripherally to the muscle (e.g., soleus). Because the stimulus causes impulses to travel within a mixed motor and sensory neuron, the latency reflects the integrity of both sensory and motor fibers in the reflex loop. A slowed latency with otherwise normal distal NCS parameters is indicative of abnormal proximal function and is specifically useful in the investigation of nerve root involvement. H-reflex latency and amplitude changes are also used in research to monitor segmental motor excitability and motor control in healthy individuals and following various neurologic conditions (e.g., SCI, polyneuropathy, stroke, or TBI), to include during gait and balance activities.[121–123]

Repetitive nerve stimulation (RNS) is a supplemental motor NCS that is used to assess the health of the neuromuscular junction (NMJ). In particular, it is performed if there is suspected presynaptic (e.g., Lambert-Eaton myasthenic syndrome, LEMS) or postsynaptic (e.g., myesthenia gravis [MG]) neuromuscular dysfunction. Patients with NMJ disease typically report fatigue that progress to weakness in ocular, bulbar, and/or proximal greater than distal extremity muscles. Questions related to specific areas of fatigue and weakness and detailed strength/endurance testing are critical as the presentation of LEMS and MG varies. Specifically, patients with LEMS typically present with LE weakness and less involvement of ocular/bulbar muscles, whereas MG most often impacts ocular, bulbar, and proximal UE muscles. The diagnosis of NMJ may be delayed as MMT with one repetition is often normal, and strength may briefly increase secondary to increased mobilization of acetylcholine and binding. In contrast, having patients perform multiple repetitions or sustained activities (e.g., squatting, shoulder shrugs, looking upward) in involved muscles may result in identified weakness, difficulty speaking/swallowing, and partial ptosis.[117]

RNS studies quantify periodic weakness and fatigue and assist in the diagnosis of NMJ disease by assessing changes in CMAP amplitudes after 5 to 10 low-rate (2 to 5 HZ) repetitive supramaximal stimulation (see Fig. 5.19). If initial decrements of greater than 10% are identified between the first and fourth or fifth trials, an additional 5 to 10 stimuli are conducted after 10 seconds of brief isometric exercise to determine if an increase in amplitude occurs, suggesting postactivation facilitation (PAF). Finally, a series of 5 to 10 trials is conducted after 30 to 60 seconds of isomeric exercise or fast rate (20 to 50 Hz) stimulation to mimic tetany, as well as every 30 to 60 seconds for up to 5 minutes to determine postactivation exhaustion. In MG, RNS shows a normal to mildly reduced initial CMAP amplitude, with a greater than 10% decrement by the fourth to fifth trial. Following PAF, the amplitude may return to baseline, but within 2 to 4 minutes of a brief isometric contraction, decrements return and maybe more pronounced. In comparison, patients with LEMS demonstrate an abnormal reduced CMAP amplitude that is exponentially increased (>60% to 100%) with a brief isometric contraction. The postactivation facilitation of the CMAP with isometric exercise is a highly sensitive (97%) and specific (99%) finding for LEMS. The identification of LEMS is critical as 60% of patients with LEMS have small cell lung cancer. Although it is a noninvasive technique that provides excellent capability for the diagnosis of NMJ disorders, RNS has limitations. Some patients may not be able to tolerate the repetitive supramaximal stimulation, and RNS has limited sensitivity for assessing ocular myasthenia.[9,117,124] Additional details regarding nerve conduction, long latency, and RNS procedures, and relevant findings, are located on the online module at F.A. Davis.

Electromyography

Rehabilitation professionals utilize different types of EMG in clinical practice and research, including diagnostic and kinesiologic EMG. This section will focus on

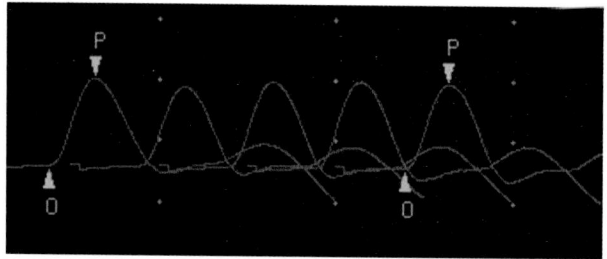

Figure 5.19 Repetitive nerve stimulation of ulnar nerve.

diagnostic EMG, but it is important to point out that kinesiologic EMG is fundamental to movement science and rehabilitation. Kinesiologic EMG has, and continues to make, extensive contributions to our understanding of neuromuscular activation during individual joint and functional movements. For more information on kinesiologic EMG, the reader is referred to a review by McManus et al.[125]

Diagnostic EMG is complementary and typically performed with NCS. It is used to assess the function and integrity of the components of the motor unit (see Figure 5.5) and has the ability, unlike NCS and RNS, to confirm axonal degeneration, regeneration, and chronicity. EMG also allows for direct evaluation of muscle and myopathic conditions. Similar to NCS, EMG serves as an extension of the patient history and clinical examination. EMG is typically performed after and builds on information obtained during nerve conduction testing.

When performing a diagnostic EMG, a small needle electrode is inserted into a specific muscle to identify potential abnormal electrical activity at rest, as well as motor unit electrical characteristics while the patient slowly builds up force (see Fig. 5.20). The examiner will assess the selected muscle(s) under four conditions: (1) insertional activity, (2) resting activity, (3) motor unit morphology and recruitment during minimal contraction, and (4) motor unit temporal and spatial summation toward full recruitment. Each condition provides unique information to the health of the motor unit and peripheral nervous system.

Needle insertion and resting activity are assessed while the patient is completely relaxed. Normal needle insertional activity is extremely brisk and stops within 200 milliseconds (ms) of cessation of needle movement. Insertional activity is described as normal, reduced, or increased. In the case of axonal degeneration or muscle disease, the muscle membrane will be irritable and insertional activity will be increased (see Fig. 5.21). Reduced or decreased insertional EMG activity generally represents chronic neuropathy or myopathy, in which there has been significant atrophy of muscle and/or infiltration of fat and connective tissue within the muscle. To improve diagnostic accuracy, the needle electrode is moved slightly to nearby areas and depths within the

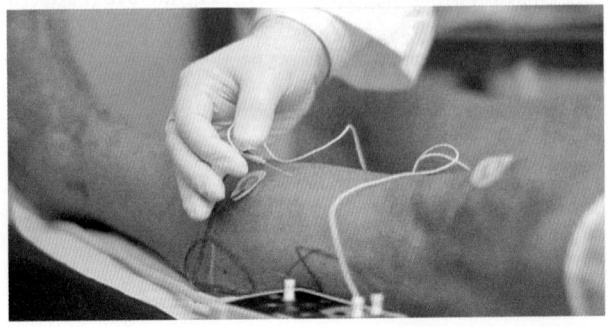

Figure 5.20 Needle EMG of the anterior tibialis.

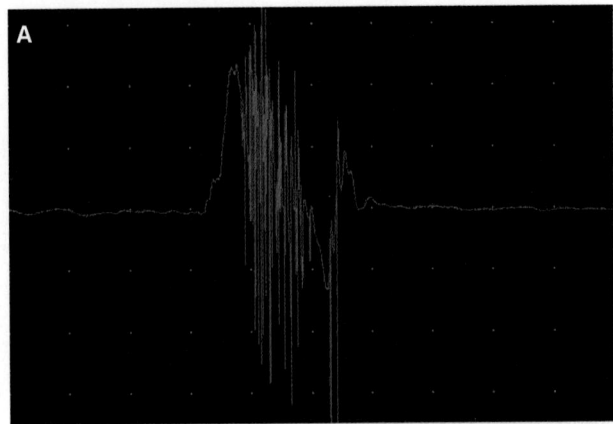

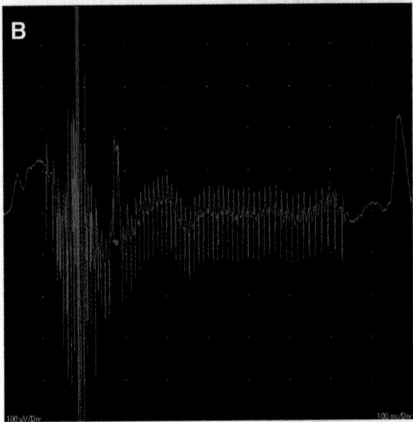

Figure 5.21 Insertional activity. (A) Normal insertional activity. (B) Increased insertional activity.

examined muscle, thus allowing multiple assessments of insertional and resting activity.[117]

While the needle is at rest between insertions, the examiner will look and listen for abnormal spontaneous activity. Abnormal spontaneous activity from individual muscle fibers includes fibrillations and positive sharp waves. Fibrillation and positive sharp waves (PSWs) are the most commonly seen abnormal spontaneous potentials and are observed following axonal degeneration (see Fig. 5.22). They occur in various neuropathic disorders, such as peripheral nerve lesions, anterior horn cell disease, radiculopathies, and polyneuropathies, and they verify axonal loss. They are also found in muscle degenerative conditions such as some myopathies (e.g., muscular dystrophy, dermatomyositis, polymyositis) and less frequently in MG. Fibrillations and PSWs may be seen on EMG within a week but may require up to 3 weeks following axon loss injury to become more widespread. Other forms of abnormal spontaneous activity include complex repetitive discharges and fasciculation potentials. Complex repetitive discharges (CRDs) often occur with chronic neuropathy and myopathy. Fibrillations, PSWs, and CRDs are not visible to the patients. Because fasciculation potentials involve discharge of the motor unit, patients may see and feel fasciculations

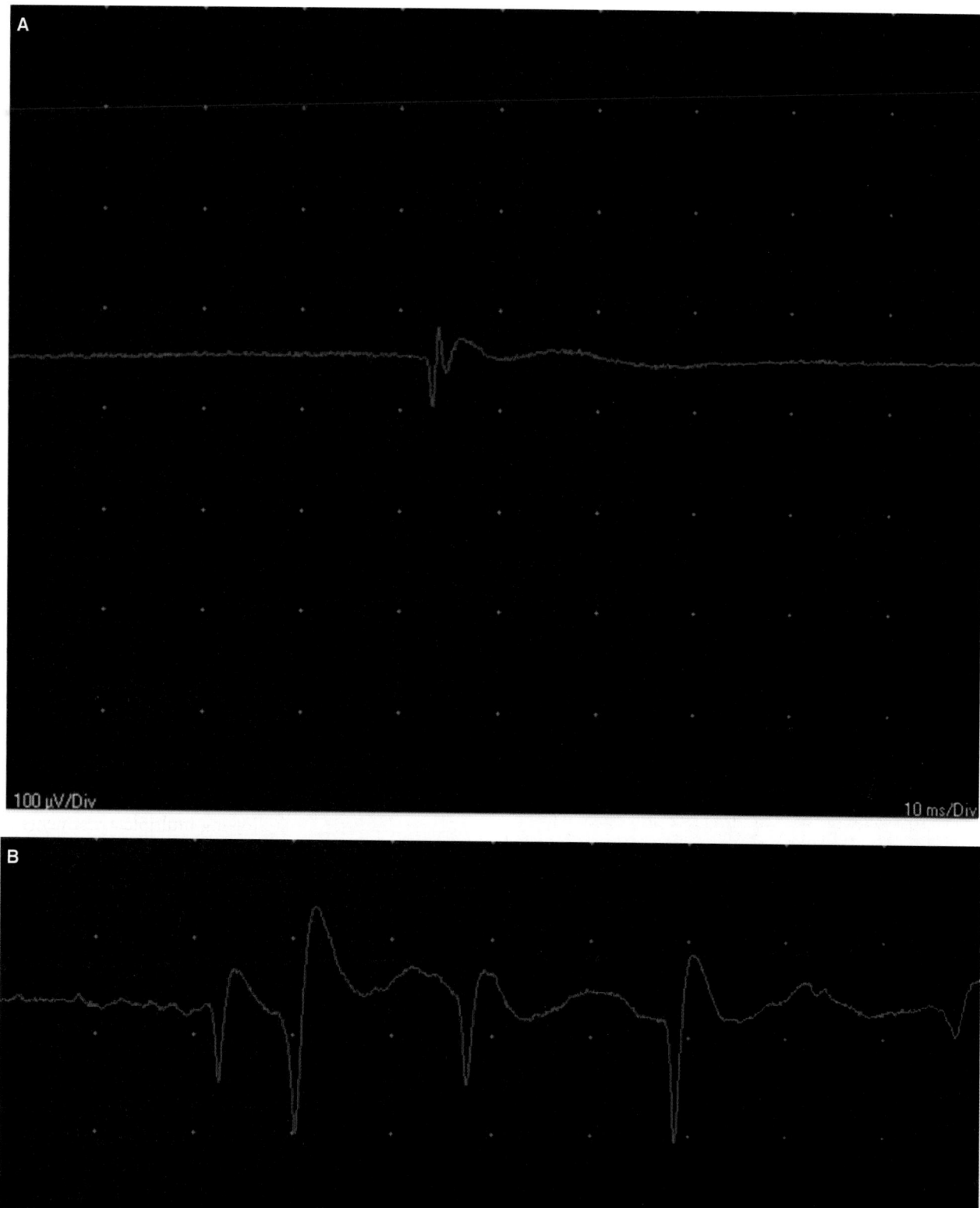

Figure 5.22 Abnormal resting potentials. (A) Fibrillation. (B) PSWs.

and report them as "muscles spasms or twitches." Fasciculations may be seen or felt infrequently by healthy individuals, are not pathologic by themselves, and often occur following exercise or fatigue. If they occur more frequently, are in multiple muscles, and are seen with other LMN signs and EMG changes, they warrant attention. Fasciculations are associated with several neuropathic and myopathic conditions, including motor neuron disease (ALS), radiculopathies, polyneuropathy, and entrapment mononeuropathies.[6,117]

After observing the muscle at rest, the patient is asked to contract the muscle minimally. When a muscle is contracted to produce force, a single axon conducts an impulse to all its muscle fibers, causing them to depolarize at relatively the same time. This depolarization produces electrical activity that is manifested as a motor unit action potential (MUAP) and can be recorded and displayed graphically. A MUAP is the summation of electrical potentials from all the fibers of that unit close enough to the electrodes to be recorded. MUAPs are examined with respect to morphology (amplitude, duration, shape) and frequency of firing. These parameters are the essential characteristics that distinguish normal from abnormal potentials. Normative values for motor unit size and shape are established. In normal

muscle, the peak-to-peak amplitude of typical MUAP may range from 300 microvolts (μV) to 5 millivolts (mV). The duration of the potential is a measure of time from onset to cessation of the electrical potential, typically from 3 to 12 milliseconds (see Fig. 5.23A). The typical shape of a MUAP is biphasic or triphasic and generally does not display more than four phases.[117]

Polyphasic potentials, which are MUAPs having five or more phases, are generally considered abnormal when seen in large numbers (see Fig. 5.23B). Polyphasic motor units reflect neuroplastic peripheral changes and, specifically, collateral sprouting from an intact and neighboring axon to denervated muscle fibers. This phenomenon is probably due to the difference in the length of the terminal branches and immature myelin in the sprouting axons extending to each muscle fiber. The result is a MUAP with a larger number of phases and longer duration than a normal motor unit. As the collateral sprouts mature and an increased number of motor fibers are integrated into the motor unit, the MUAP will increase in amplitude, creating a larger than normal (5 mV) or giant MUAP (see Fig. 5.23C). Large-amplitude MUAPs are typically seen in chronic neuropathic conditions such as long-standing radiculopathies or focal nerve entrapments such as carpal tunnel syndrome.[117]

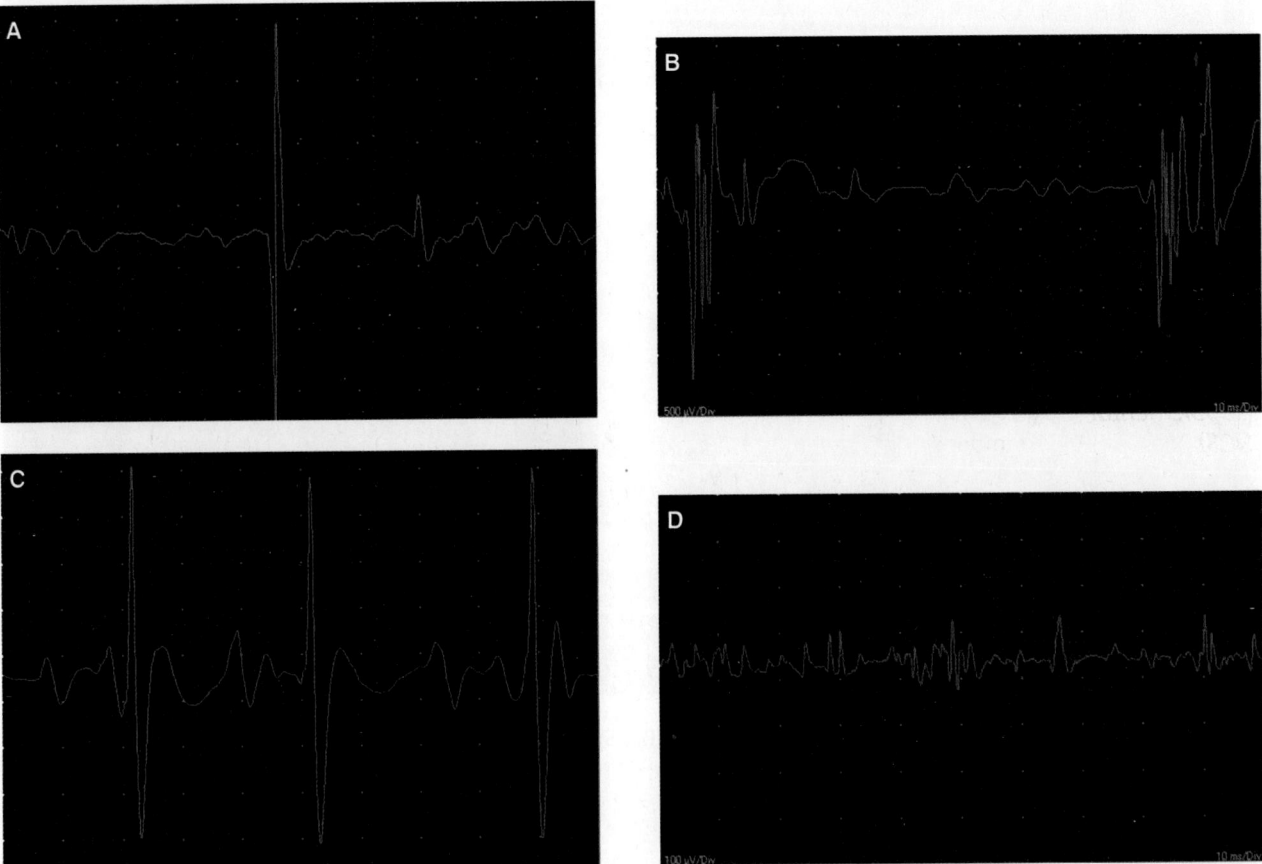

Figure 5.23 Motor unit morphology and recruitment. (A) Normal motor unit. (B) Polyphasic motor unit. (C) Larger than normal amplitude motor unit with neuropathic recruitment. (D) Short duration, low-amplitude motor units with myopathic recruitment.

The clinician ends the EMG examination of that specific muscle by assessing recruitment. The patient is asked to gradually increase force to allow for investigation of the normal transition from temporal (i.e., one motor unit increasing frequency) to spatial summation (i.e., multiple motor units firing). In normally innervated and healthy muscle, recruitment should progress from one motor unit increasing its firing rate to 12 to 15 Hz (temporal summation) prior to bringing in other motor units (spatial summation). If innervated muscle has axonal loss, it will be forced to increase the frequency of the remaining long-duration polyphasic or larger than normal amplitude motor units resulting in reduced and fast-firing frequencies (>15 Hz) consistent with *neuropathic recruitment* (see Fig. 5.9C). In contrast, patients with myopathy will have polyphasic potentials of small amplitude and short duration secondary to the loss of muscle fibers within the motor units (see Fig. 5.23D). Since the total availability of motor axons remains normal, but muscle degeneration results in fewer muscles fibers and less force, spatial summation of MUAP will occur more rapidly than normal, resulting in low-amplitude, short-duration polyphasia with *early or myopathic recruitment* (see Fig. 5.23D).[6] Table 5.12 provides a summary of the advantages, disadvantages, and clinic uses of EMG. Additional details regarding EMG procedures are also located on the online module at F. A. Davis.

Table 5.12 Characteristics of Electrophysiological Techniques				
Electrophysiology Technique	Physical Principles	Advantages	Disadvantages	Typical Use
Standard NCS	Electrical stimulation of motor/sensory nerves recorded from surface electrodes	Excellent temporal resolution (ms); physiological assessment of sensorimotor myelin and collective axonal health	No direct visualization of nerve/muscle; does not assess small nerve fiber pathology; cannot confirm motor axonal loss (Wallerian degeneration) or chronicity; may result in patient discomfort	**Clinical:** Localize and categorize (mild, moderate, severe) nerve entrapments and polyneuropathy; **Outcome:** Remyelination and overall sensorimotor axonal recovery
F-wave (supplemental NCS)	Distal supramaximal stimulus results in signal traveling to the anterior horn cell and back to the distal muscle	Examines overall and more proximal peripheral motor nerve pathways (plexus and root)	Not a stand-alone technique; does not assess sensory pathways; potential discomfort	**Clinical:** Diffuse motor fiber demyelination (Guillain-Barré syndrome); brachial plexus injuries or multilevel radiculopathies
H-reflex (supplemental NCS)	Distal submaximal stimulus creates monosynaptic reflex	Assess sensorimotor reflex arch, specific nerve root(s), and segmental motor excitability	Not a stand-alone technique; potential discomfort	**Clinical:** S1, C6–C7 and L3–4 radiculopathies **R/MC:** Segmental motor excitability and motor control/learning to include during movement (e.g., balance/gait)
RNS (Supplemental NCS)	Supramaximal RNS (5–10 stimulus per second) examined at rest, after exercise or high-rate stimulus, and recovery	Examines patient fatigue/weakness; neuromuscular junction health and dysfunction	Not a stand-alone technique; potential discomfort; limited sensitivity for DX ocular myasthenia	**Clinical:** Presynaptic (e.g., Lambert-Eaton myasthenic syndrome) and postsynaptic (e.g., MG) neuromuscular dysfunction

(Continued)

Table 5.12	Characteristics of Electrophysiological Techniques—cont'd			
Electrophysiology Technique	Physical Principles	Advantages	Disadvantages	Typical Use
EMG	Indwelling electrode (needle) provides precise PNS axonal and muscular assessment during needle insertion, rest, and motor unit recruitment	Excellent temporal resolution (ms); determines motor axonal degeneration, neuroplasticity (i.e., collateral sprouting) and motor unit recruitment (normal vs. myopathic vs. neuropathic)	No direct visualization of nerve/muscle; does not assess myelin health or sensory nerve fiber pathology; patient discomfort	**Clinical:** Axonal loss (axonotmesis/neurotmesis); localization of nerve entrapments, radiculopathy, and plexopathies; determine chronicity; PNS motor axonal recovery and prognosis
EEG	Surface electrodes on scalp detect fluctuating voltages	Excellent temporal resolution (ms); assess brainwave activity; may include evoked (e.g., somatosensory-evoked potentials) or event-related potentials; can pair with imaging (e.g., MRI, fMRI)	No visualization of CNS unless paired with imaging; standard EEG limited to cortical activity; low risk of seizure	**Clinical:** Localize and classify seizures; assist DX and management of CNS conditions; neuromonitoring in ICU and during surgeries; brain death determination **R/MC:** Functional neural network connectivity; localize hemisphere dominance, white matter changes and cortical reorganization
TMS	Magnetic stimulation activates cortical neurons. Signals recorded by EEG or NCS.	Excellent temporal resolution (ms); measures and modulates cortical/subcortical and spinal tract activity; treatment modality; can pair with EEG/NCS and imaging (MRI, fMRI)	No visualization of the CNS unless paired with imaging; low risk of seizures or headache; contraindicated if metal is in/on the head or face	**Clinical:** Examine and RX of various neurological and mental health conditions; localize cortical functions **R/MC:** Assess cortical/subcortical reorganization and neural networks; influence of excitatory/inhibitory mechanisms

Note: Nerve conduction and EMG are complementary techniques that are most often completed and analyzed at the same time.

RNS = repetitive nerve stimulation; EMG = electromyography; MG = myesthenia gravis; MRI = magnetic resonance imaging; fMRI = functional magnetic resonance imaging; DX = diagnosis; R/MC = research/motor control; EEG = electroencephalography; NCS = nerve conduction studies; TMS = transmagnetic stimulation; CNS = central nervous system; TMS = transmagnetic stimulation; RX = treatment

Electroencephalography

EEG is the most common, long-standing, and noninvasive method to assess temporal cortical activity and functional CNS network connectivity. The power of EEG lies in its ability to provide real-time assessment of neurophysiological activity between spatially remote brain areas. EEG employs surface electrodes placed on the scalp to record spontaneous, evoked (e.g., somatosensory, visual, auditory), or event-related potentials and neuronal oscillations (i.e., brain waves). EEG involves cortical brain wave assessment and serves as the reference standard for the diagnosis and localization of seizures. EEG is also used to assist in the diagnosis and management of various brain cortex–related health conditions including, but not limited to, epilepsy, TBI, stroke, brain tumors, encephalopathies, cognitive disorders (e.g., dementia), mental health conditions (e.g., schizophrenia), attention disorders, developmental delay, and sleep disorders. EEG that includes evoked potentials (e.g., somatosensory evoked potentials) also allows sensitive assessment of cortical and subcortical ischemia during intraoperative monitoring and intensive care. Clinical utilization of EEG also includes monitoring of comatose patients and ultimate determination of brain death.[126,127]

EEG-related clinical research has contributed invaluable information on neuroplastic changes following cortical lesions and subsequent rehabilitation. Various EEG studies involving patients with poor outcomes following stroke have found increased acute inhibitory EEG responses within and near the lesion, suggesting potential ischemia and/or secondary cell death. Poststroke hemisphere asymmetries with increased excitatory EEG activity in the contralateral motor area compared to the involved hemisphere are also associated with less favorable outcomes. Of interest, a decrease in the contralesional motor area EEG signal (i.e., improved hemisphere symmetry) is seen following UE and gait rehabilitation and correlates to improved clinical outcomes. Overall, EEG is established as a consistent means to characterize cortical recovery mechanisms, and growing evidence supports its use to assess treatment response to experimental therapies for various health conditions. It also holds promise as a biomarker and outcome measure in motor control research involving healthy individuals. Specifically, EEG has the added benefit of being able to be combined with other imaging (e.g., MRI) and electrophysiological techniques (e.g., TMS), thus maximizing both spatial and temporal resolution. Although EEG is a noninvasive technique, there is a small risk of seizures and headaches with testing.[126,127]

Transmagnetic Stimulation

Transmagnetic stimulation (TMS) is a noninvasive and safe technique to activate, measure, and modulate cortical neurons. TMS involves electromagnetic induction of targeted cortical neurons that are directly measured

in the brain via EEG and/or peripherally as compound motor action potentials. TMS can also be cortically measured indirectly via fMRI and provides spatial resolution and structural correlation. The primary benefit of TMS lies in its ability to evaluate cortical pathways within (e.g., arcuate fasciculus for language) and between cerebral hemispheres (e.g., corpus callosum), as well as the corticospinal pathway to a specific muscle or muscle group. TMS may involve single, paired, or repetitive pulses, with each providing unique benefits. Single pulse TMS (spTMS) examines the speed of neural pathways and assists mapping specific functional areas to include defining an individual's motor homunculus. Paired pulsed TMS results in excitatory and inhibitory facilitation of intra- and intercortical areas, thus allowing exploration of cortical neural network functional connectivity and neuroplasticity. Repetitive TMS (trams) is applied at various frequencies to modulate brain function that may last minutes to hours beyond stimulation. In particular, low-frequency (≤1 Hz) rTMS typically decreases cortical excitability, and high frequency (≥5 to 20 Hz) increases excitability. The lasting excitatory and inhibitory effects of rTMS reinforce its capability to induced synaptic neuroplastic mechanisms and its therapeutic potential.[99,128]

Although all forms of TMS have been used as clinical and research examination and outcome measures, spTMS is most often employed. Previous research has shown the value of TMS in capturing cortical level changes at different stages (acute, subacute, and chronic) and for various impairments (motor, spasticity, cognition, language, and spatial neglect) in patients following a stroke. Studies have also demonstrated the predictive validity of TMS-evoked potentials following stroke with present or improved motor responses and/or hemisphere balance in acute and subacute stages, which are seen as positive indicators for long-term functional recovery. Additional research regarding the use of TMS as an outcomes measure and its responsiveness for various neurological and mental health conditions is needed.[127,128]

The use of rTMS as a treatment modality for neurological and mental health conditions has vastly expanded over the past decade. In fact, rTMS is widely accepted as an evidence-based and insurance-approved treatment option for depression and obsessive-compulsive disorders. It also has Level A evidence as part of neurorehabilitation after stroke and for patients with neuropathic pain.[128,129] Future investigation involving rTMS for patients with postconcussion syndrome, MS, PD, dystonia, AD, and epilepsy are mixed with positive improvements most often linked to specific impairments or secondary health conditions (e.g., the patient with PD with predominate motor symptoms and/or depression). The disadvantages of TMS are minimal and primarily include a low risk for seizure or headaches, and patients with metal on or in their head or face region cannot undergo TMS protocols.[127,128] Table 5.12 provides a summary of physical principles, advantages, disadvantages, and typical use of different types of electrophysiologic techniques.

■ EVALUATION AND DIAGNOSIS

Evaluation refers to the clinical judgments therapists make based on the data gathered from the examination. Numerous factors influence the judgments therapists make when working with patients with impairments of motor function, including complexity and understanding of the nervous system, clinical findings (signs and symptoms), psychosocial considerations, and overall physical function and health. Therapists evaluate data in terms of severity of problems (activity limitations, participation restrictions, impairments) and level of recovery or chronicity. Therapists must also consider the consequences of failure to intervene appropriately when the patient is at risk for additional impairments or prolonged activity limitations. Potential discharge placement and resources also influence evaluation of the data and development of the POC. There is a clear need for the therapist to focus on those problems that directly affect function and can be successfully remediated.

The *physical therapy diagnosis* is determined from evaluation of the patient examination findings and is based on the results of relevant history, systems review, and qualitative and quantitative assessments. Activity limitations, participation restrictions, and impairments of body structure and function are identified and analyzed. The therapist also considers the patient's motor learning capabilities, problem-solving abilities, motivation, and learning styles, as well as information from other health professionals. A physical therapy diagnosis describes the impact of the condition on function at the level of the *movement system* and at the level of the *whole person*. The primary dysfunction toward which the therapist directs treatment is identified and becomes the focus of the physical therapy POC.[12] See the discussion in Chapter 1, Clinical Decision-Making.

Novice therapists can gain understanding and insights into the complex examination and practice issues facing therapists from mentoring by experienced, senior therapists. Keeping up with the scientific literature is also key to expanding abilities. Based on signs and symptoms, Table 5.13 summarizes the differential diagnosis of UMN and LMN syndromes. Tables 5.14 and 5.15 summarize the differential diagnosis of major types of CNS disorders and neuromuscular degenerative diseases, respectively.[130]

Table 5.13	Differential Diagnosis: Comparison of Upper Motor Neuron (UMN) and Lower Motor Neuron (LMN) Syndromes	
	UMN Lesion	**LMN Lesion**
Location of lesion, Structures involved	CNS cortex, brain stem, corticospinal tracts, spinal cord	Cranial nerve nuclei/nerves Spinal cord: anterior horn cell, spinal roots Peripheral nerve
Diagnosis/pathology	Stroke, TBI, spinal cord injury	Polio, Guillain-Barré Peripheral nerve injury Peripheral neuropathy Radiculopathy
Tone	Increased: hypertonia Velocity dependent	Decreased or absent: hypotonia, flaccidity Not velocity dependent
Reflexes	Increased: hyperreflexia, clonus Exaggerated cutaneous and autonomic reflexes, +Babinski	Decreased or absent: hyporeflexia Cutaneous reflexes decreased or absent
Involuntary movements	Muscle spasms: flexor or extensor	With denervation: fasciculations
Strength	Weakness or paralysis: ipsilateral (stroke) or bilateral SCI Corticospinal: contralateral if above decussation in medulla; ipsilateral if below Distribution: never focal	Ipsilateral weakness or paralysis Limited distribution: segmental or focal pattern, root-innervated pattern
Muscle bulk	Disuse atrophy: variable, widespread distribution, especially of antigravity muscles	Neurogenic atrophy: rapid, focal distribution, severe wasting
Voluntary movements	Impaired or absent: dyssynergic patterns, obligatory mass synergies	Weak or absent if nerve interrupted

TBI = traumatic brain injury; SCI = spinal cord injury.
From O'Sullivan and Siegelman[123(p153)] with permission.

Table 5.14 Differential Diagnosis: Comparison of Major Types of CNS Disorders				
Location of Lesion	Cerebral Cortex Corticospinal Tracts	Basal Ganglia	Cerebellum	Spinal Cord
Diagnosis/ pathology	Stroke	Parkinson disease	Tumor, stroke	Trauma, tumor, vascular insult: complete, incomplete SCI
Sensation	Impaired or absent: depends on lesion location; contralateral sensory loss	Not affected	Not affected	Impaired or absent below the level of lesion
Tone	Hypertonia/spasticity velocity-dependent; clasp-knife Initial flaccidity: cerebral shock	Lead-pipe rigidity: increased, uniform resistance Cogwheel rigidity: increased, ratchet-like resistance	Normal or may be decreased	Hypertonia/spasticity below the level of the lesion Initial flaccidity: spinal shock
Reflexes	Hyperreflexia	Normal or may be decreased	Normal or may be decreased	Hyperreflexia
Strength	Contralateral weakness or paralysis: hemiplegia or hemiparesis Disuse weakness in chronic stage	Disuse weakness in chronic stage	Normal or weak: asthenia	Impaired or absent below the level of the lesion: paraplegia or paraparesis; tetraplegia or tetraparesis
Muscle bulk	Normal during acute stage; disuse atrophy in chronic stage	Normal or disuse atrophy	Normal	Disuse atrophy
Involuntary movements	Spasms	Resting tremor	None	Spasms
Voluntary movements	Dyssynergic: abnormal timing, coactivation, fatigability	Bradykinesia: slowness of movement Akinesia: absence of movement	Ataxia: intention tremor, dysdiado-chokinesia, dysme-tria, dyssynergia nystagmus	Above level of lesion: intact (normal) Below level of lesion: impaired or absent
Postural control	Impaired or absent, depends on lesion location Impaired balance	Impaired: stooped (flexed) Impaired balance	Impaired: truncal ataxia Impaired balance	Impaired below level of lesion Impaired balance
Gait	Impaired: gait deficits due to abnormal weakness, synergies, spasticity, timing deficits	Impaired: shuffling, festinating gait	Impaired: ataxic gait deficits, wide-based, unsteady	Impaired or absent: depends on level of lesion
Imaging	CT-acute stroke MRI-enhanced imaging and prognostic indicator; DTI/fMRI to supplemental DX/PX	PET/SPECT assist in DX/PX of PD	MRI: DX (cerebellar tumor, stroke, and MS lesions)	CT-acute trauma; DX MRI: DX and PX
Electrophysiology techniques	EEG/TMS: supplemental for DX/PX; EEG used DX poststroke seizures; TMS may be used for RX	EEG used for sleep/seizure disorders; TMS/EEG research	EEG and seizures; TMS/EEG research	TMS motor-evoked potentials and SSEP supplemental for DX/PX of SCI and assessment spinal pathways

CT = computed tomography; DX = diagnosis/diagnostic; EEG = electroencephalography; fMRI = functional MRI; MRI = magnetic resonance imaging; MS = multiple sclerosis; PD = Parkinson disease; PET = positron emission tomography; PX = prognosis/prognostic; RX = treatment; SCI = spinal cord injury; SPECT = single photon emission computed tomography; SSEP = somatosensory evoked potentials; TMS = transmagnetic stimulation.
From O'Sullivan and Siegelman,[123(p152)] with permission.

Table 5.15 Differential Diagnosis: Comparison of Major Types of Neuromuscular Diseases

Location of Lesion	Corticospinal tracts, anterior horn cells, cranial motor nuclei and corticobulbar tracts	Multiple distal peripheral axons/myelin	Multiple peripheral nerves/nerve roots and cranial nerves	Postsynaptic receptors/cleft of the neuromuscular junction
Disorder	Amyotrophic lateral sclerosis	Diabetic polyneuropathy Chronic polyneuropathy	Guillain-Barré syndrome Acute polyradiculo-neuropathy	Myasthenia gravis
Cranial nerve involvement	Yes	No	Yes	Yes; partial ptosis often first sign: Ice pack test positive
Sensation	Typically normal; may have pain in lateral stages secondary to immobility	Glove and stocking: Often starts as burning pain/tingling and moves to numbness/loss of proprioception	Sensory impairments typically not as severe as motor impairments	Normal
Strength	Early: Asymmetric weakness of hand and leg muscles → to all muscles. One third of patients with initial bulbar weakness (worse prognosis).	Weakness/atrophy of foot muscles → to legs/fingers hands	Progressive weakness if GBS is not treated. Rapid progression of nerve roots/nerve/CNs may result in global weakness and need for respiratory support.	Fatigue; overt weakness after several repetitions; weakness in ocular/bulbar muscles → proximal extremity → distal muscles
Tone	Mixture of hypo/hypertonia secondary to LMN and UMN involvement	Hypotonia	Hypotonia	Typically, normal at rest; may see low tone in severe cases or with repetitive testing
Reflexes	Asymmetric hypo- and hyperreflexia	Hyporeflexia	Hyporeflexia	Normal
Involuntary movements	Marked fasciculations and/or spasticity	Possible periodic and distal fasciculations	Typically, none or limited since initial impact is on myelin	None
Voluntary movements	Absent/delayed (LMN) or dyssynergic (UMN)	Impaired distally and improved with visual feedback	Reduced or absent for multiple movements and typically worse with repetition	Normal with one repetition; reduced with multiple repetitions
Balance	Typically lacks ankle strategy early and progresses to poor hip/trunk control and inability to sit; balance gets worse over time	Difficulty with eyes closed or unlevel surface; uses hip/step strategy	Similar to amyotrophic lateral sclerosis but a much more rapid progression of sitting/standing impairments if not medically treated	Overall normal but with prolonged standing/severe disease may demonstrate decreased hip strategy

Table 5.15	Differential Diagnosis: Comparison of Major Types of Neuromuscular Diseases—cont'd			
Gait	Asymmetric foot slap/foot drop and equinus gait deformities; gait deteriorates with repetition secondary to weakness/fatigue	Ataxic; worse on unlevel surfaces or dimly lit areas; foot slap/drop in more severe cases	Initial presentation is often difficulty with running/jumping that rapidly → inability to walk without assistance	With prolonged walking/severe disease may demonstrate Trendelenburg
Imaging	Spinal and brain MRI used to rule out other conditions (e.g., radiculopathy/ stenosis); spinal MRI-nerve roots may show changes as disease progresses	Standard MRI used to rule out other conditions; advanced MRI techniques (DTI, fMRI) for clinical research	Imaging normal in the early part of the disease; spinal MRI-nerve roots may show changes as disease progresses	Imaging normal; used to rule out other conditions
Electrophysiology techniques	EMG identifies axonal loss and hallmark fasciculations; EMG for DX/PX; NCS will shows amplitude changes as disease progresses	NCS/EMG: DX and categorization of sensorimotor myelin and/or axonal changes	NCS key to assess myelin loss; F-waves sensitive indicator of global myelin loss and disease progression; EMG and NCS axonal changes occur as weakness progresses	Standard NCS/EMG normal with mild to moderate MG; RNS aids in DX and in the capture of early changes

CN = cranial nerves; DX = diagnosis/diagnostic; EMG = electromyography; LMN = lower motor neuron; NCS = nerve
   conduction studies; RNS = repetitive nerve stimulation; UMN = upper motor neuron; → = progresses.
From O'Sullivan and Siegelman, with permission.

SUMMARY

Examination of motor function is a challenging process that requires the physical therapist to accurately determine and categorize findings. An understanding of normal motor control and motor learning is essential to this process. Determining the causative factors responsible for abnormal movement patterns and behaviors is based on comparison of expected or normal responses (norm-referenced behaviors) with the patient's abnormal ones. This can best be achieved by a systematic and thorough approach to examination. Emphasis should be on the use of valid, reliable, and responsive measurement tools and outcome measures. The assessment of electrophysiological properties of nerve and muscle provides essential information to understand neuromuscular disease or trauma, the location of a lesion in the PNS, and prognosis or rate of healing or decay.

Examination of systems yields valuable information about the integrity of individual components (e.g., neuromuscular, musculoskeletal, cognitive). It is important to recall that normal motor control and motor learning are achieved through the integrated action of the PNS and CNS. The therapist must therefore also focus on integrated function evidenced through an examination of movement at the functional level. Success in rehabilitation also depends on our ability to understand the patient's goals and expected level of participation upon discharge. The motivation and learning abilities of the patient and potential strategies important for cognitive engagement and practice must also be considered. Our theoretical understanding of the CNS, motor control, and motor learning processes is both incomplete and imperfect. Therapists must, therefore, be constantly aware of the changing knowledge base in neuroscience and in neurological rehabilitation to incorporate new ideas into their examination and POC.

Questions for Review

1. Differentiate between recovery of function and compensation.

2. Describe the examination of consciousness and arousal. How can the levels of consciousness and arousal influence the motor function examination?

3. Differentiate between selective attention and alternating attention. How should each be examined?

4. Differentiate between spasticity and rigidity. How should each be examined?

5. Describe the examination of a hyperactive patellar deep tendon reflex. What scores are used to document an increased DTR?

6. A patient with stroke exhibits abnormal control of eye muscles and is unable to move the eyes smoothly in all directions. Cranial nerve testing should include which nerves and tests?

7. What are the issues of validity for using MMT as part of the examination of a patient with UMN syndrome (stroke) who exhibits strong spasticity and strong obligatory synergies?

8. A patient with MS reports fatigue as the number one symptom that impairs functional independence in the home environment. How should this patient's fatigue be examined and documented?

9. Define *stability*. How should it be examined?

10. Differentiate between the use of performance observations and retention tests in providing evidence of motor learning.

11. What imaging technique would be most appropriate to assist with the diagnosis and management of a patient with suspected PD?

12. Differentiate NCS from EMG and explain how each contributes to the physiological (functional) assessment of nerve and muscle integrity.

13. A patient with a primary diagnosis of diabetes for 10 years and low back pain (LBP) for 3 years is referred to physical therapy with LBP and diffuse LE weakness, burning pain, and numbness distal to the bilateral knees. What imaging and electrophysiological techniques may assist in patient assessment and management?

14. A patient has extreme fatigue in the proximal UEs and LEs and partial ptosis. These findings are most consistent with what health condition? What clinical examination items and electrophysiological technique would assist in the diagnosis?

15. What health conditions are most appropriate for rTMS?

CASE STUDY

The patient is a 17-year-old female who is 6 months post–motor vehicle accident (MVA). At the time of admission to the hospital, she was comatose and decerebrate. A CT scan revealed intracranial bleeding into the right occipital horn. She received a tracheostomy and a gastrostomy. Two months post-MVA, she was transferred to a *long-term care facility* specializing in TBI.

On initial admission she was able to open her eyes to verbal and tactile stimuli but was unable to visually track. She withdrew her UEs and LEs in response to stimulation but was not able to move them on command. She was alert but confused and was unable to carry on a conversation. ROM was within normal limits, except for right elbow flexion (20° to 100°) and right knee flexion (10° to 110°). She demonstrated increased tone in her left UE (LUE), 3 on MAS, 4 on MAS in her right UE (RUE), and 4 in both LEs (BLEs). She exhibited 4+ bilateral ankle clonus. She was unable to sit unsupported. While supported sitting in the wheelchair, her head and trunk control was poor, with persistent posturing to the left side.

She is now 6 months post-MVA and is currently being examined for transfer to active rehabilitation status.

PHYSICAL THERAPY EXAMINATION FINDINGS
Consciousness/Arousal

Fully awake; responds appropriately to varying stimuli.
Oriented to person; some confusion with orientation to place and time.
Can become agitated with minimal stimulation, especially when tired.

CASE STUDY—cont'd

Cognition/Behavior
Demonstrates difficulty with concentration and attention.
Able to follow simple instructions (one-level commands) but occasionally forgets what is asked of her.
Reaction time slows as the number of choices increase.
Easily forgets what she is doing.

Sensory Integrity
Aware of sensory input (pinprick, vibration, light touch) to all extremities.
Unable to discern common objects placed in either hand for stereognosis discrimination.

Joint Integrity and Mobility
RLE: plantarflexion contracture (40° to 50°); flexion contractures at the hip (10° to 120°) and knee (10° to 120°).
RUE: flexor contracture at the elbow (10° to 110°).
Full passive ROM in the LUE and LLE.

Tone
Increased bilaterally (R > L).
On Modified Ashworth Scale: RUE and RLE 3; LUE and LLE 2.

Reflex Integrity
Hyperactive, 3+ DTRs RUE, RLE.
Seven-beat nonsustained right ankle clonus.

Cranial Nerve Integrity
Cranial nerves 2–7,11–12 intact; dysphagia and dysphonia are present.

Muscle Performance
Strength is decreased in the RUE, RLE, and trunk (unable to test with MMT).
She is unable to sustain R knee extension while standing.

Voluntary Movement Patterns
RUE moves in partial range, obligatory mass flexor synergy pattern only.
RLE moves in flexor and extensor synergy patterns with no variation.
LUE and LLE demonstrate full voluntary control with isolated joint movements. Coordination is decreased. Unable to reach directly to an object that is held out to her and demonstrates foot placement problems with the LLE in sitting or in standing.
Demonstrates problems with coordinating limb and trunk movements.

Postural Control and Balance
Demonstrates good head control in all positions.
Sitting: can sit independently for up to 5 minutes. Demonstrates difficulty in maintaining weight equally on both buttocks. Tends to list to the right side while placing weight primarily on her left buttock. Able to reach to the left and forward; demonstrates loss of balance with minimal reaching to right.
Standing: able to stand in parallel bars with minimal assistance of 1 (Min A × 1) for up to 2 minutes. Must be reminded to place weight on RLE. Tends to lose her balance easily if she moves quickly; associated with brief episodes of dizziness and vertigo.

Functional Mobility Skills
Rolling: requires supervision and occasional Min A ×1 with rolling to the right; she requires maximal assist (Max A × 1) when rolling to the left.
Supine-to-sit: able to come to sitting by rolling to the L side and pushing up with her LUE; requires Min A × 1.
Transfers: able to perform stand pivot transfers with Min A × 1.
Gait: does not initiate ambulation on her own. Can ambulate the length of the parallel bars (2 m or 6 ft) with maximal assistance of two persons. Requires posterior splint to stabilize R knee.
Propels wheelchair by using the LUE and both feet for pushing; requires supervision for safety.

Motor Learning
Demonstrates profound deficits in short-term memory; unable to remember new information presented during therapy. Her memory for events and learning that occurred before the MVA is good.

(Continued)

CASE STUDY—cont'd

GUIDING QUESTIONS

Based on your evaluation of the data presented in the case history and the physical therapy examination, answer the following questions:

1. How has this patient's level of consciousness/arousal changed from admission to the long-term care facility to the current evaluation? How might this influence the examination of motor function?

2. Develop a physical therapy problem list. Categorize the patient's problems in terms of (1) direct impairments, (2) indirect impairments, and (3) activity limitations.

3. Prioritize the problems in terms of this patient's needs for the POC.

4. Determine the physical therapy diagnosis for this patient.

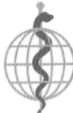

For additional resources, including answers to the questions for review, new immersive cases, case study guiding questions, references, and more, please visit **https://www.fadavis.com/product/physical -rehabilitation-fulk-8**. You may also quickly find the resources by entering this title's four-digit ISBN, 4691, in the search field at **http://fadavis.com** and logging in at the prompt.

Examination of Coordination and Balance

Dennis W. Klima, PT, MS, DPT, PhD, GCS, NCS
Thomas J. Schmitz, PT, PhD
Susan B. O'Sullivan, PT, EdD

Chapter 6

LEARNING OBJECTIVES

1. Describe the purposes of performing an examination of coordination and balance.
2. List the types of data generated from the examination.
3. Describe the common coordination and balance deficits associated with lesions of the central nervous system.
4. Discuss the primary age-associated changes that affect coordination and balance.
5. Provide a rationale for the preliminary patient observation before performing an examination.
6. Identify the motor task requirements and movement capabilities addressed during an examination of coordination and balance.
7. Differentiate between tests used to examine coordination, balance, and fear of falling.
8. Using the case study example, apply clinical decision-making skills pertinent to application of coordination and balance examination data.

CHAPTER OUTLINE

EXAMINATION OF COORDINATION *181*
OVERVIEW OF THE MOTOR SYSTEM *183*
  The Motor Cortex *183*
  Descending Motor Pathways *184*
  Cerebellum *184*
  Basal Ganglia *185*
  Dorsal (Posterior) Column–Medial Lemniscal Pathway *186*
FEATURES OF COORDINATION IMPAIRMENTS *186*
  Cerebellar Pathology *186*
  Basal Ganglia Pathology *188*
  Dorsal (Posterior) Column–Medial Lemniscal Pathology *189*
AGE-RELATED CHANGES AFFECTING COORDINATED MOVEMENT *191*
COORDINATION TESTS *192*
ADMINISTERING THE COORDINATION EXAMINATION *192*
  Preparation *192*
  Examination *193*
  Documentation *194*

OUTCOME MEASURES: UPPER EXTREMITY COORDINATION *196*
OVERVIEW OF POSTURAL CONTROL AND BALANCE *199*
  Postural Alignment and Weight Distribution *199*
  Sensory Strategies for Balance *201*
  Motor Strategies for Balance *204*
OUTCOME MEASURES: POSTURAL CONTROL AND BALANCE *206*
  Primary Balance Performance-Based Tests *207*
  Balance and Gait Combination Tests *209*
  Fear of Falling and Balance Confidence Measures *211*
  Fall Risk and Floor-to-Stand Examination *212*
SUMMARY *213*

■ EXAMINATION OF COORDINATION

A key component of motor function, coordination is the ability to execute smooth, accurate, controlled movement. "Coordinated movement involves multiple joints and muscles that are activated at the appropriate time and with the correct amount of force so that smooth, efficient, and accurate movement occurs. Thus, the essence of coordination is the sequencing, timing, and grading of the activation of multiple muscles groups."[1(p121)]

The ability to produce these responses is dependent on sensory information from the body and environment, visual and vestibular input, and fully intact musculoskeletal and neuromuscular systems. Coordinated movements are characterized by appropriate speed, distance, direction, timing, and muscular tension. In addition, they involve appropriate synergistic influences (muscle recruitment), easy reversal between opposing muscle groups (appropriate sequencing of contraction and relaxation), and proximal fixation to allow distal motion or maintenance of a posture.[2] Schmidt and Lee define coordination as the "behavior of two or more degrees of freedom in relation to each other to produce skilled activity."[3(p494)] Awkward, extraneous, uneven, or inaccurate movements characterize *coordination impairments*.

Two terms often associated with coordination are *dexterity* and *agility*.[4] *Dexterity* refers to skillful use of the fingers during fine motor tasks.[5] *Agility* refers to the ability to rapidly and smoothly initiate, stop, or modify movements while maintaining postural control.

There are several general types of coordination. *Intralimb* coordination refers to movements occurring within a single limb[6–9] (e.g., alternately flexing or extending the elbow, using one upper extremity [UE] to brush the hair, or motor performance of a single lower extremity [LE] during a gait cycle). *Interlimb* (bimanual) coordination refers to the integrated performance of two or more limbs working together[10–16] (e.g., alternately flexing one elbow while extending the other, bilateral UE tasks as required during transfers or dressing activities, or between-limb movements of the LEs and/or UEs during walking). *Visual motor* coordination[17–21] refers to the ability to integrate both visual and motor abilities with the environmental context to accomplish a goal (e.g., tracing over a zigzag line, writing a letter, riding a bicycle, or driving an automobile). A subcategory of visual motor coordination with important implications for activities of daily living (ADL) is *eye–hand coordination,*[22–26] such as required for using eating utensils, personal hygiene, or reaching for a visual target (e.g., a book from a shelf). Eye–hand coordination is perhaps more aptly termed *eye–hand–head coordination* because movement of the head is typically required for the eyes to fixate on a target or object.

Physical therapists and physical therapist assistants are frequently involved in the management of patients with coordination impairments. Data from the examination of coordination identify existing impairments. These deficits are often associated with activity limitations and participation restrictions that are related to, and indicative of, the type, extent, and location of central nervous system (CNS) pathology. Some CNS lesions present very classic and stereotypical impairments, but others are much less predictable. Diagnoses associated with coordination impairments include traumatic brain injury (TBI), Parkinson disease (PD), multiple sclerosis (MS), Huntington disease, cerebral palsy, Sydenham chorea, and vestibular pathology. Coordination impairments are also associated with some neoplasms such as astrocytoma and ependymoma that have an affinity for occurrence in the cerebellum and posterior fossa.

In the Test and Measure Categories, the *American Physical Therapy Association (APTA) Guide to Physical Therapist Practice*[4] includes impaired coordination among the examples of clinical indications for mobility (including locomotion), gait, balance, motor function, and cranial and peripheral nerve injury. Measurement of dexterity, coordination, and agility is indicated to characterize or quantify motor function as well as neuromotor development and sensory processing. Coordination exercises are included among therapeutic exercises performed by physical therapists and physical therapist assistants.

The purposes of performing a coordination examination are presented in Figure 6.1. In addition, data from the coordination examination assist the therapist with establishing the diagnosis of underlying body structure/function deficits, activity limitations, and participation restrictions (disability) along the

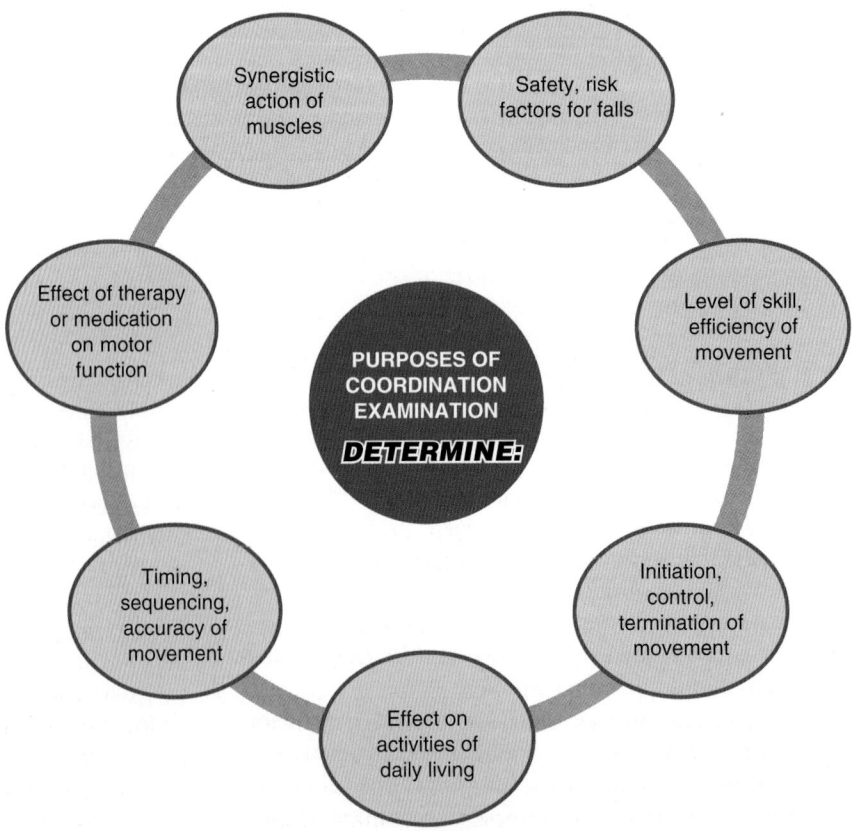

Figure 6.1 Purposes of performing a coordination examination.

International Classification of Functioning, Disability, and Health (ICF) trajectory.[4] Coordination findings also assist with establishing goals to remediate body/structure impairments, formulate expected outcomes, and direct interventions for activity and participation restrictions. Therapists may need to explore alternative strategies for performing functional activities when coordination deficits associated with degenerative diseases cannot be reversed.

■ OVERVIEW OF THE MOTOR SYSTEM

The motor system can be grossly divided into *peripheral* and *central* elements. The peripheral somatic motor system includes muscles, joints, and their sensory and motor innervation.[27] The central elements can be divided into three hierarchical levels to assist understanding their organization as well as delineating the contribution of each neuroanatomical structure. However, this does not imply a strictly top-down control of coordinated movement, as each level of the nervous system can influence other levels (above and below) depending on task demands (i.e., flexible hierarchical theory). Bear et al.[27(p452)] provide a practical description of the three hierarchical levels relative to their functional contributions to motor control: "The highest level, represented by the association areas of the neocortex and basal ganglia of the forebrain, is concerned with *strategy:* the goal of the movement and the movement strategy that best achieve[s] the goal. The middle level, represented by the motor cortex and cerebellum, is concerned with *tactics:* the sequences of muscle contractions, arranged in space and time, required to smoothly and accurately achieve the strategic goal. The lowest level, represented by the brain stem and spinal cord, is concerned with *execution:* activation of the motor neuron and interneuron pools that generate the goal-directed movement and make any necessary adjustments of posture."[27(p452)]

The motor system can also be viewed as having a *parallel arrangement.* For example, information is conveyed not only from the motor cortex to the spinal cord but also directly from premotor areas. Although the cerebellum and basal ganglion are involved in movement, they have no direct output to the spinal cord. Instead, their effect on movement is provided via connections to the motor cortex.[28] This elaborate communication network reflects a systems approach to motor control.

The critical role of sensory input on the motor system cannot be overemphasized. The integration of sensory input provides an internal representation of the environment that informs and guides motor responses.[2] These sensory representations provide the foundation on which motor programs for purposeful movements are planned, coordinated, and implemented. Sensory input to the motor system guides selection and adaptation of motor responses and shapes motor programs for corrective action. For example, the somatosensory

system provides the needed information to adjust walking when moving from a smooth surface to uneven terrain, to maintain standing balance on a moving bus, or to make the required adjustments when throwing a ball from a stable sitting surface (chair) versus an unstable one (therapy ball or foam cushion). To rule out sensory impairments as a contributing factor to coordination impairments, examination of sensory function (see Chapter 3, Examination of Sensory Function) should *precede* the coordination examination.

The Motor Cortex

The principal brain area involved in motor function is the motor cortex, which comprises cortical (Brodmann) areas 4 and 6, located in a demarcated area of the frontal lobe called the *precentral gyrus* (see Chapter 5, Examination of Motor Function: Motor Control and Motor Learning, Fig. 5.1). However, planning coordinated movement to accomplish a task involves many areas of the neocortex as it requires knowledge of the body's position in space, the location of the intended target, selection of an optimum movement strategy (i.e., which joints, muscles, or body segments will be used), memory storage until time of execution, and specific instructions to implement the movement strategy selected (where to move or what to do).[28,29]

Brodmann area 4 is designated the *primary motor cortex,* as it is the most specific cortical motor area containing the largest concentration of corticospinal neurons.[30] This area is electrically excitable, and stimuli of low intensity evoke a motor response. It lies anterior to the central sulcus on the precentral gyrus and controls contralateral voluntary movements. Brodmann area 6 is also electrically excitable but requires stimuli of higher intensities to cause a motor response.[31] It lies just anterior to area 4 and is subdivided into the superiorly placed *supplementary motor area* (SMA) and the inferiorly positioned *premotor area* (PMA).[31]

The SMA gives rise to axons that directly innervate motor units involved in initiation of movement, simultaneous bilateral grasping movements, sequential tasks, and orientation of the eyes and head. The PMA provides input to the reticulospinal neurons innervating motor units that control trunk and proximal limb movements and contributes to anticipatory postural changes.[27,32] Stimulation of area 4 typically results in uncomplicated movements of a single joint, whereas stimulation to the premotor areas (area 6) evokes more intricate coordinated movements involving multiple joints.[29]

The somatotopic organization of the motor cortex is similar to that of the sensory cortex. The motor homunculus schematically illustrates the amount of cortical area devoted to motor control of a given body part or region (see Chapter 5, Examination of Motor Function: Motor Control and Motor Learning, Fig. 5.3). Beginning on the lateral aspect of the homunculus, the mouth and facial areas are represented; moving upward are areas devoted to the hands, trunk, LEs, and feet. Note that areas requiring finer gradations of control such as the fingers, hand, and face (including muscles of speech) occupy a disproportionately larger representation (approximately half) in the motor cortex. The SMA and PMA are similarly somatotopically organized.

The motor cortex receives information from three primary sources: the *somatosensory cortex* (peripheral receptive fields), the *cerebellum,* and the *basal ganglia.* Somatosensory input is relayed directly to the primary motor cortex from the thalamus (e.g., cutaneous tactile sensations, joint and muscle receptors). The thalamus also relays information to the motor areas from the cerebellum and the basal ganglia. These connections allow for integration of motor control functions of the motor cortex, cerebellum, and basal ganglia (i.e., to carry out the appropriate course of motor action).[33]

Descending Motor Pathways

The most important descending pathway of the motor system is the corticospinal (pyramidal) tract that transmits signals from the motor cortex directly to the spinal cord. It is among the longest and largest CNS tracts. It originates primarily in areas 4 and 6 and passes through the internal capsule and the brain stem. A majority of fibers then cross to the opposite side in the medulla and descend through the lateral corticospinal tracts of the spinal cord. The fibers that do not cross at the medulla form the ventral corticospinal tracts, but a majority of these eventually cross to the opposite side in the cervical or upper thoracic regions. All fibers of the corticospinal tract terminate on the interneurons of the cord gray matter. The corticospinal tract is concerned with skilled, fine motor control, especially of the distal limbs.[33] The other major descending motor pathways that control neurons innervating muscle include the following:

- Corticobulbar tract: Some fibers project directly to motor cranial nerve (CN) nuclei (e.g., trigeminal, facial, hypoglossal) and others to the reticular formation before reaching CN nuclei.
- Tectospinal tract: This relatively small tract projects to motor neurons in the cervical cord. Fibers influence neurons innervating neck muscles as well as the spinal accessory nucleus (CN XI). It is important in guiding head movements during visual motor tasks.
- Reticulospinal tract (medial and lateral): This tract projects to the anterior horn of the spinal cord and is an important influence on muscle tone and reflex activity via influence on muscle spindle activity (increasing or decreasing sensitivity). The pontine (medial) reticulospinal tract facilitates extension of the LEs (excitation of extensor motor neurons) augmenting antigravity reflexes of the spinal cord and is an important influence on posture and gait. The medullary (lateral) reticulospinal tract has the reverse effect (excitation of flexor motor neurons).

- Vestibulospinal tracts (medial and lateral): The lateral vestibulospinal tract descends to all levels of the spinal cord and is an important contributor to postural control and movements of the head (facilitates axial extensors, inhibits axial flexors). The medial vestibulospinal tract projects primarily to the ipsilateral cervical spinal cord, which is also involved in coordinated head and eye movements.
- Rubrospinal tract: This tract merges with the corticospinal tract in the cervical region. Its role in human motor control is considered insignificant. It is believed that during primate evolution the role of this tract was completely taken over by the corticospinal tract.

Cerebellum

The primary function of the cerebellum is regulation of movement, postural control, and muscle tone. Although all of the mechanisms of cerebellar function are not clearly understood, lesions have been noted to produce typical patterns of impaired motor function and balance and decreased muscle tone (see the "Cerebellar Pathology" section).

Several theories of function of the cerebellum in motor activity have been established. Among the more widely held is that the cerebellum functions as a *comparator* and *error-correcting mechanism.*[29,34] The cerebellum compares the commands for the *intended* movement transmitted from the motor cortex with the *actual* motor performance of the body segment. This occurs by a comparison of information received from the cortex with that obtained from peripheral feedback mechanisms (termed *feedforward control*). The motor cortex and brain stem motor structures provide the commands for the intended motor response (internal feedback).[34] Peripheral feedback during the motor response is provided by muscle spindles, Golgi tendon organs, joint and cutaneous receptors, the vestibular apparatus, and the eyes and ears (external feedback). This feedback provides continual input regarding posture and balance as well as position, rate, rhythm, and force of slow movements of peripheral body segments. If the input from the feedback systems does not compare appropriately (i.e., movements deviate from the intended command), the cerebellum supplies a counteractive influence. This effect is achieved by corrective signals sent to the cortex, which, via motor pathways, modifies or corrects the ongoing movement (e.g., increasing or decreasing the level of activity of specific muscles). The cerebellum also functions to modify cortical commands for subsequent movements.[34]

This CNS analysis of movement information, determination of level of accuracy, and provision for error correction is referred to as a closed-loop system. Schmidt and Lee define this model as "a control system employing feedback, a reference for correctness, a computation of error, and subsequent correction in order to maintain a desired state."[3(p493)] It should be noted that not all movements are controlled by this system. Stereotypical movements (e.g., gait activities) and rapid, short-duration movements, which do not allow sufficient time for feedback to occur, are theorized to be controlled by an open-loop system, defined as "a control system with preprogrammed instructions to a set of effectors; it does not use feedback information and error-detection processes."[3(p497)] In this system, it is believed that control originates centrally from a motor program, which is a memory or preprogrammed pattern of information for coordinated movement. The motor system then follows the established pattern largely independent of feedback or error-detection mechanisms. Motor programs can be called up in their entirety, modified, or reassembled in a new order. They provide the important function of freeing higher executive levels from attending to all aspects of a motor response. See Chapter 10, Strategies to Improve Motor Function, for a more thorough discussion of motor control and motor learning.

Basal Ganglia

The basal ganglia are a group of nuclei located at the base of the cerebral cortex (Fig. 6.2). The three main nuclei of the basal ganglia are the *caudate nucleus,* the *putamen,* and the *globus pallidus.* These nuclei have close anatomical and functional connections with two other subcortical nuclei that are also frequently considered as part of the basal ganglia: the *subthalamic nucleus* and the *substantia nigra.*[28]

Although the influences of the basal ganglia on movement are not understood as clearly as those of the cerebellum, there is evidence that the basal ganglia play an important role in several complex aspects of movement and postural control. These include the initiation and regulation of gross intentional movements, planning and execution of complex motor responses, facilitation of desired motor responses while selectively inhibiting others, and ability to accomplish automatic movements and postural adjustments.[33,35,36] In addition, the basal ganglia play an important role in maintaining normal background muscle tone. This is accomplished by the inhibitory effect of the basal ganglia on both the motor cortex and lower brain stem. The basal ganglia also are believed to influence some aspects of both perceptual and cognitive functions.[36]

The motor portion of the basal ganglia assumes a somatotopic organization. The anatomical positioning of the basal ganglia provides insight into its contribution to motor performance. The areas of the brain associated with movement (primary motor cortex, SMA, PMA, and the somatosensory cortex) form dense projections to the motor portion of the putamen. Output of this pathway forms the *motor circuit* of the basal ganglia, which is directed back to the SMA and the PMA. These two areas and the primary motor cortex are all interconnected, and each has descending projections to the brain stem motor centers and spinal cord. This anatomical arrangement indicates that the influence of the basal ganglia on motor function is indirect and mediated by descending projections from the cortical motor areas.[36,37]

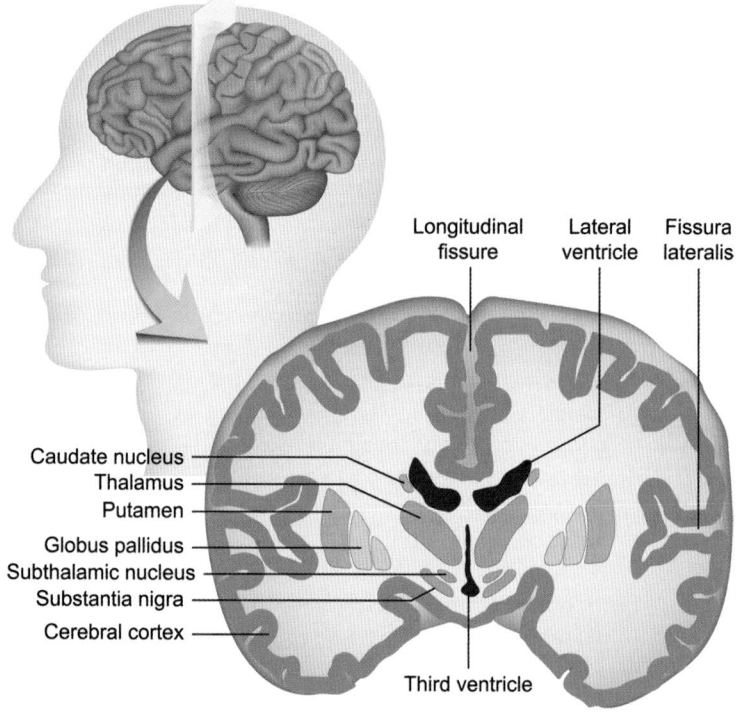

Longitudinal fissure

Lateral ventricle

Fissura lateralis

Caudate nucleus
Thalamus
Putamen
Globus pallidus
Subthalamic nucleus
Substantia nigra
Cerebral cortex

Third ventricle

Figure 6.2 The basal ganglia are composed of nuclei located deep within the cerebral hemispheres. *(Source: Getty/medical stocks/1141370738)*

Dorsal (Posterior) Column–Medial Lemniscal Pathway

Regulation of movement is dependent on sensory afferent information. Peripheral somatosensory receptors and pathways provide information about the status of the environment, the body, and the body in relation to the environment.[3] This information is encoded and conveyed to various parts of the CNS. The data are processed based on peripheral feedback and memory, which leads to selection (or modification) of a movement strategy appropriate to the task demands and environmental conditions.

The dorsal column–medial lemniscal (DCML) pathway is particularly important to coordinated movement, as it is responsible for the afferent transmission of discriminative sensations. Sensory modalities that require fine gradations of intensity and precise localization on the body surface are mediated by this system. Sensations transmitted by the DCML pathway include discriminative touch, stereognosis, tactile pressure, barognosis, graphesthesia, recognition of texture, kinesthesia, two-point discrimination, proprioception, and vibration.

This system is composed of large, myelinated, rapidly conducting fibers. After entering the dorsal column, the fibers ascend to the medulla and synapse with the dorsal column nuclei (nuclei gracilis and cuneatus). From here they cross to the opposite side and pass up to the thalamus through bilateral pathways called the *medial lemnisci*. Each medial lemniscus terminates in the ventral posterolateral thalamus. From the thalamus, third-order neurons project to the somatic sensory cortex.

■ FEATURES OF COORDINATION IMPAIRMENTS

As the cerebellum, basal ganglia, and DCML pathway provide input to, and act together with, the cortex in the production of coordinated movement, lesions in any of these areas affect higher level processing and execution of coordinated motor responses. Although it is incorrect to assign all problems of incoordination to one of these sites, lesions in these areas are responsible for many characteristic motor deficits seen in adult populations. The following sections present an overview of common clinical features associated with lesions in each of these areas.

Cerebellar Pathology

A number of specific motor impairments that affect coordinated movement are associated with cerebellar pathology.[38–42] Examples of conditions associated with cerebellar impairments include stroke, Friedreich ataxia, and MS. Glial neoplasms, including those having an affinity for the posterior fossa such as medulloblastoma and astrocytomas, may result in cerebellar deficits following surgical resection (Fig. 6.3). Many of these impairments either directly or indirectly influence the patient's ability to execute accurate, smooth, controlled movements. The motor deficits identified emphasize the crucial influence of the cerebellum on equilibrium, posture, muscle tone, and initiation and force of movement. *Ataxia* is perhaps the most common term used to describe motor impairments of cerebellar origin. Cerebellar ataxia is a general, comprehensive

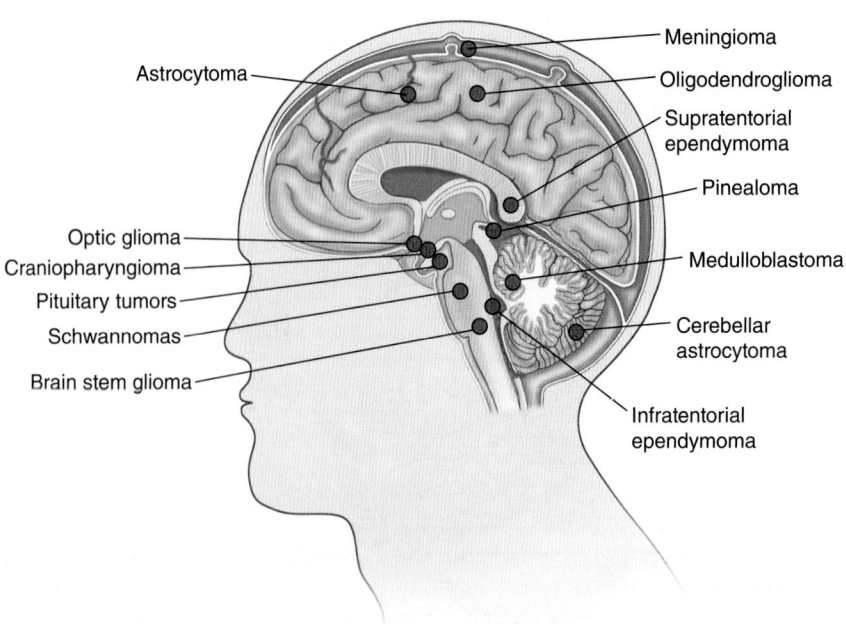

Figure 6.3 Various tumors tend to appear at different locations in the central nervous system. Astrocytoma and medulloblastomas have an affinity for the cerebellum. *(Source: from Hoffman 36-3)*

term used to describe loss of muscle coordination as a result of cerebellar pathology. Ataxia may affect gait, posture, and patterns of movement and is linked to difficulty initiating movement as well as errors in the rate, rhythm, and timing of responses.

Perlman[43] provides an adept summary of the motor impairments associated with each of the major anatomic regions of the cerebellum as follows: "The cerebellum has three anatomic divisions that account for the three types of dysfunction commonly seen: (1) the midline (vermis, paleocerebellum), which underlies titubation, truncal ataxia, orthostatic tremor, and gait imbalance; (2) the hemispheres (neocerebellum—right controlling the right side of the body and left controlling the left side), which contribute to limb ataxia (e.g., dysdiadochokinesia, dysmetria, and kinetic tremor), dysarthria, and hypotonia; and (3) the posterior (flocculonodular lobe, archicerebellum), which also influences posture and gait as well as causing eye movement disorders (e.g., nystagmus, vestibulo-ocular reflex disruption)."[43(p216)] Figure 6.4 illustrates the midline position of the vermis separating the cerebellum into two hemispheres.

The following motor impairments are manifestations of cerebellar pathology:

- *Asthenia* is generalized muscle weakness associated with cerebellar lesions.
- *Dysarthria* is a disorder of the motor component of speech articulation. The characteristics of cerebellar dysarthria are referred to as scanning speech (often described as having a *one-word-at-a-time* quality or words may be broken into separate syllables). This speech pattern is typically slow and may be slurred, hesitant, with prolonged syllables and inappropriate pauses. Word use, selection, and grammar remain intact, but the melodic quality of speech is altered.[34,39,44]
- *Dysdiadochokinesia* is an impaired ability to perform rapid alternating movements. This deficit is observed in movements such as rapid alternation between pronation and supination of the forearm. Movements are irregular, with a rapid loss of range and rhythm especially as speed is increased.[39]
- *Dysmetria* is an inability to judge the distance or range of a movement. It may be manifested by an overestimation (hypermetria) or an underestimation (hypometria) of the required range needed to reach an object or goal.
- *Dyssynergia (movement decomposition)* describes a movement performed in a sequence of component parts rather than as a single, smooth activity. For example, when asked to touch the index finger to the nose, the patient might first flex the elbow, then adjust the position of the wrist and fingers, further flex the elbow, and finally flex the shoulder.
- *Asynergia* is the loss of ability to associate muscles together for complex movements.

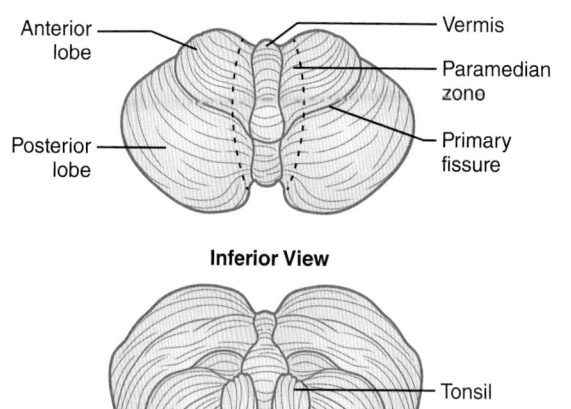

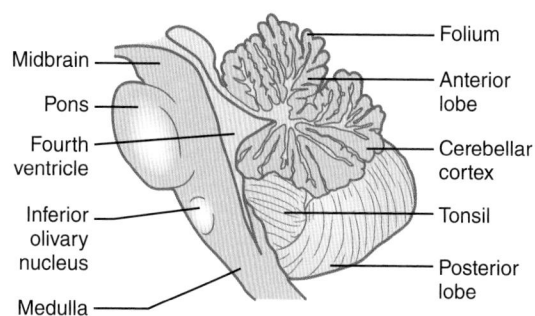

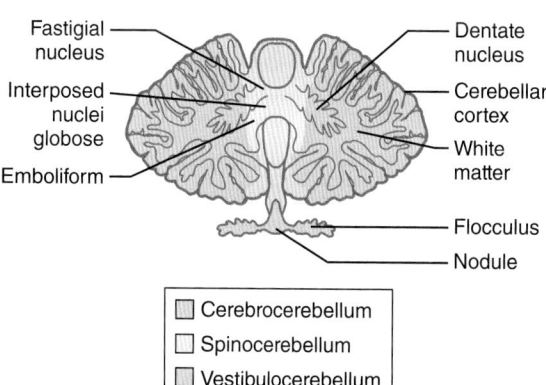

Figure 6.4 The cerebellum lies posterior to the brain stem and fourth ventricle. Lesions affecting the vermis of the cerebellum result in trunk ataxia and gait instability. *(Source: From Fell Fig 21-3)*

- *Gait ataxia* involves ambulatory patterns that typically demonstrate a broad base of support (BOS). Upright stance stability is often poor, and the arms may be held away from the body to improve balance (high-guard position). Stepping patterns are irregular in direction and distance. Initiation of forward progression of an LE may start slowly, and then the extremity may unexpectedly be flung rapidly and forcefully forward and audibly hit the floor.[45] Gait patterns tend to be generally unsteady (postural instability), irregular, and staggering, with deviations from an intended forward line of progression (veering to one side, swaying or pitching in different directions).

- *Hypotonia* is a decrease in muscle tone. It is believed to be related to the disruption of afferent input from stretch receptors and/or lack of the cerebellum's facilitatory efferent influence on the fusimotor system. A diminished resistance to passive movement will be noted, and muscles may feel abnormally soft and flaccid. Diminished deep tendon reflexes also may be noted.[34]

- *Nystagmus* is a rhythmic, quick, oscillatory, back-and-forth movement of the eyes. It is typically apparent as the eyes move away from midline to fix on an object in either the medial or lateral field (i.e., extremes of temporal or nasal vision).[46] The patient has difficulty holding the gaze on the object in the peripheral field. An involuntary drift back to midline with immediate return to the object may be observed. Nystagmus causes difficulty with accurate fixation and vision and is believed to be linked to the cerebellum's influence on synergy and tone of the extraocular muscles.

- *Rebound phenomenon*, originally described by Holmes, is the loss of the check reflex,[45] or check factor, which functions to halt forceful active movements when resistance is eliminated. Normally, when application of resistance to an isometric contraction is suddenly removed, the limb will remain in approximately the same position by action of the opposing muscle(s). For example, in applying resistance to an isometric contraction in the middle range of elbow flexion and then releasing it without warning, the intact subject will "check" or stop the motion quickly through activation of the opposing triceps as well as feedback regarding joint position and force required to prevent further motion. With cerebellar involvement, the patient is unable to stop the motion, and the limb will move suddenly when resistance is released. The patient may strike themselves or other objects when the resistance is removed.

- *Tremor* is an involuntary oscillatory movement resulting from alternate contractions of opposing muscle groups. Different types of tremors are associated with cerebellar lesions. An intention tremor, or kinetic tremor, occurs during voluntary motion of a limb and tends to increase as the limb nears its intended goal or when speed is increased.[34] Intention tremors are diminished or absent at rest. Postural (static) tremor may be evident by back-and-forth

oscillatory movements of the body while the patient maintains a standing posture. Postural tremors also may be observed as up-and-down oscillatory movements of a limb when it is held against gravity. *Titubation* typically refers to rhythmic oscillations of the head (side-to-side or forward-and-backward movements, or the movements may have a rotary component); however, the term is also less frequently used to refer to axial involvement of the trunk.

In addition to these characteristic clinical features of cerebellar involvement, a greater length of time may be required to initiate voluntary movements (delayed reaction time). Difficulty may also be observed in stopping or changing the force, speed, or direction of movement, prolonging movement time.[28] Motor learning will also be affected. Recall that the cerebellum compares the intended movement (internal feedback) with the actual movement (external feedback). For subsequent movements, the cerebellum generates corrective signals to reduce the errors (feedforward control). Lack of this feedforward control is responsible for deficits in motor learning and coordination. Recent evidence suggests cerebellar pathology can also present with cerebellar affective syndrome where patients have executive function and visuospatial deficits.[47]

Basal Ganglia Pathology

Patients with lesions of the basal ganglia typically demonstrate several characteristic motor deficits. These include (1) poverty and slowness of movement; (2) involuntary, extraneous movement; and (3) alterations in posture and muscle tone.[32,37] Thus, patients with basal ganglia involvement present on a continuum of motor behavior from severely diminished as seen in advanced PD to excessive extraneous movements apparent with Huntington disease.[37]

The following motor impairments are manifestations of basal ganglia pathology:

- *Akinesia* is an inability to initiate movement and is seen in the late stages of PD. This deficit is associated with assumption and maintenance of fixed postures (freezing episodes). A tremendous amount of mental concentration and effort is required to perform even the simplest motor activity.

- *Athetosis* is characterized by slow, involuntary, writhing, twisting, "wormlike" movements. Frequently, greater involvement in the distal UEs is noted;[48] this may include fluctuations between hyperextension of the wrist and fingers and a return to a flexed position, combined with rotary movements of the extremities. Many other areas of the body may be involved, including the neck, face, tongue, and trunk. The phenomena are also referred to as *athetoid movements*. Pure athetosis is relatively uncommon and most often presents in combination with spasticity, tonic spasms, or chorea. Athetosis can be a clinical feature of some forms of cerebral palsy.

- *Bradykinesia* is a decreased amplitude and velocity of voluntary movement.[49] It may be demonstrated in a variety of ways, such as a decreased arm swing; slow, shuffling gait; difficulty initiating or changing direction of movement; lack of facial expression; or difficulty stopping a movement once begun. Brady-kinesia is characteristic of PD.
- *Chorea* is characterized by involuntary, rapid, irregular, and jerky movements involving multiple joints. Choreiform movements demonstrate irregular timing, are most apparent in the UEs, and cannot be voluntarily inhibited; it is associated with Huntington disease.[50,51]
- *Choreoathetosis* is a term used to describe a movement disorder with features of both chorea and athetosis.
- *Dystonia* (dystonic movements) involves sustained involuntary contractions of agonist and antagonist muscles,[37,51] causing abnormal posturing (*dystonic posture*) or twisting movements. It is most common in trunk and extremity musculature but also may affect the neck, face, and vocal cords. Torsion spasms also are considered a form of dystonia, with spasmodic torticollis being the most common.[45]
- *Hemiballismus* involves large-amplitude sudden, violent, flailing motions of the arm and leg of one side of the body. Primary involvement is in the axial and proximal musculature of the limb. Hemiballismus results from a lesion of the contralateral subthalamic nucleus.[28,31]
- *Hyperkinesis* is abnormally increased muscle activity or movement; *hypokinesis* is a decreased motor response, especially to a specific stimulus.
- *Rigidity* is an increase in muscle tone causing greater resistance to passive movement. It tends to be more pronounced in the flexor muscles of the trunk and extremities, causing activity limitations in such areas as dressing, transfers, speech, eating, and postural control.[1] Two types of rigidity may be seen: *lead-pipe* and *cogwheel*. Lead-pipe rigidity is a uniform, constant resistance felt by the examiner as the extremity is moved through a range of motion (ROM). Cogwheel rigidity is considered a combination of the lead-pipe type with tremor. It is characterized by a series of brief relaxations or "catches" as the extremity is passively moved.
- *Tremor* is an involuntary, rhythmic, oscillatory movement observed at rest (resting tremor).[52] Resting tremors typically disappear or decrease with purposeful movement but may increase with emotional stress. Tremors associated with basal ganglia lesions (e.g., PD) are frequently noted in the distal UEs in the form of a "pill-rolling" movement, where

it looks as if a pill is being rolled between the first two fingers and the thumb. Motion of the wrist, and pronation and supination of the forearm, may be evident. Tremors also may be apparent at other body parts as well, such as the jaw; this is characteristic of PD. Table 6.1 provides a summary of common coordination impairments associated with pathology of the cerebellum and basal ganglia.

Dorsal (Posterior) Column–Medial Lemniscal Pathology

Coordination impairments associated with DCML lesions are somewhat less characteristic than those produced by either cerebellar or basal ganglia pathology. Lesions of the DCML typically result in coordination and equilibrium impairments related to the patient's lack of joint position sense and awareness of movement and impaired localized touch sensation. Recall that this ascending pathway carries the peripheral (external) feedback required for feedforward control. It mediates sensations critical to coordinated movement such as proprioception, kinesthesia, and discriminative touch.

Disturbances of gait are a common finding with DCML pathology. The gait pattern is usually wide based and swaying, with uneven step lengths and excessive lateral displacement. The advancing leg may be lifted too high and then dropped abruptly with an audible impact. Watching the feet during locomotion is typical and indicative of a proprioceptive loss. Another common deficit seen with DCML pathology is dysmetria. As mentioned, this is an impaired ability to judge the required distance or range of movement and may be noted in both the UEs and LEs. It is manifested by the inability to place an extremity accurately or to reach a target object. For example, in attempting to lock a wheelchair brake, the patient may inaccurately judge (overestimate or underestimate) the required movement needed to reach the brake handle. Fine motor skills may also be impaired owing to alterations in discriminative tactile and object recognition abilities.

Because vision can assist in guiding movements and maintaining balance, as well as improve accuracy of discriminative tasks, visual feedback can be an effective mechanism to compensate partially for DCML pathology. Thus, coordination and/or balance problems will be exaggerated when vision is occluded or when the patient's eyes are closed. The inability to maintain standing balance with the feet together when the eyes are closed is termed a positive *Romberg sign* and is usually indicative of proprioceptive loss. Visual guidance will also reduce the manifestations of dysmetria and diminished tactile perception. However, some noticeable slowing of movements may be observed as visually guided motions are generally more accurate when speed of movement is reduced.

Table 6.1	Common Coordination Impairments Associated With Pathology of the Cerebellum and Basal Ganglia
Coordination Impairments	**Associated Pathology**
Cerebellar Pathology	
Asthenia	Generalized muscle weakness
Asynergia	Loss of ability to associate muscles together for complex movements
Delayed reaction time	Increased time required to initiate voluntary movement
Dysarthria	Disorder of the motor component of speech articulation
Dysdiadochokinesia	Impaired ability to perform rapid alternating movements
Dysmetria	Inability to judge the distance or range of a movement
Dyssynergia	Movement performed in a sequence of component parts rather than as a single, smooth activity; decomposition
Gait disorders	Ataxic pattern; broad base of support; postural instability; high-guard position of UEs
Hypotonia	Decrease in muscle tone
Hypermetria	Overestimation of distance or range needed to accomplish a movement
Hypometria	Underestimation of distance or range needed to accomplish a movement
Nystagmus	Rhythmic, quick, oscillatory, back-and-forth movement of the eyes
Rebound phenomenon	Inability to halt forceful movements after resistive stimulus removed; patient unable to stop sudden limb motion
Tremor • Intention (kinetic) • Postural (static)	Involuntary oscillatory movement resulting from alternate contractions of opposing muscle groups Oscillatory movement during voluntary motion; increases as the limb nears target; diminished or absent at rest Exaggerated oscillatory movement of the body in standing posture or of a limb held against gravity
Titubation	Rhythmic oscillations of the head; axial involvement of the trunk
Basal Ganglia Pathology	
Akinesia	Inability to initiate movement; associated with fixed postures
Athetosis	Slow, involuntary, writhing, twisting, "wormlike" movements; frequently greater involvement in distal UEs
Bradykinesia	Decreased amplitude and velocity of voluntary movement
Chorea	Involuntary, rapid, irregular, jerky movements involving multiple joints; most apparent in UEs
Choreoathetosis	Movement disorder with features of both chorea and athetosis
Dystonia (dystonic movements)	Sustained involuntary contractions of agonist and antagonist muscles
Hemiballismus	Large-amplitude sudden, violent, flailing motions of the arm and leg of one side of the body
Hyperkinesis	Abnormally increased muscle activity or movement
Hypokinesis	Decreased motor response especially to a specific stimulus
Rigidity • Lead-pipe • Cogwheel	• Increase in muscle tone causing greater resistance to passive movement; greater in flexor muscles • Uniform, constant resistance as limb is moved • Series of brief relaxations or "catches" as limb is passively moved
Tremor (resting)	Involuntary, rhythmic, oscillatory movement observed at rest

UEs = upper extremities.

■ AGE-RELATED CHANGES AFFECTING COORDINATED MOVEMENT

Alterations in the ability to execute smooth, accurate, controlled motor responses occur with aging. The importance of understanding the basis of these changes is reflected in the large body of literature devoted to examining various aspects of motor performance in older adults.[53–71] This section presents an overview of the most salient age-associated changes affecting coordinated movement. For a more comprehensive perspective on the physiological, neurological, and musculoskeletal changes associated with aging, refer to the work of Guccione, Wong, and Avers[69]; Saxon, Etten, and Perkins[70]; and Robnett, Chop, and Brossoie.[71]

Decreased strength. Diminished strength is a well-documented finding in older adults.[55,60,62,63,72] *Sarcopenia* refers to an age-associated loss of skeletal muscle mass (decreased cross-sectional area) as well as changes in the ability of muscle tissue to regenerate.[65–68] This loss has a direct impact on strength, endurance, mobility, and the ability to perform smooth, controlled motor responses. A combination of factors is believed to contribute to this loss of muscle mass, including nutritional deficiencies, decreased ability to synthesize protein, neurological decline, altered endocrine function, lack of exercise (inactivity), and the presence of a chronic disease (comorbidity). Other contributing factors to decreased strength include a loss of alpha motor neurons (decreased number of functional motor units), loss or atrophy of fast-twitch fibers (most notably type IIb), reduced number and diameter of muscle fibers,[73] diminished oxidative capacity of exercising muscle, and a subsequent reduction in ability to produce torque.[72,74] In general, there is greater loss of strength in antigravity muscles of the back and LEs (e.g., latissimus dorsi, hip extensors, quadriceps) as compared to UEs and greater loss in proximal than in distal muscles.

Slowed reaction time. Older adults typically move more slowly. This is particularly evident for tasks that require both speed and accuracy; speed will decrease to ensure greater accuracy (speed–accuracy trade-off).[75] In general, the time interval between application of a stimulus and initiation of movement is increased.[3] This finding is also linked to degenerative changes in the motor unit. In addition, *premotor reaction time* (time interval between onset of a stimulus and initiation of a response) and *movement time* (time interval between the initiation of movement and the completion of movement) are lengthened with normal aging.[64] Evidence also suggests that greater cognitive resources are required to accomplish a task, especially tasks involving fine motor skills and dual-task performance.[76]

Decreased ROM. Investigations examining subjects from various age groups have found reduced ROM in older adults. Decreases in ROM with advancing age have been found for multiple joints, including the ankle;[77,78] elbow, forearm, shoulder, hip;[72,78] and knee.[78] James and Parker[79] found consistent declines in both active and passive ROM for 10 LE joints in a population of 80 healthy adults older than 70 years of age. Increased joint tightness tends to be most evident toward the end of ROM and may affect the overall skill in performing coordinated movements. Decreased ROM has been linked to biological aging of joint surfaces,[79] degenerative changes in collagen fibers, decreased strength, dietary deficiencies, and sedentary lifestyle.

Postural changes. A straight line projecting through the ear, acromion, greater trochanter, posterior patella, and lateral malleolus represents the lateral view of normal postural alignment. Examples of common postural changes seen with aging include forward head, rounded shoulders (kyphosis), altered lordotic curve (either flattened or exaggerated), and slight increase in hip and knee flexion. The trunk may be held anterior to the hips with a widened BOS. Neurological and musculoskeletal decline (e.g., diminished disk height, decreased strength and ROM), as well as inactivity and prolonged sitting, may contribute to poor postural alignment. The presence of comorbidities (e.g., osteoporosis, arthritis) often exacerbates these postural changes. Of particular importance is the potential loss of ability to fully accomplish preparatory postural adjustments before execution of a movement.

Changes affecting coordinated movement in the older adult may be accentuated further by decreased balance and increased postural sway (oscillating movements of body over feet),[80,81] reduced postural limits of stability (LOS), degenerative joint changes, reduced flexibility, altered sensation (see Chapter 3, Examination of Sensory Function), impaired perception (see Chapter 27, Cognitive and Perceptual Dysfunction), and diminished vision and hearing acuity. Knowledge of these anticipated age-related changes improves the therapist's ability to establish effective communication to optimize patient performance as well as assists with interpretation of test results. The potential presence of these changes has important implications for how the therapist communicates with, and provides directions to, the patient during the coordination examination. Sensitive and accurate communication that enhances the therapeutic interaction is central to the role of the physical therapist. This involves conveying information in a language or context that is meaningful and intelligible to the patient and communicates trust, respect, and compassion.

Changes in skilled motor performance are a predictable aspect of normal aging. However, this information should not negate or undermine the importance of treatment strategies to improve functional performance and quality of life. An important consideration in treatment planning is that the aging neuromuscular system maintains its physiological adaptive response to training stimuli.[82] Physical therapy intervention is highly effective in promoting and sustaining a more successful approach to aging. This is an important consideration as the population ages. It is estimated that by the year 2030, 20% of U.S. residents will be aged 65 years and over, as compared with 13% in 2010 and 9.8% in 1970.[83]

■ COORDINATION TESTS

Coordination tests generally can be divided into two main categories: gross motor movements and fine motor movements. *Gross motor movements* include body posture, balance, and extremity movements involving large muscle groups. Examples of gross motor activities include reaching, crawling, kneeling, standing, walking, and running. *Fine motor movements* involve utilization of small muscle groups that allow skillful, controlled manipulation of objects. Examples of fine motor activities include finger dexterity tasks such as buttoning a shirt, turning pages, typing, and writing.

> **Clinical Note.** During the systems review, examination of ROM, strength, and sensation typically precede the coordination examination because impairments in any of these areas may influence the ability to produce smooth, accurate, controlled motor responses. However, it is also important to note that coordination impairments may occur in the presence of normal ROM, strength, and intact sensation. As with all examination procedures, knowledge of the patient's cognition, language, and communication ability is prerequisite.

Coordination tests focus on movement capabilities in the following key areas:

- *Reciprocal motion,* which is the ability to reverse movement between opposing muscle groups
- *Movement composition,* or synergy, which involves movement control achieved by synergistic muscle groups acting together
- *Movement accuracy,* which is the ability to gauge or judge distance and speed of voluntary movement
- *Fixation or limb holding,* which addresses the ability to hold the position of an individual limb or limb segment

Coordination and balance (discussed in the following section) tests address capabilities in four basic areas of functional task requirements: transitional mobility, stability (static postural control), dynamic postural control (controlled mobility), and skill. See Chapter 5, Examination of Motor Function: Motor Control and Motor Learning, and Table 5.10, Measures of Motor Performance.

Coordination tests are ordered based on increasing challenge to the patient and typically utilize the following sequence: (1) unilateral tasks, (2) bilateral symmetrical tasks, (3) bilateral asymmetrical tasks, and (4) multilimb tasks (these constitute the highest level of difficulty).

■ ADMINISTERING THE COORDINATION EXAMINATION

Before initiating the coordination examination, the testing environment should be identified and prepared, needed equipment gathered, and patient considerations addressed. Preliminary patient observation will provide valuable insight into motor function and inform test selection.

Preparation
Testing Environment/Equipment

The coordination examination should be administered in a quiet, well-lit treatment area. Ideally, the room should be equipped with two standard chairs and a mat or treatment table. A watch or timer (for timed components of the examination) as well as a method of occluding vision should be available.

Patient Considerations

The coordination examination should be administered when the patient is well rested. A full explanation of the purpose of the testing should be provided. Each coordination test is described and demonstrated individually by the therapist before actual testing. Such demonstrations should be attended to carefully, as lack of clarity will negatively affect motor responses. Because testing procedures require mental concentration and some physical activity, fatigue, apprehension, or fear may adversely influence test results.

Preliminary Observation

Observation is an essential skill in clinical decision-making. Accurate and careful patient observation provides a rich source of preliminary information before performing a coordination examination. Depending on the practice environment, the patient might be observed performing any number of functional activities. In an outpatient setting, the patient may be observed walking to a treatment area, unbuttoning and removing an outer garment, maintaining a standing position, moving from standing to sitting, maintaining a sitting posture, and signing related forms. In an inpatient setting, observation may also include bed mobility, self-care activities, transfers, handling of eating utensils, and assuming the standing position. Use of appropriate patient guarding techniques is indicated during observations. Careful observation will provide insight into areas of impairment and provide the following general information:

- Overall level of skill in each activity and amount of assistance or assistive devices required
- Occurrence of extraneous limb movements, oscillations; specific extremities involved
- Postural sway or unsteadiness
- Distribution: proximal and/or distal musculature, unilateral or bilateral
- Situations or occurrences that alter (increase or decrease) impairments
- Amount of time required to perform an activity
- Level of safety, fall risk

Examination

Guided by information from the preliminary observation of functional activities, tests should be selected to address the required movement capabilities of interest for the individual patient.

Table 6.2 presents sample coordination tests performed in sitting and supine positions. Although multiple tests are presented, a single test is often appropriate to examine several different movement capabilities simultaneously to conserve time. For example, the finger-to-nose test can be used to examine reciprocal motion, movement composition, as well as the presence of intention tremor. The tests presented are intended as examples and are not all inclusive. Other activities may be developed that are equally effective in examining a particular impairment

Table 6.2 Coordination Tests*	
Coordination Tests	Description
1. Finger-to-nose	The shoulder is abducted to 90° with the elbow extended. The patient is asked to bring the tip of the index finger to the tip of their nose. Alterations may be made in the initial starting position to observe performance from different planes of motion.
2. Finger-to-therapist's finger	The patient and therapist sit opposite each other. The therapist's index finger is held in front of the patient. The patient is asked to touch the tip of their index finger to the therapist's index finger. The position of the therapist's finger may be altered during testing to observe ability to change distance, direction, and force of movement.
3. Finger-to-finger	Both shoulders are abducted to 90° with the elbows extended. The patient is asked to bring both hands toward the midline and approximate the index fingers from opposing hands.
4. Alternate nose-to-finger	The patient alternately touches the tip of their nose and the tip of the therapist's finger with the index finger. The position of the therapist's finger may be altered during testing to observe the ability to change distance, direction, and force of movement.
5. Finger opposition	The patient touches the tip of the thumb to the tip of each finger in sequence. Speed may be gradually increased.
6. Mass grasp	An alternation is made between opening and closing the fist (from finger flexion to full extension). Speed may be gradually increased.
7. Pronation/supination	With elbows flexed to 90° and held close to the body, the patient alternately turns the palms up and down. This test also may be performed with shoulders flexed to 90° and elbows extended. Speed may be gradually increased. The ability to reverse movements between opposing muscle groups can be examined at many joints. Examples include active alternation between flexion and extension of the knee, ankle, elbow, or fingers.
8. Rebound test	The patient is positioned with the elbow flexed. The therapist applies sufficient manual resistance to produce an isometric contraction of biceps. Resistance is suddenly released. Normally, the opposing muscle group (triceps) will contract and "check" movement of the limb. Many other muscle groups can be tested for this phenomenon, such as the shoulder abductors or flexors and the elbow extensors.
9. Tapping (hand)	With the elbow flexed and the forearm pronated, the patient is asked to "tap" the hand on the knee.
10. Tapping (foot)	The patient is asked to "tap" the ball of one foot on the floor without raising the knee; heel maintains contact with floor.

(Continued)

Table 6.2	Coordination Tests*—cont'd
Coordination Tests	**Description**
11. Pointing and past pointing	The patient and therapist are opposite each other. Both patient and therapist bring shoulders to 90° of flexion with elbows extended and index fingers of both hands extended. The therapist's and patient's index fingers are lightly touching. The patient is asked to fully flex the shoulder (fingers will be pointing toward ceiling) and then return to the horizontal position and "point" (lightly touch) the therapist's index finger (target) (see Fig. 6.5). A normal response consists of an accurate return to the starting position. In an abnormal response, there is typically a "past pointing" or movement beyond the target. Several variations to this test include movements in other directions such as toward 90° of shoulder abduction or toward 0° of shoulder flexion (finger will point toward floor). After each movement, the patient is asked to return to the initial horizontal starting position and "point" to the target.
12. Alternate heel-to-knee; heel-to-toe	From a supine position, the patient is asked to touch the knee and big toe alternately with the heel of the opposite extremity.
13. Toe-to-examiner's finger	From a supine position, the patient is instructed to touch the great toe to the examiner's finger. The position of the finger may be altered during testing to observe the ability to change distance, direction, and force of movement (to stabilize lower back, the opposite hip and knee may be flexed).
14. Heel-on-shin	From a supine position, the heel of one foot is slid up and down the shin of the opposite LE.
15. Drawing a circle	The patient draws an imaginary circle in the air with either UE or LE (a table or the floor also may be used). This also may be done using a figure-eight pattern. This test may be performed in the supine position for the LE.
16. Fixation or position holding	UE: The patient holds arms horizontally in front (sitting or standing). LE: The patient is asked to hold the knee in an extended position (sitting).

*Tests should be performed first with eyes open and then with eyes closed. Abnormal responses include a gradual deviation from the "holding" position and/or a diminished quality of response with vision occluded. Unless otherwise indicated, tests are performed with the patient in a sitting position.
LE = Lower extremity; UE = upper extremity.

and may be more appropriate for an individual patient; one such example is shown in Figure 6.5. As noted, performance in any variety of functional skills (e.g., ADL, wheelchair skills, transfers, locomotion) is also an effective means of examining many aspects of movement capabilities. Table 6.3 includes selected impairments and suggested tests appropriate for the clinical problem.

Attention should be directed to carefully guarding the patient during testing. During testing, the following questions can be used to help direct the therapist's observations:

- Is there an observed tremor at rest or with movement?
- Are movements direct, precise, and easily reversed?
- Do movements occur within a reasonable or normal amount of time?
- Does increased speed of performance affect quality of motor activity (speed–accuracy trade-off)?
- Can continuous and appropriate motor adjustments be made if speed and direction are changed?

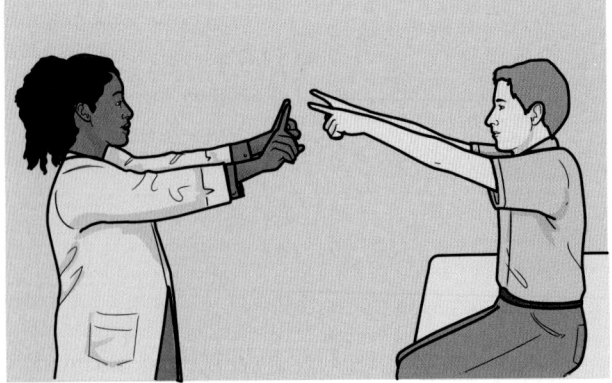

Figure 6.5 Coordination test for pointing and past pointing. From bilateral shoulder flexion, the subject (left) is returning to the start position to "point" (lightly touch) the examiner's index fingers (target). Both arms should be tested, either separately or simultaneously. The test can be performed either sitting or standing.

Table 6.3	Sample Tests for Selected Coordination Impairments
Impairment	**Suggested Tests**
Dysdiadochokinesia	Finger-to-nose Alternate nose-to-finger Pronation/supination Knee flexion/extension Walking, alter speed or direction
Dysmetria	Pointing and past pointing Drawing a circle or figure eight Heel on shin Placing feet on floor markers; sitting, standing
Dyssynergia	Finger-to-nose Finger-to-therapist's finger Alternate heel-to-knee Toe-to-examiner's finger
Hypotonia	Passive movement Deep tendon reflexes
Tremor (intention)	Observation during functional activities (tremor will typically increase as target is approached or movement speed is increased) Alternate nose-to-finger Finger-to-finger Finger-to-therapist's finger Toe-to-examiner's finger
Tremor (resting)	Observation of patient at rest; limb or jaw movements Observation during functional activities (tremor will diminish significantly or disappear with movement)
Tremor (postural)	Observation of steadiness of normal posture; sitting, standing
Asthenia	Fixation or position holding (upper and lower extremity) Application of manual resistance to determine ability to hold
Rigidity	Passive movement Observation during functional activities Observation of resting posture(s)
Bradykinesia	Walking, observation of arm swing and trunk motions Walking, alter speed and direction Request that a movement or gait activity be stopped abruptly Observation of functional activities: timed tests

Table 6.3	Sample Tests for Selected Coordination Impairments—cont'd
Impairment	**Suggested Tests**
Disturbances of posture	Fixation or position holding (upper and lower extremity) Displace balance unexpectedly in sitting or standing (perturbation) Standing, alter base of support (e.g., one foot directly in front of the other; standing on one foot)
Disturbances of gait	Walk along a straight line Walk sideways, backward March in place Alter speed and direction of ambulatory activities Walk in a circle

- Can a position or posture of the body or specific extremity be maintained without swaying, oscillations, or extraneous movements?
- Are placing movements of both UEs and LEs accurate?
- Does occluding vision alter the quality of motor activity?
- Is there greater involvement proximally or distally?
- Is there greater involvement on one side of the body versus the other?
- Does the patient fatigue rapidly?
- Is there a consistency of motor response over time?

Documentation

Approaches to documentation of examination data vary among institutions and individual therapists. The format for recording also varies among electronic software programs. Within the section on motor function, some programs include entries for coordination and dexterity and/or hand function. Others include checkbox options for specific coordination impairments based on body segment location, while others provide sections for narrative descriptions of motor function. Alternatively, an observational examination form can be used to record findings and subsequently scanned into the electronic health record.

Observational examination forms are useful in providing a composite picture of coordination impairments. These forms are often developed within clinical settings and address patient populations unique to the facility, such as those with brain injuries. They can include a rating scale in which level of performance is weighted using a numeric scale with descriptors for each score. A comments section allows for additional narrative descriptions of patient performance. For example, a coordination deficit such as dysmetria or dysdiadochokinesia may be noted as a positive (+) observed finding together with the side (left or right), location, and activity during which it occurred (e.g., + left UE dysmetria observed during finger-to-nose test). In general, these forms are *not standardized* and *lack reliability testing*. However, they provide a systematic method of data collection and documentation. In addition, use of the same form for periodic reexamination facilitates ease of comparison of changes over time.

Measuring the length of time required to complete a motor or functional task provides an important quantitative measure of movement capability. Because accomplishing an activity in a reasonable amount of time is an important criterion of performance, the length of time required to accomplish certain tasks has important implications for both function and safety. For example, assume a patient with a spinal cord injury who uses a wheelchair plans to return to school but requires 2.5 hours to complete dressing activities. The time element here would not be considered functional, especially if attempting to make an early morning class. Consider also an ambulatory patient with an ataxic gait unable to cross a street in the allotted time provided by the traffic signal. This time requirement presents a considerable patient safety issue and, as such, would also not be considered functional. Standardized timed gait measurements may be considered as a measure of functional performance.[84] To track progress of a patient with a degenerative condition (e.g., MS), the International Cooperative Ataxia Rating Scale (ICARS) or Scale for the Assessment and Rating of Ataxia (SARA) can provide increased detail for symptom grading.[85] Although they require more time to administer, these tools can track important changes in cerebellar function (e.g., response to medication).

Periodic video recording of patient performance can be used effectively to document coordination impairments and monitor progress over time. For some patients, such recordings can provide the basis for self-analysis and generating suggestions about altering movement strategies to improve function and direct attention to safety precautions. Viewed in sequence over time, the visual record can also improve patient motivation to attain further gains.

■ OUTCOME MEASURES: UPPER EXTREMITY COORDINATION

Standardized outcome measures are available to examine arm–hand and eye–hand coordination, as well as fine motor dexterity of the fingers, through use of function-based tasks or activities. Scoring is frequently based on time required for task completion and on quality of performance. Many of these measures include normative data to assist with interpretation of test results.

The examining therapist should be knowledgeable about testing guidelines and interpretation of results. Adherence to the prescribed method of administration is particularly important. Any deviations from the established protocol will affect the validity and reliability of the measures and subsequently make comparisons with published norms invalid. Importantly, standardized tests provide objective measures of patient progress over time.

Table 6.4[86–111] includes examples of outcome measures designed to examine arm, hand, and finger coordination. Additional examples are visually depicted in Box 6.1.[112–121] Many other standardized and commercially distributed tests are available. Selection of outcome measures should be based on the strength of available data addressing *reliability* (e.g., test–retest, intrarater, and interrater), *validity* (concurrent, criterion related, and predictive), and *sensitivity to change* (responsiveness, minimally detectable change [MDC], and minimal clinically important difference [MCID]). Additional considerations in selection include the availability of normative data, the type of impairments the instrument was designed to measure, and the intended population (general application or diagnosis specific).

Table 6.4	Outcome Measures: Arm, Hand, and Finger Coordination		
OM and ICF Category	**Description**	**Scoring**	**MDC; MCID**
OM: BBT[86–93] **ICF:** 1	Examines manual dexterity. A rectangular box with a central divider creates two compartments. One compartment contains 150 colored wooden blocks. As many blocks as possible are moved, one at a time, from one compartment to the other in 60 seconds.	Blocks transferred are counted. Higher scores indicate better manual dexterity. Normative values are available based on sex and age.[90]	For a 2-week training program, MDC = 4 blocks per minute; 6-month follow-up MDC = 6 blocks per minute (patients with chronic stroke, n = 17).[93] MDC: 5.5 blocks per minute (change: 18%) (patients with acute and chronic stroke, n = 62).[87]

Table 6.4	Outcome Measures: Arm, Hand, and Finger Coordination—cont'd		
OM and ICF Category	**Description**	**Scoring**	**MDC; MCID**
OM: WMFT[94-99] **ICF:** 1	Examines UE motor ability using 15 function-based tasks and two strength items.	Scores based on performance time (WMFT-TIME) and WMFT-FAS using a 6-point ordinal scale (0 = does not attempt with the involved arm, to 5 = arm does participate; movement appears to be normal). Maximum time to complete an item is 120 seconds. Maximum score is 75. Normative data are available based on age.[98]	MDC[95]: 0.7 second (average WMFT) MDC[95]: 0.1 points (average for WMFT-FAS) (patients with hemiplegia, n = 96)[94] MDC[90]: 4.36 seconds for WMFT MDC[90]: 0.37 points for WMFT-FAS MCID: 1.5–2 seconds for WMFT MCID: 0.2–0.4 points for WMFT-FAS (patients with stroke, n = 57)[95]
OM: ARAT[97,100-105] **ICF:** 1	Examines UE function using a 19-item measure divided into four subscales: grasp, grip, pinch, and gross arm movement.	Scores are based on a 4-point ordinal scale (0 = can perform no part of test to 3 = performs test normally).	MCID: 5.7 points (10% of total range of the scale) (patients with chronic stroke, n = 20)[104]
OM: 9HPT[87,100,106-108] **ICF:** 1, 2	Measure of finger dexterity. One at a time, pegs are moved from a container and placed, as quickly as possible, into holes on a board. Pegs are then individually removed from holes and returned to container.	Score based on time (seconds) required to complete the task. Alternatively, the number of pegs placed within 50 or 100 seconds is counted and recorded as pegs placed per second. Normative values are available.[107]	MDC: 32.8 sec (change: 54%) (patients with acute and chronic stroke, n = 62)[87] MDC: 2.6 seconds (dominant hand) MDC: 1.3 seconds (nondominant hand) (patients with PD, n = 262)[106] Minimum detectable change of 2.6 seconds for the dominant hand and 1.3 seconds for the nondominant hand Minimum detectable change of 2.6 seconds for the dominant hand and 1.3 seconds for the nondominant hand
OM: SHFT[109-111] **ICF:** 1, 2, 3	Examines hand grips while performing 20 tasks using common items encountered in ADL (e.g., coins, buttons, pen, cup, screwdriver, telephone) within 60 seconds.	Performance is timed; scored on a 5-point scale from 0 = task cannot be performed at all to 4 = task is completed without any difficulty within 20 seconds and the prescribed hand-grip of normal quality. The 20 subtest task scores are added for a total maximum score of 80.	MDC: 6.7–6.9 (patients with hand burns, n = 21)[110]

ICF CATEGORY: 1 = Body structure/function; 2 = Activity; 3 = Participation.

ADL = Activities of daily living; ARAT = Action Research Arm Test; BBT = Box and Blocks Test; ICF = International Classification of Functioning, Disability and Health; OM = outcome measure; MCD = minimally detectable change; MCID = minimal clinically important difference; 9HPT = Nine Hole Peg Test; PD = Parkinson disease; SHFT = Sollerman Hand Function Test; WMFT = Wolf Motor Function Test; WMFT-FAS = Wolf Motor Function Test Functional Ability Scale; UE = upper extremity.

Box 6.1 Examples of Outcome Measures: Upper Extremity Coordination

The *Jebsen-Taylor Hand Function Test* (Fig. A) examines hand and finger coordination using seven subtests of functional skills (e.g., writing, card turning, picking up small objects, simulated eating, stacking). Scored on time required to complete task. Normative data are available based on age, sex, maximum time, and hand dominance.[106,112–114] (*Courtesy of Sammons Preston Rolyan, Bolingbrook, IL 60440-3593.*)

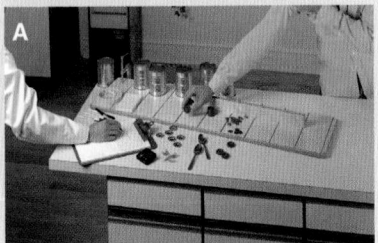

Minnesota Manual Dexterity Test (Fig. B) consists of two operations, *placing* and *turning,* and requires use of a board with wells and round disks. After a practice trial, scores are based on the time required to complete each of four trials for each operation. Normative data are available. An expanded variation of this test is the Minnesota Rate of Manipulation Test, which includes five operations: placing, turning, displacing, one-hand turning and placing, and two-hand turning and placing.[115–117]

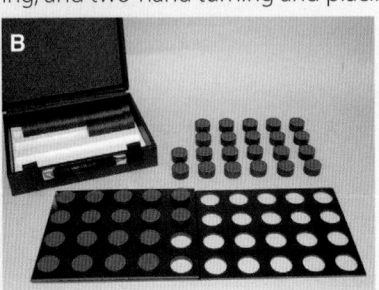

The *Purdue Pegboard Test* (Fig. C) examines coordination of the arm/hand/fingers by placement of pins, collars, and/or washes on a pegboard. There are several categories of subtests, including right-hand prehension, left-hand prehension, prehension test with both hands, and assembly. Scores are based on the number of assemblies completed within either a 30- or 60-sec period. Normative values are available.[118–121]

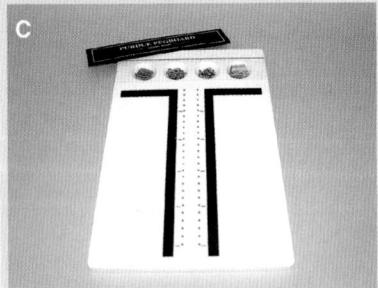

The *O'Connor Tweezer Test* (Fig. D, *left*) and the *Finger Dexterity Test* (Fig. D, *right*) examine the ability to rapidly manipulate small objects. The Tweezer Test emphasizes eye–hand and fine motor dexterity using tweezers to place a single pin in each 1/16th-inch-diameter hole. The Finger Dexterity Test also addresses fine motor dexterity through manual placement of three pins per hole. Scoring is based on time required to complete task.

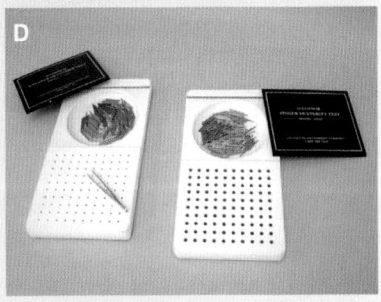

The *Hand Tool Dexterity Test* (Fig. E) utilizes ordinary tools to examine coordinated movement of arm/hand/fingers during a functional task. The test frame consists of a flat board to which two side uprights are attached. The test requires disassembly of the nuts and bolts on one upright using the appropriate tools and reassembling them on the opposite upright. The test is timed, and normative data are available. (*Courtesy of Lafayette Instrument Co., Lafayette, IN 47903.*)

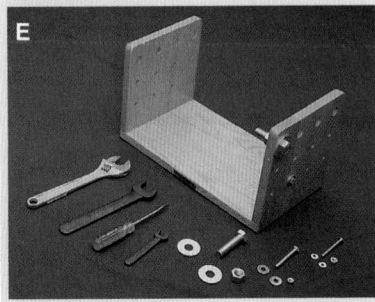

The *Roeder Manipulative Aptitude Test* (Fig. F) examines arm/hand/finger coordination as well as eye–hand coordination. Test materials consist of a high-density plastic board with four wells for washers, rods, caps, and nuts; a T-bar for placement of washer–nut assemblies; and rows of sockets for installing nuts. The test includes four timed operations: dominant hand rod–cap assembly and T-bar washer–nut assembly using both hands, right hand, and left hand. Normative data are available. (*Courtesy of Lafayette Instrument Co., Lafayette, IN 47903.*)

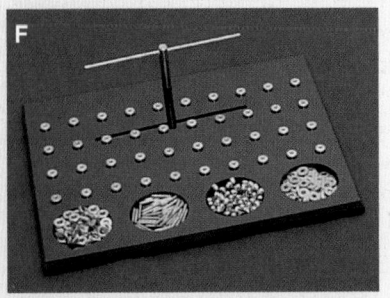

■ OVERVIEW OF POSTURAL CONTROL AND BALANCE

Postural control involves maintained orientation of the relative positions of body parts with respect to each other and gravity. Balance is the condition in which all the forces acting on the body are balanced such that the *center of mass* (COM) is within the stability limits, the boundaries of the BOS. The overall goals of the postural control system, stability and function, are achieved through integrated CNS systems of control. *Reactive postural control* occurs in response to external forces acting on the body (e.g., perturbations) displacing the COM or moving the BOS (e.g., moveable platform, therapy ball). Feedback systems provide the sensory inputs required to initiate corrective responses. *Proactive (anticipatory) postural control* occurs in anticipation of internally generated, destabilizing forces imposed on the body's own movements (e.g., catching a weighted ball). An individual's prior experiences allow the various elements of the postural control system to be pretuned or readied for upcoming movements using feedforward mechanisms. Postural requirements vary depending on the characteristics of the task and the environment. *Adaptive postural control* allows the individual to modify postural responses to changing task and environmental demands. Balance emerges from a complex interaction of (1) sensory systems responsible for the detection of body position and motion, (2) motor systems responsible for organization and execution of motor synergies, and (3) higher level CNS processes responsible for integration and action plans. An examination of balance must therefore focus on each of these three areas.

Postural Alignment and Weight Distribution

Normal postural alignment in standing can be examined by observing skeletal alignment using a plumb line (or posture grid). More sophisticated analysis can be achieved using motion analysis systems with light-emitting signals, photography, and electromyography. In standing, the COM occurs at a point about two-thirds of the body height above the BOS. Static posture in standing is examined by positioning the patient with the feet apart, normal stance width. When viewed from the side (sagittal plane alignment), the plumb line is positioned just in front of the lateral malleolus. The vertical *line of gravity* is expected to fall close to most joint axes: slightly anterior to the ankle and knee joints, at or slightly posterior to the hip joint, through the midline of the trunk, just anterior to the shoulder joint, and through the external auditory meatus (Fig. 6.6).

Natural spinal curves are present but flattened in upright stance, depending on the level of postural tone, lumbar and cervical lordosis, and thoracic or dorsal kyphosis. The pelvis is held in neutral position, with no anterior or posterior tilt. When viewed from the front

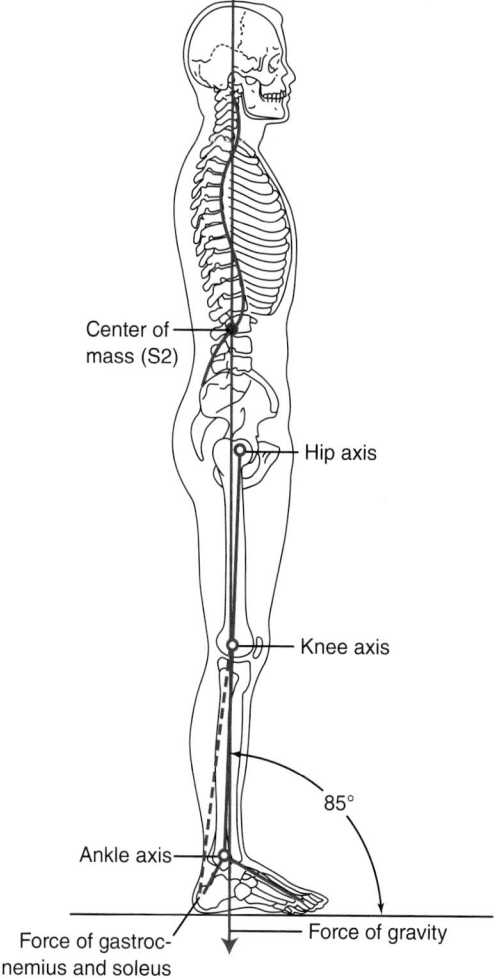

Figure 6.6 Normal postural standing alignment in the sagittal plane. In optimal alignment, the line of gravity passes through the identified anatomical structures.

or back (frontal plane analysis), the feet are positioned equidistant from the plumb line. The examiner looks for equal weight distribution between feet and symmetry of the trunk and extremities. Normal alignment minimizes the need for active muscle contraction during standing. Muscles that are tonically active at low levels during quiet stance include tibialis anterior and gastrocnemius-soleus; tensor fascia latae, gluteus medius, and iliopsoas; and abdominals and erector spinae.[122]

In sitting when viewed from the side, head and trunk are vertical. Natural spinal curves are present, and the pelvis is maintained in a neutral position (Fig. 6.7). When viewed from the front or back, the trunk and head are held in a midline orientation with symmetrical weight-bearing on both LEs (buttocks, thighs, and feet).[122]

LOS is defined as the maximum distance an individual is able or willing to lean in any direction without loss of balance or changing the BOS. Thus, in standing, an individual can shift forward and backward or side to side without losing balance or taking a step.

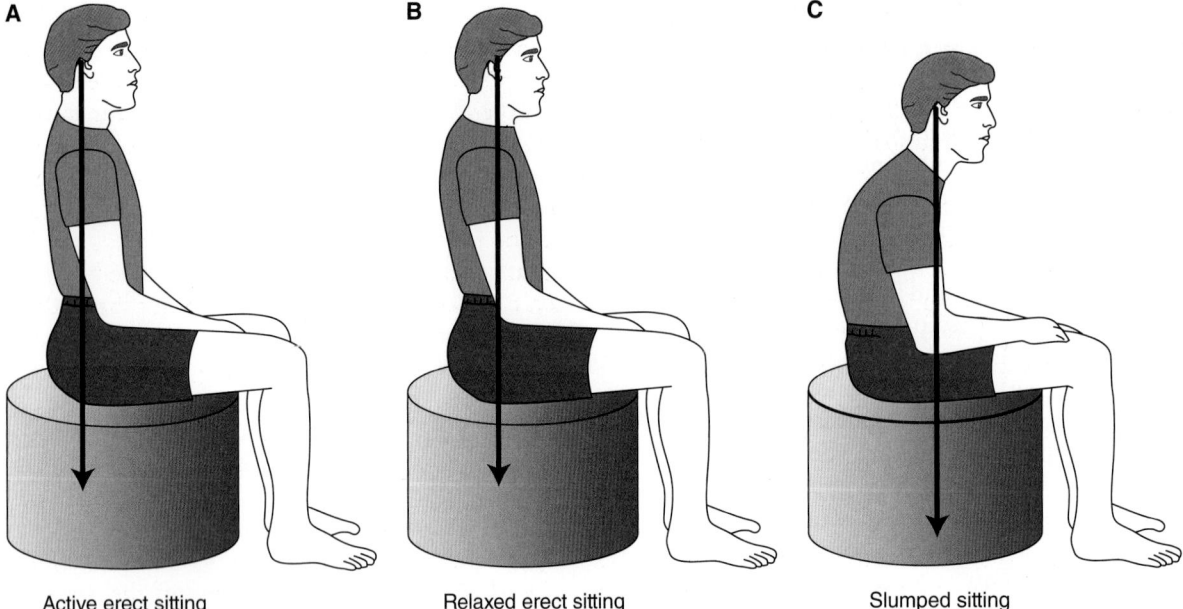

Active erect sitting   Relaxed erect sitting   Slumped sitting

Figure 6.7 Normal sagittal plane postural alignment in sitting: (A) In optimal alignment, the line of gravity passes close to the axes of rotation of the head and neck, and trunk. (B) During relaxed sitting, the line of gravity changes very little, remaining close to those axes. (C) During slumped sitting, the line of gravity is well forward of the spine and hips. *(From Bezkor EW, O'Sullivan SB, Schmitz TJ.* Improving Functional Outcomes in Physical Rehabilitation. *3rd ed. FA Davis; 2022.)*

LOS is influenced by a number of factors, including individual characteristics such as height and foot length for anterior–posterior (AP) LOS and distance between the feet and height for medial–lateral (ML) LOS.[123] Both COM position and movement (velocity and displacement) influence LOS.[124] The midpoint of LOS is termed the *COM alignment. Steadiness* refers to the ability to maintain a given posture with minimum movement (sway).[125] During standing, an individual normally exhibits small range postural shifts (*postural sway*), cycling intermittently from side to side and from heel to toe. *Sway envelope* refers to the path of the body's movement during standing. During walking, there are minimal COM movements up and down and side to side, resulting in a smooth sinusoidal curve. In sitting, the BOS is larger and COM lower (just above the support base), resulting in greater LOS.

Examination of Postural Alignment

Postural alignment and sway can be examined using visual inspection with the patient standing against a postural grid.[126] More sophisticated instrumentation, dynamic posturography, utilizes force plates to measure and quantify ground reaction forces, either center of force (COF) measures or center of pressure (COP) measures. COF is calculated using only vertical forces, and COP is calculated using both vertical and horizontal shear forces. The weight of each foot is determined, forces are calculated, and this information is converted into a visual image (Fig. 6.8). Software analysis provides

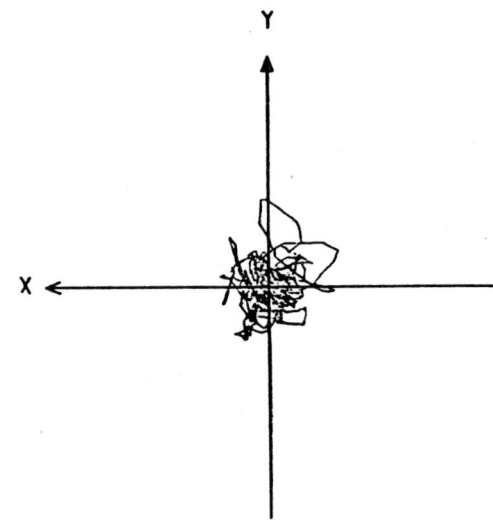

Figure 6.8 Postural sway. Recording of the movement of the center of pressure for 60 seconds in a subject standing on a balance platform. Values: mean amplitude of sway path in inches = 0.13 × 0.15; length of path = 32.2; and velocity = 0.45 in./sec. *(From Smith L, et al.* Brunnstrom's Clinical Kinesiology. *5th ed. FA Davis; 1996:406, with permission.)*

data on initial stance position (center of alignment), mean sway path, total sway excursion (LOS), and the zone of stability. These findings are valid and reliable measures of postural control.[127,128]

Using this information, the therapist can objectively determine the patient's postural symmetry, which reflects the amount of weight placed on each foot. Patients with asymmetry may present with the COP positioned away from midline. For example, the patient with stroke typically stands with most of the weight on the less affected limb. Steadiness can be determined by using postural sway measures. A large sway path is evidence of postural unsteadiness. Another example is the patient with ataxia who typically demonstrates hypermetric responses, with excessive sway, uncoordinated movements, and limited postural steadiness. The patient with PD presents with the opposite problem, hypometric responses with diminished sway and excessive stabilization.[129,130] LOSs are determined by asking the patient to actively shift weight in any direction as far as possible without losing balance or taking a step. Patients with deficits in motor control typically have reduced LOS (reduced COP excursion). For example, the patient with stroke demonstrates reduced stability limits to the more affected side. The patient with PD typically demonstrates reduced LOS overall with significant anterior stability limits if a stooped posture is evident. LOS and COM alignment are also typically altered in other pathological states (e.g., muscle weakness, skeletal deformity, and tonal abnormalities). Re-examination after training using force platform biofeedback has been used to document recovery of postural control following stroke.[131,132] It has also been used to demonstrate the effectiveness of training using biofeedback force platform training devices.[125,130,133]

Sensory Strategies for Balance

The sensory systems (vision, somatosensory, and vestibular) provide the CNS with important information about postural control and balance, including information about the results of our own actions and the surrounding environment. The CNS integrates these inputs and initiates both goal-directed, conscious actions and automatic, unconscious adjustments in posture and movements. Each individual sensory system provides unique and important information, and no one system provides all the information needed.

The visual system serves as an important source of information for the ability to perceive movements and detect the relative orientation of body segments and orientation of the body in space. This ability has been termed *visual proprioception*.[134] Two separate functional visual systems have been identified: (1) *focal vision* (also called cognitive or explicit vision) and (2) *ambient vision* (also called sensorimotor or implicit vision). Focal vision plays a major role in localizing features in the environment and in our conscious reaction to visual events. In contrast, ambient vision utilizes the entire visual field to provide information on the localizing features about the environment and to guide movements using largely nonconscious awareness.[3] Thus, each visual system has a unique functional significance. For example, the patient with brain injury who has a condition called *optic ataxia* can recognize an object using focal vision but cannot use visual information to accurately guide the hand to reach and grasp an object in the environment (impaired ambient vision). The opposite occurs in a patient with stroke experiencing *visual agnosia*. The patient cannot recognize common objects or people but can use the ambient visual system to navigate the environment. Vision also contributes to righting reactions of the head, trunk, and limbs (optical righting reactions).

Visual acuity (focal vision) can be examined using a Snellen eye chart. A distance acuity poorer than 20/50 will have a significant effect on postural stability.[135] Whereas focal vision is detected by the central retina only, ambient vision is detected by the entire visual field (central and peripheral vision). Patients with loss of peripheral vision (e.g., a patient with stroke and hemianopsia or a patient with glaucoma) may demonstrate deficits in visual proprioception and functional performance. Peripheral vision can be examined using the *confrontation method*. The patient sits in front of the therapist and is instructed to focus gaze on the therapist's nose. The therapist then slowly brings a target (moving finger or pencil) into the patient's field of view from the right or left side. The patient is instructed to indicate (point or declare) when and where the target is detected. Ambient vision can be examined by instructing the patient to navigate across the busy physical therapy gym. The abilities to navigate safely, localize features in the environment, and anticipate changes necessary to avoid obstacles and successfully reach the target area are determined. Patients with stroke who exhibit *topographical disorientation* will have difficulty navigating their environment and understanding the relationship of one place to another.

Somatosensory inputs include cutaneous and pressure sensations from the body segments in contact with the support surface (e.g., the feet in standing; the buttocks, thighs, and feet in sitting) and muscle and joint proprioception throughout the body. Light touch contact from the hands on a stable surface is also a form of somatosensory input used as a balance aid.[136] This provides information about the relative orientation and movement of the body in relation to the support surface. Cutaneous sensation (touch and pressure) of the feet and ankles and proprioception of the feet and ankles and hips are particularly important in maintaining upright standing balance. Sensory examination of the extremities and trunk is therefore essential (see Chapter 3, Examination of Sensory Function).

The vestibular system is an important source of information for postural control and balance. The semicircular canals (SCCs) detect angular acceleration and deceleration forces acting on the head, whereas the otolith organs detect linear acceleration and orientation of the head with reference to gravity. The SCCs are sensitive to fast (phasic) movements of the head, and the otoliths respond to slow head movements and positional change referenced to gravity. The vestibular system functions to stabilize gaze during head movements via the *vestibulo-ocular reflex,* and to assist in the regulation of postural tone and postural muscle activation via the *vestibulo-spinal reflexes.* Tests for vestibular function include positional and movement testing. The patient is observed for symptoms of vestibular dysfunction (e.g., dizziness, vertigo, nystagmus).[137] See Chapter 21, Vestibular Disorders, for a complete discussion of this topic.

During stance, all sensory inputs contribute to the maintenance of posture. Sensory weighting theory specifies that the CNS weights the various sensory inputs depending on the specific sensory environment and task.[138–141] *Quiet stance* is defined as standing with a stable support surface and surroundings. *Perturbed stance* is defined as standing during a brief displacement of the support surface (moving surface) or displacement of the COM over BOS (perturbation). In intact adults during quiet stance, the CNS places greater weight on somatosensory inputs. During an unexpected perturbation, somatosensory inputs are more quickly activated and provide much of the early restabilizing control, whereas vision and vestibular inputs with slower processing speeds contribute to later components of the postural restabilizing response.[142] If somatosensory inputs are impaired (e.g., peripheral neuropathy) or if somatosensory conflict is introduced (e.g., standing on dense foam), vision assumes a greater role. If both somatosensory and visual inputs are impaired or absent, vestibular inputs are critical to maintaining posture and resolving sensory conflict. CNS use of sensory inputs is flexible. Balance responses are task and context dependent and triggered by CNS weighting based on availability, timing, and accuracy of specific sensory inputs.

Because sensory inputs are redundant, stable balance can be maintained with significant impairment, on unstable surfaces, or in sensory conflict situations. However, if more than one sensory system is deficient, substantial deficiencies in postural control and balance will be evident.[143] For example, the patient with chronic diabetes who has significant diabetic neuropathy (loss of somatosensory inputs from the feet and ankles) and significant diabetic retinopathy (impaired vision) will demonstrate significant postural instability and increased fall risk. In addition, the cognitive system plays an important role in attending to and interpreting the information for CNS planning of effective postural responses. Attentional demands vary depending on the task (new learning versus familiar response) and the environment (open versus closed or dual tasking). Patients with impairments in cognition or attention demonstrate increased fall risk, especially for those activities with high stability demands.

Examination of Sensory Strategies
Romberg Test

The *Romberg test* is one of the oldest tests used to examine sensorimotor control and was developed to diagnose tabes dorsalis, a form of neurosyphilis.[144] During the test, the patient is instructed to stand with feet together (touching each other), eyes open (EO), unaided for 20 to 30 seconds. If the patient demonstrates significant sway or instability with EO, the test is over. The patient is then asked to stand with eyes closed (EC). The test is negative if the patient is stable and well balanced with either EO or EC. The test is positive if the patient is able to stand with EO but demonstrates significant instability (significant postural sway or loss of balance) with EC. During testing, it is important to tell patients you are prepared to catch them in the event of a fall. The patients should not be given any clues to help orient and stabilize posture. A positive Romberg test is indicative of severe loss of proprioception (e.g., *sensory ataxia*) that occurs with posterior column lesions in the spinal cord (e.g., cervical spondylosis, tumor, degenerative spinal cord disease, tabes dorsalis). Patients with mild vestibular or midline cerebellar lesions can usually compensate with the use of vision (EO). With severe lesions, truncal instability and loss of balance occur with EO (e.g., the patient with cerebellar ataxia). In the sharpened Romberg test, the feet are placed in tandem (heel-to-toe position) and the EO to EC conditions imposed. Individuals who are older or obese may have increased difficulty with the sharpened Romberg test. The findings of the Romberg test are qualitative, and as such it has more value as a screening tool than as a definitive test.

Sensory Organization Test

The *Sensory Organization Test* (SOT), originally known as the *Clinical Test of Sensory Interaction in Balance* (CTSIB), is based on the work of Nashner[138,139] and is used to examine the sensory contributions to postural control and balance. It examines body sway during quiet standing under six different sensory test conditions (Fig. 6.9). Dynamic posturography equipment is used to provide a moving platform that introduces mechanical perturbations (sliding or tilting movements). A moving visual surround screen is sway referenced and introduces visual conflict. Both the surround and force plate are referenced to the patient by means of hydraulic mechanisms. Test Condition 1 provides accurate somatosensory, visual, and vestibular information and is the baseline reference. Each of the other five conditions systematically varies sensory inputs, increasing the level of sensory conflict and postural difficulty (Table 6.5).

Conditions 1 to 3 are all performed with the patient standing on a stable support surface, feet shoulder width apart, providing accurate somatosensory inputs. Visual inputs are varied: Condition 1 uses EO (baseline condition), and Condition 2 uses EC. Condition 3 uses a moving visual surround (screen) referenced to body sway, thus providing inaccurate visual information. Conditions 4 through 6 repeat the visual conditions but with an altered support surface (moving platform) that provides inaccurate somatosensory information. In Conditions 5 and 6, maintenance of posture depends

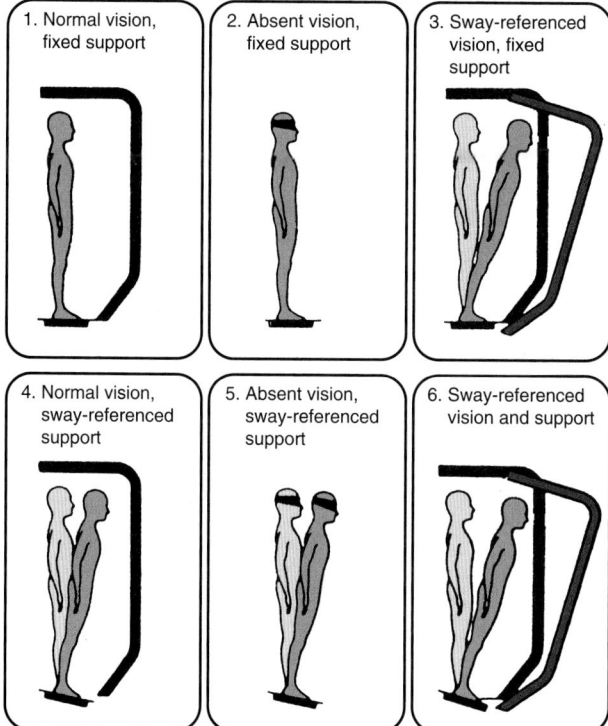

Figure 6.9 The Sensory Organization Test.

Table 6.5	Test Conditions: Sensory Organization Test/Clinical Test of Sensory Interaction and Balance
Test Condition	**Sensory Input**
Condition 1 Eyes Open, Stable Surface (EOSS)	All sensory systems available, unaltered (baseline condition)
Condition 2 Eyes Closed, Stable Surface (ECSS)	Vision absent Somatosensory unaltered Vestibular intact
Condition 3* Visual Conflict, Stable Surface (VCSS)	Vision altered Somatosensory unaltered Vestibular intact
Condition 4 Eyes Open, Moving Surface (EOMS)	Vision unaltered Somatosensory altered Vestibular intact
Condition 5 Eyes Closed, Moving Surface (ECMS)	Vision absent Somatosensory altered Vestibular intact
Condition 6* Visual Conflict, Moving Surface (VCMS)	Vision altered Somatosensory altered Vestibular intact

*Conditions omitted in the modified Clinical Test of Sensory Interaction in Balance.

on availability and accuracy of vestibular inputs with the reduction of both vision and somatosensory inputs. The patient is asked to maintain each position for 20 seconds; three trials are used for each condition.

Dynamic posturography equipment (standing on a forceplate) provides objective measurement of postural sway and COP. Composite equilibrium scores and weighted averages of scores are computed for each of the six conditions. The *Equilibrium Score* (100% maximum) quantifies how well the patient performed during each of the six conditions in terms of sway or postural stability. Ratios comparing one condition to another provide information regarding reliance on one sensory system over another. Center of gravity is computed for its position relative to the center of the BOS. Additional analyses of motor coordination using electromyography (EMG) can be used to provide information about the relative level of individual muscle activity as well as overall muscle recruitment patterns during each of the test positions. As in all testing of postural control and balance, patient safety is an important consideration. During posturography, the patient wears an overhead safety harness to prevent falls. UE support is not allowed during the test. However, the equipment includes handrails that can be used as an additional element of safety. Multiple posturography equipment devices are now available to administer the SOT, including virtual systems.

A shorter modified CTSIB (mCTSIB) is available that uses four of the six original sensory conditions and a static forceplate. Conditions 3 and 6 are omitted (see Table 6.5).[145–147] The patient stands on a stable forceplate for Conditions 1 and 2. Dense foam is used to replicate the compliant forceplate for Conditions 3 and 4 (Figure 6.10). Eyes remain open for Conditions 1 and 3 and are closed for Conditions 2 and 4. Time to administer is less than 10 minutes. Sway velocity is calculated based upon the aggregate balance performance in a final composite score.

Interpreting the Results of the Sensory Organization Test and the Clinical Test of Sensory Interaction in Balance

Interpreting the results of the SOT and CTSIB requires an understanding of how the sensory conditions are manipulated (see Table 6.5). Patients who are visually dependent for postural control will demonstrate instability in Conditions 2, 3, 5, and 6 (EC or visual conflict). Patients who are surface or somatosensory dependent will demonstrate instability in Conditions 4, 5, and 6 (standing on a moving platform [SOT] or foam [CTSIB]). Patients with vestibular dysfunction will demonstrate instability in Conditions 5 and 6 (inability to rely on vision or somatosensory inputs). Patients who demonstrate sensory selection problems and adaptive reweighting deficits present with abnormal findings in Conditions 3 through 6.

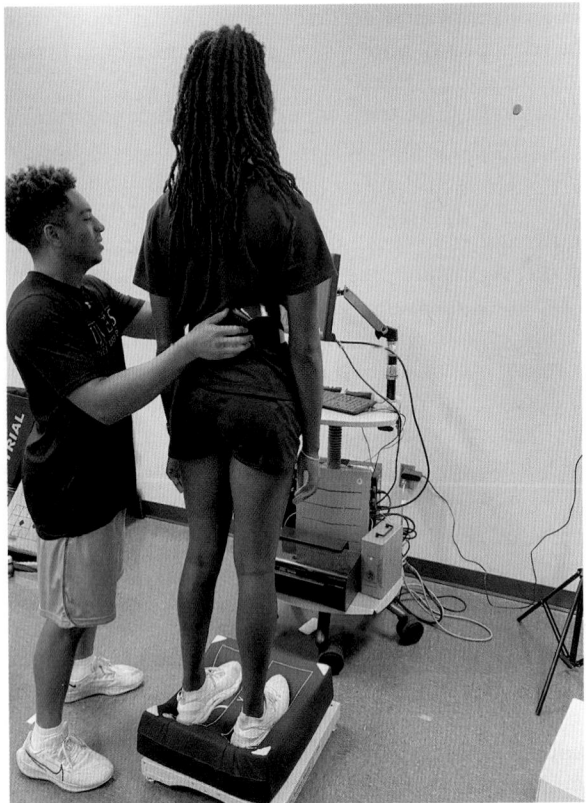

Figure 6.10 The Modified Clinical Test for Sensory Interaction in Balance.

A number of research studies have examined sensory interaction and balance with different populations. For example, studies have investigated the responses of community-dwelling adults with a history of falls[148,149] and patients with stroke,[150,151] Alzheimer disease,[152] PD,[153,154] vestibular dysfunction,[155–157] and TBI.[158]

Motor Strategies for Balance

In observational studies of infants and young children and lesioned animals (decerebration experiments), righting and equilibrium reactions comprise the *postural reflex mechanism*. Automatic *righting reactions* (RRs) orient the head in space (optical RR, labyrinthine RR, body-on-head RR) and the body in relation to the head and support surface (neck-on-body RR, body-on-body RR). *Equilibrium reactions* include tilting reactions and parachute or protective reactions. In normal adults, however, postural adjustments are far more complex and demonstrate a high degree of adaptability in response to both task and environmental context demands. Postural adjustments vary from the simple stretch reflex responses to the activation of specific movement strategies (synergistic patterns). Muscles closest to the BOS are particularly important to the maintenance of balance. As the LOS is reached with a COM disturbance, the magnitude of the postural response is increased.

Fixed Support Strategies

The term *fixed support strategies* refers to those movement strategies used to control the COM over a fixed BOS (in-place strategies). In standing, the *ankle strategy* involves shifting the COM forward and back by moving the body (legs and trunk) as a relatively fixed pendulum about the ankle joints (Fig. 6.10). Muscles are activated in a distal-to-proximal sequence. With forward sway, gastrocnemius is activated first, followed by hamstrings, then paraspinal muscles. With backward sway, the anterior tibialis is activated first, followed by quadriceps, then abdominals. The ankle strategy is commonly used when sway frequencies are low and disturbances of the COM are small and well within the LOS.

The *hip strategy* involves shifts in the COM by flexing or extending at the hips (see Fig. 6.11). It has a proximal pattern of muscle activation before distal activation. With forward sway, abdominals are activated first, followed by quadriceps. With backward sway, paraspinal muscles are activated first, followed by hamstrings. Hip strategies provide primary control for mediolateral stability. Hip muscles (abductors and adductors) are activated to control lateral sway. The hip strategy is typically recruited with faster sway frequencies (greater than 1 Hz) and larger disturbances of the COM or when the support

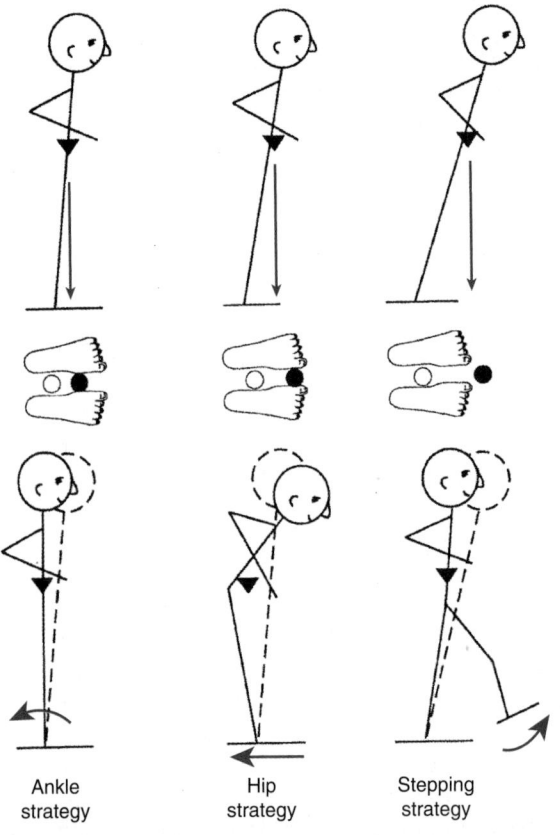

Figure 6.11 Strategies for correcting balance perturbations.

surface is small (less than the size of the feet) or compliant (e.g., standing on foam).[159,160]

Change-in-Support Strategies

Change-in-support strategies are defined as movements of the lower or upper limbs to make a new contact with the support surface. The *stepping strategy* realigns the BOS under the COM by using rapid steps or hops in the direction of the displacing force, for example, forward or backward steps. In instances of lateral destabilization, the individual takes a side step or a cross step to bring the BOS back under the COM. The stepping strategies are typically recruited in response to fast, large postural perturbations when ankle and hip strategies are not adequate to recover balance (e.g., when the COM exceeds the BOS) (see Fig. 6.10). Change-in-support movements of the upper limbs (reach or grasp) can also assist in stabilizing the COM over the BOS and serve as a protective function in absorbing impact and protecting the head in a fall event. *Reaching movements* assist in extending the BOS and stabilizing posture. These reactions were found to be prevalent in destabilization situations, occurring in 85% of trials. Stepping strategies were also frequent, leading researchers to suggest that change-in-support strategies should not be viewed just as strategies of last resort. They are often initiated well before the COM nears or exceeds the LOS, contrary to the traditional view.[160,161]

Studies have examined stepping strategies in older adults. Fallers require a greater number of recovery steps than nonfallers when perturbed through waist-pull or surface translation devices.[162] Young adults can often recover from a perturbation with a single step, whereas older adults must take multiple steps and can have collisions between the swing and support LEs.[162] Lateral step recovery is particularly challenging for older adults. When observing for compensatory stepping responses during the examination, the physical therapist should note both the timing and number of recovery steps during perturbation recovery.

Although these movement strategies have been investigated individually as distinct movement patterns, research has also shown that during normal balance combinations of strategies are used.[159] Control of movement strategies should be viewed on a continuum. The CNS quickly moves between patterns, depending on the control demands of the activity and environment. Thus, a destabilizing force may yield an initial ankle strategy that progresses quickly to a hip strategy as increased control is warranted to recover balance. When the displacement is large and ankle and hip strategies prove inadequate, a stepping strategy may be necessary to prevent a fall.[163] The CNS uses continuous sensory feedback monitoring to achieve flexibility and adaptability of movement strategies for multidirectional postural control.

Strategies in Sitting

In sitting, the BOS is composed of the thighs and buttocks and the feet if in contact with the support surface. Postural strategies in sitting to maintain balance include movement of the trunk about the hips. Backward sway elicits primary responses in hip flexors along with activity of the abdominals and neck flexors. In forward sway, extensor muscles of the hips are activated along with the extensors of the neck and trunk. If the feet are in contact with the floor, the tibialis anterior is recruited during forward reaching movements of the arm, and the gastrocnemius is recruited to brake forward movements and return the body to erect sitting.[164] Somatosensory inputs from backward rotation of the pelvis may have an important role in triggering postural strategies in sitting.[165] In frontal plane movements, activity of the hip abductors and adductors along with the quadratus lumborum is important for providing mediolateral stability.

Examination of Movement Strategies
Standing Control

An examination of movement strategies should begin with biomechanical and musculoskeletal elements (ROM, postural tone, and strength). Weakness and limited ROM in the ankles will influence successful use of an ankle strategy, whereas weakness and limited ROM about the hips will influence the hip strategy. Limitations of neck ROM can be expected in patients with primary vestibular disorders. Available movement strategies in response to AP and ML destabilizations should be determined.

Dynamic posturography provides an effective way to study movement patterns during standing. The *Movement Coordination Test*, developed by Nashner,[160] provides information about postural responses to control the COM when the platform moves, including symmetry of weight-bearing and forces generated, latency of postural responses, amplitude of response in relation to the stimulus size, and strategy utilized (ankle or hip). EMG monitoring can reveal specific muscle activation patterns and latencies. The main disadvantage of this equipment is limited use in the clinic due to expense and lack of portability (e.g., it is typically found in specialized balance or vestibular dysfunction clinics). Correlation with performance during functional tasks (e.g., walking) is also lacking.

During perturbed stance, the direction of perturbations can be varied (AP and ML). The movement strategies utilized and success of restabilization efforts should be examined and documented. Specific directional instability may be evident. Patients may demonstrate an absence or decreased use of one strategy with increased dependence on another. For example, older adults with somatosensory loss in the feet and ankles typically forgo the ankle strategy and utilize an early hip strategy. The sequencing of movement synergies should be examined and a determination of the pattern of activation made. For example, the ascending pattern of activation (distal–proximal) may be absent in patients with strong spasticity. The therapist is likely to see a proximal-to-distal activation pattern with strong co-activation of spastic muscles in the hips and knees.

Seated Control

Seated postural control and balance should be examined. During quiet sitting, the degree and direction of sway should be determined. During perturbed unsupported sitting, the available movement strategies to prevent destabilization should be examined and documented.[165] Grasp strategies (holding on to the edge of the seat) or LE hooking strategies (the foot and leg hook around the platform mat leg) are common strategies in the presence of significant instability. Seated instability is common in many patients with neurological dysfunction. For example, patients with stroke may demonstrate increased sway, problems activating trunk muscles (e.g., voluntary trunk flexion and extension), limited extent and direction of reaching, and altered postural alignment with greater weight placed on the less affected side.

For both standing and seated control, the therapist determines and documents if the movement strategies are (1) present and normal, (2) present but limited or delayed, (3) present but inappropriate for the particular context or situation, (4) abnormal, or (5) absent. The ability to modify postural strategies and adapt movements to changing task conditions should also be documented. For example, the patient can be asked to stand first with normal stance width, then with a narrowed BOS (feet together, in tandem, or single leg stance). Table 6.6 presents criteria that can be used to document functional balance with descriptors that define both static and dynamic control in sitting and standing. Time in balance is a frequent measurement parameter (e.g., patient is able to maintain steady balance in sitting without handheld support for up to 5 min).

Anticipatory Postural Control

Anticipatory postural control, the ability to activate postural adjustments in advance of destabilizing voluntary movements, should be examined. For example, the therapist asks the patient while standing or sitting to raise both arms overhead or catch a weighted ball. Changes in postural stability control are examined and documented during the performance of the voluntary activity. Impaired anticipatory postural control is found in many individuals with impairments in motor function, including patients with stroke,[166,167] PD,[168] and TBI.[169]

Dual-Task Control

Dual-task control should be examined. This is the ability to perform a secondary task (motor or cognitive) while

Table 6.6	Documenting Functional Balance
Status	Description
Normal	Patient able to maintain steady balance without handhold support (static) Patient accepts maximal challenge and can shift weight easily within full range of limit of stability in all directions (dynamic)
Good	Patient able to maintain balance without handhold support, limited postural sway (static) Patient accepts moderate challenge; able to maintain balance while picking up object off floor (dynamic)
Fair	Patient able to maintain balance with handhold support; may require occasional minimal assistance (static) Patient accepts minimal challenge; able to maintain balance while turning head/trunk (dynamic)
Poor	Patient requires handhold support and moderate to maximal assistance to maintain position (static) Patient unable to accept challenge or move without loss of balance (dynamic)
Absent	Patient unable to maintain balance

maintaining standing or seated control. For example, while standing, the patient is asked to count backward from 100 by 7 (simultaneous verbal–cognitive task) or to pour water into a glass (secondary motor task). Patients with PD have been shown to demonstrate significant impairment in dual-task control.[170,171] Patients with TBI and stroke have also been shown to demonstrate problems with dual-task control.[172,173]

■ OUTCOME MEASURES: POSTURAL CONTROL AND BALANCE

This section reviews selected postural control and balance outcome measures in common use. Individual tests can utilize a number of different postures (e.g., sitting, standing) and activities (e.g., sit-to-stand, walking, stair climbing) that challenge control. Tests typically include items that challenge both static or steady-state control and dynamic control. Asking the patient to maintain a steady posture in sitting or standing without handheld support tests static control. Test items can vary the BOS (e.g., the patient is asked to stand with double-limb support, single-limb support, tandem standing). Superimposing movement tests dynamic control (e.g., sit-to-stand, UE reach, stepping, step-ups). Walking test items challenge dynamic control and can include items of changing directions (e.g., forward, backward, sideward, pivoting), walking with head turns, or walking around obstacles.

Before starting, the clinician should analyze each test to determine what aspects of postural control and balance are being examined (e.g., static or dynamic control, proactive or reactive control, sensory interaction). The patient's unique body structure and function (impairment) deficits and activity limitations will help determine which test is the most appropriate to use in terms of postures and activities included. Some tests are diagnosis specific and developed for a specific population. For example, the Berg Balance Scale was initially validated for use with older adults and patients with stroke.[174] Others were developed with a more generalized purpose. For example, the Tinetti Performance-Oriented Mobility Assessment was developed to examine older adults with a propensity to fall.[175] Often, these instruments have been generalized for use with different populations and in different settings.

The patient should be instructed that a variety of functional activities will be used during testing. Some activities will be more difficult than others and may result in instability. The patient should be assured that the therapist will at all times protect them from a fall. During testing, all safety precautions should be observed, including close or contact guarding and use of a safety belt as indicated. When examining a patient with loss of balance (marked as "fall") during forceplate testing, the therapist should record the event with appropriate categorical deductions.

Scoring systems vary and can include an ordinal scale (e.g., 4-point or 5-point) as well as timed components. Some scale items are anchored with specific performance and time criteria (e.g., for single-leg stance, able to lift leg independently and hold for greater than 10 sec) while others use more general terms (e.g., unable or loses balance, unsteady, or steady). Tests and measures also vary in the time required to administer. Some are relatively short (e.g., 5 to 10 min), while others are quite comprehensive and lengthy (e.g., 30 to 40 min). In observing patient performance, the clinician may determine additional qualitative comments are necessary. These comments can address patient safety and fall risk, extraneous movements, excessive time requirements, alterations in speed, need for verbal cueing and assistive devices, and impact of the environment on test results. Many standardized outcome measures designed to examine postural control and balance are available. Selection of outcome measures should be based on the strength of available data addressing *reliability* (e.g., test–retest, intrarater, and interrater), *validity* (concurrent, criterion related, and predictive), and *sensitivity to change* (responsiveness, MDC, and minimal clinically important difference [MCID]). Additional considerations in selection include the availability of normative data, the type of impairments the instrument was designed to measure, and the intended population. The reader is referred to the

Rehabilitation Measures Database (https://www.sralab.org/rehabilitation-measures), the APTA's *Academy of Neurologic Physical Therapy Outcome Measures*, Edge files (https://www.neuropt.org) for additional information, and APTA Tests and Measures resources (https://www.apta.org/patient-care/evidence-based-practice-resources/test-measures).

Primary Balance Performance-Based Tests

Function in Sitting

The *Function in Sitting Test* (FIST) developed by Gorman et al.[176] is a 14-item test that examines a person's ability to maintain sitting balance during static sitting (hands in lap) with eyes open and eyes closed, as well as during dynamic challenges to balance. Reactive challenges include nudges (anterior, posterior, and lateral). Anticipatory challenges include moving the head side to side, lifting the foot, turning and picking an object up from behind, performing a forward and lateral reach, picking up an object from the floor, and scooting (anterior, posterior, and lateral). The FIST is scored on a 5-point ordinal scale: 0 = complete assistance, 1 = needs assistance to complete the task, 2 = UE support required to complete the task, 3 = verbal or tactile cues or extra time required to complete the task, and 4 = independent. Descriptors accompany each of the scores. Time to administer is less than 15 minutes. The FIST was developed by a panel of experts and tested on adults with acute stroke (within 3 months of insult). It demonstrates excellent reliability (test–retest, interrater–intrarater) and good to excellent predictive or concurrent validity.[177,178] Researchers have reported minimal detectable change for patients with acute stroke and adults with sitting balance dysfunction.[250] Recent work by Abou and colleagues demonstrates appropriate validity and test–retest reliability of the instrument for persons with spinal cord injury.[179]

Functional Reach Test

The *Functional Reach Test* (FRT) is a single-item test developed by Duncan et al.[180,181] to provide a quick screen of balance problems in older adults. It has been shown to be a marker of physical frailty.[182] Functional reach is the maximal distance one can reach forward beyond arm's length while maintaining a fixed BOS in the standing position. The test uses a level yardstick mounted on the wall and positioned at the height of the patient's acromion. The patient stands sideward next to the wall (without touching), feet normal stance width, and weight equally distributed on both feet. The shoulder is flexed to 90° and elbow extended with the hand fisted. An initial measurement is made of the position of the third metacarpal along the yardstick. For forward reach, the patient is instructed to lean as far forward as possible without losing balance or taking a step. A second measurement is then taken using the third metacarpal for reference. This measurement

Table 6.7	Functional Reach Reference Values (NORMS) by Age	
Age	Men (inches)	Women (inches)
20–40	16.7 (±1.9)	14.6 (±2.2)
41–69	14.9 (±2.2)	13.8 (±2.2)
70–87	13.2 (±1.6)	10.5 (±3.5)

From Duncan et al.[180–181]

is then subtracted from the initial measurement. See Table 6.7 for normative values of FRT. Time to administer is 5 minutes. Several studies have examined the metric support and ability of the FRT to detect change in patients with PD.[183–185]

The *Multidirectional Reach Test* (MDRT), developed by Newton,[186] evolved from the earlier FRT and measures how far an individual can reach in the forward, backward, and lateral directions using a yardstick affixed to a tripod stand. For backward reach, the test position is the same as functional reach with the yardstick position reversed to detect posterior movements. For lateral reach, the patient faces away from the wall and reaches sideways to the right (and then to the left) as far as possible. One practice trial is allowed before the start of three test trials. The therapist records functional reach in inches for all three trials and then averages the three trials. The amount of reach is influenced by several factors, including the size and height of the individual, sex, age, and health. The movement strategy used during a reach test should be documented (i.e., ankle or hip strategy, trunk rotation, scapular protraction). See Table 6.8 for normative MDRT values for older adults. Reliability has been studied in persons with stroke and spinal cord injury.[187,188] The *modified Functional Reach Test (mFRT)* incorporates forward and lateral reach to each side in sitting and has been shown to be a reliable measure.[189]

Berg Balance Scale

The *Berg Balance Scale* (BBS) developed by Berg et al.[190,191] is an objective measure of static and dynamic balance abilities in sitting, sit-to-stand, and standing. There are six static balance items and eight dynamic balance items, with the first six items considered a measure of basic balance ability. The test is scored using a 5-point ordinal scale (0 to 4) with detailed descriptors for each score. Some items are timed. Average time to administer is 14 to 20 minutes. The test demonstrates strong inter-rater–intrarater reliability.[192] Threshold cut-off scores have been a point of controversy. Score reduction on the BBS reflects a fall risk gradient.[193–195] Between the 54 and 56 score range, every point drop was linked to a 3% to 4% fall risk. Between 46 and 54, fall risk escalates to 6% to 8% for each point deduction. Finally, scores below 36 are associated with near 100% risk of falls.[194] The BBS demonstrates strong psychometric support for older adults and patients with stroke.[196] Using individual item analysis, data from community-dwelling elders and those with chronic stroke revealed that selected BBS items may have greater accuracy than the total BBS in identifying individuals with high fall risk. These items include picking an object up off the floor and standing on one leg, as well as turning 360°, placing alternate foot on stool, and tandem stance.[197] Minimal detectable change of the BBS has been reported for older adults, along with age-related performance values.[198–201]

Fullerton Advanced Balance Scale

The Fullerton Advanced Balance Scale (FABS) was developed by Rose at the University of California–Fullerton as an option for measuring higher level balance in older adults with more challenging tasks.[202] Ten balance tasks are included, and each item is graded on a 0 to 4 ordinal scale. Forty total points are available, and higher scores represent better performance. The FABS demonstrates significant convergent validity with the BBS (ρ = 0.75) and high test–retest reliability (0.96).[202,203] Activities include reaching for an object, two-foot jumping, and a backward lean task. Scores at or below 25 designate fall risk.[204] The instrument is particularly appropriate for higher level older adults and can be used at community balance and fall risk screening sessions. The FABS has been used to measure balance ability among person-specific diagnoses, including those with acute TBI.[205]

Table 6.8	Multidirectional Reach Test (MDRT) Reference Values		
REACH–MDRT	Mean (Inches) Standard Deviation Mean Age, 74 Years	Above Average (inches)	Below Average (inches)
Forward	8.9 ± 3.4	>12.2	<5.6
Backward	4.6 ± 3.1	>7.6	<1.6
Right lateral	6.2 ± 3	>9.4	<3.8
Left lateral	6.6 ± 2.8	>9.4	<3.8

From Newton.[186]

Balance Evaluation Systems Test

The *Balance Evaluation Systems Test* (BESTest) was developed by Horak and colleagues[206] as a comprehensive examination of postural control and balance. It includes 27 tasks (36 items since several tasks are performed on the left and right sides) that examine six subsystem categories of postural control: biomechanical constraints (five tasks), stability limits/verticality (three tasks), transitions/anticipatory postural responses (five tasks), reactive postural responses (five tasks), sensory orientation (two tasks), and stability in gait (seven tasks). Table 6.9 summarizes the subsystem categories and test items. It incorporates some tasks from earlier tests (i.e., functional reach, mCTSIB, Timed Up and Go [TUG], Dynamic Gait Index [DGI]). The BESTest uses a 4-point ordinal scale (0 to 3) with 0 = severe impairment to 3 = no impairments and specific descriptors for each score. The total score is 108 points with subscores available in each of the previous categories. A percent score is also calculated. Some items are measured (functional reach), and some are timed (TUG). Time to administer is 30 minutes. Training is required (training manual, workshops, online resources available). Subjects are tested wearing flat-heeled shoes or with shoes and socks off. They are allowed to use an assistive device if needed but are scored 1 point lower for that item; if they require physical assistance, a score of 0 is assigned for that item. Test–retest and interrater–intrarater reliability are excellent, as is predictive–concurrent and construct validity.[206] The BESTest demonstrates appropriate clinometric support for community-dwelling adults with and without balance dysfunction[206] and for persons with PD[207–209] and subacute stroke.[210]

A shortened version of this test is available, the Mini-BESTest. This version contains 14 tasks grouped into four categories: anticipatory postural adjustments (three items), reactive postural control (three items), sensory orientation (three items), and dynamic gait (five items).[211] Time to administer is 10 to 15 minutes.

Balance and Gait Combination Tests
Timed Up and Go Test

The *Get Up and Go (GUG) test* was developed by Mathias et al.[212] as a quick measure of composite dynamic balance and mobility. The patient is seated comfortably in a firm chair with arms and back resting against the chair. The patient is then instructed to rise and walk as safely as possible for 3 meters (10 feet), cross a line marked on the floor, turn around, walk back, and sit down. The patient is allowed to use an assistive device typically used but must complete the test without manual assistance. Time to administer is less than 5 minutes. Performance on the original GUG test used a 5-point ordinal scale ranging from 1 = normal (no risk of falls) to 5 = severely abnormal (high risk of falls). The subjective nature of the grades yielded only limited reliability.

Table 6.9	Components of the Balance Evaluation Systems Test (BESTest)[206]
Subsystem Categories	**Test Items**
Biomechanical constraints	Base of support Center of mass alignment Ankle strength and range Hip and lateral trunk strength Sit on floor and stand up
Stability limits/verticality	Sit, vertical and lateral lean, L and R Functional reach forward Functional reach lateral, L and R
Transitions/anticipatory postural adjustment	Sit to stand* Rise to toes* Stand on one leg L and R* Alternate stair touching Standing arm raise
Reactive postural control	In-place response—forward In-place response—backward Compensatory stepping—forward* Compensatory stepping—backward* Compensatory stepping—lateral, L and R*
Sensory orientation (mCTSIB)	Standing, EO, firm surface* Standing, EC, firm surface Standing, EO, on foam Standing, EC, on foam* Standing, EC, on incline*
Stability in gait	Walk, level surface Walk with change in gait speed* Walk with horizontal head turns* Walk with pivot turns* Walk and step over obstacles* Timed Up and Go Timed Up and Go—cognitive*

*Items included on the Mini-BESTest.[211]

EC = eyes closed; EO = eyes open; L = left; mCTSIB = modified Clinical Test of Sensory Interaction in Balance; R = right.

Complete BESTest copies and training materials are available at https://www.bestest.us.

Efforts by Podsiadlo and Richardson[213] to improve the objectivity and reliability resulted in the TUG test, which is widely used today. Timing with a stopwatch begins when the patient is instructed with "go" and ends when the patient returns to the start position seated in the chair (Fig. 6.12). Healthy adults are generally able to complete the test in less than 10 seconds. An assistive device may be utilized. Older adults (ages 60 to 80 years) have also been shown to average scores less than 10 (mean of 8).[214,215] Common threshold scores for fall risk include the 12-second benchmark used by

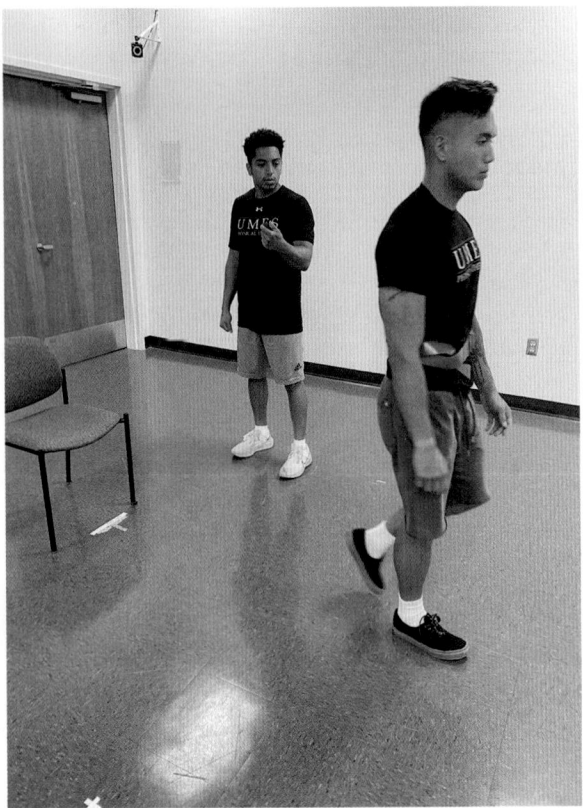

Figure 6.12 The Timed Up and Go Test.

the Centers for Disease Control and Prevention and 13.5 seconds.[216,217]

The TUG has been used to examine functional mobility deficits in patients with stroke[218,219] and PD.[220,221] Minimal detectable changes have been reported for people with PD.[222] Variations of the TUG include the *TUG cognitive* (TUGcog) in which the individual is asked to perform a simultaneous cognitive task (e.g., count backward from 100 by threes) or *TUG manual* (TUGman) in which the individual performs a simultaneous manual task (e.g., holds a cup filled with water). Researchers noted mean scores for dual tasking on the TUG can be expected to increase slightly (e.g., TUG 8.4, TUGman 9.7, TUGcog 9.7) for community-dwelling adults.[217]

Tinetti Performance-Oriented Mobility Assessment

The *Performance-Oriented Mobility Assessment* (POMA), developed by Tinetti and Ginter,[223] provides a measure of both static and dynamic balance. It was developed for use with the frail elderly, especially nursing home residents with a propensity to fall. Items are organized into two subtests of balance (16 points) and gait (12 points). Balance test items include static sitting balance, sit-to-stand and stand-to-sit, standing balance (static, with sternal nudge, EC), and dynamic standing balance (turning 360°). Gait test items include initiation of gait, path, missed step (trip or loss of balance), turning, and timed walk. Some items are scored on a 2-point scale (0 or 1) and some on a 3-point (0 to 2) scale. Average time to administer is 10 to 15 minutes. The POMA scale has a total possible score of 28. Test–retest and interrater–intrarater reliability are excellent, as are predictive and concurrent validity.[224–226] Patients who score less than 19 are considered at high risk for falls, and those who score between 19 and 24 are at moderate risk for falls. Studies have analyzed the tool's utilization in persons with stroke,[226] PD,[227,228] and amyotrophic lateral sclerosis.[229]

Dynamic Gait Index

The *DGI*, developed by Shumway-Cook et al.,[194] examines a patient's ability to perform steady-state walking and variations on command. Items include changing speed, walking with head turns (looking right or left, looking up or down), walking and pivot turn, walking while stepping over or around obstacles, and stair climbing (up and down). A 4-point scale (0 to 3) includes specific descriptors of normal control: 3 = no gait dysfunction, 2 = minimal impairment, 1 = moderate impairment, and 0 = severe impairment, with a maximum possible score of 24. Time to administer is less than 10 minutes. The DGI appears to be sensitive in predicting likelihood for falls with older adults (a score below 19 is indicative of increased fall risk).[194] Test–retest and interrater–intrarater reliability are excellent, as are predictive or concurrent and construct validity.[230–233] Minimal detectable change has been established for community-dwelling older adults[234] and individuals with stroke,[235] MS,[236] and vestibular conditions.[237] The Functional Gait Assessment is an extension of the DGI (with seven of the tool's original items) and includes three more difficulty tasks (e.g., backward walking and tandem walk). Thirty points are available.[238]

Four-Square Step Test

The Four-Square Step Test was developed with unique constructs of quadridirectional stepping and obstacle clearance.[239] Four canes are positioned in a square matrix with the handles facing outward. Beginning in the bottom left square of the cane course, the patient negotiates the four quadrants while facing forward the entire time as safely as possible (Fig. 6.13). Upon return to the original square, the sequence is reversed, and the patient returns to the original starting position. Use of a unilateral assistive device is permitted. The test demonstrates high interrater reliability (0.99) and convergent validity with the TUG (r = 0.88). Scores slower than 15 seconds classify the individual at risk for multiple falls.[239]

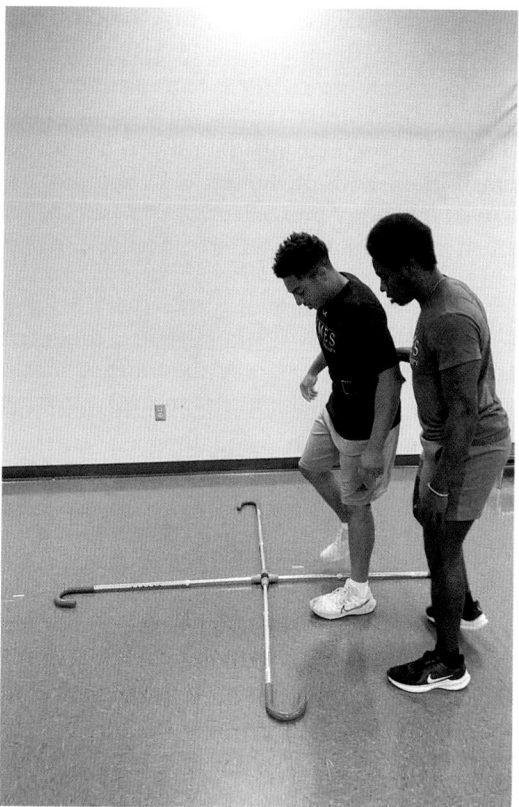

Figure 6.13 The Four-Square Step Test examines dynamic balance during negotiation of the four-quadrant cane matrix.

Walking While Talking Test

The *Walking While Talking (WWT) Test* is a dual-task measure that can be used to determine the effects of divided attention by introducing a secondary task, talking while walking.[240] The patient walks at a self-selected comfortable speed for a distance of 20 feet (6 m), turns, and returns (total distance of 40 ft [12 m]). Cognitive tasks are superimposed on the motor activity. The patient is asked to recite the alphabet (WWT-simple) or recite every other letter (WWT-complex). The time required to complete the test is recorded. This test is predictive for falls in community-dwelling older people.[241] Individuals who require a time of 20 seconds or longer (WWT-simple) or a time of 33 seconds or longer (WWT-complex) are at high risk for falls. Performance changes can be documented, including hesitations or stops, postural instability, and increased walking variability (steps off path). Cognitive changes (number of errors, mental slowing) can also be documented. Patients with impaired attention and automatic postural control can be expected to demonstrate difficulty on this test.[242] Dual-task performance impairments have been found in multiple patient poplulations.[243–246] Alternate forms of this test exist.[247] For example, the Stops Walking While

Talking Test includes initiating a conversation while the patient is walking. The test is positive if the individual stops walking while talking.[247,248]

Fear of Falling and Balance Confidence Measures

The fear of falling syndrome has gained momentum with national initiatives and clinical priorities to examine and reduce fall risk among older adults. A fall episode can lead to significant fear of falling.[249] Instruments that examine fall efficacy can generally be separated to reflect bimodal constructs: fear (or concern) about falling and balance confidence. Fear of falling refers to the phobic response aligned with fall risk, whereas balance confidence denotes a level of security perceived when performing household or community tasks.[250]

Tinetti Falls Efficacy Scale

The *Falls Efficacy Scale* (FES) developed by Tinetti et al.[251] is a self-report measure that examines how confident a person feels performing 10 ADLs without falling. The items on the test include both basic ADL (getting dressed and undressed, taking a bath or shower) and instrumental ADL (cleaning house, preparing simple meals, simple shopping). The functional mobility items include getting in and out of a car, going up and down stairs, walking around the neighborhood, reaching, and hurrying to answer the phone. The individual is asked to rate their confidence level on a 1 (very confident) to 10 (not confident at all) scale. Total scores can range from 10 (best possible) to the highest score 100 (not confident at all). The length of the test is 10 to 15 minutes. Test–retest reliability is moderate to excellent.[251,252]

Falls Efficacy Scale International

An extension of the FES, the Falls Efficacy Scale International (FES-I) was revised from the original Tinetti FES to include more challenging household and community tasks.[253] The FES-I was developed through the Prevention of Falls Network Europe (PROFANE) initiative where international researchers strategically examined tools related to falls and fear of falling. The instrument has 16 categories, and each item is graded on an ordinal scale denoting level of concern about falling during the task (1 = not concerned at all, 2 = somewhat concerned, 3 = fairly concerned, 4 = very concerned). The FES-I contains a variety of tasks at both the activity (e.g., going up and down steps) and participation (e.g., going out to a social event, visiting a friend) levels of the ICF framework. The instrument demonstrates excellent internal consistency (0.96) and test–retest reliability (0.96).[254,255] The FES-I is available in several languages, along with a validated 7-item short version of the tool, and can be particularly useful to the clinician working with patients who do not speak English.[255] In addition, measurement properties of the FES-I are supported for persons with cognitive impairment using an interview-based format delivery.[256]

Activities-Specific Balance Confidence Scale

The *Activities-Specific Balance Confidence (ABC)* scale developed by Powell and Meyers[257] is a 16-item self-report measure that asks individuals to rate their overall level of self-confidence in performing both household and community activities. Household activities include walking around the house, walking up and down stairs, picking up a slipper off the floor, and several reaching activities (reach at eye level, reach on tiptoes, stand on chair to reach). ICF community activities include walking to a car, getting in and out of a car, walking on various surfaces (parking lot, ramp) and in various

environments (crowded mall, icy sidewalk), and riding an escalator. The individual is asked to rate confidence on a scale from 100% (complete confidence) to 0% (no confidence). The overall score is calculated by adding all scores and dividing by 16 (total number of items). The length of the test is 20 minutes or less. Test–retest reliability is excellent.[257,258] Researchers have identified the minimal detectable change for patients with PD.[255]

Fall Risk and Floor-to-Stand Examination

Current approaches for fall risk examination include balance, strength, and fear of falling assessments. For example, the Stopping Elderly Accidents, Deaths, and Injuries (STEADI) initiative by the Centers for Disease Control and Prevention (Fig. 6.14) endorses a fall risk algorithm to screen older adults age 65 years

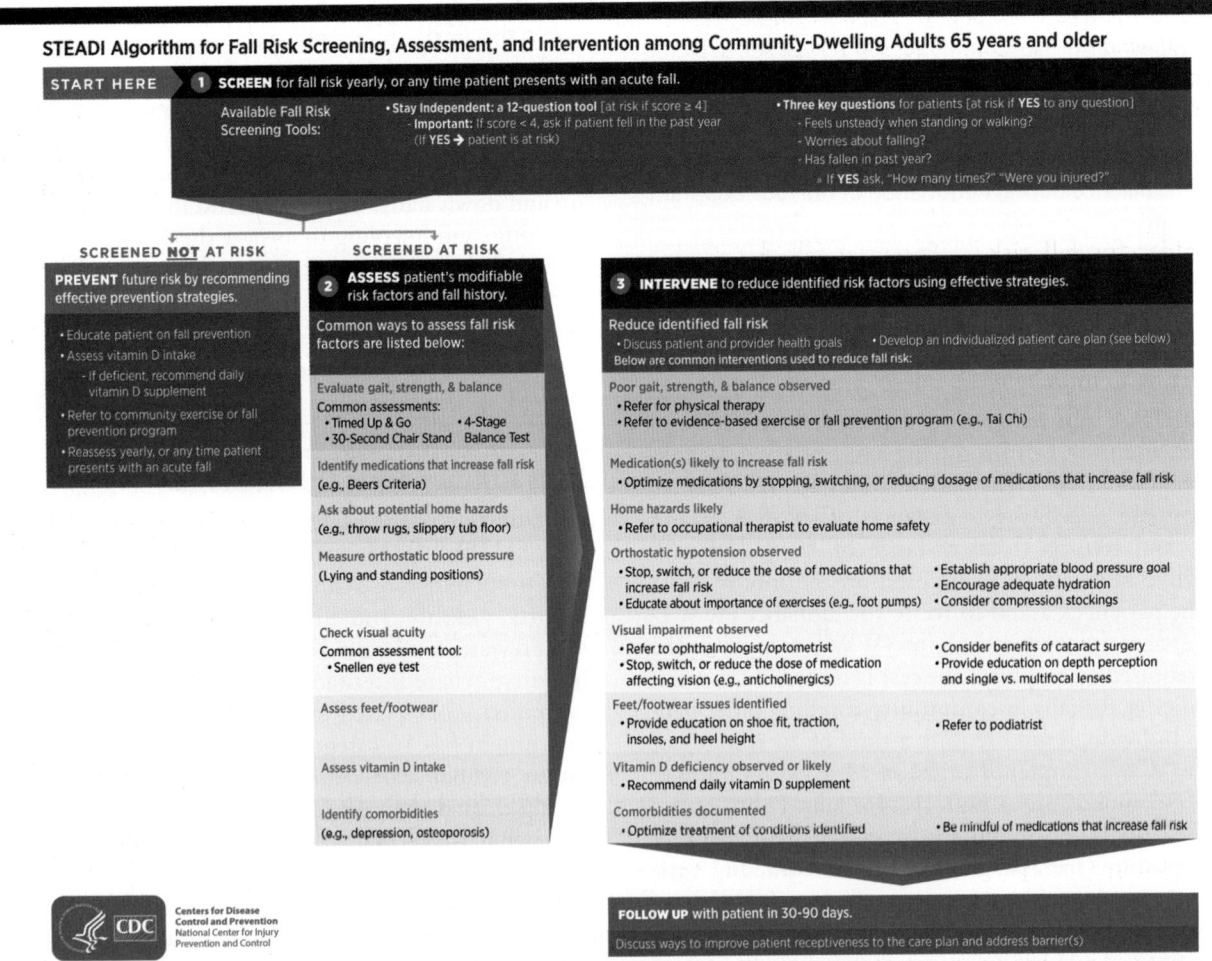

Figure 6.14 The STEADI Algorithm for Assessing Fall Risk. *(Source: https://www.cdc.gov/steadi/index.html)*

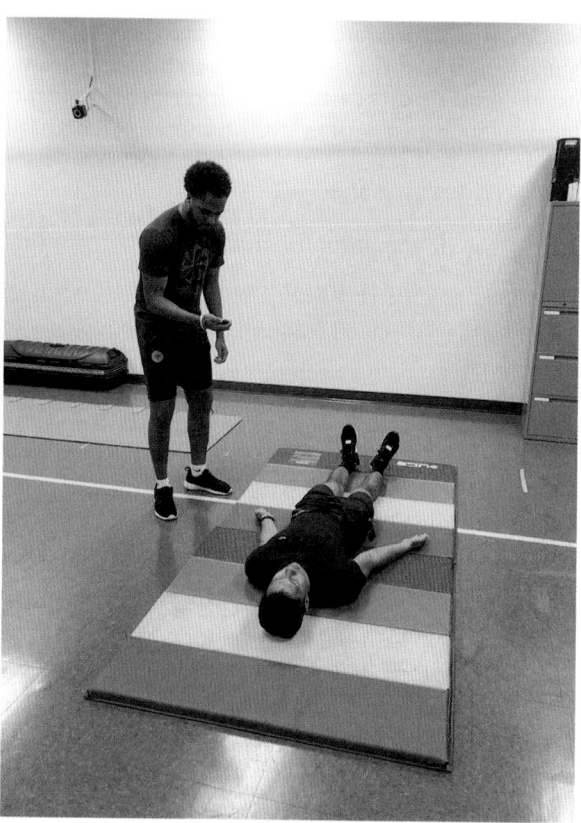

Figure 6.15 Examining floor rise ability during the timed supine-to-stand test. The patient begins in the supine position and, following the "Go" command, stands at a self-selected speed. Stopwatch timing ceases when no movement is observed.

and older for fall risk.[259] Potential fall risk is discerned using three questions related to falls in the past year, worry about falls, and perceived unsteadiness when walking. Older adults determined at risk proceed with more extensive screening, including the 30-Second Chair Rise Test and the Four-Stage Balance Test.[259]

During fall risk screening, clinicians may want to examine their patients' ability to rise from the floor in a supine-to-stand test.[260] The floor recovery transition has become increasingly important in clinical management given adverse events that can occur should an older adult remain on the floor for hours after a fall.[261] The timed supine-to-stand test requires strength, flexibility, and balance to execute. Generally, the patient assumes the supine position on a floor mat and following the command "Go" rises to stand. Timing begins on the initial verbal command and ceases when the patient assumes stable stance without movement (Fig. 6.15). The timed supine-to-stand test demonstratives convergent validity with age, sit-to-stand ability, and TUG performance.[260,262]

SUMMARY

An examination of coordination and balance provides important information about motor and sensory function. Evaluation of examination data allows the therapist to establish the diagnosis and identify underlying impairments, activity limitations, and participation restrictions. The therapist then formulates the plan of care including goals, prognosis, interventions, and expected outcomes.

A variety of outcome measures for coordination and balance have been identified. Selection should be based on the strength of available data addressing their *reliability, validity,* and *sensitivity to change*. Additional considerations in selection include the availability of normative data, the type of impairments (body structure and functions), activity limitations, and participation restrictions the instrument was designed to measure, and the intended population (general application or diagnosis specific).

Documentation should include the type, severity, and location of the impairments, as well as factors that alter the quality of performance. Emphasis has been placed on the variety of influences that affect movement capabilities. As such, evaluation of test results must be considered with respect to findings from other examinations such as sensation, ROM, muscle strength, muscle tone, and functional status.

Questions for Review

1. What are the purposes of performing a coordination examination of motor function?

2. What are the contributions (functions) of the cerebellum to coordinated movement?

3. How is peripheral feedback provided during a motor response?

4. Differentiate between motor impairments associated with cerebellar pathology and basal ganglion pathology. Provide at least five characteristic impairments for each area.

5. What predictable aspects of normal aging may affect coordinated movement?

6. Accurate and careful patient observation is an important source of preliminary information before performing a coordination examination. What type of activities would you select for the observation? What information will the observation provide?

7. Assume you are about to initiate a coordination examination. What screenings would be appropriate?

8. Identify three UE and three lower extremity coordination tests that could be used to examine a patient with severe ataxia as a result of TBI.

9. Differentiate between coordination tests for intention tremor and postural tremor.

10. What are the sensory conditions examined in the CTSIB? How should the results be interpreted?

11. Differentiate between the BBS and the POMA (Tinetti) in terms of components of balance tested.

12. The BESTest was developed to examine multiple aspects of postural control and balance. What are the six systems that items are grouped into? How is it scored?

CASE STUDY

Your patient is a 78-year-old male patient who has cerebellar deficits secondary to a vermal astrocytoma surgical resection 3 weeks ago. Prior to his retirement, he owned his own construction company. A neurological workup revealed significant coordination deficits following surgery. He lives in an assisted living facility with his wife, who assists with some caregiving activities. Prior to his surgery, the patient enjoyed attending weekly church services and visiting his son locally to see his two grandchildren.

The patient requires close supervision in ambulation with a standard walker. He demonstrates considerable trunk ataxia that worsens when his fear heightens, particularly when ambulating in confined spaces around the house. He requires contact guarding when negotiating stairs with a right handrail with a step-to-step pattern. He is afraid of falling, and his wife reports he has nearly fallen twice over the past week. You are seeing the patient in the home health setting for gait training, therapeutic exercise, and functional mobility training.

GUIDING QUESTIONS

1. Describe this patient's motor impairments and activity limitations.

2. Explain the clinical manifestations of ataxia. What are potential clinical correlates of vermal damage?

3. How might the patient's cerebellar deficits interfere with ICF participation activities?

4. What balance tests might you administer with this patient? Select the coordination tests you would use to examine the patient's movement capabilities in sitting and standing.

5. What are the requirements for documentation?

6. What fear of falling or balance confidence test would you select for this patient? Why?

7. What balance test examines stair negotiation ability?

8. What does a DGI score of 14 indicate?

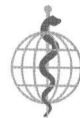

For additional resources, including answers to the questions for review, new immersive cases, case study guiding questions, references, and more, please visit **https://www.fadavis.com/product/physical -rehabilitation-fulk-8**. You may also quickly find the resources by entering this title's four-digit ISBN, 4691, in the search field at **http://fadavis.com** and logging in at the prompt.

Examination of Gait

Chapter 7

Judith M. Burnfield, PT, PhD
Guilherme M. Cesar, PT, PhD

LEARNING OBJECTIVES

1. Define terms used to describe normal gait.
2. Describe variables that are examined in each of the following types of gait analyses: kinematic qualitative analysis, kinematic quantitative analysis, and kinetic analysis.
3. Describe and provide examples of some of the most commonly used types of gait profiles.
4. Compare and contrast the advantages and disadvantages of kinematic qualitative and kinematic quantitative gait analyses.
5. Using the case study example, apply clinical decision-making skills in evaluating gait analysis data.

CHAPTER OUTLINE

PURPOSES OF GAIT ANALYSIS *216*
SELECTION OF APPROACH TO GAIT ANALYSIS *217*
GAIT TERMINOLOGY *217*
   The Gait Cycle *217*
   Phases of Gait *218*
TYPES OF GAIT ANALYSES *220*
   Kinematic Qualitative Gait Analysis *220*

Kinematic Quantitative Gait Analysis *244*
Kinetic Gait Analysis *261*
Summary of Kinematic and Kinetic Gait Analysis *265*
Gait Pattern Classification *265*
Energy Cost Analysis During Gait *266*
SUMMARY *268*

One of the major purposes of rehabilitation is to help patients achieve the highest level of function given their specific impairments so they can participate optimally in activities of interest. Human ambulation, or gait, is one of the basic components of independent function commonly affected by either disease or injury. Consequently, the desired outcome of many physical therapy interventions is to restore or improve a patient's ambulatory status. *Gait,* defined as the manner in which a person walks (e.g., cadence, step length, stride length, speed and rhythm) differs from *locomotion,* which refers to an individual's capacity to move from one place to another.[1] Although there are many specific reasons for performing a gait analysis, all of them require some information about the walking capacity of either an individual or a group of people with a particular disability. Because there are multiple approaches to gait analysis, ranging from very simple to extremely complex, the therapist must carefully consider how information obtained from a gait analysis is to be used. General as well as specific clinical indications for conducting a gait analysis may be found in the *Guide to Physical Therapist Practice 3.0,*[1] some of which are included below.

■ PURPOSES OF GAIT ANALYSIS

1. To assist with understanding the gait characteristics of a particular disorder. This includes the following:
   - Obtaining accurate descriptions of gait patterns and gait variables typical of different conditions
   - Identifying and describing gait deviations present, or typically present, in specific disorders
   - Determining balance, endurance, energy expenditure, and safety
   - Determining the functional ambulation capabilities of the patient in relation to functional ambulation demands of the home, community, and work environments
   - Classifying the severity of disability
   - Predicting a patient's future status
2. To assist with movement diagnosis by:
   - Identifying and describing gait deviations and describing the differences between a patient's performance and the parameters of normal gait
   - Analyzing gait deviations and identifying the mechanisms responsible for producing them
   - Examining balance, endurance, energy expenditure, and safety and determining their impact on gait

3. To inform selection of intervention(s) by guiding the therapist in:
- Proposing appropriate treatment of impairments that may improve gait performance
- Determining the need for adaptive, assistive, orthotic, prosthetic, protective, or supportive devices or equipment

4. To evaluate the effectiveness of treatment and guide the therapist in:
- Determining how interventions such as therapeutic exercise, endurance activities, developmental activities, strengthening or stretching, electrical stimulation, balance training, surgical procedures, and medication will affect gait
- Determining the effectiveness and fit of devices or equipment selected in providing joint protection and support, correcting deviations and dysfunctions, reducing energy expenditure, and promoting safe locomotive function

Many examples illustrating these purposes are found in the literature: descriptions of the differences between a patient's performance and the parameters of normal gait,[2–12] identification of the mechanisms causing dysfunction,[13,14] determination of either the need for, or the effectiveness of, a prosthetic device,[13,15] comparison of the effects of different types of assistive devices,[16,17] determination of either the need for, or the effectiveness of, an orthotic device,[18–22] determination of the effects of treatment interventions,[23–28] determination of energy expenditure,[15,16,29] and prediction of future status.[30–32]

SELECTION OF APPROACH TO GAIT ANALYSIS

The type of gait analysis that is selected depends on the purpose of the analysis; the type of equipment available and the experience, knowledge, and skills of the therapist. The equipment necessary for performing a specific type of gait analysis, in turn, depends on the purpose of the analysis, equipment availability, and the amount of time the therapist can expend. Equipment used in a gait analysis may be as simple as a pencil, paper, and stopwatch,[33] or as complex as an electronic imaging system with force plates embedded in the floor and electromyography electrodes placed on the client.[34–37] To select the appropriate method, the therapist must be aware of the types of analyses available and be able to determine which methods are reliable and valid. Much of the information about gait characteristics of particular disorders, as well as the mechanisms responsible for producing them, has been obtained in clinical research settings using complex instrumentation often not available for general patient use. However, given a firm understanding of the biomechanics of normal gait, including characteristic joint motions and muscle demands, a therapist can use fewer complex methods to identify variations in movement patterns from normal

and problem-solve likely causes. Efficacious treatment approaches can then be employed to address underlying causes.

Regardless of the method, a gait analysis of individual patients should provide reliable and valid data that can be used as a basis for describing present status (performance limitations and strengths), planning, and implementing interventions, evaluating effectiveness and progress over time, evaluating outcomes, and in some instances, predicting future status.

GAIT TERMINOLOGY
The Gait Cycle

The fundamental unit of walking is the *gait cycle,* which has both spatial (distance) and temporal (time) parameters. In normal walking, a gait cycle begins when the heel of the reference extremity contacts the supporting surface and ends when the heel of the same extremity contacts the ground again. In some abnormal gaits, the heel may not be the first part of the foot to contact the ground, so the gait cycle may be considered to begin when some other portion of the reference limb contacts the ground. The cycle ends with the next ipsilateral contact of that same portion of the foot with the ground.

The gait cycle is divided into two periods, *stance* and *swing* (Fig. 7.1). In normal gait at a comfortable walking speed, *stance* constitutes approximately 60% of the gait cycle and is defined as the interval in which the reference foot is in contact with the ground. *Swing* comprises approximately 40% of the gait cycle and occurs when the reference limb is not in contact with the ground. A single gait cycle includes periods of stance and swing for both the right and left limbs. During gait, body weight is smoothly transferred from one limb to the next during two intervals of double limb stance in the gait cycle when both limbs are in contact with the ground at the same time. *Initial double limb stance* occurs at the beginning of the gait cycle as weight transfers onto the outstretched reference limb from the trailing limb. *Terminal double limb stance* occurs at the end of stance as body weight transfers from the trailing reference limb to the lead limb. Initial double limb stance on the reference limb corresponds with the contralateral limb's terminal double limb stance. *Single limb support,* arising between the two double limb stance periods, is the portion of the gait cycle where only one limb supports body weight. The duration of each of these variables may be measured; for example, *cycle time, stance time* (right and left), *swing time* (right and left), initial *double limb stance time, terminal double limb stance time,* and *single limb support time.*

Two steps, a right step and a left step, form a *stride,* and a stride is equal to a gait cycle. Step and stride may be defined in two dimensions: distance and time. *Step length* is the distance from the point of heel strike of one extremity to the point of heel strike of the opposite

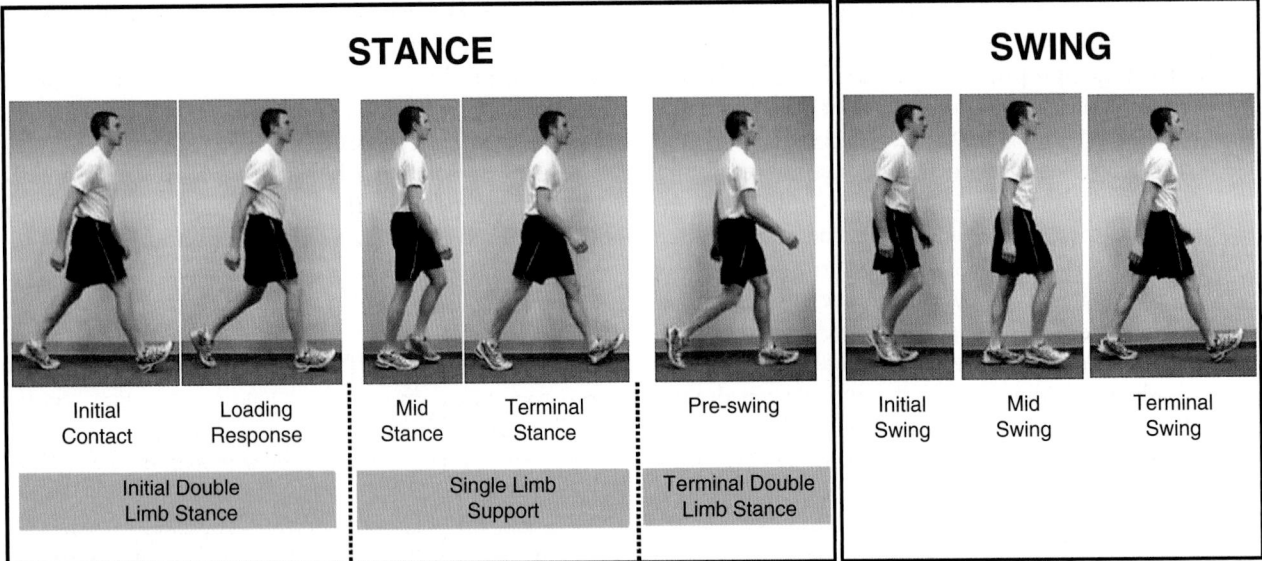

Figure 7.1 The eight phases of the gait cycle. Stance, the period when the reference limb is in contact with the ground, is comprised of the following five phases: initial contact, loading response, midstance, terminal stance, and pre-swing. Swing, the period when the limb is off the ground, is comprised of the following three phases: initial swing, midswing, and terminal swing. In addition, there are two periods in gait when both limbs are in contact with the ground: initial double limb stance (initial contact and loading response) and terminal double limb stance (pre-swing). Also, there is one period, single limb support, in which only one limb is in contact with the ground. Single limb support includes the phases of midstance and terminal stance. Note that the contralateral limb is in swing during the reference limb's single limb support. *(Courtesy of Movement and Neurosciences Center, Institute for Rehabilitation Science and Engineering, Madonna Rehabilitation Hospitals, Lincoln, NE 68506).*

extremity, whereas stride length is the distance from the point of heel strike of one extremity to the next point of heel strike of the same extremity. An alternative portion of the foot that consistently contacts the ground can be used as a reference point if the heel is not the first point of contact, as with some abnormal gait patterns. *Stride time* and *step time* refer to the length of time required to complete a step and a stride, respectively (Fig. 7.2).

Phases of Gait

Early terminology describing the phases of gait included descriptors for both stance (i.e., heel strike, foot flat, midstance, heel off, and toe off) and swing (i.e., acceleration, midswing, and deceleration). Though useful for describing normal gait, the traditional terminology is sometimes confusing in the presence of pathology. For example, many individuals with pretibial weakness or severe plantarflexion contractures lack a heel-first contact at "heel strike." Some individuals with plantarflexor spasticity maintain their heel off the ground throughout stance, not just during heel off. Others with profound plantarflexor weakness may fail to achieve a period of heel off and instead lift the full foot from the ground at the end of stance.

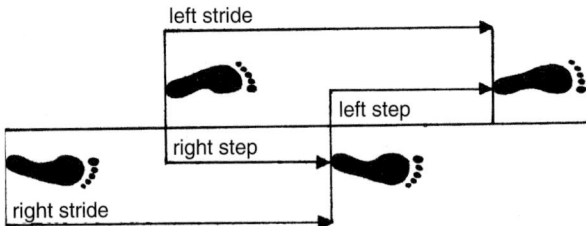

Figure 7.2 A right stride and a left stride. Right stride length is the distance between the point of contact of the right heel (at the lower left corner of the diagram) and the next contact of the right heel. Left stride length is the distance between the point of contact of the left heel (at the top left of the diagram) and the point of contact at the next left heel. Each stride contains two steps, but only the steps in the left stride are labeled. The left stride contains a right step and a left step. The right step length (shown in the middle of the diagram) is the distance between the left heel contact to the point of the right heel contact. Left step length is the distance between the right heel contact and the next left heel contact. Step and stride times refer to the amount of time required to complete a step and to complete a stride, respectively.

To avoid the confusion associated with earlier terminology, Perry and colleagues from Rancho Los Amigos National Rehabilitation Center developed a generic terminology to describe the eight functional phases of gait.[37,38] The first five phases constitute stance: initial contact, loading response, midstance, terminal stance, and pre-swing. The latter three comprise swing: initial swing, midswing, and terminal swing. The similarities and differences between the two terminologies are presented in Table 7.1.

The first stance phase, *initial contact*, represents the moment in time when the outstretched limb first hits the ground. During the next phase, *loading response,* body weight is rapidly accepted onto the outstretched limb. A small wave of knee flexion helps dissipate the impact forces associated with body weight loading onto the limb. Initial contact and loading response are the two phases that constitute *initial double limb stance,* which is sometimes referred to as *weight acceptance.*[37] Initial double limb stance ends when the foot opposite the reference limb lifts from the ground for swing.

During the next two phases, *midstance* and *terminal stance,* body weight progresses forward over a single stable limb. By terminal stance, the heel rises from the ground, the leg achieves a "trailing limb" posture, and the trunk advances well in front of the reference foot. Another term for the combined phases of midstance and terminal stance is *single limb support,* reflective of only one limb being in contact with the ground.[37]

Pre-swing, the last phase of stance, is sometimes referred to as *terminal double limb stance* or *push-off.* During pre-swing, body weight transfers from the trailing limb to the contralateral lead limb, which is experiencing initial contact and loading response. As the proportion of body weight supported by the trailing limb diminishes, residual energy stored in the Achilles tendon during mid- and terminal stance rapidly plantarflexes the ankle despite a lack of significant plantarflexor muscle activity.[37,39–41] The knee flexes to 40°, over half of the 60° required for foot clearance during the subsequent phase.

Table 7.1 Comparison of Gait Terminology

	Rancho Los Amigos[37,38]	Traditional
Stance	*Initial Contact:* Beginning of stance when heel or some other portion of foot contacts ground. Component of initial double-limb stance.	*Heel Strike:* Beginning of stance when heel first contacts ground.
	Loading Response: Body weight rapidly loads onto lead limb from trailing limb. Hip remains stable, knee flexes to absorb shock, and forefoot lowers to ground. Immediately follows initial contact and is final component of initial double-limb stance. Ends when opposite limb lifts from ground for swing.	*Foot Flat:* Immediately follows heel strike when sole of foot contacts floor.
	Midstance: Trunk progresses from behind to in front of ankle over single stable limb. First half of single limb support. Starts when contralateral foot lifts from ground for swing.	*Midstance:* Point at which body passes directly over reference extremity.
	Terminal Stance: Trunk continues forward progression relative to foot. Heel rises from ground, and limb achieves trailing limb posture. Second half of single limb support. Ends with contralateral initial contact.	*Heel Off:* Point following midstance when reference limb's heel leaves ground.
Swing	*Pre-swing:* Body weight rapidly unloads from reference limb and reference limb prepares for swing during this terminal double-limb stance period. Starts with contralateral initial contact and ends at ipsilateral limb toe off.	*Toe Off:* Point following heel off when only the reference limb's toe is contacting ground.
	Initial Swing: Starts when reference foot lifts from ground. Hip, knee, and ankle rapidly flex for clearance and advancement during this initial one-third of swing.	*Acceleration:* Beginning portion of swing from reference limb toe off to point when reference limb is directly under the body.
	Midswing: Thigh continues advancing, knee begins to extend, and ankle achieves neutral posture during this middle one-third of swing.	*Midswing:* Portion of swing when reference limb passes directly below body. Extends from the end of acceleration to beginning of deceleration.
	Terminal Swing: During this final one-third of swing, knee achieves maximal extension and ankle remains at neutral in preparation for heel first initial contact. Ends when foot contacts ground.	*Deceleration:* Portion of swing when reference limb is decelerating in preparation for heel strike.

GC = gait cycle.

Lifting of the foot from the ground reflects the onset of the first phase of swing, *initial swing*. Rapid flexion of the knee and hip ensue. During *midswing*, the thigh continues to advance into flexion, achieving a peak of approximately 25° relative to vertical. The knee begins to extend, and the tibia achieves a characteristic vertical position by the end of midswing. The ankle reaches neutral (0° dorsiflexion). During *terminal swing*, further thigh flexion is curtailed; however, the knee continues to extend until it observationally appears neutral. The ankle remains at neutral in preparation for a heel-first initial contact.

Characteristic features of normal gait are presented in Tables 7.2, 7.3, and 7.4. The gait phases, as well as normative values for joint motions, internal moments of force, and muscle activity, are presented in the first four columns of these tables. Familiarity with the normal motion patterns provides the therapist with a basis of comparison to identify deviations from standard. The internal moments (or torques) at each joint reflect the forces generated by muscles' contractile and non-contractile components, as well as ligaments and joint capsules. Internal moments counterbalance the external moments that are created by forces such as gravity and inertia acting on the body segments. In this chapter, we will describe internal joint moments, as this appears to be the more common reference point used in published literature. However, knowledge of the external moments (and thus the internal moments) is helpful for interpreting the characteristic patterns of muscle activation that contribute to stability, forward progression, shock absorption, and limb clearance throughout the gait cycle. For example, during the single limb support period of normal gait, a progressively increasing external dorsiflexion moment occurs as body weight progresses anterior to the ankle joint. Without a counteracting force from the plantarflexors, the ankle would collapse into dorsiflexion. The force generated by the plantarflexors contributes to an internal plantarflexor moment that prevents tibial collapse while simultaneously allowing controlled forward progression. Thus, the internal plantarflexor moment generated by the plantarflexors resists the external dorsiflexion moment created in large part by the force of gravity on the body.

Abnormalities in timing (e.g., activity that is premature or delayed) and amplitude (either too much or too little) can disrupt normal gait patterns. Familiarity with the muscle activity and function associated with normal gait allows therapists to identify potential causes of deviations. The last two columns of Tables 7.2, 7.3, and 7.4 present the possible effects of muscle weakness and potential compensations. The purpose of the tables is to identify components of normal gait that must be considered when observing gait and to provide an example of how to analyze the causes of an atypical gait pattern or particular deviation.

■ TYPES OF GAIT ANALYSES

The types of analyses in use today can be classified under two broad categories: *kinematic* and *kinetic*. Kinematic gait analysis is used to describe movement patterns without regard for the forces involved in producing the movement. A kinematic gait analysis consists of a description of movement of the body as a whole and/or body segments in relation to each other during gait. Kinematic gait analysis can be either *qualitative* or *quantitative*. Kinetic gait analysis is used to determine the forces involved in gait. In some instances, both kinematic and kinetic gait variables may be examined in one analysis. In addition to examining kinematic and kinetic variables, physiological variables such as heart rate, oxygen consumption, energy cost, and muscular activation patterns (electromyography) may be considered.

Kinematic Qualitative Gait Analysis

The most common method used in clinical settings is a *qualitative gait analysis*. This method usually requires only a small amount of equipment and a minimal amount of time. The primary variable examined in a qualitative kinematic analysis is *displacement*, which includes a description of patterns of movement, deviations from normal body postures, and joint angles at specific points in the gait cycle.

Observational Gait Analysis

Few clinical settings have the resources (space, money, or time) required to complete an instrumented gait analysis on every patient. As a result, observational gait analysis (OGA) often serves as an essential component of many physical therapy examinations. The results of an OGA are used to identify structural and activity limitations, plan an intervention, and assess the outcomes. While physical therapists seek an easy-to-administer tool to identify gait abnormalities, guide treatment approaches (e.g., need for orthotic devices), and assess progress,[42] the validity and reliability of existing scales remain less than optimal. This section highlights tools/approaches that clinicians may consider using.

The *Rancho Los Amigos Observational Gait Analysis* system is probably the most common OGA system used by physical therapists.[37,38] The Rancho Los Amigos OGA method involves a systematic examination of the movement patterns of key body segments (foot, ankle, knee, hip, pelvis, and trunk) during each phase of the gait cycle. The system uses a recording form comprising 45 descriptors of common gait deviations such as toe drag, excess plantarflexion and dorsiflexion, excess knee varus or valgus, pelvic hiking, and forward or backward trunk leans (Fig. 7.3). The observing therapist must determine whether a deviation is present and note the occurrence and timing of the deviation on the special form.[38]

Table 7.2	Ankle and Foot: Normative Sagittal Plane Data and Impact of Weakness[37,38]				
Phase	Characteristic Joint Position	Internal Joint Moment	Normative Muscle Activity	Effect(s) of Weakness	Possible Compensation(s)
Initial Contact	Neutral (0° dorsiflexion)	Dorsiflexor moment achieves peak during loading response.	Pretibial muscles (tibialis anterior, extensor digitorum longus, extensor hallucis longus) decelerate forefoot lowering and draw tibia forward following initial contact.	Borderline weakness (3+/5) may be accompanied by a foot slap following a heel first initial contact. Profound weakness (2+/5 or less) may result in foot flat or forefoot initial contact if pretibial strength is insufficient for achieving neutral ankle.	With borderline weakness, may slow gait to decrease demands on pretibial muscles during loading response. Alternatively, may contact ground with excess plantarflexion to decrease demands on pretibial muscles.
Loading Response	5° plantarflexion				
Midstance	5° dorsiflexion	Plantarflexor moment reaches peak during terminal stance.	Plantarflexors (gastrocnemius, soleus, flexor digitorum longus, flexor hallucis longus, tibialis posterior, peroneus longus, and peroneus brevis) progressively increase activity throughout two phases to allow controlled forward progression of tibia. Elastic energy is stored in Achilles tendon.	Excess dorsiflexion, uncontrolled tibial advancement, delayed or absent heel-off. However, if vastii are weak (vastus intermedius, vastus lateralis, vastus medialis longus, and oblique) may avoid excess dorsiflexion as it would contribute to excess knee flexion and high demand on weakened vastii.	Shortened step length and slower velocity to reduce demands on calf muscles.
Terminal Stance	10° dorsiflexion				
Pre-swing	15° plantarflexion		Calf muscles cease in early pre-swing. Stored elastic energy in Achilles tendon contributes to rapid plantarflexion as limb unloads.	Low or no heel-off and lack of rapid plantarflexion.	Use of more proximal muscles to prepare limb for advancement and clearance.
Initial Swing	5° Plantarflexion	Low dorsiflexor moment	Pretibial muscles elevate foot to neutral by midswing and then maintain in that posture.	Excess plantarflexion and foot drag, particularly in midswing. Poor posture for subsequent initial contact.	Hip hike, excess hip flexion or abduction to assist with limb clearance, or contralateral vault (excessive plantarflexion) to facilitate reference limb clearance.
Midswing	Neutral				
Terminal Swing	Neutral				

Table 7.3	Knee: Normative Sagittal Plane Data and Impact of Weakness[37,38]				
Phase	Characteristic Joint Position	Internal Joint Moment	Normative Muscle Activity	Effect(s) of Weakness	Possible Compensation(s)
Initial Contact	Appears fully extended	Brief flexor moment	Low amplitude hamstring activity (semi-membranosus, semitendinosus, biceps femoris [long head]) resists knee hyperextension.	Reliance on posterior capsule to stabilize joint and to prevent hyperextension.	*Shading represents column heading information not applicable to the identified phase of gait.*
Loading response	20° flexion	Extensor moment	Eccentric vastii activity (vastus intermedius, vastus lateralis, vastus medialis longus, and oblique) allows knee flexion for shock absorption but prevents collapse.	Unable to stabilize knee during flexion leading to limb collapse.	Avoid knee flexion (as flexion increases vastii demand) by use of (1) excess plantarflexion or (2) forward trunk lean to lessen knee extensor moment.
Midstance	Appears fully extended	Extensor moment transitions to flexor moment	Vastii activity ceases by middle of midstance.		
Terminal Stance	Appears fully extended	Flexor moment			
Pre-swing	40° flexion	Extensor moment	Rectus femoris modulates rate of knee flexion.		
Initial Swing	60° flexion		Biceps femoris (short head), gracilis, and sartorius contribute to knee flexion.	Limited knee flexion for foot clearance.	Compensatory hip hike, excess hip flexion, or abduction to assist clearance.
Midswing	25° flexion	Flexor moment	Hamstrings modulate rate of knee extension (and thigh advancement).		
Terminal Swing	Appears fully extended		Hamstrings continue activity and vastii become active in preparation for demands of initial double limb stance.	With profound vastii weakness (less than 2+/5) may see inadequate knee extension in terminal swing.	Past retract of thigh or extension thrust of knee to ensure full knee extension.

	Table 7.4	Hip: Normative Sagittal Plane Data and Impact of Weakness[37,38]			
Phase	**Characteristic Joint Position (Thigh Relative to Vertical)**	**Internal Joint Moment**	**Normative Muscle Activity**	**Effect(s) of Weakness**	**Possible Compensation(s)**
Initial Contact	20° flexion	Extensor moment	Single joint hip extensors and abductors contract vigorously to stabilize pelvis and trunk over femur. Hamstring activity diminishing.	Difficulty stabilizing pelvis and hip joint, leading to anterior tilt and increased hip flexion in sagittal plane. If abductors weak, contralateral pelvic drop may occur.	Decrease terminal swing hip flexion to limit demands on weak hip extensors during initial contact and loading response. Posterior trunk lean to reduce extensor moment. For weak abductors, may lean trunk laterally toward stance limb to reduce abductor demands.
Loading Response	20° flexion				
Midstance	Neutral	Extensor moment transitions to flexor moment	Residual hamstring activity assists with hip extension at the beginning of phase. Low-level abductor activity stabilizes pelvis.	Contralateral pelvic drop.	May lean trunk laterally toward stance limb to reduce abductor demands.
Terminal Stance	20° apparent hyper-extension (anatomical hip joint does not allow 20° extension, but hip appears to be extended 20° due to the combined impact of hip extension, backward pelvic rotation, and anterior pelvic tilt on thigh angulation relative to vertical).	Increasing flexor moment	Low-amplitude tensor fascia lata activity.	Contralateral pelvic drop.	May lean trunk laterally toward stance limb to reduce abductor demands.
Pre-swing	10° apparent hyperextension	Flexor moment	Rectus femoris assists with early thigh advancement.		
Initial Swing	15° flexion	Flexor moment	Iliacus, adductor longus, gracilis, and sartorius actively advance thigh.	With profound hip flexor weakness (less than 2/5), may exhibit limited hip flexion, thigh advancement, and foot clearance.	To facilitate limb clearance, may compensate with ipsilateral hip hiking, excess hip abduction, or contralateral limb vaulting (excessive plantarflexion).

(Continued)

Table 7.4   Hip: Normative Sagittal Plane Data and Impact of Weakness[37,38]—cont'd

Phase	Characteristic Joint Position (Thigh Relative to Vertical)	Internal Joint Moment	Normative Muscle Activity	Effect(s) of Weakness	Possible Compensation(s)
Midswing	25° flexion	Extensor moment	Increasing hamstring activity at end of phase restrains further thigh advancement.		
Terminal Swing	20° flexion	Extensor moment	Hamstrings continue to control thigh posture, while single joint hip extensors and abductors rapidly increase activity in preparation for demands of next phase of gait.	Failure to achieve optimum limb position prior to initial contact.	Alter speed.

Considerable training and practice are necessary to develop the observational skills needed for performing any OGA. Therapists who wish to learn the Rancho method can study the *Rancho Los Amigos Observational Gait Analysis Handbook.*[38] Practice gait videos, useful for developing and improving one's observational skills and for learning how to use the recording forms, may be obtained by visiting the Rancho Research Institute website (www.ranchoresearch.org/shop) or by writing to Rancho Research Institute at Rancho Los Amigos National Rehabilitation Center, 7601 East Imperial Highway, Trailer F3, Downey, CA 90242.

Podiatrists have developed their own unique OGA system.[43] A biomechanical gait analysis form for podiatrists was described by Southerland.[43] This form is used in conjunction with a static quantitative analysis that includes measurements of range of motion (ROM) of all joints from the hip to the toes and measurements of limb length. Detailed information is also collected on both the dorsal and plantar surfaces of the feet such as callus formation and corns. The examiner is expected to document abnormalities such as hallux valgus and hammer toes. The dynamic qualitative component of the analysis uses a shorthand system for recording the details of the OGA. The acronym GHORT (*G*ait, *H*omunculus, *O*bserved, *R*elational, and *T*abulator) is used to assist in recording information gathered from the observational analysis. Following completion of the dynamic portion, the rater's qualitative impressions of the patient's gait are compared with the results of the static analysis to verify the accuracy of the findings and determine the causes of abnormal function. The author states that after the first five analyses, a new rater's results are the same as or similar to those of other raters; however, the author did not reference any reliability and/or validity studies.[43] In general, these observational protocols provide the therapist with a systematic approach to OGA by directing the observer's attention to a specific joint or body segment during a given point in the gait cycle.

The advantages of OGAs are that they require little or no instrumentation, are inexpensive to use, and can yield general descriptions of gait variables. The disadvantages are that the observational method, being dependent on both the therapist's training and observational skills, is subjective and has only low to moderate reliability,[44] and validity has not been demonstrated.[45] Difficulties involved in observing and making accurate judgments about motions occurring simultaneously at numerous body segments, and inadequate training in OGA methods, are thought to contribute to the low reliability. Also, therapists differ in their observational skills. A drawback to using the Rancho Los Amigos OGA technique is that reliability and validity of the method have not been published.

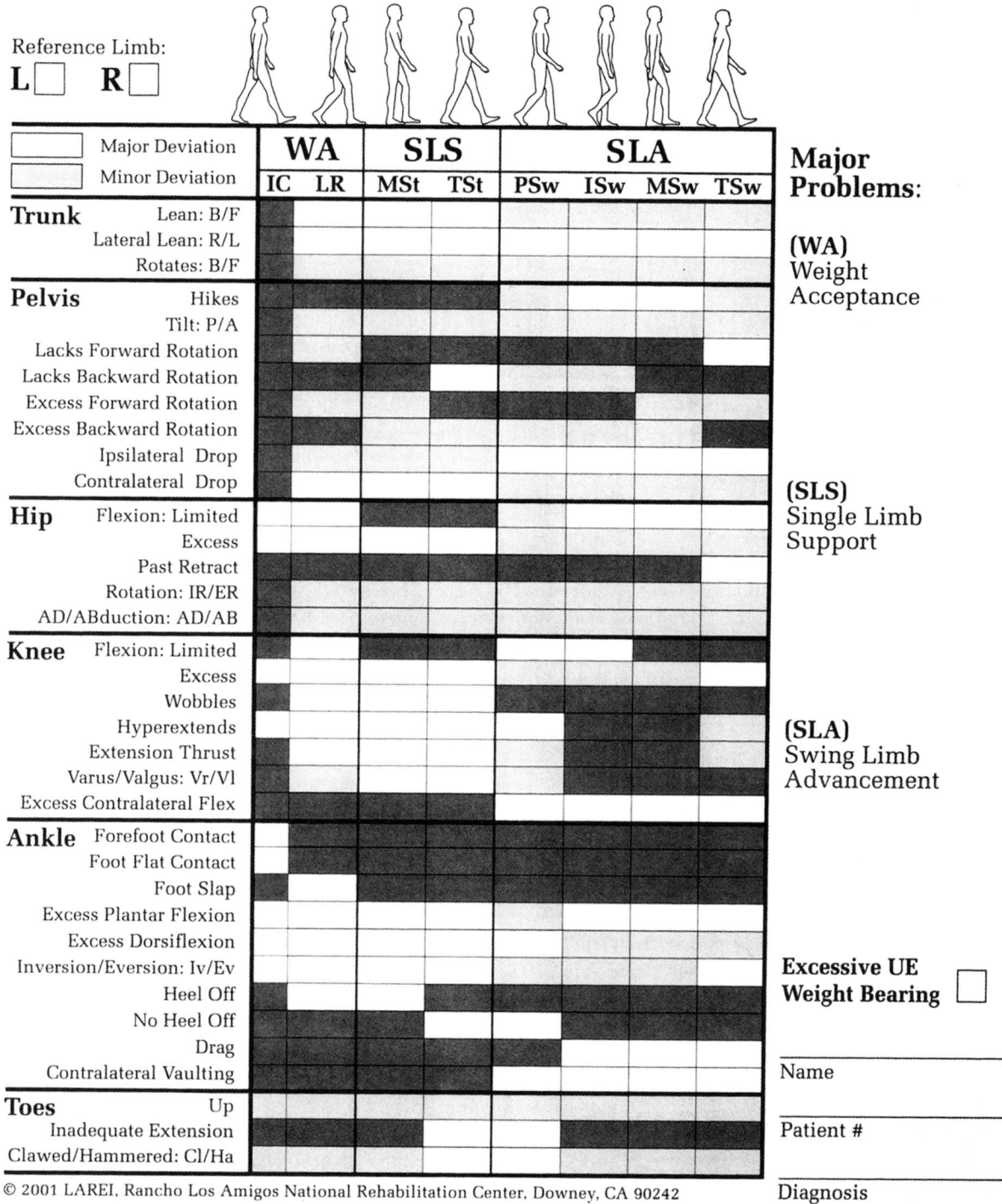

Figure 7.3 Full Body Gait Analysis Form. *(From Observational Gait Analysis Handbook,35, with permission.)*

Digital Video Recording

If therapists decide to use an OGA method, they should consider using a digital video recorder (DVR) that has the capability of slowing or stopping motion. A visual record is especially important when using the Rancho Los Amigos format because of the time involved in examining a large number of variables at six body parts. Most patients cannot walk continuously for the length of time required to complete a detailed, full-body observational analysis. Furthermore, the observers cannot rate or score a large number of variables while a subject is walking. Digital records of a patient's initial performance that can be replayed in slow motion allow therapists the time needed to make judgments about gait events. After activating the DVR pause feature, a goniometer, aligned with body segments displayed on the video monitor, can be used to assess (validate) joint angles during critical phases. This may also help refine the therapist's observational skills.

Although the use of DVRs may provide an opportunity for observers to determine the reliability of their scoring, reliability will probably remain low to moderate[46–49] unless therapists are knowledgeable about normal gait parameters and variables and are adequately trained to use the measuring instrument. Russell et al.[50] found that when observers were trained in the scoring of a Gross Motor Function Measure, a significant improvement occurred following training compared with the observers' pretraining scoring of the videotape. Brunnekreef and colleagues[51] identified higher interrater reliability among expert raters of orthopedic gait disorders (intraclass correlation coefficient [ICC] = 0.54) when using a form developed by the experts than the values documented for experienced (ICC = 0.42) and inexperienced (ICC = 0.40) raters using the same form. On the other hand, Eastlack et al.[52] found only low to moderate interrater reliability among 54 practicing physical therapists who rated 10 gait variables while observing the videotaped gait of three patients. These therapists had reported that they were comfortable performing observational gait analyses. The lack of agreement among raters found in this study, as well as the raters' lack of knowledge of normal gait parameters and terminology, has serious implications for patient treatments based on the results of observational gait analyses.[52] Krebs[53] argues that OGA is impossible to perform in a clinical setting. However, in a study using OGA, physical therapists were able to make accurate and reliable judgments of scored push-off power in the videotaped gait of subjects following stroke. This study suggests that focused analysis on specific gait parameters may be more reliable than general analyses.[54]

Specialized video analysis software may improve interrater reliability of gait measures compared to traditional video viewing methods. Borel et al.[55] reported increased measurement agreement between two raters when using Dartfish, a program that allows users to measure joint angles, distance, and time variables directly from digital videos. (*Note*: For this chapter, all manufacturer contact information is presented in Appendix 7.C [online].) Raters used Windows Media Player and Dartfish to perform the measurements required to determine Observational Gait Scale scores for 20 videos of children with cerebral palsy (CP). Dartfish has been commonly used with the athletic population.[56,57]

Interrater agreement values increased for select variables (knee position midstance, foot contact midstance,

timing of heel rise, hindfoot midstance, and the composite total score) when using the digital goniometer and the line drawing and temporal tools of Dartfish. One potential negative was that it took longer to complete the analysis using Dartfish than Windows Media Player (18 minutes versus 10 minutes per video, respectively). Additionally, this study did not determine whether the more consistent values also were valid. If OGA is employed, it should be used in conjunction with quantitative measures. Digital video recordings or videotape can provide a permanent record of the patient's gait. However, as with other patient data, it is critical to ensure confidential storage of such video.

Videography may also be used to examine joint range of motion (ROM) at the hip, knee, and ankle by taking goniometric measurements directly from the paused screen. Stuberg et al.[58] found no significant differences between goniometric measurements calculated from videotaped gait and measurements generated using a digitizer in 10 children with CP and nine typically developing children. Six blue markers, placed over key anatomical locations of the lower extremity (LE) and shoulder, guided measurements. The use of markers to guide measurements emphasizes the importance of ensuring that joints (or apparent axes of rotation) are clearly visible to facilitate measurements with the eye or a goniometer.

Mobile Device Software Applications

Program applications (apps) for mobile devices such as *smartphones* and *tablets* are being used in health care and athletic settings to assess gait. Spark Motion and Kinovea are examples of apps used for movement assessment. Videos recorded with these apps can be watched in slow motion. The clinician also has the option to overlay prior videos, integrate grids and drawings to assist with visual analysis, and calculate approximate joint angles on the videos/images for subsequent comparison.[59] Although clinically appealing, validity and reliability of such systems are just emerging.[60–63] Further validation with patients is still needed for clinical application.[64–66]

Observational Gait Analysis Process

The purpose of this section is to introduce the process involved in an OGA. The first step in the process involves the identification and accurate description of the patient's gait pattern and any existing deviations. The second step involves a determination of the causes of the deviations. To properly identify and describe a patient's gait, the therapist must have good knowledge of gait terminology and an accurate mental picture of normal gait postures and normal displacements of the body segments during each gait phase and in each plane of analysis (sagittal, coronal, and transverse). To determine the causes of a patient's gait pattern and specific deviations, the therapist must understand the normal roles and functions of muscles used during gait and the normal forces involved.[37,38,67,68]

Deviations occur because of an inability to perform the tasks of walking in a normal fashion. For example, a patient with paralysis of the dorsiflexors (which causes a foot drop) cannot attain the normal neutral position of the ankle necessary to complete the task of clearing the floor during swing. Therefore, the patient must use some other method to clear the floor. The patient could compensate for inadequate dorsiflexion by increasing the amount of hip and knee flexion, by circumduction of the entire limb, or by hiking the hip. The type of compensation that a particular individual selects depends on the specific disability. Increased hip and knee flexion may be used if the patient has an isolated problem in the ankle and adequate muscle strength and ROM in the extremity. Circumduction or hip hiking may be used if the patient has either a stiff knee or extensor thrust, which prevents use of increased knee flexion to raise the plantarflexed foot above the floor.[7] The therapist must be aware that patients may use a variety of methods to compensate for joint or muscle deficits.

Overview of Common Deviations and Underlying Causes

Tables 7.5 to 7.8 present common gait deviations and possible causes for the deviations. Given that muscle demands vary across phases of gait, the causes of a specific deviation also frequently vary based on the phase. For example, a common cause of excess plantarflexion during swing is weak pretibial muscles. However, this is not a common cause of excess plantarflexion during midstance and terminal stance, as the pretibial muscles are not normally active during this period. Instead, excess plantarflexion during mid- and terminal stance would more likely arise from the influence of plantarflexor spasticity or contractures on joint motion during this period. Thus, detective work is required to link the observed gait deviations with the specific demands of a phase in order to determine the most likely cause(s). Accurate determination of the impairments leading to the gait deviation is essential for guiding treatment interventions.

Appendix 7.A (online), Recording Form for Observational Gait Analysis, provides a sample gait analysis recording form. Check marks (√) are used to indicate observation of a specific deviation. The two columns on the far right are used to record possible causes and findings from the clinical analyses. To guide the OGA process, note that the form presented in Appendix 7.A (online) has been formatted similarly to Tables 7.5 through 7.8. If the reader decides to use the gait analysis recording forms presented in this text, reliability tests should be conducted because these forms are presented only as guides and have not been evaluated.

Table 7.5   Common Ankle and Foot Deviations[37,38]

Deviation	Phase(s)	Description	Possible Causes	Analysis
Toes or forefoot contact	Initial contact	Toes or forefoot are first point of contact with ground instead of heel.	Leg length discrepancy; plantarflexion contracture or spasticity; profound dorsiflexor weakness; painful heel; excessive knee flexion when combined with any impairment that limits ability to achieve neutral ankle.	Examine ROM and leg lengths, and examine for hip and/or knee flexion contractures and/or ankle plantarflexion contractures. Examine muscle tone and timing of activity in plantarflexors. Examine pretibial strength and for heel pain.
Foot flat contact	Initial contact	Entire foot simultaneously touches ground at initial contact.	Plantarflexion contracture; weak dorsiflexors; knee flexion contracture that prevents optimal tibial alignment prior to initial contact.	Examine ROM at ankle and knee and strength of pretibial muscles.
Foot slap	Loading response	Forefoot "slaps" the ground following a heel-first initial contact.	Weak dorsiflexors or reciprocal inhibition of dorsiflexors.	Examine strength. Evaluate muscle activation timing of pretibial muscles.

(Continued)

Table 7.5	Common Ankle and Foot Deviations[37,38]—cont'd			
Deviation	Phase(s)	Description	Possible Causes	Analysis
Excess plantarflexion	Midstance and/or terminal stance	Ankle fails to achieve 5° dorsiflexion at midstance and/or 10° dorsiflexion at terminal stance.	Plantarflexion contracture; overactivity or spasticity of the plantarflexors; could be intentional to avoid ankle and knee collapse if plantarflexors and vastii are weak.	Examine ROM and tone for plantarflexion contracture and plantarflexor tone (spasticity); examine strength of calf muscles and vastii. Evaluate if deviation may be intentional due to dual areas of weakness.
Excess dorsiflexion	Midstance and/or terminal stance	Ankle collapses into more than 5° dorsiflexion at midstance and/or more than 10° dorsiflexion at terminal stance.	Inability of plantarflexors to control tibial advance. Knee flexion or hip flexion contractures.	Examine ROM and plantarflexor strength and for hip and knee flexion contractures.
Early heel rise	Midstance	Heel comes off ground in midstance.	Spasticity or contracture of plantarflexors.	Examine ROM and tone for plantarflexor spasticity and contractures.
No heel off	Terminal stance and/or pre-swing	Heel fails to elevate from ground appropriately during terminal stance.	Weak plantarflexors; weak invertors that fail to lock midfoot in terminal stance; inadequate toe extension ROM; painful forefoot or toes.	Examine strength of plantarflexors and tibialis posterior; toe extension ROM, particularly the first metatarsal phalangeal joint; and for forefoot pain.
Toe clawing	Stance	Toes flex and "grab" floor.	Spasticity of toe flexors; excessive activation of toe flexors to compensate for weakness of the gastrocnemius and soleus; plantar grasp reflex that is only partially integrated; positive supporting reflex.	Examine tone of toe flexors, strength of plantarflexors, and presence of primitive reflexes.
Excess inversion or eversion	Stance or swing	Subtalar joint is excessively inverted or everted in contrast to expected position.	Excessive inversion: overactivity or contracture of invertors; reduced activity of evertors; primitive extensor pattern. Excessive eversion: overactivity or contracture of evertors; reduced activity or strength of invertors; primitive flexor pattern.	Examine strength and timing of LE movements and tone and for contractures.
Drag	Swing	Some portion of reference foot contacts ground during swing.	Pretibial muscle weakness; plantarflexor spasticity or contractures; inadequate knee or hip flexion.	Examine ROM of ankle, knee, and hip; strength of muscles critical for limb clearance.

LE = lower extremity; ROM = range of motion.

Table 7.6	Common Knee Deviations[37,38]			
Deviation	Phase	Description	Possible Causes	Analysis
Excess knee flexion	All phases	Knee is in greater flexion than expected for the given phase.	Knee flexor spasticity or contracture that exceeds position required for given phase; painful or effused knee; proprioceptive loss at knee; shorter LE on contralateral side. In addition, consider weak calf or hip flexion contracture if it occurs during single limb support.	Examine tone, spasticity, and ROM (contractures) and for pain, effusion, and proprioceptive loss at knee; leg length discrepancy.
Limited knee flexion	Loading response	Knee achieves less than expected 20° flexion.	May be intentional to decrease demands on weak quadriceps; secondary to plantarflexor or quadriceps tone, spasticity, or contracture; or proprioceptive impairment at knee.	Examine strength, tone, spasticity, of plantarflexors and quadriceps; plantarflexion and knee extension ROM; knee proprioception.
	Pre-swing and initial swing	Knee achieves less than expected flexion for given phase (i.e., 40° and 60° flexion, respectively).	May be secondary to plantarflexor tone, spasticity, or contracture that limits forward tibial progression in terminal stance; quadriceps tone, spasticity; proprioceptive impairment at knee; knee pain or effusion; calf weakness or hip flexion contracture that limits ability to achieve the trailing limb posture in terminal stance (a critical precursor to rapid knee flexion during pre-swing and initial swing). During initial swing, weakness of knee flexors also may contribute.	Examine tone and spasticity of plantarflexors, vastii, and rectus femoris; ROM and knee proprioception. Examine for pain and effusion. Examine plantarflexor strength and for hip flexion contracture. Evaluate if these factors may be inhibiting achievement of optimum limb posture.
Knee hyperextension	Stance	Extension of knee beyond anatomical neutral.	Structural abnormality may develop over time in presence of flaccid/weak quadriceps, which is compensated for by excess plantarflexion and/or posterior pull on thigh by gluteus maximus; quadriceps spasticity, accommodation to a fixed plantarflexion deformity, or impaired proprioception, can contribute to hyperextension if knee is exposed to deforming forces for extended duration.	Examine strength of vastii; tone, spasticity of plantarflexors and quadriceps; ROM and knee proprioception.
Wobble	Stance	Alternating flexion and extension at knee joint.	Consider proprioceptive impairments or alternating spasticity of knee flexors and extensors.	Examine knee for proprioceptive impairments and spasticity.

LE = lower extremity; ROM = range of motion.

Table 7.7	Common Hip Deviations[37,38]			
Deviation	**Phase(s)**	**Description**	**Possible Causes**	**Analysis**
Excess flexion	Initial contact and loading response	Hip positioned in greater flexion (thigh relative to vertical) than expected for given phase.	Single joint hip extensor weakness (gluteus maximus, adductor magnus) with compensation by hamstrings; severe hip and/or knee flexion contractures; hypertonicity of hip or knee flexors.	Examine single joint hip extensor and hamstring strength; hip and knee flexion ROM, tone, and spasticity.
	Midstance through pre-swing		Hip flexion or knee flexion contractures or spasticity; weak plantarflexors failing to control excess tibial advancement	Examine tone and spasticity of hip and knee flexors; ROM of hip and knee; strength of plantarflexors and hip for joint pain.
	Swing		Painful or effused hip; may be compensatory to assist with limb clearance if limb is functionally too long; flexion synergy during swing resulting in too much flexion.	Examine for compensation, determine if ankle and knee of reference limb are achieving correct joint positions. Examine contralateral limb to determine if deviations are occurring on opposite side (e.g., excess stance dorsiflexion) and could contribute to clearance problems on reference side.
Limited flexion	Initial contact, loading response, initial swing, midswing, terminal swing	Hip positioned in less flexion (thigh relative to vertical) than expected for given phase.	May be intentional to limit demand on weak hip extensors during loading response; weak hip flexors, or single joint hip extensor; hamstring spasticity or contracture limiting terminal swing advancement prior to initial contact.	Examine strength of hip flexors and extensors; ROM of hip and for spasticity of hip extensors and hamstrings.
Circumduction	Swing	Lateral circular movement of limb consisting initially of abduction, external rotation, followed by adduction and internal rotation in latter portion of swing.	Compensation for weak hip flexors or for inability to shorten leg for limb clearance.	Examine strength of hip flexors, knee flexors, and ankle dorsiflexors; ROM in hip and knee flexion, and ankle dorsiflexion and for abnormal extensor pattern.
Internal rotation	All phases	Internal rotation of femur.	Spasticity or contractures of internal rotators; weakness of external rotators; excessive forward rotation of contralateral pelvis.	Examine tone, internal rotation ROM, and strength of external rotators.

Table 7.7 Common Hip Deviations[37,38]—cont'd

Deviation	Phase(s)	Description	Possible Causes	Analysis
External rotation	All phases	External rotation of femur.	Spasticity or contractures of external rotators; weakness of internal rotators.	Examine tone, external rotation ROM, and strength of internal rotators.
Abduction	All phases	Abducted position of femur relative to vertical.	Contracture of the gluteus medius or iliotibial band; during swing, could be used to assist with foot clearance.	Examine hip abductor range of motion and for any factors that would necessitate compensatory assistance with clearance.
Adduction	All phases	Adducted position of femur relative to vertical.	Hip adductor spasticity/contracture. Excess contralateral pelvic drop.	Examine tone of hip flexors and adductors; muscle strength of hip abductors.

ROM = range of motion.

Table 7.8 Common Pelvic and Trunk Deviations[37,38]

Deviation	Phase(s)	Description	Possible Causes	Analysis
Backward trunk lean	Stance or swing	Posterior lean of the trunk relative to vertical	Purposeful to reduce demands on weakened stance limb gluteus maximus or to assist with limb advancement when hip flexion capability is limited.	Examine hip extensor and flexor strength.
Forward trunk lean	Primarily stance	Anterior lean of trunk relative to vertical	Compensation for quadriceps weakness. Forward lean reduces knee extensor moment and thus demand on vastii. May also be used to accommodate hip or knee flexion contractures.	Examine quadriceps strength and hip and knee for contractures.
Ipsilateral trunk lean	Most commonly occurs during reference limb stance	Lateral trunk lean toward reference extremity	Most commonly occurs during reference limb stance. Compensation for ipsilateral hip abductor weakness, hip joint pain, iliotibial band tightness or scoliosis.	Examine ipsilateral gluteus medius strength; hip pain and ipsilateral iliotibial band tightness and for trunk ROM.
Contralateral trunk lean	Most commonly occurs during reference limb swing	Lateral trunk leans toward opposite extremity	May be used to assist with pelvic elevation to ensure foot clearance if reference limb is functionally too long (owing to deviations or leg length discrepancy). Compensation for contralateral hip abductor weakness, hip joint pain, iliotibial band tightness, or scoliosis.	Examine contralateral gluteus medius strength, hip pain, for iliotibial band tightness, and for trunk ROM. Examine for factors contributing to swing limb being too long (e.g., limited knee flexion or excess plantarflexion during initial swing or a leg length discrepancy).
Contralateral pelvic drop	Stance	Drop of contralateral iliac crest below ipsilateral iliac crest	Ipsilateral hip abductor weakness, hip adductor spasticity, or hip adduction contracture.	Examine strength, flexibility, and tone of ipsilateral hip abductors and adductors.

(Continued)

Table 7.8   Common Pelvic and Trunk Deviations[37,38]—cont'd

Deviation	Phase(s)	Description	Possible Causes	Analysis
Ipsilateral pelvic drop	Swing	Drop of ipsilateral iliac crest below contralateral iliac crest	Contralateral hip abductor weakness, hip adductor spasticity, or hip adduction contracture.	Examine strength, flexibility, and tone of contralateral hip abductors and adductors.
Pelvic hike	Swing	Elevation of ipsilateral iliac crest above contralateral iliac crest	Action of quadratus lumborum to assist with limb clearance when hip flexion, knee flexion, and/or ankle dorsiflexion are inadequate for limb clearance.	Examine strength and ROM at knee, hip, and ankle; examine muscle tone at knee and ankle.

ROM = range of motion.

Guidelines for Performing an OGA

Guidelines for performing an OGA are presented below.

1. Select the area in which the patient will walk and measure the distance that you want the patient to traverse.
2. Position yourself to allow an unobstructed view of the subject. If digitally recording, the cameras should be positioned to view the patient's entire body (LEs as well as the head and trunk) from both the sagittal and coronal perspectives. To avoid errors in estimating the amplitude of joint angles due to angle parallax,[37,58] it is important to perform measurements on paused digital images only when the patient's LEs or body are in the same plane as the image view. Out-of-plane views can lead to distorted angle measurements.
3. Select the joint or body segment to be observed first (e.g., ankle and foot), and mentally review the normative joint positions and muscle activity for the phase of the gait period being observed (e.g., initial contact).
4. Select the plane of observation that will be used first, either the sagittal plane (view from the side) or the coronal plane (view from the front and/or back), and which side of the patient's body (either right or left) will be observed first.
5. Observe the selected body segment at a specific phase (e.g., initial contact) and make a decision about the segment's joint position. Note any deviations from normal.
6. Observe either the same body segment during the next phase or another segment at the same phase (e.g., initial contact) of the gait period. As described in number 5, again make a decision about the segment's joint position. Note any deviations from normal.
7. Repeat the process described in number 6 until you have completed an observation of all segments across all phases of the gait cycle in both the sagittal and coronal planes. Remember to concentrate on one body segment or joint at a time during one phase of the gait cycle. Do not jump from one segment to another or from one phase to another.
8. Always perform observations on both sides (right and left). Although only one side may be involved pathologically, the other side of the body may be affected.
9. Hypothesize likely causes of gait deviations (e.g., impairments in strength, ROM, or spasticity).
10. Confirm likely causes of gait deviations based on physical therapy clinical evaluation.
11. Develop and implement a treatment plan to address key underlying causes of gait dysfunction.
12. Periodically use OGA to reassess the patient's gait and determine response to treatment.

OGA in Neuromuscular Disorders

The gait patterns of individuals with neuromuscular deficits are influenced primarily by impaired motor function and motor control, weakness, abnormalities in muscle tone and synergistic organization, influences of nonintegrated early reflexes, diminished influence of righting and balance reactions, and dissociation among body parts. If proximal stability (e.g., co-contraction of the postural muscles of the trunk) is threatened by atypically low, high, or fluctuating muscle tone, controlled mobility is lost. In gait, a loss of control over the sequential timing of muscular activity may result in asymmetrical step and stride lengths. In addition, deviations may occur such as forward or backward trunk leaning, excessive or decreased hip or knee flexion, or altered dorsiflexion or plantarflexion.

In the presence of multiple muscle involvement or neurological deficits that affect balance, coordination, and muscle tone, the deviations observed, and the analysis of these deviations will be more complex than indicated in the tables. Examples of gait patterns associated with impaired motor function, spasticity, and hypotonus follow.

An individual with spasticity (e.g., an individual with diplegic CP) may have a posteriorly tilted pelvis, forward flexion of the upper trunk, protracted scapulae, and somewhat excessive neck extension. Excessive hip flexion, with adduction and internal rotation (scissoring) may be observed during stance and may be accompanied by either excessive knee flexion or hyperextension. During late stance, plantarflexor weakness may allow the ankle to collapse into excess dorsiflexion and the knee into excess flexion. Alternatively, the ankle may be positioned in excess dorsiflexion in late stance as a means of accommodating a knee flexion contracture or hamstring tightness/spasticity.

In other individuals with hypertonia, hyperextension at the knee occurs in stance and may be accompanied by plantarflexion and inversion at the ankle and foot. Electromyographic (EMG) recordings may show prolonged activity in the quadriceps and in the gastrocnemius-soleus muscle group. The hamstring, gluteal, and dorsiflexor muscle groups may be reciprocally inhibited.

In individuals with low muscle tone (hypotonia) in the trunk, core stability (tonic extension and co-contraction of axial muscles) is diminished. The pelvis may be anteriorly tilted so that the upper trunk is slightly extended. The scapulae may be retracted, and the head may be forward. During stance, the hip may be flexed and the knee hyperextended, accompanied by ankle plantarflexion. The foot may be pronated, with the majority of body weight borne on the medial border. Frequently, these individuals show diminished longitudinal trunk rotation and sluggish trunk balance reactions. They tend to rely on protective extension reactions of the limbs to maintain balance. The staggering or stepping reactions of the LEs may be pronounced, stride length and step length may be uneven, and gait may be wide based and unsteady.

Although neurological gait patterns may be complex and an analysis of the causes may be difficult, a detailed OGA can provide valuable data. Generally, to analyze gait patterns in persons who have sustained neurological damage, the following preliminary questions must be asked:

1. What is the influence of abnormal tone (hypertonicity, hypotonicity, fluctuating tone) on joint position and movement?
2. How does the position of the head influence muscle tone, position, and movement?
3. How does weight-bearing influence muscle tone, position, and movement?
4. What is the influence of abnormal (obligatory) synergistic activity on position and movement?
5. What is the impact of weakness (paresis) on position and movement?
6. How do coordination impairments affect position and movement?
7. What is the influence of impaired balance reactions on position and movement?
8. How do contractures alter position and movement?
9. What is the impact of sensory loss (e.g., proprioceptive, visual, vestibular) on position and movement?
10. How do medications impact muscle tone and weakness throughout the day?
11. What is the impact of inappropriately timed activation of a muscle on walking (e.g., how does premature onset of the tibialis anterior or delayed cessation of the gastrocnemius impact foot clearance and forward progression during gait)?

Ambulation Profiles and Scales

Profiles and rating scales constitute types of gait analyses that often include both qualitative (observational) and quantitative (spatial and temporal) measures. Profiles and scales are used for a variety of reasons, such as examination of ambulation skills,[69,70] determination of the patient's need for assistance, identification of a change in a patient's status,[70] screening for identification of the patient's need for physical therapy,[71] and identification of individuals (e.g., older adults) who are at risk for falling.[30,31] Gait analyses of one type or another may be either the sole focus of a profile, or the gait analysis may constitute only a small portion of a broad examination profile that includes balance skills and other functional activities. One particular advantage of some of these profiles is that subordinate gait skills such as standing balance may be examined in individuals who may be unable to walk independently. Since many of these profiles were developed for use with specific populations, comparative data may be available to the therapist.

The following profiles have been selected for review in this chapter because they are in current use and have been examined for reliability and/or validity: the Functional Ambulation Profile;[69] the Emory Functional Ambulation Profile[72] and the Modified Emory Functional Ambulation Profile;[73] the Iowa Level of Assistance Score;[74] the Functional Independence Measure;[75] the Functional Independence Measure plus the Functional Assessment Measure;[76,77] the Community Balance and Mobility Scale;[70,78,79] the Gait Abnormality Rating Scale (GARS)[80] and the Modified GARS;[30] the Dynamic Gait Index;[81–83] the Functional Gait Assessment;[84–88] the High-Level Mobility Assessment Tool;[89–94] the Fast Evaluation of Mobility, Balance, and Fear;[95] the Figure-of-8 Walk Test;[96] the Tinetti Performance Oriented Mobility Assessment;[97] and the Walking Index for Spinal Cord Injury II.[98,99] Thresholds for clinical importance, including the minimal clinically important difference (MCID; i.e., the smallest change in an outcome considered important by a patient/clinician) and the minimal detectable change (i.e., the smallest level of change within a measure that corresponds with a change in ability) for select functional assessments of gait capability are provided in Table 7.9.

Table 7.9   Outcome Measures: Select Functional Assessments of Gait Capability

Outcome Measure and ICF Category	Description and Scoring	MCID/MDC
TUG **ICF: 2 (Activity)**	Test evaluates time (in seconds) required for individuals to rise from chair, walk 3 meters, turn around, walk back to the chair, and sit down. Test is completed with individuals wearing regular footwear and any assistive device normally used for ambulation. **Scoring:** NA	**Alzheimer Disease**[308] Average age 81 (9) years; mild to severe Alzheimer disease. MDC: 4.09 seconds **Children with Down Syndrome**[309] MDC: 1.26 seconds **Children with Cerebral Palsy**[310] Age range: 3–10 years. *By motor function* MDC, GMFCS I: 1.4 seconds MDC, GMFCS II: 2.87 seconds MDC, GMFCS III: 8.74 seconds MCID, GMFCS I: 1.12 seconds MCID, GMFCS III: 4.65 seconds *By age* MDC, 3–5 years old: 1.59 seconds MDC, 6–10 years old: 0.95 seconds **Chronic Stroke**[178] Average age 58 (6) years; 6–46 months poststroke. MDC: 2.9 seconds Smallest Real Difference: 23%[158] **Lower-Extremity Amputation**[311] Average age 66 (13) years; individuals greater than 2 years postunilateral amputation. MDC: 3.6 seconds **Parkinson Disease**[111, 312, 313] Average age 65 (8) years (range 40–80 years); Hoehn-Yahr stages I to III. MDC: 4.85 seconds[313] Average age 68 (12) years; Hoehn-Yahr stages I to III. MDC: 3.5 seconds[111] Average age 71 (12) years; Hoehn-Yahr stages I to IV; mean disease duration 14 (6) years. MDC: 11 seconds[312] **Pregnant Women with Pelvic Girdle Pain**[314] Average age 31 (2) years; week of pregnancy 28.7 (7.4). MDC: 1.16 seconds **Spinal Cord Injury**[124, 315] Acute traumatic or ischemic SCI; American Spinal Injury Association (ASIA) classification level A, B, C, D; C2–L1. MDC: 10.8 seconds or 30% **Total Knee Arthroplasty**[316, 317] Average age 69.6 (8.1) years. MCID, 12 months postsurgery: 9.5 seconds[317] Average age 65.6 (9.7) years. MDC, Hospital for Special Surgery knee score of 78.3 (12.1) for right and 82.3 (11.2) for left lower extremities: 2.27 seconds[316]
10MWT **ICF: 2 (Activity)**	Test evaluates walking speed as individuals walk 10 meters (32.8 feet) without assistance. Time is measured only in middle 6 meters to allow for acceleration and deceleration.	**Older adults**[318] Average age 78 (8) years. MCID: Small meaningful change: 0.05 m/s Substantial meaningful change: 0.10 m/s

Table 7.9	Outcome Measures: Select Functional Assessments of Gait Capability—cont'd	
Outcome Measure and ICF Category	**Description and Scoring**	**MCID/MDC**
	Alternatively, individuals can traverse 14 meters with middle 10 meters timed. Speed calculated by dividing distance covered by time required for individual to walk given distance. Test can be performed at pre-ferred walking speed or at fastest possible speed. Assistive devices may be used if normally required for ambulation. **Scoring:** NA	***Hip Fracture***[319] Average age 79 (8) years (range 64–95 years). MDC: 0.17 m/s ***Parkinson Disease***[312] Average age 71 (12) years; Hoehn-Yahr stages I to IV; mean disease duration 14 (6) years. MDC, comfortable gait speed: 0.18 m/s MDC, fastest gait speed: 0.25 m/s ***Pregnant Women with Pelvic Girdle Pain***[314] Average age 31 (2) years; week of pregnancy 28.7 (7.4). MDC: 0.47 seconds ***Spinal Cord Injury***[124, 315, 320–322] Incomplete SCI (<12 months postinjury); C2–L1. MDC: 0.13 m/s[124, 315, 320, 321] Chronic motor incomplete SCI (greater than 6 months postinjury); average age 42 years. MCID: 0.06 m/s[322] ***Stroke***[323, 324] Acute stroke (≤45 days); average age 64 (13) years. MCID, comfortable gait speed: 0.16 m/s[323] Acute stroke (average of 35 [18] days poststroke); average age 67 (14) years MDC: All participants: 0.30 m/sec[324] Those who required physical assistance to walk: 0.07 m/sec[324] Those who could walk without assistance: 0.36 m/sec[324] *Speed measured over middle 5 meters of a 9-meter walk at comfortable pace Subacute stroke; average age 70 (10) years. MCID: Small meaningful change: 0.06 m/s[318] Substantial meaningful change: 0.14 m/s[318] ***Traumatic Brain Injury***[325, 326] Median age 23 years (range 15–50 years). MDC: 0.05 m/s[326] MCID, comfortable gait speed: 0.15 m/s[325] MCID, fastest gait speed: 0.25 m/s[292]
6MWT ***ICF: 2 (Activity)***	Test evaluates walking endurance and aerobic capacity as individuals cover as far a distance as possible over 6 minutes. Assistive devices may be used if normally required for ambulation. **Scoring:** NA	***Alzheimer Disease***[308] Average age 81 (9) years; mild to severe Alzheimer disease. MDC: 33.5 m (109.9 ft) ***Chronic Inflammatory Demyelinating Polyradiculoneuropathy***[327] Average age 54.1 (16.4) years; disease duration 8.5 (10.2) years. MCID: 20 m (65.6 ft) ***Chronic Obstructive Pulmonary Disease***[328,329] Average age 67 years. MDC and MCID: 54 m (177.2 ft) ***Older Adults***[318] Three groups of older adults with average age 78 (8), 74 (6), and 70 (10), last group comprised of stroke patients. MDC: 50 m (164 ft)

(Continued)

Table 7.9   Outcome Measures: Select Functional Assessments of Gait Capability—cont'd

Outcome Measure and ICF Category	Description and Scoring	MCID/MDC
		Intermittent Claudication[330] Average age 72 (7.4) years. MDC: 46 m (150.9 ft) ***Lower-Extremity Amputation***[311] Average age 66 (13) years; individuals greater than 2 years postunilateral amputation. MDC: 147.5 m (483.9 ft) ***Osteoarthritis, Hip or Knee***[331] Average age 64 (11) years MDC: 61.3 m (201.1 ft) ***Parkinson Disease***[312] Average age 71 (12) years; Hoehn-Yahr stages I to IV; mean disease duration 14 (6) years. MDC: 82 m (269 ft) ***Spinal Cord Injury***[315, 320, 321] Incomplete SCI (<12 months postinjury); C2–L1. MDC: 45.8 m (150 ft) or 22% change ***Stroke***[178,332,333] Average age 67 (10) years; average time since onset 1.8 (0.9) years. MCID: 34.4 m (112.9 ft)[332] Average age 58 (6) years; average time since onset 6–46 months. MDC: 36.6 m (120 ft) or 13% change[178] Average age 61.3 (12.8) years; average time since onset 63.6 (8.1) days.[333] MCID with Modified Rankin Scale as anchor: 71 m (233 ft) MCID with Stroke Impact Scale as anchor: 65 m (213 ft)
2MWT *ICF: 2 (Activity)*	Test evaluates walking endurance and aerobic capacity as individuals walk as far as possible in 2 minutes. Assistive devices may be used if normally required for ambulation. **Scoring:** NA	***Adults with Neurological Disorders***[175] Average age 47 (13) years; time since onset of disease 6 (7) years; 12 different diagnoses, including myelopathy, stroke, tumor, Huntington disease, and head injury. MDC: 16.4 m (53.8 ft) ***Children with Disabilities***[334] Children aged 6–12 years with neuromuscular disorders, including cerebral palsy and muscular dystrophy. MCID: Entire group: 23.2 m (76.12 ft) Children walking with aids: 15.7 m (51.51 ft) Children walking independently: 16.6 m (54.46 ft) ***General Population***[335] Average age 46 (18) years (range 18–85 years). MDC: Men and women combined: 42.5 m (139.44 ft) Men only: 47.2 (154.86 ft) Women only: 33.4 m (109.58 ft) ***Older Adults***[336] Average age 87 (6) years (range 76–95 years); long-term care residents. MDC: 12.2 m to 14.7 m (40 ft to 48.2 ft) ***Lower-Extremity Amputation***[311] Average age 66 (13) years; individuals greater than 2 years postunilateral amputation. MDC: 112.5 m (369.1 ft)

Table 7.9	Outcome Measures: Select Functional Assessments of Gait Capability—cont'd	
Outcome Measure and ICF Category	Description and Scoring	MCID/MDC
		Multiple Sclerosis[337] Average age 66 (13) years; Expanded Disability Status Scale 1.5 to 6.5. MDC: 19.2 m (63 ft) ***Stroke***[338] Chronic stroke, average time since onset 40.2 (34.3) months, range from 6–145 months; average age 63.5 (10) years. MDC: 13.4 m (44 ft) ***Ankle Plantarflexor Tone*** Modified Ashworth Scale 0: 14.1 m (46.26 ft) Modified Ashworth Scale 1 to 1+: 13.4 m (43.96 ft) Modified Ashworth Scale 2: 13.1 m (42.98 ft) ***Total Knee Arthroplasty***[316, 317] Average age 69.6 (8.1) years. MCID, 12 months postsurgery: 12.7 m (41.7 ft)[317] Average age 65.6 (9.7) years. MDC, Hospital for Special Surgery knee score of 78.3 (12.1) for right and 82.3 (11.2) for left lower extremities: 15.0 m (49.2 ft)[316]
DGI ***ICF: 2 (Activity)***	Test evaluates gait ability and dynamic balance. Individuals perform eight walking tests. Tasks include: 1. Walk at steady state. 2. Walk and change speeds. 3. Walk with horizontal head turns. 4. Walk with vertical head turns. 5. Walk and pivot turn. 6. Walk and step over obstacles. 7. Walk and step around obstacles. Climb stairs. Assistive devices may be used if normally required for ambulation. **Scoring:** A 4-point ordinal scale, ranging from 0–3, is used to rate each task; 0 indicates lowest level of function. Total Score = 24 Interpretation <19/24 = predictive of falls in the elderly >22/24 = safe ambulators	***Community-Dwelling Older Adults***[339, 340] Average age 76 years (range 59–88 years); history of falls or near falls in previous 12 months. MDC: 2.9 points[339] Average age 76 (7) years. MCID: Total sample: 1.90 points[340] Those with initial scores less than 21/24: 1.80 points[340] Those with initial scores ≥21/24: 0.60 points[340] ***Multiple Sclerosis***[112] Average age 42 (13) years; time since onset of disease 8.7 (8.8) years. MDC: 4.19–5.54 points ***Parkinson Disease***[111] Average age 67.5 (11.6) years; Hoehn-Yahr stages I to III; disease duration between 2 months and 15 years. MDC: 2.9 points or 13.3% ***Stroke***[88] Average age 61 (13) years; median time since stroke onset of 9 months (range 3–36 months). MDC: 4 points or 16.6% ***Chronic Stroke***[82] Average age 62 (13) years; mean time since stroke onset of 4 (8) years (range 0.5–35 years). MDC: 2.6 points ***Vestibular Disorders***[341, 342] Average age 52 (13) years; time since onset of disease 28 (59) months; peripheral vestibular disorders. MDC: 3.2 points[341] *MDC calculated from information provided in the article. Average age 60 (18) years (range 18–95 years); balance and vestibular disorders. MDC: 4 points[342]

(Continued)

Table 7.9 Outcome Measures: Select Functional Assessments of Gait Capability—cont'd

Outcome Measure and ICF Category	Description and Scoring	MCID/MDC
Modified DGI **ICF: 2 (Activity)**	Test evaluates gait ability and dynamic balance. Individuals perform eight walking tests. Tasks include: 1. Walk at steady state. 2. Walk and change speeds. 3. Walk with horizontal head turns. 4. Walk with vertical head turns. 5. Walk and pivot turn. 6. Walk and step over obstacles. 7. Walk and step around obstacles. 8. Climb stairs. Assistive devices may be used if normally required for ambulation. **Scoring:** A 4-point ordinal scale (ranging from 0–3) is used to rate gait pattern and time required to complete task, and a 3-point ordinal scale (ranging from 0–2) is used to rate level of assistance. The score 0 indicates lowest level of function. Total Score = 64	**Gait Abnormality**[343] Average age 80 years (range 52–94 years). MDC, total score: 6.3 points MDC, gait pattern: 3.9 points MDC, time: 2.8 points MDC, level of assistance: 2 points **Individuals without Disabilities**[343] Average age 66 years (range 20–99 years). MDC, total score: 5.5 points MDC, gait pattern: 3.2 points MDC, time: 2.5 points MDC, level of assistance: 1.9 points **Neurologic Disorders**[344] Average age of group 63 (12) years. Diagnoses included: multiple sclerosis, 57 (10) years old; Parkinson disease, 71 (8) years old; stroke, 66 (12) years old. MCID, total score: 6 points MCID, gait pattern: 4 points MCID, time: 2 points MCID, level of assistance: 1 point **Parkinson Disease**[343] Average age 71 years (range 41–88 years). MDC, total score: 6.8 points MDC, gait pattern: 3.7 points MDC, time: 3 points MDC, level of assistance: 1.5 points **Stroke**[343] Average age 64 years (range 24–93 years). MDC, total score: 7.4 points MDC, gait pattern: 3.8 points MDC, time: 3.4 points MDC, level of assistance: 2.8 points **Traumatic Brain Injury**[343] Average age 54 years (range 15–91 years). MDC, total score: 7.4 points MDC, gait pattern: 4.1 points MDC, time: 3.4 points MDC, level of assistance: 2.7 points **Vestibular Disorders**[343] Average age 67 years (range 23–94 years). MDC, total score: 7.2 points MDC, gait pattern: 3.9 points MDC, time: 3.6 points MDC, level of assistance: 2.3 points
Functional Gait Assessment **ICF: 2 (Activity)**	This modification of DGI also evaluates gait ability and dynamic balance. Individuals perform 10 walking tests.	**Older Adults**[345] Community-dwelling adults referred to physical therapy for balance training; average age 79 (7) years (range 60–96 years). MCID: 4 points

Table 7.9 Outcome Measures: Select Functional Assessments of Gait Capability—cont'd

Outcome Measure and ICF Category	Description and Scoring	MCID/MDC
	Tasks include: 1. Walk at steady state. 2. Walk and change speeds. 3. Walk with horizontal head turns. 4. Walk with vertical head turns. 5. Walk and pivot turn. 6. Walk and step over obstacles. 7. Walk with narrow base of support. 8. Walk with eyes closed. 9. Walk backward. 10. Climb stairs. Assistive devices may be used if normally required for ambulation. **Scoring:** A 4-point ordinal scale, ranging from 0–3, is used to rate each task; 0 indicates lowest level of function. Total Score = 30	**Parkinson Disease**[346] Average age 72 (9) years; Hoehn-Yahr stages I to III; average falls reported over 6 months 1.4 (1.5). MDC: 4 points **Stroke**[88] Average age 61 (13) years; median time since stroke onset of 9 months (range 3–36 months). MDC: 4.2 points or 14.1%; clinically: 5 points **Vestibular Disorders**[342] Average age 60 (18) years (range 18–95 years); balance and vestibular disorders. MDC: 6 points
Tinetti Performance Oriented Mobility Assessment ***ICF: 2 (Activity)***	Test evaluates gait and balance ability. It composes a nine-item balance portion and a seven-item gait portion. Gait tasks include assessment of walk initiation; step characteristics (e.g., length, height, symmetry, and continuity); walking path; trunk motion and posture; and walking stance. Assistive devices may be used if normally required for ambulation. **Scoring:** Items assessed using 3-point (0–2) or 2-point (0–1) scale; highest score indicates independence with each test item. Total assessment score = 28; gait assessment score = 12.	**Knee Osteoarthritis**[347] Average age 51 (6) years; onset of disease 3.7 (2.4) years. MDC, total assessment: 0.97 points MDC, balance portion: 0.75 points MDC, gait portion: 0.63 points **Older Adults**[348] Average age 83 (7) years; individuals residing in long-term self-care and nursing care facilities. MDC, individual assessment: 4–4.2 points MDC, group assessment: 0.7–0.8 points **Stroke**[122] Acute stroke (average of 8 [5] days poststroke); average age 75 (11) years. MDC: 6 points

(Continued)

Table 7.9	Outcome Measures: Select Functional Assessments of Gait Capability—cont'd	
Outcome Measure and ICF Category	Description and Scoring	MCID/MDC
Walking Index for SCI **ICF: 2 (Activity)**	Index measures walking function of individuals with acute or chronic spinal cord injury by scoring ability to walk 10 meters. **Scoring:** Index ranges from 0–20, where 0 represents most severe impairment. Scores increase as individuals are able to walk with a combination of independence from use of unilateral or bilateral orthotics, 1 or 2 assistive devices, and physical assistance from 1 or 2 helpers.	**Chronic SCI**[126] Average age 43 (14) years; time since injury 6 (6) years MDC: 1 point

DGI = Dynamic Gait Index; ICF = International Classification of Functioning and Disability; MDC = minimal detectable change; MCID = minimal clinically important difference; 6MWT = 6-minute Walk Test; SCI = spinal cord injury; 10MWT = 10-meter Walk Test; TUG = Timed Up and Go Test; 2MWT = 2-minute Walk Test.

Functional Ambulation Profile and Modifications

The *Functional Ambulation Profile* (FAP), developed by Arthur J. Nelson, PT, PhD, FAPTA, is designed to examine gait skills on a continuum from standing balance in the parallel bars to independent ambulation.[69] A stopwatch is used to measure the amount of time required either to maintain a position or perform a task. The test consists of three phases. In the first phase, the patient is asked to perform three tasks in the parallel bars: bilateral stance, uninvolved leg stance, and involved leg stance. In the second phase, the patient is asked to transfer weight from one LE to the other as rapidly as possible. In the third phase, the patient is asked to walk 20 feet (6 meters) in the parallel bars, with an assistive device, and, if possible, independently. Wolf et al.[72] evaluated the tool's reliability and validity in a study of 56 adults (28 with stroke and 28 without). The authors reported high interrater reliability (≥0.997) between two examiners who rated subjects' test performance. Construct validity was supported based on the test's ability to distinguish between those with and those without a stroke. Concurrent validity was demonstrated by strong correlations with participants' outcomes on the Timed 10-meter Walk Test (10MWT).

Test and the Berg Balance Scale

A more recent version of the FAP developed at Emory University is called the *Emory Functional Ambulation Profile* (EFAP).[72] This profile differs from the original FAP in that five environmental challenges have been added. The individual may negotiate the environmental challenges with or without the use of orthotics or assistive devices.[100]

The *Modified Emory Functional Ambulation Profile*[73] (mEFAP) incorporates manual assistance into the EFAP. Subtasks include 16.4 feet (5 meters) walking on a hard floor and on a carpeted floor, rising from a chair, completing a 9.8 foot (3 meter) walk and sitting back down, negotiating a standardized obstacle course, and ascending and descending five stairs.[101,102] Liaw et al.[103] evaluated the psychometric properties of the mEFAP in 40 individuals during the early phase of stroke recovery and 20 individuals with chronic strokes. The authors concluded that the mEFAP had good reliability, validity, and responsiveness for assessing walking function in patients with stroke undergoing rehabilitation.

Iowa Level of Assistance Scale

The *Iowa Level of Assistance Scale* (ILAS)[74] examines four functional tasks: getting out of bed, standing from bed, ambulating 15 ft (4.57 m), and walking up and down three steps. The patient's performance on the tasks is rated according to the following seven levels: (1) not tested for safety reasons; (2) activity attempted but not completed; (3) maximum assistance (therapist applies three or more points of contact); (4) moderate assistance (therapist applies two points of contact); (5) minimal assistance (therapist provides one point of contact); (6) standby assistance (no therapist contact but therapist not comfortable leaving patient); and (7) independence (therapist comfortable leaving room). Shields et al.[74] examined the reliability, validity, and responsiveness of the ILAS in 86 inpatients recovering from total hip or knee replacements and reported good intratester (k = 0.79 to 0.90) and moderate intertester (k = 0.48 to 0.78) reliability. Scores on the tool correlated highly with Harris Hip Rating Scale scores (r - -0.86).

Functional Independence Measure

The *Functional Independence Measure (FIM)* was created as part of a project funded by the National Institute of Handicapped Research and was designed to develop the Guide for a Uniform Data Set for Medical Rehabilitation.[104] The FIM is an 18-item measure that examines elements of a patient's physical, psychosocial, and social function. The FIM is now proprietary and is the trademark of the Uniform Data System for Medical Rehabilitation, a division of the University of Buffalo Foundation Activities (see Chapter 8 for further

discussion of the FIM). The FIM Locomotion: Walk/Wheelchair Guide is the portion of the document titled *The FIM System Clinical Guide, Version 5.2* that is related to gait and includes a seven-point level of assistance rating scale ranging from complete independence to total assistance (Table 7.10). A study designed to evaluate the accuracy of clinical judgments of patient functioning found that bias and poor judgment of a patient's functional level played a significant role in 50 rehabilitation professionals' ratings of patient functioning. The authors of the study suggested that blind ratings of the FIM and training in eliminating bias would improve accuracy.[105]

Functional Assessment Measure

The 12-item *Functional Assessment Measure (FAM)* was developed by a multidisciplinary group of clinicians at Santa Clara Valley Medical Center, San Jose, California,[76,106] to provide a measure of disability that

---

Table 7.10   The Functional Independence Measure Instrument Seven-Level Scoring System for Locomotion—Version 5.2

LOCOMOTION: WALK/WHEELCHAIR: Includes walking, once in a standing position, or if using a wheelchair, once in a seated position, on a level surface. Performs safely. Indicate the most frequent mode of locomotion (Walk or Wheelchair). If both are used about equally, code: "Both."

NO HELPER

7 Complete Independence—Subject *walks* a minimum of *150* ft (50 m) without assistive devices. Does not use a wheelchair. Performs safely.

6 Modified Independence—Subject *walks* a minimum of *150* ft (50 m) but uses a brace (orthosis) or prosthesis on leg, special adaptive shoes, cane, crutches, or walkerette; takes more than reasonable time or there are safety considerations. *If not walking,* subject operates manual or motorized wheelchair independently for a minimum of *150* ft (50 m); turns around; maneuvers the chair to a table, bed, toilet; negotiates at least a 3% grade; maneuvers on rugs and over door sills.

5 Exception (Household Ambulation)—Subject walks only short distances (a minimum of *50* ft or 17 m) *independently* with or without a device. Takes more than reasonable time, or there are safety considerations, or operates a manual or motorized wheelchair independently only short distances (a minimum of *50* ft or 17 m).

HELPER

5 Supervision

If walking, subject requires standby supervision, cueing, or coaxing to go a minimum of *150* ft (50 m).

If not walking, requires standby supervision, cueing, or coaxing to go a minimum of *150* ft (50 m) in wheelchair.

4 Minimal Contact Assistance—Subject performs 75% or more of locomotion effort to go a minimum of *150* ft (50 m).

3 Moderate Assistance—Subject performs 50%–74% of locomotion effort to go a minimum of *150* ft (50 m).

2 Maximal Assistance—Subject performs 25%–49% of locomotion effort to go a minimum of *50* ft (17 m). Requires assistance of one person only.

1 Total Assistance—Subject performs less than 25% of effort, or requires assistance of two people, or does not walk or wheel a minimum of *50* ft (17 m).

Comment: If the subject requires an assistive device for locomotion: wheelchair, prosthesis, walker, cane, AFO, adapted shoe, etc., the Walk/Wheelchair score can never be higher than level six. The mode of locomotion (Walk or Wheelchair) must be the same on admission and discharge. If the subject changes mode of locomotion from admission to discharge (usually wheelchair to walking), record the admission mode and scores based on the *more frequent mode of locomotion at discharge.*

AFO = ankle-foot orthosis; FIM = Functional Independence Measure.

reflected the communication, psychosocial adjustment, and cognitive functions of populations of individuals who sustained traumatic brain injury (TBI) and stroke. The 12 items are swallowing, car transfer, community access, reading, writing, speech intelligibility, emotional status, adjustment to limitations, employability, orientation, attention, and safety judgment. The FAM uses a 7-point rating scale modeled after the FIM to examine the individual's level or degree of independence, amount of assistance required, use of adaptive or assistive devices, and percentage of tasks completed successfully.[76,106]

The 12 items of the FAM have been combined with the 18-item FIM to produce the FIM + FAM with the intent of providing more detailed data for populations with TBI[77] and stroke. The FIM and FIM + FAM total scales are psychometrically similar measures of global disability, whereas the Barthel Index, FIM, and FIM + FAM motor scales are similar measures of physical disability.[107] However, in a study of 376 patients with stroke in Canadian inpatient rehabilitation units who were concurrently given the FIM and the FAM, the results of a Rasch analysis showed that in the motor domain, only the FAM community access item was more difficult for subjects to accomplish than were the FIM items. In the cognitive domain, the only FAM item that extended the range of the FIM was the one assessing employability. In light of the results, Linn et al.[108] concluded that adding the FAM items to the FIM reduced test efficiency and provided only minimal protection against ceiling effects of the FIM.

Community Balance and Mobility Scale

The *Community Balance and Mobility Scale*[70] was developed to evaluate balance and mobility skills in individuals who have experienced mild to moderate TBI. The scale consists of 13 items that include opportunities to assess multitasking (e.g., walking and looking at a target placed to the right or left), sequencing of movements (crouching to pick up an object from the floor and then continuing to walk), and complex motor skills (laterally and rapidly moving sideways by crossing one foot over the other and having to respond to unexpected commands to change direction). Six items are performed on both the right and left side, each of which is rated on a 6-point scale from 0 (poorest performance) to 5 (best performance).[70,78] Although the tool was developed specifically to assess individuals who have sustained mild to moderate TBI, it also has been used to measure balance and mobility in community-dwelling individuals following a stroke and in those with varying severity of chronic obstructive pulmonary disease.[70,78,79]

Gait Abnormality Rating Scale and Modifications

The *Gait Abnormality Rating Scale* (GARS)[80] was designed to distinguish nursing home residents with a recent history of two or more falls from a control group

of residents without a recent fall history. The test developers selected 16 features of the gait cycle and a scoring system in which the features are scored on a 0 to 3 rating scale (0 = normal, 1 = mildly impaired, 2 = moderately impaired, and 3 = severely impaired). Among the 16 features rated, arm-swing amplitude, upper extremity (UE) and LE synchrony, and guardedness best distinguished fallers from other subjects. The distinguishing features could be used to identify residents at risk of falling. Time, space, and resources are often very limited in nursing homes, and the only expenses involved in administering the GARS include purchase of a digital video recorder, recording media, and the therapist's time to film, review, and rate the digital recordings. However, the GARS does not provide information regarding the type of falls (trips, slips, losing balance) sustained by this population.[80] Therefore, it is not helpful in determining the cause of falls.

The *Modified GARS (GARS-M)* is a seven-item version of the GARS and contains the following variables: (1) variability, (2) guardedness, (3) staggering, (4) foot contact, (5) hip ROM, (6) shoulder extension, and (7) arm–heel strike synchrony. These variables were selected for inclusion because they were found to be the most reliable in the original GARS. Scoring is the sum of the seven items; the total score represents a rank ordering for risk of falling based on the number of gait abnormalities recognized and the severity of any abnormality identified. A higher score is associated with a more abnormal gait. Similar to the GARS, the GARS-M scores distinguished between older adults with a history of falling and those individuals who had no fall history. The GARS-M has been deemed a good predictor for persons at risk for falls.[30]

Dynamic Gait Index

The *Dynamic Gait Index* (DGI) was designed to examine the ability to adapt gait to changes in task demands. The tool was initially developed for use in community-dwelling older adults with balance and vestibular disorders[109] but has since been used across a variety of ages and patient populations.[110] The DGI uses a 0 (severe impairment) to 3 (normal) scale to rate performance on eight items, including gait on even surfaces, gait while changing speeds, gait and head turns in a vertical or horizontal direction, stepping over obstacles, and gait with pivot turns and steps. Whitney et al.[109] evaluated DGI scores and fall history in adults with vestibular disorders and reported that the odds of falling within the past 6 months were 2.58-fold higher with DGI scores of 19 or lower.[109] The tool has been used to evaluate dynamic gait and balance in a variety of patient populations, including individuals with Parkinson disease,[111] stroke,[82] multiple sclerosis,[112] cerebellar ataxia,[113] and children with CP.[114]

The DGI was further revised to enhance measurement capability. The modified DGI includes the same eight tasks as the DGI but integrates an evaluation of three facets of performance for each task: gait pattern (24 total points), level of assistance (16 total points), and time required to complete each task (24 total points). This modification enables monitoring of changes in any of the three facets of walking performance, in contrast to the original scoring system based on gait pattern alone. The three facets can also be combined into a single total modified DGI score. Shumway-Cook et al.[115] reported that the modified DGI score explained approximately 80% of the total variance in walking performance in a large population of patients with impaired mobility due to varied neurological disorders and also individuals without known disabilities.

The *Four-Item Dynamic Gait Index* consists of only half of the original eight DGI items (i.e., gait on level surfaces, changes in gait speed, and horizontal and vertical head turn activities).[83] It is faster to administer and displays adequate capacity to differentiate between individuals with and without balance and vestibular disease.

Functional Gait Assessment

The *Functional Gait Assessment* (FGA) is another modification of the original eight-item DGI. It was developed to address some of the ceiling effect attributes of the DGI when used with individuals with vestibular disorders and to clarify instructions and operational definitions associated with administering the tool.[87] Seven of the eight original DGI tasks were preserved, and three new items were added: gait with a narrow base of support, ambulating backward, and gait with eyes closed. In a study assessing age-referenced norms for FGA performance in independently living adults between the ages of 40 and 89 years, the tool was found to have excellent interrater reliability (ICC = 0.93).[86] In addition, intrarater and interrater reliability were deemed adequate given seven physical therapists' and three physical therapist students' repeated ratings of six patients with vestibular disorders (total FGA score reliability: intrarater = 0.83; interrater = 0.84).[87] Use of a threshold FGA score of 20/30 or less correctly predicted the unexplained falls experienced by six participants during a 6-month follow-up period in a study of community-dwelling 60- to 90-year-olds.[85] However, the authors recommend use of a threshold score of 22/30 or less as a more conservative criterion for those at risk for falls. The FGA has been used in studies of specific patient populations, including Parkinson disease[84] and stroke.[88]

High-Level Mobility Assessment Tool

The *High-Level Mobility Assessment Tool* (HiMAT) was designed to measure high-level mobility skills required for employment and social roles, as well as for leisure and sporting activities for younger adults recovering from a TBI.[91] The tool consists of 13 items and to complete requires only a stopwatch, a 14-step staircase,

a brick-sized object, and a tape measure.[89,116] Tasks assessed include walking (forward, backward, on toes, over an obstacle, in a figure eight), running, a run stop, skipping, hopping forward, bounding (affected and nonaffected), and going up and down stairs with and without a railing. All items are marked on a 5-point scale (0 = unable to perform to 4 = performing item normally) except for two stair items that are rated on a 6-point scale (0 to 5). The maximum achievable score is 54. The tool is appropriate only for patients who can ambulate independently for at least 20 meters without an assistive device. Thus, it is most appropriate for higher functioning patients, such as those in the latter stages of an inpatient rehabilitation program or already living in the community. Interrater reliability and test-retest reliability are high (both ICCs = 0.99).[92] Between-day testing scores demonstrated a small improvement over the 24 hours (1 point), which is suggestive of improved performance with test familiarity. This highlights the importance of allowing patients an opportunity to practice the test at least once before scoring.

The original 13-item HiMAT has been revised to a shorter, faster-to-administer version that includes only eight items: walk (forward, backward, toes, obstacle), run, skip, hop, and bound on the nonaffected LE.[94] One key difference between the two versions is that stair items were eliminated. This addresses a challenge clinicians experience when trying to administer the 13-item HiMAT test in environments lacking a 14-step staircase. Because it was the easiest item on the original scale, elimination of stairs is not expected to influence assessment of high-level mobility skills. However, it is possible that the tool may be more susceptible to a floor effect because it is less able to distinguish between abilities of more severely disabled individuals.

Fast Evaluation of Mobility Balance and Fear

The *Fast Evaluation of Mobility, Balance, and Fear* (FEMBAF) is another instrument designed to identify risk factors, functional performance, and factors that hinder mobility.[95] It consists of a 22-item risk factor questionnaire and an 18-item performance component, which includes, among other measures, stair ascent and descent, stepping over an obstacle, and one-legged standing. Di Fabio and Seay[95] reported that the FEMBAF served as a valid and reliable measurement of risk factors, functional performance, and factors that hinder mobility in their study of 35 community-dwelling older adults.

Figure-of-8 Walk Test

Many measures of overground walking focus primarily on gait performed along a straight path (e.g., the 5-meter Walk Test). In contrast, the Figure-of-8 Walk Test (F8W)[96] was developed to assess both curved- and straight-path walking in older adults with walking difficulties. The number of steps, total time, and smoothness of movement are examined as an individual completes a single figure-of-8 walk around two cones spaced 5 ft apart (Fig. 7.4). In a study of performance on the F8W in 51 older community-dwelling adults with walking difficulty, Hess et al.[96] reported significant correlations between the time to complete the F8W and overground gait speed, the GARS-M score, select physical function and efficacy measures, step length and width variability, and measures of executive function (i.e., the Trail Making Test B [Trails B]). The number of steps required to complete the F8W correlated significantly with gait speed, select physical function and efficacy measures, step width variability, and performance on the Trails B. Movement smoothness correlated significantly only with step-width variability. Given the administration of F8W is simple and the evaluation can provide important information regarding mobility and dynamic balance, this test has been used with distinct patient populations, such as individuals with CP,[117] osteoarthritis,[118] lower limb loss,[119] and Parkinson disease.[120]

Tinetti Performance Oriented Mobility Assessment

The Tinetti Performance Oriented Mobility Assessment (POMA) was initially developed to be administered to older adults but has since been used with different patient populations, such as those with Parkinson disease[121] and stroke.[122] The test consists of gait and balance items and takes approximately 15 minutes to administer. The gait assessment evaluates body posture (i.e., trunk motion); step characteristics; and walking initiation, path, and stance while individuals walk across the examination room or a hallway at a self-selected pace, as well as at a faster speed using usual assistive devices/orthoses.

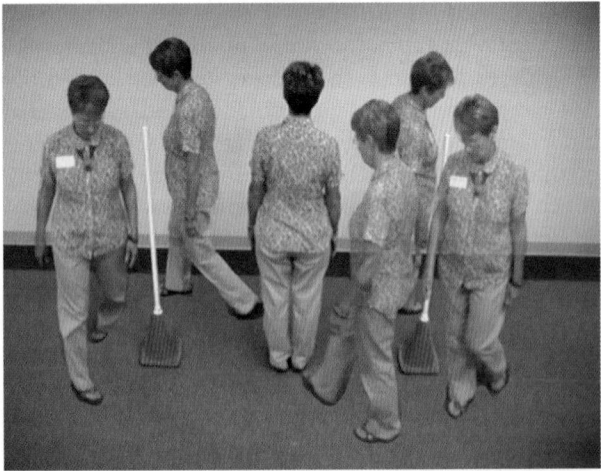

Figure 7.4 Individual performing the Figure-of-8 Walk Test, a tool developed to quantify walking ability in older adults with mobility disorders. Time to complete, number of steps, and smoothness of movement are used to score an individual's walking performance of a single figure-of-8 path around two cones spaced 5 feet apart.

Walking Index for Spinal Cord Injury II

The Walking Index for Spinal Cord Injury II (WISCI II) is a valid and reliable tool that was created to evaluate walking ability of adults and children with spinal cord injury (SCI) (paraplegia and tetraplegia) based on the extent and nature of assistance (combination of orthoses, assistive devices, and physical assistance) required to walk 10 meters at self-selected speed.[123–128] The test takes up to about 15 minutes to administer, depending on the individual's capacity and the need to don orthoses. The WISCI II is generally used in conjunction with other measures (e.g., 10MWT) to provide a more comprehensive quantification of walking function in individuals with SCI.[129–131]

Kinematic Quantitative Gait Analysis

Kinematic quantitative gait analysis is used to obtain information on spatial and temporal gait variables, as well as motion patterns. The data obtained through these analyses are quantifiable and therefore provide the therapist with baseline data that can be used to plan treatment programs and evaluate progress toward goals or goal attainment. The fact that the data are quantifiable is important because third-party payers are demanding that therapists use measurable parameters when examining patient function, establishing treatment strategies, and documenting outcomes.

Spatial and temporal measures may be critical factors in determining a patient's independence in ambulation. For example, in a study by Graham et al.[132] of 174 ambulatory adults aged 65 years and older who were admitted to a medical-surgical unit, a walking velocity (69 ft/min [21 m/min]) was identified as a meaningful threshold to differentiate those capable of independent ambulation in a hospital setting from those requiring assistance. When considering community environments, an individual may need to attain a certain gait speed to cross a local street within the time allotted by a crossing light or may need to walk a certain distance to shop in the local supermarket.

In a study of walking capability of individuals greater than 3 months poststroke, Perry et al.[133] established that walking speed was a valid predictor of community walking status. Speeds of less than 79 ft/min (24 m/min) predicted household walking, and speeds between 79 and 157 ft/min (24 and 48 m/min) predicted limited community walking status. The ability to walk faster than 157 ft/min (48 m/min) predicted unlimited community walking. It is interesting to note that the mean velocity of the community ambulators was only 60% of the 262 ft/min (80 m/min) average velocity of typical, nondisabled adults.[37] This slower velocity is sufficient for many typical activities that individuals recovering from a stroke may need to perform, yet it is less than the normal capacity required to cross a wide commercial street within the traffic signal time.[134] More recent research by Fulk et al.[135] demonstrated that the gait speed values developed by Perry et al. may overestimate actual walking activity in the home and community. The authors reported that for stroke survivors, a comfortable gait speed of 96 ft/min (29 m/min) discriminated between home and community ambulators, and a comfortable gait speed of 183 ft/min (56 m/min) discriminated between limited community and full community ambulators.[135]

Therapists need to survey the community to determine the distance and time requirements for accessing stores and public buildings before making a judgment about a patient's functional ambulation status. Considering the large footprints of many supermarkets, club warehouses, and hardware stores, individuals should be able to ambulate for a minimum of about 2,000 feet (600 meters) without sitting down in order to independently ambulate in the community.[136] Robinett and Vondran[137] found that target goals on a sample of gait analysis forms were low compared to distance and velocity requirements for crossing the street found in a community survey. Walsh et al.[138] reported that individuals 1 year after total knee arthroplasty achieved more than 80% of the normal walking speeds of their age- and gender-matched

counterparts. However, for 62% of the females and 25% of the males, the normal walking speed attained would not be sufficient to cross a street intersection safely.

Spatial and Temporal Variables

The variables measured in a quantitative gait analysis are listed and described in Table 7.11. Because spatial and temporal variables are affected by a number of factors such as age,[139–143] sex,[144,145] height and weight,[146,147] level of physical activity,[148,149] and level of maturation,[150] attempts have been made to take some of these factors into account. Ratios, such as stride length divided by functional leg length, may be used to normalize for differences in patients' leg lengths. Step length divided by the subject's height is a method sometimes used to normalize differences among patients' heights. In an attempt to control for both height and weight, body weight is divided by standing height to yield the body mass index. Other ratios are used to assess symmetry, for example, right swing time divided by left swing time and swing time divided by stance time. Sutherland et al.[150] listed the ratio of pelvic span to ankle spread as one way to determine development of mature gait in children.

Table 7.11	Gait Variables: Quantitative Gait Analysis
Variable	Description
Speed	A scalar quantity that has magnitude but not direction.
Free speed	A person's normal walking speed.
Slow speed	A speed slower than a person's normal speed.
Fast speed	A rate faster than normal.
Cadence	The number of steps taken per unit of time (e.g., steps/minute). $$Cadence = \frac{number\ of\ steps}{time}$$ A simple method of measuring cadence is by counting the number of steps taken in a given amount of time. The only equipment necessary is a stopwatch, paper, and pencil. The average cadence of adult women (117 steps/min) is slightly higher than of adult men (111 steps/min).[37]
Velocity	A measure of a body's motion in a given direction.
Linear velocity	The rate at which a body moves in a straight line.
Angular velocity	The rate of rotation of a body segment around an axis.
Walking velocity	The rate of linear forward motion of the body. This is measured in either centimeters per second or meters per minute. To obtain a person's walking velocity, divide the distance traversed by the time required to complete the distance. $$Walking\ velocity = \frac{distance}{time}$$ Walking velocity may be affected by age, level of maturation, height, gender, type of footwear, and weight. Also, velocity may affect cadence, step, stride length, and foot angle as well as other gait variables. The average self-selected walking velocity of 20- to 85-year-old males (86 m/min) is slightly faster than similar-aged females (77 m/min).[37]

(Continued)

Table 7.11 Gait Variables: Quantitative Gait Analysis—cont'd

Variable	Description
Acceleration	The rate of change of velocity with respect to time. Body acceleration has been defined by Smidt and Mommens[349] as the rate of change of velocity of a point posterior to the sacrum. Acceleration is usually measured in meters per second per second (m/s^2).
Angular acceleration	The rate of change of the angular velocity of a body with respect to time. Angular acceleration is usually measured in radians per second per second ($radians/s^2$).
Stride time	The amount of time that elapses during one stride; that is, from one foot contact (heel strike if possible) until the next contact of the same foot (heel strike). Both stride times should be measured. Measurement is usually in seconds.
Step time	The amount of time that elapses between consecutive right and left foot contacts (heel strikes). Both right and left step times should be measured. Measurement is in seconds.
Stride length	The linear distance between two successive points of contact of the same foot. It is measured in centimeters or meters. The average stride length for normal adult males is 1.46 meters.[37] The average stride length for adult females is 1.28 meters.[37]
Swing time	The amount of time during the gait cycle that one foot is off the ground. Swing time should be measured separately for right and left extremities. Measurement is in seconds.
Double support time	The amount of time spent in the gait cycle when both lower extremities are in contact with the supporting surface. Measured in seconds.
Cycle time (stride time)	The amount of time required to complete a gait cycle. Measured in seconds.
Step length	The linear distance between two successive points of contact of the right and left lower extremities. Usually a measurement is taken from the point of heel contact at initial contact of one extremity to the point of heel contact of the opposite extremity. If a patient does not have a heel strike on one or both sides, the measurement can be taken from the heads of the first metatarsals. Measured in centimeters or meters.
Width of walking base (step width)	The width of the walking base (base of support) is the linear distance (in the frontal plane) between one foot and the opposite foot. Measured in centimeters or meters.
Foot angle (degree of toe out or toe in)	The angle of foot placement with respect to the line of progression. Measured in degrees.
Bilateral Stance time (for the FAP)	The length of time up to 30 seconds that a person can stand upright in the parallel bars bearing weight on both lower extremities.
Uninvolved stance time (for the FAP)	The length of time up to 30 seconds that an individual can stand in the parallel bars while bearing weight on the uninvolved lower extremity (involved extremity is raised off the supporting surface).
Involved stance time (for the FAP)	The length of time up to 30 seconds that an individual can stand in the parallel bars on the involved lower extremity (uninvolved lower extremity is raised off the supporting surface).
Dynamic weight transfer rate (for the FAP)	The rate at which an individual standing in the parallel bars can transfer weight from one extremity to another. Measured in seconds from the first lift-off to the last lift-off.
Parallel bar ambulation (for the FAP)	Length of time required for an individual to walk the length of the parallel bars as rapidly as possible. Two trials are averaged to obtain this measurement. Measurement is in seconds.

FAP = Functional Ambulation Profile.

Measurement of Spatial and Temporal Variables

The techniques and equipment required for measurement of spatial and temporal variables range from simple to complex. The time requirements also vary, and the therapist must be familiar with different methods of examining these variables in order to select the method most appropriate to each situation. Before selecting a measurement method, the therapist must understand the variable in question and how that variable is related to the patient's gait.

Simple Methods of Measuring Spatial and Temporal Variables

Measurement of spatial variables such as degree of foot angle, width of base of support (BOS), step length, and stride length can be determined simply and inexpensively by recording the patient's footprints during gait. Simple methods of recording footprints include either the application of paints, ink, or chalk to the bottom of the patient's foot or shoe. For example, ink-soaked patches[151] and felt-tipped markers[152] have been attached to the bottom or back of patient's shoes to measure variables such as step length, stride length, step width, and foot angle.

Another way of obtaining step length and stride length data is by placing a grid pattern on the floor.[153] Masking tape is placed on the floor to create a straight-line grid pattern about 1 foot (30 cm) wide and 32 feet (10 meters) long. The tape is marked off in 1-in. (3-cm) increments for its entire length, and the segments are numbered consecutively so that the patient's heel strikes can be identified. The therapist then calls out the heel strike locations from the numbers on the grid pattern into a tape recorder.

Many variables, such as velocity, stride length, step length, and cadence, may be calculated by using a stopwatch to measure the elapsed time required for a patient to walk a known distance and recording the number of right and left steps during that same period (see Table 7.11). If assessing variables across a short distance (e.g., 20 or 30 feet [6 or 10 meters]), patients are often positioned a few steps before the "start line" so that they can achieve a steady state for the data collection.[93,151] They are also encouraged to walk a few steps beyond the "finish line." The "rolling start and finish" mitigates the influence of slow velocities at the initiation and termination of a walk on overall values compared to the "standing start and finish."[93]

Todd et al.[143] tested 84 typically developing children (41 girls and 43 boys) aged 13 months to 12 years and analyzed data from more than 200 other children aged 11 months to 16 years. A two-dimensional gait graph was developed that provides a visual record of a child's walking performance. Although the gait graph is similar in appearance to graphs used for height and weight, it shows norms for gait dimensions of cadence and stride length adjusted by height.

Two relatively simple and standardized methods that have been used to quantify walking speed in the clinical setting are the 6-minute Walk Test (6MWT) and the 10MWT. A stopwatch and tape measure are the tools required to complete the tests. See Table 7.9 for MCID and MDC values for the 6MWT and 10MWT. A form for recording temporal and spatial gait parameters is presented in Appendix 7.B (online).

6-MINUTE WALK TEST

In the 6MWT,[154,155] the distance covered walking for 6 minutes is determined. Whereas the tool was initially used as a measure of endurance and exercise capacity for individuals with cardiac and pulmonary pathology,[154,155] it has since been used to assess walking endurance in clients with a variety of underlying conditions, including Parkinson disease,[156] acquired brain injury,[157] stroke,[158] and CP.[159] One protocol for performing the 6MWT includes asking clients to walk as far as they can at their usual pace for 6 minutes while using their customary assistive devices and orthotics.[160] Clients walk in a tight oval path around two chairs spaced 18 meters apart, facilitating calculation of the overall distance traveled. Another protocol, used by the American Thoracic Society, emphasizes walking "as far as possible" while clients walk on a straight line and pivot around cones placed 30 meters apart.[161] Participants stop and rest as needed, but the stopwatch continues. Standardized encouragement is provided periodically. The final distance walked (in meters) is divided by either 6 to determine average speed in meters per minute or by 360 if reporting as meters per second.

This simple test, used in combination with other physical performance and impairment measures (e.g., ROM and muscle strength), can either monitor decline or evaluate improvement associated with treatment interventions. Mossberg[157] found that the 6MWT was a reliable measure of functional ambulation (distance walked) for patients with acquired brain injury. Fulk et al.[158] identified that the 6MWT score served as a significant predictor of the average number of steps taken per day by community-dwelling individuals with chronic stroke, accounting for 46% of the variance in community walking activity.

Numerous prediction equations have been developed to estimate the expected 6-minute walk distance based on factors such as height, age, weight, and heart rate; however, these equations have accounted for only 20% to 78% of the variance in 6MWT distances in individuals without known disability.[162–169] Variations in the procedures used across studies, as well as variability in the ages studied, likely contributed to differences in predicted outcomes for the distance walked in 6 minutes. Factors that appear to improve reliability between testing sessions include standardizing the instructions given to the patient, the type and amount of verbal encouragement, and the location of testing (e.g., a long corridor or a circular track).[93,162,170] These factors, as well as other patient characteristics such as age, height, weight, and even ethnicity,[162,166,169] should be considered when comparing a patient's value to normative data.

Fulk et al.[135] reported that distance traversed during the 6MWT was the strongest predictor of home versus community ambulation performance and limited versus full/unlimited community ambulation status in a secondary analysis of walking activity data from two stroke trials. A 6MWT distance of at least 205 meters discriminated between home and community ambulators, while the capacity to walk farther than at least 288 meters differentiated between limited and unlimited community ambulators.

Alternative tests for individuals with limited endurance include the 1-minute Walk Test,[171–173] 2-minute Walk Test (2MWT),[174,175] and 3-minute Walk Test.[81] A 12-minute Walk Test also is available for individuals with greater endurance.[155,174]

TIMED WALK TESTS (5 METERS, 10 METERS, AND 30 METERS)

Timed walked tests measure how long it takes to walk a specified distance and then use these data to calculate an average walking speed. Different distances have been used, including 5 meters,[176,177] 10 meters,[175,178–180] and 30 meters.[180] One common protocol for performing a 10MWT is to have the client ambulate across a 14-m walkway using their traditional assistive and LE orthotic devices.[160] The time (seconds) required to traverse the middle 10 meters of the walkway is recorded with a stopwatch. Two repetitions are completed at the client's preferred comfortable speed and at a fast pace. Speed (m/sec) is calculated by dividing 10 meters by the time (in seconds) required to traverse the path. To determine speed in m/min, the previously calculated speed is multiplied by 60. Average cadence and stride length also can be calculated by recording the number of steps required to traverse the 10 meters. Physiological responses (e.g., heart rate, blood pressure, respiratory rate) can be monitored immediately before and after the walking trial.

Despite efforts to standardize the test, some variability still is evident in the published literature, including the path taken (i.e., straight line versus a turn), use of assistive devices, speed (self-selected comfortable versus fast), and use of a rolling start and finish (i.e., capacity to take a few steps before and after start and finish lines, respectively) versus a standing start and finish.[93] Thus, when comparing a patient's speed to published normative data, consideration should be given to procedures used.

Low-Cost Instrumentation for Quantifying Spatial and Temporal Variables

ACCELEROMETERS

During walking, the body generates forces that can be measured using an accelerometer. These data can then

be used to calculate spatial and temporal gait features such as cadence, step symmetry, step duration, and stride duration. The methods for measuring the acceleration forces vary widely (e.g., strain gauge, piezo-resistive, capacitive, and piezoelectric), but in general, many of these devices provide an affordable, noninvasive, easy-to-apply means for quantifying select gait characteristics over extended periods (days to weeks) in the home and community.[181]

Triaxial accelerometers have been attached to the trunk in order to measure mean acceleration, cadences, and step and stride lengths.[182–186] Accelerometers have also been attached to the head and pelvis to determine acceleration patterns of these anatomical regions while subjects walked on different surfaces.[187] Simultaneous use of multiple accelerometers has enabled successful differentiation of locomotor activities for both patient and nonpatient populations,[188–191] as seen with the use of Opal sensor-based analysis system. For example, one system used five accelerometers (one on each foot and thigh and one on the sternum) to differentiate walking speeds (slow, medium, and fast) and types of activities (e.g., walking, stair negotiation, running, and jumping) with a high level of accuracy (greater than 94%) in 69 participants free of any known impairments of the locomotor system.[192]

The accuracy of accelerometer data can be impacted by many factors.[181,192,193] Devices need to be oriented correctly in relation to the manufacturer's specifications; otherwise the acceleration signals may not correspond correctly with the direction of movement, and interpretation will be confounded. Significant adipose tissue, UE movement to use assistive devices, or excessively loose mounting of the device can introduce movement artifact into the signal, again confounding interpretation. Finally, in patient populations, the acceleration signals may be altered if pathology disrupts normal foot-floor contact patterns or contributes to abnormal alignment of body parts (e.g., the impact of a persistent forward trunk lean on a trunk-mounted accelerometer in an individual with Parkinson disease).[181]

The StepWatch Activity Monitor (SAM) is one example of a commercially available accelerometer.[194–198] It records the number of strides taken in 1-minute intervals during daily activities for up to 15 consecutive days. The SAM includes a sensor (custom accelerometer) that measures 3 × 1.9 × 0.55 in (75 × 48 × 14 mm) and weighs approximately 1.4 oz (41 g; Fig. 7.5). The battery provides 35 to 41 days of normal use.[199,200] The case is contoured to fit just above the lateral malleolus and is attached by an elastic strap. A personal computer is used to set up the SAM for monitoring and also for downloading data to a computer. Michael et al.[195] used the SAM to evaluate the walking capacity of adults in the chronic phase of stroke recovery and identified significantly reduced step frequency (mean = 2,837 steps/day) compared to sedentary older adults (5,000 to 6,000 steps/day).

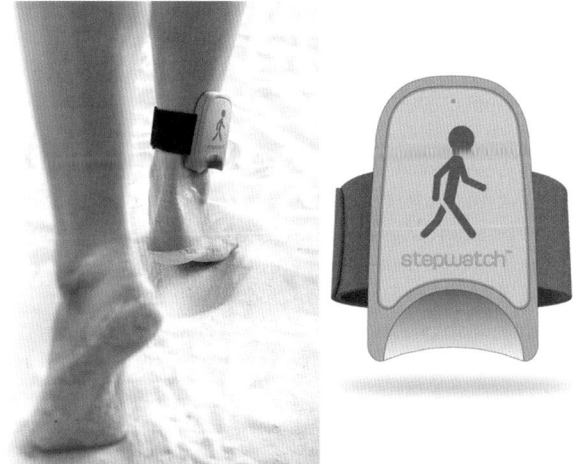

Figure 7.5 The StepWatch Activity Monitor 4 (SAM) is worn at the ankle for long-term monitoring of gait function. *(Courtesy of Modus Health, Edmonds, WA 98020.)*

Consumer-oriented activity/step-count monitors may be useful for characterizing stepping capacity in select clinical populations, particularly given findings that individuals with disabilities and older adults often have low step counts.[201] For example, Fitbit activity monitors have been used with a variety of populations to evaluate step count in laboratory and real-world environments.[202–208] Steps counted using the Fitbit (One and Zip) demonstrated excellent agreement (ICC = 0.88) with the number of visually counted steps during a 2MWT in a study of 32 community-dwelling older adults without known pathology.[209] Fulk et al.[210] compared steps recorded during a 2MWT using the Fitbit Ultra to those documented from videotaped recordings of the same test and reported that in high-functioning people with chronic stroke and TBI, the Fitbit Ultra might provide a low-cost alternative for measuring step activity compared to other, more expensive, activity-monitoring devices. Although the Fitbit Ultra's step count accuracy (ICC [2,1] = 0.73) exceeded those of other consumer-oriented activity monitors tested, including the Yamax Digi-Walker SW-701 (ICC [2,1] = 0.42) and the Nike+ FuelBand (ICC [2,1] = 0.20), the accuracy was below that of the SAM (ICC [2,1] = 0.97). On average, all devices (including the SAM) underestimated the actual number of steps taken.

When considering the pediatric population with disabilities, the Fitbit technology has provided adequate interpretation of stepping when validated against video recordings.[211,212] For children 11.8 ± 3.1 years old with impaired gait (Gross Motor Function Classification Levels I to III) due to CP (*n* = 8) and brain injury (*n* = 4), excellent mean absolute percent errors (MAPEs; values ≤5% are considered excellent, and ≥10% are considered poor) were identified with the Fitbit Zip used at the manufacturer's recommended hip location (median 2.0%, average 3.9%). Interestingly, similar MAPEs were observed when the device was used at the ankle (median 2.7%, average 3.0%), a location not suggested by the manufacturer. Of note, two children who exhibited the lowest functional characteristics (average modified Timed Up and Go Test of 19.4 seconds, average walking speed of 0.67 m/s, and average Pediatric Balance Scale of 9.5 of 56) compared with the other participants demonstrated the poorest MAPEs for both hip (17.3% and 10.4%) and ankle (8.9% and 6.2%).[212] The Fitbit technology was also analyzed with the Fitbit Charge in which its standard recommended placement is on the wrist. Children (average age 12 ± 3 years) with impaired gait due to CP (n = 6), brain injury (n = 5), stroke (n = 2), and acute transverse myelitis (n = 1) performed walking activities with the device placed on both involved and noninvolved sides. Considering the entire group of participants (28 wrists), the Fitbit Charge demonstrated excellent accuracy with MAPE of 3.2%. When step count was analyzed only from the participants' involved side (n = 20 wrists), acceptable accuracy was detected with MAPE of 7.7%.[211] Fitbit may be an appropriate wearable technology to track step count, even when used on the involved side, of children and adolescents with neurologic-induced gait impairment.

GYROSCOPES

Another type of instrument that may be used to estimate spatial and temporal gait parameters are *gyroscopes*. These devices measure the Coriolis acceleration of a vibrating triangular prism. The signal from the prism is proportional to the angular velocity. The instruments are light, portable, and relatively inexpensive. A single uniaxial gyroscope attached on the skin surface of the lower leg can provide data for calculating cadence, determining number of steps, and estimating stride length and walking speed.[213]

Kotiadis et al.[214] developed an integrated system that included accelerometers, gyroscopes, and customized inertial algorithms to replace the footswitches often used to trigger drop foot stimulators. Testing and refinement were performed for an individual after stroke who used a footswitch-driven drop foot stimulator. The combination of accelerometer and gyroscope data was sufficient for defining gait phases and controlling the drop foot stimulator during walking and stair-negotiation activities.

Instrumented Systems for Determining Spatial and Temporal Gait Parameters

Commercially available walkways (e.g., GAITRite, Strideway, Zeno) and footswitch systems (e.g., Krusen Limb Monitor, Stride Analyzer) can be used to measure spatial and temporal gait variables. Manufacturer contact information for select equipment is presented in Appendix 7.C (online).

WALKWAYS

Compared to more complex systems that require cameras and footswitches, instrumented walkways provide a reliable, valid, and relatively affordable means for rapidly quantifying spatial and temporal gait parameters.[215–221] These portable devices are used by clinics and research facilities to help classify and quantify the severity of a patient's disability and to guide and assess the effectiveness of treatment interventions. Two walkways widely available are the GAITRite and the Zeno Walkway.

The GAITRite is one example of a commercially available walkway system (Fig. 7.6). The 1/8-in.-thick, 2-foot-wide, 16-foot-long portable walkway in this system contains 18,482 sensors embedded between a sheet of vinyl and a layer of rubber. Spatial and temporal parameters can be measured, as can dynamic pressure mapping of footprints during walking. The pressure parameters measured include peak pressure, pressure time, and sectional integrated pressure over time. The walkway system can be used with or without shoes, orthoses, or walking aids, and the GAITRite software is capable of calculating spatial and temporal parameters and displaying them in graphs and tables.

In general, the GAITRite provides a valid means for reliably documenting many gait-related temporal and spatial parameters.[217,218,220] Bilney et al.[220] reported high correlations between values recorded on the GAITRite mat and those recorded using the Clinical Stride Analyzer for walking speed (0.99), stride length (0.99), and cadence (0.99) for 25 healthy adults walking at three speeds (self-selected, slow, and fast). The reliability of repeated measures appears to be better at self-selected and fast speeds compared to slower speeds.[220] Decreased consistency across measurements was documented for BOS[218,219] and toe in and toe out variables,[218,219]

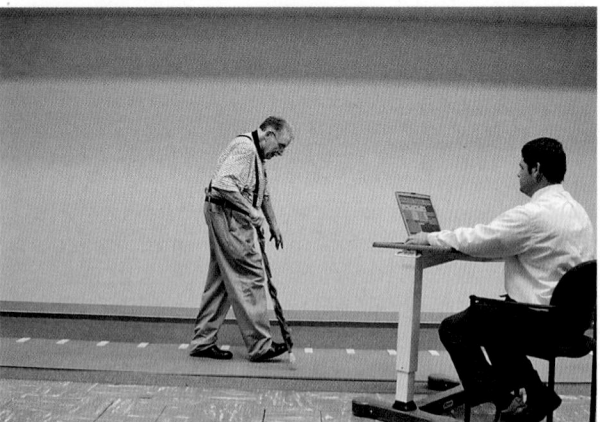

Figure 7.6 Individual with Parkinson disease walking across the GAITRite mat while temporal and spatial gait characteristics are recorded, including walking velocity, stride length and duration, cadence, and step length and duration. *(Courtesy of Movement and Neurosciences Center, Institute for Rehabilitation Science and Engineering, Madonna Rehabilitation Hospitals, Lincoln, NE 68506.)*

particularly in older adults.[219] Strong concurrent validity also has been reported for temporal and spatial gait measures recorded in outpatients recovering from strokes, even when the UE was engaged in using an assistive device.[216] The Evidence Summary Table (Table 7.12) provides an overview of selected reliability and validity studies performed using the GAITRite mat.

The portable Zeno Walkway system (Fig. 7.7) is available in 8- to 52-foot lengths and varying widths (2, 3, or 4 feet). One key feature relative to other commercially available instrumented walkways is the availability of wider mats that allow use with gait tests requiring turning maneuvers. The Zeno walkway integrates 16 levels of pressure sensors (each 1 cm in diameter) to detect gait characteristics. Spatial (e.g., step length, step width, toe in/out angle) and temporal (e.g., velocity, single limb, and double limb support time) parameters can be displayed side by side with videos and images from an integrated video camera system. The software can also be used to calculate an estimated center of mass and to detect pressure applied through an assistive device (e.g., walker or cane). Humphrey et al.[222] reported moderate to high ICC values of spatial and temporal variables recorded between the Zeno Walkway and the GAITRite with 30 older adults (average age 75 ± 6 years) without known disabilities walking across both systems at self-selected comfortable (e.g., step length ICC = 0.892; stride length ICC = 0.899; single support % ICC = 0.835) and fast speeds (step length ICC = 0.921; stride length ICC = 0.919; single support % ICC = 0.877). The Zeno system/software has been used across a variety of patient populations, including studies focused on freezing of gait in Parkinson disease,[223] as well as gait initiation[224] and termination[225,226] in individuals with multiple sclerosis. The Evidence Summary Table (Table 7.12) provides an overview of one selected validity study performed using the Zeno Walkway system.

FOOTSWITCHES AND FOOTSWITCH SYSTEMS

Footswitches are pressure-sensitive switches placed either on the patient's feet or the inside or outside of the shoes. The switches do not require a walkway, but the patient usually has to carry or wear a data collection device. Footswitches consist of transducers and a semiconductor and are used to signal such events as the heel contacting the ground. One type of footswitch device used to examine both temporal and loading variables is the Krusen Limb Load Monitor.[227] This device consists of a pressure-sensitive force plate that can be worn in a patient's shoe. It can be connected to a strip chart recorder to yield a permanent record of temporal and spatial gait variables.[227]

The Stride Analyzer is a footswitch system with special insoles containing four pressure-sensitive switches placed under the heel, the heads of the first and fifth metatarsals, and the great toe. The parameters measured by this system include stride length, velocity, cadence,

Table 7.12	Evidence Summary Table

Reliability and Validity of GAITRite System's Temporal and Spatial Gait Variables

Bilney et al. (2003)[220]
Adults Without Disabilities

Subjects	• 12 females and 13 males, age 40.5 ± 17.2 years (range 21–71 years)
Approach	• Concurrent validity between GAITRite and Clinical Stride Analyzer • Self-selected slow, comfortable, and fast speeds • Variables: speed, cadence, stride length, single support time, double support
Results	• Excellent agreement between the two systems for speed, cadence, and step length during all three walking speed conditions • Double support showed largest mean difference between two systems • Correlations between two systems for single leg support time were moderate to high
Conclusion	• GAITRite exhibited strong concurrent validity and test–retest reliability for selected spatial and temporal variables in normal adults

Cho et al. (2014)[350]
Adults With Stroke

Subjects	• 23 females and 20 males, age 52 ± 4 years, 7 ± 0.9 months poststroke
Approach	• Self-selected comfortable walking speed (single task) • Self-selected comfortable walking speed while counting backward (dual task) • Variables: speed, cadence, step and stride length, and single limb support period
Results	• Single-task condition: ICC values were high (0.99) for all variables with lowest ICC recorded for paretic leg stride length (0.98) • Dual-task condition: ICC values ranged from 0.69 (cadence) to 0.90 (paretic leg step length)
Conclusion	• GAITRite test–retest reliability for spatial and temporal gait parameters under single- and dual-task conditions was good to very good

Cleland et al. (2019)[351]
Adults With Chronic Stroke

Subjects	• 24 females and 53 males, age 59 ± 9 years (range 41–80 years), 5.8 ± 5.2 years (range 0.5– 32.8 years) poststroke
Approach	• Concurrent validity between GAITRite and 10MWT • Walking at self-selected comfortable and fast speeds • Variable: speed
Results	• Poor to good agreement for comfortable walking speed (ICC = 0.77 [95% CI: 0.46, 0.89]) • Excellent agreement for maximal walking speed (ICC = 0.94 [95% CI: 0.91, 0.96])
Conclusion	• 10MWT and GAITRite measures may not be used interchangeably • Conducting 10MWT and GAITRite tests at fast walking speeds may allow for more accurate comparison between measures

Graser et al. (2016)[352]
Children With Neurological Gait Disorders

Subjects	• Nine girls and 21 boys, age 13 ± 3.6 years, inpatient rehabilitation due to cerebral palsy, stroke, traumatic brain injury, demyelination of central nervous system, astrocytoma, postinfectious encephalopathy, medulla blastoma, transverse myelopathy, and ataxia
Approach	• Test–retest reliability • 10MWT at *self-selected comfortable and fast speeds*, and 6MWT • Variables: speed, cadence, double support, step length, speed normalized to leg length, step-extremity-ratio (ratio of leg and step length), and step time

(Continued)

Table 7.12	Evidence Summary Table—cont'd

Reliability and Validity of GAITRite System's Temporal and Spatial Gait Variables

Graser et al. (2016)[352]
Children With Neurological Gait Disorders

Results	• Median ICC from all GAITRite variables was 0.93 • Lowest ICCs for step length on less affected side during 10MWT at fast speed (0.61), for step time on more affected side during 10MWT at comfortable speed (0.81), and for extremity-step-ratio (for less affected side) during 10MWT at comfortable speed (0.81) • Highest ICC for step length symmetry during 10MWT comfortable speed (0.95) and for step length (most affected side and left side) during 6MWT (0.97)
Conclusion	• Reliable timed walking tests and spatiotemporal gait parameters obtained from GAITRite system

Menz et al. (2004)[219]
Young and Older Adults Without Disabilities

Subjects	• 18 females and 12 males, age 28.5 ± 4.8 years (range 22–40 years) • 18 females and 13 males, age 80.8 ± 3.1 years (range 76–87 years)
Approach	• Test–retest reliability • Self-selected comfortable speed • Variables: speed, cadence, step length, base of support, toe in/out
Results	• Excellent reliability (ICCs 0.82–0.92) for walking speed, cadence, and step length for young and older adults • High reliability (ICCs 0.49–0.94) for base of support and toe in/out; however, high variability for young (coefficient of variation 8.3%–17.7%) and older adults (coefficient of variation 14.3%–33%)
Conclusion	• GAITRite displayed excellent reliability for most temporal and spatial gait parameters for both groups • Base of support and toe in/out angles should be interpreted cautiously in older adults

Peters et al. (2014)[353]
Adults With Stroke Grouped by Ambulatory Capacity

Subjects	• HA: 4 females and 8 males, age 59.6 ± 11.4 years, 30 ± 29.7 months poststroke, self-selected walking speed <0.4 m/s • LCA: 4 females and 20 males, age 64.5 ± 10.3 years, 42 ± 35.8 months poststroke, self-selected walking speed 0.4–0.8 m/s • CA: 11 females and 15 males, age 62.6 ± 14.9 years, 26.7 ± 21.4 months poststroke, self-selected walking speed of >0.8 m/s
Approach	• Concurrent validity and reliability between GAITRite and 3MWT • Self-selected walking speed
Results	Average walking speed differed between GAITRite and 3MWT for all groups: • HA: GAITRite 0.25 (0.11) m/s, 3MWT 0.27 (0.11) m/s • LCA: GAITRite 0.56 (0.11) m/s, 3MWT 0.52 (0.10) m/s • CA: GAITRite 1.03 (0.16) m/s, 3MWT 0.89 (0.15) m/s Excellent within-session reliability for walking measurements: • GAITRite, ICC of 0.97 for HA, 0.89 for LCA, 0.93 for CA • 3MWT, ICC of 0.97 for HA, 0.91 for LCA, 0.85 for CA
Conclusion	• Although both 3MWT and GAITRite exhibited highly reliable measures of walking speed, the two measures did not demonstrate concurrent validity • Tests should not be used interchangeably in this population

Roche et al. (2018)[354]
Children and Young Adults With Friedreich Ataxia

Subjects	• 18 females and 18 males, age 16.4 ± 4.5 years (range 7.1–24.7 years), age at onset 9.1 ± 4.0 years (range 2.0–16.4 years)

Table 7.12	Evidence Summary Table—cont'd

Reliability and Validity of GAITRite System's Temporal and Spatial Gait Variables

Roche et al. (2018)[354]

Children and Young Adults With Friedreich Ataxia

Approach	• Reproducibility of gait spatio-temporal parameters • Self-selected walking speed (barefoot) • Variables: speed, speed normalized by leg length, cadence, step and stride length, step and stride time, base of support, percent of gait cycle in swing and stance phase and in single and double support phase, foot progression angle, GVI, and Functional Ambulation Performance
Results	• Most parameters showed high and very high reproducibility (ICC >0.8) except foot progression angle (ICC = 0.71) and base of support (ICC = 0.74) • Perfect agreement for stride time (ICC = 1.00) • Poor or fair reproducibility was not observed for any of the parameters
Conclusion	• Reliable in young patients affected by Friedreich ataxia • Some parameters are more clinically relevant (speed, cadence, double support, step length, and GVI) and deserve further investigation • Foot progression angle and base of support were weakest parameters, attributed to the software automatic errors and ankle laxity noted in every patient

Schmitz-Hübsch et al. (2016)[189]

Adults With Spinocerebellar Ataxia Type 14

Subjects	• Three females and five males, age 53 years (range 29–70 years), disease duration 18 years (range 5–33 years)
Approach	• Reliability and validity between GAITRite and Opal inertial sensor–based system • Walking pace at very slow, slow, comfortable, fast, and maximal speeds • Variables: cadence, gait cycle time, stride length, stride speed, double support time, coefficient of variance of stride time and stride length, stride length/cadence ratio
Results	• Accuracy and repeatability of gait measurements were not compromised by ataxic gait disorder • Accuracy of spatial measures was speed-dependent and direct comparison of stride length from both devices most reliable at comfortable speed • Measures of stride variability had low agreement between methods
Conclusion	• Accuracy of spatial measures was speed-dependent and a direct comparison of stride length from both devices is most reliable at comfortable walking speed

Stokic et al. (2009)[216]

Individuals Without Disabilities and Adults With Chronic Stroke

Subjects	• Without disability: 23 females and 29 males, age 47 ± 15 years (range 23–87 years) • Stroke: nine females and 11 males, age 58 ± 20 years (range 16–90 years), 4 ± 7 years poststroke
Approach	• Agreement between GAITRite and 3D video-based motion capture system • Self-selected comfortable walking speed • Variables: speed, stride time and length, step length, single support, total support
Results	• Mean differences between two methods were ≤1.5% of mean values calculated for each group
Conclusion	• GAITRite and motion analysis system provided comparable temporal and spatial measures

Van Uden and Besser (2004)[218]

Adults Without Disabilities

Subjects	• Nine women and 12 men, age 34 years (range 19–59 years)
Approach	• Test–retest reliability • Self-selected comfortable and fast speeds • Variables: speed, step length, stride length, base of support, step time, stride time, swing time, stance time, single and double support times, toe in/toe out angle

(Continued)

Table 7.12	Evidence Summary Table—cont'd

Reliability and Validity of GAITRite System's Temporal and Spatial Gait Variables

Van Uden and Besser (2004)[218]
Adults Without Disabilities

Results	• During comfortable walking speed, all measurements exhibited ICCs ≥0.92 except base of support (ICC = 0.80) • During fast walking speed, all measurements exhibited ICCs >0.89 except base of support (ICC = 0.79)
Conclusion	• Good to excellent test–retest reliability

Webster et al. (2005)[355]
Adults With Unicompartmental Knee Replacement

Subjects	• Five females and five males, age 66.5 years (range 54–83 years), >10.1 years postsurgery
Approach	• Concurrent validity between GAITRite and Vicon motion analysis system • Self-selected and fast walking speeds • Variables: speed, cadence, step length, step time
Results	• Excellent level of agreement between systems for all variables
Conclusion	• GAITRite is valid for measuring averaged and individual step gait variables

Wong et al. (2014)[356]
Adults With Sub-Acute Stroke

Subjects	• 14 females and 32 males, age 68 ± 14 years (range 35–94 years), 27 ± 15 (range 8–90) days poststroke
Approach	• Inter- and intrarater reliability • Self-selected comfortable walking speed • Five raters independently processed gait data, including speed, step time, step length, and step width • Three raters reprocessed data after delay of at least 1 month
Results	• Interrater reliability: High ICC (0.94–0.99) for all variables with lowest values for left (0.81) and right (0.84) step width • Intrarater reliability: Highest ICCs for speed and right step length (0.99–>0.99), with largest range of ICC values observed for left step width (0.74–0.97) and right step width (0.96)
Conclusion	• Reliable to quantify spatial and temporal characteristics of gait in individuals attending inpatient stroke rehabilitation • Further recommendation involves same rater processing all data

Reliability and Validity of Zeno Walkway System's Temporal and Spatial Gait Variables

Vallabhajosula et al. (2019)[357]
Older Adults With Fall Risk

Subjects	• Low-risk group: 19 females and 11 males, age 75.1 ± 6.3 years, no falls 6 months prior to study, three falls 12 months prior to study • High-risk group: 13 females and four males, age 81.1 ± 8.3 years, seven falls 6 months prior to study, 12 falls 12 months prior to study
Approach	• Concurrent validity between Zeno Walkway System and GAITRite • Walking at self-selected comfortable and fast speeds • Variables: speed, cadence, step length and time, stride length and width, stride speed, stance time, swing time, single and double support time, stance phase, swing phase, single support phase, total double support phase

Table 7.12	Evidence Summary Table—cont'd

Reliability and Validity of GAITRite System's Temporal and Spatial Gait Variables

Vallabhajosula et al. (2019)[357]

Older Adults With Fall Risk

Results	• Low-risk group, comfortable speed:
	  • Spatial parameters exhibited ICCs between 0.72 (stride width) and 0.92 (step length)
	  • Temporal parameters exhibited ICCs between 0.45 (step time) and 0.85 (stance phase, swing phase, single support phase)
	• Low-risk group, fast speed:
	  • Spatial parameters exhibited ICCs between 0.84 (stride width) and 0.94 (step length)
	  • Temporal parameters exhibited ICCs between 0.78 (swing time, single support time) and 0.96 (gait speed, stride speed)
	• High-risk group, comfortable speed:
	  • Spatial parameters exhibited ICCs between 0.85 (cadence) and 0.92 (gait speed, stride speed)
	  • Temporal parameters exhibited ICCs between 0.96 (stride width) and 0.97 (stride length)
	• High-risk group, fast speed:
	  • Spatial parameters exhibited ICCs between 0.95 (stride width) and 0.98 (stride length)
	  • Temporal parameters exhibited ICCs between 0.85 (single support phase) and 0.95 (stride speed)

Conclusion	• Acceptable concurrent validity between both systems

CA = community ambulators; CI = confidence interval; GVI = Gait Variability Index; HA= household ambulators; ICC = intraclass correlation coefficient; LCA = limited community ambulators; 10MWT = 10-minute Walk Test; 3MWT = 3-minute Walk Test; 6MWT = 6-minute Walk Test.

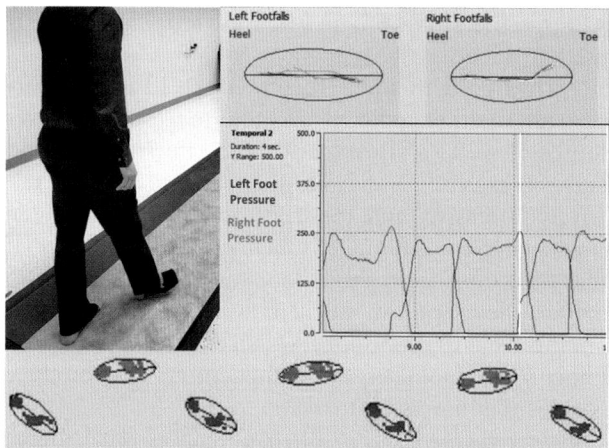

Figure 7.7 Example of data generated with ProtoKinetics software following walking trial performed on Zeno Walkway by individual with right meniscal tear. Right top graph indicates center of pressure excursion under each foot with red line representing the average excursion. Note the shortened excursion under right foot and toe-out pattern. Middle graph displays pressure pattern over time for three successive complete left footfalls (red line) and two right footfalls (blue line). Note the shortened stance time and peak pressures on affected (right) limb compared to unaffected (left) side. Bottom graph displays pressure pattern and relative foot angle across successive steps (left foot in green, right foot in purple). *(Courtesy of Movement and Neurosciences Center, Institute for Rehabilitation Science and Engineering, Madonna Rehabilitation Hospitals, Lincoln, NE 68506.)*

cycle time, single and double limb support time, swing time, and stance time. These measurements are recorded automatically, and the information is transmitted to a computer that analyzes the data. The computer can also provide graphic displays of foot–floor contact patterns. Times are presented in seconds and as a percentage of the gait cycle. The computer analysis also includes a percentage of normal using a built-in database (Appendix 7.D [online]). The advantages of the Stride Analyzer system are that measurements from both feet are available, the system is easy to move from place to place, and normative data comparisons are available because it has been used by a large number of physical therapists with different populations.[14–16,21,71,228–236]

The Stride Analyzer is suitable for use with various age groups as well as for patients with neurological or orthopedic involvement. For example, in a study by Mulroy et al.,[19] footswitches were taped to the shoe bottoms of 30 individuals recovering from a stroke to assess the effects of three ankle-foot orthosis (AFO) designs on walking and to determine whether an ankle plantar-flexion contracture influenced response to the orthoses. The conditions assessed included walking with usual footwear using three different AFOs, each with unique settings: (1) dorsiflexion assist with a dorsiflexion stop, (2) plantarflexion stop with free dorsiflexion, and (3) a rigid (solid) ankle. The footswitches were used to compare stride characteristics across conditions and to help define gait phases for subsequent analysis of joint kinematics and muscle activation patterns (electromyography [EMG]). Gait parameters were compared across the orthotic conditions and between participants with and without moderate ankle plantarflexion contractures. The authors reported that individuals without a contracture benefited from AFO designs that allowed stance phase dorsiflexion mobility (e.g., the plantarflexion stop with free dorsiflexion or the dorsiflexion assist with a dorsiflexion stop), as the rigid (solid) ankle inhibited forward progression of the tibia. Those with quadriceps weakness benefited from an AFO with plantarflexion mobility during loading response (i.e., the dorsiflexion assist with a dorsiflexion stop), as knee flexion motion was diminished compared to the other two AFO conditions.

Powers et al.[228] used the Stride Analyzer in an analysis of 22 individuals with transtibial amputations to determine the relationship between isometric muscle force and temporal and spatial gait parameters. Mean walking speed was limited to only 59% of normal, owing to reductions in both cadence (83% normal) and stride length (69% normal). Hip extensor torque of the residual limb served as the only predictor for both free and fast walking speeds. Hip abductor torque of the sound limb was the only predictor of cadence for free and fast walking speeds.

Evaluation of Joint Kinematics (Motion)

Electrogoniometers

Joint displacement can be measured relatively simply by using an electrogoniometer. Early electrogoniometer designs included two rigid links connected by a potentiometer that converted movement into an electrical signal that was proportional to the degree of movement. The rigid links or arms of the electrogoniometer were attached to the proximal and distal limb segments. More recent designs use a flexible shaft and two small end blocks that are affixed to the proximal and distal segments of the joint. The new design allows electrogoniometers to be worn under clothing for extended periods of recording time. Biometrics produces a wide variety of electrogoniometers, including twin-axis designs that simultaneously measure joint motion in multiple planes. Lam et al.[237] used these devices to study hips (abduction/adduction) and knees (flexion/extension) during corrective stumbling responses to mechanical perturbations applied to the foot of healthy infants during treadmill stepping. The authors reported that perturbations to the dorsum of the foot during swing resulted in an increase in flexor EMG activity and an increase in knee flexion during swing. Electrogoniometers provide an affordable means of measuring joint motion during walking.[37,238,239]

Video-Based Motion Analysis Systems

Two-dimensional (2D) and three-dimensional (3D) video-based motion analysis systems are available for gait analysis; however, their use is limited due to challenges with providing accurate data. Two-dimensional video-based systems use a single digital video camcorder to track subject motion. Computer software programs then assist with identifying points of reference. Unfortunately, joint angles that are out of plane (either because of rotation of the limb or due to the position of the individual relative to the camera) will not be calculated accurately. Three-dimensional video-based motion analysis systems use two or more digital video camcorders to gather 3D coordinate data. Hardware is used to synchronize data recorded from the various cameras, and postprocessing is used to identify points of reference either automatically or manually. Markers can be affixed to the skin to help identify anatomical landmarks. Though portable in nature, the accuracy of 2D and 3D video-based systems is a limitation.

Optical Marker-Based Motion Analysis Systems

Imaging-based systems are the most sophisticated and expensive methods of determining joint displacement and patterns of motion. In computerized motion analysis systems, markers placed on body segments, such as the hip, knee, and ankle, are tracked by automated systems. Motion analysis systems primarily use either *active* or *passive* markers for tracking motion.[36] *Active markers* are usually light-emitting diodes (LEDs) that flash at given frequencies.[240] Each marker is placed over a prespecified location, and its individual frequency is used to identify the marker as it moves across space at each instant in time. To power the LED, the participant is either tethered by cable to a central power source or wears a power pack. Fine cables then extend between each LED and the power unit. LEDs are relatively expensive, and the thin cables can break. One challenge to the automated labeling of active markers is that reflections from shiny floor surfaces can confound marker identification, particularly for markers located on the feet. Codamotion, Qualisys, PhaseSpace, and Phoenix Technologies are manufacturers that produce systems that use active markers.

Passive markers (Fig. 7.8) require an external source of illumination that may be provided by external light sources or by a ring of infrared-emitting diodes located around the camera lens. In the latter case, the diodes on the camera pick up the infrared light reflected by the markers that they can "see," which means that a large number of cameras are necessary for obtaining unrestricted views of markers. Qualisys, Vicon, and Motion Analysis are three manufacturers that produce systems that use passive markers.

When the systems were first developed, visualization of passive markers was problematic, but now markers are automatically tracked and a computer performs thousands of computations. However, passive marker systems require many cameras, are expensive, and require training to operate the hardware and software. Figure 7.9 provides an example of a computer-generated display of kinematic data recorded using

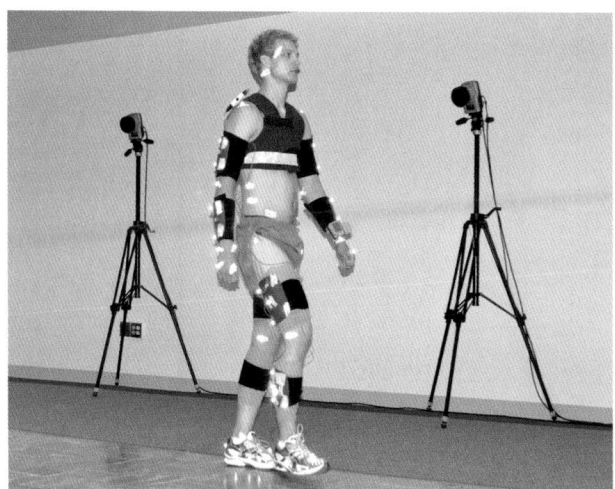

Figure 7.8 Qualisys Oqus Series-3 cameras track motion of passive reflective markers placed over known anatomical landmarks and in clusters on body segments as subject walks along a 6-meter walkway. Marker data will be used to reconstruct joint motions of the UEs, trunk, and lower extremities throughout the gait cycle. *(Courtesy of Movement and Neurosciences Center, Institute for Rehabilitation Science and Engineering, Madonna Rehabilitation Hospitals, Lincoln, NE 68506.)*

passive markers (Qualisys Motion Analysis system) as well as signals recorded from EMG sensors. In Figure 7.10, the degrees of motion for the knee and ankle are plotted against time (A) and are plotted as a percentage of a time-normalized gait cycle (B), where 0% corresponds to initial contact of the reference limb and 100% represents the next ipsilateral limb initial contact. In Figure 7.11, stick figures are shown with accompanying knee angles.

A number of important problems exist when using both active and passive marker systems. Obstruction of markers by body segments, skin/soft tissue motion, marker vibration, and improper placement of markers in relation to the joint center of motion can introduce potential errors. Determining the location of the hip joint center is particularly problematic. The ball-and-socket anatomy means that the center of the hip joint is located in the center of the femoral head. Difficulty palpating the femoral head makes accurate marker placement elusive. Radiographic studies have been performed to develop and refine algorithms that can be used to calculate the hip joint center relative to palpable landmarks (e.g., the anterior superior iliac spine, pubic tubercle).[241] Finally, inconsistencies in marker placement have been identified as one of the leading

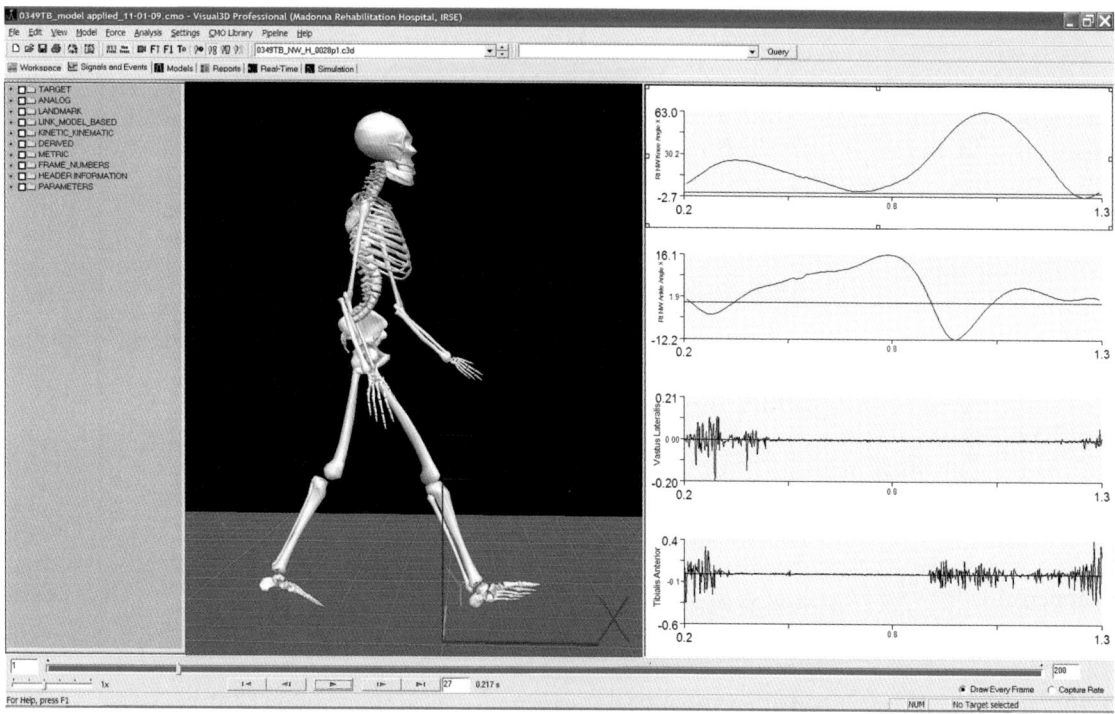

Figure 7.9 Visual 3D computer display of kinematic data recorded using the Qualisys Motion Analysis System and surface electromyographic data recorded using the MA-300 EMG system during overground gait for a 31-year-old male. Reflective markers, applied over known locations provided the anatomical reference for displayed skeleton and for subsequent analysis of joint motions. To the right of the skeleton, sagittal plane joint motions for the knee and ankle are displayed in the top two rows while surface EMG data for the vastus lateralis and tibialis anterior are displayed in the bottom two rows. *(Courtesy of Dr. Yu Shu, Movement and Neurosciences Center, Institute for Rehabilitation Science and Engineering, Madonna Rehabilitation Hospitals, Lincoln, NE 68506.)*

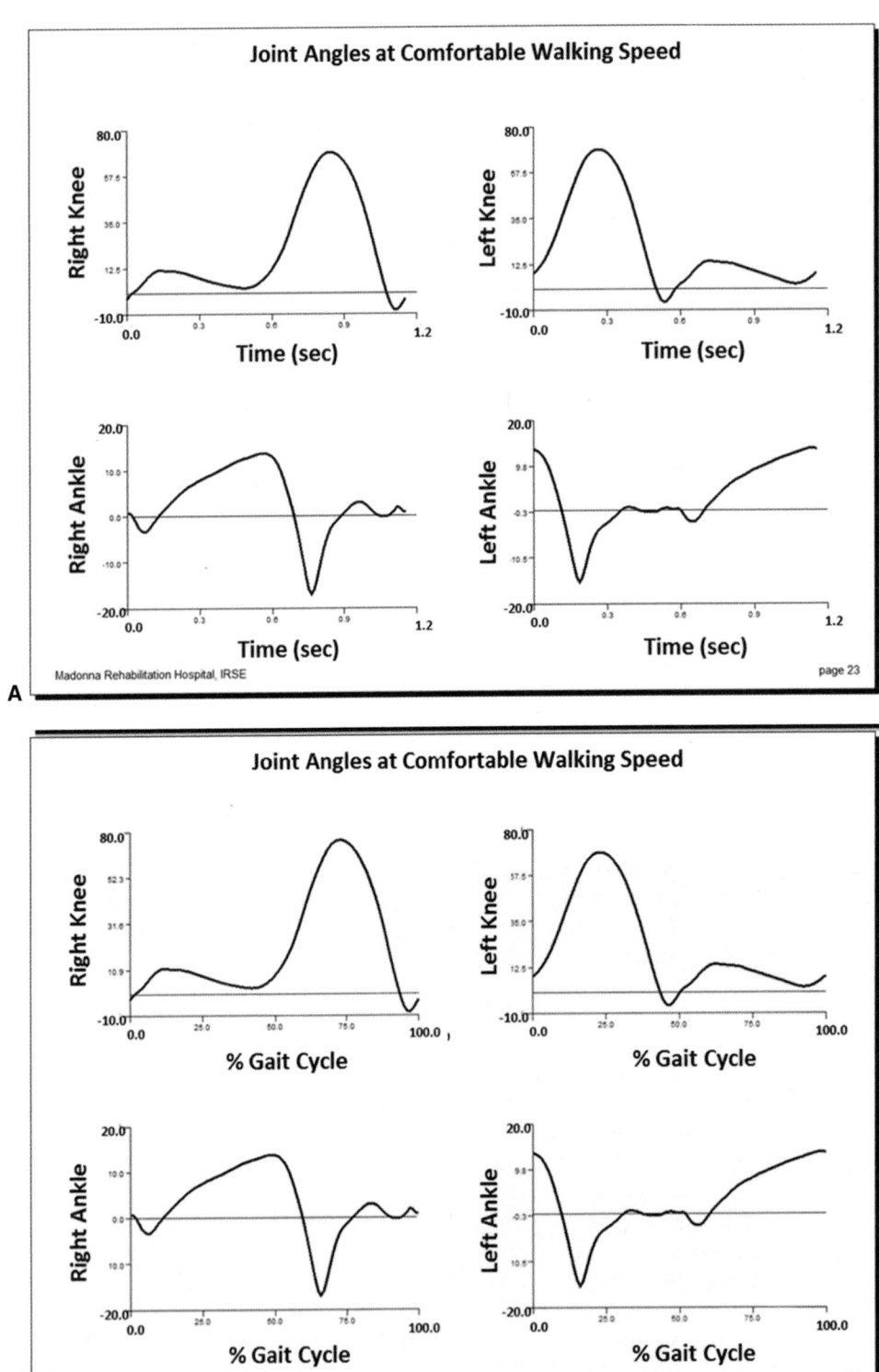

Figure 7.10 Typical graphs generated using Visual 3D software from data acquired using a Qual-isys motion analysis system. The graphs show bilateral knee and ankle range-of-motion patterns recorded during a full right lower extremity gait cycle plotted against time (A) and as a percent-age of the gait cycle (B). Note that left foot's initial contact occurred at approximately 0.6 seconds (approximately 50% gait cycle). *(Courtesy of Thad Buster, Movement and Neurosciences Center, Institute for Rehabilitation Science and Engineering, Madonna Rehabilitation Hospitals, Lincoln, NE 68506.)*

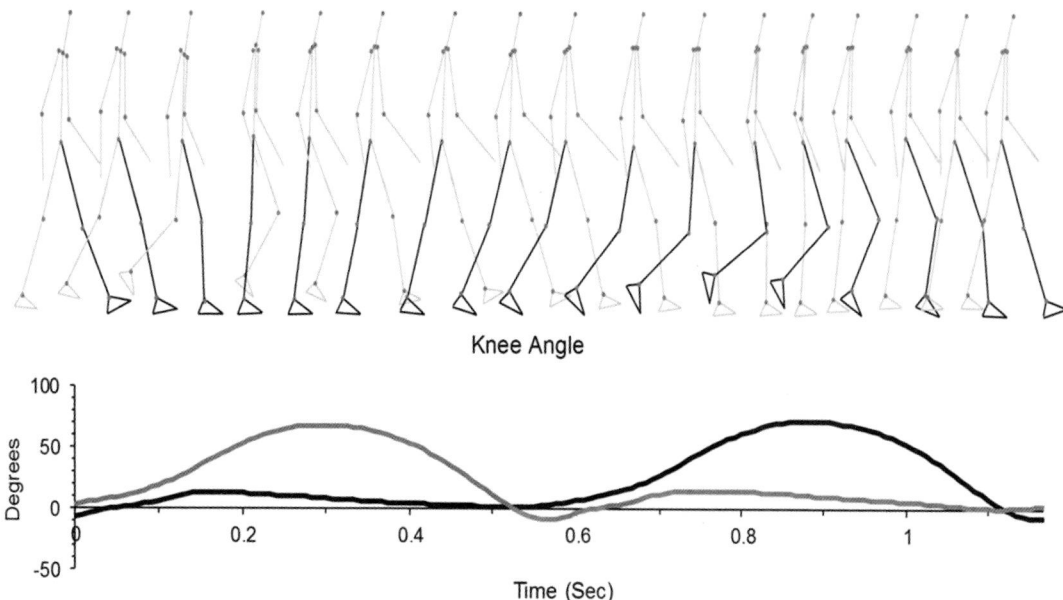

Knee Angle

Figure 7.11 Another format for presentation of the data from a motion-analysis system is computer-generated stick figure representations of one complete gait cycle. In this particular case, the pattern of knee motion is graphically presented below the stick figures. Note that the right knee (darker lower extremity in top figure and darker line in lower figure) is hyperextended at initial contact. *(Courtesy of Movement and Neurosciences Center, Institute for Rehabilitation Science and Engineering, Madonna Rehabilitation Hospitals, Lincoln, NE 68506.)*

sources of variability in kinematic findings.[242] Following implementation of a standardized protocol for marker placement, Gorton et al.[242] reported a 20% average decrease in the standard deviation of seven of nine kinematic measures recorded by 24 examiners in 12 motion analysis laboratories using two different camera systems.

As affordable computer processing and storage capabilities rapidly expand, the varying motion analysis products on the market are also evolving. Many video-based systems are able to track markers to within 0.04 in. (1 mm) of accuracy, enabling relatively precise tracking of the markers.[243] Most systems have the capacity to integrate with other technology, enabling simultaneous acquisition of relevant gait data such as footswitches to identify foot-floor contact patterns and stride characteristics, EMG systems to examine muscle activation patterns, and force plates to determine ground reaction forces. EMG, when recorded simultaneously with stride characteristics data, can be used to identify the particular portion of the gait cycle in which the muscle activity occurs. Figure 7.12 depicts how EMG and kinematic data can be used to explore factors contributing to abnormal gait patterns. The person depicted experienced difficulty with foot clearance during swing owing, in part, to excess plantarflexion during mid- and terminal swing. Out-of-phase activity of the gastrocnemius during late swing contributed to the excess plantarflexion and foot clearance challenge. In addition, the individual walked with a "stiff-legged" gait pattern with the knee excessively extended throughout much of the

gait cycle compared to the anticipated motion profile. Inappropriately timed activity of the vastus lateralis contributed, in part, to the observed knee deviations. Refer to Chapter 5, Examination of Motor Function: Motor Control and Motor Learning, for a more detailed discussion of EMG.

Key differentiating features among motion analysis systems include price, marker system options (e.g., active, passive, or both active and passive), and the capabilities and efficiency of postprocessing software. A number of systems provide manufacturer-generated analysis software that is relatively easy to learn; however, it may be difficult to modify/customize the software to meet the needs of more elaborate studies. Report-generating capabilities differ notably across systems as well and should be considered, depending on the expectations of the laboratory or clinic (e.g., need to produce rapid, easily interpretable reports for inclusion in patient charts versus export of data for statistical analysis for research purposes). Appendix 7.C (online) includes a list of gait analysis software and hardware manufacturers and their contact information. Given the evolving nature of technology, the reader is encouraged to visit the websites provided for the most up-to-date information about the capabilities of different systems.

Electromagnetic Motion Analysis System

One challenge with optical tracking systems is that the motion analysis cameras need to be able to "see" the markers to track their position and subsequently

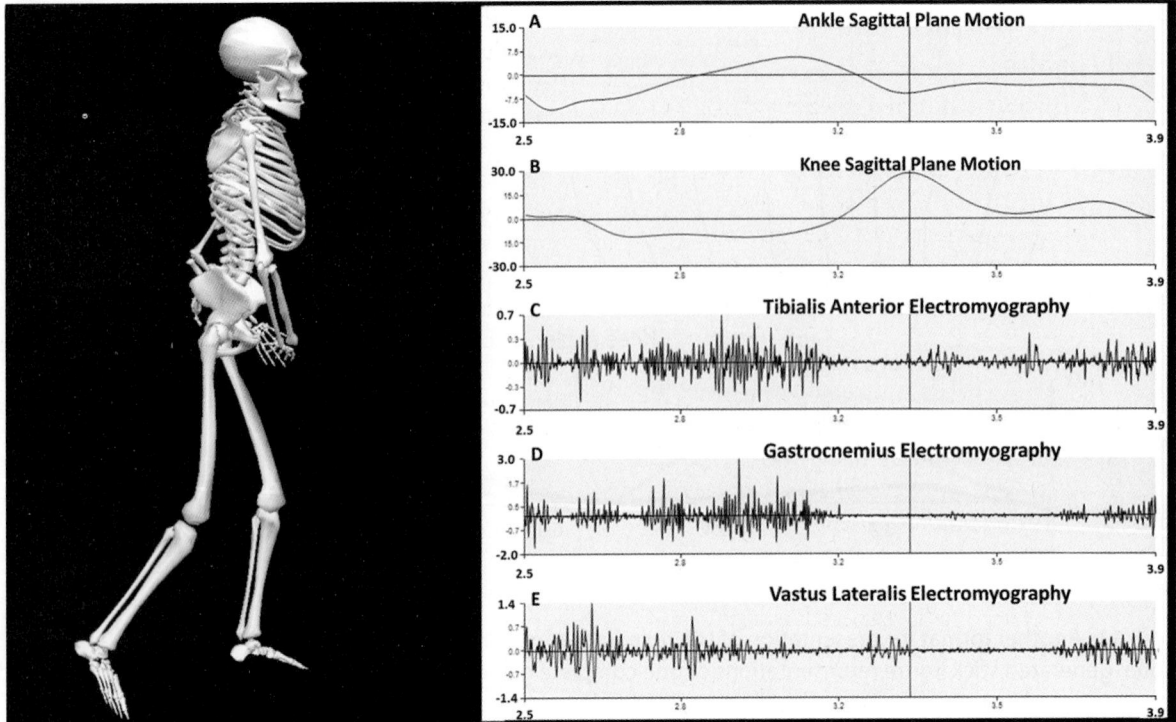

Figure 7.12 Skeleton image of individual with post-brain injury walking. Graphs display data from a single right lower extremity stride (i.e., right initial contact to next ipsilateral initial contact), including sagittal plane motion of ankle (A) and knee (B), as well as corresponding EMG from right gastrocnemius (C) and vastus lateralis (D). Right ankle demonstrates excess plantarflexion during mid- and terminal swing and at initial contact. Premature out-of-phase activity of the right gastrocnemius from midswing through loading response contributed to the excess plantarflexion, despite tibialis anterior activity during swing. Individual does not achieve normal 60° of knee flexion during initial swing, resulting in challenges with limb clearance. Loading response knee flexion is also curtailed, leading to reduced shock absorption. The knee is postured in hyperextension throughout single limb support. Out-of-phase activity of vastus lateralis during pre-swing contributed to limited knee flexion during pre-swing and initial swing. Foot flat initial contact arising from premature activity of gastrocnemius during swing reduced heel rocker and contributed to limited knee flexion during loading response. Prolonged vastus lateralis activity during single limb support contributed to sustained knee hyperextension. Prolonged activity of tibialis anterior throughout single limb support contributed to frontal plane instability of subtalar joint. *(Courtesy of Thad Buster, Movement and Neurosciences Center, Institute for Rehabilitation Science and Engineering, Madonna Rehabilitation Hospitals, Lincoln, NE 68506.)*

calculate kinematic data. This can be difficult when clients use multiple assistive devices or require substantial physical assistance from one or more therapists to navigate the walkway. An alternative motion analysis technology employs electromagnetic tracking capabilities to determine the 3D coordinates of location and angulation of each sensor. FASTRAK (manufactured by Polhemus) is an example of electromagnetic motion analysis technology. To date, a small number of studies have been published that used electromagnetic motion analysis technology to study gait-related activities.[244–248]

The equipment has garnered a following in the virtual-reality environments and animation industry.

Optical Markerless Motion Analysis System

In contrast to optical marker-based tracking and electromagnetic motion analysis systems, optical markerless motion analysis software (e.g., Theia) allows capture of 3D motion data without applying any markers/sensors to the patient. This facilitates more rapid data collection in the clinical setting but can compromise accuracy of estimations of 3D joint motion.[249,250]

Kinetic Gait Analysis

Kinetic Variables

Kinetic gait analyses are directed toward determination and analysis of the forces involved in gait, including ground (floor) reaction forces (GRFs), joint torques, center of pressure (COP), center of mass (COM), mechanical energy, moments of force, power, support moments, work, joint reaction forces, and intrinsic foot pressure (Table 7.13). Although in the past kinetic gait analyses have been used primarily for research purposes, at the present time they are being used clinically as well. Given the risk of foot pressure injuries arising from high plantar pressures in individuals with diabetic sensory neuropathy, some clinicians are using special pressure-mapping insoles to determine if clients may be at risk for developing a pressure injury. A patient walks while wearing the special insoles, and the pressures are recorded. If high pressures are identified on the bottom of the foot, patients may be referred to have special orthotics and/or shoes fabricated to help redistribute the pressures.

The instrumentation required to examine kinetic variables is complex and expensive because derivation of kinetics requires knowledge of all forces acting on the body part being analyzed (e.g., the foot or the thigh). The analysis usually starts with the forces being applied to the foot, which is determined by a force plate embedded in the floor. These plates contain load transducers that measure the COP, COM, and GRFs during gait. Typically, the force plates are based on either strain gage or piezoelectric technology.

Calculation of kinetic variables at the ankle requires knowledge of the forces acting on the foot, body mass, and location of the COM (derived from standard anthropometric tables), as well as knowledge of the acceleration of the COM. Once this knowledge is obtained, equations can be developed to calculate the net forces and net moments occurring at the ankle at that particular instant in time in order for the foot to have moved with those particular accelerations. Once forces and moments at the ankle are determined, similar equations can be applied to the adjacent proximal segment (lower leg). One then knows, for each instant in time, whether the dominant internal moment is being caused by the dorsiflexors or the plantarflexors. If the internal moment for each instant in time is multiplied by the net angular velocity between the ankle and the lower leg, the result is knowledge of the net power being produced by the muscles across the ankle. Concentric contractions add power to the limb (power generation), and eccentric contractions reduce power (power absorption). Variations in expected patterns of power generation and absorption are particularly useful in identifying deficiencies and in determining treatment goals. Unfortunately, a detailed explanation of the calculation of COM, COP, and moments and power is beyond the scope of this chapter. Readers interested in learning more about these concepts are referred to David Winter's book, which is included on the supplemental reading list.

The GRF is defined as the net vertical and shear (or horizontal) forces acting between the foot and the supporting surface. The force is three-dimensional

Table 7.13	Gait Variables: Kinetic Gait Analysis
GRFs	Vertical, anterior-posterior, and medial-lateral forces created as a result of foot contact with the supporting surface. These forces are equal in magnitude and opposite in direction to the force applied by the foot to the ground. Ground reaction forces are measured with force platforms in newtons (N) or pound force.
Pressure	Pressure = force per unit area. In gait analysis, the parameters that are usually measured include the peak pressure, the pressure-time integral, and the overall pattern of pressure distribution under the foot.
COP	The point of application of the resultant force. Movement of the COP as a function of time is used as a measure of stability of a subject who is either standing or walking on a force plate.
Torque (moment of force)	The turning or rotational effect produced by the application of a force. The greater the perpendicular distance from the point of application of a force from the axis of rotation, the greater the turning effect, or torque, produced. Torque is calculated by multiplying the force by the perpendicular distance from the point of application of the force and the axis of rotation. Torque = force × perpendicular distance or moment arm.

COP = center of pressure; GRF = ground reaction force.

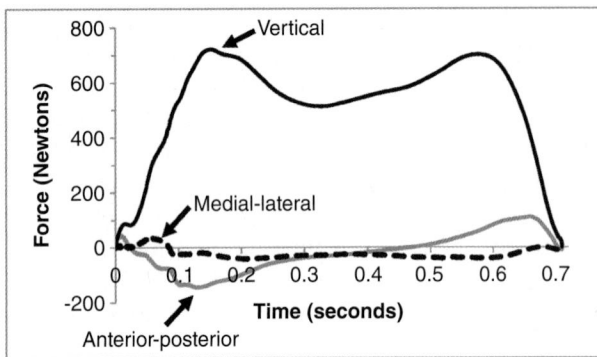

Figure 7.13 Computer-generated graph of the vertical, anterior-posterior, and medial-lateral components of the ground-reaction force obtained as an adult walks across an AMTI force plate. *(Courtesy of Movement and Neurosciences Center, Institute for Rehabilitation Science and Engineering, Madonna Rehabilitation Hospitals, Lincoln, NE 68506.)*

and can be resolved into three components: vertical, anterior–posterior, and medial–lateral (Fig. 7.13). Each component varies throughout the gait cycle and is affected by velocity, cadence, and body mass. The averaged waveforms of the vertical and anterior–posterior force components, presented as a percentage of body weight, show consistent patterns across individuals without pathology for loading rate, peak force, average force, and unloading rate. The vertical force waveform shows a characteristic double hump. The anterior–posterior force has a characteristic negative phase (representing deceleration of the body's mass after the foot hits the ground) followed by a positive phase (reflecting acceleration as body mass moves forward in late stance). In the frontal plane, an initial laterally directed GRF peaks shortly after initial contact. This is most commonly followed by an extended medially directed GRF.

Friction is required while walking and acts in the opposite direction of the desired motion. For example, during loading response, the foot imparts forward (anterior) shear force onto the floor as body weight loads onto the limb. Friction resists the tendency of the foot to slip forward. An individual's friction needs during walking, sometimes referred to as *utilized* or *required friction*, can be measured as an individual walks across a force plate. It is calculated as the ratio of the individual's shear (resultant of the anterior–posterior and medial–lateral forces) and vertical GRF components. When an individual's walking friction needs exceed the friction available at the foot–floor interface, a slip is likely to occur.[12,32,251] A tribometer is a device used to measure the friction available on different floor surfaces and in the presence of contaminants (e.g., water or oil). Some floor manufacturers will report on the slip resistance of the surfaces they distribute (e.g., different types of tile). Floor surfaces with a higher available friction

(as measured by a tribometer) are generally more slip resistant.

Instruments for Measuring Kinetic Variables
Force Plate Technology

Force plates, such as those produced by Kistler Instrument Corp., Advanced Mechanical Technology, Inc. (AMTI), and Bertec are capable of measuring the GRF, as well as calculating the COM, acceleration, velocity, *displacement, power,* and *work.* A graphic display is possible showing the waveforms of the GRF. A growing number of treadmills are capable of measuring the GRF and COP during both walking and running, including the Gaitway (Kistler Instrument Corp), C-Mill (Motek Medical), and Rehawalk (h/p/cosmos). In addition to graphical presentation and statistical functions, the treadmill systems can calculate temporal and spatial parameters.

Cook et al.[11] used a force plate to investigate the effect of a knee flexion restriction (using a brace) and walking speed on the GRF. The authors concluded that the application of a brace to restrict knee flexion for the purpose of protection after injury or while surgically repaired structures were healing may actually increase the stress on both the braced and unbraced limbs.

Hesse et al.[252] compared the trajectories of the COP and the COM in 10 healthy individuals and 14 subjects with hemiparesis. They found that the healthy subjects showed no differences in the behavior of the COP, COM, temporal parameters, and step length when initiating gait with either the right or left extremity. In comparison, patients with hemiparesis showed pronounced asymmetric behavior, depending on which limb was the starting limb (affected vs. less affected). Whereas patients who initiated gait with the affected limb were similar to healthy subjects, patients who started gait with the less-affected limb showed inconsistent movement of the COP and were incapable of producing directional movement of the body's COM. This suggests that therapists should be cautious about promoting that type of gait initiation because the affected leg may be too weak to support starting gait with the less affected leg. Rossi et al.[8] investigated the COM, COP, and GRF in a study of gait initiation in patients with transtibial amputations. These authors found that the patients consistently loaded the intact limb more than the prosthetic limb regardless of which limb initiated gait.[8]

Force plates may be used either as part of, or in combination with, motion analysis systems, and temporal and spatial analysis systems, as well as in conjunction with EMG and electrogoniometry, for a comprehensive analysis of kinematic and kinetic gait variables. Perry et al.[14] incorporated simultaneous recording of GRFs, joint motions, and LE muscle activation patterns to explore an apparent paradox related to the efficiency of toe walking and potential need for therapeutic intervention. Previous researchers identified a lower internal plantarflexor moment during toe walking compared to traditional heel-toe gait and suggested that the plantarflexed foot provided a potential compensatory advantage by reducing the need for plantarflexor strength.[253] However, the earlier researchers had not included measurements of muscle activation (EMG) in their study. The inclusion of EMG into Perry and colleagues' follow-up study[14] as well as subsequent modeling studies[254,255] of the biomechanical demands of toe walking highlighted the source of the apparent paradox. Although the internal moments were lower,[14] plantarflexor muscle activation (mean and peak) actually increased because of the biomechanically inefficient position associated with maintaining a plantarflexed foot (less than optimal length/tension of the plantarflexors).[254] The plantarflexed foot also created the need for compensatory adjustments in muscle activation at more proximal joints.[255] This series of studies highlights a potential limitation of using only kinematic and kinetic data to interpret muscle activation patterns; that is, various patterns of muscle coactivation can create the same internal moment. In addition, when a muscle is at an inefficient position on the length–tension curve, it may require greater activation to generate the same internal moment compared to the demands when more optimally aligned.

Plantar Pressure Measurement Systems

Pressure measurement systems may also be used with force plates. Pressure is equal to force divided by area and is measured by pressure sensors. Therefore, pressure is equal to the force on the sensor divided by the area of the sensor. Plantar pressure measurements are used most commonly in gait analysis to determine the pressure distribution under the foot: foot-to-ground contact, foot-to-shoe contact, and shoe-to-ground contact. Pressure measurements may be used to determine orthotic efficacy, pressure injury risk in diabetes, and for regulating weight-bearing following surgery. Many different types of measurement techniques have been developed for measuring contact pressures.

Novel Electronics' pedar and emed pressure-mapping systems provide a means for examining pressures. The pedar system consists of insoles (in a variety of lengths and widths) that can be placed inside shoes to measure plantar pressures. Each pressure insole consists of a 0.08-in. (2-mm)-thick array of 99 capacitive pressure sensors used to calculate a variety of measures, including peak pressures, mean pressures, contact area, and pressure–time integral. An example of the type of information obtained from the pedar system is presented in Figure 7.14.

Beyond shod walking, the pedar insoles can be used to measure a variety of other gait-related activities. For example, the insoles have been used to measure barefoot pressures by securing them to the foot with a thin

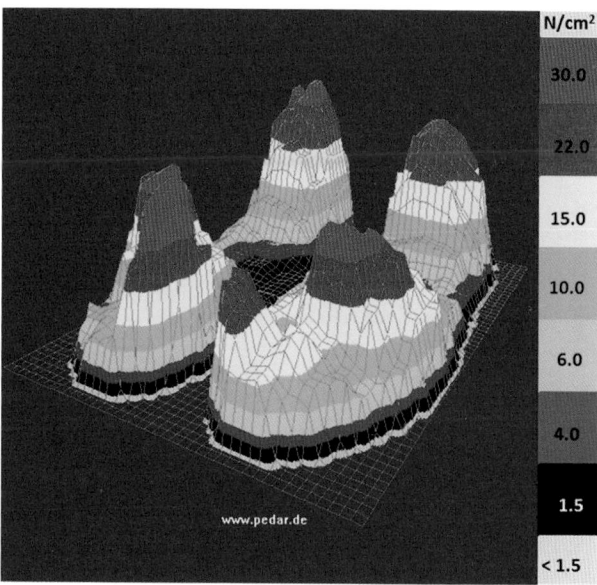

Figure 7.14 Magnitude and location of peak pressure during a left and right step of a young adult with shoes and without disability walking overground at self-selected comfortable speed. Images from both feet are placed side by side for comparison. The highest pressures (displayed in pink) occurred under the heel, metatarsal heads, and right great toe. Relatively low pressures (displayed in black, blue, and teal) were documented under the midfoot regions. *(Courtesy of Thad Buster, Movement and Neurosciences Center, Institute for Rehabilitation Science and Engineering, Madonna Rehabilitation Hospitals, Lincoln, NE 68506.)*

pair of nylon stockings.[256] Burnfield et al.[256] used the pedar system to study plantar pressures patterns in older adults walking barefoot and with shoes at three predetermined velocities (187, 262, and 295 ft/min [57, 80, and 97 m/min]). Compared to slower speeds, fast walking was associated with higher peak pressures under the heel, central and medial metatarsals, and toes, whereas walking barefoot was associated with greater peak pressures under the heel and central metatarsals compared to walking with shoes (Fig. 7.15). These findings suggest that when protection of the plantar surface of the heel and forefoot is important (e.g., with diabetic sensory neuropathy), patients should be encouraged to use shoes and avoid walking at fast speeds for prolonged periods. Subsequent work comparing barefoot walking and walking while wearing shoes examined plantar pressures when walking on grass, carpet, and concrete. Walking barefoot on concrete showed particularly high pressures.[257] Burnfield et al.[258] focused on understanding how plantar pressures in young and middle-aged adults vary across common forms of cardiovascular exercise, including treadmill walking, treadmill running, elliptical training, stair stepping, and recumbent cycling. The authors concluded that when protection of the forefoot is important (e.g., diabetic foot neuropathies), biking

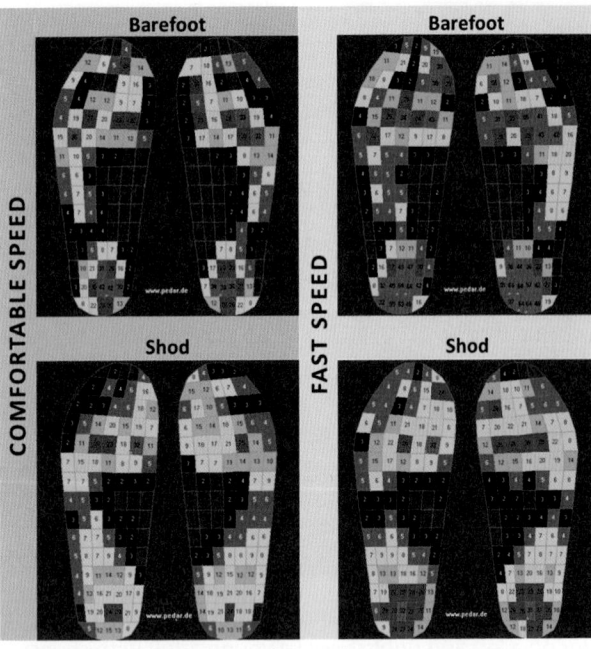

Figure 7.15 Illustrates using pedar (Novel, Inc.) pressure mapping while a 29-year-old male walked barefoot (top row) and in shoes (bottom row) at self-selected comfortable (left column) and fast (right column) speeds revealed higher pressures under the heel, metatarsal heads, and great toe during barefoot walking at a fast speed compared to the relatively low pressures while walking in shoes at a comfortable speed. Numbers within each square represent the peak pressure (N/cm²) experienced during the walking trial. *(Courtesy of Adam Taylor, Movement and Neurosciences Center, Institute for Rehabilitation Science and Engineering, Madonna Rehabilitation Hospitals, Lincoln, NE 68506.)*

and stair climbing offer optimal pressure reductions; however, in situations where protection of the heels from high pressures and forces is warranted, recumbent biking, stair climbing, and elliptical training provide greater relief.[258]

The emed pedography platform is a portable device used to record and evaluate pressure distribution under the foot in static and dynamic conditions. Semple et al.[259] used the emed system to examine COP progression as individuals with rheumatoid arthritis (RA) and individuals without known foot pathology walked. Clients with RA displayed reduced loading of painful regions of the foot as evidenced by delaying progression of the COP across the less painful midfoot followed by rapid progression of the COP across the deformed and painful forefoot.

Tekscan's system, the F-Scan Bipedal In-Shoe Plantar Pressure/Force Measurement System, measures bipedal plantar pressures using paper-thin disposable

pressure sensors placed in a patient's shoes. The sensor is ultrathin, flexible, and can be trimmed to fit; it includes 960 sensing locations distributed across the entire plantar surface. Reliability of the F-Scan System was determined by Randolph et al.[260] to be sufficient for the purpose of designing corrective measures to relieve excessive pressures on the foot. Another system produced by Tekscan is called the Mat-Scan System, which is a pressure-sensing floor mat that allows the clinician to identify barefoot pressures. Mueller et al.[261] used the F-Scan System to determine how footwear design impacted plantar pressures in 30 individuals with transmetatarsal amputations who were at risk for additional amputations owing to a history of diabetes. Though all footwear designs reduced plantar pressures under the distal portion of the residual foot compared to traditional footwear with a toe filler, the most effective design included a full-length shoe with a total contact, custom-molded Plastazote insert, and a rigid rocker-bottom sole. This work has important clinical implications given the high incidence of additional amputations in those with diabetes who have already lost a portion of one limb.[262] Armstrong et al.[263] found that patients who have high plantar pressures and wounds greater than 3.12 in. (8 cm) took significantly longer to heal than did other patients.

Isokinetic and Isometric Torque Measurement Systems

Simple handheld dynamometers and isokinetic dynamometer systems can be used to obtain static and dynamic peak torques before obtaining temporal and spatial measures. Connelly and Vandervoort[149] found that in older women, decreases in isometric and dynamic quadriceps strength led to significant decreases in fast-paced and self-selected speed. In a study examining the relationship between sagittal plane LE isokinetic muscle torques and stride characteristics for a group of elderly ambulatory men, maximal isokinetic hip extensor torque was identified as the only significant independent predictor of stride length, cadence, and free walking velocity.[264] These latter findings highlight the importance of maintaining hip extensor strength in older sedentary males.

Software for Processing, Analyzing, and Displaying Kinematic and Kinetic Data

The Visual 3D, innovative software for biomechanical analysis and modeling, is used to process a variety of gait analysis data (e.g., kinematics, EMG, force plates, gyroscopes). It works with nearly all motion-capture systems and has an integrated report generator. It allows users to expand beyond manufacturer predetermined marker sets and analysis rules. However, to fully appreciate the versatility and robustness of the Visual 3D software, it is beneficial to have access to someone with programming skills.

Summary of Kinematic and Kinetic Gait Analysis

Based on the history of gait analysis, one may expect that many gait analysis systems will continue to evolve, and more innovative methods of quantifying human gait will be created. However, the most important issues for physical therapists is the reliability and validity of the information and how information can be used to fulfill the four purposes for gait analysis (see the "Purposes of Gait Analysis" section of this chapter) as described in the *Guide for Physical Therapist Practice 3.0*.[1] In brief, these purposes are to assist with understanding the gait characteristics of a particular disorder, to assist with movement diagnosis, to inform selection of intervention(s), and to evaluate the effectiveness of treatment.

The primary advantages of temporal and spatial measures are that they can be determined simply and inexpensively and that they yield objective and reliable baseline data that can be used to formulate anticipated goals and expected outcomes and to evaluate the patient's progress. For example, gait patterns displayed by patients with arthritis often are characterized by a reduced rate and range of knee motion and a slower gait velocity compared to subjects without known pathology. Brinkmann and Perry[265] found that following joint replacement for arthritis, the rate and range of knee motion and gait velocity increased above preoperative levels but did not reach normal levels.

Usually, increases in measures such as cadence and velocity indicate improvement in a patient's gait. However, comparisons with normal standards are appropriate only if the goal of treatment is to restore a normal gait pattern (e.g., for a patient recovering from a meniscectomy). Comparison with normative standards may not be appropriate for a patient who has had a cerebral vascular accident. The appropriate norms for examining the gait of a patient with hemiplegia may be either a population of patients with hemiplegia who are of similar age, gender, and involvement or the patient's pretreatment gait.

Therapists must be cautious when selecting a norm or standard by which to measure patient progress. Significant age, gender, weight, and activity level–related differences have been found in both temporal and spatial measures.[266–268] Himann et al.[267] found that an older group (63 to 102 years) of 289 subjects had a significantly slower self-selected walking speed and smaller step length compared with a younger group. Age was a significant determinant of walking speed after age 62, but height was a significant determinant before age 62. Step length has been found to be significantly shorter, and the double limb support stance period significantly increased in an elderly sample compared to a database of young adults.[139] Cho et al.[269] found a number of gender differences in kinematic and kinetic gait variables.

For example, females had shorter stride lengths and narrower step widths, a more anteriorly tilted pelvis, greater hip flexion and internal rotation, greater knee valgus, and smaller ankle joint moment compared to males. Some of these changes were attributed to the anatomically wider female pelvis.[269]

Few disadvantages exist regarding kinematic quantitative gait analysis, except for the possible expense involved in instrumentation, the time required to apply the markers accurately to ensure valid and reliable data, and the fact that a certain amount of uncertainty exists about how to normalize for leg length, height, age, gender, weight, level of maturation, and disability. The interpretation of motion patterns obtained through motion analysis systems usually involves comparisons of an individual's data with a mean curve for normal subjects using a standard deviation (SD) for boundaries. Sutherland et al.[270] suggest that motion patterns cannot be fully analyzed without consideration of all points along the curve. They propose the use of prediction regions (multiples of the SD above and below the mean curve of data for each point in the gait cycle). Within a prediction region (Fig. 7.16), if any point along the curve of joint motion falls outside of the defined region, the patient's gait is considered to be abnormal.

Gait Pattern Classification

Identification of gait parameters that deviate widely from a norm is a fairly simple outcome of gait analysis. However, identification of groups or clusters of gait deviations that characterize a known disorder is more complicated and represents one of the very urgent

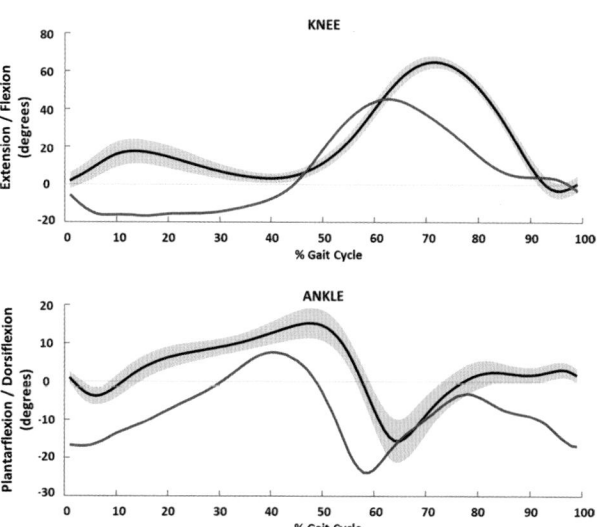

Figure 7.16 Prediction regions of sagittal plane knee and ankle kinematics of an adult with traumatic brain injury (red line) in comparison with age-matched normative data (black line with gray-shaded standard deviation).

needs in gait analysis. In an attempt to classify gait disorders, a number of statistical techniques are being used for both kinematic and kinetic gait variables. The bootstrap technique[271] is used to establish the boundaries (prediction regions) about the mean curve for healthy control subjects in order to establish the limits of normal variability. *Discriminant analysis* is used to recognize gait patterns of healthy people and persons with gait deviations. *Principal components analysis* is useful to reduce the large quantities of data acquired in a gait analysis to a set of features that accurately describe gait patterns. *Cluster analysis* is used to place subjects in homogeneous groups, or clusters, based on specified input parameters.

Normalcy Index

Principal components analysis was used to develop the normalcy index (NI), which quantifies the amount of deviation in a subject's gait compared to the gait of an average unimpaired person.[272] The NI is sensitive enough to distinguish unimpaired subjects from idiopathic toe walkers and to distinguish between involved and less involved limbs of subjects following stroke. However, the gait pathology of nonindependent walkers was not well categorized. The authors suggested that perhaps the inclusion of kinetic variables along with kinematic variables might be helpful.

The principal components method derived the NI by assigning weighted factors inversely proportional to the amount of variation exhibited by each gait measure in the unimpaired population. However, since the data come from a motion analysis system, they are subject to sources of error, such as soft tissue artifacts and marker misplacement.[272]

Cluster Analysis

Cluster analysis is a commonly used statistical technique in the social sciences that has also been used to create an objective classification system of gait patterns. Cluster analysis has been used to classify gait patterns of patients with stroke based on temporal and spatial parameters for each phase of the gait cycle. Four clusters of gait patterns were identified: *fast, moderate, flexed,* and *extended*.[273] The authors suggested that clinicians use critical parameters to categorize patients with stroke so that intervention programs could be more specifically targeted to underlying impairments.

Energy Cost Analysis During Gait

Walking at constant speed is a cyclical activity that requires the body to add energy by means of concentric contractions and to absorb energy by means of eccentric contractions. These energy transfers and exchanges are cleverly designed to make walking efficient.[29] Generally, conditions that affect either the motor control of gait and posture or conditions that affect joint and muscle structure and function will increase the energy cost of gait.[15,274-278] The type of footwear,[279] use of assistive devices, and speed of gait affect energy expenditure as well.[280] Energy expenditure is an important consideration in gait analyses, particularly in neurological conditions in which muscular resources may be low. There are three general approaches in determining energy costs: *physiological measurement, mechanical energy analysis,* and *heart rate data.* The selection of a particular approach should be done for the purpose of taking the measure and the relative importance of test characteristics outlined in the "Types of Gait Analyses" section of this chapter.

Physiological Energy Cost Measures

Physiological cost measures estimate the heat (energy) produced by a subject at rest and during exercise by using indirect calorimetry, based on the assumption that all energy-using reactions of the body depend on oxygen uptake. The most common method of measuring oxygen uptake during walking is open-loop spirometry in which exhaled air is sampled and analyzed for its oxygen content, using the Douglas bag method.[29] Stationary or moving metabolic carts or lightweight portable devices perform breath-by-breath oxygen and carbon dioxide analysis.

Two parameters of prime interest are *oxygen cost* and *oxygen rate.* One may be interested in the oxygen cost or energy expenditure per unit of distance walked (mL/kg/m), which relates to the physiological work involved in the task and reflects gait efficiency. Alternatively, the oxygen rate, or energy expenditure per unit of time (mL/kg/min), reflects the power of walking and is interpreted using knowledge of walking speed.[275,281] Perry et al.[15] used a modified Douglas bag assembly to compare the energy expenditure required for an individual with bilateral transfemoral amputations and bilateral transradial (below elbow) amputations to walk at a self-selected speed using different prosthetic devices. When wearing the microprocessor-controlled C-Leg prostheses, the subject walked farther and faster compared to the traditional non–microprocessor-controlled articulating prostheses and stubbies (nonarticulating, short prosthetic limbs). The overall rate of oxygen consumption and oxygen cost was lower while using the C-Leg compared with walking with either of the other prostheses. Cesar et al.[27] identified improved walking efficiency (as evidenced by a 30% reduction in oxygen cost) in an adolescent with CP and autism following participation in a 24-session moderate- to vigorous-intensity intervention on the ICARE, a motorized-elliptical trainer. The participant also walked farther on the 2MWT and faster during self-selected comfortable and fast walking tests.

Physiological cost analysis methods are most useful for comparing the energy cost of walking with normal values or an individual's maximum capacity and for determining the effects on energy costs of interventions such as the use of orthoses, prostheses, or assistive devices. Physiological cost analyses reflect overall costs of walking with respect to time or distance, but they cannot discern the possible causes. If insight into the particular movements is needed, mechanical energy analysis can be helpful.

Mechanical Energy Cost Determination

There are two methods of obtaining mechanical energy costs. In the first method, kinematic data alone are required, using estimates of masses of body parts and of the COM locations of these parts. By employing a spatial motion analysis system with basic equations of motion and anthropometric constants for masses of body parts, the potential energy and translational and rotational kinetic energy levels of each body part can be calculated. The differences between values obtained at each time increment indicate energy cost. Various equations are used to combine the costs across body parts to yield the total body cost. The large head, arms, and trunk (HAT) segment shows excellent exchanges between kinetic and potential energy types, providing the body with energy efficiency. When the body is at its highest position (midstance), it is also moving most slowly, but as the HAT "rolls down the hill" into initial contact of the foot, this potential energy is changed into kinetic energy, and the HAT picks up speed. In this way, a great deal of energy is saved, and the movement is efficient. However, if the person walks very slowly or very quickly, or has a stiff knee and has to lift one side of the body excessively to clear the floor, the energies are no longer complementary in size and shape; less energy exchange can take place.[282] These modes of walking are less efficient than normal walking.

The second method of obtaining mechanical energy costs uses a kinetic approach. Briefly stated, the energy changes in a body part between subsequent instants in time are calculated (1) from the product of the forces on each end of the joint and the velocity of the point of application and (2) from the muscle powers, which are the product of each muscle moment and the angular velocity of the body part. In some cases, the muscle is adding energy to the part (generation), and in other cases, it is absorbing energy. There are a number of different methods of handling the calculations of mechanical energy, exchanges, and transfers, but a sound approach is described by McGibbon et al.[283]

Heart Rate Data

A third general approach to determining the relative energy cost of gait is by measuring the heart rate (HR) during ambulation. Relative energy consumption has been found to be highly correlated with HR, and

absolute level of energy consumption has been found to be highly correlated with HR and maximum walking speed. The most accurate way to determine HR is to use a telemetry system that produces beat-by-beat information as well as electrocardiographic activity. Many inexpensive HR monitors are also available, and some are designed to download stored information to a computer (see Chapter 2, Examination of Vital Signs). HR responses to ambulation can also be determined by palpation of the radial or carotid arteries, although more error may be present.

HR measures have been shown to be adequately sensitive for some applications. For example, simple measures of HR and maximum ambulatory velocity allowed accurate prediction (r = 0.89) of energy consumption in children with myelomeningocele based on measures recorded from 21 children treadmill walking, 8 children using wheelchairs, and 5 children using both modes.[284] However, Herbert et al.[276] found no difference in HR between children with transtibial amputations and those with intact LEs, even though energy consumption was 15% higher in the children with amputations. Perhaps because the conditions were more disparate, Waters et al.[274] found that in patients with hip arthrodesis, oxygen consumption was 32% greater than normal and that HR was significantly greater than normal.

An energy index based on HR, called the Physiological Cost Index (PCI), was developed specifically to determine the relative costs of walking per unit of distance walked.[285] Calculated as the difference between the walking HR and the resting HR divided by the average speed, it is expressed in beats per meter. The reliability of PCI has been investigated in individuals without known pathology,[286–288] children with CP,[289] as well as people with spinal cord[288,290] and brain injuries.[157] The index has been used to quantify improvements following an intervention in individuals with SCI,[291,292] RA,[293] and stroke.[294–296] For example, PCI was used as a key outcome measure in a study assessing the effects of a 12-week intervention that combined functional electrical stimulation with conventional rehabilitation to manage dropfoot in individuals recovering from a stroke.[296] While walking speed increased 38.7% between the initiation and end of the trial, PCI decreased 34.6%, suggesting improved function and efficiency.

The relationship between PCI and oxygen consumption has been studied across a variety of populations, including individuals with amputations,[297] individuals with SCIs,[290] and individuals without known disabilities.[286] Some researchers have found oxygen uptake measures to be more repeatable and less variable than PCI.[287,290,298,299] One concern that has been raised is that HR measures may be affected by altered vagal or sympathetic regulation due to brain injury[300–303] or medication.[304]

The Total Heart Beat Index provides an alternative approach for determining the relative energy efficiency of walking. It is calculated by dividing the total (cumulative) number of heartbeats during exercise by the total distance traveled in a given time period.[288] It has been used to study walking efficiency in individuals with diabetic foot pressure injuries and amputations,[305] chronic incomplete SCIs,[306] and intellectual and developmental disabilities.[307] Reliable and valid use of the measure with populations with blunted HR responses requires study.

SUMMARY

This chapter has provided an overview of select methods for kinematic and kinetic gait analyses. Many of the common variables examined in gait analyses have been defined and described, and examples of studies using gait analyses have been presented. OGA and temporal and spatial variables have been emphasized because they appear to be the most common types of analyses used in the clinical setting. A brief overview of some of the motion analysis systems has been provided. Readers are encouraged to investigate the capabilities of individual motion analysis systems and to consult the gait literature for reliability and validity studies regarding these systems. The ability to perform a gait analysis that accurately describes a patient's gait will provide important quantifiable information necessary for optimal treatment planning and outcomes assessment.

Questions for Review

1. Describe the three different types of gait analyses (kinematic qualitative, kinematic quantitative, and kinetic), and list the variables examined in each type. Identify at least one variable from each type of analysis and describe a technique/technology that could be used to examine the variable.

2. Compare the advantages and disadvantages of a kinematic qualitative gait analysis with the advantages and disadvantages of a kinematic quantitative analysis.

3. Describe how a therapist would determine the concurrent validity of temporal and spatial gait measures recorded using the Zeno instrumented mat with values calculated using the Stride Analyzer.

4. A new client is referred to physical therapy with gait dysfunction arising from severe diabetic sensory and motor neuropathy. The patient has a history of bilateral recurrent pressure injuries under his first metatarsal heads, which have impaired his ability to stand/walk at work for prolonged periods of time. He recently received a new pair of custom-molded orthotic shoe inserts and was instructed to use them in his shoes to help reduce plantar pressures. Unfortunately, he is unable to feel whether they are fitting or not, secondary to the sensory neuropathy. What technology could be used to assess the effectiveness of the inserts at reducing plantar pressures? What activities should be assessed and why?

5. A person walks with excessive dorsiflexion, no heel-off, and limited toe extension in terminal stance. Hip and knee analysis reveals excess flexion during stance with absence of the normal "trailing limb" posture characteristic of terminal stance. Identify potential causes for these deviations. What additional tests or measures should be performed?

6. A person reports falling two to three times per week since a recent exacerbation of multiple sclerosis. Observational gait analysis reveals excess hip flexion, knee flexion, and ankle plantarflexion in midswing. The individual uses a past retract pattern to diminish hip and knee flexion in late swing, but plantarflexion remains excessive. Following a foot flat initial contact, the ankle remains excessively plantarflexed, and knee flexion is limited. Identify potential causes for these deviations. What additional tests or measures should be performed?

7. Identify methods that can be used to determine the energy costs that a patient incurs while walking.

8. How could a gait analysis of temporal parameters be used to demonstrate a patient's progress or lack of progress?

CASE STUDY

HISTORY

This 65-year-old woman is 5 days post right total hip arthroplasty. The surgery was performed following a femoral neck fracture incurred during a fall on the ice in front of her home. She has had daily bedside physical therapy for the past 3 days and now is independent in transfers. However, she needs to be independent in walking before she goes home.

She has a past history of diabetes mellitus (onset age 50), which is controlled with daily insulin injections. She has a recurrent history of foot pressure injuries and has been hospitalized on two occasions to manage infected foot pressure injuries. She denies any history of "heart problems." She does not participate in any regular exercise program and spends a great deal of time sitting during her work as a seamstress. She is alert and oriented to time and place and has a pleasant demeanor. She is 5 feet 3 inches tall and weighs 160 pounds.

Goniometric Examination of Passive Range of Motion (Degrees)

Lower Extremities

Joint	Motion	Left	Right
Hip	Flexion	WFL	15–40*
	Extension	WFL	0–10*
	Abduction	WFL	0–20*
	Adduction	WFL	0–10*
	Medial rotation	WFL	Not tested*
	Lateral rotation	WFL	0–20*
Knee	Flexion	WFL	0–120
Ankle	Dorsiflexion	WFL	0–15
	Plantarflexion	WFL	0–45
	Inversion	WFL	0–5
	Eversion	WFL	0–20

*Painful with movement.
WFL = within functional limits.
Upper extremities: All ROM measurements are WFL.

Manual Muscle Test

Lower Extremities

Joint	Movement	Left	Right
Hip	Flexion	G	F
	Extension	G	P
	Abduction	G	P
	Adduction	G	F+
	Lateral rotation	G	F+
	Medial rotation	G	F+
Knee	Flexion	G	F+
	Extension	G	F+
Ankle	Dorsiflexion	F	P
	Plantarflexion	F	F
	Inversion	F	F
	Eversion	F+	F
Toes	Flexion	F	F
	Extension	P	P

Upper extremities: All muscle grades are within the G to G range.

(Continued)

CASE STUDY—cont'd

Sensory Examination

	Plantar Aspect Left Foot	Plantar Aspect Right Foot
Sharp/dull	5	5
Light touch	5	5
Temperature	5	5
Proprioceptive sensation	4	4

NUMERIC VALUES REFER TO THE SENSATION SCALE BELOW.

SENSATION SCALE

1. Intact: normal, accurate
2. Decreased: delayed response
3. Exaggerated: increased sensitivity
4. Inaccurate: inappropriate perception of stimuli
5. Absent: no response
6. Inconsistent or ambiguous

INSPECTION

Patient has a pressure injury on the medial aspect of the right plantar surface that is 0.7 × 6.0 cm in diameter and 1.5 mm deep.

FUNCTIONAL EXAMINATION

Locomotion
FIM level = 5
Transfers
FIM level = 7
Activities of Daily Living
Eating: FIM = 7
Bathing: FIM = 7
Dressing: FIM = 7

GUIDING QUESTIONS

1. Develop a physical therapy problem list.
2. Complete the sample OGA form for the right LE based on the information presented (see Appendix 7.A [online]). What deviations would you expect to see for the right LE, and why? How might gait change if the client is instructed to not bear weight on the right forefoot secondary to the plantar pressure injury?
3. Present your recommendations for physical therapy intervention.

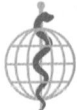

For additional resources, including answers to the questions for review, new immersive cases, case study guiding questions, references, and more, please visit **https://www.fadavis.com/product/physical -rehabilitation-fulk-8**. You may also quickly find the resources by entering this title's four-digit ISBN, 4691, in the search field at **http://fadavis.com** and logging in at the prompt.

Examination of Function

David A. Scalzitti, PT, PhD

Chapter 8

LEARNING OBJECTIVES

1. Discuss the concepts of health, function, activity, participation, disability, impairment, activity limitations, and participation restrictions.
2. Define *function* and discuss the purposes and components of the examination of function.
3. Select activities and roles appropriate to an individual's particular characteristics and condition to guide examination of function.
4. Compare and contrast characteristics of various tests of function, including performance measures and self-report measures.
5. Identify factors to consider in the selection of instruments for testing function.
6. Compare and contrast various scoring methods used in instruments to measure function.
7. Discuss the issues of reliability, validity, and responsiveness as they relate to the measurement of function.
8. Using the case study example, apply clinical decision-making skills in evaluating data from the examination of function.

CHAPTER OUTLINE

A CONCEPTUAL FRAMEWORK *272*
EXAMINATION OF FUNCTION *276*
  Purpose *276*
  General Considerations *276*
  Testing Perspectives *276*
  Types of Instruments *277*
  Instrument Parameters and Formats *278*
  Response Formats *280*
INTERPRETING TEST RESULTS *281*
  Determining the Quality of Instruments *282*
  Considerations in Selection of Instruments *284*
SINGLE-DIMENSIONAL VERSUS MULTIDIMENSIONAL MEASURES OF FUNCTION *286*

SAMPLE INSTRUMENTS TO ASSESS FUNCTION *287*
  The Functional Independence Measure *287*
  The Outcome and Assessment Information Set *288*
  The *36-Item Short-Form Health Survey 289*
  Activity Measure for Post-Acute Care *289*
  The Patient-Specific Functional Scale *289*
SUMMARY *290*

Function is a broad construct that incorporates performance at the level of body systems, the person, and society, or a combination of these. A clinician needs to consider the reasons for obtaining the measurement in deciding which aspects of function to measure and which measure of function to use. For example, is the measure to describe a specific activity limitation or an individual's overall level of function? Will the measure be used to evaluate an individual's current status or assess the outcomes of an episode of care? Will the measure be used to determine the destination at discharge, obtain reimbursement, meet regulatory requirements, communicate across health-care settings, or some combination of these reasons?

The ultimate objective of any rehabilitation program is to return the individual to a lifestyle that is as close to their previous level of function as possible or, alternatively, to maximize the current potential for function and maintain it. For an otherwise healthy person with a fractured arm, this may be a reasonably simple process: improving impairments in body function, such as range of motion (ROM) and strength, will generally correlate positively with the reestablishment of skills related to the performance of activities, such as dressing and feeding. However, considering the person with a stroke, the task is much more complex because the problems are much more extensive, complicated, and interwoven. The overall framework to assess function, however, is broadly similar for both examples. In both instances, the therapist begins by describing the problem in functional terms obtained from the history, performing a review of body systems and detailed examination using selected tests and measures, evaluating the data, establishing a diagnosis and prognosis, implementing interventions to reduce or eliminate the problems identified, and documenting the progress toward the desired functional outcome.[1]

Every individual values the ability to live independently. The construct of function encompasses all those tasks, activities, and roles that identify a person as an independent adult or as a child progressing toward adult independence. These activities require the integration of both cognitive and affective abilities with motor skills. Functional activity is a patient-referenced concept and is dependent on what the individual self-identifies as essential to support physical and psychological well-being as well as to create a personal sense of meaningful living. Function is not totally individualistic, however; there are certain categories of activities that are common to everyone. Eating, sleeping, elimination, and hygiene are major components of survival and protection common to all animals. Particular to humans are the evolution of bipedal locomotion and complex hand activities, which permit independence in the personal environment. Working and participating in recreational activities are examples of human functional activities in a social context.

This chapter presents a conceptual framework for examining functional status based on the International Classification of Functioning, Disability, and Health (ICF; see also Chapter 1, Clinical Decision-Making). The chapter presents an overview of the purposes of the examination of function and the range and rigor of formal test instruments currently available to clinicians and researchers. Considerations in test selection and principles of administration are also presented.

■ A CONCEPTUAL FRAMEWORK

Chronically ill and disabled persons represent a large segment of the population in the United States. In 2020, approximately 64 million Americans (25%) were considered to have a disability (limited in their usual activities due to one or more physical, mental, or emotional conditions).[2] Traditionally, persons with disabilities may have been categorized or classified according to their medical diseases or conditions. Medical procedures such as physical examination, laboratory tests, and imaging are the primary tools to delineate the problems created by disease. Strict focus on a biomedical model, with its emphasis on the characteristics of *disease* (etiology, pathology, and clinical manifestations), may contribute to reducing patients to their *medical labeling*, for example, referring to people by the condition they have rather than as individuals with these conditions. This model virtually ignores the equally important psychological, social, and behavioral dimensions of the illness that accompany the condition. *Illness* refers to the personal behaviors that emerge when the reality of having a condition is internalized and experienced by an individual. Factors related to illness often play a key role in determining the success or failure of rehabilitation efforts well beyond the nature of the medical condition that prompted a patient's referral to physical therapy. In helping the individual with a condition, physical therapists come to understand each person's illness as well.

A broad conceptual framework is necessary to fully understand the concept of health and its relationship to function and disability. Terms such as *well-being, health-related quality of life,* and *functional status* are often used interchangeably to describe health status. The most global definition of health has been provided by the World Health Organization (WHO), which defined health as "a state of complete physical, mental, and social well-being, and not merely the absence of diseases and infirmity."[3] Although such global definitions are useful as philosophical statements, they lack the precision necessary for measurement by clinicians or researchers.

In order to describe the components of health and provide a unified and standard language and framework for the description of health and health-related states, the ICF was endorsed by WHO in 2001.[4] The ICF complements other classifications of WHO such as the *International Statistical Classification of Diseases, 10th revision (ICD-10)*[5] as well as the more recently released *International Classification of Diseases, 11th revision (ICD-11)*.[6] Whereas the *ICD-10* and *ICD-11* are classifications of diseases, disorders, and other health conditions, the ICF attempts to provide a meaningful description of the components of health and its relationship to a person with a health condition. *Function* in the ICF is an umbrella term encompassing all body functions and structures, activities, and participation, whereas *disability* is a term that encompasses impairments in body functions and structures, activity limitations, and participation restrictions. Both function and disability are represented in the ICF to provide for the description of a continuum of the components of health from positive aspects to items an individual is not able to perform or is able to perform in a limited manner or with assistance.

The ICF framework consists of two parts: the first describes components of function and disability in the context of health, and the second describes contextual factors that may interact with components of the first part (Fig. 8.1). These components of the ICF do not model a process of disablement; rather, the ICF enables one to classify function and disability from multiple perspectives. The relationship between components and parts of the ICF does not imply causality. A bidirectional relationship exists between the components of the ICF. For example, a health condition such as angina may influence aspects of mobility such as gait, whereas at the same time increasing one's mobility by performing a regular walking program may influence the management of the health condition. In addition, a limitation in one component of the framework does not imply limitations in other components.

Body functions are defined by the ICF as the physiological functions of body systems, and *body structures* are parts of the body such as organs, limbs, and their components. *Impairment* is the term used to refer to problems in

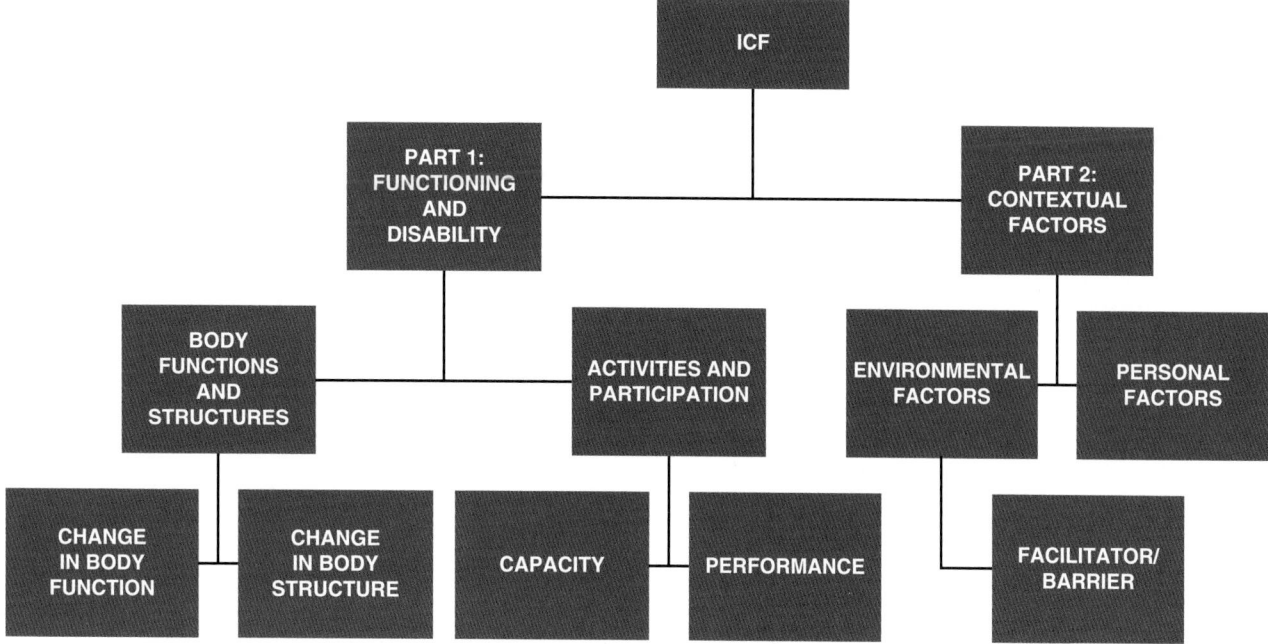

Figure 8.1 Structure of the International Classification of Functioning, Disability, and Health model of functioning and disability. *From APTA Guide to Physical Therapist Practice. (Introduction to the Guide to Physical Therapist Practice. Alexandria, VA: American Physical Therapy Association; 2014. Accessed March 1, 2022. http://guide.apta.org/)*

body function or structure. Although body functions and structures are classified in separate sections of the ICF, the classifications are designed to be used together. For example, the chapter titled "Neuromuscular and Movement-Related Functions" in the body functions classification corresponds with the chapter titled "Structures Related to Movement" in the body structures classification. Hence, for a person with rheumatoid arthritis, a clinician may use aspects of the body functions classification to describe ROM of the interphalangeal joints and muscle performance of the hand intrinsic muscles and the body structures classification to describe the integrity of the joints of the hand. The headings for the chapters in the ICF classification of body functions and structures are listed in Table 8.1.

The ICF defines *activity* as the execution of a task or action by an individual and *participation* as involvement in a life situation. The terms used to describe problems in these domains are *activity limitations* and *participation restrictions*. Through the definitions of activity and participation, an attempt is made to differentiate what a person can do because of characteristics of the individual and those of society. In the ICF, however, a single list covers both activity and participation. Instead of separate lists, the ICF allows users to differentiate activities and participation. Possible operational definitions suggested in the ICF include (1) designating some domains as activities and others as participation with no overlap, (2) designating some domains as activities and others

as participation allowing for overlap, (3) designating all detailed domains as activities and the broad categories as participation, and (4) using all domains as both activities and participation.[4(pp234–237)] To date, no standard exists for the distinction of the classification of activity and participation, and physical therapists should be aware of the potential uses of the classification for practice and research.[7]

The headings for the nine chapters in the ICF classification of activities and participation and examples of classification within a chapter are presented in Figure 8.2. The chapters are considered the first level of classification and can be used to categorize positive and negative aspects of function. The second level of classification includes categories of different actions, tasks, and activities. Subcategories provide additional detail for the main categories. For example, moving around is a category within the mobility domain of the ICF, and crawling is a subcategory of the moving around category. These subcategories allow for more specific description of the categories (second- and third-level classifications).

Contextual factors are included in the ICF model to represent the complete background of an individual's life. These factors may interact as facilitators or barriers to the health condition and to the components of function. The consideration of each contextual factor as either a *barrier* or a *facilitator* is made from the perspective of the individual whose situation is being described. Contextual factors are distinguished as *environmental factors*,

Table 8.1	International Classification of Functioning, Disability, and Health—Body Functions and Body Structures	
Body Functions	**Body Structures**
Mental functions	Structures of the nervous system
Sensory functions and pain	The eye, ear, and related structures
Voice and speech functions	Structures involved in voice and speech
Functions of the cardiovascular, hematological, immunological, and respiratory systems	Structures of the cardiovascular, immunological, and respiratory systems
Functions of the digestive, metabolic, and endocrine systems	Structures related to the digestive, metabolic, and endocrine systems
Genitourinary and reproductive functions	Structures related to the genitourinary and reproductive systems
Neuromusculoskeletal and movement-related functions	Structures related to movement
Functions of the skin and related structures	Skin and related structures

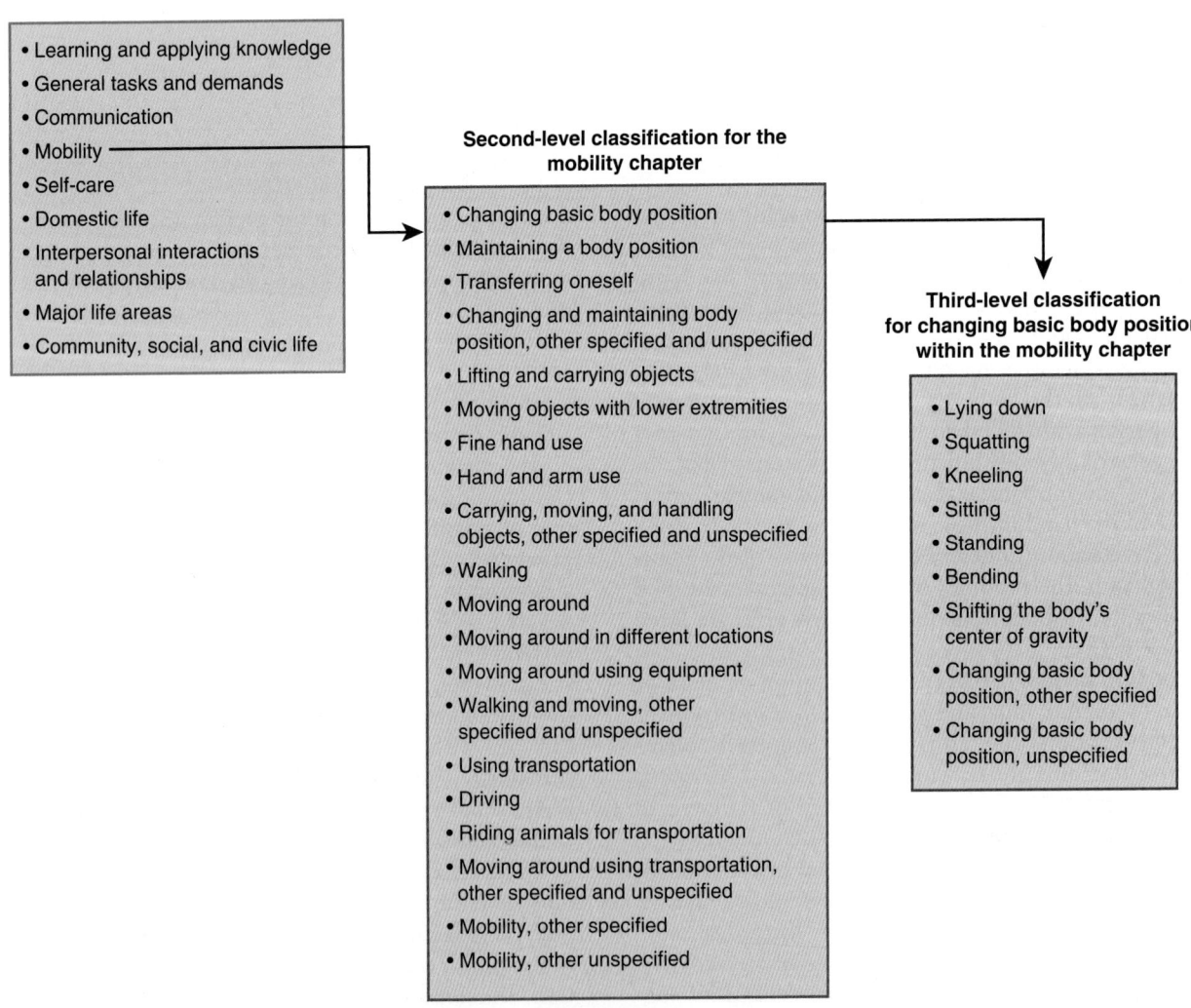

Figure 8.2 International Classification of Functioning, Disability, and Health classification of activities and participation including selected second- and third-level classifications for mobility.

which are external to the individual and can have positive or negative influence on performance, and *personal factors,* which are features of the individual that are not part of the given health condition or health state. In some cases, personal factors may be modifiable, such as fitness and education, whereas other personal factors such as age and race are not modifiable. Due to the bidirectional nature of the ICF framework, contextual factors may interact with the components of part 1. Environmental factors are classified by the ICF (Table 8.2); however, a classification of personal factors is notably omitted.

The ICF emphasizes the interaction between the person and the environment as critical to understanding functioning and disability. Physical therapists can help change discriminatory social attitudes and environmental restrictions such as architectural barriers that stigmatize individuals and restrict participation in all aspects of society. The modification of factors that are barriers and incorporation of factors that are facilitators is as important to functioning as the amelioration of activity limitations.[8]

In addition to providing a framework for the classification of function, the ICF provides a classification scheme for coding, which, although not in widespread use by clinicians, may be particularly intriguing in its delineation of actions, tasks, and activities in an implicit hierarchy of functioning. Within this hierarchy, actions (e.g., rolling, bending, sitting, standing, lifting, and reaching) are constituents of tasks and activities (e.g., bathing, dressing, and grooming). Tests and measures of actions are particularly relevant to physical therapist practice, as they capture the complex integration of systems that permits an individual to maintain a posture, transition to other postures, or sustain safe and efficient movement. Coding of body functions

and structures may incorporate qualifiers describing the extent, nature, and location of the impairments. The coding of activities and participation may incorporate qualifiers that describe the performance of the activity and the capacity to perform the activity. The activities and participation qualifiers may also incorporate how the task may be performed differently with and without assistance.

Although typical patterns of deficits in body functions and problems in activities may exist in certain disease categories, the exact empirical relationship between a particular set of impairments in body functions and structure and activity limitations is not yet known.[9] Impairments may be associated with activities and participation, but one must remember that correlation does not equal causation. As one example from the literature, the correlation between different impairment measures and function in persons with low back pain is small.[10] Instead, the relationship between an impairment and an activity limitation is most often inferred in the clinic through observation and plausible explanations. For example, physical therapists may assume that the reason a patient cannot transfer independently is causally linked to the fact that the individual has lost enough lower extremity (LE) ROM at the hip (e.g., hip flexion contractures) to prevent balancing in a fully upright posture. The return of activity following remediation of the impairment of joint mobility is then considered clinical evidence of a relationship between the impairment and the limitation. One should be aware, however, that activity may be restored without complete resolution of the impairments of body function and structures, and vice versa. Therefore, it is important that the physical therapist measure all the appropriate components of an individual's function.

Table 8.2	Environmental Factors in the International Classification of Functioning, Disability, and Health
First-Level Classification	**Examples**
Products and technology	Medications, clothes, prosthetics, walking devices, scooters, hearing aids, ramps, assets
Natural environment and human-made changes to environment	Geography, climate, light, air quality
Support and relationships	Immediate family, extended family, friends, persons in positions of authority, personal assistants, domesticated animals, health professionals
Attitudes	Individual attitudes of immediate family members, individual attitudes of health professionals, societal attitudes
Services, systems, and policies	Housing, transportation, legal, associations, health, education, political

■ EXAMINATION OF FUNCTION

Purpose

Analysis of function focuses on the identification of pertinent activities and measurement of an individual's ability to successfully engage in them. In essence, functional testing is used to measure how a person does certain tasks or fulfils certain roles in the various dimensions described by the ICF. Application of selected functional tests and measures yields data that can be used as (1) baseline information for setting function-oriented goals and outcomes of intervention; (2) indicators of a patient's initial abilities and progression toward more complex functional levels; (3) criteria for placement decisions (e.g., the need for inpatient rehabilitation, extended care, or community services) as well as communication between settings; (4) manifestations of an individual's level of safety in performing a particular task and the risk of injury with continued performance; (5) evidence of the effectiveness of a specific intervention (medical, surgical, or rehabilitative) on function; and (6) documentation to support payer requirements of change in functional status during an episode of care.

General Considerations

Physical therapists possess a unique body of knowledge related to the identification, remediation, and prevention of movement dysfunction. Thus, they have traditionally been involved in the examination of physical function. Other members of the rehabilitation team, including the occupational therapist, speech-language pathologist, nurse, rehabilitation counselor, and recreational therapist, are also typically involved in administering and interpreting functional tests. Some formal instruments were designed to be completed collectively by the team. Other tests are compiled in separate sections by specific health professionals and housed together in the patient's chart. Where teams exist, physical therapists are typically responsible for the testing of aspects of function related to mobility, such as bed mobility, transfers, and locomotion (wheelchair mobility, ambulation, negotiation of stairs and graded elevations, walking for longer distances in the community, and so forth). Instruments to measure activities of daily living (ADL) may be administered by a physical therapist alone or cooperatively with other health professionals. When overlap among team members exists (e.g., the performance of toilet transfers), the data may be collected by the physical therapist, an occupational therapist, or a nurse. In these instances, testing should be coordinated to reduce duplication and unnecessary patient stress. In noninstitutional settings or when there is no team, the physical therapist is often responsible for determining all aspects of these instruments.

Testing Perspectives

Function tests can utilize two highly divergent perspectives on what is to be tested or measured by the physical therapist. The therapist must determine in advance whether data are needed to describe the *habitual performance* of a patient's ability to do certain tasks and activities in their home and community environment or to identify the patient's *capacity* to perform certain tasks and activities measured in a clinical environment, whether the patient habitually performs up to that level or not, or even performs them at all. These perspectives are incorporated within the ICF by the constructs of performance and capacity, and the ICF allows for the separate coding of both constructs.

These divergent viewpoints directly affect what types of tests and measures should be chosen and what parameters of measurement are appropriate to yield data useful to making clinical judgments. For example, the focus on capacity or performance may influence the selection of either a performance-based measure such as the 10-meter Walk Test (10MWT) that measures the time it takes the patient to walk 10 meters, which physical therapists use to infer walking performance in the real world, or a self-report measure such as the Stroke Impact Scale, which has a section on which patients self-report their walking performance. Activity monitors, such as fitness watches, provide a numeric measure of habitual walking performance (i.e., steps/day). Most important, physical therapists must consider the differences between capacity for function and performance of habitual function in determining the prognosis for rehabilitation and estimating the likelihood of the success of an intervention. Patients accept a therapist's recommendations regarding the anticipated goals of treatment only if there is the perceived need and motivation to function habitually at the highest level of ability. Understanding the difference between what a person actually does and what that person potentially could do is an essential component of designing realistic, and achievable, functional goals. For example, even though a person might have the capacity to climb stairs, there may not be any willingness or opportunity to ever do so. Ultimately, physical therapists must abide by each patient's own decision regarding which tasks and activities will be incorporated into a daily routine and what is a meaningful level of function, regardless of the therapist's professional opinion.

Regardless of the particular instrument used, there are several basic considerations to keep in mind. The setting chosen must be conducive to the type of testing and free of distractions. Instructions should be precise and unambiguous. Testing may be biased by fatigue. If a patient performs best in the morning but tires by afternoon, an accurate determination of functional ability must consider variation in the patient's performance. Therapists should be aware of patients whose energy fluctuates during the day and interpret the data accordingly. In general, information related to body functions and body structure, activities, and participation, as well as personal and environmental factors, should be generated during the initial examination (or as soon as feasible) so the information may be considered together to develop a picture of a patient's function. Retesting should occur at regular intervals during treatment to document progress and before discharge from the episode of care.

Types of Instruments
Performance-Based Tests

A performance-based test involves observing the patient perform an activity. Generally, the therapist who chooses a performance-based test is searching for an indication of what a person can do under a specific set of circumstances, which may or may not be similar to their natural environment. If a performance-based test is chosen with the intention of making inferences about how the patient will perform in a different setting, such as the home or the community, the conditions and setting should be as similar as possible to the actual environment in which the patient usually performs the tasks and activities. This is an important distinction between assessments of the *capacity to function* in one setting as compared to their *ability to perform* the tasks in a different setting. A performance-based approach may be used either to describe the patient's current level of function or to identify the maximum level of function possible.

During the administration of the test, each task is presented, and the patient is asked to perform it. For example, to examine current level of function in wheelchair mobility, a patient would receive this instruction: "Push your wheelchair over to that red chair and stop." To determine the patient's maximum level of function in this activity, the instruction might specify a particular manner of performance: "Push your wheelchair over to that red chair *as quickly as you can* and stop." Understanding the difference between these two instructions, even though both are observation-based performance of wheelchair mobility, is essential to sound clinical decision-making. Data from the first example identify only what the patient can do under specific circumstances but do not support the inference that the patient will be able to wheel across a busy intersection in the short time span allotted at a typical crosswalk. The form of the instruction determines whether an inference can be made about the patient's maximal level of function in formulating the goals for intervention and the plan of care.

In either case, patients are given no additional instructions or assistance unless they are unable or unsure of how to perform. Then only as much direction or assistance as is needed is given and documented. Appropriate safety precautions should be taken during the session so that patients do not attempt tasks that are potentially dangerous.

Many tests have been considered as functional performance measures of capacity, including the *6-minute Walk Test* (6MWT),[11] the *Physical Performance and Mobility Examination*,[12] the *Functional Reach Test*,[13,14] the *Get Up and Go Test*,[15] the *Timed Up and Go Test* (TUG),[16] and the *Short Physical Performance Battery*.[17] A performance instrument of this sort typically measures either a

complex integration of impairments, the performance of actions, or a combination of both by direct observation. Overall, the tests provide some insight into the individual's capabilities to maintain a posture, transition to other postures, or sustain safe and efficient movement. The data from such a test, gathered under controlled conditions, characterize a person's limitations as a result of impairments and may purport to predict the success or failure of an individual in performing goal-directed tasks or activities under natural conditions, using a score that summates the combined effects of impairments throughout and across systems on movement dysfunction. Each of these tests can contribute to an understanding of an aspect of a person's function, but they should not be used to represent all aspects of function. Although these tests employ the method of direct observation of performance, they most often do not measure the task or activity as it might be accomplished in the "real" world of the patient, which is also influenced by motivation and habit, as well as external distractions.

Self-Reports

In contrast to the method of direct observation, useful data on how a person functions may also be gathered by *self-report,* in which the patient is asked directly by either the therapist or a trained interviewer (*interviewer report*) or via a *self-administered report* instrument. These may also be referred to as *patient-reported outcome measures.* Self-administered reports may be provided in a paper-and-pencil format or as an electronic version. The patient may complete these reports during the therapy visit or outside of the treatment session. The critical issue for a self-report to capture function correctly and completely lies in providing clearly worded questions without bias, concise directions on completing the questions, and a format that encourages accurate reporting of answers to all questions. Self-report is a valid method of determining function and may be preferable or equivalent to performance-based methods in some circumstances.[18,19] Self-reports should be designed so that questions are asked in a standard format, and answers are recorded as specified by the predetermined choices. For example, a paper-and-pencil test may be difficult for those with upper extremity (UE) impairments to complete.

Clinical personnel who act as interviewers must be trained to administer a questionnaire. Interviewers should practice until they have reached a high degree of agreement with expert examiners of the same cases. Periodic retraining may be necessary if interviewers do not have frequent practice administering the instrument. The interview should be scheduled with the patient in advance and conducted in an environment conducive to complete concentration. Interviews may be conducted by phone or in person, but the mode of administration should be kept consistent if comparisons of the data are to be made. Ad lib prompting by the interviewer or caregivers for answers is discouraged because these intrusions into the patient's self-report tend to bias results. If the patient has had help in filling out a form or responding to questions, this should be noted. Similarly, if a spouse, family member, or caregiver has provided the data, this should be documented as well.

The distinction in perspectives on function that was discussed regarding performance-based measures of function also holds for self-reports. It is extremely important to distinguish between questions that indicate a person's habitual performance (e.g., "*Do* you cook your own meals?") and those that identify a person's perceived capacity to perform a task (e.g., "If you had to, *could* you cook your own meals?"). It may also be important to distinguish between an individual's performance of an activity and their confidence/self-efficacy in performing an activity. For example, confidence and performance for 21 items are measured in separate scales in the American Physical Therapy Association (APTA)'s *Outpatient Physical Therapy Improvement in Movement Assessment Log* (OPTIMAL).[20]

The time frame provided in the directions is also a relevant consideration. A therapist should decide in advance if the relevant "window" on a person's self-report of function is the past 24 hrs, the previous week, the previous month, or the previous year. One can easily imagine how the same person might respond differently regarding the same functional activity depending on the frame of reference. Instruments that examine only short-term objectives may not relate well to the long-term objectives of a rehabilitation program.

Instrument Parameters and Formats

Performance-based and self-report instruments grade performance on a number of different criteria in a variety of formats. There is no one parameter or format that is perfect for every type of clinical encounter or research need. It is particularly important that documentation of a patient's progress not be blunted by *floor* or *ceiling* effects. For example, if a therapist wishes to measure changes in function among generally well older patients and the most advanced functional activity on an instrument measures "independent ambulation on level surfaces," there would be no room to demonstrate either progression or decline except around ambulation on level surfaces. Similarly, a patient who was severely debilitated might improve in transfers from needing the maximum assistance of two persons to maximum assistance of one. If the instrument only measures change from "maximum assistance" to "moderate assistance," this patient's real improvement will not be recorded.

Descriptive Parameters

Therapists should use descriptive terms that are well defined and unambiguous. Meanings of descriptive terms should be clear to all others using the medical record. Box 8.1 provides a sample set of acceptable terms and definitions. Please note that although in widespread clinical usage, there is little empirical evidence for the definitions provided for terms such as *minimal assistance* or *moderate assistance*. The definitions presented here are at best one operational definition to describe these terms. Additional terms used to qualify function include *dependence* and *difficulty*. Most often, the term *independent* refers to the complete absence of a need for human or mechanical assistance to accomplish a task, but some scoring systems consider reliance on devices and aids as a modified form of independence when used without the help of another person. The use of equipment during the performance of a functional task should be explicitly noted; for example, "independent in ambulation with axillary crutches" or "independent in dressing with adapted clothing and a long-handled shoehorn."

Difficulty is a hybrid term that suggests an activity poses an extra burden for the patient, regardless of dependence level. It is unclear whether it is a measure of overall perceptual-motor skill, coordination, endurance, or efficiency, or a combination of measures. Difficulty can be measured in two ways. One approach assumes that difficulty is likely to be present and quantifies the degree of difficulty that the individual experiences while performing the activity (e.g., "How much difficulty do you have while doing household chores? None, some, or a great deal?"). The other approach quantifies the frequency that the difficulty is encountered (e.g., "How often do you have difficulty putting on your shoes? Never, sometimes, very often, or always?").

Often it is helpful to qualify a person's performance by linking observations with nonspecific indicators of impairments such as the energy consumption required to complete the functional task and the degree to which patients must exert themselves to engage in the activity. Simple measurements of a patient's physiological response to activity generally include heart rate, respiratory rate, blood pressure, and oxygen saturation, obtained at rest (baseline measurements), during (as possible), or immediately after completion of the most stressful elements of the activity. For example, "Heart rate increased to 100 beats per minute with independent ambulation on stairs; no increase in respiratory rate." In addition, the patient's perceived fatigue, rating of perceived exertion, and overt signs of physiological stress, such as shortness of breath, also should be noted. These notations may assist the therapist in a quick identification of some obvious impairments that limit the functional task, which should be followed by more specific tests and measures of impairment.

Additional descriptors frequently used to qualify functional performance further include (1) pain, (2) fluctuations according to the time of day, (3) medication level, and (4) environmental influences. Any factors that modify a patient's function should be carefully noted and considered by the physical therapist evaluating examination data.

Box 8.1   Functional Examination and Impairment Terminology

Definitions

1. **Independent (I):** Patient is able consistently to perform skill safety with no one present.
2. **Supervision (S):** Patient requires someone within arm's reach as a precaution; low probability of patient having a problem requiring assistance.
3. **Close guarding (CloseG):** Person assisting is positioned as if to assist, with hands raised but not touching patient; full attention on patient; fair probability of patient requiring assistance.
4. **Contact guarding (ContactG):** Therapist is positioned as with close guarding, with hands on patient but not giving any assistance; high probability of patient requiring assistance.
5. **Minimum assistance (MinA):** Patient is able to complete majority of the activity without assistance.
6. **Moderate assistance (ModA):** Patient is able to complete part of the activity without assistance.
7. **Maximum assistance (MaxA):** Patient is unable to assist in any part of the activity.

Descriptive Terminology

A. Bed Mobility
1. Independent—no cuing* is given
2. Supervision
3. Minimum assistance } may require cues
4. Moderate assistance
5. Maximum assistance

B. Transfers, Ambulation
1. Independent—no cuing is given
2. Supervision
3. Close guarding
4. Contact guarding } may require cues
5. Minimum assistance
6. Moderate assistance
7. Maximum assistance

C. Functional Balance Grades

1. Normal	Patient is able to maintain steady balance without support (static). Accepts maximal challenge and can shift weight easily and within full range in all directions (dynamic).
2. Good	Patient is able to maintain balance without support, limited postural sway (static). Accepts moderate challenge; able to maintain balance while picking object off floor (dynamic).
3. Fair	Patient is able to maintain balance with handhold support; may require occasional minimal assistance (static). Accepts minimal challenge; able to maintain balance while turning head/trunk (dynamic).
4. Poor	Patient requires handhold and moderate to maximal assistance to maintain posture (static). Unable to accept challenge or move without loss of balance (dynamic).
5. No balance	

*Types of cues: verbal, visual, or tactile. In some instances (e.g., a person with a memory deficit, short attention, learning disability, visual loss), a decrease in the number of cues may represent treatment progress, even though the level of dependence remains the same. Interim progress notes can denote these changes by citing frequencies (e.g., two out of three tries) or an arbitrarily defined rank-order scale (e.g., always/occasionally/rarely).

Quantitative Parameters

The time it takes to complete a series of activities is often used to enhance a therapist's quantification of function when a given speed of performance is required or an improvement in performance speed is expected. A common example of timed functional skills is found in premedication and postmedication performance of individuals with Parkinson disease who are placed on levodopa medication. Examples of activities that may be timed include (1) walking a set distance, (2) writing a signature, (3) donning an article of clothing, and (4) crossing a street during the time of a "walk" light. Scores of timed tests should not be taken as absolute but rather as one dimension of performance. Although the ability to complete a particular activity in a specified period of time does provide one kind of important data on a patient's overall ability, it may not always be correct to conclude that what is being measured as "quicker" can be interpreted as "better." For example, the patient may get dressed quickly (within seconds) but does so with poorly coordinated movements and a haphazard outcome. When the task is slowed down, the movements may become more coordinated, with a more satisfactory functional outcome, even though the time taken to do the task increases. Similarly, certain medical conditions that affect energy expenditure may require that the patient properly pace a functional activity to complete it successfully. Thus, time scores alone do not always yield the complete functional picture. When interpreted in light of other aspects of the patient's clinical presentation, they provide an added dimension to the evaluation of data collected during examination of a function.

Response Formats

Function can be measured with tests that report data as nominal, ordinal, interval, and ratio measures. The clinician should consider the uses of the measure when deciding which format to use. In cases where the clinical decision is nominal, such as if the patient is ready for discharge to home, a nominal measure such as whether the patient can or cannot independently ascend 10 stairs may be adequate. When a numeric value is obtained, such as the score from the Berg Balance Scale,[21] the clinician may interpret the score as a dichotomous measure related to the decision (e.g., Does the patient have or not have adequate balance for discharge to home?). In cases where the clinical decision is more complex, such as the amount of assistance a patient needs with activities, nominal measures cannot be used, and the measure should reflect the type and amount of information needed for the decision.

Nominal Measures

One of the simplest formats in functional tests uses a nominal level of measurement by presenting a checklist of various functional tasks on which the patient is simply scored as able to do/not able to do, independent/dependent, completed/incomplete, or the like. The results are not particularly descriptive of the exact nature of an individual's limitations and usually require further examination before interpretation. Nominal measures, however, may be helpful in making dichotomous decisions. For example, knowledge of the ability to perform ADL skills by themselves is important in deciding if a patient can be discharged to living independently at home.

Ordinal Measures

A few tests use descriptive scales that describe a range of performance or the degree to which a person can perform the task. Most commonly, the scales are ordinal or rank-order scales; for example, "no difficulty," "some difficulty," or "unable to do"; or "always," "sometimes," "rarely," or "never." (For additional examples, consider the levels of assistance terminology and functional balance grades in Box 8.1.) Scales may be graded in ascending or descending order. The primary drawback in using such a system to score function is that these grades do not define categories that are separated by equal intervals. For example, it is not possible to tell whether the patient who went from maximal to moderate assistance changed as much as a patient who also went one level between moderate and minimal assistance.

Summary or additive measures grade a specific series of skills, award points for part or full performance, and sum the subscores as a proportion of the total possible points, such as 60/100 or 40/56. These summary measures may be considered as interval measures if the scores on the scale represent equal intervals; otherwise, these measures may be considered as ordinal measures. One method to determine if the points on the scale represent equal intervals is through the use of Rasch analysis.[22] Although these summative scales typically may include a score of zero, this value represents a floor effect of the scale and not necessarily the absence of the construct. An example of a summary measure, which may be used to measure functional mobility and activities of self-care, is the Barthel Index.[23]

Some formal, standardized instruments for testing function summarize detailed information about a complex area of function into an overall index score. Use of these instruments facilitates the interpretation of complex data and enables the clinician to compare function across conditions, settings, and populations. Caution must be exercised in considering only summated scores, however, because potentially important individual differences in functional ability can be masked.[24] A patient who is limited in only a few of the many tasks covered on a functional test will most likely score well, despite what could be substantial limitations in discrete functional activities that are pertinent to the physical therapist's anticipated goals of treatment. Similarly, two patients with the same numeric score might be quite different in their functional deficits, having gained (or lost) their points on different activities. Although these measures yield a "hard number," which is regarded statistically as an interval level of measurement, the degree to which "points" are truly equal intervals or only ordinal should be carefully scrutinized.

Interval/Ratio Measures

Interval and ratio measures in rehabilitation include performance-based measures, such as the 6MWT[11] and the TUG,[16] where the results are reported in meters and seconds, respectively. Characteristics of interval measures include the ordering of an ordinal scale and that the intervals between values are equal and known. Ratio measures include equal intervals between values and

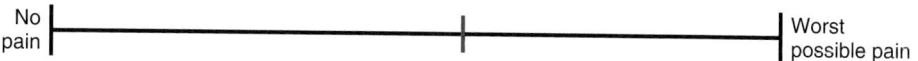

Figure 8.3 A visual analog scale for measuring pain. The patient is instructed to mark the line at the point that corresponds to the degree of pain they are experiencing. For visual analog scales that measure symptoms besides pain, the labeling of the anchors is changed to reflect the symptom being measured.

include a true zero that represents the absence of the phenomenon being measured.

Visual analog scales attempt to represent measurement quantities in terms of a 10-cm or 100-mm straight line placed horizontally or vertically on paper (Fig. 8.3). The endpoints of the line are labeled with descriptive terms to anchor the extremes of the scale and provide a frame of reference for any point in the continuum between them. Some scales will also use descriptors or numeric intervals between the endpoints to assist the individual in grading responses. The patient is asked to mark the line at a point representing a self-reported position on the scale. The patient's score is then obtained by measuring the distance in centimeters (or millimeters) from the zero mark to the mark made by the patient.

Examples of the use of visual analog scales in rehabilitation settings may be to measure pain, dyspnea, function, or satisfaction with care. Since visual analog scales include a true zero and the units are in equal intervals (e.g., millimeters), some may consider the scale as a ratio measure; however, the perception of a person completing the scale may reflect a more ordinal interpretation.[25–27] As an alternative to visual analog scales, some clinicians may use a numeric rating scale (e.g., rate your function on a scale from 0 to 10) to measure similar impairments. Although a numeric rating may be quicker to obtain in a clinical setting, scores obtained may not represent interval or ratio data, as these scales do not provide units of the measurement, and the reporting of numeric values may not represent equal intervals. For example, a four reported by one patient may not represent twice as much function as a two reported by another patient. This is due to the nature of interval and ratio scales because a ratio scale allows for the comparison of scores using addition, subtraction, multiplication, or division, and an interval scale allows for the comparison of scores using addition or subtraction. These mathematical functions cannot be performed with ordinal or nominal scores.

Knowledge of the level of measurement is important in analyzing data from groups of patients, such as a rehabilitation unit wishing to summarize the functional status of patients admitted during a specified time period. For interval and ratio measures, means and standard deviations may be calculated (assuming the data follow a normal distribution). For ordinal measures, medians and interquartile ranges are appropriate, whereas nominal measures may be represented by modes or by frequency counts. The distinction in the level of measurement is also important in the decision to use either parametric or nonparametric statistics to analyze data obtained from groups of patients.

INTERPRETING TEST RESULTS

Clearly, the single most important consideration in examining functional status is using the test results correctly to establish and revise the anticipated goals and expected outcomes of intervention and the plan of care. The therapist should carefully delineate the contributing factors that result in the functional deficit. When diminished ability is evident, the therapist must attempt to ascertain the cause of the problem. Some important questions to ask include the following:

1. What are the normal movements necessary to perform the task?
2. Which impairments inhibit performance or completion of the task? For example, do factors such as poor motor planning and execution, decreased strength, decreased ROM, or altered joint integrity impede function? Does fatigue hamper functional ability?
3. Are the patient's functional deficits the result of impaired communication, perception, vision, hearing, or cognition?

Examples of the kinds of questions a therapist must pose to assess function and integrate findings into a comprehensive treatment program are found using the case vignettes in Table 8.3.

Although the activity limitation in each case is identical, the contributing factors, goals and outcomes, and interventions would be markedly different. In Case A, the patient's inability to transfer can reasonably be attributed to decreased strength. When ameliorated, it is likely that the patient will go on to achieve an outcome of independent ambulation with a prosthesis. The patient in Case B has factors that cannot be addressed solely through physical therapy. In addition, it may be difficult to determine whether it is the paralysis or the aphasia that compromises efforts to assess and improve function. Although a similar goal of independence in wheelchair mobility and transfers may be proposed, reexamination throughout

Table 8.3	Sample Case Vignettes	
Patient Information	**Case A**	**Case B**
Patient description	36-year-old male construction worker	72-year-old female homemaker
Diagnosis	Traumatic right transtibial amputation following fracture left femur	Cerebral vascular accident with right hemiplegia with global aphasia
Partial examination findings	**Motor Control and Muscle Performance**	
	Decreased in all extremities following prolonged immobilization	Flaccid paralysis right extremities
	Activity Limitations	
	Unable to transfer from bed to wheelchair	Unable to transfer from bed to wheelchair

the episode of care may demonstrate that functional deficits persist, despite improvement in motor function. In that case, the impairments in comprehension and language function may be the more important factors contributing to functional limitation. Thus, the design of rehabilitation programs is based on the impairments that presumably underlie the functional deficits. If remediation of the impairment does not solve the functional problem, the therapist needs to reexamine the initial clinical impression by looking for other potentially causative factors.

Some functional tasks may need to be analyzed more precisely. Activities can be broken down into subordinate parts, or subroutines. A *subordinate part* is defined as an element of movement without which the task cannot proceed safely or efficiently. For example, bed mobility includes the following subordinate parts: (1) scooting in bed (changing position for comfort or skin care and getting to the edge), (2) rolling onto the side, (3) lowering the legs, (4) sitting up, and (5) balancing at the edge of the bed. A functional loss of independent bed mobility may result from an inability to perform any or all of these subroutines. These are not only checkpoints for examining patients, but they also later represent the anticipated goals of various interventions. The more involved the patient, the slower the learner, or the more complex the task, the more the functional task may need to be broken down into subordinate parts.

Determining the Quality of Instruments

Within the rehabilitation setting, many tools exist for the measurement of function or its components. A number of excellent sources are available on the Internet to learn about the psychometric properties of functional measures (see Appendix 8.A [online]). In many cases, the sources include links to the instruments or information on how to perform or obtain the measures. In deciding which measure to use, the instrument's *reliability, validity,* and *responsiveness* should be considered. If the reliability and validity of an instrument have not

been established, little faith can be put in the results obtained or in the conclusions drawn from the results. Responsiveness of an instrument is important in determining if the change in a patient's score on two different occasions truly represents a change in their function. In light of the fact that the viability of physical therapy as a reimbursable service rests on the demonstration of functional outcomes, the importance of these concepts to functional testing becomes clear. In accordance with the APTA's Standards of Measurement, physical therapists should use only those instruments whose reliability and validity are known.[28] Although no instrument will have perfect psychometric properties, therapists must be able to gauge the certainty of their data and the appropriate scope of inferences drawn from the data. Systematic reviews of patient-reported outcome measures (i.e., self-reports) may utilize the consensus-based standards for the selection of health measurement instruments (COSMIN) to appraise the quality of the psychometric properties.[29]

Reliability

A reliable instrument measures a phenomenon dependably, time after time, accurately, predictably, and without variation. If a functional test is not reliable, the patient's initial baseline status or the true effect of treatment can be concealed. A self-report or performance-based instrument with acceptable *test–retest reliability* is stable and will not indicate change when none has occurred. For performance-based measures where items are rated by the clinician, the reliability of the examiner is also important. In other words, tests performed by the same therapist of the same performance should be highly correlated (*intrarater reliability*). Tests should also have strong *interrater reliability*, or agreement among multiple observers of the same event. If a patient is examined by several therapists in the course of treatment, or reexamined over time to determine long-term change, the reliability of these measurements must be known. To use functional tests with maximum accuracy, (1) scoring criteria must be defined clearly and must be mutually exclusive, (2) criteria must be strictly applied to each clinical situation, and (3) all therapists in a facility must be retrained periodically in the use of the instrument to ensure similarity.

Values for reliability coefficients have been provided; however, disclaimers are generally added that these should not be considered absolute cutoffs. For example, Portney suggests point estimates of coefficients less than 0.50 as poor reliability, 0.50 to 0.75 as moderate reliability, above 0.75 as good reliability, and greater than 0.90 as excellent.[27(p491)] In interpreting these values, the clinician needs to consider the precision of the measurement and how the results of the test will be applied in practice. A clinician should use these values only as guidelines, and not as absolutes, in determining the accuracy of the measurement and needs to consider the purpose of using the instrument. If high precision is needed in the instrument for clinical decision-making, values of a reliability coefficient higher than the minimal threshold for "good" reliability should be used. In addition to the value of the reliability coefficient, the clinician should consider the precision of the measurement that may be expressed through values such as a confidence interval.

Validity

Validity is a multifaceted concept and established in many different ways. Questions regarding an instrument's validity attempt to determine (1) whether an instrument designed to measure function truly does just that, (2) what the appropriate applications of the instrument are, and (3) how the data should be interpreted. First, the valid instrument should, on the face of it, appear to measure what it purports to measure (*face validity*).[27,28] For example, an instrument claiming to measure balance should appear to measure some aspect of balance. Another critical dimension is whether the assessment instrument measures all the important or specified dimensions of function (*content validity*). According to COSMIN, content validity of patient-reported measures includes components of relevance, comprehensiveness, and comprehensibility.[29] If there were a gold standard (an unimpeachable measure of a phenomenon, such as a laboratory test with normative values), then a new instrument could be tested against the results of this standard (*criterion-related validity*). Such a gold standard does not exist for functional instruments. New functional measurement tools can, however, be compared to existing ones that are accepted measures of the same functional activities. The degree to which the two instruments agree helps to establish *concurrent validity*. Concurrent validity can also be demonstrated by showing that an instrument corresponds appropriately to measures of other phenomena. This method is particularly relevant for self-report instruments. The concurrent validity of some self-report instruments has

been determined by comparison with clinician ratings and other clinical findings; for example, a person's level of function as indicated by an instrument correlates directly with clinician's ratings of improvement and inversely with the patient's reports of pain.

In the comparison of a test of function to another existing instrument, one should be concerned with the ability of the measure to make an accurate classification. *Sensitivity* of a test refers to the proportion of individuals with a limitation in function (as identified by the gold standard or existing instrument) who are correctly classified. In other words, sensitivity is an indication of how well a test identifies persons who should have a positive finding on the test. In contrast, *specificity* of a test refers to the proportion of individuals who do not have a limitation in function who are correctly classified. Additional properties of a test are the positive predictive value and the negative predictive value. The *positive predictive value* is the proportion of people who have a positive finding on a test who actually have a limitation in function as classified by the comparison test; the *negative predictive value* is the proportion of people who have a negative finding on a test who do not have a limitation in function.

Both sensitivity and specificity are expressed as values between zero and one. Ideally, both sensitivity and specificity should be as close to one as possible, but this is very rare in reality. Different tests, however, will be better at identifying those with the condition, and others will be better at identifying those without the condition. This will be reflected in the magnitude of their sensitivity and specificity scores. When values of sensitivity or specificity are very close to 1.0, the SpPIn and SnNOut acronyms may help with interpretation.[30,31] The acronym SpPIn (**sp**ecific test when **p**ositive, rules **IN** disease) refers to tests that have very high specificity: a positive finding helps to rule in the condition. SnNOut (**s**ensitive test when **n**egative, rules **OUT** disease), on the other hand, refers to tests that have very high sensitivity: a negative finding helps to rule out the condition.

Sensitivity and specificity values may be combined to obtain a likelihood ratio (LR) with the equations in Box 8.2. The calculation of LRs may be helpful in determining how much the test result influences the identification of a patient's condition or limitation in function. This is especially helpful in cases when sensitivity and specificity are not high enough to apply the SpPIn and SnNOut rules.

The larger the value of a positive LR, the more helpful the finding of a positive test is in identifying the condition. Likewise, the smaller the value of a negative LR (e.g., close to zero), the more helpful the finding of a negative test is in ruling out the condition. In contrast, a positive or negative LR close to 1.0 is not helpful in identifying the condition. Likelihood ratios can be helpful in determination of post-test odds through

---

Box 8.2 Formulas to Determine Likelihood Ratios From Sensitivity and Specificity Values

Positive LR = (Sensitivity)/(1 − Specificity)
Negative LR = (1 − Sensitivity)/(Specificity)

where Sensitivity = (Number of True Positives)/(Number of True Positives Plus the Number of False Negatives)
  and Specificity = (Number of True Negatives)/(Number of True Negatives Plus the Number of False Positives)

LR = Likelihood Ratio

---

their application in Bayes theorem (i.e., the pretest odds × LR = the post-test odds).[30,31]

There is also the *predictive validity* of a test or measure, which indicates the likelihood of a subsequent phenomenon or event (e.g., return to work) on the basis of a prior phenomenon (e.g., a baseline measure of function). Finally, the degree to which an instrument measures abstract concepts such as physical mobility or social interaction can be established over time (*construct validity*). Construct validation, using a variety of statistical procedures, is a never-ending process as our understanding of the construct is further refined as instruments are developed to measure it.

Responsiveness

In addition to reliability and validity, a measure of functional status should be sufficiently sensitive to reflect *responsiveness* or a meaningful change in a patient's status. The change should exceed the *minimally detectable change* (MDC) of the instrument and a *minimal clinically important difference* (MCID). The MDC may be described as the smallest amount of change in a measurement that exceeds the measurement error of the instrument in patients who are unchanged.[27,32] A physical therapist should be aware of published MDC values for the instruments used to measure function. A sample of MDC values for the 6MWT, the TUG, and gait speed are presented in Table 8.4. It is important to keep in mind that MDC values are specific for the patient population in whom the instrument was investigated.

In cases where MDC values may not exist in the literature, values may be calculated if the reliability coefficient, such as an intraclass correlation coefficient (ICC), and a measure of its variability are known, such as the standard deviation (SD). Box 8.3 provides equations that present the relationship between the MDC_{95} (the amount of change with 95% confidence beyond measurement error) and the standard error of measurement (SEM). The second equation can be used to determine the SEM if the value of the reliability coefficient

and the SD from one of the groups used to determine reliability is known. Note that because the ICC and the SD are from a specific sample, the calculated SEM and MDC_{95} are only generalizable to persons with similar conditions. Also, note that these calculations are based on test–retest studies in which the patients are unchanged.[32] Other approaches to determining a threshold from change include diagnostic test methodology[33] and item response theory.[34]

For example, if a test–retest reliability study of unchanged persons after total knee arthroplasty reported an ICC of 0.75 and a SD of 5.0° for passive knee flexion as measured with a goniometer, the SEM is equal to 2.5°. Using this value in the first equation, the MDC_{95} is 6.925°. In other words, the measure of knee flexion would need to change more than 7° to have 95% confidence that this change was due to something other than measurement error.

The MCID is the smallest difference in a measured variable that signifies an important rather than trivial difference in the patient's condition.[27,32] The value of the MCID should exceed the value of the MDC; in other words, the MCID needs to exceed the measurement error. For example, a 50-meter change in distance on the 6MWT may be beyond measurement error; however, is the ability to walk 50 meters within 6 minutes meaningful to an individual patient's function? A number of different ways have been suggested to determine values for the MCID.[27(pp503–505)] No universal method exists. Controversies exist among the strategies to determine MCID based on the perspective of what is meaningful, as well as issues related to measurement.[35,36] The clinician should consult the literature for recommended values of the MCID for measures of function. Like the interpretation of the MDC, in consulting published values for the MCID for a measure of function, the clinician needs to consider the sample for which the values were established and the anchor for what is described as "important."

Considerations in Selection of Instruments

Many instruments have been developed to assess and classify function. Given the plethora of instruments that currently exist, it is quite reasonable to ask how these instruments compare with one another. It is important to remember that no instrument is perfect for all patients or in all situations. No instrument can measure all the items potentially relevant to a particular individual and provide the perfect composite picture. For example, one instrument may provide an extensive measure of ADL but not deal with psychological or social dimensions of function. Another instrument may investigate social functioning while omitting some ADL tasks. Many items overlap from instrument to instrument. For example, a question on the ability to ambulate is a common item found in most physical

Table 8.4 Examples of Minimal Detectable Change for the 6-minute Walk Test, the Timed Up and Go Test, and Gait Speed in Five Different Clinical Populations

Test	Population of Interest	MDC	Reference
6MWT	Total hip and knee arthroplasty	61.34 m	Kennedy et al., 2005[91]
	Older adults	65 m	Mangione et al., 2010[92]
	Alzheimer disease	33.5 m	Ries et al., 2009[93]
	Stroke (inpatient rehabilitation)	54.1 m	Fulk et al., 2008[94]
	Multiple sclerosis	88 m*	Learmonth et al., 2013[95]
TUG	Total hip and knee arthroplasty	2.49 sec	Kennedy et al., 2005[91]
	Older adults	4 sec	Mangione et al., 2010[92]
	Alzheimer disease	4.09 sec	Ries et al., 2009[93]
	Stroke (outpatient)	7.84 sec*	Hiengkaew et al., 2012[96]
	Multiple sclerosis	10.6 sec*	Learmonth et al., 2012[97]
Gait speed	Total hip and knee arthroplasty (tested as fast self-paced walk time to complete 40 meters)	4.04 sec	Kennedy et al., 2005[91]
	Older adults	0.19 m/sec	Mangione et al., 2010[92]
	Alzheimer disease	0.094 m/sec	Ries et al., 2009[93]
	Stroke (outpatient)	0.18 m/sec*	Hiengkaew et al., 2012[96]
	Multiple sclerosis	0.26 m/sec*	Paltamaa et al., 2008[98]

MDC = minimal detectable change; 6MWT = 6-minute Walk Test; TUG = Timed Up and Go Test.
*Note these values are MDC_{95}, whereas all other values are MDC_{90}.

Box 8.3   Formulas to Determine Minimal Detectable Change From a Reliability Coefficient

$$MDC_{95} = 1.96 \times SEM \times \sqrt{2}$$

$$where\ SEM = SD \times \sqrt{1-ICC}$$

---

function instruments. Although instruments may cover the same kind of activity, the questions posed about the performance of the same activity may be quite different. For example, one instrument may investigate the degree of difficulty and of human assistance required to "dress yourself, including handling of closures, buttons, zippers, snaps." Another may ask, "How much help do you need in getting dressed?" As discussed, differences also may exist in the time frames sampled in the various instruments. Critical questions to ask in selecting an instrument are presented in Box 8.4.

Extrapolating items from a variety of instruments may provide the kind of data desired but should be considered with extreme caution because this process changes reliability or validity of the measurements. Factors such as the theoretic orientation of the user, the purpose for using the instrument, and the relevance of particular functional items to certain patient

---

Box 8.4   Critical Questions to Ask in Selecting an Instrument

1. What are the domains or categories that the assessment instrument focuses on?
2. How adequately does the instrument measure the domain or domains being sampled?
3. What areas of physical function are included? Does the instrument measure activities of daily living? Does the instrument measure instrumental activities of daily living, for example, more advanced skills such as managing personal affairs, cooking, and driving? Mobility skills?
4. What aspect of function is being measured? Is the level of dependence–independence considered? What is the length of time required to complete the functional task? Degree of difficulty? Influence of pain?
5. What is the time frame sampled in the instrument?
6. What is the mode of administration?
7. What type of scoring system is used?
8. Are multiple instruments necessary to provide a more complete picture of functional status?
9. Who completes the instrument—the clinician, the patient (self-report), or family member (proxy)?
10. How long does the instrument take to complete?

populations all enter into the decision-making process. In the final analysis, the choice of instrument may be dictated by practical considerations. For example, self-report instruments, which rely on information from the patient, are limited in use to mentally competent individuals. Time and resources for administration also may influence test selection, or some rehabilitation facilities may adopt the use of a specific instrument for all patients. In any case, many suitable instruments are available for assessing functional status.

■ SINGLE- VERSUS MULTIDIMENSIONAL MEASURES OF FUNCTION

Among the factors to consider in selecting a measure of function is whether a single- or a multidimensional measure should be used. For example, *single-dimensional measures* may include a specific activity such as balance, gait, or reaching, whereas multidimensional measures would include a combination of these constructs or items from different domains of the ICF (e.g., impairments, activity limitations, and participation restrictions). As an example of a single test, gait speed as obtained during a 10MWT may be used to represent function. This test may frequently be used in clinical settings because it requires a minimal amount of time to perform and little equipment other than a stopwatch and a hallway free of obstructions. For the test, the time in seconds for the patient to ambulate 10 meters is recorded, and speed is calculated as distance divided by time (m/sec). Although this is a test of a specific mobility item (walking), one might make inferences to a patient's function based on this test. The clinician, however, is responsible to check with the literature to determine if the inferences are supported by evidence, because there are some specific populations where gait speed may be representative of a patient's ability to function. For example, in a study of persons after hip arthroplasty, it was demonstrated that gait speed measured in the laboratory was more representative of the capacity to ambulate compared to performance of walking speed in the real world. When the patients were tested in real-world environments using an activity monitor to measure gait speed, their gait speed was slower than in the clinic (capacity) compared to in the real world (performance). In this case, the measure of capacity versus performance was moderately correlated ($\rho = 0.440$).[37] Another study conducted with older persons suggests that the measure of gait speed is highly related to overall health.[38] For populations that have not been tested, however, a clinician should be cautious in using gait speed to make inferences regarding function.

Other tests may use multiple items to measure a single dimension, such as the 14 items in the Berg Balance Scale to calculate a balance score.[21] A clinician is justified using these instruments to describe the dimension of interest related to the patient's problem. However,

unless data exist, they should not be used to make inferences regarding other impairments, activity limitations, or participation restrictions. Other instruments specific to those dimensions should be used as appropriate to the patient's presentation.

Alternatively, a clinician may take an approach to understand a patient's health status in a number of domains. Further instrument development has resulted in the emergence of *multidimensional health status instruments* to measure the spectrum of health status more comprehensively. Used in conjunction with traditional clinical methods of examining signs and symptoms, multidimensional functional status instruments can add an important comprehensive view of a patient's function to the overall health status. In this respect, they add a crucial, and previously missing, component in evaluating the health of individuals.

Many comprehensive instruments have been developed to measure multiple dimensions of the ICF to present an overall view of a person's function. Specifically, several *ICF Core Sets* have been introduced for specific patient conditions, such as stroke,[39] or for settings such as post-acute rehabilitation.[40] Each core set includes items related to body functions, body structures, activities, participation, and contextual factors important to the specific condition or setting. These core sets were developed using expert opinion and have undergone testing to determine if representative items are included.[41,42] These core sets potentially may allow a clinician to focus on the most relevant items from the myriad of specific items in the ICF classification. A clinical practice guideline with recommendations for core sets of specific outcome measures related to functioning in persons with neurological conditions in a variety of settings is available.[43]

The final section of this chapter briefly presents four multidimensional instruments a physical therapist may use in practice and research. In addition, another instrument, the Patient-Specific Functional Scale (PSFS), is included to represent a measure of aspects of function important to an individual patient. Many other instruments exist, some of which were mentioned previously in this chapter and some of which are included in other chapters. For additional measures, please review the websites in Appendix 8.A (online).

For the purposes of illustration, four multidimensional instruments, the Functional Independence Measure (FIM), the Outcome and Assessment Information Set (OASIS), the 36-Item Short Form Health Survey (SF-36), and the Activity Measure for Post-Acute Care (AM-PAC), are presented. The choice of a multidimensional instrument carries the same caveats mentioned for single-dimensional instruments.[44] No instrument measures all potentially relevant items. In addition, depending on how an item is worded, items that may appear to measure the same aspect of function may be measuring different aspects of performance.[45] Table 8.5 presents a comparison of items covered by three of these

Table 8.5	Items Covered in Selected Multidimensional Functional Assessment Instruments		
	FIM	SF-36	OASIS
Symptoms		+	+
Physical function			
Transfers	+	−	+
Ambulation	+	+	+
ADL			
Bathing	+	+	+
Grooming	+	−	+
Dressing	+	+	+
Feeding	+	−	+
Toileting	+	−	+
IADL			
Indoor home	−	+	+chores
Outdoor home	−	+	+chores/shopping
Community	−	+	+travel/drive car
Work/school	−	+	−
Affective function			
Communication	+	−	+
Cognition	+	−	+
Anxiety	−	+	+
Depression	−	+	+
Social function			
Interaction	+	+	−
Activity/leisure	−	+	−
General health	−	+	−perceptions

ADL = activities of daily living; FIM = Functional Independence Measure; IADL = instrumental activities of daily living; OASIS = Outcome and Assessment Information Set; SF-36 = 36-Item Short Form Health Survey.

instruments. In the area of physical function, questions on the ability to ambulate are the only items these instruments have in common. Aspects of physical function not covered in any of these instruments include bed mobility and dexterity. The FIM and the OASIS include more ADL items than the SF-36. The SF-36 investigates work performance, whereas the FIM and the OASIS do not. This is not surprising, given that the FIM was originally developed as a tool for the inpatient rehabilitation setting, and the OASIS was expressly designed for home health agencies, both generally serving older patients.

In contrast, the development of the SF-36 was focused on younger adult populations in ambulatory care. Anxiety and depression are addressed as areas of psychological function in the SF-36 and the OASIS but not in the FIM. The OASIS does not explore social function, in contrast to the other two. Finally, only the SF-36 records general health perceptions.

■ SAMPLE INSTRUMENTS TO ASSESS FUNCTION
The Functional Independence Measure

The FIM[46,47] is an 18-item measure of physical, psychological, and social function that is part of the Uniform Data System for Medical Rehabilitation (UDSMR; Table 8.6).[48] The UDSMR collects data from participating rehabilitation facilities and issues summary reports of the records that have been entered into the UDSMR database. The FIM uses the level of assistance an individual needs to grade functional status from total independence to total assistance. A person may be regarded as independent if a device is used, but this is recorded separately from "complete" independence. A 7-point scale is used based on the percentage of active participation from the patient. Complete independence for an item is scored as a 7, and a 1 is defined as total assistance required to perform the activity or the item is not testable. Precise definitions are provided for each level of assistance. The instrument lists six self-care

Table 8.6	Categories and Items of the Functional Independence Measure
Self-care	A. Eating B. Grooming C. Bathing D. Dressing–Upper E. Dressing–Lower F. Toileting
Sphincter control	G. Bladder H. Bowel
Transfers	I. Bed, Chair, Wheelchair J. Toilet K. Tub, Shower
Locomotion	L. Walk/Wheelchair M. Stairs
Communication	N. Comprehension O. Expression
Social cognition	P. Social Interaction Q. Problem-Solving R. Memory

Additional information on the Functional Independence Measure is available from www.udsmr.org/

activities: feeding, grooming, bathing, upper body dressing, lower body dressing, and toileting. Bowel and bladder control, aspects of which some may consider as impairments rather than function, are categorized separately. Functional mobility is tested through three items on transfers. Under the category of locomotion, walking and using a wheelchair are listed equivalently, whereas stairs are considered separately. The FIM also includes two items on communication and three on social cognition.

The FIM measures what the individual does, not what that person could do under certain circumstances. The interrater reliability of the FIM has been established at an acceptable level of psychometric performance (ICCs ranging from 0.86 to 0.88).[47] The face and content validity of the FIM, as well as its ability to capture change in a patient's level of function, have also been determined. Any clinical worker can administer the FIM after appropriate training in using the response set for each item.

Rasch analysis has been applied to the scale scores of the FIM, which are ordinal measures, in order to create interval scale measurements.[49] In addition, the *WeeFIM*, an 18-item instrument based on the FIM, has been developed for use for children between the ages of 6 months and 18 years.[50]

The FIM had been widely used in inpatient rehabilitation settings and in rehabilitation research. However, in efforts to standardize data across post-acute care settings including inpatient rehabilitation, skilled nursing, home health care, and long-term care, the Centers for Medicare and Medicaid Services (CMS) implemented the collection of GG codes in place of the FIM.[51] These codes are the self-care and mobility items from the Continuity Assessment Record and Evaluation (CARE) item set.[52] Each item is scored on a 6-point scale from 01 (dependent) to 07 (independent). One difference between the rating scale of the FIM and GG codes is that the modified independent score in the FIM is not used in scoring GG codes. Instead, the scoring of the items with GG codes allows for their completion with or without assistive devices.

The Outcome and Assessment Information Set

The OASIS was designed to ensure the collection of pertinent data on the adult patient in the home care setting that would allow home health agencies to assess the quality of care by measuring the outcomes of care.[53,54] Since 1999, home health agencies have been mandated to use the OASIS as a *Condition of Participation* in the Medicare program by the Health Care Financing Administration. The current version of OASIS, known as OASIS-D, contains core items covering sociodemographic characteristics, environmental factors, social support, health status, and functional status.[55] This version of the instrument was approved in 2019 and represents an update from preceding versions. The OASIS-D includes GG codes to standardize items with other post-acute care settings. A draft of OASIS-E is available, but this version has not yet been finalized. Once finalized and approved, the OASIS-E is expected to be implemented in 2023. OASIS is not designed to be a comprehensive examination of a patient or an "add-on" measurement. OASIS items are meant to be integrated into the clinical record to highlight various aspects of a patient's status that identify particular needs for care on admission to the home health service, at follow-up every 60 days, and at discharge. The OASIS was intended to be a discipline-neutral record, administered by any health professional, including physical therapists.

Ease of administration increases with familiarity with the instrument. Unlike most other instruments, the response sets that accompany each item are specifically matched to the item. Some response sets have only two possible descriptions of the behavior, whereas others have as many as nine possible descriptions of the behavior. Therefore, the user must be familiar with the possible response set to each item and anticipate that comfort level in using this instrument will increase over a learning curve. Items from the ADL/instrumental ADL (IADL) section of the OASIS-D are listed in Table 8.7. In this section, the items have response sets that range from three possible responses to seven possible responses. Note in the proposed OASIS-E the majority of these items are in Section G, which is labeled Functional Status.

Table 8.7	Outcome and Assessment Information Set: Items From the Activities of Daily Living/Instrumental Activities of Daily Living Section of the OASIS-D

Grooming

Current Ability to Dress Upper Body

Current Ability to Dress Lower Body

Bathing

Toilet Transferring

Toileting Hygiene

Transferring

Ambulation/Locomotion

Feeding or Eating

Multifactorial Falls Risk Assessment

Additional information on the Outcome and Assessment Information Set is available from https://www.cms.gov/Medicare/Quality-Initiatives-Patient-Assessment-Instruments/HomeHealthQualityInits/OASIS-Data-Sets

The 36-Item Short Form Health Survey

The SF-36 contains 36 items based on questions used in the RAND Health Insurance Study. These 36 items were culled from the 113 questions used by RAND in the *Medical Outcomes Study* (MOS) to explore the relationship between physician practice styles and patient outcomes.[56] Thus, it was named the SF-36, because it was a short form of the MOS instrument with only 36 questions. The MOS provided important data on the functional status of adults with specific chronic conditions[57] and the well-being of patients experiencing depression compared to subjects with a chronic medical condition.[58] The SF-36 demonstrated high reliability and validity (correlation coefficients ranging from 0.81 to 0.88).[59–62] Normative data for these self-report items have been collected.[63]

All but one of the 36 questions of the SF-36 are used to form eight different scales: vitality, physical functioning, bodily pain, general health perceptions, physical role functioning, emotional role functioning, social role functioning, and mental health (Table 8.8). Items are scored on nominal (yes/no) or ordinal scales. Each possible response to an item on a scale is assigned a number of points. The total points for all items within a scale are then added and transformed mathematically to yield a percentage score, with 100% representing optimal health. The SF-36 has been used in a number of studies that describe the health status and physical functioning of patients with a variety of impairments receiving physical therapy services.[64–69]

A shortened version has been developed that uses a subset of items from the SF-36.[70] This version, known as *SF-12*, includes items from each of the eight concepts represented in the SF-36 and allows for the calculation of physical and mental subscale scores. An advantage to using fewer questions is that less time is required to complete the survey. This, however, may be at the expense of having a less precise score that may not be as sensitive to change for an individual patient.[71] The development of

the SF-36 stands as the premier example, to date, of a complete and published exploration of the psychometric properties of an instrument as an essential part of its development, and a testament to the responsibility of its creators in verifying the quality of the SF-36 as a scientific tool.

Activity Measure for Post-Acute Care

The AM-PAC is a self-report measure that was developed to assess activity limitations as described by the ICF.[72,73] As the name implies, this measure was designed to be used across settings from acute care to different post-acute care settings, as well as for many different patient conditions. The AM-PAC includes 269 items in three main domains: basic mobility, daily activities, and applied cognitive. Short-form versions of the AM-PAC consisting of items selected to match the level of patients' function in specific settings have been developed.[74,75] These versions have demonstrated the ability to predict discharge destination.[76,77] In addition, a computerized adaptive test (CAT) version of the AM-PAC is available which utilizes the item banks to customize item selection to assess an individual's function.[78] Items are selected for the CAT based on the responses to previous items. The short-form versions and the CAT minimize the time for completion and provide an accurate classification of activity.

The Patient-Specific Functional Scale

Measures have been developed to measure aspects of function for patients seen in outpatient settings. Among the measures that are in common use and have been validated among specific patient groups with musculoskeletal conditions are the *Neck Disability Index*,[79] the *Oswestry Low Back Pain Questionnaire*,[80] the *Disabilities of the Arm, Shoulder, and Hand* (DASH),[81] the *Lower Extremity Functional Scale* (LEFS),[82] and the *Foot and Ankle Ability Measure* (FAAM).[83] These measures include items for common functional tasks specific to certain patient groups. For example, the LEFS includes items related to the use of the LEs such as walking, going up and down stairs, and running. These items represent common functional items for most patients with similar conditions.

In contrast to the use of functional measures that use a list of standardized items, a clinician may be interested in assessing specific functional items that are most important to each individual patient and to the patient's goals. The PSFS can be used by a patient to identify the three most important activities to them, quantify the limitation, and measure change on follow-up visits.[84] Specifically, the patient is asked to identify up to three important activities they are unable to perform at their previous level due to their health condition. Each of the activities is given a score on a 0 to 10 scale, where 0 represents being unable to perform the activity and 10 represents the ability to perform the activity at the same level before the onset of

Table 8.8 Domains of the 36-Item Short Form Health Survey
Physical Functioning
Role Limitations Due to Physical Problems
General Health Perceptions
Vitality
Social Functioning
Role Limitations Due to Emotional Problems
General Mental Health
Health Transition

Additional information on the 36-Item Short Form Health Survey is available from www.rand.org/health/surveys_tools/mos/36-item-short-form.html

the condition. The total score on the PSFS is obtained by adding each activity score and dividing by the number of activities. For example, a college student who sprained an ankle playing intramural basketball may identify the following three activities as limited: walking to class with crutches, standing for chemistry labs, and running. This student may provide initial scores for these three items as 5, 3, and 0, respectively, which results in a total PSFS score of 2.7 [(5 + 3 + 0)/3]. On follow-up visits, a patient is asked to score the same three activities to assess the change in his functional status. In the example provided, the student may no longer require crutches for walking and reports this item as a 10. However, he still has pain with prolonged standing, which he scores a 7, and he has not resumed running for playing basketball, so he scores this a 5. This results in a total score of 7.3 (22/3). This value exceeds the published value for the MDC_{90} for the PSFS of two points.[84] Note, however, that this value for the MDC was determined in a sample of persons with low back pain.

Another benefit of the PSFS is that it can be used with patients with different musculoskeletal conditions, making it a useful tool for practice. Populations tested include those with low back pain, cervical dysfunction, knee conditions, UE problems, joint replacement, and lower-limb amputations.[85–89] In addition to use with individual patients, the validity of the PSFS has been shown for group data, which supports its use in clinical research.[90]

SUMMARY

This chapter presents a conceptual framework for understanding function and for the examination of functional status. The traditional medical model, with its narrow focus on disease and its symptoms, fails to consider the impact of the condition on the person, as well as the broader social, psychological, and behavioral dimensions of illness. All these factors have an impact on an individual's activity and participation. Although individual aspects of function may be assessed, examination of functional status must be viewed as a broad, multidimensional process. Finally, specific aspects of functional examination have been discussed, including purpose, selection of instruments, aspects of test administration, interpretation of test results, and determination of instrument quality.

Questions for Review

1. How does the measurement of function relate to health?

2. What criteria can be used in the selection of a functional instrument?

3. Discuss the uses, advantages, and disadvantages of performance-based instruments, interviewer reports, and self-administered reports.

4. Your rehabilitation facility uses the FIM. How can the instrument be administered to ensure that the results can be used with confidence in both treatment planning and research?

5. Explain how environment, fatigue, and other related issues affect measurement of function. Suggest ways to control these factors in the clinic.

6. Identify the major types of scoring systems used in functional instruments. What are some common errors in interpretation of testing results?

7. Review Tables 8.6, 8.7, and 8.8. Hypothesize a caseload in a particular setting and indicate how and when you could use each of these instruments with the proposed population. Describe the advantages and disadvantages of each. Imagine that you are looking to follow the progress of these same patients to another setting. Which instruments would you choose?

8. Using one of the instruments, develop a set of results and use them to identify treatment goals and outcomes and to formulate a plan of care.

9. For each of the following, identify particular physical tasks relevant to that individual's functional status:
   • A 22-year-old female file clerk
   • A 31-year-old male physical therapist assistant
   • A 39-year-old female homemaker with children
   • A 45-year-old male construction worker
   • A 56-year-old female schoolteacher
   • A 65-year-old male journalist

10. Discuss the relationship among disease, body structures, body functions, activity, participation, environmental factors, and personal factors.

CASE STUDY

A 78-year-old woman with a diagnosis of osteoarthritis was admitted for a right total hip replacement. The patient reported a long-standing history of discomfort. She described the hip pain as radiating posteriorly to the buttock and low back and exacerbated by weight-bearing and stair climbing. Over the past 12 months, she has experienced a very marked increase in pain and stiffness. Radiographic findings demonstrated degenerative changes of both the acetabulum and femoral head consistent with osteoarthritis. The surgical intervention replaced the right femoral head and neck with a metallic prosthesis, and the acetabulum was resurfaced with a plastic cup. Past medical history is unremarkable.

SOCIAL HISTORY

The patient is a retired manager of a small accounting firm that she and her husband established. Her husband is deceased. She has three grown children who all live in neighboring communities. Before the functional limitations imposed by the hip pain, the patient had been independent in all ADL and IADL. She also volunteered her accounting services 1 day per week to a local charity that provides meals to homebound individuals. She was a regular participant in family outings; enjoyed going to the theater, concerts, and special museum events; and was an active member of the community's historical preservation society. Recently, these activities had to be curtailed owing to the increased hip discomfort. She essentially had no activities outside the home for 3 months before admission and used a walker to minimize weight-bearing and reduce pain. She also required the assistance of a home care aide 4 hrs a day two times per week (primarily for shopping, errands, and some household management tasks). She expressed considerable distress at being unable to take a bath and having to rely on the assistance of another person for some basic care activities. She had been using aspirin for its analgesic and anti-inflammatory effects. However, the pain experienced in recent months was not alleviated by the aspirin and other conservative measures. She has been instructed to use local applications of heat, periodic rest intervals, and gentle ROM exercises. The patient has extensive medical insurance coverage and is without financial concerns.

POSTSURGICAL RIGHT HIP PRECAUTIONS

No hip flexion beyond 90°.
Avoid crossing one leg or ankle over the other.
Avoid internal rotation of right LE.

REVIEW OF SYSTEMS

Communication, Affect, Cognition, Learning Style: Fully communicative and oriented × 3. Cooperative and motivated. Hearing intact. Wears corrective lens; experiences "night blindness," which she describes as seeing poorly in dim light and her eyes take several seconds longer than normal to adjust from brightness to dimness.

Cardiopulmonary: Heart rate (HR) = 84 beats/min; blood pressure (BP) = 130/78 mm Hg; respiratory rate (RR) = 16 breaths/min; no appreciable increases with activity.

Integumentary: Surgical wound healing well; staples removed.

Strength: UE gross ROM is within normal limits. Gross strength generally good to normal, except hands. Left hip, knee, and ankle at least good on break test. Partial weight-bearing on right LE.

Joint Integrity and Mobility: Patient reports some sporadic episodes of wrist and finger stiffness on awakening in the morning and after periods of immobility. Crepitus noted in right knee. Heberden nodes noted at the distal interphalangeal (DIP) and proximal interphalangeal (PIP) joints of the left index finger.

Range of Motion: Right knee and ankle within functional limits; right hip not tested.

Muscle Performance: Grip strength is reduced bilaterally.

Pain: Patient denies pain in wrist or fingers, or right hip.

Gait, Locomotion, and Balance: The patient is ambulating on level surfaces with supervision using bilateral standard aluminum axillary crutches with partial weight-bearing on the right LE. Stair climbing also requires minimal assistance. It is anticipated that the patient will be independent with ambulation on level surfaces at time of discharge from the hospital.

Functional Status: Impaired bed mobility (modified independence device), sit-to-stand, transfers (minimum assistance).

(Continued)

CASE STUDY—cont'd

Home Environment: The patient lives alone in a fifth-floor apartment in a building with an elevator. The living space is a one-bedroom apartment on a single level.

Patient Goals: The patient is extremely motivated to once again be an independent manager of her personal care and household management needs. The prosthetic replacement has successfully relieved much of the pain experienced in the hip before surgery (most of her current discomfort is described as minor and associated with the surgical incision). She would also like to return to her family, volunteer, social, and leisure activities. She is very determined to discontinue the home care assistance as soon as possible.

GUIDING QUESTIONS

1. Based on the findings of the initial examination, discuss the links between the condition, impairments in body structures and body functions, activity limitations, participation restrictions, and contextual factors using the ICF model.

2. Identify the specific ADL and IADL skills that would need to be examined to return this patient to the highest level of function and achieve the patient's goals for rehabilitation. Discuss the appropriateness of the instruments presented in this chapter for measuring her function and documenting the outcomes of patient management.

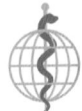

For additional resources, including answers to the questions for review, new immersive cases, case study guiding questions, references, and more, please visit **https://www.fadavis.com/product/physical -rehabilitation-fulk-8**. You may also quickly find the resources by entering this title's four-digit ISBN, 4691, in the search field at **http://fadavis.com** and logging in at the prompt.

Examination and Modification of the Environment

Kevin M. Parcetich Jr., PT, DPT, NCS
Thomas J. Schmitz, PT, PhD

Chapter **9**

LEARNING OBJECTIVES

1. Identify the role of the physical therapist in examination of the physical environment.
2. Understand the importance of environmental accessibility in optimizing patient function.
3. Identify common home, work life, and community environmental factors that affect patient function.
4. Describe strategies used to examine environmental impact on patient function.
5. Identify the general categories of tests and measures, tools used for gathering data, and data used in documenting examination of environmental factors.
6. Identify strategies to improve patient function through environmental modifications.
7. Describe the scope of adaptive equipment and assistive technology available for individuals with disability.
8. Recognize the importance of an examination of the environment within the context of a comprehensive rehabilitation plan of care.

CHAPTER OUTLINE

PHYSICAL ENVIRONMENT *294*
UNIVERSAL DESIGN *294*
   Principles of Universal Design *295*
DISABILITY ACCESS SYMBOLS *295*
PURPOSE OF EXAMINATION *295*
EXAMINATION STRATEGIES *295*
   Interview *297*
   Self-Report and Performance-Based Measures of Function *298*
   Environmental Factors Outcome Measures *298*
   Description of Physical Environment *298*
   On-Site Visits *298*
EXAMINATION OF THE HOME *300*
   Preparation for On-Site Visit *301*

ADAPTIVE EQUIPMENT *317*
ASSISTIVE TECHNOLOGY *317*
EXAMINATION OF THE WORKPLACE *318*
   Job Requirements *318*
   Functional Capacity Evaluation *320*
   On-Site Visit *321*
COMMUNITY ACCESS *322*
   Transportation *323*
   Access to Community Facilities *324*
DOCUMENTATION *324*
FUNDING SOURCES *326*
LEGISLATION *326*
SUMMARY *327*

Addressing the environment in which an individual will live and function is crucial to a comprehensive physical therapy plan of care (POC), especially for those recovering from accident or illness or transitioning from rehabilitation facilities. A well-developed POC that allows a wheelchair user to freely access their home and achieve independence in all activities of daily living (ADLs) will fall short if the home's entrance is obstructed by stairs or if a bathroom is inaccessible. As a patient progresses through rehabilitation, the living environment should be carefully considered, as returning to a familiar home and community is a high priority for most patients. This is particularly true for older adults who function best in

familiar surroundings and may be attached to a home setting that holds memories of important family events experienced over a lifetime.

Disability or disease places new emotional, caregiving, and financial demands on the family. While adjusting to these demands, the unexpected challenge of addressing needed costly modifications to a beloved home is often overwhelming. The physical therapist is part of an interdisciplinary team that advocates for the patient and family by providing education, counseling, environmental analysis, and training to aid in the successful transition to the discharge setting. Physical therapists have expertise in examining and determining the impact a patient's health condition, bodily structure

293

and function restrictions, activity and participation constraints, and personal and environmental variables will have on the ability to return to or maintain functional independence in the home, community, school, and workplace. As such, a thorough rehabilitation POC will also address examination of community accessibility, reliable transportation options, and workplace, school, or higher education settings.

This chapter addresses how the surrounding physical environment affects functional independence for patients impacted by injury, illness, or disease. It presents strategies to examine the home, workplace, and community physical settings; reviews current guidelines for public building and transportation access; and makes recommendations for environmental modifications to increase accessibility and reduce hospital readmission risk.

■ PHYSICAL ENVIRONMENT

The World Health Organization's International Classification of Functioning, Disability, and Health (ICF) recognizes disability and functioning as an outcome of the dynamic interaction between health conditions and contextual factors (personal and environmental).[1] Examples of *personal factors* include sex, age, coping styles, and other characteristics that may influence how an individual experiences disability. *Environmental factors* are defined as all external factors that influence participation either as barriers or facilitators. These factors include a variety of both built and natural objects. Built objects refer to buildings and structures created by humans; natural objects include other humans, as well as geographical objects such as vegetation, mountains, rivers, uneven terrain, and so forth. The environment encompasses a substantial range of components that affect human function and includes the individual's home, neighborhood, community, and method(s) of transportation, in addition to the individual's educational, workplace, entertainment, commercial, and natural settings.[1–3]

Barriers are environmental factors that, through their presence or absence, prevent optimal function and create disability.[3,4] Included among the identified risk factors for barriers encountered in routine daily environments is diminished access to home, school, work, or community.[3,4]

Accessibility is the degree to which an environment affords use of its resources with respect to an individual's level of function.[5] *Accessible design* typically refers to structures that meet prescribed standards for accessibility.[5] In the United States, these standards are available from the American National Standards Institute, the Fair Housing Amendments Act of 1988, and the Uniform Federal Accessibility Standards.[6–8] Requirements for public and commercial buildings are regulated by the guidelines of the Americans with Disabilities Act (ADA) Standards for Accessible Design.[9]

■ UNIVERSAL DESIGN

Universal design (UD) refers to the design of environments and products that can be used by all people to the greatest extent possible regardless of age, ability, or disability. This design concept emphasizes social inclusion by creating products and environments that are usable by a wide range of individuals of different ages, statures, sizes, and abilities, and it addresses the changing needs of human beings across the life span.[10] Other terms associated with this design concept include *inclusive design, accessible design, life span design, aging-in-place design,* and *sustainable design.*

UD has been identified as an outgrowth of the disability rights movement in the 1960s, although earlier recognition of the concepts has been identified. Its foundational elements of ensuring equal opportunity and eliminating discrimination based on disability have been embraced in many parts of the world.[11,12] The design principles provide a human-centered framework for creating spaces, furniture, landscapes, products, and services that can seamlessly accommodate diverse ability levels across generations.[13–15]

Evidence-based design (EBD) supports and informs UD. EBD is defined broadly "as basing decisions about the built environment on credible and rigorous research and linking facility design to quality outcomes."[16] It emphasizes use of research to influence the design process and evaluate design innovations. Traditionally associated with health-care architecture, EBD now supports design decisions for many structures in the built environment, including schools, office spaces, performance centers, restaurants, museums, and prisons.[14]

Although UD is both accessible and free of barriers, it is not the same as bringing existing buildings or structures into compliance with the ADA Standards for Accessible Design or other building codes or laws. Applying such standards to existing structures often results in important but selective accessibility. In contrast, UD is applied from the *inception* of a building design plan (new construction) versus eliminating barriers in existing structures. For example, the need to retrofit an existing structure with a ramp or accessible bathrooms would not be needed had the original design plan considered the needs of all users.

Incorporated into initial planning, UD elements are essentially "invisible" as compared to adaptations or add-ons made to existing structures. They apply to all features and spaces of a dwelling. Several examples of UD elements include stepless entrances, wide hallways and doorways, level transitions between rooms (no doorway thresholds), use of nonslip floors, lever door handles, rocker light switches, single-handle sink faucets, and no-step shower access. Reinforced walls capable of supporting handrails or grab bars and large closets aligned from floor to floor that are suitable for housing a residential elevator are examples of UD elements intended to meet the future needs of residents.

Principles of Universal Design

The principles of UD (Appendix 9.A [online]) were developed at the Center for Universal Design at North Carolina State University by a group of experts that included architects, product designers, engineers, and environmental design researchers.[17] The principles provide guidance for the design of products and environments. They are also intended to educate designers and consumers about characteristics that increase usability for everyone. Key elements of the principles include the following:

- *Equitable use.* The design is useful and marketable to people with diverse abilities.
- *Flexiblity in use.* The design accommodates a wide range of individual preferences and abilities.
- *Simple and intuitive.* Use of the design is easy to understand, regardless of the user's experience, knowledge, language skills, or current concentration level.
- *Perceptible information.* The design communicates necessary information effectively to the user, regardless of ambient conditions or the user's sensory abilities.
- *Tolerance for error.* The design minimizes hazards and the adverse consequences of accidental or unintended actions.
- *Low physical effort.* The design can be used efficiently, comfortably, and with a minimum of fatigue.
- *Size and space for approach and use.* Appropriate size and space are provided for approach, reach, manipulation, and use regardless of the user's body size, posture, or mobility.

■ DISABILITY ACCESS SYMBOLS

Reflective of the importance of *environmental accessibility,* an internationally recognized *wheelchair symbol* identifies buildings accessible to individuals with a disability. The Rehabilitation Act of 1973 (Sections 503 and 504) requires that all organizations receiving federal funding provide accessible programs and activities. The ADA (1990) expanded accessibility to the private sector to improve employment opportunities as well as environmental access to retail businesses, cultural events, movie theaters, restaurants, travel, and so forth. Other access symbols identify the availability of assistive listening devices, telephones with interactive text capabilities (TTY), which allow the user to communicate using a keyboard and visual display, volume-controlled telephones, availability of sign language interpretation, and so forth. The disability access symbols are presented in Figure 9.1. These symbols are prominently displayed to identify and make public the availability of accessible services.

■ PURPOSE OF EXAMINATION

A primary outcome of rehabilitation is for the patient to be fully functional in a former environment and lifestyle. To achieve this outcome, continuity of accessibility must exist within the individual's environmental context. With full accessibility as a goal, examination of the environment addresses the *patient–environment relationship* relative to accessibility, safety, usability, and function. The purposes of an environmental examination are multiple and serve to

1. Determine the degree of patient safety and level of function in the physical environment.
2. Identify barriers that may affect usability or compromise performance of customary tasks or activities.
3. Make realistic recommendations regarding accessibility, barriers, modifications, and safety to the patient and family as needed, to the employer, to government agencies or other potential funding sources, and to third-party payers.
4. Determine the need for adaptive equipment or assistive technology to support and promote function.
5. Assist in preparing the patient and family for the patient's return to a former environment and help determine whether further services may be required (e.g., outpatient treatment, home care services, and so forth).

■ EXAMINATION STRATEGIES

Physical therapists use a variety of tests and measures to examine physical impediments (e.g., safety hazards, access problems, design barriers) affecting the patient–environment relationship. The data generated are used to recommend modifications to the environment, guide selection of adaptive equipment and assistive technology, and/or propose alternative approaches to performing a task or activity (e.g., improve safety, conserve energy) to promote optimum function. The *Guide to Physical Therapist Practice*[18] includes environmental factors among test and measure categories used by physical therapists. Table 9.1 presents examples of the tests and measures used, data-gathering tools, and types of data generated.

Depending on the nature of the patient's disability, data collection tools used for examination of the environmental may include (1) interviews; (2) self-reports (checklists, questionnaires) and performance-based measures (observation) of function; (3) measures of environmental impact on function; (4) visual depictions (photographs, video recordings) and dimensions of physical space (structural specifications); (5) views of the environment from a remote site; and (6) on-site visits.

A combination of two or more of these strategies may be warranted to generate all needed data. Cost containment has placed restrictions on time and travel allocations for on-site visits. In such situations, several data collection alternatives (e.g., interview, self-report, performance-based measures and simulations, use of photographs and/or diagrams [floor plan with

	Symbol for Accessibility The wheelchair symbol should only be used to indicate access for individuals with limited mobility, including wheelchair users. For example, the symbol is used to indicate an accessible entrance, bathroom, or that a phone is lowered for wheelchair users. Remember that a ramped entrance is not completely accessible if there are no curb cuts, and an elevator is not accessible if it can only be reached via steps.
	Access (Other Than Print or Braille) for Individuals Who Are Blind or Have Low Vision This symbol may be used to indicate access for people who are blind or have low vision, including a guided tour, a path to a nature trail or a scent garden in a park, and a tactile tour or a museum exhibition that may be touched.
	Audio Description A service for persons who are blind or have low vision that makes the performing arts, visual arts, television, video, and film more accessible. Description of visual elements is provided by a trained Audio Describer through the Secondary Audio Program (SAP) of televisions and monitors equipped with stereo sound. An adapter for non-stereo TVs is available through the American Foundation for the Blind, (800) 829-0500. For live Audio Description, a trained Audio Describer offers live commentary or narration (via headphones and a small transmitter) consisting of concise, objective descriptions of visual elements (e.g., a theater performance or a visual arts exhibition).
	Telephone Typewriter (TTY) This device is also known as a text telephone (TT), or telecommunications device for the deaf (TDD). TTY indicates a device used with the telephone for communication with and between deaf, hard of hearing, speech impaired, and/or hearing persons.
	Volume Control Telephone This symbol indicates the location of telephones that have handsets with amplified sound and/or adjustable volume controls.
	Assistive Listening Systems These systems transmit amplified sound via hearing aids, headsets, or other devices. They include infrared, loop, and FM systems. Portable systems may be available from the same audiovisual equipment suppliers that service conferences and meetings.
	Sign Language Interpretation The symbol indicates that Sign Language Interpretation is provided for a lecture, tour, film, performance, conference, or other program.
	Accessible Print (18 pt. or Larger) The symbol for large print is "Large Print" printed in 18 pt. or larger text. In addition to indicating that large print versions of books, pamphlets, museum guides, and theater programs are available, you may use the symbol on conference or membership forms to indicate that print materials may be provided in large print. Sans serif or modified serif print with good contrast is important, and special attention should be paid to letter and word spacing.
	The Information Symbol The most valuable commodity of today's society is information; to a person with a disability, it is essential. For example, the symbol may be used on signage or on a floor plan to indicate the location of the information or security desk, where there is more specific information or materials concerning access accommodations and services such as "LARGE PRINT" materials, audio cassette recordings of materials, or sign interpreted tours.
	Closed Captioning (CC) This symbol indicates a choice for whether or not to display captions for a television program or videotape. TV sets that have a built-in or a separate decoder are equipped to display dialogue for programs that are captioned when selected by the viewer. The Television Decoder Circuitry Act of 1990 requires TV sets (with screens 13" or larger) to have built-in decoders as of July 1993. Also, videos that are part of exhibitions may be closed captioned using the symbol with instruction to press a button for captioning.
	Opened Captioning (OC) This symbol indicates that captions, which translate dialogue and other sounds in print, are always displayed on the videotape, movie, or television program. Open Captioning is preferred by many including deaf and hard-of-hearing individuals, and people whose second language is English. In addition, it is helpful in teaching children how to read and in keeping sound levels to a minimum in museums and restaurants.
	**Braille Symbol** This symbol indicates that printed material is available in Braille, including exhibition labeling, publications, and signage.

The Disability Access Symbols were produced by the Graphic Artists Guild Foundation with support and technical assistance from the Office for Special Constituencies, National Endowment for the Arts. Special thanks to the National Endowment for the Arts. Graphic design assistance by the Society of Environmental Graphic Design. Consultant: Jacqueline Ann Clipsham, with permission.

Figure 9.1 Disability access symbols.

dimensions] of the physical space) can be implemented to achieve the goals of the environmental examination.

Telehealth offers considerable potential to provide medical care outside the traditional in-person visit to a provider including the ability to examine a person's living environment remotely using video streaming technology (e.g., Skype, Zoom). A large and expanding body of literature, accelerated by global pandemics, addresses the extensive application of telehealth in providing health-care services,[19-29] including physical

| Table 9.1 | Examination of the Environment: Examples of Tests and Measures, Data-Gathering Tools, and Data Used in Documentation |

The physical therapist uses tests and measures to determine whether the individual's environment is adequate to enable optimal participation in their various roles. Responses monitored at rest, during activity, and after activity may indicate the presence or severity of an impairment, activity limitation, or participation restriction.

Tests and Measures	Data-Gathering Tools	Documentation
Assistive technology needs (e.g., observations, questionnaires, videographic assessments) Caregiver capacity (e.g., assessment of caregiver and caregiver resources) Current and potential barriers (e.g., checklists, interviews, observations, questionnaires, safety assessment) Physical space and environments routinely encountered (e.g., accessibility survey, observations, photographic assessments, questionnaires, videographic assessments) Quality of life (e.g., scales, surveys)	Cameras and photographs Equipment trial and simulation Structural specifications (e.g., blueprints or building plans) Tape measures Universal design criteria Video cameras and video recordings	Clinical rationale to justify need for appropriate assistive technology or reasonable accommodations Description of environmental factors that create barriers to activity and participation (e.g., lack of access to workplace due to long distance from parking area to main entrance) Description of features of home, work, school, or community physical environments Descriptions of physical space, including doorway widths, floor surfaces, distances of required travel, maneuvering space, and accessibility of bathrooms Level of compliance with regulatory standards (e.g., compliance of public buildings with ADA)

From *Guide to Physical Therapist Practice*,[18] with permission. APTA is not responsible for the translation from English.
ADA = Americans with Disabilities Act.

therapy.[30–37] The American Physical Therapy Association (APTA) has disseminated a position statement supporting the following:[38]

- Inclusion of physical therapist services in telehealth policy and regulation on the national and state levels to help society address the growing cost of health services, the disparity in accessibility of health services, and the potential impact of health workforce shortages.
- Advancement of telehealth practice, education, and research within the physical therapy profession to enhance the quality and accessibility of physical therapist services.
- Expansion of broadband access to enable all members of society to receive services delivered via electronic means.

A recent study examined the feasibility of telehealth home modification interventions using participant-owned smartphones, tablets, or computers. A pretest–post-test design (*n* = 4) demonstrated improvement in home safety and perception of performance of daily activities. Participants reported satisfaction with the mode of intervention, citing ease of use and reduction in client and caregiver burden.[39]

Interview

Exploration of the environment is typically initiated by interviewing the patient and family. If the patient's impairments and activity limitations affect only isolated tasks or activities or if accessibility issues involve limited physical environmental factors, an interview may be all that is needed to identify the barriers and provide recommendations and suggestions to improve performance and resolve access problems. In the presence of more formidable disability, the interview may be the first of several strategies used to collect data about the patient's environment. The interview can be used to establish the general characteristics of the environment (number of levels, stairs, railings, and so forth), identify any special problems previously encountered by the patient, alert the therapist to potential safety hazards, and determine the need for further tests and measures to obtain essential information. The interview process also provides the therapist an opportunity to gain knowledge of family/carepartner characteristics, including (1) attitude toward the patient; (2) the extent of their desire to have the patient return to their environment; (3) their carepartnering goals and capabilities; and (4) attitude toward rehabilitation team members, which may influence receptivity to suggested environmental modifications.

Self-Report and Performance-Based Measures of Function

Self-report measures involve asking the patient to provide information about the ability to perform certain tasks and activities in specific environments (see Appendix 9.B [online]). Administration can be either in a paper-and-pencil format, via mobile device, or by interview. An inherent shortcoming of self-report instruments is that an individual may over- or underestimate performance capabilities or the impact of environmental barriers.[40] Accuracy of reporting can be improved by requesting that the patient (1) focus the performance information on a recent time interval (e.g., *within* the previous week) and (2) distinguish between *actual* performance of an activity (e.g., *daily* use of shower for bathing) versus *perceived* ability in the absence of consistent execution of the task.[40]

Performance-based measures address classification of functional abilities and identification of activity limitations and participation restrictions. The therapist administers these measures while observing patient performance of an activity. Recommended for adults with neurological conditions, the APTA's Academy of Neurologic Physical Therapy has developed a minimum core set of performance-based outcome measures to quantify function within the constructs of balance, walking speed, walking endurance/distance, and transfer ability.[41] The core measures used to examine balance, mobility, and fall risk include the Berg Balance Scale, Functional Gait Assessment, Activities Specific Balance Confidence Scale, 10-m Walk Test, 6-min Walk Test, and the Five Times Sit to Stand Test.[41] Each outcome measure includes an accompanying document addressing setup of the environment to optimize effectiveness of administration. Interpretation of results is typically guided by comparison to normative data. These measures yield information about the impact of impairments on function and help predict patient performance within their natural environment. Performance-based tests and self-reports of function are also discussed in Chapter 8, Examination of Function. A useful additional resource for outcome measures is the Shirley Ryan Ability Lab Rehabilitation Measures Database (https://www.sralab.org/rehabilitation-measures).

Environmental Factors Outcome Measures

The environment directly affects the ability to perform tasks and activities that support physical, social, and psychological well-being. Environmental factors can either *constrain* or *promote* patients' abilities to perform customary actions within their social/cultural contexts. A variety of instruments have been developed that address the impact of environmental determinants on function and participation. Table 9.2 includes examples of outcome measures designed to examine environmental factors.[42–62]

Description of Physical Environment

The therapist may request that family members provide a description of the physical environment. This can effectively be accomplished via visual depictions (e.g., streaming video using a computer, smartphone, or tablet, photographs, videotapes, diagrams, floor plans) in combination with actual dimensions (structural specifications obtained with a tape measure) of the setting in which the patient is expected to function.

Suggestions for modifications can be made from the visual representations and measured dimensions of the patient's environment. Such environmental information will allow the therapist to simulate aspects of the patient's surroundings (before discharge) for practicing tasks while directing attention to maximizing safety and function. This will also assist the therapist to determine the need for assistive or adaptive equipment.

On-Site Visits

On-site visits require that one or more rehabilitation team members together with the patient travel to the physical location where the patient will be required to function (home, community, and/or work or school). A major advantage of the on-site visit is that it allows observation of performance in the actual environment in which the activities must be accomplished. On-site visits are often useful in reducing patient, family, caregiver, and/or employer apprehension concerning the patient's ability to function within the environment. The on-site visit also provides an important opportunity for the therapist to identify safety hazards and make recommendations regarding specific environmental barriers. During the visit, patient activity should be interspersed with adequate rest intervals to ensure that fatigue is not an influencing factor. A study by Lockwood et al. found a decreased incidence of falls when a home evaluation was completed prior to patient discharge.[63] However, others have found inconclusive evidence about the benefits of a home evaluation prior to discharge based on ADL performance, quality of life, mobility, fear of falling, falls, and hospital readmission.[64]

Whichever examination strategy or combination of strategies is applied, the scope and breadth of the information gathered will be enhanced by involvement of patient and family members. Because it is usually not feasible for the therapist to examine all aspects of the patient's total environment, involvement of other individuals can be instrumental in ensuring that the goal of maximum accessibility, function, and participation is met. This is particularly important for addressing community access. The therapist can direct and guide an investigation of community recreational, educational, and commercial facilities, as well as availability of public

Table 9.2	Outcome Measures: Examination of Environmental Factors		
Outcome Measure and ICF Category	**Description**	**Scoring**	**MDC and MCID**
HACE[42] ICF: 3	Examines six domains: home mobility, community mobility, basic mobility devices, communication devices, transportation factors, and attitudes	Self-report, 36 total items. Requires 6 to 30 minutes to complete. Instrument available in the work of Keysor et al.[43]	**NA**
CHART[44] ICF: 2, 3	Designed to examine an individual's function within their societal context using six domains of function: physical independence, cognitive independence, mobility, occupation, social integration, and economic self-sufficiency.	Each area is scored based on a range of 0 to 100 points (600 points maximum) with greater levels of participation receiving higher scores. The CHART Short Form (CHART-SF)[45,46] is a 19-item shortened version of the CHART. Available online.[47]	**NA**
CHIEF[48,49] ICF: 3	Rates frequency and impact of 25 items across five domains that prevent functioning within the home and community; also includes social, attitudinal, and policy barriers; response items carry numeric values. A CHIEF short form (CHIEF-SF) contains 12 items from the original inventory.[50]	Scores calculated by multiplying frequency of occurrence (0 = never to 4 = daily) by magnitude (big problem = 2 or little problem = 1) to provide an *impact score*. Higher scores indicate greater impact of environmental factors.[50] Available online.[51]	**NA**
FABS/M[52] ICF: 2, 3	Self-report examining environmental facilitators and barriers to participation for individuals with mobility impairments; includes 61 questions, 133 items.	Scores based on frequency of encounter and magnitude of impact on participation within six domains: mobility device, built features of homes, built/natural features in community, community destination access, community facilities access, and community support network. Available in the work of Gray et al.[52]	**NA**
SAFER tool[53]	A comprehensive functional and environmental examination tool designed for use with older adults in the home setting.	Examines 97 items including living situation, mobility, kitchen, fire hazards, eating, household, dressing, grooming, bathroom, medication, communication, wandering, memory aids, and general. A percentage score is calculated by dividing the number of problem items by the number of items addressed minus the number of N/A items and multiplied by 100.[54]	**N/A**
WeHSA[55]	Identifies hazards in the home for older adults at risk for falling.	Seventy-two fall risk hazards are examined (e.g., living area, seating, bedroom, bathroom, kitchen, laundry, footwear). Items scored as relevant or not relevant; items rated relevant are deemed a hazard or not a hazard.[54,55]	**N/A**
HAP[57,58]	A performance-based measure that examines how an individual functions in the home environment. The individual is observed performing functional activities in the home and is rated on person–environment interactions along a hazardous scale.[57,58]	Scored from 0 to 2 (0 = no hazard, 1 = mild hazard, and 2 = moderate to severe hazard). The person–environment interactions are also rated on frequency (0 = never; 5 = several times daily). The hazard score is multiplied by frequency score for a sum total. A higher score indicates greater risk for falls.[57,58]	**N/A**

(Continued)

Table 9.2	Outcome Measures: Examination of Environmental Factors—cont'd		
Outcome Measure and ICF Category	Description	Scoring	MDC and MCID
Cougar Home Safety Assessment[59]	Examines environmental safety, not the performance of individuals in the home setting.	Seventy-four criteria are examined through observation, questioning, and testing of home items (e.g., fire hazards, flooring/hallways, kitchen, bedroom, bathroom(s), closets/storage areas, parking areas, entrances, and disaster preparedness).[60] Criteria are rated as "safe" or "unsafe."	**N/A**
I-HOPE[61] *and I-HOPE Assist*[62]	Administered and scored by a trained clinician, the I-HOPE examines the person–environment fit of older adults for healthy aging in place. The I-HOPE Assist examines the person–environment fit for caregivers. Both tools can be used to determine the effects of home modifications.	For the I-HOPE, the individual rates perceived difficulty of 44 in-home activities that are then prioritized for intervention; last, tasks are performed to determine influence of barriers on performance. Results provide four sub-scores: activity, performance, satisfaction, and total barrier severity.[61] The I-HOPE Assist adapts the I-HOPE and examines the effect of completing the same activities from the caregiver perspective.[62]	**N/A**

ICF CATEGORY: 1 = Body Structure/Function, 2 = Activity, 3 = Participation.

CHART = Craig Handicap Assessment and Reporting Technique; CHIEF = Craig Hospital Inventory of Environmental Factors; FABS/M = *Facilitator and Barriers Survey* of environmental influences on participation among people with lower limb *Mobility* impairments and limitations; HACE = Home and Community Environment; HAP = Home Assessment Profile; ICF = International Classification of Functioning, Disability, and Health; I-HOPE = In-Home Occupational Performance Evaluation; I-HOPE Assist = In-Home Occupational Performance Evaluation for Providing Assistance; MCID = Minimal clinically important difference; MDC = minimal detectable change; N/A = not available (not established); SAFER tool = Shkuratova Assessment of Falls-Risk in Rehabilitation; WeHSA = Westmead Home Safety Assessment.

transportation. Guidance can also be provided in the essential role of exploring funding sources for needed modifications (potential funding sources are addressed later in this chapter).

Data from an examination of the environment are used to evaluate the need for specific recommendations and interventions. Corcoran and Gitlin[49] identify five major areas of intervention strategies: (1) *assistive or adaptive devices* such as grab bars, long-handled reachers, adapted eating utensils (e.g., rocker knife), canes, or walkers; (2) *safety devices,* such as lighting, smoke detectors, or sensing devices; (3) *structural alterations,* which include widening doors, installing railings or ramps, or removing a doorway threshold; (4) *modification or altered location of environmental objects,* such as disabling a stove, using extension levers on door handles, removing throw rugs, or moving furniture; and (5) *task modification,* such as use of visual, auditory, or other sensory cuing, work simplification, and energy conservation or joint preservation techniques.

The following sections offer suggestions for examination and modification of the home and workplace environment. The information presented is neither exhaustive nor inclusive of the needs of every patient. The environmental considerations are intended to direct attention to some of the more common access, usability, and safety concerns.

■ EXAMINATION OF THE HOME
Preparation for On-Site Visit

Before an on-site visit to the patient's home, occupational and physical therapy treatment sessions should be scheduled that include participation from family and caregivers. These visits serve several functions. They provide an opportunity to become familiar with the patient's capabilities and activity limitations. They give the family/caregivers time to learn safe methods (e.g., proper body mechanics, guarding techniques) for assisting with locomotion, transfers, exercise, and/or functional activities. During these sessions, the occupational and physical therapists will have an opportunity to provide instruction in the use of assistive devices, adaptive equipment, and/or assistive technology. The time spent in family and caregiver education is often pivotal in facilitating the patient's successful return to the home, community, and/or work or school environments. Based on patient need, family and caregiver treatment sessions with the speech-language pathologist prior to the home visit may also be warranted.

> **Clinical Note.** Although often restricted by reimbursement issues, when feasible, a day or weekend patient visit to the home should be encouraged and arranged before the on-site visit. An advantage of such visits is that problems not previously anticipated by the therapist, patient, or family may be uncovered. Following the visit, the patient's immediate assessment of their ability to function within the environment should be obtained. This can be accomplished using a self-report instrument designed to gather perceptions about environment features that either constrain or promote activity performance (see Appendix 9.B [online]). Emphasis can then be placed on initial development of a plan to resolve identified problems before the on-site visit and the patient's actual return to the environment.

Preceding the on-site visit, information should be gathered about several important areas that will influence both the preparation for and the types of recommendations made during the visit. This information includes the following:

- Information about the patient's present level of function (e.g., communication skills, bed mobility, transfers, and locomotion); data should be gathered from all involved disciplines (occupational therapist, physical therapist, speech-language pathologist, etc.).
- Knowledge of physical assistance or verbal cuing required for performance of functional activities.
- Characteristics and dimensions of required adaptive or assistive devices and equipment (e.g., walker, crutches, raised toilet seat, commode, hospital bed).
- Information about predicted level of function or improvement (expected outcomes).
- Nature of the activity limitations or participation restrictions (i.e., static or progressive).
- Insurance coverage, financial resources, and availability of potential funding sources (in terms of capacity to modify environment or obtain needed adaptive and assistive devices or assistive technology).
- Knowledge of the patient's future plans (household management, family care, employment outside the home, school, vocational training, etc.).
- Knowledge of whether the house or apartment is owned or rented; the type and ownership of the home can affect or even preclude the type of modifications the patient may require. However, it should be noted that the Fair Housing Act requires landlords to allow individuals with disabilities to make reasonable access modifications to both personal living space and common space such as entryways.
- Information about the relative permanence of the dwelling; if the patient has plans to move in the near future, it will influence the type of modifications recommended (e.g., installing permanent ramps versus removable ones or paving a gravel driveway).

This information can be obtained from a variety of sources, including the patient, rehabilitation team conferences, patient/family and caregiver conferences or interviews, health record documentation from all disciplines involved, and social service interviews. Once this information is gathered, decisions can be made concerning what adaptive or assistive devices will be needed and the appropriate team members to accompany the patient on the visit.

> **Clinical Note.** Although social workers are key members of the team throughout the rehabilitation process, they play a particularly important role in planning for transition to home and community. Discharge plans are enhanced and facilitated by the social worker's collaborative role as patient advocate and knowledge of community resources such as referral sources (home care, medical follow-up, legal assistance), accessible housing, available transportation, and potential financial assistance or funding resources.

Ideally, given their complementary expertise and skills, both the physical and occupational therapist accompany the patient on the home visit. They assume shared responsibility for examining the patient–environment interface. Depending on the specific needs of the patient and family, a speech-language pathologist, social worker, or nurse also may be among the rehabilitation team members visiting the home. For purposes of organization and structure, home visits are often divided into two global elements: (1) accessibility of the dwelling's *exterior* and (2) examination of the home's *interior*. Photographs are useful for providing images of environmental factors posing barriers to accompany letters of justification for needed modifications. A tape measure and home examination form are also important tools during the visit. Many rehabilitation departments develop their own home examination forms to meet the particular needs of their patient population. The forms (or checklists) help to organize the visit and are useful in directing attention to all necessary details. An example of a Home Examination Form is provided in Appendix 9.C (online). This form can be expanded or modified, depending on the specific needs of the individual or patient population. Some caution must be used in interpreting data from home examination forms that have not been standardized or examined for reliability.

On-Site Visit

On arrival at the home for the on-site visit, the patient may need to rest for a short while before beginning the home examination. This is an important consideration, because patients may become very excited or emotional when returning to a home environment after a lengthy absence. This may be true even if a day or weekend visit occurred before the formal home visit.

One method of gathering data about the interior of the home is to begin with the patient in bed as though it were morning. Simulation of all daily tasks and activities, including dressing, grooming, bathroom activities, and preparation of meals, can ensue. The patient should attempt to perform all transfer, exercise, locomotion, self-care, and home-making activities as independently as possible. This will provide an additional opportunity to teach the family and caregivers how and when to assist the patient.

Exterior Accessibility

Route of Entry

1. If there is more than one entry to the dwelling, the most accessible should be selected (closest to driveway, most level walking surface, fewest stairs, available handrails, etc.).
2. Ideally, the driveway should be a smooth, level surface with easy access to the home. Walking surfaces to the entrance should be carefully examined. Cracked and uneven surfaces should be repaired or an alternate route selected.
3. The route to entrance should be level and well lit, and it should provide adequate cover from adverse weather conditions. Package shelves near the entrance are useful for freeing hands to unlock and/or open doors.
4. The height, number, and condition of stairs should be noted. Ideally, steps should not be greater than 7 in. (180 mm) high with a minimum depth of 11 in. (280 mm).[6] *Nosings*, also referred to as "lips," are the 0.5 in. (13 mm) curved overhangs on the front edge of stairs. These overhangs are often problematic because they can cause a patient's toe to catch and prevent smooth transition to the next step. Nosings should be removed or reduced, if possible. Installing small wood bevels under the overhangs that taper down toward the lower step and provide a smoother contour can minimize nosing (Fig. 9.2A). The steps also should have a nonslip surface to improve traction. This can be accomplished by adding abrasive strips (Fig. 9.2B).
5. Handrails should be installed, if needed. In general, handrail height should measure between a minimum of 34 in. (865 mm) and a maximum of 38 in. (965 mm) high for stairs (Fig. 9.3A), ramps, and level walking surfaces. This range in handrail height allows for modifications to accommodate needs of particularly tall or short individuals. At least one handrail should extend a minimum of 12 in. (305 mm) beyond the foot and top of the stairs (Fig. 9.3B). Outside, cross-sectional diameter of circular handrails should be between a minimum

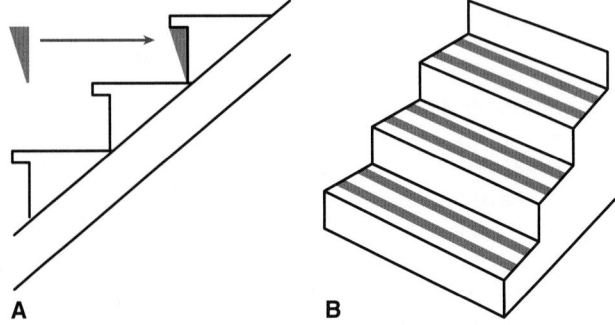

Figure 9.2 (A) Wood bevels placed under nosings minimize the danger of "toe-catching" during transition to the next step. (B) Abrasive strips of a contrasting color improve traction and depth perception.

of 1.25 in. (32 mm) and a maximum of 2 in. (51 mm). If mounted adjacent to a wall, clearance between the handrail and wall should be a minimum of 1.5 in. (38 mm).[6,9]
6. Installation of a ramp requires adequate space. Materials used to construct large ramps include durable steel, wood, wood alternative composite decking materials (combination of wood and plastic), and concrete; smaller ramps can be made from aluminum or fiberglass. The minimum ramp grade (incline or slope) for a wheelchair ramp is that for every inch of threshold height there is a corresponding 12 in. (305 mm) of ramp length (a running slope of 1:12).[6] Outdoor ramps exposed to inclement weather such as snow or ice formation require a more gradual running slope of approximately 1:20. Ramps should be a minimum of 36 in. (915 mm) wide, with a nonslip surface. The overall rise of any ramp should be no greater than 30 in. (760 mm). Handrails also should be included on the ramp with a minimum height of 34 in. (865 mm) and a maximum height of 38 in. (965 mm) and extend 12 in. (305 mm) beyond the top and bottom of the ramp (Fig. 9.3C).[6,9] Small, commercially available ramps can be used for traversing curbs and small step heights (Fig. 9.4).
7. Vertical platform lifts and stairway lifts are commercially available and may be a consideration when inadequate space is available for a ramp. *Vertical platform lifts* (Fig. 9.5) travel approximately 8 feet (243.84 cm) straight up and down. Both open and enclosed models are available. Platform lifts are often installed adjacent to stairs with an upper landing and are available in a variety of dimensions, with lengths ranging from 54 to 60 in. (137.16 to 152.4 cm) and widths ranging from 34 to 42 in. (86.36 to 106.68 cm). The lift brings the wheelchair user from the ground level to the landing level to access the entrance to the home (these lifts can be used indoors as well). *Stairway lifts* are installed directly onto existing outdoor stairways; however, they are

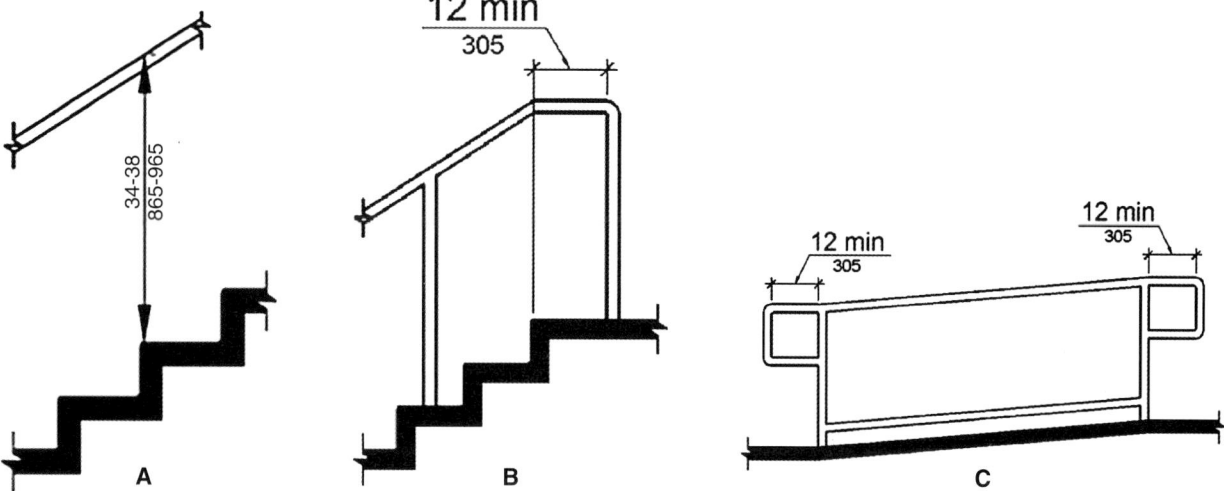

Figure 9.3 (A) Handrail height for stairs. (B) Handrail extension at top of stairs. A similar handrail extension of 12 in. (305 mm) is placed at bottom of stairs; (C) Handrail extensions should run a minimum of 12 in. (305 mm) beyond the top and bottom edge of ramp. *(From 2010 ADA Standards for Accessible Design[9] [A, p. 154; B, p. 157; C, p. 175].)*

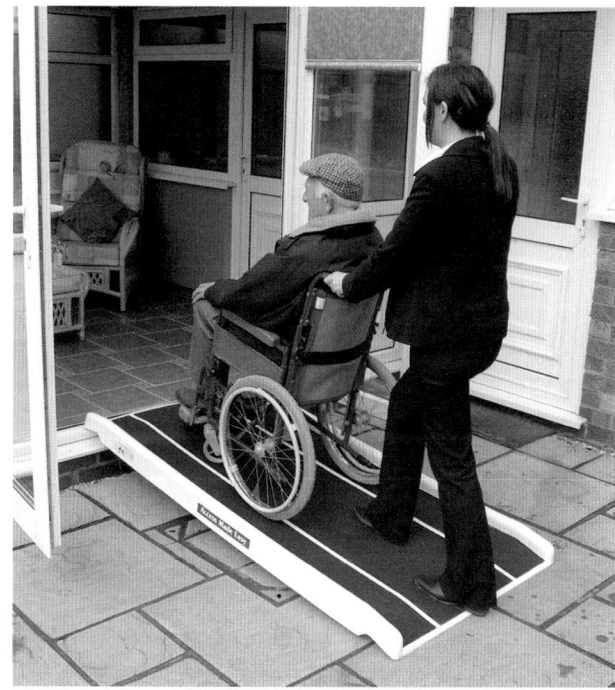

Figure 9.4 Lightweight, portable ramps are available for navigating small inclines. They are often constructed of aluminum, available in variety of lengths to accommodate different elevations, and some include a folding mechanism. *(Courtesy of AMODI, 78450 Chavenay – France.)*

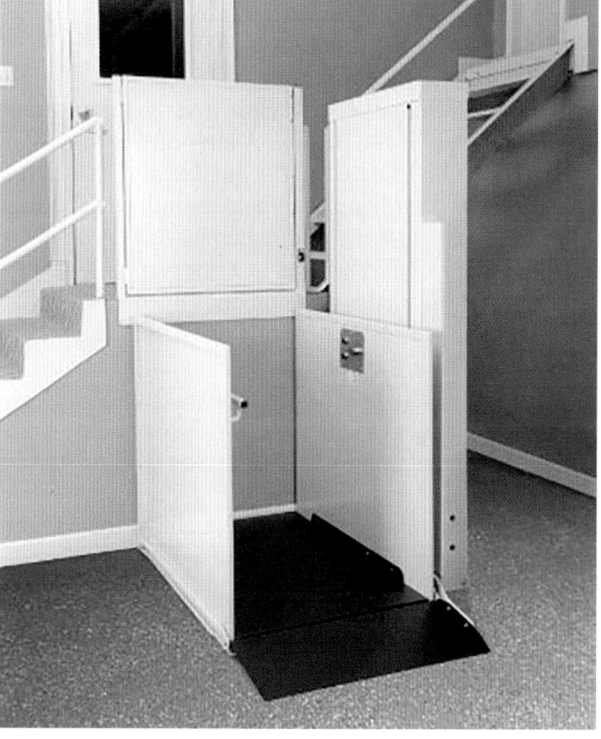

Figure 9.5 Powered residential vertical lift. This lift has a 750-lb weight capacity. The platform measures approximately 36 in. wide and 48 in. deep (91.44 × 121.92 cm). *(Courtesy of Symmetry Elevating Solutions, Peoria, IL 61615.)*

more frequently used indoors. The stairway lifts are mounted on runners that traverse the length of the stairs and slightly beyond. Many models allow the platform to fold up against an adjacent wall to allow free stair access for others entering the home (see Interior Accessibility: General Considerations, *Stairs*).

Entrance

1. For individuals using a wheelchair, the entrance should have a platform large enough to allow the patient to rest and to prepare for entry. This

platform area is particularly important when a ramp is in use. It provides for safe transit from the inclined surface to the level surface. If an individual using a wheelchair is required to open a door that swings out, this area should be at least 5 × 5 ft (153 × 153 cm). If the door swings in and away from the patient, a space at least 3 feet (91.5 cm) deep and 5 feet (153 cm) wide is required.

2. The door locks should be accessible to the patient. The height of the locks should be determined, as well as the amount of force required to turn the key. Alternative lock systems (e.g., voice-, card-, or fob-activated locks; fingerprint and facial recognition locks; remote-controlled locks; keypad electronic security systems; push-button padlocks) may be an important consideration for some patients. Particular attention should be directed toward ensuring that the locking mechanism on the door is sufficiently illuminated.

3. The door handle should allow for one-hand operation and be turned easily by the patient. Rubber doorknob covers (that stretch over a round doorknob and provide a textured grip) or lever-type handles are often easier to use for patients with limited grip strength. Lever handles do not require the same strength or range of motion (ROM) needed for traditional round doorknobs.[10]

4. The door should open and close in a direction that is functional for the patient. A long canvas "door strap" may be attached to the outside of the door (or around the door handle) to help an individual using a wheelchair close the door when leaving. A long, sturdy belt can also be used as a door strap.

5. Remote-controlled automatic door openers are available that attach to existing doors that can open, close, and lock the door; some are equipped with customized "stay-open" features to accommodate the time required to enter or exit. A handheld remote control or a touch pad can be used to activate these devices.

6. Installation of an intercom system allows the patient to see and/or hear who is at the door. Many allow remote-controlled opening of a door from any location in the home.

7. If there is a raised threshold in the doorway, it should be removed. If removal is not possible, the threshold should be lowered to no greater than 1/2 in. (13 mm) in height, with beveled edges;[7] alternatively, a threshold ramp may be installed (see Interior Accessibility: General Considerations, *Doors*). If needed, weather-stripping the door will help prevent drafts.

8. The doorway width should be measured. Generally, 32 to 34 in. (81 to 86 cm) is an acceptable doorway width to accommodate most wheelchairs. Bariatric chairs require increased width.

9. If the door is weighted to aid in closing, the pressure should not exceed 8 lb (3.6 kg) to be functional for the patient.

10. A kickplate (metal guard) may be added to doors frequently entered by individuals using a wheelchair or ambulatory assistive devices. The kickplate should measure 12 in. (30 cm) in height from the bottom of the door.

> **Clinical Note.** Several distinct considerations are required to address the environmental needs of patients who are overweight or obese, generally defined and classified using body mass index (BMI)[65] (Table 9.3). Data from the 2021 National Health and Nutrition Examination Survey indicate that greater than 42% of adults and 19.3% of youth are obese.[66,67] An overview of the unique environmental needs of this population is presented in Box 9.1.

Interior Accessibility: General Considerations
Furniture Arrangement and Features

1. Sufficient room should be made available for maneuvering a wheelchair or ambulating with an assistive device. An initial strategy is to move as much furniture as possible against the walls to increase clearance and stability (i.e., prevent sliding of furniture during movement transitions). Further stability can be achieved by placing rubber cups (floor guards) under the legs of sofas and chairs. Items such as coffee tables, footstools, or electrical wires should not obstruct access to furniture.

2. Clear passage must be allowed from one room to the next.

3. Typically, overstuffed sofas and chairs do not provide the needed support for sit-to-stand movement transitions. Although generally not the case, ideally, living room chairs should have double armrests, a firm seating surface, and an upright back. Sometimes a suitable chair can be found in a different location within the home and moved to the living room. Another option is to modify the current furniture by placing a fitted wooden board under the seat cushion and behind the seat back (if removable). If a new chair is to be purchased, recommended features of the chair should be provided to the patient and family (e.g., the height of the seat should allow the knees to flex approximately 90° with the feet flat on the floor, a firm cushioned seat, a firm cushioned back that provides adequate upright support, and double armrests).

4. Use of any unstable furniture such as rocking chairs should be discouraged for most patients. Chairs that provide mechanized elevation of the back of the seat are commercially available but should be used with caution. It may be difficult for a patient to stabilize the feet as the seat is elevating. This causes the feet (and pelvis) to slide forward, with potential for a fall.

Table 9.3   Classification of Overweight and Obesity by Body Mass Index, Waist Circumference, and Associated Disease Risks

			Disease Risk* Relative to Normal Weight and Waist Circumference	
	BMI	Obesity Class	Men 102 cm (40 in.) or less Women 88 cm (35 in.) or less	Men Greater Than 102 cm (40 in.) Women Greater Than 88 cm (35 in.)
Underweight	Less than 18.5		—	—
Normal	18.5–24.9		—	—
Overweight	25–29.9		Increased	High
Obesity	30–34.9	I	High	Very high
	35–39.9	II	Very high	Very high
Extreme Obesity	Greater than 40	III	Extremely high	Extremely high

* Disease risk for type 2 diabetes, hypertension, and cardiovascular disease.
\+ Increased waist circumference also can be a marker for increased risk, even in persons of normal weight.
From *National Institutes of Health.*[65]
BMI = Body Mass Index.

Electrical Controls

1. Unrestricted access should be provided to wall switches and electrical outlets. Power strips (surge protectors) can be used to increase the number of outlets as well as improve access. Outlets may need to be raised and wall switches lowered. For individuals using a wheelchair, use of pull-cord extensions may allow control of high electrical switches.

2. Some patients may benefit from replacement of standard toggle wall switches controlling overhead lights or fans with rocker switches that require less fine motor skill and can be activated with a fisted hand, lateral aspect of hand, or distal forearm. Rocker switches are available with illuminated surfaces and with occupancy (motion) sensor devices that automatically turn on or off. The plates surrounding wall switches come in a variety of colors and will be easier to see if they contrast with the existing wall color. For example, in rooms with light-colored walls (white, off-white, beige), darker electrical outlet and light-switch plates can be selected. Voice- and noise-activated (clapping) lighting controls are also available. A ground fault circuit interrupter (GFCI) should be installed in wet locations such as bathrooms to prevent against electrical shock. A GFCI outlet acts as a monitor for current imbalance between the hot and neutral wires and breaks the circuit if that situation occurs (e.g., faulty appliances, worn cords, or appliance contact with water). In new home construction, GFCI installation is now required; they must be retrofitted in older homes.

3. For some patients, vision may be enhanced by use of higher wattage bulbs, fluorescent lighting, full-spectrum bulbs, daylight bulbs, or high-intensity halogen lamps. Long-life, energy-efficient LED lightbulbs reduce the frequency of required bulb changes.

4. Inexpensive, programmable electrical timers can be used to regularly turn lights on and off throughout the day and night.

5. Inexpensive night-lights can be placed in strategic locations to provide additional illumination. Some are available with motion sensors.

6. Dimmer switches with touch pads (or small sliding levers) can be used to activate lamps. The dimmer module is plugged into a wall outlet and the lamp attached to the module. The lamp can be turned on or off and the level of brightness changed by touching the pad or moving the lever. Voice-activated dimmers are also available.

7. Inexpensive remote-controlled units can be used in any room of the home to control lights or small appliances. The simplest designs of these remote-controlled units send signals through existing wires (receiver modules are plugged into existing outlets and appliances are plugged into the receiver and controlled by a handheld remote); others are wireless. Receiver modules can also be wired directly into the electrical system of the dwelling. Remote-controlled units are available with large-print buttons and numbers.

Clinical Note. Many cellular phone apps are available to remotely control an expanding variety of smart appliances such as thermostats, televisions, fans, smoke/carbon monoxide alarms, garage doors, home theater systems, water heaters, door locks, and lighting and security systems.

Box 9.1   Bariatric Considerations

Patients who are obese often require specialized equipment when being lifted, moved, transferred, or transported. Bariatric equipment is space consuming, which is sometimes exacerbated in smaller homes or apartments and by older homes that were designed and built when adult height and weight statistics were lower than today. The following are environmental considerations unique to this population.

- *Training for Patients, Families, and Carepartners:* Specific training in the use of bariatric equipment and patient handling is essential. Patients who are obese frequently require assistance with numerous basic activities throughout the day (e.g., positional changes, supine-to-sit and sit-to-stand transitions, bathing, toileting, and dressing). These care requirements highlight the importance of highly trained carepartners able to promote safety and injury prevention for both the patient and themselves. When possible, the patient should be encouraged to take the lead in directing those in charge of the care provided.
- *Physical Assistance:* More than one individual may be required to assist the patient. There may be situations where as many as three or four people are needed for patient handling. When multiple people are assisting, a "leader" should be designated to direct and provide verbal cues during the activity. Third-party payers challenge reimbursement for more than one support person in the home simultaneously (duplication of services). This may require involvement from extended family members and/or require the patient and family to seek creative funding sources to meet this need (see section titled "Funding Sources").
- *Bariatric Equipment:* Inherent to its purpose, bariatric equipment is oversized, is designed for increased weight capacity, and is generally heavier and costlier than its standard adult equivalent. Bariatric equipment is extensive and includes beds (some with built-in scales), bariatric mattresses with high weight capacities, bedside commodes, standard and overhead lifts, reclining chairs, steel-framed chairs, powered lift chairs with a 1,000-lb (453.59-kg) weight capacity, bathroom equipment, adaptive equipment, wheelchairs (widths up to 48 in. [121.92 cm]), scooters, and ambulatory assistive devices. Providers of durable medical equipment typically offer patient, family, and caregiver in-home instruction. Some provide ongoing support should additional caregivers require training.
- *Risk of Pressure Injuries:* Patients who are obese are at increased risk for developing pressure injuries secondary to their size and immobility. They may be unable to effectively change positions, creating excess pressure on susceptible areas for long periods. This may require use of a specialized mattress (e.g., low air loss with alternating pressure). Excessive skin folds, moisture, or perspiration may contribute to ulcer formation. Frequent examination of the integumentary system is advised.
- *Care Environment:* Large beds (e.g., 42 to 54 in. [106.68 to 137.16 cm] wide, 80 to 90 in. [203.2 to 228.6 cm] long, and up to 1,000-lb [453.59-kg] weight capacity), lifts, and other large bariatric equipment require larger room dimensions. Passage of bariatric equipment generally requires a door width of 60 in. (152.4 cm). A large window may need to be temporarily removed to allow passage of oversized items. Ample floor space is also needed for caregivers to interface with the patient in and around the equipment. Five feet of clear floor space is recommended on each side and at the foot of the bed. The floor surface and support structures beneath need to be carefully examined. They must be able to support a patient weight ranging from 500 to 1,000 lb (226.8 to 453.59 kg) together with all needed equipment and supplies. Often space is made available on the first level of a dwelling (versus navigating patient and equipment up a narrow staircase to a small second-floor bedroom). This may require conversion of the living room to a patient care area. An environmental control unit is an important consideration.
- *Bathroom:* Space is a primary concern in gaining access to a standard residential bathroom. Sufficient door width is needed to accommodate patient size, an assistive device, and/or the individual(s) guarding the patient. A 60-in. (152.4-cm) door width and turning radius is recommended. To place a bariatric commode with armrests over a toilet or allow a two-person assist, ample space of 24 in. (60.96 cm) is needed on each side with a 44-in. (111.76-cm) front clearance. A bidet may be recommended to assist cleansing. The toilet and sink should be floor mounted with a 1,000-lb (543.59-kg) weight capacity. Longer than typical grab bars with a 1,000-lb (543.59-kg) weight capacity should be installed on reinforced walls. The shower stall should be a minimum of 4 × 6 ft (1.22 × 1.83 m) and include a level entrance, a bariatric shower seat, a shower hand sprayer, and grab bars with a 1,000-lb (543.59-kg) weight capacity. The use of shower curtains is recommended over solid doors to facilitate caregiver assistance.

Floors

1. Floors should be nonslip and level; hard-surfaced floors (e.g., engineered or solid hardwood, laminate) are ideal. When carpeting is used, a dense, low pile (0.25 to 0.5 in. [0.64 to 1.27 cm]), low-level loop generally provides for easiest movement of a wheelchair or ambulatory assistive device. Industrial-style or indoor/outdoor carpeting typically meet these requirements. High-pile carpeting and carpet padding increase roll resistance (e.g., wheelchair, rolling walker); firmer carpeting decreases roll resistance. Carpeting with bold

patterns of mixed colors may be visually confusing and impair judgment of spatial distances.[68,69] Padding under carpet is generally not recommended; if used, it should be very firm. Floor coverings may need to be secured to the floor to prevent bunching or rippling under wheelchair use.

2. Floors should be examined for uneven or unlevel areas. This may be particularly problematic with older wooden floors. Joints in wood flooring should be shallow and no more than 0.25 to 0.5 in. (0.64 to 1.27 cm) wide. Deep joints wider than 0.75 in. (1.9 cm) will cause wheelchair casters to turn and lodge, blocking movement.[68,69] Optimally, problem areas should be repaired or replaced. If restoration is not possible, several other solutions might be recommended: (1) establish a path of movement for the patient that eliminates use of the problematic area, (2) place a piece of furniture over the offending area, or (3) place brightly colored tape along the borders of the area to continually remind the patient to avoid this area of potential danger.

3. Scatter rugs should be removed; larger area rugs can be secured with a good-quality carpet tape. Use of nonskid waxes should be encouraged.

4. If flooring is to be replaced, matte finishes should be recommended to reduce glare. Patients with visual impairments will benefit from a contrasting color border along the perimeter of the room to help mark the boundaries of the space. Wide, color tape can also be used effectively.

Doors

1. Raised thresholds should be removed to provide a flush, level surface. If structural elements prevent removal, small permanent threshold ramps (transition wedges) can be installed (Fig. 9.6A). Portable, folding designs are also available (Fig. 9.6B).

2. Doorways may need to be widened (if less than 32 in. [815 mm] wide) to allow clearance for a wheelchair or assistive device. Doors may have to be removed, reversed (e.g., to open outward for easier exit, especially in the case of an emergency), or replaced with folding doors. Several other options are available to increase door clearance:

   • Pocket doors, which slide into the adjacent wall when not in use, are an option for new construction. However, they cannot be easily installed in existing structures. Alternatively, where adjacent wall space permits, a sliding door can be installed on the outside of the door frame that requires minimal structural changes. The top of the door is attached to a long glide rail installed above the doorframe extending along the upper portion of the bordering wall to allow the door to slide open. Commercially, these are referred to as "barn doors."

   • Removal of the wood strips on the inside of a door frame will add approximately 0.75 to 1 in. (2 to 2.5 cm) of clearance.

   • Use of *offset* hinges (also called *swing-clear hinges*), which swing the open door clear of the frame, provide approximately 2 in. (5 cm) of additional space.

   • Removal of the door with installation of a curtain (inexpensive spring-loaded curtain rods and a fabric or plastic shower curtain can be used); if used for a bathroom door, this option is less than optimal because it compromises privacy.

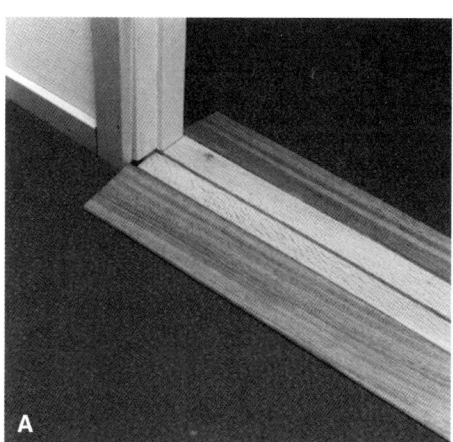
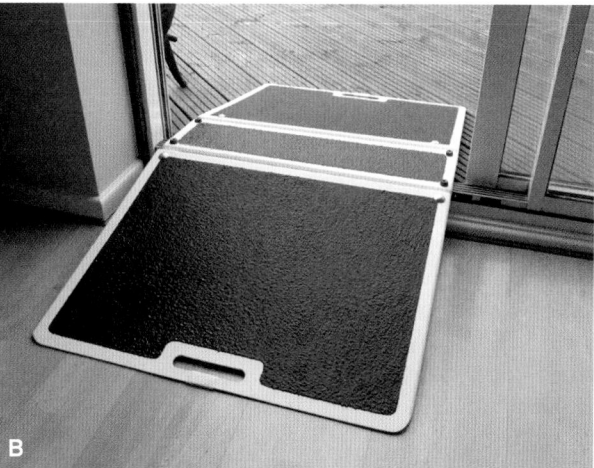

Figure 9.6 Threshold ramps can be permanently installed (A) or portable (B). Common materials used for threshold ramps are wood (A), rubber, and aluminum typically with a nonslip surface. Some portable threshold are designed to fold (B). They can be used between rooms, if a threshold cannot be removed. *([A] Courtesy of Guldmann, Inc., Tampa, FL 33634; [B] Courtesy of AMODI, 78450 Chavenay – France)*

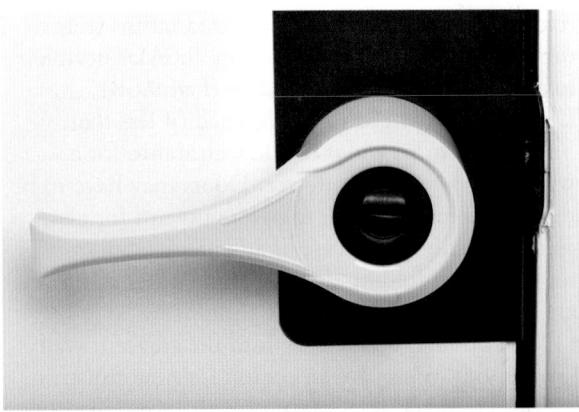

Figure 9.7 A doorknob lever adapter can be used to convert a standard doorknob into a lever handle. They can be fitted to either interior or exterior doors. *(Courtesy of Freedom Distributors, Crystal Springs, MS 39059.)*

3. As mentioned in regard to exterior doors, handles inside the home should also be examined. Rubber doorknob covers or lever-type handles may be important considerations. An adapter placed over a standard doorknob can be used to create a lever handle (Fig. 9.7). Knurled (roughened) surface door handles are used on interiors of buildings and dwellings when frequented by persons with visual impairments. These abrasive, knurled surfaces provide tactile clues that the door leads to a hazardous area and alerts the individual to danger. (Note: Brightly colored roughened areas are also used on flooring to indicate potential danger; for example, the edge of a train or subway platform.)

Windows

1. To reduce glare, window films can be installed; frosted films are effective at diffusing light without appreciably reducing ambient light.
2. Heavy draperies (with appropriately sized drapery pull rods) or shades can also be used with the added benefit of absorbing internal background noise to improve hearing and conversation.
3. Remote-controlled systems for closing or opening window coverings either partially or fully are commercially available.
4. Although not frequently seen in older dwellings, casement windows provide several important features for individuals using a wheelchair or for patients with limited upper extremity function. Casement windows open using a crank-style handle and can be locked with a single-lever locking mechanism located near the bottom of the window. Automatic openers are available on these windows.

Stairs

1. All indoor stairwells should have handrails and should be well lighted. Ideally, handrails should extend a minimum of 12 in. (305 mm) past the top and bottom of the stairs for added safety[6,9] (see Fig. 9.3B). Battery-operated touch lamps are a practical supplement where electrical light sources are unavailable. Inexpensive track lighting provides multiple adjustable lamps and requires only a single electrical source. Lighting should be bright with glare and reflection minimized. Motion detection lights that automatically turn on when the patient approaches the stairs (or other area of the home) can also be an important safety consideration.
2. Stairs should be free of clutter. Rather than climbing the stairs to move a single item to the next level, patients sometimes "store" or collect items on the stairs. This creates several safety hazards: (1) initially bending down to pick up the items before stair climbing can alter postural stability; (2) negotiating stairs holding several objects can impair balance and limit use of the handrail; and (3) other household members may not see the item(s), precipitating a fall. As an alternative, a chair or small table placed near the stairs can be used to hold a canvas sling bag or small "stair basket" with handles (that can be held in one hand) to collect items until the patient is ready to move to another floor level.
3. For individuals with decreased visual acuity or age-related visual changes, adhesive, light-reflective *tactile warning strips* provide contrasting textures on the surface of the top and bottom stairs to alert them that the end of the stairwell is near. They can also be used on each step to identify its edge. Circular bands of tape also can be placed at the top and bottom of the handrail for the same purpose. Tactile warning strips placed on the floor can be used to signal a change in level of the walking surface or entrance to another area or room of the dwelling.
4. Many patients with visual impairment will benefit also from bright, contrasting color tape on the border of each stair. Warm colors (reds, oranges, and yellows) are generally easier to see than cool colors (blues, greens, and violets).
5. For patients unable to negotiate stairs who require access to the second floor of a dwelling, a motorized stair lift may be an option (Fig. 9.8). These units are available with a variety of options such as swing-away arms for wheelchair transfers, wide adjustable seat width (22.5 to 25.5 in. [57 cm to 64 cm]), and remote call/send controls. Outdoor models are also available, as well as units to accommodate curves or turns in the stairwell. Standard residential elevators are another, more costly option; they require construction of an enclosed shaft. If the residence has "stacked" closets (same position on different floors), these closet spaces may be combined to form an elevator shaft. An alternative to standard elevators is compact shaftless home elevators (Fig. 9.9) that allow movement between two floors. They are

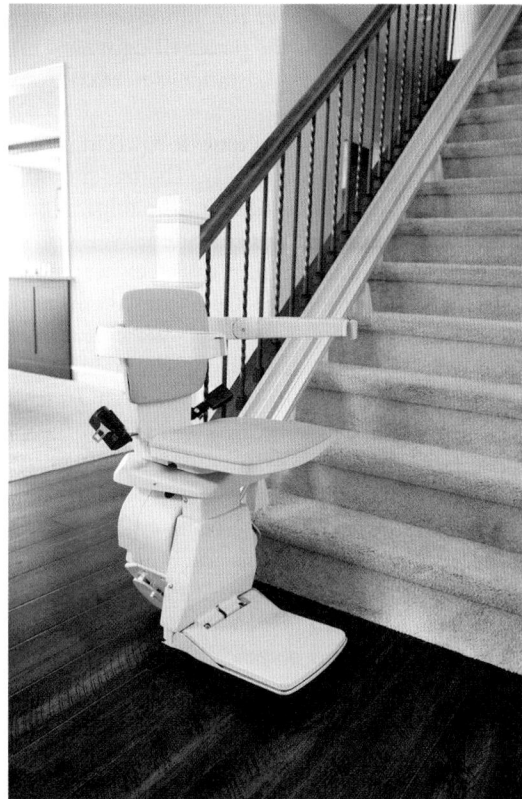

Figure 9.8 Powered stairlift with a 300-lb lift capacity is operated using armrest controls or a wireless remote control and includes obstruction sensors and retractable seatbelt. The seat swivels up to 90° at top of stairs for safe exit. When not in use, the arms, seat, and footrest fold. *(Courtesy of Bruno Independent Living Aids, Oconomowoc, WI 53066.)*

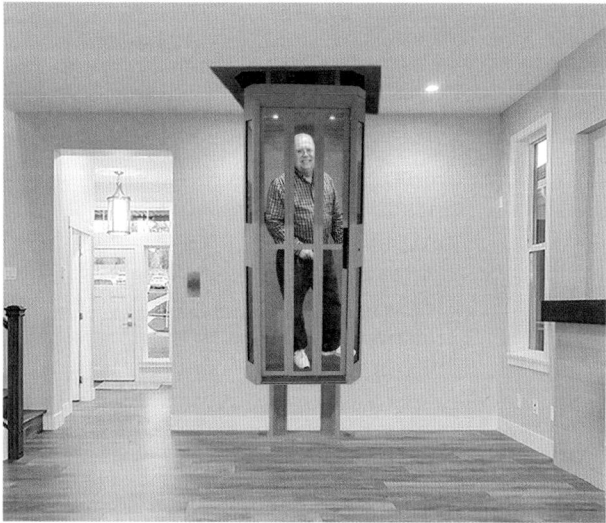

Figure 9.9 Residential shaftless elevator. This residential elevator has a 400-lb weight capacity with a car size approximately 33 in. wide, 35 in. deep, and 76 in. high (84 × 89 × 193 cm) *(Courtesy of Symmetry Elevating Solutions, Peoria, IL 61615.)*

freestanding and do not require bordering walls for installation. The car moves along a rail system adjacent to a wall. Some are battery powered that allow use during a power outage. They are typically equipped with push-button controls, a fold-down seat, and internal lighting.

Heating Units

1. All radiators, heating vents, and hot water pipes should be appropriately screened off or insulated with pipe covers to prevent burns, especially for patients who have sensory impairments. Adaptations may be required to allow patient access to heat controls (e.g., remote thermostat control, use of long-handled reachers or enlarged, extended, or adapted handles on heat control valves).
2. The heating source should be clear of combustible material and clutter. Use of space heaters should be discouraged.

Smoke and Carbon Monoxide Alarms

Smoke and carbon monoxide alarms should be in the home and checked regularly. Many models include voice warning announcements ("Fire" or "Low Battery") and allow testing the alarm using a remote control or cell phone app. At least one alarm should be on every level of the home, and ideally, one in the kitchen and each bedroom and one outside each sleeping area. Interconnected alarms enable wireless communication with each other and provide better full-home protection. Regularly scheduled battery replacement is recommended (e.g., daylight saving time change, New Year's Day). For patients with hearing impairments, the alarm can also be attached to a signaling system that activates a high-volume audible and strobe light response, to visually warn of danger. (These signaling systems also can be used to activate flashing lights in response to a doorbell, knock on the door, telephone ring, or burglar alarm.)

Clinical Note. A frequent gap in accomplishing home access is that the patient and family are provided recommendations with no community contacts to actually install the recommendations. To provide effective guidance, the therapist should be knowledgeable about licensed contractors experienced in home modifications for individuals with disability. Information about qualified contractors may be acquired from consultation with local contractors, online research, interviews with local community experts, and by visiting completed home modification sites. The identified contractor should be available for consultation and communication with the patient, family, and rehabilitation team members throughout the planning and implementation process.

Interior Accessibility: Individual Room Considerations

Bedroom

1. The bed should be stationary and positioned to provide ample space for transfers. Stability may be improved by placing the bed against a wall or in the corner of the room (except when the patient plans to make the bed). Additional stability may be achieved by placing rubber cups under each leg.

2. The height of the sleeping surface must be optimal for transfers. Furniture risers can be used to raise bed height. Wooden and high-density rubber furniture risers are commercially available in a variety of heights with routed depressions to hold each leg of the bed (or other furniture such as chairs or tables). The use of an extra-thick mattress or box spring can also provide additional height to the bed. To lower bed height, reduced-height box springs are available, or the box spring can be completely removed and a platform bed board used to support the mattress.

3. The mattress should be carefully examined. It should provide a firm, comfortable surface. If the mattress is in relatively good condition, a firm bed board inserted between the mattress and box spring may suffice to improve the sleeping surface adequately. If the mattress is badly worn, a new one should be suggested.

4. A bedside nightstand (or small table) should be available; it can be used to hold a lamp, telephone (preferably cordless with a memory dial for frequently used numbers or emergency phone numbers; cell phones have the added advantage of always remaining with the patient), necessary medications, and call bell if assistance is needed from a carepartner.

5. The closet clothes bar may require lowering to provide wheelchair accessibility. The bar should be lowered to 52 in. (132 cm) from the floor. Non-slip hangers are often recommended. Wall hooks also may be a useful addition to the closet area and should be placed between 40 in. (101.6 cm) and 56 in. (142.2 cm) from the floor. *Wardrobe lifts* can increase closet storage capacity while maintaining accessibility. They consist of a clothes bar attached by hinged supports; using an extended handle (Fig. 9.10A), the bar is manually pulled down and out to access clothing. Powered wardrobe lifts (Fig. 9.10B) are also commercially available. With height based on the patient's reaching capability, shelves can be installed at various levels in the closet. Clothing and grooming articles frequently used by the patient should be placed in the most easily accessible bureau drawer. Freestanding modular closet units are also available in a variety of dimensions. These units typically provide clothes bar, shelves, and drawers that can be adjusted to meet the needs of the user. Figure 9.11 illustrates the basic dimensions of an accessible bedroom.

Bathroom

1. If the door frame prohibits passage of a wheelchair, the patient may transfer at the door to a chair with

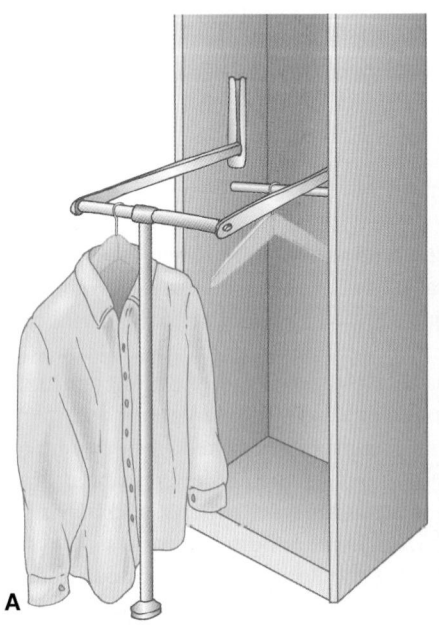
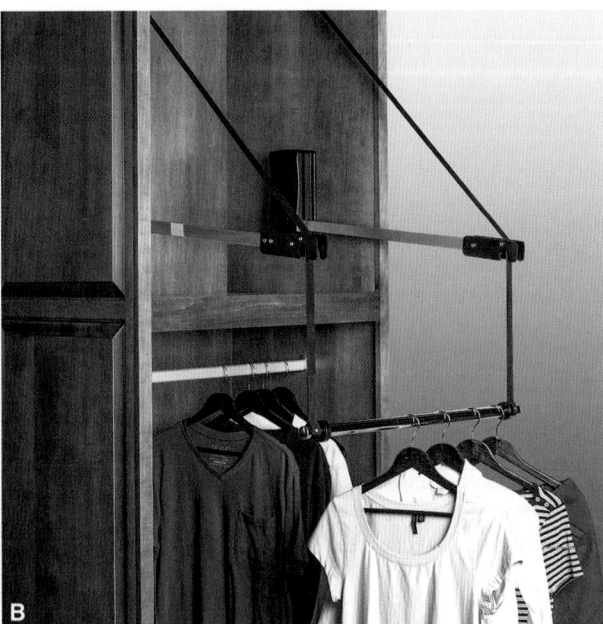

Figure 9.10 Both manually operated (A) and powered (B) wardrobe lifts are available. Powered units are typically operated via remote control. Available in a variety of sizes, wardrobe lifts lower the closet rod to allow access to clothing from a wheelchair seated position. *([B] Courtesy of Häfele America, Archdale, NC 27263.)*

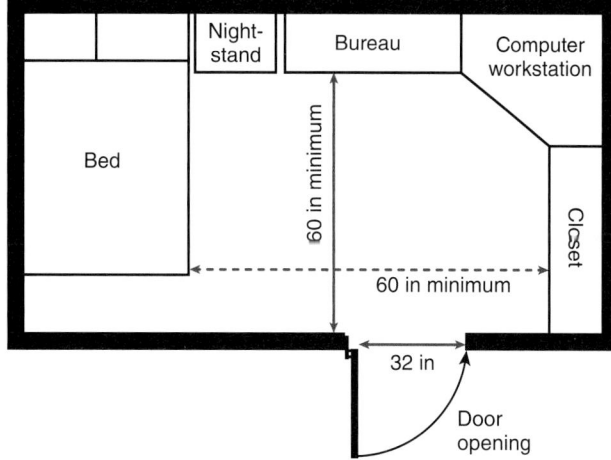

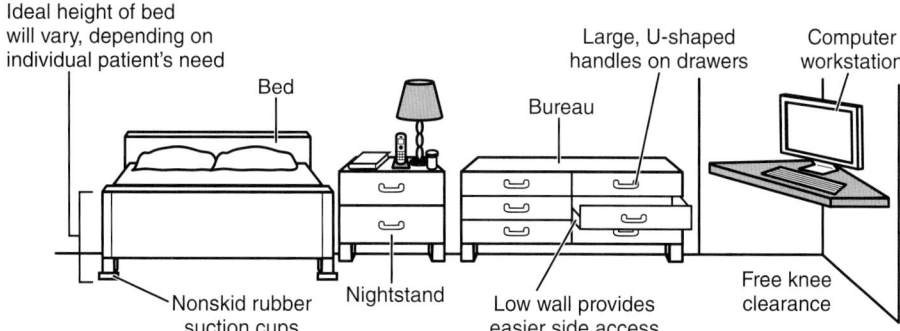

Figure 9.11 Sample dimensions of an accessible bedroom.

casters attached. As mentioned, several other solutions are available to address the problem of narrow door frames (see Interior Accessibility: General Considerations, *Doors*).

2. For many patients, an elevated toilet will facilitate transfers. The simplest approach is use of a portable raised seat attachment. Some models allow the height to be custom adjusted, whereas others provide a fixed height elevation. They are also available with hand bars on each side. Base risers can be installed to elevate the entire toilet (Fig. 9.12). Finally, a standard height toilet (14 to 15 in. [36 to 38 cm]) can be replaced with a comfort (convenient) height (17 to 20 in. [43 to 51 cm]) model. Also available are power-lift toilet seats with grab bars designed to assist the patient to standing (elevation initiated from the posterior aspect of the seat). This is a costlier option and poses potential safety risks. As with other types of mechanized seat elevators, it may be difficult to stabilize one's feet as the seat is elevating (especially in an area with the potential for a wet floor surface). For new construction, a wall-mounted toilet may be recommended that can be placed at the optimum height for the user and provide more floor space for transfer positioning. Based on patient size, weight capacity of wall-mounted units needs to be considered.

3. Grab bars securely fastened to a reinforced wall will assist in both toilet and tub transfers. Grab bars

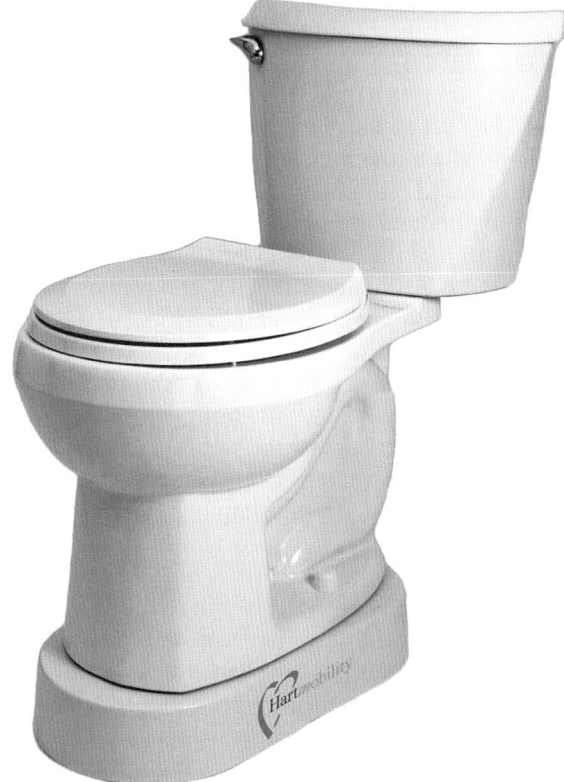

Figure 9.12 Base risers positioned between the floor and bottom of toilet increase the height of the entire toilet to facilitate transfers. *(Courtesy of Hartmobility, Zebulon, Georgia 30295.)*

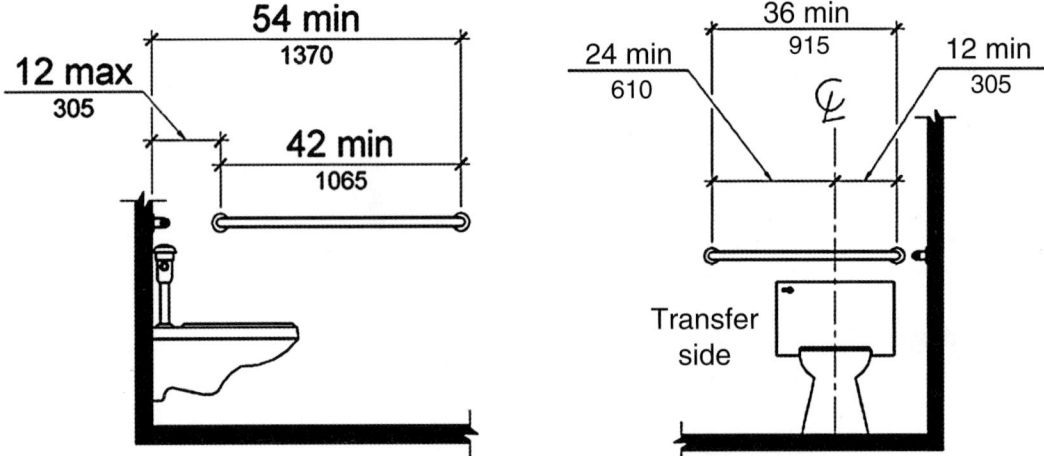

Figure 9.13 Location and dimensions of bathroom grab bars. Values denoted in inches and millimeters. The bars should be mounted horizontally 33 in (840 mm) to 36 in (915 mm) from the floor. *(Left)* The sidewall grab bar is 42 to 54 in. wide placed at a maximum of 12 in. (305 mm) from the rear wall. If anchored on or near the rear wall, it should extend 54 in. (1,370 mm) from the wall. *(Right)* The rear-wall grab bar is 24 to 36 in. wide (36 in. is considered minimum if wall space allows). When 36 in. long, 24 in. of the bar (from center of toilet) is placed toward the side used for transfers. *(From 2010 ADA Standards for Accessible Design,* Left, *p. 163,* Right, *p. 164.)*

should have a circular cross-sectional diameter of 1.25 in. (32 mm) minimum and 2 in. (51 mm) maximum and be knurled. For use in toilet transfers, the bars should be mounted horizontally 33 to 36 in. (840 to 915 mm) from the floor. The length of the grab bars should be between 42 and 54 in. (1,065 and 1,370 mm) on sidewall and between 24 and 36 in. (610 and 915 mm) on the back wall (Fig. 9.13). Ideally, two grab bars are secured horizontally to the back wall for use in tub transfers. One is placed 33 to 36 in. (840 to 915 mm) from the tub floor and the second 9 in. (230 mm) above the top rim of the bathtub. Grab bars may also be mounted horizontally at the foot-end wall of the bathtub (recommended length is 24 in. [610 mm] with placement at the front edge of the bathtub) and at the head-end wall of the bathtub (recommended length is 12 in. [305 mm] with placement at the front edge of the bathtub) (Fig. 9.14). Knurled surfaces are typically used on grab bars to improve grasp and prevent slipping.

4. A tub transfer bench (tub seat) may be recommended for bathing. Many types of commercially produced benches are available. In selecting a tub transfer bench (tub seat), function and safety are primary considerations. The bench should provide a wide base of support (some are designed with suction feet, and some provide height adjustment), a backrest, and an appropriate seating surface to facilitate transfers in and out of the tub. Tub transfer benches with relatively long seating surfaces are typically positioned with two legs in the tub and

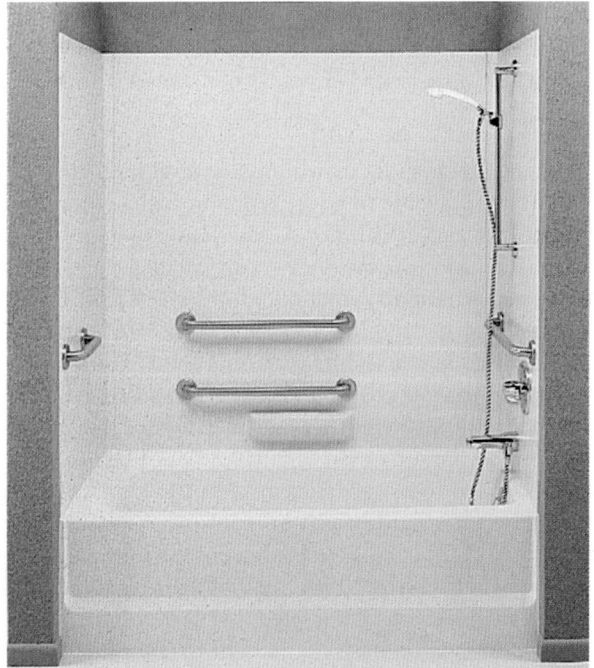

Figure 9.14 Bathtub with grab bars secured to back, foot-end, and head-end walls. The hand-spray faucet attachment facilitates control of water flow direction from a sitting position. *(Courtesy of the Swan Corporation, St. Louis, MO 63101.)*

two legs on the floor adjacent to the tub (Fig. 9.15). Smaller benches are available that require all four legs to be placed inside the bathtub. Individuals who are unable to transfer successfully with a

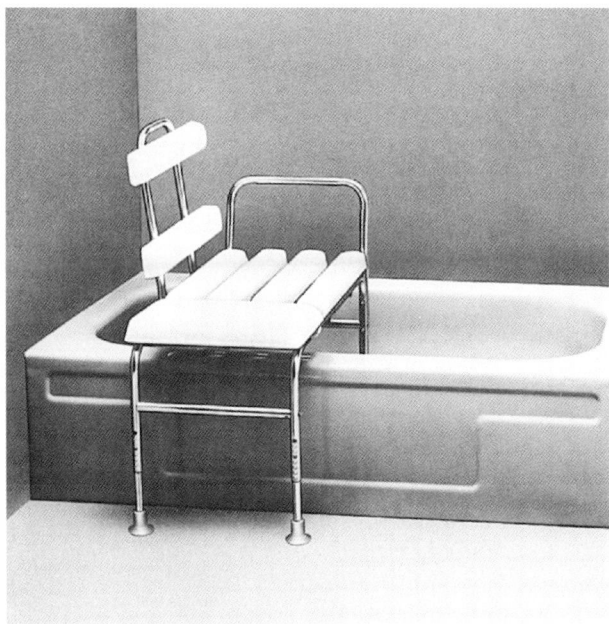

Figure 9.15 Bathtub transfer bench providing a wide base of support, a secure back rest, and a long seating surface to facilitate transfers. *(Courtesy of Lumex, Inc., Bay Shore, NY 11706.)*

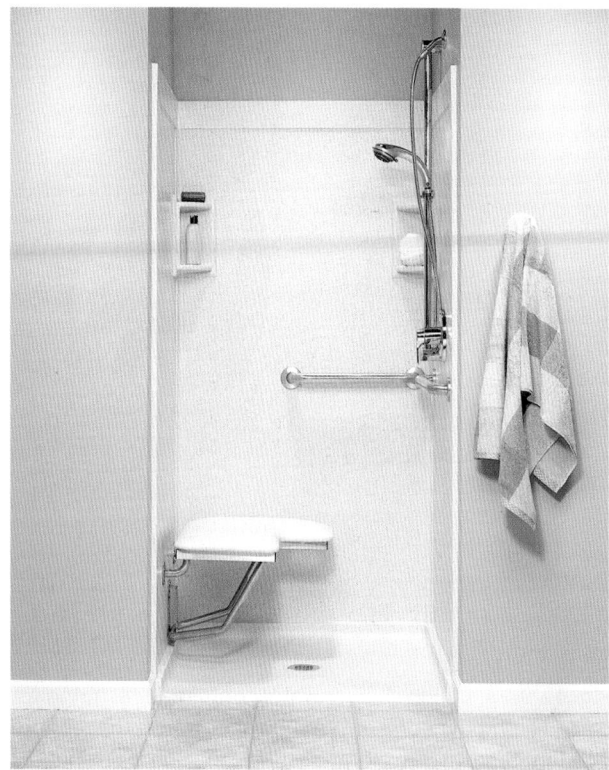

Figure 9.16 Shower stall with collapsible shower seat, grab bars, and hand-spray attachment. *(Courtesy of Swan Surfaces, Centralia, IL 62801.)*

traditional tub transfer bench may benefit from a sliding transfer bench with a swivel seat. For safety, a model should be chosen with a swivel seat able to lock every quarter turn as well as at the end of the slide rails. Individuals with postural instability should be guarded carefully to prevent loss of balance or falls when the seat is moving.

5. In shower stall areas, a collapsible seat may be permanently attached to the wall (Fig. 9.16). When not in use, it folds flat against the wall, allowing easy shower access from a standing position as well. Many newer shower designs incorporate a permanent, built-in seat.

6. Nonskid adhesive strips may be placed on the floor of the tub or shower area.

7. Additional bathroom considerations may include a hand-spray attachment to the bathtub or shower faucet (see Fig. 9.14 and Fig. 9.17), anti-scald valves to prevent water temperature from rising above a preset limit (also called *scald-guard valves* or *high-temperature stops*), water volume–control mechanisms (to prevent a sudden surge of water with resultant change in temperature), enlarged faucet handles on the tub or sink (single-lever system faucets are optimal owing to their ease of use), motion-sensor faucets, a spray attachment at the sink (allows washing hair without entering the bathtub or shower), a towel rack and small shelf for toiletry articles, and a call bell within easy reach of the patient.

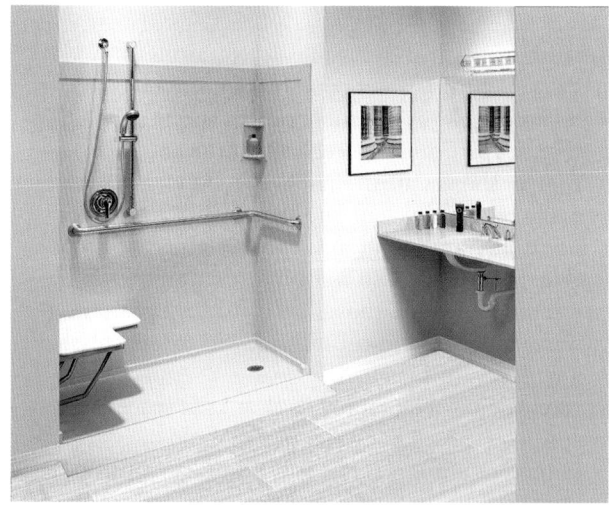

Figure 9.17 Accessible bathroom with knee clearance below sink and insulated piping. The shower entrance includes a small ramp to accommodate a difference in floor surface heights. Note that the shower hand-spray is held by a vertical slide-bar (to change height) allowing for a seated shower. Alternately, the hand-spray can be handheld to direct water flow to specific areas. *(Courtesy of Swan Surfaces, Centralia, IL 62801.)*

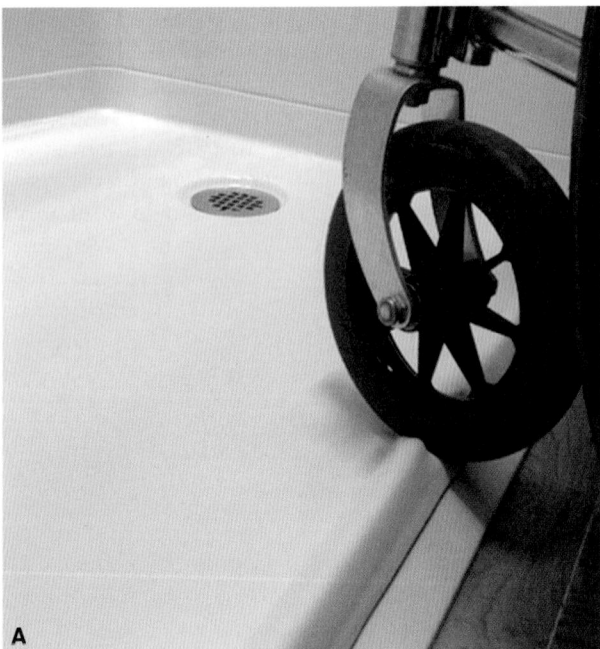
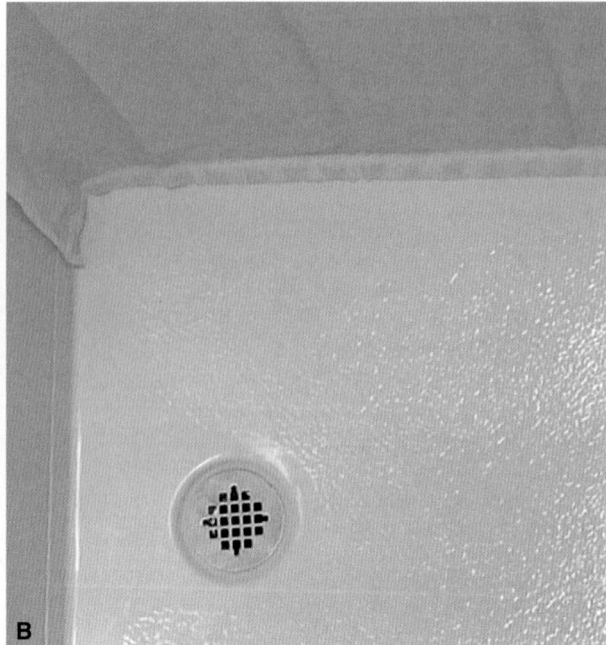

Figure 9.18 Roll-in shower water containment strategies: (A) collapsible water threshold dam placed along the edge of the shower entrance that adheres with a strong self-adhesive water-resistant tape. (B) A weighted shower curtain is designed with heavy tape weights along the bottom hem to help minimize water leakage. *(Courtesy of KR Specialties, Kingston, MA 02364.)*

Clinical Note. To prevent injury in the presence of sensory impairments, patient, family, and caregiver education should include testing water temperature before bathing.

8. With wheelchair-accessible–level (curbless) shower entries, water containment methods may be necessary. A collapsible rubber threshold dam (Fig. 9.18A) can be placed along the entrance edge of shower area. These water stoppers collapse easily by a wheelchair and then return to upright position. Shower curtains with weighted bottoms (Fig. 9.18B) can also assist in preventing water escaping from the shower stall. To help prevent water leakage from corners, shower corner splash guards can be installed.

9. Ideally, sinks should provide clear knee space below, and any exposed hot water pipes should be insulated to prevent burns (see Fig. 9.17). In new construction, shallow sinks may be installed to increase knee clearance with faucets placed on the side for easier access. Storage space lost from beneath the sink can be partially compensated for by an under-the-sink rollout cabinet that can be easily moved for wheelchair access. An enlarged mirror over the sink with the top tilted away from the wall facilitates use from a sitting position in a wheelchair (Fig. 9.19). Forward-tilting mirrors are also available with adjustable hinges for alternating placement against and away from the

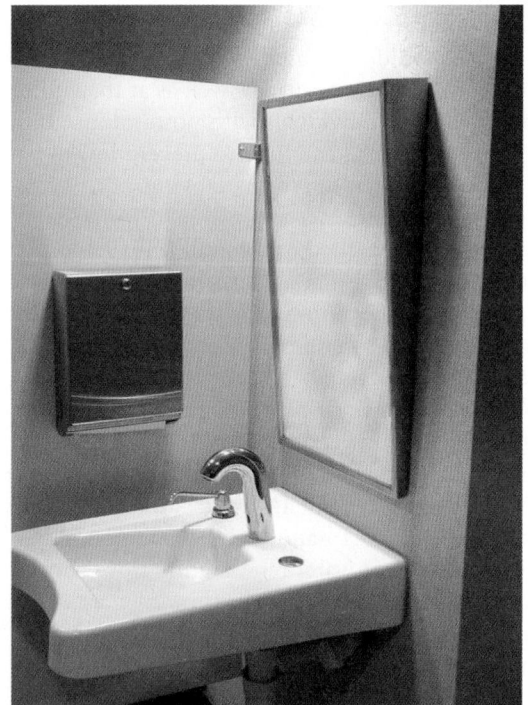

Figure 9.19 Over-sink mirror with top tilted away from wall to allow use from a seated position.

wall. Hinged-wall, gooseneck, or accordion fold-up mirrors (with one side magnified) are also helpful for close work. Figure 9.20 illustrates the minimum space requirements of a wheelchair-accessible bathroom.

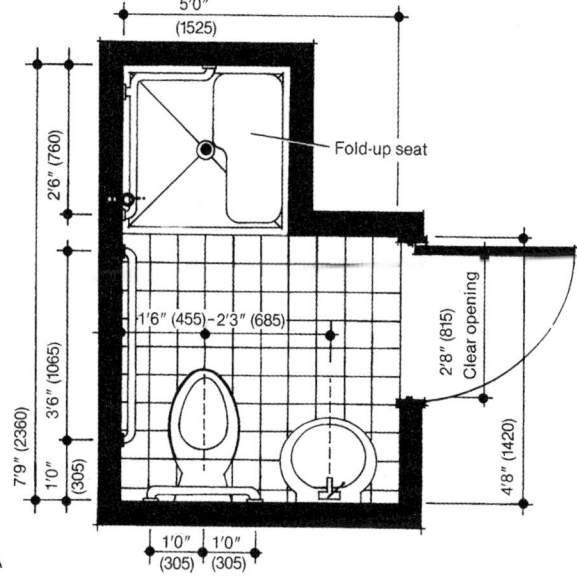

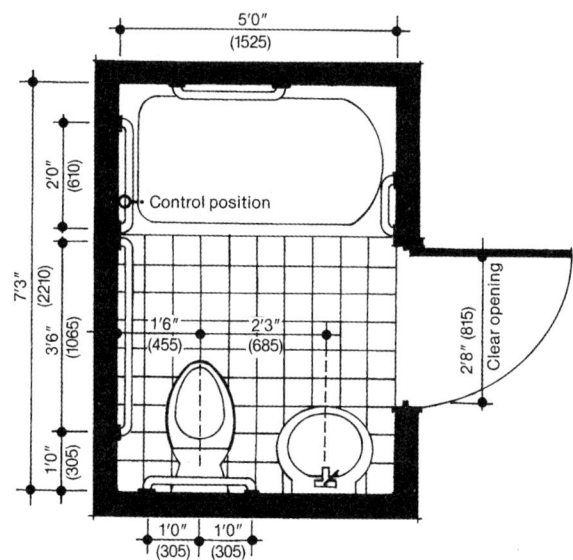

Figure 9.20 Minimum space requirements of a residential bathroom with (A) a shower stall and (B) a bathtub. The dotted line indicates lengths of wall that require reinforcement to receive grab bars or supports. *(From Nixon V, Spinal Cord Injury: A Guide to Functional Outcomes in Physical Therapy Management. Aspen Systems Corporation; 1985: 186. With permission.)*

Kitchen

1. The height of countertops (workspace) should be appropriate for the individual. When using a wheelchair, the armrests should be able to fit under the working surface. In new construction, the ideal height of counter surfaces should be no greater than 31 in. (79 cm) from the floor with a knee clearance of 27.5 to 30 in. (70 to 76 cm). Counter space should provide a depth of at least 24 in. (61 cm). All surfaces should be smooth to facilitate sliding

of heavy items from one area to another. Slide-out counter spaces are useful in providing an over-the-lap working surface (Fig. 9.21). A section of base cabinetry can be removed to provide a seated countertop workspace. For patients who are ambulatory, stools (preferably with back and footrests) may be placed strategically at the main work area(s). For patients with visual impairments, placing color tape along the border of the countertop that contrasts sharply with the color of the counter surface will help identify boundaries of the workspace. Under-the-counter cabinets with glide-out height-adjustable shelves improve access to storage areas (Fig. 9.22).

2. Improved function and safety may be provided by a sink equipped with large blade-type handles or a single-lever style faucet, scald-guard valves, or electronic sensors that allow hands-free operation by automatically turning water off and on. A spray-hose fixture allows filling heavy pots without needing to lift them from a sink. Pressure-balanced valves can be used to equalize hot and cold water; other faucets allow preprograming desired water temperature. Hot water dispensers are helpful for preparing coffee or tea and instant soups or cereals, minimizing the need for using the stove. Shallow sinks 5 to 6 in. (12 to 15 cm) deep will improve knee clearance below. Providing sink access to an individual using a wheelchair may require removal of under-the-sink cabinets. As in the bathroom, hot water pipes under the kitchen sink should be insulated to prevent burns. In new construction, motorized adjustable sinks can be mounted against a wall between two stationary cabinets with free

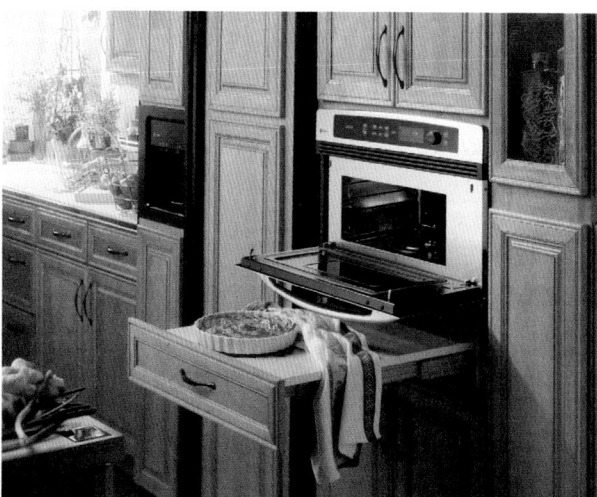

Figure 9.21 Slide-out counter spaces provide over-the-lap working surfaces. Positioned here below a built-in wall oven, the pullout surface allows for ease of transfer of hot dishes. *(Courtesy of General Electric, Appliance Park, Louisville, KY, 40225.)*

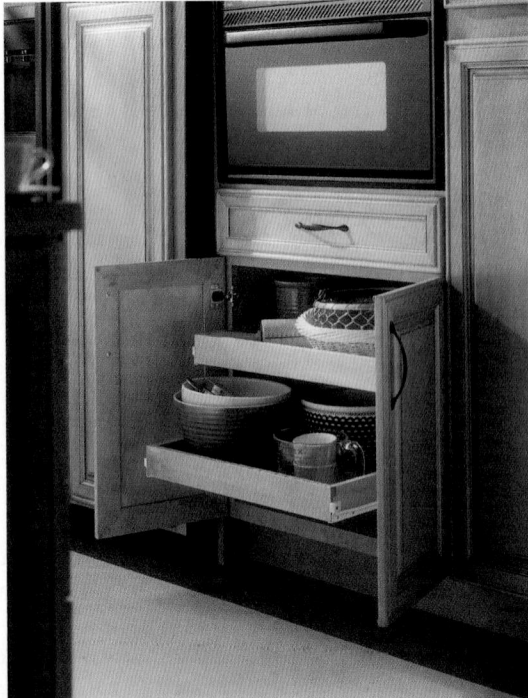

Figure 9.22 Glide-out under-cabinet shelves improve ability to see and access stored items. *(Courtesy of General Electric, Appliance Park, Louisville, KY, 40225.)*

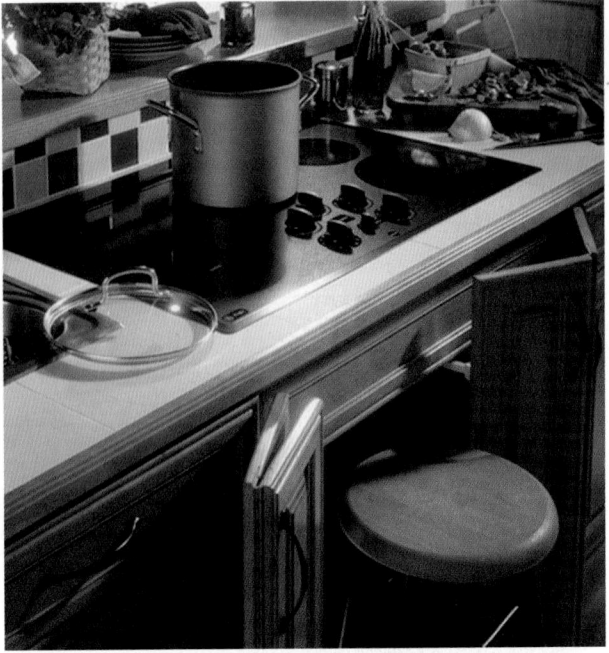

Figure 9.23 Cooktop with front-mounted controls and smooth surface that allows sliding (rather than lifting) from burner to heat-resistant countertop. Knee clearance beneath is accessed by folding doors. *(Courtesy of General Electric, Appliance Park, Louisville, KY, 40225.)*

space beneath. By activating the control switch, the sink height can be adjusted for the individual user whether seated in a wheelchair or standing.

3. A small cart with casters may be helpful to improve ease of moving articles from refrigerator to counter or table.

4. The height of tables also should be checked, and the tables may have to be raised or lowered.

5. Equipment and food storage areas should be selected with optimum energy conservation in mind. All frequently used articles should be within easy reach, and unnecessary items should be eliminated. Additional storage space may be achieved by installation of open shelving or use of pegboards for pots and pans. If shelving is added above the countertop, adjustable shelves are preferable, allowing optimal height placement for the individual patient.

6. Electric stoves are generally preferable to open-flame gas burners. For optimum safety, controls should be located on the front or side border of the stove to eliminate the need for reaching across the burners. Burners that are placed beside each other provide a safer arrangement than those placed one behind the other. A heat-resistant burn-proof counter surface adjacent to the burners will facilitate movement of hot items once cooking is completed. Smooth, ceramic cooktop surfaces also reduce the amount of lifting required while cooking (Fig. 9.23). If cooktops provide knee clearance beneath, exposed or potential contact surfaces must be insulated.

Induction (electromagnetic) stoves are also available that heat food without flames or heating elements.

7. For patients with visual impairments, large-print label-making devices and large-print stencil overlays can be used to enlarge appliance control indicators and dials (e.g., on/off or temperature indicators on thermostats, microwaves, stoves, and ovens). Timers, wall clocks, and telephones with large-print numbers are also available.

8. Wall-mounted ovens (separate from the stove) should be placed 30 to 34 in. (76 to 102 cm) from the floor with a side-opening door. These cooking units are generally more easily accessible than a single, low-level combined oven and burner unit. Oven units should be self-cleaning.

9. For many individuals, a countertop microwave oven is essential for food preparation.

10. Dishwashers should be elevated 9 in. (23 cm) and be front-loading, with pullout shelves and front-mounted controls (Fig. 9.24). Elevated (9 in. [23 cm]) side-by-side clothes washers and dryers should also be front-loading with front-mounted controls (Fig. 9.25).

11. Access to the refrigerator will be enhanced by use of a side-by-side (refrigerator–freezer) model.

12. One or more easily accessible, portable fire extinguishers should be available. It is generally recommended that fire extinguishers be mounted in open view near an exit and away from cooking appliances.

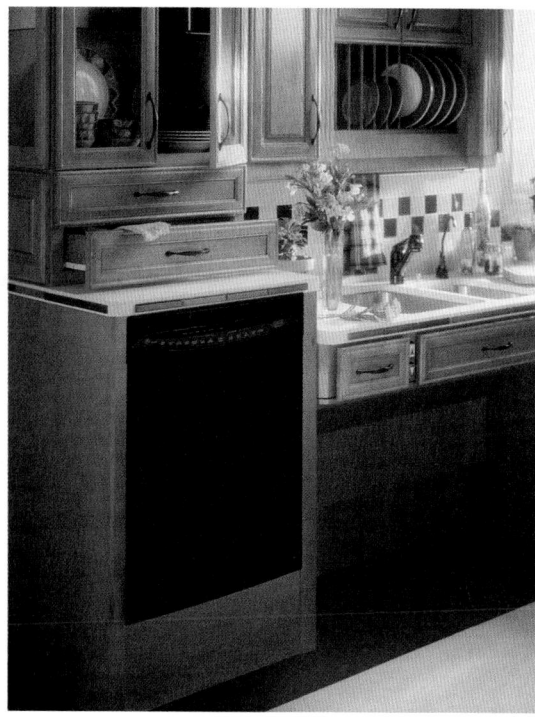

Figure 9.24 Front-loading dishwasher elevated 9 in. (23 cm) with front-mounted controls. *(Courtesy of General Electric, Appliance Park, Louisville, KY, 40225.)*

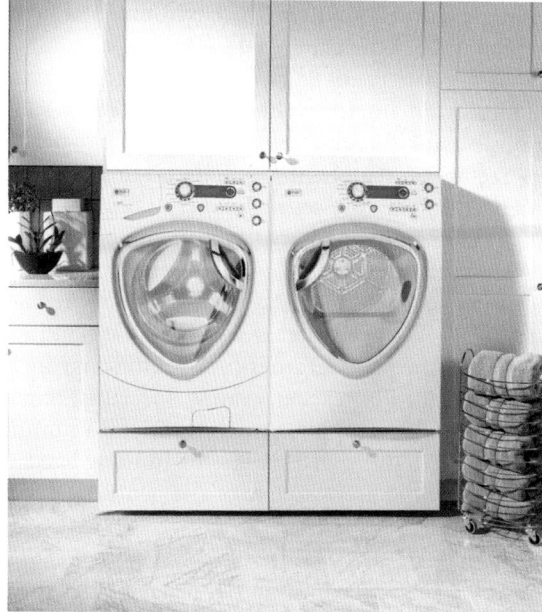

Figure 9.25 Front-loading clothes washer and dryer elevated 9 in. (23 cm) with front-mounted controls. *(Courtesy of General Electric, Appliance Park, Louisville, KY, 40225.)*

Clinical Note. For some older adults, specific areas of the home have been found to present greater hazards than others.[70] In the older adult population, over 50% of all falls occur inside the home.[70] The bathroom, kitchen, and bedroom have been identified as areas of increased fall risk.[71] Unmodified bathrooms with a high tub, the absence of grab bars, a low toilet, and potentially slippery floor conditions are environmental issues that create a high risk for falls. The dynamic nature of kitchen activities and movements performed (e.g., reaching, bending/stopping, stepping forward/backward) may result in awkward body mechanics and unsteady postures increasing the risk for falls. Fall risk reduction is an important component of examination and modification of the environment.

■ ADAPTIVE EQUIPMENT

Recommendations for *adaptive equipment* and training in their use is an area of expertise of the occupational therapist. A large variety of adaptive equipment is commercially available to increase independence, speed, skill, and efficiency in performing ADLs. Adaptive equipment is available to assist performance in such areas as bathing, personal care, dressing, meal preparation, and general household tasks (e.g., built-up handles on eating utensils and personal care items, suction devices to stabilize bowls and dishes, long-handled

reacher, sponge, duster, dustpan and brush, rocker knife, adapted cutting board). Use of adaptive equipment is typically considered a component of a *compensatory training approach* that focuses on achieving the highest level of function possible by using remaining abilities. This approach involves considering alternative ways to accomplish a task, use of intact segments to compensate for those lost, use of energy conservation and joint preservation techniques, and adapting the environment to optimize performance.

■ ASSISTIVE TECHNOLOGY

In the Assistive Technology Act of 2004, an *assistive technology device* is defined as "any item, piece of equipment, or product system, whether acquired commercially, modified, or customized, that is used to increase, maintain, or improve functional capabilities of individuals with disabilities."[72] Assistive technologies can be simple mechanical or mobility devices, but the term usually denotes some type of electronic, computer (e.g., hardware, software, peripherals), tablet application, or microprocessor-based (e.g., prosthetic knee control) device.

Assistive technologies (ATs) enable individuals with disabilities to perform daily activities by compensating for lost or impaired function. They promote greater independence and typically improve quality of life by assisting in such areas as communication, education, environmental accessibility, and work or recreational activities. Three important considerations in determining the need for ATs are (1) the individual's available function, (2) the nature of the tasks or activities that will be performed, and (3) the environmental context in which it will be used.

A large variety of ATs are commercially available. Ideally, an interdisciplinary rehabilitation team is responsible for examination, evaluation, and prescription recommendation for specific items. Although influenced by the care setting and type of AT required, participating individuals typically include the patient and family, physical and occupational therapists, a speech-language pathologist, and an *assistive technology professional* (ATP; see later discussion). Depending on the needs of the patient, other contributors may include a special education teacher, seating specialist, rehabilitation technology supplier, augmentative communication specialist, and social worker or funding specialist. Box 9.2 provides an overview of the general categories of AT.

An ATP or *rehabilitation technology specialist* is responsible for analyzing the AT needs of the patient. Through the systematic application of technology and engineering principles, this individual addresses the patient's needs in multiple contexts, including, but not limited to, education, employment, independent living, transportation, and recreation/leisure activities. The ATP recommends and guides selection of appropriate AT and educates the patient, family, and caregivers in use of the technology. The ATP or rehabilitation technology specialist may hold a degree in areas such as AT engineering, AT and human services, physical or occupational therapy, engineering, human factors and ergonomics, or another related field. In addition, they typically hold a certificate in AT. Many such certification programs have developed across the country. An example of such a certification program is the Rehabilitation Engineering and Assistive Technology Society of North America's ATP certification program.

Environmental control units (ECUs) are an important example of how ATs can enhance function and improve independence. ECUs are electronic interfaces that allow the user to control a variety of appliances and devices (e.g., telephones, bed controls, various components of an entertainment unit, room temperature and lighting, open and close curtains, open doors). These devices combine operation of all appliances into a central control panel, providing increased independence for individuals with severe disability.

The three main components of an ECU are (1) the input device, (2) the control unit, and (3) the appliance. The *input device* controls the ECU using whatever voluntary movement the individual has available (e.g., joystick, control panel, keypad, keyboard [ECU computer software programs are available], a series of switches, touch pads and screens, light pen, optical pointers, brain implants [e.g., patients with high-level spinal cord injuries] and voice, mouth-stick, and eye control). The *control unit* is the central processor that translates the input signal to an output signal to regulate the target

appliance. The *appliance* can be virtually any device that can be controlled electronically.

■ EXAMINATION OF THE WORKPLACE

An investigation of the workplace is an important component of a comprehensive examination of the environment. It is used to explore the *worker–job–environment relationship* and to determine the feasibility of returning to a former job or if reasonable accommodations will provide the needed support to resume work. The tests and measures used by physical therapists to examine work life address patient capabilities in three key areas: the ability to (1) return to work activities with or without AT, (2) obtain access to the work environment, and (3) safely perform required work activities.[18] Table 9.4 presents the tests and measures used by physical therapists to examine the patient's work life together with the tools for data-gathering and the data used in documentation.

Job Requirements

Determining the patient's ability to safely return to previous employment requires detailed information about the functional requirements of the job. If available, this information can be obtained from an existing job analysis developed by the employer when the position was first created. If a job analysis for the patient's position is not available, one will need to be created. A job analysis is a detailed description that identifies and describes the specific requirements of a job. It typically includes (1) the essential functions (fundamental duties) of a job and relative time spent on each; (2) the physical environment in which the essential functions are performed (e.g., indoors, outdoors, temperature fluctuations, noise levels); (3) the physical requirements (e.g., lifting, push/pull activities, bending, reaching); (4) the skills needed (cognitive processes, language, writing, or computer skills); and (5) the social context of the job (level of supervision, independent, contact with the public). Together with knowledge of the patient's functional capabilities, the job analysis provides an important basis for determining ability to return to work and for making recommendations for reasonable accommodations.

If a job analysis is not already available, the data can be gathered using a structured interview with the employer and patient. The interview should be designed to gather information about job requirements and tasks performed while on duty (e.g., duration of performance; weight and distance of items lifted, carried, or pulled; body positions used; repetitive exertions required on a regular basis), as well as the characteristics of the physical space in which the individual is required to work. Interview questions are developed based on the type of employment (e.g., assembly work, food service tasks, clerical work, motor vehicle operation, manual material handling, factory work).

Box 9.2 Categories of Assistive Technology

Aids for Daily Living

Aids or devices that enhance performance of activities of daily living and level of independence in such activities as eating, meal preparation, dressing, personal hygiene, bathing, or household management.
Examples: Grab bars, ramps, stairlifts, lowered counters, bathtub seats, adapted doorknobs, eating utensils, personal hygiene items, nonslip surface to stabilize dishes or other objects, and alternative doorbells.

Augmentative and Alternative Communication

Devices used to enhance personal expressive and receptive communication.
Examples: Communication enhancement devices (electronic), book holders, communication boards, eye-gaze boards, electric page turners, head wands, mouth sticks, light pointers, reading machines, personal voice amplification, signal systems, and telephone adaptations.

Computer Applications

Hardware, software, and devices to enhance computer access.
Examples: Modified, chording, expanded or alternate keyboards; voice recognition software; alternate workstations (electrically powered height and tilt adjustments); Braille translation software (conversion from print and Braille); Braille printers; access aids (head-control sticks, light pointers, eye gaze input); alternative switches (minimal pressure, voice activated) and cursor (mouse) control; voice synthesizers, large-print software that allows user to alter background and text colors (e.g., electronic books, magazines, and newspapers); magnification screens, touch screens, onscreen keyboard, screen reader; keyguards, forearm supports; text-to-speech software; speech-to-text software; optical character recognition system that scans written text to a computer and is read by a speech synthesis/screen review system; and robotic wheelchair mounting to support a laptop computer.

Environmental Control Units

Electronic systems that enhance ability to control various devices.
Examples: Electronic control of appliances, lights, doors, and security systems in the home.

Hearing Technology

Devices designed to enhance receptive communication (assistive listening devices).
Examples: Closed captioning, FM amplification systems (isolate and amplify a sound source), hearing aids, infrared amplification systems, personal amplification systems, TDDs/TTYs, television amplifiers, telephone adaptations, and visual and tactile alerting systems.

Mobility Technology

Devices designed to provide an alternative means for walking or moving within the environment.
Examples: Manual or powered wheelchairs; powered scooters; vehicle modification (driving adaptations, hand controls, wheelchair lifts); stairlifts; bus lifts; kneeling buses; and ambulatory assistive devices.

Seating and Positioning

Wheelchair (or other seating system) interventions to improve postural alignment, stability, and head control and reduce skin pressure.
Examples: Custom-fitted wheelchair (reclining back, elevating leg rests), tilt-in-space wheelchair, custom-molded seating surface, pressure-relieving seat cushions, head and neck supports, lateral thigh supports, medial knee/thigh support, lumbar supports, lateral trunk supports, and pelvic and foot supports.

Vision Technology

Devices designed to enhance interaction with the environment for individuals with visual impairments.
Examples: Talking devices (clocks, watches, calculators, thermometers, scales, handheld spell checkers, dictionaries, and thesauruses), magnifiers, speech output devices, large-print screens, mini pocket tape recorders, voice-activated daily planners, large-button phone, large-print books, magazines, and newspapers, audio books, and books on disc (can be loaded onto a computer and read to user with a voice synthesizer).

Table 9.4	Work Life: Examples of Tests and Measures, Data-Gathering Tools, and Data Used in Documentation

Work life integration or reintegration is the process of assuming or resuming activities and roles in work settings. It requires abilities such as negotiating environmental terrain, gaining access to appropriate work settings, and participating in essential activities for work.

The physical therapist uses tests and measures to make judgments as to whether an individual is prepared to assume or resume work-related roles, including ADL and IADL, or to assess the need for assistive technology or environmental adaptations.

Tests and Measures	Data-Gathering Tools	Documentation
Ability to assume or resume work-related activities with or without assistive technology (e.g., developmental capacity tests, activity profiles, disability indexes, functional status questionnaires, IADL scales, observations, physical capacity tests) Ability to gain access to work environments (e.g., needs assessment, barrier identification, interviews, observations, physical capacity tests, transportation assessments) Safety in performing work-related activities (e.g., ergonomic assessments, diaries, falls risk assessments, interviews, logs, observations, videographic assessments)	Cameras and photographs Equipment needed to perform developmental and physical capacity test Video cameras and video recordings	Ability to participate in a variety of work environments Clinical rationale to justify need and appropriate assistive technology Developmental level of motor ability Functional capacity for work Level of safety in work-related activities Physiological responses to work-related activities Results of ergonomic assessment

From *Guide to Physical Therapist Practice*,[18] with permission. APTA is not responsible for the translation from English.

ADL = activities of daily living; IADL = instrumental activities of daily living.

Functional Capacity Evaluation

Typically, the most effective means of examining the worker–job–environment interface is an on-site visit. However, a variety of standardized functional capacity evaluation (FCE) instruments are commercially available that can be used to gather preliminary data before an on-site visit. FCEs are a series of performance-based tests designed to determine current physical capacity to perform work-related activities. FCEs are used to inform work ability recommendations for people with work-related or other disabilities.[73] Depending on the job task requirements, the FCE may be all that is needed to determine ability to return to a previous job or to assume alternative job placement. The FCE provides a series of objective tests and measures designed to identify both work-related capabilities and activity limitations. Measurement parameters typically include endurance, ROM, flexibility, strength, force generation, posture, coordination, manual dexterity, and consistency of performance.[73–77]

The FCE is used to measure performance in specific components of work-related tasks. The specificity of the job will dictate the functional movements required. FCE instrument capabilities are then selected based on these requirements in order to examine the specific group of skills that comprise the employment tasks (e.g., lifting, stooping, trunk rotation, reaching). Computer-integrated FCE systems (Fig. 9.26) allow replication of physical task demands required of an individual's work environment using either standardized testing protocols or customized physical tests. A variety of tasks can be simulated, including, but not limited to, lifting, pushing, pulling, carrying capacity, turning a valve, and using a variety of tools (e.g., swinging a hammer, using a paint roller, using a manual saw). The systems may also be used for strengthening and retraining using task-specific strategies that simulate requirements of the client's real environment.

Software programs allow comparison of FCE data with normative values such as strength and ROM. Data from the FCE assist the physical therapist with the following tasks:

- Predicting the individual's work capacity and ability to safely return to work
- Identifying parameters of the physical environment needed to optimize function and prevent further injury (reasonable accommodations)
- Identifying extent of activity limitations
- Matching abilities to appropriate job placement

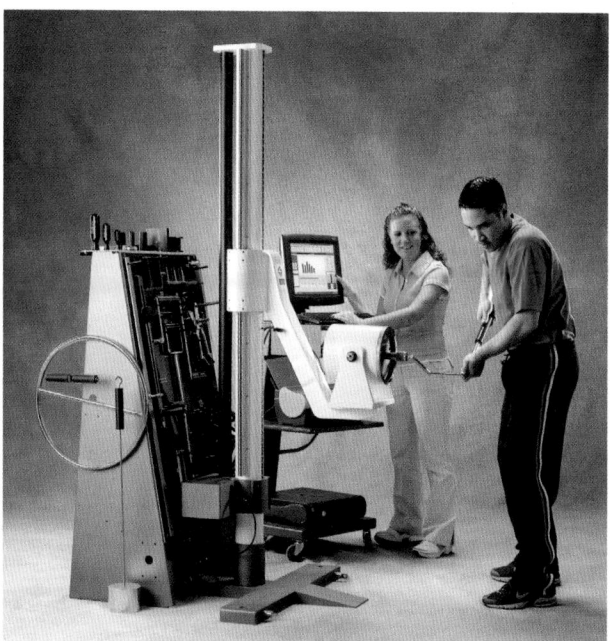

Figure 9.26 Simulator II Functional Capacity Evaluation System. *(Courtesy of BTE Technologies, Inc., Hanover, MD 21076.)*

An additional resource is the *Occupational Information Network* (O*NET) available from the U.S. Department of Labor.[78] It provides a database of occupational job requirements (e.g., required skills and knowledge, how and where the work is performed) and worker attributes. The O*NET system includes the O*NET database (files available as free downloads for application development), O*NET OnLine (access to O*NET information), and the O*NET Career Exploration Tools (career investigation and assessment tools).

On-Site Visit

The on-site visit to the workplace typically includes (1) analysis of the physical space, (2) observation of the patient/client performing work tasks within the environment in which they must be accomplished, (3) identification of safety issues, and (4) determination of the immediate or predicted risks of musculoskeletal injury for an individual worker. Data gathered during the on-site visit, information from the job analysis, and knowledge of functional abilities allow the therapist to determine if job requirements can be met and whether the patient can safely return to their previous employment. If return to work is feasible with modifications, these data also inform the therapist about establishing a *plan for risk reduction* with recommendations to eliminate the potential for injury, and to develop a *plan to optimize function* that includes suggestions for better fitting the job to the individual's anatomical and physiological characteristics in a way that enhances efficiency and performance. The principles of energy conservation, ergonomics, applied biomechanics, and anthropometrics provide the foundation for both prevention of injury and maximizing efficiency.

Many of the areas examined, recommendations made, and adaptive strategies employed in the home may be used in the work environment as well. Several considerations specific to the work setting are described in the following sections.

External Accessibility

A parking space should be available within a short distance of the building if the individual plans to drive to and from work. For wheelchair users, parking spaces should be a minimum of 96 in. (244 cm) wide, with an adjacent access aisle 60 in. (152 cm) wide. The location should be clearly marked as a reserved parking area. ADA-compliant curb cuts should be present between the parking lot and the sidewalk. In addition, the sidewalk leading to the building entrance should be a minimum of 36 in. (91 cm) wide with a maximum cross-slope ratio of 1:48.[10] Additional aspects of external accessibility of the building should be addressed using the same guidelines as those presented for home exteriors.

Internal Accessibility

The immediate work area should be carefully examined. This includes lighting; temperature; seating surface (if other than a wheelchair); the height and size of the workstation (some patients may benefit from a variable height or tilting work surface); and exposure to noise, vibration, or fumes. Access to supplies, materials, or equipment should be considered with respect to the patient's vertical and horizontal reaching capabilities. Access to drinking fountains, dining areas, and bathrooms should also be addressed.

Given the prevalence of computer workstations in many employment settings, recommendations may likely be required to optimize efficiency and reduce the potential for trauma or repetitive stress injury from poorly designed work areas. A fully adjustable chair is an integral component of an ergonomic workstation.[79] The foundational requirements for workstation chairs are depicted in Figure 9.27. Although parameters vary for each individual, the general principles for positioning at a computer workstation include screen slightly below eye level, body centered directly in front of monitor and keyboard, forearms level or tilted slightly upward, wrists free while typing, lower back well supported, thighs horizontal on seating surface, and feet resting flat on the floor (Fig. 9.28).[79,80] Height-adjustable desks and workstations are an important consideration for the prevention of health risks associated with maintaining prolonged static postures as they allow an individual to alternate between sitting and standing throughout the workday. In settings where multiple workers use the same workstation or desk, height-adjustable options

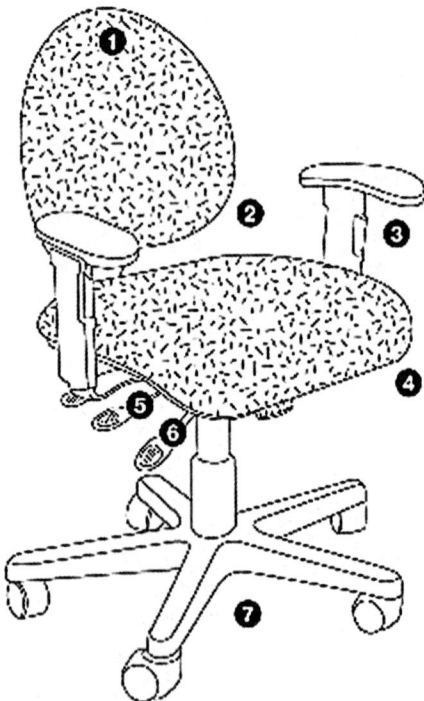

Figure 9.27 Overview of recommended features of workstation chair: (1) breathable, medium-texture upholstery; (2) adjustable lumbar support that moves up/down; (3) adjustable armrests; (4) seat with rounded front border (waterfall design); (5) adjustable seat that moves up and down and tilts forward and backward; (6) a tilt mechanism that tilts forward and backward; and (7) a five-caster base with a full 360° swivel. *(From Workplace Ergonomics Reference Guide, p. 4.)*[80]

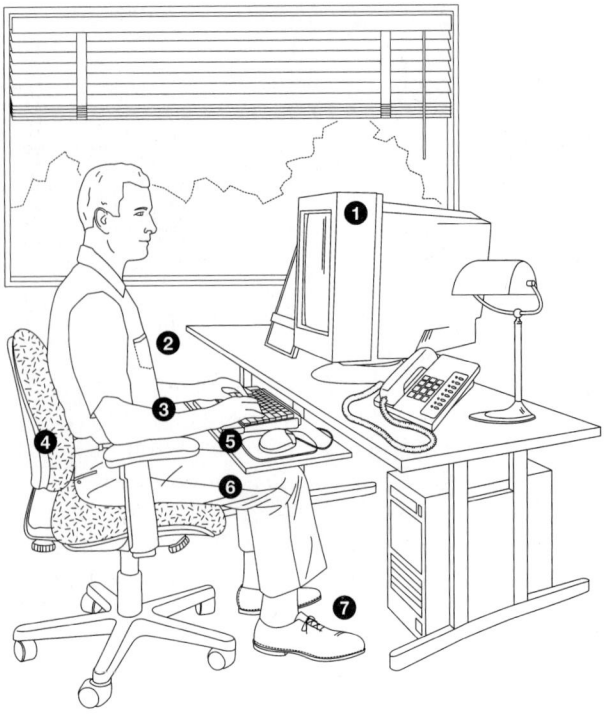

Figure 9.28 Overview of positioning recommendations for computer workstations: (1) monitor screen top slightly below eye level; (2) body centered in front of the monitor and keyboard; (3) forearms level or tilted-up slightly; (4) lower back supported by chair; (5) wrists free while typing; (6) thighs horizontal; and (7) feet resting flat on the floor. *(From Workplace Ergonomics Reference Guide, p. 6.)*[80]

allow each employee to make modifications based on their individual needs.

During examination of workstations for individuals using a wheelchair, functional sitting reach is an important consideration. From an upright wheelchair sitting position, the unobstructed high forward reach is a maximum of 48 in. (1,220 mm) from the floor, and the low forward reach is a minimum of 15 in. (380 mm) from the floor (Fig. 9.29A). When the high forward reach is over a work surface of not greater than 20 in. (510 mm), the maximum reach distance is 48 in. (1,220 mm) from the floor (Fig. 9.29B). Progressively deeper work surfaces will alter the forward reach accordingly. For example, a work surface depth between 20 and 25 in. allows a maximum forward reach of not greater than 44 in. (1,120 mm) (Fig. 9.29C). With a floor obstruction of 10 in. (255 mm), the high side reach is a maximum of 48 in. (1,220 mm) and the low side reach is 15 in. (380 mm) minimum (Fig. 9.29D). With an obstruction of a maximum of 24 in. (610 mm), the high side reach is a maximum of 46 in. (1,170 mm).[10] For individuals with good trunk control, reaching capacity will be increased.

Detailed resources are available to guide examination of the workplace. These include the *ADA Regulations and Technical Assistance Materials*,[81] the *ADA Accessibility Guidelines* (ADAAG),[82] and the *2010 ADA Standard for Accessible Design*.[9] These documents are freely available and include the technical requirements for accessibility to buildings and facilities by individuals with disabilities under the ADA of 1990. A comprehensive source of information about the ADA is provided at the U.S. Department of Justice's ADA home page.[83]

■ COMMUNITY ACCESS

To attain the goal of full accessibility, community resources, services, and facilities must be investigated. When direct involvement by the therapist is not possible, this may best be accomplished by providing the patient and family with guidelines for exploring access to local facilities.

An important consideration is to refer the patient and family to community organizations such as the Arthritis Foundation, National Easter Seal Society, Multiple Sclerosis Society, mayor's office, chamber of commerce, or Veterans Administration. These groups can provide information on services available to individuals with a disability who reside in the community. Individuals returning to school should be encouraged to contact the campus Office of Disability Resources or the Center for

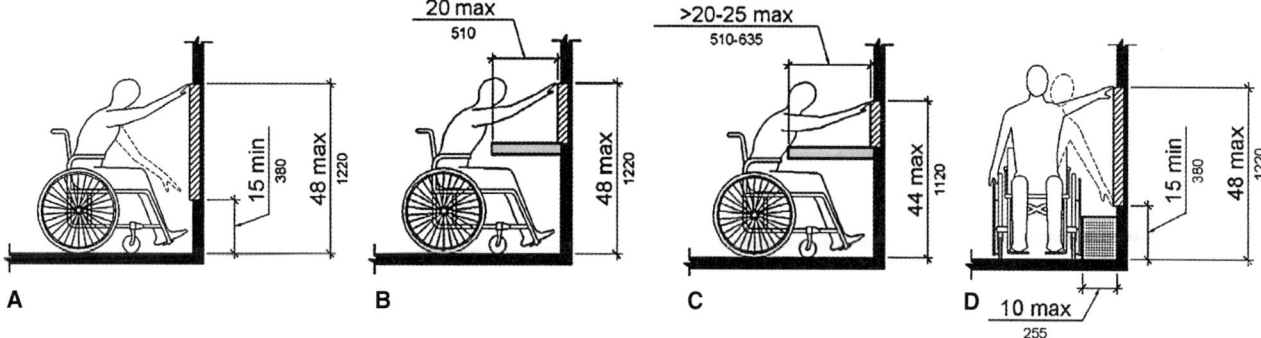

Figure 9.29 (A) Unobstructed high forward reach is a maximum of 48 in. (1,220 mm) from the floor, and the low forward reach is a minimum of 15 in. (380 mm) from the floor. (B) High forward reach over a 20-in.-deep (510-mm-deep) work surface is a maximum of 48 in. (1,220 mm) from the floor. (C) A work surface depth of 20 to 25 in. (510 to 635 mm) allows a maximum forward reach of not greater than 44 in. (1,120 mm) from the floor. (D) For a reach depth of 10 in. (255 mm), the high side reach is a maximum of 48 in. (1,220 mm). With a floor obstruction of 10 in. (225 mm), the high side reach is a maximum of 48 in. (1,220 mm) and a low reach of 15 in. (380 mm) minimum. Values denoted in inches and millimeters. *(From 2010 ADA Standards for Accessible Design, pp. 114–115.)*[9]

Student Accessibility (names vary by campus), which function to ensure appropriate and reasonable accommodations are available to facilitate an optimal learning environment for students with disabilities. Information is typically available on accessible housing and transportation, and general campus resources.

Transportation

The availability of accessible public transportation varies considerably among geographical areas. As such, careful exploration by the patient and family will be needed to determine what resources are obtainable in specific locales. Many communities provide at least part-time service of partially or completely accessible buses. These include the so-called kneeling buses equipped with a hydraulic unit that lowers the entrance to curb level for easier boarding and those designed with hydraulic lifts at the center of the bus to allow direct entry by an individual using a wheelchair (Fig. 9.30). Other design features include flip-out ramps combined with a kneeling feature for wheelchair access positioned at the side (Fig. 9.31) entrance to the bus and internal space allocation to safely position a wheelchair (Fig. 9.32).

Not all public transportation systems in the United States allow use by individuals who are nonambulatory or by those with limited ambulatory capacity. However, many urban transit systems are gradually making accommodations for individuals with mobility impairments (e.g., installation of elevators, alternatives to turnstile entrances, identified space for wheelchair riders). In many areas where public transportation is unavailable, door-to-door accessible van transportation is provided to residents with disabilities. Again, availability of such services may be limited in some rural locations.

Some patients will want to master driving an adapted automobile or van. This, of course, will significantly

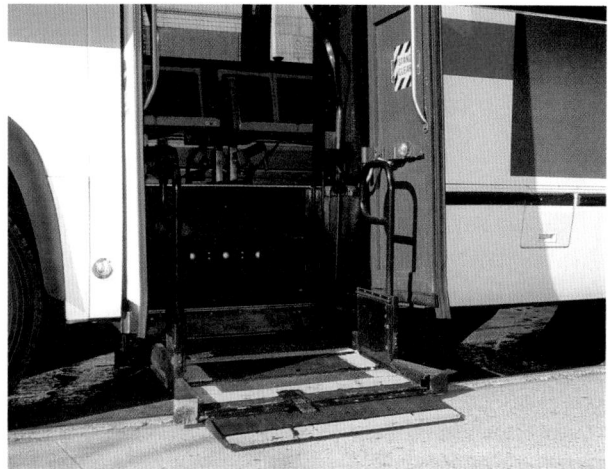

Figure 9.30 Bus lifts with extending ramps are able to accommodate wheelchairs and motorized scooters. The international wheelchair symbol for accessibility is often displayed on the doors of the bus.

improve opportunities for community travel. Motor vehicle adaptations are selected based on the physical capabilities of the individual. Common adaptive equipment includes hand controls to operate the brakes and the accelerator; control panels mounted directly on steering wheel to control windshield wipers, turn indicators, and high/low beams; steering wheel attachments, such as knobs or universal cuffs, for individuals with limited grip strength; lifting units to assist with placement of the wheelchair into the vehicle; and, for patients with tetraplegia or high-level paraplegia, self-contained lifting platforms for entry to a van while remaining seated in a wheelchair. Driver training programs are often taught by occupational therapists and offered in most large rehabilitation centers.

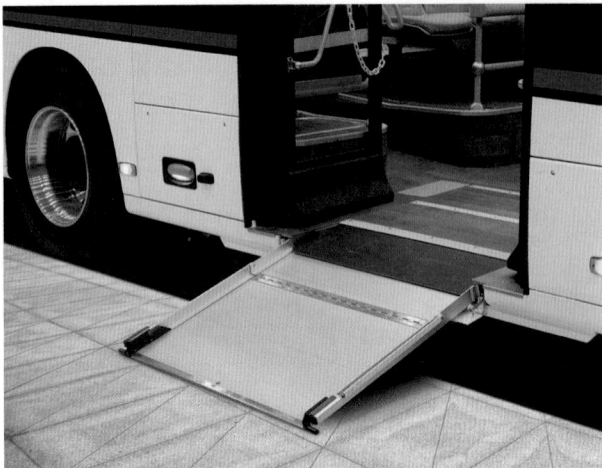

Figure 9.31 Combined boarding ramp and kneeling system allows wheelchair users to safely board bus. The kneeling system also assists general passengers to enter the bus. *(Courtesy of Hyundai Motor America, Fountain Valley, CA 92708.)*

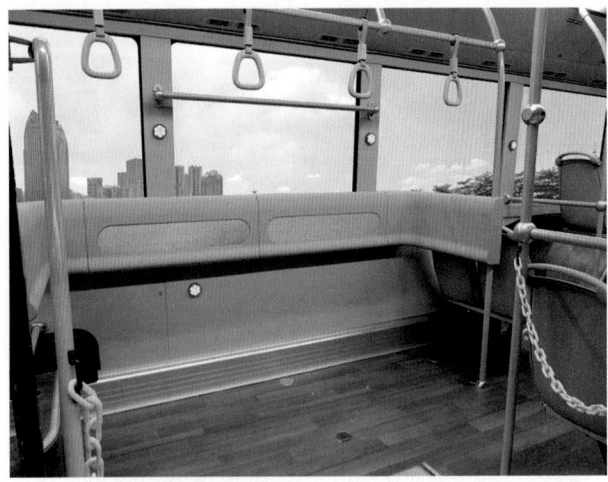

Figure 9.32 Space allocation inside bus to safely position wheelchair during transit. When not in use by a wheelchair user, the space serves as a hip rest for standing passengers. *(Courtesy of Hyundai Motor America, Fountain Valley, CA 92708.)*

For patients whose capacity for long-distance ambulation is limited and/or whose endurance is low, community-going battery-powered scooters (Fig. 9.33) may be a practical alternative for travel within a reasonable proximity of the home.

Access to Community Facilities

Area facilities used by the patient should be explored for the availability of appropriate parking areas; beveled curbs; external and internal structural accessibility of buildings; and availability of accessible drinking fountains, bathrooms, and restaurants. Theaters, auditoriums, and lecture halls must be considered with respect to accessible seating areas. Many such public presentation spaces are designed with accessible aisles leading to open floor space (sufficiently wide to accommodate two wheelchairs side by side) interspersed within rows of standard seats. This allows the individual using a wheelchair the option of either sitting next to a person who is ambulatory or someone using a wheelchair. In addition to these general considerations, stores and shopping areas should also be inspected for access to merchandise (especially for individuals using a wheelchair), appropriate aisle widths, and adequate space at checkout counters.

Some theater companies offer "touch tours" for individuals who are blind or have impaired vision, allowing them to learn about the visual elements of the production. These multisensory experiences supplement for the lack of detail provided by a live performance and are led by cast, crew, and/or management. They provide an opportunity for participants to touch and handle theater pieces while tour guides explain the significance of individual pieces.[84]

Another useful source of information on community access is the guidebook offered by many larger cities (often funded by the mayor's office or as a community service by local businesses). These guides provide information on accessibility of local cultural, civic, and religious institutions; government offices; theaters; hotels; restaurants; shopping areas; transportation; and social and recreational facilities. These publications usually can be obtained from the city's chamber of commerce, the mayor's office, or the office of tourism. Many of these guides are available online. Combined use of such guides and phoning ahead for details of accessibility will facilitate travel both within and outside the local community.

■ DOCUMENTATION

Once examination of the environment is complete, a final report is prepared that includes information from each participating team member. This report consists of information obtained from the home and, if applicable, the workplace or school setting. Information should also be included about the measures taken to explore general community accessibility. Data used in documentation are included in Tables 9.1 and 9.4.

Additional information should include (1) a description of the methods used to assist the patient in functional mobility (ambulation or wheelchair), (2) identification of the type and quantity of adaptive equipment required (including source and cost), and (3) explanation of recommended modifications with precise specifications for needed changes. AT recommendations, if utilized, should also be included. If an examination form, survey, or checklist was used during the on-site visit, it should be included with documentation or the data summarized in narrative form.

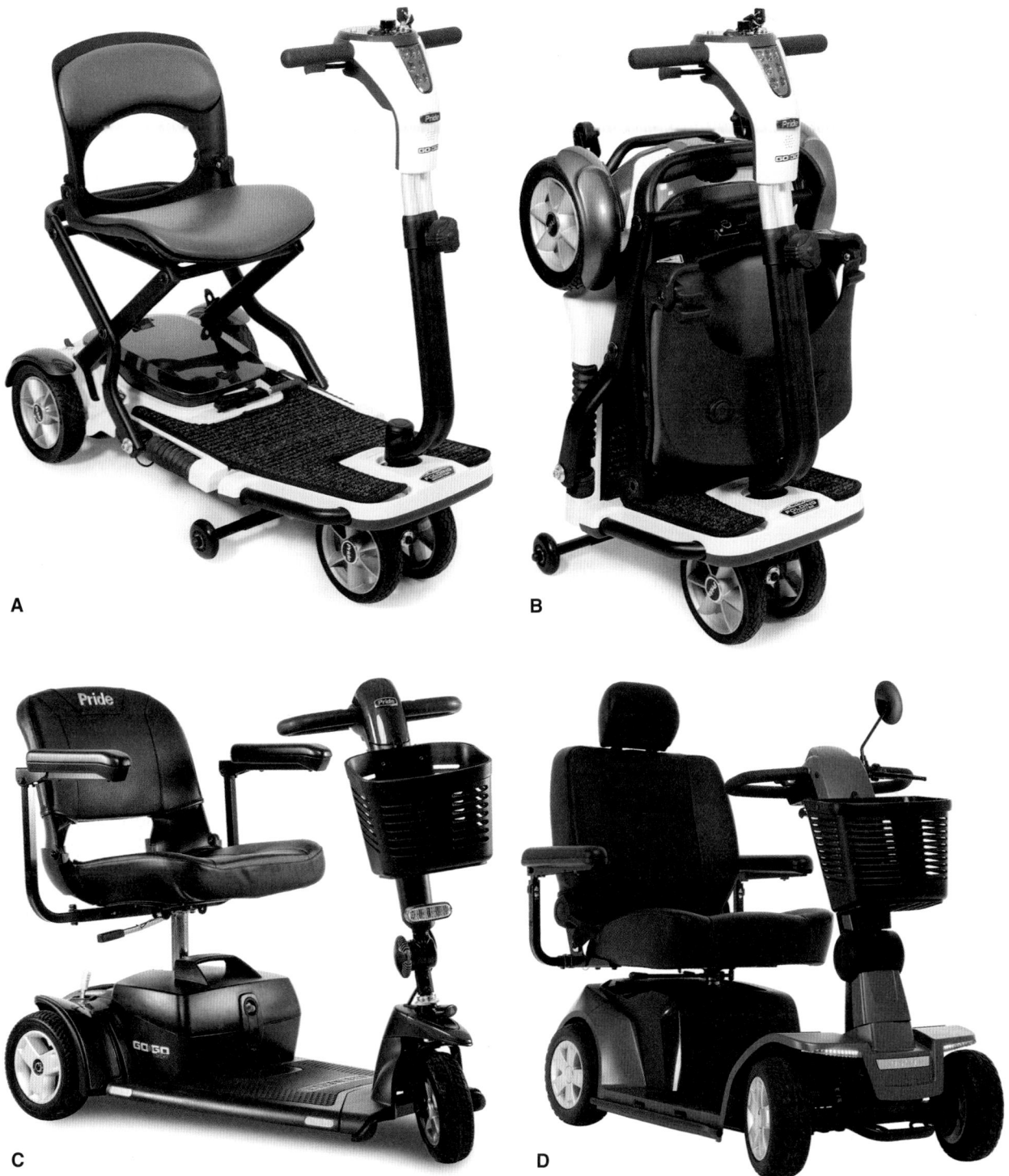

A

B

C

D

Figure 9.33 Motorized scooters are available with a variety of features and vary from lightweight folding to heavy duty designs. (A/B) This compact, lightweight four-wheel scooter is collapsible (B), a feature often important for individuals who travel, has a speed of up to 4 mph, a turning radius of 32 in. (81 cm), and a weight capacity of 250 lb (133 kg). (C) This three-wheel scooter has a maximum speed of 4.7 mph with a turning radius of 36 in. (91 cm), and a maximum weight capacity of 325 lb (147 kg). (D) This four-wheel heavy duty scooter has a maximum speed of 5.8 mph, a turning radius of 53 in. (135 cm), and a maximum weight capacity of 500 lb (227 kg). *(Courtesy of Pride Mobility, Exeter, PA 18643.)*

Documentation related to community access should include verification of the patient's knowledge of available community resources. The sources of this information, as well as whether team members were directly or indirectly involved in the community investigation, should be reported.

The completed report is then included in the patient's health record. Copies of the report are typically submitted to the patient and family, the physician, third-party payer(s) or other potential funding sources, and any community-based health-care or social service agencies that will be providing care.

■ FUNDING SOURCES

Modifications to the physical environment and acquisition of needed AT or adaptable equipment are typically very costly. With consideration to financial resources, the patient and family will need guidance to achieve optimal accessibility and function. Funding is often scarce, and securing needed financial support can be a formidable challenge. The social worker is an important source of information about state and local resources. The Internet is also a rich source of funding information and offers socially based fundraising opportunities; however, many of these online fundraising groups require a fee. Many states maintain websites that provide information on loan and grant programs as well as financing sources for accessible housing.

Other potential sources of funding include home equity or other types of bank loans, the Veterans Administration, the Division of Vocational Rehabilitation, and the Workers' Compensation Commission. Local chapters of national civic groups (e.g., Kiwanis International, Veterans of Foreign Wars, Masons/Shriners Lodges, Lions International) or diagnosis-specific organizations (e.g., Muscular Dystrophy Association, American Stroke Association, National Multiple Sclerosis Society, Parkinson's Foundation) can also be a valuable source of funding.

An important consideration is that not all patients will have current housing that is amenable to modification (e.g., an individual who previously lived in a third-floor walk-up apartment and now uses a wheelchair). In such instances, the local Housing and Urban Development Office will be an important resource. This office can provide a listing of accessible housing within the community.

Finally, creative funding for specific items (such as specialized adaptive equipment not covered by other resources) may be available through private organizations or foundations. Considerable time, research, and perseverance may be required in locating a receptive organization. General suggestions that might be considered in seeking assistance include contacting local businesses or corporate giving offices, civic or service clubs, churches or synagogues, labor unions, Jaycees, and the Knights of Columbus.

■ LEGISLATION

Much federal attention has been focused on the importance of environmental accessibility. Through legislation and a variety of private organizations, significant strides have been made in this area. In 1990, the *ADA* was signed into law. This legislation is among the most comprehensive of the civil rights laws enacted for individuals with disabilities. It guarantees civil rights protection and equal opportunity in the areas of government services, employment, public transportation, privately owned transportation available to the public, telephone service, and public accommodations.[85] This law requires that all "public places of accommodation" be made accessible to people with a disability unless it imposes "undue hardship" to the establishment. This law specifies that restaurants, movie theaters, hotels, professional offices, retail stores, and so forth make reasonable accommodations.

With respect to an individual, disability is defined in the ADA as "a physical or mental impairment that substantially limits one or more major life activities of such an individual; a record of such impairment; or being regarded as having such impairment."[85] Undue hardship includes excessive direct cost of adapting the environment, limited resources of the establishment, or situations where these changes would fundamentally alter the nature or daily operation of a business. The ADA also provides a federal tax credit incentive for measures taken by businesses to comply with this law.

The law further requires that public places allow service animals to accompany persons with disabilities within their establishments (Fig. 9.34). Service animals are defined by Title II and Title III of the ADA as "any dog that is individually trained to do work or perform tasks for the benefit of an individual with a disability, including a physical, sensory, psychiatric, intellectual, or other mental disability." Emotional support animals, comfort animals, and therapy dogs are not service

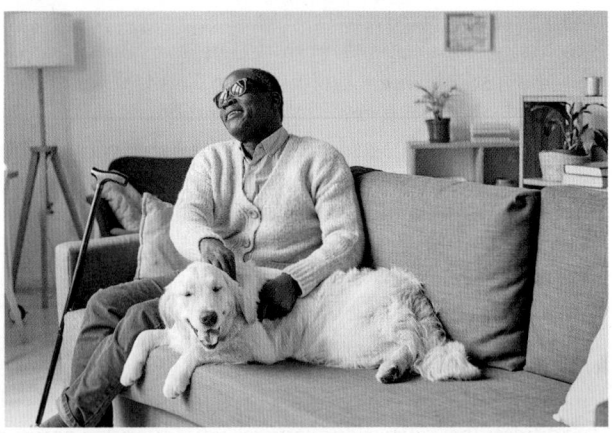

Figure 9.34 Person with impaired vision and a service dog.

animals under Title II and Title III of the ADA.[86] Some states, local governments and airlines may have broader definitions for service animals. The ADA also requires public establishments to allow the presence of miniature horses that do work or tasks for a person with disabilities. The establishment must comply if it can accommodate the horse's size and weight, if the horse is housebroken and under the owner's control, and the horse does not pose a threat with operational safety.[86]

The *Fair Housing Amendment Act of 1988* prohibits discrimination in housing on the basis of race, color, religion, gender, disability, familial status, and national origin.[87] The act includes private housing, state and local government housing, and any housing that receives federal financial support. The act requires that accessible units be included in all new multiple-dwelling buildings with four or more units. It requires landlords to allow individuals with disabilities to make reasonable, access-related modifications to their living space, as well as common areas of the building. However, the landlord is not required to pay for these modifications. To promote adherence, the Fair Housing Amendment Act also provides accessible construction standards for multifamily housing units built for first occupancy after March 1991.

The *Rehabilitation Act of 1973* provided that access must be established in all federally funded buildings and transportation facilities constructed after 1968. The law prohibits discrimination in federal employment, stipulates accessibility within federal buildings, and established the Architectural Transportation Barriers and Compliance Board. Because many federally funded institutions provided low compliance with the 1973 Rehabilitation Act, an amendment was passed in 1978. The *Comprehensive Rehabilitation Services Amendments* (P.L. 95-602) of 1978 strengthened the enforcement of the original 1973 Rehabilitation Act. The Architectural and Transportation Barriers Compliance Board is the governing body responsible for enforcing this legislation.

The *Architectural Barrier Act of 1968* (P.L. 90-480) provided that certain buildings that were financed by federal funds be designed and constructed "to insure that physically handicapped persons will have ready access to, and use of, such buildings."[88] Another important item of legislation related to environmental accessibility is the *Public Buildings Act of 1983,* which functioned to establish public building policies for the federal government. This act (Section 307) provided several amendments to the Architectural Barrier Act of 1968 to further strengthen and delineate the importance of accessibility. The term *fully accessible* in this act was defined as

> the absence or elimination of physical and communications barriers to the ingress, egress, movement within, and use of a building by handicapped persons and the incorporation of such equipment as is necessary to provide such ingress, egress, movement, and use and, in a building of historic, architectural, or cultural significance, the elimination of such barriers and the incorporation of such equipment in such a manner as to be compatible with the significant architectural features of the building to the maximum extent possible.[89]

The *Telecommunications Act of 1996* applies to all telecommunication equipment and services. It stipulates that manufacturers of "telecommunications equipment or customer premises equipment shall ensure that the equipment is designed, developed, and fabricated to be accessible to and usable by individuals with disabilities, if readily achievable."[90] The act also provides a similar accessibility directive to providers of telecommunications services.

Despite the gains made in environmental accessibility, barriers continue to exist. Inasmuch as most public transportation systems were built before 1968, accessibility is not required by law. However, the ADA indicates that all concerns that offer public transit along a fixed route must also provide buses that are accessible to individuals with disabilities, including access by wheelchairs. Other areas that continue to be problematic include revolving doors, the design of many supermarkets and shopping areas (barriers imposed by checkout areas and items displayed on high shelves), lack of available parking spaces, multiple levels of stairs at the entrance to some buildings, and the design of some theaters and auditoriums that do not have specifically designated areas for individuals using a wheelchair.

The ADA home page[83] provides an extensive listing of links to available ADA publications, as well as links to federal resources. Appendix 9.D (online) provides Web-based resources for clinicians, patients, and families.

SUMMARY

Examination of the environment is an important factor in facilitating the patient's transition to the home, work, and community. The rehabilitation team uses the data to determine the level of patient access, safety, and function within the environment. The information is also used to determine the need for ATs, environmental modifications, outpatient services, and adaptive equipment. In addition, the examination assists in preparing the patient, family, and/or work colleagues and employer for the individual's return to a given setting.

This chapter presented a sample approach to examination and modification of the environment. Common features of the physical environmental that typically warrant consideration have been highlighted. Inasmuch as a return to a former environment is often a primary goal of rehabilitation, early consideration of these issues is warranted. Collaboration among team members, the patient, family, and caregivers will ensure an optimum and highly individualized patient–environment interface.

Although increasing numbers of residential spaces and public buildings are designed to provide accessibility, this area warrants further involvement from therapists. Physical therapists are particularly effective advocates for individuals with disability. They are also well prepared to assume leadership roles in ensuring compliance with existing and new laws as well as providing valuable input to planning barrier-free environments and modification of existing structures.

Questions for Review

1. Differentiate among the terms *barriers, accessibility, accessible design,* and *UD*.

2. What are the purposes for performing an examination of the environment?

3. What types of tests and measures are used for examination of environmental factors?

4. Identify an inherent shortcoming of self-report instruments designed to gather information about functional performance within the respondent's environment. How can accuracy of reporting be improved?

5. Assume you are preparing for an on-site visit to examine a patient's home environment. What preliminary information is needed that may influence the type and extent of recommendations?

6. During a home visit, you find that a wheelchair user's bathroom door width measures 31 in. wide (77.74 cm). The patient owns the 50-year-old home and plans to remain in the dwelling. What options are available to modify the environment by increasing the bathroom door width?

7. An initial aspect of examining a patient's ability to return to previous employment involves determining the functional job requirements. Describe the information required.

8. What is an FCE? How are data from the FCE used (i.e., what decisions are informed by the data)?

CASE STUDY

An 81-year-old right-handed female was admitted to an acute care hospital status post right pontine and left caudate nucleus ischemic strokes. She reported left side sensory and motor deficits, slurred speech, weakness, and headaches persisting for several days prior to admission. She denied any history of falls or other trauma. On admission to the emergency room, it was determined that she was not a candidate for tissue plasminogen activator (tPA) due to her current anticoagulation status and time of symptom onset (greater than 4.5 hr). Following a week in the acute care setting she was deemed medically stable and transferred to an inpatient rehabilitation facility. Her past medical history includes a previous myocardial infarction, breast cancer, left total knee replacement, chronic kidney disease, type 2 diabetes mellitus with peripheral neuropathy, deep vein thrombosis, and essential hypertension.

SOCIAL HISTORY

The patient is a retired accountant. She currently serves as a volunteer treasurer for her local gardening society. Her husband is deceased. She has four grown children who all live in neighboring communities. Prior to the current hospital admission, she was independent with all ADLs and IADLs. She was driving prior to admission, was a regular participant in family gatherings, and she enjoyed gardening both at home and at the community garden. The patient has medical insurance coverage and is without financial concerns.

REVIEW OF SYSTEMS

COGNITIVE FUNCTION: Oriented to person, place, and time. The patient scored 21 (maximum score = 30) on the Montreal Cognitive Assessment.

COMMUNICATION: Dysarthria present.

CASE STUDY—cont'd

VISION: Wears corrective lenses full time, visual tracking within normal limits. She reports experiencing night blindness that she describes as seeing poorly in dim light.

HEARING: Age-related decline, intact.

Range of Motion (passive)

Upper Extremities
- Left: Within functional limits (WFL) throughout
- Right: WFL throughout

Lower Extremities
- Left: WFL throughout
- Right: WFL throughout

Strength

Upper Extremities
- Left (gross measures): shoulder 2/5, elbow 2/5, forearm/wrist 1/5, digits/grasp 1/5
- Right: 4/5 throughout

Lower Extremities
- Left (gross measures): hip flexion 2/5, knee flexion 2/5, knee extension 2/5, ankle dorsiflexion 2/5, ankle plantarflexion 2/5
- Right: 4/5 throughout

Tone: Diminished (moderate) in the left upper and lower extremities throughout.

Coordination: Impaired motor coordination of the left upper and lower extremities when compared to the right side; rated as severely impaired during finger-to-nose test, finger/thumb opposition test, foot tapping test, and heel to shin test.

Balance:
- Static sitting balance: Good, able to maintain sitting posture with noted posterior pelvic tilt and slight left lateral lean.
- Dynamic sitting balance: Good, able to maintain sitting posture during anticipatory and reactive postural control tests (e.g., Modified Functional Reach test, perturbation testing).
- Static standing balance: Fair, requires minimal assistance to maintain static standing with decreased weight-bearing on the left LE.
- Dynamic standing balance: Poor, requires maximal assistance to prevent falling when attempting to rise on toes, for single limb stance or to retrieve an object from the floor.

Sensation: Intact bilaterally to light touch, sharp/dull, and temperature sensation. Initial reports of sensory impairments have resolved.

Functional Mobility:
- Bed mobility: Requires moderate assistance to complete supine-to-sit and sit-to-supine transitions due to left side weakness and impaired coordination of the left upper and lower extremities.
- Transfers: Requires maximum assistance to complete a stand pivot transfer from hospital bed to a standard wheelchair (WC) due to poor weight acceptance on the left LE.
- Gait: Requires maximal assistance to ambulate 18 feet with a rolling walker (RW) using a left grip adapter. While ambulating with therapist, another person followed with a WC for safety. She demonstrated diminished left stance phase, poor left foot clearance during swing, decreased trunk extension, and poor management of the RW. Assistance was required to advance the left LE and RW. Stair climbing was delayed owing to safety concerns.

PATIENT GOALS

"I would like to maintain my independence and not be a bother to my children." The patient is extremely motivated to be independent in personal care and household management. She reports getting "stronger each day" as she recovers from the strokes. She has been approved for 3 weeks of inpatient rehabilitation and feels she will be able to return home with her daughter providing additional support. She would like to return to her volunteer work sometime in the next year. It is anticipated the patient will require a RW and minimal assistance for household ambulation on level surfaces at time of discharge from the rehabilitation facility.

(Continued)

DISCHARGE PLANS

The patient's daughter lives a 5-min drive away and is able to provide physical assistance and supervision as directed by rehabilitation team members. The daughter will stay at the patient's home for several weeks upon discharge. The occupational therapist has recommended a bedside commode be ordered prior to discharge.

DISCHARGE STATUS

The patient is able to complete bed mobility activities independently with the head of bed raised 20°. Transfers from bed to WC require supervision owing to left LE motor control impairments and postural instability in standing. Occasional minimum assistance is required to ambulate 133 feet with a RW using a left grip adapter. Assistance is no longer required to advance the left LE. Occasional minimum assist is required to negotiate eight standard height steps without an assistive device using a step-to pattern with right side railing support. The patient is able to independently propel a WC on smooth level surfaces using the right upper and lower extremities. Upon discharge, it was advised that the patient not ambulate in the home unsupervised.

HOME ENVIRONMENT

The patient lives alone in a split-level home with one step to enter. In the home, there are six steps with a right side railing to access the upper level that includes a kitchen with dining area, living room, and primary bedroom with full bathroom. From the entry level, there are six steps with a right side railing to access the lower level, which has a half bathroom, small den/sitting area, a guest bedroom, and a utility room with a standard washer and dryer. At your request, one of the patient's daughters has provided dimensions of door frames and height of sleeping and seating surfaces together with several photographs. The physical dimensions and photographs provide the following additional information:

Upper Level

- Primary Bedroom: two small area rugs, a nightstand with an alarm clock, a bureau, a wooden four-poster bed in the middle of room with a sleeping surface 3 feet (91.4 cm) from the floor, and a ceiling lamp fixture controlled by a switch adjacent to the door. The doorway entrance is 36 in. (91.4 cm) wide.
- Primary Bathroom (off primary bedroom): an area rug, standard toilet and sink, bathtub with a standard, fixed shower head and shower curtain to contain water. A shower chair (previously acquired following total knee replacement) is placed outside of the shower with towels and washcloths stored on the seat. The doorway entrance is 30 in. (76 cm) wide.
- Kitchen: polished linoleum floors, adequate counter space, and a dining table in the center of the room with standard kitchen chairs (floor to seat height 17 in. [43.18 cm]).
- Living room: overstuffed upholstered furniture with low seating surfaces (20.5 in. [52.07 cm]), a favorite rocking recliner, a large carpet that appears to ripple in several areas, a centered coffee table, a cordless telephone placed on the coffee table, a remote-controlled television, two end tables, and a bookcase.
- Hallway (between the kitchen/dining area and the primary bedroom): poorly lit with a long, narrow area rug.

Lower Level

- Small den/sitting room: Two large rocker reclining chairs are positioned in front of a large entertainment unit. The room is overcrowded with limited space between the chairs and the entertainment unit resulting in limited floor space. A ceiling fan with lights is operated by a remote control, and the room has heavy thick carpet.
- Utility Room: A top loading washer and dryer are present. The area has limited space but is able to accommodate a standard chair with adequate remaining floor space. There is a utility sink and overhead cabinets above the washer and dryer.

GUIDING QUESTIONS

With general knowledge of the patient's living space, what environmental modifications, adaptive equipment, or additional instruction would you suggest or provide to optimize safety and function in each of the following areas of the home?

1. Stairs
2. Primary bedroom

CASE STUDY—cont'd

3. Primary bathroom

4. Kitchen

5. Living room

6. Hallways

7. Small den/sitting area

8. Utility room

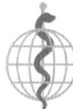

For additional resources, including answers to the questions for review, new immersive cases, case study guiding questions, references and more, please visit **https://www.fadavis.com/product/physical -rehabilitation-fulk-8**. You may also quickly find the resources by entering this title's four-digit ISBN, 4691, in the search field at **http://fadavis.co**m and logging in at the prompt.

Supplemental Readings

Bantham A, Taverno Ross SE, Sebastião E, Hall G. Overcoming barriers to physical activity in underserved populations. *Prog Cardiovasc Dis*. 2021;64:64–71.

Carnemolla P, Bridge C. A scoping review of home modification interventions—mapping the evidence base. *Indoor Built Environ*. 2020;29(3):299–310.

Carnemolla P, Bridge C. Housing design and community care: how home modifications reduce care needs of older people and people with disability. *Int J Environ Res Public Health*. 2019;16(11). doi:10.3390/ijerph16111951

Dos Santos HM, Pereira GS, Brandão TCP, et al. Impact of environmental factors on post-stroke disability: an analytical cross-sectional study. *J Stroke Cerebrovasc Dis*. 2022;31(4):106305.

Heinemann AW, Miskovic A, Semik P, et al. Measuring environmental factors: unique and overlapping International Classification of Functioning, Disability and Health coverage of 5 instruments. *Arch Phys Med Rehabil*. 2016;97(12):2113–2122.

Hwang NK, Shim SH. Use of virtual reality technology to support the home modification process: a scoping review. *Int J Environ Res Public Health*. 2021;18(21). doi:10.3390/ijerph182111096.

Keglovits M, Stark S. Home modifications to improve function and safety in the United States. *J Aging Environ*. 2020;34(2):110–125.

Khalili M, Jonathan C, Hocking N, Van der Loos M, Mortenson WB, Borisoff J. Perception of autonomy among people who use wheeled mobility assistive devices: dependence on environment and contextual factors. *Disabil Rehabil Assist Technol*. Published online October 7, 2021:1–8.

Null R, ed. *Universal Design: Principles and Models*. CRC Press; 2017.

Nussbaumer LL. *Human Factors in the Built Environment*. 2nd ed. Fairchild Books; 2018.

Richman L, Pearson J, Beasley C, Stanifer J. Addressing health inequalities in diverse, rural communities: An unmet need. *SSM Popul Health*. 2019;7:100398.

Tepper D. Making a house an accessible home: the role of PTs. APTA. Published September 1, 2016. Accessed March 28, 2022. https://www.apta.org/apta-magazine/2016/09/01/making-a-house-an-accessible-home-the-role-of-pts

Intervention Strategies for Rehabilitation

Strategies to Improve Motor Function

Tina M. Stoeckmann, PT, DSc
Susan B. O'Sullivan, PT, EdD

Chapter **10**

LEARNING OBJECTIVES

1. Utilize a hybrid model for clinical decision-making that integrates current concepts of function and disability with key considerations for motor control and motor learning.
2. Link types of skilled movements to the motor control strategies that coordinate them.
3. Pair key motor learning factors to the respective neural networks that support them.
4. Apply principles of neuroplasticity to the design and implementation of effective, evidence-based treatment plans.
5. Categorize constraints on motor function as being associated with the individual, task, or environment and determine intervention strategies based on that assessment.
6. Identify individuals' stage of motor learning based on descriptions of skill performance and incorporate appropriate instruction, practice, and feedback principles into therapeutic activities.
7. Analyze and interpret patient data, anticipate outcomes, formulate goals, and develop a plan of care that presents an integrated approach to treatment for individual cases.

CHAPTER OUTLINE

INTRODUCTION *334*
    Foundational Concepts/Theoretical Models *334*
MOTOR CONTROL *334*
    Systems Underlying Motor Control *334*
    Different Learning Networks *337*
    Neuroplasticity *338*
    Constraints on Motor Function *339*
MOTOR LEARNING *340*
    Types of Learning *340*
    Motor Learning Theories *340*
    Stages of Motor Learning *341*
    Instruction: Introducing Skill, Setting Up, Guiding Practice *341*

Practice Considerations *342*
Feedback *345*
Patient Populations: Special Considerations for Learning *346*
INTERVENTIONS TO IMPROVE MOTOR FUNCTION *347*
    Individual: Body Structure and Function *350*
    Task *358*
    Environment *363*
    Technology *364*
    Patient/Client-Related Education *364*
SUMMARY *364*

■ INTRODUCTION

As physical therapists, we focus on our patients and their ability to produce functional, goal-directed movement. Our primary role is to teach people to move in new or better ways through effective instruction, practice, and feedback, and to develop meaningful and challenging, yet achievable, goals to benchmark progress and provide motivation. We must address the limitations and resources of each person and understand the demands of the tasks and the environmental context in which they will be performed. We also need to understand the processes involved in learning and producing movement, regardless of diagnosis.

Section One in this textbook covers the examination of the body structures and functional systems in detail. This chapter will focus on key motor control features and motor learning principles involved in performing, acquiring, and improving movement skills. These considerations form the clinical decision-making framework for realistic goal-setting and effective treatment planning that broadly considers *all* movement factors, not just those associated with the performer.

Foundational Concepts/Theoretical Models

The World Health Organization's (WHO's) International Classification of Function, Disability and Health (ICF) Model,[1] introduced in Chapter 1, Clinical Decision-Making, provides a framework for describing and organizing information on function and disability. It recognizes the role of environmental factors in the creation of disability, as well as the relevance of associated health conditions and their effects. These components align well with Newell's model of constraints that influence the learning and production of movement skills: the individual's capacity for movement, the requirements of the task or activity, and the environmental situations in which the activity is performed.[2] Figure 10.1 represents a hybrid model incorporating the overlapping principles of these two concepts and provides the framework for the rest of this chapter.

Physical therapists use a patient-centered approach to frame our clinical evaluations and decision-making, as outlined in the *APTA Guide to Physical Therapist Practice*.[3] We consider the impact of our patient's injury or illness on their body structure and function, including personal factors that may influence their ability to participate optimally in therapy. This process includes identifying barriers and resources available to the patient to accomplish the task/activity and meet their participation goals: What challenges do they face? What assets do they have to work with? These issues cannot be adequately addressed without the therapist also having a clear understanding of the tasks and environmental demands as well. Table 10.1 provides an overview of these key concepts, and later in this chapter,

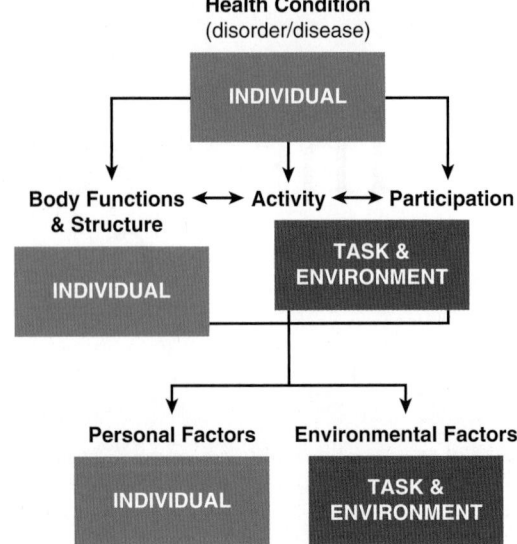

Figure 10.1 Theoretical model: hybrid of ICF and Newell's constraints. Integrating the WHO ICF categories[1] of functioning, disability, and health domains (black font) with Newell's conceptual model[2] of individual, task, and environmental constraints (text boxes) on motor skill learning and performance.

an example is provided of the task and environmental features for a farmer hoping to return to driving his tractor (Fig. 10.6, 10.7)

■ MOTOR CONTROL

Motor control has been defined as "the ability to regulate or direct the mechanisms essential to movement."[4(p3)] The body uses multiple control strategies to produce a wide range of movements from simple to incredibly complex, consciously directed to automatic. The reader is referred to the work of Schmidt and Lee[5] and Shumway-Cook and Woollacott[4] for excellent reviews of this topic.

Systems/Processes Underlying Motor Control

Motor control involves making accurate predictions of our abilities, the task requirements, and the influence of the environment in order to move successfully. This section will briefly examine the sensory, cognitive, and motor systems involved in this complex process.

Sensation/Perception

Detecting sensory information (sensation) and interpreting it appropriately (perception) is critical for evaluating initial conditions for motor planning, concurrent monitoring of movement production, and evaluation of performance outcome. The key feedback systems related to movement assessment are discussed here.

Vision plays a powerful role in identifying relevant environmental features needed for object recognition,

Table 10.1	Newell's Model of Constraints		
Individual	Task	Environment
Focus: What does the patient have to work with or work around? Assets and constraints	**Focus:** What is necessary for success? Key features of an object or activity that need to be incorporated into an action plan for success. Regulatory features	**Focus:** What is going on around the patient during their task performance? Interactions or distractions
Physical resources/barriers: strength/weakness, ROM, sensory, coordination, endurance, etc.	**Physical requirements:** object properties, forces required, excursion, timing, sequencing of components in space/time. Accurate perception is needed.	**Physical parameters:** spatial dimensions, surfaces, potential interactions, relevance of other activities. Accurate discernment is needed.
Cognitive and emotional factors: prior plus or minus experiences, insight, understanding, motivation	**Cognitive demands:** attentional focus, complexity of the task, perceptual requirements including predicting moving or unstable features of an object	**Cognitive demands:** ability to resist distraction, monitor or focus on most relevant features of the surroundings, accurately predict time to contact

ROM = range of motion.

manipulation, and environmental navigation: *depth perception* for spatial dimensions (how far away is the step, how high is the toilet); *optic flow* to estimate movement trajectories and time-to-impact (catching, avoiding traffic, timing); and *contrast sensitivity* to discern surface textures, contour, and stability (ice on sidewalk, finding the wheelchair brakes). All contribute to our ability to anticipate and monitor our body's orientation, movement timing, and sequencing, while monitoring the environment to accomplish goals.

Somatosensory feedback informs the brain about our body's "state" or status: *proprioception* for our current alignment/joint positions (posture, stair height, treadmill cadence) and *cutaneous* inputs, particularly *pressure and light touch,* connect us to our environment (is my foot on the step, is the chair behind me, is the object in my hand?).

Vestibular feedback provides us with information about *head position* relative to gravity and self-motion via changes in linear or rotational *acceleration* (am I swaying, is my head tilted?).

Cognition: Decision-Making

An incredible amount of information is continuously available to the nervous system, but the brain has limited attentional capacity to process it. Decisions about which information to attend to and what it means for movement production are critical cognitive aspects of skill.

The initial cognitive stage of information processing is known as *stimulus identification.* Based on a person's interpretation of their particular circumstance, a choice is made about whether to move: a "Go/No Go" decision. This decision may require inhibiting an automatic

response if it is not appropriate, like whether or not to step out of the elevator when the door opens. A "Go" decision is followed by *response selection:* choosing a general motor plan for *what* to do, like how to get out of bed following postsurgical precautions. Decision-making during this stage is sensitive to the number of different movement alternatives possible. More options slow reaction time (Hick's law), and a natural or well-learned association between a stimulus and response (S-R compatibility) improves reaction time, but it may also interfere with learning new motor responses.[6] For example, when crossing at a streetlight, an individual easily responds to the green light by moving forward. If a crossing guard signals the individual to move forward even though the light is red, the individual is likely to be more hesitant in responding. Once a general movement plan is chosen, *response programming* involves adding the specific details for the current situation, like specific forces, directions, timing, duration, and extent of movement. This parametric specification is based on an accurate understanding of the resources and constraints of the individual, the requirements of the task, and the status of the environment. Making accurate predictions are key goals of physical practice. See Box 5.7, Questions Examining the Patient's Ability to Problem Solve in Chapter 5, Examination of Motor Function, for strategies to assess the patient's ability to detect, interpret, plan, and execute goal-directed movements.

Motor Performance: Execution

Our movement repertoire ranges from reflexive, automatic, and habitual movements to highly focused, cognitively demanding activities such as precarious balance activities, tightly constrained timing and precision skills, or highly complex tasks such as driving. Each category of movement complexity suggests a different control strategy.

Reflexive/Automatic Movements

The original reflex and hierarchical theories of motor control described movement that is triggered and guided by sensory feedback, reflecting a "closed loop" model of control. It is organized in a top-down fashion from higher (cortical) to lower (spinal) centers. Sensory information from the body ascends in the dorsal columns and spinothalamic tracts through the brainstem to the cerebellum for unconscious processing of the body's state, as well as through the thalamus for distribution to the various cortical regions for conscious awareness and further integrative processing (see Chapter 3, Examination of Sensory Function). Reflexes like blinking, deep tendon reflexes, and the vestibulo-ocular reflex are triggered by sensory input and provide rapid, predictable, unconscious motor responses (see Chapter 5, section on Reflex Testing, Tables 5.6, 5.7, 5.8). Brainstem level descending pathways, including vestibulospinal, rubrospinal, and reticulospinal tracts, contribute to synergistic control of movement and posture, including balance reactions and proximal stabilization (see Chapter 6, Examination of Coordination and Balance). Self-sustaining neural circuits in the spine and brainstem, called central pattern generators, allow for fairly automatic continuous, rhythmic, repetitive synergistic motor patterns involved in locomotion such as running and walking,[7,8] as well as scratching,[9] etc. While voluntarily initiated and terminated once the goal is reached, the central pattern generator output is sustained primarily by ongoing sensory feedback throughout the movement cycle, requiring little cognitive oversight. All these mechanisms allow our limited conscious attention to be focused more externally on monitoring the task performance and environment.

Voluntary/Cortically Controlled Movement

The descending corticospinal tract (CST) is the only descending pathway involved in the control of voluntary isolated muscle contractions for individuated or fractionated movement (see Chapter 5, Table 5.2, Positive and Negative Features of Upper Motor Neuron Syndrome, and Table 5.11, Differential Diagnosis). Neurons in the primary motor strip give rise to the CST and are labeled *upper motor neurons* (UMNs). They descend to synapse on the alpha or lower motor neurons in the ventral horn of the spinal cord, whose axons exit at each vertebral level and combine in the plexuses to become peripheral motor nerves.

Although feedback plays a critical role in the shaping and correction of ongoing movements, deafferentation studies have shown that we can also move reasonably well in the absence of sensation.[10] *Feed forward control* involves preprogramming the movement ahead of time if it will occur too quickly for feedback-based correction.[5] This is an *"open loop"* control model; success depends on accurate prediction of task demands. For example, skilled piano playing occurs too rapidly to benefit from feedback for accuracy and is therefore an open-loop control system; balance responses can be fired in anticipation of the impending instability of a known task.

The complexity of human movement negates any simplistic model of movement control. Schmidt and Lee[5] propose a blending of both open-loop and closed-loop control processes in an *intermittent control hypothesis*. *Generalized motor programs* (GMPs), or "schema," provide the general formula for the movement category rather than having every specific version of the movement stored in the brain. Feedback about initial conditions and actual performance is used to refine and perfect movements.[11] GMPs include both fixed and flexible movement characteristics. *Invariant characteristics* are the fixed movement rules that define a movement category, like the algebraic rules that define a triangle versus a rectangle. GMPs include the relative force, relative timing, and order of movement components required for a specific task category, like the combinations of single versus double limb stance and flight phases that differentiate walking from running, hopping, and skipping. *Movement parameters* are the flexible features that are tweaked to match the specific task demands, like the values you put into the formula to get triangles of different sizes and dimensions. These parameters typically include overall force, size, and duration of the movement, such as taking longer, higher, or faster steps. These adjustments can change walking performance (speed) but not the basic pattern: it's still walking.[5] GMPs ensure flexibility by requiring fewer stored programs while providing significant adaptability of movement based on variable parameter values.

Dynamic Systems

Movement is an emergent phenomenon[12] that is not limited to biological systems. A dynamical system is any system that changes its "state" or status over time; the human body is a great example. Such systems are characterized by a diversity of elements (muscles, bones, nerves, etc.), connections (segmental linkages, neural networks), interdependence of elements (muscle activity triggers neural signaling, muscle contraction impacts skeletal structures), and adaptation (capacity for change, learning). In such a model, the entire system gravitates toward optimal stability and effectiveness. These stable states, or "attractors," are the preferred arrangements/activities that keep the components working together to meet the individual's goals.[13] A disruption to the individual, task, or environment may change the situational demands and trigger the emergence of a new motor behavior in response to the change. This is known as a "phase shift" and is often spontaneous, resulting from the self-organization of all the system's components around the goal of reestablishing stability in the new situation.[14] An injury or illness (amputation, paralysis), a change in task demands (using a sliding board or crutches) or the environment (walking on ice or a split belt treadmill) disrupts the system, triggering the need for a different motor behavior to meet the goal (mobility) under the new circumstances. According to this model, learned behaviors that are successful and efficient in meeting the movement goal become strong attractors/habits.[6] In this framework, the nervous system is no longer the top of a hierarchy or the sole source of movement production. It is just one component of a complex system, and movements emerge from the system's state rather than being preprogrammed. The implications of this model for learning new skills will be discussed further in the sections on motor learning and interventions later in this chapter.

Different Learning Networks

The multiple parallel motor control systems discussed above suggest overlapping yet specialized information processing responsibilities for learning and controlling various motor skills. This is reflected in specialized regions and complex connections in the brain that contribute to acquiring and retaining new abilities, which will be briefly outlined here.

Multiple cerebral cortices analyze various sensory inputs, maintaining a concise representation of the body, environmental context, and action demands critical for motor planning.[15] The primary *motor strip* acts as the controller, sending the commands directly or indirectly to motor neurons via the CST to execute specific actions with high speed and precision. It allows flexible synergy development for novel tasks or object manipulation requiring cognitive oversight.[16]

The premotor *mirror neuron* system is involved in interpreting the actions of others. It interacts with vision, proprioception, and motor commands to play a key role in observational learning and mental imagery[17] through action recognition.[18] It has been associated with promoting cortical reorganization and functional recovery poststroke.[19]

The *basal ganglia,* particularly the dopaminergic nucleus accumbens, is associated with predicting reward and is, therefore, involved with reinforcement-based learning, choosing movement strategies based on perception of reward versus cost.[20] It also contributes to internally generated (memory-guided) movement (see Fig. 10.2). The *limbic system* receives information from the frontal cortex about reward-based outcomes, which is paired with spatial and action-related information from parietal cortical areas for action–outcome learning. Since rewards trigger emotional responses, success positively influences the learning associated with movement production that achieves a meaningful goal. In addition, limbic outputs to the *hippocampal* system, where new memories are encoded, also contribute to learning.[21] The hippocampus itself is involved in recognition, spatial memory, and explicit, declarative learning for things such as postsurgical precautions or a home exercise program (HEP). The survival of newly generated cells in the hippocampus is strongly linked to learning experiences that are new, effortful, and successful.[22] The *amygdala* is also involved in memory processing and is influenced by stress hormones, making emotionally arousing events more likely to be remembered. Taking some risk by making practice challenging amplifies the impact of success and strengthens learning.[23,24] Easy success and passive tasks quickly become boring, while constant failure leads to frustration, anxiety, and depression. But surprising or hard-won successes are highly

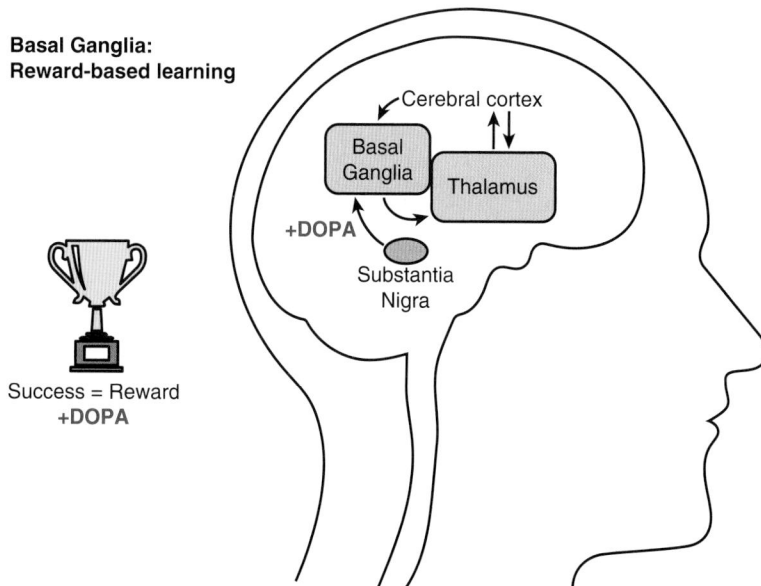

Basal Ganglia: Reward-based learning

Success = Reward
+DOPA

Figure 10.2 Learning networks: basal ganglia. Basal ganglia learning is based on predicting reward. *(Adapted from Doya.)*[15]

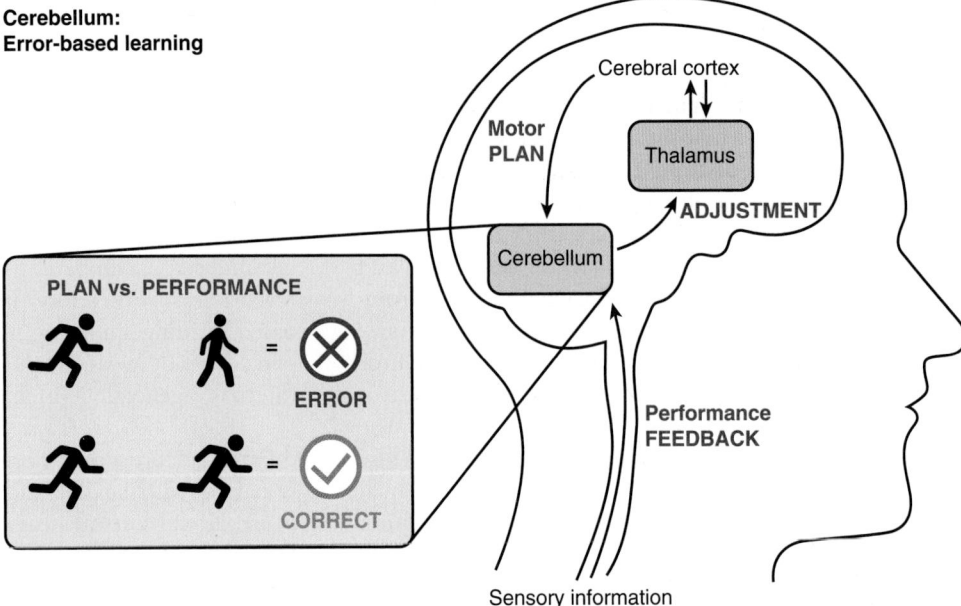

Figure 10.3 Learning networks: cerebellum. Cerebellar learning is based on detecting errors. *(Adapted from Doya.)*[15]

rewarding. Providing just the right amount of challenge is personal and will be discussed further in the "Intervention" section of this chapter.

The climbing fibers of the *cerebellum* contribute to error-based learning, which is associated with motor adaptation seen during discovery learning (see Fig. 10.3). It works by calibrating the brain's prediction of how we will move, including internal models of the body and environment. These references need to be continually updated to account for temporary but predictable changes on task demands for flexible motor control.[25] The cerebellum is responsible for procedural learning, movements that are externally driven or guided, and the timing and rhythm of body dynamics.

Lastly, other circuits are also involved at various stages of learning: corticobasal ganglia loops are differentially involved in early versus late stages of learning; a prefrontal loop involving the *prefrontal* cortex, *presupplementary* motor area, and *caudate* is involved in learning new movement sequences in the cognitive stage; a motor loop including the *supplemental motor area* and *putamen* is involved in executing well-learned movements representing the autonomous stage. These areas of the brain are also involved in mental imagery, sensory discrimination, planning and attention, rule-based learning, and spatial navigation.[15]

Neuroplasticity

The nervous system has the capacity to change in response to experience or injury across the life span—a process known as *neuroplasticity*. Motor learning is a complex and dynamic process, with plasticity occurring at many levels, driven by changes in behavioral, sensory,

and cognitive experiences and involving multiple cellular, network, and biochemical processes. Short-term plasticity has been associated with improved neuronal signaling for temporary behavioral changes lasting seconds to minutes, such as brief responses to sensory inputs, transient behavioral states, and short-term memories. The neurophysiology behind these adaptations includes improved synaptic efficiency or unmasking of new, redundant neuron pathways or "silent synapses" that permit cortical map reorganization and restoration of function. Longer-lasting changes associated with long-term potentiation (LTP) or long-term depression are associated with structural changes such as dendritic branching, spine density growth or loss, and axonal sprouting or dying back.[16,26] Positive changes associated with LTP reflect fast, efficient, reliable neuronal connections and serve as a basis for learning and memory.[27–30] Pathways in the brain are formed and reinforced through repetition, consistency, and causal relationships, summarized by the adage "neurons that fire together, wire together," referring to neural adaptation that occurs during repeated practice.[31] These changes may be adaptive and lead to improved function, but they can also be maladaptive, like compensatory motor behaviors. The primary rehabilitation principles that drive experience-dependent neuroplasticity[32] are summarized in Table 10.2.

Nerve growth factors such as brain-derived neurotrophic factor (BDNF) have been shown to have a key role in neuronal sprouting and repair processes and are associated with activity-dependent (exercise-induced) synaptic plasticity.[33] Strong emotional experiences can trigger the release of hormones and neurotransmitters

Table 10.2 Principles of Neuroplasticity	
Principle	Description
Use it or lose it, **and** *use it to improve it.*	The body does not maintain systems that aren't used. Delayed or absent rehab can limit recovery and can result in neural degradation and learned non-use. If you want a system to get better, it needs to be actively challenged; passive activity does not drive change.
Specificity	Task-specific training: Practice the actual tasks being targeted as closely as possible; if you want to get better at walking, you need to walk. Do not assume improving components will automatically integrate into function.
Repetition	Focus on sufficient practice trials to stimulate brain reorganization. Hundreds to thousands of repetitions are needed for permanent improvement. Practice beyond the therapy session is needed.
Salience	Make tasks and goals meaningful and relevant to the patient; relate to patient-identified activities and participation goals for motivation.
Intensity	Focus on sufficient training effort to stimulate brain reorganization—patients need to work hard. Get their heart rate up, add cognitive challenge, ensure exertion is required for success. Monitor your patient's response for safety and adequate level of effort.
Timing	Different neural processes are involved at the various stages of recovery and learning. Neuroprotective effects can reduce the impact of degeneration or injury. Very early training may be detrimental in some cases of neural injury. Neural reorganization after injury is robust initially but levels off within 3–6 months, after which significant effort is needed to drive change.
Age	Training-induced plasticity occurs more readily in younger brains; older adults typically require more repetitions for slower, smaller changes.
Transference	Prime the brain to learn. Exercise increases general neural excitability and stimulates neurotrophic factors. Choose challenging tasks for potential "reverse transfer" (hard to easy) benefit.
Interference	Plasticity in one experience can interfere with acquisition of other behaviors. Examples: Compensations can interfere with return of more normal movement patterns; explicit instructions can interfere with implicit learning.

Adapted from Kleim.[32]

that can strengthen memory, making salience, motivation, and reward important drivers of learning.

Constraints on Motor Function
Individual

Constraints restrict movement possibilities. Many impairments impact voluntary movement production. Impaired force production (weakness or paralysis) can limit both strength and power generation, and it can interfere with people's ability to move themselves and/or interact with objects in their environment effectively and efficiently. Limited range of motion (ROM) reduces the amount of excursion available and therefore the available/accessible workspace for personal activities such as putting on shoes or emptying the dishwasher. Endurance limitations/fatigue impacts the ability to sustain performance to complete repetitive or prolonged activities necessary for life roles and community engagement. Increased stiffness or resistance to passive

stretch (spasticity or rigidity) interferes with the ability of a muscle to be passively lengthened during dynamic activity, such as hamstrings during the swing phase of gait or biceps/triceps while brushing teeth or combing hair. Added resistance for any reason increases the effort needed to move, subsequently reducing the efficiency and smoothness of performance.

Coordination deficits also have significant negative effects on accuracy, specificity, and fluidity of movement. For example, stereotypic synergy patterns seen with UMN lesions are incompatible with individuated muscle activities and interfere with the ability to generate different combinations of muscle/movement patterns. Co-contraction may be an effective stability strategy in some situations, but other circumstances require directional and proportional responses (anterior-posterior or lateral perturbations) as exhibited by the limited balance responses seen in people with advanced Parkinson disease (PD). Slowness/smallness of activation (brady- and hypokinesia) also result in less power production, which limits momentum generation for transitional movements such as getting out of bed or rising from a chair. Excessive or unrestrained motion such as ataxia, dyskinesia, or chorea can also reduce accuracy and efficiency of movement production. Old movement habits are very hard to overcome and may continue to dominate movement efforts even when the individual's system has changed for the better (pain is gone, increased flexibility, stronger), or worse (new injury and still moving the old way, not following protocol), or the task has been modified (no longer using cane but still walks the same, not using a newly installed grab bar). Constraints also include impairments in sensory/perceptual and/or cognitive/behavioral systems as discussed in Chapter 3, Examination of Sensory Function, and Chapter 27, Cognitive and Perceptual Dysfunction.

Task and Environment

Healthy individuals perform a wide variety of movement tasks related to daily function, work, and social interests. *Motor skills* are defined as highly coordinated movement sequences for the purposes of attaining an action goal.[4] Skilled behaviors exhibit both variability and consistency. They are adapted and organized by the task goal and environment, and they are the direct result of practice and experience. Examples of skills are included in Table 10.3 later in the chapter. Categories reflect common goals or control strategies that highlight the challenges that learners face, which therapists must consider when setting up task practice. Categories can represent a single dimension such as gross versus fine motor or high motor versus high cognitive demand. Temporal organizational categories reflect different control strategies discussed above, including discrete, serial, and continuous tasks. *Discrete* skills are relatively brief, having a clear beginning and end, and are typically thought to be controlled by motor programs. *Serial* skills link together a sequence of discrete skills for one overall goal, like getting up from the floor or getting dressed. *Continuous* skills are rhythmic, cyclic skills that are repeated over and over until the performer decides to stop. They include locomotor skills and are often run by central pattern generators. For more examples, see Chapter 5, Box 5.4, Categories of Motor Skills.

The design of a successful plan of care (POC) requires careful examination of the individual's body structure and functional limitations and resources, and a strong understanding of how they relate to the demands and goals of the task, including the environment in which they will be performed. Applying these concepts to therapy practice is the focus of the next section.

■ MOTOR LEARNING

Motor learning has been defined as "a set of internal processes associated with practice or experience leading to relatively permanent changes in the capability for motor skill."[5(p497)] Motor learning is not directly observable in

practice, but rather is inferred from changes in motor behavior over time (see Chapter 5, Table 5.10, Measures of Performance). It is a process that involves three stages: acquisition, consolidation, and retention. The initial acquisition phase involves attending to and encoding sensory information from early movement experiences, providing an initial stored representation of the experience in working memory. For this information to persist longer than a few minutes, it needs to be consolidated through conscious attention and practice. In the final retention phase, an unconscious offline process of strengthening and stabilizing the information results in the formation of a long-lasting memory.[16,34-36] Sleep has been shown to play an important role in the consolidation and enhancement of procedural memories.[37]

Memory is also classified according to information content and whether it is accessed by conscious recollection. *Declarative* memory is *explicit* information that can be *consciously* recalled and stated, like the instructions and verbal cues you give your patient. *Procedural* memory is *implicit*, involves unconscious recall of motor skills, and is reflected in improved *performance* over time.[34,38] Procedural memory typically requires an extensive acquisition phase with lots of practice trials compared to declarative memory.[39] Patients with brain injury may have very poor declarative memory, yet still show improvements in motor skills with practice, even when they can't remember what they did.

Types of Learning

Nonassociative learning occurs when a single stimulus is given repeatedly with the goal of learning the characteristic of that signal and the appropriate response to it. *Habituation* results in decreasing sensitivity to a stimulus, and it is used therapeutically in vestibular rehabilitation, in patients with hyperalgesia, and in children with sensory-processing disorders. *Sensitization* involves becoming more attuned to certain sensory stimuli for things such as balance training and stereognosis.

Associative learning involves linking ideas and experiences together, allowing patients to make predictions about cause and effect; it is essential for being adaptable to changing or novel situations. *Classical conditioning* involves developing a *subconscious* response to a stimulus, which contributes to automaticity, but it can also be detrimental if the wrong cue becomes the movement trigger, like the patient sitting up straight because the therapist walks in the room. *Operant conditioning* links a *deliberate* choice to a consequence. After an injury, compensations provide immediate functional success, with failed efforts not typically repeated. Both processes involve *predicting reward.*[40]

Motor Learning Theories

Different theories of motor learning reflect various perspectives about how practice leads to lasting change in skill performance and offer guidance for providing instruction, setting up practice and the environment, and optimizing feedback for learning.

Adams' *closed-loop theory*[10] of motor learning is based on a feedback model of motor control with two key components: a *memory trace* that chooses and initiates a movement based on previous experience, and a *perceptual trace* that develops based on sensory feedback from the current performance. The memory trace provides a *reference of correctness* for error detection and performance adjustment. Practice creates new or strengthens current memory traces, implying that correct practice is imperative to avoid reinforcing the poor performance as reflected in Vince Lombardi's adage: "Only perfect practice makes perfect." This perspective has been a foundational principle of traditional rehabilitation approaches and technologies, which focus on reinforcing normal movement kinematics and errorless learning. It may relate to learning that occurs during slow, feedback-guided responses, but not for rapid, pre-planned movements (open-loop control) or learning that can occur in the absence of sensory feedback (deafferentation studies).

Schmidt's *schema theory*[11] is based on the open-loop or feed-forward motor control concept of the GMP or schema. Schema incorporate short-term memory factors such as initial conditions (body position, weight of objects, and so forth), relationships between movement elements (timing, sequencing), movement outcome, and sensory feedback of movement. This theory also includes two memory processes: recall and recognition. *Recall schema* are used to *select and define* the movement relationships based on *past* parameter choices. It is similar to Adam's memory trace but is a general movement category rather than a specific movement. *Recognition schema* evaluate movement *responses* and relationships produced by the current situation and parameter choices, like Adam's perceptual trace. This information is then abstracted to form implicit, procedural (motor) memory. With practice, most movements can be performed fairly automatically, with little attention or conscious oversight. Clinically, the schema theory suggests that "we learn skills by learning rules about the functioning of our bodies—forming relationships between how our muscles are activated, what they actually do, and how these actions feel."[5(p448)] Variable practice, including making mistakes, improves learning through increased understanding of the cause-and-effect relationships between programming factors (initial set up, amount of force, timing, etc.) and outcomes associated with those choices (failure to produce enough or producing too much force or excursion, inappropriate timing or sequencing). It also enhances our understanding of how novel and open skills in changing environments are learned.

The *dynamical systems*[6] approach also emphasizes variable practice and learning through self-discovery. Therapists work to enhance patients' intrinsic resources by addressing impairments. They set up and modify the task and environment for appropriate challenge and help highlight the key features. In this model, practice is about the patient exploring movement production and the use of personal and environmental resources to develop new *strategies* to accomplish their goals. The therapist does not necessarily provide a specific solution but instead provides a safe environment for trial-and-error learning.

Stages of Motor Learning

Learning is a continuum, but it has been divided into a framework of stages for organizing training strategies to improve motor skills (see Table 10.3). Fitts and Posner[41] developed a three-stage model of motor learning that focuses on observed motor behavior and cognitive load. It uses the terms *cognitive, associated,* and *autonomous* to describe these stages from new learner to skilled performer. Their model is described in Chapter 5.

The dynamical systems[6] model provides another perspective to this same learning continuum, focusing instead on efforts to manage the body's many degrees of freedom (DOF). New learners in the cognitive stage are *novices* whose performance appears stiff due to co-contraction to initially "freezing out" most DOF. Movement is consciously directed and limited in capacity. With practice and increasing understanding of the task demands, the learner demonstrates *advanced* performance as some movement components become habitual and more DOF are incorporated, creating a more fluid, effective performance. *Expert* performers have learned to optimize their body, properties of objects, and the environment for efficient performance for things like utilizing momentum to come to transfer or using the energy-storing properties of a dynamic brace.

Instruction: Introducing Skill, Setting Up, Guiding Practice

A person in the cognitive stage is trying to figure out what to do, what to pay attention to, how to move their body, and what is needed for success. Typically, instruction is provided by demonstration with verbal cues regarding the overall scope of the movement and key regulatory features that shape that movement (excursion, timing, sequence, segments). Mirror neurons[17,18] help patients internalize what they see during such action-observation. Watching a skilled performer helps patients appreciate the overall performance and outcome. Watching a peer who is just learning the skill can also provide meaningful information about common challenges, mistakes, and consequences. The problem-solving approach inherent in discovery learning allows patients to find successful movement strategies that work for them. Manual guidance for learning a new skill can help provide *initial* kinematic feedback and a safe environment for early practice where errors are potentially large, but such guidance should be reduced by the associative stage.[5] By then, the patient generally

Table 10.3   Stages of Motor Learning

Fitt's and Posner's Stages

Cognitive	Associative	Autonomous
• Just trying to understand the nature of the task—*what* to do • Developing strategies • *High cognitive effort* required • Errors large and frequent, but rapid improvement • Dependent on *visual* feedback • Performance is *deliberate* and variable	• Task is better organized but not automatic—focus on *how* to do it well • Less cognition required • Fewer, smaller errors; improvement slows down • Becoming more dependent on *proprioceptive* feedback	• Movement requires little attention—can perform *dual task* • Less dependence on visual and proprioceptive feedback and *feedforward* • Errors small and infrequent • Performance good in a *varying* environment

Clinical implications: Provides guidance on how to structure *practice* sessions and the *environment* based on the *stage of learning*.

Dynamical Systems Stages

Novice	Advanced	Expert
• Learner simplifies the movement to reduce the DOF by *constraining* multiple joints to move together. • The cost is reduced efficiency and flexibility. • Performance looks *stiff*.	• Learner *begins to release* additional DOF, allowing more joints to contribute to performance. • Joints can be controlled independently as necessary. • Co-contraction is reduced. • *Synergies* are used to create well-coordinated movement that is more adaptable.	• Learner has *released all* DOF needed to perform in the most *efficient* way. • Learned to take advantage of body/task *mechanics* and object/environment properties to optimize efficiency.

Clinical implications:
• Explains *co-contractions* in the early stage of motor learning as a normal strategy.
• Supports the importance of providing external support, easier postures, and simplified tasks during *early* skill development to reduce DOF.

DOF = degrees of freedom.

understands what is needed and is now learning how to refine, optimize, and automate their performance. Practice continues toward efficient automaticity of performance under variable conditions including open environments and dual tasks.

Practice Considerations

Practice drives learning. Therapists must consider the cognitive and physical resources of patients and the complexity of the environment and tasks to be learned in determining how to set up practice. Clinical decisions include the following:

• Should mistakes be avoided or embraced?
• How should practice activities and rest periods be spaced (*distribution and order of practice*)?
• When should practice be varied?
• How should the environment be structured (*closed vs. open*)?
• What tasks can be practiced in *parts vs. simplified* but kept as whole-task training?

New learners have limited capacity to deal with significant information-processing demands or task complexity compared to experienced performers. The *challenge point theory*[42] provides a framework for matching practice variables and feedback parameters within the context of task difficulty and individual skill level to optimize learning. It is represented as the intersection of two overlapping line graphs. One graph is a bell curve of task difficulty from easy to impossible related to the potential *learning* benefit of practicing at given levels of difficulty (Fig. 10.4a). The top of the curve reflects optimal learning, and it does not occur when the task is easiest; rather, the middle or moderate range of difficulty provides intermittent success. The second consideration is a logarithmic curve representing level of task difficulty related to level of *performance* errors, reflecting that performance declines (more errors) as the task becomes more difficult (Fig. 10.4b). The intersection of these two lines represents the *challenge point*, the ideal level of task difficulty at which to practice for optimal learning (Fig. 10.4c). It is not error-free practice.

Appropriate challenges create some degree of failure but lead to hard-won, long-term success, which motivates continued effort. Practice challenges beyond this critical point overtaxes the learner, leading to a negative cycle of stress. The ideal level of demand is *learner specific* and *dynamic*, shifting across tasks and stages of learning.[43]

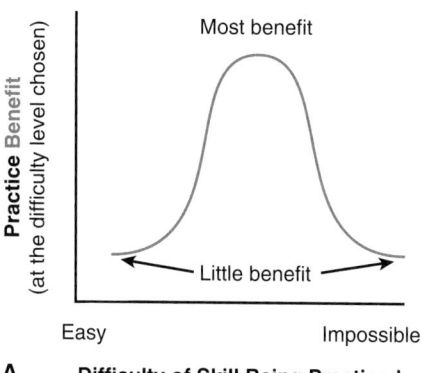

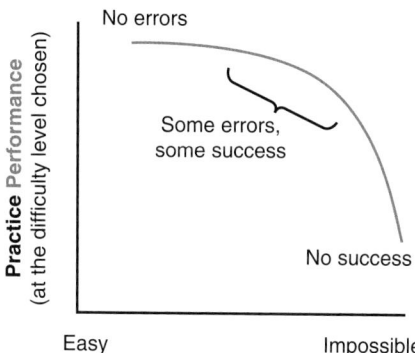

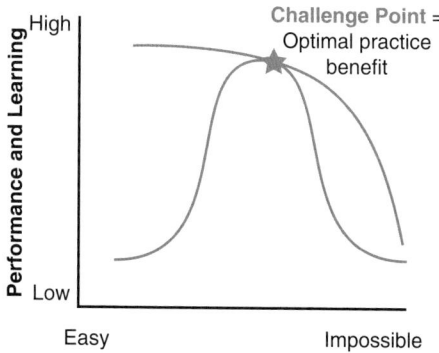

Figure 10.4 Challenge point theory. (A) Practice benefit vs. skill difficulty. Optimal skill learning occurs when the task is moderately difficult and results in intermittent success. (B) Skill difficulty vs. performance. Performance declines and more errors occur as skill difficulty increases. (C) Optimal skill learning. The intersection of skill difficulty and learner performance is the challenge point, reflecting the level of practice difficulty for optimal learning. Note that it is not error-free practice. *(Adapted from Guadagnoli.)*[42]

Since mistakes ultimately help us improve, can increasing the magnitude of error increase learning? Research technology has been used to manipulate performance environments and feedback to magnify errors for reaching and stepping tasks in efforts to enhance learning. This treatment paradigm is called *error augmentation* or *error enhancement*. Results to date have been mixed, with improvements demonstrating surprising capacity for adaptation despite neurological deficit, but they are only of modest duration and have limited carryover.[44-49]

Massed vs. Distributed Practice = Work-to-Rest Ratio

Massed practice refers to "a sequence of practice and rest times in which the rest time is much less than the practice time."[5(p497)] *Distributed practice* refers to "a sequence of practice and rest periods in which the practice time is often equal to or less than the time at rest."[5(p494)] Although learning occurs with both, distributed practice can result in better learning per training time depending on the type of skill, but the total session time is increased, creating a dilemma for therapists. Rest breaks provide an opportunity to self-evaluate, debrief with the therapist, and recharge physically and emotionally for subsequent attempts. Robust evidence indicates that high repetition and intensity are needed to drive neuroplasticity for motor learning, yet episodes of care reflect decreasing lengths of stay and dwindling therapy visits. Fatigue contributes to deterioration in performance and potential risk, but it does not necessarily interfere with learning. It is also a significant factor for many patients, who need to learn to manage it. Central or neuromuscular fatigue does require some special consideration and is addressed in the "Intervention" section of this chapter.

Blocked vs. Random Practice = Different Skills Practice

Typically, a variety of skills are practiced within a training session. For example, a typical therapy session may include transfers, walking, stairs, and balance tasks. *Blocked practice* (also called *drills*) refers to "a practice sequence in which all of the trials on one task are done together, uninterrupted by practice on any of the other tasks."[5(p493)] Blocked practice allows small trial-to-trial adjustments for rapid performance improvement within a session. It is helpful for new learners who are just trying to get the basics down and learn the relationship between performance adjustments and outcome effects. However, retention of performance improvement is limited in later learning stages because less cognitive processing is required.

Random practice refers to "a practice sequence in which the tasks being practiced are ordered randomly across trials."[5(p498)] The constant changing of tasks provides high *contextual interference* when switching from one activity to another by forcing the learner to forget what they just did when they move on to the next skill. When returning to the first skill later, they must actively retrieve it from the memory stores. This recall process increases the depth of cognitive processing and can be applied to other task variations or environments. Although improvements are seen with both practice schedules, random practice has been shown to have superior long-term retention effects despite an initial delay in acquisition compared to blocked practice.[50–52]

Constant vs. Variable Practice = Same Skill Practice

Another consideration for task practice is whether to change the task demands or environment *of a particular skill* across practice trials. *Constant practice* means the task is practiced the same way every time. This is appropriate for a closed skill performed in a closed environment where nothing changes, like a toilet or tub transfer in the patient's home. However, many skills are performed under different circumstances, requiring adaptation based on appropriate assessment of the new situation. *Adaptation* requires movement calibration for novel situations, incorporating modifiability into performance.[25] Open tasks and environments and closed tasks where the set up may be different each time (*intertrial variability*) require *variable practice*. Changing key features can subtly alter task demands, requiring accurate perception and adjustments necessary for success each time.

Mental Practice

Mental practice is "a practice method in which task performance is imagined or visualized without overt physical practice."[5(p497)] The mirror neuron system activates underlying motor programs for movement at a subthreshold level. Mental practice has consistently been found to facilitate the acquisition of motor skills.[53–57] When combined with physical practice, mental practice has been shown to increase the accuracy and efficiency of movements at significantly faster rates than physical practice alone.[58] It may be particularly useful for patients who fatigue easily, and it is also effective in alleviating anxiety associated with early practice. It can be done during rest breaks and as part of an HEP but should not be prioritized over physical practice. It is effective only if the patient has some idea of the movement to begin with. And it may be ineffective in patients with profound cognitive, communication, and/or perceptual deficits.

Part Task Practice

Complex motor skills are often modified or broken down into component parts for practice, but the benefit of doing this depends on the type of skill. Practice of *lead-up* or preparation activities has been commonly used in physical therapy to prepare learners for a more complex activity.[5(p496)] Typically, the subtasks involve performing movement components in easier postures with fewer DOF, such as practicing activities in kneeling, half-kneeling, or plantigrade before standing. However, part task practice is most effective with *serial* skills that have highly independent parts, such as wheelchair setup for a transfer, dressing, or getting up from the floor. It is not as effective for continuous movement tasks (e.g., walking) or for complex discrete tasks with highly coordinated, integrated parts that require spatial and temporal sequencing of elements. Parts must be integrated into the *whole task* so that the learner develops the complete movement plan; delaying this practice can interfere with transfer effects and learning.[5] However, task performance is often not simply a sum of its component parts, so carryover from part to whole task performance may be limited.

Simplification

An alternative to part task training is task simplification, which involves practicing an easier, scaled-back version of a skill while keeping its basic structure, allowing for *whole task* training in *early learning* but with less demand or complexity.[6] Typically, it involves external control of some DOF such as providing postural support with a device or harness, or reducing the timing or instability component of an open task such as propping open a swing-shut door, or adding training wheels to a bike. However, some of these changes may inherently change the task demands, reinforcing a different strategy for success. For example, the therapist can facilitate forward weight shift for sit-to-stand by encouraging the patient to reach forward with clasped hands, which precludes a trunk rocking, a momentum strategy to load the feet prior to rising.

Transfer of Training/Generalizability

Carryover of performance beyond the PT session is both a goal of practice and a strategy used to assess for motor learning. Logic suggests that foundational building blocks of movement at the body structure and function level of the ICF model (strength, flexibility, tone, coordination) are necessary to meet the requirements for skilled performance; without them, the movement changes. As such, rehab typically focuses on addressing these missing movement components with impairment-based treatment for restoration or compensation of function. Similarly, the maturational stages of motor development reflect a progression of increasingly complex upright movements as a hierarchy from easy to hard, which has also encouraged clinical practice to start with lower-level lead-up activities prior to full task practice. However, research suggests that these approaches of working from easy to hard or complex often do not optimize recovery and function or reduce well-learned compensatory behaviors.[59–61]

For example, leg strength has a nonlinear relationship to walking velocity after stroke; it seems to be a threshold phenomenon: once an adequate level is reached, additional strength gains may not further increase function.[19] Adding strength training to body weight support treadmill training did not improve leg strength in the Step Training Effectiveness Post Stroke (STEPS) study[62] (see Table 10.9 later in the chapter). Emerging research on high-intensity step training[63] actually found a *reverse transfer* effect from a high-level, difficult task (intensive gait training) to easier untrained tasks, including static balance measured by the Berg Balance Scale and leg strength assessed by the Five Times Sit to Stand test. These principles of practice organization and strategies are summarized in Table 10.4.

Feedback: Mode, Intensity, and Scheduling

The vast body of motor learning literature affirms the critical role of feedback in promoting motor learning. Clinical decisions about feedback include the following issues:

- What *type* of feedback should be employed (*mode*)?
- *How much* feedback should be used (*intensity*)?
- *When* should feedback be given (*scheduling*)?

Feedback Mode = Type to Give

Intrinsic feedback is the information provided by the body's own sensory systems. *Extrinsic* or *augmented* feedback is supplemental performance information that comes from external sources such as sensors,

Table 10.4	Practice Parameters	
Practice Organization		
Work-to-rest ratio	Massed practice	Practice time is greater than rest • More reps of practice in each session period • Risk of overwork, mindless repetition
	Distributed practice	Rest time is greater than practice • More time to reflect, maintain performance quality • Less time on task
Sequence of multiple skills to practice in a session	Blocked practice	A practice sequence organized for individual tasks to be performed repeatedly before moving on to the next task (e.g., AAAABBBBCCCC), also known as "drills." Can be hybrid serial blocks (e.g., ABCABCABC). • Appropriate for *new or cognitively impaired* learners and *closed* skills.
	Random practice	A practice sequence in which a variety of tasks are ordered randomly within the practice session (e.g., ABCBCBAAC). Provides *contextual interference*. • Appropriate for *advanced* learners.
Practice of single skill	Constant practice	Practicing the same skill, the same way every time (i.e., sit to stand from the wheelchair only). • Appropriate for new learners and closed skills.
	Variable practice	Practicing the same skill differently by changing aspects of the task or performance goals (i.e., sit to stand from the toilet, bed, car, bench, holding a tray). • Appropriate for *advanced* learners, *open* skills, or those with *intertrial variability*.
Practice Strategies		
	Mental practice	A practice strategy in which performance of the motor task is imagined or visualized without overt physical practice.
	Part vs. whole task practice	Component parts of a task are practiced before practice of the whole task. Works best for serial tasks; less evidence supporting use with continuous or discrete tasks. Simplification (below) may be better.
	Simplification	Easier versions of the whole task are practiced, for example, slower movement, BWS provided, remove secondary task; preserves the dynamics of continuous motions that may be disrupted with part task training.
	Transfer of training	Carryover/generalizability of performance to other task situations or versions of the movement in each skill category.

BWS = body weight support.

timers, video, wearable technology, therapist cues, etc. Augmented feedback can help the learner make associations between movement parameters and resulting action.[5] Information about the nature of the movement *outcome* in relation to the goal is considered *knowledge of results* (KR). Information about the nature or quality of the movement *pattern* is *knowledge of performance* (KP).[5] Although both are important, the relative usefulness of KP and KR can vary according to the skill being learned and the availability of feedback from intrinsic sources.[64-68] For example, precision tasks are highly dependent on focused attention for intrinsic visual and kinesthetic feedback (KP). In gross motor tasks, which tend to be more automatic and outcome-focused, KR provides key information about how to shape the overall movement. Performance cues (KP) should focus on key task elements and regulatory features for success.

Therapist's cues and performance feedback primarily tend to be in regard to quality of movement (KP), which encourages patients to develop an *internal* focus of attention on their body and how it is moving. Such direct cognitive oversight of specific performance parameters represents the cognitive stage of learning. However, complex skills are organized around movement goals or schema, which suggests attention should ultimately be focused *externally* on the goal and the movement outcome (KR). Research suggests that encouraging patient focus on intrinsic KP information may actually interfere with the development of autonomous performance.[69,70] This distinction and examples are highlighted in the "Interventions" section.

Feedback Intensity = How Much to Give

Frequent augmented feedback (e.g., given after every trial = 100%) quickly guides the learner to improved performance during practice but slows retention and overall learning by fostering dependence on the external source if maintained beyond the initial cognitive stage. Conversely, intermittent feedback may slow initial skill acquisition, but improves retention.[71-75] This is most likely due to the increased depth of cognitive processing involved in self-assessment and interpreting performance. Patients in the cognitive stage need more frequent feedback while initially getting the idea of the movement, but it should be gradually reduced by the associative stage. A faded frequency schedule that decreases the amount of feedback with improving performance is ideal for most patients. It can be tailored to the patient's specific performance using a bandwidth approach in which feedback is provided only when performance falls outside an acceptable target range (see Table 10.4).

Feedback Scheduling = When to Give

Feedback takes time to process. Inexperienced individuals perform better during both practice and retention if they are initially given more immediate feedback. However, as a learner improves, optimal learning occurs when feedback is delayed.[43] Care must be taken by the therapist not to preclude the patient's own information processing when giving feedback.[76,77] Winstein[78] points out that this provision of immediate feedback may explain why many studies on the effectiveness of therapeutic approaches cite minimal carryover and limited retention of newly acquired motor skills. It may also contribute to the benefit seen with distributed over massed practice studies. Interestingly, most augmented feedback technology provides 100% immediate, extrinsic feedback despite evidence that less feedback enhances learning. Table 10.5 summarizes the types and uses of augmented feedback.

Patient Populations: Special Considerations for Learning

Early learners struggle to deal with multiple task elements, so they may initially need part-task or simplified whole-task practice, reduced practice variability (blocked, constant), and more frequent, immediate, shorter summary KR.[42] Based on the neural networks associated with acquisition and consolidation of procedural information, it is not surprising that certain patient populations have impairments in particular aspects of motor skill learning.[79] Therefore, some patient populations may benefit from exceptions to the skill progressions discussed above. For example, patients with basal ganglia stroke have difficulty with *implicit* motor learning sequences,[80] and PD is associated with reduced cognitive flexibility, efficiency, and increased context-specificity of motor learning.[81] Traumatic brain injury (TBI) and stroke also interfere with acquisition and retention of new information through explicit learning much more significantly than implicit procedural learning.[82] In fact, providing explicit instructions may even interfere with implicit motor learning.[83] These individuals also learn best by doing, and they may benefit from errorless learning when deficits are severe.[82] Cerebellar lesions interfere with *adaptation*.[25] People with Alzheimer disease (AD) remain visually dependent for training and performance, but they can still learn implicitly through repeated exposure under constant, blocked practice conditions.[84] Minimal interference paradigms (errorless learning) have been successfully applied to memory-impaired populations, including patients with anterograde amnesia and mild cognitive impairment, patients with mild to moderate AD, and healthy older adults.[39] Even spinal cord activity can adapt with practice.[85]

Table 10.5   Feedback

Mode (type) = what?	Intrinsic vs. extrinsic	Intrinsic: one's own *internal* sensory feedback Extrinsic: supplemental, *augmented* feedback from outside sources, including therapist cues
	KP vs. KR	KP: quality of movement; kinematics, biomechanics KR: outcome of movement; results such as speed, number of errors, etc.
Scheduling (timing) = when?	*Before* movement	Preteaching or priming: cuing for set up, anticipating key features of movement; especially important for fast, open tasks.
	During movement	Concurrent feedback: *augmented* KP information is provided during closed or continuous tasks. Use with caution: patient is also getting intrinsic feedback that they should attend to. Highlight information not readily available or needed for active problem-solving.
	After movement completion: immediate vs. delayed feedback	Feedback given after a *brief delay* allows the learner time for *self-assessment*. Immediate feedback from the therapist can interfere with this process, degrading learning and leading to dependence on the therapist for performance appraisal.
Intensity (amount) = how much/how often?	Frequency: 100% = every trial; 50% = every other trial; 25% = every fourth trial	New learners (cognitive stage) need more frequent feedback, close to 100% initially, but feedback should decrease as the learner improves (autonomous stage). *Faded frequency:* Schedule over time.
	Bandwidth KR feedback	Feedback given only when performance deviates outside the boundaries of correct performance; error range is predetermined by therapist. Provides a *natural faded frequency* schedule based on individual performance.
	Average/Summary feedback	Feedback given after a set number of trials (e.g., after every second trial or every fifth or every 20th trial). It can be about each trial (summary) or an overview of performance (average). Both create a *natural delay* in providing feedback but still can give feedback about all trials.

KP = knowledge of performance; KR = knowledge of results.

■ INTERVENTIONS TO IMPROVE MOTOR FUNCTION

Neurorehabilitation for the management of patients with disorders of motor function is evolving over time. Clinicians need to keep abreast with evidence-based research that updates and validates therapeutic interventions. A growing number of *Clinical Practice Guidelines* on specific topics are available through the specialty sections and academies within the American Physical Therapy Association[86] to help summarize the research and provide action items for implementation.

An important aspect of clinical decision-making, especially for individuals with neurologic deficits, is determining the time course and level of recovery that is possible. For degenerative disorders, therapy may only slow the decline; acute lesions may stabilize but never return to baseline. A key role of the therapist is to determine whether to focus on *recovery of normal function* or to teach *compensation* for a permanent loss for setting appropriate goals and optimizing limited therapy time.[87,88] Therapy goals should be measurable and functionally relevant, providing a roadmap and timeline for the POC. General health status and prognosis inform treatment frequency, intensity, and duration decisions for short- and long-term goals. When possible, standardized *outcome measures* should be used to create goals incorporating minimal detectible change (MCD) or minimal clinically important difference (MCID) values to reflect objective, meaningful improvement. See Table 10.6 for examples with categories adapted from the *Guide to Physical Therapist Practice 3.0*[2] and

Table 10.6   Measuring Outcomes and Writing Objective Goals

Category	Outcome Measure Examples	Samples of Goals
Pathology or Health Condition	• General Health Questionnaire • Modified Cumulative Illness Rating • Brief Symptom Inventory–18 • NIHSS	Global health measures used to represent long-term goal of improving, maintaining, or slowing decline of health condition (physician over therapist focus) • NIHSS score less than 14 to qualify for inpatient rehabilitation admission
Impairments in body functions and structures	• ROM • MMT • MAS • MMSE • CTSIB • Five Times Sit to Stand	Whenever possible, *write goals related to the activities* on which these limitations impact rather than just change in MMT or ROM measurements • Increase from 7–10 sit-to-stand reps in 30 sec, which reflects functional leg-strength improvement (MCID +2.)
Activity limitations	• BBS • FGA • ABC • 10MWT	*Time* functional tasks **Speed:** More skillful, efficient performance is faster • *Supine to stand in less than 12 sec (normative data)* **Endurance:** longer sustained activity • *Client will walk >50 ft farther (MCID) during a 6MWT to allow her to get her mail*
Participation restrictions	• Physical Activity Scale for the Elderly • SIS • DHI • ABC	Accuracy: reduce object collisions, acquire more challenging targets during reaching or stepping. Consistency = number or percentage of successful trials • *Reduce number of steps with knee hyperextension from 50%–10%* • *Only one cue needed to reach back to sit 4/5 trials, three visits in a row*
Risk reduction/ prevention	• BBS • FES • DGI	• BBS score less than 45 for reduced *risk of falling* • Independent w/*pressure reliefs* • Independently initiates leg exercises prior to rising to prevent *orthostatic blood pressure*
Health, wellness, and fitness	• Geriatric Depression Scale • Assessment of Life Habits • FIS	*Fitness tracker* data can be used to set goals and measure progress (steps, time, heart rate, oxygen saturation) *More time* spent in personal, social, or work activities. • *PT fatigue score will reflect a 20% reduction in symptoms affecting ADL performance (MCID)*
Patient or client satisfaction	• Satisfaction with Life Scale • Goal Attainment Scale • Life Satisfaction Questionnaire 9	Improved *self-report*/rating based on MCD/MCID score • *PDQ-39 score for mobility section will improve less than 12 points (MCD) reflecting true change in QOL.*

ABC = Activity Balance Confidence; ADL = activities of daily living; BBS = Berg Balance Scale; CTSIB = Clinical Test of Sensory Integration in Balance; DGI = Dynamic Gait Index; DHI = Dizziness Handicap Index; FES = Falls Efficacy Scale; FGA = Functional Gait Assessment; FIS = Fatigue Impact Scale; MCID = minimal clinically important difference; MAS = Modified Ashworth Scale; MDC = minimal detectible change; MMT = manual muscle testing; NIHSS = National Institute of Health Stroke Scale;; PDQ-39 = Parkinson's Disease Quotient; QOL = quality of life; ROM = range of motion; SIS = Stroke Impact Scale; 6MWT = 6-minute Walk Test; 10MWT = 10-meter Walk Test.

outcome measures from the Rehabilitation Measures Database–Shirly Ryan Ability Lab.[89]

The rest of this chapter organizes intervention targets by individual, task, and environmental considerations, with additional sections on technology and patient education. While there are some overlapping concepts, the framework ensures that therapists consider all aspects contributing to function and provides breadth and depth for the development of therapeutic exercise and progression. See Table 10.7 for an overview with examples.

Table 10.7   Interventions to Improve Motor Control

INDIVIDUAL: Body Structure and Function
What does the patient have to work with and what are their limitations?

Musculoskeletal	Improve capacity: *strength, flexibility, ROM,* as much as possible within the limitations of their health condition (see text). If return to "normal" is not possible, explore alternative, *compensatory* movement strategies. *Prevent* secondary complications from inactivity.
Neuromuscular	Drive *neuroplasticity* with *intense, repetitive, meaningful* activity. Incorporate coordination challenges that include appropriate *timing, sequencing, and power* production within tasks (see below). Manage *spasticity* if limiting active movement through PROM/stretching, reciprocal inhibition, or medication through physician.
Cognitive/Perceptual	(Chapter 27) Structure environment, tasks (see below) and practice (see text) based on *stage of learning. Attention, perception, and prediction* are key abilities for learning and improving motor skills. When necessary, provide *compensatory or substitution* strategies such as using other sensory systems, scanning, verbalization, and supplemental cues feedback, and memory aids such as setting reminders, written instructions, etc.
Cardiopulmonary	(Chapters 12 and 13) Incorporate *physical and aerobic exercise* and the *ACSM guidelines.*
Integumentary	(Chapter 14) *Monitor* skin in individuals with mobility limitations. *Prevent* secondary complications by addressing pressure relief, circulation, skin care.
Behavioral/Psychosocial	(Chapters 19 and 26) Frame therapy sessions to enhance *motivation, autonomy, and expectation of success* as they are strongly associated with improved outcomes. Refer the patient when mood or psychological or social barriers interfere with participation.

TASK: Activity
What is required for success (regulatory features)?

Stability and Mobility	*Static* balance: maintaining steady COM within BOS • Progress from large BOS and low COM (4 point, sitting) → smaller BOS and higher COM (standing, tandem stand, SLS) • Add UE movement, external perturbation, unstable surface, close eyes, dual task *Dynamic* balance: moving COM over BOS (weight shifts) • Same positions and progressions as above • Reaching close vs. far, overhead or to the floor, planar vs. rotation • Stand → squat or up on toes *Mobility = Moving BOS:* transitions (coming to sit, standing up, walking), locomotion • supine → sit; sit → stand; floor → chair or stand • walking, multidirectional stepping, running, stairs
Open vs. closed	Identify the *regulatory features* needed and *affordances* available to perform the activity. Is this a *self-paced (closed)* or *externally paced (open)* activity? Therapist cues the *new learner,* more advanced should self-identify. • Transfers: Recognize surface height and if armrest or rails available, identify proper alignment for initial set up (scoot forward, feet back), initiate timing and sequencing of body segments to bring COM forward (trunk forward via hip flex), then up (hip and knee extended). *Progressing* task challenge can include interacting with moving, changing, or unstable objects (externally paced). • Kick a stationary ball → kick a rolling ball. • Hold/carry an empty cup → half full → full cup without spilling.

(Continued)

Table 10.7	Interventions to Improve Motor Control—cont'd
TASK: Activity *What is required for success (regulatory features)?*	
Object Manipulation	Typically requires conscious *attention* and can be used to create *dual task* challenges if performed as part of a stability or mobility activity. *New learners* should explore the object's properties in a low demand posture, but progress to more challenging situations: • Add postural challenge as above: manipulate in supported sitting → unsupported sitting → standing → tandem/on foam → walking • Progress object features/complexity: wheeled walker vs. standard walker vs. crutches; gross vs. fine motor; one vs. two hands needed
Level of Challenge	Adjust the *challenge pressure* for optimal effort: consider time constraints, DOF, postural control demands, simplification, or part task training. For new learners • Control some DOF: Bracing for foot or wrist drop, work in easier postures such as sitting, tall kneeling, or allowing UE support • Modify postural demands with support (manual, harness, device) • Break up serial skills to work on individual components (floor transfer). To *advance performance,* increase complexity, postural challenge, or pressure by incorporating more DOF, adding a secondary task or high-stakes goal/reward • Crossing the street before the light changes • Will be safe and independent to live alone
ENVIRONMENT: Participation *What is going on around the patient during performance?* *What is available to use (affordances)?*	
Open vs. Closed	Similar considerations for open vs. closed tasks. • *New learners:* quiet space, limit distractions • *Advancing performance:* add activity to the surroundings during task performance that may be *distracting,* then add components that may *interfere* with performance. Environmental monitoring as a component of *dual task:* walking or propelling in empty hall → busy hall or cafeteria → include route finding or attending to signage.

ACSM = American College of Sports Medicine; BOS = base of support; COM = center of mass; DOF = degrees of freedom; PROM = passive range of motion; ROM = range of motion; UE = upper extremity.

Individual: Body Structure and Function

This section addresses building an individual's *capacity* for improved motor performance with impairment-specific interventions. The top section of Table 10.7 briefly summarizes the primary concerns for each major body system, but rehabilitation practices for all are best addressed within the context of functional activities whenever possible. Using body structure, function evaluation, and task analysis (see Chapter 5), the therapist hypothesizes links between impairments and limitations in functional performance. The therapist also needs to determine whether the impairments can be remediated by therapy or if compensatory strategies are indicated. It is important to remember that resolution of impairment may not yield the desired improvement in functional performance without specific task practice.

Interventions to Improve Flexibility

Joint ROM and muscle flexibility must be adequate to allow for normal functional excursions of muscle and biomechanical alignment. Many factors may contribute to limitations in available range, including prolonged periods of disuse or immobility or changes in neuromusculoskeletal health. Proactive preventive measures are often necessary to maintain joint and tissue flexibility for positioning and functional mobility, maintain good circulation for tissue health, and prevent or reduce pain. Preventive measures include ROM exercises and stretching, with active modes providing the added benefits of incorporating autonomy, self-efficacy, muscle recruitment, and reciprocal inhibition. For details on how to perform ROM, stretching, and joint mobilization techniques, see *Therapeutic Exercise* by Kisner and Colby.[90] Limitations in range due to contracture likely require low-load prolonged stretching through dynamic or adjustable splinting, serial casting, or possible surgical procedures for tendon lengthening or releases.[91–93]

A warm-up period of exercise, such as calisthenics, walking, or easy cycling, or preliminary therapeutic heat modality increases muscle temperature, elasticity, and collagen extensibility, enhancing the safety of stretching. Cold modalities may decrease muscle spasm and pain if they are limiting motion.

If spasticity is a limiting factor, passive ROM (PROM) can provide temporary reduction in passive resistance, which may be helpful for applying bracing or improving positioning. Functional electrical stimulation (FES) cycling has been shown to temporarily reduce spasticity.[94] Proprioceptive neuromuscular facilitation (PNF) techniques of hold-relax; contract-relax; and contract-relax, agonist-contract utilize spindle and/or Golgi tendon organ input to reduce muscle overactivity to increase range.[95,96] Botox injections are quite effective for reducing focal spasticity for a few months, but they need to be repeated and have dosing limitations. Oral medications such as baclofen can address spasticity systemically but may have undesirable central nervous system (CNS) side effects, particularly drowsiness. Baclofen can also be provided directly to the spinal cord with an intrathecal pump, significantly reducing the dosing and CNS side effects but adding risks associated with an implantable drug delivery system.[97]

Interventions to Improve Strength, Power, and Endurance

Muscle strength is the "force exerted by a muscle or a group of muscles." *Muscle power* is "the work produced per unit of time or the product of strength and speed." *Muscle endurance* is "the ability to sustain forces repeatedly or to generate forces over a period of time."[2] Muscle performance is regulated by biomechanical and physiological factors. Biomechanical factors include initial muscle length and tension, moment arm, muscle fiber composition, fuel storage and delivery, and speed and type of contraction. Neuromuscular factors include motor unit recruitment (number, type), motor neuron firing patterns, and efficiency of cooperative synergistic patterns. Techniques that optimize these factors while addressing specific impairments and the demands of the task will yield maximum functional outcomes.

Strength Training

The effectiveness of strength training depends on achieving an adequate training stimulus and the generalizability of the improvements in force production to functional applications. *Isometric* holding contractions are used for stability and maintaining positions against external perturbations like gravity, centripetal forces, etc., while *concentric* (shortening) and *eccentric*

(lengthening) contractions help initiate and control the movement of body segments. The mode or type of exercise reflects specific features of performance. In *open chain* movements, the distal segment (hand, foot) moves freely, while in a *closed chain* movement, the distal segment is fixed, often as part of the base of support (BOS), while the proximal segment moves over it. *Plyometrics* focus on building power through high-intensity skills requiring speed and explosive force production. *Interval training* targets specific work-to-rest ratios to maintain a level of intensity to build endurance. *Circuit training* involves brief bouts of different activities targeting multiple muscle groups within a practice session.

While there are many ways to load muscles, the point of peak resistance generation depends on the properties of the load. *Elastic* loads, like elastic bands or springs, provide increasing resistance as the material is stretched, resulting in the highest force at the end of the motion where the muscle is the shortest. The *viscous* resistance of water depends on movement velocity, where faster movement creates higher resistance but is the same throughout the movement if the speed is constant. *Inertial* loads, like free weights, medicine balls, and kettle bells, initially require higher force to start, often with less force during the movement due to momentum. Typically an antagonistic force is required to stop the movement, depending on movement speed and relationship to gravity.[98] *Manual* resistance can be modulated to match variable performance throughout the movement, but it is difficult to objectively report. *Intensity* is often determined as a percentage of 1 repetition maximum (rep max) force (1RM), the total number of repetitions one is able to perform, or the amount of time spent on an exercise. Resistance is typically 60% to 80% 1 rep max, but very weak individuals can start at ~50% 1RM and do fewer reps. Perception of effort should feel like 8 out of 10 difficulty where 10 is the hardest effort you can give; the last rep should be difficult to complete. Intensity should be reduced if there is a sudden onset of fatigue/exhaustion or prolonged and severe delayed onset muscle soreness. *Good exercise practice* includes a brief warm-up and cool-down period, controlled performance without Valsalva, and consideration of medications and other health conditions on exercise tolerance. For more details on strength training, see Kisner and Colby.[90] Resistive strengthening for individuals with profound weakness (manual muscle test [MMT] = < 3/5) is not indicated, but active assisted ROM may be appropriate. Guidelines for strength training are presented in Table 10.8, with asterisks denoting the 2019 American College of Sports Medicine's (ACSM) recommendations for resistance training for health[99] and hashtags denoting ACSM's 2016

Table 10.8 Guidelines for Strength Training

Determine	Parameters of Exercise
Type of contraction	• Concentric, eccentric, isometric
Mode of exercise	• **Open chain:** distal segment moves freely (barbells, kettlebells) • **Closed chain:** distal segment fixed, weight-bearing exercises (e.g., step-ups, squats, planks) • **Stability:** maintaining a position–co-contraction (e.g., body blades, PNF's rhythmic stabilization) • **Plyometrics:** using speed and force of high-intensity skill movements to build power (jumping, pushups, kicking, throwing) • **Interval training:** specific work-to-rest ratio; can be done with any type of resistance* (more cardio focus) • **Circuit training:** shifting between exercises (more musculoskeletal focus)
Type of resistance	• **Elastic** loads: resistance increases with excursion–elastic bands or tubing, Bowflex machine • **Inertial** loads: resistance to start and stop motion depending on orientation to gravity–free weights, medicine balls, kettle bells • **Viscous** loads: resistance increases with movement speed–water, hydraulic machines • **Manual** resistance: modulated to patient performance
Intensity	• Resistance is typically 60%–80% 1RM but very weak individuals can start at 50% 1RM and do fewer reps. • Resistance should feel like 8 out of 10 difficulty where 10 is the hardest effort you can give; the last rep should be difficult to complete.* • Reduce intensity if sudden onset of fatigue/exhaustion or prolonged and severe delayed onset muscle soreness.
Repetitions	• Initial frequency is typically 2–3 sets of 8–12 reps each as tolerated* • Chronic disease: One set 8–12 reps
Exercise Duration and Frequency	• Total training time: ~15–30 minutes per session or as tolerated or 8–10 multijoint exercises that stress the targeted muscle groups* • Typically 2–3 days/week, depending on intensity and level of impairment/disease*#
Warm-up and cool-down	• Include 5–10 min of warm-ups (calisthenics, stretching, ROM exercises) and 5–10 min of cool-down (muscle relaxation, stretching). • RPE <3/10 for 10–15 min in chronic conditions#
Additional considerations	• Exercises should be performed in a controlled manner: 2 sec each up and down* • Regular breathing pattern should be maintained, while avoiding straining/Valsalva. • Consider the interactions of exercise and medications. • Resistive exercise is contraindicated with muscle grades less than 3/5.
Outcomes	• Focus on *function* for goals and performance assessment—don't assume increasing weights or reps automatically improves task performance

PNF = proprioceptive neuromuscular facilitation; RM = rep max; RPE = rate of perceived exertion.
*ACSM 2019 Recommendations for Resistance Training for Health and Fitness[98]
#ACSM 2016 Exercise Management for Persons with Chronic Diseases & Disability Basic Recommendations.[99]

recommendations for exercise management for persons with chronic diseases and disability.[100]

Electromyographic Biofeedback

For patients with severe weakness, surface electromyographic biofeedback (EMG-BFB) has been used to assist in neuromuscular recruitment and re-education. The EMG signal is amplified and converted to audio and/or visual form, providing information about muscular activity, although not force.[101] The majority of research focuses on the effects of biofeedback in stroke, with EMG-BFB shown to improve both UE (upper extremity; hand and shoulder)[102–104] and leg function.[105–107] Patients who exhibit weak (trace, poor, or fair) muscle grades or deficient sensory feedback systems will benefit the most. In a Cochrane Review of the effects of EMG-BFB for motor function recovery following stroke (13 trials, 269 participants), Woodford et al. concluded that EMG-BFB plus standard physical therapy produced improvements in motor power, functional recovery, and gait quality when compared to standard physical therapy alone, although the trials were small, generally poorly designed, and utilized varying outcome measures.[108] The therapist must carefully structure the use of biofeedback with active task practice. Such augmented feedback focusing on muscle activity must transition to active movement monitoring as recovery progresses.

Typically, maximum strength is not required for most activities; "functional" strength implies it is adequate to perform most daily activities. Interactions with real loads in real environmental situations are relevant and therefore meaningful. Consider manipulating the task and environmental demands to progress functional strength training. The neuromuscular system is wired for muscles to work in synergy, automatically, with sensory inputs linked to perception and performance. Consider cross-training for transference and adaptability.

Neuromuscular Endurance and Fatigue

Patients with deconditioning and deficits in motor function may demonstrate poor muscular endurance and fatigue. *Fatigue* is the inability to contract muscle repeatedly or sustain activity over time. Debilitating fatigue can arise from neuromuscular disease affecting the CNS as in multiple sclerosis, the peripheral nerves as in Guillain-Barré syndrome, or the neuromuscular junction as in myasthenia gravis. The Fatigue Scale for Motor and Cognitive Function[89] is a standardized measure with good psychometric properties. It is designed to assess the effects of fatigue in people with MS and can be used for assessment and goal setting. The challenge of exercise training with these patients is the risk of *acute exercise overdose*, producing exhaustion and possible injury. *Overuse weakness* is often seen in these patients and presents as prolonged weakness and fatigue following rigorous exercise; the patient does not recover with rest. The patient may be unable to get out of bed the next day or perform their normal activities of daily living (ADL). *Overtraining*, resulting from chronic overdosing of exercise, is associated with both psychological and physiological decompensation, as well as musculoskeletal injury. Even a simple conditioning program should be personalized, carefully monitored, and progressed slowly to avoid overexertion and injury.[100]

ACSM's Exercise Management for Persons with Chronic Diseases and Disabilities, 4th edition, is particularly helpful for therapists, as it discusses exercise guidelines for several different disease categories including cardiovascular, cancer, pulmonary, neuromuscular, immunological, and others.[100] Patients with chronic or central fatigue may require a discontinuous exercise protocol that carefully balances exercise with rest, like performing multiple 10-minute sessions throughout the day to achieve the total target time. Effective management includes the implementation of ergonomic changes and energy conservation techniques like sitting for meal preparation, using precut vegetables, pacing activity, implementing lifestyle changes, planning regular rest

periods, and getting good sleep. An activity log can be used to help the patient identify activities that are particularly exhausting as well as the effectiveness of rest. Patients can monitor their level of general fatigue using Borg's Rating of Perceived Exertion (RPE) scale[109] and should aim to keep their exercise activities at an RPE level of "somewhat hard" (14 or lower using the 6 to 20 RPE scale). Additionally, stress management should be included in their educational program.

Aerobic Conditioning

Aerobic training produces positive changes in maximal oxygen uptake (VO_2 max) and metabolic changes to enhance endurance.[110,111] An aerobic training program is determined based on the patient's level of deconditioning and specific health condition and symptoms. Aerobic training can utilize ergometry (two-limb or four-limb), a recumbent stepper, elliptical, group exercise, aquatics, walking, and more. In general, moderate intensities of exercises have been recommended for most patients undergoing active rehabilitation or with a chronic disease and disabilities (e.g., 40% to 70% of maximal oxygen consumption, three to five times per week for 20- to 60-min per session) with high intensities considered to be contraindicated. However, this conservative approach may be underestimating people's capacity, resulting in *underdosing* our interventions and limiting recovery in patients with neurologic disorders. Holleran and colleagues compared high- (70% to 80% Heart Rate Reserve [HRR]) and low- (30% to 40% HRR) intensity gait training after stroke and found that not only were patients able to tolerate higher intensities of practice, but it was also associated with better outcomes.[112] Woodard et al. found that heart rate response during fast walking velocity resulted in higher cardiovascular response than during standard treatment, which was unrelated to level of disability.[113] They also found a high prevalence of cardiac abnormalities without clinical symptoms, reinforcing the need to monitor activity tolerance in our patients. The 2019 Aerobic Exercise Recommendations to Optimize Best Practices in Care After Stroke (AEROBICS) update[114] provides evidence-based recommendations for screening and providing aerobic exercise prescription after stroke. Also see Chapter 15, Stroke, and ACSM's *Exercise Management for Persons with Chronic Diseases and Disabilities* for more details.[100]

Aerobic training, as a method of *motor priming* prior to skills practice, can also aid in recovery of motor function and motor learning.[115] In 2013, Mang summarized evidence of exercise-induced release of BDNF involved in neuroprotection, neurogenesis, and angiogenesis.[116] In a 2016 Cochrane Database Systematic Review (58 trials, 2,797 patients), researchers found that cardiorespiratory training reduced disability during or after usual stroke care, including improvements in walking capacity, speed, and balance. They concluded that further trials were needed to investigate cognitive changes, optimal exercise prescription, and long-term benefits.[117]

Neuromuscular Reeducation Considerations

When patients present with significant deficits in muscle activation, therapists should consider optimizing biomechanical principles and techniques for enhancing recruitment. For example, place the limb in a *gravity-eliminated* position for MMT less than 3/5, like side-lying with the top leg on a powder board for active flexor and extensor exercise. Position the target muscle to maximize its *length-tension* relationship for the strongest contraction, like pulling the hip into full extension prior to active flex hip flexion in side-lying. Superficial muscles can be tapped or lightly resisted to facilitate contraction via supplemental sensory input.

Neuromuscular electrical stimulation uses surface electrodes to deliver high-intensity intermittent current to stimulate a contraction in neurologically intact muscles that might be weak from disuse or orthopedic conditions. FES uses a moderate intensity stimulation cycle with increasingly sophisticated microprocessors to recruit muscles in a preprogrammed synergistic sequence. Advancements in technology are driving the development of more complex training units with up to 12 EMG channels and a library of preprogrammed functional tasks with the appropriate timing and sequencing of the major muscles involved. In a 2021 systematic review, FES cycling exercise was found to improve lower body muscle health in adults with spinal cord injury (SCI) and may increase power output and aerobic fitness.[118] In contrast, a 2020 systematic review of FES in subacute stroke found no added benefit.[119] Other FES devices, called *neuroprosthetics*, are used to help restore muscle activity during specific functional tasks, like dorsiflexion during gait or wrist extension for grasp.[120,121] (See Chapter 15, Stroke; Chapter 16, Multiple Sclerosis; Chapter 19, Traumatic Brain Injury; and Chapter 20, Traumatic Spinal Cord Injury, for diagnosis-specific details.) Typically, techniques to stimulate or "jump-start" weak or poorly coordinated muscles should be reduced or transitioned once active movement emerges.

Interventions to Address Coordination

Coordination is the ability to execute quick, smooth, accurate, and controlled movements. Different aspects of coordination are impaired based on neurological lesion location and can include impaired timing or sequencing including co-contraction and ataxia, brady-, hypo-, and dyskinesia, and loss of fractionated (isolated) movement or the presence of stereotypic synergy.

Ataxia refers to an inability to coordinate muscles, joints, or limbs for smooth, accurate movement. It is typically the result of cerebellar disease, lesions to cerebellar pathways, or profound sensory loss. The reader is referred to Chapter 6 for the examination and associated impairments of the cerebellum. Patients with significant ataxia and postural instability often require hands-on support and assistive devices to ensure safety and prevent falls. Traditional therapy has focused on weighting of limbs and/or trunk for proprioceptive loading, with movements being performed slowly, reciprocally, and with supplemental feedback. More recently, however, interventions have shifted toward intense functional task training. In 2014, a systematic review of allied health interventions for ataxia concluded that despite a lack of high-quality studies (many were case reports), conventional physical therapy that focused on more than one domain may lead to improvements in symptoms and daily life functions.[122] Another systematic review of assessment and treatment of postural disorders in cerebellar ataxia found some benefit for virtual reality (VR), biofeedback, treadmill exercise with body weight support, and torso weighting, although the specific efficacy for torso weighting needed further investigation.[123] That same year, Bastian and Keller had 14 patients participate in a 6-week home balance exercise program that included progressive sitting and standing exercises 20 min/day for 4 to 6 days a week, which led to improved walking speed, Timed Up and Go (TUG), Dynamic Gait Index (DGI), and some gait kinematic parameters, with all improvements but the TUG remaining a month later. They concluded that the *level of challenge was more important than duration* of exercise in producing these positive effects.[124] A 2018 systematic review concluded that 4 weeks of inpatient rehabilitation improves ataxia and functional abilities for individuals with isolated degenerative ataxias, that adding pressure splints provides no additional benefit, and that there was not enough information to support or refute whole body vibration.[125]

Coordination deficits associated with *basal ganglia* disorders include slow, small movements labeled as brady- and hypokinesia, respectively. Treatment has increasingly focused on task training over impairment-based approaches. External cuing has long been used for brady- and hypokinesia and freezing episodes in gait. A 2018 narrative review of cuing for freezing of gait (FOG) supports immediate benefits of external cuing for FOG severity, gait parameters, and arm movements, but not long-term or transfer effects.[126] A 2020 systematic review and meta-analysis of PT treatment modalities for people with PD supports conventional physiotherapy to significantly improve motor symptoms, gait, and quality of life.[127] Interventions including resistance and treadmill training improved gait; strategy training improved gait and balance; dance, Nordic walking, martial arts, balance, and gait training all improved motor symptoms, balance, and gait, with dance also improving quality of life (QOL); hydrotherapy improved balance; and dual task training did not significantly improve any of the outcomes. For more details on specific PD interventions, see Chapter 18, Parkinson Disease.

Corticospinal impairments that impact coordination include weakness (poor motor recruitment) and the presence of stereotypic synergies. Traditional approaches like PNF and neurodevelopmental treatment have focused heavily on techniques to encourage normal, out-of-synergy patterns and reduce synergistic co-contraction, but there is little evidence supporting sustained improvement. Interventions incorporating strengthening to "overpower" synergy also have not been particularly effective.[128] Botox can effectively reduce spasticity's antagonistic resistance to weak muscles but does not address the inappropriate activation or timing of the agonist muscle itself. Spinal cord stimulation has had some limited success in reactivating remaining intact neural networks after SCI.[129,130] Multichannel FES systems (discussed above) and robotic systems offer opportunities to practice moving out of synergistic patterns in simulated tasks and games. For details of these and other treatment approaches, see Chapters 15, 16, 19, and 20.

Motor Control Considerations for Individuals

Treatment planning includes using system-based interventions discussed above to increase patients' capacity for better movement. The *hierarchical control model* reminds us that sensory/perceptual inputs are important triggers for and modifiers of movement and learning, particularly for slower movements and those controlled by central pattern generators. *Systems models* suggest learners need to learn relationships between movement planning and the outcomes produced, particularly for fast, feedforward, and automatic skill performance; mistakes are opportunities for learning. Regardless of the task or strategy, it is the therapist's first responsibility to assess learner's knowledge of the skill and identify the resources and barriers to performance.

Neuroplasticity principles outlined in Table 10.2 provide guidance to optimize practice for learning, which includes making *errors*, being *rewarded* with intermittent success, and making *associations* between perception, planning, and action. Set up patients for hard work and goal attainment by setting expectations (*priming*) of *effortful achievement* for positive change.[115,131] Engage the *mirror neuron* system through observational learning of skill demonstration and subsequent mental practice. Ensure *active engagement* through personal problem-solving, outcome monitoring, and self-reflection.[132] Provide activities that are personally meaningful (*salient*) to the patient, and ultimately practiced for hundreds to thousands of *repetitions* both during and outside of therapy.[133]

How do we keep people motivated to remain engaged in repetitive practice? The seminal theoretical review paper on Optimizing Performance Through Intrinsic Motivation and Attention for Learning (OPTIMAL) outlines a few key strategies based on decades of research.[134] This model suggests that action-specific perception helps individuals prepare for task performance. *Expectations* for success alert the dopamine system to anticipate a *reward*, influencing personal goals and effort expenditure. This *external focus* on movement outcome is critical since an internal self-focus can interfere with movement automaticity and limit learning. Performance success creates a positive feedback loop, encouraging higher expectations, increased *motivation*, and enhancing *self-efficacy*, which contribute to *consolidation* of learning, as illustrated in Figure 10.5.

Patient *autonomy* is supported by giving patients choices during therapy, such as the order of exercises, extent of practice/feedback, which piece of equipment to use, etc. Encourage attention to key *regulatory features* of the task and environment to prepare to move, and to evaluate the success of the patient's attempt. Data/scores from objective measures provide feedback

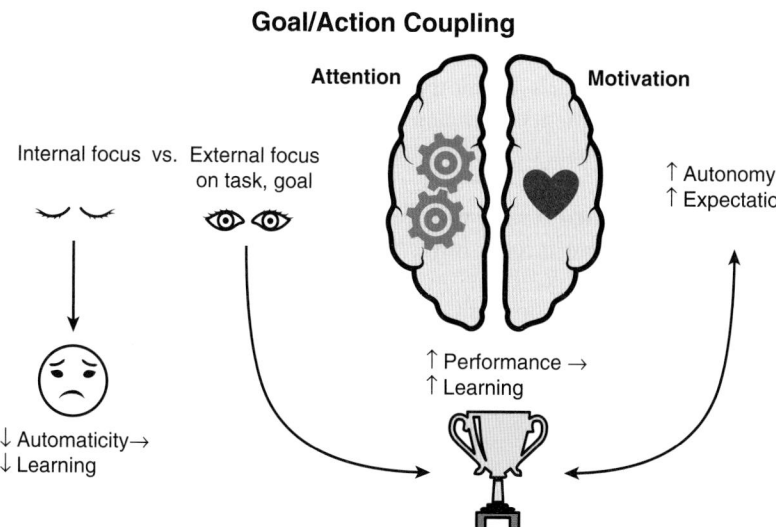

Goal/Action Coupling

Attention

Motivation

Internal focus vs. External focus on task, goal

↑ Autonomy →
↑ Expectations

↓ Automaticity→
↓ Learning

↑ Performance →
↑ Learning

Figure 10.5 Importance of motivation and attention for learning. The OPTIMAL theory of motor learning highlights motivational and attentional factors that link goals with actions, specifically an expectation of success and external focus for performance. *(Adapted from Wulf.)*[133]

that can be empowering and motivating. For example, in the International Stroke Inpatient Rehab with Reinforcement of Walking Speed (SIRROWS) study, individuals recovering from stroke who were given feedback on daily gait speed performance walked significantly faster at discharge and at 3 months postdischarge than did the control group who did not receive that feedback.[135] Progressing activity challenges helps develop functional variability, allowing patients to make appropriate adjustments for changing conditions. Variable practice also reduces attentional demands, speeds up learning, and facilitates automaticity over time.

How hard should patients be pushed? What is the appropriate balance between success and failure? Stress alerts the body to work harder and pay more attention, which improves performance. The frequency, intensity, time (duration), and type (FITT) *principle* (Chapter 1, Clinical Decision-Making, Box 1.7) has been used to help determine the appropriate level of frequency, intensity, time (duration), and type of intervention for traditional musculoskeletal exercise. However, the concept of intensity has evolved to have broader applications than just the number of repetitions or time on task. In addition to changing the cardiovascular or activity demands (harder, faster, more resistance), task difficulty can be increased by increasing the cognitive load (dual or multitasking, increasingly difficult targets or manipulation tasks), or incorporating additional pressures on performance (time limits, score attainment, critique by others). According to the *challenge point model*,[42] the therapist's goal is to set up "desirable difficulty" within task practice so that patients work hard for intermittent success. See Table 10.8 for examples of task considerations to match activities to a patient's current level of skill. A task that is too easy does not incentivize or drive change; one that is too difficult is overwhelming. Focusing on more challenging tasks also provides a potential *reverse transfer* benefit by also improving easier tasks that were not specifically practiced.

Acknowledgment of the patient's challenges and struggles reflects empathy, builds trust, and can increase the impact of positive feedback from success. Therapists should allow adequate time for patient self-reflection before providing feedback; active engagement in self-monitoring, problem identification, and generating solutions builds autonomy. Key questions to promote active decision-making and autonomy are presented in Box 10.1. The neuroplasticity principle of timing also cautions us to be mindful of *when* we are seeing our patients within their life span and episode of care. Evidence suggests that very early intense training after an acute brain lesion may increase vulnerability to additional damage, for example, within 24 hours after stroke[136] and during acute recovery from concussion.[137]

Motor Learning Considerations

New learners and individuals who are cognitively impaired are initially just trying to get the idea of a

---

Box 10.1   Key Questions to Promote Active Patient Decision-Making and Autonomy

- What is the goal of the intended movement?
- Did you accomplish the goal? If not, does the goal need to be modified?
- Did you move as planned? If not, what problems were encountered during the movement?
- What do you need to do to correct the problems in order to achieve movement success?
- For complex movements, what are the component parts or steps of the task? How should the component parts be sequenced?
- What aspects of the environment led to the success (or failure) of reaching the goal of the intended movement?
- What motivates you to keep trying?
- How confident are you in your abilities to move on your own? To be safe in your home and community environments?

---

new skill and are using a trial-and-error approach for developing movement strategies, making frequent and often large mistakes. The *therapist's role* is to facilitate task understanding through instruction and to organize early practice for optimal learning.

Instruction

Effective instruction typically involves demonstration with verbal cues that highlight regulatory features like object properties (dimensions, position, speed/trajectory of movement) and KR information regarding movement outcome. KP information about biomechanics (position, alignment, timing of body and movement segments) also helps clarify key set up and movement features necessary for success. Live or recorded demonstrations are internalized via the mirror neuron system. Skilled individuals with disabilities can serve as peer models to motivate and enhance self-efficacy in new patients. Developing a library of resources (websites, links, patient mentors) ensures availability and consistency of demonstration. Watching other patients working on similar skills within a clinic or therapy gym can also inform learning by illustrating common mistakes and fostering the patient's own problem-solving process to accomplish the desired outcome.[138]

Practice

The therapist's role in setting up therapy sessions is to establish safe yet challenging practice opportunities. Practice has a multitude of effects on behavior, including increasing the speed and efficiency of performance (skill), including reducing cognitive load by habituating successful motor behavior.[139] Initial *blocked, constant* practice is appropriate for early learning and closed skills. *Guided movement* involves physically assisting the learner through the activity and can have positive effects during the early period of skill acquisition.[140–142] Manual or robotic assistance allows the learner to identify the feedback associated with the movement, ensures safety to build confidence, and can simplify complex tasks by controlling some DOF. However, these supplemental inputs are also part of the perceptual experience, so they should be used sparingly. Manual guidance is most effective for initial KP information about alignment, weight shifting, and timing/sequencing of body segments or components of movement and are less effective during rapid or ballistic tasks. Prolonged or excessive use of guided movements limits active participation and is likely to limit autonomous performance.

Feedback

Regardless of the task, during initial practice the therapist should provide concise, relevant feedback, highlighting information critical for movement success. Do *not* attempt to correct all the numerous errors that characterize early learning; be mindful of wordy instructions or excessive information. Celebrate success and intervene when movement errors become consistent or safety is an issue. Consider the cognitive and physical resources of individual patients, the goal and complexity of the tasks, and the environment when determining how to prioritize and incorporate feedback. If an intrinsic sensory system is absent or provides distorted or incomplete information (e.g., impaired proprioception with diabetic neuropathy), use of alternative sensory systems (e.g., vision, cutaneous) should be emphasized. Supplemental feedback can help focus attention, evaluate performance and outcome, and enhance learning.

Kinematic feedback about the movement of body segments is typically provided visually. A tall mirror is a simple way to help someone self-evaluate their alignment, movement, and relationship to objects in their environment. Most people have cell phones with video capabilities that can be used for dynamic motion analysis from any perspective and provides a way to evaluate and archive performance over time. Care must be taken to respect privacy and confidentiality of others in the clinic background. A 2015 systematic review and meta-analysis of the effectiveness of the Nintendo Wii after stroke revealed lower dropout rates than traditional exercise, suggesting that kinetic feedback technology enhances engagement.[143] Advances in gaming and VR technology provide increasingly complex, realistic and real-time feedback about movement timing and coordination in 3D space for simple to highly complex simulated tasks.[144]

Kinetic feedback about center of pressure (COP) location and motion can also be provided visually using force plates or pressure mapping materials. Posturography is a classic example of how COP feedback is used to enhance standing symmetry, steadiness, and explore stability limits. Research evidence demonstrates the effectiveness of force platform training for improving in-place standing balance.[145–150] It can be an effective training mode for patients with problems in force generation or control, such as hypometria in PD, hypermetria in ataxia, or asymmetry after amputation or hemiplegia. In a Cochrane Database Systematic Review (seven trials, 246 participants), researchers found that force platform feedback improved standing balance but did not improve balance during active functional activities, nor overall independence.[151] Given the neuroplasticity principles of *specificity* and *reverse transfer*, this is not a surprising finding.

The learner's need for and use of feedback shifts across the stages of learning. New learners and patients with somatosensory deficits rely heavily on *visual* feedback. As the learner gets the idea of the movement and begins to perform with less conscious direction, proprioception plays a more dominant role, allowing the learner to focus more on monitoring the environment. Provision of augmented feedback over time should reflect a *faded frequency* schedule for which more feedback is provided in early learning but is gradually transitioned to the patient's self-assessment. The timing of feedback provision should follow a *slight delay*, rather than be provided immediately, to allow the learner a chance to analyze their own performance first. Immediate augmented feedback can interfere with this process, limiting autonomy and creating dependence on the therapist for error identification and correction. Simply asking the patient how they felt did encourage self-assessment and problem-solving, allowing the therapist to determine the patient's level of self-awareness and insight, and provide more specific follow-up.

As learners develop an understanding of the task demands, continued practice is about refining the skill to meet the specific environmental demands. Consider a farmer who wants to return to driving his tractor, as shown in Figures 10.6 and 10.7. These images help illustrate the importance of considering task- and environment-specific variables (regulatory features, affordances for movement) for generalization of training and adding salience to treatment interventions. Variable practice becomes important for problem-solving and learning predictive relationships between movement parameter adjustments and resultant outcomes, particularly for open tasks, variable layouts, and situations that can't be replicated in a therapy clinic. The therapist's role includes adjusting practice progression with task and environmental constraints to facilitate adaptability. It also includes delaying and diminishing feedback, encouraging intrinsic self-assessment by the patient. The focus is on function with personally challenging but meaningful goals. Therapist-guided movements are counterproductive at this stage, interfering with the development of autonomous performance. Successful incorporation of distracters or dual task challenges yields far more complex, flexible skills, reflecting

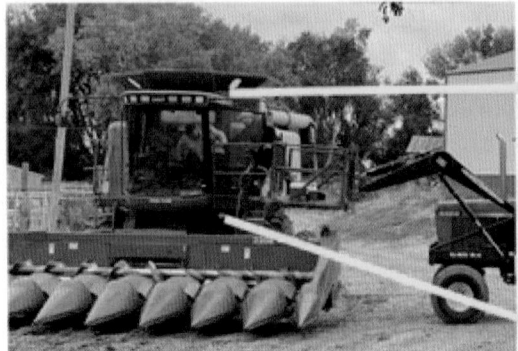
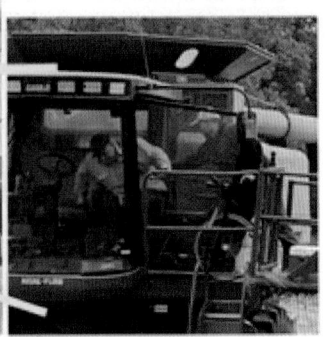

Figure 10.6 Importance of environmental considerations. Task and environmental considerations for a seated transfer into the cab of a farm tractor. Barriers include height of the cab, stairs up to cab deck, gap between wheelchair and driver's seat. Resources include forklift with platform, extended-length sliding board with cutout for modified grasp.

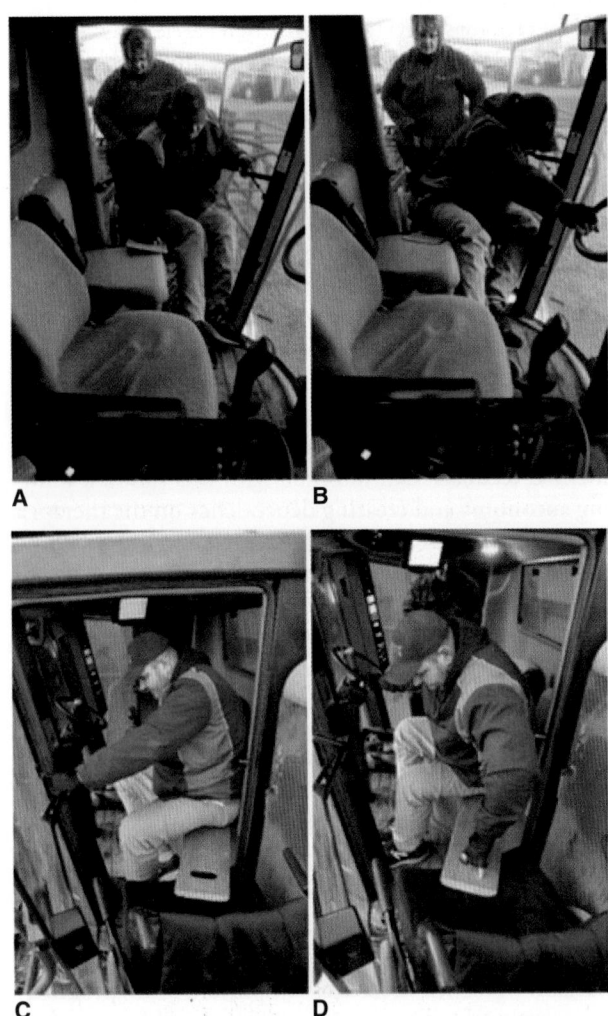

Figure 10.7 Task analysis and problem-solving. Task analysis: An individual with tetraplegia attempting a seated transfer into (A and B) and out of (C and D) the cab of a farm tractor: a closed task with multiple affordances, including the sliding board, door check, steering wheel.

progress toward autonomous control. It is important to remember that some patients may not reach this final stage of learning. For example, some patients with severe TBI may reach consistent performance only within closed, consistent, structured environments.

Task

In addition to appreciating the body structure and function resources and limitations of patients, therapists also need to understand the biomechanical and perceptual–motor requirements and environmental constraints of the tasks our patients perform. By adulthood, most functional movements have been so well practiced that they are fairly automatic, requiring little cognitive monitoring unless something unusual happens. Pain, weakness, altered sensation, poor coordination, and so on can derail our well-learned motor habits, triggering the need to develop new strategies to accomplish our goals. Tasks targeted during early rehabilitation include basic ADLs (e.g., feeding, dressing, hygiene, and so forth) and functional mobility skills (e.g., bed mobility, transfers, locomotion). Later on, instrumental ADLs, such as home chores, shopping, community mobility, recreation, and work activities are addressed, depending on the patient's level of recovery and discharge placement. The next section will focus on applying our understanding of motor control organization and motor learning principles for evidence-based rehabilitation considerations for *task analysis*.

Task-Specific Training: Focus on Function

Movement is purposeful even when subconscious; we move to accomplish goals including stability, mobility, and manipulation.[152] Rather than focusing only on impairments, neuroplasticity principles encourage us to focus on meaningful, effortful, task-specific practice early and throughout the recovery process. Balance is a great example of the complex, multilevel sensorimotor control strategies incorporated into functional tasks as a dynamic, flexible process.[153–156] It will be used to demonstrate the application of the individual, task, and environmental framework to therapeutic activities and progression[157] (see Table 10.7). The reader is also referred to the work of Shumway-Cook and Woollacott[4] for a more complete discussion of postural control and its development, assessment, and treatment.

To maintain postural control, *the individual* must have accurate perception (sensation plus cognition) of their BOS and stability limits, and their center of mass (COM) position and motion. The key sensory systems contributing to balance control are the visual, vestibular, and somatosensory/proprioceptive systems (see Chapter 6, Examination of Coordination and Balance). To maintain alignment and control (the COM), individuals also need to generate appropriate forces in the right direction, at the right time. Balance responses are directional motor synergies and include in-place strategies (ankle and hip), which maintain the COM within the fixed BOS, and change-in-support strategies (stepping and reaching to touch, lean, or grab), which change or extend the BOS for stability. In standing, *ankle strategies* are used for small perturbations on stable surfaces and represent the body swaying over the ankles like an inverted pendulum. If the ankle strategy is ineffective, if the challenge is large, or if the patient is unable to safely step or reach out to keep their balance, the individual will use a *hip strategy.* The hip strategy involves activation of hip and trunk muscles in the plane and opposite direction of the COM movement: flexion and extension during anterior–posterior shifts, abduction during lateral shifts.[158] With lateral displacements, the typical stepping response is a crossover step (87%) versus multiple corrective steps or straight side-stepping,[159] which is an important consideration for older adults who experience falls. Stepping or reaching responses are preferred when possible because the in-place hip strategy produces significant hip and trunk torques and destabilizes body motion.[159,160] These strategies can be activated reflexively by sensory information (*reactive*), or in anticipation of destabilizing activity as (*proactive*) postural readiness. If any of these components is not functioning optimally, the individual experiences instability.

How do we use this information to develop appropriate intervention strategies? Consider the patient's resources, barriers, and prognosis, then improve what can be changed and develop alternate strategies for what cannot. Consider components such as strength or reaction time for better motor responses, compensatory strategies for permanent deficits, such as providing a cane for supplementary feedback and wider BOS, or encouraging counterbalancing with the arms and head for sitting balance after SCI. Endurance includes maintaining alignment and stability for prolonged periods of time, especially in distracting or dual-tasking conditions. It is also important for patients to fluidly prioritize different sources of sensory feedback, depending on which is most accurate in various environmental conditions. Research evidence demonstrates the effectiveness of altering sensory contexts in improving sensory selection and organization for balance.[161-165] Patients should practice maintaining balance under reduced sensory feedback conditions. For example, therapists can reduce visual input with petroleum jelly–coated goggles, blinders, a visual surround, or having the patient close their eyes. Somatosensory or proprioceptive input for balance can be reduced by standing or sitting on soft surfaces or

inclines that change the orientation and pressure feedback about upright posture. Vestibular input for balance is reduced with different head positions or movement, like looking up or to the side, or performing head turns while walking. For more details specific to vestibular rehabilitation, see Chapter 21, Vestibular Disorders.

Understanding the *task* demands also guides decision-making for the appropriate level of challenge and task progression as outlined in Table 10.7. Consider the BOS size: a larger base sitting on a seat with back and feet supported is easier than if the trunk is unsupported and the feet are dangling. Standing in a wide, staggered stance is much more stable than with a smaller base like tandem or single leg standing. The farther away the COM is from the BOS and the more DOF that need to be controlled, the more challenging the task: standing is harder than tall kneeling or sitting. Create opportunities for patients to explore their stability limits by maintaining or moving their COM in different positions with leaning and reaching tasks. Reduce surface stability with squishy or slippery materials, reconfigure or move the BOS.

Maintaining balance involves both anticipatory and reactive systems.[157] *Reactive* balance requires appropriately timed and matched motor responses to the level of perturbation experienced. Slow reaction time, reduced power production, and difficulty grading muscle force to match the task demands can all contribute to ineffective balance responses. *Anticipatory* balance involves activating postural muscles ahead of instability by predicting what will happen and getting posturally "set" prior to the dynamic task. Expectations are developed through experience: lifting a heavy backpack, opening a swing-shut door, stepping up into a truck all involve a level of postural challenge that necessitates proximal muscle activity in advance of the movement initiation to remain stable throughout performance.

In a healthy system, the balance strategies used should match the level of challenge presented: small challenges should elicit an ankle strategy; larger challenges trigger a step or a grab unless the goal is stay in place, like staying on a curb, step stool, or balance beam, which would instead elicit a hip strategy. Excessive, exaggerated responses or stiff co-contraction are examples of ineffective strategies. The therapist must interpret whether the patient's balance response matches the level of challenge provided. Stepping or reaching to catch one's balance is a normal response to large perturbations and needs to be activated quickly, with accurate hand or foot placement and limb stability to accept the weight of the body. Patients often need to be given permission to take steps to keep their balance when doing challenging tasks such as standing in tandem or walking on a narrow beam. All strategies are needed under different circumstances, so all should be practiced. Variable practice allows the patient the opportunity to explore different challenges and match them with the appropriate postural response.

Research evidence demonstrates the effectiveness of training in improving balance control.[166–171] In a Cochrane Database Review (94 studies, 9,821 participants), researchers found positive effects of exercise on balance outcome measures. Different categories of exercise were included, such as gait, balance and functional task training, strengthening exercise, Tai Chi, physical activity programs (walking, cycling), computerized balance training using visual feedback, vibration platform, and multiple exercise types (combinations of programs). Programs typically ran three times a week for 3 months and involved dynamic exercise in standing with few adverse effects reported. They concluded that more high-quality research is needed to identify best types and intensity of training.[168]

Experiencing instability is very scary for the patient. The therapist is responsible for providing a safe practice environment by being always within reach of the patient. A gait belt is essential, and an overhead harness is ideal if available, especially for patients with poor insight, significant weakness, or slow reaction time. Assistive devices and discussion of appropriate footwear can also address patient safety and prevent falls. See Box 10.2 for additional balance safety considerations.

Task-Specific Training to Improve Gait and Locomotion

Traditional conceptualization and treatment of gait problems have focused primarily on kinematic and kinetic assessment of the gait cycle (see Chapter 7, Examination of Gait) and subsequent impairment-based treatments with part task training focusing on subcomponents of the gait cycle. However, this perspective fails to consider the organization of neurologic control and continuous nature of gait production (see Shumway-Cook[4] for a more complete discussion). As such, conventional impairment-based treatment approaches often have not resulted in the anticipated carryover to gait, particularly in neurological patients.[172]

Barbeau[173] summarized early attempts to apply neuroplasticity and motor learning principles to neurologic gait rehabilitation by focusing specifically on whole task locomotor training for challenging posture and adaptation (over ground and on treadmills), appropriate sensory inputs (hip extension, weight-bearing), forcing leg "reuse." Incorporation of pharmacology, FES, or body weight support (BWS) interventions promoted the reemergence of the locomotor pattern, while the walking training shaped it. Questions of optimal intensity, duration, and the significance of stage of recovery were already being raised.[173] This initial work led to subsequent landmark clinical trials to address some of these issues including the STEPS,[62] Locomotor Experience Applied Post-Stroke (LEAPS),[174] and Variable

---

Box 10.2   Compensatory Strategies to Promote Safe Balance

If the patient is a fall risk, consider the following:

- Rely on intact senses, heightening patient's awareness of what is available.
- Allow light touch support or a cane to increase somatosensory inputs about postural sway through the hand.
- Focus vision on a stationary visual target rather than a moving target.
- Minimize head movements during more difficult balance tasks requiring gaze stabilization (sensory conflict situations).
- Widen the BOS when anticipating destabilizing situations like turning, preparing to sit down, or in the direction of an expected force (e.g., step position).
- Lower the COM when greater stability is needed (e.g., crouching when a threat to balance is imminent).
- Wear comfortable, well-fitting shoes with rubber soles for better friction and gripping (e.g., athletic shoes).
- Consider an assistive device (e.g., a cane or walker) to provide a larger BOS.
- Recognize potentially dangerous environmental situations and modify as appropriate (e.g., focus on adequate lighting, supportive furniture, arrangement of furniture, removal of small scatter rugs, use of handrails and grab bars).

BOS = base of support; COM = center of mass.

Intensity Early Walking Post-Stroke (VIEWS)[175] studies (see Table 10.9 later in the chapter) as well as the development of the 2020 Clinical Practice Guideline for Locomotor Training.[176] Promising research targeting cardiovascular intensity (>70% HRmax) of stroke survivors during practice of challenging stepping repetitions has demonstrated superior locomotor outcomes compared to low-intensity conventional PT, including frequent improvements in the nonlocomotor domains of transfers and standing balance, despite not being explicitly practiced.[177,178] This *reverse transfer* effect reflects the neuroplasticity principle of *transference*, suggesting that patients can significantly improve walking outcomes without sacrificing improvements in other pre-gait tasks, thereby improving their clinical efficiency.

The bottom line is that gait is a high-level, complex dynamic balance task maintained primarily within a central pattern generator by the ongoing sensory feedback generated during the rhythmic cycle of stepping. This method of control requires little cortical oversight, allowing our conscious attention to be directed elsewhere. Sensory feedback linked to synergistic motor outputs suggests that similar individual, task, and environmental

Table 10.9	Major Research Studies Focusing on Principles of Neuroplasticity and Motor Learning

EXCITE (Extremity Constraint-Induced Therapy Evaluation)[179]

Design	Prospective, single, blind, multicenter (seven facilities) RCT Level of evidence = 1
Subjects	Adults (222) with subacute (3–9 mo) first-time, predominantly ischemic stroke, with at least 10° wrist, finger, and thumb extension
Intervention	Usual stroke care vs. 14 consecutive days of CIMT involving wearing a mitt on the less-affected hand 90% of waking hours while engaging in 6 hr/day repetitive task practice, behavioral shaping with the hemiplegic hand, plus two to three daily tasks at home.
Results	CIMT group showed significantly better and clinically relevant immediate improvements in quality, speed, and amount of use. Improvements persisted for 12 mo.
Comments	Behavioral training applied motor learning principles of adaptive/part task training of *functional tasks* with *high repetition*.

ICARE (Interdisciplinary Comprehensive Arm Rehab Evaluation)[180]

Design	Phase 3, parallel three-group, single-blind, multicenter (seven facilities) RCT. Level of evidence = 1.
Subjects	361 subjects with moderate motor impairment demonstrating at least minimal hand and finger extension from 14–106 days poststroke.
Intervention	Usual dose-equivalent OT care vs. structured, task-oriented UE training vs. monitoring only. Interventions were provided as 1-hour sessions 3 × wk for 10 weeks; monitoring not specified.
Results	No group differences in UE performance at 12 months, despite providing more than double the dosing and task-oriented therapy.
Comments	Investigational intervention described as "principle based, *impairment* focused, *task* specific, *intense, engaging, collaborative, self-directed*, and patient-centered."

Spinal Cord Injury Locomotor Trial[181]

Design	Single-blinded, multicenter (six facilities) RCT. Level of evidence = 1.
Subjects	Adults (146) within 1 week of rehab admission and 8 wks of incomplete SCI, C5 to L3 levels, ASIA B, C, or D. FIM-L score less than 4.
Intervention	One-hour sessions 5 × wk for ~12 weeks of equal time of BWSTT or overground mobility training.
Results	No significant difference between groups at 6 months, but both groups for ASIA C & D subjects achieved walking abilities beyond what had been expected.
Comments	Both intervention groups aimed to progressively increase *task* difficulty, be *repetitive*, maintain *attention*, and reinforce successful *skill acquisition*.

STEPS (Step Training Effectiveness Post-Stroke)[62]

Design	Phase 2, single-blinded multicenter (three facilities) RCT Level of evidence = 1
Subjects	80 ambulatory adults 4 months–5 years after unilateral stroke, able to ambulate at least 14 m with assistive or orthotic device and assist of 1 person
Intervention	4 interventions (1) BWSTT, (2) resistive leg cycling = CYCLE, (3) progressive-resistive leg exercise = LE-EX, (4) arm ergometry = UE-EX, were used to develop exercise pairs: BWSTT/UE-EX, CYCLE/UE-EX, BWSTT/CYCLE, and BWSTT/LE-EX. Everyone exercised 4 days/wk, with exercise type on alternate days; all participated in the same number of sessions.

(Continued)

Table 10.9 Major Research Studies Focusing on Principles of Neuroplasticity and Motor Learning—cont'd

STEPS (Step Training Effectiveness Post-Stroke)[62]

Results	BWSTT was more effective at improving and maintaining walking speed gains for 6 months vs. resisted cycling. Leg strength also improved with BWSTT; adding daily alternating leg strengthening did not provide additional benefit.
Comments	Improvements attributed to *specificity* and *intensity* of training.

LEAPS (Locomotor Experience Applied Post-Stroke[174]

Design	Phase 3, single-blinded, multicenter (6 facilities) RCT Level of evidence = 1.
Subjects	408 adults who had a moderate to severe stroke 2 months earlier who had the ability to walk ~10 ft with assist and self-selected velocity of less than 0.8 m/s
Intervention	3 training groups: (1) BWSTT at 2 months, (2) BWSTT at 6 months, (3) HEP at 2 months. All groups exercised for 36 sessions of 90 min each for 12–16 wks.
Results	At 1 year, 52% of all participants had increased their functional walking ability, but there were no significant differences between the groups.
Comments	Study was targeting *task-specific*, *high-repetition* step training compared to general exercise, as well as *timing* (2 vs. 6 months).

SIRROWS (Stroke Inpatient Rehab With Reinforcement of Walking Speed)[135]

Design	Phase 2, single-blinded, international multicenter (18 facilities) RCT Level of evidence = 1.
Subjects	Adult subjects (179) with hemiparesis from stroke, who could walk at least 5 steps with no more than maximum assistance of 1 person.
Intervention	Daily feedback about self-selected fast walking speed vs. no reinforcement of walking speed. All received the sites' usual stroke care plus daily 10-m walk (or shorter until feasible). The experimental group's walk was timed, and they were provided feedback on their performance; the control group's walk was not timed, and they got no feedback about it.
Results	Feedback about walking speed led to significantly faster speed at discharge.
Comments	This study focused on the effect of simple *feedback*.

AVERT (A Very Early Rehabilitation Trial)[136]

Design	Parallel-group, single blind, RCT at 56 acute stroke units in five countries. Level of evidence = 1.
Subjects	2,104 adults with ischemic or hemorrhagic stroke, first or recurrent
Intervention	Usual stroke care vs. very early (within 24 hr) mobilization + usual care. Mobilization included earlier, more frequent, higher doses of sitting, standing, and walking activity.
Results	Usual care had more favorable 3-month outcomes than early mobilization, despite the early mobilization group having less than 8% mortality at 3 months, less than 25% being older than 80, and 45% having a moderate or severe stroke.
Comments	The last in a series of studies challenging the principles of *time* (earlier initiation) and *intensity* (more frequent and challenging mobility). By this time, initial mobilization was within 24 hr for *both* groups because it had become the standard of care, with the difference being less than 5 hours.

VIEWS (Variable Intensity Early Walking Post-Stroke)[175]

Design	Single-blinded RCT Level of evidence = 1
Subjects	32 adults 1–6 months poststroke

Table 10.9	Major Research Studies Focusing on Principles of Neuroplasticity and Motor Learning—cont'd
VIEWS (Variable Intensity Early Walking Post-Stroke)[175]	
Intervention	Usual care vs. stepping practice at high cardiovascular intensity (70%–80% heart rate reserve) in varying contexts. All participants had up to 40 1-hour training sessions over 10 weeks. Experimental group applied perturbations to augment errors with minimal focus on kinematics and did not specifically address balance or transfers.
Results	Variable intensive step training resulted in three- to fourfold greater improvements in walking ability (velocity and distance), exceeding MCID values. Equivalent but significant changes were found in the Berg and Five Times Sit-to-Stand tests for both groups.
Comments	This study focused on *variable, high-intensity, task-specific* training and supported the *reverse transfer* of training effect.

ASIA = American Spinal Injury Association; BWSTT = body weight–supported treadmill training; CIMT = constraint-induced movement therapy; FIM = functional independence measure for locomotion; MCID = minimal clinically important difference; OT = occupational therapy; RCT = randomized control trial; SCI = spinal cord injury; UE = upper extremity.

considerations, and activity progression as described for balance tasks would be appropriate for gait training as well. See Chapter 11, Strategies to Improve Locomotor Function; Chapter 15, Stroke; Chapter 18, Parkinson Disease; and Chapter 20, Traumatic Spinal Cord Injury for more specific implementation details.

Research Applying Neuroplasticity and Motor Learning Principles Across Tasks

As our knowledge base of motor learning and neuroplasticity principles has grown, therapeutic interventions for patients with neurological injuries have greatly evolved. Several landmark papers have highlighted the importance of *high-intensity, high-repetition,* and *task-specific training* in enhancing functional recovery after CNS injury, triggering a paradigm shift away from focusing solely on traditional impairment-based, low-intensity, errorless learning. These studies and the main motor learning principles they targeted are summarized in Table 10.9. It is important to note that not all of them resulted in significant changes between groups (although most did), and several had surprising findings that challenged the conventional wisdom of the time. However, all have helped shape our current understanding of foundational intervention principles based on factors known to drive change in the nervous system, informing clinical practice and research going forward.

Of the studies listed in Table 10.9, EXCITE[179] (Extremity Constraint-Induced Therapy Evaluation) and ICARE[180] (Interdisciplinary Comprehensive Arm Rehab Evaluation) focused on UE recovery after stroke. EXCITE was the first study to show that *chronic* stroke survivors with some residual hand function could still improve their function with intense task practice, revealing that neuroplasticity occurs even in older adults and after neurological injury. ICARE revealed that both traditional occupational therapy (OT) and the experimental "principle based, impairment focused, task specific, intense, engaging, collaborative, self-directed,

and patient-centered" training approach for the UE after stroke resulted in equivalent improvements. This result suggests that we still may not fully appreciate the complexities of UE control. The studies leading up to and including AVERT[136] moved up the time course for initiating early mobility after stroke. The SIRROWS[135] study demonstrated the powerful effect of simply measuring and providing feedback on walking speed. The consecutive STEPS[62] and then LEAPS[174] studies focused initially on a potential additive benefit of impairment-based interventions to supplement body weight support treadmill training (BWSTT), and then the optimal timing for the BWSTT intervention (2 months vs. 6 months after stroke). SCILT[181] (Spinal Cord Injury Locomotor Trial) applied BWSTT parameters found to benefit individuals with stroke to individuals with SCI and found similar results. VIEWS[175] focused on and extended the concept of intensity during locomotor training. Several of these studies are also discussed further in Chapters 15, Stroke, and Chapter 20, Traumatic Spinal Cord Injury.

Environment

It is important to know what is going on around us while we are performing our tasks. Are our surroundings quiet and stationary or bustling with activity that needs to be monitored? Recognizing *affordances*, or features that support movement, is a key perceptual skill to successfully navigate new environments. Therapists incorporate or remove affordances in the practice environment to support or challenge patients, such as adding or removing grab bars, door stops, step stools, or sliding boards. Typical easy-to-hard progressions are from closed to more open or variable environments. Therapists need to provide both anticipatory and reactive activity challenges such as walking on smooth terrain (sidewalks) with no traffic and uneven terrain, predictable moving surfaces (escalator, elevator), dual tasking, and ultimately busy environments requiring an external focus, divided attention, and anticipation. Simulated environments (e.g., Easy Street, VR systems) are found in some rehabilitation centers and can serve as an intermediate practice environment before the patient returns to the home or community setting. It is important to remember that some patients (e.g., the patient with severe TBI or dementia) may never be able to function in anything but a highly structured closed environment. Modification of the home environment may be necessary to promote safety (see Chapter 9, Examination and Modification of the Environment).

Technology

While it is beyond the scope of this chapter to discuss all the new technologies currently available, therapists are increasingly considering their value in clinical practice. Promising therapies like deep brain stimulation, noninvasive brain stimulation, neuropharmacology, cognitive training, or feedback using real-time functional magnetic resonance are all based on our current understanding of neuroplasticity.[26,182] Research demonstrates effective results of neurostimulation techniques, aerobic fitness, and video games in cortical reorganization inducing neural plasticity toward motor recovery, improvement of executive functions, and transfer of spatial knowledge.[183] Most rehabilitation devices have been developed to incorporate principles of motor learning and neuroplasticity and are promoted as such: Wearables and VR provide an incredible amount, precision, and fidelity of real-time augmented feedback. Robotic exoskeletons provide structural support and complex programming for kinematically correct stepping or reaching, allowing many repetitions of practice. But the ultimate question is whether these practice and feedback strategies transfer to function beyond the research lab and clinic, and whether there is generalization of improvement to functional tasks that is meaningful and lasting.

Patient/Client-Related Instruction

Patients with deficits in motor function need to recognize the importance of repetitive practice both in therapy and out of therapy to increase movement capacity and bring about meaningful recovery. It is critical for the therapist to establish impactful and safe parameters for practice outside of therapy. Specific goals and strategies should be established with a HEP that includes targeted tasks of sufficient intensity and repetition to drive change. Relevant tools to ensure high levels of practice include a daily schedule, an activity log or home diary, specific activities according to FITT principles, and a behavior contract if necessary. Patient skills in self-evaluation, problem-solving, and decision-making should be promoted to foster independence. Such empowerment improves QOL and prepares the patient for the lifelong adjustments that will be needed. If independence is not possible because of the complexity of deficits and limitations in recovery (e.g., the patient with severe TBI or high-level SCI), education of family, friends, and caregivers is of paramount importance.

SUMMARY

This chapter has presented a conceptual framework for rehabilitation of the patient with deficits in motor function based on a hybrid model that integrates the ICF model of function and disability with an understanding of the normal processes of motor control, motor learning, and task analysis. Clinical decision-making is based on a thorough understanding of the patient's barriers and resources related to their desired activities and social roles. The unique problems of each patient require that the therapist also recognize several interrelated factors, including individual needs and changing status, motivation, goals, concerns, and potential for independent function. Broad categories of interventions have been presented, with a major emphasis on driving neuroplasticity, motor learning strategies, and task-oriented training. Interventions should remediate specific impairments when correctable, modify tasks and teach compensations when deficits are permanent, and promote adaptability for success in real-world environments. Patients deserve the best care we have to offer; it should not depend on who they are seeing or where they are being treated. To honor this commitment, therapists must utilize treatment approaches that have strong evidence of effectiveness (when available) and take into consideration other situational factors such as patient-specific features, treatment efficacy, ability to deliver care, patient priorities, etc. With dwindling numbers of therapy visits and increasingly shorter lengths of stay, HEPs that are practical, personalized, and principle-based are critical for the significant repetitions of practice and carryover needed to drive and maintain positive change in our patient's lives.

Questions for Review

1. Relate the WHO's ICF model to Newell's model of constraints on learning and skill.

2. Differentiate between reflexive and voluntary movements. How do central pattern generators and dual tasking fit in?

3. Compare the processes used by the basal ganglia versus the cerebellum to facilitate motor learning during task practice.

4. Provide some examples of constraints on motor function related to the individual, task, and environment.

5. Differentiate between the terms *motor control* and *motor learning*. How can impairments in motor control be distinguished from those of motor learning?

6. Compare and contrast the three stages of motor learning as outlined by the Fitts & Posner vs. Bernstein models. How do training strategies differ across stages and models? (See Table 10.3.)

7. Incorporate neuroplasticity principles in the design and implementation of patient-specific treatment plans. (See Table 10.2.)

8. Associate practice parameters with stages of learning and type of task being learned. (See Table 10.4.)

9. Associate properties of feedback provision with stages of learning. (See Table 10.5.)

10. Develop functional, measurable, and meaningful goals that reflect improved motor skills. (See Table 10.6.)

11. Progress/regress a functional therapeutic activity based on patient status and task analysis of the task and environmental demands. (See Table 10.7.)

CASE STUDY

HISTORY

The patient is a 36-year-old man who sustained a TBI following a motorcycle crash. Imaging revealed a left frontal skull fracture with underlying contusion, as well as right basal ganglia contusion and generalized brain edema. Admission Glasgow Coma Scale (GCS) = 7. His acute hospital course was complicated by increased intracranial pressure and severe spasticity. A gastric tube (G-tube) was inserted. During his acute care stay, the patient's neurological status showed some minor improvement (GCS = 10), so after 4 weeks he was transferred to a rehabilitation facility for a trial of intensive therapies.

PART I: PHYSICAL THERAPY EXAMINATION FINDINGS (INITIAL ADMISSION TO REHAB, 4 WEEKS AFTER INJURY)

Behavior/Cognition/Communication:
Coma Recovery Scale-Revised = 21/23

The patient is functioning at Rancho Levels of Cognitive Functioning (RLOCF) Level V Confused–Inappropriate. The patient is able to respond to simple commands fairly consistently. With increased complexity of commands or lack of any external structure, responses are nonpurposeful, random, or fragmented. The patient is easily frustrated, disinhibited (swearing and name calling), and highly distractible. Agitated Behavior Scale = 24/56 (mild). His memory is severely impaired, and he often shows inappropriate use of objects. Refer to speech and language pathology and occupational therapy (OT) for detailed assessment.

Observation:
Skin: Multiple healed lacerations on the knees and calves and pressure sores bilaterally on the lateral malleoli and calcanei from bivalve positioning splints.
Posture/positioning: Supine in bed, patient with bivalved positioning splints on B ankles. Right upper extremity (RUE) postured in extension synergy. Left upper extremity (LUE) postured in flexion synergy. Occasionally curls into side-lying fetal position. Foley catheter, adult diaper, and G-tube present.
Sensation: Localizes to pinprick with withdrawal, otherwise difficult to assess due to poor comprehension.
Passive range of motion: All within normal limits (WNL) except R elbow 0–70°, L elbow 10–100°; R > L ankles in equinovarus, R dorsiflexion (df) to −15°, L to −5°.

Motor Control
Reflexes and tone (Modified Ashworth Scale [M-AS] grades): Patient presents with hyperreflexia and spasticity throughout all four extremities
• clonus R 3–4 beats, L 1 beat.
• Babinski + (upgoing) R and equivocal on L.
• Bilateral extensor tone in LEs (scissoring at times), M-AS = 3(R), 2(L).
• UEs with mixed presentation: R elbow ext M-AS = 3, L flexors M-AS = 3

(Continued)

CASE STUDY—cont'd

Coordination/voluntary movements: Patient is observed to move all four extremities in synergy patterns when restless or agitated.
- Bilateral UEs also inconsistently demonstrate some isolated control out-of-synergy when calm and focused on a meaningful, functional activity.
- Bilateral LEs are dominated by strong, symmetric extensor synergy unless flexion synergy is triggered for rolling or getting into hook-lying.

Function

Balance requires UE support and moderate assistance for supported sitting due to limited head and trunk control; flexed posture including sacral sitting.
- Trunk Impairment Scale = 0

Standing requires maximal assist of two persons to stand in the parallel bars, R > L foot inverted and plantarflexed, LUE postured in flexion.
- Functional activities: Disability Rating Scale = 20/30
- Functional Assessment Measure (FAM): Dependent or max assist in all ADL and basic mobility (FAM = 0–1)

PART I: (QUESTIONS 1–4)

1. Identify and prioritize the problems in motor function presented in this case in terms of impairments and activity limitations based on initial admission data (4 weeks after injury).

2. Identify goals that reflect level of independence or amount of assistance needed for this patient at this point in his recovery (initial admission). All goals are to be achieved within 4 weeks.

3. Consider the standardized outcome measures data provided. Determine which could be used to develop goals reflecting measurable and meaningful improvement.

4. Identify the patient's likely stage of motor learning, appropriate practice and feedback strategies incorporated into two treatment interventions for this patient at this point in his recovery (initial admission).

PART II: REEXAMINATION 12 WEEKS AFTER INJURY

Social (for discharge planning): Married with no children. Wife is a registered nurse and very supportive of her husband. Lives in a ranch-style home with two steps to enter, no railing.

Behavior/cognition/communication: The patient is now functioning at RLOCF Level VII Automatic–Appropriate. He appears appropriate and oriented within the rehab setting, going through his daily routine automatically with minimal to no confusion. With structure, he is able to initiate social and recreational activities. He shows carryover for new learning but at a decreased rate and with shallow recall of activities; judgment remains impaired. Agitated Behavior Scale = 16/56. Speech is dysarthric and delayed, but it is usually intelligible. The patient is able to follow multistep commands.

Observation: Lacerations are healed. G-tube removed but Foley remains.

Sensation:
- LUE: Absent sensation.
- LLE: Impaired light touch and proprioception.
- RUE and RLE: Intact.

Range of motion:
- UEs: WNL except R elbow ROM 0° to 90°; elbow ROM 5° to 110°
- LEs: WNL except for R ankle df to 0°

Motor function:

Reflexes and tone: Exhibits strong associated reactions in LUE with stressful activities. Clonus and Babinski still + but responses less robust.
- RUE and RBLE: Extensor tone, M-AS = 1
- LUE: Flexor tone, M-AS = 2

Coordination/voluntary movements:
- RUE Demonstrates purposeful, full, isolated motions through available ROM. Strength is grossly 3+/5
- LUE: Limited voluntary movement; flexor synergy predominates.
- BLE: Movement is purposeful with some isolated control emerging but still slow responses; strength is grossly 4/5 F.

CASE STUDY—cont'd

Functional Activities:

Balance: Patient is able to sit unsupported with loose supervision >2 min; able to reach without loss of balance and reach in near workspace. He requires UE support for static standing and reaching, and Mod A with device for dynamic stepping.

- Trunk Impairment Score = 9
- Modified (sitting) Functional Reach Test (using R arm) = 25 cm
- Disability Rating Scale = 10
- Functional Assessment Measure (FAM):
  - Bed mobility: Rolls to right and left with supervision, FAM = 6 (increased time).
  - Supine-to-sit: FAM = 4 (min A) to R = 3 (mod A) to L
  - Sit-to-stand, transfers (bed, chair, toilet, tub bench): FAM = 3 (Mod A)
  - Wheelchair locomotion: FAM = 5 close supervision for safety
  - Gait: FAM = 0 (distance); Walks in parallel bars 10 ft with Mod A × 1
- Feeding and grooming: FAM = 4
- Dressing and bathing: FAM =3

PART II: (QUESTIONS 5–8)

5. Identify and prioritize this patient's motor function problems in terms of impairments and activity limitations (12 weeks after injury).

6. Identify goals that reflect level of independence or amount of assistance needed for this patient at this point in his recovery (12 weeks after injury). All goals are to be achieved within 4 weeks.

7. Consider the standardized outcome measures data provided. Determine which are still appropriate to use to develop goals reflecting measurable and meaningful improvement.

8. Identify the motor learning strategies and two treatment interventions appropriate for this patient at this point in his recovery.

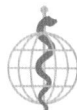

For additional resources, including answers to the questions for review, new immersive cases, case study guiding questions, references, and more, please visit **https://www.fadavis.com/product/physical-rehabilitation-fulk-8**. You may also quickly find the resources by entering this title's four-digit ISBN, 4691, in the search field at **http://fadavis.com** and logging in at the prompt.

Strategies to Improve Locomotor Function

Chapter 11

George D. Fulk, PT, PhD, FAPTA
Lee Dibble, PT, PhD, ATC, FAPTA

LEARNING OBJECTIVES

1. Select appropriate outcome measures to use with a client whose primary goal is to improve locomotion function.
2. Interpret change in walking ability using gait speed as an outcome measure.
3. Develop a practice schedule for locomotor interventions that enhances motor learning.
4. Utilize feedback during locomotor interventions to facilitate motor learning.
5. Explain how feedback can be used to enhance patient motivation.
6. Organize interventions to promote the recovery of locomotor function based on principles of neuroplasticity.
7. Develop a plan of care to improve locomotor function that targets moderate- to high-intensity stepping training.
8. Describe how to provide variable practice when utilizing a treadmill to improve locomotor function.
9. Develop a task-specific strengthening and dynamic balance exercise program that incorporates exercise guidelines and principles of neuroplasticity to improve locomotor function.
10. Design a circuit-training locomotor intervention that incorporates motor learning and neuroplasticity principles.

CHAPTER OUTLINE

EXAMINATION OF WALKING FUNCTION 368
REHABILITATION INTERVENTIONS TO PROMOTE RECOVERY OF LOCOMOTOR FUNCTION 370
General Principles 370
Task-Specific Walking Training/Treadmill Training 371
Virtual Reality and Exergaming 373
Augmenting Muscle Force Production 374
Balance and Dynamic Postural Control During Overground Walking 375
Circuit Training 377
Motor Imagery 377
Emerging Interventions 378
Performance vs. Capacity vs. Patient-Reported Outcomes 379
Gait Training With Assistive Devices 379
SUMMARY 379

The recovery or improvement of walking ability is a primary goal for people with many different health conditions who seek the services of a physical therapist.[1–4] Initially, approximately two-thirds of people who experience a stroke cannot ambulate or require assistance to walk.[5] Three months later, one-third of those with a stroke still require some level of assistance to walk. People with Parkinson disease (PD) often have impaired postural control and limited walking ability.[6] Approximately 50% of people with multiple sclerosis (MS) require assistance to walk within 15 years of their diagnosis.[7,8] Individuals with low back pain, lower extremity (LE) amputations, and a host of other health conditions often present with limited walking ability. Improving walking ability is an important goal because people who can walk independently are likely to have a lower burden of care, be able to participate in expected social roles and desired recreational activities, have a higher quality of life, be more physically active, and have improved health status.[2,3,6,9–12]

◼ EXAMINATION OF WALKING FUNCTION

Physical therapists use a variety of tests and measures to assess locomotor function. Evaluation of gait and functional walking ability assists the physical therapist in selecting appropriate interventions, measuring change, and setting goals. The major requirements for successful walking include the following: (1) support of body mass by the LEs, (2) production of locomotor rhythm, (3) dynamic postural control of the moving body, (4) propulsion of the body in the intended direction, and (5) adaptability of the locomotor response to changing environmental and task demands. Physical therapists use observational gait analysis (OGA) as a preferred method to examine gait kinematics. One instrument used clinically is the Rancho Los Amigos (RLA) OGA System. The RLA OGA instrument gathers data on the cyclical movements of walking that occur from one stride cycle to the next. The gait cycle is divided into *stance* and *swing* phases. The physical therapist visually analyzes a patient's walking pattern, looking for asymmetries and deviations from normal. Based on these observations, the physical therapist gains insight into which body structure/function impairments may be the cause of the deviations.

Clinic-based measures of walking capacity that physical therapists commonly use include gait speed measured over a short distance (5-meter or 10-meter Walk Test [10MWT]),[13] the 6-minute Walk Test (6MWT),[13] Functional Gait Assessment (FGA),[13] Community Balance and Mobility Scale,[14] Walking Index for Spinal Cord Injury,[15] Amputee Mobility Predictor,[16] and the High-Level Mobility Assessment Tool.[17] A variety of outcome measures such as the Functional Independence Measure and the Unified Parkinson Disease Rating Scale, which assess overall function, contain items that measure walking ability. See Chapter 7, Examination of Gait, for additional information on outcome measures and greater detail on examination of gait.

Gait speed is likely the most widely used parameter to measure and assess walking capacity across many different patient populations, including cerebrovascular accident (CVA), PD, MS, incomplete spinal cord injury (SCI), total joint replacement, vestibular dysfunction, traumatic brain injury (TBI), individuals with LE amputation, older adults, and many others. Gait speed should be used with all patients for whom recovery of walking ability is a goal. It is valid, reliable, and responsive, and there are established cut-off values to assist with prediction and other clinical decisions.[13,18] The minimal clinically important difference (MCID) of gait speed has been established for a variety of patient populations and is useful for goal setting and interpreting change during rehabilitation. For people with stroke, the MCID ranges from 0.13 to 0.17 m/s;[19–21] for older adults, it is estimated to be 0.13 m/s;[22] for individuals who have sustained a hip fracture, it is estimated to be 0.10 m/s;[23,24] for people with chronic obstructive pulmonary disease, it is estimated to be 0.11 m/s;[25] and for patients receiving inpatient rehabilitation with a variety of health conditions (e.g., total knee arthroplasty, fracture, stroke, congestive heart failure, infection, total hip arthroplasty) it ranges from 0.12 to 0.18 m/s[26] (Table 11.1). These values differ slightly, likely due to differences in the patient populations, acuity of the

Table 11.1 Estimates of Minimal Clinically Important Difference of Comfortable Gait Speed		
Patient Population	**MCID**	**Anchor of Importance**
Stroke	0.17 m/s[19]	Patient perception of important change in walking ability
Stroke	0.16 m/s[20]	1-point improvement on modified Rankin Scale
Stroke	0.13 m/s[21]	Decrease in physical assistance required to walk
Older adults	0.13 m/s[22]	Change in SF-36 mobility questions; walk one block and climb one flight of stairs Patient perception of important change in general mobility
Women with hip fracture	0.10–0.17 m/s[23]	Change in SF-36 mobility questions; walk one block and climb one flight of stairs
Older adults with hip fracture	0.10 m/s[24]	Change in Timed Up and Go Expert opinion
Patients with chronic obstructive pulmonary disease	0.08–0.11 m/s[25]	Change on the incremental shuttle walk Patient self-report of feeling of improvement
Patients undergoing inpatient rehabilitation (total knee arthroplasty, stroke, congestive heart failure, total hip arthroplasty, and others)	0.10–0.18 m/s[26]	Patient perception of walking ability Decrease in physical assistance required to walk Change to less-supportive assistive device Change in gait speed categories

MCID = minimal clinically important difference; SF-36 = 36 Item Short Form.

health condition, and differences in the anchor of importance across studies.

Self-report measures of walking ability are important as they provide information related to the patient's perceptions of the impact of their health condition. An example of such a measure is the Multiple Sclerosis Walking Scale,[27] which is a self-report measure that was originally designed for people with MS but has been used with other patient populations.[28,29] Activity monitors that incorporate accelerometers are useful and accurate measures of walking performance in the home and community.[30,31] Findings from these various tests and measures of walking ability (OGA, clinic-based, self-report, and activity monitors), as well as findings from other components of the initial examination, can be used to identify what aspects of locomotion are challenging for the patient, to select specific interventions, provide feedback to the patient, and to measure change.

■ REHABILITATION INTERVENTIONS TO PROMOTE RECOVERY OF LOCOMOTOR FUNCTION

General Principles

Moderate- to high-intensity locomotor training, treadmill (TM) training, task-oriented circuit training, virtual reality and exergaming, dance, strengthening exercises, dynamic balance exercises, motor imagery, and behavioral change are some of the primary interventions physical therapists use to promote recovery of walking ability in patients and clients.[32-38] The specific type of intervention(s) selected will depend on the health condition of the patient, stage of recovery, and patient preference. However, there are some general principles related to exercise, learning, and neuroplasticity that should be incorporated as a part of any specific intervention designed to improve walking ability. *Exercise* is a planned, structured, and repetitive body movement(s) designed to improve fitness.[39] *Motor learning* is a set of processes associated with practice and experience that leads to relatively permanent changes in the ability to perform movement.[40] Within the context of motor function interventions, *neuroplasticity* refers to changes that occur within the central nervous system (CNS) as a result of behavioral and environmental stimuli.[41]

Intensity

Prescribing the optimal dosage of the intervention is critical. The training dosage should follow the FITT principle (frequency, intensity, time, type). Although the frequency and time vary across studies, there is growing evidence in people with acute onset neurological health conditions that the intensity of walking training (measured by indirectly by heart rate [HR]) is a key component in facilitating improvement in walking capacity.[42] Guidelines for exercise training for people

with stroke recommend an intensity of 11 to 14, using Rating of Perceived Exertion scale, or 55% to 80% of maximal HR.[43,44] Increasing the intensity of the training can be done by increasing the speed of stepping or load (e.g., stepping with a weighted vest or with ankle weights). Vitals should be continuously monitored during training with all patient populations.

Motor Learning

Two key contributors to motor learning are *practice* and *feedback*. For learning to occur, enough practice of the task must be done. In animal models examining neuroplastic changes and in human motor learning studies, upward of 500 to 600 repetitions of the task are performed per session in order to demonstrate improvement in motor behavior.[45-47] Unfortunately, observational studies of physical therapy practice reveal that patients likely do not typically receive sufficient amount of practice to optimally promote motor learning. Lang and colleagues[48] found that patients receiving outpatient physical therapy on average performed 33 active LE movements, 6 passive LE movements, 8 purposeful movements, and took 292 steps.

The structure and conditions of practice have an impact on motor learning. *Variable* practice leads to improved retention and motor learning compared to *constant* practice. In relation to locomotor interventions, an example of variable practice would be walking on a TM at different speeds (instead of at a constant speed) or ambulating on varying surfaces. Constant practice would encompass walking on the TM at the same speed throughout the intervention session. Variable practice may lead to improved motor learning compared to constant practice because functionally the task of walking requires people to vary their walking speed or gait pattern depending on the environment and goal. *Random* practice, where several different tasks are practiced in a random order, instead of *blocked* practice, where all trials on one task are practiced together in a block, can also lead to improved motor learning of movement tasks.

Feedback related to performance and task completion can also be used to promote motor learning. Feedback can be *intrinsic*, that is, feedback that comes to the performer through their sensory systems (i.e., proprioceptive, visual), or *extrinsic*, feedback that is provided (usually by the physical therapist) to augment intrinsic feedback. *Knowledge of results* (KR) is terminal, extrinsic feedback about the results of the outcome of the movement. Knowledge of results feedback can be delivered in a variety of ways: immediately following every trial, after a period of delay between completion of the trial and provision of KR, fading the amount of KR over successive trials, or providing summary KR after a certain number of trials. Reducing the amount of KR feedback through faded or summary feedback is more effective for motor learning than providing feedback after every trial. Observational research on how much feedback is provided during treatment sessions suggests that physical therapists may provide too much feedback, which may inhibit motor learning.[49]

Dobkin and colleagues[50] provided daily KR feedback on gait speed for people with stroke who were undergoing inpatient rehabilitation. Participants performed a daily timed 10-meter walk. Participants in the experimental group were told that they had done well and their specific time. If it was faster than the day before they were told by how much; if the time was the same, they were told they were holding their own; and if it was slower, they were encouraged by being told that soon they would walk faster. Both the experimental and comparison groups received the same type and amount of physical therapy. The only difference was that the comparison group did not receive KR feedback on their gait speed. The group that received KR feedback demonstrated a significant difference in gait speed at discharge compared to the comparison group, 0.91 m/s vs. 0.72 m/s. These results illustrate the impact of feedback and its motivational potential.

Wulf and Lewthwaite[51] summarized the importance of focus of attention, motivation, and autonomy on motor learning. In a series of studies, they report that an external focus of attention (concentrating on the intended effect of the movement) rather than an internal focus of attention (concentrating on how the body is moving) was more beneficial for motor learning. For example, when balancing on a platform, subjects that were instructed to minimize the movement of the platform demonstrated better motor learning than subjects who were instructed to minimize the movement of their feet.[52] In addition to providing information related to task goal completion, feedback can be an effective motivator as well. Positive feedback after successful trials and ignoring unsuccessful trials can enhance motor learning.[53] Providing pretask feedback to increase a patient's confidence can positively impact motor learning.[54] Enhancing patient autonomy by providing increased choice and control over the intervention can also be beneficial for motor learning. For example, participants who were allowed to decide if they wished to use an assistive device during a balance task demonstrated greater motor learning on the balance task than participants who were not given a choice.[55] Increasing motivation, self-confidence, and autonomy promote greater engagement in the task and enhance motor learning. Chapter 10, Strategies to Improve Motor Function, provides more detail on strategies to promote motor learning.

Neuroplasticity

Neuroplastic changes can occur at the cellular level and synapse all the way up to cortical maps and networks. Kleim and Jones[41] suggest that neuroplasticity is the means through which the brain learns new behaviors and damaged brain relearns motor behaviors. Intensive,

task-oriented practice drives neuroplastic changes within the CNS, which in turn promotes improved movement and functional recovery.[41,56–59] Task specificity, repetition, intensity, and salience are a few of the critical principles of experience-dependent neuroplasticity.[41]

Interventions that are valued by the patient, specific to the task being (re)learned, provided at a high dosage at a moderate to high intensity, with feedback that promotes motor learning and challenging are likely to be associated with beneficial neuroplastic changes and improvements in walking ability. Box 11.1 summarizes some of the important principles of motor learning and neuroplasticity that may be incorporated into locomotor interventions. See Chapter 10, Strategies to Improve Motor Function, for a more detailed discussion on motor learning and neuroplasticity.

Task-Specific Walking Training/ Treadmill Training

There is a considerable body of research that supports the use of task-specific walking training on a TM and overground in a variety of clinical populations. These include individuals with LE amputations, joint arthroplasty, and neurological diagnoses (CVA, SCI, PD, MS).[32,60,61] Outcomes from these studies suggest that TM training may result in improvements in gait speed, gait endurance, gait symmetry, and aerobic fitness. Neurologically, TM walking may provide a sensorimotor environment that facilitates the recruitment of spinal cord and brainstem circuits that compose central pattern generators. The recruitment of these circuits helps to produce the rhythmic, reciprocal muscle activity necessary for a coordinated gait pattern. As a strategy to improve locomotor function, using a TM provides such task-specific training while allowing the clinician to closely monitor and supervise the patient in a controlled,

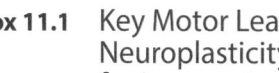

Box 11.1   Key Motor Learning and Neuroplasticity Principles for Locomotor Rehabilitation

- Task-specific practice with a high number of repetitions is critical.
- Variable and random practice promotes motor learning.
- Summary and faded knowledge of results feedback promotes motor learning.
- Feedback is beneficial for motivational purposes.
- Provide external focus of attention.
- Provide control and autonomy to the patient.
- Ensure the task is high intensity.
- Ensure the task is challenging and engaging for the patient.
- Ensure the task is goal directed and meaningful to the patient.

stable environment. From a metabolic/cardiorespiratory physiological perspective, TM training provides a controllable moderate- to maximal-intensity exercise stimulus that, when performed chronically, contributes to increased bio-energetic efficiency required during ambulation in everyday life.

Task-specific walking training, whether overground or on a TM, should incorporate the guiding principles outlined above. From an intensity standpoint, the following parameters may be varied to manipulate the intensity of the exercise stimulus: speed (when overground, the patient can be encouraged to walk as fast as possible or when on the TM, the speed can be increased); incline (TM belt can be inclined or when walking overground it can be done on an incline [ramp] or over stairs); load (the patient can don a weighted vest or ankle weights); and overall training time. Practice and feedback can be manipulated to enhance motor learning. For example, variable practice can be introduced by varying the speed of the TM. Feedback on speed, distance, and time can be provided in summary form and for motivational purposes.

The biomechanical characteristics of TM training make it a convenient and useful clinical tool. During overground walking, gait speed and other spatial and temporal features may vary from step to step. In contrast, successful TM walking requires that the participant's gait speed matches that of the TM belt. The TM imposes external spatial temporal constraints on the gait pattern, acting as an external pacemaker. Treadmill walking as an external pacemaker has been used in people with PD to improve gait rhythm and stability and may improve the symmetry of stride length as well as the consistency of cadence.[62]

For people with chronic stroke, SCI, and TBI, the current best evidence strongly recommends task-specific, moderate- to high-intensity walking training (targeting 60% to 80% of heart rate reserve [HRR] or 70% to 85% of maximum HR) on a TM and overground.[32] There is also evidence to support moderate- to high-intensity stepping practice in people at the subacute stage of recovery after stroke[63,64] and for people with PD.[65] Step training performed on a TM should use an overhead safety harness to reduce fall risk. The use of body weight support (BWS) from the harness system may be needed initially or with patients with severe paresis who cannot fully weight bear through the affected LE. The amount of BWS should be minimized and reduced during training. Heart rate should be continuously monitored using a HR monitor that can be strapped on the patient's chest, upper arm, or wrist. The speed of the TM is increased gradually so the patient is training at a moderate- to high-intensity level. The patient can also walk backward and sideways on the TM. Manual assistance to move the limbs and control the trunk is minimized.

It is important to also incorporate overground walking as part of the intervention in addition to stepping on the TM. An overhead harness can also be used during overground training for safety. During overground training, the patient is encouraged to walk fast to achieve targeted intensity levels. Specific walking skills can also be performed such as backward walking, sidestepping, stepping over obstacles, walking while carrying objects, and providing unexpected perturbations to the patient while walking. The load while walking overground can be manipulated by having the patient wear a weighted vest, ankle weights, and incorporating elastic bands to facilitate stepping at a moderate- to high-intensity level. See Figures 11.1 to 11.3.

The Academy of Neurologic Physical Therapy (ANPT) has developed online resources guided by the findings of the Clinical Practice Guideline to Improve Locomotor Function following Chronic Stroke, Incomplete Spinal Cord Injury, and Brain Injury[32] to support physical therapists as they implement walking interventions at a moderate- to high-intensity level. These are available at the ANPT website: https://www.neuropt.org/practice-resources/best-practice-initiatives-and-resources/intensity_matters. Additionally, ANPT has developed video cases that highlight different interventions delivered at a high- to moderate-intensity level for people with various neurological health conditions, including SCI. These are available at the ANPT YouTube site: https://www.youtube.com/playlist?list=PLH8hBAd9u40lSIGbP9s3dz2BiveybZKW7.

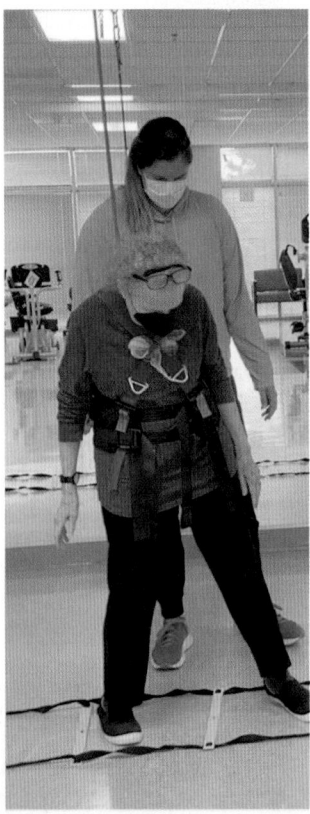

Figure 11.1 Overground locomotor training: sidestepping.

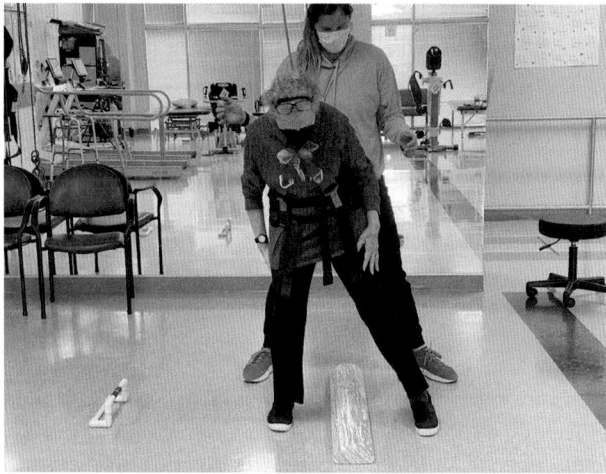

Figure 11.2 Overground locomotor training: sidestepping over an object.

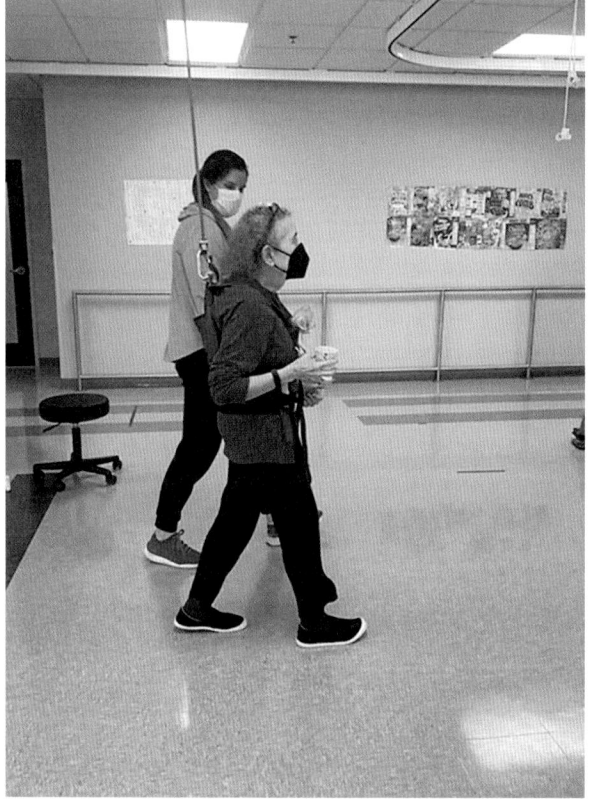

Figure 11.3 Overground locomotor training: walking and carrying an object.

High-intensity interval training (HIIT) walking on the TM and overground is another strategy to train stepping at a high intensity. HIIT strategy involves short bursts (30 seconds) of walking on the TM and overground at maximal tolerated speeds, followed by 30 to 60 seconds of rest for a total of 20 minutes of stepping on the TM and 20 minutes overground. An average HRR of ~70% is targeted.[66,67]

To ensure patient safety, the patient's response during and after moderate- to high-intensity training should be closely monitored. HR should be continuously monitored, and blood pressure (BP) should be taken periodically after training intervals. Patients should be monitored for signs or symptoms of cardiorespiratory issues (angina, cyanosis, pallor), new onset neurological symptoms, and orthopedic injury. If during training the patient's systolic BP drops by more than 10 mm Hg from resting level, systolic BP is greater than 240 mm Hg, diastolic BP is greater than 110 mm Hg, the patient experiences chest pain or angina, new onset neurological symptoms, claudication pain, or severe fatigue or shortness of breath, then training session should be stopped and the patient's physician notified.

Virtual Reality and Exergaming

A critical factor that promotes motor learning and generalization of acquired skills to untrained tasks is the variability of practice. Although strategies to improve locomotor function such as training using a TM or walking overground in the clinic are effective, they are limited in their ability to provide varied practice environments and task challenges. In addition, adherence to basic TM training programs may pose a clinical challenge due to participants' lack of interest or boredom with the undistracted task of walking on a TM.

Virtual reality (VR) interventions provide a viable option that may address the barriers created by environmental restrictions, time demands, and participant lack of interest.[68,69] For the purposes of this chapter, VR is defined broadly to include the use of video or other gaming systems that allow the participant to immerse themselves, partially or fully, in a computer environment that mimics real-world activities. Examples of partially immersive systems include Microsoft Kinect or Nintendo Wii together with a screen.[70] Fully immersive systems include head-worn goggles or virtual environments in which video projectors provide images to between three and six sides of a room-sized environment (see Fig. 11.4).[71,72]

Regardless of the health condition, systematic reviews, and meta-analyses of the effects of VR on walking and mobility outcomes, such as gait speed, stride and step length, and composite mobility (e.g., Timed Up and Go) suggest that there is a significant benefit for VR interventions.[68–70,73] Additionally, the Clinical Practice Guideline to Improve Locomotor Function Following Chronic Stroke, Incomplete Spinal Cord Injury, and Brain Injury recommends VR interventions coupled with walking training to improve walking capacity.[32]

Examples of commercially available VR systems that have been utilized and have shown benefit include games involving weight shifting in static stance on a Nintendo Wii balance board or dance video games on

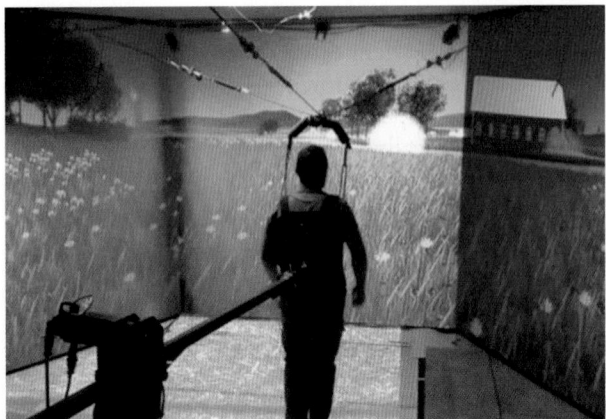

Figure 11.4 An example of a VR environment for gait training. In this VR environment, the participant walks on a treadmill and is provided visual input on four sides (anterior, both sides, and on the ground) that is synchronized with gait speed on the treadmill.

the Microsoft Kinect. Interventions from 15 to 45 minutes in duration delivered one or two times per week appear to provide benefit. VR interventions provide the opportunity to incorporate many of the guiding principles discussed earlier in the chapter. For example, the games are engaging and challenging. Random practice of different gait-related tasks can be set up through the gaming system. The system can also provide feedback for motivational purposes that can be tracked over time. Interaction with the VR environment provides an external focus of attention as well. The potential benefits of this technology, which allows task-specific training that cognitively engages the participant while remaining in the clinical setting or increasing practice time as part of a home program, warrant consideration for use in locomotor rehabilitation programs. VR interventions can be delivered in a telerehabilitation format also.[74,75]

Augmenting Muscle Force Production

A key strategy for improving muscle force production is to combine resistance training with task-specific practice. This requires repetitive practice of tasks that are *specific to the outcome* (i.e., locomotion) and *meaningful to the patient* in terms of function. Biomechanical studies of gait have demonstrated that there are three main muscle groups that contribute to the power required for forward propulsion during gait (hip extensors during early stance, ankle plantarflexors during late stance, hip flexors during early swing). In addition, there are two muscle groups that contribute to power absorption during gait (knee extensors during early stance, knee flexors during late swing). Although muscle-specific resistance training (e.g., progressive resistance, isokinetic equipment) may also be indicated and complementary to locomotor rehabilitation, training of muscles involved in locomotion within the context of tasks that are

specific to the positions and modes of contraction utilized during gait will optimize transfer of strength gains to locomotor skills.[76–78]

Training the muscle groups critical to power production and power absorption during gait in the mode of contraction in which they are utilized will maximize the benefits of resistance training interventions to gait. Given that the portions of the stance phase prior to mid-stance require eccentric contractions of the LE to decelerate the body's momentum, and the portions of stance phase subsequent to mid-stance require concentric contractions to accelerate the body forward, strengthening exercises must include task-specific functional activities. For example, task-specific functional activities that focus on concentric and eccentric LE extensor muscle control might include partial wall squats, step-ups and step-downs, sit-to/from-stand transfers, and first bilateral, then single-limb heel rises to strengthen ankle plantarflexors.

During normal unimpaired gait, hip extensor and ankle plantar flexor muscle actions during the stance phase of gait are concentric in nature and occur at high angular velocities (greater than 200 degrees/second) over a short period of time.[79] Such movement demands suggest that training of these muscles with more ballistic concentric contractions may be warranted.[80,81] An example of strengthening of the hip extensors and ankle plantar flexors in this manner is the use of a leg press or leg sled using hopping movements (Fig. 11.5).

While a focus on extensors and flexors is appropriate for sagittal plane progression during gait, a focus on frontal plane stability requires attention to the musculature on the medial and lateral portions of the LE. Examples include strengthening of hip abductors and adductors using side-stepping, cross-stepping, and braiding (manual contact or resistive bands can be used for resistance). See Figure 11.6.

The goals of locomotor rehabilitation may also dictate the intensity of the resistance. For example, increases in locomotor speed or the ability to tolerate and improve walking on inclined surfaces or ascending stairs may require increases in muscle power (high muscle force delivered in a short period of time). Resistance training for this purpose should be delivered at a high intensity relative to an individual's one repetition maximum or performed in an explosive manner.[82] In contrast, sustained coordinated production of ambulation on level surfaces requires a reduced intensity of muscle contractions, but these contractions may be required over minutes to hours. Resistance training for this purpose should be delivered at intensities lower than 60% one-Repetition Max but performed for durations of time rather than counting repetitions. The overall objective is to improve the oxidative capacity of the muscle. Owing to the varied demands of ambulation in the home and community, individuals should be trained for both muscular power and endurance.

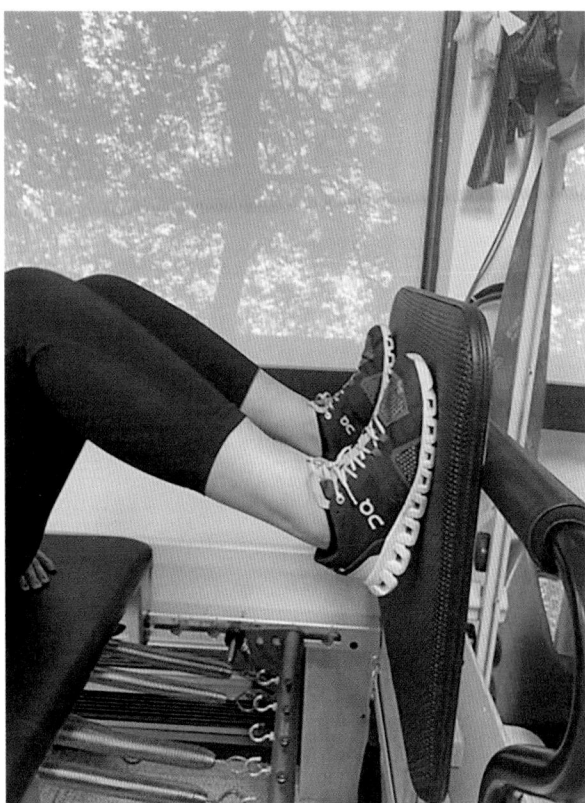

Figure 11.5 Using a sled to ballistically perform ankle PF. Can progress to single leg with knee and hip extended.

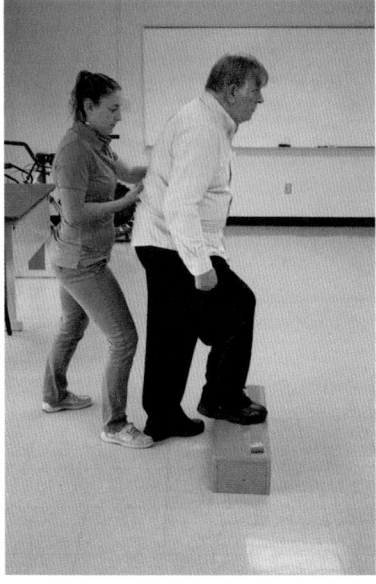

Figure 11.6 Step up onto a 4-inch step.

Balance and Dynamic Postural Control During Overground Walking

Adequate standing balance and control of the COM are integral components of locomotion. As continuous postural adjustments are needed during locomotion, intervention strategies to improve balance should be selected that impose similar demands. Locomotion requires the ability to maintain upright stance (stability) and dynamic postural control (controlled mobility) to control movements while standing (e.g., weight shifting, LE stepping). Examples of interventions to improve standing balance and dynamic postural control follow; balance interventions are also discussed in Chapter 10, Strategies to Improve Motor Function.

Initial standing activities may require a widening of the BOS through the touch-down support of the hands and can be performed in the parallel bars, between two treatment tables, or next to a wall or corner of a room (corner standing). The patient is first directed to stand tall and hold steady in the posture. Enhanced postural awareness and practice of COM control can be achieved with limits of stability (LOS) training during weight shifting and in response to anticipated and unanticipated perturbations (anticipatory and reactive postural control). Active exercise to improve standing balance may include activities that require COM control while reducing the BOS (e.g., heel raises, toe-offs), transitions to and from single-limb stance (back-kicks and sidekicks, hip and knee flexion, hip flexion with knee extension, marching in place), and tasks that change the height of the COM (partial squats). These exercises can also be performed in a pool. Adding ankle cuff weights, further alteration of the BOS (e.g., feet apart, feet together, tandem stance), upper extremity position (e.g., arms overhead, reaching), and support surface (e.g., inflated disc, wobble board) can all impose greater challenge.

Engagement of ankle and hip strategies to control the COM can be promoted using incremental shifts in COM alignment and postural sway movements. Challenges can be enhanced using unstable surfaces or alterations in sensory inputs. Examples include using a foam cushion to degrade somatosensory input, modifying visual input by progressing from eyes open to closed, modifying the stability of the support surface (using split foam rollers [flat side down progressing to flat side up], and wobble boards), or changing the static position of the head position to alter vestibular inputs. Self-imposed or externally provided large COM shifts in all directions beyond the LOS will promote stepping strategies. Balance control can be further enhanced using manual perturbations, resistive band around pelvis during stepping (forward, backward, sideward), and using mobile and compliant surfaces with alterations in BOS (feet together, tandem standing, and single-limb stance). See Box 11.2 and Figures 11.7 and 11.8.

Previous research suggests that there is a limited transfer of static standing balance activities to dynamic stability during gait.[83] For this reason, if improvements in stability during gait are desired, overground walking must be trained with the incorporation of dynamic postural control activities during gait. Examples of overground walking activities with dynamic postural control

Box 11.2   Balance and Dynamic Postural Control During Overground Walking

- Stationary Base of Support/Static Center of Mass Activities
  - Static standing in wide stance, progressed to narrow or tandem stance
    - Eyes open/eyes closed, stationary head/looking up/head turns
  - Stabilization against expected and unexpected perturbations
- Stationary Base of Support/Dynamic Center of Mass Activities
  - Tai Chi forms with feet stationary
  - Anterior/posterior/lateral/rotational UE reaching
  - Picking objects up off the floor (progress from light to heavy objects)
  - Throwing and catching objects (progress from light to heavy objects)
- Moving Base of Support/Dynamic Center of Mass Activities
  - Stepping in different directions: backward, forward, side stepping, braiding
  - Sit to from stand from various surfaces
  - Standing heel and toe lifts
  - Transitions to single-limb stance
  - Forward, lateral, and backward step-ups/downs
  - Walking on different surfaces/ascend and descend curbs, ramps, stairs
  - Walking with horizontal or vertical head turns
  - Walking while performing cognitive or motor secondary tasks
  - Obstacle course: different surfaces (carpet, mat, grass, gravel, ramp), stepping over/around objects, curbs, carrying object, varying speed, heel/toe walking, tandem walking

UE = upper extremity

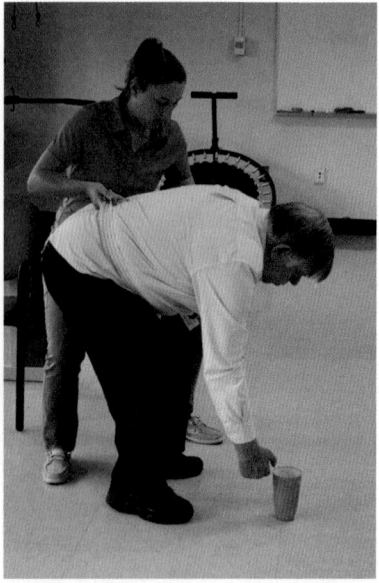

Figure 11.7 Picking up an object from the floor.

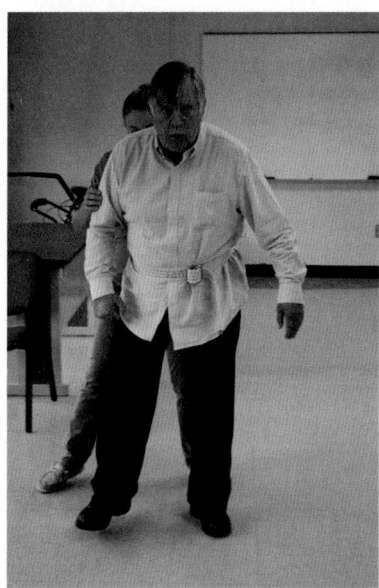

Figure 11.8 Sidestepping.

demands includes the modification of sensory inputs (walking on compliant surfaces, compromising vision, or asking for vertical or horizontal head movements to alter vestibular input); practicing rapid accelerations and decelerations of the COM to perform rapid starts, stops, and turns during gait; and practicing the avoidance of apparent and suddenly appearing obstacles in the gait path. Studies that have examined such interventions have some gait outcome improvements in varied patient populations.[84–86] Observational research suggests that the repetition of balance tasks during rehabilitation may be inadequate; therefore, consideration of increasing the practice dosage of these tasks is warranted.[87]

Although TM walking and overground walking practice may provide benefits in terms of dynamic balance, adherence to such programs over the long term may limit the overall effects. For this reason, alternative forms of exercise that provide similar benefits to gait and balance training that are more engaging are worthy of consideration. Dance is one such form of exercise. From a dynamic balance standpoint, many dance forms require repetitions of backward walking, turning, and changing speeds, all of which require the individual to control the COM (and provide variable task practice). If performed to music with a non-balance-impaired partner, additional benefits include auditory cueing, safety, working memory, and cognitive sequencing practice, and the social connection that occurs with the partner. Recent studies document improvements in measures of dynamic balance and gait as a result of dance interventions.[88–90] Tango and ballroom dance have been studied most often, although other forms have research support also. Studies have examined the effects of dance interventions performed between 1 to 7 days per week, 30 minutes up to 75 minutes per session, and between 8 weeks and 18 months in overall duration.[88,91]

Circuit Training

Task-oriented locomotor circuit training involves setting up a variety of different task-oriented intervention stations, some of which are discussed in the above sections (e.g., augmenting force production, TM training, dynamic postural control during overground walking). At each station, the patient performs the indicated number of task repetitions or for a specific duration (at a certain intensity) and then moves on to the next station, with a short rest between stations.[92–94] A Cochrane systematic review concluded that there is moderate evidence that circuit training can improve mobility in people with stroke.[95]

Specific training stations include tasks or activities such as standing and reaching, standing on different surfaces, walking through an obstacle course, transitioning from supine to sitting to standing, walking and carrying objects, walking and picking up objects from the floor, walking in different directions, walking with head turns, stepping up and down off a step, walking at varying speeds and over varying surfaces, and standing and kicking a ball. Adding ankle weights, a weighted vest, or having the patient walk against the resistance of a resistance band can vary the intensity of the task. Strength and balance exercises (described earlier) can also be incorporated into the circuit. As patient performance improves, the specific tasks are progressed by increasing the complexity and difficulty. For example, strategies to progress performance in an obstacle course might include increasing speed, carrying an object while walking through it, or stepping over higher/wider objects. A dual cognitive task can be added to the activity to increase the difficulty as well. See Box 11.3 and Figures 11.9 through 11.11.

Motor learning and neuroplasticity principles can effectively be incorporated to enhance motor learning and promote recovery. Variable and random practice is inherent to the circuit set up and different walking-related tasks at the various stations. KR feedback can be provided, for example, by informing the patient how long it took to complete the obstacle course, motivating the patient to improve on that time. An external focus of attention can be provided by instructing patients to step to or over objects instead of providing verbal instructions to lift the foot up higher when stepping (these instructions promote an internal focus of attention). Autonomy can be provided by allowing the patient to select the tasks that will be performed in the circuit, to select different objects to walk around/

Box 11.3   Circuit Training Activities

- Obstacle course: different surfaces (carpet, mat, grass, gravel, ramp), stepping over/around objects, curbs, carrying object, varying speed, heel/toe walking, tandem walking
- Walking and picking up objects
- Stepping in different directions: backward, forward, sidestepping, braiding
- Sit to/from stand from various surfaces
- Walking on different surfaces
- Stair, curbs
- Forward, lateral, and backward step-ups/downs
- Standing and reaching
- Standing on different surfaces (firm, foam, carpet, grass, gravel, incline) with varying base of support (wide/narrow base of support, tandem, one foot on step and one foot on ground), and visual (eyes open/eyes closed) input
- Walking with horizontal and vertical head turns
- Walking on balance beam
- Walking on heels/toes, tandem walking
- Standing/walking and kicking ball
- Dual task: walking and carrying and/or walking with cognitive task (subtract serial 7s)
- Standing heel and toe lifts
- Walking against resistance of resistance band or with ankle weights or weighted vest
- Provide unexpected perturbations while walking
- Strength and balance exercises (see Box 11.2)

over in the obstacle course, to determine the height of a step-up/down surface, and to choose what objects to carry while walking. People with chronic stroke are also able to achieve moderate intensity levels (>40% HRR) while performing circuit training that involves functional mobility tasks.[96,97]

Motor Imagery

Motor imagery (MI) is the mental rehearsal of a movement without the movement actually occurring.[98] Motor imagery activates some of the same cortical structures that are activated during actual movement, which may be the mechanism for improving behavioral performance.[99] Using MI as an intervention may involve either *visual imagery*, where the individual visualizes performing the activity from the perspective of third person, or *kinesthetic imagery*, where the individual imagines the sensory experience of the activity as it might normally occur from a first person perspective.[98]

In the context of locomotion, MI is the mental practice of walking. Mental imagery practice should be relatively short (10 to 20 minutes).[98] An MI session is performed in a comfortable position (often sitting) with

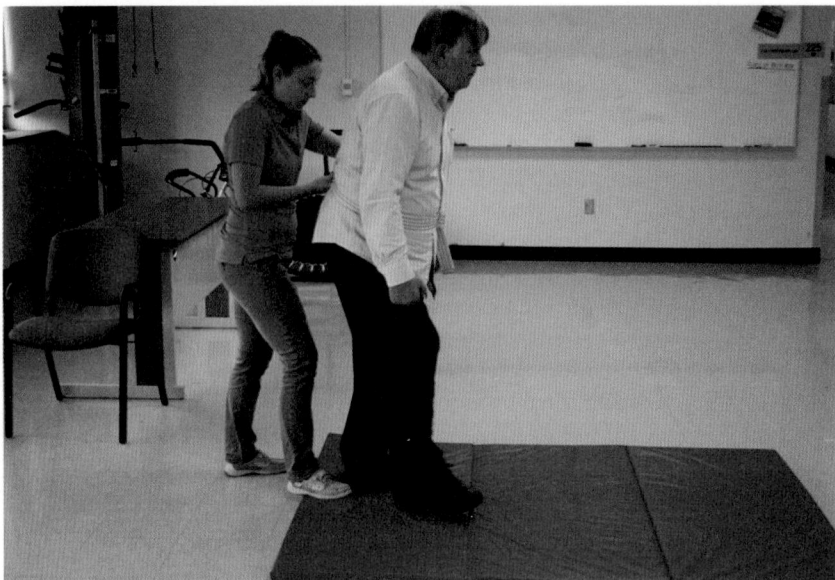

Figure 11.9 Walking on foam/ uneven surface.

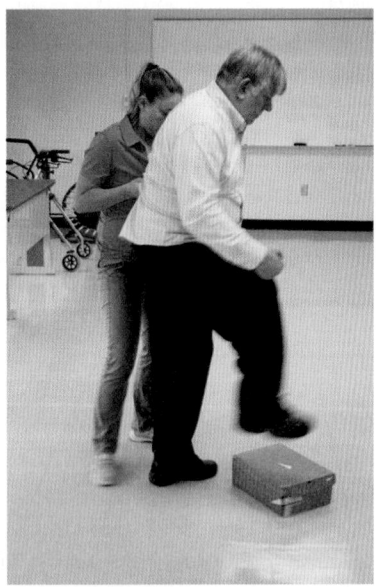

Figure 11.10 Stepping over an object while walking.

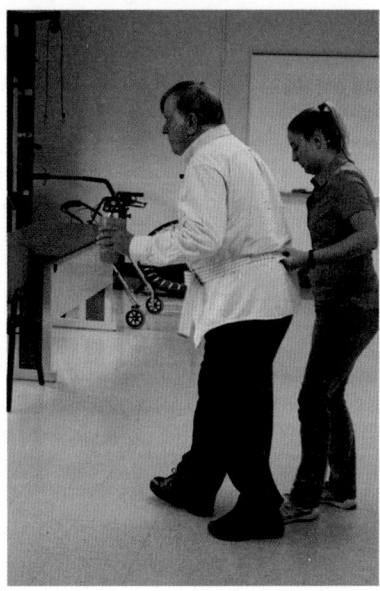

Figure 11.11 Walking while performing a motor dual task, carrying an object.

a short period of guided relaxation prior to initiation. The therapist guides the individual through a detailed, specific visual or kinesthetic mental rehearsal of the walking task. The tasks that are mentally rehearsed can be very specific (e.g., see how your left foot pushes down and backward, then lifts up off the ground). Dunsky and colleagues[100] and Dickstein and colleagues[101] provide examples of specific MI sessions that incorporate both visual and kinesthetic imagery. A metronome can be added to provide auditory cues for the cadence of the imagined steps.[100] MI should be done in combination with physical practice of the task[102,103] and can be done as part of a group intervention,[104] as well as through telerehabilitation.[105] Research supports the use of MI combined with other interventions to improve walking

ability in people with stroke,[101,102,104,106] PD,[98,107] total knee arthroplasty,[108] and lower limb amputations.[109]

Emerging Interventions
Support for Behavioral Change

Early studies that incorporate the use of activity monitors, telehealth-supported exercise, and methods to support behavior change that engage patients to overcome barriers to walking are promising.[110,111] Patients wear an activity monitor that captures activity data such as steps/day, which can then be relayed to the patient and physical therapist. The information is used to set goals to increase stepping activity, provide motivating feedback, and to problem-solve ways to overcome barriers to increasing walking activity. Mobile technologies to provide feedback on and increase physical activity in this manner with neurologically intact individuals can positively influence physical activity levels.[112] Preliminary findings indicate that this strategy may support increased walking activity in people with stroke and PD.[111,113]

Neuromodulation

In the context of individuals with cortical injuries that contribute to impairments in their walking patterns, the use of noninvasive brain stimulation (NIBS), such as repetitive transcranial magnetic stimulation (rTMS) and transcranial direct current stimulation (tDCS) has been utilized. The proposed mechanism of the observed effects is the modulation of cortical neural processing that counteracts maladaptive neural plasticity after cortical injury.[114,115] Meta-analyses of NIBS on gait-related outcomes in people poststroke suggest that there may be positive effects on gait, although the effects depend on stimulation type (rTMS vs. tDCS), stimulation parameters (frequency, intensity, duration), neural structures stimulated (hemisphere, specific neural center), and individual specific factors (type and extent of stroke, time since stroke).[116] Further research is needed to best determine the optimal combination of NIBS with task-specific training to optimize outcomes in individuals with neurological injury.

Exoskeleton

In those individuals with substantial gait impairments that severely limit their ambulation ability or result in substantial asymmetry, wearable powered exoskeleton devices may hold promise for improving gait. These devices may be unilateral or bilateral and most commonly provide mechanical assistance to hip motion. Bilateral devices may be able to be tuned to provide greater assistance to the more impaired extremity. In studies on individuals poststroke, these devices are effective at increasing paretic and nonparetic limb step lengths.[117] Small studies in individuals with moderate PD have shown modest effects on walking endurance and physiological cost.[118]

Performance vs. Capacity vs. Patient-Reported Outcomes

Regardless of the types of interventions used to improve gait, standardized outcomes are needed to quantify the benefits of training. In addition, in the context of progressive conditions, such outcomes are necessary to identify declines that may signal the progression of disability. While in-clinic measures of gait speed (10MWT), gait endurance (6MWT), or dynamic stability during gait (FGA) are useful capacity measures, they do not accurately represent the performance that an individual demonstrates during their daily life activities. In addition, such in-clinic measures may not reflect how an individual perceives changes in their gait. In order to provide a full-spectrum view of gait-related disability and potential improvements in gait function, clinicians should employ:

1. objective in-clinic valid and reliable measures of gait (such as those summarized at the Rehabilitation Measures Database housed as Shirley Ryan Ability Lab [https://www.sralab.org/rehabilitation-measures])
2. measures of multiday ambulatory activity (such as those available on commercially available smartwatches or specifically designed pedometers)
3. patient-reported outcomes, such as Patient-Reported Outcomes Measurement Information System [PROMIS] measures designed to allow individuals to subjectively evaluate their gait-related functional limitations to daily activities imposed by their condition.

Gait Training With Assistive Devices

Appendix 11.A (online) contains detailed information on different types of assistive devices, gait patterns with assistive devices, and gait training with assistive devices techniques.

SUMMARY

Recovery of independent walking ability is an important goal for many patients who require the services of a physical therapist. It is a functional skill that directly affects performance of expected roles within the patient's social, cultural, and physical environment. A variety of interventions are available, including moderate- to high-intensity task-specific step training, TM training, VR, strengthening, dynamic balance, circuit training, and MI. Principles of motor learning, neuroplasticity, and exercise prescription guidelines should inform the development of the plan of care to improve locomotor function.

Questions for Review

1. When interpreting change in a patient's gait speed over the course of your intervention, how much should the patient's gait speed change in order for you to be confident that the patient exhibits clinically meaningful improvement in locomotor function?

2. Describe key motor learning and neuroplasticity principles that should be incorporated into any specific locomotor rehabilitation intervention.

3. Describe intensity guidelines for moderate- to high-intensity locomotor training, and list safety concerns that should be monitored.

4. What variables can be manipulated to increase the intensity of locomotor training when using a TM?

5. Describe two task-specific interventions to increase muscle force production that would improve stance and swing phase of gait in the coronal plane.

6. List overground walking activities that promote dynamic postural control demands.

7. Describe three stations you could use in a circuit training intervention designed to promote recovery of locomotor function.

CASE STUDY

PART A

You are working with a 58 y/o woman who had a left CVA 4 weeks ago in an outpatient facility. She was recently discharged home after spending 2 weeks in an inpatient rehabilitation facility. She lives alone on the fourth floor of an apartment building. She returned to work this week as an administrative assistant at a bank and takes public transportation to work. She can walk independently in her home and short distances in the community. She uses an off-the-shelf ankle foot orthosis (AFO) and straight cane. She reports her primary goal is to improve her walking ability. She has difficulty crossing the street in the city, making it on time to work because she cannot walk quickly enough to catch the bus, and has fallen once at home while walking at night to the bathroom.

GUIDING QUESTIONS PART A

1. What tests and measures would you use with this patient?

2. What locomotion-related tests and measures would you perform to gain more specific insight into this patient's locomotor function?

PART B

You find the following during your initial examination:

1. Motor Function: Fugl-Meyer LE motor function section, 29/34. Full score on all items except:

   a. Movement combining synergies: knee flexion and ankle dorsiflexion, both 1/2
   b. Movement out of synergy: knee flexion and ankle dorsiflexion, both 1/2
   c. Normal reflexes: 0/2
   d. Coordination: speed: 1/2

2. Sensory integrity: proprioception of right ankle is normal.

3. Muscle performance: right ankle dorsiflexion 22 lb of force (normative values for women 50 to 59; dominant side: 43.7 lb).

4. Balance: Mini-Balance Evaluation Systems Test: 19/28; test findings indicate difficulty with anticipatory postural control, postural responses to perturbation, dynamic balance during gait, and dual task.

5. Self-Care/Domestic Life and Work Life: Stroke Impact Scale 16: 68%

6. Specific locomotor function tests:

   a. Gait speed: 0.80 m/s (normative values for women 50 to 59: 1.31 m/s)
   b. 6MWT: 318 meters (normative values for women 20 to 59: 674 meters)
   c. Community Balance and Mobility Scale: 34/96; test findings indicate difficulty with support of body mass by the right lower extremity, dynamic postural control of the moving body, propulsion of the body in the intended direction, adaptability of the locomotion to changing environmental and task demands and with stairs.
   d. Multiple Sclerosis Walking Scale: 75%; self-report outcome measure indicates that patient has difficulty with stairs, running, walking endurance, speed of walking, and need to concentrate more while walking.

CASE STUDY—cont'd

GUIDING QUESTIONS PART B

1. Based on the findings from the initial examination, outline an intervention session that addresses the major locomotor impairments and limitations with which the patient presents.

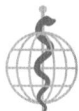 For additional resources, including answers to the questions for review, new immersive cases, case study guiding questions, references, and more, please visit **https://www.fadavis.com/product/physical -rehabilitation-fulk-8**. You may also quickly find the resources by entering this title's four-digit ISBN, 4691, in the search field at **http://fadavis.com** and logging in at the prompt.

Chronic Pulmonary Dysfunction

Pei-Tzu Wu, PT, PhD, CCS
Julie Ann Starr, PT, DPT, CCS, FAPTA

Chapter 12

LEARNING OBJECTIVES

1. Define the disease processes (including definition, etiology, pathophysiology, clinical presentation, and clinical course) of chronic obstructive pulmonary disease, asthma, cystic fibrosis, and restrictive lung disease.

2. Describe examination procedures (including patient interview, vital signs, observation, inspection, palpation, auscultation, and laboratory tests) for a patient with pulmonary disease.

3. Identify the anticipated goals and expected outcomes of pulmonary rehabilitation.

4. Describe the rehabilitative management of a patient with chronic pulmonary dysfunction.

5. Value the therapist's role in the management of a patient with chronic pulmonary dysfunction.

6. Analyze and interpret patient data, formulate realistic goals and outcomes, and develop a plan of care when presented with a clinical case study.

CHAPTER OUTLINE

RESPIRATORY PHYSIOLOGY 383
CHRONIC LUNG DISEASES 384
  Chronic Obstructive Pulmonary Disease 384
  Asthma 389
  Cystic Fibrosis 390
  Restrictive Lung Disease 391
  Coronavirus Disease 2019 (COVID-19) 392
MEDICAL AND SURGICAL MANAGEMENT 393
  Smoking Cessation 393
  Pharmacological Management 393
  Supplemental Oxygen 395
Surgical and Interventional Management of Chronic Pulmonary Disease 396
PHYSICAL THERAPY MANAGEMENT 396
  Goals and Outcomes 396
  Examination 397
  Exercise Prescription 400
  Pulmonary Rehabilitation 402
  Home Exercise Programs 407
  Multispecialty Team 407
  Patient Education 408
  Secretion Removal Techniques 408
SUMMARY 412

Years ago, patients with chronic pulmonary disease were given a standard prescription for rest and avoidance of exercise.[1] The stress imposed by exercise was considered deleterious to people with pulmonary disorders. A pivotal study by Pierce et al. provided the impetus to change direction in the treatment of pulmonary dysfunction. Exercise training effects of decreased heart rate (HR), respiratory rate (RR), minute ventilation, oxygen consumption, and carbon dioxide production at submaximal exercise levels were documented in their subjects with chronic obstructive pulmonary disease (COPD). Increased maximal aerobic capacity was also documented.[2] Reconditioning of patients with pulmonary disease was found to be possible. Pulmonary rehabilitation has emerged since that time as a multidisciplinary comprehensive program of care for patients with chronic pulmonary disease to optimize physical functioning, enhance social participation and quality of life, minimize disease symptoms, and reduce hospital admissions and health-care costs.[3]

COPD, asthma, and cystic fibrosis (CF) are the most common chronic obstructive lung diseases for which pulmonary rehabilitation is provided. Patients with chronic restrictive lung diseases have also demonstrated improvement in functional abilities following pulmonary rehabilitation.[4] It is clear that pulmonary rehabilitation is of value for all patients in whom respiratory symptoms have resulted in a decreased functional capacity or a decreased quality of life.[3]

In this chapter, the most common chronic pulmonary diseases encountered in pulmonary rehabilitation programs are discussed as well as the physical therapy examination and treatment of patients with chronic pulmonary disease. A brief review of ventilation and respiration is warranted for a better understanding of the disease pathologies and for understanding the rationale of the physical therapy procedures.

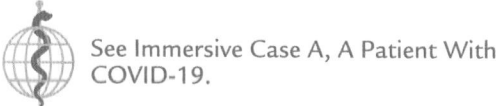

See Immersive Case A, A Patient With COVID-19.

■ RESPIRATORY PHYSIOLOGY

Air is inspired through the nose or mouth through all of the conducting airways until it reaches the distal respiratory unit, which contains the respiratory bronchiole, alveolar ducts, alveolar sacs, and alveoli (Fig. 12.1). The movement of air through the conducting airways is termed *ventilation*. At full inspiration, the lungs contain their maximum amount of air. This volume of air is called *total lung capacity* (TLC), which can be divided into four separate volumes of air: (1) tidal volume, (2) inspiratory reserve volume, (3) expiratory reserve volume, and (4) residual volume. Combinations of two or more of these lung volumes are termed *capacities*. Figure 12.2 illustrates the relationship of lung volumes and capacities.

The amount of air inspired or expired during normal resting ventilation is termed *tidal volume* (TV or V_t). As this TV of air enters the pulmonary system, it travels through the conducting airways to reach the respiratory units. TV is about 500 mL/breath for a young, healthy, male of European descent, and approximately 400 mL/breath for a healthy female. Asian and African American people have lower lung volumes with a reduction of 6%

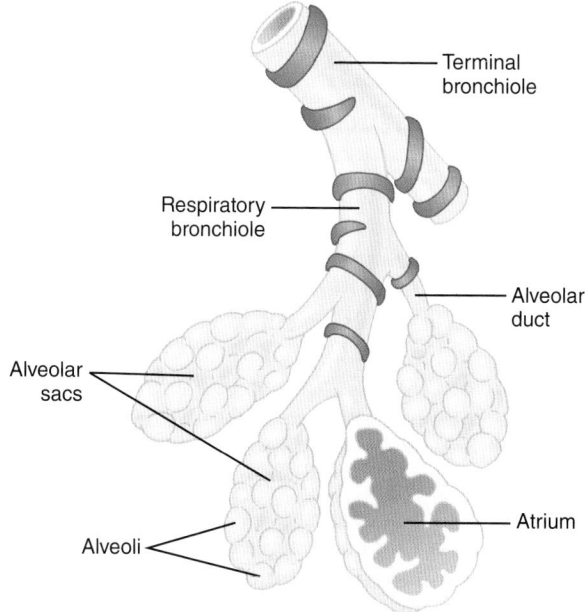

Figure 12.1 Anatomy of the distal conducting airway, the terminal bronchiole and the respiratory unit, the respiratory bronchiole, alveolar ducts, alveolar sacs, and alveoli.

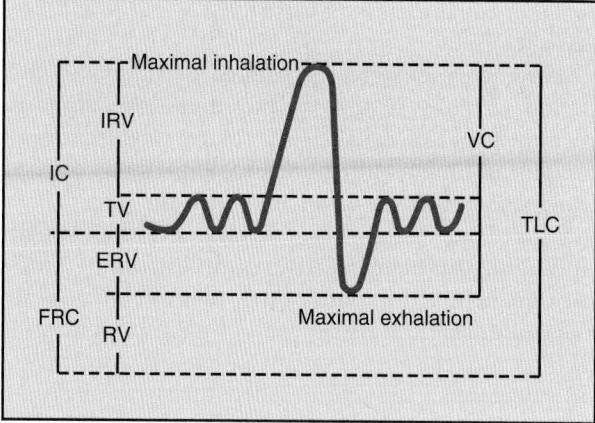

Figure 12.2 Lung volumes and capacities. (ERV = expiratory reserve volume; FRC = functional residual capacity; IC = inspiratory capacity; IRV = inspiratory reserve volume; RV = residual volume; TLC = total lung capacity; TV = tidal volume; VC = vital capacity.)

to 7% and 12%, respectively, when compared to people of European descent.[6-8] The amount of inspired air that actually reaches the distal respiratory unit and takes part in gas exchange is about 350 mL of that 500 mL total of the tidal breath. The remaining 150 mL of the inhaled tidal breath remains in the conducting airways and does not take part in gas exchange, termed *anatomical dead space*.[5] When only a tidal breath occupies the lungs, there is "room" for additional air that can be further inhaled. This inspiratory volume in excess of that used in tidal breathing is the inspiratory reserve volume (IRV). Aptly named, it is the volume of air that can be inspired when needed but is usually kept in reserve. There is a quantity of air that can potentially be exhaled beyond the end of a tidal exhalation. Although it is usually kept in reserve, the volume of air that can be exhaled in excess of tidal breathing is called the *expiratory reserve volume* (ERV). The lungs are never completely emptied of air even after maximally exhaling the ERV. The volume of air remaining within the lungs when ERV has been exhaled is called the residual volume (RV).

The sum of two or more volumes is referred to as *capacity*. TV plus the IRV is known as the *inspiratory capacity*. This refers to the volume of air that can be inspired beginning from a tidal exhalation. The combination of RV and ERV is the functional residual capacity (FRC). FRC is the volume of air that remains in the lungs at the end of a tidal exhalation. The sum of IRV, TV, and ERV is called the *vital capacity* (VC). It is all of the possible volume of air within the lungs that is under volitional control. The common method of measuring VC is to achieve maximal inspiration, then forcibly exhale as hard and fast as possible into a measuring device until ERV has been exhausted. Because this is a forced expiratory maneuver, it is termed the *forced vital capacity* (FVC). As stated earlier, all volumes together equal total lung capacity: TV + IRV + ERV + RV = TLC.

Flow rates measure the volume of air moved in a period of time. Expiratory flow rates, therefore, are measurements of exhaled gas volume divided by the amount of time required for the volume to be exhaled. Flow rates reflect the ease with which the lungs can be ventilated, the state of the airways, and the elasticity of the lung parenchyma (tissue). An important airflow measurement is the volume of air that can be forcefully exhaled during the first second of an FVC maneuver. This is called the *forced expiratory volume in 1 sec* (FEV$_1$). This flow rate is thought to reflect the status of the airways of the lungs. In healthy individuals, FEV$_1$ is 70% or more of the total FVC (FEV$_1$/FVC > 70%).[9] *Peak expiratory flow* (PEF) is the greatest flow rate generated during a maximal forced expiratory maneuver. Individuals with COPD often measure PEF on a daily basis with a handheld peak flow meter to track their pulmonary status. Daily peak flow rates are compared to the patient's own "best" test value.[10] A drop in a patient's peak flow rate indicates airway narrowing and may indicate the need for a physician visit and/or change in medication regimen.

Inspiratory mechanics can also be helpful in understanding a patient's pulmonary disease. *Maximum inspiratory pressure* (PI$_{max}$) reflects the greatest static inspiratory effort that can be generated from RV. It is measured as a pressure in millimeters of mercury or centimeters of water and reflects the strength of the muscles of inspiration. The maximal pressure is defined as the highest negative pressure that the patient can sustain for 1 second during the testing procedure.[11]

Lung volumes, capacities, flow rates, and mechanics depend on the size and configuration of the thorax. Therefore, height, gender, and race influence static and dynamic lung measurements. Any alteration in the properties of the lungs or chest wall due to the aging process or a disease process will also change the lung volumes, capacities, flow rates, and/or mechanics.

Respiration is a term used to describe the gas exchange within the body. This should not be confused with *ventilation,* which describes only the movement of air. External respiration is the exchange of gas that occurs at the alveolar capillary membrane between atmospheric air and the pulmonary capillaries. Internal respiration takes place at the tissue capillary level between the tissues and the surrounding capillaries. The following discussion traces the course of gas exchange, specifically that of oxygen and carbon dioxide, during both external and internal respiration (Fig. 12.3).

For external respiration to take place, there must first be an inhalation of air from the environment through the conducting airways and into the respiratory bronchioles and alveoli. Oxygen diffuses through the walls of the respiratory unit, through the interstitial space, and through the pulmonary capillary wall. Most of the

oxygen (98.5%) then travels through the blood plasma into red blood cells where it occupies one of the gas-carrying sites of hemoglobin. A small portion of dissolved oxygen (1.5%) is carried in the plasma.

The now-oxygenated blood in the pulmonary capillaries travels to the left side of the heart via the pulmonary veins. From there it is pumped into the aorta, then through a network of connecting arteries, arterioles, and capillaries, until its destination, the tissue, is reached. Internal respiration begins when the arterial blood reaches the tissue level. Oxygen diffuses from the gas-carrying sites of hemoglobin, out of the red blood cell, out of the capillary, through the cell membranes, and into the mitochondria of the working cells.

Carbon dioxide (CO_2), which is produced at the tissue level as a by-product of metabolism, diffuses out of the working cells into the blood in the capillaries. Carbon dioxide is then transported to the venous system and into the right side of the heart. Once the carbon dioxide–laden blood makes its way through the right atrium, the right ventricle, the pulmonary artery, and the pulmonary capillaries, it diffuses out through the capillary membrane, through the interstitial space, and into the alveoli, where, during external respiration, it is finally exhaled into the atmosphere.

When the cycle of external and internal respiration has occurred, oxygen has been extracted from the environment and provided to the body tissues. Meanwhile, carbon dioxide has been removed from the body tissues and released into the external environment. Of course, this system is dependent on an intact cardiovascular system to pump the blood through the lungs and deliver it to the working cells, and then return it back from the working cells to the lungs, all in a timely fashion.

■ CHRONIC LUNG DISEASES
Chronic Obstructive Pulmonary Disease

COPD is the most common chronic pulmonary disorder. It is one of the top three causes of mortality in the world, and it is projected to increase in coming decades.[9]

The *Global Initiative for Chronic Obstructive Lung Disease (GOLD)* is an ongoing collaborative work of the National Heart, Lung, and Blood Institute (NHLBI) and the World Health Organization (WHO). In its initial report of 2001, GOLD set out to increase worldwide awareness of COPD, to advocate for its prevention as well as to decrease morbidity and mortality from the disease. According to GOLD, COPD is defined as a preventable and treatable disease. The pulmonary component of COPD is characterized by airflow limitation caused by chronic inflammation of the small airways and air spaces in response to significant exposure to noxious particles or gases. Mucociliary dysfunction is also a characteristic of the disease. COPD is usually progressive. Additional significant extra pulmonary effects, such as a decrease in body mass index (BMI), decreased

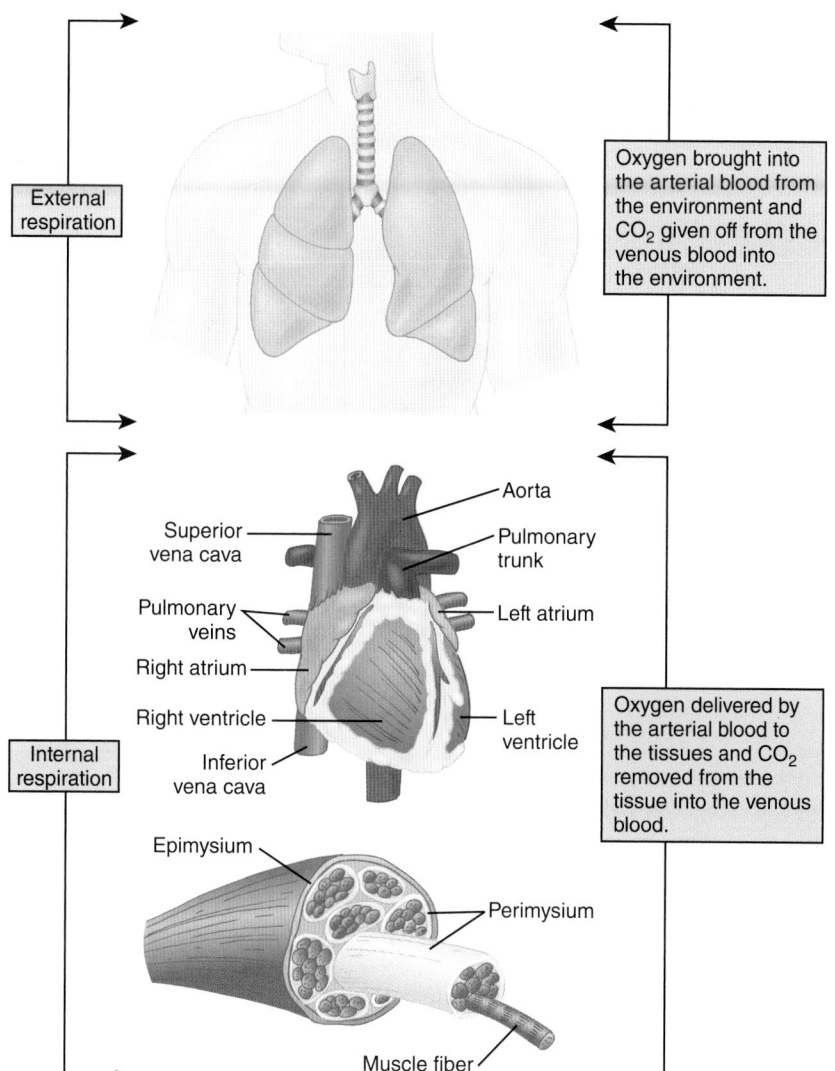

External respiration

Oxygen brought into the arterial blood from the environment and CO_2 given off from the venous blood into the environment.

Aorta
Superior vena cava
Pulmonary trunk
Pulmonary veins
Left atrium
Right atrium
Right ventricle
Left ventricle
Inferior vena cava

Internal respiration

Oxygen delivered by the arterial blood to the tissues and CO_2 removed from the tissue into the venous blood.

Epimysium
Perimysium
Muscle fiber

Figure 12.3 The process of external and internal respiration.

muscle strength, and exercise intolerance, contribute to the symptomology of COPD in individual patients.[9] The severity of COPD was classified based on the patient's airflow limitation (i.e., Grade 1: mild, $FEV_1 \geq$ 80% predicted; Grade 2: moderate, $50\% \leq FEV_1 < 80\%$ predicted; Grade 3: severe, $30\% \leq FEV_1 < 50\%$ predicted; Grade 4: very severe, $FEV_1 < 30\%$ predicted). Airflow limitation in conjunction with symptoms (e.g., dyspnea) and history of moderate/severe exacerbation (e.g., prior hospitalizations), also known as the ABCD assessment tool, help evaluate prognosis and guide therapeutic strategies for a patient with COPD (Fig. 12.4).[9] Refer to the case study at the end of this chapter for use of this classification system.

Risk Factors

Risk factors for the development of COPD include both environmental factors and host factors. Cigarette smoking is the major environmental causal agent in the development of COPD.[9] Smoking history is quantified in units of *pack-years*, the number of packs per day times the number of years smoked. Passive exposure to cigarette smoke (e.g., secondhand smoke) also contributes to COPD. Other environmental factors that contribute to the development of COPD include occupational exposures (e.g., organic and inorganic dusts), indoor pollutants (e.g., smoke from wood-burning fireplace), and outdoor pollutants (e.g., air pollution).[9]

Host factors that would make a person more susceptible to the development of COPD include hyperreactivity of the airways, overall lung growth (the amount of lung tissue developed during childhood, which is partially determined by nutritional status, health status, height, and exposure to pollutants), and genetics. It is perplexing that less than 15% of smokers go on to develop COPD in their lifetime.[12] There are a number of ongoing studies investigating the potential for a genetic influence in the development of COPD.[13,14]

Pathophysiology

COPD is characterized by pathological changes that can be found throughout the pulmonary system—in

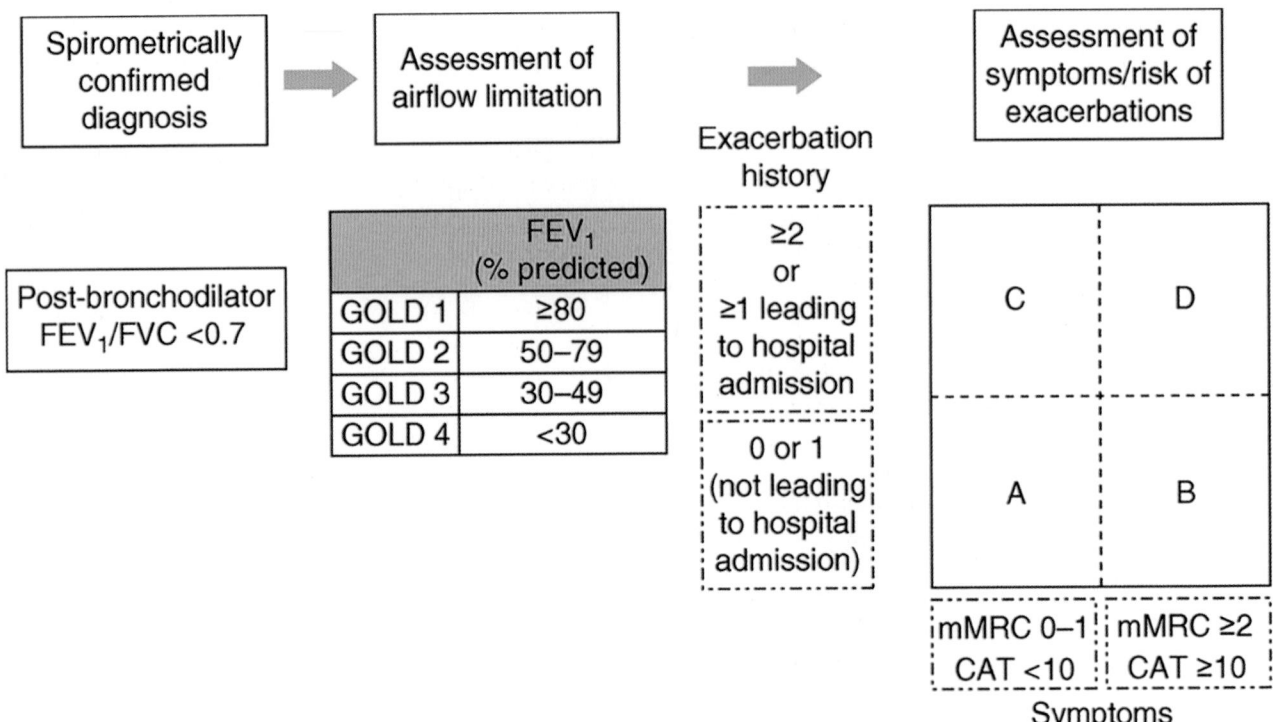

Figure 12.4 The ABCD assessment tool from the Global Initiative for Obstructive Lung Disease (GOLD). The results of spirometric assessment will categorize patients into a grade of 1 through 4. The results of the exacerbation history and the assessment of symptoms further categorize patients into a group of A through D. (Global Initiative for Obstructive Lung Disease [GOLD], with permission.)

the airways, airspaces, and pulmonary capillaries. Chronic inflammation, including an increase in neutrophils, macrophages, and T lymphocytes, damages the endothelial lining of the airways. Airway inflammation causes airway narrowing, which is worsened by an imbalance of proteases/antiproteases and oxidants/antioxidants in patients with COPD.[9] Disruption in the normal tissue repair process also leads to airway remodeling and destruction of fragile lung parenchyma. These airway changes appear to be most pronounced in the smaller peripheral airways (bronchioles).[9] These changes result in the loss of the normal elastic recoil properties of the lung tissue. Endothelial changes in the pulmonary vasculature are altered early in the development of COPD and result in thickening of the vessel walls. In advanced stages of the disease, there is destruction of the pulmonary capillary bed. Mucus hypersecretion, resulting in a chronic productive cough, is present due to an increase in the size of submucosal glands and the number of goblet cells within the bronchial walls. Decreases in ciliary function and alterations in physiochemical characteristics of bronchial secretions impair airway clearance and contribute to airway obstruction. Damaged and inflamed mucosa shows an increased activation of epidermal growth factor receptors within the bronchial walls, which in turn cause bronchial hyperreactivity.[9]

During normal inspiration, the lungs and the airways are pulled open, increasing the diameter of the airway lumen. During normal exhalation, as the thorax returns to its resting position, the airways decrease in size. In patients with COPD, during inspiration, the airways are pulled open by thoracic expansion, allowing air to enter. During exhalation, the airways, already narrowed by inflammation, remodeling, and in some cases excessive secretions, close prematurely, trapping air in the distal airways and airspaces. This air trapping causes hyperinflation, which is defined as an abnormal increase in the amount of air within the lung tissue at the end of a tidal exhalation (increased FRC).

Ventilation in the alveoli and *perfusion* in the capillary membrane are no longer well matched, resulting in *hypoxemia,* a condition of decreased amount of oxygen in the arterial blood to the tissues. As the disease progresses and more areas of the lungs become involved, hypoxemia will worsen, and *hypercapnea,* a condition of an increased amount of carbon dioxide within the arterial blood, will develop. Increased pulmonary vascular resistance secondary to capillary wall damage and reflex vasoconstriction in the presence of hypoxemia results in pulmonary hypertension, defined by a mean pulmonary artery pressure greater than 35 to 40 mm Hg, and right ventricular hypertrophy, termed *cor pulmonale.*[15] *Polycythemia,* an increase in the number of circulating red blood cells, occurs in order to potentially increase the oxygen-carrying capacity of the blood.

Clinical Presentation

Patients with COPD usually present with a history of cigarette smoking. The most characteristic symptom of COPD is dyspnea. Dyspnea may be first evidenced during exertion. As the disease progresses, dyspnea worsens so that it occurs at progressively lower levels of activity. Severely involved patients may feel dyspneic even at rest. In a portion of patients with COPD, there is also a slow and insidious development of chronic cough and expectoration. On physical examination, the thorax appears enlarged owing to hyperinflation and the loss of lung elastic recoil properties. The anterior–posterior diameter of the chest increases, and a dorsal kyphosis results. These anatomical changes give the patient a barrel-chest appearance (Fig. 12.5).

As the resting position of the thorax is now held in a more inspiratory mode, the available range of thoracic motion is limited—that is, there is decreased thoracic excursion. There are morphological changes to the ventilatory muscles due to a greater demand, both in frequency of contraction and in the power needed to move this altered thorax. The muscles of ventilation hypertrophy as a result. Figure 12.6 shows many of the accessory muscles of ventilation that may be recruited for breathing. In severe disease, these muscles are recruited even

at rest to aid in the work of breathing. The length–tension relationship of muscles of ventilation is altered as the thorax increases in size with chronic hyperinflation. There are also changes in the alignment of muscle fibers, especially the fibers of the diaphragm. With hyperinflation, the diaphragm cannot return to its domed shape on exhalation. In severe disease, the diaphragm fiber alignment may become more horizontal than vertical (i.e., flatter, potentially resulting in an inward motion of the lower ribs during a diaphragm muscle contraction of inhalation) (Fig. 12.7).

Auscultation of the chest may demonstrate decreased intensity of both breath and heart sounds. Partially obstructed bronchi and bronchioles may result in an expiratory *wheeze,* described as a musical, whistling sound. *Crackles* are an intermittent bubbling or popping sound that may also be present from secretions in the airways. Pursed-lip breathing, cyanosis, and digital clubbing may all be present in the advanced stages of COPD. (See "Examination" in the "Physical Therapy Management" section for clarification of terms.)

Significant and progressive airway limitation is reflected in altered pulmonary function tests. Lung volumes and capacities, especially RV and FRC, are increased from normal values due to air trapping. Figure 12.8 shows the changes in lung volumes and capacities that typically occur in obstructive pulmonary disease.

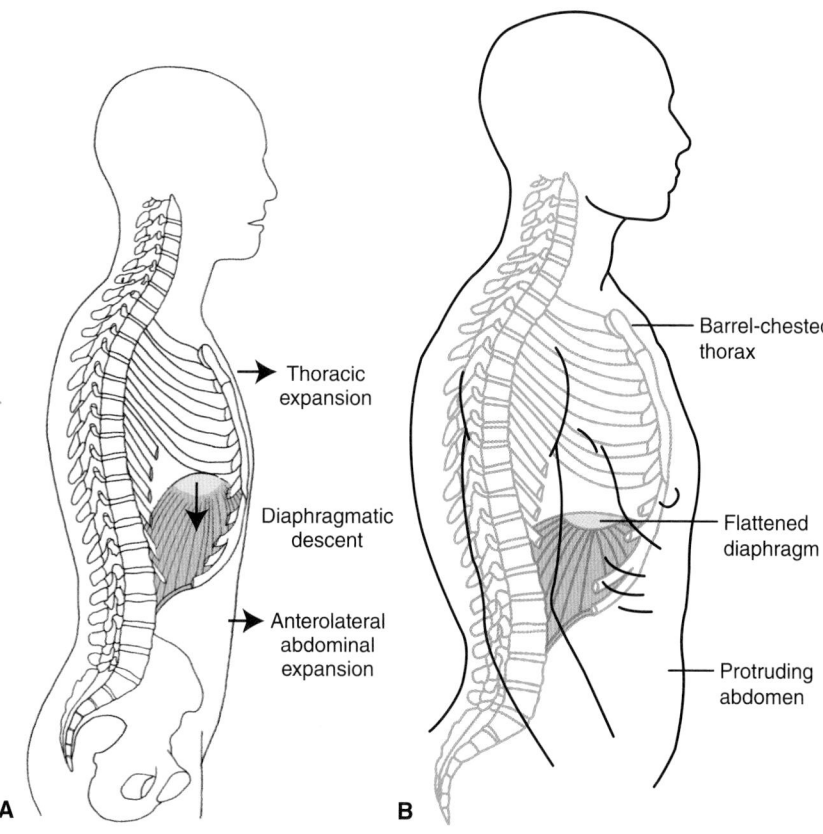

A

B

Figure 12.5 (A) Normal thoracic configuration. (B) Changes in the configuration of the thorax with chronic obstructive pulmonary disease.
(Adapted from Levangie P, Norkin C. Joint Structure and Function: A Comprehensive Analysis. 5th ed. F.A. Davis; 2011, p. 202, with permission.)

Thoracic expansion

Diaphragmatic descent

Anterolateral abdominal expansion

Barrel-chested thorax

Flattened diaphragm

Protruding abdomen

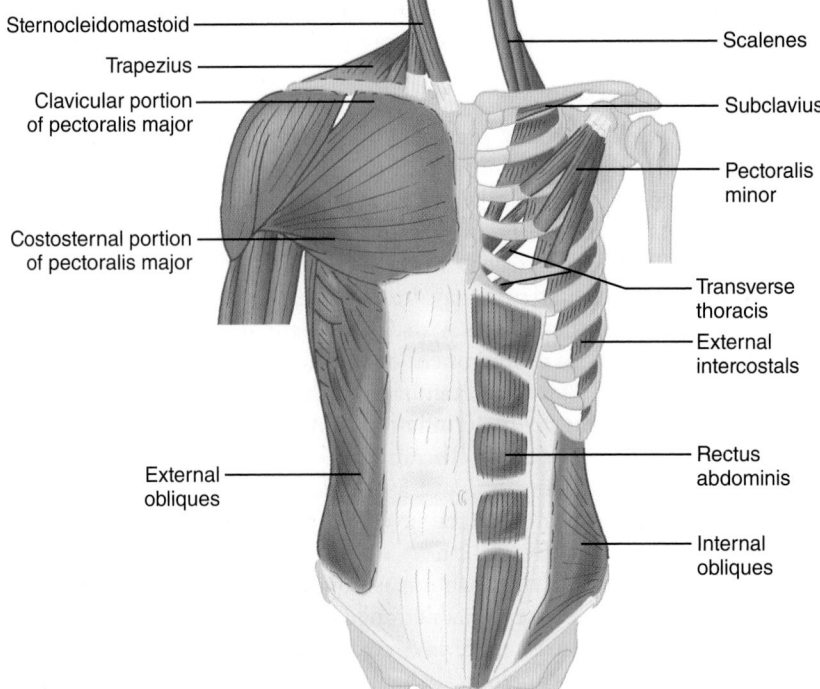

Figure 12.6 Accessory muscles of ventilation are those used during times of increased ventilatory demand. The right side of the figure shows some of the anterior superficial muscles of the thorax that can be accessory muscles of ventilation, and the left side of the thorax shows the deeper accessory muscles of ventilation.

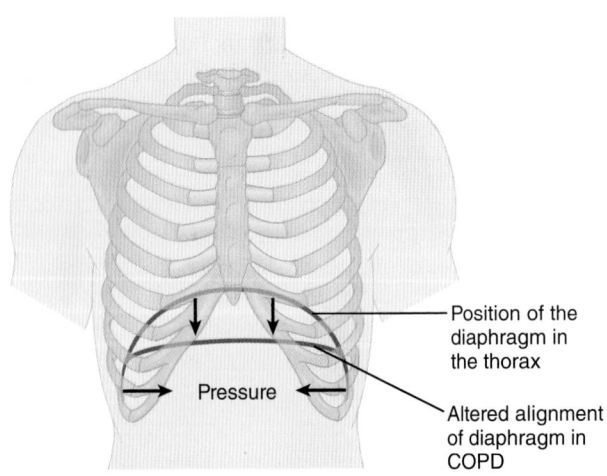

Figure 12.7 Alteration in alignment of fibers of the diaphragm due to hyperinflation. *(Adapted from Levangie P, Norkin C. Joint Structure and Function. 5th ed. F.A. Davis; 2011, p. 202, with permission.)*

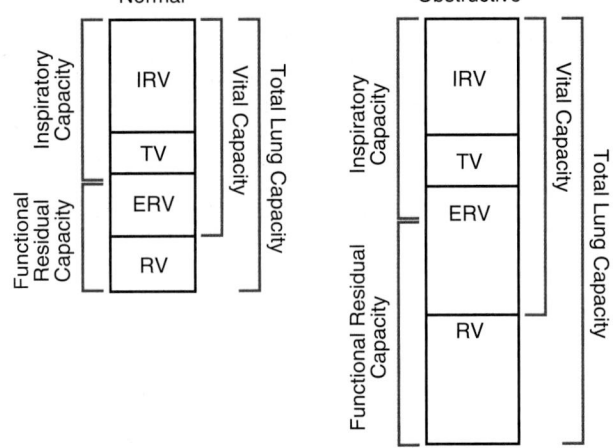

ERV: Expiratory reserve volume
IRV: Inspiratory reserve volume
RV: Residual volume
TV: Tidal volume

Figure 12.8 Lung volumes of a healthy pulmonary system compared with the lung volumes found in obstructive disease. *(Adapted from Roy S, Wolf S, Scalzitti D. The Rehabilitation Specialist's Handbook. 4th ed. F.A. Davis; 2013, with permission.)*

Expiratory flow rates, especially FEV_1, are decreased. The ratio of FEV_1 to FVC is decreased to less than 70%.[9] These changes in pulmonary function do not show a major reversibility in response to pharmacological agents.

Arterial blood gas analyses may reflect hypoxemia in the early stages of COPD and hypercapnea a bit later as the disease progresses. With disease progression, chest radiographs show several characteristic findings, including flattened, less domed, hemidiaphragms, alterations in pulmonary vascular markings, hyperinflation of the thorax, hyperlucency reflecting a decreased tissue density, elongation of the heart, and right ventricular hypertrophy.

The inflammatory reaction in the airways of patients with COPD can also affect other organ systems.[15] Therefore, COPD is not only a pulmonary disorder but also has extrapulmonary (i.e., systemic) effects, including changes to skeletal muscle mass and function, cardiovascular disease, osteoporosis, and depression.[16]

Course and Prognosis

The clinical course of COPD has an insidious onset with a disease progression that can develop over many years. Early identification of individuals at risk for the development of COPD has been elusive. Although smoking is the most prevalent risk factor for development of disease, not all smokers develop clinically significant lung disease. Therefore, a smoking history alone is not predictive for the development of COPD. The *BODE* index has been developed as a prognostic indicator for mortality risk in patients with COPD.[9] The index uses four domains to calculate mortality risk: BMI (B), airflow obstruction (O), dyspnea (D), and exercise capacity (E).[17] This index can be found at http://reference.medscape.com/calculator/bode-index-copd. The higher the score on the BODE, the greater is the mortality risk. Leading causes of death in patients with COPD are respiratory failure, lung cancer, and cardiovascular disease.

Asthma

Asthma is a common chronic pulmonary disease, affecting 20 million adults and 5.1 million children in the United States.[18] The *Global Initiative for Asthma* (GINA) is a collaborative work of the NHLBI and WHO. Since its launch in 1993, GINA's goal has been to reduce asthma prevalence, morbidity, and mortality. According to GINA, asthma is a disease of variable expiratory airflow limitation with symptoms of wheezing, shortness of breath, chest tightness, and cough.[19] The disease is characterized by chronic airway inflammation associated with airway hyperresponsiveness (bronchospasm) to direct or indirect stimuli. Asthma exacerbations may improve spontaneously or with medical intervention and are interspersed with symptom-free intervals.

Diagnosis

The diagnosis of asthma is clinically based on a history of episodic wheezing, shortness of breath (SOB), tightness in the chest, and coughing, which may be worse at night and early morning in the absence of any other obvious cause. The FEV_1 during exacerbations will be less than 80% of the predicted value. After inhalation of a rescue drug used to quickly relieve acute symptoms (e.g., inhaled short-acting beta-2 agonist), an improvement of at least 12% (or 200 mL) in FEV_1 indicates reversibility of the airway limitation consistent with a diagnosis of asthma.[10,19]

Etiology

A number of different phenotypes of asthma have been identified. Historically, the two types of asthma that have been described are *allergic asthma* and *nonallergic asthma*. The most common phenotype of asthma is allergic (or extrinsic) asthma. Allergic asthma has an immunologic (immunoglobulin E [IgE]–mediated) response to certain environmental triggers (dust mites, pollen, mold, animal dander). Induced sputum from this group of individuals shows eosinophilic inflammation, which causes the common symptoms and pathophysiological findings of asthma. *Atopy*, or allergic sensitivity, is the strongest feature of the phenotype of allergic asthma.

Nonallergic (or intrinsic) asthma is a less common form of asthma. There are no clinical findings of atopy in nonallergic asthma; however, an inflammatory response, which is eosinophilic, neutrophilic, or both, results from exposure to an irritant such as smoke, fumes, infections, or cold air.[19] Viral infections have been suggested to play a role in both the development and exacerbation of asthma.[20] Symptoms of asthma may begin at any age.

Pathophysiology

The major physiological manifestation of asthma is inflammation of the bronchial mucosa, leading to narrowing of the airways, bronchospasm, and increased bronchial secretions, all in response to a trigger (Fig. 12.9). The narrowed airways increase the resistance to airflow and cause air trapping on exhalation, leading to hyperinflation. These narrowed airways also provide an abnormal distribution of ventilation to the alveoli. Even during periods of remission, some degree of airway inflammation is present.

Clinical Presentation

The clinical symptoms of asthma *during an exacerbation* may include cough, dyspnea on exertion or at rest, and wheezing. The chest is usually held in an expanded

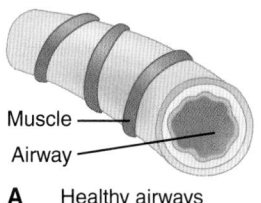

A Healthy airways

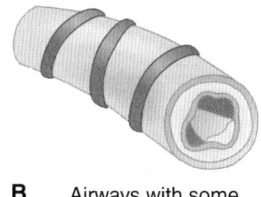

B Airways with some inflammation in stable asthma

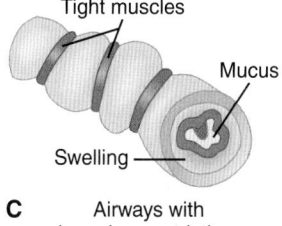

C Airways with bronchoconstriction, inflammation, and secretions in an exacerbation of asthma

Figure 12.9 Small airways (A) of a healthy pulmonary system, (B) of a person showing the chronic inflammation of asthma, and (C) of a person in an exacerbation of their asthma.

position, indicating that hyperinflation of the lungs has occurred. Accessory muscles of ventilation may be required for breathing, even at rest. Intercostal, supraclavicular, and substernal retractions (visible inward motion of the soft tissue) may be present during inspiration. While expiratory wheezing is characteristic of asthma, crackles may also be present. With severe airway obstruction, breath sounds may be markedly decreased owing to poor air movement, and wheezing may be present not only during exhalation but also heard on inspiration.

Chest radiographs taken during an asthmatic exacerbation usually demonstrate hyperinflation, as evidenced by an increase in the anterior–posterior diameter of the chest and hyperlucency of the lung fields. Less commonly, chest radiographs may reveal areas of infiltrate or *atelectasis* from the bronchial obstruction. Chest radiographs may be read as normal between asthmatic exacerbations.

The most dramatic clinical presentation during an exacerbation of asthma is a decreased FEV_1. RV and FRC are increased because of air trapping at the expense of VC and IRV, which are reduced. The reversibility of these pulmonary function test abnormalities is characteristic of asthma. During remission, the patient with asthma may have normal or near-normal pulmonary function tests.

The most common arterial blood gas finding during an asthmatic exacerbation is mild to moderate hypoxemia. Usually some degree of hypocapnia is present secondary to an increased minute ventilation. With severe asthma exacerbations, hypoxemia will be more pronounced and hypercapnia may occur, indicating that the patient is experiencing decreased alveolar ventilation. Ventilator muscle fatigue and respiratory failure may follow.

Clinical Course

By the time adulthood is reached, many children with asthma no longer have symptoms of the disease. When the onset of asthma symptoms begins later in life, the clinical course is usually more progressive, showing changes in pulmonary function tests even during periods of remission. Airway remodeling in response to chronic airway inflammation is thought to be responsible for the progressive nature of the disease.

Cystic Fibrosis

CF is a chronic disease that affects the excretory glands of the body. Secretions made by these glands are thicker, more viscous than usual, and can affect a number of systems of the body, including the pulmonary, pancreatic, hepatic, sinus, and reproductive systems. Dysfunction of the pulmonary system is the most common cause of morbidity and mortality in patients with CF. Other presentations may occur due to the effect of this disease on other organ systems, such as failure to thrive, diabetes, sinusitis, biliary disorders, and infertility.

Etiology

CF is an autosomal recessive genetically transmitted disorder (Fig. 12.10). There are currently 35,000 people living with CF in the United States.[21]

The CF gene (cystic fibrosis transmembrane conductance regulator [*CFTR*]) has been identified on the long arm of chromosome 7. The *CFTR* functions to transport electrolytes and water in and out of the epithelial cells of many organs in the body, including lungs, pancreas, and digestive and reproductive tracts. Defective transport of sodium, potassium, and water leaves the mucus made by excretory glands thickened and difficult to move and can often obstruct the lumen of its excretory gland. Over 1,700 mutations of this gene have been described thus far.[22]

Pathophysiology

The chronic pulmonary component of CF is related to the abnormally viscous mucus secreted in the tracheobronchial tree, which impairs the function of the mucociliary transport system. The altered secretions result in airway obstruction and hyperinflation. Exaggerated and sustained neutrophilic airway inflammation in response to infection is also a feature of this disease.[23] Partial or complete obstruction of the airways reduces ventilation

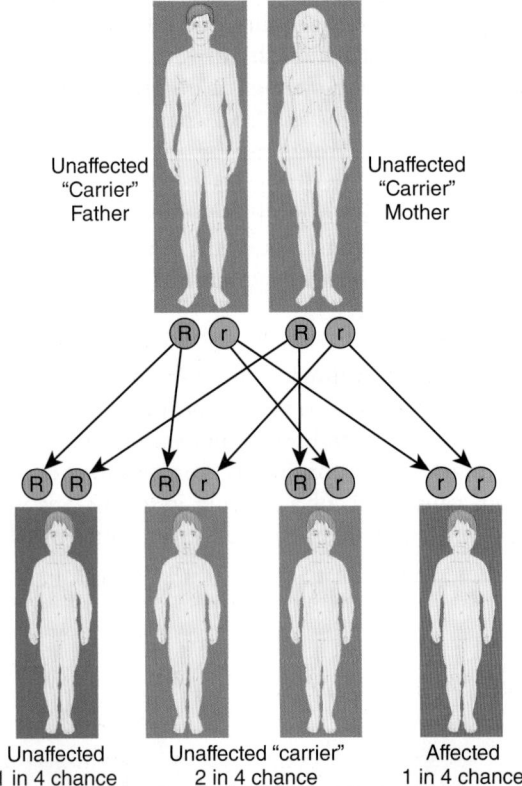

Figure 12.10 Autosomal recessive trait (Mendelian) requires that both parents be carriers of the disease or have the disease in order for their child to have the disease.

to the alveolar units. Ventilation and perfusion within the lungs are not matched. Fibrotic changes are ultimately found in the lung parenchyma.

Diagnosis

Infant screening for CF was instituted in all 50 U.S. states and the District of Columbia by 2010. The diagnosis of CF may be suspected in patients who were not screened as an infant, who present with a positive family history of the disease, who present with recurrent pulmonary infections from *Staphylococcus aureus, Pseudomonas aeruginosa,* or both, or who have a diagnosis of malnutrition or failure to thrive. A simple sweat test can be performed to rule out or confirm the diagnosis. A chloride ion concentration of ≥60 mEq/L found in the sweat of children is a positive test for the diagnosis of CF.[22] Genotyping for the most common *CFTR* mutations can also be done.

Clinical Presentation

The clinical presentation of CF can be related to any number of involved systems. Failure to thrive due to gastrointestinal dysfunction, diabetes due to pancreatic dysfunction, or frequent pulmonary infections and chronic cough due to pulmonary dysfunction are all possible presentations of the disease.

With pulmonary involvement, a patient presents with thick bronchial secretions that may be difficult to clear. With advancing disease, the chest wall will become barrel shaped with an increased anterior–posterior (AP) diameter and an increased dorsal kyphosis due to loss of the elastic recoil properties of the underlying lungs and chronic hyperinflation. There is a resultant decrease in thoracic excursion. Breath sounds may be decreased with adventitious sounds of crackles and wheezes. Hypertrophy of accessory muscles of ventilation, pursed-lip breathing, cyanosis, and digital clubbing may all be present.

Pulmonary function studies show obstructive impairments, including decreased FEV_1, decreased PEF, decreased FVC, increased RV, and increased FRC. The abnormal ventilation–perfusion relationship within the lungs results in hypoxemia and hypercapnea, demonstrated by arterial blood gas analysis. As the disease progresses, destruction of the alveolar capillary network causes pulmonary hypertension and cor pulmonale. In advanced disease, chest radiographs show diffuse hyperinflation, increased lung marking, and atelectasis.

Course and Prognosis

Sixty-three percent of new cases of CF in 2020 in the United States were diagnosed by mandatory infant testing.[24] The course of the disease, while quite variable, has been linked to *CFTR* genotype, modifier genes, and environmental factors.[25,26] Life expectancy continues to improve owing to early diagnosis and improved medical management. Although some patients unfortunately

die in early childhood, 57.2% of all patients diagnosed with CF are currently older than 18 years of age.[24] The predicted median survival age of patients with CF was 50 years between 2016 and 2020, a remarkable improvement from a mean survival age of 16 years, 50 years ago.[24] Respiratory failure is the most frequent cause of death in patients with CF. Therefore, treatment of the pulmonary dysfunction, including removal of the abnormally thick secretions and prompt treatment of pulmonary infections, is important to the management of CF. Gastrointestinal dysfunction from CF can be aided by proper diet, vitamin supplements, and replacement of pancreatic enzymes. Habitual exercise has been linked to higher aerobic capacity, increased quality of life, and improved survival.[27] Nutritional status is also a powerful predictor of prognosis.[28]

Restrictive Lung Disease

Restrictive lung diseases are a group of diseases referred to collectively as *interstitial lung diseases,* with differing etiologies that result in difficulty expanding the lungs and a reduction in lung volumes. These disorders are grouped together as they have similar clinical presentations.

Etiology

This group of disorders is often divided into two groups: those with a known cause and those that are idiopathic. Rheumatic diseases, oxygen- or drug-induced toxicity, inhalation of organic and inorganic dust, inhalation of noxious gases, radiation exposure, asbestos exposure, and infection can cause damage to the pulmonary parenchyma and pleura and result in restrictive pulmonary disease. The most common restrictive lung disease is idiopathic pulmonary fibrosis (IPF), also termed *usual interstitial pneumonia.*

Pathophysiology

The changes occurring within the lung parenchyma and pleura depend on the etiologic factors of restrictive disease. Many of the disorders begin with parenchymal changes due to chronic inflammation and thickening of the alveoli and interstitium. As these diseases progress, distal airspaces become fibrosed, making them more resistant to expansion (i.e., less distensible). Consequently, lung volumes are reduced. A reduced pulmonary vascular bed eventually leads to hypoxemia and cor pulmonale. Asbestosis (asbestos-induced pulmonary fibrosis) is a type of restrictive lung disease that shows both parenchymal and pleural fibrosis.[29,30]

Clinical Presentation

Dyspnea with activity and a persistent nonproductive cough are the classic symptoms of interstitial lung diseases. Signs of restrictive lung disease include rapid, shallow breathing; limited chest expansion; inspiratory crackles, especially over the lower lung fields; digital clubbing; and cyanosis.[30]

The plain chest radiograph reveals fine interstitial markings in a reticular, or netlike, pattern. Reduction in overall lung volume and radiographic evidence of pleural involvement, when present, can also be seen on plain chest radiographs, although their diagnostic and prognostic abilities are limited. High-resolution computed tomography is a radiological test for the diagnosis of IPF that typically shows basilar subpleural changes in a reticular pattern along with traction bronchiectasis (misshapen airways due to a pulling by fibrotic tissue on the airway wall) and honeycombing.[30,31]

Pulmonary function tests reveal a reduction in VC, FRC, RV, and TLC. Expiratory flow rates may be somewhat normal. The ratio between FVC and FEV_1 may be normal or even increased. Figure 12.11 shows the changes in lung volumes and capacities that occur in restrictive pulmonary parenchymal disease.

Arterial blood gas studies show varying degrees of hypoxemia and hypocapnia. Exercise may significantly lower oxygenation, even for patients with normal oxygenation at rest.

Course and Prognosis

Restrictive pulmonary diseases may have a slow onset, but they are relentlessly progressive. Survival depends on the type of restrictive disease, the etiologic factor, and the available treatments. Predictors of mortality include age, smoking history, BMI, radiological findings, pulmonary function tests, level of oxygenation, and distance walked on a 6-minute Walk Test.[31-34]

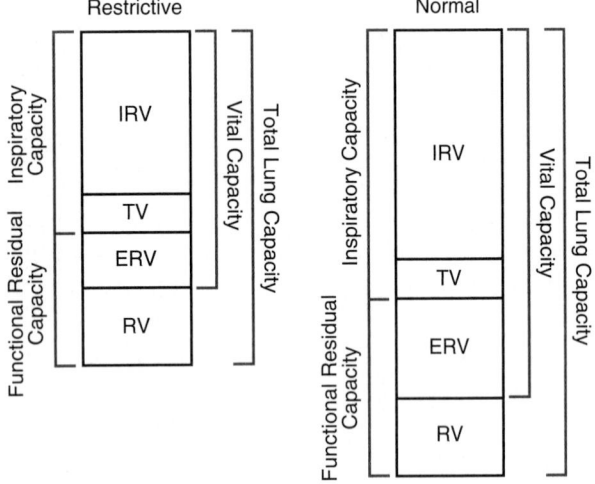

ERV: Expiratory reserve volume
IRV: Inspiratory reserve volume
RV: Residual volume
TV: Tidal volume

Figure 12.11 Lung volumes of a healthy pulmonary system compared with the lung volumes found in restrictive disease. *(Adapted from Roy S, Wolf S, Scalzitti D. The Rehabilitation Specialist's Handbook. 4th ed. F.A. Davis; 2013, with permission.)*

Coronavirus Disease 2019 (COVID-19)

In the past two decades, infectious diseases, such as the severe acute respiratory syndrome (SARS), the Middle East respiratory syndrome, and the coronavirus disease 2019 (COVID-19), have had catastrophic impacts on global health.[35] COVID-19, in fact, has become the third leading cause of death in the United States in 2020 after heart disease and cancer.[36] Severe acute respiratory syndrome coronavirus 2 (SARS-CoV-2), the virus that leads to COVID-19, primarily infects the respiratory system. The most common clinical presentation includes diffuse pneumonia, acute respiratory distress syndrome, and respiratory failure, one of the leading causes of death in COVID-19 patients.[37] The SARS-CoV-2 respiratory infection is contained within the interstitial compartment, which leads to diffuse interstitial-base abnormalities such as impaired diffusing capacity.[38] Patients with COVID-19 present with alterations in lung function, exercise capacity, and symptoms similar to individuals with interstitial lung disease.[39]

The post-acute sequelae of COVID-19 have been described as "long COVID"[40,41] or "post-COVID conditions,"[42,43] which is commonly used to refer to signs and symptoms that continue or develop after acute COVID-19. Long COVID includes both ongoing symptomatic COVID-19 (from 4 to 12 weeks) and post-COVID-19 syndrome (12 weeks or more).[44] The risk factors and pathophysiological mechanisms contributing to long COVID are not yet well understood.[45] However, research demonstrates that long COVID can impact people regardless of length of hospitalization or severity of acute COVID-19.[46-48] Long COVID can affect the respiratory, cardiac, renal, endocrine, and neurological systems, and the most common symptoms include fatigue, chest tightness, SOB, headache, and cognition dysfunction.[44,49] Symptoms may be singular, multiple, constant, transient, or fluctuating, and can change in nature over time.[46]

It is currently not well known when and what amount of physical activity is safe or beneficial for people living with long COVID. Physical activity prescription in long COVID should be approached with caution and vigilance to ensure safety and provide longer-term recovery.[45] People with long COVID may experience postexertional symptom exacerbation, defined as the triggering or worsening of fatigue or exhaustion following activity that could previously be tolerated. Pacing and close monitoring of vital signs (e.g., HR) during and after physical activity is recommended. To accommodate symptom fluctuations in long COVID, symptom-titrated physical activity, instead of fixed activity prescription or graded exercise therapy, is also recommended. Another common long-term effect of infection with SARS-CoV-2 is exertional oxygen desaturation. It is suggested that pulse oxygen saturation drops more than 3% during or after mild exertion, when compared to that before physical activity, requiring immediate attention. People with long COVID should also be screened for cardiac impairment and autonomic nervous system dysfunction before rehabilitation interventions and with continued monitoring for signs and symptoms of exercise intolerance (e.g., orthostatic hypotension, chest pain, dizziness, palpitations, breathless, presyncope, syncope) during any physical activity interventions.[44,45]

■ MEDICAL AND SURGICAL MANAGEMENT

Medical management of chronic pulmonary disease includes smoking cessation, pharmacological agents, and use of supplemental oxygen. Surgical and interventional management is a consideration for select patients with severe lung involvement. The following discussion provides an overview of these interventions.

Smoking Cessation

Smoking is the major causal agent in the development of COPD as well as a contributing cause to many other disease processes. The Global Initiative for Chronic Obstructive Pulmonary Disease states that "smoking cessation has the greatest capacity to influence the natural history of COPD."[9] The addictive properties of smoking and the withdrawal symptoms of smoking cessation make it difficult for smokers to quit. A majority of smokers who try to quit do so on their own. Unfortunately, 80% of smokers who try to quit on their own return to smoking within 1 month. Smokers report an average of six to nine attempts at smoking cessation before they are successful.[50] Using a structured smoking cessation program can increase the success of a person attempting to quit smoking.

There are two general types of smoking cessation programs: behavioral therapy and pharmacological therapy. *Behavioral therapy* includes education on the benefits of being a nonsmoker, counseling, and support through the arduous process of withdrawing from smoking. Acupuncture and hypnosis are considered part of a behavioral therapy approach because the purpose is to change smoking behavior. *Pharmacological therapy* includes the use of nicotine replacement therapy such as nicotine gum, lozenges, patches, sprays, or inhalers, and non-nicotine replacement medications such as bupropion (Zyban) and varenicline (Chantix) to assist in the cessation of smoking. Nicotine replacement therapy decreases the withdrawal symptoms linked to nicotine, such as craving for tobacco products, anger, irritability, anxiety, depression, and concentration problems[51,52] and increases the likelihood of quitting by 50% to 60%.[52]

Smoking cessation without any support has a long-term success rate of approximately 6%. Intense behavioral therapy has an improved smoking cessation rate compared to no behavioral therapy. A Cochrane Review in 2016 found that the use of intense behavioral therapy along with pharmacological therapy was the most effective method for smoking cessation, with a success rate of up to 25%.[53] Recommendations for smoking cessation need to be tailored to the individual patient as access to counseling may be difficult to obtain, and adverse medication reactions may be encountered. For example, nicotine replacement therapy can be beneficial in a comprehensive smoking cessation program; however, it is not recommended following a cardiovascular event. The regional offices of the American Lung Association and the American Cancer Society are good resources for local smoking cessation programs.

Pharmacological Management

Pharmacological agents provide relief from the symptoms of chronic lung disease and improve the health and functional status of individuals with lung disease. Each patient with a chronic pulmonary diagnosis will require a tailored plan of care. It is not unusual for patients to be on a combination of drugs for the management of their pulmonary disease. This discussion will provide information on both maintenance drugs and rescue drugs used in the care of patients with pulmonary disease. Table 12.1 provides foundational information on the pharmacological management of lung disease. Table 12.2 includes recommendations from GINA for pharmacological control of asthma symptoms.[19]

Maintenance Drugs

Maintenance drugs are used to reduce or minimize pulmonary symptoms throughout the day. These drugs are taken on a regular schedule to keep respiratory symptoms at bay. Maintenance drugs for patients with chronic pulmonary disorders include corticosteroids, long- and short-acting muscarinic antagonists (anticholinergics), long-acting beta-2 agonists, phosphodiesterase 4 inhibitors, and leukotriene antagonists. Methylxanthines, nonselective phosphodiesterase inhibitors, are bronchodilators that are less frequently prescribed as a maintenance drug, as safer medications are available. While these maintenance drugs are available for use, each disorder uses these drugs in a different order or combination. For example, inhaled anti-inflammatories are the mainstay of medical management of the chronic inflammation of asthma. Inhaled bronchodilators, like anticholinergics or long-acting beta agonists, are commonly prescribed for patients with COPD. And antibiotics and inhaled mucolytics may be the first-line drugs to treat the respiratory symptoms that accompany CF.

Routes of administration of maintenance drugs are usually inhalation or ingestion. Inhalation is the advisable route of administration, when possible, as it limits systemic side effects of the drug. However, improper use of the inhalation device is a barrier to disease control. Studies reported that 74.8% of patients did not use their inhalation device correctly,[54] and the high prevalence of poor inhaler technique was not associated with

Table 12.1	Common Drugs Used in the Medical Management of Patients With Chronic Pulmonary Disease			
Use	Drug Category	Example Name	Action	Adverse Reactions
Maintenance	Anticholinergic LAMA	Tiotropium (Spiriva)	Bronchodilation	Throat irritation Drying of tracheal secretions Tachycardia Palpitations
Maintenance	LABA	Salmeterol (Serevent)	Bronchodilation	Tachycardia Palpitations GI distress Nervousness Tremor Headache Dizziness
Maintenance	Corticosteroids	Fluticasone (Flovent)	Anti-inflammatory effects	Increase BP Sodium retention (edema) Muscle wasting Osteoporosis GI irritation Atherosclerosis Hypercholesterolemia Increased susceptibility to infection
Maintenance	Phosphodiesterase 4 inhibitor	Roflumilast (Daxas)	Anti-inflammatory effects	GI distress Depression Headache Insomnia Rhinitis/sinusitis Urinary tract infection
Maintenance	Leukotriene receptor antagonist	Montelukast (Singulair)	Blocks allergic reaction	GI distress Sore throat Upper respiratory tract infection Dizziness Headache Nasal congestion
Maintenance	Mucolytics	Dornase alfa (Pulmozyme)	Thins secretions	Voice changes Sore throat Runny nose or eyes Rash
Rescue	Short-acting beta-2 agonist	Albuterol (Ventolin)	Bronchodilation	Tachycardia Palpitations GI distress Nervousness Tremor Headache Dizziness

BP = blood pressure; GI = gastrointestinal; LABA = long-acting beta-2 agonist; LAMA = long-acting muscarinic antagonist.

device type.[55] Even with specific training and learned correct use, Melani et al.[56] reported increased errors in the use of the inhalation device over time that reduced control over the symptoms of lung disease.

Rescue Drugs

Rescue drugs are used for immediate relief of *break-through* symptoms of bronchoconstriction (symptoms that "break through" and become apparent even with

Table 12.2	Suggested Pharmacological Management of Patients With Asthma			
Track 1	**Steps 1–2**	**Step 3**	**Step 4**	**Step 5**
Controller and preferred reliever. Using ICS-formoterol as reliever reduces the risk of exacerbations compared with using a SABA reliever.	As-needed low-dose ICS-formoterol	Low-dose maintenance ICS-formoterol	Medium-dose maintenance ICS-formoterol	Add-on LAMA Refer for phenotypic assessment ± anti-IgE, anti-IL5/5R, anti-IL4R Consider high-dose ICS-formoterol

Reliever: as-needed low-dose ICS-formoterol

Track 2	**Step 1**	**Step 2**	**Step 3**	**Step 4**	**Step 5**
Controller and alternative reliever. Before considering a regimen with SABA reliever, check if the patient is likely to be adherent with daily controller	Take ICS whenever SABA taken	Low-dose maintenance ICS	Low-dose maintenance ICS-LABA	Medium-/high-dose maintenance ICS-LABA	Add-on LAMA Refer for phenotypic assessment ± anti-IgE, anti-IL5/5R, anti-IL4R Consider high-dose ICS-LABA

Reliever: as-needed short-acting beta-2 agonist

ICS = inhaled corticosteroids; IgE = Immunoglobulin E; IL5 = interleukin 5; IL4R = interleukin 4 receptor; IL5R = interleukin 5 receptor; LABA = long-acting beta-2 agonist; LAMA = long-acting muscarinic antagonist; SABA = short-acting beta-2 agonist. Step 1 is for everyone with a diagnosis to gain and maintain control of their asthma symptoms. If Step 1 is insufficient in keeping asthma symptoms at bay, the patient needs to move to the next step(s) in order to control their asthma. Treatment may be stepped up or down within a track using the same reliever at each step, or switched between tracks, according to the patient's needs and preferences. *Adapted from Global strategy for asthma management and prevention; Update 2022, with permission.*[19]

careful management). Inhaled short-acting beta-2 agonists are used for this purpose. Patients are advised to use their prescribed inhaled short-acting beta-2 agonist on an as-needed basis. If a patient reports an increased frequency in the use of a rescue drug, it is indicative of a flaw in the maintenance drug regimen or a change in the patient's pulmonary status.

Antibiotics

Pulmonary infections are frequent in patients with chronic pulmonary diseases. They can be devastating to the patient and cause major setbacks in pulmonary rehabilitation efforts. The early signs of an infection are often noted by changes in the patient's baseline status (i.e., a change in exercise ability, peak flow rates, dyspnea, or color or amount of sputum, or an increase in the use of rescue inhalers). Antibiotics are used to either kill the bacteria outright (bacteriocidal) or interfere with the growth and/or proliferation of bacteria (bacteriostatic). There are many categories of antibiotics (e.g., penicillins, cephalosporins, tetracyclines) that are effective on different infecting organisms. It is important to identify the infecting organism in order to prescribe the appropriate antibiotic. Prophylactic use of antibiotics has not demonstrated a significant decrease in hospital admissions, changes in lung function, clinically significant quality of life, or mortality.[57]

Supplemental Oxygen

The long-term use of supplemental oxygen (greater than 15 hr/day) has been shown to prolong the survival of patients with COPD whose resting arterial partial pressure of oxygen (PaO_2) is 55 mm Hg or less, which correlates with an oxygen saturation (SaO_2) of 88% or less.[9,58] In patients with right heart failure or erythrocytosis, the cutoff is less than 60 mm Hg.[9] In patients whose resting SaO_2 is greater than 88% but their exercise abilities are limited by exertional dyspnea, supplemental oxygen during exercise may be helpful in reducing this symptom.[59] The amount of oxygen used should be titrated individually to maintain an SaO_2 of at least 90%, if possible. The long-term use of oxygen in patients with moderate oxygen desaturation (SaO_2 = 89% to 93%) at rest or with exercise did not result in quality of life or distance walked on the 6-minute Walk Test.[60] Various supplemental oxygen delivery methods are available; continuous flow, pulsed flow, and reservoir are among the most common.

Surgical and Interventional Management of Chronic Pulmonary Disease

There are few surgical options for the patient with pulmonary disease. Criteria used to determine the appropriateness of an intervention include the distribution of emphysema throughout the lungs, the presence of large bullae, the presence or absence of interlobar collateral ventilation, and the severity of the lung disease.

Lung volume reduction surgery (LVRS) is a surgical technique that removes nonfunctional, overdistended lung tissue to restore more normal biomechanics to the thorax. LVRS may be indicated in patients with heterogeneous areas of hyperinflated, relatively nonfunctional lung tissue (with or without collateral ventilation) alongside of relatively functional lung tissue. The surgical procedure removes approximately 20% to 35% of the most diseased lung tissue, relieving the more normal lung tissue of its burden. This surgical procedure reduces RV and FRC (i.e., decreases hyperinflation), allowing for a more normal resting position of the diaphragm, an increased diaphragmatic excursion, and a more normal chest wall motion.[9] Research has shown postoperative results of increased exercise capacity, lung function, quality of life, and gas exchange in patients with moderate *upper lobe* lung disease.[9,61–63] Patients with severe pulmonary disease whose distribution is in non-upper-lobe areas of the lung show only slight improvement in functional abilities and quality-of-life scores along with a high mortality rate.[9,61,62,64]

Minimally invasive, endobronchial lung volume reduction interventions are becoming available to treat the hyperinflation of emphysematous lung tissue without surgery. The placement of an endobronchial one-way valve in an airway reduces airflow into that designated area of the lung while allowing air and secretions to be expelled. The valve decreases hyperinflation of that area of the lung, allowing improved function to the healthier adjacent lung tissue. A second means of minimally invasive lung volume reduction is by deploying lung coils into an airway to occlude the airway and collapse the lung tissue distal to the obstruction. A third approach is to inject into overdistended areas of the lungs a substance that causes localized inflammation leading to atelectasis, scarring, and remodeling of that area. The result of all of these bronchoscopic interventions is to reduce areas of hyperinflation, allowing the more normal lung tissue room to function.[65,66]

Lung transplantation for end-stage pulmonary disease has an overall survival rate of 92.6% at 3 months, 85.5% at 1 year, 83.2% at 3 years, and 70.6% at 5 years.[67] The goals of lung transplantation are to restore normal lung function, restore normal exercise capacity, and prolong life.[9] People awaiting a lung transplant include patients with COPD, CF, IPF, and pulmonary hypertension. The number of patients awaiting lung transplantation continues to grow, far exceeding the number of organs available for transplantation, making transplantation a reality for only a small number of individuals.[68]

■ PHYSICAL THERAPY MANAGEMENT

Chronic pulmonary diseases and their associated dysfunction have a slow, yet progressive course. The person with pulmonary dysfunction often avoids activities that result in the uncomfortable sensation of dyspnea. A slow but steady decrease in these patients' functional activities follows, resulting in progressive aerobic deconditioning. It is common for someone with pulmonary disease to have lost many functional abilities before ever seeking medical help. The intended outcome of pulmonary rehabilitation is to interrupt this downward spiral of physical inability, improve exercise performance, decrease the symptom of dyspnea, and improve quality of life.[69,70]

Goals and Outcomes

The *Guide for Physical Therapist Practice*, available through the American Physical Therapy Association, provides a general framework for physical therapy intervention for patients with chronic pulmonary diseases. Tests and measures for patients with chronic pulmonary disorders include, but are not limited to, categories of aerobic capacity/endurance, circulation, ventilation and respiration, and community, social, and civic life.[71] Examples of goals and outcomes for the individual patient with pulmonary dysfunction are presented in Box 12.1.

Box 12.1 Examples of Goals and Outcomes for Patients With Chronic Pulmonary Dysfunction

- Patient/client, family and caregiver understanding of disease process, expectations, goals, and outcomes is enhanced.
- Cardiovascular endurance is increased.
- Strength, power, and endurance of peripheral muscles are increased.
- Performance of physical tasks, both basic activities of daily living and instrumental activities of daily living, is improved.
- Strength, power, and endurance of ventilator muscles are increased.
- Independence in airway clearance is improved.
- Patient/client decision-making ability regarding the use of health-care resources is improved.
- Patient/client self-management of symptoms and self-management of pulmonary disease are enhanced.

Examination

The examination of a patient's pulmonary status has several purposes: (1) to evaluate the appropriateness of the patient's participation in a pulmonary rehabilitation program, (2) to determine the therapeutic interventions most appropriate for the participant's plan of care (POC), (3) to monitor the participant's physiological response to exercise, and (4) to appropriately progress the participant's POC over time.

Patient History

A patient interview should begin with the chief complaint and the patient's perception of why pulmonary rehabilitation is being sought. The chief complaint is often SOB, loss of function, or both. A medical history contains pertinent pulmonary symptoms specific to that patient: cough, sputum production, wheezing, and SOB severity. Occupational, social, medication, smoking, and family histories should also be obtained and documented.

Laboratory Tests

Various laboratory studies to examine patients with pulmonary disease may be performed and interpreted. These include radiology, pulmonary function tests (PFTs) including flow rates, arterial blood gas analysis, SaO_2 measurements, and electrocardiograms (ECGs).

Tests and Measures
Vital Signs

HR, BP, RR, SaO_2, temperature, and presence of pain (usually associated with SOB) should be examined and documented (see Chapter 2, Examination of Vital Signs). An individual's height should be measured, as there is a direct relationship between height and lung volumes. Weight, for its use as a prognostic indicator, should be measured on a standard scale, and each subsequent measurement should be performed on the same scale.

Observation, Inspection, and Palpation

By observing the neck and shoulders of a patient with pulmonary disease, the use of accessory muscles of ventilation can be observed (see Fig. 12.6). A normal configuration of the thorax reveals a ratio of anteroposterior (AP) to lateral diameter of 1:2. Destruction of the lung parenchyma results in an increase in the AP diameter and a reduction of this ratio (up to 1:1) (see Fig. 12.5). During inhalation and exhalation, both sides of the thorax should move symmetrically; any asymmetries should be noted and documented.

Cyanosis is a bluish discoloration of the skin that can be observed periorally, periorbitally, and in nailbeds; it indicates acute tissue hypoxia. An indicator of more chronic tissue hypoxia is digital clubbing of the fingers and toes. In digital clubbing, there is an increase in the angle created by the distal phalanx and the point where

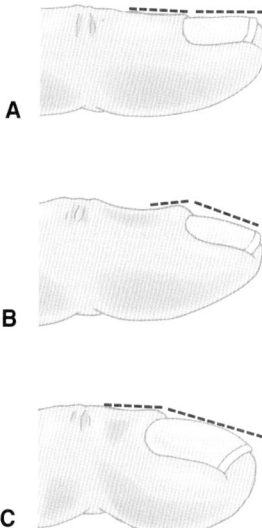

Figure 12.12 Digital clubbing is a sign of chronic tissue hypoxia. (A) Normal. (B) Early clubbing with angle present between nail and proximal skin. (C) Advanced clubbing.

the nail exits from the digit. The tip of the distal phalanx becomes bulbous (Fig. 12.12).

Auscultation of the Lungs

Auscultation involves listening over the chest wall as air enters and exits the lungs. To perform auscultation of the lungs, a stethoscope is placed firmly on the patient's thorax anteriorly, laterally, and posteriorly (Fig. 12.13). The patient is asked to inspire fully through an open mouth, then to exhale quietly. Inhalation and the beginning of exhalation normally produce a soft rustling sound. The end of exhalation is normally silent. This characteristic of a normal breath sound is termed *vesicular.* When a louder, more hollow and echoing sound occupies a larger portion of the ventilatory cycle, the breath sounds are referred to as *bronchial.* When the breath sounds are very quiet and barely audible, they are termed *decreased.* These three terms—*vesicular, bronchial,* and *decreased*—allow the listener to describe the intensity of the breath sound.

In addition to the description of the intensity, there may be additional sounds and vibrations heard during auscultation. These are called *adventitious* breath sounds. These sounds are superimposed on the already-described intensity of the breath sound. According to the American College of Chest Physicians and the American Thoracic Society, there are two types of adventitious sounds: crackles and wheezes.[72] *Crackles,* previously termed *rales* and *rhonchi,* sound like the rustling of cellophane and have a multitude of potential causes (tissue fibrosis, secretions in the airways, pulmonary edema, etc.). *Wheezes* have been described as high-pitched, coarse, whistling sounds. A decrease in the size of the lumen of the airway will create a wheezing sound, much like

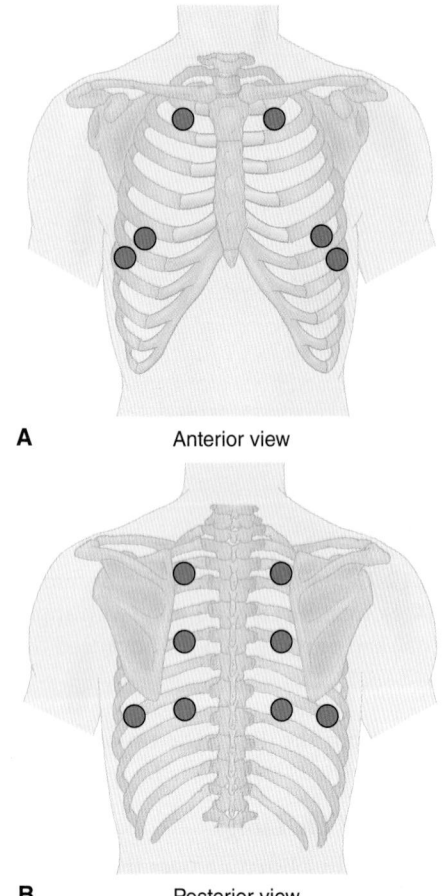

A Anterior view

B Posterior view

Figure 12.13 Auscultation of the lungs. A global assessment of lung sounds requires that the therapist listens through a stethoscope, which is placed anteriorly, posteriorly, and laterally on the upper, middle, and lower thorax.

stretching the neck of an inflated balloon narrows the passageway through which air must escape, producing a whistling sound.

Measurement of Dyspnea and Quality of Life

There are many scales that can be used to quantify dyspnea. Measurements at the beginning and the end of a rehabilitation program and during periods of exacerbation can be accomplished using the clinically practical *Modified British Medical Council (mMRC) Dyspnea Scale*.[73] The *Baseline Dyspnea Index* (BDI) is another dyspnea scale that is encountered more in the research literature than in clinical practice.[74] While both these scores are reliable and valid, they are not interchangeable.[75] Quality-of-life (QOL) measures that are specific to chronic pulmonary dysfunction include the *Chronic Respiratory Questionnaire* and the *St. George's Respiratory Questionnaire*.[76,77] Shorter disease-specific QOL measures such as the *COPD assessment test* (CAT) and the *COPD Control Questionnaire* (CCQ) may be more clinically useful in determining the patient's baseline

health-related QOL.[78–80] These outcome measures may be helpful in demonstrating improvement made with physical therapy intervention. Table 12.3 presents information regarding dyspnea and QOL outcomes measures.

Measurement of Strength and Endurance

Patients with pulmonary disease may show peripheral and ventilatory muscle weakness due to deconditioning, malnutrition, steroid use, and the systemic inflammation of the disease process.[16,81–83] Muscle weakness can contribute to exercise limitations and an inability to perform activities of daily living (ADL). Therefore, measurement of peripheral muscle strength and inspiratory muscle strength will determine the need for strength training during rehabilitation. The use of *manual muscle testing* (MMT) may not be the best choice for strength assessment. The maximal effort that is required during MMT makes it likely that patients will produce a *Valsalva maneuver* while performing the test. In patients with pulmonary disease, the increased intrathoracic pressure from a Valsalva maneuver closes off the small airways, causing SOB, and therefore limits full participation in the test. A *Five Times Sit to Stand Test* might be a better choice to assess functional lower extremity strength in patients with pulmonary disease.[84–86] The *6-Minute Pegboard and Ring Test* is a measurement of upper extremity function that has been shown to be a reliable and valid measurement tool.[87]

Inspiratory muscle strength is determined by measuring the patient's ability to create a *negative inspiratory pressure* (PI_{max}). The standard starting patient position for the test is seated with nose clips in place. The person is asked to let out all their air before beginning the test (i.e., start the test at RV). The person is then asked to "breathe in" against an occluded mouthpiece. The negative pressure is recorded using an aneroid manometer.[88] The result of this test is the negative pressure, reported in millimeters of mercury or centimeters of water, that was generated and sustained after 1 second of effort. Normative values for inspiratory pressure are related to a person's characteristics of age and sex.[89] This ability to generate a negative inspiratory pressure reflects the strength of the muscles of inspiration.

Exercise Testing in Patients With Pulmonary Disease

An *exercise tolerance test* (ETT) can provide objective information to (1) document a patient's functional abilities, (2) document a patient's symptomatology, (3) prescribe safe exercise, (4) document changes in oxygenation during exercise and determine the need for supplemental oxygen, and (5) identify any changes in pulmonary function during exercise performance.

An ETT protocol gradually increases exercise intensity in order to stress the patient with pulmonary dysfunction to their point of limitation. Incremental cycle

Table 12.3	Outcome Measures: Dyspnea and Quality of Life		
Outcome Measure	**Description**	**Scoring**	**MCID**
Modified Medical Research Council Dyspnea Scale[73] ICF: Body structure and function	A simple self-assessment tool that measures dyspnea ranging from 0: I only get breathless with strenuous exercise to a 4: I am too breathless to leave the house.	Score of 0–4; a higher score signifies greater dyspnea.	N/A
Baseline Dyspnea Index[74] ICF: Participation	A self-administered 24-item questionnaire covering three domains of functional impairment, magnitude of task, and magnitude of effort.	Score of 0–12; a lower score signifies greater impact on overall health.	N/A
Chronic Respiratory Questionnaire[76] ICF: Participation	A self-administered 20 items over four domains of dyspnea, fatigue, emotional function, and mastery.	Score of 20–140; a higher score signifying greater impact on overall health.	0.5 points
St. George's Respiratory Questionnaire[77] ICF: Participation	A self-administered questionnaire of 50 items regarding three domains, symptomatology, activity, and impact	Score of 0–100; higher scores indicating greater impact on overall health.	4 units
COPD assessment test[78] ICF: Participation	A self-administered tool that measures health-related quality of life and physical limitations using eight questions to identify the impact of pulmonary disease	Score of 0–40; a higher score signifies lower quality of life.	2 points
Clinical COPD Questionnaire[79,80] ICF: Participation	A self-administered tool that measures health-related quality of life using 10 questions divided into three domains: symptoms, functional state, and mental state	Score of 0–60; a higher score signifies a lower quality of life.	0.4 points

MCID = minimal clinically important difference

ergometry testing is widely used in clinical practice for patients with chronic pulmonary disorders. The *American Thoracic Society* and *American College of Chest Physicians* recommend a protocol that begins with 3 minutes of rest, 3 minutes of unloaded pedaling, and then an increase of 5 to 25 W every minute until the patient reaches exhaustion, followed by a recovery phase of at least 2 to 3 minutes.[90,91]

HR, blood pressure, ECG, RR, rate of perceived exertion (RPE), rate of perceived dyspnea (RPD), and SaO_2 are monitored during the test. Documentation of peak HR, peak RPD, peak RPE, and peak workload can be used to appropriately prescribe exercise. Peak VO_2 is also a measurement that can be collected during an ETT but requires equipment not always found in the clinical setting. PFTs performed before and after an exercise test document the effects of exercise on lung function. A reduction of greater than or equal to 20% in FEV_1 is an indication that exercise provoked airway hyperresponsiveness.[92] Criteria for stopping a pulmonary ETT are presented in Box 12.2.

The *6-minute Walk Test* (6MWT) is a functional performance measure that asks a patient to walk as far as possible in 6 minutes. The patient is allowed to stop and rest during the administration of the test. Total distance walked is the recorded result of the test. The 6MWT has been shown to have a good correlation with a patient's functional abilities.[93]

The *Incremental Shuttle Walk Test* (ISWT) is another functional performance measure that uses a recorded audio signal to dictate incrementally increasing walking speeds over level ground. Two destination points are placed 9 meters apart, so that the walking path is 10 meters. The person is asked to reach each destination point by the time the increasingly frequent audio signal sounds. The test is terminated when the person can no longer keep up with the increasing tempo of the signals, meaning that the person is more than 0.5 meters from the cone at the time of the audio signal and cannot catch up during the next shuttle. Recording of SaO_2, HR, and RPD occurs at the beginning and end of the test. The results of the ISWT are the number of shuttles that the person completes.[94] These results have a positive correlation with maximal oxygen consumption (VO_{2max}).[93]

Gait speed is an easy-to-perform outcome measure, needing only a stopwatch and a length of corridor.[95] Performing the test requires a 20-meter course. The acceleration leg of the course is the first 5 meters, the deceleration leg of the course is the last 5 meters, and the timed section of the course is the middle 10 meters. The person is asked to begin at the start of the 20-meter course and walk at a comfortable pace for the length of

Box 12.2   Indications for Terminating a Symptom-Limited Maximal Exercise Test

Absolute indications

1. ST elevation (**greater than** 1 mm) in leads without preexisting Q waves
2. Drop in systolic blood pressure of **greater than** 10 mm Hg
3. Moderate-to-severe angina
4. Central nervous system symptoms (e.g., ataxia, dizziness, or near syncope)
5. Signs of poor perfusion (cyanosis or pallor)
6. Sustained ventricular tachycardia or other arrhythmia (e.g., second- or third-degree atrioventricular block)
7. Technical difficulties monitoring the ECG or systolic blood pressure
8. The individual's request to stop

Special considerations in individuals with chronic pulmonary disease

1. Moderate-to-severe chronic obstructive pulmonary disease may exhibit oxyhemoglobin desaturation with exercise. It is recommended to monitor the partial pressure of arterial oxygen (PaO_2) or percent saturation of arterial oxygen (SaO_2) during the exercise testing.
2. In addition to standard termination criteria, exercise testing may be terminated because of severe arterial oxyhemoglobin desaturation (i.e., $SaO_2 \leq 80\%$).

Adapted from ACSM's Guidelines for Exercise Testing and Prescription.[148]

the course. The therapist measures the time it takes to traverse the middle 10 meters. The result of this outcome measure is gait velocity reported in either meters per second or feet per second.

Data from these functional tests can be used to determine disability, predict hospital discharge disposition and mortality, assess the ability to perform ADL, quantify health-related quality of life, determine home and community walking abilities and the need for oxygen therapy, demonstrate the effectiveness of medication changes, and determine the prescription of exercise.[17,92,93,95]

Examining a patient's functional capabilities should be used as an outcome measure to document functional improvements following physical therapy intervention, even if an ETT has been performed. The 6MWT is easy to administer and requires minimal equipment, making it the most commonly used outcome measurements to demonstrate changes in a patient's abilities following pulmonary rehabilitation.[96] The clinically significant change from a 6MWT is between 25 and 35 meters.[97] The clinically significant change for the ISWT is 47.5 meters.[98] The clinically significant change in gait speed is 0.05 meters/second.[95] Table 12.4 presents information regarding these functional mobility outcomes measures.

Exercise Prescription

Exercise prescription for aerobic training incorporates four variables that together allow the therapist to develop a patient-specific exercise prescription designed to produce an increase in functional capacity. These variables are *mode, intensity, duration,* and *frequency.*

Table 12.4	Outcome Measures: Functional Mobility		
Outcome Measure	Description	Scoring	MCID
6-min Walk Test[93,97] ICF: Participation	The participant is asked to cover as much distance as possible in 6 min. Assistive devices can be used. Individuals can rest as needed, although the timer does not stop. This is a self-selected walking speed that has a good correlation to performance of ADL.	Distance walked in 6 min.	25–35 m
Incremental Shuttle Walk Test[94,98] ICF: Participation	Two cones are set to identify a 10-m walking course. The participant is told to walk between cones to a walking speed dictated by an audio signal. The starting gait speed is 0.5 m/sec and increases each minute by 0.17 m/sec. The test is finished when the subject is unable to maintain the required speed and fails to complete two consecutive shuttles in the time imposed.	Distance covered from the completed number of shuttles traversed.	48 m
Gait speed[95] ICF: Participation	Walking speed is measured by a walking course that has a 5-m acceleration leg, a 10-m timed leg, and a 5-m deceleration leg.	Gait speed is calculated in m/sec.	0.05 m/sec

ADL = activity of daily living; MCID = minimal clinically important difference

Mode

Any type of sustained *aerobic exercise* can be used for pulmonary rehabilitation. Lower extremity (LE) activities, including walking and cycling, are often used to improve exercise tolerance. Specificity of training remains an important factor in the choice of exercise modes so that training translates into functional abilities.[99] Upper extremity (UE) aerobic exercise (e.g., arm ergometry) can also be included. Many programs utilize a circuit approach (combining a variety of resistive and aerobic exercises) to train different muscle groups, in different ways, with interspersed rest periods.

Intensity

There are several ways to prescribe exercise intensity: oxygen consumption, HR, RPE, RPD, and a percent of peak workload. Following is a discussion of each means of prescribing exercise intensity.

Exercise Intensity as a Percent of VO$_{2peak}$

Moderate intensity exercise can be prescribed using approximately 45% to 60% of the peak VO$_2$ achieved on an ETT. Vigorous intensity exercise would be approximately 65% or greater of the peak VO$_2$ achieved on an ETT.[77] Patients with mild to moderate pulmonary disease may be able to exercise for a period of time at these intensities to produce a training effect. While using a percentage of VO$_2$ may be the most accurate method of prescribing exercise from a graded exercise test, assuming that peak VO$_2$ was measured, it does not give the clinician a means to monitor exercise intensity during the actual performance during an exercise session.

Exercise Intensity as a Percentage of Heart Rate

There is a relationship between increasing workloads, increasing VO$_2$, and increasing HR, making exercise HR a more practical choice for prescribing and monitoring exercise intensity in the clinical setting.[100]

Patients with mild to moderate pulmonary disease may not have a pulmonary limitation to their ability to perform exercise; therefore, their exercise test may have the expected cardiovascular endpoint. If these patients have no other concomitant diseases, have no musculoskeletal or neurological constraints, and are committed to exercise, 65% to 85% of their highest HR achieved on the ETT could be used to prescribe exercise intensity.[100] It should be emphasized that when prescribing exercise intensity by HR, a heart rate range should be given, rather than a single number.

Exercise Intensity by Rating of Perceived Exertion or Rating of Perceived Dyspnea

In patients with severe pulmonary impairments, dyspnea may be the limiting factor to exercise performance. Patients with severe pulmonary impairment will likely approach their ventilatory maximum on an ETT before their cardiovascular maximum is reached; that is, their peak exercise HR may be lower than their maximum HR owing to pulmonary constraints. For these patients, prescribing exercise intensity using a percentage of the peak HR may underestimate their exercise abilities. The rating of perceived dyspnea obtained from an exercise test can be used to prescribe exercise intensity for patients with COPD (Table 12.5).[101-104] A perceived dyspnea rating of up to 3 (moderate SOB) corresponds approximately to 50% of VO$_{2max}$. A rating of about 5 to 6 corresponds to approximately 80% of VO$_{2max}$. The use of RPD, especially when levels of exercise are in the vigorous intensity range (greater than 80% peak VO$_2$), has been shown to be a valid and reliable means of prescribing exercise.[101]

The RPE is often used as a means of prescribing exercise intensity for patients with cardiovascular and pulmonary diseases.[100,105] Using the RPE scale allows the patient to self-regulate exercise intensity based on the perception of exertion. RPE has been correlated with

Table 12.5	Rating of Perceived Exertion: The Borg CR10 Scale	
The Borg CR10 Scale		
0	Nothing at all	"No P"
0.3		
0.5	Extremely weak	Just noticeable
1	Very weak	
1.5		
2	Weak	Light
2.5		
3	Moderate	
4		
5	Strong	Heavy
6		
7	Very strong	
8		
9		
10	Extremely strong	"Max P"
11		
12	Absolute maximum	Highest possible

Note: For correct usage of the scale, the exact design and instructions given in Borg's folders must be followed. The scale with correct instructions can be obtained from Borg Perception (see the Borg Perception website at https://borgperception.se). *Adapted from BorgPerception AB*[149]; *Update 2022, with permission.*

VO_2, making it a useful means of prescribing and monitoring exercise intensity. Perceived exertion ratings of 12 to 13 and 14 to 17 on the 6 to 20 RPE scale were correlated with 40% to 60% and 60% to 90% of VO_{2max}, respectively[100] (see additional discussion in Chapter 13, Heart Disease, and Table 13.14).

Exercise Intensity as a Percentage of Peak Workload

Clinicians often prescribe exercise intensity by utilizing a combination of physiological parameters (e.g., HR, RPE, and RPD), as these measures allow for the day-to-day variations in a participant's physiological state. Using a percentage of peak workload, while not a physiological parameter, may be helpful when prescribing exercise intensity for patients with severe pulmonary disease. In this population, the exercise intensity needed to allow for a usual exercise session duration may be so low as to produce little or no training effect.[106,107] Rather, exercise using short bursts of high-intensity activity, interspersed with low-intensity exercise or rest periods (i.e., high-intensity interval training [HIIT]) has been suggested.[108–117] In fact, HIIT has been considered as a preferable training option, compared to continuous exercise training, in patients with chronic lung disease, given its superior effect on improving exercise capacity and lessening exercise-induced dyspnea.[118] According to the *Guidelines for Pulmonary Rehabilitation* from the *American College of Chest Physicians* and the *American Association of Cardiovascular and Pulmonary Rehabilitation*, an exercise intensity that uses a high percentage of the patient's peak exercise capacity is well tolerated, and physiological training effects have been documented.[119] There is a dose relationship between exercise intensity and training outcomes, meaning the higher the exercise intensity, the greater the training.[100] They do caution, however, that lower intensity exercise may be associated with better adherence.[119] Current research on interval training versus continuous exercise training is presented in Table 12.6.

It may be the case that a 6MWT is the only functional measurement available for a given patient. The 6MWT has been determined to be a moderate to vigorous intensity for patients with pulmonary dysfunction, and the results can be used to predict Peak VO_2.[120,121] Therefore, the results of the 6MWT can be used to prescribe exercise intensity. The common workload intensity associated with a 6MWT is 80% of the average walking speed performed on the test.[122]

Duration

Exercising within prescribed exercise intensity for at least 20 to 30 minutes is recommended.[100] The duration of the training session varies according to patient tolerance, with some participants not being able to maintain continuous exercise for 20 to 30 minutes. Oscillating between high-intensity and low-intensity exercise or rest periods can be used to accomplish a total of 20 to 30 minutes of discontinuous exercise.

Frequency

The frequency of exercise refers to the number of sessions performed on a weekly basis during the exercise training period. The frequency of exercise is often dependent on the intensity that can be achieved and the duration that can be maintained. If 20 to 30 minutes of continuous aerobic exercise can be accomplished using a moderate intensity, three to five evenly spaced workouts per week are recommended. More frequent exercise sessions are recommended for patients with lower functional abilities. One to two daily sessions are advisable for patients with very low functional work capacities.

Pulmonary Rehabilitation
Exercise Training

A pulmonary rehabilitation exercise session includes the following components: check-in, warm-up, exercise at the prescribed intensity, and cool-down. The check-in period is a time to obtain baseline data, including resting HR, RR, BP, oxygen saturation, auscultation of the lungs, and weight. It is also the time to discuss medication schedules, any problems the patient may have encountered since last visit, and any changes that need to be addressed by a member of the pulmonary rehabilitation team, such as a change in expiratory flow rates, cough, or sputum production. PFTs assessed with a handheld device may be performed pre- and postexercise during a pulmonary rehabilitation session to assess the impact of the maintenance medication. Patients who use a rescue inhaler should carry this with them during the exercise session. If a patient was found to have a significant decrease in oxygenation on their exercise test, supplemental oxygen should be readied before initiation of physical activity.

The warm-up component is a time to slowly increase the HR and BP to ready the cardiovascular, pulmonary, and musculoskeletal systems for aerobic exercise. For those patients with mild to moderate lung disease who had a cardiovascular endpoint to their exercise test, the warm-up is usually accomplished by performing the same mode of exercise that will be used in the aerobic portion of the program but at a lower intensity, with an emphasis on controlled breathing. For example, cycling with no resistance could be used as a warm-up activity for a biking program. The warm-up for patients performing continuous exercise lasts approximately 5 minutes. For patients with severe lung disease who are prescribed short bursts of high-intensity exercise, there is little opportunity for a warm-up.

The exercise portion of the pulmonary rehabilitation session consists of a mode or modes of activity at the appropriate intensity for the advised duration. This portion of the program lasts for at least 20 minutes of either continuous or discontinuous activity. Participant

Evidence Summary Table 12.6   Exercise Training Intensity: Interval Versus Continuous Exercise

Design	Subjects	Interventions	Results	Comments
Louvaris et al. (2016)[109]				
Randomized controlled study	128 patients with COPD, 85 in the interval training group, 43 in the usual care group who did not participate in pulmonary rehabilitation.	12-week high-intensity exercise training exercise cycle 3x/week at 130% of baseline peak work for 30 sec of exercise and 30 sec of rest for 45 min, resistance training, breathing retraining, diet and education.	Training group increased their number of steps per day, 27% over baseline, increased the time spent in nonsedentary activities while the control group declined in the number of steps per day. These effects persisted 12 weeks after the cessation of the program.	High-intensity interval training not only increased the exercise potential of patients with COPD, but also there was a carryover to ADL that persisted after the cessation of the rehab program.
Nasis et al. (2015)[110]				
Nonrandomized controlled parallel group study	36 participants with stable COPD, Stages II–IV, mean age 69 years. Participants were divided into two groups. Group 1: those who demonstrated dynamic hyperinflation during exercise testing, and Group 2: those who did not.	Group 1 was trained with three sessions/week for 12 weeks using 30 sec of 100% workload peak and 30 sec rest for 45 min. Total workload increased 5% weekly.	After training, Group 1 showed an increase in peak workload, increase in VO$_2$ peak, decrease in SBP, HR, and V$_E$ at submaximal levels and a decrease in dynamic hyperinflation during exercise. Group 2 showed increase in peak workload, VO$_2$ peak, and an increase in cardiac output.	Pulmonary rehabilitation induces cardiovascular training effects in both groups. The study used a noninvasive device to measure cardiac output in participants with COPD.
Santos et al. (2015)[112]				
Randomized controlled trial	34 subjects with stable mild to very severe COPD were divided into two treatment groups. Mean age 67 years.	Group 1: 30 minutes 3x/week of treadmill training at 60% of workload max for 20 sessions. Group 2: 30 min, 3x/week at 80% of workload max for 20 sessions. Both groups also performed strength training and flexibility training and attended education sessions.	Both groups improved in quality of life, dyspnea, endurance, and strength greater than the known MCID for each outcome measure. There was not a statistically significant difference between the two groups.	The high-intensity workload was continuous, not interval, treadmill training at 80% of workload max found on a CPET. Other studies used discontinuous 100% to 120% of workload on a CPET. This study found that both moderate (60%) and high-intensity (80%) exercise improved quality of life, symptom control, and exercise tolerance.

(Continued)

Evidence Summary Table 12.6 Exercise Training Intensity: Interval Versus Continuous Exercise—cont'd

Design	Subjects	Interventions	Results	Comments
		Gruber et al. (2014)[113]		
Nonrandomized parallel group study	43 patients with cystic fibrosis. Interval training group included participants with SaO_2 values less than 90% at rest or at low levels of exercise. Standard exercise group included participants with SaO_2 values greater than 90% Mean age 26 years; mean BMI 17	Interval training was 10 intervals of 30 sec of exercise and 60 sec of rest, totaling 16-min sessions, 5×/week for 6 weeks. Intensity was a comfortable walking pace of 3–4 km/hr at an incline of 50% max grade on steep ramped exercise test. Standard exercise program was 45 min of treadmill and sports participation at approximately 60%–70% of VO_2 from a cycle exercise test 5×/week for 6 weeks.	Absolute and relative VO_{2peak}, and VE_{peak} significantly increased in both groups. Standard exercise program had a longer exercise time per session and had a superior improvement in VO_{2peak} and peak work.	The participants assigned to the IT group had more severe lung disease and were deemed inappropriate for the usual pulmonary rehabilitation program. In this more compromised group, interval training was shown to be effective in improving their functional abilities.
		Butcher et al. (2013)[114]		
Randomized cross-over design	14 subjects with moderate to severe COPD, 49–78 years, BMI 23–33, FEV_1 46%–75% predicted	SRAT versus CPET for prescription of exercise intensity.	Exercise intensities that used SRAT results found peak work rates to be 204% of the work rates using the results of the CPET. Participants in using the HIIT protocol had an increase of 170% of time and 95% of work over the constant workload protocol.	Usual cardiopulmonary exercise testing using an increase of 5–15 W/min underestimates the peak work possible in patients with moderate to severe COPD.
		Klijn et al. (2013)[115]		
Randomized controlled study	110 subjects with severe and very severe COPD, mean ages 61 years, mean FEV_1 % predicted 32, mean BMI 25 were divided into two groups.	Exercise program 3×/week for 10 weeks. Group 1: NLPE, including high-volume, low-intensity exercise at 50%–60% work max and low-volume, high-intensity exercise at 100%–120% of work max. Group 2 began with 10 min of 30% work max and progressed to 24 min at 75% work max.	Improved cycle time, improved dyspnea, decreased fatigue, and increased CRQ scores in both groups, significantly greater improvement in the NLPE group. Fat free mass increased minimally but significantly in the NLPE group.	Participants with severe and very severe COPD and low fat free body mass benefit from a tailored training program to improve muscle efficiency and preserve muscle mass, improve endurance, decrease dyspnea, and increase quality-of-life scores.

Evidence Summary Table 12.6   Exercise Training Intensity: Interval Versus Continuous Exercise—cont'd

Design	Subjects	Interventions	Results	Comments
		Mador et al. (2009)[111]		
Randomized controlled study	48 patients with COPD, 21 in the interval training group, 20 in the continuous training group.	All patients exercised 3×/week for 8 weeks. Interval training: 1 min at 150% and 2 min at 75% of the estimated target for 20–40 min. Continuous training: 50% of peak power on the cycle ergometer (or 80% of 6MWT average speed) for 20–40 min.	Both groups improved in 6MWT distance, maximal work capacity, endurance exercise time, quality of life, and dyspnea. No significant difference in the extent of improvement between the two intervention groups.	Compared with continuous training, interval training was well tolerated and produced similar improvements in exercise capacity and quality of life. Participants in the interval training were exercised on both the treadmill and cycle ergometer; however, there is lack of scientific evidence to support these two modalities being complementary.
		Brønstad et al. (2013)[117]		
Randomized controlled trial	17 patients with stable COPD, GOLD stage 2 and 3, and were randomized to two isocaloric protocols.	All patients were trained of uphill treadmill walking for 3×/week for 10 weeks. Aerobic interval training: Four 4-min intervals at 90%–95% of peak HR separated by 3 min at 50%–70% of peak HR. Moderate continuous training: 70% peak HR.	Both groups similarly improved in exercise capacity (VO$_2$ peak and work economy) and systolic cardiac function. No significant difference was observed between groups.	The small sample size could prevent possible differences being detected between two groups.

ADLs = activities of daily living; BMI = body mass index; COPD = chronic obstructive pulmonary disease; CPET = cardiopulmonary exercise test; CRQ = Chronic Respiratory Questionnaire; FEV$_1$ = forced expiratory volume in 1 sec; GOLD = *Global Initiative for Chronic Obstructive Lung Disease*; HIIT = high-intensity interval training; HR = heart rate; IT = interval training; MCID = minimal clinically important difference; NLPE = nonlinear periodized exercise; SBP = systolic blood pressure; 6MWT = 6-minute Walk Test; SRAT = steep ramp anaerobic test; V$_E$ = minute ventilation; VO$_2$ = volume of oxygen consumed.

monitoring can be accomplished using RPE and RPD scales and measures of HR, RR, and SaO$_2$ (oximetry).

The training period should be followed immediately by a cool-down period consisting of a slow decline in exercise intensity after the patient completes the exercise duration prescribed. This may consist of 5 to 10 minutes of low-level activities that slowly return the cardiovascular system to near pre-exercise levels or ramping down of the intensity of short bouts of exercise.

Finally, stretching exercises are performed to maintain joint and muscle integrity and to help prevent injury. Stretching exercises should be performed during exhalation to prevent a Valsalva maneuver, which would worsen a participant's pulmonary capabilities and put undue stress on the cardiac system. Patients often use accessory muscles of ventilation during the exercise program; therefore, the muscles of the neck and UEs should be incorporated into the stretching program.

Strength Training

Extremity Strength Training

While cardiopulmonary endurance training through continuous or discontinuous exercise is the mainstay of pulmonary rehabilitation, generalized strength training has been found to counter the systemic effects of COPD that result in peripheral and ventilatory muscle weakness. Strength of both UEs and LEs has been shown to increase with appropriate training. Weight training of the targeted muscle groups has been prescribed in a variety of ways. Vonbank et al.[122] improved work capacity by using a training load that allowed for 8 to 15 repetitions before fatigue. A number of strengthening methods have been used, including free weights, isokinetic devices, stair climbing, high resistance on a cycle ergometer, and Theraband.[123,124] Regardless of the mode used for strengthening, patients should be encouraged to perform these exercises during the exhalation phase of ventilation, thus refraining from a Valsalva maneuver that may impair ventilation and affect exercise performance.

Inspiratory Muscle Training

Patients with COPD may have weak inspiratory muscles that translate into breathlessness and exercise limitations.[119] In the presence of inspiratory muscle weakness, defined as a PI_{max} of less than 60 mm Hg, many research studies have demonstrated the ability to increase inspiratory muscle strength using threshold loading devices.[125–132] Inspiratory muscle training devices provide resistance to the inspiratory phase of ventilation in order to increase the strength of these muscles. Figure 12.14 shows one type of inspiratory muscle training device (Philips Healthcare, Andover, MA). Inspiratory muscle training has also been studied for its ability to alter the perception of dyspnea. A number of researchers have demonstrated a decrease in the severity of dyspnea during the performance of ADL and exercise with inspiratory muscle training.[127,129,131,132] The use of inspiratory muscle training should be considered based on the patient's type of disease, severity of disease, presence of inspiratory muscle weakness, level of dyspnea, and motivation to participate.[119] Just as there are

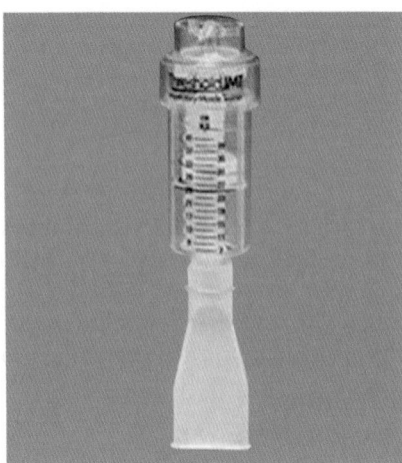

Figure 12.14 A threshold inspiratory muscle trainer for use in improving strength and endurance of the muscles of inspiration. *(Courtesy of Philips Healthcare, Andover, MA 01810.)*

continuous and interval training for the general exercise portion of pulmonary rehabilitation, these two options have also been reported for inspiratory muscle training. Continuous inspiratory muscle training uses a submaximal training load, as low as 10% of the patient's PI_{max} for a prolonged duration of up to 20 to 30 minutes. Progression of this exercise prescription is to slowly increase the training load over time, upward to 60% of the initial IP_{max}.[125] Interval training uses a higher load, up to maximum load tolerable, for short bursts of 2 to 3 minutes of exercise interspersed with rests of 1 to 2 minutes.[132] Both types of protocols have shown improvements in respiratory muscle function and decreases in dyspnea. There is also literature that shows an increase in functional mobility with training of the inspiratory muscles.[132]

Exercise Progression

Exercise progression is appropriate when the individual perceives the exercise session to be easier (lower RPE or RPD) or when the same exercise workload is performed with a lower HR—that is, when physiological adaptation to exercise has occurred.

Exercise progression should first be directed toward increasing the number of continuous minutes of exercise and decreasing the amount of time spent in low-intensity exercise or rest periods. When 20 minutes of continuous activity can be accomplished, an increase in exercise duration or intensity can be proposed. Frequency should be adjusted as necessary, based on duration and intensity.

Program Duration

Improved exercise tolerance can occur in multiple settings: an inpatient rehabilitation hospital program, an outpatient pulmonary rehabilitation program, or a home-based program.[3] Because of the limited length of stay for many inpatient rehabilitation hospital admissions, most increases in functional capacity occur in an outpatient or home pulmonary rehabilitation program. Generally, conditioning exercises are conducted up to three times per week over a course of 6 to 12 weeks.[119] At the end of the rehabilitation program, QOL measurements, dyspnea measurements, and functional assessments (6MWT or ISWT) should be readministered to assess the benefits of pulmonary rehabilitation for each participant. Exercise abilities gained in a pulmonary rehabilitation program have been found to gradually decline over 12 to 18 months following completion of the program. Pulmonary rehabilitation programs that last longer than 12 weeks have shown greater sustained benefits than shorter programs.[119]

An unfortunate reality is that patients with pulmonary dysfunction often have decreased exercise ability following an exacerbation of their disease. There is evidence to support a reduction in dyspnea in patients who repeat pulmonary rehabilitation after an acute exacerbation of their COPD.[133]

Home Exercise Programs

A home exercise program (HEP) should begin while the participant is enrolled in a pulmonary rehabilitation program. When deemed appropriate (based on exercise response and laboratory data), the participant can be assigned home exercise activities. The patient uses an exercise log to record parameters such as exercise HRs, RPEs, RPD, exercise workloads, and any questions that may arise about the HEP (Fig. 12.15). At regular intervals, the therapist analyzes the data and adjusts the HEP as necessary. Progression to an independent HEP is an important rehabilitation goal to promote a participant's lifelong commitment to exercise.

Multispecialty Team

Although exercise training is integral to pulmonary rehabilitation, participants may require additional services and information to optimize their exercise capability

and to improve quality of life. The pulmonary rehabilitation team may consist of a number of health-care providers. While professional roles may overlap, each team member brings their own level of expertise to the participants in a pulmonary rehabilitation program. Team members may include nurses, for their expertise with medication regimens; respiratory therapists, for their knowledge of oxygen delivery systems and independent secretion removal devices; occupational therapists to teach energy conservation during the performance of ADL; dieticians for nutritional support; social workers for community resources and counseling; exercise physiologists for exercise prescription and implementation; and physicians for overall care management. All of these professionals may not be present at each session of a pulmonary rehabilitation program, but the ability to refer participants to these professionals will improve overall care. The following sections address other elements of a pulmonary rehabilitation program: patient

Activity Log

Week of: _____

Aerobic exercise

	Monday	Tuesday	Wednesday	Thursday	Friday	Saturday	Sunday
Mode							
Average HR							
Average RPE							
Average dyspnea							
Start time							
End time							
Comments:							

Strengthening exercise:

	Monday	Tuesday	Wednesday	Thursday	Friday	Saturday	Sunday
Type							
Weight							
# of reps							
Comments:							

Figure 12.15 An exercise log that can be used to follow a patient's ability to exercise both during and independent of the pulmonary rehabilitation program.

education, secretion removal techniques, and *activity pacing*. Smoking cessation should also be considered as a component of pulmonary rehabilitation. (See the section on smoking cessation in the medical management section of this chapter.)

Patient Education

The concept of self-management is promoted in the individual and group educational sessions of a pulmonary rehabilitation program.[119] Participants are given individual, one-on-one time to identify their own needs and address issues that are particular to themselves. Benefits from group discussions include support from peers regarding the patient's feelings or needs, learning from others' experiences and questions, and socialization that only a group can provide. Key components of a patient's education program are presented in Box 12.3.

Education makes it possible for patients to assume responsibility for their own wellness. A patient will carry out the required activities to produce the desired outcome only if the patient knows what to do, knows how to do it, and also wants to do it. This theory of self-efficacy for the patient with pulmonary disease begins with a daily routine that includes self-assessment, adherence to a medication schedule, performance of airway clearance techniques, ADL with pacing, and an appropriate HEP.

Self-assessment is used to recognize the first signs of an exacerbation of the disease: increased dyspnea; decreased exercise tolerance; and change in pulmonary flow rates, sputum color or consistency, pedal edema, or any other significant change from baseline. An *exacerbation protocol* is an individually devised set of instructions consistent with the participant's disease and abilities. These instructions may include the use of airway clearance techniques, the use of pacing techniques, or a change in the exercise prescription, as well as contact with the primary care physician for a review of symptoms and pharmacological management.

Once the patient has completed a pulmonary rehabilitation program, continued support through community exercise groups is essential to maintaining the new level of physical activity obtained with pulmonary rehabilitation.[3] Access to new information and continued support is possible through groups such as the *Better Breathing Club*, sponsored by the American Lung Association. See Appendix 12.A (online), Web-Based Resources for Clinicians, Families, and Patients With Chronic Pulmonary Dysfunction.

Secretion Removal Techniques

Secretion retention can interfere with ventilation and the diffusion of oxygen and carbon dioxide in some patients with pulmonary disease. Patients with secretion retention may improve their exercise performance if proper secretion removal techniques have been performed before the physical activity. An individualized program for secretion removal directed to the areas of involvement can optimize ventilation and therefore gas exchange capabilities. Secretion removal techniques include programs that rely on a caregiver (postural drainage, percussion, and shaking) or independent programs, such as the active cycle of breathing technique (ACBT) and autogenic drainage (AD); positive expiratory pressure (PEP) devices, such as the TheraPEP PEP Therapy System (Smiths Medical, Dublin, OH); airway oscillation devices, such as the Flutter (Cardinal Health, Dublin, OH) or the Acapella (Smiths Medical, Dublin, OH); or high-frequency chest compression (HFCC) devices, such as the Vest System (Hill-Rom, St. Paul, MN).

Manual Secretion Removal Techniques
Postural Drainage

Positioning a patient so that the bronchus of the involved lung segment is perpendicular to the ground is the basis for *postural drainage*. Using gravity, these positions assist the mucociliary transport system in removing excessive secretions from the tracheobronchial tree. Standard postural drainage positions are presented in Figure 12.16. Although these postural drainage positions are optimal for gravity drainage of specific lung segments, such positioning may not be realistic for some patients. Modification of these standard positions may prevent any untoward effects yet still enhance secretion removal. Box 12.4 lists precautions that should be considered before instituting postural drainage with patients with signs and symptoms of increased daily pulmonary secretions. These are not absolute contraindications but relative precautions. The list is not meant to be inclusive; however, it does provide a range of considerations that should be addressed before instituting postural drainage.

Box 12.3 Education Topics

Anatomy and physiology of respiratory disease
Airway clearance techniques
Nutritional guidelines
Energy-saving techniques
Stress management and relaxation
Benefits of being smoke free
Impact of environmental factors on COPD
Pharmacology/use of MDIs
Oxygen delivery systems
Psychosocial aspects of COPD
Diagnostic techniques
Management of COPD
Community resources
Exercise: Effects, contraindications, adherence

COPD = chronic obstructive pulmonary disease; MDIs = metered dose inhalers.

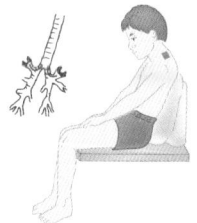

UPPER LOBES Apical Segments

Bed or drainage table flat.

Patient leans back on pillow at 30° angle against therapist.

Therapist claps with markedly cupped hand over area between clavicle and top of scapula on each side.

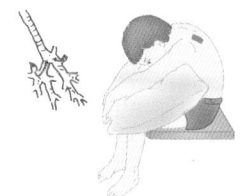

UPPER LOBES Posterior Segments

Bed or drainage table flat.

Patient leans over folded pillow at 30° angle.

Therapist stands behind and claps over upper back on both sides.

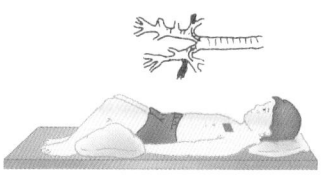

UPPER LOBES Anterior Segments

Bed or drainage table flat.

Patient lies on back with pillow under knees.

Therapist claps between clavicle and nipple on each side.

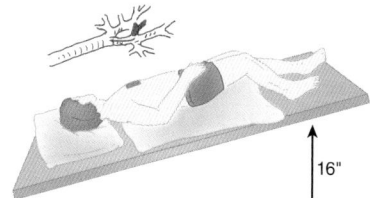

16"

RIGHT MIDDLE LOBE

Foot of table or bed elevated 16 inches.

Patient lies head down on left side and rotates 1/4 turn backward. Pillow may be placed behind from shoulder to hip. Knees should be flexed.

Therapist claps over right nipple area. In females with breast development or tenderness use cupped hand with heel of hand under armpit and fingers extending forward beneath the breast.

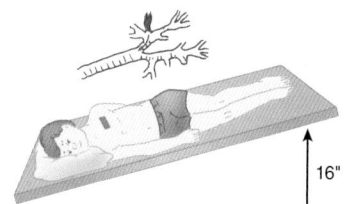

16"

LEFT UPPER LOBE Singular Segments

Foot of table or bed elevated 16 inches.

Patient lies head down on right side and rotates 1/4 turn backward. Pillow may be placed behind from shoulder to hip. Knees should be flexed.

Therapist claps with moderately cupped hand over left nipple area. In females with breast development or tenderness use cupped hand with heel of hand under armpit and fingers extending forward beneath the breast.

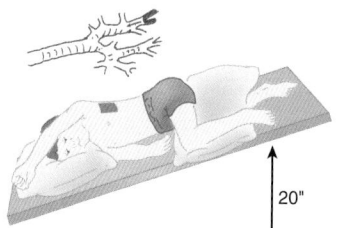

20"

LOWER LOBES Anterior Basal Segments

Foot of table or bed elevated 20 inches.

Patient lies on side, head down, pillow under knees.

Therapist claps with slightly cupped hand over lower ribs. (Position shown is for drainage of left anterior basal segment. To drain the right anterior basal segment, patient should be on the left side in same posture.)

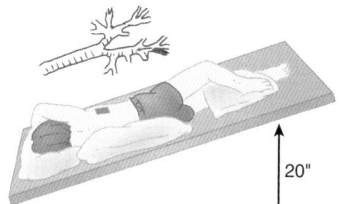

20"

LOWER LOBES Lateral Basal Segments

Foot of table or bed elevated 20 inches.

Patient lies on abdomen, head down, then rotates 1/4 turn upward. Upper leg is flexed over pillow for support.

Therapist claps over uppermost portion of lower ribs. (Position shown is for drainage of right lateral basal segment. To drain the left lateral basal segment, patient should lie on the right side in the same posture.)

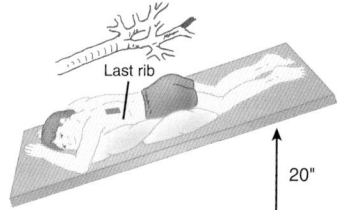

Last rib

20"

LOWER LOBES Posterior Basal Segments

Foot of table or bed elevated 20 inches.

Patient lies on abdomen, head down, with pillow under hips.

Therapist claps over lower ribs close to spine on each side.

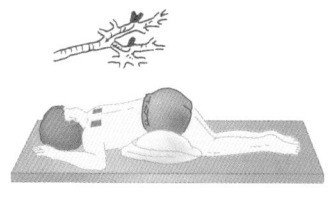

LOWER LOBES Superior Segments

Bed of table flat.

Patient lies on abdomen with two pillows under hips.

Therapist claps over middle of back at tip of scapula on either side of spine.

Figure 12.16 Positions used for postural drainage. *(Adapted from Roy S, Wolf S, Scalzitti D. The Rehabilitation Specialist's Handbook. 4th ed. F.A. Davis; 2013, with permission.)*

Percussion

Percussion is a force rhythmically applied with the therapist's cupped hands to the patient's chest wall. The percussion technique is applied to specific areas on the thorax that correspond to an underlying involved lung segment. The technique is typically administered for 3 to 5 minutes over each involved lung segment. Percussion is thought to release the pulmonary secretions from the wall of the airways and into the lumen of the airway. By coupling percussion with the appropriate postural drainage position for a specific lung segment, the probability of secretion removal is enhanced. Because percussion is a force directed to the thorax, there are conditions that would necessitate caution with this technique, such as a fractured rib, flail chest, osteoporosis, elevated coagulation studies, or decreased platelet count. These examples are by no means inclusive, but they provide some patient presentations that might require modification (a gentler force applied to the thorax) or elimination of the percussion technique.

Box 12.4   Precautions for Postural Drainage

Precautions for the use of the Trendelenburg position

Circulatory: congestive heart failure, hypertension
Pulmonary: pulmonary edema, shortness of breath made worse with Trendelenburg position (head of bed lower than foot)
Abdominal: obesity, abdominal distention, hiatal hernia, nausea, recent food consumption

Precautions for the use of the side-lying position

Vascular: axillofemoral bypass graft
Musculoskeletal: arthritis, recent rib fracture, shoulder bursitis, or tendonitis, any conditioning that would make appropriate postural drainage positioning uncomfortable

Shaking

Following a deep inhalation, a bouncing maneuver is applied with the therapist's open hands to the rib cage throughout the expiratory phase of breathing. This *shaking* is applied to a specific area on the thorax that corresponds to the underlying involved lung segment. Five to seven deep breaths with shaking on exhalation are appropriate to hasten the removal of secretions via the mucociliary transport system. Shaking is commonly used following percussion in the appropriate postural drainage position. Because this technique consists of a force applied to the thorax, the same circulatory and musculoskeletal considerations are needed as in the application of percussion.

Airway Clearance

Once the secretions have been mobilized with postural drainage, percussion, and shaking, the task of removing the secretions from the airways is undertaken using an airway clearance technique. *Coughing* is the most common and easiest means of clearing the airway. However, it should be noted that high intrathoracic pressures, such as those generated during coughing, could force the closing of small airways in some patients with obstructive pulmonary diseases. By trapping air behind the closed airway, the forced expulsion of air during a cough becomes ineffective in clearing secretions. *Huffing* is an alternative method of airway clearance that is useful for patients with obstructive pulmonary disease. A huff uses many of the same steps of coughing, without closing the glottis, and thus does not create the high intrathoracic pressures. The patient is asked to take a deep breath and then rapidly contract the abdominal muscles while forcefully saying "HA HA HA." This allows a forced expiration through a stabilized open airway and makes secretion removal more effective.[134]

Active Cycle of Breathing Techniques

ACBT is an independent breathing exercise program the patient can perform to clear secretions from the airways. This technique includes three phases: (1) a breathing control phase, (2) a thoracic expansion phase, and (3) a forced expiratory technique. ACBT begins with a few minutes at the breathing control phase, defined as relaxed, diaphragmatic, TV breathing. From this breathing control phase, the patient determines what to do next. If secretions need to be loosened, the patient will perform three to four thoracic expansion exercises, defined as three to five deep inhalations with a 3-second hold followed by a passive exhalation. A return to the breathing control phase follows, which can last for a few seconds to a few minutes, while the patient assesses themselves and makes a decision of what is next needed. If the patient feels that there are secretions ready to be moved more proximally, then the forced expiratory technique completes the cycle. The forced expiratory technique, defined as one or two huffs from TV down to low lung volumes, is used to move secretions into the larger, more proximal airways. The forced expiratory technique is followed by a period of breathing control for rest and reassessment. If secretions are not ready to be expelled, the patient may return to thoracic expansion exercises. Using ACBT, secretions are "milked" from smaller to larger airways. Once the secretions have moved into the larger airways, huffs from mid or high lung volumes remove the secretions from the airways. This independent technique has been demonstrated to be as effective as postural drainage, percussion, and shaking.[135] Figure 12.17 emphasizes that the patient begins at breathing control and always returns to breathing control for rest and the patient's own assessment of

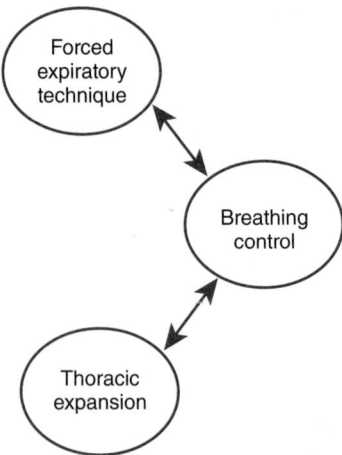

Figure 12.17 Active cycle of breathing begins with breathing control. All choices are made from the breathing control phase. After each choice is made, thoracic expansion or forced expiratory technique, the patient returns to breathing control to rest and make the next choice.

their status before moving to either thoracic expansion with breath hold or the forced expiratory technique.

AD is a three-phase breathing exercise that improves airway secretion clearance from peripheral to central airways. The three phases include (1) unstick, (2) collect, and (3) evacuate. AD begins with loosening peripheral secretions by breathing at low lung volumes for at least three breaths. As the crackle of secretions starts to become louder, the collect secretion phase begins with breathing at low-to-middle lung volumes for at least three breaths. When ready to evacuate the airway secretion from the central airways, the patient begins breathing at middle-to-high lung volumes for at least three breaths. The AD technique can improve lung function by increasing oxygen saturation and peak expiratory glow rate;[136] however, it requires effort and commitment from the individual, which makes it a challenging technique for some populations (e.g., pediatric patients).[137]

Oral Airway Oscillation Devices

Airway oscillation devices, such as the Flutter or the Acapella (Fig. 12.18), alter the exhaled airflow throughout the airways. The patient first inhales a normal size breath. During active exhalation through the device, the exhaled air causes an intermittent backward air pressure that oscillates the airways. The usual procedure is to exhale 10 or so breaths through the device, followed by two large, exhaled volumes through the device and finally a huff or cough to clear mobilized secretions. This routine is repeated until secretions are cleared from the lungs. An airway oscillation device has been shown to help in the removal of secretions from airways.[138,139]

Positive Expiratory Pressure

PEP devices have a valve to regulate expiratory resistance (Fig. 12.19). Inhalation of a normal size breath through the mask or mouthpiece is unresisted. Active exhalation is against a PEP measuring 10 to 20 cm H_2O. A treatment session lasts approximately 10 to 20 min with frequent pauses to remove the mask or mouthpiece so that the patient can cough or huff to

clear secretions. The session is completed when all secretions have been cleared from the airways. PEP has been shown to be as effective as postural drainage, percussion, and shaking.[140,141]

High-Frequency Chest Compression Devices

The HFCC device uses an inflatable vest with air channels that is worn over the patient's thorax (Fig. 12.20). The vest is attached to an air compressor that rapidly delivers small air volumes in and out of the vest. The inflation of the vest causes compression to the chest wall, and the deflation allows the chest wall to recoil back to its resting position. The patient assumes a comfortable seated position for treatments lasting between 20 and 30 minutes. Secretions may be cleared at any time throughout the treatment. HFCC has been shown to be as effective as other secretion removal techniques.[142,143]

Breathing Exercises

Pursed-lip breathing involves an unresisted inspiration followed by an active oral exhalation through a narrowed (or pursed) mouth opening. When pursed-lip breathing is used by patients with COPD, it may delay or prevent airway collapse, allowing for better gas exchange.[144,145] Most patients demonstrate this strategy during periods of dyspnea and rarely need to be taught the technique.

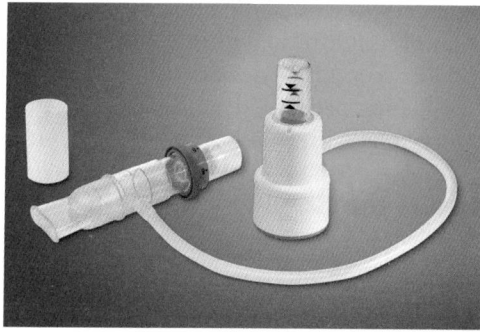

Figure 12.19 The positive expiratory pressure system for an independent program of secretion removal. *(Courtesy of Smith Medical, Dublin OH, 43017.)*

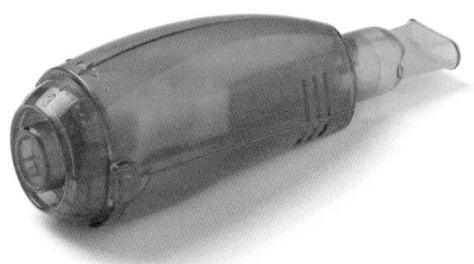

Figure 12.18 The Acapella device used for an independent program of secretion removal. *(Courtesy of Smith Medical, Dublin, OH 43017.)*

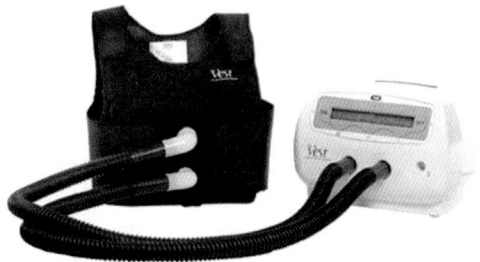

Figure 12.20 The high-frequency chest wall compression device (the Vest) can be used for an independent program of secretion removal. *(Courtesy of Hill-Rom, St. Paul, MN 55126.)*

Although diaphragmatic breathing has been taught to patients with chronic pulmonary dysfunction for years, there is little evidence to support its use to improve pulmonary mechanics.[145] Some patients require the use of accessory muscles with exercise, with exacerbation of their disease, or with periods of dyspnea. Strengthening accessory muscles of ventilation may be a more effective treatment program than encouraging the use of an ineffective diaphragm with little ability to generate muscle force and/or limited muscle excursion. In patients with very flattened diaphragms, focusing on diaphragmatic breathing may even be detrimental.

Activity Pacing

Activity pacing refers to the performance of any activity within the limits or boundaries of that patient's breathing capacity. For example, an activity that usually causes dyspnea needs to be broken down into component parts such that each component can be performed at a rate that does not exceed breathing abilities. By breaking activities down into component parts and interspersing rest periods between each component, the total activity can be completed without dyspnea or undo fatigue. For example, patients often find that climbing stairs causes a great deal of dyspnea and discomfort. Rather than climbing the entire flight of stairs (usually done too fast and with a breath hold), the patient might be instructed as follows: "Take a deep breath. Now, on exhalation, walk up one (or two or three) stair(s). Now recover. Take in another good breath and walk up the next one (or two or three) stair(s) and recover. Repeat this technique until the flight of stairs is completed." The patient is able to reach the top of the stairs without becoming dyspneic and without undue fatigue. Pacing can and should be part of every activity that would otherwise cause dyspnea. Pacing should be used when performing ADL, ambulation, stair climbing, and other daily tasks. Pacing is not a technique to be used during the aerobic portion of a pulmonary rehabilitation program. During exercise, some SOB is expected to occur.

SUMMARY

Pulmonary rehabilitation is a well-established treatment for patients with chronic pulmonary disease. Components of these programs typically include exercise training, strength training, education, secretion removal instruction, and psychosocial support. Outcomes of pulmonary rehabilitation may include increased aerobic capacity, increased skeletal muscle strength, reduced dyspnea during exercise and ADL, and an increase in the perception of health-related quality of life. Gains made in pulmonary rehabilitation programs can make the difference between a lifestyle of dependence and one of independence. Physical therapists have the important role of evaluating patients, determining their potential, and through exercise prescription and exercise programs, ensuring that rehabilitation goals and outcomes are realized.

Questions for Review

1. How does the clinical presentation of obstructive lung disease differ from the clinical presentation of restrictive lung disease?

2. Explain how altered airway structure leads to airflow limitation.

3. (a) What would be the expected breath sounds of a patient with COPD? Describe intensity and adventitious sounds. (b) What would be the expected breath sounds of a patient with asthma during an exacerbation? Describe intensity and adventitious sounds.

4. Identify the tests and measures required to determine the extent of pulmonary disease.

5. What are the pulmonary endpoints to a symptom-limited graded exercise test?

6. How does exercise prescription differ for a patient with mild pulmonary disease as compared to a patient with severe pulmonary disease?

7. (a) How do you know when to progress a patient's exercise program? (b) What is the nature of that progression? (c) Do you need a new ETT to progress a patient's exercise workload?

8. How would you respond to a patient's comment that it would take longer to climb stairs with pacing than without?

9. Design a secretion removal treatment plan for a patient with CF that can be carried out independently before coming to pulmonary rehabilitation.

10. What evidence is presented in the current literature regarding the benefits of pulmonary rehabilitation?

CASE STUDY

PATIENT WITH COPD

A 67-year-old white female was admitted to the hospital with a COPD exacerbation. She was treated with noninvasive ventilation for 2 days, inhaled bronchodilators, and intravenous antibiotics and corticosteroids. After the acute care hospital stay of 7 days, the patient was transferred to an inpatient rehabilitation facility for 7 days. She is now referred to outpatient pulmonary rehabilitation.

PAST MEDICAL HISTORY

COPD with exacerbations numbering two per year for the past 3 years, s/p lumpectomy of right breast 8 years ago, smoking history of 45 pack-years; quit on the day of this admission to hospital for acute bacterial pneumonia.

MEDICATIONS

2 L/min of oxygen by nasal cannula. Maintenance: Spiriva (Tiatroprium, a long-acting muscarinic antagonist [anticholinergic] [LAMA]), Serevent (Salmeterol, a long-acting beta agonist [LABA]), Flovent (fluticasone, an inhaled corticosteroid). Rescue: Albuterol (short-acting beta-2 adrenergic [SABA]).

OCCUPATION

Secretary, works 32 hr/week. Presently on medical leave.

SOCIAL AND ENVIRONMENTAL

Lives with husband in own home. Three steps to enter home, 12 stairs within the home.

OBJECTIVE FINDINGS

Interview

Mental status: awake, alert, talks in three- to four-word sentences. Adequate historian. Chief complaint: SOB limiting function. Patient is able to walk 120 ft before needing to rest to catch her breath. No complaints of increased secretions. Patient is dependent in shopping, house cleaning, and laundry.

Dyspnea and Quality-of-Life Measures

mMRC grade 3
CAT score of 28

Patient Goal

Patient's desired functional outcome is to be oxygen free and able to care for grandchildren without SOB.

Resting Vital Signs

HR 72, BP 96/74, SaO_2 at rest 86% on room air, 93% on 2 L/min pulsed O_2 on 1 pulse/breath, RR 32, temperature 98.5°F.

Observation, Inspection, Palpation

Thin, frail-looking female wearing nasal cannula; kyphosis noted. Patient uses posture of forward sitting with arms supported on chair arms to enhance ventilatory accessory muscle use. Increased AP diameter of thorax, accessory muscle use at rest; labored, symmetrical breathing pattern with pursed-lip breathing. No venous distention, no edema, no cyanosis, minimal clubbing evident.

Auscultation

Decreased breath sounds throughout both lung fields, especially at bases. End expiratory wheezes at left lateral base.

Strength

The Five Times Sit to Stand test resulted in 24.3 seconds.

Bilateral shoulder elevation, abduction, and extension, elbow flexion and extension area are all graded as greater than or equal to a 3/5, tested in the upright sitting position. Patient unable to lie prone or supine for further testing secondary to orthopnea. Maximal resistance was not applied in order to avoid Valsalva.

Maximal inspiratory effort (PI_{max}) was 42 mm Hg.

Exercise Test Data

Patient performed a 5-minute, staged exercise test using a cycle ergometer. The test began with 3 minutes of rest sitting on the cycle. The exercise began with stage 1: 3 minutes of unresisted pedaling. Each subsequent stage was 1 minute with an increase of 15 W. Max workload was 30 W. ECG was within normal limits. The distance covered for the 6-minute Walk Test was 200 m on 2 L O_2 by nasal cannula.

(Continued)

CASE STUDY—cont'd

	Rest	Peak
HR (beats/min)	84	121
BP (mm Hg)	128/76	156/80
RR (breaths/min)	24	36
Tidal volume (L)	0.32	0.99
SaO_2 on 2-L nasal cannula	98%	93%
RPE on 0–10 scale	1	7
RPD on 0–10 scale	3	8
FEV_1 (L/sec)	1.107 (45% predicted)	1.074
FVC (L)	1.76 (64% predicted)	1.68
FEV_1/FVC	62%	
Predicted MVV (L/min)	38.7	
Actual V_E (L/min)	7.68	35.64

BP = blood pressure; FEV_1 = forced expiratory volume in the first second; FVC = forced vital capacity; HR = heart rate; MVV = maximal voluntary ventilation; RPD = rating of perceived dyspnea; RPE = the Borg rating of perceived exertion; RR = respiratory rate; SaO_2 = oxygen saturation; V_E = minute ventilation.
*Predicted MVV was calculated using the following equation[146,147]: MVV = FEV_1 × 35

GUIDING QUESTIONS

1. In what stage of airflow limitation does this patient present?

2. Did the pulmonary system or cardiovascular system stop her exercise test?

3. (a) Identify this patient's impairments, functional limitations, and disability restrictions. (b) Identify general anticipated treatment goals and expected outcomes for a 3-month (12-week) pulmonary rehabilitation program. (c) Identify outcome measures that will be used to assess the effectiveness of a pulmonary rehabilitation program.

4. (a) Formulate a physical therapy POC for week 1. Patient will be seen three times/week for this first week of therapy. (b) Briefly describe exercise progression for the first month of the program.

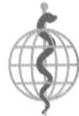 The reader is referred to Immersive Case B: A Patient With Acute COVID-19, an interactive case that guides users through the interview, examination, diagnosis, and writing of goals and the plan of care for a patient with acute COVID-19, available online at **fadavis.com**.

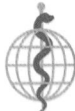 For additional resources, including answers to the questions for review, new immersive cases, case study guiding questions, references, and more, please visit **https://www.fadavis.com/product/physical -rehabilitation-fulk-8**. You may also quickly find the resources by entering this title's four-digit ISBN, 4691, in the search field at **http://fadavis.com** and logging in at the prompt.

Chapter 13

Konrad J. Dias, PT, DPT, PhD, CCS

LEARNING OBJECTIVES

1. Describe the etiology, pathophysiology, symptomatology, and sequelae of coronary heart disease.
2. Describe the etiology, pathophysiology, symptomatology, and sequelae of congestive heart failure.
3. Identify and describe the examination procedures used to evaluate patients with heart disease and establish a diagnosis and plan of care.
4. Describe the role of the physical therapist in assisting the patient in recovery from heart disease in terms of interventions, patient-related instruction, coordination, communication, and documentation.
5. Identify and describe strategies of intervention during various phases of cardiac rehabilitation.
6. Analyze and interpret patient data, formulate realistic anticipated goals and expected outcomes, and develop a plan of care when presented with a clinical case study.

CHAPTER OUTLINE

INTRODUCTION AND EPIDEMIOLOGY OF HEART DISEASE 415
CARDIAC ANATOMY AND PHYSIOLOGY 416
  Heart Tissue 417
  Coronary Arteries 417
  Heart Valves 418
  Cardiac Output and Cardiac Index 418
  Cardiac Cycle 419
  Blood Flow and Hemodynamic Values 419
  Electrical Conduction of the Heart 420
  Neurohormonal Influences on the Cardiovascular System 421
  Myocardial Oxygen Supply and Demand 422
  Laboratory Values 422
CARDIOVASCULAR RESPONSES TO AEROBIC EXERCISE 423
  Measures of Energy Expenditure 423
  Normal Responses 423
  Abnormal Responses 426
CARDIAC PATHOLOGIES AND PHYSICAL THERAPY IMPLICATIONS 426

Hypertension 426
Acute Coronary Syndrome 428
Heart Failure 438
Valvular Heart Disease 444
Electrical Conduction Abnormalities 444
Heart Transplantation 450
EXAMINATION OF THE PATIENT WITH HEART DISEASE 450
  Medical Record Review 450
  Patient Interview 450
  Tests and Measures 451
PHYSICAL THERAPY INTERVENTION FOR PATIENTS WITH HEART DISEASE 454
  Therapeutic Exercise 454
  Cardiac Rehabilitation 454
  Interventions for Patients With Heart Failure 457
EDUCATION FOR PATIENTS WITH HEART DISEASE 461
PSYCHOLOGICAL/SOCIAL ISSUES 464
PRIMARY PREVENTION OF CORONARY ARTERY DISEASE 465
SUMMARY 465

■ INTRODUCTION AND EPIDEMIOLOGY OF HEART DISEASE

Cardiovascular disease (CVD) encompasses a group of disorders of the heart and blood vessels and includes coronary artery disease (CAD), cerebrovascular disease, hypertension, heart failure, and other conditions. The global burden of CVD is enormous with approximately 18.6 million deaths around the world attributed to CVDs in 2019.[1] CAD, also called coronary heart disease (CHD), refers to the pathological process of atherosclerosis, specifically affecting the coronary arteries. CAD includes the diagnoses of angina pectoris, myocardial infarction (MI), silent myocardial ischemia, and sudden cardiac death.

The pathophysiological conditions that underlie CVD are atherosclerosis, altered myocardial muscle mechanics, valvular dysfunction, arrhythmias, and hypertension (HTN). Atherosclerosis is a disease in which lipid-laden plaque (lesions) is formed within the intimal layer of the blood vessel wall of moderate- and large-size arteries. Over time the plaque may extend into the lumen causing a decreased luminal diameter. Atherosclerosis is also a primary contributor to cerebrovascular disease (cerebrovascular accident [CVA]) and peripheral vascular disease (PVD).

Alteration in myocardial muscle mechanics involving the systolic and/or diastolic properties of the myocardium results in an impairment of left ventricular (LV) function. Heart failure (HF) is a clinical diagnosis caused by impaired LV functioning and is referred to as congestive heart failure (CHF) when it is accompanied by signs and symptoms of edema (i.e., congestion). There are many causes of HF, including myocardial scarring and remodeling as a result of an MI; cardiomyopathy involving an enlarged, thickened, and/or hardened heart muscle from various causes; or impaired valvular function, especially within the mitral and aortic valves.[2]

Arrhythmias are caused by a disturbance in the electrical activity of the heart, resulting in impaired electrical impulse formation or conduction. Arrhythmias may present as benign or malignant (i.e., life threatening). Examples of malignant arrhythmias are sustained ventricular tachycardia (V-tach) and ventricular fibrillation (V-fib). An example of a common benign arrhythmia in older adults is atrial fibrillation (A-fib) with a controlled ventricular response involving a ventricular rate between 60 and 100 beats per minute (bpm).

HTN is the most prevalent CVD in the United States and one of the most powerful contributors to cardiovascular morbidity and mortality.[3] Revised guidelines from the American Heart Association (AHA) and American College of Cardiology (ACC) define HTN as a systolic blood pressure consistently greater than 130 mm Hg or diastolic blood pressure equal to or greater than 80 mm Hg.[3]

CVD remains the leading cause of death and disability in the United States. According to the AHA's Heart Disease and Stroke Statistics 2021 Update, an estimated 126.9 million Americans have one or more types of CVD. In 2018, CHD was the leading cause (42.1%) of deaths in the United States, followed by stroke (17%), high blood pressure (11%), HF (9.6%), diseases of the arteries (2.9%), and other CVD (17.4%).[1] Heart disease is also the number one killer of women, taking more lives than all forms of cancer combined. On average, heart disease strikes an individual every 39 seconds. The direct and indirect costs of CVD and stroke including health expenditure and lost productivity total more than $363.4 billion.[1]

This chapter begins with a review of normal anatomy and physiology of the cardiovascular system and its relevance to physical therapist practice, along with normal cardiovascular responses to exercise. Additionally, various cardiovascular pathologies and pertinent physical therapy implications are discussed. The contemporary management of CVD in 2022, as discussed in this chapter, not only reflects specific physical therapy management considerations for the treatment of each condition but more importantly highlights preventive strategies to be incorporated to reduce the overall burden of heart disease in society. Elements of the patient examination, evidence-based interventions, goals, outcomes, cardiac medications with relevant physical therapy implications, patient education, and appropriate Internet resources provide the reader with a holistic management for patients with heart disease.

■ CARDIAC ANATOMY AND PHYSIOLOGY

The heart lies within the left thoracic cavity. The base of the heart is located superiorly, approximately between the second and third ribs; the apex is located inferiorly, approximately at the level of the fifth rib (Fig. 13.1). In this position, the heart is rotated in the sagittal plane so that the right ventricle (RV) is positioned anterior to the left ventricle (LV) and tipped anteriorly, bringing the apex closer to the chest wall. In the posterior–anterior view of a chest x-ray, the RV occupies a significant portion of the frontal plane. The right atrium (RA) is generally located in the area of the second intercostal space and the *angle of Louis*. When one palpates the sternum, the angle of Louis is the "bump" that demarcates the manubrium from the body of the sternum. The second intercostal spaces are lateral and slightly below the angle of Louis. The right and left second intercostal spaces are important auscultatory landmarks. The right space

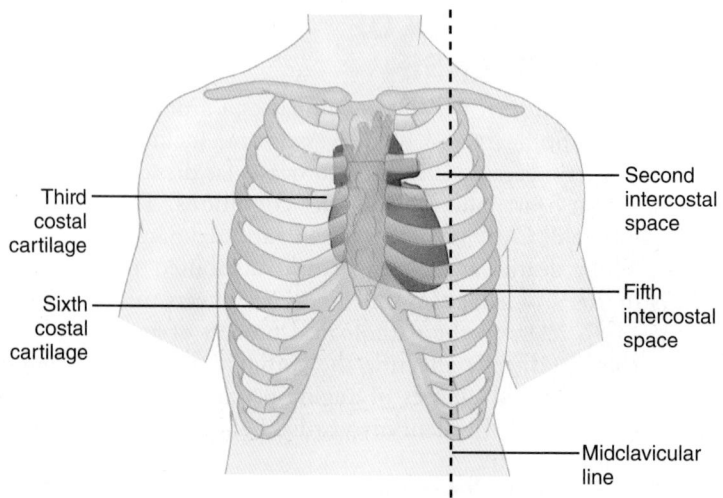

Figure 13.1 Surface anatomy of the heart.

is known as the *aortic area,* while the left is designated as the *pulmonic area.* The apex of the normal heart is in the fifth intercostal space at the midclavicular line. In a healthy heart, this area, known as the *point of maximal impulse (PMI),* is where the contraction of the LV is most pronounced.

Heart Tissue

The heart wall is made up of three tissue layers (Fig. 13.2). The outermost layer of the heart is a double-walled sac called the *pericardium.* The two layers of the pericardium include an outer tough, fibrous layer of dense, irregular connective tissue called the *parietal pericardium* and an inner thin *visceral pericardium.*[4] The visceral pericardium is also called the *epicardium.* Between the two pericardial layers is a closed space filled with 10 to 20 mL of clear pericardial fluid. This fluid serves as a lubricant allowing the two surfaces to slide over each other.

Clinically, patients may develop an infection with resultant inflammation of the pericardium called *pericarditis.* The clinical signs that accompany this pathology and are used to differentially diagnose pericarditis include a *pericardial friction rub* (an audible grating sound suggesting irritation of the pericardium) that can be auscultated with each heartbeat, sharp constant pericardial chest pain, possible fever and shortness of breath, and electrocardiographic changes including a saddle-shaped elevation of the ST-elevation with or without depression of the PR interval.[5] In some patients with pericarditis, the excessive fluid accumulation within the closed pericardial space may lead to a secondary condition known as *cardiac tamponade.* Tamponade involves compression of the heart caused by fluid buildup in the space between the myocardium and pericardium. In this state, patients demonstrate compromised cardiac function and contractility due to the excess fluid within the closed space pushing against the heart.[5]

The muscular middle layer of the heart is called the *myocardium.* It is the layer that facilitates the pumping action of the heart to move blood to the entire body. Myocardial cells may be categorized into two groups based on their function—mechanical cells contributing to mechanical contraction and conductive cells contributing to electrical conduction.

Alterations in the muscular wall of the heart are called cardiomyopathies. There are three common classifications of cardiomyopathies: *dilated, hypertrophic,* and *restrictive.*[6] Dilated cardiomyopathy is evidenced by ventricular dilation and altered cardiac muscle contractile function. CAD is the prime cause of *dilated cardiomyopathy,* causing mitochondrial dysfunction and resultant myocardial damage. Myocarditis (inflammation of the heart muscle) and alcohol abuse are additional causes of dilated cardiomyopathy. *Hypertrophic cardiomyopathy* presents as diastolic dysfunction or altered ventricular filling ability with concomitant increases in ventricular mass. Chronic HTN and aortic stenosis are conditions that lead to the development of hypertrophic cardiomyopathy. *Restrictive cardiomyopathy* also presents as diastolic dysfunction with limited relaxation and filling ability owing to the presence of an excessively rigid ventricular wall. The connective tissue changes of the heart associated with diabetes are an example of a restrictive cardiomyopathy. Damage to myocardial cells from cardiomyopathies and various other etiologies lead to cardiac muscle dysfunction and resultant HF, which is discussed in detail later in this chapter.

The innermost layer of the heart is called the *endocardium.* The tissue of the endocardium forms the inner lining of the chambers of the heart and is continuous with the tissue of the valves and the endothelium of the blood vessel. Because the endocardium and valves share similar tissue, patients with infections of the endocardium are at risk for developing valvular dysfunction.[7] Endocardial infections can spread into valvular tissue, developing vegetations (a mixture of bacteria and blood clots) on the valve.[7] In patients with newly developed vegetations, bronchopulmonary hygiene procedures including percussions and vibrations must be used with extreme caution as these procedures may cause the vegetation to dislodge and move as emboli resulting in an embolic stroke.

Coronary Arteries

The coronary arteries originate in the sinus of Valsalva located in the wall of the aorta near the aortic valve.[8] There are three major vessels that supply the heart with oxygenated blood. These three vessels include the right coronary artery, the left anterior descending artery, and the left circumflex artery (Fig. 13.3).

The right coronary artery originates from the area near the right aortic leaflet, and the left main coronary

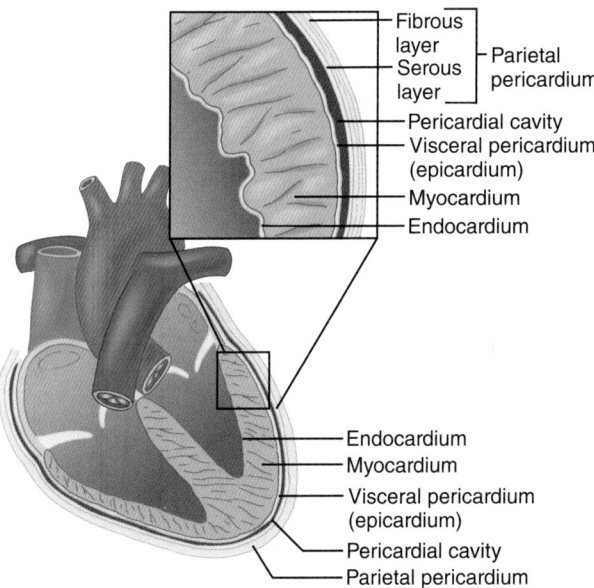

Figure 13.2 Layers of the heart.

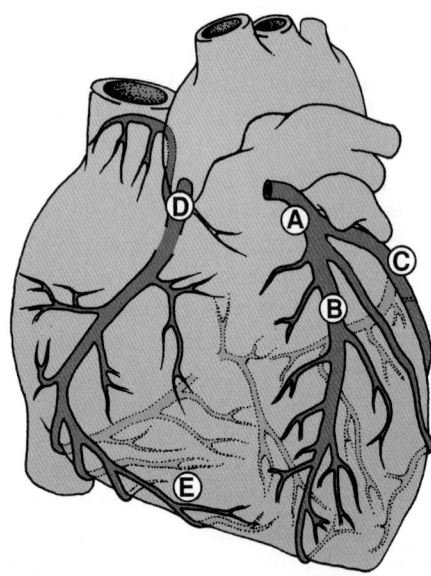

Figure 13.3 Coronary circulation: (A) left main (LM); (B) left anterior descending (LAD); (C) left circumflex (CX); (D) right coronary (RCA); (E) posterior descending (PDA). The branches of the LAD are known as diagonals; the branches of the CX are known as marginals.

artery arises from the area near the left aortic leaflet. When the aortic valve is open during systole, the origins of the coronary arteries are located behind the aortic leaflets within the wall; when the aortic valve is closed during diastole, the openings of the coronaries are clearly exposed, allowing them to be easily perfused. The coronary arteries therefore receive the majority of their blood flow during diastole, unlike the other arteries of the body that are perfused during systole.[8]

The left main coronary artery branches into the left anterior descending (LAD) and the circumflex. The LAD may have further divisions, known as diagonal branches that come off the primary LAD. The LAD and its diagonal branches primarily supply the anterior and apical surfaces of the LV, as well as portions of the interventricular septum. The circumflex may also have branches, known as marginal branches. The circumflex and its marginal branches supply the lateral and part of the inferior surfaces of the LV and portions of the left atrium (LA). The right coronary artery (RCA) supplies the RA, most of the RV, part of the inferior wall of the LV, portions of the interventricular septum, and the conduction system. The posterior descending artery (PDA) is most commonly a branch of the RCA and perfuses the posterior heart. If the RCA does not perfuse the posterior heart, the left circumflex (CX) will supply this area. When the PDA comes from the RCA, the anatomy is referred to as being right dominant; if the PDA comes from the CX, the anatomy is referred to as being left dominant. For physical therapists, there is no clinical importance to whether the anatomy of the myocardium is either left or right dominant.[9]

Reduced blood flow within any of the coronary arteries will result in ischemia and possible infarction of cardiac tissue. In addition, coronary arteries may present in spasm. In this condition, the smooth muscle contraction within the walls of the artery suddenly spasms, resulting in a profound narrowing of the coronary artery. Cigarette smoking is a major risk factor for vasospastic angina.[10] Further, there exists evidence of changes in autonomic activity detected by heart rate variability shortly before an episode of coronary spasm. Finally, guidewire or balloon dilatation at the time of a percutaneous coronary intervention is a risk factor of coronary spasm.

Heart Valves

Four heart valves ensure one-way blood flow through the heart. Two atrioventricular (AV) valves are located between the atria and ventricle. The AV valve, positioned between the RA and RV, is called the *tricuspid valve*; the left AV valve is the *mitral valve* (also known as the bicuspid valve). This valve is located between the LA and LV. The *semilunar valves* lie between the ventricles and arteries that emerge from the ventricles. These valves are named based on the vessels they correspond with (i.e., *pulmonic valve* on the right in association with the pulmonary artery, and aortic valve on the left relating to the aorta).

Flaps of tissue called *leaflets or cusps* guard the heart valve openings. The right AV valve has three cusps and is therefore called *tricuspid*, whereas the left AV valve has only two cusps and hence is called *bicuspid*. These leaflets are attached to the papillary muscles of the myocardium by chordae tendineae. The primary function of the AV valves is to prevent backflow of blood into the atria during ventricular contraction or systole, while the semilunar valves prevent backflow of blood from the aorta and pulmonary artery into the ventricles during diastole. Opening and closing of each valve depend on pressure gradient changes within the heart created during each cardiac cycle.

Patients with cardiopulmonary disease commonly present with nonspecific signs and symptoms of dyspnea and fatigue. The etiology of these vague signs and symptoms can potentiate from various sources, one of which is valvular dysfunction. Therefore, auscultation of the four heart valves is a useful first step in determining valvular dysfunction that leads to atypical symptomology of shortness of breath and fatigue. The auscultation of valves is discussed later in the chapter within the examination process.

Cardiac Output and Cardiac Index

The goal of the heart is to provide adequate cardiac output (CO) to generate aerobic energy to meet the metabolic demands of the body. Because the energy demands of the body are constantly changing, the heart's CO must also be able to dynamically adapt to the changing energy demands of the body as well as its own myocardial oxygen needs. CO is defined as the amount of blood leaving the LV of the heart per minute (expressed in L/min). Normal CO at rest is approximately 4 to 6 L/min. It is influenced by heart rate (HR) (expressed as beats per minute [bpm]) and *stroke volume* (SV), which is the volume of blood ejected out of the heart per contraction (expressed in milliliters of blood [mL]). Physiologically, CO at any given point of time is the product of HR and SV.

Clinically, especially in critical care settings, the concept of cardiac index (CI) is often preferred to CO. CI expresses the CO in relationship to the body surface area (BSA) expressed in meters such that CI = CO/BSA.[11] The normal CO range at rest is 4 to 6 L/min; the normal CI range is 2.5 to 3.5 L/min/m².[11] CI provides a more complete determination of the adequacy of an individual's CO than CO alone. For example, in comparing a 6-ft-tall individual and a 5-ft-tall individual, each with a CO of 3 L/min, the 5-ft-tall person will have a higher CI and therefore better tissue perfusion because there is less BSA to be perfused by the 3 L of CO.

SV is the volume of blood ejected with each myocardial contraction and is influenced by three factors: (1) *preload,* the amount of blood filled in the ventricle at the end of diastole (also known as *left ventricular-end diastolic volume [LVEDV]*); (2) *contractility,* the ability of the ventricle to contract; and (3) *afterload,* the force the LV must generate during systole to overcome aortic pressure and open the aortic valve.[11] Afterload may also be described as the load against which the LV contracts during left ventricular ejection.

Throughout the cardiac cycle, diastole and systole place different demands on the ventricles. During diastole, the ventricles must be compliant, able to stretch to accommodate the blood entering the ventricles (preload). During systole, the ventricles must be able to contract adequately to eject the SV. The principle of Starling's length–tension relationship is applicable to the myocardium and the relationship between the properties of diastole and systole.[12] During diastole, as muscle length increases (e.g., the ventricular chamber size increases), the ability of the myocardium to develop force is increased, up to a point. Beyond a certain length, however, force development is impaired owing to the inadequate alignment of the actin and myosin filaments (Fig. 13.4).

In general, SV will increase with an increase in preload or contractility and will decrease with an increase in afterload. Normally about 55% to 75% of the preload is ejected as the SV. The *ejection fraction* (EF) demonstrates this relationship between SV and LVEDV such that EF = SV ÷ LVEDV. This value represents the ratio of the volume of blood ejected by the LV per contraction relative to the volume of blood received by the LV following diastole.[13] Normal EF is approximately 55% to 75%

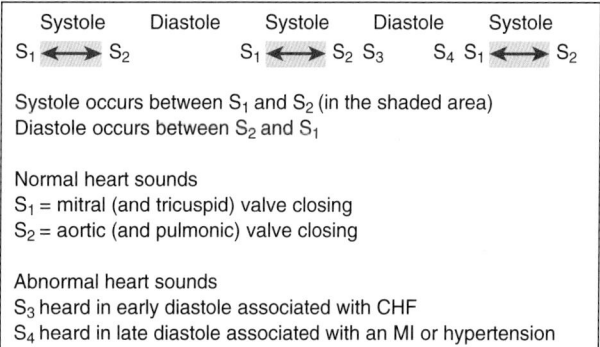

Figure 13.4 Left ventricular (LV) function curves. (A) With normal LV function, as the left ventricular volume increases, stroke volume will also increase. (B) With LV function impairment, the curve will shift to the right, and for any given length, stroke volume is decreased compared with normal (point *b* has a deceased SV compared with point *a*). (C) When normal LV function experiences an increase in sympathetic activity, the curve will shift to the left, and SV will increase (note that point *c* is greater than point *aa*).

(67% ± 8%) and is widely used clinically as an index of contractility.[13]

Cardiac Cycle

The cardiac cycle consists of two interrelated phases: *systole,* the contraction phase, and *diastole,* the filling phase. During diastole, the ventricles fill with blood from the atria via opening of the AV valves. The AV valves lie between the atria and the ventricles and include the tricuspid valve on the right and mitral valve on the left. The first two-thirds of ventricular filling is passive; during the last one-third, the atria contract and push the blood into the ventricles. This contraction is known as the *atrial kick.*[14] After the atrial kick, diastole ends, and the AV valves close. Systole begins with both the AV and semilunar valves closed. An initial *isovolumetric contraction,* like an isometric contraction of striated muscle, increases the pressure within the ventricles, and the semilunar valve opens. The LV then undergoes a concentric contraction, causing a volume to be ejected, called the SV. After the SV is ejected, the aortic valve closes, and systole is complete. The cardiac cycle is defined by the presence of normal heart sounds, S_1 and S_2. Heart sounds are associated with valvular closings; S_1 is associated with AV valve closure, and S_2 is associated with semilunar valve closure. Systole occurs between S_1 and S_2, and diastole occurs between S_2 and S_1 (Fig. 13.5).

Blood Flow and Hemodynamic Values

Blood enters the heart via the superior and inferior vena cava into the RA. Blood moves forward from the RA

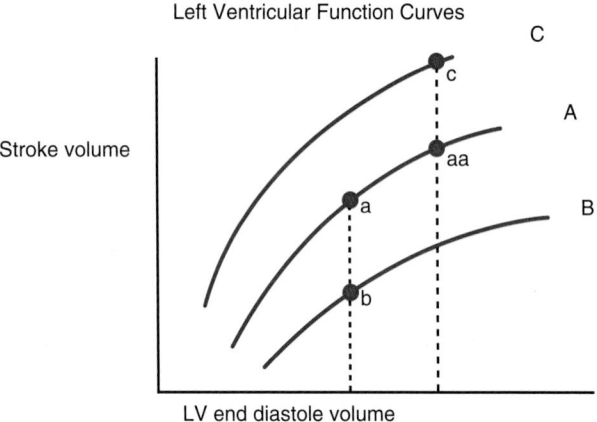

Figure 13.5 Heart sounds of the cardiac cycle.

Table 13.1	Hemodynamic Variables
Right-Sided Heart Catheterization	**Normal Ranges**
Central venous pressure	0–8 mm Hg
Right atrial (mean)	0–8 mm Hg
Pulmonary artery	Systolic 20–25 mm Hg Diastolic 6–12 mm Hg Mean 9–19 mm Hg
Pulmonary capillary wedge pressure	6–12 mm Hg
Left-Sided Heart Catheterization	**Normal Ranges**
Left ventricular end-diastolic pressure	5–12 mm Hg
Left ventricular peak systolic pressure	90–140 mm Hg
Systemic arterial pressure	Systolic 110–120 mm Hg Diastolic 70–80 mm Hg Mean 82–102 mm Hg
Cardiac output	4–5 L/min
Cardiac index (Cardiac output ÷ Body surface area)	2.5–3.5 L/min
Stroke volume	55–100 mL/beat
Systemic vascular resistance	800–1,200 dynes/sec/cm^{-5}

Adapted from Braunwald E, Zipes D, Libby R. *Heart Disease: A Textbook of Cardiovascular Medicine.* 11th ed. Saunders; 2018.

through the tricuspid valve to the RV and through the pulmonic valve to the pulmonary artery (PA) and pulmonary capillaries. The capillaries perfuse the alveoli, and the alveolar–capillary membrane is the site of gas exchange. Newly oxygenated blood within the pulmonary veins (PVs) travels to the LA and passes through the mitral valve into the LV. Blood within the LV travels down to the apex, where it is squeezed in a wringing motion during systole and moved from the apex to the LV outflow tract and finally out through the aortic valve to the aorta.

Blood volume in any chamber or vessel generates a pressure. The normal pressure recordings for the cardiovascular system are presented in Table 13.1. Owing to the relationship between blood volumes and pressures, a direct measure of blood volumes within the heart is accomplished by invasive monitoring of the intravascular or chamber pressures. In *right-sided heart catheterization,* an invasive catheter known as a Swan-Ganz catheter or PA catheter, with pressure-sensitive recording ability, is inserted into the internal jugular or subclavian vein and progressed antegrade through the right side of the heart.[15] Common measurements taken with a right-sided heart catheterization are RA pressure, PA pressure, and *pulmonary capillary wedge pressure (PCWP).* The PCWP is an indirect measure of the *left ventricular end-diastolic pressure (LVEDP),* one of the most sensitive measures of LV function.[15] An advantage of right-sided heart catheterization is the ability to monitor filling pressures not only on the right side but also on the left side, by estimation, without the need for the more difficult and risky LV catheterization.[15] The procedure of left-sided heart catheterization involves placing a catheter into the femoral or radial artery and advancing it retrograde to the flow of blood through the aorta, across the aortic valve, and into the LV where LVEDP can be directly monitored. The LV catheter lies within a high-pressure system (the left side of the heart and the aorta) and therefore can stay in place for only a short period of time (e.g., 1 hr) because of the difficulties associated with cannulation (catheter insertion)

within a high-pressure system. In contrast, the right-sided heart catheter, which lies within a relatively low-pressure system (the right side of the heart), provides continuous monitoring of pressures and can be kept in place for several days.

Electrical Conduction of the Heart

It is important to note that mechanical contraction of the ventricles only occurs with appropriate electrical conduction through the heart. Effective contraction depends on an intact electrical conduction system that results in depolarization of the myocardium and timely repolarization. In *normal sinus rhythm,* the impulse begins in the sinus node and travels through the atria, the AV node, bundle of His, Purkinje fibers, septum, and ventricles.

Electrical conduction can be viewed via the electrocardiogram (ECG) complex (Fig. 13.6). Each component of the complex reflects a certain phase of the conduction pathway:

- The P wave depicts sinus node activation and atrial depolarization.

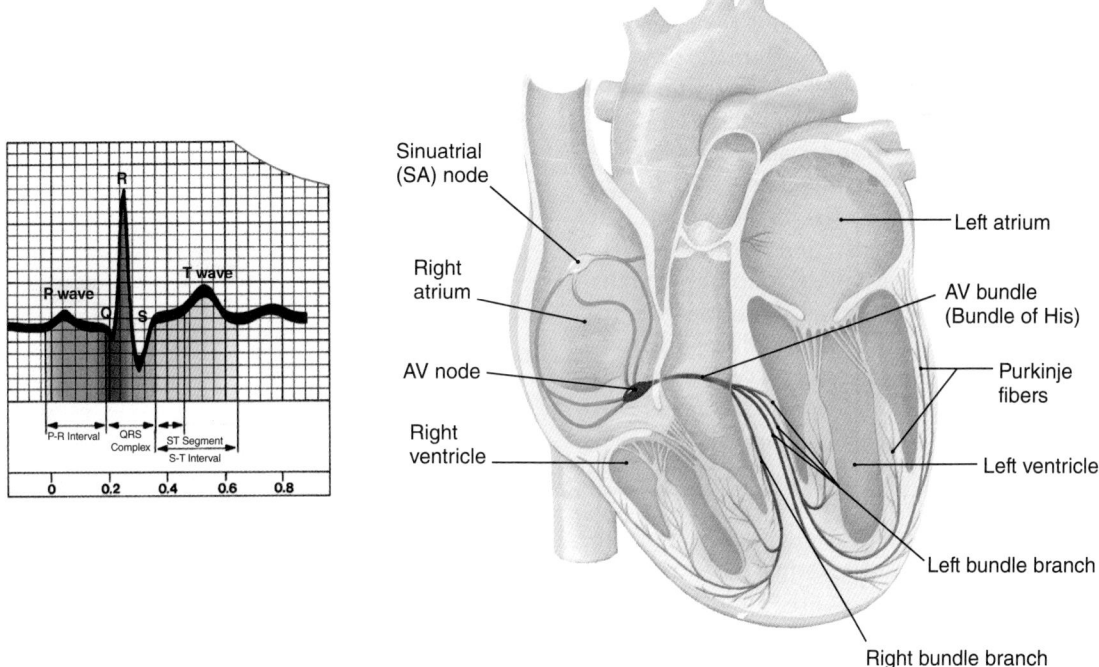

Figure 13.6 The heart and normal cardiac electrical activity. The ECG is the body surface manifestation of the depolarization and repolarization waves of the heart. The P wave is generated by atrial depolarization, the QRS by ventricular muscle depolarization, and the T wave by ventricular repolarization. The PR interval is a measure of conduction time from atrium to ventricle, and the QRS duration indicates the time required for all ventricular cells to be activated. The QT interval reflects the duration of the ventricular action potential. *(Adapted from* Taber's Cyclopedic Medical Dictionary. *21st ed. F.A. Davis; 2005, p. 1022, with permission.)*

- The PR segment demonstrates conduction through the AV node.
- The QRS complex denotes electrical flow through the ventricles causing ventricular depolarization.
- The ST segment describes the initiation of ventricular repolarization.
- The T wave illustrates the completion of ventricular repolarization.

Each ECG complex represents one cardiac cycle or one heartbeat. In a series of ECG complexes representing sinus rhythm, each QRS complex should be preceded by a P wave, and the QRS complexes should be equally spaced apart, indicating a regular rhythm. ECG interpretation enables the clinician to differentially diagnose the cause of reduced CO that may occur from a true mechanical problem versus that occurring from an electrical problem disrupting mechanical activity of the heart.

Neurohormonal Influences on the Cardiovascular System

The autonomic nervous system influences the heart and blood vessels through direct neural and indirect neurohormonal mechanisms. The heart has dual direct innervation from the sympathetic and parasympathetic nervous systems. The sympathetic receptors of the heart are primarily beta-adrenergic receptors and are located on the sinus node and within the myocardium. Stimulation of the receptors by the neurotransmitter norepinephrine (noradrenaline) increases the overall activity of the heart by increasing the HR (*chronotropy*) and force of contraction (*inotropy*), and this results in coronary artery dilation. Sympathetic stimulation of the alpha-adrenergic receptors on peripheral blood vessels causes vasoconstriction and an increase in *peripheral vascular resistance.*

The sympathetic nervous system may also stimulate the adrenal cortex to secrete the catecholamine epinephrine. This blood-borne hormone has sympathetic effects that at times may be even more long lasting and potent than direct sympathetic activation. Epinephrine is released as part of the normal exercise response, especially when exercise is continued beyond a few minutes. The increase in HR and contractility noted with exercise is in part due to this hormonal influence.

The normal parasympathetic influence on the cardiovascular system is via the vagus nerve. Parasympathetic stimulation results in a depression of HR, decreased force of atrial contraction, and decreased speed of conduction through the AV node. Vagal fiber innervation to ventricular myocardium is relatively small; therefore, the effect on LV function is minimal. During exercise, the effects of the sympathetic nervous system and catecholamine release significantly override any effect from the parasympathetic system. The impact of direct parasympathetic influence on peripheral blood vessels is limited to a vasodilatory effect on the bowel, bladder, and genitals.

The catecholamine role in myocardial functioning during exercise is especially crucial for the patient who has lost direct sympathetic activation to the heart. The majority of patients who have undergone a heart transplant remain completely denervated during the first 6 to 12 months following transplantation with some reinnervation found during the second year after transplantation.[16] Sympathetic influence on the denervated heart is therefore solely dependent on catecholamine stimulation of thc beta-adrenergic myocardial receptors to increase HR and contractility.[16] Clinically, the patient with a denervated heart following transplantation will present with elevated resting HRs to achieve normal CO, delayed elevation in HRs with exercise due to circulating catecholamines, decreased maximum HR responses, and slower decreases in HR values during the recovery phase of exercise.[17]

Myocardial Oxygen Supply and Demand

Myocardial oxygen supply and myocardial oxygen demand must be in balance. *Myocardial oxygen supply* depends on the delivery of oxygenated blood through the coronary arteries, the oxygen-carrying capacity of arterial blood, and the ability of the myocardial cells to extract oxygen from the arterial blood. *Myocardial oxygen demand* (MVO_2), the energy cost to the myocardium, is dependent on many factors. Clinically, MVO_2 is calculated as the product of HR and systolic blood pressure (SBP), known as the *rate pressure product (RPP)* or double product. Any activity that increases HR and/or blood pressure (BP) will increase MVO_2. Therefore, any increase in systemic oxygen demand (e.g., exercise) will increase the energy cost of the heart and increase MVO_2.

The myocardium is routinely very efficient at extracting oxygen from its blood supply. Therefore, during times of increased energy demand, very little increase in extraction can occur. The primary mechanism for increasing myocardial oxygen supply during times of increased demand is by increased *coronary blood flow.* In general, there is a linear relationship between coronary blood flow and MVO_2. During exercise, coronary blood flow may increase five timcs above resting level in response to the increased demand. Unlike skeletal muscle, which has the capability of both aerobic and anaerobic metabolism, the heart muscle (myocardium) is essentially dependent on aerobic metabolism and has very limited anaerobic capacity.

Laboratory Values

When managing patients with heart disease, certain laboratory values are particularly important. Table 13.2

Table 13.2	Laboratory Tests and Reference Values	
Test	**Reference Value**
Sodium	135–145 mEq/L
Potassium	3.5–5.0 mEq/L
Chloride	95–105 mEq/L
Calcium	9–11 mg/dL
BUN	10–20
Creatinine	0.5–1.2 mg/dL
Glucose	70–110 mg/dL
Carbon dioxide	20–29 mEq/L
Magnesium	1.5–2.5 mEq/L
Hgb (g/dL)	Adult female: 12–16 Adult male: 13–18
HCT (%)	Adult female: 36–46 Adult male: 37–49

BUN = blood urea nitrogen; HCT = hematocrit; Hgb = hemoglobin.

provides reference values for various laboratory tests. The hemoglobin and hematocrit levels depict the oxygen-carrying capacity within the system. Each gram of hemoglobin carries approximately 1.34 mL of oxygen within arterial blood. A normal hemoglobin level is approximately 12 to 14 g/100 mL of blood in adult males and 14 to 16 g/100 mL of blood in adult women. For example, for a hemoglobin level of 15 g/100 mL of blood, the oxygen-carrying capacity is approximately 20 mL O_2/100 mL of blood ($15 \times 1.34 = 20$). Now, considering a patient with a hemoglobin level reduced to 7.5 g/100 mL of blood, the oxygen-carrying capacity is reduced by half and is approximately 10 mL of O_2/100 mL of blood. With reduced oxygen-carrying capacity, the heart is forced to work harder to compensate for low oxygen levels to provide sufficient oxygen to the peripheral tissue. During HF, increased workload placed on a failing heart will exacerbate the failure. A general rule of thumb is to use caution and lower the intensity when exercising patients with cardiovascular disease and hemoglobin levels less than 8 g/100 mL of blood.

Electrolyte levels are also important to consider before treating patients with heart disease. Appropriate levels of potassium, calcium, and magnesium allow for normal electrical conduction through the heart.[18] *Hypokalemia*, low potassium (usually less than 3.5 mEq/L), produces arrhythmias with flattened T waves, depressed ST segments and U waves, as well as bilateral lower extremity (LE) muscle cramping. An inverted U wave may also be noticed on the ECG. *Hypocalcemia* (low blood serum calcium levels) and *hypomagnesemia* (low magnesium in blood) have the potential of increasing ventricular ectopy within the heart. In addition, calcium enhances contractile function of muscle cells. Patients with hypocalcemia have reduced cardiac contractility, whereas those with hypercalcemia present with erratic heartbeats.

Renal function tests are done to determine kidney function and examine *blood urea nitrogen* (BUN) and *creatinine* levels. These levels are especially important to review in patients with HF and patients prescribed diuretics.[18] Finally, many patients with heart disease also have diabetes; therefore, it is important to review blood glucose levels before exercise.

■ CARDIOVASCULAR RESPONSES TO AEROBIC EXERCISE

Measures of Energy Expenditure

An individual's cardiorespiratory fitness is best defined by measurement of the *maximal oxygen consumption* (VO_2max). Oxygen consumption is measured when performing aerobic activity with increasing intensity using large muscle groups until maximum capacity. The VO_2max reflects the maximum amount of oxygen consumed per minute when the individual has reached maximum effort. Routinely, it is expressed relative to the body weight as milliliters of oxygen consumed, per kilogram body weight, per minute (mL/kg/min). Fick's equation defines two major factors that influence the oxygen uptake. These two factors include the CO and the arterial–venous oxygen difference. Increases in CO during activity reflect appropriate functioning of the central cardiovascular system in increasing exercise capacity. The arterial–venous oxygen difference is the difference between oxygen content of arterial and venous blood and provides the clinician with the oxygen extraction capabilities at the level of the peripheral muscle. The arterial–venous oxygen difference reflects the involvement of the peripheral muscle in increasing exercise capacity.

Energy expenditure at rest and during activity is also important to consider in the management of patients with cardiovascular disease. Energy expenditure is commonly computed from the amount of oxygen consumed at rest or while performing any given activity. Units that best quantify energy expenditure include kilocalorie (kcal), absolute volume of O_2 consumed per unit of time during an activity (mL/min), volume of O_2 consumed during an activity relative to body weight (mL/kg/min), and metabolic equivalents (METs).

A single MET is defined as the amount of oxygen consumed at rest per unit of body weight for 1 minute.[19] The quantity of oxygen consumed in a minute per unit body weight at rest provides a measure of the energy expenditure to run bodily functions while the individual is at rest. Approximately 3.5 mL of oxygen per kilogram body weight is consumed to run bodily functions at rest and is often quantified as 1 MET.[19]

During participation in an activity, the amount of oxygen consumed in a minute per unit body weight reflects the energy expenditure required to participate in that activity. Activity intensity, based on the corresponding MET level, can range from light to vigorous. The MET levels for a variety of activities have been determined in past research investigations and compiled within the Compendium of Physical Activities.[20] This compendium is a useful resource for clinicians in determining the energy expenditure of any given activity. Activities are usually categorized as being light intensity when MET levels are less than 3 METs, moderate intensity if MET levels are between 3 and 6 METs, and vigorous intensity if the activity is over 6 METs.[20] Knowledge of systemic energy requirements is important in prescribing exercise and activity guidelines, as well as in exercise testing for patients with cardiac impairments. Table 13.3 provides estimated MET levels for a variety of occupational and recreational tasks.

Normal Responses

HR and oxygen uptake increase with increasing workload. There is a direct, almost linear relationship between HR and external workload (Fig. 13.7). There is usually a 10-bpm increase in HR per MET level increase in exercise intensity. Therefore, if the physical therapy intervention requires an increase in systemic oxygen consumption, then HR should also increase. It is worth noting that some cardiac medications, particularly the beta blockers, suppress the sympathetic nervous system's effect on the heart and limit the linear increase in HR. Failure of the HR to increase with increasing workloads (chronotropic incompetence) must be evaluated. Other physiological parameters may be useful to examine, including BP, respiratory rate, skin color, and temperature, as well as the patient's level of cognition and perceived exertion. An adverse response in any of these parameters is an indication of the patient's inability to hemodynamically respond to the given intensity of work.

BP should be taken before and immediately after exercise with the patient in the same position (i.e., supine, sitting, standing) and from the same arm each time. Ideally, BP should be taken during exercise to determine the actual hemodynamic response to the increased workload. However, depending on the type of exercise modality, this may be technically difficult. In these cases, HR and BP must be taken immediately after exercise. As with HR, a linear increase in systolic pressure is expected with increasing levels of work (see Fig. 13.7).

Arm ergometry and leg ergometry are common modes of exercise used in clinical practice for exercise testing and prescription. A recent study investigated the relationship of the HR with SBP, diastolic blood pressure (DBP), and workload (WL) during arm ergometry and leg ergometry exercise.[21] The findings of this study

Table 13.3   Metabolic Equivalent Chart

Intensity (70-kg person)	Endurance Promoting	Occupational	Recreational
1.5–2 METs 4–7 mL/kg/min 2–2.5 kcal/min	Too low in energy level	Desk work, driving auto, electric calculating machine operation, light housework, polishing furniture, washing clothes	Standing, strolling (1 mph), flying, motorcycling, playing cards, sewing, knitting
2–3 METs 7–11 mL/kg/min 2.5–4 kcal/min	Too low in energy level unless capacity is very low	Auto repair, radio and television repair, janitorial work, bartending, riding lawn mower, light woodworking	Level walking (2 mph), level bicycling (5 mph), billiards, bowling, skeet shooting, shuffleboard, powerboat driving, golfing with power cart, canoeing, horseback riding at a walk
3–4 METs 11–14 mL/kg/min 4–5 kcal/min	Yes, if continuous and if target heart rate is reached	Brick laying, plastering, wheelbarrow (100-lb load), machine assembly, welding (moderate load), cleaning windows, mopping floors, vacuuming, pushing light power mower	Walking (3 mph), bicycling (6 mph), horseshoe pitching, volleyball (six-person, noncompetitive), golfing (pulling bag cart), archery, sailing (handling small boat), fly fishing (standing in waders), horseback riding (trotting), badminton (social doubles)
4–5 METs 14–18 mL/kg/min	Recreational activities promote endurance; occupational activities must be continuous, lasting longer than 2 min	Painting, masonry, paper hanging, light carpentry, scrubbing floors, raking leaves, hoeing	Walking (3.5 mph), bicycling (8 mph), table tennis, golfing (carrying clubs), dancing (foxtrot), badminton (singles), tennis (doubles), many calisthenics, ballet
5–6 METs 18–21 mL/kg/min	Yes	Digging garden, shoveling light earth	Walking (4 mph), bicycling (10 mph), canoeing (4 mph), horseback riding (posting to trotting), stream fishing (walking in light current in waders), ice or roller skating (9 mph)
6–7 METs 21–25 mL/kg/min 7–8 kcal/min	Yes	Shoveling 10 times/min (4.5 kg or 10 lb), splitting wood, snow shoveling, hand lawn mowing	Walking (5 mph), bicycling (11 mph), competitive badminton, tennis (singles), folk and square dancing, light downhill skiing, ski touring (2.5 mph), water skiing, swimming (20 yards/min)
7–8 METs 25–28 mL/kg/min 8–10 kcal/min	Yes	Digging ditches, carrying 36 kg or 80 lb, sawing hardwood	Jogging (5 mph), bicycling (12 mph), horseback riding (gallop), vigorous downhill skiing, basketball, mountain climbing, ice hockey, canoeing (5 mph), touch football, paddleball
8–9 METs 28–32 mL/kg/min 10–11 kcal/min	Yes	Shoveling 10 times/min (5.5 kg or 14 lb)	Running (5.5 mph), bicycling (13 mph), ski touring (4 mph), squash (social), handball (social), fencing, basketball (vigorous), swimming (30 yards/min), rope skipping
10+ METs 32+ mL/kg/min 11+ kcal/min	Yes	Shoveling 10 times/min (7.5 kg or 16 lb)	Running (6 mph = 10 METs, 7 mph = 11.5 METs, 8 mph = 13.5 METs, 9 mph = 15 METs, 10 mph = 17 METs), ski touring (5+ mph), handball (competitive), squash (competitive), swimming (greater than 40 yards/min)

From Fox SM, et al. Physical activity and cardiovascular health: 3. The exercise prescription: Frequency and type of activity. *Mod Con Cardiovasc Dis.* 1972;41:26, with permission.

MET = metabolic equivalent; mph = miles per hour.

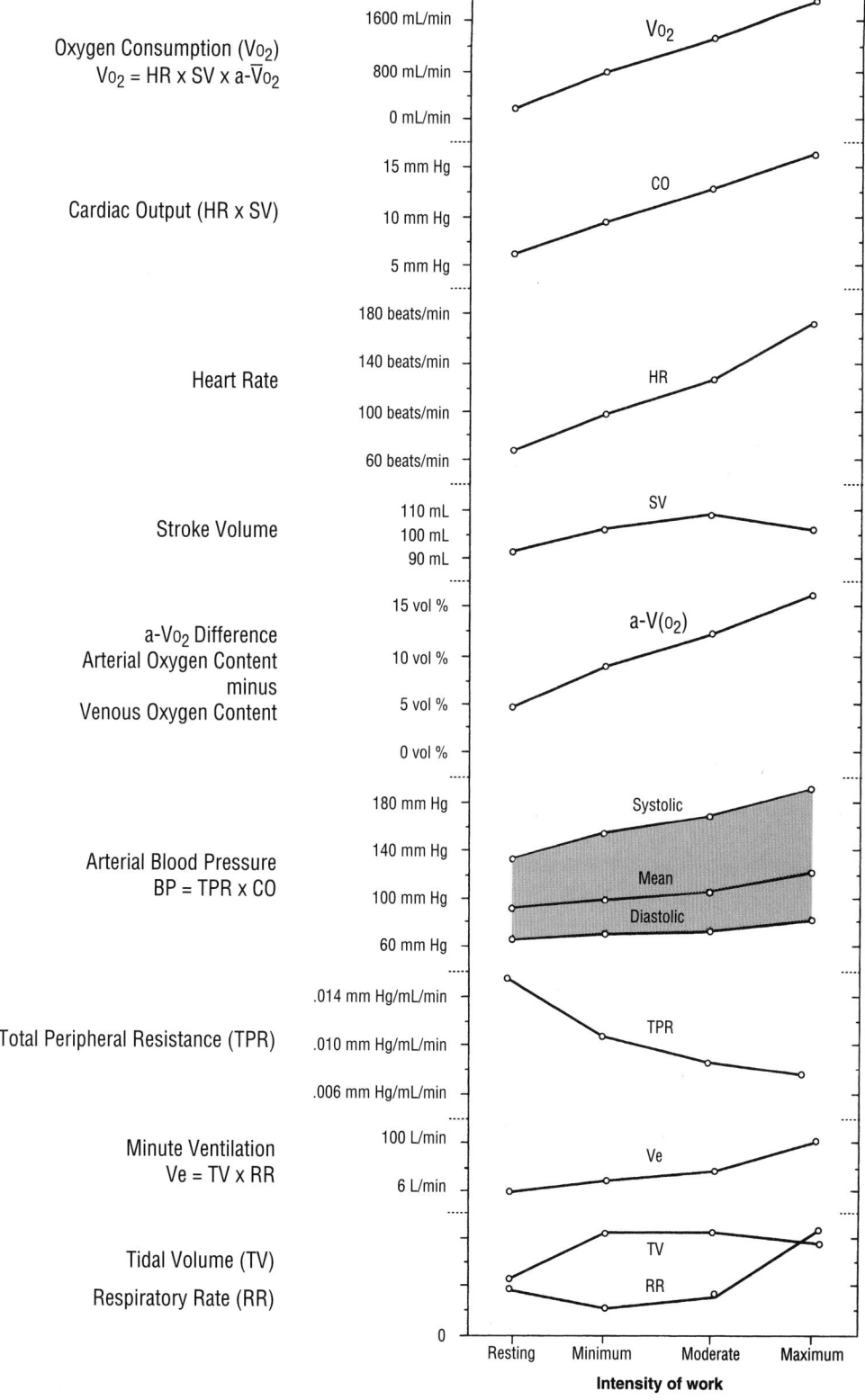

Figure 13.7 Cardiopulmonary response to acute aerobic exercise. *(Adapted from Berne RM, Levy MN. Cardiovascular Physiology. 5th ed. CV Mosby; 1986, p. 237; Zadai CC. Clinics in Physical Therapy, Pulmonary Management in Physical Therapy. Churchill Livingstone; 1992, p. 27; and McArdle WD, et al. Essentials of Exercise Physiology. Lea & Febiger; 1994, p. 230.)*

revealed a larger increase in SBP, WL, and WL relative to body mass during leg exercise compared to arm exercise at any given absolute HR.[21] The findings from this investigation inform physical therapists that higher SBP, lower DBP, and higher WL are achieved at any given submaximal HR during leg ergometry compared with arm ergometry.

Abnormal Responses

Signs and symptoms of exercise intolerance are presented in Box 13.1. If a patient experiences any of these symptoms, the activity should be stopped and the patient stabilized. It is also important to inform patients that some responses may be delayed for as long as several hours after exercise (e.g., prolonged fatigue, insomnia, sudden weight gain due to fluid retention). Observation of the patient throughout the physical therapy intervention provides a mechanism for ongoing examination. The therapist must be alert to subtle changes in the patient's facial expression, skin color, tone of voice, or cognitive status because these may indicate activity intolerance and may require immediate patient examination and modification of the intervention. In addition to the patient's subjective complaint of fatigue or discomfort, there are other responses that warrant termination of an exercise session. These abnormal responses are included in Box 13.1.

Box 13.1   Indications of Exercise Intolerance That Warrant Modification or Termination of an Exercise Session

Signs and Symptoms

- Moderately severe or increasing angina
- Marked dyspnea
- Dizziness, light-headedness, or ataxia
- Cyanosis or pallor
- Excessive fatigue
- Leg cramps or claudication

Other Abnormal Responses

- Failure of the systolic pressure to rise as exercise continues
- A hypertensive blood pressure response, including a systolic pressure of greater than 200 mm Hg and/or a diastolic pressure greater than 110 mm Hg
- A progressive fall in systolic pressure of 10–15 mm Hg
- A significant change in cardiac rhythm detected either by palpation or by ECG monitoring (e.g., arrhythmias, ST-T wave changes).

Adapted from the American College of Sports Medicine's *Guidelines for Exercise Testing and Prescription*. 11th ed. Lippincott Williams & Wilkins; 2021.

■ CARDIAC PATHOLOGIES AND PHYSICAL THERAPY IMPLICATIONS

The pathophysiological conditions that underlie heart disease include HTN, atherosclerosis within the coronary arteries, altered myocardial muscle mechanics, valvular dysfunction, and arrhythmias. The clinical presentations of CVD are diverse and depend on the source of the alterations in structure and function within the cardiovascular system including altered perfusion of coronary arteries, reduced contractility of the LV, or alterations in electrical activity. Common signs and symptoms associated with heart disease are chest pain, dyspnea, fatigue, syncope, and palpitations. However, although these clinical manifestations are strongly associated with heart disease, they are not exclusive for heart disease. Therefore, taking a thorough patient history and performing an appropriate examination and evaluation are crucial to establishing the physical therapy movement diagnosis, goals, outcomes, and plan of care (POC).

Another important consideration is that the extent of an individual's activity limitations cannot solely be based on the cardiac diagnosis and pathology. Individuals with similar cardiac pathologies may experience different degrees of activity limitations. Activity limitations are influenced by multiple factors beyond cardiac dysfunction. These factors include the degree of peripheral muscle strength, the extent of compensatory mechanism activated within the body that allow cardiac functioning to continue for a length of time before the patient becomes symptomatic, and the pharmacological management provided to the patient. The following section delineates the major pathologies affecting heart function, medical management of these conditions, and pertinent implications for physical therapist practice.

Hypertension

Hypertension (HTN) is currently the most prevalent cardiovascular disease in the United States. It has also routinely been referred to as one of the most powerful contributors to cardiovascular morbidity and mortality. Traditionally, HTN has been defined as BP values greater than 140/90 mm Hg. In 2017, the ACC and the AHA published revised guidelines that aimed to incorporate new information from studies regarding BP-related risk of cardiovascular disease (CVD), research on ambulatory BP monitoring, home BP monitoring, and appropriate threshold values to initiate antihypertensive drug treatment.[3] These new guidelines reference BP as normal, elevated, or stages 1 or 2. Normal BP is defined as less than 120/less than 80 mm Hg; elevated BP as 120 to 129/less than 80 mm Hg; hypertension stage 1 as 130 to 139 or 80 to 89 mm Hg, and hypertension stage 2 as greater than 140 or greater than 90 mm Hg.[3] The primary reason for the lowering of BP parameters within the 2017 guidelines is due to the results of the landmark SPRINT trial published in the *New England Journal of Medicine* in 2015.[22] The results of this large multicenter randomized controlled trial revealed a 25% significant reduction in all-cause mortality and a 27% significant reduction in cardiovascular events at 3-year follow-up in individuals who received more aggressive pharmacological management to maintain SBP under 120 mm Hg compared to controls who received less aggressive BP control and maintained a SBP between 135 and 139 mm Hg. This study validates that lowering SBP has beneficial effects in reducing death and cardiovascular events. It is also important to ensure that the average BP to deem an individual hypertensive be based on greater than two readings obtained on more than two occasions of measurement. The guidelines additionally state that it is appropriate for clinicians to advocate for out-of-office and self-monitoring of BP measurements to confirm the diagnosis of hypertension. In some patients, BP is not consistently elevated and fluctuates between hypertensive and normal values. This is called *labile HTN* and is diagnosed following the evaluation of elevated BP values over a more prolonged length of time.

Hypertensive individuals may have elevations in both systolic and diastolic values; however, in older adults, isolated systolic hypertension (ISH) is commonly noted with elevations in SBP above 140 mm Hg with diastolic BPs under 90 mm Hg.[23] ISH can be caused by underlying conditions such as artery stiffness, an overactive thyroid gland, diabetes, valvular dysfunction, or obesity. ISH warrants pharmacological management and healthy lifestyle changes to reduce the likelihood of stroke, heart disease, and chronic kidney disease.

It is also worth noting that although somewhat controversial, home readings correlate more closely with the results of daytime ambulatory measurements of BP than with BP taken in the clinician's office. This is especially true in individuals with *white coat hypertension* defined as BP that is consistently elevated at medical practitioner office readings but does not meet diagnostic criteria for hypertension based on out-of-office home readings. The 2017 guidelines recommended that clinicians screen for white coat syndrome in adults with an untreated SBP greater than 130 but less than 160 mm Hg or DBP greater than 80 but less than 100 mm Hg, using either ambulatory or home monitoring devices.[3]

Broadly, HTN may be divided into two major categories: *primary (or essential)* HTN and *secondary (or nonessential)* HTN. *Primary or essential HTN* is diagnosed when there is no known cause for the elevation in BP values and exists in approximately 90% to 95% of all patients with HTN. Genetic factors, environmental influences (including dietary sodium intake), stress, obesity, excessive alcohol consumption, and other risk factors (including age, lack of exercise, and glucose intolerance) have implications on the occurrence of essential

HTN.[24] Regardless of the underlying cause, the pathophysiology of essential hypertension depends on the primary or secondary inability of the kidney to excrete sodium at a normal blood pressure with overall reductions in control mechanisms responsible for lowering BP.[24] *Secondary or nonessential HTN* occurs in approximately 5% to 10% of the hypertensive population and is caused by an identifiable medical problem such as primary renal disease, illicit drug use, renovascular disease, obstructive sleep apnea, Cushing syndrome, endocrine disorders, coarctation of the aorta, and more.[25]

Uncontrolled elevated BP levels produce a variety of additional complications, including HF, renal failure, dissecting aneurysms, PVD, retinopathy, and stroke. These negative consequences are directly related to the level of BP. Because of this, the 2015 U.S. Preventive Services Task Force (USPSTF) guidelines indicate that all individuals 18 years or older should be screened for elevated BP.[26] The USPSTF guidelines indicate once-a-year screening for hypertension in adults 40 years or older and for adults at increased risk for hypertension. These include African Americans, persons with high-normal BP, or persons who are overweight or obese with body mass index (BMI) greater than 27. Less frequent screening (i.e., every 3 to 5 years) is appropriate for adults aged 18 to 39 years and not at increased risk for hypertension and with a prior normal BP reading.

Management of Hypertension and Physical Therapy Implications

Treatment for individuals with hypertension involves a combination of nonpharmacological therapies involving lifestyle changes coupled with antihypertensive drug therapy. Physical therapists can play an integral role in assisting patients with necessary lifestyle changes including weight loss, adopting the *Dietary Approaches to Stop Hypertension* (DASH) eating plan, reducing sodium intake, increasing physical activity, and moderating alcohol consumption.[3] The benefits of these lifestyle changes include lowering the dosage of medications and reducing the occurrence of adverse side effects.

Empirical evidence has documented reductions in systolic BP values with each of the lifestyle changes mentioned earlier. Maintenance of a normal body weight evaluated by a BMI between 18.5 and 24.9 is important for all individuals. Further, it is important to recommend patients follow the recommendations of the DASH diet, eating fruits, vegetables, low-fat dairy products, and a reduced content of saturated fat and total fat. In addition, it is important to note that the AHA recommends no more than 2,300 milligrams (mg) of sodium per day and an ideal limit of no more than 1,500 mg per day for most adults, especially for those with high blood pressure.[3] Adopting a dietary plan based on DASH guidelines has been shown to decrease SBP by about 6 to 11 mm Hg. Finally, alcohol consumption must be limited to no more than two drinks per day in most men and no more than one drink per day in women and lighter-weight individuals.[3]

Research documented in a review of meta-analyses reveals that aerobic exercise training reduces BP by 5 to 7 mm Hg, while dynamic resistance training lowers BP by 2 to 3 mm Hg.[27] In general, studies have demonstrated a reduction in blood pressure when prescribed at a frequency of three to four sessions per week of moderate intensity with a duration of approximately 40 minutes for a period of 12 weeks. The physiological factors responsible for the potential drop in BP values with aerobic exercise are incompletely understood. Most research theorizes the antihypertensive effects of exercise to be related to a reduction in sympathetic activity and an overall improvement in endothelial function.

Dance therapy may also be utilized as an alternate modality of physical activity in managing patients with hypertension. A 2016 systematic review and meta-analysis investigated the effects of dance therapy in patients with hypertension. The review included four studies that met the inclusion criteria. Dance therapy resulted in a significant reduction in SBP (WMD −12.01 mm Hg; 95% CI: −16.08, −7.94 mm Hg; $P < .0001$) when compared with control subjects. Significant reductions in DBP were also found (WMD −3.38 mm Hg; 95% CI: −4.81, −1.94 mm Hg; $P < .0001$), compared with control group.[28] Additionally, the authors documented significant improvements in overall exercise capacity and quality of life with the use of dance therapy.

Pharmacological intervention is the most common form of medical management for patients with HTN. Six classes of medications currently exist: beta-adrenergic blockers, angiotensin-converting enzyme (ACE) inhibitors, angiotensin II receptor blockers, diuretics, vasodilators, and calcium channel blockers. Table 13.4 provides details on common categories of cardiovascular medications and relevant physical therapy implications. It is ideally recommended that patients be evaluated routinely every month after initial antihypertensive therapy is initiated and reevaluated every 3 to 6 months thereafter to ensure the achievement of adequate BP control. In addition to pharmacology, it is important for clinicians to educate patients and clients diagnosed with HTN on lifestyle modifications, including weight reduction, sodium restriction, moderation of alcohol intake, and regular aerobic exercise.

A growing body of new research provides compelling evidence on the association between BP control and cognitive decline. Research from the SPRINT-Mind Trial published in 2019 indicates that more aggressive BP control to achieve a SBP level of less than 120 mm Hg reduced the incidence of mild cognitive impairment by 19% in ambulatory people older than 50 years during a median follow-up of 5.1 years.[29] An additional study shows evidence for changes in biomarkers within the brain evaluated on imaging. The study showed that aggressive BP control under 120 mm Hg was significantly associated with a smaller increase in cerebral white matter lesion volume.[30] These studies collectively provide valuable insight on the importance of BP control to reduce cognitive decline. It is useful for physical therapists to advocate that patients and clients seek routine assessment and control of BP to not only achieve optimal cardiovascular outcomes but also reduce the likelihood for cognitive decline.

Acute Coronary Syndrome

Acute coronary syndrome (ACS) is the new terminology for ischemic heart disease or CAD. It involves a spectrum of entities ranging from the least involved condition on the spectrum (unstable angina) to the worst involved condition (sudden cardiac death). Additional entities on the spectrum include non–Q-wave myocardial infarction (NQMI), non–ST-segment elevation myocardial infarction (NSTEMI), and Q-wave myocardial infarction (QMI), also referred to as ST-segment elevation myocardial infarction (STEMI). The hallmark sign for any patient presenting with any condition on the spectrum is ischemic chest pain because of a dyssynchrony between the myocardial oxygen supply and demand. A discussion of physical therapy interventions for managing patients with ACS is delineated later in this chapter.

Pathophysiology of Acute Coronary Syndrome

The primary pathophysiological event in ACS is an imbalance of myocardial oxygen supply to meet the myocardial oxygen demand (MVO_2). The decrease in supply results from a narrowing of the lumen of the coronary artery, usually due to a fixed atherosclerotic lesion. Atherosclerosis is a disease in which lipid-laden plaque (lesions) is formed within the intimal layer of the blood vessel wall of moderate- and large-size arteries; over time the plaque may extend into the lumen causing a decreased luminal diameter. The lesion results from an initial endothelial dysfunction that causes changes within the intima of the blood vessel and progresses to luminal narrowing.[31] Several risk factors have been identified that are associated with an increased risk for the formation of an atherosclerotic lesion. Table 13.5 provides a summary of known risk factors, their pathophysiological association with endothelial dysfunction, and relevant physical therapist implications for assessment of each risk factor.

Clinical Manifestations

Occlusions may occur in coronary arteries and not produce symptoms. In general, symptoms of CAD are not experienced until the lumen is at least 70% occluded. There are, therefore, many patients who are unaware of their subacute occlusions. It is important that an individual's risk factors are known and that interventions

Table 13.4   Cardiovascular Medications and Physical Therapy Implications

Medication Class	Generic and Trade Name	Primary Effect of Medication	Side Effects	Physical Therapy Implication
Antiarrhythmics	• Pacerone (Amiodorone) • Diltiazem (Cardizem) • Flecainide • Quinidine	Rate and rhythm control	• Fatigue • Nausea • Alterations in liver, kidney, pulmonary, and thyroid function.	• Monitor for hepatic impairment. • Assess vital signs. • Watch for fatigue, malaise. • Monitor alterations in metabolism that may indicate thyroid dysfunction.
Anticoagulants	• Xarelto (Rivaroxaban) • Fragmin (Dalteparin) • Heparin (various) • Eliquis (Apixaban) • Coumadin (Warfarin) • Pradaxa (Dabigatran etexilate) • Fondaparinux (Arixtra)	Slows down the body's process of making clots.	• Bleeding—gums, hematuria, heavy menses, nose-bleeds, hemoptysis. • Warfarin (Coumadin) is unsafe during pregnancy.	• Monitor INR for patients on Warfarin. Generally, INR of 2–3 is therapeutic. Values greater than 5 indicate bleeding risk and values less than 1 indicate subtherapeutic levels. • Diet: Avoid supplements with vitamin K. • Routinely check INR when the patient is on antibiotic therapy.
Antiplatelet Agents	• Aspirin • Plavix (Clopidogrel) • Brilinta (Ticagrelor)	Inhibits platelet aggregation	• Bleeding, hemorrhage, pruritis	• Assess balance and fall risk. • Monitor signs and symptoms of gastrointestinal bleed, bruising, hematuria. • Monitor elevations in BP which may increase the possibility for hemorrhage.
ACE Inhibitors	• Benazepril (Lotensin) • Captopril (Capoten) • Enalapril (Vasotec) • Fosinopril (Monopril) • Lisinopril (Zestril) • Moexipril (Univasc) • Perindopril (Aceon) • Quinapril (Accupril) • Ramipril (Altace) • Trandolapril (Mavik)	• Decrease the production of angiotensin II which helps decrease vascular vasoconstriction. • Decrease sodium retention in kidney.	• Dry cough • Dizziness • Hypotension • Fatigue • Risk of angioedema	• Watch for signs of angioedema—rashes, raised patches of skin, burning itching skin, facial swelling. • Monitor blood pressure closely.

(Continued)

Table 13.4	Cardiovascular Medications and Physical Therapy Implications—cont'd			
Medication Class	**Generic and Trade Name**	**Primary Effect of Medication**	**Side Effects**	**Physical Therapy Implication**
ARBs	• Azilsartan (Edarbi) • Candesartan (Atacand) • Eprosartan • Irbesartan (Avapro) • Losartan (Cozaar) • Olmesartan (Benicar) • Telmisartan (Micardis) • Valsartan (Diovan)	Reduces vascular resistance.	• Hypotension (dizziness, light-headedness, fainting) • Angioedema • Hyperkalemia	• Watch for signs of angioedema—rashes, raised patches of skin, burning and itching skin, facial swelling. • Monitor blood pressure closely
ARNI	Sacubitril and valsartan (Entresto)	• Valsartan blocks the action of angiotensin II causing vasodilation. • Sacubitril blocks the breakdown of natriuretic peptides causing diuresis.	• Hypotension • Angioedema • Hyperkalemia	• Assess renal function. • Ensure patients are not talking ARB with ARNI as the risk of angioedema increases. • Watch for signs of angioedema. • Monitor BP closely.
Beta-Andrenergic Blocking Agents	• Acebutolol (Sectral) • Atenolol (Tenormin) • Betaxolol (Kerlone) • Bisoprolol (Zebeta, Ziac) • Carteolol (Cartrol) • Carvedilol (Coreg) • Labetalol (Normodyne, Trandate) • Metoprolol (Lopressor, Toprol-XL) • Nadolol (Corgard)	Decreases sympathetic activity thereby reducing heart rate, blood pressure, myocardial oxygen demand, and controlling tachydysrhythmias.	• Orthostatic hypotension • Bradycardia • Blunted heart rate response with activity	• Monitor vital signs. • Use rate or perceived exertion in conjunction with heart rate to determine exercise intensity. • Assess orthostatic hypotension. • Monitor for signs and symptoms of reduced cardiac output (fatigue, dizziness, weakness).
Calcium Channel Blockers	• Amlodipine (Norvasc, Lotrel) • Bepridil (Vascor) • Diltiazem (Cardizem, Tiazac) • Felodipine (Plendil) • Nifedipine (Adalat, Procardia) • Nimodipine (Nimotop) • Nisoldipine (Sultar) • Verapamil (Calan, Isoptin, Verelan)	Blocks the inward movement of calcium into the heart and vascular smooth muscle cells, thereby reducing blood pressure, myocardial oxygen demand, controlling tachydysrhythmias.	• Reduced cardiac output and bradycardia. • Constipation • Peripheral edema • Light-headedness • Headaches	• Monitor vital signs. • Use rate or perceived exertion in conjunction with heart rate to determine exercise intensity. • Assess orthostatic hypotension. • Monitor for signs and symptoms of reduced cardiac output—fatigue, dizziness, weakness.

Table 13.4   Cardiovascular Medications and Physical Therapy Implications—cont'd

Medication Class	Generic and Trade Name	Primary Effect of Medication	Side Effects	Physical Therapy Implication
Diuretics	• Amiloride (Midamor) • Bumetanide (Bumex) • Chlorothiazide (Diuril) • Chlorthalidone (Hygroton) • Furosemide (Lasix) • Hydrochlorothiazide (Esidrix, Hydrodiuril) • Spironolactone (Aldactone)	Decrease vascular volume and congestion.	• Dehydration • Dizziness • Electrolyte imbalances • Headache • Upset stomach	• Monitor vital signs • Assess orthostatic hypotension. • Check electrolyte levels. • Assess skin turgor.
Inotropes/Pressors	• Adrenalin (Epinephrine) • Digoxin • Dobutamine • Primacore (Milirone) • Levophed (Norepinephrine) • Neo-Synepthrine (Phenylephrine)	• Increase myocardial contractility. • Increases vasoconstrictive activity on the vasculature.	• Hypertension • Tachycardia/bradycardia • Headache • Palpitations • Dyspnea	• Monitor for extravasation necrosis for patients on Levophed. • Close monitoring of vital signs with mean arterial pressure greater than 60 mm Hg.
Mineralocorticoid Receptor Antagonists	• Aldactone (Spironolactone)	Decreases fluid volume and thereby reduces blood pressure.	• Potassium-sparing diuretic causes hyperkalemia. • Anorexia, nausea, vomiting, diarrhea, abdominal cramps.	• Monitor for dehydration (skin turgor). • Check for electrolyte imbalance. • Assess vital signs.
Statins (Cholesterol-Lowering Medications)	• Atorvastatin (Lipitor) • Lovastatin (Mevacor) • Simvastatin (Zocor) • Rosuvastatin (Crestor)	Inhibits the action of HMG CoA reductase, thereby reducing the synthesis of cholesterol.	• Headache • Dizziness • Insomnia • Weakness • Muscle pain and damage • Liver damage	• Assess for signs of rhabdomyolysis including muscle pain, tenderness, weakness. • Monitor liver function test enzymes.
Vasodilators/Nitrates	• Gonitro (Nitroglycerin) • Sublingual Notrostat • Extended-release capsules Nitrogard • Nitroglycerin transdermal	Increases coronary blood flow by dilating coronary arteries and improving collateral flow to ischemic myocardial regions.	• Dizziness • Headache • Hypotension • Tachycardia • Syncope	• Avoid interventions that cause systemic vasodilation (hot shower). • Assess for orthostatic hypotension. • Closely monitor blood pressure and symptoms of decreased cardiac output. • Ensure patient carries nitroglycerin for all therapy appointments.

ACE = angiotensin-converting enzyme; ARB = angiotensin receptor blocker; ARNI = angiotensin receptor neprysilin inhibitor; BP = blood pressure; INR = International Normalized Ratio.

Table 13.5   Risk Factors for Endothelial Dysfunction and Atherosclerosis

Risk Factor	Pathophysiology	Physical Therapy Clinical Assessment
Diabetes and metabolic syndrome	Causes overexpression of growth factors and/or cytokines, and oxidative stress.	Assess blood glucose levels and glycated hemoglobin levels.
Hypercholesterolemia	Increases oxidative lipoproteins in blood.	Assess blood cholesterol and triglyceride levels.
Hypertension	Angiotensin II promotes endothelial damage.	Assess resting and exercise blood pressure values.
Environmental toxins	Nicotine, tobacco, and other air pollutants increase oxidative stress.	Assess smoking/vaping history.
Infectious agents	Bacterial and/or viral toxins promote endothelial damage.	Assess white blood cell count and presence of infection.
Age	Aging promotes cell senescence.	Assess age of patient/client.
Sex hormonal imbalance	Estrogen deficiency promotes endothelial dysfunction.	Regard postmenopausal women at increased risk.

and monitoring are adjusted according to the individual needs of the patient.

The clinical conditions resulting from atherosclerosis of the coronary arteries are due to inadequate myocardial oxygen supply to meet the myocardial oxygen demand (MVO_2). Myocardial oxygen demand reflects the amount of oxygen that the heart needs to maintain the metabolic demands of the body. The myocardial oxygen supply reflects the amount of oxygen provided to the heart by the blood which is controlled by the coronary arteries. This imbalance between myocardial oxygen supply and demand is reflected in three common clinical presentations of ACS including angina, injury, and infarction and is discussed in the following section.

Angina

Angina, or cardiac-related chest pain, is due to ischemia. Ischemia is characterized by reduced blood flow to the myocardium. Ischemia is a temporary condition due to the imbalance between the myocardial oxygen supply and demand. On restoring the balance between oxygen supply and demand, ischemia will be reversed, and the angina will disappear.

There are three major types of angina: unstable, stable, and variant angina. *Unstable angina* is sometimes referred to as preinfarction angina or crescendo angina. In patients with unstable angina, chest pain typically occurs at rest without any obvious precipitating factors or with minimal exertion.[32] In addition, chest pain increases in severity, frequency, and duration and is therefore called crescendo angina. Chest pain in the unstable state is refractory to treatment. Unstable angina usually warrants immediate medical intervention, because the patient is at impending risk for further complications such as an MI or a lethal arrhythmia such as ventricular tachycardia or ventricular fibrillation.

The term *stable angina* is used when angina occurs during exercise or activity. Chest pain is experienced at a certain intensity of exercise when the myocardial oxygen demand exceeds the blood supply to the myocardium and is alleviated by decreasing the MVO_2.[33] As mentioned earlier, the MVO_2 is calculated as the product of HR and SBP, known as the RPP. When patients experience episodes of stable angina, exercise must be terminated, and HR and BP need to be taken to determine the RPP (RPP = HR × SBP). Research demonstrated the substantial prognostic power in utilizing the RPP over both age-predicted maximum HR and percentage of HR reserve in predicting cardiovascular events in individuals with a negative stress test for myocardial ischemia.[34] In patients with stable angina, termination of exercise and nitroglycerin can reduce the MVO_2. It is noteworthy that patients experiencing stable angina often describe the sensation as an intensity less than 5 out of 10, which improves to 0 out of 10 when the oxygen supply is able to balance the demand. It is important to remember that any report of angina requires intervention; the clinician cannot ignore the symptoms even when the patient describes the sensation as light (1 to 2 out of 10). Finally, some patients may experience dyspnea as their anginal equivalent; that is, they do not have the typical chest discomfort often associated with ischemia but instead experience shortness of breath (SOB).[35] For these patients, treatment should be immediate and follow the guidelines for ischemia.

The third type of angina is *variant* or *Prinzmetal angina* and is caused by a vasospasm of coronary arteries in the absence of occlusive disease. Coronary arteries can spasm as a result of exposure to cold temperatures, stress, medications that vasoconstrict blood vessels, smoking, or cocaine use. Patients with this type of angina respond to nitroglycerin for short-term management of their chest pain. Additionally, patients must be educated on removing precipitating factors that trigger vasospasm of the coronary arteries.

Injury and Infarction

Injury represents the presence of a new acute MI. The term *injury* is used because the myocardial tissue is being acutely injured during a sudden heart attack. Acute injury to the myocardial tissue then progresses to irreversible, dead infarcted tissue. Thus, the term *injury* illustrates the presence of a new MI, whereas the term *infarction* depicts an old heart attack with irreversibly dead tissue.

Individual myocardial cells may differ in their tolerance for ischemia; however, irreversible changes start to appear minutes to hours from the onset of myocardial ischemia. The actual process of injury and infarction evolves over a period of hours. Angina commonly precedes a MI, but the intensity of the symptoms is dramatically increased when the patient is moving into having a heart attack. Patients frequently describe their discomfort as 10 out of 10 on a pain scale during an acute MI. While ischemia is due to a partial blockage of the coronary artery, an infarction results from complete occlusion of the vessel. This complete occlusion commonly results from a rupture of a vulnerable plaque with resultant formation of a thrombus. The type of plaque, more so than the size, will influence the risk of rupture. Lipid-rich and soft plaques are more vulnerable to rupture than collagen-rich and hard plaques. Angiographically, large plaque lesions are not necessarily more susceptible to rupture than smaller lesions. Because atherosclerosis begins within the walls of the artery, many vulnerable plaques are invisible via angiogram or appear smaller than their actual size.

The effects on the ventricle because of the infarction often extend beyond the acute infarction period. These long-term effects occur primarily in ventricles that have sustained a moderate to large MI. As the ventricle heals, a process of *remodeling* occurs because of the presence of the infarcted tissue and subsequent dilation. Over time, this reengineering process produces an alteration in ventricular size, shape, and function. Thus, the resultant ventricle often operates at an increased myocardial energy cost due to its inefficient muscle mechanics. Often pictured as three concentric circles (although not absolutely histologically correct), the area of infarction would be at the center of the circle surrounded first by an area of injury and then an outside area of ischemia (Fig. 13.8).

Although most MIs heal initially without incident, complications may occur. The major complications following a MI are recurrence of ischemia, LV failure, and ventricular arrhythmias. Therefore, when a patient is said to have had a *complicated MI,* it is indicative that ischemia, LV failure, or significant ventricular arrhythmias have developed in the acute post-MI period.

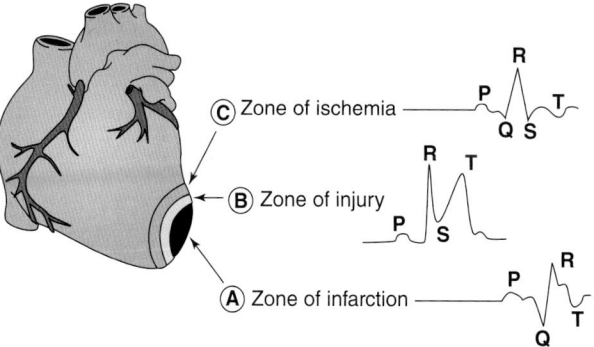

Figure 13.8 ECG following a myocardial infarction. (A) *Zone of infarction:* when infarction occurs through the full thickness of the myocardium (transmural), an abnormal Q wave usually appears. (B) *Zone of injury:* ST elevation occurs in the area of injury. (C) *Zone of ischemia:* ST depression and/or T-wave inversion occurs in an area of decreased perfusion (ischemia).

Ischemia after MI is particularly important because it indicates that there may be vulnerable myocardium with a reduced oxygen supply that may go on to infarct and thereby potentially enlarge the MI.

The ultimate complication following an acute MI is cardiogenic shock characterized by inadequate CO and insufficient arterial BP to perfuse the major organs because of severe LV failure.[36] This condition necessitates extraordinary medical interventions such as the *intra-aortic balloon pump (IABP).*[36] The IABP facilitates CO, decreases MVO_2, and increases coronary artery perfusion. The IABP is a balloon catheter placed within the aorta that inflates during diastole, thereby increasing coronary artery perfusion, and deflates during systole, thereby decreasing afterload. The IABP may be used in other conditions besides post-MI cardiogenic instability. Some examples include patients with hemodynamic decompensation awaiting heart transplantation, those with unstable angina, those with malignant arrhythmias such as ventricular tachycardia or ventricular fibrillation, and patients with severe hemodynamic instability post-cardiac surgery.

Evaluation of Patients With Acute Coronary Syndrome (the Evaluation Triad)

In addition to history taking and review of systems, the evaluation of patients with ACS places emphasis on three major components: evaluating patient subjective reports, ECG changes, and cardiac enzyme levels (Fig. 13.9). These three components are sometimes referred to as the evaluation triad. Two of the three components of the triad must be positive to rule a patient as having a MI. Patients with chest pain accompanied by ECG changes are said to have a STEMI or QMI. Patients without ECG changes who report chest pain and have elevated cardiac enzymes are said to have an

NSTEMI, also known as NQMI. Finally, patients who do not present with any chest pain but have positive findings on the ECG and elevated cardiac enzymes are said to have a silent MI. The following narrative discusses each component in more depth.

Reported Symptoms in Acute Coronary Syndrome

Most patients with myocardial ischemia will present with classic chest pain referred to as *angina pectoris*. Classic angina pectoris is diffuse, retrosternal, and described as a pressure, heaviness, tightness, or constriction in the center or left of the chest. Pain is usually precipitated by exertion and relieved by rest.[37] It is important for therapists to evaluate factors that provoke chest pain. These may include activities that increase myocardial oxygen demand, including physical activity, emotional stress, or sexual intercourse.

The patient may report an intense pressure like "an elephant sitting on the chest." Further, angina may present as a referred pain due to involvement of a neural reflex pathway via the thoracic and cervical nerves. This results in chest pain not being felt in a specific spot but usually as a diffuse discomfort that may be difficult to localize. It may radiate to anywhere in the upper extremities (UEs) and thorax, most specifically to the left arm and left jaw.[37] Figure 13.10 delineates common areas for referred patterns of chest pain.

The hallmark approach to differentially diagnosing ischemic chest pain from nonischemic chest pain is to observe for accompanying signs and symptoms of compromised CO.[37] These signs and symptoms include dizziness, light-headedness, weakness, diaphoresis (sweating), and fatigue. Thus, cardiac chest pain during ischemia or an infarction will be accompanied by signs of compromised CO, but chest pain from other etiologies, including pulmonary chest pain, pleural pain, gastrointestinal-related chest pain, or musculoskeletal pain of the thorax, will not precipitate the classic signs and symptoms of compromised CO.[37]

Electrocardiographic Changes in Acute Coronary Syndrome

MIs are identified by 12-lead ECG findings.[38] The ECG (also referred to as EKG) is used to examine HR, rhythm, conduction delays, and coronary perfusion. Two of the most common types of ECG are the single-lead and the 12-lead ECG. In the single-lead ECG, only one area of the heart (e.g., anterior, lateral, or inferior) may be viewed at a time. This area may be changed, however, by altering the location of the electrodes. In the 12-lead ECG, 12 areas are viewed.

The single-lead ECG is sensitive to rate and rhythm changes and is commonly used for monitoring patients during ambulation and activity. Continuous monitoring is accomplished either via telemetry (radio transmission), allowing the patient freedom to move around when wearing this portable device, or by hardwire, where the patient is attached to the monitor by a cable approximately 15 ft long, therefore limiting mobility. A variation of the single-lead ECG is the three-lead ECG and is used for monitoring in an inpatient setting. It can be worn continuously throughout an entire treatment session or throughout the entire hospitalization. Unlike the single-lead or three-lead system, the 12-lead ECG

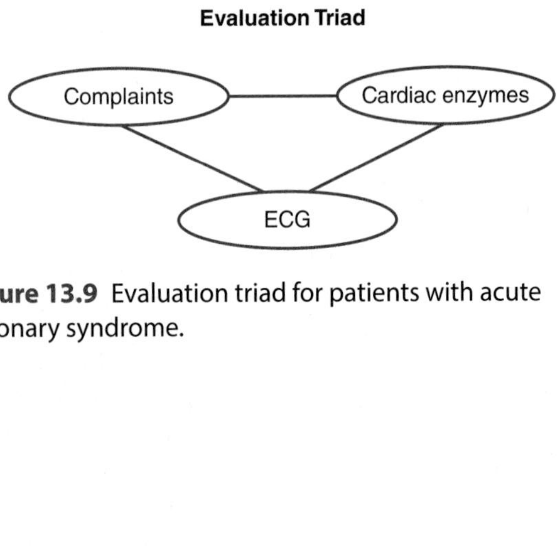

Evaluation Triad

Figure 13.9 Evaluation triad for patients with acute coronary syndrome.

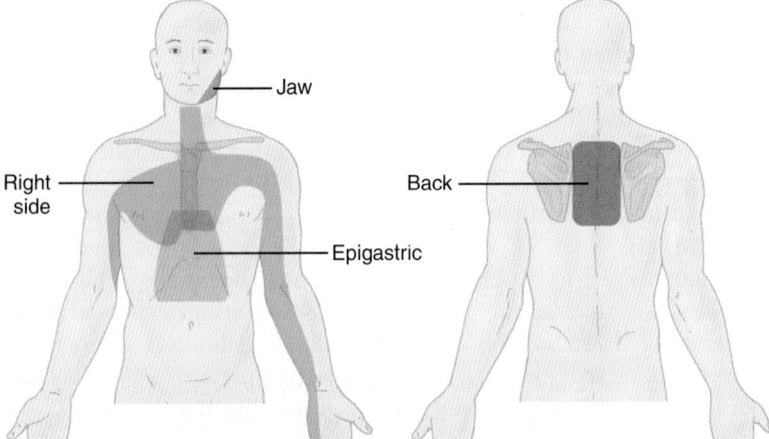

Usual Distribution of Pain with Myocardial Ischemis

Figure 13.10 Referral pattern for chest pain.

does not provide continuous monitoring, except during an exercise tolerance test (ETT) completed on a treadmill or stationary bicycle ergometer. Two common uses for the 12-lead ECG are the resting ECG taken with the patient quietly supine and during exercise during an ETT. Twelve-lead ECGs are invaluable in identifying perfusion impairments in the coronary arteries and in assisting with arrhythmia detection. During the ETT, the ECG is continuously monitored to determine the presence of ischemia or arrhythmias with each increase in workload. The 12-lead ECG is sensitive to changes in perfusion as well as rate, rhythm, and conduction. Each coronary artery is represented by a cluster of leads that, although not absolutely correlated with each individual's anatomy, gives a general schema for myocardial perfusion.

During the examination of a 12-lead ECG, the ST segment is clinically useful in identifying the presence of impaired coronary perfusion, either ischemia or injury.[38] The *J point,* the point where the S wave turns into the ST segment, is the point of reference for interpreting the ST segment.[38] If ischemia is present, the ST segment will be depressed two small boxes or more beyond the J point, and/or the T wave may also be inverted (flipped). Ischemic changes are present only while the ischemia is present; when the ischemia has resolved, the ECG will return to normal.[38] Conversely, a large acute MI, with subsequent injury to the myocardial tissue, will produce ST-segment elevations on the 12-lead

ECG (see Fig. 13.11). Elevation of the ST segment signifies acute injury to the myocardium termed a STEMI. In light of acute injury to heart muscle, the patient is not stable and needs immediate medical intervention. Large STEMI will subsequently produce pathological Q waves hours to days following the acute process.[38] Therefore, a QMI represents a large MI that occurred hours to days earlier. A QMI was formerly known as a *transmural MI* because they usually involved the full thickness of the ventricular wall. Conversely, an acute MI may be relatively smaller and not cause acute injury to the myocardial tissue. In this case, ST segments are not seen on the ECG, and the MI is called an NSTEMI or an NQMI. An NQMI formerly known as a *nontransmural* or *subendocardial MI* does not involve the entire thickness of the myocardial wall but rather affects tissue primarily below the endocardium.

Anatomical classifications for MIs are based on the surfaces of the LV and not the anatomical heart. An anterior MI involves the anterior surface of the LV, an inferior MI involves the inferior surface of the LV (the diaphragmatic region), a lateral MI involves the lateral surface of the LV, a septal MI involves the septum, and a posterior MI involves the LV posterior wall.[39] MIs to different aspects of the ventricle result from compromised levels of blood flow within specific vessels. The RCA supplies blood to the inferior and posterior aspects of the LV and therefore is responsible for producing an inferior- or posterior-wall MI. The anterior and septal

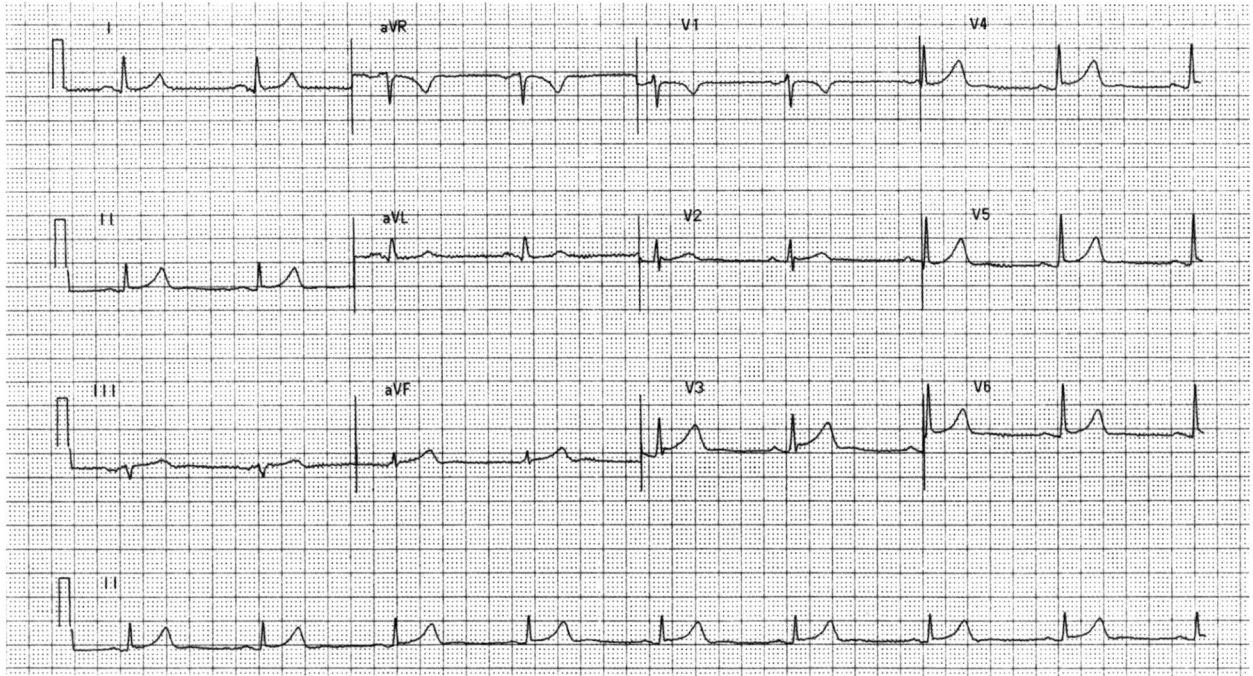

Figure 13.11 Normal 12-lead ECG from 50-year-old woman; slight ST elevation is insignificant. Twelve leads are presented; at the bottom of the page is a rhythm strip from lead II. Heart rate from the rhythm strip is approximately 52 (there are 5.8 large boxes between complex 3 and 4; therefore 300/5.8 = 52).

aspects of the LV are perfused by the LAD; therefore, LAD occlusions are likely to produce anterior or septal MIs. The CX artery supplies blood to the lateral wall of the LV and thereby produces a lateral infarction when it is occluded. The involvement of occlusion within specific vessels can be determined by a 12-lead ECG.[39] RCA involvement is most likely depicted on leads II, III, and aVF (augmented voltage to a unipolar limb lead). LAD pathology will be illustrated in chest leads V1, V2, V3, and V4, whereas CX pathology will most likely be demonstrated in leads I, aVL, V5, and V6 (see Fig. 13.12).

Cardiac Enzymes in Acute Coronary Syndrome

Blood work also helps determine the presence of an MI. The most frequently used markers include cardiac troponins I and T as well as the MB isoenzyme of creatine kinase (CK-MB).[34] Creatine kinase MB subunit (CK-MB), an isoenzyme, is released into blood and elevates with intracellular myocardial damage.[40] Creatine kinase (CK) is found in many tissues besides the myocardium, especially striated muscle, brain, and liver. Injury to these areas will elevate total CK. To differentiate the type of tissue injured, use of CK-MB will isolate the source to the myocardium. Troponin levels should not be elevated in the setting of striated muscle trauma. Other markers that may be used to diagnose an acute MI are the proteins troponin I, troponin T, and myoglobin. Total CK-MB, troponin I, and troponin T have a high sensitivity for the diagnosis of an MI.[40] Today, many hospitals have replaced conventional troponin assays with the new fifth-generation high-sensitivity troponin I and T tests that can detect troponin at concentrations 10- to 100-fold lower than conventional assays. In essence, high-sensitivity troponins facilitate

I Lateral Circ	aVR	V1 Septal LAD	V4 Anterior LAD
II Inferior RCA	aVL Lateral Circ	V2 Septal LAD	V5 Lateral Circ
III Inferior RCA	aVF Inferior RCA	V3 Anterior LAD	V6 Lateral Circ

Figure 13.12 Anatomical pathology and ECG interpretation. Leads I, aVL, V5, and V6 depict problems in the lateral aspect of the left ventricle due to occlusion of blood flow within the circumflex artery. Leads II, III, and aVF depict problems in the inferior aspect of the left ventricle due to occlusion of blood flow within the RCA. Leads V1 to V4 depict problems in the anterior aspect of the left ventricle due to occlusion of blood flow within the LAD artery.

earlier exclusion of an acute MI.[40] It is prudent for physical therapists to assess each of these biomarkers documented in the medical record to determine if the patient is ruling in for an acute MI.

Medical Management of Acute Coronary Syndrome

Once the diagnosis of a MI has been reached (i.e., the patient is "ruled in" for an MI), the subsequent goal of medical management is to keep the patient hemodynamically stable and optimize the healing of the injured myocardium. Two major categories of medical interventions including revascularization procedures and pharmacological interventions are addressed in the following sections.

Percutaneous Transluminal Coronary Angioplasty

Percutaneous transluminal coronary angioplasty (PTCA) uses a balloon and collapsed stent (stainless steel "cage-like" tube with multiple slots) on the tip of a catheter, inserted into the radial or femoral artery and advanced retrograde along the aorta to the openings of the coronary arteries. The catheter is inserted into the coronary artery until the site of the lesion is reached. The balloon is then inflated, and the stent expands, compressing the plaque against the interior artery walls, thereby increasing the luminal area. The balloon is deflated and removed, and the stent holds the lumen open. The stent is commonly coated with a drug (e.g., paclitaxel [Abraxane]).[41] Drug-coated stents (collectively referred to as *drug-eluting stents*) are used to prevent endothelial cell proliferation that may occur in response to endothelial trauma and the presence of a foreign object placed within the coronary artery and result in restenosis (recurrence of stenosis).[41]

The surgical and catheterization reports identify which vessels were revascularized and which vessels have less than 70% lesions and were therefore not revascularized. Because a vessel is not currently a candidate for revascularization does not guarantee that it will not be problematic later, either by rupturing or continuing to demonstrate progressive atherosclerosis. It would be shortsighted to assume that a patient who has had a revascularization procedure cannot become ischemic.

Coronary Artery Bypass Graft

A *coronary artery bypass graft (CABG)* uses a donor vessel to bypass the lesion (narrowed lumen) and establish an alternate improved blood supply. The donor vessel may be the radial artery of the nondominant UE, the saphenous vein, or the internal mammary artery. The patient's harvested saphenous vein or radial artery must be completely detached from both its proximal and distal insertions; the graph is sutured proximally into the aorta and distally into the involved artery beyond the occlusion. When the internal mammary artery is used, it maintains its native proximal attachment while the distal segment is reattached below (bypass) the area of occlusion. Bypass surgery techniques are constantly evolving; traditionally, the full sternum was cut and retracted, but newer minimally invasive techniques called *minimally invasive direct coronary artery bypass* have emerged that involve less sternal cutting, and some techniques involve no sternal cutting at all but access the heart via the intercostal space.[42]

Most CABG procedures involve placing the patient on an artificial heart–lung machine (bypass pump), which maintains the oxygenation and circulation of the blood while the heart is stopped during the surgical procedure. Because of the bypass pump, patients may have additional fluid weight gain following surgery and may feel fatigued, and some patients may have transient atrial fibrillation and cognitive changes. Newer techniques have facilitated the use of *off-pump procedures* to limit the time on the bypass pump. During this procedure, the surgeon operates on a beating heart for the entire or part of the procedure to limit time on the heart–lung machine and reduce the negative sequelae that result from excessive pump time.[43] The evidence concludes that the off-pump CABG procedure is a less invasive method for coronary revascularization with definite patient benefits including less manipulation of the aorta, avoidance of complications associated with cardiopulmonary bypass, fewer blood transfusions, shorter hospital length of stay, shorter duration on intubation, reduced pulmonary complications, and reduced cost, all of which may prove superior to conventional CABG in appropriately selected patients.[43]

Physical Therapy Clinical Implications

For patients who have had bypass surgery (e.g., CABG), recovery is somewhat slower than for patients who have been revascularized through a PTCA procedure. This is because of the complexity of the surgical procedure and the incisional healing. Further, prolonged time in the crucifix position during surgery may predispose individuals to developing an ulnar nerve palsy after surgery.[44] Examination of sensation and manual muscle testing are indicated to rule out the potential for brachial plexus injuries.

The number and location of incisions depend on the surgeon's technique (i.e., either a full sternal cut, partial sternal cut, or intercostal approach). The donor graft site may require additional incisions: a leg incision if the saphenous vein is used, a nondominant arm incision if the radial artery is used, or no additional incision if grafted with the internal mammary artery. Physical therapy intervention should address any soft tissue impairments associated with the incision to maintain appropriate tissue extensibility and range of motion (ROM), with awareness that patients often indicate soreness and/or discomfort around the donor site. Further, radial pulses cannot be obtained on the extremity where a radial graft artery was grafted for the bypass procedure.

If a sternal wound is present, appropriate posture, scapula retraction, and functional shoulder movements should be encouraged. Proprioceptive neuromuscular facilitation (PNF) UE diagonal patterns often work well, as do the traditional cardinal plane ROM exercises. Patients should be reminded that only a few repetitions at a time throughout the day are better tolerated than more intensive repetitions completed once a day, with the latter regimen potentially resulting in incisional soreness.

Sternal precautions are commonly applied to reduce dehiscence of the incision. Cited risk factors for dehiscence include diabetes, pendulous breasts, obesity, and COPD.[45] Interestingly, there is no direct evidence that links the use of arm movements or activity to an increased risk of sternal complications after surgery. Interestingly, robust evidence supports early implementation of upper body activity and exercise in patients recovering from median sternotomy while minimizing risk of complications.[46] Sternal precautions vary greatly by physician, institution, and type of surgery performed. It is important to develop a professional collegial relationship with the surgical team to discuss surgical techniques and mobility concerns to ensure the best outcome for the patient. Cahalin, LaPier, and Shaw developed an algorithm delineating sternal precaution guidelines for patients with high, moderate, or low risk for sternal complications.[45] They presented guidelines based on the risk of the patient. General considerations in sternal precaution guidelines include the following:

- Lifting, pushing, pulling objects greater than 10 lb
- Performing shoulder and/or flex greater than 90° when UE is weighted
- Encouraging shoulder active ROM in pain-free range
- Avoiding scapular retraction past neutral
- Avoiding trunk flex and rotation with supine to sit transfers
- Minimizing or avoiding UE use with sit to stand
- Applying sternal counterpressure (splinting) with cough
- Limiting driving

Adams and colleagues proposed an approach that applies standard kinesiologic principles in the management of patients with a sternotomy.[47] The paper presents pictures and guidelines on teaching patients how to perform load-bearing movements in a way that avoids excessive stress to the sternum by keeping movement constrained within an imaginary tube around the thorax. To avoid sternal discomfort, all patients will benefit from splinting the incision with a hand or pillow when laughing, coughing, or sneezing.[45]

Early ambulation and mobility beginning the first day after surgery will assist in the patient's physical and emotional recovery. Even though the heart function is perhaps the best it has been in quite some time, the effects of major surgery on energy level and mobility must be emphasized. The impact of fatigue on the patient's sense of well-being may be profound, and it is important that patients understand the need for rest as well as ambulation. Patients will benefit from information regarding energy conservation and rest periods.

Pharmacological Management

Cardiovascular pharmacological agents are critical in the medical management of patients with CAD. There are a variety of drugs designed to reestablish the balance of myocardial supply and demand, with new drugs being added all the time. The major anti-ischemic categories are beta blockers, calcium channel blockers, and nitrates. *Beta blockers* decrease beta-sympathetic activity on the heart, resulting in a decrease in HR and contractility and therefore reduced energy demand. *Calcium channel blockers* reduce BP and therefore decrease the work of the heart. Calcium channel blockers are also somewhat unique in preventing coronary smooth muscle spasm and thereby may increase myocardial blood supply. *Nitrates,* one of the oldest categories of drugs, are potent vasodilators that decrease preload and afterload and therefore decrease myocardial work and dilate coronary arteries. *Afterload reducers,* particularly those that affect the renin–angiotensin–aldosterone system, such as *ACE inhibitors* and *angiotensin receptor blockers (ARBs),* are frequently used to normalize BP and reduce workload on the heart. Table 13.4 provides details on common categories of cardiovascular medications and relevant physical therapy implications.

Heart Failure

HF is a high-prevalence syndrome characterized by impaired cardiac pump function, resulting in inadequate systemic perfusion and an inability to meet the body's metabolic demands.[48] Being a syndrome, patients in HF present with an array of signs and symptoms. This section presents the epidemiology, causes and types of HF, pathophysiological and clinical presentation of HF, medical management, and evaluation for this patient population. A discussion of physical therapy interventions for managing patients with HF is delineated later in this chapter.

Epidemiology of Heart Failure

With the marked improvement in anti-ischemic medications, increased knowledge and management of CAD risk factors, availability of sophisticated monitoring, and revascularization techniques, more patients are living longer with coronary disease than similar patients 20 or 30 years ago. New technology and medications continually improve the understanding and management of CAD; however, an undesired effect of long-term CAD may be the increased prevalence of HF, also known as congestive heart failure (CHF). Technology and other advances in medicine are reducing mortality with a concomitant increase in morbidity. Therefore, patients with HF are less likely to die and more likely to live longer with the worldwide prevalence and incidence of HF approaching epidemic proportions.

Recent statistics show that the prevalence of HF continues to markedly increase with approximately 6 million individuals over age 20 years diagnosed with HF.[49] The overall prevalence of HF is projected to steadily increase by 46% from 2012 to 2030, affecting more than 8 million adults in the United States.[49] HF has surpassed MI as the leading cause of cardiac deaths in the United States and is the most frequent cardiac diagnosis for hospital admissions and readmissions.

Causes of Heart Failure

The most common cause of HF is cardiac muscle dysfunction. *Cardiac muscle dysfunction* is a general term describing altered systolic and/or diastolic activity of the myocardium that usually develops because of an underlying abnormality within the cardiac structure or function. HF may be caused by diseases of the myocardium, pericardium, endocardium, heart valves, or coronary vessels, or by metabolic disorders.[48] Several reasons exist for the development of cardiac muscle dysfunction. Box 13.2 presents potential precursors and risk factors for the development of cardiac muscle dysfunction.

Types of Heart Failure

HF is categorized from a structural and functional perspective. From a structural perspective, HF is described as *left-sided heart failure* or *right-sided heart failure.* Left-sided HF occurs with LV insult. Pathology of the LV reduces the CO, leading to a backup of fluid into the LA and lungs. The increased fluid in the lungs produces the two hallmark pulmonary signs of left-sided HF: SOB and cough.[50] Primary right-sided HF occurs from direct insult to the RV caused by conditions that increase PA pressure. Increased pressure within the PA subsequently increases the afterload, thereby placing greater demands on the RV and causing it to go into failure.[50] With RV failure, blood is not effectively ejected from the RV and backs up into the RA and venous vasculature, producing two hallmark peripheral signs: jugular venous distention and peripheral edema. Often, left-sided HF may be severe as seen in patients experiencing a HF exacerbation. With severe LV pathology, fluid from the LV backs up into the lungs, increasing PA pressure and causing fluid to back up into the right side of the heart and the systemic venous vasculature. This is called *biventricular failure.* Therefore, patients with biventricular failure will present with both pulmonary and systemic signs of HF. Table 13.6 provides hemodynamic pressures noted with left, right, and biventricular failure.

From a functional perspective, HF is described as systolic or diastolic dysfunction.[51] *Systolic dysfunction,*

Box 13.2   Causes of Cardiac Muscle Dysfunction

Precursors	Description
Hypertension	Increased peripheral arterial pressure contributes to increased afterload and pathological hypertrophy of the left ventricle
Coronary artery disease	Acute injury to myocardial tissue damages ventricular contractility causing systolic dysfunction. Scar formation seen in infracted tissue alters relaxation and may lead to diastolic dysfunction.
Cardiac dysrhythmias	Normal electrical conduction through the heart allows for normal mechanical contraction of the ventricles. Altered electrical conduction alters the mechanical activity of the ventricles exacerbating heart failure.
Valve abnormalities	Cardiac valve pathology (stenosis or regurgitation) causes structural changes to the chamber behind the valve resulting in cardiac muscle dysfunction and failure.
Pericardial pathology	Pericarditis (fluid in the pericardial space) with resultant cardiac tamponade compresses the ventricles leading to cardiac muscle dysfunction and heart failure.
Cardiomyopathies	Damage to the myocardial cells from various pathological processes alters the systolic and/or diastolic function of the ventricles.

Table 13.6   Example of Hemodynamic Pressures Associated With Heart Failure

An increase in PAP and/or PCWP is associated with LV failure; an increase in CVP is associated with RV failure; and increases in CVP, PAP, and PCWP are associated with biventricular failure.

Pressure (Norms)	LV Failure	RV Failure	Biventricular Failure
CVP (0–8 mm Hg)	6 mm Hg	12 mm Hg	12 mm Hg
PAP (9–19) mm Hg	22 mm Hg	16 mm Hg	22 mm Hg
PCWP (6–12) mm Hg	18 mm Hg	10 mm Hg	18 mm Hg

CVP = central venous pressure; LV = left ventricle; PAP = pulmonary artery pressure; PCWP = pulmonary capillary wedge pressure; RV = right ventricle.

also known as *heart failure with reduced ejection fraction (HFrEF)* is characterized by compromised contractile function of the ventricles causing reductions in the SV, CO, and EF. Patients with systolic dysfunction will usually present with compromised EFs less than 40%.[51] *Diastolic dysfunction*, also known as *heart failure with preserved ejection fraction*, is characterized by compromised diastolic function of the ventricles. With this condition, the ventricles cannot relax and fill appropriately during the relaxation (diastolic) phase of the cardiac cycle. The impaired ability to fill the ventricles with blood reduces the volume of blood ejected with each contraction (the SV) and the overall volume of blood ejected per minute (the CO). EF is unaltered and remains normal between 50% and 75%.[51] No reduction in the ratio is noted because there is no change in the contractile ability of the ventricles. However, there is a low volume of blood being ejected with each contraction, as less blood entered the ventricle before the contraction phase. The 2022 Heart Failure Guidelines from the ACC, AHA, and the Heart Failure Society of America now present a new category of HF for those individuals with an EF between 41% and 49%.[52] Patients with EFs in this category are termed to have heart failure with mild reduction in ejection fraction (*HFmrEF*). This category is especially meaningful for individuals who demonstrate an improvement in heart function achieved with medical treatments to achieve an EF greater than 40%, thereby indicating an improvement in prognosis transitioning them from a state of HFrEF to HFmrEF.

Pathophysiology of Heart Failure

HF involves a complex series of events involving pathophysiological and compensatory factors in response to cardiac muscle dysfunction.[48] When the myocardium is dysfunctional, compensatory mechanisms are activated with the goal of maintaining adequate CO. Neurohormonal mechanisms including activation of the sympathetic nervous system are triggered to increase HR and maintain CO at rest. Thus, patients experiencing an acute bout of HF are very likely to be unstable and tachycardic at rest. Clinically, to assess stability, it is important to not only assess the absolute resting HR but also evaluate resting HR relative to the patient's baseline resting HR values.[53] In other words, a patient with a resting HR that is usually 60 beats/min and presents on a given day with a resting HR that is 80 beats/min would need further assessment of other signs and symptoms that indicate the possibility of the patient moving into a state of decompensated HF.

When patients are in HF and the ventricle is ejecting low blood volumes, blood begins to accumulate within the ventricles, causing congestion. This congestion increases the LVEDV and contributes to an elevation in LV pressure. The increased pressure is transmitted retrograde toward the LA and the PVs. This increase in hydrostatic pressure in the PVs causes fluid to move from the veins into the interstitial space of the lung, resulting in pulmonary edema.[54]

It is also important to consider kidney function for patients with HF. Low blood volume pumped out of the heart causes less blood to perfuse the kidney and is likely to put the kidney in failure.[54] Patients experiencing an acute HF exacerbation often go into renal failure. It is therefore crucial for therapists to monitor BUN and plasma creatinine levels. An increase in urea production, elevated BUN and creatinine levels, and decreased urine output indicate renal dysfunction.

From a musculoskeletal standpoint, patients with HF often present with skeletal muscle wasting and weakness, myopathies, and osteoporosis. These negative sequelae are associated with inactivity and prolonged bedrest.[50] Several studies have investigated the effects of HF on skeletal muscle abnormalities and found reductions in the size and number of type I and type II muscle fibers. It is therefore imperative that the physical therapy POC place emphasis on interventions to improve overall muscle function and functional mobility in this patient population.

Clinical Manifestations of Heart Failure

The clinical presentation of the patient with CHF depends not only on the amount of LV failure but also on the status of compensatory mechanisms and the impact of drug therapy. Over time, the energy cost of the compensatory mechanisms proves to be too much for the impaired myocardium. The patient then begins to present with signs and symptoms of CHF and now moves from being asymptomatic to symptomatic. Although the terminology may be somewhat confusing, it is important to note that when a patient is referred to as being in *compensated HF*, the patient's congestive symptoms can be relieved by medical intervention. A patient who is *decompensated* is showing signs and symptoms of congestion and requires medical and pharmacological readjustment. Felker and colleagues defined decompensated HF as the presence of new or worsening signs/symptoms of dyspnea, fatigue, or edema that lead to hospitalization or unscheduled medical care (doctor visits or emergency department visits).[55] An expert consensus decision-making pathway published by the AHA provided an understanding of the many signs of decompensation and effective ways to manage these symptoms noted during an acute HF exacerbation.[56]

The hallmark signs of decompensation are related to increased congestion and increased ventricular filling pressures.[57] Common signs and symptoms of CHF include fatigue, dyspnea, edema (pulmonary and peripheral), weight gain, presence of an S_3 heart sound, and renal dysfunction.[55,57] Pulmonary edema may be evident by chest x-ray and auscultation of adventitious sounds. Peripheral edema may be evident in gravity-dependent LEs by the presence of indentations in the skin when pressure is applied, that is, pitting edema. Pitting edema associated with CHF is usually bilateral and may extend from the foot to the pretibial area. Documentation should include a numerical grade based on the duration of indentation after fingertip pressure. See Chapter 14, Vascular, Lymphatic, and Integumentary Disorders, for Palpation/Pitting Scale. Weight gain and peripheral edema are among the signs of systemic volume overload.

On auscultation of the heart and lungs, characteristic sounds are heard with CHF. The usual abnormal heart sound associated with CHF is an S_3 heart sound. This is a low-frequency heart sound heard in early diastole and occurs due to poor ventricular compliance and subsequent turbulence of blood within the ventricle. The S_3 heart sound is correlated with increased LVEDP and PCWP with sensitivity of 30% to 50% and specificity of 80% to 90%.[58] Heart murmurs (extra heart sounds), especially those of mitral regurgitation, may also be present owing to the effect of the enlarged LV pulling on the mitral valve. Lung auscultation for patients with HF reveals the presence of crackles or rales.[54] These are crackling/bubbling sounds suggesting fluid in the lung. The sounds are usually heard during inspiration and represent the movement of fluid in the alveoli and subsequent opening of the alveoli that were previously closed because of the excess fluid. Negi and colleagues in 2014 discovered that pulmonary crackles and an S_3 heart sound were present in more than 50% of all patients admitted to the emergency department for HF decompensation.[59] Further, the authors reported that patients with crackles and S_3 heart sound had higher readmission rates than those without these signs: odds ratio for pulmonary crackles was 2.8; odds ratio for S_3 heart sound was 2.6.[59]

Dyspnea is one of the most common symptoms experienced with left-sided CHF. The SOB is associated with pulmonary edema.[55] When fluid accumulates in the lungs, gas exchange is altered at the alveolar–capillary interface. Gas exchange (respiration) will occur at the alveolar–capillary interface only when ventilation within the alveoli is matched with perfusion within the pulmonary capillary (V/Q matching). Excessive amounts of fluid within the pulmonary parenchyma cause a ventilation/perfusion mismatch, thereby reducing the amount of oxygen delivered to blood and causing dyspnea.[55]

Three other symptoms reported by patients in CHF are paroxysmal nocturnal dyspnea, orthopnea, and bendopnea.[57] Paroxysmal nocturnal dyspnea (PND) is characterized by sudden episodes of SOB occurring in the night. Orthopnea is increased SOB in the recumbent position. The severity of orthopnea is often crudely documented by observing the number of pillows a patient needs to keep the upper body in an upright or semirecumbent position. Therefore, a patient with three- or four-pillow orthopnea suggests a greater severity of HF when compared with a patient with one-pillow orthopnea. Physiologically, as patients assume a recumbent position from an upright position, with their legs elevated to the same horizontal level as their trunk, fluid moves back to the heart causing an increase in preload. A failing heart cannot keep up with the additional preload and excess fluid returning to the heart, therefore causing a backup into the lungs producing increased symptoms of SOB.

Bendopnea, a relatively new sign, was discovered in 2014 by Thibodeau and colleagues. This sign involves the presence of increased SOB when the patient bends forward.[60] In a prospective study of 102 patients with systolic HF, the authors measured the time to onset of bendopnea. The researchers found that bendopnea occurred in 28% of subjects with a median time to onset of 8 sec. Further, patients with bendopnea had higher supine right atrial pressures, PCWP, PND, orthopnea, and dyspnea on exertion compared with patients without bendopnea.[60]

One of the common complaints of patients with CHF is early onset of muscle fatigue.[61] The cause of the muscle fatigue may be multifactorial, including a decrease in peripheral blood flow, changes within the peripheral vascular beds, peripheral vasoconstriction, atrophy of muscle fibers, and increased utilization of anaerobic metabolism for energy production.

Patients with HF will present with decreased exercise tolerance owing to a culmination of the pathophysiological and compensatory events associated with HF.[62] It is difficult for patients to exercise when they have gained weight, have SOB, and have a rapid HR. There are a variety of methods to measure exercise tolerance in patients with HF. In regard to classifying the severity of HF, the AHA/ACC and New York Heart Association (NYHA) have created two complementary classification systems that address structural and functional limitations in HF[48] (see Figure 13.13). From a structural perspective, HF is staged from Stage A to Stage D, based on the extent of structural damage to the myocardium. This classification system represents the irreversible progression of disease severity. Clinicians also utilize the NYHA and Functional Classification Scale (see Fig. 13.13). Classification is based on the development of symptoms and the amount of energy required to provoke them. Patients in class I have mild HF and relatively better exercise tolerance compared with patients in class IV with severe CHF and poor exercise tolerance.

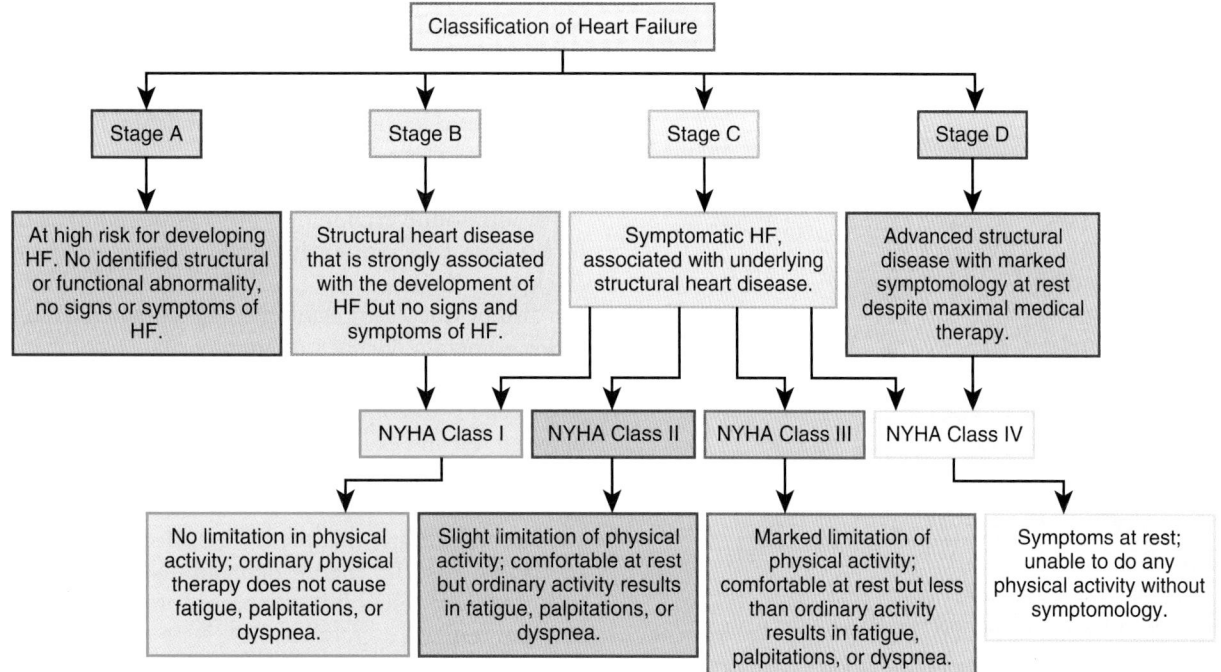

Figure 13.13 Classification of heart failure.

Medical Examination and Evaluation of Heart Failure

Medical interventions include a variety of tests to identify the etiology and evaluate the severity of HF. Following an examination of signs and symptoms of HF in a patient, several key tests are typically performed. These include the chest x-ray, electrocardiogram analysis, laboratory tests, echocardiography, and nuclear imaging studies.

Radiological Findings in Heart Failure

Three hallmark characteristics of the chest x-ray help confirm the diagnosis of CHF (Fig. 13.14):

1. An enlarged cardiac silhouette: The enlargement of the heart in patients with CHF occurs secondary to congestion of fluid in the lungs and possible pathological hypertrophy of the ventricles. This is often termed cardiomegaly.[63]
2. Opacities (white areas) in the lung field with interstitial and parenchymal edema.[63] This occurs when excessive fluid collects in the lung when LV end-diastolic pressures exceed 25 mm Hg.
3. Blunting of the costophrenic angle. The lower ribs meeting the diaphragm creates this sharp image observed on chest x-ray. In patients with CHF, fluid settles to the lower, dependent aspect of the lung, producing an opaque appearance, and blunts the costophrenic angle.

Electrocardiogram Changes

ECG changes in patients with acute decompensated HF may identify underlying predisposing or precipitating conditions for HF. These changes may include LV hypertrophy, left atrial abnormalities, myocardial ischemia or infarction, or the presence of atrial fibrillation.[64]

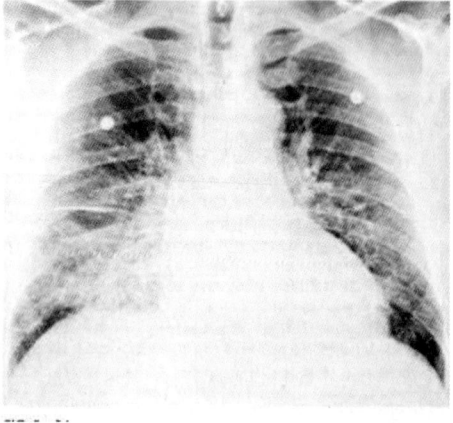

Figure 13.14 Radiographic examination to confirm heart failure.

Laboratory Findings in Heart Failure

Significant laboratory data include blood counts, markers of renal function, cardiac enzymes, and B-type natriuretic peptide (BNP) and N-terminal pro-BNP (NT-proBNP) assays. Analyses of blood counts assist the clinician in identifying the presence of infection or anemia that may have precipitated the event. An assessment of cardiac enzymes is important to consider in an effort to evaluate potential myocardial injury. Finally, *natriuretic peptide assays* supplement clinical judgment when the cause of a patient's dyspnea is uncertain. Natriuretic peptides including BNP and NT-proBNP are released from ventricular myocytes in response to volume overload within the respective chambers.[65] These chemicals are cardiac neurohormones that target the kidney when released, to increase diuresis and decrease the overall volume of fluid within the vasculature and chambers of the heart. Circulating levels of BNP are elevated in plasma in patients with HF.

BUN and serum creatinine concentrations may be used as markers of reduced CO or elevated right-sided pressures that potentiate renal venous congestion.[64] There is no level of BNP that perfectly separates patients with and without HF. Normal levels of BNP are less than 100 pg/mL.[64] Values above 500 pg/mL are generally considered to be positive for HF. In some patients, the BNP level provides an indication of the extent of HF, where higher BNP levels without renal failure indicate worsening failure of the ventricles. Therefore, a patient with a BNP of 1,000 pg/mL has more significant HF than a patient with a BNP of 500 pg/mL when there is no renal dysfunction present. However, in a patient with renal dysfunction, extremely high BNP levels may be noted due to an inability to respond to the BNP released from the heart. For these patients, the levels of BNP are not indicative of the extent of HF exacerbation. Therefore, results of BNP and NT-proBNP should be interpreted in the context of all available clinical data.

Echocardiography and Nuclear Imaging

With ultrasound technology, echocardiography is used to examine wall motion integrity, valvular status, wall thickness, chamber size, and LV function.[66] The EF can also be calculated using the data obtained from the echocardiogram. Echocardiography may accompany a stress test and is known as a *stress echo*. The purpose of a stress echo is to compare LV function and wall motion between rest and exercise when an increased VO_2 results in an increased MVO_2. A positive stress echo indicates a worsening of LV function as activity increases; a negative stress echo indicates that the LV has adequately adapted to the increase in energy demand. Nuclear imaging (e.g., thallium sestamibi) compares coronary perfusion between rest and exercise. If there is no decrease in perfusion with increasing workloads, the test is negative; if there is a decrease, the test is considered positive.

Nuclear imaging (e.g., thallium sestamibi) compares coronary perfusion between rest and exercise. If there is no decrease in perfusion with increasing workloads, the test is negative; if there is a decrease, the test is considered positive.

When a patient is unable to perform an exercise test because of limitations such as musculoskeletal or neurological impairments, a pharmacological stress test such as a *persantine thallium* test is often recommended.[67] Persantine, when given intravenously, decreases coronary vascular resistance by causing arterioles to vasodilate and therefore increases the blood flow through the capillary beds. If an artery is atherosclerotic, its arteriole may have gradually dilated over time to increase capillary blood flow by means of pressure autoregulation. Therefore, when persantine is given, the diseased arteries may have a limitation in the amount of further arteriolar dilation that can occur. In comparison to the nondiseased arteries, there will be a relative decrease in blood flow through the capillary beds of the diseased arteries. Imaging studies will thus detect a relative decrease in blood flow to the area of the myocardium that is perfused by the diseased artery compared with that perfused by a nondiseased artery. Adenosine, which is a coronary and peripheral vasodilator (as well as an antiarrhythmic), has similar effects as persantine and may be used instead.[67]

Finally, coronary computed tomography angiography (CCTA) uses an injection of iodine-containing contrast material and CT scanning to examine the coronary arteries and determine whether they are constricted. The 2021 ACC/AHA Guidelines reflect growing support for the use of CCTA and highlight a higher diagnostic accuracy in assessing coronary ischemia compared to other noninvasive diagnostic tests.[68]

Pharmacological Management of Heart Failure

With the advent of new medications such as ACE inhibitors, diuretics, and angiotensin receptor neprilysin inhibitors, the symptoms of volume overload are more effectively managed. Table 13.4 provides details on common categories of cardiovascular medications and relevant physical therapy implications. The principles of drug management for patients with HF are twofold: (1) to increase the contractility or pumping ability of the heart to relieve congestion and (2) to decrease the workload on the heart by reducing either the total volume of fluid in the system (the preload) or the vascular resistance (the afterload).[48] Drugs that increase contractility are known as *positive inotropes;* the common drug in this category is digoxin. Diuretics decrease preload, thereby decreasing LVEDV. Patients are often on a sliding scale dosage of diuretics depending on the amount of fluid weight gain; they are instructed to weigh themselves daily and adjust diuretics accordingly. Afterload reducers, particularly those that block the effects of

the renin–angiotensin system (e.g., ACE inhibitors or ARBs), are often a critical component of drug management in this population.[69] By blocking salt and water retention through aldosterone suppression, preload is decreased; by blocking vasoconstriction through angiotensin II suppression, afterload is reduced.[69] A new medication known as an angiotensin receptor neprilysin inhibitor (ARNI) combines two antihypertensive drugs (sacubitril and valsartan) and has become a hallmark medication in the management of chronic HF.[70] Valsartan blocks the action of angiotensin II, thereby decreasing vasoconstriction. Sacubitril blocks the breakdown of natriuretic peptides, allowing sodium and water to be excreted. The combined effects of these two medications reduce the work on the heart and improve outcomes in patients with HF. Finally, the increase in sympathetic activity that accompanies HF causes an increase in MVO_2 (from beta-receptor stimulation), peripheral vasoconstriction, and resultant reduction in peripheral blood flow (from alpha-receptor stimulation). Drugs that combine both beta-receptor blockade and alpha-receptor blockade minimize these affects. Beta blockade will result in a decrease in MVO_2, and alpha blockade will result in decreased afterload due to suppression of peripheral vasoconstriction.

Mechanical and Surgical Support

For the symptomatic patient in NYHA class III/IV, there are dramatic surgical options that may improve function, such as heart transplant, left ventricular assist devices (LVADs), myoplasty, and biventricular pacing. It is beyond the scope of this chapter to discuss in detail the complexity of each of these procedures. Heart transplantation involves replacing the patient's heart with a donor heart. The donor heart will be denervated; therefore, it will not have any direct sympathetic or parasympathetic connection and will be dependent on the intrinsic pacemaker of the SA node and hormonal stimulation to increase HR. The patient with a heart transplant requires careful pharmacological management. Immune-suppressing drugs are used to prevent the body from rejecting the organ as well as for careful control of infection.

The LVAD is a temporary pump inserted into the patient to perform the work of the LV or to augment the function of the failing heart. The patient is connected to an external energy source but also has the option of wearing a battery pack that allows freedom of movement for hours, in which the patient can go shopping, go to the movies, and so forth. It is important for the therapist to consider the effects of a 6-lb mass (created by the external energy source) resting below the diaphragm that is likely to alter ventilator performance. Finally, gentle progression of exercise intensity must be utilized. Therapists must be vigilant to check for flow limitations (10 to 12 L/min) or changes in cardiovascular function that may occur secondary to use of a mechanically driven pump. *Myoplasty* is a surgical procedure in which an enlarged LV undergoes a size reduction by removing dilated, scarred myocardium that is ineffective in contributing to contractility. A new class of pacemaker, the biventricular pacer, includes an intraventricular conduction delay (e.g., left bundle branch block on the ECG) for patients with severe CHF. This pacer coordinates the contraction of the right and left ventricles and in doing so provides a more effective LV contraction and increased CO.

Valvular Heart Disease

The prevalence of valvular heart disease is rapidly increasing in the United States and worldwide. Valvular heart disease increases with age with more than one in eight people aged 75 and older presenting with moderate or severe valve disease. Broadly, three major disorders encompass valvular dysfunction of one or more of the four heart valves. These include stenosis, prolapse, and regurgitation:

1. *Stenosis* involves narrowing of a heart valve limiting the flow of blood through the valve. As the pathological condition progresses, the chamber behind the valve pathologically hypertrophies to pump against the obstruction.
2. *Prolapse* involves enlarged valve cusps that become floppy and bulge backward. When the cusps and support mechanisms of the valve are destroyed, the valve droops down. As the disease progresses, prolapse may progress to regurgitation.
3. *Regurgitation* refers to the forward and backward movement of blood resulting from incomplete valve closure. During certain phases of the cardiac cycle, valves must close appropriately to prevent blood from flowing in a retrograde fashion. In a regurgitant valve, the valve does not close properly, leading to regurgitation of blood into the chamber behind the pathological valve.

Valve replacements are often used for treating valvular disease. Patients with stenosis or regurgitation of the aortic or mitral valves are prime candidates for valve replacement surgeries. A median sternotomy is the route to access the heart. Two major types of valves are used for valve replacement procedures: (1) mechanical valves and (2) biological valves derived from cadavers, porcine tissue, or bovine tissue.[71] Mechanical valves are preferred in patients younger than age 65 years because of their durability and long life. However, the major disadvantage is that they tend to be thrombogenic. Patients who receive a mechanical valve must be on lifelong anticoagulation therapy. For this reason, patients who have a history of a prior bleed, wish to become pregnant, or have poor medication adherence may not be candidates for a mechanical valve. For these patients, biological valves may be more appropriate. The postoperative care for patients with a valve replacement is similar to that for patients who have had a CABG. In addition, neurological monitoring must be continuous postoperatively owing to the potential for an embolic stroke that may occur during or after the procedure. Finally, recent developments in minimally invasive procedures have advanced therapeutic choices for older adults. Currently a transcatheter aortic valve implantation can be performed for patients with severe symptomatic aortic stenosis who are considered inoperable for open surgical aortic valve replacement.[71] This procedure involves the replacement of the aortic valve via a transfemoral access, subclavian access, or direct aortic transapical access. Transfemoral access is the most commonly used access route performed in 95% of patients who have this procedure.

Electrical Conduction Abnormalities

Arrhythmias are any alteration in the electric conduction of the heart from the normal beat (see Fig. 13.15). They are caused by a disturbance in the electrical activity of the heart, resulting in impaired electrical impulse formation or conduction. Arrhythmias may present as benign or malignant (i.e., life threatening). Examples of *malignant arrhythmias* are sustained ventricular tachycardia (V-tach) and ventricular fibrillation (V-fib). An example of a common *benign arrhythmia* in older adults would be atrial fibrillation (A-fib) with a controlled ventricular response. This section reviews a few conduction abnormalities and relevant implications for the physical therapist.

Ectopic Beats

A beat that originates from a site other than the sinus node is known as an *ectopic beat*. The common ectopic beats are atrial (*premature atrial contractions [PACs]*) and ventricular (*premature ventricular contractions [PVCs]*). PVCs may occur either by themselves or in groups such as couplets (two PVCs) or triplets (three PVCs) or alternating with sinus beats such as bigeminy (every other beat a PVC) or trigeminy (every third beat a PVC).

A PAC is an ectopic beat that originates in the atria and may present as an irregular rhythm (Fig. 13.15B). It may be difficult to distinguish a PAC from a premature junctional contraction (PJC), an ectopic beat that originates within the area around the AV node. Usually, PACs or PJCs will not compromise CO, and physical therapy intervention may be appropriate if accompanied by adequate hemodynamic responses. The presence of ectopic beats results in an irregular rhythm. Usually, ectopic beats are transient, and their severity depends on their impact on CO. It is certainly common to have a few PVCs even in a normal heart. Many people may have ectopic beats during times of stress or with stimulants such as nicotine and caffeine. Even though this may be a common response in a normal heart, it is important to educate patients with myocardial pathology who may have ectopic beats or irregular rhythms to

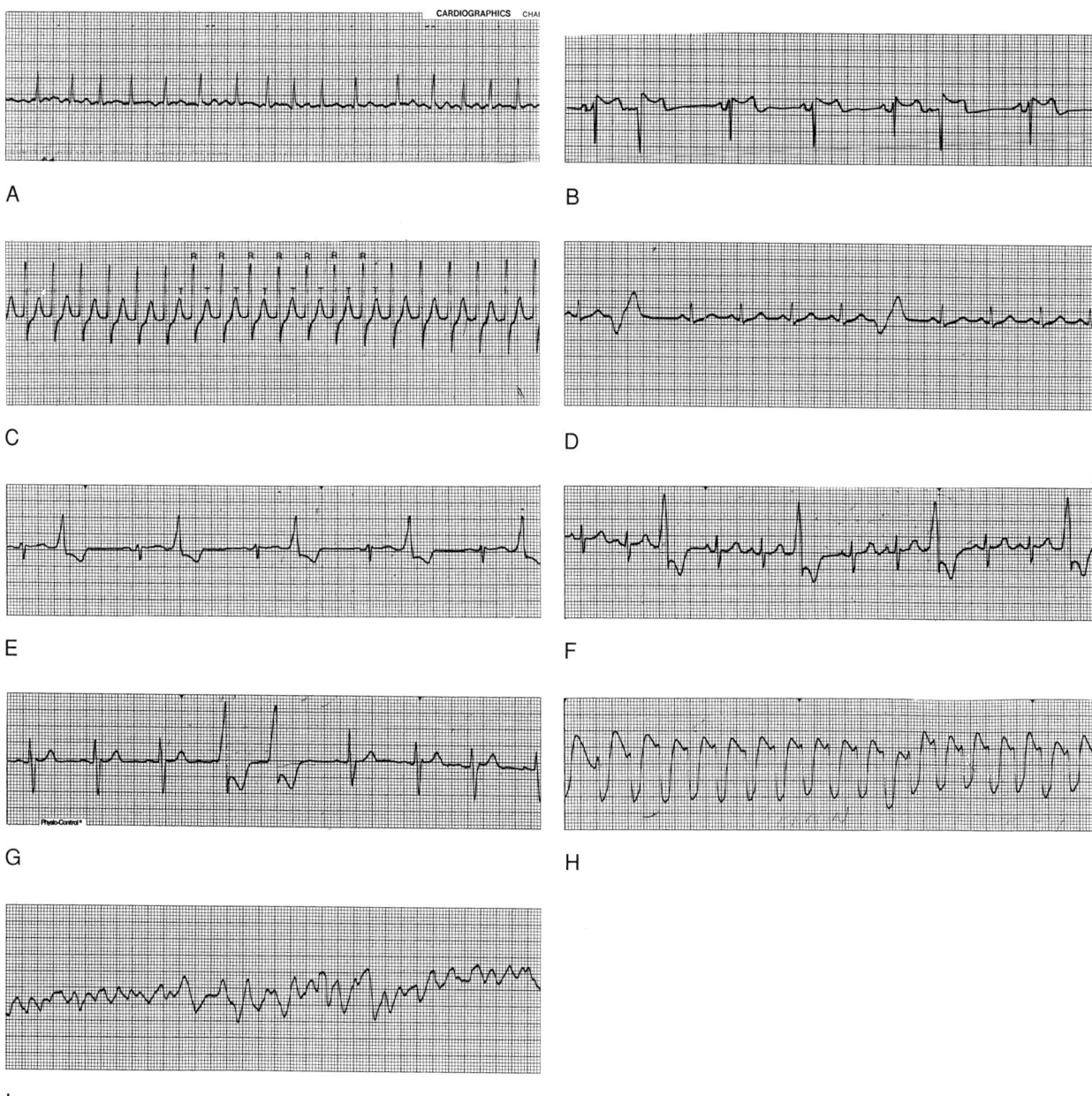

Figure 13.15 Examples of ectopy and arrhythmias. (A) Atrial fibrillation. (B) Atrial premature beat, also known as premature atrial contraction (PAC) (note third complex). (C) Supraventricular tachycardia (SVT). (D) Premature ventricular contraction (PVC) (note third complex). (E) Bigeminy (note second, fourth, and sixth complexes are PVCs). (F) Trigeminy (note second, fifth, and eighth complexes are PVCs). (G) Couplets (note fourth and fifth complexes are PVCs). (H) Ventricular tachycardia (V-tach). (I) Ventricular fibrillation (V-fib) (V-tach deteriorates into V-fib). *(From Brown K, Jacobson S.* Mastering Dysrhythmias: A Problem-Solving Guide. *F.A. Davis; 1988, p. 30, with permission.)*

avoid these aggravators. An increase in ectopy is undesired. Although the specific time frame a patient may be at risk for increased ectopy is not clearly known, a good rule of thumb may be abstinence from caffeine or smoking for at least 2 hours either before or after exercise. Patient education on wellness strategies and removal of ectopy aggravating factors is always useful for any patient with cardiovascular disease.

Supraventricular Ectopy

Supraventricular ectopy involves the rapid firing of an ectopic focus that originates in any location above the ventricles (atrial or junctional area). Examples of supraventricular ectopy include (1) paroxysmal atrial tachycardia and (2) supraventricular tachycardia. A sudden run of PACs occurring at a fast rate (100 to 200 bpm) is known as *paroxysmal atrial tachycardia.* A run of either PACs or PJCs at a rate of 150 to 250 bpm is known as supraventricular tachycardia (SVT) (Fig. 13.15C). Patients with SVT usually respond to a carotid massage where stimulation of the baroreceptors within the carotid bodies of the carotid artery produces a parasympathetic response. Other treatment interventions to reduce HR for patients with SVT include coughing and breath-holding techniques achieved through the Valsalva maneuver or carotid sinus massage.[72] Each of these techniques is geared to increase parasympathetic drive in different ways to reduce HR.

Ventricular Ectopy

PVCs are ectopic beats that originate in the ventricle and may present as irregular rhythms. Two hallmark characteristics identify PVCs on the ECG: (1) a P wave is absent as the impulse originates in the ventricle and (2) a wide and bizarre QRS complex signifies abnormal electrical conduction through the ventricle

(Fig. 13.15D). Single PVCs will not compromise CO if usually less than seven per minute. Therefore, physical activity may be appropriate if accompanied by an adequate hemodynamic response. If the PVCs increase with activity, the activity should be stopped and the patient examined for possible signs of compromised CO. PVCs may come from the same irritable site and are called *unifocal PVCs.* If they originate from different ectopic sites within the ventricle, they are known as *multifocal PVCs* (Fig. 13.16A). Multifocal PVCs suggest a more irritable ventricle and are therefore more serious than unifocal PVCs. It is appropriate for the therapist to have the patient medically evaluated before beginning or continuing an activity. Finally, a rare type of PVC known as an *R-on-T PVC* occurs when PVC fires *very prematurely* on the T wave of the preceding cardiac cycle (Fig. 13.16B). These patients must be monitored closely because they are at an increased risk for developing a life-threatening dysrhythmia such as ventricular tachycardia or ventricular fibrillation.

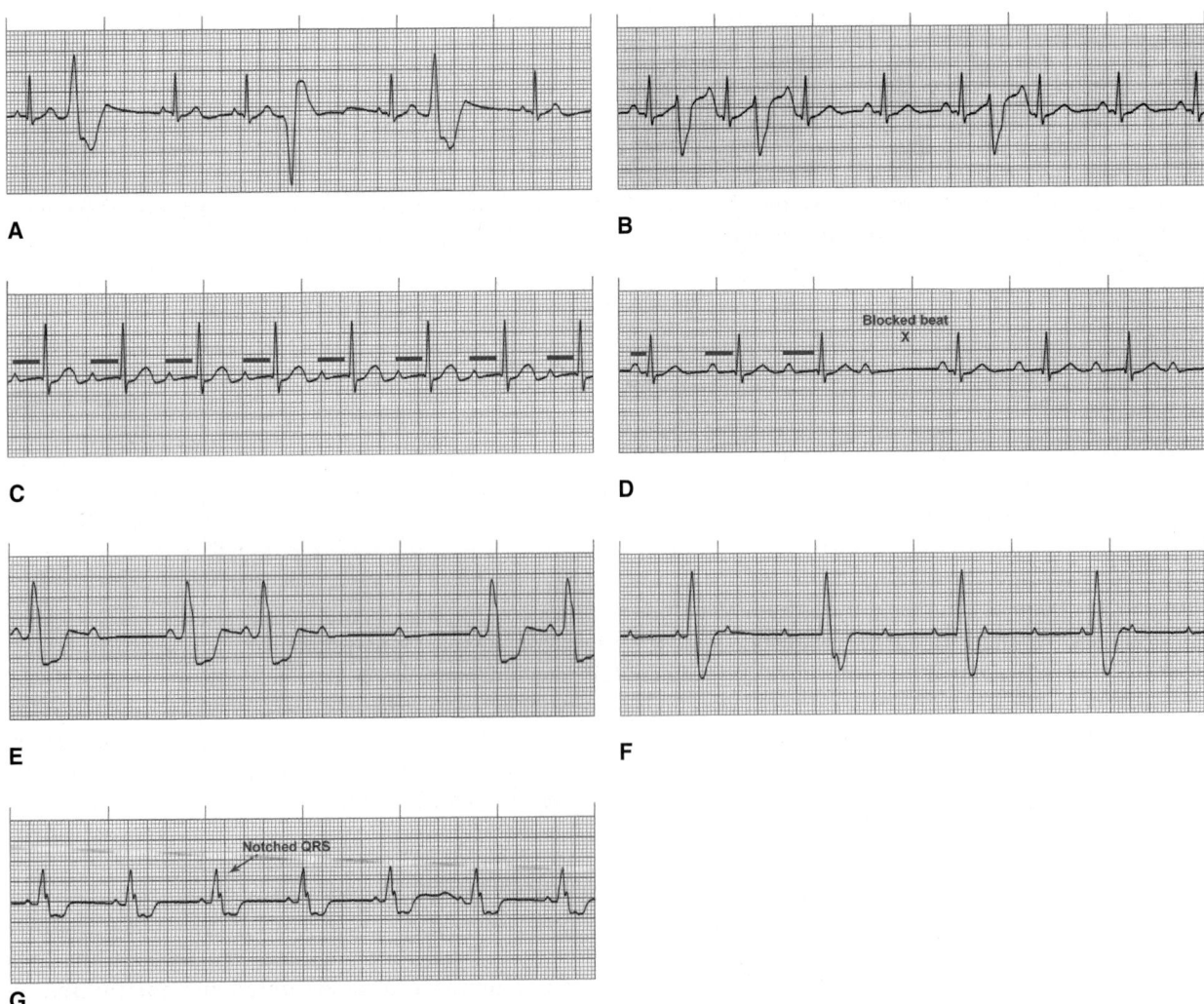

Figure 13.16 (A) Multifocal or multiform PVCs; (B) R-on-T PVC; (C) first-degree AV block; (D) Wenckebach rhythm; (E) second-degree type II; (F) third-degree AV block; (G) bundle branch block. *(From Jones S. ECG Success: Exercises in ECG Interpretation. F.A. Davis; 2008.)*

In ventricular bigeminy (Fig. 13.15E), every other beat is a PVC; in trigeminy, every third beat is a PVC (Fig. 13.15F). These rhythms occur transiently or episodically, and many patients have frequent bursts of these rhythms. If ectopy increases with activity, the activity should be immediately stopped. When two PVCs occur together, it is known as a couplet (Fig. 13.15G); when three PVCs occur together, it is known as a triplet. Couplets and triplets are important in that they suggest a high level of ventricular irritability. Altered LV function and ischemia are two of the more common causes for ventricular ectopy; therefore, medical management is directed toward improved LV function and perfusion whenever possible, as well as arrhythmia control.[73] Physical therapy intervention is conservative at best and depends on the hemodynamic stability of the patient.

Ventricular Tachycardia

A run of four or more PVCs in a row is known as V-tach (Fig. 13.15H)). V-tach may be either sustained or nonsustained. *Sustained V-tach,* by definition, occurs at an HR of at least 100 bpm and lasts for at least 30 sec. The patient may or may not have a palpable pulse and, if present, the pulse will be weak. Because of the severe decrease in CO and rapid hemodynamic deterioration associated with this rhythm, the presence of sustained V-tach is considered an emergency.[74] Medical intervention must be initiated as soon as possible. No physical therapy intervention is appropriate, except assisting the patient in stabilization, initiating cardiopulmonary resuscitation (CPR) when indicated, and activating the advanced cardiac life support (ACLS) system. V-tach may deteriorate quickly into V-fib.

Nonsustained V-tach occurs either in groups of three to five PVCs known as *salvos* or a run of six or more PVCs lasting for up to 30 sec. Nonsustained V-tach is considered a high-risk indicator for potentially lethal arrhythmias. Because the rhythm is nonsustained, the decrease in CO may not be sufficient to cause symptoms. However, until the etiology of the arrhythmia is identified and the rhythm controlled, physical therapy intervention is generally inappropriate.

Ventricular Fibrillation

V-fib is characterized by quivering of the ventricles resulting from inadequate electrical stimulation. The ECG demonstrates a sustained run of different-looking PVCs coming from different ectopic foci (Fig. 13.15I). When the ventricles do not contract but rather quiver, there is ineffective CO. The patient will arrest and die if this rhythm is not altered immediately. The treatment of choice is activation of ACLS, including electrical defibrillation and medication. Patients who survive ventricular fibrillation through defibrillation become candidates for an indwelling defibrillator placement known as an *automatic implantable cardiac defibrillator* (AICD).

Automatic Implantable Cardiac Defibrillator

The AICD is implanted in patients who have life-threatening ventricular arrhythmias (V-tach, V-fib).[75] The AICD is programmed to deliver an electrical shock if it detects an HR higher than its programmed HR limit.[75] Therefore, it is important for the physical therapist to know this limit and avoid an exercise intensity that may inadvertently activate the device. In addition to knowing the HR settings for the patient with an AICD, there are other considerations. ST-segment changes on the ECG may be common and are not specific for ischemia; therefore, other diagnostic studies must be done. In addition, UE aerobic or strengthening exercises should be avoided initially after placement of a pacemaker or defibrillator to avoid inadvertently dislodging the device or the lead wires. Checking with the physician when these exercises may be included is prudent.

Atrial Fibrillation

Atrial fibrillation (A-fib) is characterized by quivering of the atria due to inadequate electrical stimulation. A varied number of non–sinus-originating P waves (known as fibrillatory waves) exist for each QRS complex (Fig. 13.15A). The ventricular rhythm is said to be "irregularly irregular" because there is no regularity to the irregularity of the ventricular rhythm. It is important to note that effective contraction of the atria accounts for approximately 15% to 20% of CO—the *atrial kick*.[76] In patients with abnormal electrical conduction causing a quivering of the atria (A-fib), the mechanical contractile ability of the atria is reduced, resulting in a low atrial kick and compromised CO.[76]

Patients may exhibit A-fib continuously as their baseline rhythm or go in and out of this rhythm at rest or with activity. Physical therapy intervention may be appropriate for patients in A-fib who have a good ventricular rate at rest, with appropriate hemodynamic and HR increase with exercise. In patients with A-fib and rapid ventricular rates (greater than 120 bpm) at rest, exercise intensity must be lowered and hemodynamic responses monitored carefully. This is because a rapid ventricular rate in addition to the loss of atrial kick further compromises the CO and results in altered hemodynamic responses. A good rule of thumb is to avoid physical activity and seek medical consultation if the patient's resting HR is greater than 115 bpm, if the patient appears uncomfortable, or if there is an inadequate hemodynamic response. Because this rhythm is irregular, it is important to monitor the HR for a full minute rather than 15 to 30 sec to obtain an accurate pulse rate.

Typically, A-fib is medically managed in a three-pillar approach of rate control, rhythm control, and anticoagulation.[77] A significant body of new research goes beyond traditional management and has focused on lifestyle modification to lower the risk of A-fib development and progression. A recent scientific statement from the AHA calls for all clinicians to incorporate risk factor modification as the fourth and essential pillar in the overall management of A-fib.[78] Physical therapists possess the knowledge and skills to examine and treat a wide range of risk factors including obesity, hypertension, diabetes, sleep apnea, and inactivity, all of which collectively lead to A-fib. In this way, physical therapists can provide significant contribution in addressing current deficiencies in A-fib risk-factor management.

Conduction Delays and Blocks

Changes in the length of the PR interval, the width of the QRS complex, and the length of the QT interval are some of the ECG measurements indicative of conduction abnormalities.

Conduction delays through the AV node are classified as first-, second-, or third-degree heart blocks. *First-degree heart block* occurs when the conduction time through the AV node is prolonged; therefore, the ECG will have an increased length of the PR interval (Fig. 13.16C). There are two categories of *second-degree heart block:* Mobitz type I and Mobitz type II; each is hallmarked by the presence of dropped beats. Mobitz I, also known as *Wenckebach,* presents with a gradual increase in PR interval length in the preceding beats and then an eventual dropped beat (Fig. 13.16D); Mobitz II has normal PR intervals in all the beats preceding the dropped beat (Fig. 13.16E). In *third-degree heart block,* a mismatch of atrial and ventricular conduction exists, so there is no consistency between the atrial contraction and the ventricular contraction (i.e., no relationship between P waves and the QRS complex on the ECG) (Fig. 13.16). Patients in first-degree block have no limitations to exercise. Whether or not exercise is permitted with second- and third-degree blocks depends on the etiology and subsequent hemodynamic responses. It is advisable to seek medical clearance before beginning a formal exercise program.

Conduction delays through the bundle of His are known as either right bundle branch block (RBBB) or left bundle branch block (LBBB). Bundle branch blocks are not true arrhythmias because there is no change in the actual rhythm, just in the timing of conduction through the bundle of His. The heart is still depolarized from the same pacemaker; only the route of activation is changed. Bundle branch blocks present on the ECG as a distortion of the QRS complex with an increased duration (i.e., widening) (Fig. 13.16G). The presence of an LBBB on the ECG is usually permanent and indicates a pathological condition. RBBB may occur from a variety of reasons; it may be a permanent change due to underlying disease, or it may be benign. RBBB can also occur transiently. LBBB usually indicates the presence of more significant disease than RBBB.

The presence of a new bundle branch block should be medically evaluated before beginning or progressing an exercise program. Following medical clearance, there is usually no contraindication to exercise in either the RBBB or LBBB population. Because of the alteration of the QRS complex and as a result the ST segment, the sensitivity of the ECG in detecting ischemia via ST depression is lost in the patient with LBBB. Further, during exercise a fast-left bundle branch cannot be distinguished from ventricular tachycardia. In such cases, patients with an LBBB do not undergo exercise stress tests; rather, they undergo chemical stress tests to stress the heart.

Pacemakers

The use of pacemakers has increased considerably, with the most common indications for placement of a permanent pacemaker being (1) an HR that is too slow (symptomatic bradycardia); (2) an HR that fails to increase appropriately with exercise (chronotropic incompetence); or (3) an electric pathway that is blocked, resulting in AV delays or bundle branch blocks.[79]

A pacemaker is a device that is placed subdermally near the heart and consists of an implantable pulse generator and lead wires that connect the pacemaker to the myocardium. The pulse generator contains a long-life battery and circuitry for timing, sensing, and output functions. The life of the battery usually dictates the life of the pacemaker and varies depending on the type of battery and the extent to which the pacemaker is being used. In some cases, the patient is dependent on the pacemaker for every cardiac contraction and is likely to utilize the life of the battery in a shorter period. The average pacemaker battery life is between 5 and 10 years. Replacement of pacemaker batteries is done after serial assessments have confirmed a reduction in battery life. Battery life may be consumed more rapidly when the patient is more reliant on the pacemaker for maintaining an appropriate HR. In 2016, the U.S. Food and Drug Administration approved the newest miniature pacemaker. Empirical research has identified certain complications associated with conventional transvenous pacing systems related to the pacing lead and pocket. In light of these complications, a novel, self-contained, miniaturized pacemaker named Micra has been developed.[80] This pacemaker primarily does single chamber pacing and may be beneficial for some patients.

Patients are reliant on pacemakers at different levels. Some patients usually have normal electric conduction and so do not need to be reliant on the pacemaker at all times. Other patients have altered electrical conduction through the heart and may be very reliant on the pacemaker to keep them alive. Therefore, it is important for therapists to determine how reliant the patient may be on their pacemaker. When pacemakers trigger a pace due to altered electrical conduction through the heart, the ECG reveals a pacer spike. Thus, if the patient has a pacemaker and no pacer spikes are evident on the ECG, the therapist can infer that the heart is conducting normally, and the pacemaker is there for emergency needs only. Conversely, if the ECG demonstrates a pacer spike in every cardiac cycle, the therapist must understand that this patient is 100% reliant on the pacemaker and thus ensure that the pacemaker is adequately rate responsive during activity.

The basic functions of the pacemaker lead wires are to provide the pacemaker with information on intrinsic myocardial activity and pace the myocardium when intrinsic activity fails. There are four primary functions of pacemakers: (1) the ability to sense intrinsic cardiac function, (2) the ability to stimulate cardiac depolarization in response to failed intrinsic activity, (3) the ability to respond to increased metabolic demand by providing rate-responsive pacing, and (4) the ability to provide diagnostic information stored within the pacemaker.

Pacemakers have rate and rhythm sensitivity as well as the ability to override certain arrhythmias. Pacemakers may also be combined with AICD capabilities. Pacemakers are coded by either a three- or five-category system according to which chamber (atria or ventricle) is sensed, what chamber is paced (atria or ventricle), and whether the electrical stimulus will trigger a response or be inhibited (Table 13.7). Because pacemakers may fail to work properly, ECG monitoring is helpful to determine whether the pacer is working properly.

Calculating Heart Rate From Electrocardiography

HR can be determined from an ECG strip.

The ECG graph paper consists of a series of small boxes (represented by light black lines) and large boxes (represented by heavy black lines). Each large box is made up of five small boxes. The horizontal axis represents time; when the ECG paper is moving at the usual speed of 25 mm/sec, five large boxes constitutes 1 second. Knowing that time is on the x-axis, there are many ways to calculate HR from the ECG graph paper. An easy way to calculate a minute rate is to count the number of complexes in 6 seconds (i.e., 30 large boxes) and multiply by 10. Often the ECG paper will have 3-second intervals premarked on the electrocardiographic paper. An alternative approach is to identify an R wave from one ECG complex that is close to or on a heavy black line (i.e., a large box), and then assign each of the following heavy black lines (large boxes) a number in the following order: 300, 150, 100, 75, 60, 50, 40. The heavy line closest to the next R wave will provide an approximation of HR (Fig. 13.17). Finally, dividing 300 by the number of large boxes between

Table 13.7   Pacemaker Classification System

Chamber Paced	Chamber Sensed	Response	Rate-Responsive Pacing
O = none	O = none	O = none	R = rate responsive
A = atria	A = atria	I = inhibit	
V = ventricle	V = ventricle	T = trigger	
D = dual chamber	D = dual chamber	D = capacity to both inhibit and trigger	

Pacemakers are commonly identified by a three-letter code as displayed in the first three columns. Pacemakers may also have the capacity to respond to physiological stimuli to increase rate (column 4) and to override atrial tachycardia. A fifth column, for antitachycardiac function, is rarely used because of the increased sophistication of the newer implantable defibrillators/pacemakers, which renders this function unnecessary. Example: VVI pacer will provide an electrical impulse to the ventricle if it senses that there is no ventricular activity within an appropriate time frame. If there is intrinsic ventricular electrical activity, the pacemaker will be inhibited.

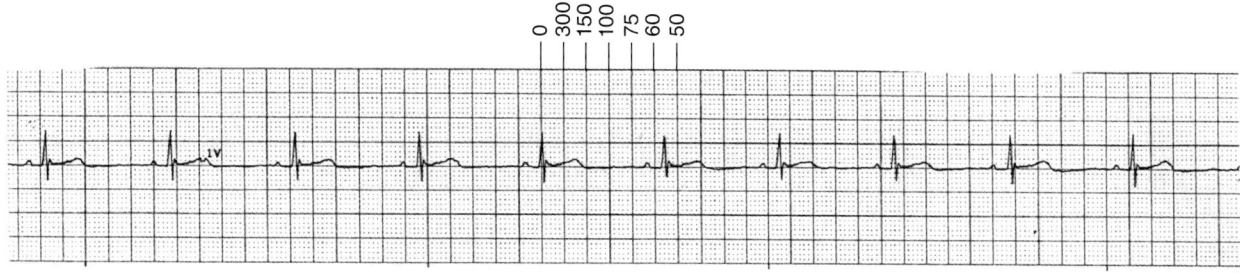

Figure 13.17 Calculation of a heart rate from a rhythm strip. Begin with the fifth complex (which falls on a large black line) and count each large black line to the right of this complex in the order of 300, 150, 100, 75, 60, 50. The sixth complex falls between two large lines (i.e., 50 and 60). There are five small lines between each large line. Between 50 and 60 there are 10 beats; therefore, each small line in this case would be two beats. The heart rate would be 60 – 4 = 56. An alternate method would be to count the number of complexes in a 6-sec strip and multiply by 10.

two R waves will also indicate the HR. If the rate is regular, any of the preceding strategies will work. If the rate is irregular, however, the complexes will need to be counted over a long time, and a minimum of a 6-second strip should be used.

Heart Transplantation

Patients who have undergone a heart transplantation may present with the following: (1) calf cramps owing to the immunosuppressive drug cyclosporine; (2) decreased LE strength; (3) obesity owing to long-term corticosteroid use; (4) increased risk of fracture owing to osteoporosis associated with long-term, high-dose corticosteroids; and (5) increased probability of developing atherosclerosis in the coronary arteries of the donor heart after the first postsurgical year. Because the heart is denervated, HR alone provides a limited measure of exercise intensity. Therefore, BP and perceived exertion should be included in routine data collection.

■ EXAMINATION OF THE PATIENT WITH HEART DISEASE

Owing to the increasing incidence and prevalence of heart disease in our society, many patients referred to physical therapy will have cardiovascular dysfunction or may be at risk for developing CVD. The history taking, review of systems, and data from specific tests and measures will guide and inform development of the physical therapy diagnosis, goals and outcomes, prognosis, and POC. This section addresses elements of the examination and tests and measures specific to the cardiovascular system.

Medical Record Review

The medical record of a patient with a history of cardiovascular impairments may at times be overwhelming. The patient interview is typically helpful if clarification of the medical record is needed. Depending on the type of setting (inpatient, outpatient, acute rehabilitation, home care), the specific contents of the medical record may vary. Important items to note within the medical record include the following:

1. Medical problems, past medical history, physician's examination
2. Medications, including type, dosage, and schedule
3. Laboratory tests including but not limited to
   a. Blood tests for specific cardiac enzymes that may indicate an MI has occurred
   b. Electrolytes, including potassium, magnesium, and calcium if ventricular arrhythmias are present
   c. Complete blood count (CBC), which may indicate the presence of reduced oxygen-carrying capacity within the body through the hemoglobin and hematocrit values
   d. Renal and liver profile through assessment BUN, creatinine, and liver function tests
   e. Presence of CAD risk factors, such as elevated lipid values (e.g., total cholesterol, low-density lipoproteins [LDLs], triglyceride), blood sugars (glucose), C-reactive protein, and homocysteine levels
   f. Arterial blood gases for individuals in critical illness
4. Results of any diagnostic studies or interventions: chest x-ray, ECGs, ETT, cardiac catheterization, surgical reports, hemodynamic monitors (e.g., pressure readings from central line and/or arterial line)
5. Nursing and other health-care provider notes

The medical record contains information regarding what has happened to the patient as well as the status of the patient within the last 24 hours or since the last health-care provider intervention. Flowcharts, which record vital signs, temperature, oxygenation requirements, and volume status over time, provide up-to-date patient data, especially when working with the more medically challenged patient.

Patient Interview

The formal patient interview should follow the medical record review. A determination of overall cognition (e.g., orientation, memory, learning needs, comprehension) is the first step in the interview process. Additionally, information regarding the patient's lifestyle, previous level of functioning, recreational interests, work requirements, and goals are all important in establishing appropriate interventions for the patient. The International Classification of Functioning, Disability, and Health recommends the clinician evaluate environmental and personal factors that affect a patient's overall ability for activity and participation.[81] Based on this model, it is important for therapists to assess the patient's prior level of participation in addition to the prior level of activity. An assessment of both baseline activity and participation is useful in generating goals and the appropriate functional prognosis of the patient. Further, an assessment of an individual's prior level of function should not only be limited to the level of function before the most recent hospital admission. Often when a patient is asked their level of function before the most recent hospital admission, the therapist assumes that this level of function before the most recent admission is the patient's optimal level of function. This may not be true for a patient who had a higher level of function a few months earlier who now presents with a relatively lower level of function at this admission due to multiple recent readmissions. Clinically, it is useful to interview patients on their level of function over a prolonged length of time prior to their current state.

Data should also be obtained about the patient's response to health and illness, coping status, support systems, and knowledge of heart disease. It is important to note that not all the information from the interview needs to be obtained on the first session. During subsequent sessions, the patient may begin to feel better and less anxious and may therefore be able to communicate more easily. Patient education can often be woven into the interview process, either subtly or overtly. The patient should describe, in their own words, the quality and location of the symptom for which medical attention is being sought. It is common for physical therapists to ask a patient about pain; for patients with cardiac disease, one should be cautious about assuming that the patient's symptom is pain. Many patients will not use pain as their qualifier but instead describe their symptoms as pressure, heaviness, SOB (dyspnea), aching, heartburn, or general malaise, to identify a few. Knowing the symptom presentation for each individual will make patient education and activity progression easier. It is also important to identify any consistent precipitating factors and alleviators, as well as duration and frequency of symptoms.

The interview also helps to establish rapport and trust between therapist and patient, thereby creating an environment for mutual goal setting. This in turn facilitates patient adherence to the rehabilitation program. Patients who are recovering from an MI or from surgery need to understand the time frames for healing and convalescence. Education for family members and significant others is also crucial for patient adherence and understanding.

Tests and Measures

Following the International Classification of Functioning, Disability, and Health, specific examination tests and measures are presented to identify impairments in body structure and function (Table 13.8) and in functional activity limitations and participation restrictions (Table 13.9).

Table 13.8	Examination for Patients With Cardiovascular Disease
Body Structure and Function Impairment	Key Test/Measure
Baseline Hemodynamic Stability	**Resting Heart Rate and Rhythm:** These must be assessed at rest and with activity. Normal resting heart rate is 60–100 beats/min. Alterations in heart rate values from this range at rest must be evaluated to determine the stability of the patient at rest. Beyond an assessment of the absolute heart rate value at rest, it is also important to consider relative changes in resting heart rate values on a day-to-day basis to determine the relative stability of the patient.[53] In other words, a patient with a routine resting heart rate of 60 beats/min who presents on any given day with a heart rate of 80 beats/min may be demonstrating relative instability due to an exacerbation of their pathology. Finally, if the peripheral pulse is difficult to obtain, an apical pulse may be obtained by auscultating the heart at the fifth intercostal space, midclavicular line.
Baseline Hemodynamic Stability	**Heart Rhythm:** The regularity of the pulse is important to assess to determine the presence of an arrhythmia. Pulses may be felt as regular, irregular, regularly irregular, or irregularly irregular. A patient who presents with any form of irregularity in their pulses will need a follow-up ECG to confirm the dysrhythmia.
Hemodynamic Stability With Exercise	**Exercise Heart Rate and Rhythm:** An assessment of heart rate and rhythm during exercise is important to help determine the appropriateness of the cardiovascular system in meeting the metabolic needs of the body during exercise. Heart rate traditionally increases 10 beats/min per MET level increase in activity. The inability to increase heart rate sufficiently or a profound increase in heart rate with activity needs further evaluation. Further, it is important to evaluate heart rate responses with activity each day to determine the relative stability of the patient on a day-to-day basis. In other words, an assessment of the patient's relative changes in heart rate to the same absolute work is useful in identifying stability on a day-to-day basis.[53]
Hemodynamic Stability With Exercise	**Respiratory Rate:** Normal respiratory rate at rest in an adult is 12–20 breaths/min. Respiratory rates greater than 30 breaths/min at rest signify instability and will need further assessment. Further, it is important for the clinician to assess respiratory rate changes during activity at each visit to assess relative changes in stability on a day-to-day basis. A simple test is the use of a talk test where the therapist assesses the patient's ability to talk or sing while exercising. The inability to fluently talk or sing due to an elevated respiratory rate signifies that the patient is exercising at an intensity greater than the anaerobic threshold.[89]

(Continued)

Table 13.8   Examination for Patients With Cardiovascular Disease—cont'd

Body Structure and Function Impairment	Key Test/Measure
Hemodynamic Stability With Exercise	**Blood Pressure With Activity:** Arterial BP is a product of CO and TPR, where BP = CO × TPR. An increase in either of these factors will increase BP, and a decrease in either variable decreases BP. The primary factor that changes during activity is the CO and not the TPR. Therefore, clinically, a change in BP during activity is primarily due to a change in CO. Aerobic exercise of increasing intensity increases CO and concomitantly increases BP. Conversely, a drop in BP during aerobic exercise indicates a drop in CO or signifies the inability of the heart to meet the metabolic needs of the peripheral tissue. Signs of compromised CO, including fatigue, weakness, tiredness, and dizziness, usually accompany this drop in BP. Therefore, BP is essential to assess in the patient who demonstrates signs of compromised CO during activity to determine whether CO is being maintained.
Hypoxemia	**Pulse Oximetry:** Pulse oximetry is used to assess pulmonary respiration or gas exchange at the level of the alveolar–capillary interface. Pulse oximetry readings less than 90% indicate hypoxemia and warrant further evaluation. Patients with HF often present with a shunt that compromises gas exchange, thereby reducing pulse oximetry readings.
Dyspnea	**Dyspnea:** Dyspnea may be assessed by asking patients their *Perceived Level of Dyspnea* on a scale of 1–10 (0 = nothing at all; 10 = maximal). The Minimal Clinical Important Difference has not been established in heart disease but has been established as 1 point in patients with chronic lung disease.[90] An alternate method for measurement is the *Dyspnea Scale*, a 5-point ordinal scale (0 = no dyspnea; 4 = severe difficulty, cannot continue) (see Box 13.3).
Altered Breathing Patterns	**Paroxysmal Nocturnal Dyspnea:** An assessment of a patient's report of experiencing a sudden episode of SOB at night is an important sign of an exacerbation of HF. It has a sensitivity and specificity of 39%–41% and from 80%–84%, respectively.[91]
Altered Breathing Patterns	**Orthopnea:** Orthopnea is SOB that increases in the recumbent position. This sign has a reported sensitivity of 22%–50% and a specificity of 74%–77% for HF exacerbation.[91] Patients with HF require increased numbers of pillows to sleep at night to avoid symptoms of orthopnea. Therefore, clinically, the number of pillows required can be used to gauge the severity of HF.
Dyspnea on Exertion	**Dyspnea on Exertion:** Dyspnea, especially with exertion, is one of the most common symptoms of HF, and it frequently appears early in the disease. Absence of dyspnea on exertion has a sensitivity of 84%–100% in ruling out worsening heart failure.[91]
Baseline Instability in HF	**Displacement of the Point of Maximum Impulse (PMI):** The apical impulse is traditionally auscultated at the midclavicular line. An apical impulse recorded greater than 3 cm from the midclavicular line may be an accurate indicator of left ventricular enlargement with a sensitivity of 92% and a specificity of 91%.[92]
Angina	**Angina:** The classical presentation of angina is substernal chest pressure accompanied by the *Levine sign* (the patient clenching their fist over the sternum). The Levine sign has a high diagnostic accuracy for ischemia.[93] For some patients, angina does not present in the classic way but rather may present as a pain or heaviness in the shoulder, jaw, arm, elbow, or upper back between scapulae. Angina may radiate from the chest to the arm or up to the throat, or it may present as indigestion or even SOB. The patient is often asked to rank their discomfort on the *Angina Scale* (see Box 13.4).
Abnormal Heart Sounds	**Heart Auscultation:** Normal heart sounds are identified as S_1 (lub), which occurs at the time of the closure of the mitral (and tricuspid) valve and marks the beginning of systole and S_2 (dub), which occurs at the time of aortic (and pulmonic) valve closure and marks the end of systole. Figure 13.18 depicts locations on the chest for appropriate auscultation of each valve. The aortic valve is best auscultated at the second intercostal space, right sternal border. The pulmonic valve is heard at the second intercostal space, left sternal border. The tricuspid valve is auscultated at the fourth intercostal space, left sternal border, and the mitral valve is best heard at the fifth intercostal space, along the midclavicular line.

Table 13.8 Examination for Patients With Cardiovascular Disease—cont'd

Body Structure and Function Impairment	Key Test/Measure
	Murmurs are abnormal heart sounds commonly the result of valvular disorders due to the changes in blood flow around and through the altered valve. A *systolic murmur* will present as audible turbulence between S_1 and S_2, and a *diastolic murmur* will present as turbulence between S_2 and S_1. Other abnormal sounds include S_3 and S_4 sounds. The S_3, also known as a *ventricular gallop*, occurs after S_2 and is clinically correlated with increased LVEDP and PCWP during a heart failure exacerbation with sensitivity of 30%–50% and a specificity of 80%–90%.[58] S_4, also known as an *atrial gallop*, occurs before S_1 and is clinically associated with an MI or chronic HTN. Finally, a *pericardial friction rub* is a hallmark sign of acute pericarditis.[94]
Abnormal Lung Sounds	**Lung Auscultation:** Normal lung tissue produces vesicular (soft, low-pitched) sounds in the peripheral aspect of the lungs and bronchial breath (loud, high-pitched) sounds centrally along the manubrium of the sternum. Patients with LV failure often have the adventitious sounds of *crackles*. The auscultated crackles are coarse and best appreciated over the lung bases. The crackles typically occur late in inspiration. In patients admitted to the hospital with HF decompensation, pulmonary crackles and an S_3 heart sound were present in more than 50% of all patients.[59] Further, crackles and S_3 heart sound had higher readmission rates than those without these signs: odds ratio for pulmonary crackles was 2.8; odds ratio for S_3 heart sound was 2.6.[59] Figure 13.19 provides information on the location for placement of the stethoscope for lung auscultation. Additionally, the lower two illustrations in the figure demonstrates specific segments of the lung based on the location of the auscultation.
Baseline Instability Due to Increased Cardiac Filling Pressures	**Jugular Venous Distention:** Patients with HF presenting with backup of fluid into the venous vasculature should be examined for the presence of jugular venous distention. To examine for this sign, the patient is placed at a 45° semirecumbent position.[77] The patient's head is turned away from the side to be evaluated, and the clinician observes for a distention or pulsations of the jugular vein 3–5 cm above the sternum. The highest point of visible pulsation is determined, and the vertical distance between this level and the level of the sternal angle of Louis is recorded (Fig. 13.20). Elevated jugular venous pressures have been associated with an increased risk of HF hospitalization (relative risk, 1.32; 95% Confidence Interval I 1.08–1.62; $P < .01$), death or hospitalization for HF (RR, 1.30; 95% Confidence Interval I 1.11–1.53; $P < .005$).[95]
Peripheral Edema	**Pitting Edema and Weight Gain:** In patients with CHF, low SV causes a reduced blood volume perfused to the periphery. This stimulates the pressoreceptors as they sense a decrease in volume. These pressoreceptors subsequently relay a message to the kidney to retain fluid. This retention of fluid increases the hydrostatic pressure within the peripheral vasculature, thereby pushing fluid into the interstitial space, resulting in peripheral edema and weight gain. Edema can be assessed through girth measurements or by using the Palpation/Pitting Scale (Chapter 14). The severity of peripheral edema is categorized into four stages based on the time taken for the skin to rebound to its original contour after pitting. It is also important to note that edema can accumulate in the abdominal area (ascites) or sacral areas of the body. Weight gain of greater than 3 lb in 24 hours or 5 lb in a week signifies worsening HF.[50]
Peripheral Muscle Weakness	**Muscle Strength:** Standard manual muscle testing of major muscle groups in the UEs and LEs is effective if weakness is suspected below functional limits. If strength of peripheral muscles is above functional limits, assessment of functional strength can be performed with a standardized sit-to-stand test called the *Five Times Sit to Stand Test* or a timed chair rise test called a *30-Second Chair Rise Test*.
Inspiratory Muscle Weakness	**Maximal Inspiratory Pressure:** Strength of the inspiratory muscles is important in patients with HF. Empirical evidence suggests that patients with chronic HF have weak inspiratory muscles.[96] An inspiratory muscle strength of less than 60 cm H_2O traditionally depicts the presence of weak inspiratory muscles.[96]

BP = blood pressure; CHF = congestive heart failure; CO = cardiac output; HF = heart failure; HTN = hypertension;
LE = lower extremity; LV = left ventricle; LVEDP = left ventricular end diastolic pressure; MET = metabolic equivalent;
MI = myocardial infarction; PCWP = pulmonary capillary wedge pressure; RR = relative risk; SOB = shortness of breath;
SV = systolic volume; TPR = total peripheral resistance; UE = upper extremity.

Box 13.3   Dyspnea Scale

0 = No dyspnea
1+ = Mild, noticeable
2+ = Mild, some difficulty
3+ = Moderate difficulty, but can continue
4+ = Severe difficulty, cannot continue

Box 13.4   Angina Scale

0 = No angina
1+ = Light, barely noticeable
2+ = Moderate, bothersome
3+ = Severe, very uncomfortable: preinfarction pain
4+ = Most pain ever experienced: infarction pain

Heart Valves

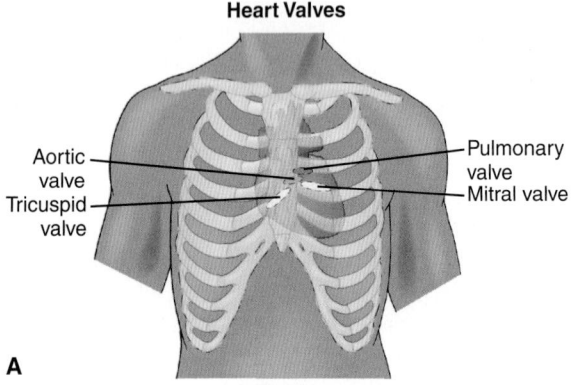

Aortic valve
Tricuspid valve
Pulmonary valve
Mitral valve

A

Auscultation Points

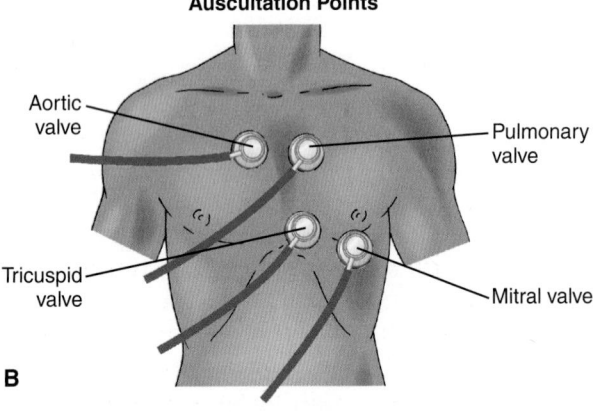

Aortic valve
Tricuspid valve
Pulmonary valve
Mitral valve

B

Figure 13.18 Anterior view of the chest wall of a man showing skeletal structures, heart, location of the heart valves, and auscultation points.

■ PHYSICAL THERAPY INTERVENTION FOR PATIENTS WITH HEART DISEASE

The goals of physical therapist interventions and education are to improve the individual's exercise capacity (being able to do more work), exercise efficiency (being able to do the same work with less cost), and exercise tolerance (being able to do the same work with less signs and symptoms); enhance self-management of their cardiac pathology; and most importantly, improve quality of life.

Therapeutic Exercise

A patient's responsiveness to functional improvement with therapeutic exercise is influenced by both central cardiovascular function and peripheral muscle weakness. Patients with greater degrees of peripheral weakness will be more responsive to exercise treatment compared with patients with greater degrees of central cardiovascular dysfunction. Additionally, the degree of improvement is variable from one individual to another and is directly dependent on the degree of purposeful exercise training that directly targets muscle weakness. Finally, a patient's presentation may differ throughout the course of treatment. For this reason, assessment of patient signs, symptoms, and hemodynamic stability must be completed at each treatment session so that interventions may be modified accordingly. For example, if a patient with HF has a relatively higher resting HR, increased weight gain, worsening lung sounds, and increased SOB, treatment will need to be modified in light of worsening stability.[53,62]

Cardiac Rehabilitation

Cardiac rehabilitation is a comprehensive exercise, education, and lifestyle modification program designed to enable participants to achieve optimal physical, psychological, social, and vocational functioning. Treatment is geared to control symptoms, improve exercise capacity and tolerance, and improve overall quality of life.

Patients, especially older adults who have been hospitalized for an ACS event such as a MI or CABG, or who have had a HF exacerbation or valve replacement surgery are at an increased risk of disability due to inactivity and bedrest. For these patients, a formal exercise prescription program is useful in improving overall activity and participation. Table 13.10 summarizes current empirical evidence on the benefits of cardiac rehabilitation. As noted in the table, evidence is controversial regarding the effect of cardiac rehabilitation on mortality in patients with CHD. However, besides mortality, cardiac rehabilitation has been found to have several beneficial effects, including an improvement in cardiovascular risk factors, exercise capacity, return to work, and overall quality of life.

Phase I Cardiac Rehabilitation

Cardiac rehabilitation is traditionally begun in the acute hospital setting. In phase I cardiac rehabilitation, physical therapy interventions focus on assessing the patient's hemodynamic responses to activity as well as increasing independence in functional mobility activities including bed mobility, transfers, ambulation, stair climbing, and

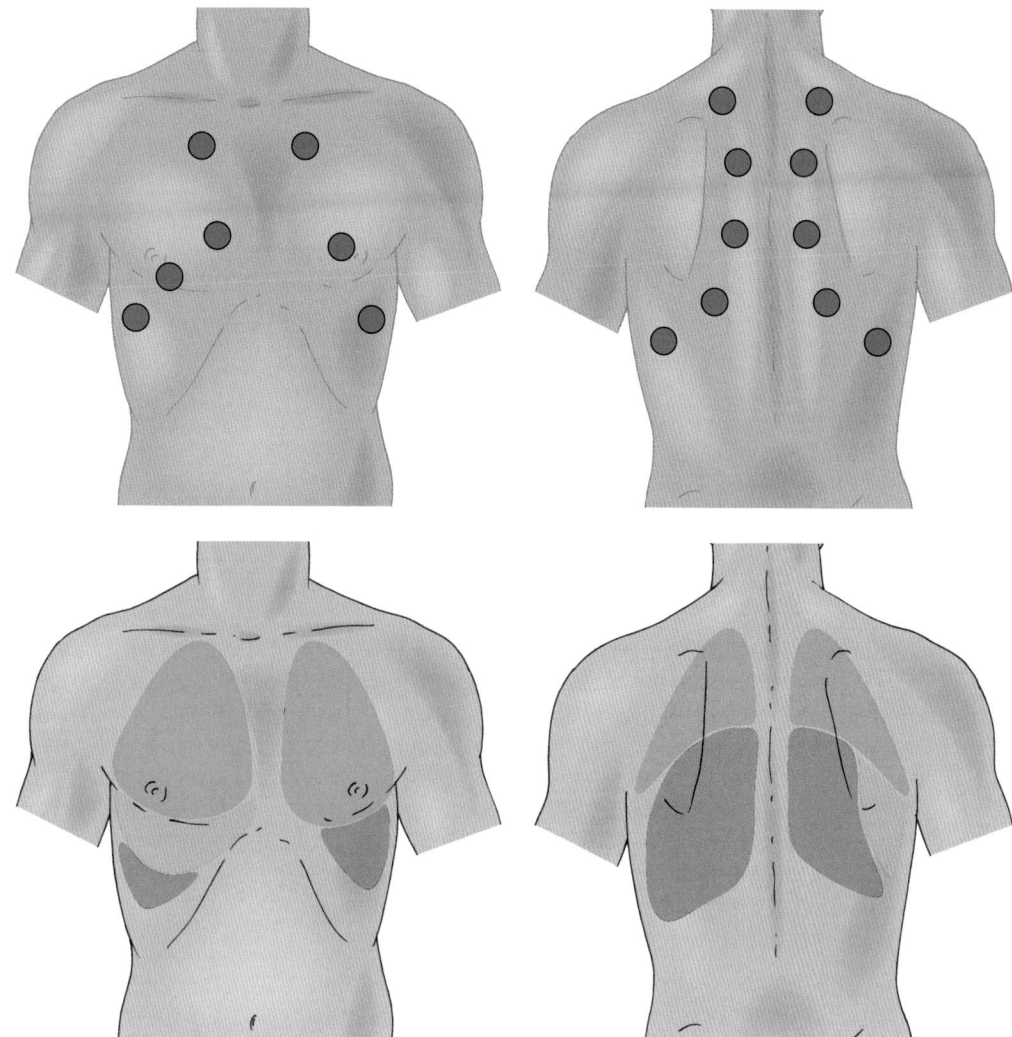

Figure 13.19 Auscultation of lungs.

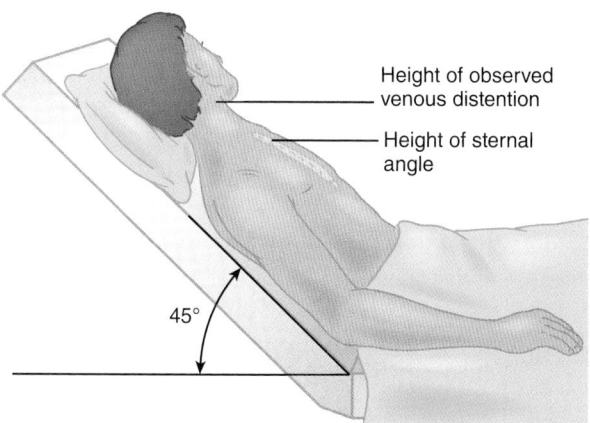

Height of observed venous distention

Height of sternal angle

45°

Figure 13.20 Examination of jugular venous distention.

activities of daily living. With a shortening of the length of stay in hospital settings, physical therapists are challenged to promote early ambulation, introduce patients to the goals of cardiac rehabilitation, and enroll patients in post-acute phase II programs. In a large observational

study involving 1,241 patients hospitalized for a cardiac event or cardiac surgery, researchers noted that a delay in the commencement of outpatient cardiac rehabilitation by more than 30 days was an independent predictor of decreased improvement in exercise performance.[82]

There are a variety of inpatient cardiac rehab programs, frequently progressive based on levels of increasing energy costs (e.g., MET levels). Each facility will establish its own levels and criteria for activity progression and education; an example of an inpatient program is shown in Table 13.11. Following are some general comments and recommendations about the various levels. It is important to note that activity progression occurs along a continuum and is not done in a rigid format. Although a patient must demonstrate the ability to sit at the bedside with appropriate hemodynamic response before ambulating in the hallway, the patient's individual response and medical history will dictate how quickly the patient is able to progress. A patient may progress through more than one level within any treatment session.

Table 13.9   Outcome Measures: Activity Limitations and Participation Restrictions in Patients With Cardiovascular Disease

Activity and Participation Limitation	Key Test/Measure
Activity—Cardiovascular Deconditioning	***Walk Tests:*** A variety of walk tests are used to assess endurance in the patients with cardiopulmonary compromise. Two such tests include the *6-minute Walk Test (6MWT)* and the *2-minute Walk Test (2MWT),* where a participant is asked to ambulate back and forth continuously on a premeasured walkway for 6 minutes or 2 minutes, respectively. **6MWT:** The American Thoracic Society has published guidelines for administering the 6MWT.[97] Shoemaker and colleagues report a minimal clinically important difference for the 6MWT in a patient with heart failure to be 45 m.[98] The researchers found that this change of 40–45 m is a change that is greater than the measurement error and correlated with improvements in aerobic capacity and health-related quality of life.[80] **2MWT:** In this test, the subject was asked to walk for 2 minutes. The total distance covered in 2 minutes is measured. The subject was allowed to use assistive devices when performing the test. Subject is asked to walk at a safe and comfortable pace. No verbal cues are provided during the test.
Activity—Cardiovascular Deconditioning	***2-minute Step Test:*** The 2MST was initially developed by Rikli and Jones when space limitation or weather prohibited the subject from performing a 6MWT or 2MWT.[99] Subjects are asked to attain a standing position near a wall, doorway, or next to a high-back chair or countertop. Because this is not a test of balance, the subject is allowed to hold on to a high countertop or chair for support. In this test, the subject is asked to step in place for 2 minutes. Stepping involved flexing the hip and the knee to a height that is midway between the iliac crest and the knee on the opposite side. Stepping on both sides, right and left, counts as a single step. The score recorded is the total number of correct height steps taken by one of the legs within 2 minutes. If the knee height can no longer be maintained, the participant is asked to stop, or to stop and rest until proper form can be regained. During rest intervals, the clock continues to run.
Activity—Cardiovascular Deconditioning	*Exercise Tolerance Tests (ETTs):* To examine the ability of the cardiovascular system to accommodate to increasing metabolic demand, an ETT, stress test, or graded exercise test is performed. The patient exercises through stages of increasing workloads, expressed in units of oxygen. Oxygen cost may be expressed in L/min, mL O_2/kg/min, kcal, or METs; the MET represents a factor of the basic systemic oxygen requirement at rest, roughly 3.5 mL O_2/kg/min. The most common modalities used in exercise testing of patients with cardiac impairments are the treadmill, bicycle, and arm ergometer (Fig. 13.21). The best indicator of an individual's aerobic capacity is through examination of the peak oxygen uptake or VO_2max and anaerobic threshold measured through use of a metabolic cart. When expensive equipment like a metabolic cart is not available, field tests such as the step test, bicycle tests, and walk tests can be useful in predicting the maximal oxygen consumption from the submaximal steady state heart rate.[53] A multitude of tests are available to quantify exercise capacity. An excellent resource for these tests is the *American College of Sports Medicine's Guidelines for Exercise Testing and Prescription.*
Activity—Decreased Balance	***Tests of Balance and Fall Risk:*** A variety of functional tests including the *Timed Up and Go Test, Berg Balance Test,* and 10-meter Walk Test measuring gait speed can be utilized in assessing a patient's balance and fall risk.
Activity—Decreased Mobility	***Activity Measure for Post-Acute Care (AM-PAC):*** The AM-PAC is an outcome measure that assesses function in three major domains: basic mobility, daily activities, and applied cognitive.[100] The primary goal for the development of this measure was to create a single measure to effectively measure function across all care settings within the continuum of care following an acute-care stay. The AM-PAC is a patient-reported outcome measure and therefore captures the patient's perspective. The measure is available in two basic formats: a computer-based version and a short-form version.

Table 13.9	Outcome Measures: Activity Limitations and Participation Restrictions in Patients With Cardiovascular Disease—cont'd
Activity and Participation Limitation	**Key Test/Measure**
Activity— Decreased Mobility	***Mobility Measures in Post-Acute Care:*** Depending on the care setting, a variety of measures exist to document a patient's activity and functional status including the *Functional Independence Measure (FIM)* commonly used in inpatient rehabilitation facilities, the *Minimum Data Set (MDS)* used in skilled nursing facilities, and the *Outcome and Assessment Information Set (OASIS)* that is primarily used in home care (see Chapter 7).
Participation— Quality of Life	***Minnesota Living With Heart Failure Questionnaire (MLHFQ):*** The MLHFQ is a patient self-assessment of how heart failure affects a patient's daily life. It was developed by Thomas Rector in 1992 and since then has been used in multiple research investigations as a measure of quality of life in patients with heart failure. The approximate time to complete the questionnaire is 5–10 minutes. The content reflects most frequent and important ways heart failure affects patients' lives. All items are assessed on a 1–5 Likert scale. Sum of item responses allows for total and individual dimension scores. The test–retest/reproducibility assessed by Rector and colleagues is a Pearson correlation of 0.87.[101] Internal consistency measured by Cronbach's alpha for all items is 0.92[101] The minimally important difference is five points on the total score.[101] In addition, the estimated standard error of the measure is six to seven points.
Participation— Quality of Life	***Seattle Angina Questionnaire (SAQ):*** The SAQ is an outcome measure that is utilized to assess the impact of angina in a patient's quality of life within the previous 4 weeks of the assessment date.[102] The survey uses 19 items to assess the severity of limitations in everyday life. There are two distinct sections of the survey—the impact of angina on the patient's ability for completing ADLs and a second section involving several questions that assess the patient's health conditions. The measure has been a validated disease-specific health status instrument for CAD with high test–retest reliability, predictive power, and responsiveness. However, its use has been limited by its length (19 items). Therefore, in 2014 a short version (seven items) was developed, tested, and validated to increase the feasibility of measuring patient-reported outcomes in patients with CAD.

ADLs = activities of daily living; CAD = coronary artery disease; MET = metabolic equivalent.

Phase II Cardiac Rehabilitation

Exercise prescription parameters traditionally utilized in phase II outpatient cardiac rehabilitation programs are presented in Table 13.12.

Interventions for Patients With Heart Failure

Exercise-based rehabilitation in the management of patients with HF continues to revolutionize in the 21st century. More recently, two seminal papers published in the *Physical Therapy Journal* collectively encapsulate the evidence related to HF rehabilitation research.[53,83] The first, a clinical practice guideline, disseminates nine systematically developed statements that assist physical therapists in making informed decisions on treatments for the management of patients with HF. Two algorithms coupled with action statements pertaining to aerobic exercise, strength training, high-intensity interval training, inspiratory muscle training, and the use of

neuromuscular electrical stimulation provide a holistic approach to the management of patients with HF.[83] Table 13.14 provides a summary of the exercise-based recommendations developed from the clinical practice guidelines.

Note that most of the exercise-based research in HF has involved patients with reduced EF in the stable state of their disease. An unfortunate mismatch exists between the phenotypic characteristics of subjects studied in clinical trials and the complex, multimorbid nature of patients typically seen in physical therapists' clinical practice.[84] In light of this mismatch, a second knowledge translation paper was subsequently published by the clinical practice guideline development group to increase the utilization of evidence in clinical practice and maximize guideline-directed care.[53]

This HF knowledge translation proposes a clinically oriented five-step ABCDE (Assessment, Behavior Modification, Cardiorespiratory fitness testing, Dosing, Education) model to assist physical therapists in

Figure 13.21 Estimated oxygen requirements for step, bicycle, and treadmill. The standard Bruce protocol begins at 1.7 mph and 10% grade (roughly 5 METs). Oxygen requirements increase with progressive increases in workload for all modalities. *(Adapted from Fletcher et al., p. 156.)*

Metabolic equivalents, step test, bicycle ergometer, and Bruce/Cornell treadmill protocols

Clinical status bands (overlapping ranges): Healthy dependent on age, activity; Sedentary healthy; Limited; Symptomatic.

Functional Class	O2 Cost ml/kg/min	METS	Step Test Height (cm)	Bicycle Ergometer KPDS	Bruce MPH	Bruce %GR	Cornell MPH	Cornell %GR
Normal and I	56.0	16			5.0	18	5.0	18
Normal and I	52.5	15					4.6	17
Normal and I	49.0	14					4.2	16
Normal and I	45.5	13			4.2	16		
Normal and I	42.0	12	40	1500			3.8	15
Normal and I	38.5	11	36	1350				
Normal and I	35.0	10	32	1200	3.4	14		
Normal and I	31.5	9	28	1050			3.0	13
Normal and I	28.0	8	24	900			2.5	12
Normal and I	24.5	7	20	750	2.5	12	2.1	11
Normal and I	21.0	6	16	600			1.7	10
II	17.5	5	12	450	1.7	10		
III	14.0	4	8	300	1.7	5	1.7	5
III	10.5	3	4	150	1.7	0	1.7	0
IV	7.0	2						
IV	3.5	1						

Bruce: 3-min stages (additional high stage MPH 5.5 / %GR 20).
Cornell: 2-min stages.
Step Test: Nagle Balke Naughton — 2-min stages, 30 steps/min, step height increased 4 cm q 2 min (height for 70 kg body weight).
Bicycle Ergometer: 1 watt = 6 kpds; for 70 kg body weight.

Balke-Ware (% grad at 3.3 mph, 1-min stages)

% grade: 26, 25, 24, 23, 22, 21, 20, 19, 18, 17, 16, 15, 14, 13, 12, 11, 10, 9, 8, 7, 6, 5, 4, 3, 2, 1

ACIP (2-min stages; first 2 stages 1 min)

MPH	%GR
3.4	24
3.1	24
3	21
3	17.5
3	14
3	10.5
3.0	7.0
3.0	3.0
2.5	2.0
2.0	0

mACIP (2-min stages; first 2 stages 1 min)

MPH	%GR
3.4	24
3.1	24
2.7	24
2.3	24
2	24
2	18.9
2	13.5
2	7
2	3.5
2	0

Naughton (2-min stages)

%GR (2 MPH)	%GR (3 MPH)	%GR (3.4 MPH)
17.5	32.5	26
14	30	24
10.5	27.5	22
7	25	20
3.5	22.5	18
0	20	16
	17.5	14
	15	12
	12.5	10
	10	8
	7.5	6
	5	4
	2.5	2
	0	

Ware (2-min stages)

MPH	%GR
3.4	14.0
3.0	15.0
3.0	12.5
3.0	10.0
3.0	7.5
2.0	10.5
2.0	7.0
2.0	3.5
1.5	0
1.0	0

Table 13.10 Research on Effectiveness of Cardiac Rehabilitation Programs

Researcher, Journal, Year	Outcomes
Buckley et al. Journal of the American Heart Association; *2021*	Exercise-based cardiac rehabilitation among patients with incident A-fib to be associated with lower odds of all-cause mortality, rehospitalization, and incident stroke at 18-month follow-up.[103]
Powell et al. British Medical Journal; *2018*	A systematic review of 22 studies including 4,834 patients with CHD found no difference in all-cause mortality (19 studies; $n = 4,194$; risk difference 0.00, 95% CI −0.02 to 0.01, $P = .38$) or cardiovascular mortality (nine studies; $n = 1,182$; risk difference −0.01, 95% CI −0.02 to 0.01, $P = .25$) in patients who participated in exercise cardiac rehabilitation compared to those who did not participate in exercise.[104]
Gabrys et al. Sports Medicine; *2021*	A German database of 54,163 patients with CHD found exercise-based phase III cardiac rehabilitation to be independently associated with reduced mortality and reduced loss in working capacity.[105]
Ekblom et al. European Journal of Preventive Cardiology; *2022*	In a total sample of 20,895 patients from the SWEDEHEART registry, exercise-based cardiac rehabilitation was significantly associated with reduced total mortality and more pronounced in women, compared with men.[106]
Lawler and colleagues, American Heart Journal; *2011*	Systematic review revealed that exercise-based cardiac rehabilitation has favorable effects on cardiovascular risk factors, including smoking, blood pressure, body weight, and lipid profile.[107]
Dibben and colleagues, Cochrane Database of Systematic Reviews; *2021*	A Cochrane Review and meta-analysis of 85 trials that randomized 23,430 people with CHD with a median follow-up of 12 months delineated that cardiac rehabilitation reduced risk of MI, a likely small reduction in all-cause mortality, and a large reduction in all-cause hospitalization, along with associated health-care costs and improved health-related quality of life up to 12 months' follow-up.[108]

CHD = coronary heart disease; CI = confidence interval; MI = myocardial infarction.

Table 13.11 Inpatient Cardiac Rehabilitation Program

CCU—Essentially Bedrest	Level 2
Level 1	1.5–2 METs
1–1.5 METs	• Sitting 15–30 min, 2–4 times/day
• Evaluation and patient education	• Leg exercises
• Arms supported for meals and ADLs	• Commode privileges
• Bed exercises and dangle with feet supported (if CK levels have peaked and patient has no complications)	• Reclining upright chair
Education	• Limited ADL
• Introduction to inpatient cardiac rehab and role of physical therapy	• Electric razor
• Education	• Limited supervised room ambulation for small uncomplicated MI
• Monitored progression of activity	Education
• Home exercise/activity guidelines/outpatient cardiac rehab	• Identification of CAD risk factors
Sitting—Limited Room Ambulation	• Concept of "healing interval" and need to pace activities
	Room—Limited Hall Ambulation

(Continued)

Table 13.11	Inpatient Cardiac Rehabilitation Program—cont'd

Level 3

2–2.5 METs
- Room or hall ambulation up to 5 min as tolerated three to four times per day
- Standing leg exercises optional*
- Sit on side of bed or in bathroom to wash (per discretion nurse/PT)
- Manual shave
- Bathroom privileges
- Independent or assisted ambulation in room or hall as advised by PT

Education
- Size of infarct and how it relates to the need for gradual resumption of activities
- Impact of exercise on reducing the patient's risk factors
- Teach use of Borg's Scale for Rating of Perceived Exertion and appropriate parameters with activity

Progressive Hall Ambulation

Level 4

2.5–3 METs
- Hall ambulation 5–7 min as tolerated three to four times per day
- Standing trunk exercises optional*
- Independent or assisted ambulation in hall as advised by PT

Education
- Teach pulse taking and appropriate parameters with activity
- Reinforce benefits of outpatient cardiac rehabilitation

Progressive hall ambulation

Level 5

3–4 METs
- Hall ambulation 8–10 min as tolerated
- Arm exercises optional*
- Standing shower
- Independent hall ambulation as advised by PT

Education
- Written home exercise/activity guidelines reviewed
- Patient given written information on outpatient cardiac rehab

Stair Climbing

Level 6

4–5 METs
- Progressive hall ambulation as tolerated
- Full flight of stairs (or as required at home) up and down one step at a time†

Education
- Answer patient's questions
- Check for understanding of activity guidelines

Patient Outcome—No Evidence of Hemodynamic Compromise With Activity Progression (All Levels)

No systolic drop in BP greater than 10 mm Hg or increase greater than 30 mm Hg
No HR increase greater than 12 if beta blocked, or no HR increase greater than 20 if not beta blocked
No complaints of dizziness, light-headedness, or angina
Perceived exertion less than 13/20

Hemodynamic Monitoring

Level 1

- HR and BP before and after supine bed exercises
- Orthostatic signs supine and dangling at bedside

Level 2

- Orthostatic signs (supine, sit, and stand) before exercises and transfer
- HR and BP after leg exercises/transfer to chair
- HR and BP after return to bed

Levels 3–6

- HR and BP in sitting and standing prior to activity
- HR and BP immediately following activity
- HR and BP 5 min after activity

From Rehabilitation Services Department, Newton Wellesley Hospital, Newton, MA, with permission.
ADL = activities of daily living; BP = blood pressure; CAD = coronary artery disease; CCU = coronary care unit; CK = creatine kinase; ETT = exercise tolerance test; HR = heart rate; MET = metabolic equivalent; MI = myocardial infarction; PT = physical therapist.
*Optional exercises are at the discretion of the PT and may be used to establish the patient's cardiovascular response in the room, prior to moving on to more challenging hallway ambulation; or in those patients who require general strengthening exercises.
†Stair climbing activities should take place after the ETT if the scheduling of the ETT permits. Otherwise, patients may, at the discretion and supervision of the PT, climb stairs on the day prior to the ETT.

Table 13.12	Exercise Prescription Parameters Utilized in Outpatient Cardiac Rehabilitation Programs
Condition	**Parameters**
Mode	Utilize large muscle groups, aerobic forms of exercise including walking, jogging, cycling, rowing, stepping, arm ergometry, and other endurance activities. Must be enjoyable to maximize compliance.
Frequency	A minimum of three times a week but preferably must be carried out most days of the week.
Duration	Variable, but most research utilizes a duration of 12 weeks of exercise training.
Components	• A 5–10-minute warm-up that involve stretching, flexibility movements, and aerobic activity is beneficial in allowing for an incremental increase in heart rate. • Conditioning phase of 30–45 minutes of aerobic exercise with a minimum 20 minutes of exercise. • A 5–10-minute cool-down phase to promote venous return and avoid adverse consequences post-activity including post-exercise hypotension, angina, ischemic ST-T changes, and ventricular arrhythmias.
Intensity	• Aim for 40%–85% of functional capacity (VO$_2$max), corresponding to 55%–90% of maximal heart rate. • THR usually determined by the Karvonen method. THR = Resting Heart Rate + % intensity (symptom limited heart rate maximum – resting heart rate). • Prescribed based on RPE based on the Borg RPE scale (Table 13.13). The Borg's RPE is a measure scale where the patient rates their level of exertion during the activity on a scale of 6–20. This scale is a validated method that most patients can learn and apply easily and is extremely valuable during bouts of unsupervised exercise.
Progression	Progression of intensity is individualized based on several factors including patient tolerance, symptoms, motivation, and goals.
Resistance Training	Resistance exercises are traditionally prescribed based on the individual's measured or estimated maximal strength or the "1RM." General strength prescription on available studies indicates a training intensity 30% and 80% of the 1RM. Exercises are performed for 12–15 repetitions per set, performed two to three times each week. Higher intensity resistance exercise (≥70% 1RM) are more effective in increasing muscular strength and neural adaptations than low-intensity exercise.[109]

1RM = one-repetition maximum; RPE = rating of perceived exertion; THR = target heart rate.

applying the evidence into patient/client management. This easy-to-use paradigm was developed in the context of other knowledge and social norms to facilitate the application of the evidence in clinical practice. In this five-step model, physical therapists are encouraged to incorporate a formal assessment of stability, address behavior modification, test cardiorespiratory fitness, select and dose skilled interventions, and educate patients on disease management during any episode of care in the holistic management of patients with HF.

■ EDUCATION FOR PATIENTS WITH HEART DISEASE

For patients with heart disease, patient and family education develops along a continuum, depending on the patient's baseline status and readiness to attend to the information. The physical therapist, along with other members of the health-care team, must determine the patient's and family's ability to understand and adhere to the information. Appropriate discharge or ongoing outpatient topics to be addressed include the following:

1. *Activity Guidelines.* Patients (and family) need to be able to understand specific activity guidelines, which include planned exercise sessions as well as leisure time and rests.
2. *Self-Monitoring.* Patients may monitor the intensity of their activity in a variety of ways; two of the more common ways are palpating a pulse and rate of perceived exertion (RPE). Because many older patients have decreased sensitivity in their palpation skills, the use of RPE may be easier and more reliable. Those patients who can take a

Table 13.13	Rating of Perceived Exertion: The Borg Rating of Perceived Exertion Scale*
6	No exertion at all
7	
8	Extremely light
9	Very light
10	
11	Light
12	
13	Somewhat hard
14	
15	Hard (heavy)
16	
17	Very hard
18	
19	Extremely hard
20	Maximal exertion

*Copyright Gunnar Borg. Reproduced with permission.
For correct usage of the scale(s), the exact design and instructions given in Borg's folders must be followed. See Borg G. *Borg's Perceived Exertion and Pain Scales.* Human Kinetics; 1998.

pulse or choose to invest in an HR monitor may prefer to use these methods. A variety of wearable devices exist to assist patients in monitoring HR and rhythm. Self-monitoring involves not only HR or the Borg RPE Scale but also awareness of other symptoms or signs that may suggest exercise intolerance, such as light-headedness, mental confusion, dyspnea, and inability to carry on a brief conversation while performing an activity. Patients with CHF commonly use the dyspnea scale and the Borg RPE Scale.

3. *Symptom Recognition and Response.* Being able to recognize their specific cardiac symptoms and know how to respond is a key component in patient education. Patients should have written information regarding the action they should take when symptoms occur, for example, when to call their physician or go to the hospital. Angina is the most common symptom associated with CHD, whereas weight gain (2 lb in 24 hours or greater than 5 lb in a week), dyspnea, LE edema, and increased pillows for sleep are common signs and symptoms for HF exacerbation. The traffic light approach developed by the Agency for Healthcare Research and Quality can be used to assist patients in recognizing relevant symptoms of decompensation and appropriate actions to take based on their symptomatology.[85]

This tool provides the patient with criteria that place them in a red, yellow, and green state based on presenting signs and symptoms. Figure 13.22 is an adaptation of this tool and provides physical therapists with a graphic that can be utilized to help patients self-assess signs and symptoms of HF decompensation and take appropriate actions based on their symptomatology. Patients in the red zone need immediate medical care, while patents in the yellow zone need to contact their physician for a possible change in medications. Absence of signs and symptoms related to HF exacerbation places patients in the green zone, where they are safe to continue activity and exercise.

4. *Nutrition.* Patients commonly meet with a nutritionist to discuss their usual dietary habits and to make recommendations when needed for a more heart-healthy diet. Most commonly, patients with heart disease are instructed to reduce fat intake; patients with CHF are instructed to monitor salt and fluid intake. Today, physical therapists are challenged to change a culture marked by incessant marketing of sugars and calorie-rich foods. Appropriate nutritional counseling and collaboration with a nutritionist can tremendously help patients reduce their weight and consume a heart-healthy diet. Berner and colleagues summarize the best known screening tools for general health, diet, and nutrition, and provide useful intervention strategies that can be used to support behavior change related to diet and nutrition.[86]

5. *Medications.* Patients receive written information regarding the desired action of their medications, potential side effects, dosage, and timing of medications. Patients should also know which nonprescription drugs such as cold, sinus, allergy, or anti-inflammatory medications they should avoid because of possible interactions with prescription drugs. Patients should also be encouraged to disclose all herbal remedies and supplements that they may be taking.

6. *Lifestyle Issues.* Many factors influence whether a patient will return to work after a cardiac event. Many patients with heart disease need to return to work if they were employed before their event.

7. *Sexual Activity.* Resumption of sexual activity may be an uncomfortable discussion for some patients. There may be many issues of concern for the patient (e.g., fear, anxiety, performance concerns, lack of libido). Patients and their partners are encouraged to verbalize their concerns to each other and seek appropriate information from their health-care team. Some medications (e.g., beta blockers) may blunt the sexual response, and it is important that patients communicate this with their physician. Often, another medication or category of medication may be better tolerated. When patients

Table 13.14   Exercise Interventions Utilized for Patients With Heart Failure

Intervention	Parameters/Dosage	Benefit
Continuous Moderate Aerobic Exercise	For patients with stable, NYHA class II–III HFrEF use the following parameters: • Time: 20–60 minutes • Intensity: 50%–80% of peak VO_2 or peak work • Frequency: three to five times per week • Duration: at least 8–12 weeks • Mode: treadmill or cycle ergometer or alternate approaches like dancing	Significant improvement in peak VO_2 proportional to training intensity where higher training intensities yield greater changes in peak VO_2, improved health-related quality of life, reduced all-cause and HF-related hospital admissions and hospital days.
High-Intensity Interval Training	For patients with stable, NYHA class II–III HFrEF use the following parameters: • Time: greater than 35 total minutes of 1–5 minutes of high intensity (>90%) alternating with 1–5 minutes at 40%–70% active rest intervals, with rest intervals shorter than the work intervals • Intensity: greater than 90% of peak VO_2 or peak work • Frequency: two to three times per week • Duration: at least 8–12 weeks • Mode: treadmill or cycle ergometer • Total weekly high-intensity exercise dose should be at least 460 kcal, 114 min, or 5.4 MET-hr	Improved peak VO_2 above that achieved with moderate-to-vigorous intensity continuous exercise training. Adverse events were not different compared to controls and other exercise training intensities.
Resistance Training	For patients with stable, NYHA class II–III HFrEF, use the following parameters: • Time: 45–60 minutes per session • Intensity: 60%–80% 1RM, two to three sets per muscle group • Frequency: three times per week • Duration: at least 8–12 weeks	Significant improvements in aerobic capacity, 6MWD, health-related quality of life, and muscle strength.
Inspiratory Muscle Training	For patients with stable, class II and III HFrEF with or without baseline inspiratory muscle weakness, use a threshold inspiratory muscle trainer or similar device: • Time: 30 min/day or less if using higher training intensity (>60% MIP) • Intensity: greater than 30% MIP • Frequency: 5–7 days/week • Duration: at least 8–12 weeks	Improved MIP, sustained MIP, exercise capacity measured by peak VO_2 and 6MWD.
Neuromuscular Electrical Stimulation	For patients with stable NYHA class II–III HFrEF using the following parameters: • Time: 30–60 minutes per session • Waveform: biphasic symmetrical pulses at 15–50 Hz • Intensity: on/off time 2/5 sec, pulse width for larger muscles of the LE should be 200–700 us and for small LE muscles 0.5–0.7 ms, 20%–30% of MVC, intensity to muscle contraction • Frequency: 5–7 days/week • Duration: at least 5–10 weeks	Improved muscle strength and endurance, Peak VO_2, 6MWD, and health-related quality of life. No adverse events attributable to the NMES intervention throughout the available evidence. Patients did experience mild self-limited cramps or muscle soreness.

6MWD = 6-min walk distance; HF = heart failure; HFrEF = heart failure with reduced ejection fraction; LE = lower extremity; MIP = maximum inspiratory pressure; MVC = maximal voluntary contraction; NMES = neuromuscular electrical stimulation; NYHA = New York Heart Association.

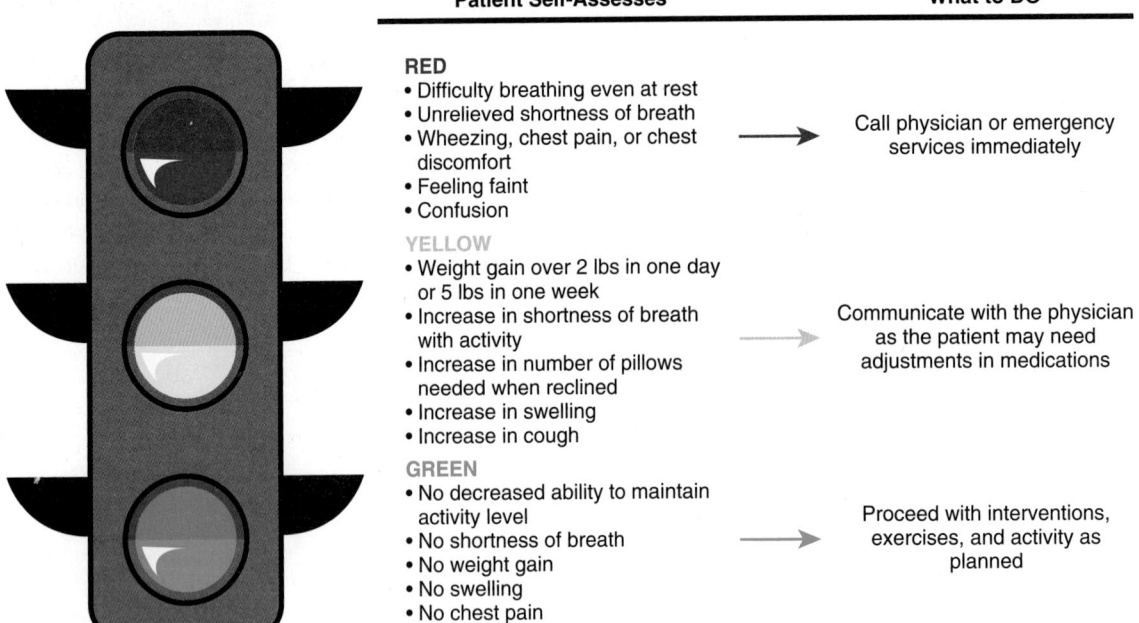

Patient Self-Assesses	What to DO
RED • Difficulty breathing even at rest • Unrelieved shortness of breath • Wheezing, chest pain, or chest discomfort • Feeling faint • Confusion	Call physician or emergency services immediately
YELLOW • Weight gain over 2 lbs in one day or 5 lbs in one week • Increase in shortness of breath with activity • Increase in number of pillows needed when reclined • Increase in swelling • Increase in cough	Communicate with the physician as the patient may need adjustments in medications
GREEN • No decreased ability to maintain activity level • No shortness of breath • No weight gain • No swelling • No chest pain	Proceed with interventions, exercises, and activity as planned

Figure 13.22 Patient self-assessment tool for heart failure decompensation.

feel ready for sex, their energy level throughout the day is satisfying for them, and they can walk outdoors and climb stairs comfortably, they are probably ready for sexual activity. It may be helpful for patients to remember that sexual activity is not unlike other physical activity with respect to energy cost, and therefore, planning, pacing, and warm-up are powerful contributors for a more comfortable outcome. In some cases, the physician may recommend taking prophylactic NTG before sexual activity.

Box 13.5 outlines suggested topics for patient, family, and caregiver education and counseling from the U.S. Department of Health and Human Services Clinical Practice Guidelines for Patients with CHF.

■ PSYCHOLOGICAL/SOCIAL ISSUES

Cardiac disease may not only create new emotional issues but also enhance some that might have existed before the cardiac event. Physical therapy practitioners need to understand the psychosocial aspects of each patient, including personality styles and coping skills. They need to recognize stages of psychosocial adaptation and help patients to progress in their own adjustment. Therapists can play an important role in reassuring patients that many of these issues are normal sequelae of their event and in encouraging patients to seek guidance and counseling in whatever arena they feel appropriate (e.g., counseling, religion).

Box 13.5 Suggested Topics for Patient, Family, and Caregiver Education and Counseling

Self-Management

- Signs and symptoms of worsening heart failure
- Plan of action if symptoms worsen
- Self-monitoring techniques including with daily weights
- Lifestyle changes

Prognosis

- Life expectancy
- Advance directives

Activity Recommendations

- Recreation, leisure, and work activity
- Exercise

Dietary Recommendations

- Sodium restriction
- Fluid restriction (if required)
- Alcohol restriction

Medications

- Effects of medications
- Dosing and Adherence
- Likely side effects and what to do if they occur
- Availability of lower-cost medications or financial assistance

In more severe cases of generalized anxiety or depression, referral to a mental health practitioner is warranted (i.e., psychiatrist, psychologist). The therapist should utilize an integrated patient-/client-centered approach, working together with patients to develop goals, outcomes, and a POC that is congruent with their needs, values, and level of functioning. See additional discussion in Chapter 26, Psychosocial Issues in Physical Rehabilitation.

■ PRIMARY PREVENTION OF CORONARY ARTERY DISEASE

In the contemporary management of patients with heart disease, physical therapists are strongly encouraged to not only treat patient impairments and mobility restrictions but also focus on public health initiatives related to primary and secondary prevention. Patients who do not have documented CAD but who have identifiable risk factors should be encouraged to adopt lifestyle behaviors that can modify their risk factors. Health education and primary prevention programs through individualized education and exercise guidelines attempt to modify an individual's risk factors and thereby prevent CAD. The AHA has a comprehensive primary prevention guideline document that provides clinicians with a simple ABCDE approach to incorporating prevention into clinical practice. These include A—Use of aspirin and other antiplatelet therapy; B—BP control; C—Cholesterol reduction and Cigarette cessation; D—Diet, weight, and Diabetes management; and E—Exercise and Economic and social factors.[87]

Patients are instructed in appropriate dietary guidelines, including low fat, adequate fiber, minerals and vitamins, and decreased salt, particularly if the patient has high BP. Besides lowering total dietary fat, patients are instructed to decrease their percentage of saturated fats and avoid trans-fatty acids. Elevated levels of the amino acid homocysteine appear to increase the risk of arterial endothelial disease. Folic acid, a B vitamin, lowers homocysteine levels. If weight loss is needed, patients are encouraged to see a nutritionist to design a sensible eating plan.

The physical therapist HF clinical practice guidelines encourage all physical therapists to advocate for a culture of physical activity.[83] In general, for patients with cardiovascular diseases, several professional organizations including the AHA and the U.S. Department of Health and Human Services recommend 150 min/week of moderate-intensity physical activity (e.g., brisk walking) or 75 min/week of vigorous-intensity physical activity (e.g., running or jogging), or an equivalent combination.[87,88]

Modification of all CAD risk factors is key to the success of any primary prevention intervention. Patients are encouraged to identify risk factors and to seek resources to assist in modifying them. There are many community-based smoking cessation programs or medically supervised programs that a patient might explore. Stress management programs are also varied and can be adapted to the individual's needs. Proper and consistent use of any medications that might be used in controlling risk factors, such as antihypertensives, antihypercholesterolemics, blood glucose–lowering agents (hypoglycemics), and antianxiety agents or antidepressants, is crucial to the success of any program.

SUMMARY

Physical activity is important for all individuals and is especially beneficial for those individuals diagnosed with CAD and HF. Individuals with heart disease should understand that a consistent exercise program is part of the management for their disease and is as necessary as their medications. Having heart disease means that the person needs to understand the parameters in which they may safely participate in activity either recreationally or as a prescribed exercise. The role of the physical therapist is to provide a safe exercise prescription for all patients.

During the time of illness, the effects of decreased activity can be devastating. A paradox exists, however, in that the less activity that is done, the less activity can be done because of a decreased work capacity. Therefore, the relative energy cost of all activity increases, and the heart works harder for any given task. Not encouraging the patient to resume activity when the patient is medically stable is a disservice. As physical therapists, our role is clear: to understand the pathophysiology of the disease process, to accurately examine the patient, and to establish a safe POC. The ultimate goals and outcomes of a successful rehabilitation program are to improve the patient's physiological response to exercise, decrease the work of the cardiovascular system, improve overall level of activity and participation, and improve quality of life.

It goes without saying that through purposeful patient education, use of behavior modification techniques, appropriate guideline-directed management, and effective partnership within the multidisciplinary team, physical therapists can achieve the vision of the American Physical Therapy Association of transforming society to improve the human experience for patients with heart disease.

Questions for Review

1. Discuss key differences between an NSTEMI and a STEMI.
2. Differentiate the three different types of angina. How would you instruct your patient in symptom recognition?
3. Discuss sternal precautions that you would instruct your patient to use following a median sternotomy procedure.
4. Describe the use of the evaluation triad in the evaluation of patients with ACS.
5. Describe differences between compensated and uncompensated CHF.
6. Discuss appropriate goals, education, and treatment interventions for patients with ACS in phase I cardiac rehabilitation.
7. Discuss appropriate goals, education, and treatment interventions for patients with ACS in phase I cardiac rehabilitation.
8. Discuss appropriate goals and treatment guidelines for patients with CHF.

CASE STUDY

A 58-year-old man presents to the local emergency department (ED) with chief complaint of SOB and difficulty sleeping last night; patient had to sit up all night to make symptoms even a little better. Patient came to the ED because he was unable to get ready for work owing to increased SOB. Patient reports that he has felt SOB off and on for a couple of months, usually associated with physical activity; symptoms, however, usually resolved with rest. Today's episode was the first related to sleeping.

PAST MEDICAL HISTORY
- CAD: anterior MI 4 years ago
- Hypercholesterolemia
- PVD

MEDICATIONS
- Digoxin, captopril, furosemide (Lasix), diltiazem, simvastatin (Zocor)

FAMILY/SOCIAL
- Patient works full time as an engineer; travels 3 to 4 days per month.
- Married, lives with his wife in a two-story home on a 2-acre lot; three college-aged children.
- Patient is an avid golfer; enjoys gardening and landscaping.

PHYSICAL EXAMINATION
- Heart sounds: S_1, S_2 normal; S_3 present, no S_4; 2/6 systolic murmur
- Lung sounds: crackles 1/3 way
- Rhythm/rate: irregular, 140 bpm
- BP: 100/60 mm Hg
- Respiratory rate: 26 breaths/min
- SaO_2: 90%
- Jugular venous distention: 5 cm
- Echocardiogram: akinetic apex, akinetic distal septum and anterior wall; dilated atria and LV
- Chest x-ray: unavailable

CASE STUDY—cont'd

LABORATORY DATA

- Enzyme pending; CBC WNL except BUN and creatinine slightly elevated.
- BNP: 900 pg/mL.
- Patient remained in the hospital for 2 days while medications were adjusted. During this time patient underwent further testing, including an ETT.

RESULTS OF ETT

- Bruce protocol: 4 min; estimated VO_2max; 20 mL O_2/kg/min (approximately 6 METs); max vital signs: 130 bpm HR; 120/60 mm Hg BP
- ECG: (–) negative for ischemia, chest pain
- Reason for stopping: absolute exhaustion
- Examination immediately post-ETT: (+) S_3
- Physical and occupational therapy were requested to assist with exercise guidelines and discharge planning

PATIENT'S GOALS

- Return to work.
- Resume hiking.
- Begin to prepare his garden for spring planting within the next 5 weeks.

PHYSICAL THERAPY INTERVENTION

- Exercise tolerance via low-level exercises sitting and standing, as well as 5-minute walk.

VITAL SIGNS

- Sitting (rest): HR 90 bpm; BP 110/60 mm Hg
- Sitting exercises: HR 108 bpm; BP 110/60 mm Hg
- Standing (rest): HR 110 bpm; BP 108/60 mm Hg
- Standing exercise: HR 116 bpm: BP 110/60 mm Hg
- 5-minute walk: 1,000 ft; HR 120 bpm; BP 116/60 mm Hg

HOME INSTRUCTIONS

- Meetings planned with patient and his family to discuss discharge guidelines over the next 4 to 8 weeks.

FOLLOW-UP

- Patient returns to his primary care provider 3 months after discharge. Echocardiogram is unchanged with EF 30%. Patient states that he has been following discharge guidelines.

VITAL SIGNS

- HR 100 bpm; BP 116/70 mm Hg (resting).
- Patient states that he feels great and just wants to get on with his life.

GUIDING QUESTIONS

1. What is a reasonable presenting diagnosis? Identify each piece of information (and how you interpreted it) that you used to make this diagnosis.

2. Explain the pathophysiology of the patient's presenting symptoms. Discuss the significance of his HR and heart rhythm in relation to his symptoms.

3. If the patient's symptoms and signs worsened, and he was admitted to the coronary care unit (CCU):
   a. What would you expect these signs/symptoms to be that would bring the patient to the CCU?
   b. What might be a reasonable cause of his signs/symptoms worsening?
   c. What other drugs/interventions might be given in the CCU?

4. What rhythm do you think the patient is in and why? What do you think might be a reason that he is in this rhythm?

(Continued)

CASE STUDY—cont'd

5. What do you think the chest x-ray would look like and why?

6. What is your interpretation of the patient's vital sign response to PT intervention? What is your plan for your next session?

7. What exercise prescription would you recommend for the patient at home (modality, intensity, duration, frequency)?

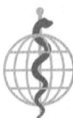

For additional resources, including answers to the questions for review, new immersive cases, case study guiding questions, references, and more, please visit **https://www.fadavis.com/product/physical -rehabilitation-fulk-8**. You may also quickly find the resources by entering this title's four-digit ISBN, 4691, in the search field at **http://fadavis.com** and logging in at the prompt.

Vascular, Lymphatic, and Integumentary Disorders

Tamara N. Gravano, PT, DPT, MSPT, EdD
Brian J. Wilkinson, PT, DPT, CHT, CLT
Deborah G. Kelly, PT, DPT, MSEd, CLT-LANA

Chapter 14

LEARNING OBJECTIVES

1. Understand basic concepts about the anatomy, physiology, and pathophysiology of the vascular, lymphatic, and integumentary systems.
2. Describe wound physiology related to normal and abnormal wound healing.
3. Recognize the characteristics and risk factors of common disorders of the vascular, lymphatic, and integumentary systems.
4. Identify the components of a comprehensive examination of a patient with a disorder related to the vascular, lymphatic, and/or integumentary systems.
5. Analyze and integrate wound examination data to complete the physical therapy evaluation.
6. Interpret the rationale for skin and wound care treatment with particular attention to moist wound healing, arterial wound hydration, venous wound compression, lymphedema treatment, and foot care for the patient with diabetes.
7. Design an appropriate plan of care for an individual with a vascular, lymphatic, and/or integumentary disorder.
8. Using the case study example, apply clinical decision-making skills and contemporary evidence to design a plan for a patient requiring advanced wound care.

CHAPTER OUTLINE

ANATOMY AND PHYSIOLOGY OF THE VASCULAR, LYMPHATIC, AND INTEGUMENTARY SYSTEMS *470*
  Vascular System *470*
  Lymphatic System *470*
  Integumentary System *471*
WOUND PHYSIOLOGY *471*
  Normal Wound Healing *471*
  Abnormal Wound Healing and Management of a Chronic Wound *476*
VASCULAR, LYMPHATIC, AND INTEGUMENTARY DISORDERS *478*
  Arterial Insufficiency and Ulceration *478*
  Venous Insufficiency and Ulceration *479*
  Lymphedema *481*
  Pressure Injuries *482*
  Neuropathy *484*

EXAMINATION AND EVALUATION *485*
  Examination *485*
  Evaluation *494*
INTERVENTION *494*
  Coordination, Communication, and Documentation *495*
  Patient-/Client-Related Instruction *495*
  Procedural Interventions *495*
  Dressings *508*
  Manual Lymphatic Drainage *512*
  Compression Therapy *512*
  Positioning *517*
  Pressure-Redistributing Devices *517*
  Exercise *517*
  Orthotics *518*
  Scar Management *519*
SUMMARY *520*

Patients and clients with disorders of the vascular, lymphatic, and integumentary systems have complex and often interrelated health problems that must be recognized by their providers before healing can occur. In recent years, options for intervention have expanded significantly, empowering the physical therapy provider with challenging and rewarding clinical treatments for clients. This chapter offers foundational material on which to build sound, evidence-based clinical decisions. Though interrelated, the systems discussed have unique characteristics and functions. This chapter facilitates understanding of the separate systems and then illustrates how the systems are intricately and essentially related. The elements of examination and the intervention strategies for all disorders are combined to ensure that the overlapping health conditions, body functions and structures, environmental factors, and personal factors will be addressed and considered in the plan of care (POC) to positively affect participation and engagement in activities. In this text, information about thermal injuries is complementary and supplemental to the information in this chapter.

ANATOMY AND PHYSIOLOGY OF THE VASCULAR, LYMPHATIC, AND INTEGUMENTARY SYSTEMS

In the microscopic world of circulation, blood and lymph vessels permeate most tissues, carrying oxygen and nutrients while removing carbon dioxide and other waste products. Not all vessels involved are the "large tubes" often associated with the circulatory system. Capillaries are woven throughout most of the tissues of the body; they are found around muscle fibers, through connective tissues, and below the basement membrane of the epithelium.[1] Since arteries and veins are too large and too thick to allow diffusion between the bloodstream and surrounding tissues, a delicate network of blood and lymph capillaries controls all chemical and gaseous exchange between blood, interstitial fluid, and lymph.[1] In the normal system, homeostatic mechanisms adjust blood flow across the capillary walls to meet the needs of adjacent peripheral tissues. Consistently, new information is uncovered each year that further elucidates the complexities of the circulatory system and how it interacts with the other systems of the body. It is essential to understand the delicate vessels that carry blood to the peripheral tissues and the typical processes to prime an understanding of the disorders discussed later in the chapter.

Vascular System

Arterial System

Arteries carry rich, oxygenated blood away from the heart, branching off into sections with smaller diameters called *arterioles,* leading ultimately to microscopic capillaries. Arteries have three-layered walls that give them strength and elasticity. The walls of arteries are generally thicker than those of veins because they have to withstand intense blood flow pressures generated by the powerful circulation influenced by the heart. Arteries are strong and durable, keeping their cylindrical shape when stretched. The movement of blood through arteries is dependent on heart function. Arteries can change in diameter when the volume of blood passing through them changes. They can also change in diameter when the sympathetic division of the autonomic nervous system is triggered, either contracting (*vasoconstriction*) or relaxing (*vasodilation*). Because they have contractile abilities, arteries do not need valves to affect blood flow. Understanding these terms and concepts is necessary as this chapter discusses peripheral vascular disease, capillary blood flow, and wound healing.

Venous System

Veins return oxygen-depleted blood from tissues and organs back to the heart. At the beginning of the venous system, superficial blood capillaries empty into venules that carry blood toward medium-sized veins (about the size of muscular arteries). Superficial veins run above the fascia of the muscles; deep veins run below the fascia. Perforating veins run between the superficial and the deep, penetrating the fascia to connect the superficial and deep vessels. Veins also have three-layered walls, but they do not need to be as muscular or elastic as arteries because the blood pressure in veins is lower than in arteries. Venous walls are so thin that they do not hold their shape well under stress, collapsing or tearing when stretched.

As blood moves through the outermost regions of the body (the peripheral vascular system), from the arteries to the veins, blood pressures decrease. The blood pressure in the medium-sized veins is so low that it cannot oppose the force of gravity without structural assistance.[1] In the limbs, medium-sized veins contain *valves* that project from the inner walls of the veins, oriented in the direction of blood flow. Under normal conditions, the valves allow blood to flow in only one direction, preventing the backflow of blood. When the valves are working normally, any movement that compresses or pulls on a vein will help with the return of blood back toward the heart. Skeletal muscle contraction will squeeze venous blood toward the heart. The act of walking helps to empty veins and move blood out of the lower extremities (LE). When the walls of veins weaken or become enlarged, the valves cannot function properly, and blood pools in the veins. Eventually, the veins become distended, leading to varicose veins. If a valve or valves do not close properly, this leads to a condition known as *venous reflux.* These terms and concepts are important as the chapter discusses chronic venous disease and LE swelling.

Lymphatic System

Although parallel and working in concert with the venous system, the lymphatic system is separate and unique. Because of its many roles and diffuse locations throughout the body, anatomists classify the lymphatic system as parts of the immune system, circulatory system, and integumentary system. The two primary functions of the lymphatic system are to protect the body from infection and disease via the immune response and to facilitate the movement of fluid back and forth between the bloodstream and the interstitium, removing excess fluid, blood waste, and protein molecules in the process of fluid exchange. *Lymphatics* are located in all portions of the body except the central nervous system and certain portions of the eye.[2] The lymphatic system includes lymph vessels (superficial, intermediate, and deep; also referred to as *lymphatics*), lymph fluid, and lymph tissues and organs (lymph nodes, tonsils, spleen, thymus, and Peyer patches).

Lymph fluid, also called *lymph,* is first absorbed at the capillary level, channeled through small vessels called *precollectors,* and finally picked up by the larger, valved vessels called *collectors.* A collector is composed of individual lymph segments known as *lymphangions.*

The collectors have contractile properties, smooth muscle, and valves. Lymphatics are even thinner and more likely to collapse under pressure than veins.[2–4] Lymph moves throughout the body by several mechanisms. Superficially, the process of diffusion and filtration moves lymph fluid. Below the dermis, intrinsic contractions within the vessels drive lymph propulsion in the deeper collectors. Drainage depends on the contraction of the valved lymph segments that create a pumping force. Classic literature reports information about lymph flow, but new knowledge about the lymphatic system is continually expanding.[4–10] The human body is wonderfully equipped to provide a variety of stimuli that have an impact on lymphangion contraction:

- parasympathetic, sympathetic, and sensory *nerve stimulation*
- *contraction of muscles* adjacent to a vessel
- *pulsation of arteries* adjacent to a lymph vessel (even precapillary arterioles have pulsation)
- abdominal and thoracic cavity pressure changes that occur during *breathing*
- *volume changes* within each lymphangion (internal receptors respond to tension and trigger a contraction)
- *mild mechanical stimulation* of dermal tissue, such as *manual lymphatic drainage* (MLD) techniques, increases frequency of lymphangion contractions

Excess lymph fluid is transported through the thoracic duct and emptied into the venous angles at the left and right jugular vein trunks. Under normal conditions, lymph flow is not adversely affected by gravity. Under abnormal conditions such as morbid obesity or *chronic venous insufficiency* (CVI), the lymphatic system may exhibit excess lymph pooling related to gravity, especially in the LE.

Integumentary System

Also referred to as an *organ,* the integumentary system, of all the body systems, is the most frequently visualized and palpated structure by a physical therapy provider. The integumentary system has a functional relationship with many other body systems. The health of this system is dependent on the normal functions of the arterial, venous, and lymphatic capillaries (dermal circulation). A thorough review of the functions of the skin illustrates the importance of even a small area of damage to this organ. The discussion on skin anatomy, with diagrams, in this textbook, supplements the overview here. The *epidermis,* the outermost layer of skin, is avascular and water resistant. It provides protection from infection, abrasion, and chemicals and assists with heat regulation, retention, and dissipation. Melanocytes, which are present in this layer, determine skin color and protect from ultraviolet radiation. The epidermis regenerates rapidly, allowing individuals to heal quickly when conditions are normal. The *dermis* follows below the epidermis and is 20 to 30 times thicker than the epidermis. It contains blood vessels and lymphatics, nerves and nerve endings, and sensory neurons that supply the epidermis. The dermis also contains hair follicles, sweat glands, sebaceous glands, and nails. All of these components project through the epidermis to the surface of the skin. These appendages are a deep source of epithelial cells needed to resurface a wound during healing. The contents of the dermis are surrounded and supported by collagen, elastin, and ground substance that provide structure, strength, flexibility, and elasticity. The *hypodermis* (also referred to as the *subcutaneous layer*) is not part of the integument but is essential in stabilizing skin over skeletal muscles and organs. It consists of loose connective tissue and fat cells and provides insulation and protection to underlying structures. The hypodermis plays a vital role in the prevention of *pressure injuries,* especially over the ischial tuberosities and greater trochanters.

When there is an injury to the integument, some or all of the components of the integument are impaired, resulting in many possible sequelae such as decreased lubrication, loss of elasticity, increased scar formation, loss of tensile strength, reduced ability to resist infection, and increased or decreased sensitivity.

■ WOUND PHYSIOLOGY
Normal Wound Healing

In the human body, an elegant sequence of events ensures that wounds will heal when an injury occurs. Within the endogenous fluids of the body, every cell and chemical mediator is programmed and ready to act when needed. When conditions are normal, the body is equipped to heal itself.

Phases of Healing

The classic model of overlapping phases of wound healing describes a continuous process, its phases not entirely distinct. This chapter uses the model to draw attention to the normal process and provide guidelines for what can be expected in normal healing. The number of days to complete each phase varies based on factors such as age, size of the wound, comorbidities, continued trauma, nutrition, blood flow, medications, stress, and infection. The repair process is the same for all wounds, but the sequence will be much quicker in more shallow wounds with less tissue loss. In all stages of healing, wounded tissues are striving to achieve homeostasis. Italicized words in the following stress important concepts during each phase.

Inflammation (Phase I)

- Inflammation is the *normal* immune system reaction to injury.
- It is the *central activity* in wound healing.
- Temporary repair is initiated by coagulation (clotting factors, platelets) and *short-term decreased* blood flow.
- *Necrosis* occurs after cells have been injured or destroyed.

- The spread of pathogens is slowed: debris and bacteria are attacked by a host of cells. If the wound is acute, some periwound edema, erythema, and drainage can be expected. If fluid accumulates at the injury site, it is called *pus*.
- Oxygen is delivered via *increased* blood flow to keep the phagocytic cells alive and functioning.
- Permanent repair is facilitated by creating a clean wound, *setting the stage* for the next phase of healing; signals are generated that reepithelialization can begin.
- The time frame is day of injury to approximately day 10.
- The rate of the inflammatory process is affected by the size of the wound, blood supply, available nutrients, and extrinsic environment.
- If this phase is interrupted or delayed, *chronic inflammation can result*, lasting from months to years (see the "Abnormal Wound Healing and Management of a Chronic Wound" section).

Proliferation (Phase II)

- *New tissue* fills in the wound as fibroblasts secrete collagen.
- Skin integrity is restored by reepithelialization or contraction (see discussion later).
- Angiogenesis occurs: new blood vessel growth from endothelial cells and fragile capillary buds grow into the wound bed; new reddish, slightly bumpy tissue is called *granulation tissue*.
- Epithelial cells differentiate into type I collagen. *Collagen synthesis* occurs, but the resulting new scar tissue is fragile and must be protected; trauma during this phase may return the wound to the inflammatory process.
- The time frame is day 3 of injury to approximately day 20.
- The rate of proliferation is affected by the size of the wound, blood supply, available nutrients, and extrinsic environment.
- If this phase is interrupted or delayed, the result may be a chronic wound.

Maturation/Remodeling (Phase III)

- Maturation or remodeling of new tissue begins while granulation tissue forms during the prior (proliferative) phase.
- Epithelial cells continue to differentiate into type I collagen.
- New skin has *tensile strength* that is 15% of normal. Scar tissue is rebuilding but reaches 80% of original tensile strength at best.
- Underlying granulation tissue is replaced by *less vascular* tissue.
- In deep wounds, dermal appendages are rarely repaired (hair follicles, sebaceous and sweat glands, nerves) but instead are replaced by *fibrous tissue*.

- Over time, the scar tissue matures, changing from red to pink to white in light-skinned individuals, or in dark-skinned individuals it may appear hyper- or hypopigmented. Over time, scars should change texture from raised and rigid to flat and flexible.
- The time frame is approximately 9 days postinjury up to 2 years.
- Rate of maturation/remodeling is affected by the size of the wound, blood supply, available nutrients, and extrinsic environment.

The Role of Oxygen in Wound Healing

The need for oxygen to sustain life is apparent at the systemic and cellular levels of human physiology. Oxygen reaches the wound bed through blood flow to the area. When oxygenated blood flows to the tissues of the body, it is called *perfusion*. Wound contraction, collagen deposition, angiogenesis, and granulation are examples of wound healing steps supported by oxygen perfusion. As a safeguard, most cells in the wound environment have an enzyme that converts oxygen to a form that allows the cell to support wound healing.[11] Wound tissue oxygenation or perfusion is so crucial that it is a sensitive indicator for the risk of postoperative infection.[11,12] A decrease in oxygen availability in any wound results in an increased likelihood of infection. Wound perfusion may be limited for a variety of reasons, but the two most common problems are edema and necrosis. The presence of edema and/or necrotic tissue can make it more difficult for oxygen to reach the wound. Since compression can reduce edema and débridement can reduce the presence of necrotic tissue, these procedural interventions are important components of most wound care. Unless contraindicated owing to arterial disease, compression and débridement will assist wound oxygenation. Peripheral vasoconstriction can also limit wound perfusion. Problems with vasoconstriction cannot always be improved readily. Interventions that will increase wound perfusion and are appropriate for all individuals include keeping the wound area warm, avoiding smoking, hydrating the individual, and controlling pain and anxiety. Improvement of oxygen levels in wound tissue alone may trigger wound healing. Adequate oxygen levels will also enhance the effectiveness of growth factors and a host of other cells that require oxygenation to maintain their function. The delivery of exogenous oxygen is discussed later in the chapter in the "Hyperbaric Oxygen Therapy" section. The nutritional status of the individual, as discussed later, will also have an impact on oxygenation since hemoglobin, iron, vitamin B_{12}, and folic acid are needed to enable red blood cells to carry oxygen to healing tissues.

The Role of Moisture in Wound Healing

In the past, the goal of wound care was to create and maintain a dry wound, packed with dry dressings, dried by heat lamps, and exposed to the air. Modern wound management is based on the concept of creating and maintaining a *moist wound environment* to facilitate wound healing. More than 50 years ago, research confirmed that a dry wound creates an environment that is hostile to wound healing. A dry wound allows the formation of wound scab and *eschar*, which inhibit migration of epithelial cells, provide food for pathogens, and affect blood flow to the wound bed. A dry wound also allows cooling of the wound surface; without a protective barrier, the surface temperature of the wound is decreased, and healing is slowed. Adhesion of gauze or other dry dressings to the wound bed causes trauma to the wound bed and pain to the individual upon removal. As the wound dries through evaporation or by the removal of dry dressings, the rich endogenous fluids that contain the elements necessary for wound healing are significantly decreased or lost.

Wound management experts agree that adequate wound hydration is the most crucial external factor responsible for optimal wound healing.[11–16] Wounds are typically covered with an occlusive or semiocclusive dressing. This type of dressing is also called a *moisture-retentive dressing* because it retains fluids on the wound bed. There are many types and styles of dressings that will facilitate a moist environment (see the "Dressings" section for further discussion). Maintaining a moist wound with an occlusive dressing includes holding an appropriate amount of endogenous fluids on the wound, preserving the cells needed for healing and keeping them in contact with the wound bed. Some chronic wound fluid may contain substances that can delay healing, so a balance must be maintained between moisture and exudate removal.[17,18] Moisture softens wound scab and eschar; under the right conditions, the body's own enzymes dissolve the eschar in a process called *autolytic débridement*. Occlusive dressings help maintain the appropriate wound surface temperature to prevent delays in healing and protect the wound surface from trauma and bacteria and other contaminants.

Basic principles of moist wound healing include covering the wound with a barrier (occlusive dressing) that preserves adequate wound hydration; limiting fluid loss from the wound surface while the dressing is in place; allowing gaseous exchange; maintaining periwound integrity; controlling heavy *exudate;* and removing the dressing when exudate begins to leak out from the edges of the dressing.

It has long been believed that occlusive dressings should not be applied over infected wounds because trapped bacteria could fulminate. Studies have produced evidence that the opposite may be true in many cases.[17–20] Because in acute wounds, and some chronic wounds, endogenous fluids have bacteria-fighting chemical elements, evidence of colonized bacteria in the wound does not automatically preclude the use of occlusive dressings. Specially selected dressings such as hydrocolloids are a good choice in this situation.

With the use of a systemic antibiotic and a close watch for signs of change in the patient's symptoms, clinicians may be able to utilize occlusive or moisture-retentive dressings over some types of wounds that are infected. The use of this dressing technique may broaden if the evidence continues to build in strength. Meanwhile, there is ongoing investigation into the contents of chronic wound exudate and its power to break down growth factors and prolong the inflammatory phase of wound healing. Information on this level should guide the use of occlusive dressings in the chronic wound healing environment.[21,22]

Despite half a century of research to support the concepts of moist wound healing, there are still practitioners who ignore the evidence and utilize outdated methods of wound management. Clinicians must strive to educate patients, families, and all wound care team members about appropriate wound care concepts.

The Role of Nutrition in Wound Healing

It is well established that nutritional status can significantly impact wound healing. Adequate protein intake is required for collagen synthesis and the formation of new blood vessels and muscle tissue.[22] Literature abounds with information about critical nutritional issues such as the role of specific nutrients in wound healing, how poor nutritional status can delay wound healing, the use of particular pharmacological interventions, and appropriate routes for nutritional support (enteral versus parenteral). Newer literature supports the classic understanding that the function of nutrients is crucial to wound healing.[22–30]

Issues related to wound healing and nutrition are present across the life span. Pediatric patients in long-term care, recovering from surgery, or with wounds, burns, or trauma are at risk for pressure injuries.[31] As with adults, adequate protein intake is essential for timely healing. Another patient population of concern is aging adults, whose tissues may be fragile and whose immune systems are more easily compromised. Nutrition plays a role in the prevention and management of pressure injuries in this population as well.[27]

Nutrients that must be present for a wound to close and heal on time include iron, vitamin B_{12}, and folic acid (essential so that red blood cells can deliver oxygen to tissues), vitamin C and zinc (essential for tissue repair), vitamin A (essential to stimulate collagen cross-linking), and arginine (enhances healing and immune function).[28,29] High protein intake provides the amino acids required to build new tissue. Protein and calorie needs vary depending on the size of the wound and the medical condition of the patient. In response to the available information and the need for more research, nutrition and metabolic support for acutely and chronically ill patients is emerging as a key branch of medicine.

As part of the wound care team, a physical therapist will contribute to the plans for nutritional support of the patient. Clinicians will collect data through medical record review, observation, history taking, and dietary examination methods. Because exercise, hydration, and improved appetite often are interrelated, a physical therapist should pay close attention to a patient's activity level, strength, conditioning, and mobility issues while encouraging fluid and nutrient intake.

Wound Characteristics

Wound characteristics describe the physical appearance of the wound but may also provide clues to the cause of the wound, phase of healing, and likelihood of closure. The characteristics of wounds may be defined as dry, wet, or granulating. Wounds can also be defined by their etiology, such as diabetic, vascular, or traumatic. Wound characteristics can provide valuable information needed to make sound clinical judgments about treatment. For example, the location of the wound may prompt the clinician to select a particular dressing, change patient positioning, or prescribe orthotic footwear. Descriptions of wound characteristics in documentation can indicate progress (or failure to progress) toward closure and healing. Wound characteristics should be identified during the initial examination and then monitored at least weekly during the wound-healing phase. Depending on the etiology and chronicity of the wound, some characteristics may not be evident on initial examination but could appear later as complications of the wound healing process. The following characteristics should be tracked and documented throughout the phases of wound healing:

- *Location:* specific location on the body
- *Size:* depth, width, and length
- *Shape:* irregular versus distinct
- *Edges:* condition and shape of wound edges, evidence of premature healing
- *Tunneling, undermining, sinus tracts:* presence and depth
- *Base:* characteristics of the wound base compared to sides and edges
- *Necrotic tissue:* eschar, slough: amount, color, texture, adherence to wound bed
- *Exudate:* amount, color, consistency, odor
- *Granulation tissue:* presence or absence, estimated amount, location
- *Epithelialization:* presence or absence, premature or as expected
- *Exposed structures:* color and condition of any visible bone(s), tendon(s), or ligament(s)
- *Periwound area:* edema, inflammation, induration, maceration
- *Pain patterns:* aggravating and relieving factors (although not an observed characteristic, it is measurable and significant to the intervention)
- *Quantity of bacteria:* amount present in a wound; referred to as the *bioburden*

The quantitative biopsy is the gold standard for obtaining a wound culture, but it is not used universally owing to cost, lack of laboratory facilities, and potential pain for the patient.[9] A swab culture is often used as an alternative, but it is limited to detecting surface contamination, not tissue infection. Clinical intuition is also important in determining if infection is probable.

The examination will include data about the wound characteristics using observation, palpation, measurement, photography, and tracing. A clinician who is new to the wound care team should remember that these skills take practice to master.

Wound Closure

Primary Intention

Healing by primary intention occurs when a qualified health-care provider closes a wound by bringing the edges together. Approximating the edges can occur through the use of sutures, staples, glue, skin grafts, or skin flaps. Wounds closed by primary intention still pass through the phases of wound healing but usually in a shorter time span. A wound closed by primary intention that later reopens due to maceration or infection has opened by the process of *dehiscence* (Fig. 14.1). Following dehiscence, a wound is almost always allowed to close by secondary intention.

Secondary Intention

Closure and subsequent healing by secondary intention occurs when a wound is left open to heal on its own. The mechanisms of healing by secondary intention are

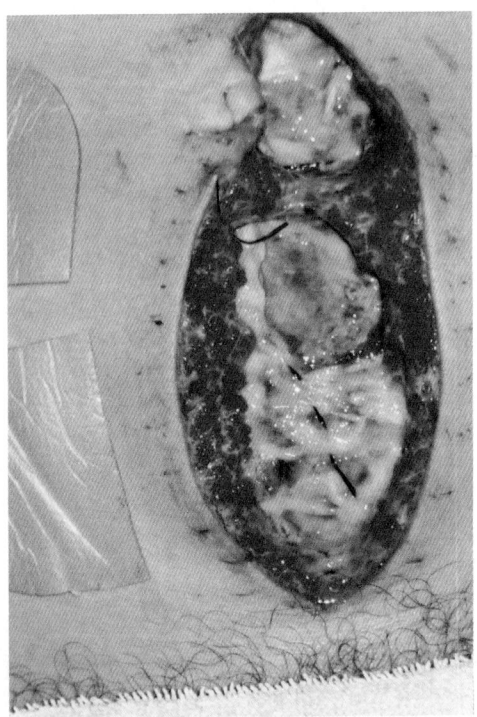

Figure 14.1 Wound dehiscence following appendectomy.

contraction, reepithelialization, or a combination of both. Deeper wounds heal by replacing injured tissue with scar tissue as collagen fills the wound bed.

Contraction occurs when growth factors trigger myofibroblasts to pull the wound edges inward. During the contraction process, existing tissue migrates, pulling the wound edges toward the center of the wound. This process forms no new tissue. New tissue may be forming in the wound simultaneously but not via contraction. Growth factors and myofibroblasts can be influenced positively or negatively by physiological factors such as the amount of oxygen and nutrients available and by mechanical factors such as external compression and the shape of the wound. Even though contraction is a normal occurrence in certain types of wound healing, it can cause disfiguring scars and impaired tissue function if it is too rapid. Since there is a centripetal movement of the entire thickness of the surrounding skin, tissue elongation may not keep up with the pace of contraction, causing significant functional and cosmetic deformity. Clinicians should intervene by applying specific types of pressure to the tissues to slow the deforming forces of contraction. (Scar management is discussed later in the chapter.)

Epithelialization is another response used by the body to close a wound. As noted in the phases of normal wound healing, chemical mediators send signals for reepithelialization to begin in phase I (the inflammatory phase). Actual repair begins in phase II when new tissue is formed to cover the wound. Growth factors stimulate specialized epithelial cells, called *keratinocytes,* to begin to migrate from the edges of the wound toward the center. In partial-thickness wounds in which the dermal appendages have not been destroyed, the cells will also migrate from the hair follicles, sebaceous glands, and sweat glands. In more minor, shallower wounds, this process may be triggered to begin as early as 12 hr after wounding. In more significant wounds, it may be 10 days or longer before the cells begin to migrate. In a chronic wound, there are many reasons why this process is not triggered or is interrupted. (See discussion under "Abnormal Wound Healing and Management of a Chronic Wound.")

When epithelial cells meet at the center of the wound, the wound is covered with new skin, migration ends, and cells will stop dividing. This is referred to as *contact inhibition.* At the time of contact inhibition or full reepithelialization, wound *closure* has occurred. Wound *healing,* however, may continue for several years beneath the surface of the skin as the tissue undergoes reorganization. A significant amount of intervention is still required to support the wound successfully from "closed" to "healed" status. A physical therapist will provide routine surveillance and specific interventions for the many possible sequelae of a wound. When a wound is closing and healing by secondary intention, the rate

of closure and the physiology of closure are impacted by a number of factors that a clinician will monitor and document:

- *Wound shape:* linear wounds (surgical) contract most rapidly; circular wounds (pressure injuries) contract most slowly.
- *Wound depth:* all things equal, the shallower the wound, the quicker is the closure.[30–32]
  - *Superficial* (loss of the epidermis): this type closes by reepithelialization.
  - *Partial thickness* (loss of the epidermis and dermis): this type closes primarily by reepithelialization with minimal contraction.
  - *Full thickness* (loss of all layers of the epidermis, dermis, and deeper structures): this type closes by contraction and scar formation; however, epithelial cells will migrate from the wound edges to assist in wound closure if the environment is homeostatic.
- *Wound location:* areas with least pressure, most perfusion (face) will close more rapidly than areas with most pressure, least perfusion (sacrum, heel).
- *Wound etiology:* least traumatic (surgery) will close more rapidly than most traumatic (pressure injury, burn).

As deeper wounds heal, the wound is filled with tissue, but the repair process does not replace lost muscle, fat, or dermis with those same tissue types. Instead, the wound is filled with scar tissue made up primarily of collagen, which is laid down in a somewhat disorganized fashion to quickly replace lost tissue and structural integrity of the skin. As the wound enters the maturation and remodeling phases, the collagen is reorganized along the lines of stress. Because the original tissue is not replaced with more of the same, a wound that is closed and finally healed does not return to its prototypical prewounded state. This concept is particularly important to understand the position on reverse staging of pressure injuries as described in the "Tests and Measurements" section. Understanding this concept is key when planning protection, positioning, patient education, footwear, and exercise programs for individuals with all types of wounds, whether they are acute, closed, healed, or chronic wounds.

Tertiary Intention

Also called *delayed primary,* this type of closure occurs when a wound is allowed to heal by secondary intention and then is closed by primary intention as the final treatment. The delay in primary closure is usually due to treatment of a present infection prior to closing the wound. Closing a wound with an infection leads to abscesses and further tissue damage beneath the skin's surface. Therefore, the infection must be resolved prior to closure.

Abnormal Wound Healing and Management of a Chronic Wound

A chronic wound results when the sequence of events that leads to normal wound closure and healing does not occur. The characteristics and causes of chronic wounds vary owing to the diverse nature of individuals with wounds, their medical histories, and the etiologies of the wounds. Even if the chronic wound moves through the classic phases of wound healing, it does so in an abnormal manner. Vital actions and reactions necessary for wound healing are interrupted, stunted, or absent in the chronic wound.

Although the characteristics of abnormal wound closure and healing may be varied, concepts can be used to illustrate the failure of a wound to pass through phases of wound healing in a timely manner. The following discussion highlights what may happen if there is an interruption to any of the classic phases of wound healing:

- *Inflammation (Phase I):* If there is inadequate blood flow and oxygen supply to support cellular life and activity, cells may not initiate the repair sequence. Debris and bacteria may collect if not removed, and pathogens spread more rapidly. Bioburden increases and may facilitate infection.
- *Clinical signs:* An increase in the amount of drainage, change in color or odor, lingering swelling, eschar/necrosis from ischemic conditions, periwound maceration, chronic inflammation, *tunneling, undermining,* and infection may develop if the host's immune system is unable to resist the impact of the bacterial load.
- *Proliferation (Phase II):* If collagen synthesis is delayed in this phase, skin integrity will be poor. If angiogenesis is delayed, there will not be enough myofibroblasts to initiate wound contraction. The need for oxygen and nutrients will be very great, and without them, available cells will be unable to reproduce rapidly, resulting in delayed epithelialization.
- *Clinical signs:* Keratinocytes do not migrate when the wound bed is not moist, healthy, clean, and granulating. Epithelial cells may attempt to migrate from the wound edges, but without a wound bed that is ready, they will build up at the wound edge and may migrate over the edge, forming a lip that curls under, called epibole. Epibole is formed via contact inhibition. Contact inhibition occurs when the migrating skin cells meet similar skin cells and stop growing. This contact inhibits further migration because the cells have reached their goal. However, with epibole, the skin cells did not traverse the wound bed but actually rolled under itself and made contact with itself. Once this occurs, the epithelialization phase ends, even though the wound is still open. Furthermore, granulation tissue is either absent, pale, or delayed; new tissue is weak and breaks down or bleeds easily; tunneling, eschar, and periwound maceration may be evident. Necrosis, if it has not

been removed, will delay angiogenesis. Changes in drainage color, amount, odor, or lingering swelling may signal a return to the inflammation stage.
- *Maturation/remodeling (Phase III):* If the synthesis and lysis of collagen are out of balance, weakened tissue will break down easily, or hypertrophic scarring will build up too rapidly.
- *Clinical signs:* Newly formed skin breaks down with little provocation, or scar tissue may build up within the outline of the original wound (hypertrophic) or beyond the margins of the original wound (keloid).

Infection in Wound Healing

Wound infection is a potential problem for any individual. Infection may turn life threatening if the patient is frail or critically ill. Regardless of the condition of the individual, wound infection is detrimental to wound closure and healing time. Bioburden has a greater impact on wound healing than most underlying medical conditions.[33] True infection is identified if the presence of bacteria or microorganisms is greater than 10^5 per gram of tissue determined by a quantitative culture. This determination can only be made with a biopsy. Surface swabs that are cultured may or may not be conclusive for actual infection since there are many types of bacteria that exist on the skin all the time.

The effects of infection include the following:

- Inefficient cellular activity, decreased collagen metabolism, chemical mediators absent or dilute, cells absent or confused by lack of direction from chemical mediators, and presence of other cells (When the bioburden is greater than 10^5 organisms per gram of tissue, epithelialization may not occur.)
- Decreased oxygen in the wound bed; insufficient oxygen to support the regeneration of tissue and to assist in the prevention of infection
- Increased rate of cell necrosis
- Overall decline of body systems; contributes to strain on the specialized cells
- Risk of wound sepsis, osteomyelitis, gangrene
- Signs of potential infection
- Change in wound drainage (amount, color, consistency, odor)
- Swelling disproportionate to wound size
- Periwound redness, darkening, or warmth (less obvious with darker skin)
- Increase in pain or tenderness
- Change in the quality of granulation tissue or failure to produce quality tissue (may be pale, soft, easily broken down)
- No measurable wound contraction within 2 to 4 weeks
- Tissue culture/punch biopsy results of greater than 10^5 organisms per gram of tissue
- Fever, nausea, fatigue, loss of appetite

Clinicians should use a structured approach to identify clinical infections. Careful identification of infection may help avoid the risk of antibiotic overuse.[34] The punch biopsy is the gold standard for confirming infection, but a physical therapist should watch for the early signs of infection: *warmth, redness/darkening, swelling, fever, malaise,* and *loss of appetite.*

Factors Contributing to Abnormal Wound Healing

The factors or triggers contributing to abnormal wound healing are varied but can be placed into broad categories for better understanding. Most abnormal wound healing will be influenced by factors from all the categories. Treatment intervention that addresses factors from one category and not the others will be incomplete.

Intrinsic Factors

Intrinsic or internal factors are conditions within the body that may contribute to abnormal healing. These factors relate primarily to the wound and periwound areas and include aging skin and inadequate blood flow or decreased oxygen supply from an underlying disease. As the integument ages, there is a decrease in moisture content leading to an increase in brittle quality and a delay in the renewal time affecting the stratum corneum. *Rete pegs,* undulations between contact layers of the epidermis and dermis (the papillary layer), become less functional with an increased risk of shearing.

Changes in the dermis include a decrease in elasticity, collagen, and mast cell production, along with a reduction in the vascularity and number of pain receptors. Available fat in the subcutaneous layer begins to resorb during aging, decreasing protection against pressure and shearing. Finally, certain comorbidities and underlying disease are intrinsic factors that may affect acute and chronic wound healing. The more common conditions known to affect healing are diabetes, cancer, circulatory insufficiencies, HIV infection, and connective tissue diseases.

Extrinsic Factors

Extrinsic or environmental factors are those influences that come from outside the body. The medical professionals caring for a person with a wound may be able to moderate the impact of extrinsic factors on the wound environment. Examples of extrinsic factors include the effects of radiation therapy or chemotherapy; incontinence; medication, smoking, recreational drugs, and alcohol (all slow or eliminate cellular reactions needed for healing); dehydration and malnutrition (both slow the delivery of oxygen to wound tissues); bioburden/infection (healing is slowed by pathogens, necrotic tissue, granulomas); and stress (negative effects of stress can lead to impaired healing).[32,35–40]

Iatrogenic Factors

Iatrogenic refers to any injury or illness that occurs as the result of medical care. Theoretically, these factors are under the control of the medical professionals who care for the patient and are therefore preventable. Factors include, but are not limited to, poor wound management, frequent disruption of the wound through inappropriate cleansing, use of inappropriate dressings and dressing techniques, use of cytotoxic topical agents that lead to inefficient cellular activity, and lack of moisture resulting in delayed or absent migration of keratinocytes. Frequent dressing changes not only disturb the fragile surface of the wound but will also slow wound healing by reducing wound temperature. It can take more than 30 minutes for a wound to return to normal temperature after a dressing change. Infection can be an iatrogenic factor when caused by cross contamination, improper use of gloves and other protective devices, inadequate use of sterile and clean technique, lack of proper hand washing, and lack of adherence to standard precautions.[41] Other iatrogenic factors that contribute to abnormal wound healing include shear injuries (skin tears) that occur during transfers and repositioning and ischemia from unrelieved pressure owing to inadequate turning schedules or absent or inadequate *pressure-redistributing devices* (PRDs).

Complications of Chronicity

A chronic wound creates a complex and serious health problem for an individual (Fig. 14.2). Chronic wounds may lead to complications, including any or all of the following: impairments of body function and structures, restrictions in activities and participation, need for assisted living or home care, decreased quality-of-life perceptions, depression, infection, malnutrition and

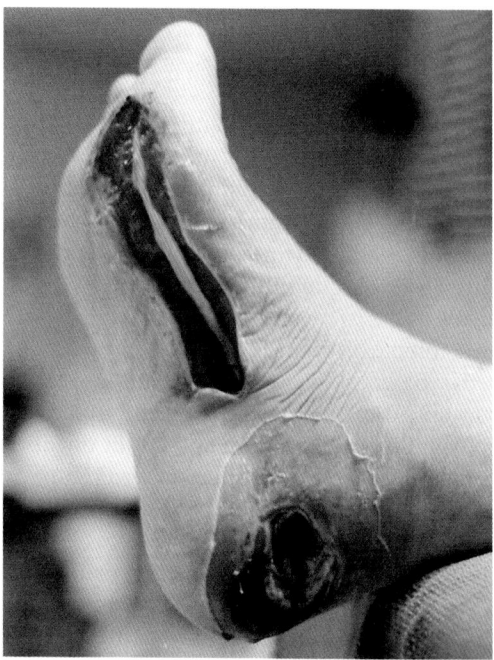

Figure 14.2 Chronic wound as a result of diabetic neuropathy.

weight loss, protein depletion, tissue fibrosis, loss of limb, and death. Every year millions of Americans are treated for chronic wounds at a cost of billions of dollars, making this type of wound one of the most costly challenges in health care. A chronic wound that fails to close and heal because of an underlying pathology will not progress readily until the cause is corrected or improved. The clinician must determine the factors contributing to abnormal wound healing and then develop an appropriate POC to overcome or address the obstacles.

■ VASCULAR, LYMPHATIC, AND INTEGUMENTARY DISORDERS

Arterial Insufficiency and Ulceration

The term *arterial insufficiency* refers to a lack of adequate blood flow to a region or regions of the body. Many different disorders may arise from arterial insufficiency and can be classified by a variety of descriptors. For the purposes of this chapter, references will pertain to arterial insufficiency owing to organic disruption of blood flow to the extremities or to *peripheral vascular disease* (PVD). PVD is a general term used to describe any disorder that interferes with arterial or venous blood flow of the extremities. PVD caused by arterial insufficiency may be related to smoking, cardiac disease, diabetes mellitus, hypertension, renal disease, and/or elevated cholesterol and triglycerides. Obesity and a sedentary lifestyle are related contributors in this disease process and its associated vessel obstruction. When several of these factors are combined, as they often can be, the possibility of health problems is considered inevitable. The damage caused by these factors is reflected in structural changes in the walls of the arteries, causing abnormal blood flow. The following is a brief overview of disorders that occur with abnormal arterial blood flow:

- *Arteriosclerosis:* thickening, hardening, and loss of elasticity of arterial walls.
- *Atherosclerosis:* the most common form of arteriosclerosis, associated with damage to the endothelial lining of the vessels and the formation of lipid deposits, eventually leading to plaque formation.
- *Arteriosclerosis obliterans:* a peripheral manifestation of atherosclerosis characterized by *intermittent claudication (IC)*, rest pain, and trophic changes. This is the arterial disease most likely to lead to ulceration. Known risk factors for development of the disease are smoking, diabetes mellitus, hypertension, hyperlipidemia, and hyperhomocysteinemia.
- *Thromboangiitis obliterans* (Buerger disease): inflammation leads to arterial occlusion and tissue ischemia, especially in young biological males who smoke.
- *Raynaud disease:* a vasomotor disease of small arteries and arterioles that is most often characterized by reversible pallor and cyanosis of the fingers.

In some cases, both the hands and feet may be affected. The cause of Raynaud disease is unknown, but attacks are usually triggered when the affected area comes into contact with a cold stimulus or during a period of emotional distress.
- *Ulceration*: a peripheral sign of a long-standing disease process; by definition, arterial ulcers are associated with arterial insufficiency.

Between 10% and 30% of LE ulcers are caused by arterial disease.[42] The incidence of arterial disease and LE ulceration is significantly lower than that for venous disease and ulceration; however, arterial wounds more frequently lead to loss of limb and death due to ischemia associated with the condition. These important facts signal the significance of taking a thorough history, performing a systems review, and conducting adequate skin inspection during the initial visit with any individual who might have arterial disease.

Clinical Presentation

- Wounds will most frequently be located on the distal LEs: lateral malleoli, dorsum of feet, toes.
- When wounds are present on an ischemic limb, atherosclerotic occlusion of the peripheral vasculature is almost always present.
- The majority of patients with arterial insufficiency also have diabetes mellitus.
- Trophic changes are present and include abnormal nail growth, decreased leg and foot hair, and dry skin.
- Skin is cool upon palpation.
- Wounds are painful, and the patient may also describe pain in the legs and/or feet (see later discussion in the "History" section). Pain may be increased when an affected extremity is elevated.
- Wound base is usually necrotic and pale, lacking granulation tissue.
- Skin around the wound may be black, mummified (dry gangrene).
- Other signs of arterial insufficiency will be evident: decreased pulses, *pallor* on leg elevation, and *rubor* when dependent.

History

Painful cramping or aching of the LEs during walking is commonly reported by patients with chronic arterial occlusion of the LEs. The pain is caused by IC that occurs when exercising muscles are not receiving the blood perfusion needed for normal function. Patients should be examined for other signs of arterial insufficiency if IC is occurring. Rest pain that develops at night, awakens the patient, or requires analgesics for relief is considered more severe than claudication. The individual with vascular dysfunction may also be diabetic. Diabetes mellitus may contribute to slower healing times and difficulty fighting infection. A wound in a distal, ischemic area is not likely to close or heal on time unless the vascular supply is enhanced or restored. Individuals with arterial disease and diabetes mellitus are more likely to have hypertension and may have previous bypass grafts or amputations of the toes, pain on ambulation or rest, pain with LE elevation, cold hands and feet, and color changes of fingers and toes. Owing to the long latency period between injury to the arterial circulation and clinical appearance of impairments, health-care providers, families, caregivers, and patients must collaborate to effectively optimize the quality of life for these patients through education, prevention, and vigilance.

Tests and Measurements

One of the most important screening tests for individuals with arterial disease is performed using a handheld Doppler ultrasound unit to measure blood flow to the LEs. The readings are calculated, and the end result is called the *ankle-brachial index* (ABI). Results provide useful information about the status and potential loss of perfusion in the LEs. Refer to "Arterial Perfusion" in the "Tests and Measurements" section under "Examination and Evaluation."

Intervention

If ulceration is present, intervention should enhance chemical and gaseous homeostasis in the wound bed, facilitate superficial blood flow to target tissues, and educate patients about the importance of facilitating blood flow to the extremities. Treatment will include appropriate wound care as well as important adjuncts to wound care. Results of the ABI will guide the therapist and referring practitioner in the appropriate use of compression. In a diagnosis of mixed arterial and venous disease, the condition that is more severe should be prioritized. If the arterial condition is worse, compression may be inappropriate even when edema is present. A nonhealing wound on an ischemic limb can lead to gangrene, amputation, further amputation, and/or loss of life (Fig. 14.3). In the most severe cases, conditions

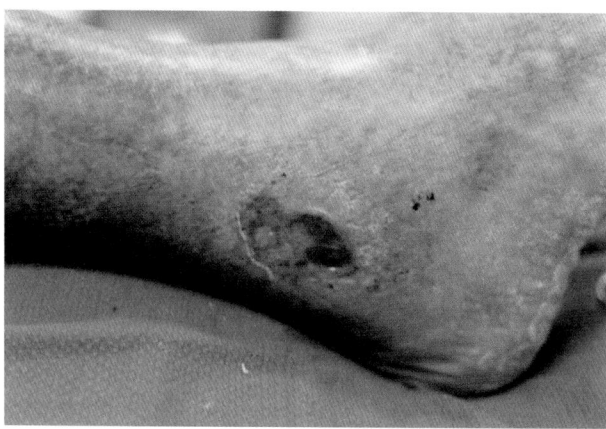

Figure 14.3 Clinical presentation of arterial insufficiency.

for wound healing are inhospitable to wound closure, and chances for closure are poor. In this case, necrotic tissue should not be debrided, since the dead tissue will not be replaced with new tissue. Skin grafts may not adhere to the virtually lifeless ischemic wound bed. Antibiotics cannot reach the wound systemically, and topical agents are too superficial to stop infection. At this point, vascular surgery may be an option for some individuals. A bypass graft may be used to restore arterial circulation to the ischemic tissue. For others, living with a chronic nonhealing wound or coming to terms with amputation are the only options. Most experts agree that the most important intervention in PVD is prevention of smoking. The second most important intervention is exercise for weight control. Exercise will also improve collateral circulation, lipid profiles, and management of hypertension. A physical therapy provider plays a crucial role in wound care for patients with arterial wounds and should address patient education and exercise in the intervention plan.

Venous Insufficiency and Ulceration

Venous insufficiency refers to inadequate drainage of venous blood from a body part, usually resulting in edema and/or skin abnormalities and ulcerations. Though there is no agreement on the definition of a chronic wound, the diagnosis of CVI refers to venous insufficiency that has been present for at least several weeks. The majority of individuals with PVD are diagnosed with CVI. An ulcer due to CVI is deemed to be chronic if it persists anywhere between 4 weeks and 3 months with stalled healing. CVI is the most common cause of LE ulcers.[43] In current literature, venous insufficiency is synonymous with venous hypertension, defining the beginning of a chain of pathophysiological events that often result in ulceration. Some authors still use the term *venous stasis ulcer,* but it has been shown that blood stasis (blood pooling) is not the cause of these wounds.[44-47] Although it is clear that ulcerations are the result of inadequate venous circulation, the mechanism by which this happens is not fully understood. Research has focused on how skin breakdown is affected by dysfunction of circulating white blood cells (WBCs), endothelial cell dysfunction, fibrin deposition, edema, and lymphatic congestion.[48,49]

The incidence of venous ulceration is much higher than that of arterial ulceration (Fig. 14.4). In fact, 80% of all LE ulcers are caused by venous disease.[42] The higher incidence is not clearly understood even though years of clinical and laboratory research have been devoted to understanding venous disease. The path from CVI to ulceration can take many turns. Aging, lack of exercise, obesity, pregnancy, long hours of sustained standing or sitting, heredity, and history of deep vein thrombosis (DVT) will predispose an individual to venous hypertension and subsequent CVI.[49]

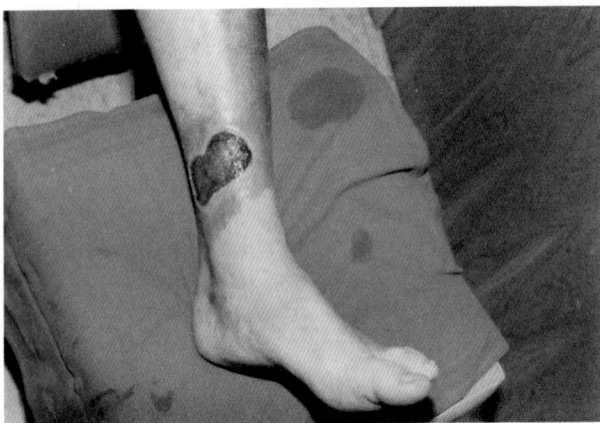

Figure 14.4 Venous insufficiency with leg ulcer.

Clinical Presentation

- Swelling of unilateral or bilateral LEs, relieved in the early stages by elevation
- Complaints of itching, fatigue, aching, heaviness in involved limb(s)
- Skin changes including *hemosiderin staining* and *lipodermatosclerosis*
- *Fibrosis* of the dermis
- Increase in skin temperature of lower legs
- Wounds:
  - Most frequently located on the LEs: proximal to the medial malleolus although can occur anywhere (arterial wounds may also occur at this location).
  - Not significantly painful; usually complaints of minor dull leg pain are relieved with elevation.
  - Granulation tissue is usually present in the wound bed.
  - Tissue is *wet* from a typically large amount of draining *exudate.*
  - Signs and symptoms of lymphedema may be present. (It is common to see the impact of chronic inflammation and fluid overload as triggers for the onset of lymphedema.)

History

Because the incidence of CVI increases with age, clinicians should be suspicious of the disease in older patients. The slow development of venous disease and ulceration usually implies a history of lingering swelling, slow healing, repeated infection, and frequent recurrence of skin breakdown. Once ulceration occurs, venous wounds can exist for years. This progression of symptoms frequently leads to a mechanical overload of the lymphatic system and subsequent development of lymphedema. If the individual is older than age 50 years, it is likely there are comorbidities such as diabetes mellitus, hypertension, congestive heart failure (CHF), or a history of DVT. Owing to the long latency period between injury to the venous circulation and clinical manifestations, health-care providers, patients, families, and caregivers must collaborate using the tools of education, prevention, and vigilance.

Tests and Measurements

With the exception of mixed arterial and venous disease, the vascular examination results for patients with venous insufficiency will show strong distal pulses and a normal ABI. On palpation, the skin temperature of the lower leg may be elevated. This sign can imply a worsening or impending complication of CVI.[50–52] The use of instrumentation to measure skin temperature can be invaluable during the examination; measuring skin temperature will be covered later in this chapter. Existing edema may decrease with elevation unless it occurs in the advanced stages of disease or in combination with lymphedema. With venous disease, pitting edema may occur in the periwound area, the foot and ankle, or anywhere on the body. Advanced edema and lymphedema are generally unaffected by elevation and require compression as part of effective management. However, before adding compression, it is important to address the possibility of an arterial component to the venous pathology. If there is arterial insufficiency, healing will be impaired, and compression may be contraindicated.[43,51] Results from the ABI give preliminary information about potential arterial insufficiency, but more sophisticated laboratory tests may be indicated to confirm or rule out arterial disease in the individual who also has venous insufficiency.

Intervention

The most important therapeutic measure for the prevention and treatment of venous LE ulcers is *compression therapy.* Compression refers primarily to specialized bandaging and specialized garments but can also include intermittent pneumatic compression. All of these treatment interventions are discussed later in the chapter. Even though edema is a natural characteristic of the first phase of wound healing, excessive edema can delay timely wound healing by slowing perfusion of tissues and facilitating the growth of bacteria.[11] Along with compression and appropriate wound care for patients with CVI, treatment includes exercise to increase mobility and positioning to support and enhance venous blood flow.[44] Compression therapy is essential for timely healing if arterial disease has been ruled out. As mentioned earlier, in a diagnosis of mixed arterial and venous disease, the more severe pathology is prioritized. Significant arterial disease will most likely preclude the use of compression. For the individual with a diagnosis of venous disease or mixed (mild) arterial/venous disease, a combination of therapeutic measures will accelerate positive outcomes.[53] These include compression bandaging and garments, gait training, MLD, and exercise, including range of motion (ROM). A wound care plan should not include whirlpool owing to the risks of dependent positioning, cross contamination, cytotoxic additives, and unnecessary costs.

Lymphedema

Lymphedema is a chronic disorder characterized by an abnormal accumulation of lymph fluid in the tissues of one or more body regions.[2,54–56] The accumulation of fluid can be caused by a number of events but is most often caused by a mechanical insufficiency of the lymphatic system. This means that some components of the lymphatic system are not functioning sufficiently to manage the lymph fluid present in the affected body region. Lymphedema can be classified as primary or secondary lymphedema. *Primary lymphedema* (Fig. 14.5) is caused by a condition that is congenital or hereditary. With primary lymphedema, lymph node or lymph vessel formation is abnormal. The most common abnormality is *hypoplasia,* a condition in which there are fewer lymphatic vessels, and they are smaller than normal. One of the more common forms of primary lymphedema appears in *Milroy disease. Secondary lymphedema* (Fig. 14.6) is caused by injury to one or more components of the lymphatic system: Some portion of the lymphatic system has been blocked, dissected, fibrosed, overloaded, or otherwise damaged or altered.

Secondary lymphedema is more prevalent than primary. In developed countries, the most common cause of secondary lymphedema is surgery and/or radiation therapy as part of breast cancer treatment. The rise in the incidence of other types of cancer and the subsequent treatments for those cancers have led to an increase in reports of lymphedema following treatment for cancer of the prostate, bladder, uterus, ovaries, and skin. Cancer is not the only causative factor for lymphedema. It is common for an individual with CVI to develop lymphedema, triggered by long-standing fluid overload in the LEs.[57] Secondary lymphedema can also be triggered by the complications of paralysis, disuse in

chronic regional pain syndrome, or trauma to regional lymph nodes following liposuction, pelvic fracture, hernia repair, and other surgical interventions where lymph nodes or lymph vessels are located.[58–61] Lymphedema is a common disease, and health-care providers can expect an increase in the number of patients with this condition over the next decade.[62]

Through the efforts of experts in the field of physical therapy, there has been compelling evidence to support a *prospective surveillance model* as the standard of care in breast cancer treatment.[62,63] Surveillance includes regular follow-up visits performed by physical therapists to identify and monitor changes that might signal adverse effects of treatment. Studies have shown that this model is more cost effective than treating the late adverse effects of treatment such as advanced-stage lymphedema.[62–65] This model should also apply to individuals undergoing treatment for other types of cancer and those at risk of developing lymphedema for other reasons. The collection of data on the incidence of non-cancer-related secondary lymphedema is limited by the lack of specific education related to lymphedema among health-care professionals and by a lack of clinical suspicion when examining individuals with a history of swelling.[66,67] In the tropical and subtropical regions of the world, secondary lymphedema is most often caused by *filariasis,* which involves a person experiencing multiple bites from mosquitoes that carry the parasite. In filariasis, microscopic nematode worm larvae live a full life cycle in the lymphatic vessels, causing inflammation and blocked lymphatic vessels.

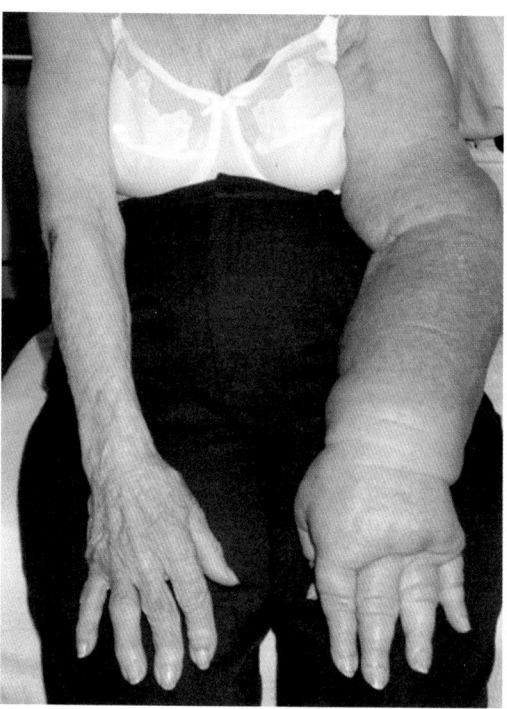

Figure 14.6 Secondary lymphedema of unilateral upper extremity.

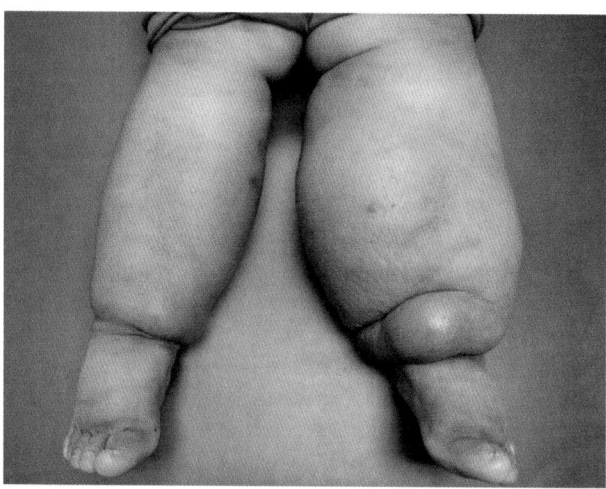

Figure 14.5 Primary lymphedema of bilateral lower extremities with one extremity more involved than the other.

Clinical Presentation

- Swelling distal to or adjacent to the area where lymph system function has been impaired
- Swelling usually not relieved by elevation
- Pitting edema in the early stages of disease; nonpitting edema in later stages, as fibrotic changes occur
- Feelings of fatigue, heaviness, pressure, or tightness in the affected region
- Numbness and tingling as swelling becomes more severe
- Discomfort varying from mild to intense
- Fibrotic changes of the dermis
- Dermal abnormalities such as *cysts, fistulas, lymphorrhea, papillomas, hyperkeratosis*
- Increased susceptibility to infection, at first local to the affected region but often becoming systemic
- Loss of mobility and ROM
- Impaired wound healing

History

A patient history consistent with lymphatic system damage or deformity is pivotal in the diagnosis of lymphedema. A patient's history might include cancer, cancer treatment, radiation therapy, lymph node disruption, CVI, trauma, surgery, or (in primary lymphedema) onset of swelling at birth or puberty. There may be a long latency period between injury to the lymphatics and clinical manifestations; thus, health-care providers and patients must adhere to prevention guidelines and be suspicious of any signs and symptoms that might suggest lymphedema. The condition can develop within a few weeks of the initial insult to the system or as long as 30 years later. Lymphedema cannot be reversed, but it can be prevented from progressing to the next stage if identified and adequate measures are taken.

Tests and Measurements

For most individuals, the diagnosis of lymphedema can be made without the use of special tests. A patient history consistent with lymph system damage or deformity, a systems review, differential diagnosis, inspection, and palpation of the integument and girth measurements is adequate for accurate diagnosis in most cases. Unique findings might include the *Stemmer sign,* skin texture changes, skin folds, fibrosis, increase in girth, *papules,* lymph leakage, and *elephantiasis.* Severity is determined by a collection of data, including the presence of fibrotic tissue changes (brawny or woody [hardened] and/or lobular [rounded projection]); the number of episodes of cellulitis; condition of the superficial integument of the lymphedematous limb (papules, leakage, fungus, venous wounds); circumference or volume differences between involved and uninvolved limbs; and quality-of-life issues (sleep, mobility, activities of daily living [ADL], relationships). A noninvasive test called *lymphoscintigraphy* is a special test using a radioactive tracer and a gamma camera to provide images of the lymphatic system. This test is useful for differential diagnosis and to characterize the severity of lymphedema.[61,66,67]

Intervention

A physical therapy provider should be cautious about the application of pressure to an edematous or lymphedematous body part. Although compression is an essential intervention, pressures that are too high will occlude superficial lymph capillaries and prevent the initial step of fluid absorption needed to control edema and lymphedema.[3,4]

Current intervention for the patient/client with lymphedema requires attention to detail and a level of expertise not often fully provided in entry-level professional educational programs. Practitioners are best served by gaining additional education to verify their competency to treat these patients. The current recommended course of care is a two-phase program of *complete decongestive therapy* (CDT).[68–71] Phase I (intensive) includes skin care, MLD, lymphedema bandaging, exercise, and compression garment at the *end* of phase I. Phase II (self-management) includes skin care, compression garment during the day, exercise, lymphedema bandaging at night, and MLD as needed.[72] A good source of information on training programs, the procedures for CDT, identifying trained therapists, and patient education related to lymphedema is the National Lymphedema Network (https://lymphnet.org).

As with many progressive, chronic disorders, the effectiveness of treatment is significantly improved by early intervention. Accurate and early diagnosis occurs when health-care professionals are sensitized to the signs and symptoms and carefully evaluate the examination data. In the POC, the number and frequency of treatments should not be determined by lymphedema staging or by circumferential differences between limbs. (The severity of the condition is not determined by these data alone.) Some individuals with lymphedema may present with more involved signs and symptoms than the measurements imply. The physical therapy provider should pay close attention to indicators such as a history of cellulitis, brawny tissue changes, increasing impairment in developing the POC, and the number of visits needed.

Pressure Injuries

Formerly termed pressure ulcer, a *pressure injury* is "localized damage to the skin and/or underlying soft tissue usually over a bony prominence or related to a medical or other device.[73] The injury can present as intact skin or an open ulcer and may be painful. The injury occurs as a result of intense and/or prolonged pressure or pressure in combination with shear. The tolerance of soft tissue for pressure and shear may also be affected by microclimate, nutrition, perfusion, co-morbidities and condition of soft tissue."[74–77] The new term *pressure injury* was agreed upon by the National Pressure Ulcer

Advisory Panel (NPUAP) in 2016 in order to be more inclusive and descriptive of wounds to both intact and ulcerated skin. In addition to the change in nomenclature, the NPUAP concurrently changed its name to the National Pressure Injury Advisory Panel to remain consistent with its own recommended terminology. Pressure injuries occur when pressure is significant enough in force or time as to cause ischemia to the soft tissues below the epidermis. As deeper vessels are occluded, decreased blood flow leads to cell death, tissue necrosis, and finally a visible wound. The superficial dermis can tolerate *ischemia* for 2 to 8 hr before breakdown occurs. Deeper muscle, connective, and fat tissues tolerate pressures for 2 hr or less. Thus, there may be significant damage to underlying tissues while initially the epidermis and dermis remain intact. The clinical implications of this phenomenon are discussed next and in the "Tests and Measurements" section. Readers can gain a greater understanding of the depth of damage to the integument by referring to Chapter 24, Burns, to view cross sections of skin, illustrating which components of the skin are lost at descending levels of damage.

Pressure injuries occur most frequently among individuals who are immobilized for long periods of time. Although pressure injuries can occur at any age during prolonged periods of immobility, they are more likely to occur in individuals who are hospitalized, elderly, incontinent, and/or underweight and among individuals of all ages following spinal cord injury (SCI).[42,69–78] Up to 25% of hospital-acquired pressure injuries may originate during surgery.[77] According to Reed et al.,[79] the presence of low albumin levels, confusion, and a *do not resuscitate* order are also pressure injury risk factors. Pressure injuries increase the risk of death for aging individuals whether at home, in a hospital, or at a long-term care setting.[78] In developed countries, the incidence of chronic wounds, including pressure injuries, is increasing as the population ages.[79,80]

Clinical Presentation

The severity of pressure injury can be estimated by observing clinical signs. A progression from least tissue damage to most severe damage is presented here.[76] More details on the challenges of identifying pressure injury depth are covered later in the chapter.

- The first clinical sign of pressure injury is *blanchable erythema* along with increased skin temperature. If pressure is relieved, tissues may recover in 24 hr. If pressure is unrelieved, nonblanchable erythema occurs. The skin may still be fully intact in the earliest stage of pressure injury formation, but it will become more fragile.
- Progression to a superficial abrasion, blister, or shallow crater indicates involvement of the dermis.
- When full-thickness skin loss is apparent, the wound appears as a deep crater. Bleeding is minimal, and tissues are *indurated* and warm. Eschar formation marks full-thickness skin loss. Tunneling or undermining is

often present. (The official staging classification for pressure injuries is covered later in this chapter.)
- The majority of all pressure injuries develop over six primary bony areas (Fig. 14.7): sacrum (Fig. 14.8), coccyx, greater trochanter, ischial tuberosity, calcaneus (heel), and lateral malleolus.

History

If an individual has a history of a period of immobility followed by the discovery of a warm, red spot over a bony prominence, a pressure injury can usually be confirmed. If the spot is unnaturally soft to the touch, sometimes referred to as "boggy," this is enough evidence to suspect that damage is deeper than the epidermis, even if the skin remains fully intact.

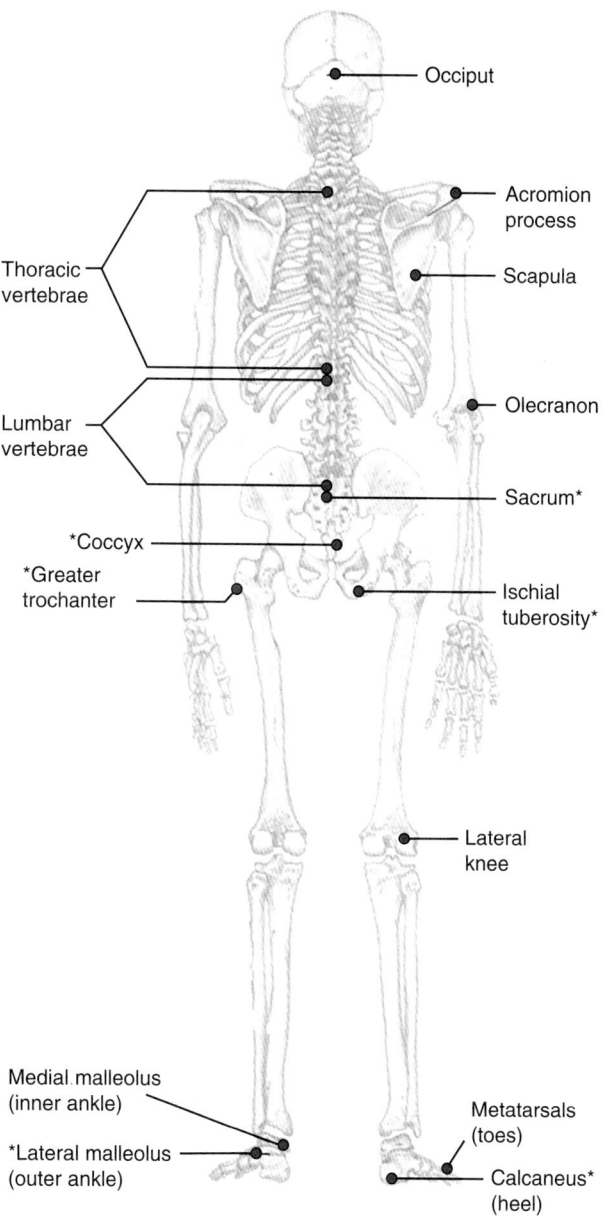

* Most common sites of pressure ulcers

Figure 14.7 Pressure points of bony prominences.

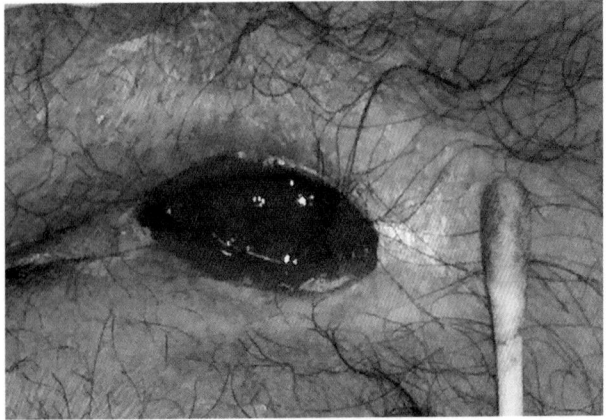

Figure 14.8 Sacral pressure injury.

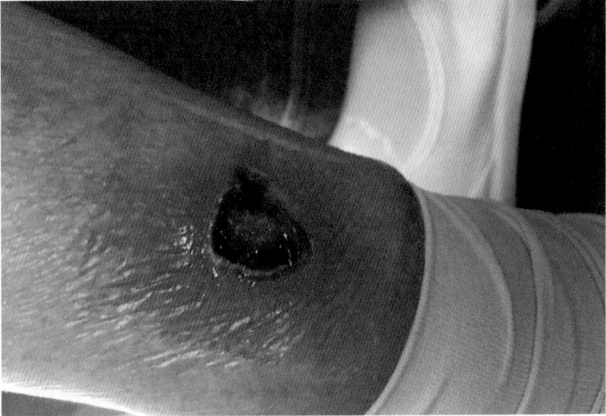

Figure 14.9 Unstageable pressure injury: obscured full-thickness skin and tissue loss.

Tests and Measurements

During examination, along with general wound characteristics, pressure injuries are classified by grading or staging systems that describe the degree of tissue damage observed. It can also be important to use a tool to measure an individual's risk of developing a pressure injury before a tissue injury exists. Refer to the "Integumentary Integrity" section for more information on risk assessment for patients with pressure injuries (Fig. 14.9).

Intervention

A physical therapy provider treats integumentary disorders that involve the epidermis, dermis, hypodermis, or below into exposed bone, tendon, muscle, and organs. For closure and subsequent healing to occur, intervention for disorders of the integument must facilitate local and regional homeostasis of the vascular and lymphatic systems. In addition to appropriate wound care, it is imperative that the underlying cause of pressure be addressed. Wounds will not close and remain healed unless the reduction of pressure and prevention of future breakdown are top priorities in the intervention plan. Pressure management is accomplished with the use of PRDs, *pressure mapping* to determine pressure loads, *positioning/turning schedules,* and *education* of the patient, family, and caregivers. Other factors that contribute to wound onset and risk for wound onset should be considered and/or addressed. These factors include shear, friction, mobility, sensation, moisture, nutrition, age, and underlying medical condition. With appropriate wound care, control of pressure, and attention to risk factors, a wound should progress in a timely manner through the phases of wound healing, showing signs of improvement in a matter of weeks.[31]

Neuropathy

Neuropathy can be defined as any disease of nerves and can include peripheral nerves, cranial nerves, and/or autonomic nerves. Neuropathy exists in many disease processes; however, the most common disease process

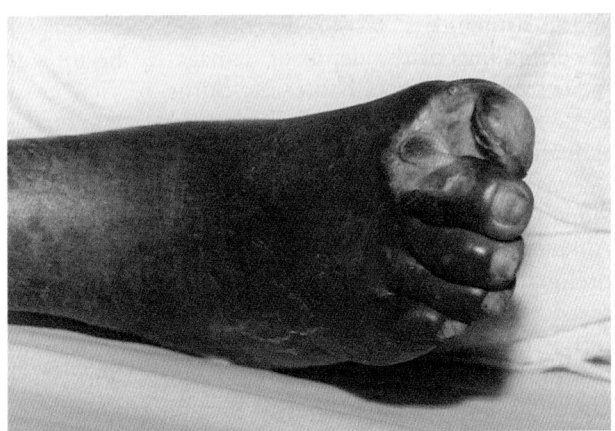

Figure 14.10 Chronic wound as a result of diabetic neuropathy.

seen with neuropathy is diabetes mellitus. For most chronic diseases, including diabetes, the effects of neuropathy are peripheral. The etiology of diabetic neuropathy is not fully understood but thought to be related to high levels of glucose in the blood over a long period of time. *Diabetic neuropathy* is a generic term for any diabetes mellitus–related disorder of the peripheral or autonomic nervous systems or the cranial nerves. The majority of symptoms from diabetic neuropathy will be located in the LE, with foot insensitivity and subsequent ulceration on the plantar surface being the most common (Fig. 14.10).

It is estimated that 15% of individuals with diabetes will develop a foot wound sometime in their life, making them almost 40 times more likely to undergo amputation because of a nonhealing wound than the nondiabetic population.[42] To complicate matters, many individuals with diabetes have coexisting arterial disease because the conditions are not mutually exclusive. Although the incidence is lower than for venous and arterial wounds in general, the underlying diabetic condition creates a difficult physiological environment in which to close a wound. The incidence of neuropathic LE wounds is likely to grow as the population ages and the incidence of diabetes continues to escalate. According to the Centers for Disease Control and Prevention (CDC), almost half of all adults now are at risk for diabetes.[81] Diabetes affects more than 37 million people of all ages in the United States. This figure represents 11.3% of the population. About 60% to 70% of people with diabetes have mild to severe forms of neuropathy, and more than 60% of the nontraumatic lower-limb amputations that are performed in the United States occur among people with diabetes.[80] If current trends prevail, the impact of diabetic neuropathy on future wound care needs for our patients will continue to expand.

Clinical Presentation

- Ulceration is usually located on the weight-bearing surfaces of the foot
- Usually anesthetic, round, over bony prominences but can be located anywhere
- Sensory neuropathy, if present:
  - Patient unable to sense pain and pressure
  - Risk of skin breakdown without patient awareness
  - Mechanical, repetitive stresses most common causative factors of wounds
- Motor neuropathy, if present:
  - Loss of intrinsic muscles
  - Hammertoe, claw-toe deformities adding to risk of breakdown owing to poor weight distribution and rubbing from shoes
  - Foot drop
- Autonomic neuropathy, if present:
  - Decreased or absent sweat and oil production leading to dry, inelastic skin
  - Increased susceptibility to skin breakdown and injury
  - Propensity for heavy callus formation
- Dysvascular symptoms, if present:
  - Usually arterial disorders but can be complicated by reduced cardiac function from autonomic causes
  - Ischemia
  - Impaired healing time (also present owing to diabetes)
  - Impaired transport of oxygen, antibiotics, and nutrients needed for healing

History

A history of diabetes is sufficient to warrant investigation of diabetic neuropathy. If the individual has had diabetes for years or has had trouble regulating insulin levels even for a few years, the presence of diabetic neuropathy is very likely. When ulceration is visible, the history will include specific details about the wound in addition to information about other symptoms.

Tests and Measurements

During the examination, every patient with diabetes should be checked, using monofilaments, for the presence of *protective sensation* in the LEs. This should be part of a systems review for patients with diabetes even when diabetes is not the primary diagnosis. Data on skin temperature of the LEs should also be recorded during the examination. Information about blood glucose levels should be obtained as part of the examination and must be considered for the safe development of the POC.[81]

Intervention

Physical therapy providers are in an ideal position to provide education and comprehensive foot care intervention for the diabetic population. In addition to appropriate wound care and maintenance of acceptable blood glucose levels, the intervention must include some method of decreasing weight-bearing stresses. Options for off-loading include crutches or walker, changes in gait patterns, walking casts or orthoses, and specialized footwear. It is common to utilize all of the off-loading options over the course of treatment for patients with foot ulceration. Intervention must include a comprehensive program, including elements of wound care, foot care, education, PRDs, orthotics, exercise, and modalities. Every effort should be made by clinicians and patients alike to improve or retain the skin integrity of the foot. (Refer to Appendix 14.A (online) for patient education information on foot care.) In addition to other medical complications of diabetes, altered circulation to the foot can complicate symptoms of diabetic neuropathy. Intervention should address the most significant problem first but with lower expectations for healing when vascular disorders coexist with neuropathy.

The five most common disorders of the vascular, lymphatic, and integumentary systems have been discussed. Other disorders caused by surgery, trauma, malignancy, hematological disease, connective tissue disease, and thermal injury *will* affect the systems discussed in this chapter. Owing to space restrictions, however, they are not discussed at this time. Interested readers should seek one of the texts mentioned in the reference list to supplement the information presented here.[1,2,32,47,55] Examination and treatment of other disorders would utilize the same tests and measurements and treatment interventions discussed in this chapter based on the patient's unique characteristics.

■ EXAMINATION AND EVALUATION

Examination

History

Many of the disorders discussed in this chapter have a slow or insidious onset, and this tends to make the assessment of a patient's history very challenging despite its high importance. A thorough history includes seeking information on systems beyond the local affected area. Physical therapy examinations for all disorders begin with gathering data from the patient, family, and other involved individuals. For the disorders discussed in this chapter, information needed from the history is similar, which makes the inclusion of these topics in one single chapter ideal.

Systems Review

It might be tempting to skip a systems review before using other tests and measurements in the examination process to save time. This step, however, is of utmost importance as physical therapists move toward greater autonomy. Results may alert the physical therapist to concerns that may require referral to another practitioner. A systems review is particularly important here because the disorders discussed in this chapter are often the result of dysfunction in other systems of the body. For example, diabetes mellitus may lead to wounds of the feet, breast cancer surgery may lead to lymphedema, heart disease may lead to arterial wounds of the LEs, and paralysis may lead to pressure injuries. A comprehensive approach to observing and examining the patient will set the stage for the investigation and data collection that follow.

Tests and Measurements

Owing to the close relationship among disorders of the vascular, lymphatic, and integumentary systems; the importance of differential diagnosis; and the likelihood of a patient or client presenting with more than one disorder, a physical therapist will use a wide variety of available tests and measurements during the examination. The tests and measurements discussed in this chapter are described in the order in which they are presented in the *Guide to Physical Therapist Practice.*[82] A review of the test and measurement categories should serve as a reminder of the responsibility of the examining therapist to document thoroughly. A physical therapist is skilled in the use of many valid and reliable tests and measurements and is often the most appropriate provider to utilize these tools to ensure that the patient receives the most patient-centered, comprehensive, and timely care. For purposes of space, only the most essential categories have been addressed. An annotated version of selected tests and measurements has been included to assist the reader in understanding the tests and conditions under examination.

Aerobic Capacity/Endurance

Aerobic capacity during functional activities is important to measure since activity is encouraged as part of long-term management of the disorders in this chapter. In addition to information obtained during the systems review, the gathering of additional data depends on the individual patient. This might include the use of angina, claudication, and dyspnea scales, pulmonary function tests, and ECG. A determination of heart rhythm sounds, as well as breath and voice sounds, may also be required.

Anthropometric Characteristics

HEIGHT AND WEIGHT

Data on height and weight are necessary to address and track normal weight values, especially for the patient with a disorder that results in abnormal fluid retention such as diabetes, edema, lymphedema, venous disease, or underlying cardiopulmonary disease.

VOLUMETRIC MEASUREMENT

Volumetrics are performed utilizing special containers that hold water and a graduated cylinder for water collection (Fig. 14.11). This method is accurate for measuring changes in body dimensions with the most common measurements taken for the hand, full upper extremity (UE), foot, or full lower leg; however, it can be time consuming, may be awkward to administer, and may be inappropriate when open wounds are present due to cross-contamination risks.

GIRTH MEASUREMENT

Girth is recorded using a tape measure to determine circumferential body dimensions (Fig. 14.12). Ideally, a tape measure specially designed to measure girth should be used. Bony landmarks are sometimes used as reference points in taking girth measurements, and the standard among experts who treat edema is to use consistent centimeter intervals. For example, in measuring the LE, circumferential measurements are taken in centimeter intervals, starting from the floor or weight-bearing surface to the groin. The smaller the interval, the better

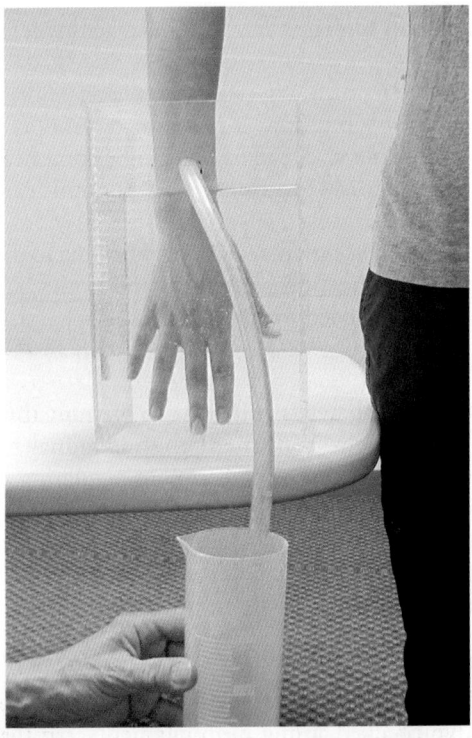

Figure 14.11 Volumetric examination for edema.

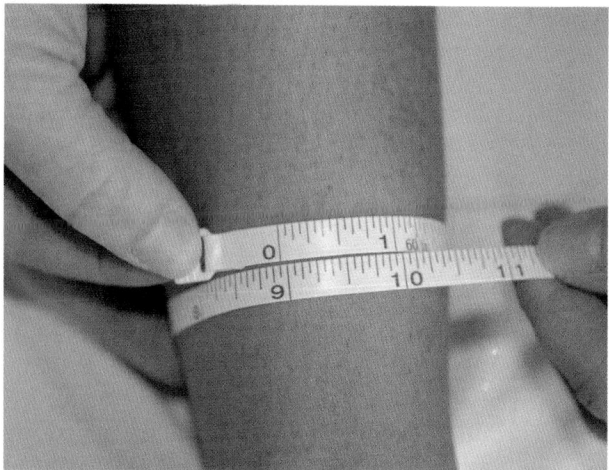

Figure 14.12 Tape measure examination for girth measurement.

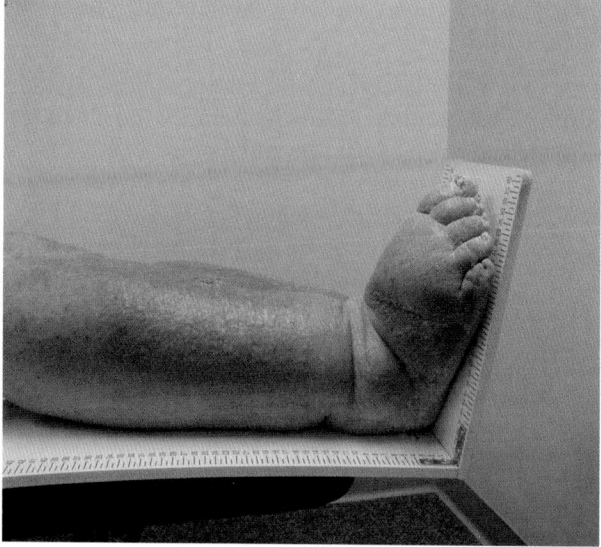

Figure 14.13 Use of footboard with ruler to establish consistent intervals for measuring lower extremity circumferences.

is the representation of body dimensions. Clinicians choose intervals of 4, 6, 8, or 10 cm. Special measuring boards (Fig. 14.13) can be obtained for measuring the LE, or a well-placed clipboard under the foot can be used to establish the beginning "floor" measurement if the patient is in supine position. A physical therapy provider must remember that girth measurements by themselves should not be used to determine severity, frequency of visits, or duration of the episode of care. Advanced fibrotic changes can occur to the dermis and underlying connective tissue without a significant increase in the girth of a limb.[2,59]

ADDITIONAL TOOLS

Data on anthropometric measurements may be collected using *tonometry* or *bioelectrical impedance*. Although not a standardized procedure, soft-tissue tonometry uses a device that measures tissue tension at the surface of the skin. Less pliable skin creates a higher tension reading, suggesting the presence of fluid and/or tissue fibrosis. Data from tonometry can be useful for subclinical evidence of edema, lymphedema, and fibrotic changes before they are visible or palpable. Bioelectrical impedance analysis provides accurate measurements to help predict the onset of lymphedema, often many months before a clinical diagnosis is possible. The technique involves passing a very small amount of alternating current (AC) through the limb to be tested and measuring the impedance to its flow at various frequencies. This technique is more sensitive than limb volume measurements in detecting changes in the extracellular fluid volume. In studies thus far, the false-negative rate has been found to be zero.[83–86]

Palpation/Pitting Scale

Palpation of soft tissues must be a regular part of vascular, lymphatic, and integumentary examinations. There is no universal pitting scale currently used by

health-care professionals. Some scales are based on how deep an indentation is left after applying fingertip pressure. Other scales are based on the perceived severity of the pitting by the examiner. The following scale, most commonly used by physical therapists and other medical providers, gives a numerical grade to the pitting based on how long it remains after fingertip pressure is applied:

1+: Indentation is barely detectable.
2+: Slight indentation visible when skin is depressed, returns to normal in 15 seconds.
3+: Deeper indentation occurs when pressed and returns to normal within 30 seconds.
4+: Indentation lasts for more than 30 seconds.

If using a pitting scale during an examination, it is wise to document an explanation of the grades or scoring system used. It is common for a physical therapist to assess pedal edema because it may be attributed to chronic wounds, inflammation, infection, cellulitis, diabetes, liver disease, renal disease, CVI, lymphedema, phlebo-lymphedema, CHF, or trauma.

Staging or Grading of Lymphedema

In an effort to categorize levels of severity, some professionals use staging or grading systems for edema and lymphedema in addition to one or more of the measurement techniques previously mentioned.[1,2] Grading or staging of edema and lymphedema is not universally used by health professionals and should be accompanied by objective information in the examination results. One of the most frequently used systems is the *International Society of Lymphology Staging*

System as described in their most recent consensus document:[56]

- *Stage 0:* Subclinical state where the peripheral swelling is not visible, but lymphatic transport is impaired. Symptoms such as achiness and tingling in the extremity and subtle tissue changes may be noted.
- *Stage I:* Early onset of swelling that is visible and subsides with elevation. Pitting may be present.
- *Stage II:* Consistent volume change with pitting present. Elevation rarely reduces the swelling, and progressive tissue fibrosis occurs.
- *Stage III:* Skin changes such as thickening, hyper-pigmentation, increased skin folds, fat deposits, and warty overgrowths occur. Tissue is very fibrotic, and pitting is absent.

Stages 0 and I are considered early stage lymphedema. Another term would be *preclinical lymphedema* as the patient begins to feel "heaviness" in the limb or body part but may not be able to see it. Stage II is considered moderate/established lymphedema. Stage III is late-stage lymphedema and often appears as elephantiasis due to the appearance of the skin.

Arousal, Attention, and Cognition

After evaluating screening results during the history and systems review, the physical therapist will decide whether there is a clinical indication for tests and measurements in this category. It is important for the therapist to understand the patient's level of motivation, orientation, attention, and ability to process instructions. Many of the disorders in this chapter, such as diabetic neuropathy, CVI, and lymphedema, require lifelong adherence to the self-care component of the treatment to retain the gains made during intervention. Most of the information regarding cognition can be obtained through interviews and observations. Additional tools would include cognitive and behavior scales, safety checklists, and learning profiles.

Assistive and Adaptive Devices

It is very likely that patients with vascular, lymphatic, or integumentary disorders will need assistive devices during the intervention and self-care phases of management. Increasing mobility is a key factor in timely recovery or symptom management of these disorders. Observation, gait analysis, functional screening, and manual muscle testing are often used to guide this determination. Adaptive devices may be issued by a physical therapist, or by an occupational therapist who is providing concurrent treatment to a patient with these types of impairments.

Circulation

Collecting data about the movement of blood and lymph through the arterial, venous, and lymphatic systems is interrelated with the tests and measurements for integumentary integrity. Tests and measurements for skin changes that may occur with impairment of the circulation are discussed under the "Integumentary Integrity" section. The presence or risk of pathology of the circulatory systems can be detected in many cases by skilled observation and palpation (e.g., temperature and pulses).

Temperature

To further examine circulation, skin temperature can be assessed by palpation. Objective data should also be collected and quantified using a *radiometer* or a *thermistor,* because superficial skin temperature changes are often indicative of pathology (Fig. 14.14). A decrease in skin temperature can indicate poor arterial perfusion. An increase can indicate infection or active disease processes such as cellulitis or a *Charcot joint.* An increase in temperature can also indicate a worsening or impending complication of CVI.[52]

Arterial Perfusion

The therapist collects data to determine whether adequate blood flow is reaching distal tissues. If blood flow is adequate, the oxygen supply will be adequate. Some noninvasive tests and measurements are designed to determine *blood flow* and *skin perfusion,* whereas others address *oxygen levels* in the tissues. Pulses should be palpated initially to provide information about possible vascular system involvement. The examination should include palpation of the following arteries: brachial and radial, femoral, popliteal, dorsalis pedis, and posterior tibialis. The following scale, commonly used by physical therapists and other medical providers, gives a

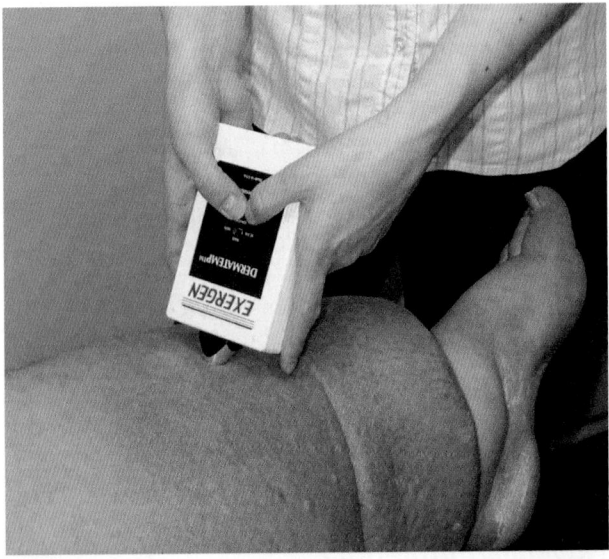

Figure 14.14 Skin temperature examination using a skin thermometer.

numerical grade and a descriptive word to describe the pulse quality:

0   = *Absent,* no perceptible pulse
1+ = *Thready,* barely perceptible
2+ = *Weak,* palpable but diminished
3+ = *Normal,* easy to palpate
4+ = *Bounding,* very strong, may imply the possibility of an aneurysm or other pathological condition

Auscultation by stethoscope of major pulse points may identify a *bruit.* If turbulent blood flow is heard, the patient may have partial blockage of the artery. Barriers to effective pulse taking include scar tissue, edema, fibrosis, and tissue induration.

Doppler ultrasound is considered an essential component of the vascular examination.[47,87,88] The examiner uses a handheld probe to direct a sound wave into the vessel to be tested. The sound wave is reflected by red blood cells moving in the vessel. The sound wave signal is changed into audible sound that is transmitted from a small, handheld unit. The ABI is the most frequently performed test using Doppler ultrasound. A blood pressure cuff is inflated to occlude blood flow temporarily and is then deflated as the examiner listens for the return of flow. Blood flow is observed on the UE at the brachial artery and on the LE at the posterior tibial and the dorsalis pedis arteries (Fig. 14.15). The ABI is a ratio of the LE systolic pressure divided by the UE pressure. Table 14.1 presents the ranges of ABI values and potential vascular indications. Obtaining an ABI provides useful information about the arterial system since the ABI is an indicator of loss of perfusion in the LE. Results will guide the therapist in decisions about the use of compression and débridement and will help predict the likelihood of timely wound closure. When the examiner cannot occlude blood flow with the blood pressure cuff, calculations may show a falsely elevated ABI. Arteriosclerosis or calcified vessels

Table 14.1	Ankle-Brachial Indexes With Corresponding Indications
Ankle-Brachial Index Ranges	**Possible Indication**
>1.2	Falsely elevated, arterial disease, diabetes
1.19–0.95	Normal
0.94–0.75	Mild arterial disease, + intermittent claudication
0.74–0.50	Moderate arterial disease, + rest pain
<0.50	Severe arterial disease

(from diabetes mellitus) can make it difficult for the cuff to compress enough to get an accurate ABI. The target arteries would be documented as *noncompressible vessels.* Test options when the vessels are noncompressible include taking toe pressures with a special cuff, proceeding with transcutaneous oxygen testing (see later), or recommending referral for a vascular laboratory workup.

Trophic Changes

Trophic changes occur in the soft tissue of the LEs when circulation is impaired by poor arterial blood flow and interruptions in nerve supply. Observation is the most accurate way to note trophic changes. Changes include dry, shiny skin (pale in individuals with lighter skin), decreased or absent leg hair, and thick toenails. It should be noted that these signs are also a predictable part of aging but not to the same degree as can be seen with trophic changes. The presence of changes indicates the need for other tests of circulation.

Pain

When related to circulation, a thorough pain history may be all that is necessary to suggest the possibility of arterial disease. Reports of pain indicate the need for further tests and measurements of the vascular system. Pain as the result of IC is described earlier in this chapter. Rest pain that develops at night, awakens the patient, or requires analgesics for relief is considered more severe than IC. Pain can be measured for severity on a visual analog scale. The degree of impairment from IC is often measured in terms of how far an individual can walk before experiencing acute LE pain or fatigue. IC can be classified objectively with a rating scale to indicate severity based on distance walked before onset of pain. The *Walking Impairment Questionnaire* is a disease-specific questionnaire commonly used to examine patients with claudication. It does not, however, measure the impact of claudication on quality of life (QOL).[89] The most

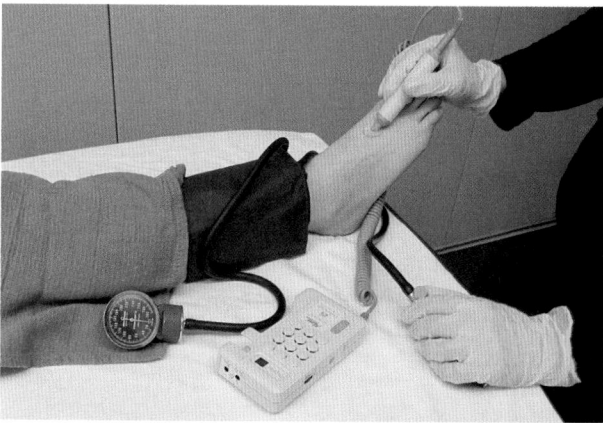

Figure 14.15 Ankle-brachial index test performed using a handheld Doppler ultrasound instrument.

extensively researched disease-specific QOL questionnaire for IC is the *Claudication Scale.*[89–92]

Special Tests

There are many other noninvasive and invasive tests used to detect, examine, diagnose, or confirm arterial disease and dysfunction. Appendix 14.B (online) presents a brief description of special tests for arterial and venous function, including *rubor of dependency, air plethysmography (APG), transcutaneous oxygen (TcPO₂)* measurement, and *skin perfusion pressure (SPP)* measurement. Although some of the tests are useful for predicting healing of ulcers and amputation wounds, they may not be readily reimbursed when performed by a physical therapist. The APG, $TcPO_2$, and SPP are used primarily for research purposes because they are time consuming to perform.

Venous Patency

Venous disease and dysfunction can be detected with a wide range of tests and measurements. The amount of time available for examination, as well as reimbursement issues, may influence decisions about which tests to use. Refer to Appendix 14.B (online) for a brief description of *Venous Filling Time, Percussion Test,* and the *Trendelenburg Test.* Owing to inconsistencies in interpretation and administration, the *Homans Test,* or Homans sign (pain in the calf when the ankle is passively dorsiflexed, which may or may not be performed with manual compression of the calf), should not be relied on to accurately detect a DVT. A physician should be contacted and a Doppler study used if an individual exhibits two of the following signs: change in skin temperature, change in skin color (darker), pain in the calf (experienced by approximately half of patients), or swelling. Many clinicians now utilize the Well Criteria for DVT because it can provide objective data based on clinical findings to assist in decision-making.[93–95]

Lymph Vessel Integrity

Patient history and clinical findings are used most often to make a diagnosis of lymphedema. Most invasive tests have lost popularity because of the risk of triggering the onset of lymphedema or an exacerbation of existing lymphedema owing to the irritation caused by dye and/or needle puncture. When invasive tests are indicated, the most common test procedure is *lymphoscintigraphy.* This test, using dye and a special camera and computer, can visualize many vital lymphatic system functions.[2,96]

Gait, Locomotion, and Balance

It is always important to utilize tests and measurements to assess and document a patient's ability to move. The importance of movement to improve blood and lymphatic flow and to facilitate the overall return to function for most individuals makes this category essential.

During the initial examination, gathering data through observation, gait analysis, and postural control tests is usually adequate. The examination results may indicate the need for additional tests such as inventories, or batteries of tests to further document safety (fall risk) or equipment needs. Individuals who are morbidly obese have unique challenges with gait that should be addressed during the examination.

Integumentary Integrity

Collection of data about skin and subcutaneous tissues is interrelated with the tests and measurements for circulation and cutaneous sensation.

Observation and Palpation

Characteristics of the skin are noted almost entirely by observation and palpation. A comparison between involved and normal integument is made with careful attention to color, moisture, texture, firmness, temperature, elasticity, symmetry, and shape. In the presence of a wound, the wound tissue, the periwound area, and the wound exudate should all be observed and data recorded regarding the observations. The location of a wound, presence of edema, and presence of lymphedema can be documented using a *body diagram.*

Trophic Changes

Because they are an important part of many disorders involving the integument, trophic changes are mentioned again under this section. Readers who are making a quick reference specifically to integumentary integrity in this chapter are reminded to refer to all sections related to trophic changes. As in the section on circulation, observation is an important approach to noting changes.

Fibrosis

The best way to detect fibrotic changes of the skin is through palpation of the affected tissue. The superficial skin and underlying tissue will feel thickened, firm, and unyielding or immobile. Fibrosis is common in later stages of CVI and lymphedema. Testing for the presence or absence of the *Stemmer sign* is an objective measurement that can be added to the examination for lymphedema and is often present starting in patients with stage 2 lymphedema. When the dorsal skin folds of the toes (normally the second toe is used) or fingers are resistant to lifting, or cannot be lifted at all, the Stemmer sign is said to be "present." The clinician must be cautious, however, because a negative or "absent" skin fold test does not fully rule out lymphedema.

Coloration

Skin color will vary based on the underlying disease. Observation is the best way to note comparisons between normal tissues and those under examination.

The most abnormal color changes include red, purple, and brown. Color changes may indicate a chronic condition such as hemosiderin staining or an acute situation such as redness associated with DVT. If color changes are intermittent, they may signal a disease such as Raynaud disease. However, skin color is determined by melanin, and depending on the amount of melanin present, darker-skinned individuals may mask certain circulation problems. For example, for those with cyanotic limbs, a bluish tint may be visible in lighter-skinned individuals, but that may not be easily seen in those with darker skin, which may appear gray.[8] For darker-skinned patients, erythema may appear purple, not red.[8] Care must be taken to consider other factors in the assessment, such as temperature and palpation.

Temperature

The temperature of the skin is most often examined by palpation, but data can be objectively collected and quantified using a radiometer or a thermistor (see Fig. 14.14). Maintenance of normal skin temperatures is essential for good wound healing. Abnormal skin temperatures can signal problems related to the dermis or other structures. A decrease in superficial skin temperature may indicate poor arterial perfusion. An increase may indicate infection or active disease processes.

Wounds

Size and Depth

A number of tools and scales are available for gathering data about wounds, edema, lymphedema, and other aspects of integumentary integrity. Wounds not classified with staging or grading can be described based on the depth of tissue damage. The descriptions used for depth of burn injury—superficial, partial, and full thickness—can also be used to describe depth in other types of wounds. Objective measures included in documentation are vital for communication about the patient. A calibrated grid, photographs used only with consent, tracings, graphs, and specifically designed forms are most commonly used to document wound size and depth.

Drainage

Drainage is usually measured by observation and is often described in terms of color and thickness. In the case of heavy drainage where suction might be needed, the liquid exudate may be collected in a canister and measured. Examining wound drainage may be very important because it may indicate a normal response to trauma (a few days) or a prolonged response to necrotic tissue, a foreign substance in the wound, or infection. The most common language for describing wound drainage is described in Table 14.2.

Staging

Pressure injuries are typically classified using a staging or grading system that gives information about the severity of the wound based on depth of tissue destruction. Both the National Pressure Injury Advisory Panel (NPIAP) and the Agency for Healthcare Research and Quality (AHRQ) support the use of the universal classification system described in Table 14.3.[97–100]

Staging can be challenging because tissue damage may be deeper than what appears on the surface, wounds cannot be staged when necrotic tissue is present, and darker skin does not always show the reddened alterations indicating stage 1. To respond to these challenges, the NPIAP has redefined the definition of a pressure injury and the stages of pressure injuries. The new terminology includes the use of Arabic numbers instead of Roman numerals for the stages. The revised stages and the change in terminology from pressure ulcer to pressure injury more accurately describe pressure injuries. These improvements describe injuries to both intact and ulcerated skin, as wounds classified as stage 1 typically present with intact skin that has become more fragile. The staging descriptions are intended for use with pressure injuries and not to describe the severity of other wound types.

Table 14.2 Descriptions of Drainage by Color and Thickness		
Drainage Type	**Color**	**Thickness**
Transudate	Clear	Thin, watery
Serosanguineous	Clear or tinge of red/brown	Thin, watery
Exudate	Creamy, yellowish	Moderate to very thick, expected with autolytic débridement
Pus	Yellow, brown	Moderate to very thick
Infected pus	Hues of yellow, blue, green	Thick, usually indicates infection (but may be normal as white blood cells macrophage necrotic cells and turn them into slough); drainage can be foul and yet the wound may not be infected

Table 14.3 Pressure Injury Staging Criteria Revised by National Pressure Injury Advisory Panel

Pressure injuries are staged to indicate the extent of tissue damage. The stages were revised based on questions received by NPIAP from clinicians attempting to diagnose and identify the stage of pressure injuries. Schematic artwork for each of the stages of pressure injury was also revised and is available for use at no cost through the NPIAP website (https://npiap.com/page/PressureInjuryStages).

Stage	Description
Stage 1 Pressure Injury: Non-blanchable erythema of intact skin	Intact skin with a localized area of non-blanchable erythema, which may appear differently in darkly pigmented skin. Presence of blanchable erythema or changes in sensation, temperature, or firmness may precede visual changes. Color changes do not include purple or maroon discoloration; these may indicate deep tissue pressure injury.
Stage 2 Pressure Injury: Partial-thickness skin loss with exposed dermis	Partial-thickness loss of skin with exposed dermis. The wound bed is viable, pink or red, moist, and may also present as an intact or ruptured serum-filled blister. Adipose (fat) is not visible and deeper tissues are not visible. Granulation tissue, slough, and eschar are not present. These injuries commonly result from adverse microclimate and shear in the skin over the pelvis and shear in the heel. This stage should not be used to describe moisture associated skin damage (MASD) including incontinence associated dermatitis (IAD), intertriginous dermatitis (ITD), medical adhesive related skin injury (MARSI), or traumatic wounds (skin tears, burns, abrasions).
Stage 3 Pressure Injury: Full-thickness skin loss	Full-thickness loss of skin, in which adipose (fat) is visible in the ulcer and granulation tissue and epibole (rolled wound edges) are often present. Slough and/or eschar may be visible. The depth of tissue damage varies by anatomical location; areas of significant adiposity can develop deep wounds. Undermining and tunneling may occur. Fascia, muscle, tendon, ligament, cartilage and/or bone are not exposed. If slough or eschar obscures the extent of tissue loss this is an Unstageable Pressure Injury.
Stage 4 Pressure Injury: Full-thickness skin and tissue loss	Full-thickness skin and tissue loss with exposed or directly palpable fascia, muscle, tendon, ligament, cartilage, or bone in the ulcer. Slough and/or eschar may be visible. Epibole (rolled edges), undermining and/or tunneling often occur. Depth varies by anatomical location. If slough or eschar obscures the extent of tissue loss this is an Unstageable Pressure Injury.
Unstageable Pressure Injury: Obscured full-thickness skin and tissue loss	Full-thickness skin and tissue loss in which the extent of tissue damage within the ulcer cannot be confirmed because it is obscured by slough or eschar. If slough or eschar is removed, a Stage 3 or Stage 4 pressure injury will be revealed. Stable eschar (i.e., dry, adherent, intact without erythema or fluctuance) on the heel or ischemic limb should not be softened or removed.
DTPI: Persistent non-blanchable deep red, maroon or purple discoloration	Intact or non-intact skin with localized area of persistent non-blanchable deep red, maroon, purple discoloration, or epidermal separation revealing a dark wound bed or blood-filled blister. Pain and temperature change often precede skin color changes. Discoloration may appear differently in darkly pigmented skin. This injury results from intense and/or prolonged pressure and shear forces at the bone–muscle interface. The wound may evolve rapidly to reveal the actual extent of tissue injury or may resolve without tissue loss. If necrotic tissue, subcutaneous tissue, granulation tissue, fascia, muscle, or other underlying structures are visible, this indicates a full thickness pressure injury (unstageable, Stage 3, or Stage 4). Do not use DTPI to describe vascular, traumatic, neuropathic, or dermatologic conditions.

Additional Pressure Injury Definitions

Medical Device–Related Pressure Injury: This describes an etiology. Medical device–related pressure injuries result from the use of devices designed and applied for diagnostic or therapeutic purposes. The resultant pressure injury generally conforms to the pattern or shape of the device. The injury should be staged using the staging system

Mucosal Membrane Pressure Injury: Mucosal membrane pressure injury is found on mucous membranes with a history of a medical device in use at the location of the injury. Due to the anatomy of the tissue these injuries cannot be staged.

Used with permission of the National Pressure Ulcer Advisory Panel, April 12, 2017. The permission granted through this process cannot be transferred to others or used for other purposes than expressed above and approved by the NPIAP. ©NPIAP
Source: https://npiap.com/page/PressureInjuryStages
DPTI = Deep pressure tissue injury.

Wound Healing Tools

A variety of tools can be utilized to document wound status and wound healing. Since there is no single wound characteristic that can be used alone to monitor healing or predict outcomes, it is best to use a tool that includes multiple characteristics as measures of wound healing. The three tools with the most well-established reliability and validity are the *Sussman Wound Healing Tool*,[32] the *Pressure Ulcer Scale for Healing*,[32,100] and the *Pressure Sore Status Tool*.[32] The *Wagner Ulcer Grade Classification* system is a tool designed for examination of a patient with a diabetic foot when neuropathy and ischemia are present.[32,101]

Risk Factor Assessment

Although all individuals may be subjected to the same intensities of pressure for similar amounts of time, they all will not develop pressure injuries. As a result, factors related to individual risk, susceptibility, or tolerance capacity should be determined. A physical therapy provider will find that data from a risk assessment can be helpful in planning cost-effective intervention strategies. As discussed earlier in the chapter, there are many factors that put individuals at risk for developing pressure injuries, such as poor peripheral circulation, diabetes mellitus, nutritional status, mobility, and continence issues, to name a few. To objectify and standardize risk assessment, a number of reliable tools have been validated by research:

- *Norton Risk Assessment Scale:* original risk assessment instrument scores individuals on physical condition, mental condition, activity, mobility, and incontinence.[102]
- *Gosnell Scale–Pressure Sore Risk Assessment:* refinement of the Norton scale includes changes to the following scoring categories: nutrition, mental condition, activity, mobility, continence, skin appearance, medication, diet, and fluid balance.[103]
- *Braden Scale for Predicting Pressure Sore Risk:* the six scoring categories of this instrument include sensory perception, moisture, activity, mobility, nutrition, and friction/shear.[104]

Muscle Performance

Muscle strength screening during the systems review and specific manual muscle testing during the examination should be included for the individual with a disorder of the vascular, lymphatic, or integumentary system. Functional muscle strength identified during an examination of functional mobility skills and ADL is also important. Lack of strength and immobility exist concurrently, often leading to problems such as pressure injuries, CVI, increased LE edema and lymphedema, varicosities, and poor control of diabetic sequelae.

Orthotic, Protective, and Supportive Devices

There are many situations in which an individual who has disorders mentioned in this chapter would need to be assessed for an orthotic, protective, or supportive device. Those individuals already using a device may need a modification. For the individual with impaired sensation of the feet, *extra-depth* shoes may be indicated. Existing shoes should be checked periodically for fit and wear. A referral to another professional for protective footwear may be needed. Supportive devices may allow an individual to increase their activity level, offsetting the risks of a sedentary lifestyle. Compression garments and bandaging, considered *supportive devices,* must be checked periodically for fit and function to ensure that they retain their effectiveness. Garments and bandages will be essential intervention choices for most individuals with edema and lymphedema. In the later stages, a patient's need for devices may provide a way to quantify the remediation of impairments or activity limitations imposed by the symptoms of the disorder. A physical therapist is skilled in selecting, fitting, and monitoring the best devices in this category. A poorly fitted device may do more harm than good.

Pain

Pain is often a cause of psychological distress for individuals with chronic wounds. The presence or absence of pain, its location and intensity, its effect on sleep, and other QOL factors should be measured (see Chapter 25, Chronic Pain). Pain scales, drawings, and maps are effective for documentation. Owing to the high incidence of comorbidity in patients with disorders of the vascular, lymphatic, and integumentary systems, the measurement of pain may also assist in making a differential diagnosis.

Posture

Indications for examination of posture include pain, heavy or large limbs, scar tissue, poor body image (e.g., following cancer treatment), obesity, and decreased sensation. Data can be obtained with the combined use of a posture grid, tape measure, observation, and palpation. A physical therapy provider will begin a posture assessment initially by observation the moment the client enters the room and will continue to assess and observe posture formally and informally during the examination and intervention.

Range of Motion

The need for adequate ROM and the impact of decreased ROM cannot be underestimated. Following ROM screening during the systems review, specific ROM measurements are often indicated, especially with persons for whom movement is an essential part of symptom management. Examples are numerous but include ankle ROM for the person with CVI, shoulder ROM following breast cancer surgery, or knee ROM in the individual with lymphedema of the LE. A universal goniometer or inclinometer and tape measure are required to obtain objective ROM data.

Self-Care and Home Management

Activity limitations and disability are common with disorders of the vascular, lymphatic, and integumentary systems. Examination, education, and training that allow the patient to safely perform self-care and home management activities are of great importance in planning and implementing the self-management phase. Descriptions and quantifications are needed for documentation and goal setting. Examination tools should include functional measures of both basic activities of daily living and instrumental activities of daily living, as well as fall risk scales (see Chapter 8, Examination of Function).

Sensation

Information from the history and systems review may indicate the need for a detailed examination of sensory function. Therapists should not rely on history alone as an indication for sensory testing, however, because many individuals are unaware of their deficits until tested. Sensory tests are particularly important when symptoms are long-standing or include complaints of numbness, tingling, or burning. Patients who should routinely be tested are those who may receive LE compression treatments, and all individuals who have a diagnosis of peripheral neuropathy, diabetes mellitus, and/or arterial disease. In addition to observation and palpation, therapists should conduct initial testing for protective sensation using filaments such as the *Semmes-Weinstein monofilaments*. The filaments are supplied in varying sizes and are each mounted on a handle. The filament is used to apply pressure to the skin until it bends. The patient is asked to report, with eyes closed, whether the filament is touching the body part. Each monofilament supplies a specific amount of force when it is placed on the test area and gently bent. The monofilaments are available in a large set, but most testing can be accomplished using a few filaments. An individual has *normal sensation* when the 4.17 monofilament (1 *g* of force) can be felt on the plantar surface of the skin. An individual has *protective sensation* intact when the 5.07 filament (10 *g* of force) can be felt (Fig. 14.16). With loss of protective sensation, the individual cannot sense trauma to the foot, often leading to foot ulceration. For the individual who has lost protective sensation, the use of special protective footwear is indicated. Lack of sensation, especially protective sensation, can be a characteristic of long-standing diabetes mellitus. Decreased sensation may signal a disorder such as *scleroderma*. To test for sharp/dull sensation, vibratory sensation, pressure, and other sensations, tools for gathering data include a pressure scale, tuning fork, and/or aesthesiometer.

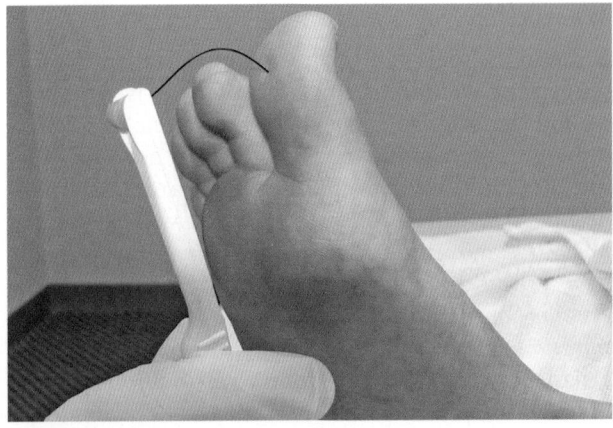

Figure 14.16 A monofilament used to assess presence of protective sensation. Bowing of the filament indicates that appropriate pressure has been applied.

Ventilation and Respiration

Tests and measures should be used to determine if the patient has adequate ventilation and respiration to meet normal oxygen demands. The presence of pathology might be indicated from a predictable source such as breath sounds or the color of nailbeds. A less predictable sign, such as swelling around the ankles, could also indicate pathology. Initial data may be gathered by examining arterial blood gases, observing the work of breathing, or utilizing a spirometer. Additional appropriate tests include the airway clearance test and use of a pulse oximeter (see Chapter 12, Chronic Pulmonary Dysfunction).

Evaluation

Diagnosis, Prognosis, and Plan of Care

Once the examination is complete, the physical therapist evaluates the data and determines the diagnosis and prognosis. The physical therapist needs to consider a number of factors, including clinical findings, overall physical function and health status, social support, multisystem involvement and comorbid conditions, and chronicity, severity, and stability of the condition. This information is outlined in the *Guide to Physical Therapist Practice*[82] and presented in this textbook. The next step is the design and implementation of the POC, including procedural interventions.

■ INTERVENTION

Physical therapist intervention for disorders of the vascular, lymphatic, and/or integumentary systems should include a variety of techniques to address the problems identified during the examination. It is common for patients with disorders in these systems to present with multiple factors contributing to the primary diagnosis. The intervention plan should reflect a holistic view of the patient. For example, an individual with signs and symptoms of venous disease may also present with poor ankle ROM, an LE wound, and lymphedema. The wound must be cleansed and dressed, but the limb should also receive compression for optimum healing. Ankle ROM must be improved because ambulation will enhance calf pump function. Another example of the need to view patients holistically would be an individual with signs and symptoms of arterial disease who also presents with decreased LE strength, diabetes, and peripheral neuropathy. Exercise is important for this person, but it must be carefully coordinated to address arterial health, diabetes management, and skin protection.

A natural component of viewing patients holistically is to be able to identify the need for interdisciplinary care. This concept may be more important for individuals with disorders of the vascular, lymphatic, or integumentary systems for the very reasons listed in the previous paragraph: These populations present with complicated, multisystem problems that are often best addressed using a team approach. Integrated care facilitates an exchange of information among all the health professionals who are involved in the care of the patient. This model of care might be delivered by a team of individuals who work together every day, or it might be coordinated by a medical provider who pulls together certain professionals for a particular patient's needs.

Coordination, Communication, and Documentation

In keeping with practice standards, the physical therapy provider coordinates intervention efforts to ensure the patient receives the highest quality of care. Critical to this goal is open communication among the health-care team, patient, family, and caregivers. The team will most likely include a physician, nurse, physical therapist, occupational therapist, dietitian, and social worker. Referrals to other health-care professionals (e.g., podiatrist, orthotist, or prosthetist) who can support the patient can also be made. Meticulous documentation will have a significant impact on issues such as continuity of care, an adequate number of visits for procedures, and a stronger working relationship with referring practitioners. Photographs, special forms for data collection, and body graphs are very effective tools to enhance communication and documentation. Appendix 14.C (online) provides an example of an examination form that might be used to document data collected for a patient with a disorder of the vascular, lymphatic, or integumentary system.

Patient-/Client-Related Instruction

Disorders of the vascular, lymphatic, and integumentary systems represent major health events for patients and their families and require lifelong management strategies. Patients and families often react with anger, despair, or confusion when learning about a condition

that may be permanent. The value of patient and family education cannot be underestimated. Patient education will be the key to preparing individuals to manage their symptoms, prevent recurrence, and remain vigilant about their condition. Information should be provided that is appropriate to the patient/family/caregiver's educational level with provisions for follow-up and repetition. Motivational strategies are important to ensure adherence to self-management. For many chronic disorders, high-quality patient education has been shown to result in positive changes in health behaviors, QOL perceptions, and adherence to home programs. Instruction for the patient should include resources, educational materials, and a home program.

Resources for patients with vascular, lymphatic, and integumentary disorders include the following:

- Community services and support groups related to the patient's diagnosis
- Counseling services, as needed, especially for assistance with QOL issues
- Internet sites
- Family member participation in care
- Educational materials
- Instructional materials, multimedia tools
- Self-management strategies
- Available resources including materials found on the Internet (see Appendix 14.D [online])
- Home program
- Skin and/or wound care; prevention practices; scar management
- Compression garment or bandage wear and care
- Exercise
- Edema control
- PRDs
- Foot care for patients with diabetes (see Appendix 14.A (online) for a foot care guide)

Outpatient or home therapy may be required for some patients. Follow-up visits at regularly scheduled intervals may be the best way to facilitate adherence to the home program and to prevent recurrence or exacerbation of symptoms.

Procedural Interventions

This section has been organized in the order in which a physical therapy provider would provide patient care. Within each section, information has been organized from most invasive/least selective (nonspecific) to least invasive/most selective (highly specific). In developing the POC, a physical therapist should select interventions that are least invasive/most selective, always trying to create an environment that is conducive to healing. The ultimate goal should be to optimize the body's opportunity to heal. Despite tremendous gains in the management of vascular, lymphatic, and integumentary disorders, there are still an alarming number of practitioners using outdated and often harmful methods to treat these disorders. Overused interventions such as povidone-iodine, wet-to-dry dressings, whirlpool, and compression pumps have been replaced for at least two decades with more advanced, biocompatible, and cost-effective methods of treatment.[105] The use of inappropriate agents can delay healing and may cause harm. Supporting literature abounds for the clinician seeking evidence-based practice. Elements of skin and wound care that are often overlooked or underestimated for their impact include PRDs, positioning, exercise, patient education, compression, and orthotics.

The physical therapy provider treating a patient with a wound should strive to establish an ideal wound healing environment. The choices made about intervention should be guided by the goal of achieving this ideal environment, described as moist, free from necrotic tissue, free from exudate, warm, protected from trauma, and protected from infection. Physical therapists may manage wound care in a primary care role or in consultation with a physician and/or other providers. Interventions involving pharmaceuticals will always require physician consultation for a prescription. "Although practice may change based on new evidence, the search for healing in the most humane way and fastest time possible persists as the goal."[106(pS1)]

Cleansing

Wound cleansing is differentiated from wound débridement, which is discussed in the next section. The wound cleansing method should be selected based on its ability to support or return a wound bed to homeostasis. Chemical and mechanical trauma should be minimized even in the presence of infection. A decision to cleanse should be made carefully because many wounds do not need to be cleansed at every dressing change. Often the negative effects to the wound from cleansing outweigh the positives. There is not only potential loss of endogenous fluids from the wound surface but also significant slowing of cellular activity for up to 3 hr after wound cleansing.[107]

Whirlpool

Since whirlpool can be classified as a means of cleansing and mechanical débridement, it is discussed in both categories of intervention. Despite at least a decade of investigation, with little evidence to support its use, whirlpool is still used by some clinicians for both nonselective mechanical débridement and wound cleansing. However, many clinicians involved in wound care have decreased their use of whirlpool significantly in response to the evolution of wound care and the subsequent publication of the Clinical Practice Guidelines of a joint panel of NPUAP, European Pressure Ulcer Advisory Panel (EPUAP), and Pan Pacific Pressure Injury Alliance (PPPIA). These guidelines state that "it is seldom used and is no longer recommended."[108]

Standards have changed with increased knowledge of the microenvironment in the wound bed and a greater understanding of the chemical mediators necessary for homeostasis.

The historical rationale for use of whirlpool was based on its use in deodorization, skin and wound cleansing, mechanical nonselective débridement, wound decontamination and infection control, and softening of adherent necrotic tissue in preparation for débridement. There is little evidence to support whirlpool as the *optimal* method for achieving these.

Evidence-based rationale for a decrease in the use of whirlpool is based on several factors. There is risk of contamination from waterborne pathogens and from patient cross contamination. The dependent position can initiate or increase venous congestion and extremity edema. With whirlpool, there is loss of endogenous fluids from the wound bed and heat loss affecting core body temperature and the local wound area. Even mild changes in core body temperature (hypothermia) have negative effects on the cells that are important to wound healing. In addition, mechanical disruption of granulation tissue, epithelial cells, and new skin grafts occurs, primarily from the use of water agitation. Immersion in a whirlpool saturates wound tissue and surrounding skin, creating the potential for maceration, skin breakdown, and temporary inactivation of normal skin defenses. Thus, there is the potential to prolong inflammation and delay wound healing. Whirlpool can also increase heart and respiratory rates. Finally, the use of whirlpool is labor intensive and costly in terms of use of water, utilities, linen, and staff.[109]

Pulsatile Lavage With Suction

Pulsatile lavage with suction (*PLWS*, also referred to as *forceful irrigation*) is a method of wound irrigation combined with suction (Fig. 14.17).[110] Pulsed irrigation and simultaneous suction remove the irrigation fluid, wound exudate, and loose debris. In use for over

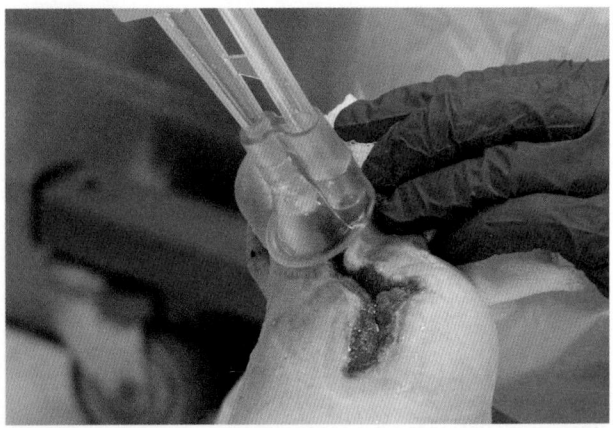

Figure 14.17 Physical therapist guides the pulsatile lavage with suction shield close to the wound surface.

several decades, this wound cleansing and débridement method has several advantages over whirlpool cleansing. PLWS uses less water, requires less staff support, and involves less treatment time and less cleanup time. PLWS can be performed bedside and in the home. (*Note*: Family or visitors should not be allowed in the room during the procedure owing to aerosolization of microorganisms.)[111-115] This type of cleansing collects wound exudate and debris efficiently and delivers topical antibiotics, antiseptics, and antibacterial solutions efficiently. PLWS speeds healing by rapid removal of contaminants and treats tunneling wounds and undermining wounds using special cannula tips (Fig. 14.18). The risk of periwound maceration and cross contamination is eliminated with use of disposable equipment.

Although the advantages are clear, there are disadvantages to using PLWS. These include risk of overuse, especially with clean, granulating wounds, and risk of trauma to newly formed tissue from plastic tips, pulsed irrigant, and/or suction. Treatment may be painful to the patient. PLWS use should be limited to experienced therapy providers who are well versed in anatomy, especially when irrigating tracts, areas of undermining, or exposed bone, tendon, blood vessels, cavity linings, grafts, or flaps. All staff involved in treatment must wear disposable personal protective equipment (PPE). Compared to other irrigation options, disposable, single-use equipment contributes to landfill burden. There is considerable cost when labor, PPE, and equipment are calculated.

Nonforceful Irrigation

As soon as possible, wound cleansing should be accomplished with minimal pressure or force on the wound bed by nonforceful irrigation. This can be accomplished by pouring a solution over a wound or using a bulb syringe or other device designed to deliver an irrigant to the wound (Fig. 14.19). There are several products that package saline specifically for wound cleansing.

Several manufacturers produce a spray container that delivers saline or a surfactant at very gentle pressures (Fig. 14.20). Infected wounds can also be effectively cleaned with nonforceful irrigation. Wounds with necrotic tissue or debris, however, may respond best to a few sessions of a more forceful type of cleansing. For wounds that are clean, with new tissue growth, cleansing should be done only to remove excess endogenous fluids or residue left by dressing products.

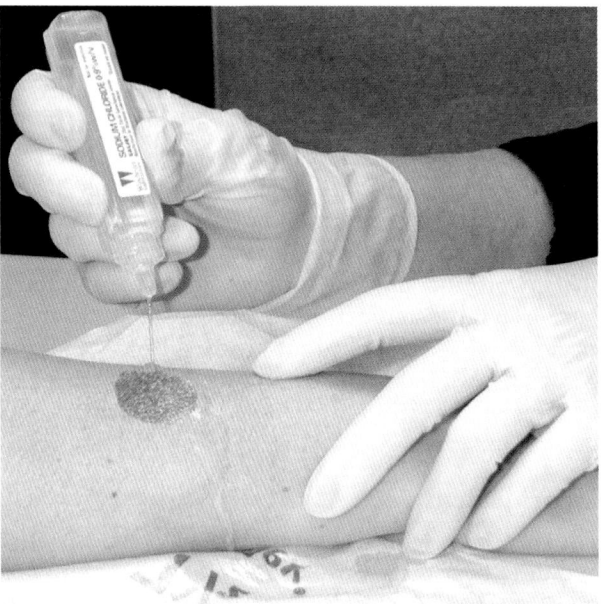

Figure 14.19 Wound cleansing with nonforceful irrigation.

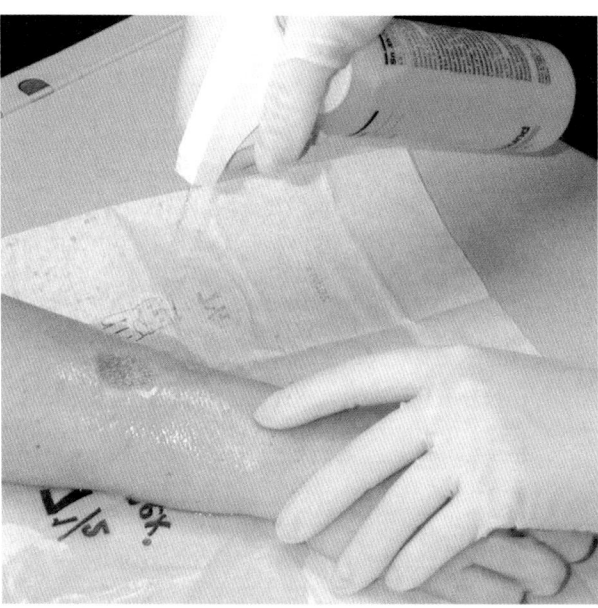

Figure 14.20 Wound cleansing with a spray cleanser.

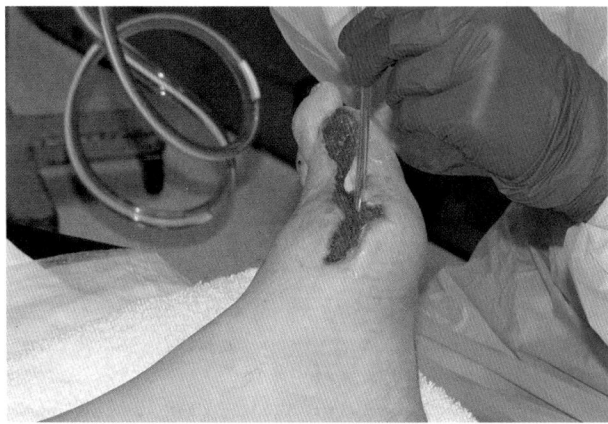

Figure 14.18 A special tip may be used to gently cleanse a deeper wound with pulsatile lavage with suction.

Commercial Skin and Wound Cleansers

There are many skin and wound cleansers designed as topical solutions and marketed to treat acute and chronic wounds. For many years, solutions have been used indiscriminately without consideration or measurement of the potential side effects on the new cells budding in the wound bed during the proliferation phase. These topical cleansers may have some antimicrobial effects, but most have significant antimitotic (inhibiting mitosis) effects as well.[115] This means that cleansers may adversely affect important cells such as fibroblasts and epidermal keratinocytes during tissue repair. The cells most affected are the all-important cells that fill and cover a wound. Information on the toxicity of the most common cleansers has been created to assist health-care providers in selecting or rejecting the use of cleansers.[115,116] It is no surprise that acetic acid is extremely cytotoxic to the cells in a wound, but of greater concern is the fact that ordinary bath soaps, even moisturizing body washes, are very cytotoxic. A physical therapy provider utilizing commercial cleansers or ordinary soap must consider the rationale behind the use of each topical agent applied to the wound and weigh the cost to the wound: some contribute to wound healing, whereas others contribute to aspects other than wound healing.

Débridement

Débridement is defined as the removal of foreign material and dead or damaged tissue. Removal of devitalized or infected tissue is a chief intervention to prevent or control bacterial growth, encourage normal cellular activity in the wound bed, and enhance the rate of tissue repair. For clarity in this chapter, *nonselective débridement* refers to techniques that remove all tissue, both necrotic and living. Methods in this category may be quick but are often painful and frequently cause damage to nearby healthy tissue. *Selective débridement* refers to techniques that remove necrotic tissue in a controlled method. Selective methods are more comfortable and gentle to the wound bed but may remove tissue more slowly.

The importance of physical therapist proficiency in sharp débridement is reflected in the *Guide to Physical Therapist Practice*.[82] In response, most professional-level programs include instruction in sharp débridement within the curriculum. In the majority of states, débridement is included in the scope of practice for physical therapists. Physical therapy providers should consult their state's practice act to ensure that débridement is within their scope of practice before providing this intervention.

When choosing a method of débridement, clinicians must consider not only the wound status but also the physiological, emotional, and financial status of the patient. Modern wound management experts avoid débridement techniques that cause the wound to bleed excessively due to the highly damaging effects to the wound tissues.

Nonselective Débridement

WET-TO-DRY DRESSINGS

A wet-to-dry (WTD) dressing consists of wet gauze applied to the wound bed and allowed to dry on the wound. Removal of the dry dressing débrides the wound, pulling away any cellular material that has adhered to the gauze. This method of débridement removes necrotic tissue as well as rich endogenous fluids, fibrin, and other cells critical to wound healing. It is frequently uncomfortable for the patient, often causing bleeding and trauma to the wound bed. There is literature to describe the use of WTD dressings for débridement, but the efficacy of the procedure has not been demonstrated.[117,118] Wound management experts agree with a multidisciplinary panel: "One of the most routinely and inappropriately used forms of non-selective mechanical débridement is the WTD dressing."[119(p28)] Once believed to be less costly than other dressing options, it has been shown that WTD gauze dressings are actually more costly than dressings made of advanced materials. There is evidence that clearly highlights the many negative aspects of WTD dressings and encourages clinicians to choose more beneficial débridement options.[120–127]

Since WTD dressings can be classified as a tool for mechanical débridement and/or a primary wound dressing, the procedure has been discussed here and in the section on dressings.

SURGICAL DÉBRIDEMENT

Surgical débridement provides rapid results when treating life-threatening necrosis, large wounds, tunneling wounds, and necrotic or infected bone. Wide excision, removing viable and nonviable tissue, is usually done in the operating room with anesthesia. Laser débridement, another form of surgical débridement, may be appropriate when an individual is not a candidate for operating room procedures. Surgical débridement is not within the scope of practice of a physical therapist.

PULSATILE LAVAGE WITH SUCTION

PLWS will provide nonselective débridement while cleansing a wound. Refer to the detailed discussion of PLWS in the "Cleansing" section earlier.

WHIRLPOOL

Whirlpool can be used for mechanical débridement through its feature of water agitation. It can also be used to soften necrotic tissue in preparation for sharp, enzymatic, or autolytic débridement. There are, however, often better methods of preparing tissue for débridement than whirlpool. See discussion in the "Cleansing" section earlier.

Selective Débridement

SHARP

Sharp débridement is defined as the removal of dead or necrotic tissue or foreign material from and around a wound using sterile instruments such as a scalpel (Fig. 14.21), scissors, and/or forceps (Fig. 14.22). Considered the *gold standard* of methods for removal of necrotic tissue, sharp débridement is a minor, tissue-sparing procedure that is performed bedside or in a procedure room. In the majority of U.S. states, it is within the scope of practice for a physical therapist to perform sharp débridement. It is incumbent on the therapist to be aware of their state practice act regarding regulations. The American Physical Therapy Association (APTA) position statement indicates that sharp débridement should be performed exclusively by physical therapists, not other personnel. For a full copy of this statement, go to https://www.apta.org/article/2020/10/30/analysis-value-physical-therapy-wound-care. Additional information can be found in the *Guide to Physical Therapist Practice*.[82] To maintain

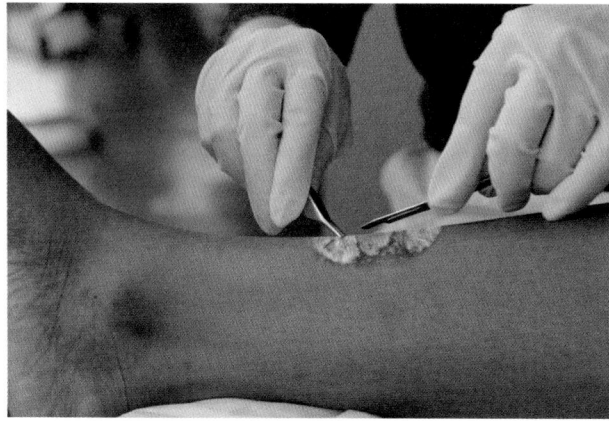

Figure 14.21 Use of scalpel and forceps for sharp débridement.

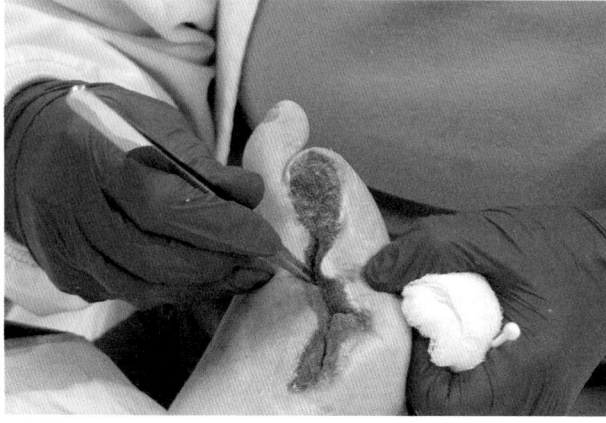

Figure 14.22 Selective débridement of necrotic tissue can be accomplished using forceps.

current standards, a physical therapist should not débride except in the presence of necrotic tissue.

Even though sharp débridement is effective for all types of necrotic tissue, there are situations in which this form of débridement is not appropriate. It is contraindicated for vascular wounds with limited blood flow where eschar may be serving as a cap or cover for a chronic open wound. Without adequate perfusion in this scenario, there is little hope of wound closure. Sharp débridement is not appropriate for wounds with tunneling (when the wound bed cannot be seen) or areas affected by dry gangrene. Patients with low platelet counts, on anticoagulants, or with other conditions that inhibit clotting are not suitable candidates. It may be contraindicated for pressure injuries on the heels covered with dry eschar. (*Note:* Some experts maintain that in this scenario, eschar provides protection as long as there is no infection present; others maintain that eschar must be removed because it inhibits epithelial cell growth.)[99]

CHEMICAL OR ENZYMATIC

Enzymatic débridement is a type of selective débridement that includes the application of a topical agent containing enzymes that act by dissolving necrotic tissue. There are several types and brands of enzymatic agents, each designed to affect a certain type of necrotic tissue. Advantages for this type of treatment are that débridement is selective, patient discomfort is minimal, and application procedures are simple. Disadvantages include the potential development of dermatitis of the intact periwound skin, frequent dressing changes disrupting the wound bed, and the need to crosshatch existing eschar with a scalpel so that the enzyme can penetrate the wound. Enzymatic débridement agents do not have an impact on pathogen levels in the wound bed and should not be considered antimicrobial. Some enzymatic débridement preparations contain the protein papain. Topical drug products containing papain were taken off the market in the United States in November 2008 because they were not approved by the Food and Drug Administration (FDA). When utilizing other types of enzymatic agents still on the market, a referral for treatment and a prescription for the enzymatic agent are currently required in most regions of North America.

BIOSURGERY

Biosurgery as a form of selective débridement is also referred to as *maggot débridement therapy* (MDT), or maggot or larval therapy (Fig. 14.23). Although it has been in use in the Western world for over 150 years, its popularity declined with the advent of antibiotics. Biosurgery is now generating new interest owing to the rise of multidrug-resistant bacteria such as methicillin-resistant *Staphylococcus aureus* (MRSA). Sterile, newly hatched larvae are placed on chronic wounds and

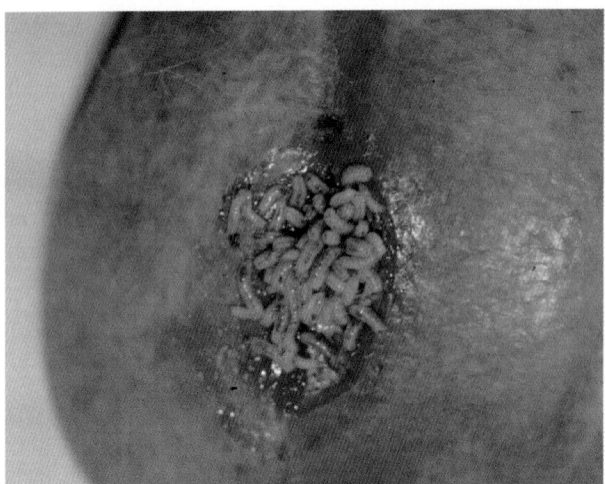

Figure 14.23 Maggot therapy for a cavity wound.
(Courtesy of the Biosurgical Research Unit, Surgical Materials Testing Laboratory, Bridgend, UK.)

held in place with dressings or a *biobag* for 2 to 5 days before removal. Biosurgery has been shown to remove devitalized tissue, decrease the risk of infection, and improve wound healing without side effects in a wide variety of wound types. Biosurgery is recommended for osteomyelitis and deep wound infections that remain unresponsive to more conventional antibiotic and surgical therapy. Although moist wound healing is compatible with biosurgery, a very wet wound environment has an adverse effect on larval survival. Certain types of moisture-retentive wound dressings are more compatible with larval survival than others.[128–137]

Medical-Grade Honey

The use of medical-grade honey as a wound dressing has been shown to enhance débridement and healing. Honey dressings are available in hydrocolloid, alginate, and liquid categories. They have been shown to facilitate autolytic débridement, decrease or eliminate wound odor, prevent biofilm (thin layer of bacteria) formation, and soften necrotic tissue.[138–143]

Autolytic Débridement

Autolytic débridement uses the endogenous enzymes on the wound bed to digest devitalized tissue and promote granulation tissue formation. In practice, the body's natural fluids are held in contact with the wound base with a moisture-retentive dressing for 3 to 7 days. By increasing the moisture content of slough and necrotic tissue with enzyme-rich body fluids, autolytic activity is facilitated. Although this method is the least invasive/most selective, as well as inexpensive, painless, and biocompatible, each patient is examined to determine if this type of débridement is best for the existing wound. The type of moisture-retentive dressing selected to promote autolytic débridement will be based on the health of the periwound tissues and the level of fungal or

bacterial loads. The presence of infection does not rule out the use of occlusive dressings, as described earlier in the discussion on moist wound healing.

Topical Agents

Current standards for chronic wound care have decreased the use of topical agents even in the presence of infection. In the literature, these agents may be referred to as *antiseptics, disinfectants,* and/or *antimicrobials.* Other topical agent categories include *antibiotics* and *analgesics.* Guidelines reveal that almost all human-made products are cytotoxic to WBCs even when diluted.[98] Many agents once thought to be safe are now known to be unsafe to healing tissue, causing adverse reactions at any concentration. Many agents once thought to be effective as antibacterial or decontaminating agents are now known to be ineffective. When striving for wound bed homeostasis, preserving cellular life in endogenous fluids is almost always more desirable than destroying it with additives. Many physicians and wound management experts use the following adage to guide in the decision-making process: "It is desirable never to put anything in the wound that cannot be tolerated comfortably in the conjunctival sac."[144] In plain terms, "If you can't put it in your eyes, don't put it in the wound." Even under Direct Access, in most states physical therapists are not permitted to prescribe medications, even over-the-counter products, for wound care. If, during the examination or intervention, a physical therapist determines that a topical agent may be indicated, the patient's physician should be contacted and the findings discussed. Consideration of topical agents should always include the risks and benefits of the topical agent in relation to potential cytotoxicity, biocompatibility, safety, and efficacy.

Antiseptics

Povidone-Iodine

Povidone-iodine (PVI) is a combination of iodine plus a polymer that provides bactericidal effects. One commonly known product name is Betadine (Purdue Products LP, Stamford, CT 06901). Used indiscriminately for many years on acute and chronic wounds, it is now recommended mainly for wounds infected with *S. aureus.* The 1994 AHRQ guidelines advised against cleansing ulcer wounds with skin cleansers or antiseptic agents (e.g., povidone-iodine, iodophor, sodium hypochlorite solution [Dakin solution], hydrogen peroxide, acetic acid).[99] Although the guidelines address pressure injuries, the wound-healing evidence is applicable to all wound treatments. In 2018, newer clinical practice guidelines also supported the avoidance of skin cleansers on intact skin.[99,108] This evidence implies that the use of PVI, as well as other antiseptics, is inconsistent with practice standards. In rare instances when such agents are recommended by a physician and are indeed appropriate, clinicians should document sound reasoning behind the use of these products because they will be held accountable to these published and respected guidelines. An example of a situation such as this would be when other, less cytotoxic treatments have failed to reduce the bacterial load in an infected wound. The literature does not provide adequate clinical or legal reasons to use PVI for managing wounds. In addition, the FDA has not approved the use of PVI solution or PVI surgical scrub solution for wounds. PVI has been shown to reduce bacterial counts in infected wounds, and currently there is no antimicrobial resistance to PVI.[143] Its use is contraindicated for the noninfected wound.[98]

SODIUM HYPOCHLORITE SOLUTIONS: DAKIN SOLUTION (BLEACH AND BORIC ACID), SODIUM HYPOCHLORITE (HOUSEHOLD BLEACH)

Sodium hypochlorite is cytotoxic even at very dilute concentrations. It damages fibroblasts and endothelial cells and causes cellular damage to granulation tissue. It is irritating to the skin and can initiate severe reactions in some individuals. It is used in the management of wounds with purulent exudate. Treatment should be discontinued when the wound is clean. Its use is contraindicated for the noninfected wound.[98,144]

ACETIC ACID SOLUTION

Acetic acid is traditionally used to inhibit bacterial infections; however, the solution has been found to be more damaging to fibroblasts than to bacteria. A common form of acetic acid is found in vinegar. It is corrosive and cytotoxic at any dilution. It has been used to manage contamination by *Pseudomonas aeruginosa*. Its use is contraindicated for the noninfected wound.[98,144]

OXIDIZING AGENTS: HYDROGEN PEROXIDE SOLUTION

When this solution comes in contact with tissue, there is a release of oxygen and temporary antimicrobial activity. Its bubbling action is used for nonselective débridement to loosen small debris. It is cytotoxic unless diluted to a very weak concentration. Its use is contraindicated for wounds that are noninfected, tunneling, or granulating.[98,144]

Antibacterials

This section includes a sample of commonly used topical antimicrobials, antibiotics, and antibacterials. Each of these topical agents is effective against a variety of bacteria and is selected by the physician based on the species cultured for an individual patient. All share a risk of similar side effects such as burning, itching, contact dermatitis, and/or allergic sensitivity. There is little evidence in the literature to show levels of cytotoxicity in these topical agents. Examples include the following:

- Bacitracin/Baciguent: associated with allergic reactions.
- Neosporin/neomycin sulfate: causes greatest incidence of allergic reactions.

- Silvadene/silver sulfadiazine: primarily for thermal injuries, silver is selectively toxic to bacteria but may inactivate topical proteolytic enzymes.[144]
- Sulfamylon/mafenide acetate: diffuses easily through eschar, primarily for thermal injuries.
- Bactroban/mupirocin ointment: currently effective against all species of staphylococcus.
- Gentamicin/Garamycin: currently effective against all species of staphylococcus and streptococcus.

Owing to the paucity of information on cytotoxicity, risk of side effects, and growing incidence of antibiotic-resistant bacteria, use of these products for chronic wounds should be considered carefully and is usually contraindicated for the noninfected wound.

CREAMS AND OINTMENTS (OVER THE COUNTER)

Some antibacterial ointments and creams such as Bacitracin and Neosporin can be purchased without a prescription. These are minimally bacteriostatic owing to their dilution. Once they lose their antibacterial strength, the ointments may trap bacteria and encourage bacterial growth from surface contamination. If ointments or creams are used, the wound should be cleansed regularly to remove potential contamination; however, frequent cleansing may disrupt the healing process. These preparations can be used to provide moisture to a dry wound, but they may create a greasy wound bed, making early epithelial cell migration difficult. A more biocompatible ointment that will provide moisture to a healing wound is Aquaphor (Beiersdorf Inc., Wilton, CT 06897).

Analgesics

The use of topical anesthetics to control wound pain is controversial in the literature. Conflicting reports and the lack of substantial research have led to concerns about the impact of anesthetics on the wound bed. This issue is further complicated by the broad profile of patients with wounds, their etiologies, and comorbidities. The more common agents used topically are lidocaine or a mixture of lidocaine and prilocaine. Amitriptyline, a tricyclic antidepressant, has local anesthetic properties and has shown promise as an option for treating wound pain when applied topically.[145] While topical anesthetics may be under scrutiny for their effects, vasoconstriction in particular, there is a need for more investigation since pain is a major issue for most patients with wounds.[145]

Growth Factors

Growth factors are substances that stimulate cell growth and proliferation. These substances serve as the messaging center to signal other cells in the area to act. They usually consist of a group of proteins but can also include hormones. Growth factors normally abound in the fluids of a wound. In most chronic wounds, the normal timetable for healing has been delayed or stopped due in part to a decrease in the amount of growth factors in the wound. Growth factors that are decreased or absent can be added topically to the wound bed. Increasingly, evidence supports the practice of adding growth factors to a wound to facilitate healing. The practice of applying exogenous growth factors in conjunction with good wound care has been accepted for over 20 years.[17,146–149] Growth factors can be isolated from an individual's own tissue, added to a liquid formula in a laboratory, and then applied to the wound. Growth factors can also be cultivated in a laboratory from human platelets and packaged in a gel form. An example of an autologous growth factor product with a name familiar to many clinicians is Aurix System (Cytomedix Inc., Gaithersburg, MD 20877).[150] Recombinant DNA technology has resulted in other products such as Becaplermin gel (Regranex Gel; Smith & Nephew Inc, Andover, MA 01810).[151] Reimbursement for the application of growth factors varies and should be checked before use. For example, Becaplermin gel is FDA approved for the treatment of LE diabetic neuropathic ulcers that extend into the subcutaneous tissue or beyond but currently may not be approved for the treatment of pressure, venous, or other nondiabetic-related wounds.

Topical Agents and Acute Wounds

The use of antiseptics and antibiotics to reduce bacterial levels in acute, traumatic wounds follows a different rationale from that of chronic wounds. The risk for contamination is high in wounds resulting from trauma or thermal injury. It is accepted practice to use cytotoxic products such as povidone-iodine or Silvadene (silver sulfadiazine) in the *early* management of acute traumatic wounds. The goal is to discontinue the use of cytotoxic agents as soon as the wounds are clean and able to produce and support endogenous fluids.

Mechanical Modalities

Procedures for use of modalities vary based on unique patient characteristics and individual patient response. Several comprehensive wound management texts such as *Wound Healing: Evidence-Based Management* by McCulloch and Kloth[152] and *Wound Care: A Collaborative Practice Manual for Health Professionals* by Bates-Jensen and Sussman have summaries of modalities protocols.[153] It is prudent to check current reimbursement and documentation guidelines when billing for these services. The decision to use mechanical modalities rests in the hands of the physical therapist unless physician authorization is required to receive reimbursement. The reimbursement requirement may vary from state to state and sometimes between payers in the same state. In some cases, individual physicians may develop their own protocols that require physical therapists to contact them before changing a POC.

Ultrasound

Therapeutic ultrasound (US) application for wound management differs from its use as a modality to treat pain. Therapeutic ultrasound also differs from diagnostic US which is used to visualize internal anatomical structures. Therapeutic ultrasound stimulates cell activity, accelerating processes such as inflammation. Once thought to target only the sluggish wound in the inflammatory stage, evidence now demonstrates that the effects can be seen throughout all wound-healing phases.[154–156] Basic scientific evidence and clinical research have established that skin repair and wound contraction can be accelerated, collagen secretion can be stimulated, and elastin properties can be affected to strengthen scar tissue. One option for the treatment is to cover the wound with a sheet of hydrogel or an application of amorphous hydrogel as a medium to transmit the signal from the US head. US is then delivered with a handheld applicator to the wound bed through the gel. Another option for treatment is to apply US transmission gel to the periwound area and treat from this region in addition to or instead of the wound bed.[154–156] The newest option for delivery of US is to use a system that provides noncontact, nonthermal, low-frequency ultrasound (Fig. 14.24). A mist of sterile saline is propelled toward the wound, and the US is transferred from the device to the patient without contact or pain. Studies have provided evidence (Table 14.4) that this type of US treatment may reduce bacterial quantity in a wound and promotes healing, especially in wounds that have been slow to heal.[157–163]

Electrical Stimulation

The use of electrical stimulation (ES) to treat chronic and, more recently, acute wounds is well documented. ES is recommended to eliminate bacterial load, promote granulation, decrease inflammation, reduce edema, reduce wound-related pain, and augment blood flow. Human skin, wounds, and the cells that facilitate wound healing all have measurable electrical currents. ES affects various types of cells and their activities by supporting, altering, or providing electrical currents

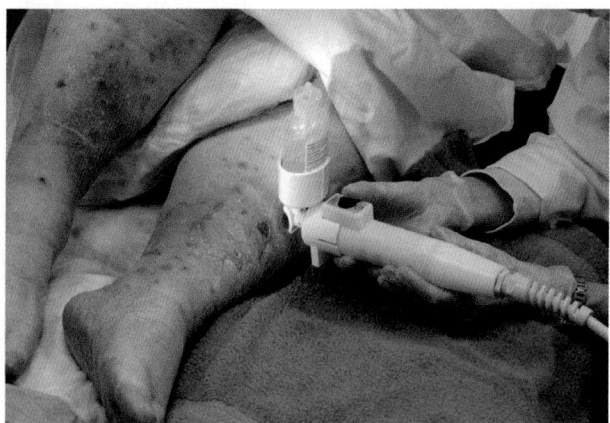

Figure 14.24 Application of noncontact, nonthermal, low-frequency ultrasound treatment to leg wounds. *(Courtesy of Alliqua Biomedical, Yardley, PA 19067.)*

Table 14.4 Evidence Summary: Does Noncontact Low-Frequency Ultrasound (MIST) Decrease the Healing Time of Chronic Wounds?

White et al. (2015)[157]

Design	RCT
Level of evidence	1
Subjects	Inclusion: Adults with chronic venous leg ulcers (≥6 weeks and ≤5-year durations, between 5 and 100 cm² area) and an ankle-brachial pressure index of greater than 0.8 Exclusion: Uncontrolled DM (HbA₁c greater than 12% in last 3 months), active infection of wound on day of inclusion, renal failure, exposed tendon/ligament/muscle/bone in the ulcer, osteomyelitis/cellulitis/gangrene in the limb, arterial ulcer, pregnant or breastfeeding women, women of childbearing age not willing to use highly effective contraception, planned surgical procedure during study period for the wound, prior skin replacement/negative pressure therapy/or ultrasound therapy to the wound 2 weeks prior, radio or chemotherapy currently or within last 3 months, ultrasound required near or on electronic implant or prosthesis, not capable of providing informed consent, enrolled in another trial currently or last 30 days.
Intervention	MIST US was applied to a clean wound bed for 3–12 minutes, dependent upon wound size, three times per week. This was followed by application of a nonadherent dressing and strong compression therapy (3×/week).
Results	Both control and NCLFU groups saw significant improvement in wound size; however, there was no significant difference between the two groups.
Comments	Limitations: difference of frequency between two treatment groups (Standard of Care: At least 1×/week versus NLFU: 3×/week).

Beheshti et al. (2014)[158]

Design	Comparative
Level of evidence	2
Subjects	Inclusion: Wound duration longer than 4 weeks and no clinical improvement after using the clinic's standard of care for healing during a 2-week period. Exclusion: Allergy to US contact gel, pregnancy, known contraindications to US, ankle or knee prosthesis, metal in lower leg, suspected or confirmed local cancers or metastatic disease and neuropathy, no evidence of infections including active cellulites, suspicious thrombophlebitis and no history of antibiotic therapy at time of enrollment, PAD, DM, or RA.
Intervention	HFU therapy was applied for 5–10 minutes around edge of the ulcer. Mist therapy delivered low-intensity (0.1–0.8 W/cm²), low-frequency (40 kHz) US energy to wound bed for 4–12 minutes.
Results	No significant difference between groups for complete wound healing duration. No significant difference in edema between groups at 2 months. Significant difference noted in edema in ultrasound groups compared to standard of care at 4 months. Significant reduction in pain in HFU and MIST groups compared to standard of care at 2 months, no significant difference between HFU and MIST.

Ennis et al. (2005)[159]

Design	RCT
Level of evidence	2
Subjects	Inclusion: Subjects over 18 years old with type 1 or 2 diabetes and a chronic diabetic foot ulcer (greater than 30 days) of Wagner grade 1 or 2 on plantar surface of foot, glycosylated hemoglobin level less than 12, no exposure of bone/ligament/tendons in the wound, no clinical signs of infection, not currently taking antibiotics.

(Continued)

Table 14.4	Evidence Summary: Does Noncontact Low-Frequency Ultrasound (MIST) Decrease the Healing Time of Chronic Wounds?—cont'd
	**Ennis et al. (2005)[159]**
Intervention	Intervention and control group both received standard of care treatment. Intervention group received US treatment for 4 min, device was held 5–15 mm away from the wound bed. Control group received a sham treatment that was designed to simulate the US treatment by providing same parameters of pressure and time to the wound bed. Both interventions were performed 3×/week.
Results	Significant reduction in exudate at 5 weeks in US group compared to control. No significant difference in granulation tissue between groups; 40.7% of US group healed compared to 14.3% of control. Significantly shorter healing time frames found in US group compared to control.
Comments	Despite no clinical evidence of infection in the tissue when evaluated, 86% of US group and 93% of control group showed presence of aerobic bacteria on biopsy. This information was not made available to the investigators during the study and may have had influence on the results.
	**Kavros et al. (2008)[160]**
Design	Retrospective
Level of evidence	2
Subjects	Inclusion: Below the knee wounds that received MIST therapy 3×/week for 90 days or until wound healed. Inclusion for compare group: Met criteria for MIST therapy but were not able to accommodate for required 3×/week treatment visits. Exclusion: Patients who did not meet criteria for US therapy 3×/week had significant discontinuity of treatments, did not complete the treatment regimen at the wound center, or had participated in a previous study of MIST therapy in the critical limb ischemia at the wound center.
Intervention	MIST therapy system utilizing noncontact US delivering low-intensity (0.1–0.8 W/cm^2) and low-frequency (40 kHz) US energy through atomized sterile saline mist to the wound bed. Treatment times ranged from 3–20 minutes based on size of wound.
Results	A faster rate of healing was noted for the patients who received MIST therapy compared to standard of care ($P = 0.002$), and a greater percentage of wounds treated with MIST therapy healed compared to standard of care ($P = 0.009$).
	**Kavros et al. (2007)[161]**
Design	Prospective, parallel, RCT
Level of evidence	2
Subjects	Inclusion: Nonhealing foot/ankle/leg wound with documented critical ischemia present for a minimum of 8 weeks. Exclusion: patients undergoing chemotherapy and patients unable or unwilling to attend three treatment sessions per week.
Intervention	MIST therapy was delivered with low-intensity (0.1–0.8 W/cm^2), low-frequency (40 kHz) US energy via saline mist to wound bed without directly contacting the body or wound. This was performed 3×/week in conjunction with standard care.
Results	Significant improvement in wound healing noted at 12 weeks in intervention group compared to standard care alone.

Table 14.4 Evidence Summary: Does Noncontact Low-Frequency Ultrasound (MIST) Decrease the Healing Time of Chronic Wounds?—cont'd

Olyaie et al. (2013)[162]

Design	RCT
Level of evidence	2
Subjects	Inclusion: Patient with a venous leg ulcer greater than 4 weeks who did not respond to standard of care treatment for 2 weeks. Exclusion: Patients who were pregnant or who had a known allergy to US gel, known US contraindications, history of antibiotic therapy at time of enrollment, RA, DM, or peripheral artery disease (ABI less than 0.8 or signs of artery disease).
Intervention	HFU: High-intensity (0.5–1 W/cm^2), high-frequency (1–3 MHz) US was applied for 5–10 minutes to skin surrounding ulcer. NCLFU: Low-intensity (0.1–0.8 W/cm^2), low-frequency (40 kHz) US was delivered to wound bed using atomized sterile saline mist without direct contact to the body or wound. Treatment time was based on total wound area ranging from 3–20 minutes.
Results	At 4-month follow-up, the HFU and NCLFU showed significant improvement in wound size ($P = 0.04$) compared to standard of care alone. Significant difference was also noted in edema and pain rating at 4-month follow-up in HFU and NCLFU compared to standard of care ($P < 0.05$).
Comments	Limitations: Small sample size and use of perpendicular axis for measurement of wound bed. Researchers note use of more precise imaging, and histopathological assessment methods may have enhanced study accuracy.

Yao et al. (2014)[163]

Design	Prospective RCT pilot study
Level of evidence	2
Subjects	Inclusion: age 18–90 years old, DM I/II, presence of chronic diabetic foot wound (0.5–15 cm^2 area) of Wagner grade 1 or 2, TcPO$_2$ greater than 30 mm Hg or ABI greater than 0.6. Exclusion: Treatment with noncontact US during the 4 weeks prior to study, LE malignancy (either limb), critical limb ischemia, local infection of limb with the target ulcer, systemic infection, pregnancy, end-stage renal disease, severe liver disease, venous leg ulcer with or without DM, or known/suspected lidocaine allergy.
Intervention	NCLFU therapy was utilized with a frequency of 40 kHZ and an intensity ranging from 0.2–0.6 W/cm^2. The transducer was held 0.5–1.5 cm away from wound bed, and US waves were delivered in a continuous mode through a sterile saline mist. Treatment duration varied with wound area with a single session lasting approximately 5 min.
Results	Subjects who received NCLFU 3×/week showed significant wound area reduction at weeks 3, 4, and 5 compared to control and those who received NCLFU 1×/week ($P < 0.05$). Biochemical and histological analyses showed trend toward reduction of proinflammatory cytokines, matrix metalloproteinase-9, vascular endothelial growth factor, and macrophages in both NCLFU groups.
Comments	Researchers of this pilot study noted the need for more research in the area to determine possible effects of NCLFU on proinflammatory cytokines.

ABI = ankle-brachial index; DM = diabetes mellitus; HFU = high-frequency ultrasound; LE = lower extremity; NCLFU = noncontact low-frequency ultrasound; PAD = peripheral artery disease; RA = rheumatoid arthritis; RCT = randomized controlled trial; US = ultrasound.

to accelerate wound healing. A clear understanding of medical electricity will assist the clinician in applying an appropriate ES treatment. The available literature on this treatment is diverse and instructive.[164–173] There are a variety of options for treatment setup, depending on the goals of treatment, the type of wound, and the condition of the patient. Standard equipment for the direct method of application includes an ES unit, treatment and nontreatment electrodes, and a substance such as saline-soaked gauze or a hydrogel dressing applied to the wound bed or cavity to enhance electrical conductivity under the treatment electrode (Fig. 14.25). For the indirect method, gel electrodes straddle the wound and interface with the periwound skin. Clinical decisions related to voltage, electrode placement, dosage, and other variables must be made on a case-by-case basis. Detailed information about treatment protocols, strength of evidence, and guidelines for treatment can be found in wound care texts.[172,173]

Thermal and Nonthermal Diathermy

Pulsed shortwave diathermy (PSWD), continuous shortwave diathermy (CSWD), and nonthermal pulsed radiofrequency stimulation (PRFS) have been used successfully to treat chronic open wounds, facilitating progress from one phase of wound healing to the next. These diathermy treatments utilize radio waves to provide thermal and nonthermal effects, respectively. All models transmit radiation from an applicator head to the target tissues. PSWD heats superficial and deep tissues. CSWD heats deep muscle and joint tissues. PRFS is nonthermal and can influence tissue at the cellular level. Individuals with arterial insufficiency are not good candidates for PSWD or CSWD because their tissues are not able to dissipate heat well enough to

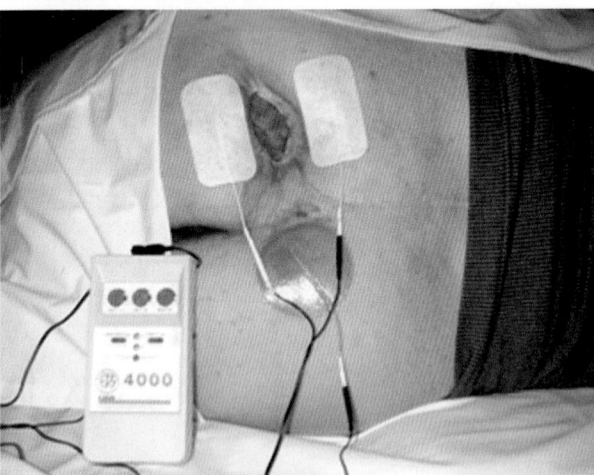

Figure 14.25 Conductively coupled bipolar treatment electrodes of opposite polarity positioned on opposite sides of a wound. *(From McCulloch and Kloth, Wound Healing: Evidence-Based Management. 4th ed. F.A. Davis, Figure 26–28, with permission.)*

avoid burns. Wound sites treated with diathermy have demonstrated increased fibroblast proliferation, collagen formation, tissue perfusion, and metabolic rate. The number of clinical studies is smaller than that of other modalities, and there are only a few well-controlled clinical studies. The evidence for the role diathermy plays in wound healing will need to be stronger for this modality to be readily utilized in clinical settings. Physical therapists have used diathermy for wound care since the publication of a number of studies regarding the nonthermal effects of pulsed diathermy and the production of smaller, more portable, user-friendly diathermy units.[174,175] Equipment needed for treatment includes a diathermy unit/electronic console and one or two applicator heads. Treatment is usually delivered without touching the skin. Wounds should be carefully prepared before treatment according to guidelines provided by the distributor.

Ultraviolet Radiation

Ultraviolet (UV) radiation energy is a form of radiation between x-ray and visible light on the electromagnetic spectrum.[176,177] UV wavelengths have been divided into wavelengths and bands. The three bands most useful for their effects on human skin are UVA, UVB, and UVC. UV has cutaneous and bactericidal effects that include increased blood flow, enhanced granulation tissue formation, destruction of bacteria, stimulation of vitamin D production, and thickening of the stratum corneum. The varied physiological effects make this treatment appropriate for a variety of skin diseases, as well as acute and chronic wounds.[154] The effects of UV radiation on antibiotic-resistant bacteria make it a potentially effective tool in wound care; however, there are only a few up-to-date, well-controlled clinical studies emerging at this time.[176,177] Early supporting literature is now quite dated, leaving room for new clinical studies to provide evidence of the efficacy of the intervention. UVC in particular has been found to be effective in the treatment of MRSA, *vancomycin-resistant enterococcus*, and some strains of *Pseudomonas aeruginosa*.[178–180] The treatment is typically delivered to a clean wound with dressings removed, using a UVB or UVC lamp. Treatment distance, dosage, frequency, and subsequent clinical outcomes will vary based on the goals of the treatment and the status of the wound.[180–182] Care must be taken when using UV lamps, as burns and injuries have occurred. Physical therapists planning to utilize UV for wound care might partner with a wound care team, a resourceful vendor, and the latest evidence to devise a comprehensive treatment plan.

Hyperbaric Oxygen Therapy

Hyperbaric oxygen therapy (HBOT) delivers 100% oxygen to an individual resting inside a sealed chamber. The oxygen is delivered at a pressure greater than the atmosphere. This *systemic* treatment increases the amount of oxygen available for cell metabolism, improving oxygen delivery to hypoxic tissue. Systemic HBOT is, however, associated with risks related to oxygen toxicity. The literature demonstrates positive responses to this treatment when used as an adjunct to other forms of wound care, but few randomized controlled trials have been completed.[154,183–186] A meta-analysis of studies on HBOT in 2018 revealed that adjuvant HBOT improves major amputation rates but not wound healing in patients with diabetic foot ulcers and peripheral arterial obstructive disease. More evidence is needed to determine effectiveness in other conditions for wound healing. Chambers to deliver *topical* oxygen have been available for at least a decade. These smaller chambers enclose a limb or a segment of the body instead of requiring coverage of the entire body.

Following physician referral, a physical therapy provider may assist or coordinate a systemic or topical treatment. Often, a trained technician will manage the equipment controls and the delivery chamber. Wound care may occur before or after the HBOT or the topical HBOT, depending on the preferences of the physician and the protocol of the facility. Discussion among investigators comparing the effects of systemic versus topical oxygen is ongoing. In some studies, topical oxygen is also referred to as *topical hyperbaric oxygen* (THBO) and *O₂ therapy*.[10,11,187] Instead of the full-body chamber used for HBOT, THBO is portable and is delivered in a localized limb chamber.[10,11,184,185] THBO has been combined with ES and also with cold laser for the treatment of pressure injuries and neuropathic foot wounds.[186] A systematic review of THBO demonstrated that topical oxygen therapy facilitates wound healing dynamics among individuals with chronic diabetic foot ulcers. Other investigations suggest that topical O_2 therapy enhances the effects of growth factors to improve perfusion in wound healing. Renewed interest by investigators should lead to more refined protocols and improved strength of evidence in the field.[187–191]

Negative Pressure Wound Therapy

Negative pressure wound therapy (NPWT) is used as an adjunct to wound healing to facilitate wound closure in acute surgical wounds as well as more challenging, slow-to-heal wounds. The procedure is known by several terms, but the most well known is *vacuum-assisted closure* or *VAC* (Kinetic Concepts, Inc., San Antonio, TX 78265). An open-cell foam dressing is placed in the wound, and a suction tube is connected from the foam to a portable pump. An airtight seal is created over the foam and the suction tube with a clear, occlusive film (Figs. 14.26, 14.27, and 14.28). A controlled amount of negative (subatmospheric) pressure is applied through the foam to the entire wound bed. Typically, for the first few days (48 hr), the negative pressure is applied continuously via the portable pump system. After a significant amount of excess wound fluid has been

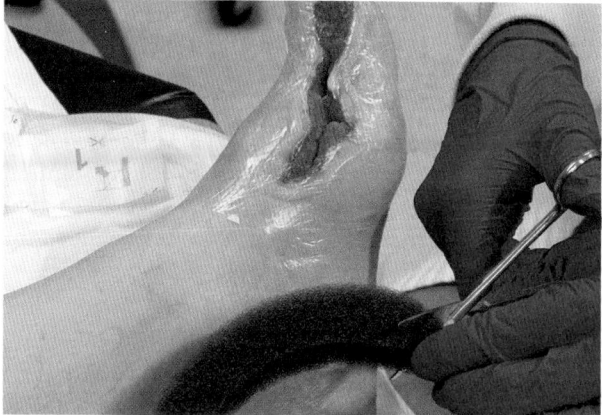

Figure 14.26 Reticulated foam dressing is cut to the shape of the wound outline in preparation for applying negative pressure wound therapy.

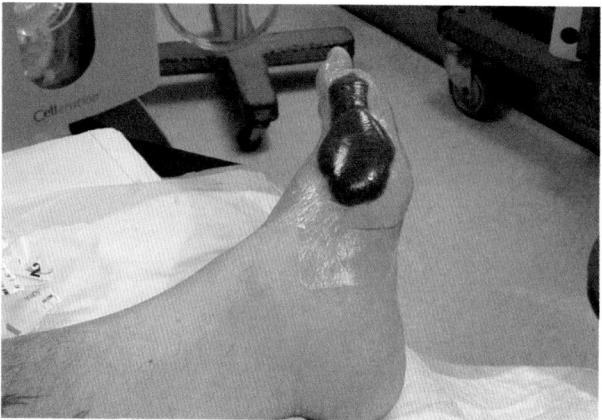

Figure 14.27 Reticulated foam dressing covered with a polyurethane sheet before tubing and suction are applied.

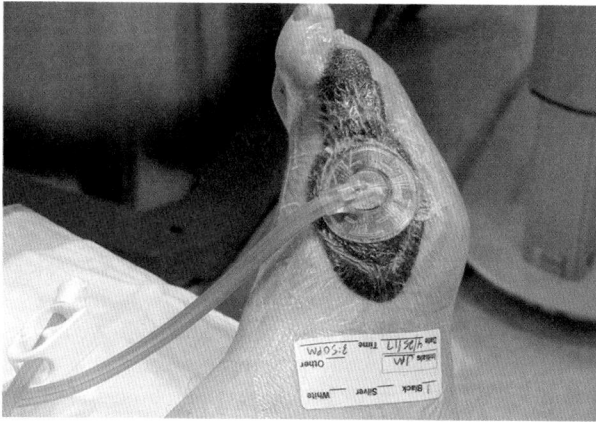

Figure 14.28 A wound treated with negative pressure wound therapy with reticulated foam dressing, tubing, and polyurethane sheet covering the entire wound to maintain the vacuum during treatment with vacuum-assisted closure.

withdrawn, the pump is programmed to apply pressure intermittently. The foam dressing is changed every 12 (infected wounds) to 48 hr or longer (clean wounds). A recent addition to the features of the wound VAC is an automated system that will rinse a wound regularly with either saline or an antiseptic or antibiotic solution and then remove the fluids with the regular suction treatment. This feature is most often recommended for severely infected orthopedic and trauma wounds.[192–194]

Evidence on the effects of this treatment is mounting. NPWT has been shown to enhance granulation tissue formation, promote wound edge approximation, remove edema from wounds, and improve oxygen levels in the wound.[189–202] Studies have also shown that with the use of NPWT, the healing time for selected wounds decreased in comparison to standard wound care.[195,196,200] One claim still under investigation is the ability of the VAC to remove bacteria from the wound bed.[201] Another study showed the ability of VAC to increase the concentration of antibiotics in the treated tissue.[202] Although a prescribing health-care provider must order this type of therapy, many are unaware of this intervention and would be responsive to an appropriate recommendation by the therapist. In different environments, physical therapy providers, nurses, or other clinical staff may administer the treatment.

Cold Laser Therapy

Cold laser is also referred to in the literature as *low-level cold laser, low-level infrared laser,* or *monochromatic infrared energy* (MIRE). Low-energy laser treatment uses light in the infrared spectrum. This therapy has been promoted for augmenting wound healing[203] and reversing the symptoms of peripheral neuropathy in individuals with diabetes.[204] It is thought that the effects of laser treatment may be to increase circulation and reduce pain by increasing the release of nitric oxide into the microcirculation. A recent meta-analysis showed that low-level cold laser therapies helped reduce the size of diabetic foot ulcers. Supportive, peer-reviewed literature is modest but growing, and more evidence is needed in this area.[203–212] Despite the term *cold laser,* light in the infrared spectrum can also be used to deliver heat as a treatment modality. Owing to the perceived lack of adequate evidence, some third-party payers do not cover cold laser treatment except when used as a heat modality.

Dressings

The type of wound dressings selected may have a profound effect on a wound's healing time. There are hundreds of choices for the discerning clinician. Information on indications, contraindications, and expected outcomes can be obtained from individual vendors listed in Appendix 14.E (online), as well as from texts devoted entirely to wound care.[152,153] Physical therapists monitoring a wound on a regular basis and knowledgeable about dressing alternatives are often the most suitable clinicians to make appropriate dressing selections. This chapter includes introductory information necessary to make clinical decisions about dressings: the characteristics of the dressing categories and the effects of the dressings on the wound bed.

A dressing applied directly to the wound is referred to as the *primary* dressing. The dressing applied over the primary dressing is referred to as the *secondary* dressing. Some advanced dressings serve as the primary and secondary, including adhesive and absorptive qualities in the same dressing. Choosing or recommending appropriate dressings should be directed by the characteristics of the wound and periwound tissues, not by what is available in the facility or clinic. A product that preserves wound hydration by limiting or controlling fluid loss is usually ideal. To understand the wide range of options and to assist in selecting the appropriate dressing, refer to Appendix 14.F (online) for a listing of dressings categorized by treatment goal (purpose) and type of wound (indication).

Gauze/Fiber

Gauze dressings (Fig. 14.29) are considered by many wound management experts to be outside the description of modern wound dressings.[117] Used and misused for decades, there are more reasons not to use gauze than there are indications for use. As a primary dressing, gauze leaves contaminating fibers in the wound, contributes to desiccation, is permeable to bacteria, can be adherent to the wound, releases excessive amounts of bacteria into the air on removal, causes a loss of normothermia, and is painful on removal if it adheres to the wound surface. Once thought to be cost effective, it has been shown in more than one study to be more costly than other dressing choices. One study of home health wound care showed that due to the longer time required to heal as compared to moist dressings, gauze dressings ended up costing more overall.[197]

Gauze ribbon can be used to maintain an opening for drainage in a tunneling wound. It can also be used successfully to gently support a cavity wound but should not be used to aggressively pack any shape of wound.

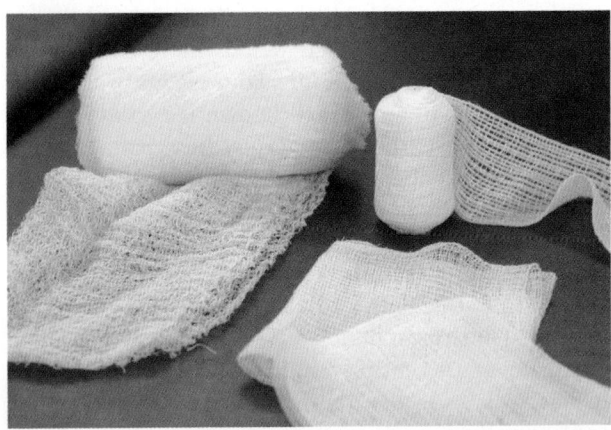

Figure 14.29 Samples of gauze dressings.

It was once thought that cavity wounds should be packed very full, but it has since been established that granulation tissue and epithelial cells do not flourish with aggressive gauze packing. The additional pressure from a tightly packed wound will impede the flow of oxygen and nutrients to the granulating wound bed. Several studies now question the traditional use of gauze to fill surgical wounds and other healing wounds, favoring instead foams, hydrocolloids, alginates, and other less irritating materials.[200] Gauze can be an effective secondary dressing, especially if the dressings will be changed frequently or if exudate is heavy. Gauze 4 × 4s and a roll of gauze are typically used to create a WTD dressing. WTD dressings were previously discussed under the section on débridement because of their nonselective removal of tissue during dressing changes. Because WTD dressings can be classified as a tool for mechanical débridement or as a primary wound dressing, they are discussed in both categories. Refer to that section of the chapter for more details.

Impregnated Gauze

Designed to be less adherent, this category includes products made of tightly meshed synthetic fibers or woven products such as cellulose acetate. Fiber materials are impregnated with a petroleum emulsion such as Vaseline, intended to prevent the gauze from sticking to the wound surface. Used as a primary dressing, this choice is minimally absorptive, provides minimal protection, does not enhance a moist environment, and may create a greasy wound bed. One of its more appropriate uses is as a primary dressing over new sutures to prevent them from catching or sticking to the dressing, with a gauze secondary dressing placed on top to hold the impregnated gauze in place.

Transparent Films

Films are made of a transparent membrane with an acrylic adhesive layer (Fig. 14.30). Transparent films do not allow bacteria or moisture into the wound. They facilitate a moist wound environment, trapping endogenous fluids in the wound bed to assist with autolytic débridement, wound bed homeostasis, and *angiogenesis*. Films assist in protecting skin from the effects of shearing, friction, and the contaminating effects of incontinence. Removal of a film dressing must be done with great caution because this can cause skin tears, especially with fragile or aging skin. Currently, few films have absorptive qualities and cannot be used on highly exuding wounds.

Foam

Foams are highly absorbent pads, sheets, or ropes of polyurethane or polyvinyl alcohol available in many sizes, with many features (Fig. 14.31). They are available with or without adhesive backing so that they can be used as a primary or secondary dressing. Foam dressings are highly absorptive but also help to create an occlusive environment for moist wound healing. They should not be used alone on a dry wound but could serve as a secondary dressing if the primary dressing was a gel product. One of the newest foam dressings is impregnated with methylene blue and gentian violet to provide broad-spectrum antibacterial protection (Fig. 14.32).

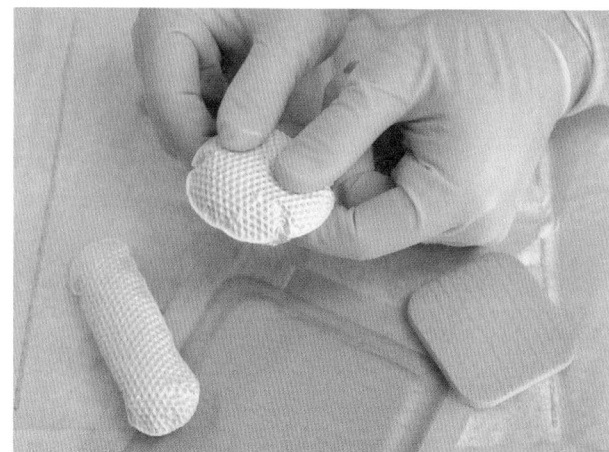

Figure 14.31 Samples of foam dressings.

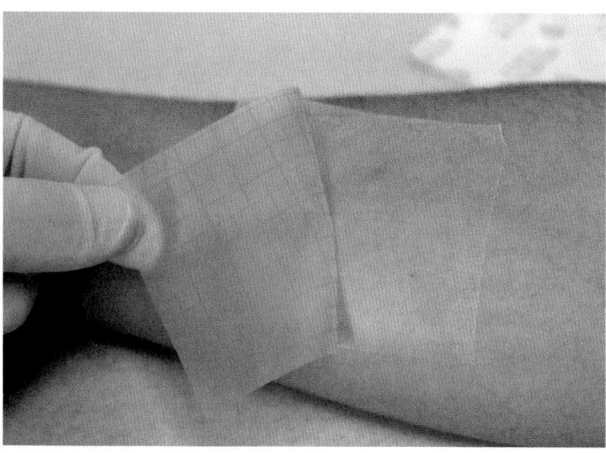

Figure 14.30 Application of a film dressing.

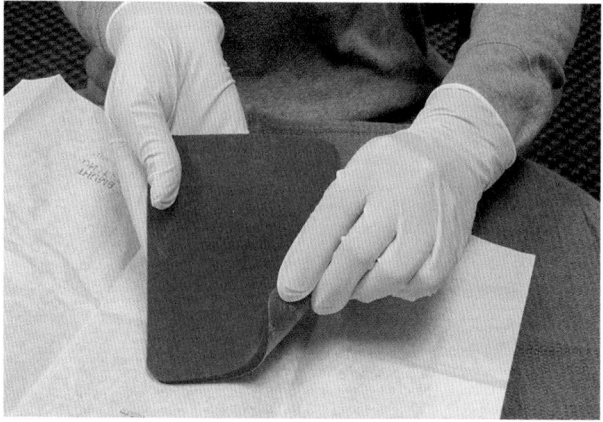

Figure 14.32 Sample of a gentian violet and methylene blue antibacterial foam dressing.

Methylene blue and gentian violet are nontoxic organic pigments that assist in controlling bioburden without the risk of being cytotoxic to living tissue. Since the blue pigments do not absorb into the skin, the dressings can be used for long periods of time as the wound closes and heals.[211,212]

Hydrogels

Hydrogels are categorized as *amorphous*, referring to a liquid-like gel, or as *sheets*, consisting of a thin, flexible sheet of polymer containing at least 90% water (Fig. 14.33). Both types are used to increase moisture in a dry wound bed, soften necrotic tissue, and support autolytic débridement. Both have some absorptive qualities and will swell slightly until they are saturated. The amorphous gel (Fig. 14.34) must be contained in the wound with a secondary dressing. The flexible sheets usually require a secondary dressing but are available through some vendors with tape attached to the borders. Patients tend to respond positively to the soothing sensation of the hydrogel application.

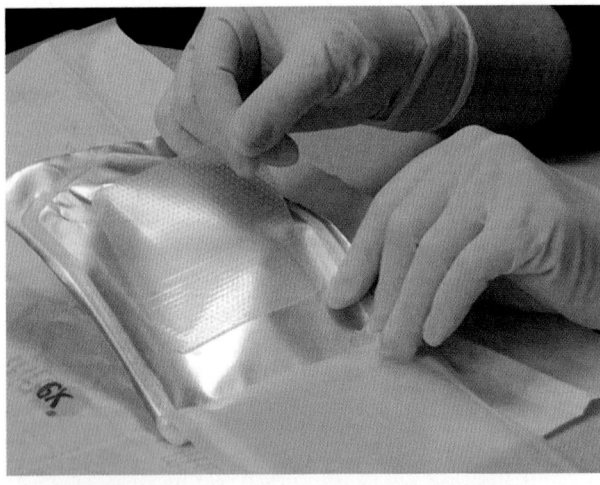

Figure 14.33 Sample of a hydrogel sheet dressing.

Hydrocolloids

Considered the most occlusive of the moisture-retentive dressings, hydrocolloids are also available in less occlusive or semipermeable styles. As with foams, these dressings come in a variety of styles and shapes, including pastes, granules, powder, and sheets. They typically consist of an absorbent colloidal material combined with a film or foam backing (Fig. 14.35). Hydrocolloid dressings work best on mild to moderate exudating wounds. When wound exudate combines with the colloidal polymer, a soft, gelatinous, often yellow, and malodorous mass is formed. Patients, families, caregivers, and other health-care providers must be informed about this harmless reaction so that infection is not assumed. Hydrocolloids have been used successfully as occlusive dressings over infected wounds without the fulmination of existing bacteria. They are also the dressing of choice to cover and protect larvae during MDT.[133–136]

Alginates

This dressing category is also known as *calcium alginate* because the dressings are manufactured using the calcium salts of alginic acid derived from marine algae and kelp (seaweed). The raw material is woven and then converted into flat sheets, ropes, or ribbon shapes (Fig. 14.36). Alginates absorb 20 to 30 times their own weight, are gentle to apply and remove, and are biocompatible with the wound bed. A chemical reaction between the dressing and wound exudate creates a gel substance that helps to maintain a moist wound environment while absorbing excess exudate. Because they are permeable, alginates do not provide a barrier against bacteria. This characteristic makes them an effective choice when an infected wound cannot be covered with an occlusive dressing. Most alginates currently require a secondary dressing to hold them in place. Several manufacturers are combining alginates with other products, such as hydrocolloids, to maximize their effectiveness. There is growing interest in the use of silver in advanced

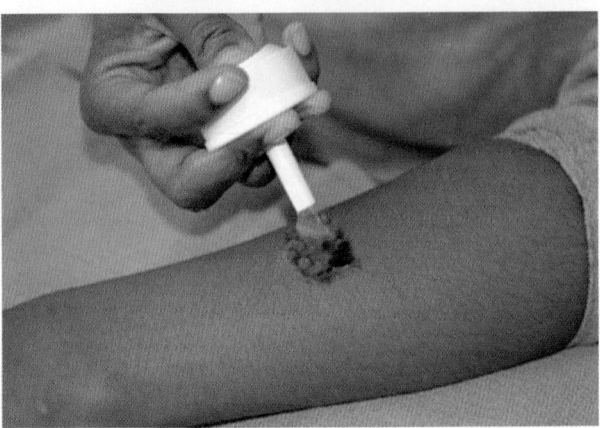

Figure 14.34 Application of an amorphous gel dressing.

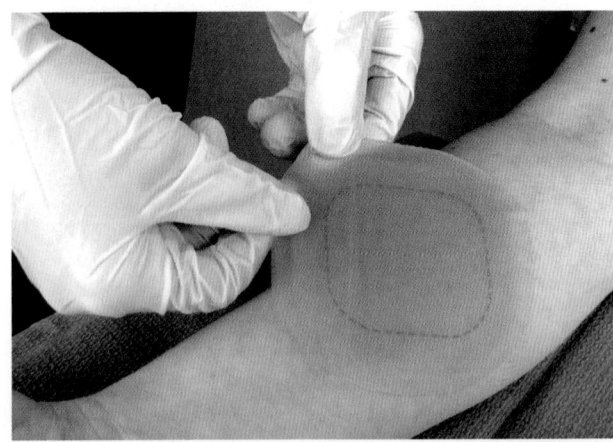

Figure 14.35 Sample of a hydrocolloid dressing.

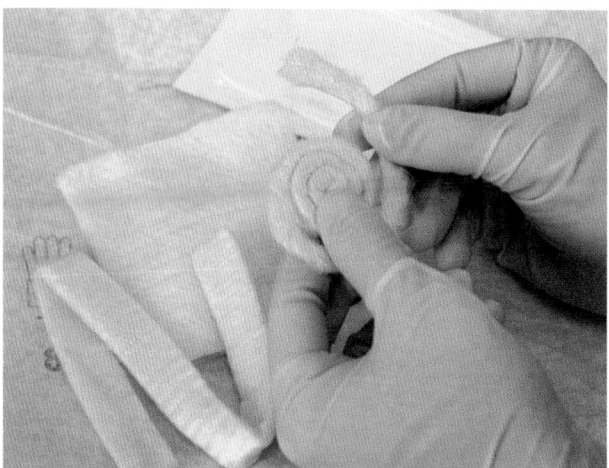

Figure 14.36 Samples of alginate dressings.

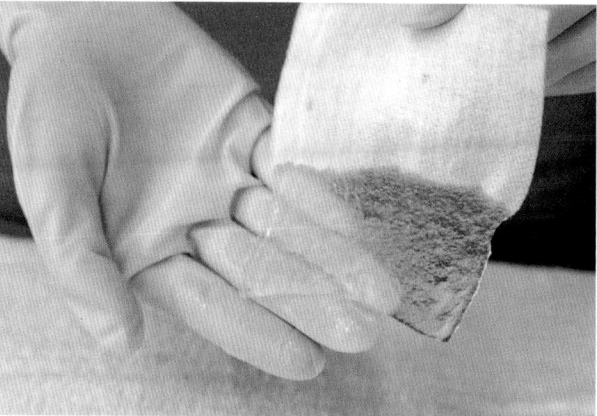

Figure 14.37 Sample of a synthetic fiber dressing simulating the change in consistency from dry to gel as wound drainage is absorbed.

dressings to combine the antimicrobial action of silver with the absorptive qualities of alginates. However, silver should only be used short term, in the presence of infection, and is not recommended in burns due to its toxicity to keratinocytes and fibroblasts.[213–215]

Hydrofibers

Hydrofiber or hydroactive dressings are designed to have a selective absorptive capacity. They have the combined positive characteristics of alginate, foam, and gel dressings. When in contact with the wound, the synthetic fibers absorb exudate and align themselves perpendicular to the wound surface. This vertical wicking process keeps debris and wound fluid contained within the dressing.[216] There is considerably less pain on removal of a hydrofiber dressing because the fibers do not stick to the wound or dry out.[216,217] Hydrofiber dressings are also flexible and suited for placement over joint surfaces.[218,219] The dressing properties allow growth factors and other peptides to survive on the wound bed. Aquacel is a spun Hydrofiber dressing that readily absorbs moisture (Fig. 14.37). Aquacel Ag adds ionic silver to the absorbent dressing (ConvaTec, Skillman, NJ 08558). Due to their relatively new status as a dressing type, there is little evidence yet of its effectiveness as compared to other dressing types, as no systematic reviews or randomized controlled trials have been published to date.[218]

Composite Dressings

Composite dressings represent a general category of wound dressings that combine different types of dressings into a single dressing. They usually have three layers that each have their own functions.[220,221] The layer closest to the wound will allow moisture to pass through and will be nonstick. The next layer will be absorbent, pulling drainage away from the wound. The outer layer will typically be waterproof so that the wound is protected

but drainage cannot leak as easily. A composite dressing could be a primary or secondary dressing. Composite dressings can be more expensive than other dressing categories, which is a consideration when choosing a POC. Studies in this area show promising results. A composite dressing of *Aloe vera*–loaded gelatin (OP-Gel) demonstrated an anti-inflammatory effect and 80% wound healing in 8 days.[222]

Biological Dressings/Skin Substitutes

Considered by some to be topical applications and by others to be dressings, human skin equivalents and bioengineered tissues are finding their place in the wound care arena. Skin substitutes are created using a variety of techniques and substances. Cells are derived from sources such as neonatal male foreskin and porcine (pig) dermal collagen. The products are produced in laboratories, shipped either frozen or cooled, and then applied to the patient's wound by a member of the wound care team. Although a physician would prescribe the use of a skin substitute, other health-care professionals can apply the product to the wound based on individual facility protocol. Skin substitutes consist of living skin applications that resemble skin structure and function and may include epidermal and dermal layers. They are useful as temporary coverage, providing skin protection for the wound bed. Some have been shown to stimulate endogenous cell activity. Most are marketed to use on wounds that have not responded to conventional therapy, such as chronic diabetic foot ulcers, venous leg ulcers, and deep burn wounds.[219] There is evidence that biological skin substitutes are more effective than traditional wound dressings at healing diabetic foot ulcers by 12 weeks.[222] Examples to look for when investigating skin substitutes are Apligraf (Novartis, East Hanover, NJ 07936), Dermagraft (Organogenesis, Canton, MA 02021), and Biobrane (Smith & Nephew, Auckland, New Zealand 1140).[222]

Innovative Dressings

New wound care products frequently enter the market as research and development continue to grow. One of the driving forces in the creation of new products is an expanding list of resistant bacterial strains. Cost is another factor that drives development as clinicians search for the most economical dressing for their patient that will establish the ideal wound environment, facilitate débridement, maintain moisture, absorb bacteria, and decrease the number of dressing changes. Some of these new products include options such as polysaccharide dressings, absorptive fillers, hydrophilic fiber, dressings that contain collagen, new skin substitutes, and dressings made with a hyaluronic acid derivative applied directly to the wound.

Manual Lymphatic Drainage

MLD is a specialized manual therapy technique that stimulates primarily superficial lymphatic circulation. It is considered to be one of the five elements of an effective treatment intervention for lymphedema, known as CDT, and many types of edema. This manual therapy provides a gentle stretch to the skin that enhances lymph capillary activity. MLD will increase the frequency of lymphangion contractions; improve lymph transport capacity; redirect lymph flow toward collateral vessels, anastomoses, and uninvolved lymph regions; and mobilize excess lymph fluid that has overwhelmed a body segment or region.[72,223] The techniques of MLD are gentle and specific, requiring specialized education to be performed accurately (Fig. 14.38). To obtain contact information for training facilities that provide specialized education in MLD as a part of CDT, refer to the special section in Appendix 14.D (online) for contact information. The benefits of this treatment are not limited to the population with lymphedema. MLD is used successfully for edema from CVI, sports injury, neurological injury, and postoperative swelling, but there is a need for more well-designed randomized controlled trials to provide high-ranking evidence.[223,224] The use of MLD is contraindicated for treating patients with cardiac-, pulmonary-, or renal-related edema because the amount of fluid that will be mobilized may overwhelm one or all of those systems when disease is present.[225,226]

Compression Therapy

Controlling edema or lymphedema is critical to all stages of healing. Edema inhibits wound healing primarily by affecting the perfusion of tissues. Unless there are red flags present, compression should be part of every treatment for individuals with lymphedema, edema, and CVI. Compression therapy should be introduced as soon as clinical signs of swelling or fibrosis appear. A physical therapist may find indications for compression therapy during the examination or later, during the intervention. In most situations, the therapist will decide what type and/or style of compression should be applied.

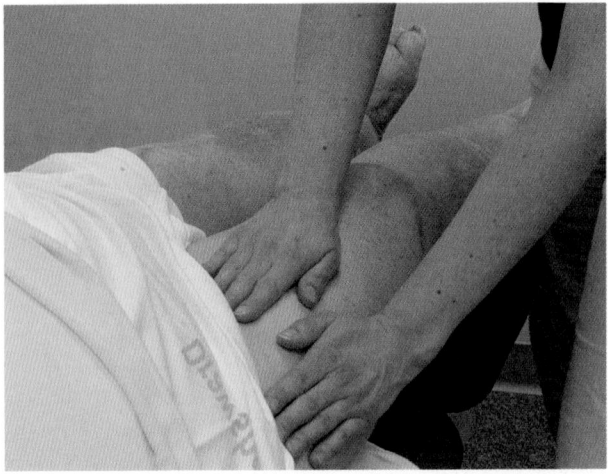

Figure 14.38 Manual lymphatic drainage on the lower extremity.

applied. Medical provider authorization, however, may be necessary for reimbursement. When LE wounds are present, compression is essential for timely wound healing. For the individual with mixed arterial and venous disease, an ABI test is indicated to provide information about the safety of using compression on the LE. A greater understanding of how the lymphatic system functions has created a paradigm shift in the way intervention for all types of swelling is planned and delivered. Aggressive compression techniques were once used to "milk" the fluid out of a limb. It is now understood that deep pressure and mechanical "milking" techniques are counterproductive and harmful to the superficial capillary network that filters lymph and interstitial fluids.[3]

Elevation

Elevation is used as a means of controlling some types of swelling and is often a precursor to compression therapy. Mild, acute swelling of the extremities may be relieved temporarily with elevation. Active ROM exercises (e.g., ankle pumps) can be performed alongside elevation to facilitate blood flow in the extremities. Patients should be educated about how to elevate safely, paying attention to positioning so that optimal venous and lymphatic circulation is facilitated. Elevation should be viewed as a temporary or complementary measure while other means of controlling swelling are employed.

Unna Boot

Compression of the LE for a patient with a venous wound can be applied using zinc paste–impregnated gauze or Unna boot. The moist gauze roll is wrapped over the wound, around the foot and ankle, and then covered with compression bandaging. It is an inexpensive means of covering a wound, providing compression, and supporting the calf pump to empty stagnant venous blood from the LE. For the appropriate patient, an Unna boot can be left in place for up to 1 week. Examples of conveniently packaged products are Medicopaste (Graham-Field, Atlanta, GA 30360), Unna-FLEX (ConvaTec, Skillman, NJ 08558), and Gelo-Cast (BSN-JOBST, Charlotte, NC 28209). Despite the abundance of materials available for applying the boot, there is little information in the literature to support the topical application of zinc for wound healing. The success of this treatment application is most likely owing to the compression. Unna boot is not appropriate for arterial or mixed arterial/venous ulcers due to the potentially negative effects of compression when arterial disease is present. Although the treatment is used frequently, there are other methods for combining compression with wound care to treat patients with venous wounds.[227,228]

Four-Layer Bandage System

Similar to the Unna boot, yet distinctive, four-layer compression bandaging systems have been designed for the management of venous leg ulcers. The systems include a wound covering with modest absorptive qualities and several layers of different types of compression bandaging. The bandage system has been shown to be comfortable and cost effective, but new literature compared four-layer systems to other types of compression and found that other options may be even more cost effective.[229,230] An example of a well-known system is Profore (Smith & Nephew, Fort Worth, TX 76107). For the appropriate patient, a four-layer bandage system can be left in place for up to 1 week. As with all compression, watch for signs of ischemia, do not use for a patient who has a documented ABI of below 0.8, and rule out arterial disease before using.

Long-Stretch and Short-Stretch Bandages

Both long-stretch and short-stretch bandages are used to control edema and supply therapeutic levels of compression to support the venous and lymphatic systems. Long-stretch bandages such as Ace (3M, St. Paul, MN 55144) bandages provide a *high resting pressure,* which means that they continue to constrict when the wearer is resting. Owing to their extensibility or stretchiness, they do not provide significant *working pressure,* the ability to resist muscle contraction during activity. Long-stretch bandages are readily available and require minimal training to apply. Short-stretch bandages, such as Comprilan (BSN Medical, Charlotte, NC 28209) and Rosidal (Lohmann & Rauscher, Topeka, KS 66619), provide *low resting pressure* and *high working pressure* (Fig. 14.39). They are less extensible or stretchy, providing a more rigid shell when applied to a limb. This feature makes short-stretch bandages more appropriate for treating edema and lymphedema. Higher working pressures increase the efficiency of the muscle pump during activity, whereas lower resting pressures make the bandages more tolerable to wear. The appropriate application of short-stretch bandages is a complex skill

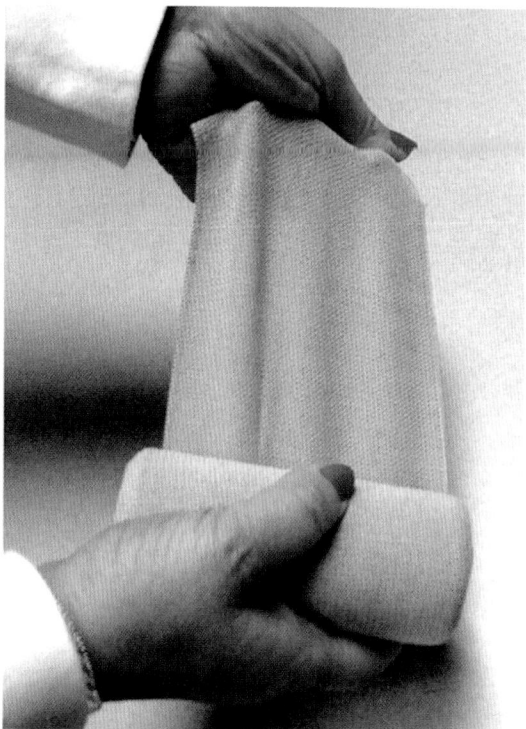

Figure 14.39 Sample of short-stretch bandage.

that requires special training to utilize safely. For a successful outcome as an intervention to reduce, support, or retain limb size, a physical therapy provider needs training, experience, knowledge, and clinical intuition. The amount of working and resting pressure delivered to a limb that is bandaged depends on several important factors: the number of layers of bandage, the age and condition of the bandages, the tension on the bandage when it is applied, and the skill of the clinician.[231]

Lymphedema Bandaging

This highly specialized form of bandaging utilizes multiple layers of unique padding materials and short-stretch bandages to create a supportive structure for edematous and lymphedematous body segments. Lymphedema bandaging provides support for tissues that have lost elasticity; facilitates a mild increase in tissue pressure, assisting lymph vessels to empty; prevents refilling of the interstitium between MLD treatments; improves the efficiency of the muscle pump during activity; and provides localized pressure where indicated to soften fibrotic tissue.

Bandaging protocols include techniques for applying compression to the head and neck, fingers and hands (Figs. 14.40 and 14.41), the UE (Fig. 14.42), and the LE (Fig. 14.43). The chest, abdomen, genital area, and back can also receive specialized support from compression products.[231]

As with MLD, the benefits of this treatment are not limited to the population with lymphedema. When compression is indicated, standard or modified

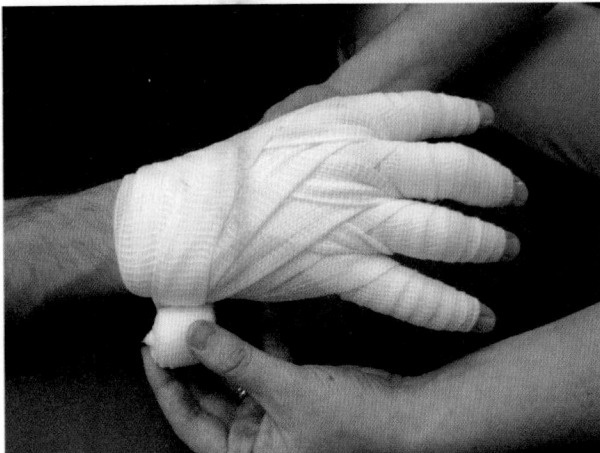

Figure 14.40 Application of lymphedema bandaging to fingers and hand.

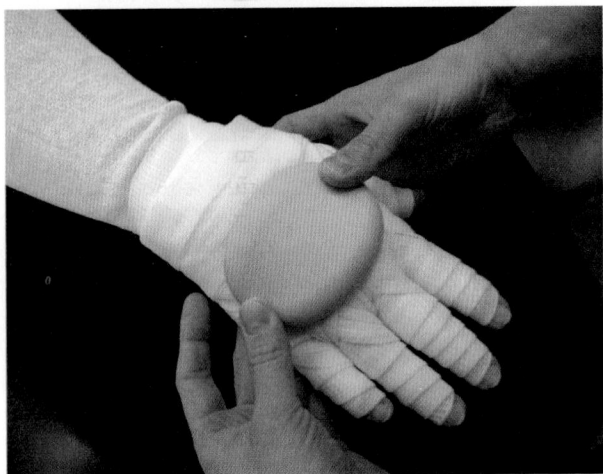

Figure 14.41 Use of foam padding to enhance the effects of lymphedema bandaging.

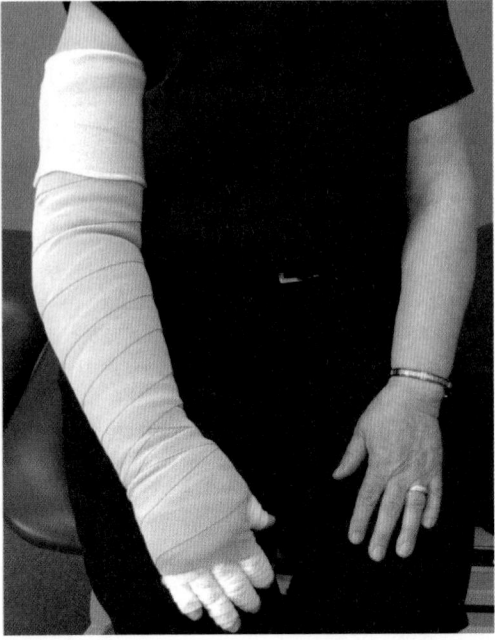

Figure 14.42 Lymphedema bandaging of the upper extremity.

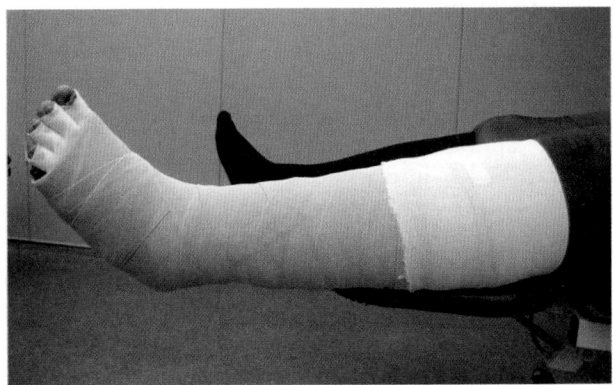

Figure 14.43 Lymphedema bandaging of the foot, ankle, and calf.

lymphedema bandaging can be beneficial to the population with edema (e.g., postoperative, CVI, venous ulcers, orthopedic injury).[232–237] To obtain contact information for training facilities that provide specialized education in bandaging as a part of CDT, refer to Appendix 14.D (online).

Compression Garments

Many patient/client populations use compression garments (Fig. 14.44). Originally designed to assist venous blood flow in the LEs, they are now specifically designed to manage burn and surgical scars, provide support to venous circulation, and prevent reaccumulation of fluid in the lymphedematous limb. There are a variety of garment styles and fabrics, custom and off the shelf, to meet the unique needs of different populations. Varying amounts of pressure are woven into the fabric during manufacturing. The amounts of pressure are conveyed as millimeters of mercury (mm Hg). Low pressure would start at 12 to 25 mm Hg, and higher pressures

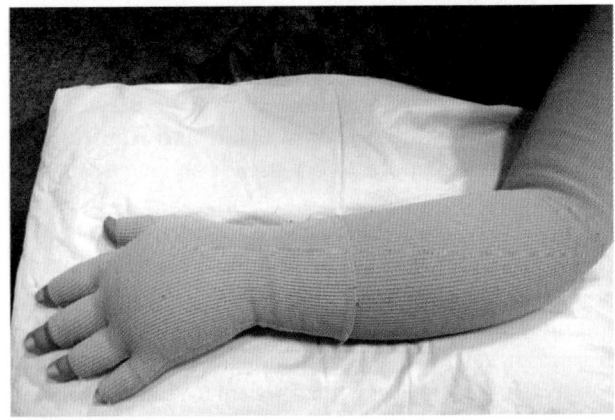

Figure 14.44 Patient wearing custom-fitted upper extremity compression sleeve and separate glove with open fingertips.

go up to 30 to 40 mm Hg. It is important to understand that garments must be appropriately selected and fitted by a trained professional. When worn correctly by a patient who has been prepared for garment wear and educated about compression, the garments serve an essential role in managing chronic, lifelong conditions such as CVI and lymphedema.[231,237]

Garments should not be used as a treatment to remove excess fluids from an extremity. If applied to an extremity that has not been adequately evacuated, the garments will be uncomfortable and may worsen the patient's symptoms.[238–240] Currently, manufacturers are participating in clinical research supporting the use of silver in compression garments. Juzo (Juzo, Cuyahoga Falls, OH 44223) adds permanently bonded silver to the textile fiber of LE garments such as stockings to inhibit bacterial growth and reduce odor.

Limb Containment Systems

Another option for some individuals is a quilted compression device or limb containment system. These unique compression options may be easier to don and doff, can be worn under short-stretch wraps or alone, and can be custom made to any part of the body (Figs. 14.45 and 14.46). This option may be useful for a person who is unable to apply a more fitted support garment independently or whose skin is compromised or fragile. The garments are often chosen by patients to wear at night instead of bandaging. There are many

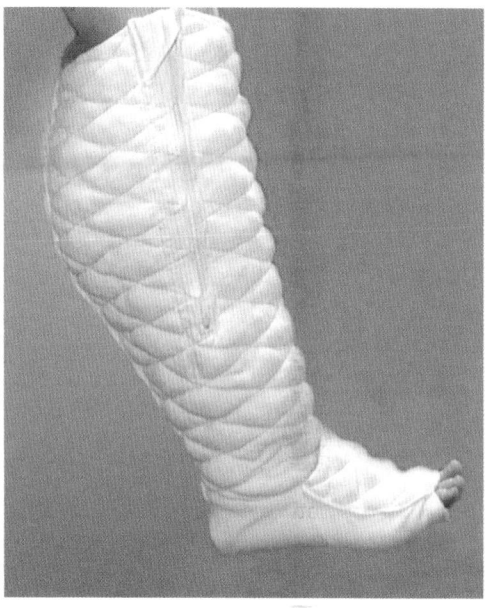

Figure 14.46 Quilted channel compression garment for venous insufficiency.

styles of therapeutic nightwear to add to a home program to help retain limb reductions achieved in physical therapy. These specialized garments can be made to support venous circulation or lymphatic drainage through altering the style and the stitching channels to complement the diagnosis. A physical therapist can consult with the leading manufacturers to get information on garment options to integrate this type of compression into the POC or the aftercare (or check out https://www.lohmann-rauscher.us or https://medical.essityusa.com/).

Compression Guidelines

Compression treatment should be customized to the characteristics of each individual. Since there is inherent risk in the application of compression, relative contraindications for compression should be evaluated, including history of DVT, acute local infection, CHF, cor pulmonale, and acute dermatitis. To assist in clinical decision-making, the following is a summary of general guidelines for compression bandaging and garments for patients with edema and lymphedema:

- *Arterial wounds:* No compression or very light compression with close involvement of the referring practitioner. Long-stretch bandaging or off-the-shelf low compression garment (12 to 25 mm Hg) can be used. Edema will not be significant and will evacuate quickly.
- *Venous wounds:* Compression is an essential component of treatment for wound healing and support of the venous system.[238,239] Short-stretch bandaging with high working pressure and low resting pressure will facilitate the effects of the calf pump during activity. A high pressure of 40 mm Hg at the ankle has been suggested.[239] Compression garments at

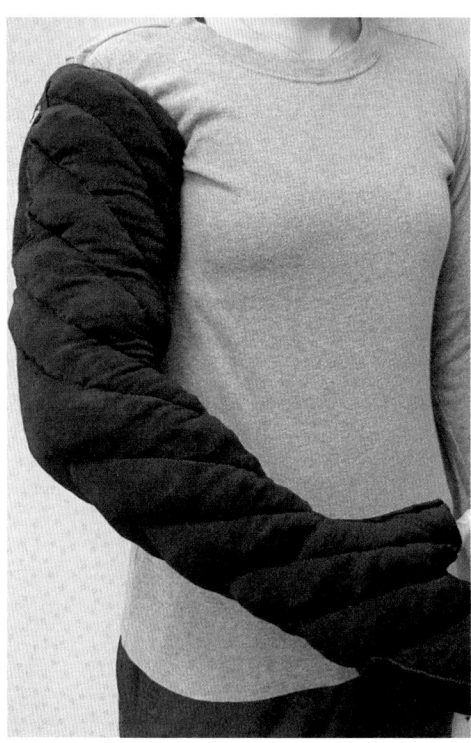

Figure 14.45 Individual wearing a quilted, custom limb containment system as part of a lymphedema management plan.

pressures of 20 to 30 mm Hg to 30 to 40 mm Hg are used depending on location and severity of swelling as well as ability of the patient to don and doff garments.

- *Neuropathic wounds:* Compression is contingent on blood flow. Fifteen percent of patients with a neuropathic condition also have an arterial component to their disease and must have an ABI calculated before compression is applied. If no arterial involvement, compress with short-stretch wrap. Follow up with compression garments for long-term use at lower compression of 12 to 25 mm Hg up to 20 to 30 mm Hg.
- *Lymphedema:* Short-stretch compression wrap worn 23 hr/day until limb reduction goal is reached, then moderate- to high-compression garments at 20 to 30 mm Hg to 30 to 40 mm Hg, depending on location and severity of swelling, as well as ability of the patient to don and doff garments.[239]
- *Edema:* Case studies and reports from the field establish that the compression treatment for patients with lymphedema also works well for patients with edema.[241] Short-stretch compression bandages are worn 23 hr/day, graduating to daytime only, decreasing as edema resolves. Off-the-shelf garments at lower levels of compression provide support for skin and help to retain reductions that therapy has achieved.

Intermittent Pneumatic Compression

Until the 1990s, intermittent pneumatic compression (IPC) was one of the few clinical interventions used to treat swelling (Fig. 14.47). Since then, new information about the physiology of edema and lymphedema, as well as lymphatic system function, has limited its value in treating some patients with edema and most patients with lymphedema. Intermittent compression pumps can facilitate venous return and may be an important adjunct to other forms of compression for the individual with a venous disorder.[3,242] A review of the evidence provided only modest support for the use of IPC for the treatment of venous leg ulcers.[237,240] Many individuals with long-standing venous insufficiency also have lymphedema. There is even less evidence and more controversy related to the use of IPC for lymphedema.[242–244] If a trial of IPC is indicated, MLD should be delivered before and after each treatment to offset the negative effects of fluid pooling that occurs adjacent to the edge of the limb sleeves. If indicated for treatment, IPC pressure settings must be kept very low to avoid collapse of the superficial lymph capillaries. Each client should be carefully examined by an experienced health-care professional before IPC is applied. Blood pressure readings should be taken before each treatment to confirm that IPC will be safe to use. Increasing total peripheral resistance with pneumatic compression will increase the work of the heart, increasing blood pressure. Pneumatic compression treatment is contraindicated for individuals with hypertension or a blood pressure reading greater than 140/90 mm Hg. Other contraindications to intermittent compression include acute inflammation or trauma, local infection, presence of thrombus, cardiac or kidney dysfunction, obstructed lymphatic channels, and impaired cognitive function.

Sequential Pneumatic Compression With Truncal Component

Advances in compression systems include more pneumatic chambers that inflate and deflate in a sequential pattern at very low pressures. The newest home use models include truncal decongestion and clearance in preparation for receiving lymph from affected areas. This appliance style mimics the benefits of MLD in the clinic setting (Fig. 14.48). Manual treatments clear the trunk proximally before treating more distal segments of the body. Stretch fabric is incorporated into the appliance design to further mimic the light stretch to the skin that is applied with MLD.[72,245–247]

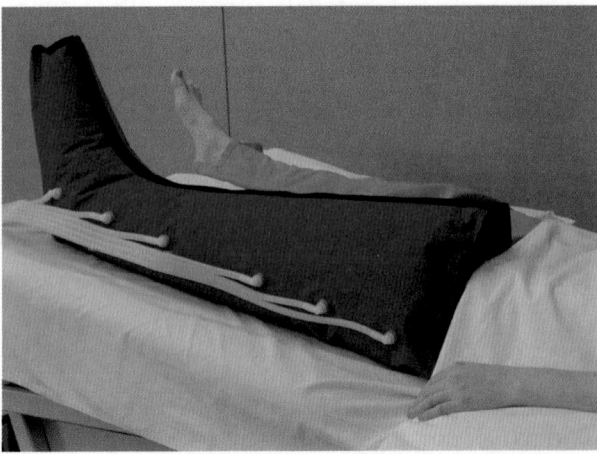

Figure 14.47 Intermittent pneumatic compression pump.

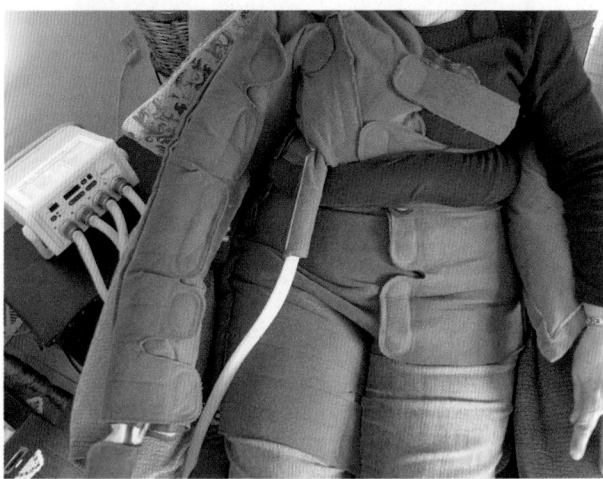

Figure 14.48 Sequential pneumatic compression with truncal component designed to retain and support the benefits of in-clinic lymphedema therapy at home.

Positioning

Positioning techniques are used to prevent or protect pressure injuries as well as other types of wounds, edema, lymphedema, and vascular disorders. This important aspect of intervention, as well as PRDs, should not be overlooked or underestimated during treatment planning. Devices and techniques selected for positioning should be compatible with the individual's health status. It is paramount that a personalized positioning and repositioning schedule be developed and prominently displayed for any patient who cannot position or reposition independently. The standard time intervals used for turning schedules (i.e., every 2 hr) are often too long for individuals who are frail, have fragile skin, or have existing wounds. A turning schedule could be as frequent as every 30 min in some cases, whereas for other individuals, every 4 hr may be enough. Suggestions for patient positioning programs include the following:[248-251]

- The patient's heels should be protected and elevated off the surface of the bed.
- The head of bed should not be elevated past 30°, unless medically necessary.
- An individualized turning schedule should be provided.
- PRDs should be used in conjunction with a turning schedule.
- Positioning with weight-bearing directly over the greater trochanter should be avoided.
- Positioning with full weight-bearing over an existing wound should be avoided.
- Donut-shaped devices for seating solutions should not be utilized.
- Pillows and wedges should be used to separate bony prominences from the bed and other body parts.

Pressure-Redistributing Devices

Pressure has a direct influence on perfusion or vascularity of a wound site. PRDs should be used to prevent skin breakdown, during the wound healing phase, and during the self-management phase, for lifelong protection and prevention. One of the most often used PRDs has adjustable air-filled cushions that mimic the pressure-relieving properties of water and aim to remove friction while sitting (Fig. 14.49). Along with positioning, patients and their caregivers must be educated about pressure redistribution and prevention of pressure-related trauma.[251] Advances in support surfaces that redistribute weight have made them more sophisticated and effective (Fig. 14.50). Experts in positioning systems are readily available to advise and instruct clinicians working with special populations.[252] Groups such as the Consortium for Spinal Cord Medicine, NPIAP, and the Department of Health and Human Services have made recommendations and algorithms for positioning and PRDs that can be used for intervention planning.[74,98,253]

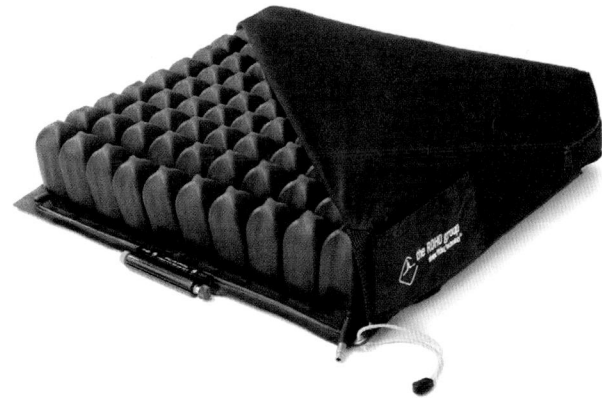

Figure 14.49 ROHO QUADTRO SELECT HIGH PROFILE cushion for pressure redistribution and skin protection. *(Courtesy of Permobil ROHO Seating and Positioning, Inc., Belleville, IL 62221.)*

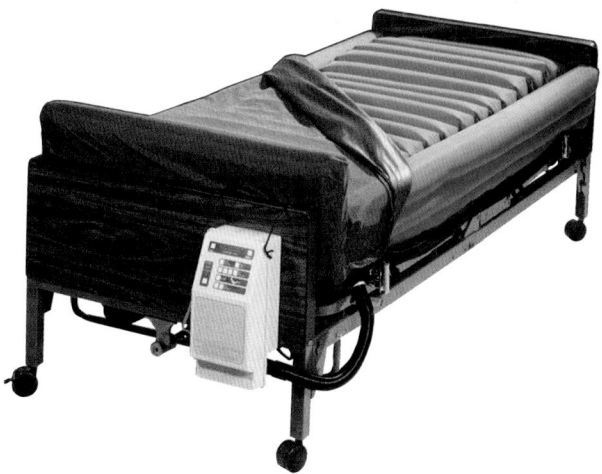

Figure 14.50 *Select*Air MAX, a low-air-loss support system for pressure relief. *(Courtesy of Permobil ROHO Seating and Positioning, Belleville, IL 62221.)*

Exercise

The powerful impact of exercise on the healing wound should be appreciated for a variety of reasons, including increased strength and joint ROM, improved quality of movement, increased ADL, improved QOL perceptions, increased blood flow to the extremities, improved calf pump activity, prevention of pressure injuries, prevention of falls, and enhanced effects of lymphedema bandaging. Too often, exercise is neglected in the intervention plan for individuals with vascular, lymphatic, and integumentary disorders, especially those with wounds or edema. In accordance with the vision statement of the APTA, members of the physical therapy profession are charged to "transform society by optimizing movement to improve the human experience."[254] As such, the physical therapist is viewed as the movement expert and should intentionally promote activities in the POC related to increasing activity levels as appropriate. There is a vast body of knowledge that supports aerobic exercise, due to its anti-inflammatory and anti-oxidative effects, in decreasing the time required for healing, notably in aging individuals, obese individuals, and the diabetic population.

Exercise prescription should be customized to the patient's needs and medical status. A walking program can benefit most individuals who are able to ambulate even short distances. Water-based exercise programs can facilitate the transition from bed or chair to land-based exercise. Individuals with wounds can participate in water-based exercise if it is appropriate to cover the wounds with occlusive dressings. The hydrostatic pressure of water contributes to support of edematous and lymphedematous body segments and creates an ideal setting for exercise for most individuals with swelling. The implementation of active exercise for individuals with lymphedema or who are at risk of developing lymphedema is under investigation. Early literature shows that specific, active exercise may help and not hurt those individuals.[255,256] Recent literature supports high-load active exercise with compression therapy as beneficial for people with lower-limb lymphedema.[257,258]

Patients should be educated about the concept that movement, activity, and formal exercise are all important for long-term management of the conditions listed in this chapter. Physical therapists introduce these concepts, provide expert instruction, and develop appropriate home exercise programs. Patients are encouraged to follow the exercise prescriptions at home and accept them as part of their everyday lives. However, some types of exercise might be contraindicated or need to be planned with caution when medical issues arise, such as the need to restrict weight-bearing on a foot wound, in the presence of unstable cardiopulmonary conditions, or related orthopedic problems that would limit activity.

Orthotics

Splinting

Patients who are immobile may benefit from resting splints to retain, or dynamic splints to regain, functional ROM. Splinting can also prevent skin breakdown by retaining normal positioning of joints during periods of immobility. Extra precautions (i.e., padding) must be taken to protect aging or fragile skin from breakdown when semirigid thermoplastic materials are used for splinting. The use of splinting to manage burn scars is an essential part of the POC for an individual with a thermal injury. Positioning and splinting information found there can also be applied to patients with other types of wounds.

Total Contact Casting

One method for the reduction of weight-bearing stresses on the foot is the application of a *total contact cast* (TCC). This method can be useful for the individual with a neuropathic ulcer on the plantar surface of the foot. After infection and swelling have been controlled, a plaster cast is applied from the toes to below the knee. A trained individual uses plaster, padding techniques, and the placement of a rubber insert on the weight-bearing part of the cast to complete the application. A TCC is usually worn for 7 to 10 days at a time, removed for skin care, and then reapplied.[259,260]

Neuropathic Walker

A removable ankle-foot orthosis can be custom fabricated or ordered prefabricated to provide weight distribution and cushioning for the individual with an insensate foot, a chronic foot ulcer, or Charcot joint (Fig. 14.51). This option is versatile in fit and allows skin checks, dressing changes, and pressure alterations as needed.[259–261]

Cast Shoes

Cast shoes or postoperative shoes can be utilized as an inexpensive, temporary alternative for wound off-loading. These shoes, however, do not provide any means of controlling foot motion and provide only little cushioning protection for the chronic wound. This option should be considered temporary. Patients wearing cast shoes for pressure distribution should be monitored closely for signs of complications.

Extra-Depth Shoes

Extra-depth shoes have a roomy toe box and a deep sole to provide shock absorption and cushion. The shoes should fit such that pressure is redirected away from bony prominences and wounds (Fig. 14.52).[261] Available in many styles, they can be purchased from an orthotist or at a specialty shoe store. Individuals with

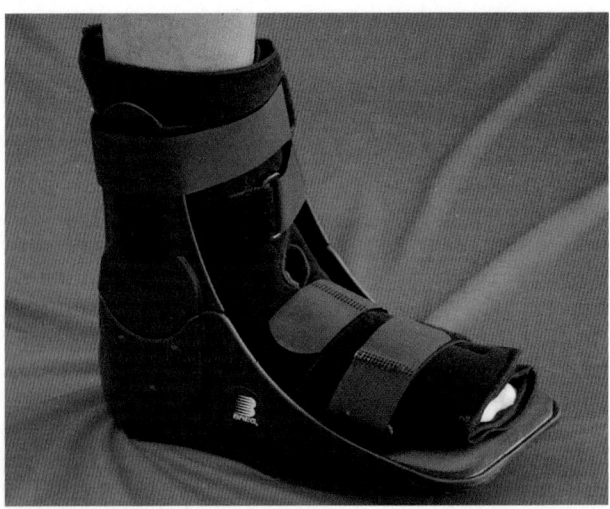

Figure 14.51 An ankle-foot orthosis specifically designed to allow distributed weight-bearing for individuals with neuropathy.

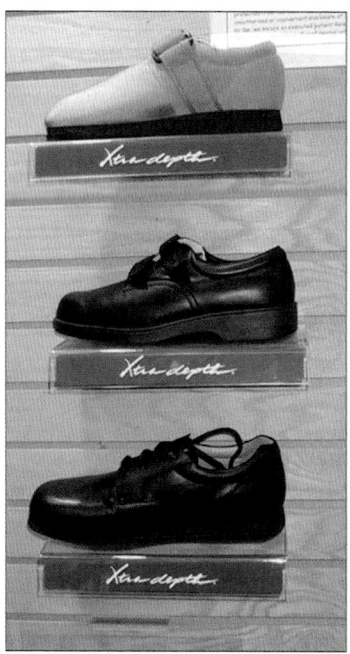

Figure 14.52 Extra-depth shoes that redirect foot pressures away from problem areas.

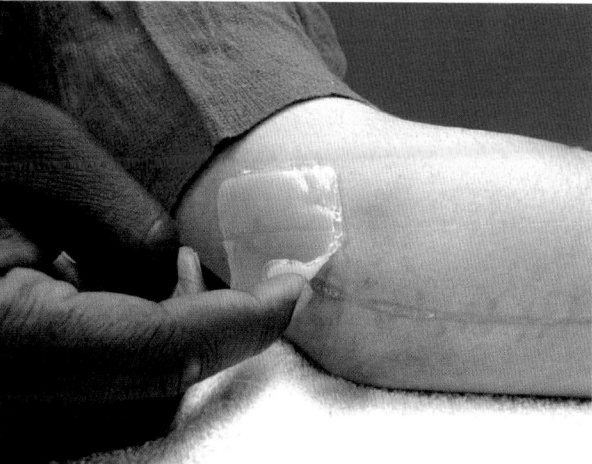

Figure 14.53 Application of a silicone gel sheet to scar tissue during the maturation phase of wound healing.

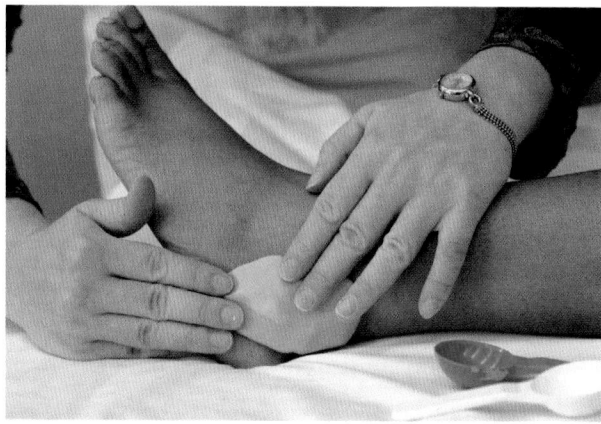

Figure 14.54 Application of elastomer putty to scar tissue during the maturation phase of wound healing.

insensate feet, with or without wounds, should strongly consider wearing this type of shoe to support skin protection and ulcer prevention.

Scar Management

As described earlier in this chapter, scar formation is an expected component of wound healing.[262–264] After the wound is filled with collagen, the tissue must be remodeled and shaped into the finely structured end product. Contraction of scar tissue can lead to disfigurement and loss of function, especially if the scar tissue is located over or near a joint surface. Issues of disfigurement and dysfunction are greatest following thermal injury. Currently, the mechanisms by which scar can be controlled are not completely understood. Although some interventions seem to help manage scar tissue effectively, there is room for further investigation into how to achieve optimal control of scar formation. Most scar tissue is managed by a physical therapy provider using compression garments, stretching exercises, orthotics, positioning, specific types of massage, and the use of topical adjuncts such as silicone gel sheets (Fig. 14.53) and elastomer putty (Fig. 14.54). Topical creams, oils, and ointments have some positive effects on scarring, but it is not known if the massaging actions used to apply the agents or the agents themselves provide the therapeutic effects. Early and adequate intervention can prevent most of the complications of scarring. Since the process of scar formation usually continues for 6 to 24 months, routine follow-up care should be part of the intervention plan. Individuals with scar tissue must learn how to safely massage the skin at home because frequent pressure applications have the greatest influence on new connective tissue orientation. When conservative measures of scar management have not controlled scarring, surgical intervention may be indicated. However, following surgery, the individual will have a new wound and subsequent new scar to manage.

SUMMARY

There is reason for enthusiasm among therapists who are interested in the care of patients with vascular, lymphatic, and integumentary disorders. Skin and wound care practices continue to advance with clinical trials, randomized controlled studies, and empirical data all contributing to the expanding collection of knowledge. New information about the microcirculation of blood and lymph has changed intervention strategies. The role of the skin as an organ has garnered new respect. It is not surprising that there is an explosion of research, literature, and products to serve the needs of individuals with disorders affecting these systems. Current and future generations are facing health-care challenges of a magnitude never before seen in our society, including an increase in the number of individuals with conditions related to the disorders discussed in this chapter. The incidence of patients with diabetes, obesity, vascular and lymphatic disease, chronic wounds, and antibiotic-resistant pathogens is on the rise. Issues compounding the challenges include a growing population of older individuals, health-care reimbursement challenges, and numerous ethical dilemmas in daily clinical practice.

This chapter provides support for clinicians in their efforts to provide robust, evidence-based patient care. Topics of particular importance include current strategies for wound management, the importance of adequate and appropriate patient education, pressure injury prevention and precautions, advanced foot care for individuals with diabetic neuropathy, optimal compression for lymphedema, the essential role of moisture in wound healing, and the importance of exercise as part of the POC.

There is great need for ongoing research to establish the level of strength of evidence for a variety of topics that may or may not be important in the world of vascular, lymphatic, and integumentary disorders. Some of the concepts that deserve a second look are the impact of bioburden on the wound infection continuum, the preparation of the wound bed, the use of exogenous oxygen applications, noncontact US, nonthermal radiofrequency stimulation, cold laser, biosurgery/maggot therapy, bioengineered tissue, exogenous growth factors, medical-grade honey, and topical silver preparations. In addition to expanding the evidence, improvements in the standardizing of wound care education are needed. The interdisciplinary nature of wound care calls for more communication among health-care professionals. Wise clinicians must keep abreast of new information and current standards of care, approaching new entries to the field with a strong sense of clinical intuition as well as a firm grasp of reputable scientific evidence.

Questions for Review

1. Discuss the differences, similarities, and relationships among the arterial, venous, and lymphatic systems. Compare anatomy, method of fluid movement, and function.

2. Outline some of the unique characteristics that can be identified clinically for disorders of the vascular, lymphatic, and integumentary systems.

3. Prepare a list of factors that contribute to abnormal wound healing. Divide the list into intrinsic, extrinsic, and iatrogenic factors.

4. Review the annotated tests and measurements included in this chapter that should be used during a physical therapy examination. Identify tests and measurements routinely performed for patients with vascular, lymphatic, or integumentary disorders.

5. Design a checklist of examination categories for examining a patient with a disorder of the vascular, lymphatic, or integumentary system.

6. Create a general list of the primary components of a POC for a patient with a wound.

7. Explain how a physical therapist should respond to the understanding that many vascular, lymphatic, and integumentary disorders have a long latency period and require a heightened level of vigilance and proactivity in order to recognize symptoms and initiate treatment as early as possible.

8. Explain the rationale for each of the following treatments in skin and wound care: moist wound healing, arterial wound hydration, venous wound compression, lymphedema treatment, and foot care for the individual with diabetes.

CASE STUDY

REFERRAL

A 78-year-old woman with a primary diagnosis of Alzheimer disease has been living in a residential facility for 10 months. The physician at the facility refers her to physical therapy. Referral is for advanced wound care of pressure injury right ischial tuberosity.

CASE STUDY—cont'd

PAST MEDICAL HISTORY

Significant for history of mild osteoarthritis of both knees, prior left total hip arthroplasty, cataracts in both eyes, and removal of colon polyps. Onset of symptoms of Alzheimer disease 3 years ago.

CURRENT MEDICAL HISTORY

Health conditions include mild hypertension controlled by medication and a stage 3 pressure injury over the right ischial tuberosity.

MEDICAL INTERVENTION PREVIOUS TO CURRENT REFERRAL

Pressure injury treated for 4 weeks (30 days) with twice daily (BID) hydrogen peroxide flushes followed by dry gauze 4 × 4s covered with gauze pad and adhesive tape. No changes in wound bed for 4 weeks. No other wound care intervention in place.

PSYCHOSOCIAL

The patient's husband also resides at the same facility and lives in the same room. He is frail but mobile and assists spouse with most ADLs. There are no children or local family in the area to help. The patient enjoys music and trips by wheelchair to the facility's activity center.

COGNITIVE

Patient disoriented to place and time. Becomes agitated during wound care. She is unable to follow weight shift and turning schedules independently and has difficulty following simple instructions.

PHYSICAL THERAPY EXAMINATION DATA

Body Structure/Function

- *Wound:* Stage 3 pressure injury over right ischial tuberosity. Measures 2.36 × 1.57 in. (6 × 4 cm) with depth of 1.57 in. (4 cm). The wound bed is 50% necrotic yellow slough and 50% red granulation tissue. Periwound tissue is intact, well defined, and shows no signs of maceration. Drainage is moderate, yellow-brown, and thin with minimal odor. The wound is currently contaminated but not infected (i.e., colonized bacteria are present but not to the level of clinical infection).
- *Strength and ROM:* Patient unable to follow commands consistently for examination of strength but appears to have functional strength and ROM of bilateral upper extremities (BUEs). Gross bilateral lower extremity strength is impaired perhaps owing to declining activity levels. Active ROM appears functional in BUEs. Bilateral hip flexion contractures of 30° can be reduced to 15° with passive ROM.

Activity Limitations—Mobility

Patient is either in wheelchair or bed 24 hr/day. Patient is unable to roll independently but can often assist using BUEs when instructed. Requires maximum assist of two to pivot transfer. The patient is unable to ambulate at this time but has front-wheeled walker available.

Participation Restrictions

Requires close supervision during social engagement due to propensity to become agitated.

GUIDING QUESTIONS

1. What are the contributing factors that have most likely led to the chronicity of this wound?
2. What other information would you like to ask about in order to formulate the best possible POC for this patient?
3. What other factors might contribute to the slow healing time of this wound?
4. What combination of interventions to clean and débride would allow removal of necrotic tissue while protecting granulation tissue?
5. Clinically, which electromodalities are biocompatible for the treatment of this wound (irrespective of payment), and how will they contribute to wound healing?
6. Other than local wound care, what intervention will be essential for wound closure?
7. Once progress has been made in wound healing, if the wound were to become dry, what dressing types could be used to create a moist wound environment?
8. If using an occlusive dressing, why should this patient be closely monitored?

(Continued)

CASE STUDY—cont'd

9. Assuming this patient's wound will close, what are the expectations for the condition of her skin over the wound site?

10. Which members of the interdisciplinary team would you want to involve in order to provide the most holistic care possible?

11. What adaptive equipment would you ideally want to provide to this patient and her caregiver (irrespective of cost and reimbursement)?

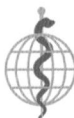

For additional resources, including answers to the questions for review, new immersive cases, case study guiding questions, references, and more, please visit **https://www.fadavis.com/product/physical -rehabilitation-fulk-8**. You may also quickly find the resources by entering this title's four-digit ISBN, 4691, in the search field at **http://fadavis.com** and logging in at the prompt.

Stroke

Judith E. Deutsch, PT, PhD, FAPTA   **Chapter 15**

LEARNING OBJECTIVES

1. Describe the epidemiology, etiology, pathophysiology, symptomatology, and sequelae of stroke.
2. Identify and describe the procedures used to examine and evaluate patients with stroke to establish a diagnosis, prognosis, and plan of care.
3. Describe the role of the physical therapist in assisting the patient in recovery from stroke in terms of interventions, patient-/client-related instruction, coordination, communication, and documentation.
4. Describe and practice clinical reasoning used to examine and evaluate client care, formulate realistic goals, and develop a plan of care for a clinical case study.

CHAPTER OUTLINE

EPIDEMIOLOGY AND ETIOLOGY *524*
RISK FACTORS AND STROKE PREVENTION *525*
PATHOPHYSIOLOGY *526*
  Management Categories *527*
  Vascular Syndromes *527*
NEUROLOGICAL SEQUELAE AND ASSOCIATED CONDITIONS *532*
  Altered Consciousness *532*
  Speech and Language Deficits *532*
  Dysphagia *535*
  Cognitive Deficits *535*
  Affective Status *536*
  Hemispheric Behavioral Differences *536*
  Perceptual Deficits *538*
  Seizures *538*
  Bladder and Bowel Dysfunction *538*
  Cardiovascular and Pulmonary Dysfunction *539*
  Deep Vein Thrombosis and Pulmonary Embolus *539*
  Osteoporosis and Fracture Risk *539*
  Disordered Sleep *539*
MEDICAL DIAGNOSIS OF THE STROKE HEALTH CONDITION *540*
  History and Examination *540*
  Tests and Measures *540*
  Cerebrovascular Imaging *540*
MEDICAL, PHARMACOLOGICAL, AND NEUROSURGICAL MANAGEMENT OF STROKE *541*
  Medical Management *541*

Pharmacological Management *542*
  Neurosurgical Management *542*
REHABILITATION *542*
  Acute Phase *543*
  Subacute Phase *544*
  Chronic Phase *544*
INTEGRATED FRAMEWORK FOR CLINICAL DECISION-MAKING *545*
EXAMINATION *545*
  Participation *547*
  Activity *548*
  Body Function and Structure *552*
PROGNOSIS AND DIAGNOSIS *557*
GOALS AND OUTCOMES *558*
PHYSICAL THERAPY INTERVENTIONS *558*
  Structure of the Intervention *559*
  Interventions to Improve Participation *561*
  Interventions to Improve Activities *561*
  Interventions to Improve Body Function and Structure *581*
  Aerobic Capacity and Physical Activity *581*
PATIENT-/CLIENT-RELATED INSTRUCTION *583*
DISCHARGE PLANNING *583*
RECOVERY AND OUTCOMES *583*
SUMMARY *584*

*S*troke *(cerebrovascular accident [CVA])* is the sudden loss of neurological function caused by an interruption of blood flow to the brain. *Ischemic stroke* is the most common type, affecting about 80% of individuals with stroke, and can be the result of thrombosis, embolism, or hypoperfusion. A thrombus is a local occlusion of a blood vessel, and an embolus is material from a distant site that either blocks or impairs blood flow, depriving the brain of essential oxygen and nutrients. Lack of oxygen and nutrients results in tissue necrosis and penumbral area where the cells may be damaged but preserved.[1] *Hemorrhagic stroke* occurs when blood vessels rupture, causing leakage of blood in or around the brain.

Clinically, a variety of focal deficits are possible, including changes in the level of consciousness and impairments of sensory, motor, cognitive, perceptual, and language functions. To be classified as stroke, neurological deficits must persist for at least 24 hr. Motor deficits are characterized by paralysis *(hemiplegia)* or weakness *(hemiparesis),* typically on the side of the body opposite the side of the lesion. The term *hemiplegia* is often used generically to refer to the wide variety of motor problems that result from stroke. The location and extent of brain injury, the amount of collateral blood flow, and early acute care management determine the severity of neurological deficits in an individual patient. Impairments may resolve spontaneously as brain swelling subsides (reversible ischemic neurological deficit), generally within 3 weeks. Residual neurological impairments are those that persist longer than 3 weeks and may lead to lasting disability. Strokes are classified by etiologic categories (thrombosis, embolus, or hemorrhage), specific vascular territory (anterior cerebral artery syndrome, middle cerebral artery syndrome, etc.), and management categories (transient ischemic attack, minor stroke, major stroke, deteriorating stroke, young stroke).

 See Immersive Case C: A Patient With Stroke

■ EPIDEMIOLOGY AND ETIOLOGY

Stroke is the fifth leading cause of death and the leading cause of long-term disability among adults in the United States. An estimated 7.6 million Americans older than 20 years of age have experienced a stroke. Each year, approximately 795,000 individuals experience a stroke; approximately 610,000 are first attacks, and 185,000 are recurrent strokes. Women have a lower age-adjusted stroke prevalence than men. However, this prevalence is reversed in older ages; women over 85 years of age have an elevated prevalence compared to men. Compared to White Americans, Black Americans have twice the risk of first-ever stroke; rates are also higher in Mexican Americans, American Indians, and Alaskan Natives. The incidence of stroke increases dramatically with age, effectively doubling in the decade after 65 years of age. Approximately 10% of all strokes occur in individuals 18 to 50 years of age. Between 5% (Black males 45–64 years old) and 22% (Black females 65–74 years old) of persons who survive an initial stroke will experience another one within 5 years. This highlights the importance of secondary prevention. Current data reveal that stroke incidence has been declining in recent years in a largely White adult cohort.[2,3]

The incidence of stroke deaths is greater than 133,000 annually, and strokes account for 1 of every 20 deaths in the United States. Death rates due to stroke have been declining since 2009. The type of stroke is significant in determining survival. Of patients with stroke, hemorrhagic stroke accounts for the largest number of deaths, with mortality rates of 37% to 38% at 1 month,

whereas ischemic strokes have a mortality rate of only 14.7% at 1 month.[2] Survival rates are dramatically lessened by increased age, hypertension, heart disease, and diabetes. Loss of consciousness at stroke onset, lesion size, persistent severe hemiplegia, multiple neurological deficits, and history of previous stroke are also important predictors of mortality.[4]

Stroke is the leading cause of *serious* long-term disability in the United States. Of ischemic stroke survivors 65 years or older, incidences of disabilities observed at 6 months include hemiparesis (50%), inability to walk without assistance (30%), dependence in activities of daily living (ADL) (26%), aphasia (19%), and depression (35%). Stroke survivors represent the largest group admitted to rehabilitation hospitals, and about a third of patients receive outpatient rehabilitation services. Another indicator of disability is the fact that approximately 26% of patients with stroke are institutionalized in a long-term care facility. Direct and indirect costs of stroke are in the tens of billions, with the most recent report in 2018 of 52.8 billion.[2]

Atherosclerosis is a major contributory factor in cerebrovascular disease. It is characterized by plaque formation with an accumulation of lipids, fibrin, complex carbohydrates, and calcium deposits on arterial walls that leads to progressive narrowing of blood vessels. Interruption of blood flow by atherosclerotic plaques occurs at certain sites of predilection. These generally include bifurcations, constrictions, dilations, or angulations of arteries. The most common sites for lesions to occur are at the origin of the common carotid artery or at its transition into the middle cerebral artery, at the main bifurcation of the middle cerebral artery, and at the junction of the vertebral arteries with the basilar artery.

Ischemic strokes are the result of thrombus, embolism, or conditions that produce low systemic perfusion pressures. The resulting lack of cerebral blood flow (CBF) deprives the brain of needed oxygen and glucose, disrupts cellular metabolism, and leads to injury and death of tissues. A thrombus results from platelet adhesion and aggregation on plaques. *Cerebral thrombosis* refers to the formation or development of a blood clot within the cerebral arteries or their branches. It should be noted that lesions of extracranial vessels (carotid or vertebral arteries) can also produce symptoms of stroke. Thrombi lead to ischemia, or occlusion of an artery with resulting *cerebral infarction* or tissue death *(atherothrombotic brain infarction [ABI]).* Thrombi can also become dislodged and travel to a more distal site in the form of an intra-artery embolus. *Cerebral embolus (CE)* is composed of bits of matter (blood clot, plaque) formed elsewhere and released into the bloodstream, traveling to the cerebral arteries where they lodge in a vessel, producing occlusion and infarction. The most common source of CE is disease of the cardiovascular system. Occasionally, systemic disorders may produce septic, fat, or air emboli that affect the cerebral circulation. Ischemic strokes may also result from low systemic perfusion, the result of cardiac failure or significant blood loss with resulting systemic hypotension. The neurological deficits produced with systemic failure are global in nature with bilateral neurological deficits.

Hemorrhagic strokes, with abnormal bleeding into the extravascular areas of the brain, are the result of rupture of a cerebral vessel or trauma. Hemorrhage results in increased intracranial pressures with injury to brain tissues and restriction of distal blood flow. *Intracerebral hemorrhage (IH)* is caused by rupture of a cerebral vessel with subsequent bleeding into the brain. Primary *cerebral hemorrhage* (nontraumatic spontaneous hemorrhage) typically occurs in small blood vessels weakened by atherosclerosis producing an *aneurysm. Subarachnoid hemorrhage (SH)* occurs from bleeding into the subarachnoid space typically from a saccular or berry aneurysm affecting primarily large blood vessels. Congenital anomalies that produce weakness in the blood vessel wall are major contributing factors to the formation of an aneurysm. Hemorrhage is closely linked to chronic hypertension. *Arteriovenous malformation (AVM)* is another congenital anomaly that can result in stroke. AVM is characterized by a tortuous tangle of arteries and veins with agenesis of an interposing capillary system. The abnormal vessels undergo progressive dilation with age and eventually bleed in about 50% of cases. Sudden and severe cerebral bleeding can result in death within hours because intracranial pressures rise rapidly, and adjacent cortical tissues are compressed or displaced as in brain stem herniation.

■ RISK FACTORS AND STROKE PREVENTION

Cardiovascular diseases affecting the brain and heart share several common risk factors important to the development of atherosclerosis. Major risk factors for stroke are hypertension, diabetes mellitus (DM), disorders of heart rhythm, high blood cholesterol and other lipids, smoking/tobacco use, and heart disease (HD). In patients with ABI, approximately 70% have hypertension, 30% HD, 15% congestive heart failure (CHF), 30% peripheral arterial disease (PAD), and 15% DM.[3] Blood pressure (BP) is a powerful determinant of risk for both ischemic stroke and intracranial hemorrhage. Individuals with BP less than 120/80 mm Hg have approximately half the lifetime risk of stroke of those with hypertension.[2(pe380)] Importantly, HTN increases the risk of recurrent stroke.[3] Patients with marked elevations of hematocrit are also at an increased risk of occlusive stroke owing to a generalized reduction of CBF. Cardiac disorders (e.g., rheumatic heart valvular disease, endocarditis) and cardiac surgery (e.g., coronary artery bypass graft [CABG]) increase the risk of embolic stroke. Atrial fibrillation is a powerful risk factor for ischemic stroke with a three- to fivefold increased risk. End-stage renal disease and chronic kidney disease

also increase the risk of stroke. Sleep apnea is an independent risk factor for stroke, almost doubling the risk of stroke or death. Control of these chronic diseases and conditions is essential in reducing stroke risk.[2,3]

Several stroke risk factors are specific to women. Women with early menopause (before 42 years of age) have twice the risk of ischemic stroke as women with later menopause. The use of estrogen alone or estrogen plus progestin increases the risk of ischemic stroke (up to 44% to 55% or higher). Pregnancy, birth, and the first 6 weeks postpartum can also increase risk of stroke, especially in older women and African Americans. Preeclampsia is an independent risk factor for stroke.[2]

Modifiable risk factors include cigarette smoking, physical inactivity, obesity, diet, and sleep. Risk of stroke is two to four times higher in current smokers than in nonsmokers or those who have quit for more than 10 years. Exposure to secondhand smoke increases the risk of stroke by 20% to 30%. Physical activity (moderate to vigorous exercise) is associated with an overall 35% reduction in stroke risk, whereas light exercise (walking) does not appear to have the same benefit. As with a cardiac risk profile, the more risk factors present or the greater the degree of abnormality of any one factor, the greater is the risk of stroke. Stroke risk factors considered nonmodifiable include family history, age, gender, and race (African American).

Lifestyle changes can greatly reduce the risk of stroke. Achieving the greatest ideal cardiovascular health metrics, including avoiding smoking and tobacco products; engaging in daily physical activity; eating a healthy diet; maintaining a healthy weight, getting enough sleep; and keeping cholesterol, BP, and glucose at healthy levels, is associated with a lower risk of stroke. Table 15.1 indicates the definitions of cardiovascular health, provided by the American Heart Association (AHA) 2020 Goals,[3,5] and updated values for physical activity, blood glucose, and non-HDL cholesterol as well as adding sleep, which is not included in the new Essential Eight recommendations.[6]

Effective stroke prevention depends on improving public awareness concerning the *early warning signs of stroke.* Only about 60% of Americans can recognize even one warning sign, and only 55% can identify one stroke symptom.[3] Early warning signs identified by the AHA and National Stroke Association are known as FAST, an acronym that stands for *F*acial dropping, *A*rm weakness, *S*peech difficulties, *T*ime.[5] *FAST* is used as a mnemonic to help improve responsiveness to stroke victims by calling out the most common warning signs. Patients and families are encouraged to call 911 immediately, even if these symptoms go away quickly or are not painful. The significance of recognizing early warning signs rests with prompt initiation of emergency care under the rule that "time is brain."

Early computed tomography (CT) is used to differentiate between atherothrombotic stroke and hemorrhagic

Table 15.1 Definitions of Cardiovascular Health[2,5,6]

	Level of Cardiovascular Health for Each Metric for Adults 20 Years of Age and Older		
	Poor	Intermediate	Ideal
Current Smoking	Yes	Never or quit >12 mo	Former ≥23 mo
BMI	≥30	25–29.9	<25
*Physical Activity**	None		
Healthy Diet Pattern, Number of Components (AHA Diet Score)‡	<2 (0–39)	2–3 (40–79)	4–5 (80–100)
*Total Non-HDL Cholesterol, mg/dL**	≥220	131–159	<130
Blood Pressure	SBP ≥140 mm Hg or DBP ≥90 mm Hg	SBP 120–139 mm Hg or DBP 80–89 mm Hg or treated to goal	<120 mm Hg/80 mm Hg
*Fasting Plasma Glucose, mg/dL and HbA$_{1c}$**	>126 HbA^{1c} >8	100–125 or treated to goal HbA^{1c} >5.7–6.4	<100 No history of diabetes
*Sleep, self-reported hours per night**	<6 hr >10 hr	6–7 hr 9–10 hr	7–9 hr

‡In the context of a healthy dietary pattern that is consistent with a Dietary Approaches to Stop Hypertension [DASH]–type eating pattern, to consume ≥4.5 cups/day of fruits and vegetables, ≥2 servings/week of fish, and ≥3 servings/day of whole grains and no more than 36 oz/week of sugar-sweetened beverages and 1,500 mg/day of sodium. The consistency of one's diet with these dietary targets can be described using a continuous American Heart Association diet score, scaled from 0 to 100. Modified from Lloyd-Jones et al.[5] with permission. Copyright © 2010, American Heart Association, Inc. *Updated with Essential Eight from Lloyd-Jones et al.[6]
AHA = American Heart Association; BMI = body mass index.

stroke. If the stroke is atherothrombotic, clot-dissolving enzymes (e.g., tissue plasminogen activator [tPA]) can be used for thrombolysis. To be effective, thrombolytic therapy such as tPA must be given within 3 to 4.5 hr of symptom onset. It cannot be given to patients with hemorrhagic stroke or patients with active intracranial bleeding (e.g., serious head trauma) because the drug may worsen bleeding. It is also contraindicated in patients with severe uncontrolled hypertension. Within this window of opportunity, the patient must recognize the situation as a medical emergency, be transported to an appropriate hospital, be evaluated by emergency department (ED) staff (including a CT scan of the brain), and be treated.[7,8] Although this treatment has been available since the mid-1990s and has been shown to be safe and to dramatically reduce death and disability, fewer than half of individuals experiencing stroke arrive at the ED within 2 hr of symptoms.[9] Women are less likely than men to arrive in time. Of those arriving at the ED within 2 hr of symptoms, only 65% received imaging within 1 hr of ED arrival.[10]

In the United States, there is a Stroke Center Network dedicated to providing the highest quality of acute stroke care. Direct access to a *comprehensive stroke center*

(CSC) is associated with a shorter onset-to-treatment time and better outcomes for ischemic stroke treated with thrombolysis.[11] Even with policy changes that allow emergency first responders to transmit individuals directly to a CSC, only about half of patients have timely access.[12] A significant predictor in successfully accessing emergency care is the "executive" spouse or significant other who is able to make the decision to seek treatment immediately. Patients who do receive tPA are at least 33% more likely to recover from their stroke with little or no disability after 3 months as compared to those who do not receive the treatment.[13] Major heart and stroke organizations currently promote the use of the term *brain attack,* comparable to heart attack, to help individuals recognize the importance of seeking immediate emergency care.

■ PATHOPHYSIOLOGY

Sudden cessation of CBF and oxygen-glucose deprivation sets in motion a series of pathological events. Within minutes, neurons die in the ischemic core tissue, while most neurons in the surrounding penumbra survive for a slightly longer time. Cell survival depends largely on the severity and the duration of the ischemic episode. For cells to survive, 20% to 25% of regular blood flow is required. Without timely reperfusion, cells in the penumbra die, neuronal activity ceases, and the infarct expands. Ischemia triggers several damaging cellular events, termed *ischemic cascade.* The release of excess neurotransmitters (e.g., glutamate and aspartate) produces a progressive disturbance of energy metabolism and anoxic depolarization, which results in an inability of brain cells to produce energy, particularly adenosine triphosphate (ATP). This is followed by excess influx of calcium ions and pump failure of the neuronal membrane. Excess calcium reacts with intracellular phospholipids to form free radicals. Calcium influx also stimulates the release of nitric oxide and cytokines. Both mechanisms further damage brain cells. Research efforts are ongoing toward development of drugs that might promote angiogenesis, restore blood supply, stimulate neuroprotective genes, and reverse the metabolic changes of the ischemic penumbral area.[14]

Ischemic strokes produce *cerebral edema,* an accumulation of fluids within the brain that begins within minutes of the insult and reaches a maximum by 3 to 4 days. It is the result of tissue necrosis and widespread rupture of cell membranes with movement of fluid from the blood into brain tissues. The swelling gradually subsides and generally disappears by 2 to 3 weeks. Significant edema can elevate intracranial pressures, leading to intracranial hypertension and neurological deterioration associated with contralateral and caudal shifts of brain structures *(brain stem herniation).* Clinical signs of *elevating intracranial pressure (ICP)* include decreasing level of consciousness (stupor and coma), widened pulse pressure, increased heart rate, irregular respirations *(Cheyne-Stokes respirations),* vomiting, unreactive pupils (cranial nerve [CN] III signs), and papilledema. Cerebral edema is the most frequent cause of death in acute stroke and is characteristic of large infarcts involving the middle cerebral artery and the internal carotid artery.

Management Categories

Transient ischemic attack (TIA) refers to the temporary interruption of blood supply to the brain. Symptoms of focal neurological deficit may last for only a few minutes or for several hours but by definition do not last longer than 24 hr. After the attack, there may be evidence of residual brain damage or permanent neurological dysfunction. It is therefore recommended that they be considered like acute strokes.[1] TIAs may result from a number of different etiologic factors, including occlusive episodes, emboli, reduced cerebral perfusion (arrhythmias, decreased cardiac output, hypotension, overmedication with antihypertensive medications, subclavian steal syndrome), or cerebrovascular spasm. The major clinical significance of TIA is as a precursor to susceptibility for both cerebral infarction and

myocardial infarction. The risk for recurrent stroke is 3.5%, 8%, and 9.2% at 2, 30, and 90 days post-TIA, respectively.[15]

Patients are classified as having a *major stroke* in the presence of stable, usually severe, impairments. The term *deteriorating stroke* refers to the patient whose neurological status deteriorates after admission to the hospital. This change in status may be due to cerebral or systemic causes (e.g., cerebral edema, progressing thrombosis). The category of *young stroke* describes a stroke affecting persons younger than age 45 years. Causes of stroke in children include perinatal arterial ischemic stroke, sickle cell disease, congenital HD, thrombophlebitis, and trauma.[3]

Vascular Syndromes

CBF varies with the patency of the vessels. Progressive narrowing secondary to atherosclerosis decreases blood flow. As in coronary HD, symptomatic changes generally result from a restriction of flow greater than 80%. The severity and symptoms of stroke are dependent on a number of factors, including (1) the location of the ischemic process, (2) the size of the ischemic area, (3) the nature and functions of the structures involved, and (4) the availability of collateral blood flow. Presenting symptoms may also depend on the rapidity of the occlusion of a blood vessel because slow occlusions may allow collateral vessels to take over, whereas sudden events do not.

CBF is controlled by numerous *autoregulatory mechanisms* (cerebral) that modulate a constant rate of blood flow through the brain. These mechanisms provide homeostatic balance, counteracting fluctuations in systolic BP (SBP) while maintaining a normal flow of 50 to 60 mL per 100 g of brain tissue per minute. The brain has high energy requirements and very little metabolic reserves. Thus, it requires a continuous, rich perfusion of blood to deliver oxygen and glucose to the tissues. Cerebral flow represents approximately 17% of available cardiac output. Chemical regulation of CBF occurs in response to changes in blood concentrations of carbon dioxide or oxygen. Vasodilation and increased CBF are produced in response to an increase in $PaCO_2$ or a decrease in PaO_2, whereas vasoconstriction and decreased CBF are produced by the opposite stimuli. Blood flow is also altered by changes in the blood pH. A fall in pH (increased acidity) produces vasodilation, and a rise in pH (increased alkalinity) produces a decrease in blood flow. Neurogenic regulation alters blood flow by vasodilating vessels in direct proportion to local function of brain tissue. Released metabolites probably act directly on the smooth muscle in local vessel walls. Changes in blood viscosity or ICP may also influence CBF. Changes in BP produce minor alterations of CBF. As pressure rises, the artery is stretched, resulting in contraction of smooth muscle in the vessel wall. Thus, the patency of the vessel is decreased, with a consequent decrease in CBF. As pressure falls, contraction lessens and CBF increases. Following stroke, autoregulatory mechanisms may be impaired.[16]

Knowledge of cerebral vascular anatomy is essential to understand the symptoms, diagnosis, and management of stroke. Extracranial blood supply to the brain is provided by the right and left internal carotid arteries and by the right and left vertebral arteries. The *internal carotid artery* begins at the bifurcation of the common carotid artery and ascends in the deep portions of the neck to the carotid canal. It turns rostromedially and ascends into the cranial cavity. It then pierces the dura mater and gives off the ophthalmic and anterior choroidal arteries before bifurcating into the middle and anterior cerebral arteries. The anterior communicating artery communicates with the anterior cerebral arteries of either side, giving rise to the rostral portion of the circle of Willis (Fig. 15.1). The *vertebral artery* arises as a branch off the subclavian artery. It enters the vertebral foramen of the sixth cervical vertebra and travels through the foramina of the transverse processes of the upper six cervical vertebrae to the foramen magnum and into the brain. There it travels in the posterior cranial fossa ventrally and medially and unites with the vertebral artery from the other side to form the basilar artery at the upper border of the medulla. At the upper border of the pons, the basilar artery bifurcates to form the posterior cerebral arteries and the posterior portion of the circle of Willis. Posterior communicating arteries connect the posterior cerebral arteries with the internal carotid arteries and complete the circle of Willis.

Anterior Cerebral Artery Syndrome

The *anterior cerebral artery (ACA)* is the first and smaller of two terminal branches of the internal carotid artery.

It supplies the medial aspect of the cerebral hemisphere (frontal and parietal lobes) and subcortical structures, including the basal ganglia (anterior internal capsule, inferior caudate nucleus), anterior fornix, and anterior four-fifths of the corpus callosum (Fig. 15.2). Because the anterior communicating artery allows perfusion of the proximal ACA from either side, occlusion proximal to this point results in minimal deficit.

More distal lesions produce more significant deficits. Table 15.2 presents the clinical manifestations of *ACA syndrome*. The most common characteristics of ACA syndrome include contralateral hemiparesis and sensory loss with greater involvement of the lower extremity (LE) than the upper extremity (UE) because the somatotopic organization of the medial aspect of the cortex includes the functional area for the LE.

Middle Cerebral Artery Syndrome

The *middle cerebral artery (MCA)* is the second of the two main branches of the internal carotid artery and supplies the entire lateral aspect of the cerebral hemisphere (frontal, temporal, and parietal lobes) and subcortical structures, including the internal capsule (posterior portion), corona radiata, globus pallidus (outer part), most of the caudate nucleus, and the putamen (Fig. 15.3). Occlusion of the proximal MCA produces extensive neurological damage with significant cerebral edema. Increased ICP typically leads to loss of consciousness, brain herniation, and possibly death. Table 15.3 presents the clinical manifestations of *MCA syndrome*. The most common characteristics of MCA syndrome are contralateral spastic hemiparesis and sensory loss of the face, UE, and LE, with the face and UE more involved than the LE. Lesions

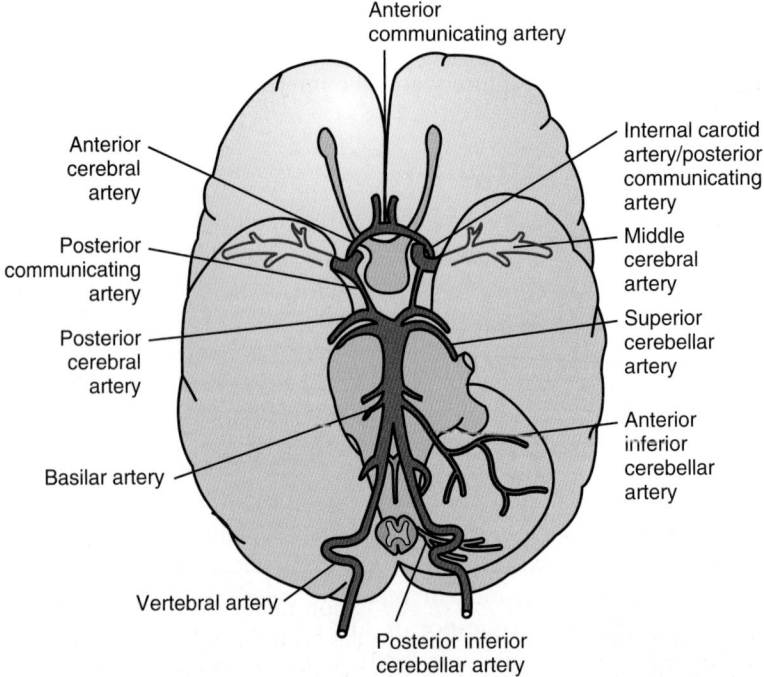

Figure 15.1 Cerebral circulation: circle of Willis.

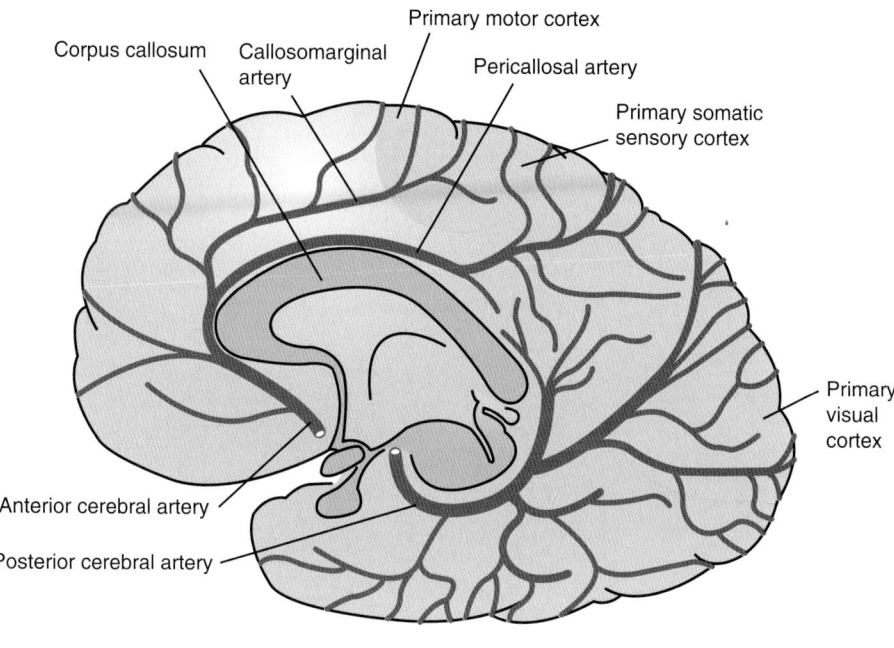

Figure 15.2 Cerebral circulation: A midsagittal view of the brain illustrates the distribution of the anterior and posterior cerebral arteries.

Table 15.2 Clinical Manifestations of Anterior Cerebral Artery Syndrome	
Signs and Symptoms	Structures Involved
Contralateral hemiparesis involving mainly the LE (UE is more spared)	Primary motor area, medial aspect of cortex, internal capsule
Contralateral hemisensory loss involving mainly the LE (UE is more spared)	Primary sensory area, medial aspect of cortex
Urinary incontinence	Posteromedial aspect of superior frontal gyrus
Problems with imitation and bimanual tasks, apraxia	Corpus callosum
Abulia (akinetic mutism), slowness, delay, lack of spontaneity, motor inaction	Uncertain localization
Contralateral grasp reflex, sucking reflex (Can be asymptomatic if circle of Willis is competent)	Uncertain localization

LE = lower extremity; UE = upper extremity.

of the parieto-occipital cortex of the dominant hemisphere (usually the left hemisphere) typically produce aphasia. Lesions of the right parietal lobe of the nondominant hemisphere (usually the right hemisphere) typically produce perceptual deficits (e.g., *unilateral neglect, anosognosia, apraxia,* and *spatial disorganization*). *Homonymous hemianopsia* (a visual field defect) is also a common finding. The MCA is the most common site of occlusion in stroke.

Internal Carotid Artery Syndrome

Occlusion of the *internal carotid artery (ICA)* typically produces massive infarction in the region of the brain supplied by the MCA. The ICA supplies both the MCA and the ACA. If collateral circulation to the ACA from

the circle of Willis is absent, extensive cerebral infarction in the areas of both the ACA and MCA can occur. Significant edema is common with possible uncal herniation, coma, and death (mass effect).

Posterior Cerebral Artery Syndrome

The two posterior cerebral arteries (PCAs) arise as terminal branches of the basilar artery, and each supplies the corresponding occipital lobe and medial and inferior temporal lobe (see Fig. 15.2). They also supply the upper brain stem, midbrain, and posterior diencephalon, including most of the thalamus. Table 15.4 presents the clinical manifestations of *PCA syndrome.* Occlusion proximal to the posterior communicating artery typically results in minimal deficits owing to

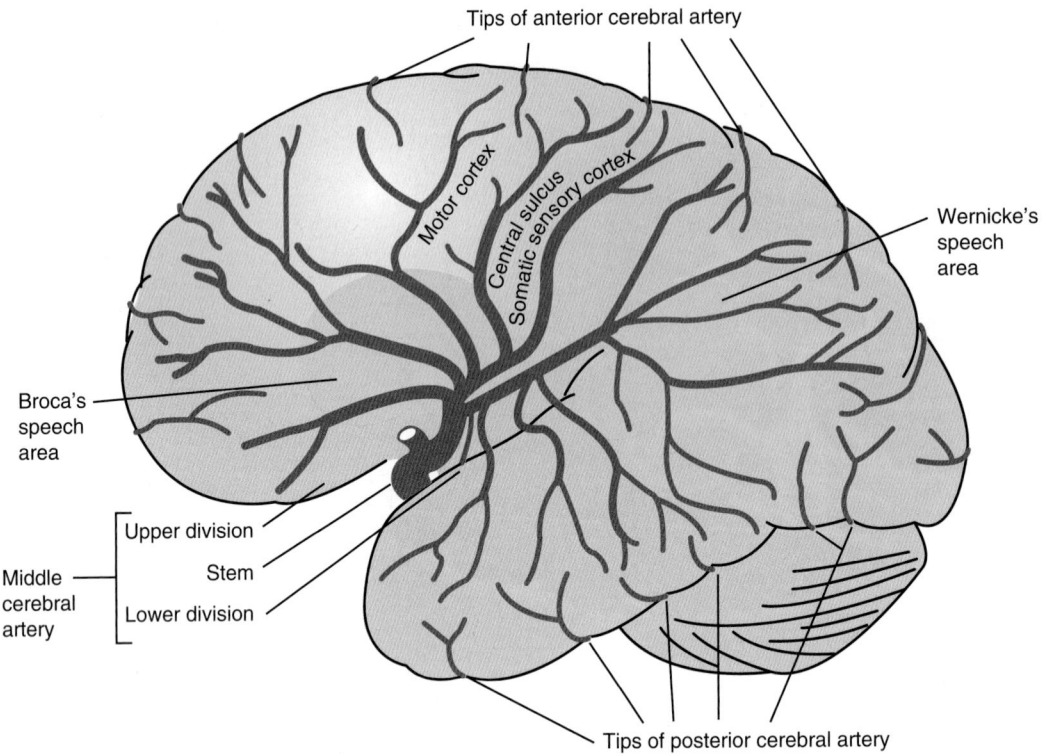

Figure 15.3 Cerebral circulation: A lateral view of the brain illustrates the distribution of the middle cerebral artery.

Table 15.3 Clinical Manifestations of Middle Cerebral Artery Syndrome	
Signs and Symptoms	Structures Involved
Contralateral hemiparesis involving mainly the UE and face (LE is more spared)	Primary motor cortex and internal capsule
Contralateral hemisensory loss involving mainly the UE and face (LE is more spared)	Primary sensory cortex and internal capsule
Motor speech impairment: Broca or nonfluent aphasia with limited vocabulary and slow, hesitant speech	Broca cortical area (third frontal convolution) in the dominant hemisphere, typically the left hemisphere
Receptive speech impairment: Wernicke or fluent aphasia with impaired auditory comprehension and fluent speech with normal rate and melody	Wernicke cortical area (posterior portion of the temporal gyrus) in the dominant hemisphere, typically the left
Global aphasia: nonfluent speech with poor comprehension	Both third frontal convolution and posterior portion of the superior temporal gyrus
Perceptual deficits: unilateral neglect, depth perception, spatial relations, agnosia	Parietal sensory association cortex in the nondominant hemisphere, typically the right
Limb-kinetic apraxia	Premotor or parietal cortex
Contralateral homonymous hemianopsia	Optic radiation in internal capsule
Loss of conjugate gaze to the opposite side	Frontal eye fields or their descending tracts
Ataxia of contralateral limb(s) (sensory ataxia)	Parietal lobe
Pure motor hemiplegia (lacunar stroke)	Upper portion of posterior limb of internal capsule

LE = lower extremity; UE = upper extremity.

Table 15.4 Clinical Manifestations of Posterior Cerebral Artery Syndrome

Signs and Symptoms	Structures Involved
Peripheral Territory	
Contralateral homonymous hemianopsia	Primary visual cortex or optic radiation
Bilateral homonymous hemianopsia with some degree of macular sparing	Calcarine cortex (macular sparing is due to occipital pole receiving collateral blood supply from MCA)
Visual agnosia	Left occipital lobe
Prosopagnosia (difficulty naming people on sight)	Visual association cortex
Dyslexia (difficulty reading) without agraphia (difficulty writing), color naming (anomia), and color discrimination problems	Dominant calcarine lesion and posterior part of corpus callosum
Memory defect	Lesion of inferomedial portions of temporal lobe bilaterally or on the dominant side only
Topographic disorientation	Nondominant primary visual area, usually bilaterally
Central Territory	
Central poststroke (thalamic) pain Spontaneous pain and dysesthesias; sensory impairments (all modalities)	Ventral posterolateral nucleus of thalamus
Involuntary movements; choreoathetosis, intention tremor, hemiballismus	Subthalamic nucleus or its pallidal connections
Contralateral hemiplegia	Cerebral peduncle of midbrain
Weber syndrome Oculomotor nerve palsy and contralateral hemiplegia	Third nerve and cerebral peduncle of midbrain
Paresis of vertical eye movements, slight miosis and ptosis, and sluggish pupillary light response	Supranuclear fibers to third cranial nerve

LE = lower extremity; MCA = middle cerebral artery; UE = upper extremity.

the collateral blood supply from the PCA (similar to ACA syndrome). Occlusion of thalamic branches may produce hemianesthesia (contralateral sensory loss) or *central poststroke (thalamic) pain*. Occipital infarction produces homonymous hemianopsia, *visual agnosia, prosopagnosia,* or, if bilateral, cortical blindness. Temporal lobe ischemia results in amnesia (memory loss). Involvement of subthalamic branches may include the subthalamic nucleus or its pallidal connections, producing a wide variety of deficits. Contralateral hemiplegia occurs with involvement of the cerebral peduncle.

Lacunar Stroke

Lacunar strokes are caused by small vessel disease deep in the cerebral white matter (penetrating artery disease). They are strongly associated with hypertensive hemorrhage and diabetic microvascular disease. Lacunar syndromes are consistent with specific anatomical sites. *Pure motor lacunar stroke* is associated with involvement of the posterior limb of the internal capsule, pons, and pyramids. *Pure sensory lacunar stroke* is associated with

involvement of the ventrolateral thalamus or thalamo-cortical projections. Other lacunar syndromes include *dysarthria/clumsy hand syndrome* (involving the base of the pons, genu of anterior limb, or the internal capsule), *ataxic hemiparesis* (involving the pons, genu of internal capsule, corona radiata, or cerebellum), *sensory/motor stroke* (involving the junction of the internal capsule and thalamus), and *dystonia/involuntary movements* (choreoathetosis with lacunar infarction of the putamen or globus pallidus; hemiballismus with involvement of the subthalamic nucleus). Deficits in consciousness, language, or visual fields are not seen in lacunar strokes because the higher cortical areas are preserved. A hypertensive hemorrhage affecting the thalamus can also produce central poststroke pain.[16]

Vertebrobasilar Artery Syndrome

The *vertebral arteries* arise from the subclavian arteries and travel into the brain along the medulla where they merge at the inferior border of the pons to form the basilar artery. The vertebral arteries supply the cerebellum (via posterior inferior cerebellar arteries) and the medulla (via the medullary arteries). The basilar artery supplies the pons (via pontine arteries), the internal ear (via labyrinthine arteries), and the cerebellum (via the anterior inferior and superior cerebellar arteries). The basilar artery then terminates at the upper border of the pons, giving rise to the two posterior arteries (see Fig. 15.1). Occlusions of the vertebrobasilar system can produce a wide variety of symptoms with both ipsilateral and contralateral signs because some of the tracts in the brain stem will have crossed and others will not. Numerous cerebellar and cranial nerve abnormalities also are present. Table 15.5 presents the clinical manifestations of *vertebrobasilar artery syndromes.*

Locked-in syndrome (LIS) occurs with basilar artery thrombosis and bilateral infarction of the ventral pons. LIS is a catastrophic event with sudden onset. Patients develop acute hemiparesis rapidly progressing to tetraplegia and lower bulbar paralysis (CNs V through XII are involved). Initially the patient is dysarthric and dysphonic but rapidly progresses to mutism (anarthria). There is preserved consciousness and sensation. Thus, the patient cannot move or speak but remains alert and oriented. Horizontal eye movements are impaired, but vertical eye movements and blinking remain intact. Communication can be established via these eye movements. Mortality rates are high (59%), and those patients who survive are left with severe impairments associated with brain stem injury.[16]

Extracranial injuries to the vertebral arteries as they travel through the cervical spine can also produce vertebrobasilar signs and symptoms. Forceful neck motions (e.g., whiplash or aggressive neck manipulations) are among the more common types of injuries.

■ NEUROLOGICAL SEQUELAE AND ASSOCIATED CONDITIONS

Altered Consciousness

An altered level of consciousness (coma, decreased arousal levels) may occur with extensive brain damage (e.g., large proximal MCA occlusion). The *Glasgow Coma Scale* developed by Teasdale and Jennett[17] is used to document the level of coma (see Chapter 19, Traumatic Brain Injury). Three areas of function are examined: eye opening, best motor response, and verbal responses. The therapist may document levels of consciousness using standard descriptive terms: *normal, lethargy, obtundation, stupor,* and *coma* (see Chapter 5, Examination of Motor Function: Motor Control and Motor Learning). Since the patient's behaviors can be expected to fluctuate, frequent repeat observations are necessary.

Speech and Language Deficits

Patients with lesions involving the cortex of the dominant hemisphere (typically the left hemisphere)

demonstrate speech and language impairments. *Aphasia* is the general term used to describe an acquired communication disorder caused by brain damage and is characterized by an impairment of language comprehension, formulation, and use. Aphasia has been estimated to occur in 30% to 36% of all patients with stroke.[4] There are many different types of aphasias; major classification categories are fluent, nonfluent, and global. In *fluent aphasia (Wernicke/sensory/receptive aphasia),* speech flows smoothly with a variety of grammatical constructions and preserved melody of speech. Auditory comprehension is impaired. Thus, the patient demonstrates difficulty in comprehending spoken language and in following commands. The lesion is located in the auditory association cortex in the left lateral temporal lobe. In *nonfluent aphasia (Broca/expressive aphasia),* the flow of speech is slow and hesitant, vocabulary is limited, and syntax is impaired. Speech production is labored or lost completely, whereas comprehension is good. The lesion is located in the premotor area of the left frontal lobe. *Global aphasia* is a severe aphasia characterized by marked impairments of both production and comprehension of language. It is often an indication of extensive brain damage. Severe problems in communication may limit the patient's ability to learn and often impede successful outcomes in rehabilitation. See Chapter 28, Neurogenic Disorders of Speech and Language, for a complete discussion of these impairments and their management.

Patients with stroke commonly present with *dysarthria* with a reported incidence ranging from 48% to 57%.[4] This term refers to a category of motor speech disorders caused by lesions in parts of the central or peripheral nervous system that mediate speech production. Respiration, articulation, phonation, resonance, and/or sensory feedback may be affected. The lesion can be located in the primary motor cortex, the primary sensory cortex, or the cerebellum. Volitional and automatic actions such as chewing and swallowing and movement of the jaw and tongue are impaired, resulting in slurred speech. In patients with stroke, dysarthria can accompany aphasia, complicating the course of rehabilitation (see Chapter 28, Neurogenic Disorders of Speech and Language).

It is important to establish a reliable mode of communication before proceeding with the examination. Close collaboration with the speech-language pathologist will aid in making an accurate determination of the patient's communication abilities. It is important to distinguish between a motor disorder (dysarthria) and a language disorder (aphasia). Preservation of receptive language functions (auditory comprehension, reading comprehension) and expressive language function (word-finding, fluency, writing) abilities will guide the communication strategy. Gestures, demonstration, communication boards, and simple language are strategies to enhance communication.

Table 15.5 Clinical Manifestations of Vertebrobasilar Artery Syndrome

Signs and Symptoms	Structures Involved
Medial medullary syndrome	Occlusion vertebral artery, medullary branch
Ipsilateral to lesion Paralysis with atrophy of half the tongue with deviation to the paralyzed side when tongue is protruded	CN XII, hypoglossal, or nucleus
Contralateral to lesion Paralysis of UE and LE	Corticospinal tract
Impaired tactile and proprioceptive sense	Medial lemniscus
Lateral medullary (Wallenburg) syndrome	Occlusion of posterior inferior cerebellar artery or vertebral artery
Ipsilateral to lesion Decreased pain and temperature sensation in face	Descending tract and nucleus of CN V, trigeminal
Cerebellum or inferior cerebellar peduncle	Cerebellar ataxia: gait and limbs ataxia
Vertigo, nausea, vomiting	Vestibular nuclei and connections
Nystagmus	Vestibular nuclei and connections
Horner syndrome: miosis, ptosis, decreased sweating	Descending sympathetic tract
Dysphagia and dysphonia: paralysis of palatal and laryngeal muscles, diminished gag reflex	CN IX, glossopharyngeal, and CN X, vagus, or nuclei
Sensory impairment of ipsilateral UE, trunk, or LE	Cuneate and gracile nuclei
Contralateral to lesion Impaired pain and thermal sense over 50% of body, sometimes face	Spinal lemniscus—spinothalamic tract
Complete basilar artery syndrome (locked-in syndrome)	Basilar artery, ventral pons
Tetraplegia (quadriplegia)	Corticospinal tracts bilaterally
Bilateral cranial nerve palsy: upward gaze is spared	Long tracts to cranial nerve nuclei bilaterally
Coma	Reticular activating system
Cognition is spared	
Medial inferior pontine syndrome	Occlusion of paramedian branch of basilar artery
Ipsilateral to lesion Paralysis of conjugate gaze to side of lesion (preservation of convergence)	Pontine center for lateral gaze (PPRF)
Nystagmus	Vestibular nuclei and connections
Ataxia of limbs and gait	Middle cerebellar peduncle
Diplopia on lateral gaze	CN VI, abducens, or nucleus
Contralateral to lesion Paresis of face, UE, and LE	Corticobulbar and corticospinal tract in lower pons
Impaired tactile and proprioceptive sense over 50% of the body	Medial lemniscus
Lateral inferior pontine syndrome	Occlusion of anterior inferior cerebellar artery, a branch of the basilar artery
Ipsilateral to lesion Horizontal and vertical nystagmus, vertigo, nausea, vomiting	CN VIII, vestibular, or nucleus

(Continued)

Table 15.5 Clinical Manifestations of Vertebrobasilar Artery Syndrome—cont'd

Signs and Symptoms	Structures Involved
Facial paralysis	CN VII, facial, or nucleus
Paralysis of conjugate gaze to side of lesion	Pontine center for lateral gaze (PPRF)
Deafness, tinnitus	CN VIII, cochlear, or nucleus
Ataxia	Middle cerebellar peduncle and cerebellar hemisphere
Impaired sensation over face	Main sensory nucleus and descending tract of fifth nerve
Contralateral to lesion Impaired pain and thermal sense over half the body (may include face)	Spinothalamic tract
Medial midpontine syndrome	Occlusion of paramedian branch of the mid-basilar artery
Ipsilateral to lesion Ataxia of limbs and gait (more prominent in bilateral involvement)	Middle cerebellar peduncle
Contralateral to lesion Paralysis of face, UE, and LE	Corticobulbar and corticospinal tract
Deviation of eyes	Abducent nerve nucleus, medial longitudinal fasciculus
Lateral midpontine syndrome	Occlusion of short circumferential artery
Ipsilateral to lesion Ataxia of limbs	Middle cerebellar peduncle
Paralysis of muscles of mastication	Motor fibers or nucleus of CN V, trigeminal
Impaired sensation over side of face	Sensory fibers or nucleus of CN V, trigeminal
Medial superior pontine syndrome	Occlusion of paramedian branches of upper basilar artery
Cerebellar ataxia	Superior or middle cerebellar peduncle
Internuclear ophthalmoplegia	Medial longitudinal fasciculus
Contralateral to lesion Paralysis of face, UE, and LE	Corticobulbar and corticospinal tract
Lateral superior pontine syndrome	Occlusion of superior cerebellar artery, a branch of the basilar artery
Ipsilateral to lesion Cerebellar ataxia of limbs and gait, falling to side of lesion	Middle and superior cerebellar peduncles, superior surface of cerebellum, dentate nucleus
Dizziness, nausea, vomiting	Vestibular nuclei
Horizontal nystagmus	Vestibular nuclei
Paresis of conjugate gaze (ipsilateral)	Uncertain
Loss of optokinetic nystagmus	Uncertain
Horner syndrome: miosis, ptosis, decreased sweating on opposite side face	Descending sympathetic fibers
Contralateral to lesion Impaired pain and thermal sense of face, limbs, and trunk	Spinothalamic tract
Impaired touch, vibration, and position sense, more in LE than UE (tendency to incongruity of pain and touch deficits)	Medial lemniscus (lateral portion)

CN = cranial nerve; LE = lower extremity; PPRF = paramedian pontine reticular formation; UE = upper extremity.

Dysphagia

Dysphagia, an inability to swallow or difficulty in swallowing, occurs in about 51% of patients with stroke. It can be seen in hemispheric stroke, brain stem stroke, or pseudobulbar and suprabulbar palsy. In brain stem stroke, the reported incidence is as high as 81%. Cranial nerve involvement results in swallowing dysfunction of the oral stage (CN V [trigeminal], CN VII [facial]), the pharyngeal stage (CN IX [glossopharyngeal], CN X [vagus], and CN XI [accessory]), or the oral and pharyngeal stages (CN XII [hypoglossal]). Dysphagia is also common in patients with multiple strokes. The most common problems seen in patients with dysphagia include delayed triggering of the swallowing reflex, reduced pharyngeal peristalsis, and reduced lingual control. Altered mental status, altered sensation, poor jaw and lip closure, impaired head control, and poor sitting posture also contribute to the patient's swallowing difficulties. Most patients demonstrate multiple problems that can include drooling, difficulty ingesting food, compromised nutritional status, and dehydration. *Aspiration,* the penetration of food, liquid, saliva, or gastric reflux into the airway, occurs in about one-third of patients with dysphagia. Aspiration can lead to acute respiratory distress within hours, aspiration pneumonia, and, if left untreated, death.[18,19]

A referral to a dysphagia specialist or multidisciplinary dysphagia team is indicated. Team members typically include the physician, nurse, occupational therapist, speech-language pathologist, and dietitian. Clinical evaluation of dysphagia includes an examination of oral-motor function, pharyngeal function, functional status (e.g., upright sitting position, use of adaptive feeding equipment), and abnormal reflexes, and a feeding trial. Instrumental testing can include a *modified barium swallow, videofluoroscopic evaluation of swallowing,* and *fiberoptic endoscopic evaluation of swallowing.*[20] If dysphagia is severe enough, patients may be placed on nothing-by-mouth (NPO) precautions. The use of tube feeding, either a nasogastric (NG) tube for short periods of time or an invasive gastrostomy (G) tube for more long-term care, is required. Nutrition can also be provided through an intravenous route (total parenteral nutrition [TPN]).

Cognitive Deficits

Cognitive deficits may include impairments in alertness, attention, orientation, memory, or executive functions. Premorbid changes associated with aging may also account for some of the limitations noted and may be determined from interviews with family, significant others, or caregivers. Difficulty with *alertness* results from lesions in the prefrontal cortex and reticular formation with the person appearing lethargic. *Disorientation* presents as the person being unable to provide information about self, time of day, physical or geographical

location, or disability and is the result of lesions affecting the prefrontal cortex, limbic system, and limbic cortex. *Attention* is the ability to select and attend to a specific stimulus while simultaneously suppressing extraneous stimuli. Attention disorders include impairments in sustained attention, selective attention, divided attention, or alternating attention. Altered attention results from lesions in the prefrontal cortex and reticular formation. *Memory* is defined as the ability to store experiences and perceptions for later recall. Immediate and short-term memory impairments are common, occurring in about 36% of patients with stroke, whereas long-term memory typically remains intact.[3] Thus, the person cannot remember the instructions for a new task given only minutes or hours ago but can easily remember events from 30 years ago. Short-term memory loss is associated with lesions of the limbic system, limbic association cortex (orbitofrontal areas), or temporal lobes. Long-term memory loss is associated with lesions of the hippocampus of the limbic system. Memory gaps may be filled with inappropriate words or fabricated stories, an impairment termed *confabulation* that also results from lesions in the prefrontal cortex. The patient may be confused, demonstrating disorientation and an inability to understand the specific context of a conversation. *Confusion* is the result of disruption of the prefrontal cortex. *Perseveration* is the continued repetition of words, thoughts, or acts not related to current context. Thus, the patient gets "stuck" and repeats words or acts without much success at stopping. Preservation results from lesions in the premotor and/or prefrontal cortex.

Executive functions, defined as those abilities that enable a person to engage in purposeful behaviors, include volition, planning, purposeful action, and effective performance. Patients with lesions of the prefrontal cortex typically demonstrate impairments in executive function including some or all of the following: impulsiveness, inflexible thinking, lack of abstract thinking, impaired organization and sequencing, decreased insight, impaired planning ability, and impaired judgment. Patients are unable to realistically appraise their environment and the people and events in it. They also demonstrate difficulty in self-monitoring and self-correcting behaviors, thereby posing safety risks.[21,22] (See Chapter 27, Cognitive and Perceptual Dysfunction, for a complete discussion of these impairments and their management.)

Multi-infarct dementia (vascular dementia) results from multiple small infarcts of the brain and is seen in 6% to 32% of patients. It is more common in individuals over age 60 and is associated with episodes of cerebral ischemia (microvascular or small vessel disease) and hypertension. Other contributing factors include arrhythmias, myocardial infarct, TIAs, diabetes, obesity, and smoking. Scattered areas of the brain are involved, evidenced by focal neurological deficits. Onset is frequently abrupt. The person exhibits impairments in memory and cognition and may fluctuate between periods of impaired function and periods of improved function. This stepwise and paroxysmal deterioration of intellectual function is in contrast to the gradual onset and steadier, widespread decline seen in Alzheimer dementia.[21]

Delirium, also known as *acute confusional state*, is seen more commonly in the acute care setting and results from a number of factors following acute stroke. Deprivation of oxygen to the brain, metabolic imbalance, or adverse drug reactions can all induce confusion. Additional contributory factors can include sensory and perceptual losses coupled with an unfamiliar hospital environment and inactivity. Delirium is characterized by a clouding of consciousness or dulling of cognitive processes and impaired alertness. Thus, the patient is inattentive, incoherent, and disorganized with fluctuating levels of consciousness. Hallucinations and agitation are also common. Nighttime may be particularly problematic. Patients with significant sensory loss following stroke may experience sensory deprivation problems evidenced by irritability, confusion, psychosis, delusions, and even hallucinations. These problems are more frequently seen in the acute phase, especially with patients who have been confined to a bed or whose bed is positioned to limit social interaction (e.g., with the more involved side toward the door). Some patients are equally unable to deal with a sensory overload, produced by too much stimulation. Altered arousal levels are implicated.

It is important to examine cognitive abilities early because they may affect the validity of other tests and measures. An examination of orientation (to person, place, time, and circumstance [e.g., awareness of event causing need for medical care]), attention (selective, sustained, alternating, divided), memory (immediate, short and long term), and ability to follow instructions (one-, two-, and three-level commands) can be made from observations of the patient's interactions and responses to specific questions. Higher cortical functions can be examined using tests of simple arithmetic and abstract reasoning (grasp of information, abstract thinking and problem-solving, calculating ability, constructional ability). The *Mini-Mental State Examination* provides a valid and reliable quick screen of cognitive function.[23] A determination of learning impairments (retention and generalization) usually requires repeat sessions with the patient before a complete picture can be ascertained. Difficulties arise in reaching an accurate determination of cognition when the person presents with impairments in communication or perception. Close collaboration with the occupational therapist, speech-language pathologist, and the rest of the team is essential.

Affective Status

Lesions of the brain affecting the frontal lobe, hypothalamus, and limbic system can produce several emotional changes. The patient with stroke may demonstrate *pseudobulbar affect* (PBA), also known as *emotional lability* or *emotional dysregulation syndrome*. PBA occurs in about 18% of cases and is characterized by emotional outbursts of uncontrolled or exaggerated laughing or crying that are inconsistent with mood. The patient quickly changes from laughing to crying with only slight provocation. The patient is typically unable to control these episodes or to inhibit the expression of spontaneous emotions. Frequent crying may also accompany depression. *Apathy* occurs in about 22% of cases and is characterized by a shallow affect and blunted emotional responses. In such patients, apathy is frequently misconstrued as depression or poor motivation. Patients can also demonstrate *euphoria* (exaggerated feelings of well-being), increased levels of irritability or frustration, and social inappropriateness. Changes in the ability to sense, move, communicate, think, or act as before are enormously frustrating by themselves and create high stress levels for the patient with stroke. Increased levels of anxiety, irritability, and frustration are the natural outcomes of high stress levels. These behaviors along with a poor perception of one's self and environment may lead to increasing isolation and social withdrawal.[22]

Depression occurs in approximately 31% of persons poststroke. It decreases to 25% and 23% at 1 and 5 years poststroke, respectively.[24] It is characterized by persistent feelings of sadness accompanied by feelings of hopelessness, worthlessness, and/or helplessness. Patients with depression may also experience a loss of energy or persistent fatigue, an inability to concentrate, and decreased interest in daily life along with changes in weight and sleep patterns, generalized anxiety, and recurrent thoughts of death or suicide. Depression is seen with lesions in the left frontal lobe (acute stage) and with lesions in the right parietal lobes (subacute stage).[25] Most patients remain significantly depressed for many months, with an average time of 7 to 8 months.[26] Depression occurs in both mildly and severely involved patients and thus is not significantly related to the degree of motor impairment. Patients with lesions of the left hemisphere may experience more frequent and more severe depression than patients with right hemisphere or brain stem strokes. These findings suggest that poststroke depression is not simply a result of psychological reaction to disability but rather a direct impairment of the CVA.[27] Anxiety can coexist with depression during any phase of recovery.[25] Prolonged poststroke depression can interfere with the success of rehabilitation and result in poorer long-term functional outcomes. Refer to Chapter 26, Psychosocial Issues in Physical Rehabilitation, for a more complete discussion of psychosocial impairments and their management.

Hemispheric Behavioral Differences

Individuals with stroke differ widely in their approach to processing information and in their behaviors.

Those with *left hemisphere lesions* (right hemiplegia) demonstrate difficulties in communication and in processing information in a sequential, linear manner. They are frequently described as cautious, anxious, and disorganized. This makes them more hesitant when trying new tasks and increases the need for feedback and support. They tend, however, to be realistic in their appraisal of their existing problems. Individuals with *right hemisphere lesions* (left hemiplegia), on the other hand, demonstrate difficulty in spatial-perceptual tasks and in grasping the whole idea of a task or activity. They are frequently described as quick and impulsive. They tend to overestimate their abilities while acting unaware of their deficits. This lack of insight and concreteness impairs the patient's ability to participate in rehabilitation. Safety is a far greater issue for patients with left hemiplegia, where poor judgment is common. These patients also require a great deal of feedback when learning a new task. The feedback should be focused on slowing down the activity, checking sequential steps, and relating them to the whole task. Patients also need help recognizing the consequences and risks of their actions. The patient with left hemiplegia frequently cannot attend to visuospatial cues effectively, especially in a cluttered or crowded environment. Table 15.6 summarizes the behavioral differences attributed to damage of the left and right hemispheres.

Table 15.6 Hemispheric Differences Commonly Seen Following Stroke

Right Hemisphere Lesion	Left Hemisphere Lesion
Left-side hemiplegia/paresis	Right-side hemiplegia/paresis
Left-side sensory loss	Right-side sensory loss
Visual–perceptual impairments: Left-side unilateral neglect Agnosias Visuospatial disorders Disturbances of body image and body scheme Difficulty processing visual cues	*Speech and language impairments:* Dominant hemisphere: • Nonfluent (Broca) aphasia • Fluent (Wernicke) aphasia • Global aphasia Difficulty processing verbal cues, verbal commands
Behavioral deficits: Quick, impulsive behavioral style Poor judgment, unrealistic Inability to self-correct Poor insight, awareness of impairments, denial of disability Increased safety risk	*Behavioral deficits:* Slow, cautious behavioral style Disorganized Often very aware of impairments, extent of disability
Intellectual deficits: Difficulty with abstract reasoning, problem-solving Difficulty synthesizing information and grasping whole idea of task Rigidity of thought Memory impairments, typically related to spatial-perceptual information	*Intellectual deficits:* Disorganized problem-solving Difficulty initiating tasks, processing delays Highly distractible Memory impairments, typically related to language Perseveration
Emotional deficits: Difficulty with ability to perceive emotions	*Emotional deficits:* Difficulty with expression of positive emotions
Difficulty with expression of negative emotions	
Task performance: Fluctuations in performance	*Task performance:* Apraxia common: difficulty planning and sequencing movements • Ideational • Ideomotor
Deficits of either hemisphere depending on lesion location: Visual field defects: homonymous hemianopsia Emotional abnormalities: lability, apathy, irritability, low frustration levels, anxiety, depression Cognitive deficits: confusion, short attention span, loss of memory, executive functions	

Emotional states and behavioral styles can best be examined through observation of the patient in a variety of situations over a number of sessions. It is important to correlate findings with those reported by other team members and by the family regarding premorbid behaviors and emotional characteristics. Families who report a "personality change" after stroke are likely responding to presenting emotional impairments and disinhibition. Episodes of euphoria and crying should be carefully documented and links to situational or environmental circumstances explored. Duration and frequency of these episodes should also be documented along with strategies that are successful in bringing about an end to the episode (redirecting strategies). The patient's response to new or stressful situations should also be carefully observed for evidence of anxiety (e.g., excessive worrying, restlessness, irritability). The therapist should examine for evidence of depression. Depressed patients can also be irritable, angry, or hostile and wish to be left alone.[22] The *Beck Depression Inventory*[28] is a useful instrument for depression screening. It consists of 21 statements that are scored on a scale from 0 to 3 (the short version has 13 questions and takes 5 min to complete).

Perceptual Deficits

Stroke can produce visual–perceptual deficits, with a reported incidence ranging from 32% to 41%.[4] They are frequently the result of lesions in the right parietal cortex and are seen more with left hemiplegia than right. These may include disorders of *body scheme/body image, spatial relations,* and *agnosias.* Body scheme refers to a postural model of the body, including the relationship of the body parts to each other and the relationship of the body to the environment. Body image is the visual and mental image of one's body that includes feelings about one's body. Both may be distorted following stroke. Specific impairments of body scheme/body image include *unilateral neglect, anosognosia, somatagnosia, right–left discrimination,* and *finger agnosia.* Spatial relations syndrome refers to a constellation of impairments that have in common a difficulty in perceiving the relationship between the self and two or more objects in the environment. It includes specific impairments in *figure–ground discrimination, form discrimination, spatial relations, position in space,* and *topographical disorientation.* Agnosia is the inability to recognize incoming information despite intact sensory capacities. Agnosias can include visual object agnosia, auditory agnosia, or tactile agnosia (astereognosis). Significant information on sensory and perceptual deficits will be gained by close collaboration with the occupational therapist. Refer to Chapter 27, Cognitive and Perceptual Dysfunction, for a more complete discussion of these deficits and their management.

Because the patient with left hemiplegia may behave in ways that tend to minimize their disabilities, it is easy for staff to overestimate the patient's perceptual abilities. For the patient with visuospatial deficits, the use of gestures or visual cues may decrease this patient's ability to perform tasks, whereas verbal cues may increase chances for success. Equally important strategies include carefully structuring the environment to minimize clutter and activity, providing adequate lighting, and providing clear boundaries and reference points.

Problems in *unilateral neglect* (lack of awareness of part of the body or the external environment) will limit movement and use of the more involved extremities (usually the nondominant left side). The patient typically does not react to sensory stimuli (visual, auditory, or somatosensory) presented on the more involved side. Careful observation of spontaneous use of affected limbs as well as specific responses to inquiries for movement on or toward the hemiplegic side will provide important information about neglect. Persistent neglect may result in bruising or trauma to the hemiplegic limbs during activity and negatively affect rehabilitation outcomes.

Seizures

Seizures occur in a small percentage of patients with stroke and are slightly more common in occlusive carotid disease (17%) than in MCA disease (11%). Seizures are common right after stroke during the acute phase (e.g., in about 15% of cases with cerebral hemorrhage); late-onset seizures can also occur several months after stroke. They tend to be of the partial motor type. Seizures are potentially life threatening if not controlled. Anticonvulsant medications may be indicated (e.g., phenytoin [Dilantin], carbamazepine [Tegretol], phenobarbital [Solfoton]).[4]

Bladder and Bowel Dysfunction

Disturbances of bladder function are common during the acute phase, occurring in about 29% of cases.[4] Urinary incontinence can result from bladder hyperreflexia or hyporeflexia, disturbances of sphincter control, and/or sensory loss. A toileting schedule for prompted voiding is often implemented to reduce the incidence of incontinence and to accommodate for factors that cause functional incontinence, such as inattention, mental status changes, or immobility. Generally, this problem improves quickly. Persistent incontinence is often due to a treatable medical condition (e.g., urinary tract infection). Absorbent pads and special undergarments or external collection devices may be used if incontinence proves refractory. Urinary retention can be controlled pharmacologically and with intermittent or indwelling catheterization. Early treatment is desirable to prevent further complications such as chronic urinary tract infection and skin breakdown. Patients who are incontinent often suffer embarrassment, isolation, and depression. Persistent incontinence is associated with a poor long-term prognosis for functional recovery.

Disturbances of bowel function can include incontinence and diarrhea or constipation and impaction. Patients who are constipated may require stool softeners and dietary/fluid modifications and medications to resolve this problem. Physical activity is also helpful.

Cardiovascular and Pulmonary Dysfunction

The majority of strokes are caused by vascular disease. Persons who have had a stroke as a result of underlying coronary artery disease may demonstrate impaired cardiac output, cardiac decompensation, and serious rhythm disorders. If these problems persist, they can directly alter cerebral perfusion and produce additional focal signs (e.g., mental confusion). Patients with stroke typically exhibit low peak VO_2 levels during exercise (about half of that achieved by age-matched healthy individuals).[29] These vary according to age, level of disability, number and severity of comorbidities, secondary complications, and medications. Cardiac limitations in exercise tolerance may restrict rehabilitation potential and require diligent monitoring and careful exercise prescription by the physical therapist.

Many persons with stroke are deconditioned and exhibit low work capacities, the result of acute illness, bedrest, and limited activity levels. Some individuals may have been inactive before the stroke. Changes in the cardiovascular system associated with deconditioning include reduced cardiac output, decreased maximal heart rate, increased resting and exercise BPs, decreased maximal oxygen uptake, and decreased vital capacity. Changes in the musculoskeletal system (e.g., decreased muscle mass and strength, decreased bone mass, decreased flexibility) and decreased glucose tolerance also affect exercise tolerance and endurance levels. Decreased activity levels may also be related to depression, a common finding in stroke.

Pulmonary function is often impaired in individuals with stroke. Decreased lung volume, decreased pulmonary perfusion and vital capacity, and altered chest wall excursion are all common findings. The decreased respiratory output is accompanied by increased oxygen demands required during activity using altered and unfamiliar movement patterns. For example, walking using an orthosis and assistive device dramatically increases the energy demands of the activity. The end result for the patient with stroke is increased fatigue and decreased endurance.

Deep Vein Thrombosis and Pulmonary Embolus

Deep vein thrombosis (DVT) and *pulmonary embolus* (PE) are potential complications for all immobilized patients. The incidence of DVT in patients with stroke is as high as 47% with an estimated 10% of deaths attributed to PE.[4] The dangers are particularly high during the acute phase when venous stasis from immobility

and prolonged bedrest, limb paralysis, hemineglect, and reduced cognitive status significantly elevate the risk. About 50% of cases do not present with clinically detectable symptoms and can be identified only by Doppler duplex ultrasonography (the gold standard for rapid screening), radiocontrast venography, or impedance plethysmography. Patients with symptoms may report calf pain and tenderness, or a tight feeling in the calf. Swelling can vary from minimal to high and typically affects the foot and ankle. Prompt diagnosis and treatment of acute DVT are necessary to reduce the risk of fatal PE. About half of patients at time of diagnosis of DVT have already had a PE. Signs and symptoms of PE include chest pain, tachypnea, tachycardia, anxiety, restlessness, and apprehension together with persistent cough. About 10% to 15% of patients with PE will die. Symptomatic treatment of DVT consists of continuous infusion or subcutaneous injections of low molecular weight heparin followed by long-term oral anticoagulants (warfarin [Coumadin]). Bedrest is instituted (up to 24 hr) until anticoagulation from medications takes effect. The patient is then mobilized out of bed and will wear compression stockings. In select cases, surgical removal of the thrombus or placement of intracaval filters is undertaken. Treatment of PE involves supplemental oxygen or intubation in severe cases, anticoagulants, and thrombolytic drugs and, in some cases, surgical intervention. Primary prevention of DVT and PE involves prophylactic administration of anticoagulants, exercising the legs to improve blood flow, early mobilization, and use of elastic support stockings.[30]

Osteoporosis and Fracture Risk

Osteoporosis, a bone disease characterized by a loss of bone mass per unit volume, is common in older adults and results from decreased physical activity, changes in protein nutrition, hormonal deficiency, and calcium deficiency. Patients with stroke who are immobilized and restricted in weight-bearing demonstrate increased risk of osteoporosis and disuse muscle atrophy. Fall risk is also increased with incidence rates ranging between 23% and 50% for individuals with chronic stroke.[31–33] Risk of falls in patients with stroke is multifactorial, arising from sensorimotor deficits, impaired balance, confusion, attention deficits, perceptual deficits, visual impairments, behavioral impulsivity, depression, and communication problems.[32–34] Increased risk of fracture, especially vertebral and hip fracture, is the natural outcome of osteoporosis and falls. In patients with stroke, osteoporosis and hip fracture are more likely on the more involved side.[35] Paradoxically, persons who receive rehabilitation are more likely to experience a fall.

Disordered Sleep

Disrupted sleep is common after stroke and can lead to poorer outcomes. The three most common sleep disorders in people with stroke are obstructive sleep apnea

(OSA), insomnia, and restless legs syndrome (RLS). OSA is a risk factor for stroke and can be a consequence as well.[36] Between 30% (severe) and 70% (mild) of people with stroke have OSA.[37] People with stroke and OSA have greater disability and poorer function than those with stroke without OSA.[38] Approximately 38% of people with stroke suffer from insomnia,[39] which can lead to lower quality of life (QOL).[40] RLS may be present in up to 15% of people with stroke and is associated with lower QOL.[41,42]

MEDICAL DIAGNOSIS OF THE STROKE HEALTH CONDITION

History and Examination

An accurate history profiling the timing of neurological events is obtained from the patient or from family members in the case of the unconscious or noncommunicative patient. Of particular importance are the exact time and pattern of symptom onset. An abrupt onset with worsening symptoms and decreasing level of consciousness is suggestive of cerebral hemorrhage. Severe headache described as "the worst headache of my life" is suggestive of SH. An embolus also occurs rapidly, with no warning, and is frequently associated with HD and/or heart complications. A more variable and uneven onset is typical with thrombosis. The patient's past history, including episodes of TIAs or head trauma, presence of major or minor risk factors, and medications; pertinent family history; and any recent alterations in patient function (either transient or permanent) are thoroughly investigated.[43] Stroke can mimic a number of other conditions that must be ruled out, including seizures, space-occupying lesions (e.g., subdural hematoma, cerebral abscess/infection, tumor), syncope, somatization, and delirium secondary to sepsis.[44]

The physical examination includes measuring vital signs (heart rate [HR], respiratory rate [RR], BP); signs of cardiac decompensation; and function of the cerebral hemispheres, cerebellum, cranial nerves, eyes, and sensorimotor system. The presenting symptoms will help to determine the location of the lesion, and comparison of both sides of the body will reveal the side of the lesion. Bilateral signs are suggestive of brain stem lesions or massive cerebral involvement.[43]

Tests and Measures

The *National Institutes of Health Stroke Scale (NIHSS)* is a valuable screening tool that focuses on initial and serial examination of impairments following acute stroke. The scale includes 11 items and uses a variable ordinal scale. Some items are scored 0 to 2 or 0 to 3 (level of consciousness, best gaze, visual fields, facial palsy, limb ataxia, sensory, best language, dysarthria, extinction, and inattention); other items are scored 0 to 4 (motor arm and motor leg). Specific descriptors are attached to each score. It was designed to be completed in 5 to 8 min. (The NIHSS and instructions on how to administer it are available at https://www.stroke.nih.gov/documents/NIH_Stroke_Scale_Booklet_508C.pdf.45) An examination scoring service for the NIHSS is maintained by the National Stroke Association. The NIHSS has been used to discriminate between stroke subtypes.[46–48] It has also been recommended as the measure for stroke severity, from acute to chronic patients, in stroke recovery research trials.[49]

A number of biomarkers can be used to help identify acute cerebral ischemia. These include inflammatory mediators such as interleukin-6, matrix metalloproteinase (MMP-9), markers of glial activation, and so forth. Biomarker assays may play an increasing role in the diagnosis of acute stroke as more research becomes available.[44] Biomarkers using neuroimaging techniques will serve as measures to predict structural and functional stroke recovery.[50]

A standardized set of blood analyses is performed, including hematological studies, serum electrolyte levels, and renal and hepatic tests. These tests are used to rule out metabolic abnormalities as well as blood, kidney, or liver conditions.

Cerebrovascular Imaging

Cerebrovascular imaging is the main tool to establish the diagnosis of suspected ischemic stroke and to rule out hemorrhagic stroke and other types of central nervous system (CNS) lesions (e.g., tumor or abscess). Advanced neuroimaging can rapidly identify the occluded artery and estimate the size of the core and the penumbra. It is also used to guide ischemic stroke therapy. Lack of imaging use is high in acute stroke primarily because many patients arrive beyond the strict 3-hr time window.[51]

Computed Tomography

CT scan is the most commonly used and readily available neuroimaging technique. CT resolution allows identification of large arteries and veins and venous sinuses. It demonstrates poor sensitivity for detecting small infarcts and infarction in the posterior fossa. Many times, CT scans during the acute phase are negative with no clear evidence of abnormalities. However, acute bleeding and hemorrhagic transformation are visible on CT scanning (Fig. 15.4). In the subacute phase, CT scans can delineate the development of cerebral edema (within 3 days), which then fades over the next 2 to 3 weeks. Cerebral infarction (within 3 to 5 days) is visible with the addition of contrast material by showing areas of decreased density. Long-term parenchymal changes consistent with scar formation are also visible on CT. It is important to remember that the extent of CT lesion does not necessarily correlate with clinical signs or changes in function.

Magnetic Resonance Imaging

MRI has evolved to become the first-line imaging in some stroke centers, whereas in other facilities it is used

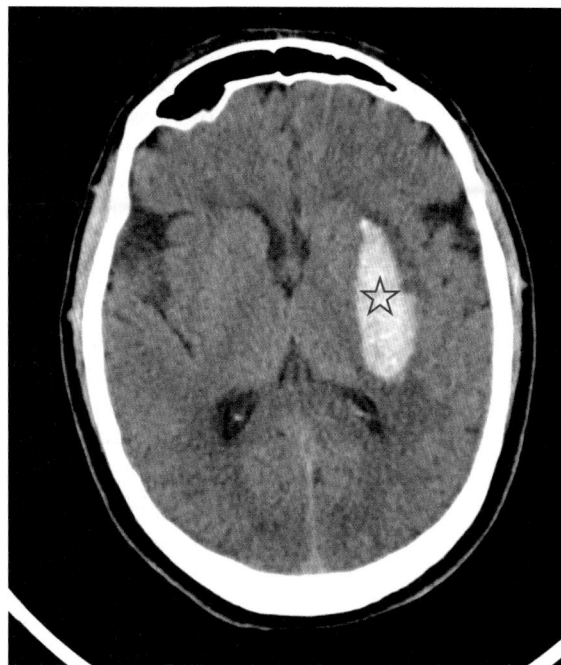

Figure 15.4 Computed tomography demonstrating an acute intracerebral hemorrhage (star). *(From Weber E, Vilensky J, Fog A. Practical Radiology: A Symptom-Based Approach. F.A. Davis; 2013, with permission.)*

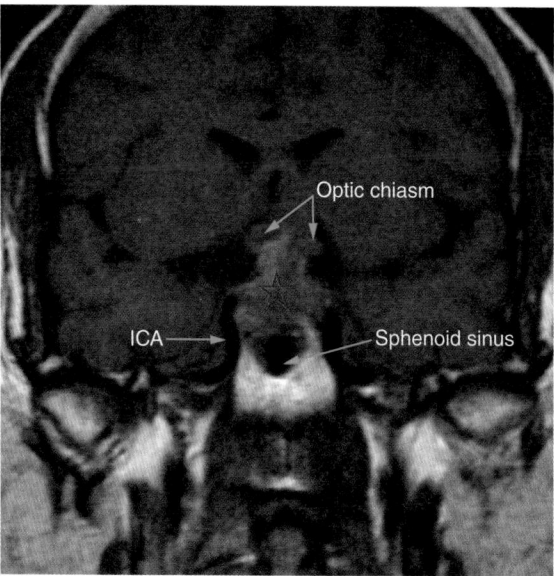

Figure 15.5 Coronal MRI without contrast enhancement on a pregnant patient with headache and visual field defect. The T1 hyperintensity of the greatly enlarged pituitary (star) indicates subacute hemorrhage. ICA = internal carotid artery. *(From Weber E, Vilensky J, Fog A. Practical Radiology: A Symptom-Based Approach. F.A. Davis; 2013, with permission.)*

when CT has not provided clear evidence of lesion location. MRI measures nuclear particles as they interact with a powerful magnetic field. MRI, especially diffusion/perfusion MRI, shows greater resolution of the brain and its structural detail than does a CT scan (Fig. 15.5). MRI is more sensitive in the diagnosis of acute strokes, allowing detection of cerebral ischemia as early as 30 min after vascular occlusion and infarction within 2 to 6 hr. It is also able to detail the extent of infarction or hemorrhage and can detect smaller lesions than a CT scan. Use of contrast enhancement allows documentation of changes in an infarct over the first 2 to 3 weeks. MRI scans cannot be performed on individuals with certain implantable devices (e.g., pacemakers) or on patients who are claustrophobic.[51]

Magnetic Resonance Angiography

Magnetic resonance angiography is a type of magnetic resonance image that uses special software to create an image of the arteries in the brain. It is used to identify vascular abnormalities (e.g., stenosis) and alterations in blood flow as a result of embolus or thrombosis. It provides similar information as classical angiography (x-ray of blood vessels following dye injection) with increased sensitivity of detection and with lowered risks.[51]

Doppler Ultrasound

Doppler ultrasound imaging is a noninvasive technique that sends sound waves into the body. Echoes bounce off the moving blood and artery and are formed into an image. Diagnostically, transcranial Doppler is used to examine the posterior circulation of the brain (the vertebrobasilar system). Carotid Doppler is used to examine the carotid arteries and typically precedes carotid endarterectomy. It is also used to examine the peripheral arteries in the diagnosis of PAD.

Arteriography and Digital Subtraction Angiography

Arteriography is an x-ray of the carotid artery with a special dye injected into an artery in the leg or arm. Digital subtraction angiography is also an x-ray of the carotid artery with less dye used. These procedures are considered invasive and carry a small risk of causing a stroke.

■ MEDICAL, PHARMACOLOGICAL, AND NEUROSURGICAL MANAGEMENT OF STROKE

Medical Management

Medical management of stroke includes strategies to achieve the following:

• Improve cerebral perfusion by reestablishing circulation and oxygenation and assist in stopping progression of the lesion to limit deficits. Oxygen is delivered via mask or nasal cannula. Patients in a coma may require intubation or assisted ventilation and suctioning.

- Maintain adequate BP. Hypotension or extreme hypertension is treated; antihypertension agents have the added risk of inducing hypotension and decreasing cerebral perfusion.
- Maintain sufficient cardiac output. If the causes of stroke are cardiac in origin, medical management focuses on control of arrhythmias and cardiac decompensation.
- Restore/maintain fluid and electrolyte balance.
- Maintain blood glucose levels within the normal range.
- Control seizures and infections.
- Control edema, intracranial pressure, and herniation using antiedema agents. Ventriculostomy may be indicated to monitor and drain cerebrospinal fluid.
- Maintain bowel and bladder function, which may include urinary catheter. Catheterization is typically short term but may be long term with the patient in coma.
- Maintain integrity of skin and joints by instituting protective positioning, a turning schedule every 2 hours, and early physical and occupational therapy.
- Decrease the risk of complications such as DVT, aspiration, pressure injuries, and so forth.

Pharmacological Management

Pharmacological interventions for completed stroke and its comorbidities are summarized in Box 15.1.[52–56]

Neurosurgical Management

Neurosurgical interventions may include the following:

- In hemorrhagic stroke, surgery may be indicated to repair a superficial ruptured aneurysm or AVM, prevent rebleeding, and evacuate a clot (hematoma). Larger, deeper intracranial or brain stem vascular lesions are generally not amenable to surgery. Surgery may also be indicated for resection of a superficial unruptured AVM when there is high risk of rupture and stroke.
- Mechanical thrombectomy is the removal of a large blood clot by sending a stent retriever to the site of the blocked blood vessel in the brain. To remove the brain clot, a catheter is threaded through an artery in the groin up to the blocked artery in the brain where the clot is removed. The procedure should be done within 6 hr of acute stroke symptoms, and only after a patient receives tPA.
- Carotid endarterectomy is a surgical procedure used to remove fatty deposits from the carotid artery. It is a useful procedure to prevent recurrent strokes or the development of stroke in individuals with TIAs. Stenosis of 60% to 99% is the typical guideline used when surgery is considered and can reduce stroke risk by as much as 55%. It cannot be performed

with acute stroke because altered pressures could subject ischemic areas to further damage.

■ REHABILITATION

Rehabilitation has an important role in increasing participation in societal roles by promoting activity and reducing body function and structure impairments. Prevention of secondary complications is an important component of rehabilitation. Patient-centered care and shared clinical decision-making facilitate goal setting to develop a *comprehensive plan of care* (POC).[57] The team of rehabilitation specialists includes the physician, nurse, physical therapist, occupational therapist, speech-language pathologist, and social worker. Additional disciplines may include a neuropsychologist, nutritionist, and recreational therapist or vocational counselor. The patient/client, family, and caregivers, as important members of the team, should be involved in all decision-making regarding the POC. Interdisciplinary communication is critical for effective team function and occurs through case conferences, informal interactions, patient care rounds, and patient/client family meetings. Effective case management also includes a coordinated education plan and accurate and effective documentation. It is critical for the team to provide a supportive environment to assist patients and their family members in their adjustment to this life-altering event.

The National Stroke Association instituted a process to certify stroke rehabilitation specialists. The designation of *clinical stroke rehabilitation specialist (CSRS)* ensures that therapists are expert stroke clinicians through a rigorous set of courses and written examination and a nationally recognized credential, the CSRS certification. Additional information can be found at https://www.stroke.org.

The overall focus for patients with moderate to severe stroke is on long-range planning, with consideration of anticipated episodes of care that typically include hospital-based care (acute care, inpatient rehabilitation, or subacute rehabilitation), outpatient rehabilitation, and home-/community-based care.

Stage of recovery and severity of the stroke will influence the setting and therapy for a person poststroke. Stages of recovery have recently been defined on the basis of links to biology.[58] These time periods are helpful in understanding the therapeutic approach one might take considering events such as cell death (in the hyperacute phase, 0 to 24 hr), period of inflammation and scarring 1 to 7 days poststroke (acute phase) and the endogenous plasticity (the nervous system's ability to repair itself) that starts in the acute phase, peaks in the early subacute phase (7 days to 3 months), and plateaus in the late subacute (3 to 6 months) through the chronic phase (more than 6 months).[58] Episodes of care may include hospital-based care (acute care, inpatient

---

Box 15.1   Medications Commonly Used to Treat Patients With Stroke[45–49]

- **Thrombolytics** (alteplase and tenecteplase [Activase or tPA]): Converts plasminogen to plasmin, degrades fibrin present in clots, dissolves clots, and reestablishes blood flow (e.g., lysis of thrombi causing ischemic stroke; also used to dissolve clots in coronary arteries, pulmonary emboli, deep vein thrombosis [DVT]).
  Possible adverse effects: The most common complication is brain hemorrhage.
- **Anticoagulants** (e.g., warfarin [Coumadin], heparin, dabigatran etexilate [Pradaxa]): Used to reduce the risk of blood clots and prevent existing clots from getting bigger by thinning the blood; indications include DVT prophylaxis, stroke prevention, peripheral vascular disease. With Coumadin, clotting times are closely monitored. Heparin is given intravenously and is faster acting.
  Possible adverse effects: Increased risk of bleeding and hemorrhage, hematomas.
- **Antiplatelet therapy** (e.g., acetylsalicylic acid [aspirin]; clopidogrel bisulfate [Plavix]; dabigatran etexilate [Pradaxa]; ticlopidine hydrochloride [Ticlid, Aggrenox, Persantine]): Prevent platelets (blood cells) from sticking together; long-term, low dose is used to decrease the risk of thrombosis and recurrent stroke; higher doses may be used in place of anticoagulants and may be recommended for patients with atrial fibrillation.
  Possible adverse effects: Increased risk of gastric ulcers and bleeding.
- **Antihypertensive agents** (e.g., ACE inhibitors, alpha blockers [Minipress], beta blockers, calcium channel blockers, direct vasodilators, diuretics, postganglionic neuron inhibitors): Used to control hypertension.
  Possible adverse effects: Dizziness, hypotension, among other symptoms.
- **Angiotensin II receptor antagonists** (telmisartan [Micardis], losartan potassium [Cozaar, Hyzaar]): Block angiotensin II, a chemical that triggers muscle contraction around blood vessels, narrowing them; enlarges blood vessels and reduces blood pressure.
  Possible adverse effects: Dizziness, hypotension, among other symptoms.
- **Anticholesterol agents/statins** (atorvastatin calcium [Lipitor], rosuvastatin calcium [Crestor], simvastatin [Zocor], lovastatin [Mevacor], fluvastatin [Lescol]): Lower cholesterol by inhibiting the enzyme in the blood that produces cholesterol in the liver; for management of hypercholesterolemia and mixed dyslipidemias.
  Possible adverse effects: Dizziness, headache, insomnia, weakness.
- **Antispasmodics/spasmolytics** (e.g., carisoprodol [Soma], chlorzoxazone [Parafon Forte], cyclobenzaprine [Flexeril], diazepam [Valium], methocarbamol [Robaxin], orphenadrine [Norflex/Norgesic]): Used to relax skeletal muscle and decrease muscle spasm.
  Possible adverse effects: May cause drowsiness, dizziness, dry mouth, among other symptoms.
- **Antispastics** (e.g., baclofen [Lioresal], dantrolene sodium [Dantrium], diazepam [Valium], tizanidine [Zanaflex]): Used to relax skeletal muscle and decrease muscle spasm.
  Possible adverse effects: May cause drowsiness, dizziness, confusion, weakness, among other symptoms.
- **Anticonvulsants** (e.g., carbamazepine [Tegretol], clonazepam [Klonopin], diazepam [Valium], phenobarbital [Luminal], phenytoin [Dilantin]): Used to control seizures; act as a generalized central nervous system depressant.
  Possible adverse effects: May cause drowsiness, ataxia, sedation, among other symptoms.
- **GABA (gamma-amino butyric acid) receptor antagonists** (e.g., baclofen [Kemstro, Lioresal]): Inhibit the action of GABA, which inhibits neurotransmitters and regulates the nervous system. May be used to manage spasticity.
  Possible side effects: Drowsiness, dizziness, or headache.
- **Neurotoxins** (e.g., botulinum toxin [Botox]): Interact with proteins in nerves to relax muscles.
  Possible side effects: Pain or swelling at site of injection, drowsiness.
- **Antidepressants** (e.g., fluoxetine [Prozac], monoamine oxidase inhibitors, sertraline [Zoloft], tricyclics [Amitriptyline]): Used to control depression.
  Possible adverse effects: May cause anxiety, tremor, insomnia, nausea.

---

rehabilitation, or subacute rehabilitation), outpatient rehabilitation, and home-/community-based care.

Acute Phase

The patient may be first seen in a neurological intensive care unit or specialized stroke care unit in a facility that also provides comprehensive rehabilitation services. Evidence supports the benefits of specialized stroke units in improving functional outcomes when compared to patients not receiving specialized care. Individuals who received this care were more likely to be alive, independent, and living at home 1 year after stroke.[59] The therapist needs to be aware of the patient's current status by reviewing the medical record and communicating with the medical team. During acute care, the therapist assists in ongoing monitoring of the patient's recovery and is alert for changes in the patient's status (e.g., changes in vital signs [HR, BP, RR], drop in

O_2 saturation levels, skin changes, alterations in mental status and consciousness). Early mobilization prevents or minimizes the harmful effects of bedrest and deconditioning. Early, frequent, short bouts of mobilization have been shown to produce better outcomes at 3 months than do long bouts. However, very early (<24 hr after stroke) more frequent mobilization is detrimental to functional outcomes.[60] Early mobilization may also increase the patient's level of consciousness and foster return to independence. Functional reorganization is promoted through early stimulation and use of the hemiparetic side. *Learned nonuse* of the hemiparetic extremities and maladaptive patterns of movement are minimized. Mental deterioration, depression, and apathy can be reduced through the fostering of a positive outlook toward the rehabilitation process. Interventions include but are not limited to functional mobility training (e.g., bed mobility, sitting, transfers, locomotion), ADL training, range of motion (ROM), splinting, and positioning.

Instruction, education, and training of patients and their families/caregivers is initiated early regarding current condition (pathophysiology, impairments, activity limitations) and risk factors for disability. It includes an overview of the recovery process, the rehabilitation POC, and expected transitions across care settings. It is important to remember that this is a highly stressful time for patients and families, and information needs to be graded in appropriate amounts and repeated and reinforced throughout the course of treatment. The therapist should establish effective communication. This includes speaking to the patient in a normal tone and volume, speaking slowly and giving the patient enough time to respond, using simple yes/no questions, and using gesture and tactile cues whenever appropriate. Controlling the environment and reducing distractions will also help to ensure the patient's attention and promote good communication. Awareness of the presence of visual field defect (homonymous hemianopsia) and perceptual changes (unilateral neglect) will influence choice of the therapist's position when interacting with the patient.

Current trends are toward shorter acute care hospital stays (average stay is about 5 days).[2] However, early discharge has resulted in an increase in the number of serious medical complications seen during subacute rehabilitation or at home. These complications may result in delays during active rehabilitation and, for some, temporary cessation of therapy or transfer back to the acute hospital until medical complications are resolved. It is important to monitor patients for potential risk of complications and medical emergencies (e.g., cardiac arrhythmias, DVT, uncontrolled BP, and recurrent stroke).

Subacute Phase

Persons poststroke with moderate or severe residual body function structure impairments or activity limitations may benefit from intensive inpatient rehabilitation provided in a freestanding rehabilitation facility or in a rehabilitation unit within the acute care hospital. Rehabilitation programs certified by the Commission on Accreditation of Rehabilitation Facilities and the Joint Commission can be expected to adhere to uniform standards and provide high-quality care.[4] They are referred to inpatient rehabilitation if they can tolerate an intensity of services consisting of two or more rehabilitation disciplines, 6 days a week for a minimum of 3 hr of active rehabilitation per day. If the patient requires less intensive services, transfer to a transitional care unit within a skilled nursing facility is instituted. Here rehabilitation services are less intense, ranging from 60 to 90 minutes of therapy services 5 days per week.[4] In this phase of rehabilitation, patients who are more dependent may respond well to electromechanical gait training.[61]

The timing of rehabilitation services is an important factor in predicting outcome. In general, a shorter onset-to-admission interval, within the first 20 days, has been shown to significantly improve functional outcomes when compared to longer intervals. Additional factors that influence the timing of rehabilitation efforts include medical stability, severity of cognitive–perceptual deficits, motivation, patient endurance, and recovery. In an era of time-limited payment for comprehensive rehabilitation services, selecting the optimal time for rehabilitation services may prevent unnecessary patient failures and improve long-term functional outcomes.

Chronic Phase

Rehabilitation services during the chronic phase, generally defined to be more than 6 months poststroke, are typically delivered in an outpatient rehabilitation facility, in a community setting, or at home. Outpatient services are prescribed for the patient who is discharged from inpatient rehabilitation, is in need of continuing rehabilitation, and can enter and exit the home with ease. Many of the interventions begun during inpatient rehabilitation are continued and progressed in order to sustain the gains made and improve functional performance. Those for walking include moderate- to high-intensity treadmill training,[62] circuit class,[63] and high dose of repetitive task practice.[64,65] Those for UE use include constraint-induced movement therapy (CIMT), mental practice,[66] mirror therapy,[67] interventions for sensory impairment,[68] and virtual reality.[69] Telerehabilitation may be used as a mode of therapy delivery as it has been found comparable to in-person delivery.[70]

Some patients with mild involvement may also benefit from outpatient rehabilitation services. A complete record of past medical and rehabilitation services should be made available to these agencies. The intensity of services provided varies but is generally less than that of inpatient rehabilitation (e.g., 60 to 90 minutes per visit, two to three times per week). The patient and family are instructed in a home exercise program (HEP) and educated about the importance of maintaining exercise levels, health promotion, fall prevention, and safety.

The patient may receive home care rehabilitation services, typically for the patient who is unable to exit the home independently. The challenges of being home can impose additional daily stresses for the patient and family. Difficulties should be addressed promptly as they arise. The therapist needs to emphasize the development of problem-solving skills to ensure successful adaptation to variable home and community environments. Fall risk factors should be eliminated or minimized as appropriate or possible. Examination of the environment and recommendations for modification of the environment are important parts of the preparation for return to home (see Chapter 9, Examination and Modification of the Environment).

Finally, the patient should be assisted in resuming participation in community and recreational activities. With increasing activity levels, it is important to monitor the patient's endurance levels carefully and provide instruction in activity pacing and energy conservation techniques as needed. Physical fitness programs (primarily cardiovascular and mixed training with walking)[71] have been shown to reduce dependence and improve cardiovascular function, strength, balance, and walking speed after stroke. A small number of stroke survivors can be evaluated and assisted in return to work. As the patient becomes successful in the home and community environments, services should be gradually phased out, but a wellness program should be in place (see Chapter 29, Promoting Health and Wellness). Follow-up visits at periodic intervals are recommended to identify problems as they develop and ensure long-term maintenance of function.

There is a large body of research on the efficacy of stroke rehabilitation with more than 25 Cochrane Systematic Reviews. However, the Cochrane researchers often conclude that further high-quality research is needed to determine the most effective interventions. Additional research is also needed to investigate the effect of rehabilitation interventions on QOL, participation, overall cost–benefit ratios, and the differential effects of stroke severity, latency, and age.

■ INTEGRATED FRAMEWORK FOR CLINICAL DECISION-MAKING

In this chapter, the examination and intervention for the person poststroke is guided by evidence-based practice resources and the integrated framework for clinical reasoning (see Chapter 1, Clinical Decision-Making).[57] Resources to guide evidence-based practice for persons poststroke include clinical practice guidelines specific for persons poststroke[72–79] and recommendations for examination tools for persons poststroke from the StrokEDGE task force.[80] There are many websites that

offer updated information on stroke management, and some of these can be found in Appendix 15.A (online). Evidence-based resources coupled with patient preferences and clinician expertise form the evidence-based triad for practice.

The integrated framework for clinical reasoning proposes shared decision-making between the clinician and patient, allowing both patient preferences and clinician expertise to collaboratively develop the POC. The framework in the *Guide to Physical Therapist Practice*[81] can be used to organize the steps in the decision-making process. The hypothesis-oriented algorithm for clinicians (HOAC) II represents the iterative process of generating and testing hypotheses at each step of the patient client management.[82] The International Classification of Functioning, Disability, and Health (ICF) provides enablement language and a structure for organizing information.[83] Standardized assessments and task analysis guide examination. The formulation of the POC, inclusive of prognosis, is informed by the individual's goals and the clinician's assessment of their ability to achieve them based on the body function structure limitations that restrict activity and participation coupled with evidence from the literature. Factored into the decision-making are the patient's abilities (assets), priorities, and resources, including family, home, and community resources. Interventions are *restorative* (aimed at improving impairments, activity limitations, and participation restrictions), *preventive* (aimed at minimizing potential complications and indirect impairments), and *compensatory* (aimed at modifying the task, activity, or environment to improve function). See discussion in Chapter 1, Clinical Decision-Making.

■ EXAMINATION

The three basic components of a comprehensive physical therapy examination include patient/client history, systems review, and tests and measures. The selection of examination procedures will vary depending on a number of factors, including patient's goals, age, location and severity of stroke, stage of recovery, phase of rehabilitation, and home/community/work situation, as well as other factors.

The purposes of the examination are as follows:

- Screen for likely benefit from rehabilitation services and the most appropriate choice of a care setting.
- Develop a specific POC, including patient and clinician goals, expected outcomes, prognosis, and interventions.
- Measure progress toward projected goals and outcomes.
- Determine if referral to another practitioner is indicated.
- Plan for discharge.

The interview that precedes the formal examination allows the clinician and the person poststroke to identify the relevant goals for this episode of care. This shared decision-making process guides the system review, screening, selection of tests and measures that inform the prognosis, diagnosis, and development of the POC. Examination findings are coordinated with other members of the rehabilitation team in order to arrive at an integrated POC. Box 15.2 presents Elements of the Examination of the Patient With Stroke, highlighting possible body function structure limitations observed in persons poststroke. Many of these examination procedures, tests, and measures are discussed in earlier chapters (see Chapters 2 through 9).

Box 15.2   Elements of the Examination of the Patient With Stroke

Patient/Client History

- Goals (emphasis on participation and activity)
- Communication and cognition screen (see details later)
- Age, sex, race/ethnicity, primary language, education
- Social history: cultural beliefs and behaviors, family and caregiver resources, social support systems
- Occupation/employment/work
- Living environment: home/work barriers
- Hand dominance
- General health status: physical, psychological, social, and role function; health habits
- Family history
- Medical/surgical history
- Medications
- Medical/laboratory test results
- Functional activity level: premorbid

Systems Review

- Neuromuscular
- Musculoskeletal
- Cardiovascular/pulmonary
- Integumentary
- Endocrine

Tests and Measures

Tests and measures are selected based on their ability to quantify or describe each of the following:

Participation: Work, community, and leisure activities: ability to assume/resume activities, safety; use of the Goal Attainment Scale or the Stroke Impact Scale

Wheelchair management and mobility: safety and endurance

Activities:

- **Postural control and balance:** sensorimotor integration, balance strategies (static and dynamic); safety PASS
  Primary impairments: altered balance, increased fall risk
- **Gait and locomotion:** speed, distance, steps, temporal-spatial description, use of assistive devices/orthotic devices, wheelchair mobility, safety. 10MWT, 6MWT, Functional Gait Assessment
- **Upper extremity use:** active isolated movement against gravity, Action Reach Arm Test, Motor Activity Log

- **Functional status and activity level:** performance-based examination of functional skills (FIM level), basic and instrumental ADL; functional mobility skills; home management skills; assistive or adaptive devices: fit, alignment, function, use; safety

Body Function Structure:

- **Level of consciousness, arousal, attention, and cognition: mental status, insight, motivation**
  Primary impairments: impaired alertness and attention, perseveration, confabulation, confusion, disorientation, distractibility, memory deficits, impaired judgment
- **Emotional status**
  Primary impairments: depression, pseudobulbar affect, apathy, euphoria
  Secondary impairments: depression
- **Behavioral style**
  Primary impairments: impulsive or cautious behavioral styles; frustration, irritability
- **Communication and language:** coordinate efforts with the speech-language pathologist
  Primary impairments: fluent, nonfluent, or global aphasia, dysarthria
- **Circulation:** cardiovascular signs and symptoms
  Common comorbidities: hypertension, coronary artery disease, congestive heart failure, diabetes, deep vein thrombosis
- **Ventilation and respiration/gas exchange:** pulmonary signs and symptoms
  Common comorbidities: chronic pulmonary disease
- **Anthropometric characteristics:** body mass index, girth, length
  Secondary impairments: edema, common in hand and foot
- **Integumentary integrity:** skin condition, pressure-sensitive areas; effectiveness of protective pressure-relieving devices
  Secondary impairments: altered skin integrity, pressure injuries
- **Pain:** intensity and location
  Primary impairments: central poststroke pain
  Secondary impairments: hemiplegic shoulder and/or hand pain
- **Cranial and peripheral nerve integrity**
  Primary impairments: visual field defects (CN II); impaired facial sensation (CN V) and facial movements

Box 15.2   Elements of the Examination of the Patient With Stroke—cont'd

(CNs V and VII); vestibular/auditory dysfunction (CN VII), dysphagia and dysarthria (CNs IX, X, XII)

- **Sensory integrity and integration**
  Primary impairments: homonymous hemianopsia, tactile/proprioceptive/kinesthetic losses, astereognosis
- **Perceptual function:** collaborate with an occupational therapist on assessment as needed
  Primary impairments: spatial relations syndrome, body scheme/body image disorders, unilateral neglect, agnosia, topographical disorientation
- **Joint integrity, alignment, and mobility:** ROM (active and passive); muscle length and soft tissue extensibility
  Secondary impairments: altered biomechanical alignment; loss of joint ROM, muscle and soft tissue length
- **Posture:** alignment and position, symmetry (static and dynamic, sitting and standing); ergonomics and body mechanics
  Secondary impairment: altered biomechanical alignment
- **Motor function: motor control and motor learning**
  Primary impairments:
  Selective capacity synergies: flexion and extension synergy patterns

Altered voluntary movement patterns: altered initiation, sequencing, timing of muscle contractions; altered force production
Altered reflex integrity: hyperreflexia, tonic reflexes, associated reactions
Abnormal tone: flaccidity initially; spasticity: spastic posturing
Altered sequencing, timing, balance, endurance
Coordination, dexterity, agility: coordination deficits
Motor planning: ideomotor or ideational apraxia

- **Muscle performance: strength, power, and endurance**
  Primary impairments: paralysis or weakness; fatigue
  Secondary impairments: disuse atrophy
- **Aerobic capacity and endurance:** functional activity testing, graded exercise testing
  Secondary impairments: decreased endurance
- **Orthotic, protective, and supportive devices:** fit, alignment, function, use, safety

Adapted from the *Guide to Physical Therapist Practice.*[81]

The order of the examination may vary. In this chapter, we propose that examination of participation and activities is done first, followed by determination of underlying body function structure limitations. We also propose that once the patient's participation goals are set there be a listing of the activities to achieve these goals. The therapist would then observe the patient's movements as they perform these activities and hypothesize and then further test possible underlying body function structure impairments (see Chapter 1, Clinical Decision-Making).

There are many standardized tests used to assess persons poststroke. The ones presented in this chapter (Table 15.7) are based on the clinical practice guidelines (CPGs) for outcome assessment[74] and a synthesis of those recommended by the Academy of Neurologic Physical Therapy's (ANPT) StrokEDGE workgroup[80] and the interdisciplinary task force on stroke recovery research.[49] The clinical practice guideline for outcome measures for persons with neurologic health conditions recommended six outcomes measures based on their psychometric properties across multiple neurologic health conditions including persons poststroke. The ANPT has developed resources to make it easier to administer and interpret each of those tests. These resources can be found on their website. The ANPT StrokEDGE workgroup reviewed 54 outcomes measures for persons poststroke. They then rated them on

the basis of their psychometric properties and clinical utility for persons poststroke. Further, they recommended, on the basis of a Delphi study, a core set of measures that entry-level PT students should learn and measures that should be used in different settings (https://www.neuropt.org/practice-resources/neurology-section-outcome-measures-recommendations/stroke). Table 15.7 is organized based on the ICF model and by practice setting.

Participation

Examination of participation begins by understanding the patient's participation goals during the interview. The *Goal Attainment Scale (GAS)* allows for customization of goals and a specific way of measuring them. The GAS requires an interview and a follow-up assessment if goals were achieved or not.[84] Information on test administration can be found at https://www.sralab.org/rehabilitation-measures. Alternatively, participation can be examined with a stroke-specific standardized test such as the Stroke Impact Scale.

Stroke Impact Scale

The *Stroke Impact Scale (SIS)* is a self-report measure developed to assess function and QOL after stroke. It is therefore both an activity and a participation measure. It includes 59 items organized into eight subgroups: strength, memory and thinking, emotions,

Table 15.7 Standardized Assessments Organized by the International Classification of Functioning, Disability, and Health and Setting

ICF Domain	Test	Acute Care	Inpatient	Out-Patient	Stroke Research	Entry-Level Education
Participation	Goal Attainment Scale		X	X		
	Stroke Impact Scale			X		X
Activity						
Posture and Balance	Postural Assessment Scale	X	X	X		X
	Functional Reach	X	X	X		X
	Berg Balance Scale*		X	X		X
	Timed Up-and-Go*	X	X	X		
Gait	6-minute Walk Test*	X	X	X		X
	10-meter Walk Test*	X	X	X	X	X
	Dynamic Gait Index					X
Upper Extremity Use	Action Research Arm Test				X	X
	Motor Activity Log		X	X		
Function	Functional Independence Measure		X			
Body Function Structure	Ashworth					X
	Fugl-Meyer Motor Performance				X	X
	Orpington Prognostic Scale	X			X	X

*Tests that are recommended in the Clinical Practice Guideline for outcome assessment.[74] Three tests not recommended by EDGE are Activities Balance Confidence Questionnaire and the Five Times Sit to Stand Test.

communication, ADL, mobility, hand function, and participation. The participation domain has eight questions covering work, social activities, quiet recreation, active recreation, role as a family member or friend, participation in spiritual or religious activities, feeling emotionally connected, and ability to help others. The final item of the SIS asks the person to rate perceived recovery on a scale of 0 to 100 with 100 representing full recovery and 0 representing no recovery. It takes about 30 minutes to complete. The SIS is a valid, reliable, and sensitive measure of change in this population.[85,86] A unique score can be calculated for the participation domain, and responses may be accurately provided by proxy.[87] The form and user agreement are available at https://www.sralab.org/rehabilitation-measures.

Activity

Activities to be examined are selected based on those required for the participation goal. Examination requires movement observation of the activities and tasks complemented by standardized tests. Activities or tasks can

be grouped according to their different motor control requirements, posture and balance, gait, and UE use. There are also tests of function, which combine the motor control requirements into whole-body ADL.

Postural Control and Balance

Postural control and balance (when measured at the activity level with the standardized tests described in this chapter) may be categorized as an activity or at the body function structure level when looking at basic features of the postural control (such as using anticipatory control, balance strategies, and sensory integration). In this chapter, they are kept together because the examination and intervention begin at the task level, then go to the body function structure level to interpret deficits. Postural control and balance are disturbed following stroke and are characterized by asymmetries in alignment and movement. Common postural alignment deviations following stroke are presented in Table 15.8. Control of balance may be impaired when reacting to a destabilizing external force (*reactive postural control*) and/or during self-initiated movements

Table 15.8 Common Postural Alignment Deviations Associated With Stroke

Body Segment	Postural Alignment Deviations
Pelvis	• Asymmetrical weight-bearing with majority of weight borne on the stronger side • In sitting, posterior pelvic tilt (sacral sitting) • In standing, unilateral retraction and elevation on the more affected side
Trunk	• With sacral sitting, a flattened lumbar curve with exaggerated thoracic curve and forward head • Lateral flexion with trunk shortening on more affected side
Shoulders	• Unequal height with more affected shoulder depressed • Humeral subluxation with scapular downward rotation and lateral flexion of trunk • Scapular instability (winging) may be present
Head/Neck	• Protraction with lateral trunk flexion • Lateral flexion of the head with rotation away from the more affected side
Upper Extremities	• More affected UE typically held in a flexed, adducted position, with internal rotation and elbow flexion, forearm pronation, wrist and finger flexion; limb is non–weight-bearing • Stronger UE used for postural support
Lower Extremities	• In sitting: More affected LE typically held in hip abduction and external rotation with hip and knee flexion (flexion synergy pattern) • In standing: More affected LE typically held in hip and knee extension with adduction and internal rotation (scissoring pattern); ankle plantar flexion • Unequal weight-bearing on feet, similar to pelvis in sitting

LE = lower extremities; UE = upper extremities.

(proactive or anticipatory postural control). Thus, the patient may be unable to maintain stable balance in sitting or standing or to move in the posture without loss of balance. Disruptions of central sensorimotor processing contribute to an inability to recruit effective postural strategies and adapt postural movements to changing task and environmental demands. Persons with stroke typically demonstrate uneven weight distribution and increased postural sway in standing. Patients with stroke often experience delays in the onset of motor activity, abnormal timing and sequencing of muscle activity, and abnormal co-contraction, resulting in disorganization of normal postural synergies. For example, proximal muscles are typically activated in advance of distal muscles or, in some patients, very late. Compensatory responses typically include excessive hip and knee movements. Corrective responses to perturbations or destabilizing forces are inadequate and result in loss of balance and frequent falls. Patients with hemiplegia typically fall in the direction of weakness.[88–92] Examination should include both the ability to hold (static) the sitting and standing positions as well as move (dynamic) in and out of the sitting and standing positions.

The patient's ability to maintain a stable position (steadiness) and position within the base of support (BOS; symmetry) is determined. Dynamic stability control can be examined by having the patient move within a given posture (weight shift) or reach within

their limit of stability (LOS). The patient is directed to shift weight in all directions, especially to the more involved side where greater impairments are expected. Functional tasks that utilize moving from one posture to another (e.g., supine-to-sit, sit-to-stand) can also be used to examine dynamic postural control.[93]

Performance-based postural control and balance scales highly recommended by the StrokEDGE group are either stroke specific, such as the *Postural Assessment Scale for Stroke Patients (PASS),* or have been validated for persons poststroke, such as the *Functional Reach, Berg Balance Scale,* and *Timed Up and Go* (the latter three can be found in Chapter 6, Examination of Coordination and Balance).

• The *PASS* examines the postural abilities in lying, sitting, and standing, and changing posture (supine-to-affected side, supine-to-unaffected side, supine to sitting, sitting to standing, and standing picking up a pencil off the floor). The 12 items are scored using an ordinal scale with descriptors ranging from "cannot perform" to "perform with little help" to "perform without help." It demonstrates good construct validity and high interrater and intrarater reliability.[94] It has been shown to be highly responsive to change in acute patients (14 to 30 days poststroke), moderately responsive to change in subacute patients (30 to 90 days poststroke), and least responsive in chronic patients (180 days poststroke) except when the latter are severe, in which case the responsiveness is high.[95] The minimal detectable change for acute patients is 2.2 points.[96] A minimal clinically important difference (MCID) is not established, but extensive predictive and criterion validity can be viewed at https://www.sralab.org/rehabilitation-measures.

Ipsilateral Pushing

Ipsilateral pushing (also known as *pusher syndrome* or *contraversive pushing*) is motor behavior characterized by active pushing with the stronger extremities toward the hemiparetic side with a lateral postural imbalance.[97] The end result is a tendency to fall toward the hemiparetic side. Ipsilateral pushing occurs in about 10% of patients with acute stroke and results from stroke affecting the posterolateral thalamus.[98,99] The result is an altered perception of the body's orientation in relation to gravity. Karnath et al.[97] found that patients experienced a misperception of subjective postural vertical position, perceiving their body as vertical when it was actually tilted about 20° toward the hemiparetic side. They also found that the visual and vestibular input for orientation perception to vertical remained intact as patients were able to align their bodies with the help of visual cues and conscious strategies. No significant association between ipsilateral pushing and hemineglect, anosognosia, aphasia, or apraxia has been found.[98]

Functional skills are significantly impaired for patients with ipsilateral pushing. During sitting, the push results in a strong lateral lean toward the weaker side; when sitting in a wheelchair, ipsilateral push often thrusts the patient over onto the wheelchair arm. In standing, a strong push creates an unstable situation with a high risk of falls because the hemiparetic LE typically cannot support the body weight. The patient shows no fear even when active pushing leads to instability and strongly resists any attempts to passively correct posture to midline, symmetrical weight-bearing. This pattern is totally opposite the expected postural deficiency seen in most patients after stroke, that is, increased weight-bearing to the stronger side to compensate for deficits on the hemiparetic side. Patients also typically demonstrate severe problems in transfers and gait. During transfers to the less involved side, the patient demonstrates increased pushback away from that side.

During walking, the patient typically exhibits inadequate extension of the hemiparetic LE with inability to transfer weight toward the less involved LE. During swing, strong scissoring (adduction) of the more involved LE is typically evident. The use of a cane during ambulation is problematic because patients use the cane to increase push to the hemiplegic side. Pedersen et al.[98] demonstrated that patients with ipsilateral

pushing behavior have poorer rehabilitation outcomes with longer hospital stays and prolonged recovery times. They also had significantly lower functional scores on admission and discharge with increased levels of dependence at discharge. However, with training, the brain can compensate well. The syndrome is rarely still evident at 6 months.[100]

Examination of the patient with ipsilateral pushing should include a focus on several criteria of behavior, including the following: (1) spontaneous body posture with tilting toward the more paretic side, (2) an increase of pushing force by the less-involved extremities evidenced by increased abduction and extension, and (3) resistance to passive correction of the posture. Broetz and Karnath[101] developed the *Clinical Assessment Scale for Contraversive Pushing*, which scores each of these three criteria in both sitting and standing. A subjective rating scale is used. The scores for each criterion range from 0 to 1. Because the criteria are examined in both sitting and standing, the maximum for each is 2 with a maximum possible overall score of 6. Patients are diagnosed with pushing behaviors if all three criteria are present and a score of 1 or more exists in each of the three criteria. Functional examination will reveal consistent difficulties with transfers to the less affected side and difficulties with independent sitting, standing, and walking.[102]

Gait and Locomotion

Gait is altered following stroke owing to a number of factors such as lack of selective capacity (ability to isolate movement), weakness, sensory loss, impaired balance, and loss of balance confidence. An examination of gait typically includes an *observational gait analysis (OGA)*. The therapist examines the movements occurring at the ankle, foot, knee, hip, pelvis, and trunk during walking (kinematic gait analysis). Gait is observed from the different planes of motion, and deviations are identified. Digital video recording of a patient's gait for subsequent OGA can improve identification of gait deviations, provides a visual record of performance, and offers a useful teaching tool (patient feedback) to assist with remediation of gait problems. Quantitative measures of distance and time, cadence, velocity, and stride times should also be obtained using measured walkways and a stopwatch. Kinetic gait analysis examines the forces involved in the production of movement during walking and requires sophisticated instrumentation (force plates). See Chapter 7, Examination of Gait.

Persons poststroke often present with slow gait that is asymmetrical. Typically, stance time on the stroke-affected side is reduced and step length is increased relative to the less affected side. There is a decreased push-off on the stroke-affected leg, which further compromises step length on the stroke-affected side. There may be a lack of dissociation between the right and left sides of the body, with the stroke-affected side moving as a unit rather than with a dissociating arm swing from the LE on forward progression.

It is recommended that measurement of gait include independence, speed, endurance, and quality.[103] The StrokEDGE recommends both a measure of gait speed, the 10-m Walk Test (10MWT), and a measure of endurance, the 6-minute Walk Test (6MWT), as well as a more global measure of gait performance, the Dynamic Gait Index (see Chapter 7, Examination of Gait). Ambulation profiles and scales can be used to determine locomotor function following stroke. These tests have been examined for reliability and/or validity and are reviewed in Chapter 7, Examination of Gait. For persons poststroke, the Functional Ambulation Category is used to measure independence.[103]

Gait speed has been found to be particularly useful in classifying a patient's ability to ambulate in different environments. Perry et al.[104] constructed a walking ability questionnaire and surveyed a group of 147 patients with chronic stroke about the effects of their limited walking ability. They then developed the *Classification of Walking Handicap After Stroke.* Functional categories (physiological walker, household walker, and community walker) provide a useful method of identifying a customary level of walking at home and in the community. For example, a *physiological walker* walks for exercise only either at home or in parallel bars during physical therapy. A *limited household walker* relies on walking to some extent for home activities and requires assistance for some walking activities, uses a wheelchair, or is unable to perform others. A *community walker* can walk unlimited distances outside.

Factors that differentiated household from community ambulators included strength, proprioception, isolated knee control (flexion and extension), and velocity.

This classification system can be used to improve communication among clinicians, treatment planning, and documentation. It also forms the basis for the *Functional Ambulation Classification Scale.*[105]

More recently, Fulk et al.[106] were able to classify walking ability based on population studies[107–109] that quantified the numbers of steps walked, walking speed, and walking endurance. This newer classification offers concrete measures to differentiate between walking categories. For example, a person poststroke who walks more than 7,500 steps/day, or 287 m on the 6MWT, can be classified as an unlimited community walker. The new scale offers the clinician the choice to examine step frequency or use the 6MWT to identify walking category. Table 15.9 compares the two classifications. Measuring walking speed and distance in a clinical setting offers the clinician a perspective on the person's capacity. Measuring steps in the community offers insight into the person's performance. When measuring performance, the clinician will also need to consider how confident the patient is as well as the influence of environmental factors such as a high area deprivation index.[110]

Upper Extremity Use

UE use poststroke is compromised and can present with no active movement to limited movement and, when resolved, as isolated selective movement. Measurement of UE function is recommended by the StrokEDGE group using a combination of the performance-based *Action Research Arm Test (ARAT)* and the self-report *Motor Activity Log (MAL).*

The ARAT has 19 UE functional tasks/movements with four subscales: grasping, gripping, pinching, and gross movement. Ordinal scoring is used for the 19 items, where 0 indicates no movement and 3 indicates

Table 15.9	Classification of Ambulation		
	Household Walker	Limited Community Walker	Community Walker
Perry et al.[104] description and criteria	• Able to walk throughout home • Does not use wheelchair in the home • Difficulty on stairs • Gait speed: <0.40 m/s	• Can enter and leave home independently • Ascends/descends curbs independently • Manages stairs • Independent walking in some (1–2) moderate community settings (i.e., visit friend in local restaurants) • Gait speed: 0.40–0.80 m/s	• Independent walking in home and all community activities • Can walk in crowded areas and on uneven terrain • Gait speed: >0.80 m/s
Fulk et al.[106] description and criteria	• 100–2,499 steps/day • Gait speed: <0.49 m/s • 6MWT distance: <205 meters	• 2,500–7,499 steps/day • Gait speed: 0.49–0.92 m/s • 6MWT distance: 205–287 meters	• ≥7,500 steps/day • Gait speed: >0.92 m/s • 6MWT distance: >287 meters

Data from Perry et al.[104(p985)] and Fulk.[106]
6MWT = 6-minute Walk Test; m/s = meters per second.

normal movement. Items in each subscale are totaled for grasping (18-point maximum), gripping (12-point maximum), pinching (18-point maximum), and gross movement (9-point maximum), with a total scale score of 57, indicating normal UE use. It takes between 5 and 20 minutes to administer the ARAT. The test is valid and reliable.[111-114] However, it does have significant floor effects at 14 days poststroke (greater than 21% of participants) and notable ceiling effects (greater than 21% of participants) at 30, 90, and 180 days poststroke.[86] The MCID of the ARAT if the dominant hand is affected is 12 points, and if the nondominant hand is affected, it is 17 points.[115]

The MAL is a self-report measure that uses a semistructured interview to assess arm function. Individuals are asked to rate quality of movement (QOM) and amount of movement (AOM) during 30 daily functional tasks (original MAL), 28 functional tasks (MAL 28), or 14 tasks (MAL 14).[116-118] Target tasks include object manipulation (e.g., pen, fork, comb, and cup) as well as the use of the arm during gross motor activities (e.g., transferring to a car, steadying oneself during standing, pulling a chair into a table while sitting). The AOM as well as QOM of the weaker arm are scored for each item on a 5-point scale ranging from no movement (0) to movement and quality comparable to before the stroke (5).[116,118] The MAL is recommended for use with people who are already in the community, and it may be scored by a caregiver.[102,103]

Functional Status

Functional measures are used to quantify activity limitations, inform the POC, monitor progress, ascertain efficacy of stroke rehabilitation efforts, and make recommendations for long-term care or placement. Instruments can include items to examine *functional mobility skills* (bed mobility, movement transitions, transfers, locomotion, stairs), *basic ADL (BADL) skills* (feeding, hygiene, dressing), and *instrumental ADL (IADL) skills* (communication, home chores). Information on functional disability following stroke is typically gained through performance-based measures. The *Barthel Index*[119] and the *Functional Independence Measure (FIM)*[120] have been extensively tested and demonstrate excellent reliability, validity, and sensitivity.

However, in order to promote consistency across settings, the Centers for Medicare and Medicaid Services replaced FIM with Section GG Functional Abilities and Goals. The Section GG Functional Abilities and Goals consists of 23 self-care and mobility tasks (and two additional wheelchair mobility tasks if the patient is nonambulatory) that are rated on a 6-point ordinal scale with scores ranging from independent to dependent. Self-care items include eating, oral hygiene, toilet hygiene, washing upper body, showering/bathing self, upper body dressing, lower body dressing, and putting on/taking off footwear. Mobility items include roll

to left and right, sit to lying, lying to sitting on side of bed, sit-to-stand, chair/bed to chair transfer, toilet transfer, car transfer, walk 10 feet, walk 50 feet with two turns, walk 150 feet, walk 10 feet on uneven surfaces, 1 step, 4 steps, 12 steps, pick up object from floor, wheel 50 feet with two turns, and wheel 150 feet. See Chapter 8, Examination of Function.

Body Function and Structure

Impairments of body function and structure may explain difficulty with activities required for participation. It is important to determine the person's cognitive and communication abilities, as this information will further influence the therapist's examination and intervention strategies. Specific body functions and structures may be examined completely or selectively based on the clinician's hypothesis of which may be limiting activity. For example, if during gait observation the clinician observes difficulty clearing of the affected LE, the clinician may hypothesize weakness of the affected LE and perform strength testing. In the event of a comprehensive examination, the clinician may want to clear passive body functions and structures such as flexibility, tone, integumentary system, and sensation before looking at active structures such as motor performance.

Flexibility and Joint Integrity

An examination of joint flexibility may be performed as a gross active screen and include passive ROM using a goniometer for limited ROM areas that will be targeted for therapy as well as examination for joint hypermobility/hypomobility and soft tissue changes (swelling, inflammation, or restriction) that could affect ROM. The shoulder and wrist should be examined closely because joint malalignment problems are common. Flaccidity will result in shoulder subluxation, which should be carefully evaluated and monitored. The UE is placed in a nonsupported position, and the gap in the glenohumeral joint is measured with a tape measure. Edema of the wrist often produces malaligned carpal bones with resulting impingement during wrist extension. Measurement may be affected by tonal changes or spasticity, so the clinician should attend to those fluctuations and standardize position for measurement. Active ROM (AROM) may be limited or impossible for the patient in early or middle recovery in the presence of paresis, spasticity, or obligatory synergies that can preclude isolated voluntary movements. ROM limitations and developing contractures should be carefully documented.

Contractures can develop anywhere but are particularly apparent in the paretic limbs. As contractures progress, edema and pain may develop and further restrict mobility. In the UE, limitations in the shoulder motions of flexion, abduction, and external rotation are common. Contractures are likely in the elbow flexors, wrist and finger flexors, and forearm pronators. In the LE, plantarflexion contractures are common.

Muscle Tone and Spasticity

Flaccidity (hypotonicity) is present immediately after stroke and is due primarily to the effects of cerebral shock. It is generally short lived, lasting a few days or weeks. Flaccidity may persist in a small number of patients with lesions restricted to the primary motor cortex or cerebellum. Spasticity (hypertonicity) emerges early in about 90% of cases and occurs on the side of the body opposite the lesion. Spasticity in upper motor neuron syndrome occurs predominantly in antigravity muscles (see Chapter 5, Table 5.4). In the patient with stroke, UE spasticity is frequently strong in scapular retractors; shoulder adductors, depressors, and internal rotators; elbow flexors and forearm pronators; and wrist and finger flexors. In the neck and trunk, spasticity may cause increased lateral flexion to the hemiplegic side. In the LE, spasticity is often strong in the pelvic retractors, hip adductors and internal rotators, hip and knee extensors, plantar flexors and supinators, and toe flexors. Spasticity results in tight (stiff) muscles. Posturing of the limbs (e.g., a tightly fisted hand with the elbow flexed and held tightly against the chest or a stiff extended knee with a plantarflexed foot) is common with moderate to severe spasticity. Spastic posturing can lead to development of painful spasms (similar to muscle cramping), degenerative changes, and fixed contractures. The automatic adjustment of postural muscles that occurs normally in preparation for and during a movement task is also impaired. Thus, patients with stroke may lack the ability to adjust and stabilize proximal limbs and trunk appropriately during movement, with resulting postural abnormalities, balance impairments, and increased risk for falls.

Passive motion testing can be used to determine the presence of hypotonicity or spasticity. Severity of spasticity can be graded on the basis of speed-dependent resistance to passive stretch using the *Modified Ashworth Scale* (see Chapter 5, Table 5.5). The position of the affected limbs at rest (resting postures) and during voluntary movements should be observed for tonal influences.

Sensation and Vision

Deficits in somatic sensations (touch, temperature, pain, and proprioception) are common after stroke. The type and extent of impairment are related to the location and size of the vascular lesion. Specific localized areas of dysfunction are common with cortical lesions, whereas diffuse involvement throughout one side of the body suggests deeper lesions involving the thalamus and adjacent structures. Impairment in touch sensation (64% to 94%), impairment in proprioception (17% to 52%), vibration (44%), and loss of pinprick sensation (35% to 71%) have been reported.[121,122] Sensory loss has

also been reported in the ipsilateral, less affected limbs, though to a lesser extent (12% to 25%). Symptoms of crossed anesthesia (ipsilateral facial impairments with contralateral trunk and limb involvement) typify brain stem lesions. Disturbances in cortical sensory modalities (two-point discrimination, stereognosis, kinesthesia, graphesthesia) are also found.[123,124] Profound sensory impairments will negatively affect motor performance, motor learning, and rehabilitation outcomes and contribute to unilateral neglect and *learned nonuse* of limbs. Sensory impairment is also associated with pressure sores, abrasions, and shoulder pain and subluxation.

The visual system should be carefully investigated, including tests for visual field defects (CN II, optic radiation, visual cortex), acuity (CN II), pupillary reflexes (CNs II and III), and extraocular movements (CNs III, IV, and VI). Ocular motility disturbances, such as diplopia, oscillopsia, visual distortions, or paralysis of conjugate gaze, may be present with brain stem strokes. Visual field defects (homonymous hemianopsia) need to be differentiated from visual neglect, a perceptual deficit characterized by an inattention to or neglect of visual stimuli presented on the involved side. The patient with pure hemianopsia is typically aware of the deficit and may spontaneously compensate by moving the eyes or head toward the side of deficit; the patient with visual neglect will be unaware (inattentive) of the deficit (see Chapter 27, Cognitive and Perceptual Dysfunction). The use of prescriptive eyeglasses should be determined before any testing; the therapist should ensure that eyeglasses are worn and clean.

Central poststroke pain (CPSP) is defined as pain arising as a direct consequence of a lesion or disease affecting the central somatosensory system and occurs in about 10% of strokes.[125] It can result from lesions at any level of the somatosensory pathways including the medulla, thalamus, and cortex. The thalamus is thought to play an important part in the underlying pathophysiology of central pain. CPSP can be severe and persistent (described as "burning," "aching"), spontaneous and intermittent (described as "lacerating" or "shooting" pain), or evoked by mechanical (stroking the skin, pressure) or thermal (heat or cold) stimuli. Symptoms may be focal, affecting the hand/arm or foot/leg, or in severe cases affecting half the body. Development of pain is typically within the first few months after stroke, though onset may be delayed for many months. Spontaneous recovery is rare and chronic suffering common. The debilitating nature of CPSP frequently limits participation in rehabilitation programs and outcomes.[126]

A sensory examination should include testing of superficial sensations (e.g., touch, pressure, sharp or dull discrimination, temperature) and deep sensations (proprioception, kinesthesia, vibration). Combined (cortical) sensations such as stereognosis, tactile localization, two-point discrimination, and texture recognition should also be examined once the integrity of the superficial sensations of touch and pressure is established. Sensory testing procedures are described in detail in Chapter 3, Examination of Sensory Function. The quality of sensory impairments experienced can range from mild altered perception to marked changes in sensory thresholds, delayed perceptions, uncertainty of responses, altered time for sensory adaptation, and sensory persistence.[121] Impairments may be evident in one sensory modality and not in others. Differences can also be expected between upper and lower hemiplegic extremities, depending on lesion location. Comparisons with the intact side should be viewed with caution because impairments may exist in the supposedly "normal" extremities due to aging and comorbidities. Sensory testing may be difficult or need to be deferred owing to cognitive or communication deficits.

Integumentary Integrity

Ischemic damage and subsequent necrosis of the skin results in skin breakdown and pressure injuries. The skin breaks down typically over bony prominences from pressure, friction, shearing, and/or maceration. Intense pressure for a short time or low pressure for a prolonged time results in pressure injuries. Friction occurs as the skin rubs or is dragged against the supporting surface, for example, when the patient slides down in bed or is pulled up. Spasticity and contractures also contribute to increased friction. Shearing occurs from sliding of adjacent structures in opposite directions (skin versus underlying bone), for example, during transfers from bed to wheelchair. Maceration is caused by excess moisture, for example, with urinary incontinence. Additional risk factors include reduced activity (bedfast or chairfast), immobility, decreased sensation, abnormal patterns of movement, poor nutrition, and decreased level of consciousness. The incidence of pressure injuries is increased with comorbid medical conditions such as infections, peripheral vascular disease, edema, and diabetes.

Daily systematic inspection of the skin is indicated for high-risk patients, particularly over areas prone to break down. The skin must be kept clean, dry, and protected from injury. Adherence to proper techniques for positioning, turning, and transferring is essential. The therapist collaborates with nursing to develop and monitor a positioning schedule and time in each position. Pressure-redistributing devices (PRDs) are used to minimize high concentrations of pressure (e.g., foam pads, alternating pressure mattress, water mattress, air-fluidized bed, sheepskin, heel and elbow protectors, multipodus boots, and seating cushions). Proper use of PRDs and positioning (seating) in the wheelchair should be closely examined.

Motor Control
Stages of Motor Recovery

Initially, flaccid paralysis is present *(stage 1)*. This is replaced by the development of spasticity, hyperreflexia,

and mass patterns of movement, termed *obligatory synergies,* all characteristic of upper motor neuron syndrome. Muscles involved in obligatory synergy patterns are strongly linked in a highly stereotyped, abnormal pattern; isolated joint movements outside the obligatory pattern are not possible. During *stage 2* (early synergy), facilitatory stimuli will elicit partial range synergies. As recovery progresses, spasticity is marked with full ROM and obligatory synergies *(stage 3)*. Synergy influence begins to decline in *stage 4* as some isolated out-of-synergy joint movements emerge. During *stage 5,* relative independence of synergy, spasticity continues to decrease, and isolated joint movements become more apparent. During *stage 6,* patterns of movement are near normal. This general pattern of recovery was initially described by Twitchell[127] and Brunnstrom[128] and confirmed by additional investigators[129,130] (Table 15.10). Progression through these stages exists, though individual recovery is highly variable. Some patients experience mild involvement with early full recovery, whereas other patients demonstrate severe involvement with incomplete recovery. The degree of recovery depends on several factors, including lesion location and severity and capacity for adaptation through training. Finally, recovery differs within patients. For example, the UE may be more involved and demonstrate less complete recovery than the LE, as is seen in MCA syndrome.

Abnormal and highly stereotyped obligatory synergies emerge with spasticity following stroke. Thus, the patient is unable to perform an isolated movement of a single limb segment without producing movements in the remainder of the limb. For example, efforts to flex the elbow also result in shoulder flexion, abduction, and external rotation. Two distinct abnormal synergy patterns have been described for each extremity: a flexion synergy and an extension synergy (Table 15.11). An inspection of the synergy components reveals that certain muscles are not usually involved in either the flexion or extension synergy. These muscles include the (1) latissimus dorsi, (2) teres major, (3) serratus anterior, (4) finger extensors, and (5) ankle evertors. These muscles, therefore, are generally difficult to activate while the patient is exhibiting these patterns. Obligatory synergies are often incompatible with normal ADL and functional mobility skills. For example, the patient with a strong LE extensor synergy will have difficulty walking owing to foot plantarflexion and inversion with hip and knee extension and adduction (scissoring gait pattern). As recovery progresses, spasticity and obligatory synergies begin to disappear, and more normal synergies with isolated joint control become possible.

Fugl-Meyer Assessment of Physical Performance

The *Fugl-Meyer Assessment of Physical Performance (FMA)* is a standardized way to test for motor recovery.[131] It is based on the work of Twitchell[127] and Brunnstrom.[128,132] This is an impairment-based test with items organized

Table 15.10   Sequential Motor Recovery Stages Following Stroke

Stage	Description
1	Recovery from hemiplegia occurs in a stereotyped sequence of events that begins with a period of *flaccidity* immediately following the acute episode. *No movement of the limbs* can be elicited.
2	As recovery begins, the basic limb synergies or some of their components may appear as associated reactions, or *minimal voluntary movement* responses may be present. At this time, spasticity begins to develop.
3	Thereafter, the patient gains *voluntary control of the movement synergies,* although full range of all synergy components does not necessarily develop. Spasticity has further increased and may become severe.
4	Some *movement combinations that do not follow the paths of either synergy are mastered,* first with difficulty, then with more ease, and *spasticity begins to decline.*
5	If progress continues, more *difficult movement combinations are learned* as the basic limb synergies lose their dominance over motor acts.
6	With the *disappearance of spasticity, individual joint movements become possible, and coordination* approaches normal. From here on, as the last recovery step, normal motor function is restored, but this last stage is not achieved by all, for the recovery process can plateau at any stage.

From Brunnstrom S. *Movement Therapy in Hemiplegia.* Harper & Row; 1970, with permission.

Table 15.11   Obligatory Synergy Patterns Following Stroke

	Flexion Synergy Components	Extension Synergy Components
Upper extremity	Scapular retraction/elevation or hyperextension Shoulder abduction, external rotation Elbow flexion* Forearm supination Wrist and finger Flexion	Scapular protraction Shoulder adduction,* internal rotation Elbow extension Forearm pronation* Wrist and finger flexion
Lower extremity	Hip flexion,* abduction, external rotation Knee flexion Ankle dorsiflexion, inversion Toe dorsiflexion	Hip extension, adduction,* internal rotation Knee extension* Ankle plantarflexion,* inversion Toe plantarflexion

*Generally the strongest component.

by sequential recovery stages. A three-point ordinal scale is used to measure impairments of volitional movement with grades ranging from 0 (item cannot be performed) to 2 (item can be fully performed). Specific descriptions for performance accompany individual test items. Subtests exist for UE function, LE function, balance, sensation, ROM, and pain. The cumulative test score for all components is 226 with availability of specific subtest scores (e.g., UE maximum score is 66, LE score 34; balance score 14). This instrument has good construct validity and high reliability for determining motor function following stroke.[133,134] The instrument requires an estimated 30 to 45 minutes to administer. A shortened version consists of combining the UE and LE sections to form the *Fugl-Meyer Motor Scale.* This version has also been shown to be a useful measure of stagewise recovery and outcomes with a shortened administration

time.[135] Both the upper and lower limb sections were recommended as a core clinical measure of body function structure in a recent Delphi study.[136] The motor section is recommended for stroke research recovery.[49] For the LE motor score, a change of greater than 5 points is required to be outside of measurement error,[137] and the estimated MCID of the UE-FM scores ranges from 4.25 to 7.25 points, depending on the different facets of UE movement.[138] This test is used in many of the studies of stroke recovery and rehabilitation.

Selective Capacity

Clinicians may use the synergies to describe movement, but examination should focus on the person's selective capacity or ability to isolate movement. Voluntary movement patterns should be examined to determine if the person has movement that is *active, isolated,* and *against gravity.* In early stages of recovery, movement can be partially active, partially isolated, and also gravity reduced. The assessment consists of asking the person to voluntarily move a limb in one direction at a specific joint (e.g., shoulder or hip flexion) and then observing the extent to which the person can move through the full available ROM without moving the other joints in that limb. For example, the person poststroke may be able to actively flex their shoulder 50% against gravity while maintaining the elbow extended and wrist/hand relaxed; after this point, the elbow and wrist may flex, and the shoulder may abduct.

While testing for active isolated movement, the clinician may observe *associated reactions,* which also typically present in patients with stroke who exhibit strong spasticity and obligatory synergies. These consist of unintentional movements of the hemiparetic limb caused by voluntary action of another limb or by other stimuli such as yawning, sneezing, or coughing. For example, when the patient vigorously contracts the elbow flexors of the stronger UE, the hemiparetic elbow also flexes; or when the patient flexes the hip to lift the hemiparetic LE in sitting, the hemiparetic UE also flexes.

Muscle Performance

If the patient demonstrates some degree of selective capacity, then testing of muscle strength is indicated. Paresis is found in 80% to 90% of all patients after stroke and is a major factor in impaired motor function, activity limitation, and disability. Patients are unable to generate the force necessary for initiating and controlling movement. The degree of primary weakness is related to the location and size of the brain injury and varies from a complete inability to achieve any contraction (hemiplegia) to hemiparesis with measurable impairments in force production.[139] Deficits on the contralateral side typically include hemiparesis (opposite UE and LE). Owing to the high incidence of MCA strokes, the UE is frequently more affected than the LE. About 20% of individuals with MCA strokes fail to regain any functional use of the affected UE. Typically, distal muscles exhibit greater strength deficits than proximal. This can be explained by the greater facilitation of distal muscles than proximal by the corticospinal system. Mild weakness also occurs on the ipsilateral, or what should be called the "less affected," side.[140,141] This can be explained by the fact that only 75% to 90% of the corticospinal fibers cross in the medulla to the contralateral side. The remainder are transmitted to the spinal cord ipsilaterally in the anterior or ventral corticospinal tract. Once in the spinal cord, some of these fibers cross while the rest remain uncrossed, thereby explaining bilateral weakness.[142] The amount of weakness experienced by the patient may also vary according to the extent and level of inactivity (disuse atrophy) and the specific functional tasks attempted. Thus, a patient may appear stronger in some tasks than others.[143]

Poststroke weakness is associated with several changes in both the muscle and the motor unit. Changes occur in muscle composition, including atrophy of muscle fibers. There is a selective loss of type II fast-twitch fibers with subsequent increase in the percentage of type I fibers (a finding also reported in older adults). This selective loss of type II fibers results in slowed force production; difficulty with initiation and production of rapid, high-force movements; and rapid onset of fatigue.[123,143–145] The number of functioning motor units and discharge firing rates also decrease. This is explained by the presence of transsynaptic degeneration of alpha motor neurons that occurs with loss of corticospinal innervation. Abnormal recruitment of motor units with altered timing occurs.[146–148] Thus, patients demonstrate inefficient patterns of muscle activation and higher levels of co-contraction. This opposing muscle activation can contribute to muscle weakness and incoordination. These impairments in force production and coordination have been reported in both paretic and less affected UEs after stroke.[149,150] Patients demonstrate increased effort and fatigability with frequent complaints of feelings of weakness. Denervation potentials on electromyography (EMG) are common, also the result of denervation changes in the corticospinal tracts. Overall reaction times are increased, a finding also reported in the less affected extremities and for older adults in general. Movement times are prolonged, a timing abnormality that contributes to impairment of coordinated motor sequences.

Although an examination of strength is necessary, the traditional manual muscle test (MMT) poses problems of validity in the presence of strong spasticity, reflex, and synergy dominance. The patient who is not able to isolate specific movements should not be examined using MMT. In this situation, an estimation of strength can be made from observation of active movements during functional activities (functional strength testing). The patient's self-report can also yield important indicators of weakness and fatigue. The patient in later recovery with improving motor control and isolated movement can be examined using traditional MMT or handheld dynamometry. Use of a computerized isokinetic dynamometer can reveal important objective data regarding forces generated, peak torque, time to peak torque, and total work normalized to body weight. See Chapter 4, Musculoskeletal Examination.

Coordination

Proprioceptive losses can result in sensory ataxia. Strokes affecting the cerebellum typically produce cerebellar ataxia (e.g., lateral medullary syndrome, basilar artery syndrome, pontine syndromes) and motor weakness. The resulting problems with timing and sequencing of muscles can significantly impair function and limit adaptability to changing task and environmental demands. Basal ganglia involvement (posterior cerebral artery syndrome) may lead to slowed movements (bradykinesia) or involuntary movements (choreoathetosis, hemiballismus).

Coordination tests can be used to examine movement control. The therapist focuses on elements of speed/rate control, steadiness, response orientation, and reaction and movement times. Fine motor control and dexterity should be examined using writing, dressing, and feeding tasks (see Chapter 6, Examination of Coordination and Balance). Although more significant impairments can be expected on the hemiparetic side, it is important to remember that subtle deficits can occur on the less involved side. Thus, it is important to examine both unilateral and bilateral movements, including symmetrical, asymmetrical, and unrelated movements. Performance may vary as the patient moves from supine to sitting to standing positions with the resultant increased postural demands and greater degrees of freedom.

Motor Planning

Motor praxis is the ability to plan and execute coordinated movement. Lesions of the premotor frontal cortex of either hemisphere, left inferior parietal lobe, and corpus callosum can produce *apraxia*. Apraxia is more evident with left hemisphere damage than right and is commonly seen with aphasia. The patient demonstrates difficulty planning and executing purposeful movements that cannot be accounted for by any other reason (i.e., impaired strength, coordination, sensation, tone, cognitive function, communication, or uncooperativeness). There are two main types of apraxia. *Ideational apraxia* is an inability of the patient to produce movement either on command or automatically and represents a complete breakdown in the conceptualization of the task. The patient has no idea how to do the movement and thus cannot formulate the required motor programs. With *ideomotor apraxia,* the patient is unable to produce a movement on command but can move automatically. Thus, the patient can perform habitual tasks when not commanded to do so and often perseverates, repeating the activity over and over. Significant information on apraxia will be gained by close collaboration with the occupational therapist. Refer to Chapter 27, Cognitive and Perceptual Dysfunction, for a more complete discussion of these deficits and their management.

Cranial Nerves

The therapist should examine for facial sensation (CN V), facial movements (CNs V and VII), and labyrinthine/auditory function (CN VIII). The presence of swallowing difficulties and drooling necessitates an examination of the motor nuclei of the lower brain stem cranial nerves (CNs IX, X, and XII) affecting the muscles of the face, tongue, larynx, and pharynx. This includes determination of motor function of the lips, mouth, tongue, palate, pharynx, and larynx. The gag reflex should be examined because hypoactivity may lead to aspiration into the airway. Adequacy of cough mechanisms should also be carefully examined. The therapist needs to be able to recognize the presence of swallowing difficulties and initiate prompt referral.

Aerobic Capacity and Endurance

A supervised exercise test with ECG monitoring may be indicated for survivors of stroke with cardiovascular disease in the subacute phase. Performance measures include significant ECG changes, HR, BP, *rating of perceived exertion (RPE)*, and other signs of ischemic intolerance. The mode of testing will depend on the individual patient and can include leg cycle ergometry, semirecumbent cycle ergometry, a combination arm-leg ergometer, treadmill (TM) walking, or a seated stepper. If balance is impaired, recumbent equipment or an overhead safety harness on a TM should be used. Test protocols are individualized and are generally submaximal with a gradual progression in intensity. An intermittent protocol with rest periods may be required for some patients. Clinical endpoints of testing are similar as for other patients with cardiovascular disease (serious dysrhythmias, greater than 2-mm ST-segment depression or elevation, SBP greater than 250 mm Hg or diastolic BP [DBP] greater than 115 mm Hg, volitional fatigue).[29]

For ambulatory patients, walking endurance can be measured using a *6- or 12-minute Walk Test* (see discussion in Chapter 7, Examination of Gait). The time, total distance, number of rest stops, and symptoms at rest stops are recorded. Shorter distances (e.g., a 2-minute Walk Test) have been used for patients with acute stroke.[151] Table 15.9 shows the value of the information gleaned from the 6MWT.

■ PROGNOSIS AND DIAGNOSIS

Formulating a POC involves weighing the person's resources and limitations, interpreting the results of the examination tests that are predictive, and consulting the literature on the health condition. For example, administering the *Orpington Prognostic Scale (OPS)* is recommended by StrokEDGE to assess the person in the first 2 weeks poststroke because it is valid and reliable, and the scores predict discharge setting.[152,153] It has four domains—balance, cognition, motor, and proprioception—which are often measured anyway. Using the OPS, the clinician can predict the discharge setting as follows: a score of less than 3.2 indicates discharge to home within 3 weeks of stroke, a score of greater than 5.2 requires long-term care, and a score between 3.2 and 5.2 requires intensive rehabilitation (see Table 15.7).[153]

Evidence from basic science is accumulating to support motor recovery poststroke, and the findings of specific tests are being recommended for inclusion in stroke recovery clinical trials. A consensus panel recommended assessing the integrity of the *corticospinal tract (CST)* using diffusion tensor imaging across the continuum of recovery. The integrity of the CST has demonstrated a moderate to strong relationship with sensorimotor recovery. Similarly, the panel recommended, for inclusion in stroke recovery trials of the UE, the use of motor-evoked potentials (MEPs), which are measured using transcranial magnetic stimulation. They propose that people with stroke be classified based on the presence of MEP (+) or absence of MEP (–) to understand how they respond to treatments. The presence of a MEP indicates a better prognosis. Once this type of information is available, the clinician will be able to select therapies based on the likelihood of motor recovery.[50]

Clinical tests may also be predictive. Strong evidence has been reported supporting the clinical measurement of the UE impairment as predictive of recovery, demonstrating that the lesser the degree of UE impairment early on, the greater is the recovery. There is a model that uses the UE Fugl-Meyer score to distinguish between five types of UE recovery.[154] Another model that uses the ARAT, finger extension, and shoulder abduction has been shown to predict UE capacity up to 6 months poststroke.[155] Independent walking at 6 months was predicted (using the Functional Ambulation Category) for persons poststroke less than 80 years old, whose knee extension strength Medical Research Council was a grade ≥3/5, and their Berg Balance Test less than 6, 6 to 15, or ≥16/56, were combined to form the TWIST prediction tool. The TWIST prediction tool was at least 83% accurate for all time points.[156]

It has also been suggested that the NIHSS be used as a measure of stroke severity with the goal of having severity guide prognosis.[49] Additional factors known to moderate prognosis are discussed under Recovery and Outcomes later in this chapter.

■ GOALS AND OUTCOMES

Examples of long-term participation and activity goals with short-term body function structure goals for patients with stroke are presented in Box 15.3 These examples illustrate the logic of having short-term goals reflect the underlying body function and structure impairment that interfere with participation and activity. The examples refer to the person who had an MCA stroke 3 weeks prior and is currently receiving physical therapy in a subacute rehabilitation facility.

■ PHYSICAL THERAPY INTERVENTIONS

Therapists select interventions based on an accurate examination and evaluation of the existing body function and structure impairments and activity limitations that interfere with activity and participation goals. The intervention is modified based on the patient's resources, capabilities, and affective state. Physical therapy can take the form of rehabilitation, compensation, or prevention (see Chapter 1, Clinical Decision-Making). Rehabilitation is indicated whenever there is the potential for structural and behavioral plasticity. In more severe cases with limited recovery potential, compensation-adaptation and prevention strategies may be employed.[57] Repetitive task-specific training based

---

Box 15.3   Example of Participation, Activity, and Related Body Function Structure Goals*

Participation Goal

Patient will participate with close supervision in their daughter's wedding ceremony and reception in 2 months.

Related Activity Goals

1. Patient will sit in a folding chair with no armrests for 30 minutes in 1 month.
2. Patient will independently transition from sit-stand-sit on a folding chair with no armrests 5 times in 20 seconds in 1 month.
3. Patient will walk escorting (arm in arm) the bride 300 meters on a level surface using a single-point cane in 2 months.
4. Patient will increase walking speed (10MWT) from 0.50–0.75 m/s in 2 months.
5. Patient will increase his Berg Balance Scale from 48–54 in 2 months.
6. Patient will safely and independently transfer in and out of his car in 1 month.

Related Body Function Structure Goals

1. Patient will increase the affected ankle dorsiflexion, eversion, and plantarflexion by half a grade in 1 month.
2. Patient will increase passive range of motion of the affected hip extension by 5° in 2 weeks.
3. Patient will respond to external perturbations in the anterior–posterior direction using an ankle or hip strategy five out of five times in 6 weeks.

*Goals refer to person who had a middle cerebral artery stroke 4 weeks prior and is currently receiving physical therapy in a subacute rehabilitation facility.

on motor learning principles coupled with exercise and physical activity are the core principles that organize the approach to intervention. PT interventions target meaningful salient goals with consideration of how to (1) structure the environment, (2) schedule practice, (3) provide feedback, (4) dose the intervention, (5) progress the program, and (6) encourage problem-solving, reflection, and self-management. If available, an algorithm may guide intervention selection based on specific criteria (see later section in this chapter, Interventions to Improve Upper Extremity Use).

Evidence-based practice (EBP) promotes the use of current best research evidence along with individual clinical expertise and the needs of the patient to reach informed decisions about patient care. EBP allows therapists to identify the best (most effective) techniques and take responsibility for evaluating their practice on an ongoing basis. The clinician who practices EBP will regularly consult the literature to select interventions based on best available evidence. Using a combination of synthesis evidence, such as CPGs and systematic reviews (SRs) with meta-analyses, is recommended as the starting point for reviewing the evidence because SRs may find limited evidence in an area where the CPG can fill the gap. This may be followed by high-quality randomized controlled trials (RCTs) that will have specific protocols for practice. It is important to note that in some instances the available evidence may be a single small study or even a case study, particularly when an area of study is new and not well developed. Then the clinician may draw upon their prior knowledge and patient preferences to make a decision about the intervention that is selected.

There is not one optimal intervention for all persons poststroke. As they are a diverse group with variable levels of function, interventions must be carefully selected on the basis of individual abilities and needs. The choice of interventions must also take into consideration a number of other factors, including phase of poststroke recovery (acute, subacute, chronic), severity of the stroke, age of the patient, number of comorbidities, cognitive abilities, communication status, affective status, social and financial resources, and potential discharge placement. Shared decision-making indicates that the patient's preferences should be considered as well.

Structure of the Intervention

Motor skill learning is based on the brain's capacity for recovery through mechanisms of neuroplasticity. An effective rehabilitation plan capitalizes on this potential and encourages active participation with the goal of acquiring skills. Activities are selected that are meaningful and important to the patient. Optimal motor learning can be promoted through attention to several factors, most importantly, (1) task and learner, (2) structuring

the environment, (3) practice schedules, (4) feedback, (5) dose, (6) progression, and (7) self-monitoring. Carr and Shepherd[157] describe many of these strategies in their book *A Motor Relearning Programme for Stroke*. The Optimal Theory proposed by Wulf and Lewthwaite stresses the importance of motivation and attention to maximize motor learning.[158] See also Chapter 10, Strategies to Improve Motor Function.

Task, Goal, and Learner

The patient's goals influence task selection. The type of task (serial, continuous) and the stage of the learner (cognitive, associative, and autonomous) also guide the intervention (see Chapter 10, Strategies to Improve Motor Function). The therapist first assists the patient in learning the desired task (cognitive stage). Explicit verbal instructions are used to direct the patient's attention to the task. Then, critical task elements and successful outcomes are identified. The desired task is demonstrated at the ideal performance speeds. The patient then begins to practice. Ideally, there should be whole task practice. If the task has a number of interrelated steps, practice of component parts may also be part of therapy (see later section Practice Schedule). The therapist should give clear, simple, and precise verbal instructions and not overload the patient with excessive or wordy instructions. There is some evidence to suggest that providing excessive information about the task can be disruptive to learning, especially for patients with MCA stroke involving the sensorimotor cortex. This interference may block formation of the implicit motor plan.[159,160] Correct performance should be reinforced, and intervention provided when movement errors become consistent (see later section Feedback). The learner is an active participant in the therapy process, reflecting on their performance while developing problem-solving strategies.

Structuring the Environment

The environment can be structured using Gentile's taxonomy.[161] Gentile's taxonomy has three organizing categories: (1) the environment conditions (open or closed environment), which also includes the environmental context (stationary or in motion: with or without intertrial variability), (2) the desired outcome of the action (body stability or body transport), and (3) manipulation (use or no use of the limbs).[145] It is a useful tool for structuring the environment relative to the task. For example, a patient practicing sitting on a plinth in a quiet room would be in a closed environment that is stationary and has no trial variability working on stability without manipulations. The addition of another support surface such as a chair or a bed would add some intertrial variability but keep the rest of the conditions the same. Giving the person a UE task in addition to the sitting would add a manipulation component.

A simplified version of the taxonomy has four categories that emphasize the environmental context and the movement goal:

1. Stationary individual in stationary environment
2. Moving individual in a stationary environment
3. Stationary individual in a moving environment
4. Moving individual in a moving environment

This hierarchy represents a guideline for progression. In the first context, a patient may be practicing sitting on a mat table in a closed treatment space; in the second, the patient may practice sitting on a therapeutic ball or the hospital bed; in the third, the patient may be sitting in a wheelchair in the PT gym; and in the fourth, the patient may be navigating the wheelchair in the PT gym. Each level increases the complexity. The first level is a stationary individual in a stationary environment with no manipulation, and in the fourth level there is a moving individual in a moving environment with manipulation.[161]

Other considerations in the environment are sounds, lighting, and interaction with other people. Persons with stroke and cognitive/perceptual deficits may initially benefit from training in a *closed environment* with limited distractions. Later, the environment can be varied, providing an appropriate level of *contextual interference*. Thus, the patient is progressed toward performing the same skill in a more *open environment*, with variable and real-life challenges. Ultimately, the closer the environmental demands of the practice setting, the greater the likelihood of transfer of skill.

Practice Schedule

Practice is essential for motor skill learning and recovery. The therapist needs to organize the patient's therapy session to ensure optimal practice. *Blocked practice* (constant repetition of a single task) is used to improve *initial* performance and motivation, especially for patients with disorganized movements. It also provides a mechanism for strengthening when you need repetition of a movement. Most hospitalized patients also initially require a *distributed practice schedule* with adequate rest periods owing to limited endurance, as both physical and cognitive fatigue can result in decreased performance. The patient should be encouraged to self-monitor practice sessions and recognize when fatigue may be setting in and rest is required. *Variable practice* (practice of more than one task within a session) using a serial or random order should begin as soon as possible. Variable practice improves performance and results in better retention of learned skills and improved ability to adapt to changing task demands. Patient, staff, and family efforts should be coordinated to ensure continued and consistent practice during off-therapy times. Practice schedules are reviewed in Chapter 10, Strategies to Improve Motor Function.

Feedback

Feedback can be intrinsic (naturally occurring as part of the movement response) or extrinsic (provided by the therapist). During early motor learning, the therapist provides extrinsic feedback (e.g., verbal cueing, manual cueing) and manual guidance to shape performance. It is important to monitor performance carefully and provide accurate feedback. The patient's attention should be directed to naturally occurring intrinsic feedback. Feedback can be provided verbally using *knowledge of performance* (KP) to address the kinematic features of the movement and *knowledge of results* (KR) to emphasize achievement of task goals. Augmented feedback can also be provided manually, using sensory input as well as manual contacts to maintain normal alignment or guide movement when the patient lacks active control or has reduced sensation. Manual techniques can be drawn from some of the neurofacilitation approaches with a clear understanding of the intent of the feedback. Great care must be taken to avoid dependence on the therapist (i.e., the patient is only able to move with the therapist's manual or verbal assistance) by providing decreasing amounts of physical guidance and augmented feedback systematically. This requires careful consideration during each treatment session. Therapists should allow the patient adequate time for introspection about the movements and available intrinsic feedback (see Table 10.5 in Chapter 10).

Dose and Progression

Therapy for persons poststroke has to be dosed with high enough intensity, be it frequency, duration, or repetitions, to achieve neuroplastic and behavioral changes.[162] The frequency, intensity, time, type (FITT) principle can guide dose considerations (see Chapters 1 and 10). Although it is challenging to achieve similar doses to those reported in the literature, the therapist has to approximate them as best as possible. Therapy needs to be challenging enough but not too difficult to discourage active participation in therapy.

Increased challenge can be achieved by using the Gentile taxonomy to progress the difficulty of the (1) environment, going from a closed to an open environment; (2) environmental context, introducing variability in the environment; (3) movement goal, from stability to mobility; and (4) manipulation, adding a manipulation component to the task. Progression can also be achieved by modifying the dose parameters of frequency, intensity, and duration. In reviewing the literature, it is important to note, where available, the dose and progression used in research studies.

Motivation and Self-Efficacy

Motivation and self-efficacy (confidence) are key to successful learning. Self-efficacy has been shown to aid in the transfer of skill from the therapeutic to the real-world setting for persons poststroke.[163] Motivational factors influence long-term engagement of the learner. This includes education about the task (purpose, effects of practice and exercise, expected outcomes) and identification of possible barriers. Providing feedback (both KP and KR, but also positive feedback) and encouragement is important to ensure motivation. Patients need to experience feelings of self-efficacy, self-control, and competence. The patient should be fully involved in collaborative goal setting from the beginning and be reminded of the goal, the task, what progress has been made, and the expected outcomes. Task salience, goal setting, and collaborative planning are key motivational techniques. Treatment sessions should include positive experiences, ensuring the patient experiences success in therapy and instilling self-confidence. Beginning and ending the therapy session on a positive note (a successful activity) is a helpful strategy. Self-efficacy ratings and summary comments can be used to monitor progress (e.g., "What successes did you achieve in therapy today?"). Supportive strategies should be discussed with family and caregivers.

Interventions to Improve Participation

Participation is best trained at the task-activity level in the environmental context where the goals are to be achieved. Often, this is not feasible, so the therapist uses the results of the movement analysis of tasks to reproduce the activities in the therapeutic setting to be as close as possible to the environmental and contextual conditions required for participation.

Participation goals may be addressed with interventions that target both cognitive and motor operations. These interventions include mental practice through motor and motivational (focusing on feelings of accomplishment) imagery, virtual environments, and dual tasking to promote cognitive motor interference.

Interventions to Improve Activities

Most of the interventions presented in this chapter are in this section on improving activities to reflect the importance of a task-based training approach. The tasks are organized as postural control and balance, locomotion and gait, UE use, functional, aerobic capacity, and physical activity. Included in this section are also relevant body function and structure interventions that support the tasks, such as increasing ROM, selective capacity of the limbs, and muscle strength. The clinician will have the patient work at the task or activity level and then move into body function and structure interventions as needed. For example, the patient will work on gait in the best environmental context and then turn to a selective LE strengthening activity or use of functional electrical stimulation as needed.

Postural Control and Balance

Postural control and balance can be viewed at both the body function and structure or the activity levels. For persons poststroke, balance training in the context of the task produces better outcomes.[162] Therefore, in this intervention section, training balance in the context of the task is illustrated along with stimulating specific postural responses that aim directly at eliciting a specific balance strategy or target a specific body function and structure impairment, such as decreased vision or proprioception.

Training at the task level begins by having the person poststroke either hold a position or move in and out of the position. Observation of the deficits will guide the intervention starting point. For example, for the person poststroke seen in an outpatient setting who is a librarian returning to work, the intervention may start with the person standing, placing books on a shelf. If that person had difficulty with the task, one intervention option is an environmental modification, lowering the height of the shelf as a way of reducing the force generation requirement for the UE and the balance demand on the LEs. The person may need additional KP cues to modify the kinematics of the movement or force generation through the LEs to modify the way the person shifts the weight. Another option would be promoting a stepping response to adjust for a loss of balance while placing the book. As a second example, for a person with a recent acute stroke, the intervention may start at the bedside observing the person's ability to hold a sitting position at the edge of the bed. The therapist focuses on identifying the patient's ability to hold the position and alignment. Often, the person poststroke may not be able to symmetrically hold or move into a position. Instruction for alignment would precede using some form of manual guidance. KP or KR is provided to guide the attainment of a safe position with the best biomechanics.

Stroke results in significant changes in postural control and balance. Patients typically exhibit delayed, varied, or absent balance responses with deficits in latency, amplitude, and timing of muscle activity. Falls and fracture can occur and lead to a loss of confidence in balance and locomotor skills.[164] It is therefore important to challenge the patient's balance while maintaining safety. The goals of training are to progressively increase the level of difficulty (e.g., range and speed of self-initiated movements) while encouraging consistency, symmetry, and maximum use of the more affected side. Supportive devices such as a posterior leg splint, gait belt, or body-weight support harness can be used to assist in early standing to promote confidence and prevent falls.

Progression for balance training can be viewed broadly as first attaining postural alignment and static stability in upright postures followed by center-of-mass (COM) control training. In sitting and standing, the patient is instructed to explore their LOS through low-frequency weight shifting. The patient learns how far in any one direction they can safely move and how to align the COM within the BOS to maintain upright stability. KP about symmetrical weight-bearing as well as activities that promote use of the more affected side are encouraged. Weight-bearing on the more affected hip (sitting) and lower limb (standing) is encouraged, while unnecessary activity of the less affected limbs (grabbing for support) is discouraged. The therapist increases the difficulty of the balance activity by manipulating the following:

- *BOS:* Sitting, Trunk training with seated balance training as well as sit-stand practice.[78] LEs uncrossed to crossed; standing, wide to narrow to tandem position; standing on one LE (beginning with less affected, progressing to more affected LE)
- *Support surface:* Sitting on a mat to sitting on a therapy ball; standing on the floor to standing on dense foam, standing on woodchips, standing on a moving surface[78]
- *Sensory inputs:* Eyes open to eyes closed; feet on firm surface or foam
- *UE position/support:* Light touchdown support; UEs extended out to the side to UEs folded across the chest
- *UE movements:* Single UE raises to bilateral UE raises (symmetrical, asymmetrical); reaching movements with emphasis to the more affected side; picking objects off table, stool, floor
- *LE movements:* Single LE support, stepping (forward-backward, side; step-ups); marching in place; foot on ball, moving ball
- *Trunk movements:* Head and trunk rotations; looking up at ceiling or down to floor
- *Destabilizing functional activities:* Sit to stand, sit down, turning, floor to standing, lunges[162]
- *Walking activities:* Forward, backward, sideward, crossed step[162,165]
- *Dual-task training (combined motor-cognitive dual tasks):* Standing while catching or kicking a ball; standing while talking; standing while holding a tray with a glass of water;[166,167] combined motor-cognitive dual tasks[168]
- *Other activities:* Tai Chi, bicycling and during the late phase of stroke complemented with virtual reality, force platform biofeedback, and aquatic balance activities[78]
- *Modifying environmental conditions:* Closed to open environments

Postural strategy training is an important component of intervention. Ankle strategies can be promoted through small-range anterior–posterior shifts or by applying a small perturbation at the hips (forward-backward). Standing on a half-foam roller or wobble board also promotes ankle strategies but may be too advanced for some patients during early rehabilitation. Hip strategies can be promoted through larger anterior–posterior shifts or stronger perturbations.

Medial–lateral hip strategies are promoted by tandem stance (on floor or half-foam roller). Stepping strategies are promoted by increased displacements of the COM (e.g., forward, backward, or sideward leans that move the COM outside of the BOS). The therapist can apply an elastic band around the hips, offering resistance to the forward lean. Resistance that is quickly released once the patient achieves the desired lean will necessitate a step to control balance. Step-ups (small step to large; foam surface) should also be practiced.

The therapist provides well-timed feedback to help the patient correct alignment and adjust postural control. During balance training, the patient should be encouraged to actively problem-solve. The patient is presented with challenges, identifies potential problems, and recruits safe strategies to maintain balance. Adaptability of skills needed for successful community reentry is promoted. Safety education about fall prevention and fall recovery is a critical factor in ensuring maintenance of the patient's hard-won functional independence.[169]

Research supports the effectiveness of balance training programs in improving balance ability for patients with stroke. Review of balance training for persons in the chronic phase poststroke showed that balance can be improved after treatment measured by the Berg Balance Scale (BBS), Functional Reach (FR), and Sensory Organization Test (SOT). Those gains were retained for the BBS but not for the SOT, suggesting that the participants may have compensated rather than changed their underlying strategy or acquired a new skill.[165] There was too much variability in the type of training to propose a dose. However, training performed in the context of the task is more efficient than balance training in isolation. Both one-on-one training and group programs have produced positive results. Finally, there is limited evidence that balance performance may deteriorate once the intervention is stopped.[170,171]

Training With Visual Feedback

The use of visual feedback has been shown to improve balance in persons poststroke. The patient's balance is detected either with a force platform represented as their center of pressure or with motion-sensing equipment represented as an avatar in a virtual environment.

Force platform biofeedback (center-of-pressure biofeedback) promotes practice of voluntary movement shifts in response to computer-generated visual feedback. Patients can also practice responding to unexpected platform tilts (perturbations) in order to improve reactive balance control. A safety harness may be required during early training; holding on with one or both hands is discouraged. Improvements with biofeedback/forceplate training have been found in steadiness (reduced sway),[172,173] postural symmetry,[172,173] and dynamic stability.[173–175] There is very limited evidence of carryover of improved balance during functional skills, specifically transfer skills and endurance,[175] FR, and measures of ADL and mobility.[173] Carryover to improved locomotor performance has not been demonstrated.[172,175] Failure to find significant correlations to gait is most likely related to specificity of training, specifically a dissimilarity between training mode and outcome measure.

Virtual reality, such as noncustom video games and customized virtual environments coupled with TMs, and video games played on a Nintendo Wii console, have been tested for rehabilitation of postural control and activity level balance.[176] They offer a form of visual feedback that is coupled with gamification. There is a small but consistent benefit for VR and video games compared to an active control when measuring balance with the BBS and the Timed Up and Go test. The improvement, however, did not reach the MCID.[177,178] In a review that compared the efficacy between off-the-shelf games and customized systems for persons in the chronic phase poststroke, it was found that customized systems are superior to noncustom VR.[177] VR and video games may be an appropriate tool to engage a subset of persons poststroke for balance training.

The Patient With Ipsilateral Pushing (Pusher Syndrome)

The patient with ipsilateral pushing presents with an entirely different set of postural control and balance problems. The patient sits or stands asymmetrically but with most of the weight shifted toward the weaker side. The patient uses the stronger UE or LE to push over to the weaker side, often resulting in instability and falls. Efforts by the therapist to passively correct the patient's tilted posture often result in the patient pushing more forcefully. Training needs to emphasize upright positions with *active* movement shifts toward the stronger side. Use of visual stimuli is effective, as patients retain the ability to correct posture with such stimuli but may not be able to do so spontaneously. Visual mirror feedback and a computer-generated interactive visual feedback both have shown their ability to reduce contraversive pushing.[179] Patients should be asked to look at their posture and see if they are upright. It is important to emphasize that the patient orient to their midline.[180] Environmental prompts can be used to assist orientation. These can include use of a mirror if visuospatial deficits are not present or vertical structures in the environment. For example, the therapist can sit on the patient's less involved side and instruct the patient to "lean over to me." Or the patient can be positioned with the stronger side next to a wall and instructed to "lean toward the wall."[102]

Therapists can provide verbal and tactile cues for postural orientation. To improve sitting posture, training activities can include sitting on a therapy ball to promote symmetry and sitting. In early standing, the weaker LE is often flexed and has difficulty supporting the body on that side. Extension can be assisted using an air splint or a posterior leg splint or by direct tapping over the quadriceps muscle. The modified plantigrade position is effective for early supported standing; however, the therapist should focus on unilateral support using the weaker UE. Again, an air splint can be used to assist extension of the weaker arm. If a cane is used, it can be shortened to encourage weight shift to the stronger side. An environmental boundary can be used to achieve symmetrical standing (e.g., standing in a doorway or corner standing). It is important to limit pushing with the sound extremities. For example, in sitting or standing, the therapist should block the stronger limb from drifting laterally into abduction and extension and pushing.[181,182] During wheelchair sitting, the patient should be assisted to maintain upright posture and midline orientation.

Motor learning strategies are very effective in reducing the effects of this disorder and enhancing recovery. In particular, the therapist should demonstrate correct orientation to vertical, provide consistent feedback about body orientation, and practice correct orientation and weight shifts. The patient should be fully involved in problem-solving. For example, the therapist should ask questions such as "What direction are you tilted?" and "What direction do you have to move in order to achieve vertical?" Karnath et al.[100] indicated that the prognosis for recovery is good with effective training.

Interventions to Improve Gait and Locomotion

Improving gait for persons poststroke can be addressed in several ways: task- and goal-oriented training, specific overground locomotor training (LT), LT using a motorized TM, TM training aided by a harness (body weight–supported treadmill training [BWSTT]), robotic-assisted LT, high-intensity stepping, functional electrical stimulation, and motor imagery (MI) and VR. Additional strategies include rhythmic auditory cueing, community-based training, circuit training, LE strengthening, management of LE spasticity, improving LE ROM, and standing balance practice. Varying levels of evidence support each approach. In this section, the approaches and supporting evidence (and wherever possible differentiating based on level of acuity) are provided.

Task- and Goal-Oriented Treadmill and Overground Locomotor Training at Moderate to High Intensity

Task-specific and goal-oriented training focuses on practicing walking to improve speed and endurance.[78,79,103] Task practice needs to be repetitive, adapted, and at a moderate to high intensity that is measured with repetitions and a target HR.[72] CPGs from multiple countries give LT at a moderate to high intensity their highest recommendation. The ANPT Guideline specifies that for persons in the chronic phase poststroke (greater than 6 months), the training take place at moderate to high intensity of 60% to 80% of HR reserve.[72] There are challenges to achieving this level of intensity, and the patient needs to be carefully monitored for safety. The ANPT has created many resources for implementing this recommendation (e.g., case scenarios, recommendations for HR monitors, and tools for tracking training). The resources can be found at https://www.neuropt.org/practice-resources/best-practice-initiatives-and-resources/intensity_matters.

In an RCT conducted with persons between 1 and 6 months poststroke, a high-intensity group was compared to a usual-care group where each received 40 sessions over 10 weeks. The first week consisted of walking on a body weight–support (BWS) treadmill with assist for the swing phase of gait. Nylon straps were used to stabilize the pelvis as necessary to ensure successful stepping. Successful stepping was defined as positive step lengths, lack of stance-phase limb collapse, and sagittal/frontal plane stability. After the second week, variability was the focus, alternating approximately every 10 minutes between speed-dependent treadmill training (TT) (at 70% to 80% HR reserve and RPE ≥14), skill-dependent (e.g., perturbations, obstacles, weights) TT, overground training (high speeds or variable tasks), and stair climbing. Walking speed and distance as well as steps in community were greater for the high-intensity group.[183] Most recently this group has compared high-intensity stepping with training in variable contexts to high-intensity stepping and forward walking and low-intensity variable training. They report that all groups increased their stepping activity. However, the group that trained at high intensity in variable contexts also saw an increase in balance confidence.[184] This type of therapy is promising, and there have been reports of it implemented in inpatient rehabilitation.[185]

Overground activities include functional, task-specific skills, such as the following:

- Walking in all directions
- Walking on different surfaces
- Stair climbing, step-over-step
- Walking in a community environment: Walking on ramps, curbs, uneven terrain, over and around obstacles
- Activities that involve coincident timing: Crossing at a streetlight, stepping on and off elevators or escalators, walking through automatic doors
- Dual-task activities: Walking while holding a ball, bouncing a ball, carrying a tray, carrying on a conversation

In a systematic review of 19 RCTs that included 1,008 persons poststroke, task-based training decreased anxiety for persons poststroke who are walking independently.[162] Outcomes for walking distance, walking ability, and balance differed depending on level of recovery. Persons in the chronic phase poststroke were able to improve walking distance and walking ability but not balance. Persons in the subacute phase were able to improve balance and walking ability but not walking distance. Persons in the acute phase did not improve at all.[162] This finding highlights the relevance of phase of recovery when selecting an intervention. Persons in the earlier recovery phases may have lacked the capacity to engage in overground walking activities. In addition, given the open-loop nature of these tasks, it may be difficult for some patients to achieve a high intensity of training. The greatest challenge with this task-based approach is to provide a high enough training intensity protocol, particularly to persons in the early recovery poststroke.

Locomotor Training Using a Treadmill Without Body Weight Support

LT on a TM without using a harness for support has been shown (in 16 RCTS with a total of 610 participants) to improve maximum gait speed and temporal-spatial parameters of gait for persons in all phases of recovery.[162] The ability to increase walking speed on the TM resulted in gait speed improvement as well as an increase in step width. The TM offers the advantage of progressing parameters of speed and distance systematically. Investigators are exploring how to best combine overground walking with TT.[186]

Locomotor Training Using Body Weight Support and Treadmill Training

BWS and motorized TT allows the clinician to use a closed-loop training environment to improve recovery of walking ability after stroke using intensive task-oriented training. Normal kinematics and phase relationships of the full gait cycle are promoted, including limb loading in midstance and unweighting and stepping during swing. Initially, manual assistance can be provided by trainers to normalize gait in the presence of muscle weakness and impaired balance. For example, one therapist provides manual assistance to foot placement during stepping movements of the weaker LE while a second therapist stands behind the patient and provides manual assistance to pelvic rotation movements (Fig. 15.6). An overhead harness is used to support a portion of the patient's weight (e.g., 30% progressing down to 20%, then 10%). The harness controls the upright position of the patient in the absence of good postural stability and reduces fear of falling. The use of a harness also eliminates the need for adaptive UE support to compensate for LE weakness (e.g., as seen with the use of a walker). As improvements in walking occur, the harness is removed, and full weight-bearing is allowed. At this point, the patient is practicing supervised walking on a TM. Initially the TM speeds are slow (e.g., 0.52 mph [0.23 m/sec]) and are gradually increased as the patient's walking ability is improved (e.g., 2.6 mph [1.2 m/sec]). Progression is to task-specific practice and overground walking.

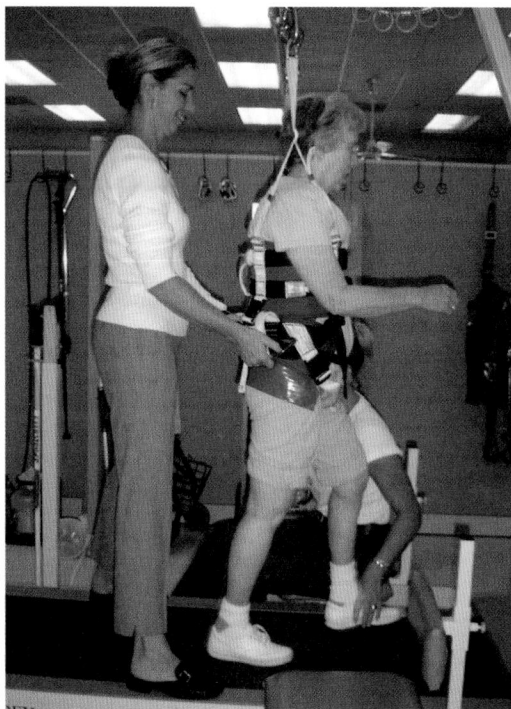

Figure 15.6 Locomotor training using body-weight support and a motorized treadmill. One therapist manually assists pelvic motions while a second therapist assists stepping of the hemiparetic left lower extremity.

TT and BWS is a relatively safe task-oriented LT activity that has been extensively studied in patients recovering from stroke in both the subacute and chronic phases.[187–193] In the stroke guidelines from Australia and New Zealand, they give the use of the treadmill with and without BWS a strong recommendation. This is based on 28 studies with a total of 1,680 participants who favor the use of the treadmill with and without BWS to increase walking endurance, and 47 studies with 4,343 participants showing improvements in gait speed.[79] A Cochrane review that informed this recommendation reported gait speed improvements of 0.06 m/s for those who needed assistance while walking and of 0.08 m/s for those who were walking independently. The authors concluded that the greatest benefits are for those individuals poststroke who are already walking.[62] Another review that compared treadmill walking to overground walking speed (0.07 m/s) and distances (18 m) were found to be similar or somewhat better for treadmill walking.[194] TT appears to be a safe intervention for patients with acute and subacute stroke as well as for chronic stroke.

Electromechanically Assisted Locomotor Training

Electromechanical, robotic-assisted LT is used in rehabilitation to improve walking after stroke, especially when participants are in the early phase of recovery and cannot engage in overground walking. In a recent Cochrane Systematic Database review, Mehrholz et al.[61] reviewed 62 trials involving 2,440 participants. They determined that when combined with conventional physiotherapy, these devices were found to increase the odds of patients becoming independent walkers. This was particularly true for patients in the first 3 months poststroke or those later on who were still not able to walk. Electromechanical-assisted gait training appears to be most beneficial for persons early in their recovery who are dependent in walking and should not be the only form of gait training.[78]

Functional Electrical Stimulation and Ankle-Foot Orthosis

The ANPT recently published a guideline on the use of functional electrical stimulation *(FES)* and ankle-foot orthoses (AFOs) for persons in the acute and chronic phases poststroke.[73] They reviewed 122 meta-analyses, SRs, RCTs, and cohort studies to make their recommendations. There were eight action statements related to their use across the ICF. AFOs and FES should be used to increase gait speed, mobility, and dynamic balance, and improve QOL. For persons in the chronic phase poststroke, FES should be used for both muscle activation and walking endurance. They stated that AFOs and FES may be used to improve walking endurance for persons in the acute phase poststroke and may be used to improve gait kinematics. Importantly, AFOs and FES should *not* be used to reduce tone or plantar flexor spasticity. Interestingly, FES may not be superior to an AFO, but it is believed to have greater therapeutic effects, while AFOs may promote greater compensatory effects. (See Box 15.4 for a summary of the recommendations.) Specific recommendations on dose for each application can be found here: https://www.neuropt.org/practice-resources/anpt-clinical-practice-guidelines/AFO_FES-post-stroke/afo-fes-action-statements.

FES can be used to stimulate dorsiflexor function and improve the gait pattern of patients with drop foot. Sufficient strength in the quadriceps muscle is needed to prevent the knee from buckling. This requirement limits the number of patients who can successfully use the device. The patient wears a small, lightweight cuff that fits just below the knee. Electrodes are positioned to stimulate the anterior tibialis and the peroneus longus muscles. A gait sensor attaches to the patient's shoe and transmits a wireless signal to the stimulator. The level of stimulation can be adjusted by a handheld remote control, which also allows the patient to turn the device off and on. The device can be used as a bridge to the recovery of normal motor function or, in the absence of recovery, can be used indefinitely as an orthotic. FES training should be paired with a comprehensive physical therapy POC. FES is theorized to have a positive effect on brain plasticity with its provision of high-level sensory-motor input into the CNS.[195]

Box 15.4 Summary of Academy of Neurologic Physical Therapy Recommendations for Use of Functional Electrical Stimulation and Ankle-Foot Orthoses

For persons with poststroke hemiplegia:

- **To Improve QOL:** Clinicians *should* provide AFO or FES for persons with foot drop as a result of *chronic* hemiplegia.
- **To Improve Gait Speed:** Clinicians *should* provide AFO or FES for persons with decreased LE motor control as a result of *acute or chronic* hemiplegia.
- **To Improve Other Mobility:** Clinicians *should* provide AFO or FES for persons with decreased LE motor control as a result of *acute or chronic* hemiplegia.
- **To Improve Dynamic Balance:** Clinicians *should* provide AFO or FES for persons with decreased LE motor control as a result of *acute or chronic* hemiplegia.
- **To Improve Walking Endurance:** Clinicians *may* provide AFO or FES for persons with decreased LE motor control as a result of *acute* hemiplegia. Clinicians *should* provide AFO or FES for persons with decreased LE motor control as a result of *chronic* hemiplegia.
- **To Improve Plantarflexor Spasticity:** Clinicians *should **not*** provide AFO or FES for persons with decreased LE motor control as a result of acute or chronic hemiplegia.
- **To Improve Muscle Activation:** Clinicians *may* provide an AFO with decreased stiffness for persons with decreased LE motor control as a result of acute or chronic hemiplegia to allow muscle activation while walking with an AFO. Clinician *should* provide FES for persons with decreased LE motor control as a result of chronic hemiplegia who have goals to improve activation of the anterior tibialis muscle while walking without FES.
- **To Improve Gait Kinematics:** Clinicians *may* provide AFO for persons with acute or chronic hemiplegia with goals to improve ankle dorsiflexion at initial contact and during swing and loading response. Clinicians *may* provide FES for persons with chronic hemiplegia with the same goals.

For more information on sources of evidence, recommended outcome measures, guidance on dose, and tips for practice, visit https://www.neuropt.org/practice-resources/anpt-clinical-practice-guidelines/AFO_FES-post-stroke/afo-fes-action-statements

AFO = ankle-foot orthoses; FES = functional electrical stimulation.

Motor Imagery and Virtual Reality

MI and *VR* using video games allow simulation of real-world environments for walking training. MI is recommended as an adjunct to LE training, and VR is recommended as an adjunct to gait training.[78] Imagining walking has been studied at the strategy level and the task level.[196–198] At the strategy level, individuals poststroke imagined walking and changing the kinematics and kinetics of their movement, for example, loading the affected LE and taking a larger step with the less affected extremity. This type of training improved gait speed.[196] In a second study, the training was done at the task level. Persons poststroke had to imagine themselves walking in different environments with an emphasis on the task. This intervention resulted in an increased gait speed but no significant increase on falls self-efficacy when compared to the active control group that engaged in an UE intervention.[197]

In a final study from the same group, the therapy was delivered in the home combining physical practice plus MI. The therapy was customized to the participant and included walking inside and outside the home. The clinician first observed the task performed and then adjusted the cues for the intervention. There were cues for movement as well as increasing self-efficacy. For example, the participant was observed walking in

their home environment that required stair climbing to get from the basement to the kitchen. On the stairs, the participant tripped and was helped by the caregiver to maintain balance. During the imagery practice, the participant imagined tripping and then successfully catching themselves without assistance. Then the participant imagined feeling good about having overcome the "tripping." This type of motivational imagery aids with increasing confidence. The therapy that was delivered using a combination of in-person and telerehabilitation sessions was found to be feasible.[198] The appeal of MI is that it is portable and low cost. To use this intervention, it is important to determine that the person poststroke is able to imagine. This can be assessed by administering the Kinesthetic and Visual Imagery Questionnaire (KVIQ), which has been validated for persons poststroke.[199,200]

As with balance training, gait training with VR has been implemented with a TM coupled to a virtual environment, off-the-shelf video games, and specialized systems.[176] A Cochrane review did not find evidence to support VR for gait speed.[69] However, other high-quality SRs have found there has been a small but consistent effect favoring VR (both semi-immersive and immersive systems) for improving gait speed.[177,201] This finding applies to persons in the subacute and chronic phases poststroke. The ANPT CPG on interventions for locomotor recovery in people with chronic neurological health conditions also strongly recommends virtual reality.[72] The challenge with this technology currently is that some of the systems are not available in the clinic. However, this is an area of rapid development, and transfer of the technology to the clinic is accelerating.

Orthotics for the Lower Extremity

Orthotics and assistive devices are compensations for lack of active control and balance. An orthosis may be required when persistent problems prevent safe ambulation (e.g., inadequate ankle dorsiflexion during swing, mediolateral ankle instability, and insufficient push-off during late stance). Orthotic prescription will depend on the unique problems each patient presents. The pattern of instability and weakness at the ankle and knee and the extent and severity of spasticity and sensory deficits of the limb are major considerations when prescribing an orthosis. Temporary devices (e.g., dorsiflexor assists) may be used during the early stages while recovery is proceeding to allow the patient to practice standing and walking. Use of a temporary orthosis also provides insight into the type of components that will most effectively address the patient's needs. Permanent devices are prescribed once the patient's status stabilizes. Consultation with a certified orthotist and clinic team is initiated if a permanent orthosis is needed.

- *Foot–ankle controls:* An *AFO* is commonly prescribed to control impaired ankle-foot function. Examples include a custom-molded polypropylene AFO *(posterior leaf spring [PLS], modified AFO, or solid ankle AFO)* or *conventional double upright/dual channel AFO.* The least restrictive AFO is the PLS used to control drop foot. An AFO of higher-density plastic that covers more surface area can provide additional control of calcaneal and forefoot inversion and eversion. A solid ankle-molded AFO provides maximum stabilization through its lateral trim lines that project more anteriorly. Movement in all planes (dorsiflexion, plantarflexion, inversion, and eversion) is limited. The conventional double upright metal AFO may be indicated for patients who cannot tolerate plastic AFOs owing to sensory impairments, girth fluctuations, or diabetic neuropathy or who require additional controls. A posterior stop can be added to limit plantarflexion, while a spring assist can be added to assist dorsiflexion (Klenzak joint). Advantages of a conventional AFO include better stabilization of the ankle, allowing improved heel-strike and push-off. Disadvantages include heavier weight, less cosmetic appearance, and increased difficulty donning and doffing. Please see the earlier section on the CPG recommendations under FES for additional guidance on application of AFOs.

- *Knee controls:* Knee instability following stroke can be controlled with an AFO by adjusting the position of the ankle. An ankle set in 5° dorsiflexion limits knee hyperextension, whereas an ankle set in 5° plantarflexion decreases the flexor moment and stabilizes the knee during midstance. A patient with knee hyperextension without foot and/or ankle instability may benefit from the application of a *Swedish Knee Cage* or strapping to protect the knee. Extensive bracing using a knee-AFO (KAFO) is rarely indicated or successful. The added weight and restrictions in normal knee joint motion significantly increase energy costs and limit independent function.

The need for an orthosis or a particular type of orthosis may change with continuing recovery. The therapist may need to recommend a change in prescription or discontinuing the use of a device. With limited reimbursements, ordering a new orthosis may prove problematic and speaks to the need to anticipate changes when ordering the initial device. For example, a good option for the patient who needs a custom-molded solid AFO is to order a hinged AFO with a plantarflexion stop. As the patient regains sufficient knee and dorsiflexor control, the device can be adjusted to remove the stop and allow the hinges to work. Orthotic training includes donning and doffing, skin inspections, and education in safe use of the device during gait. See Chapter 30, Orthotics, for a more complete description of orthotic devices, examination, and training.

Wheelchairs

Many persons poststroke require the use of a wheelchair for mobility at some point during their recovery. Persons with stroke exhibit postural asymmetries, which need to be carefully evaluated. These include the following:

- Trunk laterally flexed to the weaker side; head may also be flexed to the weaker side.
- Pelvic posterior tilt with some obliquity (lower on the unaffected side).
- LE rolled out into abduction and external rotation; if spasticity is present, increased hip extension, adduction, and internal rotation with knee extension may occur; foot is typically plantarflexed and inverted.
- UE held flexed and adducted to the trunk with increased elbow, wrist, and finger flexion. With flaccidity, the shoulder is subluxed with the hand dangling in a dependent position.

Positioning in a wheelchair needs to correct for these postural asymmetries and ensure correct sitting posture. Refer to Chapter 32, Seating and Wheeled Mobility, for a more complete discussion of general principles of prescription and wheelchair adaptations.

Interventions to Improve Upper Extremity Use

Interventions to improve the use of the UEs involve task-specific training and deliberate use of the UE with whole skills required for ADL as well as the management of musculoskeletal impairments, sensory retraining, strengthening, improvement of selective capacity, and noninvasive brain stimulation.[78] These interventions may be done in collaboration with the occupational therapist. Patients with MCA syndrome may exhibit severe sensory, motor, and functional impairments of the UE with limited recovery. These patients benefit from early mobilization, ROM, and positioning strategies. Compensatory training strategies and environmental adaptations should be considered to maximize function. For patients who achieve some recovery of voluntary movement, training strategies should focus on repetitive, task-specific practice. The tasks selected should be relevant and important to the patient (e.g., reaching and manipulation, walking with devices, stair climbing). UE training activities may be closely coordinated with the occupational therapist.

Algorithm for Selecting Upper Extremity Interventions

An international multidisciplinary group of experts in UE recovery poststroke has developed a smartphone application—the ViaTherapy app—using an algorithm to guide UE rehabilitation[202] (see Fig. 15.7). The algorithm is based on the shoulder abduction finger extension model.[203,204] This model has shown that in those persons poststroke demonstrating some voluntary finger extension and some visible shoulder abduction on day 2 after stroke had a 98% probability of achieving UE function. A number of patients do not develop the finger extension in the first 2 days but do so in the first 12 weeks poststroke. For this reason, the 12-week period poststroke is used as the first question in the algorithm (dividing interventions based on this time frame). The ViaTherapy app can be downloaded for free in the app store or found online (https://www.viatherapy.org). It guides management of the UE with task-specific training as well as management of body function and structure deficits.

Several questions guide the user on how to select interventions (see Fig. 15.7):

1. Is the person within the first 12 weeks of stroke onset? (If the answer is YES, the interventions are found in boxes 1 to 4; if the answer is NOT YET, the interventions are found in boxes 5 to 8.)
2. Does the patient have shoulder pain or is at high risk for shoulder pain?
3. The following three questions refine the search:
   a. Can the patient produce voluntary activity of the upper limb?
   b. In the seated position, can the patient produce any shoulder abduction against gravity and/or produce any elbow abduction against gravity?
   c. With the forearm prone on the table and hands and fingers unsupported, can the patient initiate finger and/or thumb extension three times within a minute?

Responses to these questions will take the user to the appropriate box containing a list of interventions that have been rated with an A if there is at least one RCT. There is also a star rating (with four being the highest rating) based on expert opinion that takes into account time, equipment required, and ease of use. Treatment dose is offered and is based on the references reviewed. The references supporting the recommendations are available in the app. Outcome measures are also suggested. To guide the clinician in deciding if the intervention is suitable for the patient, the app reports both on who has not been studied and on the exclusion criteria for specific interventions. For each intervention (e.g., strengthening), there is a description of the benefits, who the intervention is for, dose, whether it can be performed in groups and self-administered. Finally, because shoulder pain can occur with persons poststroke at many phases of recovery, management is presented in a separate box (box 9 in Fig. 15.7), which can apply to any patient.

In the absence of voluntary movement, most of the interventions are the same for the first 12 weeks after the stroke (box 1) and beyond 12 weeks (box 5). These interventions involve maintaining ROM, preventing or managing edema, sensory retraining, managing spasticity, positioning, patient education, eliciting movement by using imagery, mirror therapy and electrical stimulation, patient education, providing supportive devices, and teaching compensatory techniques. As the person poststroke acquires movement, some of the interventions are discontinued and others are added. For example, task-specific training is proposed when there is some active shoulder movement starting in boxes 3 and 7, and constraint-induced movement therapy applies only once people have some active finger movement applying only to boxes 4 and 8. Any patient who presents with shoulder pain can be managed with the recommended interventions in box 9.

Task-Specific Training for the Upper Extremity

Task-specific training is included in boxes 3, 4, 7, and 8 of the ViaTherapy app's upper limb algorithm (Fig. 15.7). This suggests that some active control is required for task-specific training of the UE. The UE can be used as a stabilizer, an assist, and a manipulator. During a reaching movement, the hand is transported by the arm. During that trajectory, the hand, as the distal effector, begins to assume the shape it needs in order to grasp an objective. Van Vliet's work has shown that a functional task modifies the kinematics of the reach and grasp in persons poststroke.[205] This suggests that reaching tasks should be done with meaningful objects.

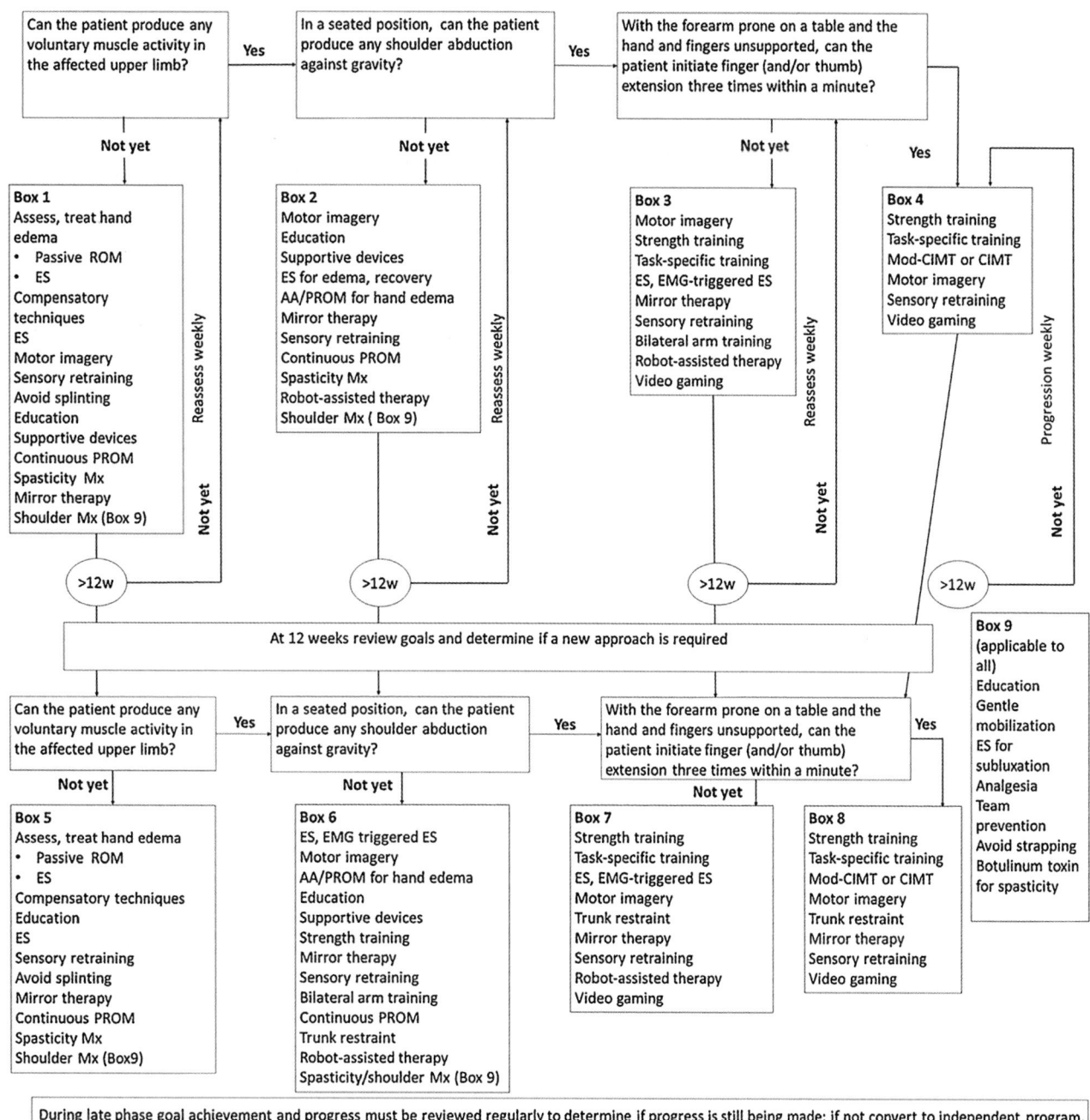

Figure 15.7 Algorithm for selecting upper extremity interventions. *(From Wolf SL, et al. Group upper extremity stroke algorithm working. Best practice for arm recovery poststroke: an international application. Physiotherapy. 2016;102(1):1, with permission.)*

Task-specific training can be done in concert with reducing the synergistic postures. This can be done by promoting a postural shift toward the more affected side using the arm as a stabilizer by weight-bearing on the extended arm and stabilized hand on a support surface. This early activity promotes proximal stabilization and counteracts the effects of excess flexor hypertonus and a dominant flexion synergy. Approximation can be used to increase activity of shoulder/scapular stabilizers. Weight-bearing activities are performed in sitting (Fig. 15.8) and standing positions. Control may progress from holding to dynamic stabilization activities. For example, the patient stabilizes with the more affected UE while performing weight shifts and functional tasks with the stronger UE (e.g., reaching). The more affected UE should also be recruited for postural assistance during functional training activities (e.g., pushing up from side-lying into sitting).[206]

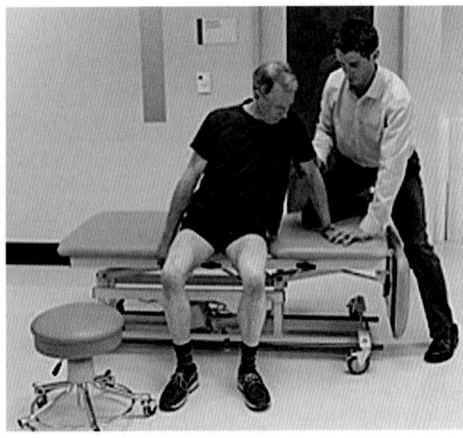

Figure 15.8 Sitting with extended arm support. The therapist assists in stabilizing the elbow and fingers in extension.

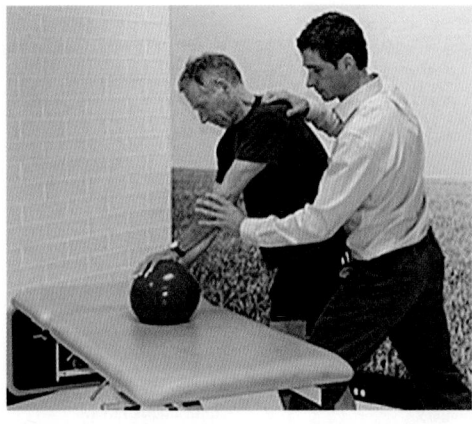

Figure 15.9 Standing in modified plantigrade with hemiparetic hand positioned on small ball. The patient practices rolling the ball from side to side; the therapist stabilizes the elbow and shoulder.

Patients with stroke have difficulty regaining control of scapular upward rotation and protraction, elbow extension, and wrist and finger extension necessary for forward reach and manipulation. Reaching and manipulation also require accurate processing and use of visual–perceptual information. Patients with limited voluntary control can practice initial reaching in a supported position (e.g., side-lying with arm supported by therapist or on a powder board, sitting with the UE resting on a tabletop). A cloth can be used to decrease friction effects as the patient practices wiping or polishing a table. The patient can also practice reaching forward and downward touching the floor. More advanced reaching activities include independent lifting and reaching forward (e.g., UE placed into a shirt sleeve). Combining reaching with increased balance challenges in modified plantigrade or standing should also be incorporated. For example, the patient can practice pushing a ball side to side or forward and backward while standing in modified plantigrade (Fig. 15.9). Or in standing, the patient can practice reaching to pick an object up off a shelf, a low stool, or the floor. Varying the height and distance reached, increasing the weight of objects held in the hand, or increasing the speed and accuracy requirements can increase difficulty. Substitution movements (e.g., trunk or head lateral movements) or excessive shoulder elevation should be discouraged.[206]

Meaningful task-oriented practice involving grasp and manipulation is important for stimulating recovery. Initial hand movements typically include gross grasp and release while advanced hand patterns (fine motor control) may not be present unless there is more advanced recovery. Voluntary release is generally much more difficult to achieve than voluntary grasp and stretching/positioning, and inhibitory techniques may be necessary to facilitate extension movements. Initial hand tasks can include using the more affected hand to stabilize (e.g., hand stabilizes paper while the stronger hand writes, hand stabilizes food while the stronger hand cuts) or holding a book with both hands for reading. The patient should be encouraged to use the weaker hand to assist in ADL (e.g., washing the upper body with a washcloth, bringing food to mouth). Forks, toothbrushes, and pens may need to have built-up handles for grasp. Task training should combine reach patterns with hand activity (e.g., picking sock up off floor, reaching for an object off a shelf). Advanced hand activities include practice of wrist and finger extension, opposition, and manipulation of objects (e.g., using utensils to eat; drinking from a cup; writing; picking up and reorienting coins, paper clips, or other objects). Pronation often predominates, whereas active supination without elbow and shoulder flexion is difficult to achieve. The therapist must observe movements carefully and assist in eliminating those aspects of movement patterns that interfere with effective and efficient control. Graded physical assist and use of mental practice/imagery techniques can be helpful to improve learning and performance.[206,207]

Constraint-Induced Movement Therapy

CIMT is a multifaceted intervention designed to promote increased use of the more affected UE. The patient is engaged in intense task-oriented practice of the more affected UE for up to 6 hr a day, performed on consecutive weekdays for 10 to 15 days (Fig. 15.10). The less affected UE is restrained from use by having the patient wear a safety mitt for up to 90% of waking hours.[208] The therapist uses shaping techniques to modify and progress performance (e.g., an object is lifted and placed at increasing distances away from the patient). Feedback, coaching, modeling, and encouragement are provided during practice. Behavioral methods designed to ensure

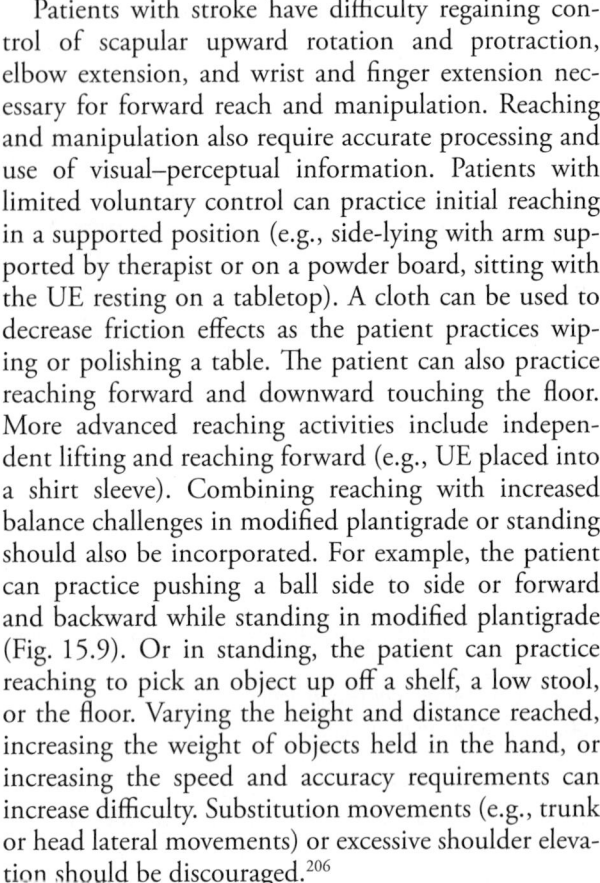

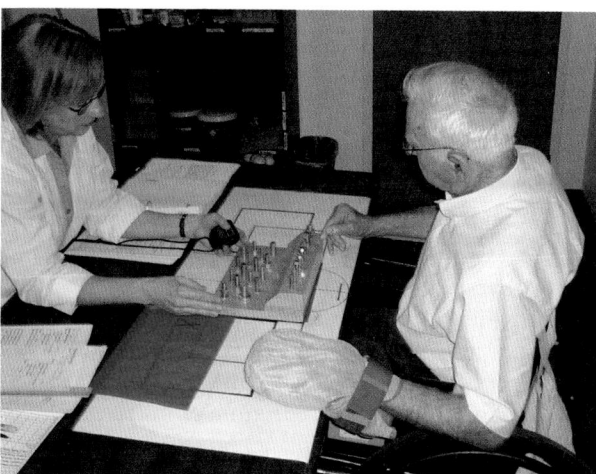

Figure 15.10 Constraint-induced movement therapy (CIMT). The patient practices a pegboard task using the hemiparetic hand while the less affected hand wears a mitt. The therapist times the activity while encouraging the patient.

adherence to exercise and develop task-oriented behaviors include engaging the patient in the following:

- Self-monitoring of target behaviors (e.g., mode of activity, duration, frequency, perceived exertion, and overall response to activity)
- Problem-solving to identify obstacles and generate potential solutions
- Behavioral contracting to engage the patient in carrying out behaviors throughout the day
- Social support strategies to educate and enlist caregivers in providing optimal support

Refer to the work of Mark and Taub[208] for a more complete description of these techniques. *Modified CIMT* (mCIMT) has also been used for patients with stroke. For example, Page et al.[209,210] used 30 minutes of functional task practice and shaping techniques 3 days per week and restraint of the less affected UE for up to 5 hr per day. Training occurred over an extended 10-week period. This outpatient protocol increased the use and function of the more affected arm.[209,210]

Limited gains in motor function but not a reduction in disability following CIMT have been demonstrated in patients with stroke.[211] The *EXCITE trial* was a large prospective, single-blind, randomized, multisite study that included 222 patients after stroke. CIMT was compared to customary care and found to significantly improve outcomes as measured by the Wolf Motor Function Test and the MAL.[212] Associated changes in brain organization with CIMT have also been demonstrated on functional magnetic resonance imaging (fMRI), including an apparent shift in motor cortical activation toward other ipsilateral areas and the contralesional hemisphere.[213] Gains have also

been reported in the patients receiving mCIMT.[209,210] It is important to note that patients were included in the studies if they had potential for recovery and some residual upper arm and hand movement (active wrist and finger extension) but tended not to use the arm. Limited pain or spasticity and absence of cognitive impairment were also inclusion criteria. Many early studies involved patients with chronic stroke (greater than 1 year). Evidence also exists for positive results with patients with subacute stroke (less than 1 year)[212] and patients with acute stroke (less than 2 weeks).[214] The Cochrane researchers in their most recent review of the literature concluded that the evidence supported limited improvements after CIMT in motor function and motor impairment, but these benefits did not reduce disability. Studies showing long-term benefits are also limited.[211]

In contrast, another review, which separated CIMT into three categories—(1) original CIMT, (2) high-intensity mCIMT, and (3) low-intensity mCIMT—reported gains. Specifically, the original CIMT (based on 41 RCTs and 1,342 participants) showed positive effects for arm–hand activities, self-reported a significant increase in amount of arm–hand use in daily life, and self-reported quality of arm–hand movements in daily life.[215(p11)] The high-intensity mCIMT (based on 17 RCTs and 512 subjects) found a significant increase in the amount of arm–hand use in daily life and self-reported arm–hand quality and quantity. These effects were found for participants early after stroke but not for those in the chronic phase.[215] For the low-intensity mCIMT (23 RCTs with 627 participants), there were positive effects for motor function of the paretic arm, arm–hand activities, self-reported amount of use, and quality in daily life and basic ADL. These findings applied to those who were early in rehabilitation and chronic but not to those in between.[162] CIMT is a therapy that has been extensively studied and has several variations. It is becoming easier to know what changes occur and where in the recovery patients benefit from the different types of CIMT therapy.

Electrical Stimulation

Electrical stimulation of the peripheral nerves and muscles with external electrodes has been applied to the UEs of persons poststroke while performing selected movements as well as task-based movements.[216] It can take the form of neuromuscular electrical stimulation (NMES) or EMG-triggered NMES, both of which have been used with persons recovering from stroke to reduce spasticity, improve sensory awareness, prevent or reduce shoulder subluxation, and stimulate volitional movements.[217–220] NMES has been shown to increase the ability of muscle to exert force by preferentially activating the fast-contracting motor units. Effective treatment results have been reported for improving function of the deltoid and supraspinatus muscles, whereby the glenohumeral alignment was improved and subluxation reduced. Optimal results have been obtained when combined with task-specific training.[219] EMG-NMES to the affected wrist and finger extensors has been shown to improve motor function of the paretic arm, arm–hand activities, and active ROM.[162] The electrical stimulation findings do not appear to differ between persons in the early or late stages poststroke. For this reason, it is included in boxes 1, 2, 3 and 5, 6, 7 of the UE algorithm of the ViaTherapy app (see Fig. 15.7). Once the person has selective capacity of the upper limb, electrical stimulation is not used.

Motor Imagery

MI is the systematic application of imagery techniques for improving motor performance and learning. It can be practiced in a visual or kinesthetic mode. The patient is instructed to either see or feel the movement as they imagine executing it. Mental practice can be facilitated through the use of audiotapes and has been successfully combined with physical practice to enhance UE improvements in both activity and impairments.[66,221] There is strong evidence that it can be used to improve arm–hand activities from the earliest stages of recovery as long as the patient is cognitively able to engage in the practice.[162] It is best when combined with physical practice. As noted in the gait section, it is important to determine that the patient has the ability to imagine by using the KVIQ or a quick mental chronometry screen. For this screen, the clinician compares the executed to imagined times for a specific task for congruence. For example, if the person executes a sequential finger movement task in 10 seconds but needs only 3 seconds to imagine the same task, there is no congruence, and perhaps the person is not able to effectively imagine.

Virtual Reality and Video Games

Video games and virtual reality interventions are recommended in the ViaTherapy app for boxes 3, 4, 7, and 8 (Fig. 15.7). Active, isolated movement of the upper limb is required to play these games, especially when they are not interfaced with a robotic device. The most recent Cochrane review by Laver et al.[69] provided support for VR-augmented therapy enhancing the use of the upper limb (UL) for persons poststroke as an adjunct to therapy. It may be an option when engagement and motivation may be facilitated by gamification and feedback. Some systems have been implemented in a self-managed telehealth model and found to be superior to in-person CIMT.[222] A new generation of immersive technologies are emerging as tools for upper limb rehabilitation. A recent study reported on the use of the HTC VIVE headset with commercial games to restore upper limb use reporting improvements in the Fugl-Meyer score.[223] There are still many questions about safety and implementation before adopting the new technologies. If a video game is incorporated into clinical practice, a clear understanding of the game and its application may enhance its efficacy. There are two games analyses that may be useful in applying video games in practice.[224,225]

Mirror Therapy

Mirror therapy is recommended as an adjunct to therapy for patients with greater severity to improve motor function.[78] *Mirror therapy (MT)* is a therapeutic intervention that focuses on moving the less impaired limb while watching its mirror reflection. A mirror is placed in the patient's midsagittal plane, presenting the patient with the mirror image of their less affected limb as if it were the hemiparetic limb. It is believed that mirror neurons help create the illusion that the affected hand is moving. It can be practiced in a unimanual or bimanual mode. It was first introduced by Ramachandran et al.[226] for individuals with UE loss. For patients with stroke, MT has been shown to improve LE recovery and ankle dorsiflexion,[227,228] UE recovery and distal motor function, as well as recovery from hemineglect.[228,229] These findings were reported in studies to which MT was added to conventional therapy.

A Cochrane review by Thieme et al.[67] included 14 studies with patients in the subacute and chronic phases poststroke with a wide range of abilities. Therapy was either unimanual (five studies) or bimanual (six studies) with 10 to 60 minutes provided 1, 2, 5, and 7 days/week for 2 to 4 weeks in an inpatient setting or the home. They found that MT improved motor function, which was retained after 5 months. There were also improvements in ADL and decreased shoulder pain.

MT is being combined with task-specific training, MI, and NMES.[230–232] It has been shown that the combination of task-specific training plus MT is better at improving upper limb use than either in isolation.[231] It is important to note that use of mirrors is contraindicated in patients with marked visuospatial perceptual impairments. A video of MT with a stroke patient can be viewed online (https://www.youtube.com/watch?v=1BnsQO7a4Og).

Simultaneous Bilateral Training

Simultaneous bilateral training involves using both arms simultaneously alone or in combination with augmented sensory feedback. Bilateral arm training with rhythmic auditory cueing is an example of this intervention.[233] It is theorized that similar movement in the less affected extremity facilitates movement in the more affected extremity. Positive results have been reported in improving motor recovery after stroke.[234–236] However, when compared to usual or conventional care, simultaneous bilateral training was not shown to be significantly better than other UE interventions in terms of improvements in ADL, arm or hand movements, or scores on motor impairment measures. The Cochrane reviewers cited lack of high-quality evidence in these findings.[237] In the most recent Canadian guidelines for poststroke rehabilitation, it is indicated that this is not better than unilateral activities.[78] Nonetheless, there are many bimanual tasks, and it is important to train those.

Robotic-Assisted Training

Robotic devices have been developed to assist the patient with moderate to severe motor impairments in improving UE function and recovery. They are used in conjunction with task-oriented training and motor learning principles. Robots work to restore lost motor function and can include pneumatic actuators (acting as muscles) to power the device or passive robotic systems using elastic bands or springs. Reach and grasp/release movements are typically targeted. They can be unilateral or bilateral. These devices are used to augment therapist–patient interventions and enable high levels of intensive practice.[236] They can target proximal, distal, and proximal plus distal UL muscles. Unilateral proximal (shoulder–elbow) robots have been found to improve motor function of the shoulder, muscle strength, and pain.[162] Bilateral elbow–wrists robots were shown to improve motor function of the paretic arm and strength.[162] Limited evidence exists of treatment efficacy that can be generalized to arm and hand use during ADL.[238] In a large randomized trial of persons with moderate to severe stroke, robotic devices were not found to be any better in improving motor function on the FMA than standards of care delivered at high intensity.[239] The high cost of equipment currently limits widespread use in the clinical setting.

Strengthening

Muscle weakness is a major impairment after stroke and contributes to significant activity limitations (e.g., walking, sit-to-stand transfers, stair climbing, UE activities). It is discussed in the UE section because it is found in boxes 3, 4, 6, 7, and 8 of the UE algorithm (Fig. 15.7). It is important as well for postural control and function and is relevant for gait and locomotion. Progressive resistive strength training has been shown to improve muscle strength in individuals with stroke,[240–243] with no evidence of a detrimental increase in spasticity or reduction in ROM.[240,241,243] A large effect is reported for persons poststroke in the chronic phase who engaged in progressive resistive strengthening using the American College of Sports Medicine (ACSM) guidelines (training should include a load of 8 to 12 repetition maximum for at least two sets, and these loads need to increase progressively). However, the carryover to activities (e.g., walking) had a smaller effect. Notably, the improvements were found for persons in the chronic phase poststroke.[242]

Combining resistance training with task-oriented functional activities may enhance carryover in terms of improving function (e.g., sit-to-stand transfers [Fig. 15.11], partial wall squats [Fig. 15.12], step-ups, stair climbing while the patient is wearing weighted cuffs). Circuit-training workstations can be used to maximize muscle training.[244] Lifting free weights or using elastic bands places added demands for postural stability in sitting and standing and is an element of training to improve postural control.

Many patients with stroke demonstrate poor hand function with no effective grasp. Specially designed gloves may be necessary to ensure maintained contact with exercise equipment (e.g., leather mitts with Velcro, wrist cuffs). Patients with impaired sensation are at increased risk for injury and should be monitored closely. Patients with postural deficits should be safely positioned to prevent falls (e.g., stable seat, corner standing while lifting free weights).

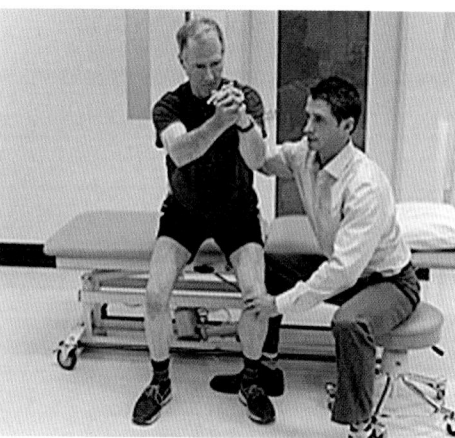

Figure 15.11 Sit-to-stand transitions. The therapist assists the patient in straightening the hemiparetic knee while bringing the center of mass forward. Hands are clasped together.

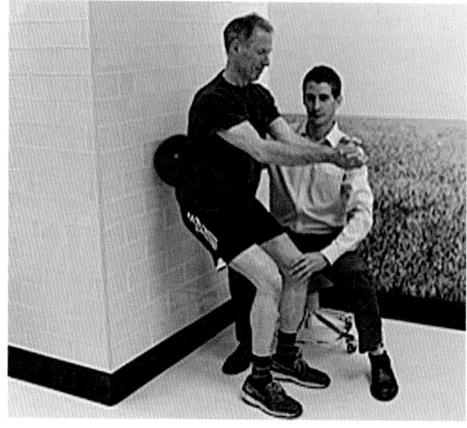

Figure 15.12 The clinician breaks from task-based training to address lower extremity strengthening in a weight-bearing position.

Clinical Note. In determining a safe exercise prescription, it is important to remember the high incidence of hypertension and cardiac disease in patients with stroke. High-intensity strengthening exercises (sustained maximal effort) are generally contraindicated in patients with recent stroke and unstable BP. Isometric exercise that is accompanied by the Valsalva maneuver and dangerous elevations in BP is also contraindicated. Dynamic exercises performed in an upright position (sitting) produce less elevations in BP than recumbent/supine exercises. For patients at risk, submaximal protocols using low-intensity exercises (e.g., 30% to 50% of maximal voluntary contraction) are appropriate for initial exercise. Varying the exercises is also an effective strategy to reduce cardiovascular risk. The therapist needs to ensure that warm-ups and cooldowns are adequate and that the overall exercise progression is gradual.

Management of Range of Motion

The Canadian Stroke Guidelines recommend placing the UE in a variety of safe positions within the patient's visual field.[78] Positioning strategies are important in maintaining soft tissue length (Box 15.5). Effective positioning of the hemiparetic extremities encourages proper joint alignment while positioning the limbs out of the good biomechanical alignment. ROM and positioning should be viewed as a whole-body intervention because the malalignment of the LEs and the trunk could then influence the position of the upper limbs. Coordination with team members, staff, family, and caregivers is essential for long-term management.[245]

In the UE, correct passive range of motion (PROM) techniques require careful attention to external rotation and distraction of the humerus, especially as ranges approach 90° of flexion or more. Mobilization of the scapula on the thoracic wall with an emphasis on upward rotation and protraction will prevent soft tissue impingement in the subacromial space during overhead

---

Box 15.5   Positioning Strategies to Reduce Common Malalignments

Supine Position

- Head/neck: Neutral and symmetrical; supported on pillow.
- Trunk: Aligned in midline.
- More affected UE: Scapula protracted, shoulder forward and slightly abducted; arm supported on a pillow; elbow extended with hand resting on a pillow; wrist neutral, fingers extended, and thumb abducted.
- More affected LE: Hip forward (pelvis protracted); knee on a small pillow or towel roll to prevent hyperextension; nothing against the soles of feet. For persistent plantarflexion, a splint can be used to position the foot and ankle in neutral position.

Side-Lying on Less Affected Side

- Head/neck: Neutral and symmetrical.
- Trunk: Aligned in midline; small pillow or towel can be placed under the rib cage to elongate the hemiplegic side.
- More affected UE: Scapular protracted, shoulder forward; arm on a supporting pillow with elbow extended, wrist neutral, fingers extended, and thumb abducted.
- More affected LE: Hip forward and flexed, knee flexed and supported on a pillow.

Side-Lying on More Affected Side

- Head/neck: Neutral and symmetrical.
- Trunk: Aligned in midline.
- More affected UE: Scapula protracted; shoulder forward; arm placed in slight abduction and external rotation; elbow extended, forearm supinated, wrist neutral, fingers extended, and thumb abducted.
- More affected LE: Hip extended and knee flexed and supported by pillows. An alternative position is slight hip and knee flexion with pelvic protraction.

Sitting in an Armchair or Wheelchair

- Head/neck: Neutral and symmetrical; head directly above pelvis.
- Trunk: Spine extension.
- Pelvis: Aligned in neutral with weight-bearing on both buttocks.
- More affected UE: Shoulder protracted and forward; elbow supported on an arm trough or lapboard; forearm, wrist neutral, fingers extended, and thumb abducted (resting splint as needed).
- Both LEs: Hips flexed to 90°, positioned in neutral with respect to rotation.

LE = lower extremity; UE = upper extremity.

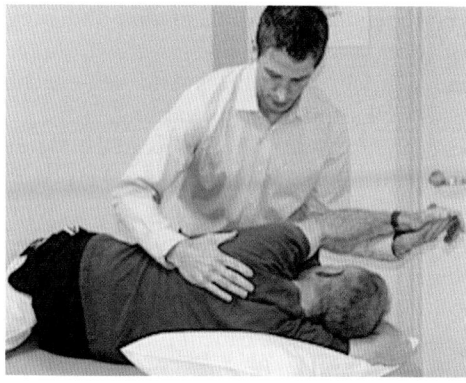

Figure 15.13 Range-of-motion exercises for the hemiparetic upper extremity. The therapist carefully mobilizes the scapula during arm elevation.

movements of the arm (Fig. 15.13) preparing the arm for forward reach patterns. The use of overhead pulleys for self-ROM is *contraindicated* because of failure to achieve the previous requirements for scapulohumeral movement. Full extension of the elbow is important because the majority of patients with stroke develop tightness in elbow flexors as a result of excess flexor spasticity. Normal length of wrist and finger extensors should also be maintained, as tightness is typical in flexion. This can be achieved functionally through sitting, weight-bearing on the extended paretic UE with the wrist extended and fingers open and extended (see Fig. 15.8). Edema and tonal changes may produce impingement with wrist extension. In this situation, grade 1 and grade 2 mobilization to the carpal bones before stretching at the wrist is indicated. Positioning the limb to reduce the likelihood of distal edema is best. Once present, the edema can also be managed with gentle retrograde massage.[245]

Strategies to teach patients safe self-ROM activities can be used to protect the joint and promote joint flexibility. Activities include the following:

- In *arm cradling,* the stronger UE cradles and lifts the more affected UE to 90° humeral flexion; the arm is moved into positions of horizontal abduction and adduction. Active trunk rotation is combined with the arm movements.
- In *tabletop polishing,* the more affected UE is positioned in humeral flexion with scapular protraction and elbow extension; both hands are positioned on a towel. The less affected hand moves the paretic hand by pulling on the towel (forward and side to side). Trunk movements and ROM are optimized by placing the chair slightly back from the table.
- Sitting, the patient leans forward and reaches both hands down to the floor. This position encourages forward flexion of the humerus with scapular

protraction, and extension of the elbow, wrist, and fingers.
- Supine, hands are clasped together and placed behind the head, the elbows fall flat to the mat. This activity should be considered only if scapular upward mobility is present. Hands clasped, self-overhead movements are contraindicated if scapulohumeral rhythm is lacking.

When sitting in a wheelchair, the patient's paretic UE can be positioned on an arm trough (shallow elbow/forearm support) attached to the armrest. The shoulder is positioned in 5° of abduction and flexion and neutral rotation; elbow in 90° flexion and slightly forward; forearm pronated; and hand in a functional resting position. Routine use of splinting is not recommended in the literature; however, it may still be evaluated on a case-by-case basis.[78]

Management of Spasticity

Patients who demonstrate spasticity (resistance to rapid stretch) can benefit from interventions designed to manage the secondary effects of spasticity (immobility, soft tissue contracture, and deformity). These include early mobilization and slow prolonged stretching to maintain the length of spastic muscles and soft tissues and promote optimal positioning. It is important to note that the methodological quality of research studies in this area is diverse and not well controlled, and available evidence about the effectiveness of stretching is inconclusive.[246,247] Once full range is achieved, the limb is positioned in the lengthened position. For example, the shoulder is extended, abducted, and externally rotated with the elbow, wrist, and fingers extended. The hand is positioned in weight-bearing to the patient's side (see Fig. 15.8) and maintained for several minutes. The benefits of *sustained stretching* include relaxation through mechanisms of autogenic inhibition. In sitting, slow rocking movements can be added to increase relaxation effects from influences of slow vestibular stimulation. Side sitting on the hemiparetic side provides sustained stretch to the spastic side flexors. The patient, family members, and caregivers should be taught safe ROM and stretching techniques.

Modalities can aid in temporarily reducing spasticity to allow task practice. These include the application of cold, massage, and electrical stimulation. Cold slows nerve conduction and decreases muscle spindle activity. These factors can lead to a temporary reduction of tone. Cold can be applied with ice packs or ice massage (duration 10 to 20 minutes). The effects of cold are short lived, generally lasting for about 20 to 30 minutes. FES can be used to target the weak antagonist muscles (e.g., peroneal nerve stimulators) and works to decrease tone through the effects of reciprocal inhibition. FES has been used with some success to decrease spasticity during the treatment time.[247] There is no evidence to support the use of airsplints around the paretic arm to reduce tone. Use of botulinum toxin injections for focal and painful spasticity are supported by the Canadian Stroke Guidelines for spasticity management of both upper and lower limb for persons poststroke.[78]

Management of Sensory Function

Patients who have significant sensory impairments may demonstrate impaired or absent spontaneous movement. The more the patient can be encouraged to use the affected side, the greater is the chance of increased awareness and function. Conversely, the patient who refuses to use the hemiplegic side contributes to the problems imposed by lack of sensorimotor experience. Without attention during treatment, this *learned nonuse* phenomenon can contribute to further deterioration.

Multiple interventions for UE sensory impairment after stroke have been described. These can be categorized into sensory retraining and sensory stimulation approaches. *Sensory retraining programs* include use of MT (described earlier), repetitive sensory discrimination activities, bilateral simultaneous movements, and repetitive task practice. *Sensorimotor integrative treatment* focuses on normalizing tone, practice of functional activity, and use of augmented sensory cues. *Sensory stimulation intervention* includes compression techniques (weight-bearing, manual compression, inflatable pressure splints, intermittent pneumatic compression), mobilizations, electrical stimulation, thermal stimulation, or magnetic stimulation. In a review of 13 studies, Cochrane reviewers[68] found significant clinical and methodological diversity, limited RCTs, generally small sample sizes with inadequate data, variability in outcome measures, and limited used of functional performance and participation outcome measures. They concluded there was insufficient evidence to support or refute the effectiveness of many of these interventions in improving sensory function. Limited evidence was found in support of the following:

- MT for improving detection of light touch, pressure, and temperature pain
- Thermal stimulation intervention for improving rate of recovery of sensation
- Intermittent pneumatic compression for improving tactile and kinesthetic sensation

The results of a systematic review of sensory retraining by Schabrun and Hillier[248] were similar with additional support found for electrical stimulation interventions. Two RCTs provided evidence of sensory retraining by matching the sensation between the hands and vision. They reported improved sensory discrimination, motor control, actual use, perceived performance, and satisfaction with upper limb tasks.[249,250] This intervention required 45 min/day for at least 10 sessions.

They recommended including graded and progressive discrimination tasks for various textures and object recognition, augmented feedback and self-checking for accuracy as well as intensity of training.[249]

Sensory retraining may be incorporated into functional training. The therapist may maximize weight-bearing and compression of the sensory-deficient limbs. Approximation can be applied with the sensory-deficient UE by weight-bearing in sitting or standing/modified plantigrade position and to the pelvis during standing activities. While sitting on a ball, the patient can practice bouncing. The compression and approximation that occur through the spine enhance activity in the postural extensors.

A safety education program should be instituted early for patients, family, and caregivers to improve awareness of sensory impairments and ensure protection of anesthetic limbs. This is particularly important for preventing UE trauma during transfer and wheelchair activities.

Hemianopsia and Unilateral Neglect

Patients with hemianopsia or unilateral neglect demonstrate a lack of awareness of the contralesional side. The impairments are more pervasive in patients with neglect and in its most severe form (anosognosia) may extend to a total unawareness of the disability or the extent of the problems. They are more common in patients with right hemisphere damage. The remediation interventions recommended in the Canadian Stroke Guidelines include visual scanning, virtual reality, MI, and MT (for inattention) with or without limb activation as well as patient and family education on neglect.[78] It should be noted, however, that a Cochrane review found the evidence to support these approaches to be low.[251]

These patients benefit from training strategies that encourage awareness and use of the environment on the hemiparetic side and use of the hemiparetic extremities. Visual scanning movements can be taught by encouraging turning of the head and axial trunk rotation to the more involved side. Cueing (e.g., visual, verbal, or motor cues) is used to direct the patient's attention. For example, a red anchor line can be taped on the floor and the patient directed to visually follow the line from one side to the other. Or a red ribbon can be attached to the patient's hemiparetic wrist and the patient directed to keep the red ribbon in sight. Scanning movements can also be stimulated using visual tracking tasks on a computer. During therapy, the therapist stimulates and encourages active voluntary movements of the neglected limbs while encouraging the patient to look at their limbs while moving. UE exercises that involve crossing the midline toward the hemiparetic side may be useful. Functional activities that encourage bilateral interaction are also valuable (e.g., pouring a drink and drinking from a cup; picking up an object with the more involved hand and placing it in the other; "dusting a tabletop" with a cloth held by both hands). MT, in particular for inattention, is better when combined with arm activation.

The therapist needs to maximize the patient's attention by optimizing visual, tactile, and proprioceptive stimuli on the more affected side. These can include stroking, brushing, tapping, or vibrating the hemiparetic limbs. The therapist also needs to consistently reorient the patient as inattention develops. Patients with very low levels of arousal are likely to be less responsive to therapy efforts.[252–254]

Supportive Devices for the Upper Extremity

The use of supportive devices is controversial. There is no evidence that support slings prevent glenohumeral subluxation or glenohumeral pain.[162] However, the practice guidelines acknowledge the need to protect the shoulder joint, especially when the UE is flaccid, during movement transitions, and when the arm is in a dependent position.[78] This is because a patient with hypotonia is at increased risk of shoulder *traction injury*. Slings may be used to prevent soft tissue stretching (e.g., supraspinatus, capsular stretching) and relieve pressure on the neurovascular bundle (e.g., brachial plexus/brachial artery). They support the weight of the arm and protect the patient. They also free up the therapist to attend to postural/trunk control during functional activities. However, slings have a number of negative features. They do little to reduce subluxation or improve shoulder function, especially if scapular and trunk malalignment are not adequately addressed. Most slings have the additional negative feature of positioning the arm close to the body in adduction, internal rotation, and elbow flexion. With prolonged use, contractures and increased flexor tone may develop. Slings also contribute to body scheme disorders and body neglect. Prolonged use of slings blocks spontaneous use of the UE and contributes to learned nonuse. Slings may also block balance reactions involving the UE. They are recommended for use when patients do not acquire active movement.

Close collaboration with the occupational therapist is important in the appropriate selection and use of slings. Gillen[206] suggests the following guidelines:

- Therapists should minimize sling use during rehabilitation.
- Slings may be useful for initial transfer and gait training.
- Slings that position the UE in flexion are less desirable and should be used only for select upright activities and only for short time periods.
- No one sling is appropriate for all patients; selection and use should be carefully evaluated and sling effectiveness carefully reevaluated.

- Effective alternatives to use of a sling should be considered: humeral taping (strapping) to facilitate or inhibit musculature surrounding the scapula and neuromuscular electrical stimulation (NMES), which has been shown to reduce shoulder subluxation.[162] The hand can also be positioned in a garment pocket.

The patient, family members, and caregivers should be instructed in and allowed to practice proper use of the support. As recovery progresses and voluntary movement emerges, spontaneous reduction of shoulder subluxation may occur, eliminating the need for a sling.

For patients using a wheelchair, an arm board or lap tray can provide support for the flaccid arm. A lateral elbow guard and/or straps may be necessary if the patient's arm slips off the side. Patients with decreased sensation are at risk for hand injury if the hand becomes stuck in the spokes of the wheelchair; elbow trauma can occur if the elbow slips off the side (e.g., the elbow hits as the patient is going through a doorway).

Management of Shoulder Pain

Shoulder pain is box 9 in the ViaTherapy app's UE algorithm (Fig. 15.7) and can apply at any point in the recovery poststroke. Several causes of hemiplegic shoulder pain have been identified that can be broadly divided into flaccid and spastic presentations. In the flaccid stage, proprioceptive loss, lack of muscle tone, and muscle paralysis reduce the support and normal seating action of the rotator cuff muscles, particularly the supraspinatus. The ligaments and capsule thus become the shoulder's sole support. The normal orientation of the glenoid fossa is upward, outward, and forward, so that it keeps the superior capsule taut and stabilizes the humerus mechanically. In the absence of supporting musculature, any abduction or forward flexion of the humerus, or scapular depression and downward rotation, reduces this stabilization and causes the humerus to sublux. Initially, the subluxation is not painful, but mechanical stresses resulting from traction and gravitational forces produce persistent malalignment and pain. Glenohumeral friction–compression stresses also occur between the humeral head and superior soft tissues during flexion or abduction movements in the absence of normal scapulohumeral rhythm *(shoulder impingement syndrome)*. During the spastic stage, abnormal muscle tone may contribute to poor scapular position (depression, retraction, and downward rotation) leading to subluxation and restricted movement. Secondary tightness in ligaments, tendons, and joint capsule can develop quickly. *Adhesive capsulitis* (intracapsular inflammation and "frozen shoulder") can occur. Poor handling and positioning of the more affected UE have been implicated in producing joint microtrauma and pain. Activities that traumatize the shoulder include PROM without adequate mobilization of the scapula (promoting normal scapulohumeral rhythm), traction or pulling on the UE during a transfer, or using reciprocal pulleys. An incorrectly aligned joint can significantly impair the patient's ability to move. Additional interventions aimed at reducing subluxation can include NMES therapy, EMG biofeedback, taping, and slings (previously discussed). Kinesiotaping in particular has been shown to reduce pain and shoulder subluxation[255] as well as improve the ability to move into flexion.[256]

Complex regional pain syndrome type 1 (CRPS-1), also known as shoulder–hand syndrome (SHS) or reflex sympathetic dystrophy, is caused by proximal trauma to the shoulder or neck or can occur with stroke and may be the result of autonomic nervous system changes. Clinical factors associated with its development include motor deficits, spasticity, sensory deficits, and initial coma.[257] Early on, pain is intermittent and limited to the shoulder. During later stages, pain is intense and involves the whole extremity. CRPS-1 is associated with a range of other symptoms. Stiffness and limitations in ROM occur. The wrist tends to assume a flexed position with intense pain likely during wrist extension movements. The elbow is not typically involved. Early *stage 1* vasomotor changes include discoloration (pale pink or cool) and alterations in temperature. The skin may be hypersensitive to touch, pressure, or temperature variations. The patient typically guards against movement attempts. *Stage 2* is characterized by subsiding pain and early dystrophic changes: muscle and skin atrophy, vasospasm, hyperhidrosis (increased sweating), and coarse hair and nails. There is radiographic evidence of early osteoporosis. In *stage 3,* the atrophic phase, pain and vasomotor changes are rare. There is progressive atrophy of the skin, muscles, and bones (severe osteoporosis is evident). Pericapsular fibrosis and articular changes become pronounced. The hand typically becomes contracted in a clawed position with metacarpophalangeal extension and interphalangeal flexion (similar to the intrinsic minus hand). There is marked atrophy of the thenar and hypothenar muscles with flattening of the hand. Chances of reversal of signs and symptoms are high for stage 1 and variable for stage 2, whereas stage 3 changes are largely irreversible.[257]

Early diagnosis and identification of factors that cause CRPS are essential. Interventions are selected on the basis of examination findings. Because of close daily contact with the patient, the physical therapist is frequently one of the first to recognize and report early signs and symptoms. A prevention protocol should be implemented. In the flaccid stage, the arm should be supported at all times. Proper positioning and handling are essential. In bed, patients should be positioned so they cannot roll onto the more affected UE, compressing it.

In supine and wheelchair sitting, the scapula/shoulder should be supported with the arm forward in slight abduction and neutral rotation. During transfers and standing, supportive devices should be considered to prevent traction injury. Interventions aimed at reducing pain and stiffness include appropriate PROM and mobilization techniques (gentle grade 1 to 2 mobilizations). PROM to the UE without scapular mobilization is *not* permitted. PROM of the shoulder should be limited to 90° during flexion and abduction or to the point of pain, not beyond the pain position. The therapist needs to ensure that everyone involved in assisting the patient (e.g., family member, caregiver, nurses, and aides) has been instructed in proper handling/mobilization of the UE and recognizes the importance of avoiding trauma and traction injuries during PROM, transfers, and wheelchair activities. Active movements of the UE are encouraged to promote shoulder ROM (e.g., pushing away a tabletop therapy ball while standing). Interventions to manage edema are also a consideration. Additional considerations include no infusions into the veins of the hemiplegic hand. Persistent pain may be managed with oral analgesics or local injection techniques (corticosteroids). Repeat steroid injections are not recommended due to likely weakening of the rotator cuff. With intractable pain, surgical nerve blocks may be considered.[258]

Functional Status

Intervention to restore functional status most often takes place in acute care, inpatient acute rehabilitation, or a subacute facility. The loss of sensory and motor function on one side will present a challenge for the patient as they relearn postural control and functional mobility. Observation of the movement will identify activity limitations and allow for hypothesizing what body function structure limitations may be incorporated into the intervention (see Chapter 1, Clinical Decision-Making). For example, when a person rolls to the less affected side, the affected arm is left behind. This could be due to weakness, incoordination, or sensory loss. The clinician needs to identify which one and work on remediating the problem in the context of the task. If it is weakness or incoordination, the task may be set up so that the movements at first are gravity assisted. If it is sensory, the patient may have to look at the limb or use a mirror. Or, at first the patient may compensate and use the other limb to assist with movement of the affected limb. If the person is unable to do the movement, they may require guided movements progressing to active assisted movement and then finally to active movement.

Persons poststroke present with asymmetrical posture and movement. Whenever possible, that should be reduced to provide better biomechanics for movement, but it cannot be the sole focus of the therapy. If they are able to change their initial conditions (posture) or the therapist can change the environment, then they may have success with the movement.

Normal function implies variability of movements. Muscles need to be activated in varied activities using varied types of contractions. All three types— eccentric, isometric, and concentric—are important to include in an exercise program. For the patient with stroke who demonstrates very weak movements, isometric and eccentric contractions should be practiced before concentric contractions because they utilize elastic elements and muscle spindle support more efficiently. For the same amount of tension, fewer motor units are required. Practice of functional tasks that utilize variations of contractions should also be implemented.

BED MOBILITY

Rolling to both sides should be practiced; rolling onto the less affected side will prove more difficult. Extremity movement patterns can be used to enhance the movement. Care must be taken to ensure the patient does not leave the more affected UE behind but rather brings it forward. This can be accomplished by having the patient clasp the hands together first. The more affected LE can be used to assist in rolling by pushing off from a flexed and neutral, hook-lying position (Fig. 15.14). Rolling onto the more affected side and into a side-lying-on-elbow position is important to promote early weight-bearing. This position has the added benefit of elongating the lateral trunk flexors, which may be shortened.

The patient practices moving from supine-to-sit leading from both sides, with an emphasis on rising with the more involved side leading (closest to the edge of bed or mat). The therapist may provide assistance from side-lying on the more affected side by shifting the LEs over the edge of the bed or mat while the patient pushes up into sitting using both UEs for support. Controlled lowering should also be practiced.

Bridging activities help develop trunk and hip extensor control important for use of a bedpan, pressure relief on the buttocks, initial bed mobility (scooting), and sit-to-stand transfers. It also develops advanced LE out-of-abnormal-synergy control (hip extension with knee flexion) and stimulates early weight-bearing through the foot (see Fig. 15.15). Bridging activities include independent assumption of the posture, holding in the posture, and moving in the posture (lateral weight shifts, bridge-and-placing hips to one side). If the more affected LE is unable to hold in a hook-lying position, the therapist will need to assist by stabilizing the foot. Lifting the less affected foot off the surface (placing it on a small ball) while maintaining the pelvis level significantly increases the difficulty and can be used to increase demands on the more affected side. Difficulty can also be increased by varying the position of the UEs, from extended and abducted at the sides to arms folded across the chest or hands clasped together overhead in a prayer position.

SITTING

Training sitting is strongly recommended in the Australian and New Zealand CPGs.[79] It is important that sitting practice extend beyond arms' length. They offer the following practical guidance:

- Give clear instructions so patient understands and agrees to treatment plans, progression, amount of practice, and goals.
- Therapists should consider safety of patients with severe weakness.
- If a patient is to do unsupervised or semi-supervised practice, ensure they can communicate with staff as needed (e.g., the call bell is near them, and patient/family know where staff are located and how to contact them).

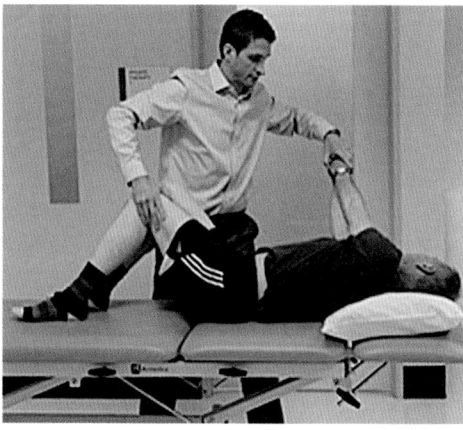

Figure 15.14 Early mobility activities: Rolling onto the unaffected side. The therapist assists the movement through contacts on the knees and clasped hands.

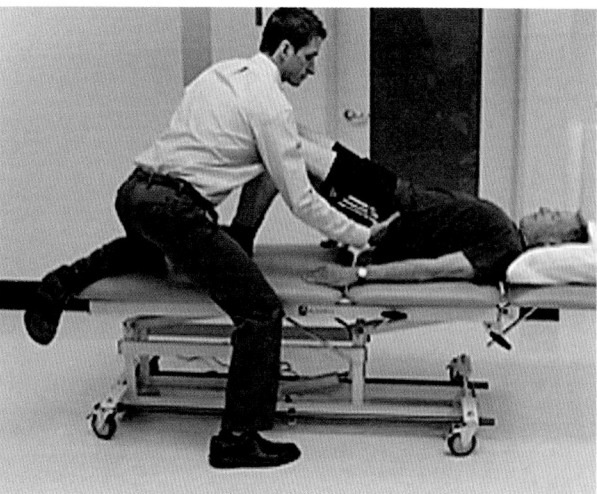

Figure 15.15 The patient practices bridging, combining hip extension with knee flexion. The therapist cues the patient to activate the hip extensors on the hemiparetic lower extremity.

- Feedback about weight transfer or reaching length should be used to continue to motivate patients.
- Consider incorporating functional training (such as reaching out to pick up a cup from a table).
- For stroke survivors with very weak leg extensors on the affected side, sitting with the person's non-affected hip, shoulder, and arm against a wall may be useful for encouraging extensor activity in the affected leg.

Aim to have the feet flat on the floor and attain a neutral pelvis and a straight spine. A good initial posture will make it easier for the person to transition to other positions. Typically, patients with stroke will sit asymmetrically with weight borne more on the less affected side, pelvis in a posterior tilt, and upper trunk flexed (kyphotic). Lateral flexion to the affected side is also common. The therapist models correct sitting position and provides verbal instruction for correction and, if needed, manual cues. Early sitting can be assisted by having the patient use the UEs for bilateral support at sides or in front on tabletop, a large ball, or the therapist's shoulders with the therapist sitting directly in front of the patient. Sitting on a therapy ball may also be used to promote pelvic alignment and mobility and trunk upright alignment (gentle bouncing). Sitting control can start with reaching beyond the BOS and then, if that is not possible, work to move in smaller ranges or practice holding the position. The patient should also practice scooting in sitting ("butt walking") to ensure mobility for dressing (putting pants on) and practice initial positioning for sit-to-stand transitions (coming to the edge of the seat to place the feet back and under the body).

Summarized data from studies training sitting balance (six RCTs, 150 participants) showed no gain in symmetry while sitting and standing. However, when data were pooled from studies that used a strategy of reaching beyond arm's length, the researcher found positive effects for sitting balance.[162]

SIT-TO-STAND AND STAND-TO-SIT TRANSFERS

Practicing sit-to-stand transfers is also strongly recommended in the Australian and New Zealand CPG.[79] This recommendation is based on two Cochrane reviews.[64,259] They offered the following practical guidance.

In individuals who are not able to independently stand up from sitting, the following approaches may be considered:

- Performing squats on a sliding or fixed tilt table[260]
- Performing reaching tasks in sitting, with emphasis on loading the more affected lower limb[260]

To progress training and provide an appropriate level of challenge, clinicians may consider the following:

- Increasing number and speed of repetitions
- Lowering the height of the sitting surface

- Altering foot position to increase load through the more affected lower limb
- Providing progressively unstable surface under the feet (e.g., foam)[260]

Other considerations for motivation, movement quality, and safety during training are as follows:

- Performing the training independently or in a group setting
- Providing visual targets (e.g., for shoulder or leg position)[260]
- Using an external device for visual or auditory feedback (e.g., on lateral symmetry)
- Monitoring or counting repetitions
- Providing hands-on or verbal feedback on QOM
- Having a wall on the unaffected side for safety or to assist vertical perception[260]
- Considering the appropriate environmental setup and level of challenge for those who may be fearful of falling

Sit-stand can be practiced with attention to symmetrical weight-bearing, coordinated muscular responses, and adequate timing. Sit-to-stand task can be viewed and in three phases. The patient first actively flexes the trunk and uses momentum to shift the body mass forward (flexion-momentum phase), then extends the hips and knees to move vertically into the upright position (extension phase), and finally stabilizes in erect standing (stabilization phase). Patients with stroke can demonstrate difficulty with each of these phases. To assist the patient in relearning this task, the patient's feet can be placed evenly side by side in mild ankle dorsiflexion to allow forward movement of the body. Placement of the UEs forward with hands clasped together also assists with the flexion-momentum stage. To assist with the extension phase, the height of the seat can be initially elevated to decrease the extensor force required; the therapist can also provide tactile and proprioceptive cues to assist hip and knee extension (see Fig. 15.11) and to guide the direction of the weight shift. Increased weight-bearing on the stronger LE can be achieved by varying the initial foot position, placing the stronger foot slightly behind the weaker foot. Performance during the stabilization stage can be initially practiced with a wider BOS and support of the hemiplegic arm to maximize trunk alignment and balance. The patient with stroke typically accomplishes sit-to-stand very slowly. With repetitive practice, the patient should be encouraged to focus on increasing the speed of the movement to retrain timing of limb movements, alignment, and balance during this task. The task of stand-to-sit requires eccentric control throughout the trunk and LEs and must also be retrained. Eccentric movements (small-range movements) can be practiced with the patient positioned back against a wall doing partial wall squats as part of a mat exercise program (e.g., bridging, low trunk rotation) or by performing scooting to the right and left while sitting at the edge of a mat.

TRANSFERS

During early transfers, the patient may require maximal assistance. Adjusting the hospital bed to the height of the chair or wheelchair will help to decrease the difficulty of the transfer. Staff often emphasize the sound side by placing the chair to that side and having the patient stand and pivot a quarter turn on the stronger LE before sitting down. Although this compensatory strategy promotes early transfers, it neglects the weaker side and may make subsequent training more difficult. The patient should be taught to transfer to both sides, with emphasis on moving toward the more affected side. Practice to both sides has functional significance, because most bathrooms are not large enough to allow positioning of the wheelchair on both sides of a tub or toilet. Also, the patient is not likely to be able to reposition the wheelchair once they transfer into bed so that a transfer toward the same direction can be achieved when getting out of bed. When transferring, the patient's affected arm can be stabilized in elbow extension and shoulder external rotation against the therapist's body. Alternatively, the patient's UEs (hands in prayer position) can be placed in front or to one side on the therapist's shoulders. The therapist can then assist by using manual contacts, either at the upper trunk or pelvis. The more affected LE may be stabilized by the therapist's knee exerting a counterforce on the patient's knee as needed. Transfer training should include practice in transferring to various surfaces and heights (e.g., wheelchair, toilet, tub seat, car).

Functional training is begun early and continued throughout the course of rehabilitation. Training activities and postures are varied according to individual needs. Advanced functional training should include practice in getting down to and up from the floor in the event of a fall. Incorporating ROM or strength training while practicing function will make the session more efficient.

Interventions to Improve Body Function and Structure

The management of body function and structure (BFS) impairments is integrated with task-level training. There is strong evidence that strength training is important to address BFS deficits in stroke rehabilitation (see Strengthening earlier in this section). Evidence to support strengthening of the LE exists for water-based exercises, neuromuscular stimulation (NMES) of the paretic leg, transcutaneous electrical nerve stimulation, strength training, mixed cardiorespiratory and strength exercises, and high-intensity practice.[162] Therefore, the clinician can work at the BFS or the task level to achieve strengthening. Other BFS may need to be addressed in preparation for task-based training, such

as increasing and maintaining ankle ROM through passive stretching, administration of pharmacological agents to reduce spasticity, and positioning in the wheelchair or bed.

A sequence for the intervention would start with joint mobilization and retrograde massage of the affected ankle in advance of sit-stand training. Increasing joint ROM and reducing edema are preparatory interventions to practice sit-stand-walk tasks that require a specific amount of ankle ROM to be performed in a biomechanically correct way. This is an example where the clinician uses BFS interventions to create initial conditions for the tasks practice that will increase likelihood of success.

Aerobic Capacity and Physical Activity

Persons poststroke are deconditioned, predisposed to a sedentary lifestyle, and at increased risk for falls and recurrence of cardiovascular disease. They require greater energy expenditure than prior to the stroke, so they are prone to fatigue. The inactive lifestyle leads to secondary complications such as reduced cardiorespiratory fitness, increased fatigability, muscle atrophy/weakness, osteoporosis, and impaired circulation to the lower extremities in stroke survivors. In addition, diminished self-efficacy, greater dependence on others for ADL, and reduced ability for normal societal interactions can have a profound negative psychological impact.[261] Therefore, physical activity (PA) and exercise are important for both rehabilitation and prevention of secondary conditions.

Individuals recovering from stroke can benefit from PA and endurance (aerobic) training to improve cardiovascular function. It is important to promote PA across the continuum of recovery. In the first 24 hr after stroke, it is *not* recommended to engage in mobility out of bed.[79] This finding is based on extensive research on the harms and benefits of the intensive activity for persons immediately after stroke.[262] It is highly recommended to minimize bedrest by having early mobilization (within 48 hr after stroke), and functional activity training is appropriate.[263] During the subacute stage, patients/clients may be able to engage in more traditional exercise training modes such as TM walking, cycle ergometry (upper and lower body ergometer), or seated stepper. Patients with balance impairments will benefit from TT or overground walking with a safety harness or from a recumbent cycle ergometer. The therapist should assess barriers and facilitators to PA.[245] To ensure safety, patients should receive a thorough examination and supervised exercise test. Stroke guidelines (2014) recommend a graded exercise test with ECG monitoring.[261] The 6MWT, although used with many diagnoses to measure cardiorespiratory fitness, should be interpreted with caution when used with persons with stroke because the correlation between distance walked and peak VO_2 test is low to moderate.[261]

Exercise prescription elements include mode (type of exercise), frequency, intensity, and duration[264] (see Chapter 13, Heart Disease). Choice of training mode depends on the individual's abilities and interests and should be customized.[71] Intensity guidelines for acute persons poststroke suggest using an RPE of 11 or less (6 to 20 category scale) and HR of 10 to 20 beats above resting.[261] For subacute persons who have greater motor ability and are more medically stable, intensity can be increased. The moderate-intensity continuous exercise guidelines are (1) 40% to 70% of V̇O²Max or heart rate reserve, (2) 55% to 80% of HR maximum, (3) 11 to 14 RPE, (4) 20 to 60 minutes, (5) 5 to 10 minutes of warm-up and cooldown, (6) 3 to 5 days a week.[261] Greater intensity may be achieved with high-intensity interval training (HIIT).

HIIT can consist of both short and long intervals. In studies by Boyne and colleagues, short intervals involved 30-sec bursts at maximum safe speed alternated with a 30- to 60-second resting recovery periods.[265] Each overground and treadmill bout started with a 60-second recovery for the first three bursts, then progressed to 30-sec recovery for the rest of the session. For bouts of long-interval HIIT, the target HR was ~90% HR$_{peak}$ for bursts and ~70% HR$_{peak}$ for recovery periods. Speed was continually adjusted as needed to achieve and maintain the target HR, by changing the treadmill belt speed or verbally cueing the participant to change overground speed. The goal was to reach the target HR zone within 1 to 2 minutes each burst. Recovery periods started with rest breaks until the HR trajectory was determined. The 20-minute treadmill bout included three 4-minute bursts with recovery durations of 3 minute, 3 minutes and 2 minutes. Each 10-minute overground bout included two 3-minute bursts with 2-minute recovery periods. They reported that short-interval HIIT was well suited to increase gait speed and that long-interval HIIT could be applied to improve gait endurance. Importantly they showed that both modalities could be achieved with overground as well as treadmill walking.[266]

The use of a training log or exercise diary is an excellent way to help the patient keep track of prescriptive elements, objective measurements (HR, BP), and subjective reactions (RPE, perceived enjoyment). Wearing a pedometer may serve as feedback and incentive for activity. Adequate supervision, monitoring, and safety education about warning signs for impending stroke and heart attack are critical components.[29,261]

Exercise Precautions

Careful monitoring of exercise is essential. For patients at risk, BP, HR, and RPE should be taken initially, during, and after each exercise. As exercise progresses, less frequent monitoring can be implemented. The therapist also needs to monitor breathing rate and pattern, ensuring that breath holding and Valsalva do not occur.

Patients should be instructed in how to measure their own HR and RPE. They should also be taught the warning signs for when to stop exercising. These include the following:

- Light-headedness or dizziness
- Chest heaviness, pain, or tightness; angina
- Palpitations or irregular heartbeat
- Sudden shortness of breath not due to increased activity
- Volitional fatigue and exhaustion

Patients who are on medications that limit cardiac output (e.g., beta blockers) will demonstrate reduced HR responses and lower peak HRs. Patients taking diuretics to reduce fluid volume may demonstrate altered electrolyte balance with resulting dysrhythmias. Patients taking vasodilators may require a longer cooldown period after exercise to prevent postexercise hypotension.[28]

Patients undergoing an aerobic conditioning program demonstrate improvements in physical fitness, functional status, psychological outlook, and self-esteem. Regular exercise may have the additional benefit of reducing risk of recurrent stroke or heart attack. Patients who participate in a regular conditioning program may be more successful in adopting continuing, lifelong exercise habits and in moving beyond the disability associated with stroke.

Physical fitness for persons poststroke was assessed in a Cochrane Database Systematic Review by Saunders et al.[71] They reviewed 75 trials with 3,017 participants and found that cardiorespiratory fitness training after stroke reduced disability as well as improved physical fitness, maximal walking speed, and preferred gait speed and balance. Their review also included mixed training (cardiorespiratory plus strengthening) and found that preferred walking speed and walking capacity as well as balance improved. Some mobility benefits persisted after training. A separate review reported that combining cardiovascular and strengthening activities has been shown to have beneficial effects for PA, walking distance, maximum gait speed, and aerobic capacity.[162] Boyne et al. confirmed these findings and added that intensity of training yielded better results, and specificity of training was relevant when training walking.[267] Clinicians may wish to combine therapies to increase their efficiency in delivering care unless their primary aerobic fitness goal is walking, in which case they should train walking.

One strategy to combine interventions of aerobic training and functional training is *circuit class training (CCT)*. When used to improve mobility of persons poststroke who were either inpatients or dwelling in the community, CCT has been found, in a Cochrane review, to be safe and effective.[63] It may also reduce inpatient length of stay. Rose[169] reported on the effectiveness of a circuit-training physical therapy (CTPT) program in the acute rehabilitation setting. Patients received a 60-minute training session, 5 days a week, using four task-specific stations. Activities were stratified and tailored to patients' specific mobility levels (nonambulatory, severe, moderate, and mild groups). In addition, a 30-minute daily session was dedicated to critical inpatient rehabilitation issues (family and home program education, wheelchair and orthotic prescription). When compared to standard physical therapy of the same intensity, the CTPT groups showed significantly greater improvements in gait speed, primarily in ambulatory patients.

An important area of ongoing study is how to reduce sedentary behavior in persons poststroke. A recent Cochrane review did not have specific recommendations but identified this as an important area to address.[268]

■ PATIENT-/CLIENT-RELATED INSTRUCTION

Stroke represents a major health crisis for patients and their families. Lack of knowledge about the cause of the illness or the recovery process and misconceptions concerning the rehabilitation program and potential outcomes can negatively influence coping responses and progress in rehabilitation. Frequently, the problems seem unmanageable and overwhelming for the family, especially when faced with alterations in the patient's behavior, cognition, and emotion. Patients may feel depressed, isolated, irritable, or demanding. Families often demonstrate reactions that include initial relief and hope for full recovery, followed by feelings of entrapment, depression, anger, or guilt when complete recovery does not occur. These changes and feelings can strain even the best of relationships. Therapists may influence this situation because of the high frequency of contact and the often close relationships that develop with patients and their families. It is important that the therapist partner with the patient and the family to improve outcomes and satisfaction with the episode of care. There are many important guidelines to follow when planning educational interventions:

- Involve the client and their family in decision-making and encourage open discussion and communication.
- Give accurate, factual information; counsel family members about the patient's capabilities and limitations; *avoid* predictions that categorically define expected function or future recovery.
- Structure interventions carefully, giving only as much information as the patient or family need or can assimilate; provide reinforcement and repetition.
- Adapt interventions to ensure they are appropriate to the educational and cultural background of the patient and family.
- Offer a variety of educational interventions: didactic sessions, books, brochures, and videotapes, and family participation in therapy (see Appendix 15.A [online]).

- Be supportive and sensitive and maintain a positive, hopeful manner.
- Assist patients and families in understanding alternatives and developing problem-solving abilities.
- Motivate and provide positive reinforcement in therapy; enhance patient satisfaction and self-esteem.
- Refer patients and families to support and self-help groups (see Appendix 15.A [online], American Stroke Association).

Psychotherapy and counseling (e.g., sexual, leisure, vocational) can assist in improving overall QOL and should be recommended as needed.

■ DISCHARGE PLANNING

Planning for discharge begins early in rehabilitation and all aspects of shared decision-making involves the patient and family. Potential placement (safe place of residence), level of family and community support, and need for continued medical and rehabilitation services should be explored. Family members should regularly participate in therapy sessions to learn exercises and activities designed to support the patient's independence. Discharge should be considered when reasonable treatment goals/outcomes are attained. Indication of the attainment of a functional ceiling can be considered when there is lack of evidence of progress at two successive evaluations. Home visits should be made, if possible, before discharge to determine the home's physical structure and accessibility. Potential problems can be identified and corrective measures initiated. (See Chapter 9, Examination and Modification of the Environment, for additional discussion.) Home adaptations, assistive devices, and supportive services should be in place before the patient is discharged to home. A HEP coupled with patient and caregiver training should be instituted. Caregiver training of gait and mobility-related function and activities has been reported to have a positive impact on improving basic ADL and reducing caregiver strain.[162] Patients with residual impairments or activity limitations who will be receiving outpatient or home therapy should be given all the necessary information concerning these services. Community services should be identified, and information should be provided to the patient and family. Long-term follow-up at regularly scheduled intervals should be initiated to maintain patients at their highest possible functional level.

■ RECOVERY AND OUTCOMES

Recovery from stroke is generally fastest in the first weeks and months after onset. Patients can continue to make measurable functional gains generally at a reduced rate for months or years after insult. Late recovery of function has been consistently demonstrated for patients with chronic stroke (defined as greater than 6 months poststroke) who undergo extensive task-specific functional training that emphasizes use of the more involved extremities. Prolonged recovery with improvements occurring over a period of years is especially apparent in the areas of language and visuospatial function. Rates of motor recovery vary across management categories: patients with minor stroke recover rapidly with few or no residual deficits, whereas severely impaired individuals demonstrate more limited and prolonged recovery. The initial grade of paresis, measured on initial hospital admission, is an important predictor of motor recovery. In the case of complete paralysis on admission, complete motor recovery occurs in less than 15% of patients.

Functional mobility skills are impaired following stroke and vary considerably from individual to individual. The ability to recover functional tasks is influenced by a number of factors. Motor and perceptual impairments have the greatest impact on functional performance, but other limiting factors include sensory loss, disorientation, communication disorders, and decreased cardiorespiratory endurance. Personal factors include high motivation, stable supportive family, financial resources, and therapy that is intensive training with repetitive practice.[269-271] Patients who are seen in a specialized stroke unit have fewer deaths, greater independence, and better health outcomes than those in a nonspecialized unit.[272] Patients who receive inpatient stroke rehabilitation (skilled occupational, physical, and speech therapy) demonstrate improved motor recovery, functional status, and QOL at discharge.[273-276] In a systematic review of the literature (151 studies), Van Peppen et al. found strong evidence in support of task-oriented exercise and intensive training. Inpatient rehabilitation admission averaged a little over 2 weeks. Approximately 80% of patients were discharged home.[275] Postdischarge outpatient treatment or home care for stroke survivors is often indicated because functional status typically is not stabilized at discharge from a rehabilitation hospital, and effects diminish over time with no treatment. Patients who demonstrate less successful rehabilitation outcomes tended to include those with (1) advanced age, (2) severe motor impairments (e.g., prolonged paralysis, apraxia), (3) persistent medical problems (e.g., incontinence), (4) impaired cognitive function (e.g., decreased alertness, poor attention span, judgment, memory, learning difficulty), (5) severe language disturbances, (6) severe visuospatial hemineglect, and (7) other less well defined social and economic problems.[273-276] Researchers who studied long-term follow-up at 2 years poststroke (148 patients) found that only 12% demonstrated a decline in mobility. Depression was cited as the single major risk factor for mobility decline.[277]

SUMMARY

Stroke results from many different vascular events that interrupt cerebral circulation and impair brain function, including cerebral thrombosis, emboli, and hemorrhage. The location and size of the ischemic process, nature and functions of the structures involved, availability of collateral blood flow, and effectiveness of early emergency medical management all influence the symptomatology that evolves. For many patients, stroke represents a major cause of disability, with diffuse problems affecting widespread areas of function. Examination using standardized assessments of participation, activity, and BFS are complemented with movement observation of tasks. Effective rehabilitation should take advantage of the brain's capacity for repair and recovery. A shared decision-making approach to rehabilitation interventions promotes recovery and independence through restitution, compensation, and prevention. Task-oriented training using motor learning constructs, coupled with exercise science, forms the basis of the intervention. Ultimately, management should be customized to address the individual as well as factors such as stroke location, stroke severity, and phase of recovery.

■ ACKNOWLEDGMENT

The author wishes to acknowledge Gerard Fluet, PT PhD, who offered advice on the content; Kathy Gill Body, who consulted on the previous edition; and my MD, PhD student, John Palmieri, who helped with research and writing of tables.

Questions for Review

1. Differentiate between ACA syndrome and MCA syndrome in terms of expected deficits.

2. Differentiate between lesions of the right and left hemispheres in terms of expected behavioral deficits.

3. What are the major types of aphasia that can result from stroke? Where are the lesions located?

4. Differentiate between the following stroke-specific instruments: the Fugl-Meyer Assessment of Physical Performance (FMA) and the SIS.

5. Describe the behaviors of the patient with stroke who demonstrates ipsilateral pushing. What is the primary focus of rehabilitation intervention?

6. Describe the steps for structuring a therapeutic session to promote motor skill acquisition.

7. What are the essential elements of constraint-induced movement therapy to improve UE function poststroke?

8. Describe high-intensity stepping and how it relates to LT and aerobic training.

9. Describe how the Orpington scale and information from the transcranial magnetic stimulation can guide prognosis.

10. What important guidelines should be followed when planning an educational program for the patient with stroke and for family members?

CASE STUDY

HISTORY
The patient/client is a 41-year-old man admitted to an acute care hospital with a diagnosis of CVA with R hemiparesis (L MCA). He was admitted to a rehabilitation facility 7 days later. His goal is to walk independently and resume his responsibilities as a spouse and provider.

PAST MEDICAL HISTORY
- History of mild hypertension well controlled with medication
- Smokes 1 pack/day; 20-year history

MEDICATIONS
- Persantine 50 mg po tid
- Tenormin 25 mg po qd
- Aspirin 10 grains po bid

SOCIAL HISTORY
Patient lives with his wife and three teenage children and was independent and active before CVA. He has a college education and has worked for 18 years as a computer programmer. There is a two-step access to a rented, single-family house.

COGNITION
- Mild disorientation to time and place
- Attention span for up to 5 minutes on task
- Difficult to examine further owing to language impairment; cognitive deficits likely

LANGUAGE/COMMUNICATION
- Auditory comprehension: Reliable yes/no
- Verbal expression: Limited to only occasional automatic words
- Reading comprehension: Can read sentences
- Written expression: To be determined
- Gestures: Spontaneous use of gestures not evident

PHYSICAL THERAPY EXAMINATION
(Not assessed in this order, documented according to facility standards)
Passive Range of Motion
- BUEs Within Normal Limits (WNL); R shoulder pain at end ranges
- BLEs WNL except R dorsiflexion 0° to 5°

Sensation
- Right upper extremity (RUE) and right lower extremity (RLE) unable to test due to communication deficits.
- Patient reports pain in RUE, end ranges of shoulder motions.

Motor Control
- RUE: Active movement (1/2 range) (shoulder and elbow flexion); unable to isolate against gravity but can isolate into flexion and extension in a gravity-eliminated position. Unable to isolate movement of the hand, which is in flexion.

(Continued)

CASE STUDY—cont'd

- RLE: Full motion in both extensor and flexor synergy patterns with extensor pattern dominating; able to isolate hip flexion and extension and knee extension in the full range in a gravity-eliminated position.

Strength
- Left upper extremity (LUE) and left lower extremity (LLE): Full isolated movement with G+ to N strength
- RUE: Poor strength in the shoulder and elbow flexors
- RLE: Fair strength in the hip flexors and extensors and knee extensors, poor strength in the ankle dorsiflexors

Coordination
- LUE and LLE intact
- RUE and RLE: Limited movements; unable to test

Postural Control/Balance
- Sitting control: Maintains balance without support and proper alignment for 10 min. Able to displace COM over BOS independently and to both sides.
- Standing control: Able to maintain independent standing in parallel bars for up to 1 minute with LUE handhold. Able to displace COM over BOS with supervision to both sides.
- BBS: 46.

Functional Status
- Rolls to R: Independent with bedrail
- Rolls to L: min assist with UE
- Scoots up in bed: Supervision
- Supine-to-sit: min assist
- Sit-to-supine: min assist
- Transfers bed to chair: Stand pivot transfer, min assist (FIM 4)
- Eating: Supervision (FIM 5)
- Bathing: mod assist RUE and RLE (FIM 3)
- Dressing: mod assist RUE and RLE (FIM 3)

Gait and Locomotion
- W/C mobility: Propels 150 ft with supervision (FIM 5); uses LUE and L foot for propulsion.
- Locomotion: Ambulates 0.4 m/s using a hemi cane and a temporary dorsiflexor assist and close supervision to contact guard. Presents step asymmetry, decreased clearance of the stroke-affected leg, decreased stance time on the stroke-affected leg. Lacks a loading response and push-off.
- Stairs: Unable to test.

Upper Extremity Control
- Using extremity as a stabilizer when positioned in sitting

Endurance
- Tolerates 3/4-hour treatment session with frequent rests

Other Tests
  Orpington Score: 3.4

PSYCHOSOCIAL
Patient is motivated and cooperative. He appears anxious about his future and exhibited a brief episode of crying during the initial therapy session. His main goal is to walk again. Family is supportive and anxious to have him home again.

GUIDING QUESTIONS
1. Identify/categorize this patient's problems in terms of
    a. participation limitations.
    b. activity limitations.
    c. body function/structure limitations.

2. Identify three activity-based long-term goals (3 weeks) and three body function structure or activity-based goals (1 to 2 weeks) for this patient.

CASE STUDY—cont'd

3. For each of the following, formulate a treatment intervention that could be used during the first 2 weeks of therapy. Provide a brief rationale that justifies your choices.
   a. To address a UE deficit
   b. To address bed mobility
   c. To address transfers
   d. To address gait and locomotion

4. Describe how you would structure the intervention for the initial physical therapy sessions with this patient.

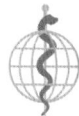 The reader is referred to Immersive Case C: A Patient With Stroke, an interactive case that guides users through the interview, examination, diagnosis, and writing of goals and the plan of care for a patient with stroke, available online at **fadavis.com**.

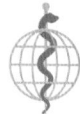 For additional resources, including answers to the questions for review, new immersive cases, case study guiding questions, references, and more, please visit **https://www.fadavis.com/product/physical -rehabilitation-fulk-8**. You may also quickly find the resources by entering this title's four-digit ISBN, 4691, in the search field at **http://fadavis.com** and logging in at the prompt.

Chapter 16

Multiple Sclerosis

Nora E. Fritz, PhD, PT, DPT, NCS
Tara L. McIsaac, PT, PhD

LEARNING OBJECTIVES

1. Describe the etiology, epidemiology, pathophysiology, signs and symptoms, diagnosis, and course of multiple sclerosis (MS).
2. Describe elements of the medical management of patients with MS.
3. Identify and describe the examination procedures used to inform the evaluation of patients with MS to establish the physical therapy diagnosis, prognosis, and plan of care.
4. Describe the role of the physical therapist in the management of patients with MS in terms of direct interventions and patient-/client-related instruction to maximize function and quality of life.
5. Describe appropriate elements of the exercise prescription for patients with MS.
6. Review current research findings concerning the rehabilitation of patients with MS.
7. Identify the psychosocial impact of MS and describe appropriate interventions.
8. Analyze and interpret patient data, formulate realistic goals and outcomes, and develop a plan of care when presented with a clinical case study.

CHAPTER OUTLINE

ETIOLOGY *589*
PATHOPHYSIOLOGY *589*
DISEASE COURSE *590*
 Exacerbating Factors *590*
SYMPTOMS *591*
 Sensory *591*
 Pain *591*
 Visual *591*
 Motor *593*
 Fatigue and Fatigability *593*
 Coordination and Balance *593*
 Gait and Mobility *594*
 Speech and Swallowing *594*
 Cognitive Impairment *594*
 Depression *594*
 Emotional Impairments *595*
 Bladder Dysfunction *595*
 Bowel *595*
 Sexual Dysfunction *595*
DIAGNOSIS *595*
MEDICAL MANAGEMENT *596*
 Management of Acute Relapses *596*
 Disease-Modifying Therapeutic Agents *597*
 Management of Symptoms *601*
FRAMEWORK FOR REHABILITATION *603*

PHYSICAL THERAPY EXAMINATION *604*
 Patient/Client History *604*
 Systems Review *606*
 Tests and Measures *606*
 Goals and Outcomes *611*
PHYSICAL THERAPY INTERVENTIONS *612*
 Management of Sensory Deficits and Skin Care *612*
 Management of Pain *613*
 Exercise Training *614*
 Management of Bladder Control *620*
 Management of Sexual Function *621*
 Management of Fatigue *621*
 Management of Spasticity *622*
 Management of Coordination and Balance Deficits *623*
 Locomotor Training *625*
 Functional Training *628*
 Management of Speech and Swallowing *629*
 Cognitive Training *630*
PSYCHOSOCIAL ISSUES *630*
PATIENT AND FAMILY/CAREGIVER EDUCATION *631*
SUMMARY *631*

Multiple sclerosis (MS) is a progressive autoimmune disease characterized by inflammation, selective demyelination, and gliosis. It causes both acute and chronic symptoms and can result in significant disability and impaired quality of life (QOL). MS affects over 900,000 persons in the United States and approximately 2.8 million people worldwide.[1] It was first defined by Dr. Jean Charcot in 1868 by its clinical and pathological characteristics: paralysis and the cardinal symptoms of intention tremor, scanning speech, and nystagmus, later termed *Charcot triad.* Using autopsy studies, he identified areas of hardened plaques and termed the disease *sclerosis in plaques.*[2]

The onset of MS typically occurs between ages 20 and 50 years with 9% having onset after the age of 50, and prevalence is highest in the age group of 55 to 64 years.[3,4] Only 3% to 5% of all individuals with MS have symptoms before the age of 16, although cases as young as 2 years have been reported.[5] The disease is more common in women than in men by a ratio of approximately 3:1, but men display a more progressive disease course and more rapid disability.[4] Interestingly, when symptoms occur after age 50 years, the prevalence is approximately equal for men and women, and approximately half of all individuals experience the progressive form of the disease.[6] Although the incidence and prevalence of MS overall have increased over the past five decades, this increase appears to be mostly related to an increased prevalence in women.[7] There are also ethnic/racial differences. Black populations have

47% increased risk of MS, and Hispanics and Asian/Pacific Islanders have 50% and 80% lower risk of MS, compared with White populations.[8] However, Black individuals tend to experience a more progressive disease course, have more frequent relapses with less recovery, are more likely to have optic nerve and spinal cord involvement, are more likely to develop greater disability over the same time period than their White counterparts, and they have the highest MS-related mortality under the age of 55 of all ethnic/racial groups.[9,10]

Epidemiological studies have established a geographical pattern of MS prevalence with areas of high, medium, and low frequency. High-frequency areas include the temperate zones of the northern United States, the Scandinavian countries, northern Europe, southern Canada, New Zealand, and southern Australia. Areas of medium frequency are closer to the equator and include the southern United States and Europe and the rest of Australia. Low-frequency areas are tropical and include Asia, Africa, and South America. Migration studies indicate that the geographical risk associated with an individual's birthplace is retained if emigration occurs after age 15 years. Individuals migrating before this age assume the risk of their new location.[1,11,12]

■ ETIOLOGY

The risk of developing MS in the general population is 0.1%, while the risk of MS is increased in persons with an affected family member. The risk is 2% for a child of a person with MS, 5% for a sibling or fraternal co-twin of a person with MS, rising to 25% for an identical co-twin.[13] Genetic studies have revealed more than 100 interacting alleles that may contribute to MS susceptibility with mutations in the human leukocyte antigen major histocompatibility complex (*MHC*) gene most strongly correlated. It appears that although individuals do not inherit the disease, they may inherit a genetic susceptibility to immune system dysfunction.[14]

When persons with a genetic susceptibility are exposed to a viral agent, the immune system responds with activated myelin-reactive lymphocytes, a concept known as *molecular mimicry*. Implicated viruses in this process under investigation include the Epstein-Barr virus, human herpesvirus-6, cytomegalovirus, human endogenous retroviruses (HERVs), *chlamydia pneumoniae,* measles, rubella, and varicella-zoster viruses; and questions remain about the role of SARS-CoV-2, though none have been definitely proven to trigger MS.[15–17] The viruses may be retained in the body, resulting in a self-perpetuating autoimmune process. Risk of MS may also be increased with vitamin D deficiency and smoking.

■ PATHOPHYSIOLOGY

In patients with MS, an abnormal immune-mediated response attacks the *myelin* nerve coating, the *oligodendrocytes* (myelin producing cells), and the nerve fibers themselves in the central nervous system (CNS). The response triggers activation of immune cells (e.g., selective activation of helper T cells and killer T cells, with a corresponding decrease in regulatory T cells, and B-cell activation) that cross the blood-brain barrier, entering the CNS and initiating a damaging inflammatory cascade of events (the *outside-in model*).[18] The *inside-out model* has been proposed in which oligodendrocyte damage and loss occur first, which then triggers immune attacks and inflammation.[19] Along with inflammation and phagocytic activity of macrophages, mitochondrial damage is thought to contribute to demyelination, oligodendrocyte loss, and axonal damage.[18,20] Myelin serves as an insulator, speeding up the conduction along nerve fibers from one node of Ranvier to another (termed *saltatory conduction*). It also serves to conserve energy for the nerve because depolarization occurs only at the nodes. Disruption of the myelin sheath and active demyelination slow neural transmission and cause nerves to fatigue rapidly. With severe disruption, conduction block occurs with resulting disruption of function.

The acute inflammatory attack on myelin gradually subsides, contributing to the pattern of fluctuations in function that characterize this disease (*relapses,* defined as periods of acute worsening of neurological function, and *remissions,* defined as periods without disease progression and partial or complete abatement of signs and symptoms). With repeat attacks, the anti-inflammatory processes become less effective and are unable to keep up. During the early stages of MS, oligodendrocytes survive the initial insult and can produce remyelination. This process is often incomplete and, as the disease becomes more chronic, stalls altogether. When the oligodendrocytes become damaged, myelin repair cannot occur. One form of MS, primary progressive MS in which relapses and remissions do not occur, appears to be closely associated with oligodendrocyte damage and neurodegeneration.[21] Demyelinated areas eventually become filled with fibrous astrocytes and undergo a process called gliosis. Gliosis refers to the proliferation of neuroglial tissue within the CNS and results in glial scars (*plaques*). The axon itself becomes interrupted, undergoes neurodegeneration, and is believed to be the main cause of permanent neurological disability. It has long been thought that MS progresses in a two-stage process: inflammatory damage with associated demyelination and some axonal damage as the first stage and degenerative changes including axonal and oligodendrocyte destruction as the second stage. Studies suggest that both neuroinflammation and neurodegeneration may occur simultaneously rather than sequentially.[20]

In advanced cases of relapsing-remitting MS and earlier in progressive forms of MS, there are both acute and degenerative lesions of varying size scattered throughout the CNS (brain, brain stem, cerebellum, and spinal cord). Lesions primarily affect white matter early, with lesions of gray matter evident in more advanced disease. Lesions may also include small perivascular areas of demyelination and pial surface lesions. Brain atrophy, the loss of axons and myelin throughout the brain, is evident even in early stages of the disease and is progressive. There are certain areas most susceptible, such as the optic nerves, periventricular white matter, spinal cord (corticospinal tracts, posterior white columns), and cerebellar peduncles.[20]

■ DISEASE COURSE

MS is highly variable and unpredictable from person to person and within a given individual over time. In 1996, the U.S. National Multiple Sclerosis Society (NMSS) Advisory Council on Clinical Trials in Multiple Sclerosis defined the clinical course descriptions (phenotypes) of multiple sclerosis.[22] These phenotype descriptions were intended to represent the spectrum of MS subtypes but were based on subjective views of the time and lacked objective biological supports that are now available. These descriptions of MS phenotypes were revised in 2013 by the International Advisory Committee on Clinical Trials of MS, eliminating one subtype (progressive relapsing MS) and adding a new subtype (clinically isolated syndrome).[23] Since 2013, the four phenotypes used to characterize MS, shown in Box 16.1, are clinically isolated syndrome (CIS), relapsing-remitting MS (RRMS), primary progressive MS (PPMS), and secondary progressive MS (SPMS). The 2013 revisions also added modifiers for each phenotype, clarified in 2017 and 2020 as *activity* (clinical relapses or new MRI activity) and *progression* (progressive accumulation of disability independent of any relapse activity), both of which should be evaluated at least annually.[23–25]

CIS refers to a first episode of inflammatory demyelination in the CNS that could become MS if additional activity occurs. CIS can be further characterized as *not active* or *active* in which case it becomes RRMS. *RRMS* is the most common course, affecting approximately 85% of patients with MS. It is characterized by discrete attacks or relapses followed by remissions and can also be further characterized as *active* or *not active*. Most people diagnosed with RRMS will eventually transition to *SPMS*. SPMS begins with a relapsing-remitting course followed by progression to steady and irreversible worsening of neurological function and accumulation of disability. As with CIS and RRMS, SPMS can be further characterized as either *active* or *not active* but is also characterized as *with progression* or *without progression*, referring to progressive accumulation of disability. *PPMS* is a less common form occurring in about 15% of cases. It is characterized by a nearly continuous worsening of the disease from the onset without distinct attacks and is further characterized as *active* or *not active* and as *with progression* or *without progression*.

Box 16.1   Four Major Clinical Subtypes of MS[23]

Clinically Isolated Syndrome (CIS)

- A single clinical episode indicating central nervous system (CNS) demyelination in a person not known to have multiple sclerosis (MS)
- Not Active
- Active

Relapsing-Remitting Disease (RRMS)

- Clearly defined relapses or exacerbations followed by partial or full recovery
- Not Active
- Active

Primary Progressive (PPMS)

- Progressive accumulation of disability from onset
- Active and with progression
- Active but without progression
- Not active but with progression
- Not active and without progression (stable disease)

Secondary Progressive (SPMS)

- Progressive accumulation of disability after initial relapsing course
- Active and with progression
- Active but without progression
- Not active but with progression
- Not active and without progression (stable disease)

Because the course of the disease may alter (RRMS to SPMS), clinicians need to be alert to changes in signs or symptoms in terms of severity, frequency, and impact on function, evaluating at least annually.[16,23–25] The 1996 category of progressive relapsing MS was eliminated since these patients are now classified as PPMS with disease activity. Box 16.1 summarizes the disease-course definitions and modifiers (clinical subtype/phenotype) of MS.

Exacerbating Factors

MS relapses (exacerbations) are defined by new and recurrent MS symptoms lasting more than 24 hr, but generally of longer duration, that are unrelated to another etiology. Several exacerbating factors have been identified. Avoiding these factors is important in ensuring the patient's optimal function. An individual whose overall health deteriorates is more likely to have a relapse than one who remains healthy. Viral or bacterial infections (e.g., common cold, influenza, urinary tract infection, sinus infection) and diseases of major organ systems (e.g., hepatitis, pancreatitis, asthma attacks) are associated with relapses of disease. There is also a modest link between stress and acute attacks. Both major stresses (divorce, death, job loss, and trauma) and minor stresses (exhaustion, dehydration, malnutrition, and sleep deprivation) can affect the immune system and an already compromised nervous system.

Pseudoexacerbation refers to the temporary worsening of MS symptoms. The episode typically comes and goes quickly, usually within 24 hr. The overwhelming majority of individuals with MS demonstrate an adverse reaction to heat, known as *Uhthoff symptom*. Anything that raises the body temperature can bring on a pseudoattack. External heat stressors include sun exposure, hot muggy environmental temperatures, or a hot bath. Internal elevations in temperature can be produced by fever or prolonged exercise; however, studies indicate exercise is a safe and essential component of health for individuals with MS.[26] The effects are usually immediate and dramatic in terms of reduced function and increased fatigue. Most pseudoattacks resolve within 24 hr of cooling off and/or the end of a fever.

■ SYMPTOMS

Symptoms of MS vary considerably, depending on the location of specific lesions within the CNS. Early symptoms typically include visual disturbances (e.g., episodes of double vision) and paresthesias progressing to numbness, weakness, and fatigability. In more advanced stages, patients demonstrate multiple symptoms with varying involvement. Common MS symptoms are presented in Box 16.2.[20,27] The onset of symptoms can develop rapidly over a course of minutes or hours; less frequently, onset is insidious, occurring over a period of weeks or months. An early remission may lead the individual to postpone initial neurological workup for months or longer.

Sensory

Complete loss of any single sensation (anesthesia) is rare. Focal deficits can produce limited areas of diminished sensation (hypoesthesia). Altered sensations are far more common and can include *paresthesias* (pins-and-needles sensation) or numbness of the face, body, or extremities. Disturbances in position sense are also common, as are lower extremity (LE) impairments of vibratory sense.[20,27]

Pain

Approximately 80% of patients with MS experience pain, with clinically significant pain occurring in about 55% of individuals; almost half experience chronic pain.[27,28] Pain in MS is often assumed to be *neuropathic* resulting from demyelinating and axonal lesions in the spinothalamic tracts or sensory roots and is described as a burning, aching, "pins-and-needles" pain. *Nociceptive pain* (activation of nociceptors in the periphery)

Box 16.2   Common Symptoms in Multiple Sclerosis

Sensory Symptoms

- Hypoesthesia, numbness
- Paresthesias

Pain

- Paroxysmal limb pain, dysesthesias
- Headache
- Optic or trigeminal neuritis
- Lhermitte sign
- Hyperpathia
- Chronic neuropathic pain

Visual Symptoms

- Blurred or double vision (diplopia)
- Diminished acuity/loss of vision
- Scotoma
- Nystagmus
- Lateral gaze palsy

Motor Symptoms

- Paresis or paralysis
- Fatigue
- Spasticity, spasms
- Ataxia: incoordination, intention tremor
- Postural tremor
- Impaired balance and gait

Fatigue

- Physical fatigue
- Cognitive fatigue
- Emotional fatigue
- Social fatigue

Coordination and Balance Symptoms

- Ataxia
- Hypotonia
- Truncal weakness
- Postural tremor
- Impaired balance

Gait and Mobility Symptoms

- Difficulty walking
- Difficulty with transfers
- Falls, fall injuries, fear of falling

Speech and Swallowing

- Dysarthria
- Dysphonia
- Dysphagia

Cognitive Symptoms

- Diminished information processing
- Short-term memory deficits
- Difficulty performing multiple tasks simultaneously

(Continued)

Box 16.2 Common Symptoms in Multiple Sclerosis—cont'd

- Diminished attention, concentration
- Diminished executive functions
- Diminished visual–spatial abilities

Affective Symptoms

- Depression, major depressive disorder
- Anxiety
- Pseudobulbar affect

Bladder and Bowel Symptoms

- Spastic bladder
- Flaccid bladder
- Dyssynergic bladder
- Recurrent urinary tract infections
- Constipation
- Diarrhea and incontinence

Sexual Symptoms

- Decreased libido
- Impaired ability to achieve orgasm
- Women: Changes in sensation, vaginal dryness
- Men: Erectile dysfunction, decreased sensation, difficulty ejaculating

Pattern of Symptoms

- Varies greatly from person to person
- Varies over time in each individual affected
- First symptoms usually transient; typically sensory and/ or visual
- Diagnosis involves evidence of damage occurring in at least two separate areas of the central nervous system and at two separate points in time at least 1 month apart (*dissemination of lesions in space and time*)

and *nociplastic pain* (altered processing; centralized pain) are not well described or understood in MS (also see Chapter 25, Chronic Pain). Survey research of MS pain phenotypes indicates that up to 23% may be nociplastic only, and another 27% a mixed type of neuropathic and nociplastic.[28] Patients often experience acute, paroxysmal pain characterized by sudden and spontaneous onset. The pains are described as intense, sharp, shooting, electric shock–like, and burning. The most common types are trigeminal neuralgia, paroxysmal limb pain, and headache. *Trigeminal neuralgia* (tic douloureux) results from demyelination of the sensory division of the trigeminal nerve innervating the face, cheek, and jaw. Eating, shaving, or simply touching the face may trigger painful episodes. A common sign of posterior column damage in the spinal cord is Lhermitte sign in which flexion of the neck produces an electric shock–like sensation running down the spine and into the LEs. Paroxysmal limb pain presents as abnormal burning, aching pain (*dysesthesias*) that can affect any part of the body but is more common in the LEs and is often worse at night and after exercise. It can be aggravated by temperature elevations. *Hyperpathia*, a hypersensitivity to minor sensory stimuli, can occur. Headache is more frequent in MS than in the general population and can be migraine or tension type. Musculoskeletal pain associated with muscle and ligament strain can develop from mechanical stress, abnormal postures, and immobility, often the result of weak muscles, powerful spasticity, and tonic spasms. Anxiety and fear can worsen pain symptoms.[27,28]

Visual

Visual symptoms are common with MS and are found in approximately 80% of patients. Involvement of the

optic nerve produces altered visual acuity; blindness is rare. *Optic neuritis,* inflammation of the optic nerve, is the initial clinical event in 25% of new cases of MS, and 50% to 70% of all patients will at some point experience optic neuritis. It produces an ice pick–like pain behind the eye with blurring or graying of vision or blindness in one eye. A *scotoma* or dark spot may occur in the center of the visual field. Neuritis rarely affects both eyes and is usually self-limiting. Vision generally improves within 4 to 12 weeks. Damage to the optic nerve will also affect light reflexes. Relative afferent pupillary defect (*Marcus Gunn pupil*) often develops in individuals with MS who have had an episode of optic neuritis. Shining a bright light into the healthy eye will produce reflex contraction in both eyes (consensual light reflex). If the light is then shone in the affected eye only, a paradoxical widening (dilation) of both pupils occurs.

Eye movements can be disturbed in a variety of ways. *Nystagmus* is common in patients with MS and results from lesions affecting the cerebellum or central vestibular pathways. This involves involuntary and rapid cyclical movements of the eyeball (horizontal or vertical) that develop when the patient looks to the sides or vertically (gaze-induced nystagmus) or when the patient moves the head. *Internuclear ophthalmoplegia* (INO) produces incomplete eye adduction (lateral gaze palsy) on the affected side and nystagmus of the opposite abducting eye with gaze to one side. It is caused by demyelination of the pontine medial longitudinal fasciculus (MLF). Additional impairments in conjugate gaze and control of eye movements may also be present with brain stem lesions affecting cranial nerves III, IV, and VI or the MLF. *Diplopia,* double vision, occurs when the muscles that control the eyes are not well coordinated. Visual disturbances frequently remit and are seldom the primary cause of disability. The effects of impaired vision on balance and movement should be carefully examined.[29,30]

Motor

Patients with corticospinal lesions demonstrate signs and symptoms of upper motor neuron (UMN) syndrome. Paresis, spasticity, brisk tendon reflexes, involuntary flexor and extensor spasms, clonus, Babinski sign, exaggerated cutaneous reflexes, and loss of precise autonomic control all characterize UMN involvement. (See discussion in Chapter 5, Examination of Motor Function: Motor Control and Motor Learning.)

Weakness

Patients with UMN syndrome demonstrate movements that are slow, stiff, and weak, the result of loss of orderly recruitment and reduced firing rate modulation of motor neurons. Reduced muscle strength, power, and endurance, along with impaired synergistic relationships, are evident. Patients with cerebellar lesions demonstrate asthenia or generalized muscle weakness along with ataxia. Patients can also experience muscle weakness secondary to inactivity. Muscle weakness can vary from a mild paresis, often transient at first, to total paralysis of the involved extremities.[27]

Spasticity

Spasticity is an extremely common problem in patients with MS; spasticity can range from mild to severe, depending on the duration of the disease, number of relapses, and worsening symptoms in recent months. It occurs in the muscles of the upper extremities (UEs) and particularly the LEs. Clinical indications of spasticity include impaired voluntary control of movement (abnormal co-contraction); increased deep tendon reflexes (DTRs); clonus; and decreased range of motion (ROM). Spasticity also results in increased fatigue, impaired functional mobility, and impaired activities of daily living (ADL). Spasticity can cause pain, disabling contractures, abnormal posturing, problems in maintaining skin integrity, and falls. For some patients, spasticity can be beneficial to sitting and standing,[31] acting to support weak musculature. Spasticity fluctuates on a daily basis and can be exacerbated by certain factors such as fatigue, stress, overheating (fever, environmental), cold temperatures, infections, or noxious stimuli (e.g., pain, bladder, renal, bowel, skin lesions/injury).[31] Certain antidepressant agents (serotonin-reuptake inhibitors such as fluoxetine, sertraline, and paroxetine) can exacerbate spasticity. Spasticity does not typically abate during spontaneous remissions. In patients with advanced disease, spasticity can be quite disabling and difficult to manage.[31,32]

Fatigue and Fatigability

Fatigue is one of the most frequent and disabling symptoms of MS. Fatigue in MS may come on abruptly without warning and worsens throughout the day.

People with MS describe four biopsychosocial experiences of fatigue: (1) physical (lack of or drained of energy, heavy limbs, feeling unable to move/paralyzed); (2) cognitive (unable to think clearly, as if in a dream, not fully present, needing more effort to concentrate on and remember information); (3) emotional (feelings of sorrow, shame, isolation, depression, fear, worry, and anxiety); and (4) social (loss of autonomy, not being understood by others).[33] Despite its prevalence, the pathophysiology of fatigue in MS is still not completely understood. Fatigue is perception measured by self-report, whereas fatigability is a measure of physical or cognitive work capacity or decline in performance over time.[34] Changes in fatigue depend on the task being performed, the environment, and the individual's mental and physical capacity.[35] Central factors contributing to fatigue in MS include inflammation, axonal conduction velocity, imbalance of neurotransmitter levels, and decreased cerebral glucose metabolism. Peripheral factors of fatigue in MS involve slowed contractile properties and decreased metabolic response of muscles.[35] A patient's level of fatigue can be influenced by physical exertion, exposure to heat and humidity, disturbed or reduced sleep, depression, anxiety, cognitive impairment, and medical conditions (e.g., respiratory infection). Side effects of medications also affect fatigue, including analgesics, anticonvulsants, antidepressants, antihistamines, antihypertensive agents, and anti-inflammatory agents.[36]

Coordination and Balance

Demyelinating lesions in the cerebellum and cerebellar tracts are common in MS, producing cerebellar symptoms. Clinical manifestations include ataxia, hypotonia, and truncal weakness. Ataxia is a general term used to describe uncoordinated movements characterized by dysmetria, dyssynergia, and dysdiadochokinesia. Progressive ataxia of the trunk and LEs is often apparent. During sitting or standing, when a limb or the body must be supported against gravity, the patient typically presents with truncal dysmetria (shaking, back-and-forth oscillatory movements) seen as a *postural tremor*. Dysmetria and ataxia of the limbs are involuntary, rhythmic, shaking movements, seen as *intention (action) tremors,* that occur when purposeful movement is attempted and results from the inability of the cerebellum to dampen motor movements. See Chapter 6, Examination of Coordination and Balance. These tremorous movements vary in severity from slight, barely perceptible quivering to wide oscillations. When severe they impose significant limitations in performance of functional activities, particularly in such areas as eating, speaking clearly, writing, personal hygiene, and walking. Dysmetria and ataxia can be exacerbated by stress, excitement, and anxiety, all adrenaline-releasing conditions producing a temporary aroused condition.[27,37,38] Severe numbness of the feet can contribute to difficulty with standing balance or walking (sensory ataxia).

Lesions affecting the cerebellum or central vestibular pathways can produce vestibular dysfunction. Patients may experience symptoms of dizziness, disequilibrium, vertigo, and nausea. Symptoms are precipitated or made worse by movements of the head or eyes. See Chapter 21, Vestibular Disorders.

Gait and Mobility

Individuals with MS have difficulty walking due to muscle weakness, fatigue, spasticity, impaired balance, impaired sensation, visual problems, and ataxia. Approximately half of patients with RRMS will require some form of assistance during walking within 15 years of their diagnosis. Weakness in one or both LEs may result in asymmetric step lengths and increased variability of gait, while severe LE extensor spasticity may produce a scissoring gait pattern. Staggering, uneven steps, poor foot placement, uncoordinated limb movements, and frequent loss of balance characterize ataxic gait. Gait and balance impairments increase the risk of falls and fall injury. Approximately 50% to 80% of patients with MS have balance and gait dysfunction, and at least 50% fall at least once each year. Three interrelated problems contribute to balance impairment in MS: smaller and slower movements to limits of stability (LOS), slowed responses to perturbations and postural movements, and decreased ability to maintain a position (ataxia). Fear of falling is associated with self-imposed restrictions in mobility and contributes to disability and social isolation.[39,40] Safe and goal-oriented walking requires higher-level cognitive processing, highlighting the strong relationship between cognitive function and gait.[41] Deficits in both walking and cognitive function are common in MS. These impairments are compounded when performing walking and cognitive tasks simultaneously (dual tasking), referred to as *cognitive-motor interference* (CMI). While walking performance declines in people with MS as a result of CMI, a systematic review and meta-analysis of 13 studies found only minimal difference in the CMI between individuals with and without MS.[42]

Speech and Swallowing

Speech problems are the result of muscle weakness, spasticity, tremor, or ataxia. As many as 44% of individuals with MS experience impairment of speech or voice after disease onset.[43,44] Dysarthria is characterized by slurred or poorly articulated speech with low volume, unnatural emphasis, and slow rate. Dysphonia is characterized by changes in vocal quality including harshness, hoarseness, breathiness, or hypernasal sounds. Poor coordination of the tongue, oral, and pharyngeal muscles can also result in dysphagia, difficulty in swallowing. Signs of swallowing dysfunction include difficulty chewing and

maintaining a lip seal, inability to swallow (ingest food), and spitting or coughing or throat clearing during or after meals. Aspiration pneumonia is a serious complication that can develop if foods or liquids are inhaled into the trachea. Signs of aspiration include coughing or throat clearing after intake, a wet voice quality with gurgling or sounds of congestion, and fever. The patient is also at risk for poor nutritional intake and dehydration and may experience weight loss. Poor coordination of breath control and posture contributes to speech and feeding difficulties.[43,45] See Chapter 28, Neurogenic Disorders of Speech and Language.

Cognitive Impairment

Cognitive impairment is common in MS and may appear in either early or later stages of the disease, with prevalence rates of up to 70%.[46] Multiple aspects of cognition are impacted by MS, most commonly in decreased information processing speed.[47] Other deficits in selective cognitive domains include impaired attention and concentration, executive functioning (concept formation, abstract reasoning, problem-solving, planning, and sequencing), visuospatial functions, verbal fluency, and working memory.[46-48] Overall intellectual functioning, long-term memory, conversational skills, and reading comprehension are typically intact. Cognitive impairments are related to the specific locations and total volume of the lesions, cerebral atrophy, third ventricle width, and corpus callosum size.[49] With increasing lesion load over time, neuroplastic changes occur to compensate and maintain cognitive function but eventually are ineffective.[49] Cognitive function is not associated with overall severity of the disease, its course, or the patient's disability status. Focal frontal lobe lesions can produce cognitive inflexibility and poor impulse control. Secondary factors that can influence cognition include depression, anxiety, fatigue, medications, and comorbid conditions (e.g., cardiovascular or cerebrovascular disease).[48,50] Level of cognitive dysfunction is a major factor in determining QOL, social functioning, employment status, and function.[48,51] See Chapter 27, Cognitive and Perceptual Dysfunction.

Depression

Depression is a common symptom of MS; indeed major depressive disorder, the most severe form, occurs in up to 50% of individuals.[50] The age-standardized incidence of depression is 71% higher and prevalence is roughly 10% higher than in the matched population.[52,53] Inflammation may be a contributing factor to depression in MS, as individuals with other neuroinflammatory diseases, such as inflammatory bowel disease and rheumatoid arthritis, also experience depression at similar rates to individuals with MS.[54] Depressive symptoms can include feelings of hopelessness or despair, diminished interest or pleasure in activities, changes in appetite and significant weight loss or gain, insomnia or hypersomnia (daytime sleepiness), feelings of lethargy or worthlessness, fatigue or loss of energy, decreased concentration, and recurrent thoughts of death and suicide.[50] Depression can occur from a complex interaction of pathological processes in MS, a preexisting or predisposition to mood disorder as a side effect of some drugs (e.g., corticosteroids, interferon), a psychological reaction to the stresses of this far-reaching and unpredictable disease, and normal grieving of the losses associated with MS.[50,55]

Other mood disorders also occur more frequently in MS; the prevalence of anxiety disorders is up to 36%, adjustment disorder is up to 22%, and bipolar disorder (alternating periods of depression and mania) is up to 13%.[50,53,56] Denial, anger, aggression, and substance abuse can also occur. Patients with MS face enormous issues related to the ambiguity of their health status, unpredictable course of disease activity, unpredictable future status, and loss of effective functioning during the prime of their lives.

Emotional Impairments

Affective disorders in MS occur as a direct result from effects of the disease on the brain and can include changes in mood, feelings, emotional expression, and control. Pseudobulbar affect (PBA), also known as *involuntary emotional expression disorder* or *emotional incontinence,* occurs in about 10% of people with MS and is characterized by sudden and unpredictable episodes of crying, laughing, or other emotional displays.[57,58] PBA may occur when the disease damages the area of the brain that controls normal expression of emotion, including the limbic system and paralimbic networks.[57] Euphoria is an exaggerated feeling of well-being, a sense of optimism incongruent with the patient's incapacitating disability, which is less common and can occur in more advanced MS or with significant cognitive changes.[59,60] Apathy is the lack of motivation affecting cognitive, emotional, and behavioral domains, which occurs in MS with a prevalence of up to 40% and is correlated to more severe cognitive dysfunction.[60,61]

Bladder Dysfunction

Urinary bladder dysfunction occurs in about 80% of patients. Demyelinating lesions affecting the lateral and posterior spinal tracts unmask the sacral reflex arc producing loss in volitional and synergistic control of the micturition reflex. Types of bladder dysfunction in MS can include a small, spastic bladder (a failure-to-store problem), a flaccid or big bladder (a failure-to-empty problem), or a dyssynergic bladder. The dyssynergic bladder represents a problem with coordination between bladder contraction and sphincter relaxation. Common symptoms include urinary urgency, urinary frequency, hesitancy in starting urination, nocturia (frequency at night), dribbling, and incontinence. The severity of bladder symptoms is associated with severity of other neurological symptoms, particularly pyramidal tract involvement. Progressive loss of functional mobility (e.g., hand skills, sitting balance and transfer skills, ambulation) contributes to personal hygiene problems, emotional distress, and functional incontinence (inability to toilet or manage dysfunction). Emptying dysfunction with large residual urine volume increases the risk of recurrent urinary tract infections (UTIs) and kidney damage from frequent UTIs.[62]

Bowel

Constipation is the most common bowel complaint in patients with MS and results from lesions affecting control of the gastrocolic reflex. It is associated with the presence of spasticity of the pelvic floor muscles and is also a frequent consequence of inactivity, lack of fluid intake, poor diet and bowel habits, depression, and medication side effects. Bowel impaction is a serious complication that requires immediate attention. Diarrhea and incontinence are less problematic but can also occur as a result of loss of rectal control, sphincter abnormalities, or other, secondary problems (e.g., gastroenteritis, inflammatory bowel disease, medication side effect).[63]

Sexual Dysfunction

Sexual dysfunction is common, affecting as many as 91% of men and 72% of women. In women, symptoms can include changes in sensation, vaginal dryness, trouble reaching orgasm, and loss of libido. In men, symptoms can include erectile dysfunction, decreased sensation, difficulty or inability to ejaculate, and loss of libido. Sexual activity is also affected by the appearance of other symptoms such as spasticity, uncontrollable spasms, pain, weakness and fatigue, bladder or bowel incontinence, losses in functional mobility, and changes in self-image. Psychological factors have a large impact on function. Sexual dysfunction has tremendous functional and psychosocial implications for both patient and partner.[64]

■ DIAGNOSIS

The early and accurate diagnosis of MS is important to take advantage of the recent advances in effective medication treatments for relapsing-remitting MS. Misdiagnosis or delayed diagnosis is not uncommon because the initial presentation of MS is highly variable, and patients can consult with a wide range of health-care professionals.[24,25] There is no definitive diagnostic test for MS. Instead, a diagnosis of exclusion is made by a neurologist based on a careful medical history, a complete neurological examination, and supportive laboratory tests. Diagnosis of MS relies on two key features determined from evidence of lesions seen on MRI: dissemination in space (*DIS*) and dissemination in time (*DIT*).

- DIS can be satisfied by at least one T2-weighted MRI lesion seen in two of the four MS typical areas of the CNS: periventricular, juxtacortical/cortical, infratentorial, or spinal cord.
- DIT can be satisfied by a single scan in a patient with a clinically silent contrast-enhancing (gadolinium) lesion and another clinically silent T2-weighted (nonenhancing) lesion at any time. Alternatively, any new T2 lesion seen after the original scan, or the presence of CSF-specific oligoclonal bands can fulfill DIT.[25]

The revised 2017 *McDonald Criteria of the International Panel on Diagnosis of MS* has resulted in earlier diagnosis of MS with improved specificity and sensitivity (TipSheet is available at https://www.nationalmssociety.org).[25] In addition, other possible diagnoses that mimic MS must be ruled out. The mnemonic **VITAMINS** is helpful in ruling out the many diseases/disorders of **V**ascular, **I**nfectious, **T**raumatic, **A**utoimmune, **M**etabolic/toxic, **I**diopathic/genetic, **N**eoplastic, and p**S**ychiatric origin that can mimic MS.[20,65,66] Among the common differential diagnoses are *acute disseminating encephalomyelitis* (*ADEM*), acute and subacute *transverse myelitis*, and *neuromyelitis optica* (NMO) spectrum disorders.[20,67]

Laboratory tests used to help confirm the diagnosis include MRI, evoked potentials (EPs), and lumbar puncture (LP) with cerebrospinal fluid (CSF) analysis. MRI is highly sensitive for detecting MS plaques/lesions in the white matter of the brain and spinal cord (Fig. 16.1). The Consortium of Multiple Sclerosis Centers in 2016 revised their guidelines for diagnostic and follow-up standardized MRI protocol.[68] A brain MRI with gadolinium (GAD) is recommended for the diagnosis of MS, because it is specifically used to see vascular structures and breakdown in the blood-brain barrier. Most new lesions are characterized by an area of GAD enhancement seen as signal hyperintensity, "bright spots," often ovoid and arranged at right angles to the corpus callosum as if radiating from this area. When seen in sagittal view, they are referred to as *Dawson fingers*, which are relatively specific to MS and may help differentiate from other conditions, such as NMO (Fig. 16.1).[69]

A spinal cord MRI is additionally recommended if the brain MRI is nondiagnostic or if the presenting symptoms are at the level of the spinal cord. Follow-up MRIs with GAD are recommended to demonstrate DIT and ongoing disease activity that is "clinically silent" (active lesion without correlated clinical signs) while on medication treatment. In addition, follow-up MRIs should be done to evaluate unexpected clinical worsening and as a new baseline prior to starting or modifying medications, with routine brain MRIs every 6 months to 2 years for all patients with relapsing MS.[68] MS lesions that appear as hypointense areas on T1-weighted MRIs, "black holes," are thought to indicate axonal loss, tissue destruction, and neurodegeneration.[70,71] Most patients with clinically defined MS have well-defined MRI changes; however, 5% of individuals with clinically defined MS do not exhibit MRI changes. Lesions seen on MRI in "silent" areas of the brain that do not cause symptoms make it difficult to correlate the MRI findings of lesion load and the individual's clinical signs and symptoms, called the clinical-radiological paradox.[72] Additionally, some healthy individuals can exhibit bright spots on MRI.[66,73]

Up to 90% of individuals with MS demonstrate abnormal EP. The presence of demyelinating lesions on visual, auditory, and somatosensory pathways produces slowed central conduction. Of the three, visual evoked potentials have been found to be the most helpful in the diagnostic process.[20,67]

Patients with MS show elevated total immunoglobulin (IgG) in CSF and the presence of oligoclonal IgG bands in response to inflammatory demyelinating lesions. Patients with PPMS have higher levels of immunoglobulins in spinal fluid than patients with RRMS.[20,67]

■ MEDICAL MANAGEMENT

A number of medications are used to help treat and prevent relapses and slow the progression of neurological disability. Medications are also given to provide symptom relief.

Management of Acute Relapses

Corticosteroid therapy (methylprednisolone) is used to treat acute disease relapses (exacerbations), shortening the duration of the episode. These drugs exert powerful anti-inflammatory and immunosuppressive effects, including diminished swelling within the CNS, decreased T-cell activation, limited immune cell penetration of the CNS, and enhanced apoptosis of activated immune cells. The drugs do not modify the disease course or degree of recovery. Typically, corticosteroids are given in high doses (500 to 1,000 mg/day), administered intravenously for a brief course (e.g., 3 to 5 days), followed by tapered dosage of oral medication over a period of 1 to 3 weeks. Potential adverse side effects include mood changes, increased blood pressure, fluid retention, hyperglycemia, acne, and insomnia. Chronic use is associated with hypertension, diabetes, aseptic femoral necrosis, osteopenia, and peptic ulcer.

Plasmapheresis (plasma exchange) may be used to enhance recovery from an acute relapse in patients who fail to respond to steroids. It is used for an exacerbation of RRMS and is not recommended for PPMS or SPMS.

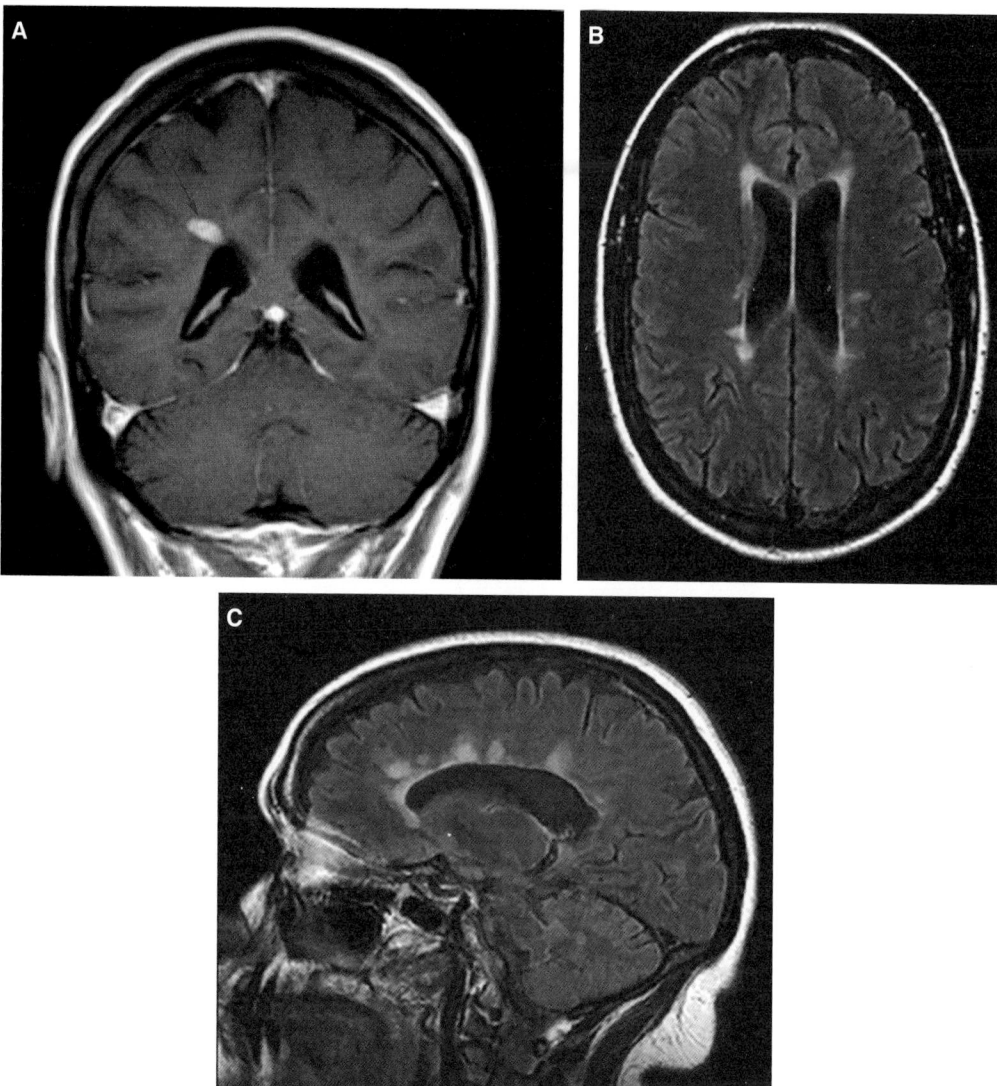

Figure 16.1 (A) Coronal contrast-enhanced T1 MRI. The contrast enhancement of a periventricular white matter lesion (arrow) indicates that this is an active MS plaque. Other (older) plaques in this case that were T2 hyperintense showed no enhancement. *(From Weber et al.,[71] with permission.)* *(B) Axial and (C) sagittal T2-weighted MRI demonstrating common periventricular lesional pattern in persons with MS. (From Raz et al.,[69] with permission.) The pattern seen in (C) is known as Dawson fingers, and indicates demyelinating plaques through the corpus callosum; this pattern of T2 hyperintensities is relatively specific to MS and may help in the differentiation between MS and other demyelinating conditions, such as neuromyelitis optica.[69]*

Disease-Modifying Therapeutic Agents

Since 1993 the U.S. Food and Drug Administration (FDA) has approved drugs to reduce disease activity in people with MS. The goal of these drugs is to prevent future disease activity, not return function that has been lost. The Multiple Sclerosis Coalition developed a consensus paper, updated in 2019, summarizing current evidence about disease modification in MS and providing support for access to disease-modifying therapies (DMTs) for people with MS in the United States.[74] The consensus paper identified four important themes from the evidence in DMTs in MS: (1) early and successful control of disease activity is important for reducing the accumulation of disability, helping individuals with MS to stay active, and protecting QOL; (2) early disease activity and progression result in physical impairments as only one aspect of disability; (3) prognosis is variable and unpredictable among individuals; and (4) treatment adherence is important to efficacy, and barriers to adherence should be identified and addressed early. The DMTs that have been approved by the FDA through August 2020 are listed in Table 16.1. Synthetic interferon drugs are injectable drugs that have substantial

Text continued on page 601

Table 16.1   Disease-Modifying Therapeutic Agents for Multiple Sclerosis[75,244]

Agent	FDA-Approved Indications	Select Side Effects	Contraindications/ Boxed Warning	Delivery System and Frequency
Alemtuzumab (Lemtrada)	Relapsing forms of MS, generally for patients who have had an inadequate response to two or more MS therapies	Infusion reactions: • Rash • Fever • Headache • Anaphylaxis • Cardiac arrhythmias • UTI • Upper respiratory infection • Diarrhea • Paresthesia • Dizziness • Nausea	Because of the risk of autoimmunity, life-threatening infusion reactions, and malignancies, alemtuzumab is available only through restricted distribution under a REMS program	IV infusion in a medical center on 5 consecutive days followed 12 months later by IV infusion on 3 consecutive days
Cladribine (Mavenclad)	Relapsing forms of MS. Because of its safety profile, generally recommended for those with inadequate response to or unable to tolerate alternative treatments	• Respiratory infection • Headache • Low WBC count	• Increased risk of cancer (malignancy) • Contraindicated in persons with cancer • Serious infections (TB, hepatitis B or C, shingles) • Hepatotoxicity • Complications with blood transfusions	Orally in two treatment courses, once per year for 2 years; each treatment course has two cycles that are 4 to 5 days long and about 1 month apart
Daclizumab (Zinbryta)	Relapsing forms of MS, generally for patients who have had an inadequate response to two or more MS therapies	• Nasopharyngitis • Upper respiratory tract infection • Rash • Depression • Increased liver enzymes • Influenza • Dermatitis	• Hepatic injury and other immune-mediated disorders • Depression and suicide	Injection, monthly
Dimethyl fumarate (Tecfidera)	Relapsing forms of MS	• Flushing • GI symptoms • Rash	• PML • Anaphylaxis • Flushing • Lymphopenia	Oral, twice daily capsule
Diroximel fumarate (Vumerity)	Relapsing forms of MS	• Flushing • Nausea, diarrhea, stomach pain, indigestion	• PML • Decreased WBC count • Liver problems • Shingles or other infections	Orally twice/day
Fingolimod (Gilenya)	Relapsing forms of MS	• Bradycardia on first dose • Headache • Influenza • Diarrhea • Back pain • Increased liver enzymes • Macular edema • Lymphopenia • Bronchitis	• Bradyarrhythmia • Infection risk • PML and other encephalopathies • Decreased pulmonary function tests • Hepatic injury • Contraindicated for recent MI, unstable angina, stroke, TIA	Oral, once daily capsule

Table 16.1 Disease-Modifying Therapeutic Agents for Multiple Sclerosis[75,244]—cont'd

Agent	FDA-Approved Indications	Select Side Effects	Contraindications/ Boxed Warning	Delivery System and Frequency
Glatiramer acetate (Copaxone) (and therapeutic equivalent Glatopa)	Relapsing forms of MS	• Injection site reactions • Lipoatrophy • Vasodilation, rash, dyspnea • Chest pain	• Immediate postinjection reactions • Lipoatrophy and skin necrosis • Potential effects on immune response	SC injection, every day or three times weekly
Interferon beta-1a (Avonex)	Relapsing forms of MS	• Flu-like symptoms • Depression • Increased liver enzymes	• Depression, suicide • Hepatic injury • Anaphylaxis • CHF • Seizures	IM injection, weekly
Interferon beta-1a (Rebif)	Relapsing forms of MS	• Flu-like symptoms • Depression • Increased liver enzymes • Abdominal pain • Hematological abnormalities	• Depression, suicide • Hepatic injury • Anaphylaxis • Seizures • Injection site necrosis	SC injection, three times weekly
interferon beta-1b (Beta-seron, Extavia)	Relapsing forms of MS	• Flu-like symptoms • Injection site reactions • Depression • Increased liver enzymes • Decreased WBCs	• Depression, suicide • Hepatic injury • Anaphylaxis • Seizures • Injection site necrosis • CHF	SC injections, every other day
Mitoxantrone (Novatrone)	Worsening relapsing forms and SPMS	• Discolored urine, sclera • Nausea • Alopecia • Amenorrhea, infertility • Infections • Cardiac toxicity	Cardiotoxicity and secondary leukemia (monitoring required long term)	IV infusion in a medical center every 3 months, (max cumulative dose of 140 mg/m²)
Monomethyl fumarate (Bafiertam)	Relapsing forms of MS	• Flushing • Abdominal pain • Diarrhea and nausea	• PML • Decreased WBC counts • Hepatotoxicity • Herpes zoster infection	Orally two times/day
Natalizumab (Tysabri)	Relapsing forms of MS	• Headache • Fatigue • UTI • Lower respiratory infection • Arthralgia • Gastroenteritis • Vaginitis • Depression • Diarrhea	Because of the risk of PML, natalizumab is available only through a restricted distribution program called the TOUCH Prescribing Program	IV infusion in a medical center monthly
Ocrelizumab (Ocrevus)	PPMS and relapsing forms	• Infusion reaction • Respiratory tract infections • Herpes infections • Infusion reaction	• Hepatitis B reactivation • Increased risk of cancers, including breast	IV infusion in a medical center every 6 months

(Continued)

Table 16.1   Disease-Modifying Therapeutic Agents for Multiple Sclerosis[75,244]—cont'd

Agent	FDA-Approved Indications	Select Side Effects	Contraindications/ Boxed Warning	Delivery System and Frequency
Ofamtumab (Kesimpta)	Relapsing forms of MS	• Upper respiratory tract infection • Headache • Injection site reactions	• Hepatitis B reactivation • Decreased immunoglobulins	SC injection at weeks 0, 1, 2 followed by once monthly starting at week 4
Ozanimod (Zeposia)	Relapsing forms of MS, and active secondary and progressive disease	• Upper respiratory tract infection • Elevated liver enzymes • Orthostatic hypotension	• Bradyarrhythmia when starting treatment • Macular edema	Orally one time/day
Peginterferon beta-1a (Plegridy)	Relapsing forms of MS	• Flu-like symptoms • Injection site reactions • Depression • Increased liver enzymes • Decreased WBCs	• Depression, suicide • Hepatic injury • Anaphylaxis • Seizures • Injection site necrosis • CHF	SC injections, every 2 weeks
Ponesimod (Ponvory)	Relapsing forms of MS	• Upper respiratory tract infection • High blood pressure • Abnormal liver tests	• Infections • Macular edema • Bradycardia or bradyarrhythmia after the first dose • New or worsening shortness of breath • Skin cancers	Orally once/day
Siponimod (Mayzent)	Relapsing forms of MS	• Headache • High blood pressure • Abnormal liver tests	• Infections • Macular edema • Bradycardia or bradyarrhythmia after the first dose • New or worsening shortness of breath • Skin cancers	Orally once/day
Teriflunomide (Aubagio)	Relapsing forms of MS	• Increased liver enzymes • Alopecia • Diarrhea • Influenza • Nausea • Paresthesia	Hepatotoxicity and risk of teratogenicity	Oral, once daily capsule

CHF = congestive heart failure; FDA = U.S. Food and Drug Administration; GI = gastrointestinal; IM = intramuscular; IV = intravenous, MI = myocardial infarct; MS = multiple sclerosis; PML = progressive multifocal leukoencephalopathy; PPMS = primary progressive multiple sclerosis; REMS = Risk Evaluation Mitigation Strategy; SC = subcutaneous; SPMS = secondary progressive multiple sclerosis; TB = tuberculosis; TIA = transient ischemic attack; UTI = urinary tract infection; WBC = white blood cell.

MS Coalition Consensus paper on DMTs available at: http://www.nationalmssociety.org/NationalMSSociety/media/MSNationalFiles/Brochures/DMT_Consensus_MS_Coalition.pdf. Information on ocrelizumab available at: https://www.mstrust.org.uk/a-z/ocrelizumab.

immunomodulating properties. These are close copies of a naturally occurring human chemical, interferon beta. Interferons slow down the immune system response by reducing inflammation, swelling, and rapid proliferation of T and B cells. They also block activated T cells from crossing the blood-brain barrier. Other disease-modifying drugs and their indications, contraindications, side effects, and delivery are also included in Table 16.1.

Recent advances have led to promising agents for treating progressive MS, including ocrelizumab (Ocrevus), a monoclonal antibody that binds to a molecule on the surface of B cells and depletes them from circulation.[75] Patients may show reduced relapses, reduced number of new lesions on MRI, and reduced severity of attack as evidenced by acquired neurological deficits. For patients with new and suspected MS (CIS), the medications may delay time to a second clinical episode and a confirmed diagnosis of MS. Continued, frequent relapses or excessive MRI activity may indicate the need to switch drug therapy to higher doses or combination therapies. These agents cannot, however, reverse existing deficits. All of these medications are contraindicated for women who are pregnant or trying to become pregnant, or who are breastfeeding.[74] The impacts of the SARS-CoV-2 virus and COVID-19 disease on people with MS are only beginning to be understood at the time of this writing. Golshani and Hrdý (2022) review studies to date that report on the efficacy, safety, and suggested timing of receiving SARS-CoV-2 vaccination for patients with MS.[76]

Common adverse effects of the injectable interferon drugs include injection site skin reactions (soreness, redness, pain, bruising, or swelling) and flu-like symptoms following injection that lessen over time (fever, chills, sweating, muscle aches, and fatigue). Injection sites are varied to reduce adverse effects. Rare and more severe adverse reactions include depression, allergic reactions, and liver reactions. Copaxone can produce similar injection site reactions and an initial flushing reaction immediately after injection (anxiety, chest pain, palpitations, shortness of breath). It has the advantage of not causing flu-like symptoms or depression.

Patients receive Novantrone by intravenous (IV) infusion in a medical facility and must be closely monitored for serious heart and liver damage. Tysabri poses serious risks for a rare brain infection (progressive multifocal leukoencephalopathy [PML]). Following the first dose of Gilenya, patients must be monitored for changes in heart and pulmonary function. An additional disadvantage is the significant annual cost of these drugs (in the thousands or tens of thousands of dollars) that may not be covered fully by private insurance plans.[74]

Problems with adherence using immunomodulating agents are well documented, especially for the injectable medications.[74] Health professionals can have a significant impact on promoting acceptance and maintenance of immunomodulating therapy. In discussions with the patient, the therapist needs to determine the patient's understanding of the treatment benefits and risks, perception of their illness, general mood and level of self-esteem, lifestyle and daily living situation, and level of family and community support. Professionals need to support the patient's hope for a positive outcome from drug therapy and emphasize the benefits of early treatment and the importance of consistency in management.[74,75]

Management of Symptoms

Pharmacological agents are used for symptomatic relief of a wide range of symptoms in MS. The clinician should have a thorough understanding of the medications the patient is taking, the expected benefit, and potential adverse reactions.

Spasticity

Management of spasticity and spasms includes the use of muscle relaxants. Oral baclofen (Lioresal) is commonly used and is highly effective in reducing muscle tone and decreasing the frequency of spasms and clonus. Dosage is progressed gradually to obtain optimal effects. Other examples of oral agents include tizanidine (Zanaflex), dantrolene sodium (Dantrium), and diazepam (Valium). The reduction in spasticity must be balanced with the possibility of adverse effects from overdosing that may include sedation (drowsiness), weakness, and fatigue. The therapist must be alert to these changes and communicate with the physician to achieve optimal dosing for rehabilitation. The therapist must also recognize that at times spasticity can be used to enhance function, substituting for lack of strength. For example, extensor spasticity can be used to assist standing during a stand-pivot transfer. Significant reduction of spasticity with medications might serve to produce loss of function. Carbamazepine (Tegretol) can be effective in reducing paroxysmal (sudden, sharp onset) spasms. Patients who do not adequately respond to standard drug treatment (e.g., those with intractable spasticity or spasms) may benefit from intrathecal administration of baclofen directly into the CSF of the lumbar spine via a catheter. A programmable implanted pump controls the dosage. Significant reduction in spasticity and spasms has been reported in the LEs and trunk with less improvement reported in the UEs. Adverse effects can include sedation, dizziness, impaired vision, and impaired speech. Pump failure, infection, programming error, and lead displacement can also occur.[77]

Botulinum toxin (BT) injections are used as the most common chemodenervation agent (neurolytic) to provide localized relief of muscle tone and spasms. Efficacy is short term and generally lasts up to 3 months. Excessive use of BT can overly weaken muscles, so it is typically reserved for patients with significant problems. Physical therapy stretching of the limb for at least

4 weeks after injection is an important adjunct. Phenol injections have also been used but are more unpredictable in degree and duration of response and are associated with sensory side effects.[77]

Surgical intervention may be considered for patients with intractable spasticity. The typical surgical candidate presents with spastic paralysis for many years resulting in a nonfunctional limb and serious complications (e.g., contractures and skin breakdown). Interventions include severing tendons (*tendonotomy*), nerves (*neurectomy*), or nerve roots (*rhizotomy*).[66,77]

Pain

A variety of drugs are available to manage pain, and clinical decisions are based on type of pain. Tricyclic antidepressants, selective serotonin and norepinephrine reuptake inhibitors (SSNRIs) (e.g., duloxetine hydrochloride [Cymbalta] and pregabalin [Lyrica]) are used to treat burning, central neuropathic pain similar to the use with peripheral neuropathic pain. Paroxysmal pain responds to carbamazepine (Tegretol), amitriptyline (Elavil), phenytoin (Dilantin), diazepam (Valium), or gabapentin (Neurontin). Dysesthesias are managed with low doses of amitriptyline (Elavil), imipramine (Tofranil), or desipramine (Norpramin). Antiepileptic drugs (carbamazepine) are used with trigeminal neuralgia. The discomfort and pain associated with spasticity and spasms may be managed with over-the-counter or prescription anti-inflammatory drugs. Sometimes pain can be managed with mild painkillers (acetaminophen or ibuprofen). Strong opioids (oxycodone, methadone, morphine) have limited effectiveness and are not typically prescribed.[20,78]

Fatigue

Amantadine (Symmetrel) and modafinil (Provigil) are used for managing MS-related fatigue, but a 2021 study showed these medications had no additional benefit over placebo and recommended behavioral therapies.[79] In patients receiving DMTs, glatiramer acetate is associated with less fatigue than interferon beta-1b.[74] Nonpharmacological approaches to managing fatigue include exercise and cognitive-behavioral therapy (CBT).[80] A meta-analysis of MS fatigue management with exercise, education, and medication found that rehabilitation interventions had stronger and more significant effects on reducing the impact or severity of self-reported fatigue than did medication.[81]

Cognitive and Emotional Impairments

Cognitive rehabilitation training has been used to improve function in patients with MS.[82] Compensatory training strategies (e.g., memory aids, organizational tools) can improve function in everyday activities together with modifying the home environment to limit distractions. Acetylcholinesterase inhibitors used for the treatment of Alzheimer disease (donepezil [Aricept], memantine [Namenda]) have been shown to provide only modest benefits in memory deficits and verbal learning in some patients.[20,48]

Depression can be managed effectively with psychotherapy and psychopharmacology. Commonly used antidepressant medications are fluoxetine (Prozac), paroxetine (Paxil), sertraline (Zoloft), duloxetine hydrochloride (Cymbalta), venlafaxine (Effexor), and bupropion (Wellbutrin). Some antidepressants can also decrease fatigue. Patients with pseudobulbar affect can be effectively treated with the antidepressant medication amitriptyline (Elavil). Complementary therapies such as mindfulness meditation, yoga, journaling, and support groups often help the patient cope with the stresses of this unpredictable disease. Exercise and an active lifestyle are important components to reduce depression and anxiety.[20,50]

Bladder and Bowel Impairments

Urinary problems require a complete urodynamic workup to identify the specific cause of the problem and to arrive at the appropriate course of treatment. Treatment for an overactive, spastic bladder (storage dysfunction) typically involves pharmacological management with anticholinergic medications (tolterodine [Detrol], oxybutynin [Ditropan], imipramine [Tofranil]) to regulate bladder emptying. Adverse effects can include dry mouth, constipation, blurred vision, dry eyes, and less commonly tachycardia. Dietary recommendations include drinking eight glasses of fluid per day (water) while limiting intake of caffeine or alcohol. A flaccid bladder (emptying dysfunction) is managed with alternate techniques for emptying, including instruction in the *Credé maneuver* (the application of manual downward pressure over the lower abdomen) or intermittent self-catheterization (ISC) performed four to five times per day. Pharmacological agents may include cholinergic stimulation with urecholine. Dietary recommendations include limiting intake of citrus and tomato products (ketchup, salsa, pizza sauce). The acidity in cranberry juice, which is often recommended for UTIs, is a bladder irritant and can worsen urgency of an already spastic bladder. A dyssynergic bladder (combined dysfunction) is managed with alpha-adrenergic blocking agents (e.g., terazosin [Hytrin], prazosin [Minipress], tamsulosin [Flomax]) and antispasticity agents (e.g., baclofen [Lioresal], tizanidine hydrochloride [Zanaflex]). On rare occasions when bladder symptoms cannot be controlled with medication and/or ISC, continuous catheterization (indwelling or Foley catheter; condom, or Texas catheter) or surgical urinary diversion (suprapubic catheter) may be necessary. For example, the patient with advanced disease and significant ataxia of the UEs may be unable to manually perform self-catheterization. UTIs result from retention of urine in the bladder and from catheterization procedures. Antibiotic therapy is the mainstay of treatment.[62,83]

Constipation is a common problem and may be associated with medications that can exacerbate constipation (e.g., antihypertensives, analgesics/narcotics, tricyclic antidepressants, anticholinergics, diuretics, sedatives/tranquilizers, antacids). It is typically managed with dietary changes including increased fluid intake (six to eight glasses daily) and fiber in the diet. Bulk-forming supplements (Metamucil, FiberCon, Citrucel, Benefiber) or stool softeners (docusate [Colace], polyethylene glycol [MiraLAX]) can also be used. Regular or continuous use of stimulant laxatives and enemas is not recommended. Bowel training may also include manual disimpaction. Incontinence management includes dietary changes such as avoidance of irritants (caffeine, alcohol); adjustment of medications used to reduce spasticity, which can contribute to the problem; or addition of medications to control bowel spasms (tolterodine [Detrol], propantheline [Pro-Banthine]).[63]

■ FRAMEWORK FOR REHABILITATION

The chronicity of this disease, along with its variable and unpredictable course, may lead some to view individuals with MS as poor candidates for rehabilitation. Although the disease or its direct impairments cannot be altered, there is strong evidence to support physical therapy rehabilitation in producing significant gains in enhancing levels of activity and participation.[84] Multidisciplinary rehabilitation, including CBT for depression and information-provision interventions for patient knowledge, shows moderate evidence for gains over a longer period at the level of activity and participation. A systematic review (SR) of 39 SR studies between 2001 and 2016 evaluated the range of rehabilitation interventions in MS. The most common interventions focused on improving strength, mobility, aerobic capacity, and QOL. There was also strong evidence for comprehensive fatigue management interventions for patient-reported fatigue, followed by cognitive/psychological intervention for depression.[84]

Rehabilitation referral should be initiated early in the disease when behavioral and lifestyle changes may be easier to implement. Social determinants of health (SDOHs) are conditions in which people are born, grow, live, learn, work, and age that affect health and lead to health disparities and health inequities.[85] The therapist must consider how the patient with MS is impacted by their SDOHs and include this as part of the assessment.[86] Referral is recommended at diagnosis for baseline assessments, education on exercise, health and wellness concerns, and early support for cognitive and work-related difficulties.[16,84,87–89] Periodic reassessment should be done at least annually to establish and revise goals and to measure outcomes.[90] Rehabilitation interventions can be effective for people with MS, but a crucial factor for success is incorporating strategies that

support behavior change.[91,92] The physical therapist is a crucial member of the health-care team in educating the newly diagnosed individual with MS and discussing healthy lifestyle, fitness, and wellness programs. See Chapter 29, Promoting Health and Wellness.

Individuals with neurodegenerative diseases such as MS benefit from *restorative intervention,* aimed at remediating or improving impairments, activity limitations, and participation restrictions. Direct CNS impairments are not responsive to intervention, whereas indirect impairments caused by evolving multisystem dysfunction from inactivity and disuse can be modified (Fig. 16.2). For example, strength training can result in meaningful improvements in balance and gait. Goals and outcome statements reflective of restorative intervention focus on remediating impairments and regaining functional independence while promoting self-management skills. As the disease progresses, important goals and outcomes also include assisting the patient in effective coping skills by promoting acceptance and adjustment to limitations and disabilities and enhancing QOL. The enhancement of QOL at every stage of the disease may in fact be the most meaningful outcome for patients in the face of chronic neurodegenerative disease.

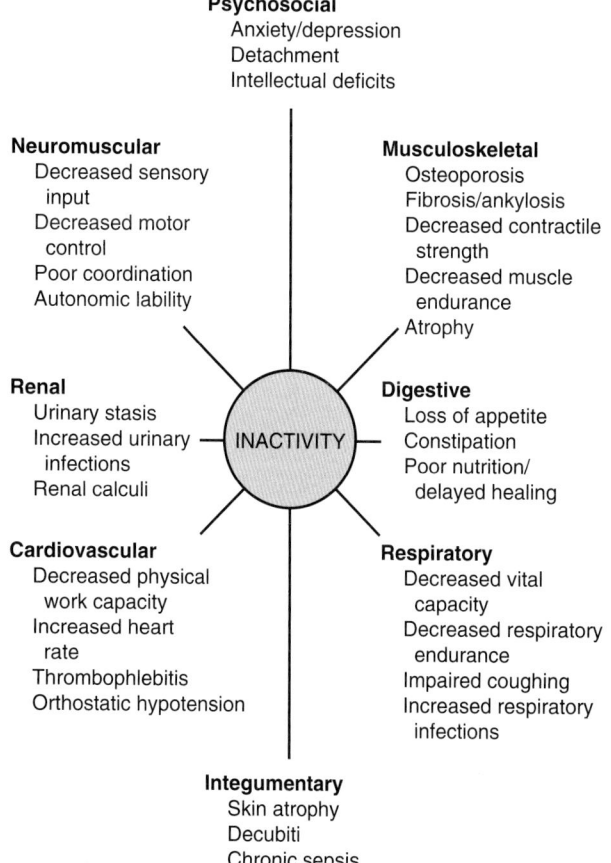

Figure 16.2 Clinical manifestations of inactivity.

Preventive intervention is aimed at minimizing potential complications, impairments, activity limitations, or disabilities at every stage of disease. Preventive interventions for the patient with MS are geared toward decreasing the duration and severity of symptoms, reducing effects of inactivity, or delaying the emergence of disease sequelae through early detection and intervention, termed *secondary prevention*. Prevention is also aimed at minimizing the degree of disability, termed *tertiary prevention*. Goal and outcome statements reflective of preventive intervention focus on promotion of health, wellness, and fitness, and preservation of optimal function.

Compensatory intervention is aimed at modifying the task, activity, or environment to maintain optimal function within the scope of existing impairments and limitations. Goal and outcome statements reflective of compensatory intervention focus on regaining/maintaining function.

Maintenance therapy is defined as a series of occasional clinical, educational, and administrative services designed to maintain the patient's current level of function. Individuals with MS who benefit from maintenance therapy typically are in the late stages of the disease (Expanded Disability Status Scale [EDSS] stages 7.0 to 9.5; the EDSS is discussed later in the section titled Tests and Measures). Maintenance programs have historically not been well funded by insurance and require careful documentation. The Centers for Medicare and Medicaid Services (CMS), which covers services for older adults and disabled individuals, covers maintenance therapy if the *professional skills of a therapist* (one having specialized knowledge and judgment) are needed to prevent or slow deterioration of a person's condition and maintain the maximal predictable level of function. As the result of a legal settlement agreement on January 24, 2013, in the case of *Jimmo v. Sibelius*, CMS issued a clarification that the coverage of skilled services does not rely on the presence or absence of a beneficiary's potential for improvement but rather on the beneficiary's need for skilled care. Providers and contractors of Medicare coverage are now directed to visit the *Jimmo* Settlement Agreement webpage (https://www.cms.gov/Center/Special-Topic/Jimmo-Center) for further details. For example, if risk of secondary impairment and loss of functional capabilities is reduced, or safety of caregivers is enhanced, then maintenance therapy should be reimbursed by CMS. A variety of interventions are used to achieve goals and outcomes, including limited direct interventions, patient-/client-related instruction, and supportive counseling. The therapist tapers the frequency of the visits as the patient or family/caregivers are able to assume independent self-management of the care plan. Indeed, recent models of rehabilitation delivery that promote routine 6- to 12-month reassessments of

function to optimize management of care in Parkinson disease may also show benefit for management of MS.[93]

A coordinated interdisciplinary team is necessary to oversee the comprehensive examination and management needed to address the patient's complex and multifaceted problems.[94] The team typically includes the physician, nurse, physical therapist, occupational therapist, speech-language pathologist, nutritionist, psychologist, and social worker. As with any team, the patient is the central figure, with family and caregivers being key members. The ideal rehabilitation program considers the patient's disease history, course, and symptoms, including impairments, activity limitations, and disability. Of equal importance are the patient's abilities (assets), priorities, and resources (e.g., family, home, community). The focus is on long-range planning with anticipated episodes of care, including hospital-based, outpatient, and home-/community-based care. Dal Bello-Haas[95] discusses a continuum of care based on disease stage (early, middle, and late) for individuals with neurodegenerative diseases. Considerations for the patient with MS are presented in Table 16.2.

■ PHYSICAL THERAPY EXAMINATION

MS may impact many different areas of the CNS; thus, it is imperative that a careful examination is performed to determine the extent of neurological and functional involvement. Subsequent reexaminations at specified intervals are used to distinguish change in status as well as effects of treatment. It may not always be possible to differentiate change in status associated with remission of symptoms from treatment outcomes. Considering the variability of symptoms of any individual patient, it is often beneficial to observe performance over a period of a few days to obtain a representative sample of baseline functioning. Fatigue and exacerbating factors should be considered when scheduling the examination.

Physical therapy examination data can be obtained through the patient's history and systems review and relevant tests and measures. The selection of examination procedures and level of inquiry are determined by the patient's unique status. The severity of problems, stage of disease (early/mild, middle/moderate, and late/advanced), age, setting of rehabilitation, and other factors must all be considered in structuring the examination. See Box 16.3 for an outline of the elements of examination of patients with MS.

Patient/Client History

Data obtained through interview with the patient/family and review of the medical record will provide information on general demographics, medical/surgical history, social and employment history, family

Table 16.2	Stages of Multiple Sclerosis: Common Impairments, Activity Limitations, and Intervention Strategies	
Stage of MS	**Common Impairments and Activity Limitations**	**Intervention Strategies**
Early/Mild	• Few/minimal impairments and activity limitations with independence maintained • Motor symptoms present but do not interfere with daily activities • Symptoms for RRMS are more variable and do not progress at the same rate as PPMS • SPMS initially presents with relapsing-remitting course followed by a more progressive course	*Preventive and Restorative* • Regular exercise to improve/maintain motor performance, strength, mobility, flexibility, ROM, balance, locomotion, endurance, and perceived QOL • Community classes to improve/maintain socialization, camaraderie, positive outlook, and life purpose *Compensatory* • Patient/family/caregiver education about disease process, rehabilitation, energy conservation • Determine need for adaptive or assistive devices • Determine need for environmental modification of home/workplace • Provide psychological support with early referral to support groups for patient and family/caregiver • Referral to other health-care professionals as needed
Middle/Moderate	• Progressive course with increasing number and severity of impairments • Minimal to moderate activity limitations, participation restrictions • ADL with modified dependence (assistance) • Difficulty with balance and gait, postural instability	*Preventive and Restorative* • Regular exercise to maintain/improve motor performance, strength, mobility, flexibility, ROM, balance, locomotion, endurance, and perceived QOL • Community classes to improve/maintain socialization, camaraderie, positive outlook and life purpose *Compensatory* • Assistive devices to maintain function • Motorized wheelchair or scooter for community mobility • Environmental modifications to home • Patient/family/caregiver education and training • Psychological support for patient and family/caregiver • Referral to other health-care professionals as needed

Late/Advanced	• Progressive course with numerous impairments with increasing severity
	• Severe activity limitations with dependence in most activities
	• Great difficulty walking; typically in wheelchair or bed most of the day
	• Assistance needed with all ADLs
	• Severe participation restrictions:
	  • Not able to live alone
	  • Typically requires full-time assistance or placement in chronic care facility
	  • Social interactions restricted
	• Cognitive problems may be prominent, including dementia, hallucinations, and delusions
		Preventive
		• Maximize upright posture, out-of-bed time
		• Maximize participation in ADLs
		• Prevention of contractures, pressure wounds, pneumonia, and so forth
		Compensatory
		• Family/caregiver education and training: safety education, transfers, positioning, turning, skin care
		• Pressure-redistributing devices
		• Hospital bed, wheelchair, mechanical lift
		• Psychological support for patient and family/caregiver
		• Referral to other health-care professionals as needed

Adapted from Dal Bello-Haas.[95]

ADLs = activities of daily living; MS = multiple sclerosis; PPMS = primary progressive multiple sclerosis; QOL = quality of life; ROM = range of motion; RRMS = relapsing-remitting multiple sclerosis; SPMS = secondary progressive multiple sclerosis.

Box 16.3 Elements of the Examination of the Patient With Multiple Sclerosis

History

- Demographic information: age, sex, race/ethnicity, primary language, education
- Social history: cultural beliefs and behaviors, family and caregiver resources, social support systems
- Occupation/employment/work information
- Living environment: home/work barriers
- Hand dominance
- General health status: physical, psychological, social, and role function, health habits
- Social and health habits (current and past)
- Family history
- Medical/surgical history
- Current conditions/chief signs/symptoms
- Medications
- Medical/laboratory/clinical test results
- Functional status and activity level: premorbid and current

Systems Review

- Cardiovascular/pulmonary
- Cognitive/affective
- Genitourinary
- Integumentary
- Musculoskeletal
- Neuromuscular

Tests and Measures

- Aerobic capacity and endurance: during functional activities and standardized exercise protocols; cardiovascular signs and symptoms in response to exercise and activity; pulmonary signs and symptoms in response to exercise and activity
- Anthropometric characteristics: body mass index, girth, length
- Assistive or adaptive devices: fit, alignment, function, use; safety
- Assistive technology
- Balance: degree of postural instability, balance strategies; safety
- Circulation: response to position change/degree of orthostatic hypotension
- Communication
- Cranial and peripheral nerve integrity
- Environment, home, and work barriers
- Functional status and activity level: performance-based examination of functional skills, basic and instrumental activities of daily living; functional mobility skills; home management skills
- Gait and locomotion: gait pattern and speed, safety
- Integumentary integrity: skin condition, pressure sensitive areas; activities, positioning, and postures to relieve pressure
- Joint integrity, alignment, and mobility: range of motion (active and passive); muscle length and soft tissue extensibility
- Mental functions: cognition, memory
- Motor function: motor control and motor learning
- Muscle performance: strength, power, and endurance
- Neuromotor development and sensory processing
- Pain: intensity and location
- Perceptual function: visuospatial skills
- Posture: alignment and position, symmetry (static and dynamic, sitting and standing); ergonomics and body mechanics
- Psychosocial function: motivation
- Range of motion
- Reflex integrity
- Self-care and domestic life
- Sensory integrity and integration
- Skeletal integrity
- Ventilation and gas exchange
- Work, community, and leisure activities: ability to participate in activities, safety

---

history, living environment, general health status, social and health habits, and disease duration. The patient's current/primary complaints and current functional status and activity level should be ascertained. Coexisting health problems and medications should also be identified. See Box 16.3 for specifics.

Systems Review

Data obtained from the history and medical record will inform the systems review and help focus selection of appropriate tests and measures. Review of the following systems is included: (1) cardiovascular/pulmonary; (2) cognitive,

affective, and communication; (3) genitourinary; (4) integumentary; (5) musculoskeletal; and (6) neuromuscular.

Tests and Measures

The following are specific areas and relevant tests and measures that can be used to examine function in patients with MS. For more detailed descriptions, see earlier chapters in this text focusing on examination. See Table 16.3 for descriptions, scoring, and minimum detectable change/minimal clinically important difference for selected tests and measures described in this section.

Table 16.3	Selected Outcome Measures for Persons With Multiple Sclerosis by International Classification of Functioning, Disability, and Health Domain		
Outcome Measure and ICF Category	Description	Scoring	MDC/MCID
Fatigue Scale for Motor and Cognitive Functions[114] *Body Function and Structure*	20-item self-report measure evaluating motor and cognitive fatigue in persons with MS	Cognitive (10 items) and motor (10 items) subscales are scored for a total score (max 20 points)	MDC: not established MCID: not established
MFIS *Activity Participation*	21-item self-report measure evaluating motor, cognitive, and psychosocial impacts of fatigue	Physical (9 items) Cognitive (10 items) Psychosocial (2 items)	MDC: 20.2 points[245] MCID: not established
Trunk Impairment Scale[246] *Body Function and Structure Activity*	A measure examining motor function of the trunk in sitting	Items are scored out of a possible 23 points with static sitting (0–7), dynamic sitting (0–10), and coordination (0–6) subscales	MDC: not established MCID: not established
Visual Analog Scale–Fatigue[247,248] *Body Function and Structure*	Single-item self-report measure for fatigue	There are various versions; two examples: • *0–10 scale:* 10 indicates major fatigue problem • *100 mm line:* right end of scale indicates extremely tired	MDC: 3.47 points on 0–10 scale (rheumatoid arthritis)[223] MCID: −0.82–1.12 for meaningful improvement and 1.13–1.26 for meaningful worsening on a 0–10 scale (rheumatoid arthritis)[249]
12-item MS Walking Scale[126] *Activity*	12-item self-report measure evaluating the impact of MS on walking ability	Items are scored 1–5, and the sum of the scores is then: [(Sum of scores −12)/48] * 100	MDC: 22 (Learmonth, 2013b)[250] MCID: not established
6MWT[251] *Activity*	Measure of distance walked in 6 minutes	Utilize a marked course and measuring wheel to obtain distance traveled in 6 minutes	MDC: ±88–92.16 m (MS)[250,252] or a change of 31.7%[253] MCID: decline of 53–55 m detects individuals with MS who are deteriorating versus individuals who are stable[252]
Nine-Hole Peg Test[254] *Activity*	Timed performance test; the individual moves nine pegs from a peg board to a well, one at a time, and then returns the pegs to the pegboard, one at a time	Time to complete this task is measured in seconds for both the dominant and nondominant hands	MDC: Dominant hand 19.4 s and 29.1% change Nondominant hand 18.6 s and 20.5% change[255] MCID: 20% change (MS)[256]
MS Quality of Life–54[140] *Activity Participation*	54-item self-report measure of health-related quality of life; contains the SF-36 and 18 additional MS-specific items	There is no overall summary score, rather there are two combined summary scores (mental health composite and physical health composite)	MDC: not established MCID: not established

(Continued)

Table 16.3 Selected Outcome Measures for Persons With Multiple Sclerosis by International Classification of Functioning, Disability, and Health Domain—cont'd

Outcome Measure and ICF Category	Description	Scoring	MDC/MCID
Rivermead Mobility Index[257] *Activity*	15-item (14 self-report items and 1 performance item) measure examining mobility	Items are scored on a 2-point scale (0 = no; 1 = yes) for a maximal score of 15 points	MDC: 3 points (stroke,[258] chronic inflammatory demyelinating polyneuropathy[259]) MCID: 2 points (MS)[257,260]
Timed 25-ft Walk[261] *Activity*	A measure of fast walking speed	Time to walk 25 ft at the individual's quickest safe speed is recorded	MDC: 2.7 sec (MS)[250] MCID: not established
Outcome Measures Balance: **Berg Balance Scale** **Functional Reach** **Dynamic Gait Index** **TUG; TUG Cognitive & Manual** **Dynamic Gait Index** **Activities-Specific Balance Confidence Scale**	*See discussion in Chapter 6, Examination of Coordination and Balance*		
CARE Tool[131,262]	*See discussion in Chapter 8, Examination of Function*		

CARE = Medicare Continuity Assessment Record and Evaluation; ICF = International Classification of Functioning, Disability, and Health; MCID = minimal clinically important difference; MDC = minimal detectable change; MFIS = Modified Fatigue Impact Scale; MS = multiple sclerosis; 6MWT = 6-minute Walk Test; TUG = Timed Up and Go.

All measures "highly recommended" or "recommended" by the MS EDGE Task Force for use across settings (acute, inpatient rehabilitation, home health, skilled nursing facility, and outpatient) *and* required at entry-level education (http://www.neuropt.org/docs/ms-edge-documents/final-ms-edge-document.pdf?sfvrsn=4 and http://www.neuropt.org/docs/ms-edge-documents/ms-edge-summary-recommendations.pdf?sfvrsn=4).

Cognition

Memory function, attention, concentration, conceptual reasoning, problem-solving, and speed of information processing should be examined as well as the effects of fatigue on cognitive performance. An expert panel convened by the Consortium of MS Centers in 2001 developed the *Minimal Examination of Cognitive Function in MS (MACFIMS)*. This 90-minute battery of seven neuropsychological tests examines processing speed/working memory, learning and memory, executive function, visual–spatial processing, and word retrieval.[96] In 2012, the *Brief International Cognitive Assessment for MS (BICAMS)* was introduced.[97] The BICAMS includes a 15-minute battery of three neuropsychological tests and is sensitive and specific to cognitive impairment defined by the MACFIMS.[98] A brief screen of cognitive function can be achieved using the *Mini-Mental State Examination (MMSE)*,[99] though many individuals with MS may experience ceiling effects. The Symbol Digit Modalities Test (SDMT) may be the most appropriate cognitive test if the examiner has less than 5 minutes available;[97] the SDMT has been shown to have excellent validity for predicting diagnosis, course, and work disability and is easy to administer.[100]

Affective and Psychosocial Function

Emotional stability should be examined. The presence of emotional lability, euphoria, emotional dysregulation, or depression (symptoms, severity, length, effect on functional performance); the level of stress and anxiety; coping strategies; and presence of sleep disorders should be documented. A useful instrument is the Beck Depression Inventory.[101] Many of these domains may also be assessed with QOL scales, which are discussed later in this chapter under General Health Measures. As previously mentioned, it is imperative that the physical therapist be familiar with the patient's medications, because numerous medications will have effects on the affective and psychosocial domain.

Sensation

Given the extent of variability in sensory deficits in individuals with MS, a detailed examination of superficial and deep sensations should be completed. See Chapter 3, Examination of Sensory Function. Additionally, sensory deficits and their effects on QOL in individuals with MS can be assessed using quantitative measures such as the *Nottingham Sensory Assessment*,[102] neurothesiometer, Semmes-Weinstein monofilaments,[103] or Vibratron.[104] Sensory function may also be assessed with the *Visual Analog Scale*[103] or *Guy's Neurological Disability Scale*,[105] a comprehensive multidimensional scale designed to assess the wide range of disability in patients with MS. Caution should be used when selecting measures, as only the neurothesiometer, visual analog scale, and Vibratron have established reliability in persons with MS.[103,104] Although vibration sensation is assessed in the neurological examination with a tuning fork, quantitative assessment of vibration with the Vibratron may be useful as it demonstrates strong correlations with balance performance and integrity of the spinal cord white matter in persons with MS.[104,106]

Pain

The presence of acute, paroxysmal pain (Lhermitte sign, dysesthesias) and chronic pain including pain behaviors and reactions during specific movements and provoking stimuli should be documented. The *McGill Pain Questionnaire*[107] or the *Neuropathic Pain Scale*,[108] developed to assess distinct pain qualities associated with neuropathic pain, can be used. See Chapter 25, Chronic Pain. The *Brief Pain Inventory*[109] assesses pain severity and pain interference and has established reliability and validity in persons with MS.

Visual Acuity

Acuity, tracking, and accommodation should be examined; the presence of visual deficits (blurred vision, field defects [scotoma], diplopia) should be documented.

Cranial Nerve Integrity

Motor and sensory cranial nerve function should be examined; the presence of deficits (optic pain [optic neuritis], oculomotor dyscontrol, dysphagia, impaired gag reflex, trigeminal neuralgia) should be documented.

Range of Motion

Passive ROM and active ROM should be examined; the presence of specific ROM impairments should be documented.

Muscle Performance

Functional strength using manual muscle testing (MMT) and dynamometers (isokinetic, grasp and pinch dynamometers) should be examined; strong spasticity may be a contraindication to standard MMT positions.

Fatigue

The frequency, duration, and severity of fatigue should be examined; precipitating factors, activity levels, and efficacy of rest attempts should be documented.[110] The *Modified Fatigue Impact Scale (MFIS)* developed by Fisk et al.[111,112] is a structured, self-report, 21-item questionnaire addressing the effects of fatigue on cognitive, physical, and psychosocial function using a 5-point ordinal scale with 0 equal to never and 4 equal to almost always. Each area (subscale) can be scored separately; the total MFIS score range is from 0 to 84.[113] An abbreviated version of the MFIS has five items (the *MFIS-5*). Additionally, the *Fatigue Scale for Motor and Cognitive Functions (FSMC)* is a 20-item scale developed as a measure of cognitive and motor fatigue for people with MS.[114] To measure fatigue during the examination and treatment process, the Visual Analog Scale—Fatigue can be used as a single-item self-report of fatigue (see Table 16.3).

Temperature Sensitivity

The degree of temperature sensitivity and its effect on fatigue and weakness should be examined. A tympanic membrane thermometer (ear thermometer) can be used before, during, and after moderate-intensity exercise. A determination of the correlation between temperature changes and worsening of neurological symptoms can be made. This transient increase in symptoms following a raise in core temperature, which may be seen with exercise, has been more accurately termed a *pseudoexacerbation* and occurs due to transient increased blockade of nerve conduction in demyelinated fibers.[66]

Motor Function

The therapist should examine for the presence of corticospinal signs (paresis, spasticity, hyperactive DTRs, positive Babinski sign, and involuntary spasms [flexor or extensor]).

Spasticity can be examined using a subjective rating scale. The *Ashworth Spasticity Scale*[115] led to the more widely used *Modified Ashworth Scale*.[116] These are ordinal scales designed to measure tone intensity; the modified Ashworth has an additional grade at the lower end allowing for more discrete rating. A determination should be made of the differences between lower limbs versus upper limbs; right and left sides; and factors that influence tone.

The therapist should examine for the presence of cerebellar signs (ataxia, intention tremor, nystagmus, dysarthria). The effects of position change (e.g., sitting to standing) may produce an increase in ataxic movements with increased demands for postural stability and should be documented.

The therapist should examine for the presence of vestibular dysfunction (dizziness, vertigo, nystagmus, blurred vision with head and body movements, and postural imbalance). See Chapter 21, Vestibular Disorders.

Posture

Static and dynamic postural control in different positions (e.g., sitting, standing) should be examined. The presence of postural abnormalities and postural tremor should be documented. Instruments can include posture grids, plumb lines, and still photography with light-emitting diodes.

Balance, Gait, and Locomotion

The therapist should examine static and dynamic balance, reactive and anticipatory control, sensory interaction, and synergistic strategies. Useful instruments include the *Clinical Test for Sensory Interaction in Balance*,[117] dynamic posturography,[118,119] the *Berg Balance Scale*,[120,121] the *Tinetti Performance Oriented Mobility Examination (POMA)*,[122] and the *Balance Evaluation Systems Test (BESTest)*.[123] Balance tests are noted in Table 16.3; additional information on the *Timed Up-and-Go, Activities Balance Confidence Scale*, and *Functional Reach* can be found in Chapter 6, Examination of Coordination and Balance.

Gait parameters and characteristics should be examined including gait speed, kinematics, stability, safety, and endurance. Examination of patients with significant ataxia can be enhanced by use of videotaped performance. Useful tests include timed walk tests (10-meter Walk Test, 6-minute Walk Test, 2-minute Walk Test, Timed 25-ft Walk, which is a component of the MS Functional Composite [MSFC] and the standard walking test included in MS Clinical Trials), the *Dynamic Gait Index;*[124] and the *Ambulation Index (AI)*.[125] Self-reported walking function can be assessed with the *Multiple Sclerosis Walking Scale-12 (MSWS-12)*,[126] and LE coordination may be assessed with the *Six Spot Step Test*.[127,128] Additional walking tests are recommended by the American Physical Therapy Association's (APTA) MS-EDGE (http://www.neuropt.org/docs/ms-edge-documents/final-ms-edge-document.pdf). See Chapter 7, Examination of Gait, for more detail.

Alignment and fit, safety, practicality, and ease of use of orthotic and assistive devices should be examined along with energy conservation and expenditure. Wheelchair skills, including functional mobility, management, safety, transfers, and energy conservation and expenditure, should be examined.

Aerobic Capacity and Endurance

Vital signs (heart rate, blood pressure, respiratory rate) and breathing patterns should be examined at rest and during and after exercise. Exertional symptoms (dyspnea; elevated blood pressure) and perceived exertion during and after activity should be documented. Useful scales include the *Rating of Perceived Exertion Scale (the Borg Ratings of Perceived Exertion [RPE] Scale)*[129] and the *Dyspnea Scale*.[130]

Skin Integrity and Condition

Skin integrity and condition should be examined. Areas of insensitivity, bruising, moisture buildup, and skin breakdown should be examined and documented, along with level of urinary continence; bed and wheelchair positioning; effectiveness of pressure-relieving compensatory strategies and pressure-redistributing devices (PRDs); and cognitive status and safety awareness.

Functional Status

An examination of functional mobility skills, basic ADL, and instrumental activities of daily living (IADL) is indicated, together with social functioning and community and work adaptive skills. A commonly used instrument for patients undergoing active rehabilitation is the *Continuity Assessment Record and Evaluation (CARE) Item Set*,[131] replacing the *Functional Independence Measure (FIM)* (see Chapter 8, Examination of Function).

Environment (Home, Community, and Work)

Physical space for barriers, access, and safety should be examined; a specific task analysis (patient performance-based examination) in relevant environments (home, work) may be included (see Chapter 9, Examination and Modification of the Environment).

General Health Measures

General health measures are used to examine outcomes across a broad spectrum of global or long-term health outcomes. Instruments involve self-report of the patient's perceptions of limitations and QOL (e.g., physical and social function, general health and vitality, emotional well-being, bodily pain, and so forth). The *Health Status Questionnaire (SF-36)*[132] is widely acknowledged as the gold standard of generic measures of health status. The properties of this instrument have been investigated in patients with MS. Freeman et al.[133] found limitations in evaluating change in moderate to severely disabled patients participating in inpatient rehabilitation with significant floor and ceiling effects in four of eight SF-36 dimensions.

Disease-Specific Measures

Disease-specific measures are designed to examine attributes common in a specific disease entity. Items are included to provide information about the disease process and outcomes, and ideally document clinically meaningful change over time. Thus, the instruments have greater responsiveness or sensitivity to change than general health measures.

Expanded Disability Status Scale for Patients With Multiple Sclerosis

In 1955, Kurtzke developed a 10-point scale for rating overall disability in MS (the *Disability Status Scale*

[DSS]),[134] which was expanded in 1983 to increase its clinical sensitivity, becoming the EDSS (https://www .nationalmssociety.org/NationalMSSociety/media/ MSNationalFiles/Brochures/10-2-3-29-EDSS_Form .pdf).[135] This scale has been widely adopted by clinicians and has been used as a standard in MS research. Based on a standard neurological examination, patients are graded on presenting symptoms in seven specific functional systems (pyramidal, cerebellar, brain stem, sensory, bowel and bladder, visual, mental). These functional system scores (FSS) are then used to calculate the overall EDSS score from 0 to 10, with 0 equal to normal neurological function and 10 equal to death owing to MS. For example, patients classified in EDSS step 2.5 demonstrate minimal disability in two FSS. The EDSS focuses on ambulation as the primary indicator of disability (see scores 3.0 through 6.5 for levels of ambulation; patients with scores 7 or greater are unable to walk). Criticisms of the EDSS include its lack of sensitivity to changes that do not include functional mobility (ambulation), problems in interrater reliability with patients whose performance is less impaired (scores in the lower ranges, ambulation less impaired),[136,137] and because high variability and nonlinearity of the scale make determination of change over time challenging.[138,139]

Multiple Sclerosis Functional Composite

The *MSFC* is a 21-item test that includes three different functional subtests: the Timed 25-ft Walk (T25FW), the Nine-Hole Peg Test, and the Paced Auditory Serial Addition Test (PASAT). The *MSFC Administration and Scoring Manual* can be obtained from the NMSS (http:// www.nationalmssociety.org/NationalMSSociety/ media/MSNationalFiles/Brochures/10-2-3-31-MSFC_ Manual_and_Forms.pdf).

Multiple Sclerosis Quality of Life–54

The *Multiple Sclerosis Quality of Life–54 (MSQOL-54)* is a multidimensional health-related quality-of-life measure that combines both generic and MS-specific items into a single instrument.[140] The generic items are from the SF-36 to which 18 items were added to provide more information regarding MS-specific issues.[132] No overall summary score is used: the MSQOL-54 consists of 12 subscales, 2 combined summary scores, and 2 single-item measures. The subscales are physical function, role limitations—physical, role limitations—emotional, pain, emotional well-being, energy, health perceptions, social function, cognitive function, health distress, overall QOL, and sexual function. The summary scores are the physical health composite summary and the mental health composite summary. The single-item measures are satisfaction with sexual function and change in health.

Multiple Sclerosis Quality of Life Inventory

The *MS Quality of Life Inventory* is a comprehensive outcomes examination that includes a battery of 10 self-report scales (138 items) that provide information about health-related QOL in MS, including the Health Status Questionnaire (SF-36), MFIS, MOS Pain Effects Scale, Sexual Satisfaction Scale, Bladder Control Scale, Bowel Control Scale (BWCS), Impact of Visual Impairment Scale, Perceived Deficits Questionnaire, Mental Health Inventory, and MOS Modified Social Support Survey. The battery can be administered in approximately 45 min in most cases. Abbreviated versions of some of the scales can reduce the set to 81 items requiring approximately 30 minutes to administer. A *User's Manual* can be obtained from the NMSS (http:// www.nationalmssociety.org/NationalMSSociety/ media/MSNationalFiles/Brochures/MSQLI_-A-User -s-Manual.pdf).

Functional Examination of Multiple Sclerosis

The *Functional Examination of MS (FAMS)* is a 59-item index of health-related QOL measures with six subscales (mobility, symptoms, emotional well-being [depression], general contentment, thinking/fatigue, and family/social well-being). The mobility subscale strongly correlates with the EDSS.[141]

Multiple Sclerosis Impact Scale

The *MS Impact Scale (MSIS-29)* measures the physical and psychological impact of MS.[142] The scale was primarily developed for community-based populations though testing with hospital-based populations (patients admitted for inpatient rehabilitation, IV corticosteroid treatment for MS relapses, and with PPMS) revealed consistency of psychometric properties.[143]

The *Academy of Neurologic Physical Therapy Multiple Sclerosis Outcome Measures Taskforce* of the APTA has compiled a list of measures for each relevant International Classification of Functioning, Disability, and Health (ICF) category together with instrument analysis, recommendations for use, and relevant references (http://www.neuropt.org/docs/ms-edge-documents/ final-ms-edge-document.pdf). Selected outcome measures are listed in Table 16.3.

Goals and Expected Outcomes

The general goals and expected outcomes for patients with progressive disorders of the CNS, adapted from the *Guide to Physical Therapist Practice,* are presented in Box 16.4. These general goals will provide the basis for development of specific anticipated goals and expected outcomes for an individual patient.

In this document, the reader will find relevant information on patient/client diagnostic classification; examination components; considerations for evaluation, diagnosis, and prognosis; and suggested interventions. Thus, the *Guide to Physical Therapist Practice* serves as a primary resource to help physical therapists design an appropriate plan of care (POC) and document the services provided and outcomes achieved.

> ### Box 16.4 Examples of General Goals and Expected Outcomes for Patients With Progressive Disorders of the Central Nervous System
>
> 1. Impact of pathology/pathophysiology is reduced.
>   - *Decrease:* risk of secondary impairment; intensity of care
>   - *Improve:* patient/client, family, and caregiver knowledge of disease, prognosis and plan of care; symptom management
> 2. Impact of impairments is reduced.
>   - *Decrease:* pain
>   - *Improve:* cognitive function, joint integrity, mobility, sensory awareness, skin integrity, motor function, muscle performance, postural control and balance, gait and locomotion, management of fatigue, aerobic capacity
> 3. Ability to perform physical actions, tasks, or activities is improved.
>   - *Improve:* independence with activities of daily living; tolerance of positions and activities; activity pacing and energy conservation; problem-solving and decision-making skills; safety of patient, family, and caregivers
> 4. Disability associated with chronic illness is reduced.
>   - *Improve:* ability to assume/resume self-care and home management; ability to assume work (job/school/play), community, and leisure roles; patient/client and family knowledge and awareness of personal and environmental factors associated with condition worsening; awareness and use of community resources
> 5. Health status and quality of life are improved.
>   - *Decrease:* stressors
>   - *Improve:* sense of well-being; insight, self-confidence and self-management skills; health, wellness, and fitness
> 6. Patient/client satisfaction is enhanced.
>   - *Improve:* acceptability of access and availability of services and quality of rehabilitation services to patient/client and family; coordination of care with patient/client, family, caregivers, and other professionals.

Adapted from the *Guide to Physical Therapist Practice.*

PHYSICAL THERAPY INTERVENTIONS

Management of Sensory Deficits and Skin Care

In patients with MS, inflammation causes a disruption in neuronal signaling, causing a variety of sensory symptoms. Strategies should be instituted to increase awareness of sensory deficits, compensate for sensory loss, and promote safety. It is important to remember that sensory deficits may remit, so ongoing examination is necessary. The success of compensatory training strategies depends on the availability of other intact sensory systems. For example, visual compensation techniques can be instituted when deficits in proprioception produce imbalance and place the patient at risk for falls. If multiple sensory systems are involved (e.g., vision is also impaired), sensory compensatory strategies are not likely to be successful.

Patients with proprioceptive losses demonstrate impairments in movement control and motor learning. They require increased use of other sensory systems, especially vision. Tapping, verbal cueing, and/or biofeedback can all be effective forms of augmented feedback. Proprioceptive loading through exercise, light tracking resistance, resistance bands or weights, and the use of a pool may heighten residual proprioceptive function and improve movement awareness.

Visual loss will interfere with movement and postural control. Blurred vision, especially at night or in low light situations, can occur after episodes of optic neuritis. When individuals with MS must stand in an upright position in the dark, the likelihood of falls increases.[144] It is therefore important to instruct the patient to maintain adequate lighting at all times (e.g., use a bright light at night) and reduce clutter to improve safety. Adding color contrast between items in the environment (e.g., stair markings) can also improve safety. Double vision is frequently the result of impaired coordination and weak eye muscles. It can be controlled by placing a patch over one eye and is an important strategy for improving reading, driving, or watching television. However, eye patching should not be used all the time, because it will prevent possible adaptation of the CNS. Eye patching also interferes with depth perception. The symptoms of visual blurring and double vision also fluctuate and can be heightened with fatigue, an increase in temperature, stress, and infection. If low vision persists, the patient should be referred to a low-vision specialist or one of the national service organizations that provide help to individuals with vision impairments (*National Association for Visually Handicapped, National Federation of the Blind, American Foundation for the Blind*).

One of the most common early sensory symptoms of MS is decreased sensitivity to touch and vibration.[145,146] This may result in reduced sensitivity on the soles of the feet and difficulty with proprioception and kinesthetic awareness. This sensory ataxia may result in difficulty with foot placement and an increased risk of falls in individuals with MS. Persons with MS are also at an increased risk of developing pressure injuries owing to the symptoms of MS, including loss of sensation, immobility, loss of bowel and bladder control, and nutritional state. Changes in skin turgor, static posturing, and prolonged pressure over bony prominences increase the likelihood of skin breakdown. Patients may not feel the discomfort of a prolonged position or may be unable to shift position because of weakness or spasticity. In addition, spasticity and/or spasms may cause friction effects between the skin and supporting surfaces. Awareness, protection, and care of desensitized parts should be taught early in the rehabilitation process and consistently reinforced by all members of the team. It has been demonstrated that patient education programs result in 50% reductions in pressure injury incidence.[147] The patient/family/caregiver should be educated in the following principles of skin care:

- The skin should be kept clean and dry. Soiled skin should be cleansed and dried promptly.
- The skin should be inspected regularly (at least once a day) and carefully, with particular attention to persistent areas of redness and over bony prominences.
- Clothing should be breathable and comfortable (soft, not too loose or wrinkled, or too tight). Seams, buttons, and pockets should not press on the skin, particularly in weight-bearing areas.
- Regular pressure relief is essential. Patients should be instructed to change their position or be changed frequently, typically every 2 hr in bed and every 15 to 30 minutes when sitting in a wheelchair.[148]

PRDs may be necessary to protect insensitive areas and should be implemented as appropriate. These can include mattresses (water, gel, air, or alternating pressure) to distribute body weight and reduce shear and friction in bed. Sheepskins, air or foam cushions, cuffs, and/or boots may be necessary to protect body areas prone to breakdown (shoulder blades, elbows, ischial tuberosities, sacrum, trochanters, knees, malleoli, or heels). Cushions (foam; fluid or air pressure–relieving cushions) are necessary for patients who spend prolonged periods of time sitting in their wheelchair. When evaluating a PRD, it is imperative that a pressure mapping system be used to determine its effectiveness and ensure that the areas of high pressure are adequately protected.[148]

Prevention is the best strategy. Important measures for maintaining skin integrity and function include maintaining good nutrition and drinking plenty of fluids. Studies suggest that for patients with MS with pressure injuries, there are increased requirements for specific nutrients; particularly zinc and iron supplementation should be considered.[149] The patient must

be cautioned against activities that might traumatize the skin. Dragging, bumping, or scraping body parts during a transfer or bed mobility activities can injure the skin. Thermal injury can result from contact with hot water or hot objects. If nonblanchable skin redness develops (lasting longer than 30 minutes), patients should be instructed to stay off the area until the redness disappears. If the redness does not disappear within 24 hr, the individual should seek medical attention. Blisters, blue areas, or open sores indicate more serious injury and require immediate attention. This may include systemic antibiotic therapy for infection and wound management techniques (cleansing and débridement, topical antibiotic agents, and protective dressings). See Chapter 14, Vascular, Lymphatic, and Integumentary Disorders, for more detailed information on skin care.

Management of Pain

Pain can be classified into four categories: (1) pain directly from MS, (2) pain secondary to other symptoms of MS, (3) pain as a result of drug treatment for MS, and (4) pain independent of MS. The management of pain depends on an accurate determination of its causes. Musculoskeletal strain or joint malalignment from chronically weakened muscles are important considerations and are responsive to physical therapy intervention. Patients may experience relief of pain with regular stretching or exercise, massage, and ultrasound. Postural retraining and correction of faulty movement patterns along with orthotic and/or adaptive seating devices can reduce malalignment and pain. Stabbing pain from Lhermitte sign may be relieved with a soft cervical collar to limit neck flexion. Hydrotherapy or pool therapy using *lukewarm* water may have a beneficial effect on painful dysesthesias. Pressure stockings or gloves can also be used to relieve pain, converting the sensation of pain to one of pressure. Neutral warmth may be an additional factor in the pain relief experienced with stockings or gloves. Patients with chronic pain may benefit from referral to a total management approach for chronic pain, for example, the *multidisciplinary pain clinic* (see Chapter 25, Chronic Pain). Stress management techniques, relaxation training, biofeedback, and meditation are often helpful in reducing both anxiety and pain. The use of transcutaneous electrical nerve stimulation to modulate pain in patients with MS has had conflicting results, with some patients experiencing improvement and some a worsening of symptoms.[78] Pain is linked to depression, fatigue, anxiety, and sleep in persons with MS,[150] so management of pain requires examination of other contributing factors. Behavioral approaches such as mindfulness,[151] self-management,[152] self-hypnosis,[153] and positive psychology[154] have demonstrated success in improving pain outcomes in persons with MS and warrant further examination.

Exercise Training

Exercise training is safe for individuals with MS; it is not associated with an increased risk of either relapses or adverse events.[155] Muscle weakness and decreased endurance are common findings in patients with MS. As a result, persons with MS may adopt a sedentary lifestyle and limit their physical activity. Thus, early education on the importance of exercise is crucial. The benefits of exercise have been firmly established in terms of producing meaningful physiological and psychological changes, improving function while lessening disability, and enhancing QOL. Khan and Amatya identified 53 systematic reviews investigating rehabilitation in MS.[84] They found strong evidence to support physical therapy to improve activity and participation domains in persons with MS as well as strong evidence to support the reduction of patient-reported fatigue. Individuals with minimal to moderate impairments (i.e., EDSS scores between 1 and 6) demonstrate the best exercise tolerance. This speaks to the need to institute exercises early in the course of the disease. Additional systematic reviews and meta-analyses demonstrate the positive effect of exercise therapy on depression,[156,157] fatigue,[158] cognition,[88,159] gait and gait endurance,[160,161] balance,[160] arm/hand function,[162] strength,[163-165] cardiorespiratory fitness,[165] respiratory function,[166] and disability in both relapsing[84] and progressive MS,[167] as well as strength, activity, and respiratory function in nonambulatory persons with MS[168] and wheelchair users.[169] Recommendations for exercise and physical activity across the disease course can guide prescription; the general recommendation is for at least 150 min/week of exercise and/or at least 150 min/week of lifestyle physical activity.[170]

The use of technology may augment rehabilitation for persons with MS. Virtual reality and gaming[171-173] may be useful and motivational alternatives or additions to traditional exercise therapy to improve arm movement and control, walking, and anticipatory postural control in persons with MS. Virtual reality is also an effective interface for wheelchair users.[174] Training programs focusing on whole-body vibration may improve muscle strength and walking endurance and reduce fall risk in persons with MS.[161,175,176]

Exercise responses of the patient with MS are influenced by a host of factors that require careful attention during exercise, including fatigue, spasticity, incoordination, impaired balance, sensory loss (numbness), tremor, and heat intolerance. As a result of exercise-induced increases in core body temperature, individuals with heat intolerance may be more tolerant to resistance exercise than endurance or aerobic exercise.[177] Additionally, depression may affect adherence to an exercise program. Therapists therefore need to provide constant reinforcement and a positive environment.

Individuals with MS will vary greatly in their responses to exercise. The focus and pace of therapy must be readjusted according to the patient's specific abilities and needs at that time. Patients with RRMS who are experiencing an exacerbation should not exercise until remission is evident. Exercise therapy can be reinstituted when the deterioration has stabilized, and no new symptoms are appearing. Patients with PPMS can exercise within the limits of their capabilities as exercise may slow further deterioration and optimize remaining function.[130] Emerging evidence suggests that body weight–supported treadmill training, total-body recumbent stepper training, and electrical stimulation cycling may be useful modalities for improving disability, fitness, and functioning in individuals with severe mobility restrictions (EDSS > 6).[178,179] Table 16.4 presents a summary of selected systematic reviews and meta-analyses related to exercise and MS.

Strength and Conditioning

Maximal muscle force during sustained isometric or isokinetic exercise is lower for persons with MS secondary to reduced ability to activate muscles (reduced force/unit muscle mass), reduced muscle metabolic responses, and muscle weakness secondary to muscle fiber atrophy, spasticity, and disuse. Determining an appropriate exercise prescription to improve strength and endurance is challenging and needs to be carefully individualized for each patient. Prescription is based on four interrelated elements: frequency of exercise, intensity of exercise, type of exercise, and time or duration (the *FITT equation*). The following guidelines can be used:[180]

- Exercise sessions should be scheduled on alternate (nonendurance) days and during optimal times, such as in the morning, when body core temperatures tend to be lowest and before fatigue sets in. Patients with greater neurological involvement may require more frequent exercise (e.g., daily exercise time).
- Resistance training modes can include weight machines, free or pulley weights, resistance bands, or isokinetic machines.
- Circuit training, in which improved work capacity is developed using different stations that alternate work between UEs and LEs, distributes the load among muscles and may prove beneficial for reducing the likelihood of fatigue.
- Sessions should involve discontinuous work, carefully balancing exercise with adequate rest periods.
- Progression is generally slower than with healthy individuals.
- Precautions should be taken to prevent the deleterious effects of overwork. Exercising to the point of fatigue is contraindicated and can result

Table 16.4	Evidence Summary of Exercise for Multiple Sclerosis		
Subjects	**Design/Intervention**	**Results**	**Comments**
	Andreu-Caravaca et al. (2021)[190]		
43 studies identified, 26 of which were RCTs	Systematic review and meta-analysis examining the benefits of aerobic training programs in persons with MS.	Aerobic training results in improvements in balance on the Berg Balance Scale and functional capacity measured with gait speed, Timed Up and Go, and walking endurance.	The greatest effects were seen when the aerobic training was delivered with continuous (as opposed to interval) training that targeted walking (as opposed to cycling or arm ergometry).
	Campbell et al. (2016)[167]		
13 studies identified	Systematic review examining the effect of physical therapy rehabilitation for persons with progressive MS	Studies were underpowered, or power analyses were not performed. Multidisciplinary rehabilitation results in improvements in disability on the FIM as well as fatigue and QOL. Inspiratory muscle training had a positive impact on maximal inspiratory and expiratory pressure in persons with progressive MS. Therapeutic standing significantly improved hip and ankle passive range of motion and reduced leg spasms. Results were inconclusive for exercise therapy, BOTOX injections, acupuncture, and BWSTT.	A large variety of interventions were considered (8 different types across 13 studies) ranging from exercise training to inspiratory muscle training to treadmill training to BOTOX injections.
	Cruickshank et al. (2015)[163]		
7 of 20 identified studies included individuals with MS	Systematic review and meta-analysis of strength training in individuals with MS or Parkinson disease.	Strength training has a positive impact on muscle strength (effect size of 0.31), fatigue, functional capacity, QOL, power, and EMG activity in persons with MS with EDSS ≤6.5.	The majority of studies examined muscle strength as the primary outcome with secondary outcomes of fatigue, QOL, or muscle power. Improvements in muscle power, fatigue, and strength may underlie improvements in functional capacity.
	Dalgas et al. (2015)[157]		
15 studies identified	Systematic review and meta-analysis of RCTs examining the effect of exercise on depressive symptoms in persons with MS	The overall effect size of −0.37 indicated a small, yet beneficial effect of exercise on depressive symptoms.	Baseline depression score, disability level, outcomes used, and intensity of exercise can influence the observed results of exercise training.
	Gil-Bermejo-Bernardez-Zerpa et al. (2021)[263]		
Five studies identified	Systematic review examining impact of motor imagery on motor performance in persons with MS.	Practicing motor imagery resulted in improvements in walking speed, walking distance, fatigue, and QOL.	Small sample size, lack of randomization and blinding, and sample limited only to persons with low disability; however, motor imagery may augment active exercise therapy approaches.

(Continued)

Table 16.4	Evidence Summary of Exercise for Multiple Sclerosis—cont'd		
Subjects	**Design/Intervention**	**Results**	**Comments**
		Gopal et al. (2021)[198]	
Eight studies identified	Systematic review and meta-analysis of physical therapy interventions to address sexual dysfunction in MS.	Physical therapy can greatly improve sexual function (d = 0.82) and emotional well-being (d = 0.78), and moderately improve sexual satisfaction (d = 0.65).	The most effective interventions were pelvic floor muscle training and mindfulness.
		Gunn et al. (2015)[160]	
15 studies identified	Systematic review and meta-analysis of randomized and quasi-randomized studies examining interventions targeting fall reduction and balance improvement in persons with MS.	General exercise programs and gait, balance, and functional training demonstrated significant improvements in balance outcomes, which may not significantly impact fall risk.	Providing intensive practice and challenging balance activities is critical for maximizing effectiveness of balance interventions.
		Heine et al. (2015)[158]	
45 studies identified; 36 studies had sufficient data for meta-analysis	Systematic review and meta-analysis examining the impact of exercise on fatigue in MS.	26 of 45 studies utilized a nonexercise control: exercise therapy produced a significant effect of fatigue (SMD −0.53; p < 0.01), particularly endurance training, mixed training, and "other" training.	The majority of studies did not include individuals with progressive MS or an EDSS greater than 6.
		Kantele et al. (2015)[161]	
Seven studies identified	Meta-analysis of RCTs examining effects of long-term whole-body vibration on mobility in MS.	Improved 2–6-minute walking endurance following long-term whole-body vibration (effect size 0.25).	There was no improvement on walking speed (effect size 0.17) or balance (effect size −0.10) with whole-body vibration. All studies targeted individuals with low disability levels.
		Khan et al. (2017)[84]	
39 studies identified; 15 of them were Cochrane reviews	Systematic review of systematic reviews investigating rehabilitation in MS.	There is "strong" evidence for physical therapy to improve the following: activity (disability), participation, depression (with CBT), patient knowledge (with information-provision interventions). There is "limited" evidence for improved patient outcomes (i.e., fatigue, spasticity) using psychological and symptom management programs.	High-quality evidence is needed to support many rehabilitation approaches. The cost-effectiveness, optimal dosage, or economic benefit of various interventions is not discussed.

Table 16.4	Evidence Summary of Exercise for Multiple Sclerosis—cont'd		
Subjects	Design/Intervention	Results	Comments
	Kjølhede et al. (2012)[164]		
16 studies identified	Systematic review of studies utilizing progressive resistance training in persons with MS at EDSS less than 6.5.	Progressive resistance training improves muscle strength in persons with MS. The results are less consistent for improvements in muscle hypertrophy and neural changes, functional capacity, balance, and self-reported fatigue, mood, and QOL.	Heterogeneity of the results may be a result of varied training protocols, sample sizes, outcome measures, and type and severity of MS.
	Martín-Valero et al. (2014)[166]		
15 studies identified	Systematic review and meta-analysis examining respiratory training interventions in MS.	Respiratory muscle training resulted in improvements in maximum inspiratory pressure and maximum expiratory pressure.	Training protocols were heterogeneous with regard to intensity, frequency, and duration.
	Platta et al. (2016)[165]		
20 studies included	Systematic review examining the effects of exercise, physical activity, and physical fitness on cognition in MS.	Exercise training results in significant changes in muscular (effect size 0.27) and cardiorespiratory (effect size 0.47) fitness outcomes.	Studies that did not include a measure of physical fitness were not included in this analysis.
	Raats et al. (2022)[264]		
16 studies included	Systematic review examining the effects of interventions targeting trunk control on trunk and upper limb performance in MS.	Interventions included generic postural interventions (n = 9) focused on abdominal muscle activation, breathing, neutral position and lower extremity movements (Pilates, Ai-Chi), and specifically developed trunk training programs (n = 7) focused on trunk strengthening and dynamic movements. Overall improvements were shown in trunk strength, stability, and coordination.	The majority of programs integrated upper limb movements into training, but only 8/16 studies included upper limb outcome measures, demonstrating improvement in upper limb function as well.
	Sandroff et al. (2016)[88]		
26 studies identified	Systematic review examining the effects of exercise, physical activity, and physical fitness on cognition in MS.	*Exercise:* Class U (inadequate or conflicting data) with four of nine studies supporting improvements in cognition with chronic exercise. *Physical activity:* Class C (possibly effective) with four of six studies supporting improvements in cognition with physical activity. *Physical fitness:* Class C (possibly effective) with seven of eight studies supporting improvements in cognitive performance with physical fitness.	Many studies included cognition as a secondary outcome and may be underpowered to detect changes.

(Continued)

Table 16.4	Evidence Summary of Exercise for Multiple Sclerosis—cont'd		
Subjects	Design/Intervention	Results	Comments
		Selph et al. (2021)[169]	
74 of 168 studies identified included persons with MS	Systematic review examining interventions to improve function in wheelchair users with MS, cerebral palsy, and spinal cord injury.	Among studies of persons with MS, walking ability may be improved with treadmill training and multimodal exercises; function may be improved with treadmill, balance exercises, and motion gaming; balance is likely improved with balance exercises and may be improved with aquatic exercises, robot-assisted gait training, motion gaming, and multimodal exercises; ADL, female sexual function, and spasticity may be improved with aquatic therapy; sleep may be improved with aerobic exercises and aerobic fitness with multimodal exercises.	No studies provided evidence for prevention of cardiovascular conditions, development of diabetes, or obesity.
		Spooren et al. (2012)[162]	
11 studies identified	Systematic review examining UE training in MS.	Motor training programs can improve arm and hand performance in MS. Effect sizes were not calculated.	10 of 11 studies included UE training in conjunction with LE training.
		Toomey et al. (2012)[168]	
16 studies identified	Systematic review examining rehabilitation interventions for nonambulatory individuals with MS.	Five of 16 studies targeted exercise (i.e., aerobic exercise, strength training, respiratory muscle training) and suggest improvements in the target muscle trained, without carryover to other activities. Four of 16 studies examined multidisciplinary rehabilitation interventions and noted improvements at impairment and activity levels. Five of 16 studies examined cooling suits and found inconclusive results on fatigue. One of 16 studies examined therapeutic standing, resulting in significant improvements in hip and ankle ROM that did not carry over to other activities.	All studies identified were low-grade; high-grade evidence is needed to improve recommendations for nonambulatory persons with MS.

ADL = activities of daily living; BWSTT = body weight support treadmill training; CBT = cognitive-behavioral therapy; EDSS = expanded disability status scale; EMG = electromyography; FIM = Functional Independence Measure; LE = lower extremity; MS = multiple sclerosis; QOL = quality of life; RCT = randomized controlled trial; ROM = range of motion; SMD = standardized mean difference; UE = upper extremity.

in worsening of symptoms, most notably temporary increased weakness. This may have additional adverse effects on the continuing motivation of the patient.

- Precautions should be taken to monitor the effects of fatigue. *Time to fatigue* varies greatly among individuals with MS and is *not* correlated with the level of physical impairment or disability.
- Precautions should be taken to manage core body temperature and prevent overheating.[181,182] Environmental temperatures should be carefully controlled. Air-conditioning is a medical necessity in many climates. Additional cooling can be achieved by using fans, wet neck wraps, spray bottles for misting the skin with cool water, and immersion in cool water with aquatic exercises. Surface cooling devices have emerged as effective tools in managing body temperatures, controlling fatigue, and improving function. These include cooling suits or vests.[183–185]
- Precautions should be taken with certain impairments. Tactile and proprioceptive losses or incoordination and tremors may make the use of some equipment (e.g., free weights) unsafe. Visual feedback, when intact, should be used to monitor exercise performance. An alternative suggestion would be to use synchronized arm/leg ergometers to control limb movements.
- Precautions should be taken with cognitive and memory impairments. Individuals may require written or posted exercise instructions/diagrams including reminders of the number of repetitions, proper form, and correct use of equipment.
- Functional training activities (e.g., closed chain exercises) can be used to promote strength and functional endurance. Individuals with ataxia and balance problems may require the use of more stable postures (e.g., modified plantigrade, quadruped, or supported sitting).
- Group exercise classes can provide valuable motivation and social support. The therapist's primary role is one of educator and group leader. Successful management of group classes requires careful, individualized examination of group members to determine specific goals and exercises.
- Outcome measures can include isokinetic dynamometry, MMT (may be unreliable if spasticity is present), functional tests (e.g., sit-to-stand), fatigue (MFIS), and QOL measures (HRQoL).

Recent work suggests that 8 weeks of individualized progressive resistance training in a group setting is sufficient to improve hip strength in persons with MS.[186]

Aerobic Conditioning

Individuals with MS demonstrate expected physiological responses to submaximal aerobic exercise; that is, heart rate (HR), blood pressure (BP), and oxygen uptake (VO_2) all increase in a linear fashion in response to increasing workloads. Respiratory responses (respiratory rate [RR] and minute ventilation) also increase. However, HR and BP responses may be blunted if cardiovascular dysautonomia is present. A direct relationship exists between the duration and extent of disease[187] and the likelihood of autonomic cardiovascular dysfunction. Patients with MS can also demonstrate respiratory muscle dysfunction (weakness, dyssynergia), contributing to reduced exercise tolerance.

Exercise tolerance and maximal aerobic power (VO_2max) are reduced in individuals with reduced cardiorespiratory fitness secondary to physical inactivity. Decreased physical work capacity, decreased vital capacity, increased HR at rest and in response to exercise, decreased muscular strength, increased fatigue, increased anxiety, and depression are common findings.

Determining an appropriate exercise prescription to improve cardiovascular conditioning needs to be carefully individualized for each patient. While predicting exercise capacity and cardiorespiratory fitness is challenging for individuals with MS, peak VO_2 and exercise capacity can be predicted through submaximal testing.[188,189] The following guidelines for *clinical exercise testing* can be used.[180]

- The preferred mode is either an upright or recumbent leg cycle ergometer. A recumbent device is indicated if sitting balance is impaired. Combination leg and arm ergometry or UE ergometry alone may be necessary in the presence of significant LE involvement. Toe clips and heel straps are recommended to control foot placement, especially in patients with spasticity, tremor, or weakness.
- Performance measures include HR, RPE, BP, and expired gas analysis (VO_2). Using the RPE scale, peripheral (muscles, joints) exertion is consistently rated as more stressful (higher) than central (cardiopulmonary) exertion.
- A continuous or discontinuous protocol (3- to 5-minute stages) can be used; the discontinuous protocol is indicated with symptomatic disease, especially fatigue.
- A submaximal test should be used. Most individuals with MS can achieve 70% to 85% of their age-predicted maximal heart rate (HRmax).
- Recommendations for increasing workloads for each stage are 12 to 25 W for LE work and 8 to 12 W for combined UE and LE work.
- Termination criteria include achievement of peak HR, peak VO_2, volitional fatigue, significant BP changes (systolic blood pressure greater than 250 mm Hg or diastolic blood pressure greater than 115 mm Hg or a hypotensive response), or a decrease in oxygen uptake with increasing work rate.

- Precautions should be taken to monitor for attenuated HR or BP responses during exercise. A category-ratio RPE scale can be used to estimate central and peripheral exertion.[108]
- Precautions should be taken to manage core body temperature and prevent overheating (e.g., use of a fan for cooling).
- Precautions should be taken to monitor the effects of fatigue.
- Precautions should be taken to prevent the deleterious effects of overwork.
- Precautions should be taken with certain medications that can affect results: amantadine hydrochloride (HCl) may temporarily reduce fatigue; baclofen and amitriptyline HCl may cause muscle weakness; prednisone can also cause muscle weakness along with reduced sweating and hypertension.
- Morning is the optimal time for testing.

Prescription is again based on the four interrelated elements of the FITT equation. Recommendations for exercise programming to improve aerobic conditioning include the following:[180]

- Recommended training frequency is 3 to 5 days/week, on alternate days. Daily exercise at lower levels of intensity is recommended for individuals with more limited exercise capacities (e.g., 3 to 5 metabolic equivalents [METs]).
- Training intensity should be limited to 60% to 85% HRpeak or 50% to 70% peak VO_2.
- Recommended duration is 30 minutes per session or, for more involved individuals, three 10-minute sessions per day.
- Type of exercise can include cycling, walking, swimming, or water aerobics.
- Circuit training may prove best for optimizing training.
- Individuals with balance problems or sensory loss will require non–weight-bearing activities.
- Exercise precautions are discussed in previous sections.
- Outcome measures include graded exercise test results, HR (which may be difficult to monitor with dysautonomia; sensory loss in the fingers may make self-monitoring difficult), tests of lung function (forced vital capacity [FVC]), body composition, RPE, fatigue (FI, MFIS), functional status, and QOL measures (HRQoL).

Patient education is particularly important because the overall success of a fitness program is influenced by the individual's level of understanding of the basic principles of training, independence in self-monitoring, and skill in decision-making relative to level of impairment and exercise modifications required, as well as lifestyle and general health and safety considerations. Aerobic training results in improvements in balance and functional capacity measured with both gait speed and gait

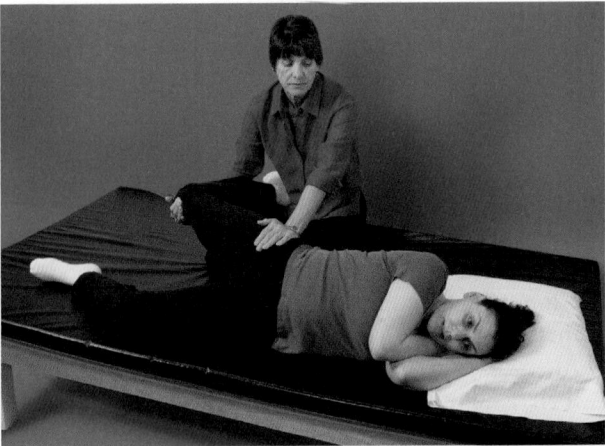

Figure 16.3 Side-lying hip flexor/rectus femoris stretch. This position allows the therapists to control the hip and ensure that excessive lumber lordosis is prevented while also modulating the amount of stretch between the iliopsoas and the rectus femoris.

endurance, with the largest effects noted when the intervention included continuous training that targeted walking.[190]

Flexibility Exercises

Stretching and ROM exercises are necessary to ensure adequate joint motion and to counteract the effects of spasticity (Fig. 16.3). Sedentary or inactive persons who are dependent on wheelchairs often develop tightness in hip flexors, adductors, hamstrings, and plantar flexors. Limited overhead ROM is seen with tightness in the pectoralis major/minor and latissimus dorsi and is associated with a slumped, forward posture. Patients confined to bed typically present with tightness in hip/knee extensors, adductors, and plantar flexors. Stretching and ROM exercises should be performed daily. For adequate stretching, holding at end range should be a minimum of 30 to 60 seconds repeated for a minimum of two repetitions. The use of orthoses or dynamic splinting is an appropriate option for prevention and in some cases reversal of contractures.[191,192] Considering the gait deviations and difficulty with transfers/bed mobility that arise from limited ROM and spasticity, it is important to also include aggressive trunk ROM to allow for full function of the core musculature, most notably the quadratus lumborum (Fig. 16.4). More active patients may benefit from Tai Chi, which provides additional important benefits of relaxation and balance training. ROM measurement using goniometry is an appropriate outcome measure.

Management of Bladder Control

The prevalence of urinary incontinence among individuals with MS is greater than 50%. Many individuals benefit from physical therapy intervention to address bladder control in conjunction with care

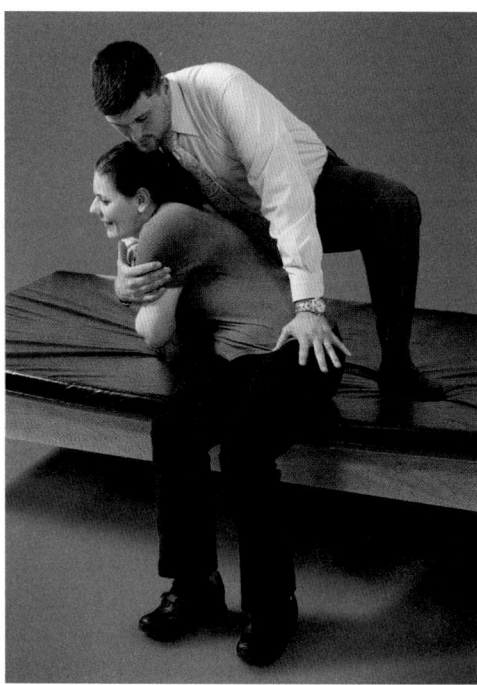

Figure 16.4 Seated trunk stretch. The pictured position allows the therapist to control the pelvis to ensure trunk stretching while maintaining control of the individual's trunk to apply the correct emphasis to the desired muscle groups.

from a urologist. Timed voiding on a schedule is useful when individuals have impaired bladder sensation, whereas fluid restriction at certain times of the day may minimize incontinence events (e.g., restrict evening fluid intake to avoid nocturia).[193] Biofeedback and physical therapy targeting the strength of the pelvic floor muscles are successful at combating urgency and nocturia, improving incontinence, and improving QOL.[83,194–196] Functional training may also assist patients who may be unsteady when hurrying to the restroom, which has been linked to increased fall risks among persons with MS.[197]

Management of Sexual Function

Emerging evidence suggests that physical therapy interventions targeting pelvic floor muscle training and mindfulness training may greatly improve sexual function, sexual satisfaction, and emotional well-being in persons with MS.[198] Routine assessment of sexual functioning and satisfaction remains low and could be a useful adjunct to therapeutic interventions targeting bladder control.

Management of Fatigue

With approximately 75% of individuals with MS describing persistent or sporadic symptoms, fatigue is among the most debilitating. Fatigue is characterized by overwhelming sleepiness, excessive tiredness, and sense of weakness that comes on suddenly and

severely. Aversion to activity for fear of bringing on fatigue is also common. The resultant lowered activity levels have important implications for diminished health status and deconditioning. Therapists are faced with a balancing act, on one hand prescribing exercise, while on the other hand avoiding overwork and the development of fatigue. Aerobic exercise training (previously discussed) and *energy effectiveness strategies (EES)* are central to any intervention plan to lessen fatigue.[36] During exercise prescription and physical therapy sessions, it is imperative that a skilled therapist recognize the difference between MS-related fatigue and the expected exercise-related fatigue. MS-related fatigue during exercise is often associated with thermal stress, which can be offset with adequate rest and the use of cooling and precooling treatments during exercise.[183–185]

Patients are instructed to keep an *activity diary* in which they record how they slept the night before, daily activities by hour, and how costly those activities were. For each activity, they can be asked to rate their level of fatigue (F), the value or importance of the activity (V), and satisfaction perceived with performance of the activity (S) by assigning a number between 1 and 10 with 1 being very low and 10 being very high. For example, the activity might be fixing lunch. Scores reported for this activity might be $F = 7$, $V = 3$, and $S = 2$. Aggravating factors associated with increasing fatigue (e.g., heat stress) and MS symptoms that appear or worsen during the day are also recorded. An *MS Daily Activity Diary* is available online (http://www.hail.ku.edu).

Based on this information, therapists can initiate training sessions, teaching EES. *Energy conservation* refers to the adoption of strategies that reduce overall energy requirements of the task and overall level of fatigue. These can include modifying the task or modifying the environment to ensure successful completion of daily activities. For example, a motorized scooter or powered wheelchair can be considered for community or home mobility to help conserve energy and maintain independence. Other mobility equipment such as walkers, crutches, or orthotics can also be considered. Activities that are difficult or have high energy needs can be broken down into component parts, requiring accurate activity analysis. *Activity pacing* refers to the balancing of activity with rest periods interspersed throughout the day. For the patient with chronic fatigue, *rest–activity ratios* are developed, with periodic rest periods planned in advance. Time-outs with complete rest should be instituted if an activity becomes exhaustive. Overall levels of energy can be improved if patients learn to set priorities and limit their activities, saving their energy for those activities that are truly important to them (e.g., activities that are enjoyable and meaningful in terms of the individual's lifestyle). The occupational therapist addresses EES and can provide valuable suggestions in terms of planning, work simplification, and developing encrgy-efficient activities for self-care and home management. The vocational rehabilitation counselor can provide useful strategies for behavioral modification and vocational rehabilitation. Team efforts with the physical therapist and others are important for consistency and reinforcement. Weekly review of activities and recommended modifications is used to evaluate progress. The MFIS should be administered on a regular basis to monitor ongoing fatigue status. Finally, stress management techniques are important components of symptom management.

The occupational and physical therapist should together complete a direct environmental examination of the home and/or job site. See Chapter 9, Examination and Modification of the Environment. A number of adaptations may be considered to improve efficiency and safety, including air-conditioning, home or work modifications, or ergonomic equipment. The patient/family/caregivers should be educated as to the importance of these recommendations for improved function. Periodic review of equipment and environmental modifications is also recommended. Additional referrals or collaboration with neuropsychology may also be useful to combat fatigue. Recent work suggests that behavioral interventions may also improve fatigue in persons with MS.[152,199]

Proper communication between the occupational and physical therapist and the patient's physician can ensure that the correct doses of the pharmacological treatments are in place, as the therapist has the unique opportunity of observing the patient in various circumstances and at various activity levels.

Management of Spasticity

Although spasticity varies greatly from person to person, muscles that typically demonstrate strong tone include the antigravity muscles. For example, in the LEs, the quadriceps, hip adductors, and plantar flexors are often spastic, while in the UEs the elbow, wrist, and finger flexors together with shoulder adductors are spastic. Individuals with MS typically demonstrate stronger spasticity in the LEs than the UEs. Spasticity is functionally limiting and contributes to the development of a number of secondary impairments such as contractures, postural deformity, and pressure injuries.

A variety of physical therapy interventions can be used, including cryotherapy, hydrotherapy, therapeutic exercise, stretching, positioning, or any combination thereof. The responses to these interventions must be monitored closely and carefully balanced with pharmacological interventions. The therapist must closely monitor the effects of the antispasticity medications prescribed and optimize physical therapy interventions with the dosing cycle. For example, patients on baclofen will respond better to stretching techniques if they are applied in the middle of the dosing cycle rather than at the end or beginning. Physical therapists must also recognize contributing factors that affect tone and rcspond appropriately. For example, infection or fever that increases tone may require a referral to the physician. It is important to reduce or eliminate all factors that can aggravate spasticity (e.g., heat, humidity, stress).

Topical cold (ice packs or wraps) or hydrotherapy (cool bath) can temporarily reduce spasticity by decreasing tendon reflex excitability and clonus and by slowing conduction of impulses in nerves and muscles. The effects of cryotherapy are relatively short lived, although some patients may experience enhanced ability to move that lasts for minutes or hours. It is important to remember that some patients, particularly those with intact sensation, may react to the unpleasant sensation of cold with *fight-or-flight* (autonomic nervous system) responses, such as increased HR, increased RR, or nausea. Cryotherapy is contraindicated in these patients.

Stretching and ROM exercises begun early in the course of the disease and continued daily can help patients maintain joint integrity and mobility in the presence of spasticity. Maintained stretch, held for 30 minutes to 3 hr, also can be used to decrease stretch reflex activity. Maintained stretch can be achieved with prolonged positioning (e.g., tilt table standing with toe wedges), low-load weights applied using skin traction, or serial casts. Air splints also provide an effective mechanism to maintain limbs in lengthened, out of spasticity positions. Patients/family members/clients should be taught stretching exercises as part of a home exercise program (HEP). Fast, ballistic stretching movements are contraindicated because spasticity is velocity sensitive. Stretching movements need to proceed slowly to gradually achieve the desired range.

Active exercises at slow or self-selected speeds should focus on expanding the available ROM. Emphasis on contracting the antagonist muscles can assist through mechanisms of reciprocal inhibition. Electrical stimulation of muscles antagonist to the spastic muscles can also be used to decrease spasticity. Movements that encourage abnormal postures should be discouraged. Patients with abnormal co-contraction may benefit from exercises focused on improving motor control (timing exercises) or biofeedback. Tai Chi, yoga, and aquatic exercises combined with cool water temperatures (less than 85°F [29.44°C]) can also be helpful in producing desired relaxation.[200]

Functional activities aimed at reducing tone should concentrate on trunk and proximal segments, because many patterns of hypertonus seem to be fixed from the action of the stronger proximal muscles. Extensor tone seems to predominate, so activities that stress LE flexion with trunk rotation are generally the most effective. For example, lower trunk rotation (LTR) in hook-lying can be effective in reducing proximal extensor tone. One very effective strategy is to position the patient in hook-lying with a therapy ball under the flexed legs and gently rock the ball back and forth. Moving from quadruped position to side-sitting can also be effective in reducing extensor tone in some patients as the activity combines LTR with prolonged inhibitory pressure on the quadriceps.[201]

For the patient with limited functional mobility (EDSS levels of 7 or above), positioning out of abnormal spastic postures is an important component of the management program. In general, prolonged or static positioning in any fixed posture can be deleterious to the patient with strong spasticity and should be avoided. For example, the patient who remains in bed all day with the LEs positioned in extension, adduction, and plantarflexion may be unable to flex enough at the hips and knees to sit in a wheelchair. Similarly, the feet will remain fixed in plantarflexion and cannot be positioned on the footrests. A positioning schedule using varied positions (in bed, chair, or wheelchair) will help keep the patient from getting stuck in any one posture. Mechanical positioning devices (e.g., resting splints, toe spreader, finger spreader, ankle splint) are helpful in maintaining position and preserving joint structures.

Management of Coordination and Balance Deficits

Cerebellar deficits (ataxia, postural instability) are common in MS. Impairments in somatosensory, visual, and vestibular systems are also common and can significantly impair coordination and balance. Spasms and muscle weakness can affect balance by changing the force and sequence of muscle contraction.[202] These combined effects result in difficulty in sustaining upright postures, walking, and other functional activities, leading to an increased risk of falls.

Interventions directed at promoting postural control should first focus on static control (holding) in weight-bearing, antigravity postures (e.g., sitting, quadruped, kneeling, modified plantigrade, and standing). Progression through a series of postures is used to gradually increase postural demands by varying the base of support (BOS), raising the center of mass, and increasing the number of body segments (degrees of freedom) that must be controlled. Dynamic postural control can be challenged by incorporating activities such as weight shifting and UE reaching (Fig. 16.5) or LE stepping. In sitting, combining UE movements with trunk movements (flexion with rotation and extension with rotation) is an excellent activity. This can be progressed to more advanced dynamic activities with the patient sitting on a therapy (Swiss) ball as opposed to sitting on a hard, flat surface (Fig. 16.6). Core musculature is engaged while the demands on ankle and knee musculature are minimized. This allows for a more focused core balance program that can progress to standing.[203]

An important goal of therapy is to promote safe and functional balance. Effective training should involve

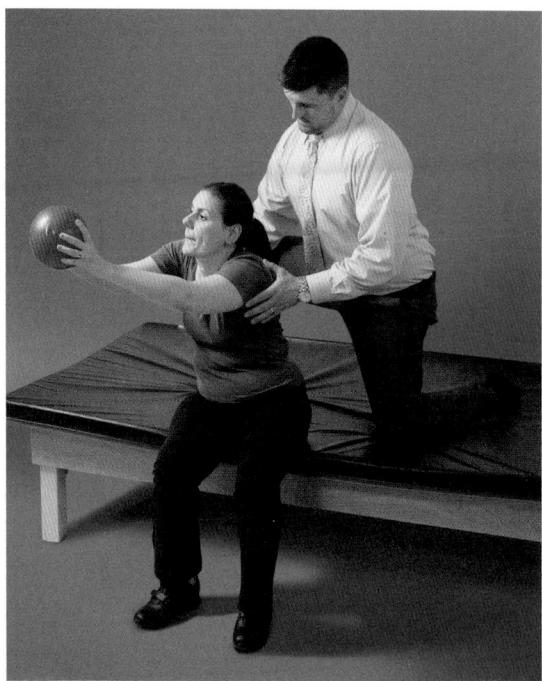

Figure 16.5 Dynamic postural control is promoted through weight shifting and upper trunk rotation to the right.

a variety of everyday functional tasks that challenge balance. Figure 16.7 demonstrates a dynamic postural control activity of combined stepping and reaching. Figure 16.8 demonstrates sit-to-stand movement transitions. As training progresses, tasks are modified (e.g., wide base to narrow base to tandem stance, stable surface to moveable surface) to promote adaptation of skills. Sensory contexts are also varied to promote adaptive control in different perceptual contexts (e.g., eyes open to eyes closed, firm surface to thick foam surface).[201] Patients with MS and central vestibular dysfunction may benefit from vestibular rehabilitation to improve impaired balance and disability due to dizziness or disequilibrium[204] (Fig. 16.9). See Chapter 21, Vestibular Disorders, for additional discussion.

The pool is an important therapeutic medium to practice static and dynamic postural control in both sitting and standing, as well as walking. Water provides graded resistance that slows the patient's ataxic movements, while the buoyancy aids in upright balance. Water aerobics have been shown to be effective in improving strength, decreasing muscular fatigability, increasing endurance, and improving overall fatigue and QOL in patients with MS.[200,205,206] When recommending aquatic exercise programs, it is imperative to assess the individual's tolerance to heat. It is commonly recommended that persons with MS exercise in a pool that is 26.66° to 29.44°C (80° to 85°F).

Biofeedback training using augmented feedback can be used to improve balance function. Augmented visual

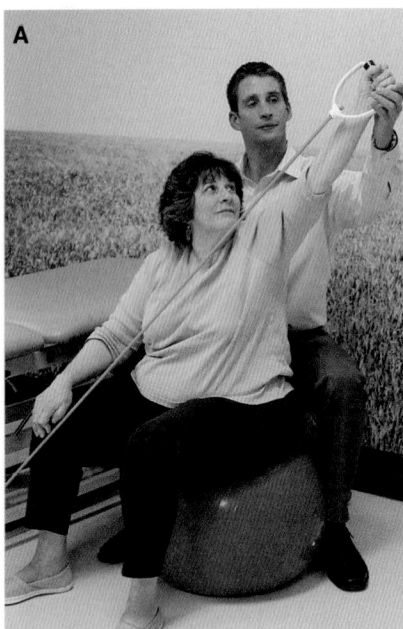 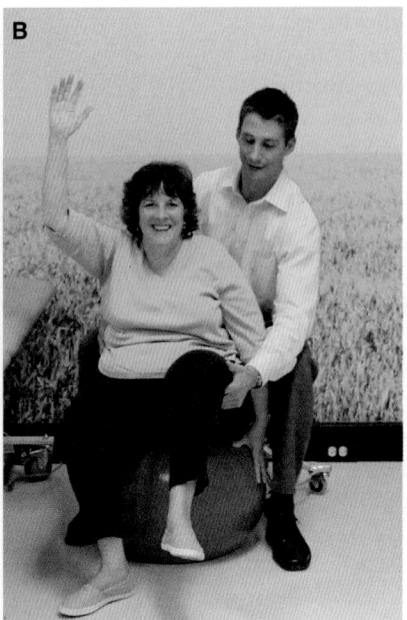 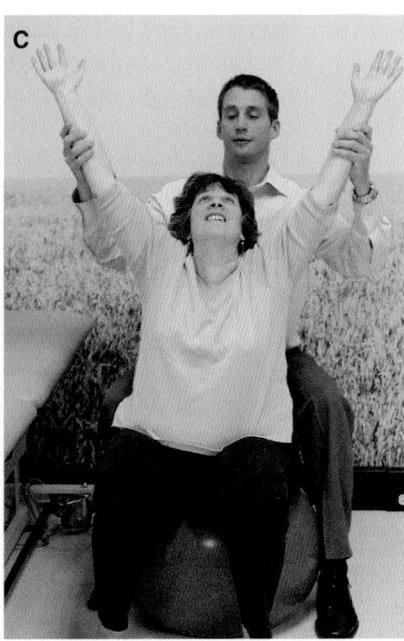

Figure 16.6 Sitting on the ball, the patient practices dynamic postural control activities: (A) unilateral resisted overhead reach, (B) reciprocal stepping and overhead arm swing, and (C) resisted overhead reaching.

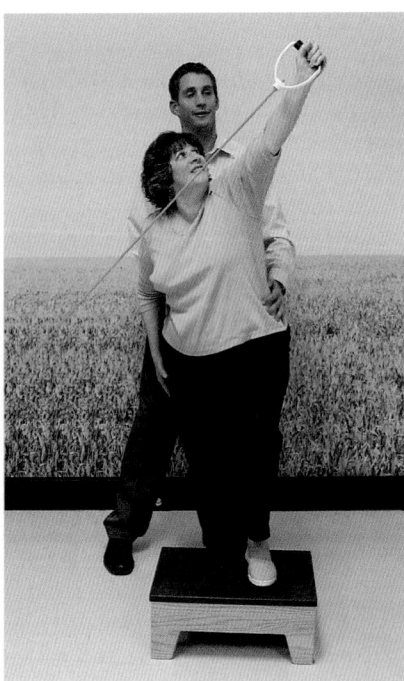

Figure 16.7 Dynamic postural control activities. This position demonstrates an advanced stepping and reaching activity with the added challenge of a resistance tube.

feedback[207] and augmented proprioceptive feedback (e.g., whole-body vibration platform training)[208] have been used to improve function in patients with MS. If available, the added biofeedback from visual and/or auditory feedback displays on force platform training machines is especially useful for patients with somatosensory deficits. The patient with ataxia needs to learn how to reduce excess postural sway (frequency and amplitude) and to control center of alignment position. Prolonged latencies (onset of responses) should be expected.

Control of ataxic limb movements (tremor and dysmetria) can be achieved through proprioceptive loading and light resistance. For example, the therapist can use dynamic reversals with light tracking resistance to modulate force output and reciprocal actions of muscles. Ataxic movements have sometimes been helped by the application of latex resistance bands or light weights to stabilize movements. Cuff weights (wrist or ankle), weighted boots, or a weighted jacket or belt can reduce tremors of the limbs or trunk. The extra weight will also increase energy expenditure and must therefore be carefully balanced against the increased fatigue the weight might cause. Weighted canes or walkers can be used to reduce ataxic UE movements that interfere with the use of an assistive device during ambulation. Weighted spoons or forks can be used to enhance eating. For patients with significant tremor, these devices may mean the difference between dependent and independent function. External devices (braces or splints) can be used to stabilize ataxic limbs but also have the undesirable effect of adding weight to limb movements. Air splints can also stabilize limb movements and should be considered, because they are lighter and less energy costly. A soft cervical collar can be used to stabilize head and neck tremors. All these strategies, however, should be viewed as temporary and compensatory. Once the

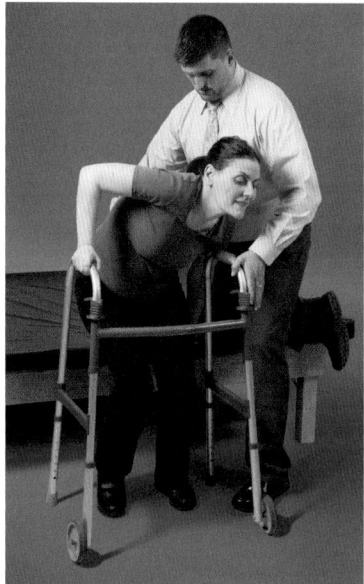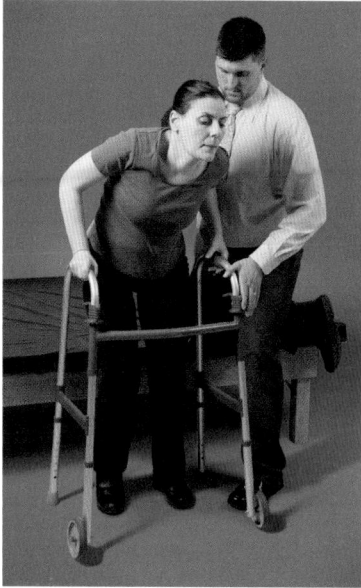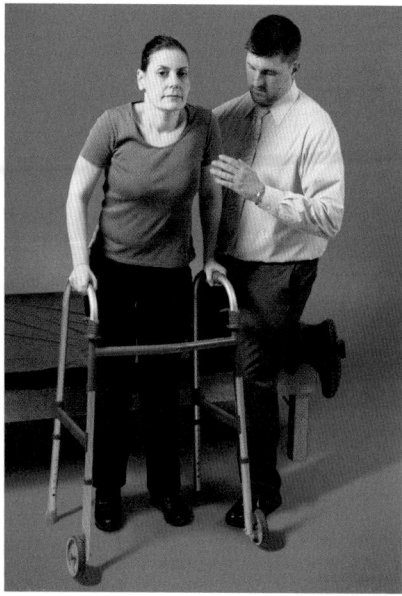

Figure 16.8 Sit-to-stand movement transition. The sit-to-stand transition is an important component of pre-gait/gait training, transfer training, and balance training.

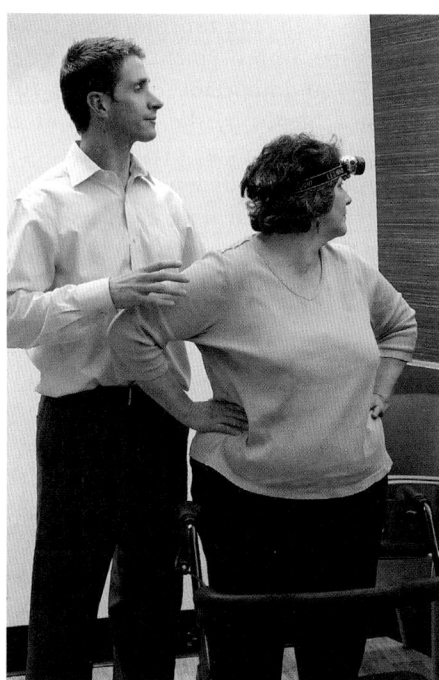

Figure 16.9 Head turns for vestibular training.

devices are removed, ataxic movements will return or in some cases may temporarily worsen.

Unwanted movements are worse under conditions of stress, anxiety, and excitement. The increased arousal, the result of adrenaline pumping through the system, increases existing tremors while decreasing function. Stress management techniques are therefore an important component of the POC. In general, patients do better in a low-stimulus environment that allows full concentration on control of movements. They benefit from augmented feedback (verbal cueing of knowledge of results and knowledge of performance; biofeedback) and repetition to improve motor learning. The patient with MS is often restricted in practice by neuromuscular fatigue and neurological deficits that impair sensory feedback, attention, memory, and concentration. The successful therapist will need to carefully identify the patient's resources and abilities and capitalize on them to maximize motor learning.

Locomotor Training

Walking ability is frequently impaired. However, at least 65% of patients with MS are still walking after 20 years.[27] Early gait problems often include poor balance and heaviness of one or more limbs. Patients frequently report difficulty lifting their legs (hip flexor weakness). Weak dorsiflexors are also common, resulting in foot drop. Problems with foot clearance may result in a circumducted gait pattern, among other gait deviations. Later problems evolve owing to clonus, spasticity, sensory loss, and/or ataxia. Weakness generally extends to include the quadriceps and hip abductors. Quadriceps weakness typically results in hyperextension of the knee and forward flexion of the trunk with increased lumbar lordosis. Hip abductor weakness results in a Trendelenburg gait pattern with a strong lateral lean to the weak side.

A well-designed exercise program of tone management, stretching, strengthening exercises, and task-specific walking training can improve walking. Standing and walking activities should stress safety and maintaining a stable BOS; maximum weight-bearing through the LEs; and adequate weight transfer and forward progression with trunk, limb, and pelvic kinematics consistent with safe walking. Verbal and manual cueing can assist the patient in the correct mechanics of gait. A variety of functional activities should be practiced. These include walking forward and backward, side-stepping, and cross-stepping (Fig. 16.10). Braiding, which combines side-stepping and cross-stepping, is a complex, higher-level walking activity. Stair climbing, negotiating curbs and ramps, navigating around obstacles, and walking on varied surfaces should also be practiced for safety in community mobility. See Chapter 11, Strategies to Improve Locomotor Function, for further discussion. As previously mentioned, the pool is an important medium that can be used to assist training of the more involved patient with ataxia while reducing tone and fatigue.

Locomotor training (LT) using an antigravity treadmill or a treadmill training (TT) with body weight support (BWS) results in improvements in muscle strength, spasticity, endurance, balance, walking speed, and QOL. Level of effort is reduced while detrimental effects on fatigue are not evident.[209,210] BWSTT is also safe and beneficial for individuals with progressive disease and results in improvements in fatigue and QOL.[211] Robot-assisted treadmill training (RATT) with BWS has also been used, and when compared with conventional BWSTT, patients in both groups experienced similar improvements in outcome measures.[212,213] When RATT

was compared with conventional gait training, no difference in outcomes was found between the groups.[214] Recent work suggests that eccentric training may be particularly useful for persons with MS; downhill treadmill walking resulted in significant improvements in fatigue, mobility, balance, and strength when compared with uphill walking.[215] Other forms of stepping, as in recumbent stepping, may be promising rehabilitation tools, particularly for individuals with progressive disease.[211] In summary, LT with BWS is an activity-dependent intervention that is feasible and safe and has the potential to result in significant improvements in function for patients with MS.

Balance and LT may also be paired with secondary cognitive or motor demands during training to target dual-task deficits. The ability to perform tasks simultaneously is frequently impaired in persons with MS due to motor and cognitive impairments. A SR of dual-task training studies in neurodegenerative disorders concluded that virtual reality training may improve dual-task performance.[216]

Orthotics and Assistive Devices

Patients with MS often require orthotic devices as ambulation skills decline. Improvements in energy efficiency and safety are also important outcomes. Ankle-foot stability can be achieved by the addition of an ankle-foot orthosis (AFO). AFOs are prescribed for foot drop, poor knee control (especially hyperextension), minimal to moderate spasticity, and poor somatosensation. The most common types used are the standard polypropylene AFO (Fig. 16.11) and the carbon fiber AFO, which are lightweight and have the added benefit of cosmesis. An AFO with an articulated joint can be prescribed to provide more rigid control for the ankle with the addition of a plantarflexion stop. Functional electrical stimulation (FES) devices have become prevalent in treatment and compensation for foot drop with improvements in walking performance and satisfaction reported. Patients also experienced fewer falls and reduced fatigue.[217–219] In order to effectively use any orthotic or FES device for foot drop, an individual must have adequate hip flexion strength. Relative contraindications to the prescription of these devices include severe spasticity, foot edema, and weakness (nonfunctional grades of LE muscles, especially hip flexors). Although knee-ankle-foot orthoses can provide additional stabilization control of the knee, they are rarely used because of the increased energy expenditure required.

Canes, forearm crutches, or a walker may be necessary to compensate for deficits in fatigue, strength, sensory loss (numbness), or balance (Fig. 16.12). For many patients, acceptance of an assistive device involves full recognition of their disability, so early discussion and introduction of these devices may smooth the transition when these devices are required. They need to be convinced that use of these devices is far safer than "wall

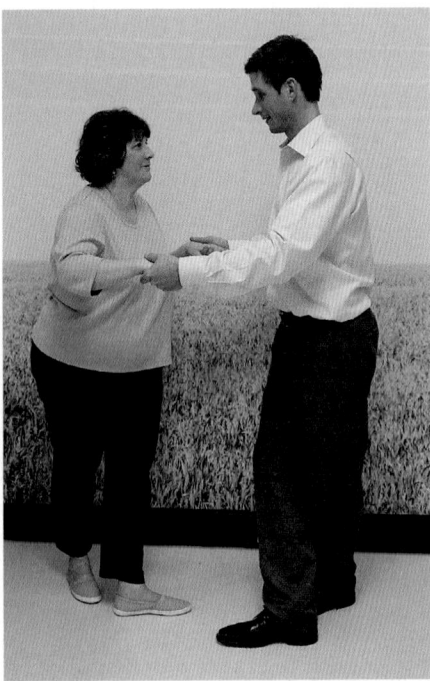

Figure 16.10 Patient practices cross-stepping. Dynamic standing activities are an integral component of an exercise program geared toward improving gait/locomotion.

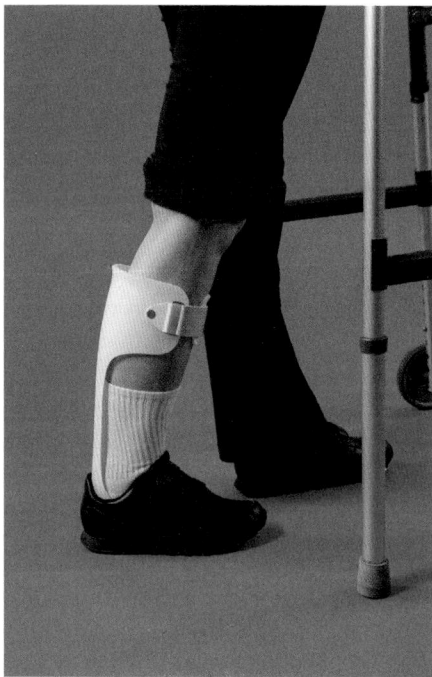

Figure 16.11 Patient is wearing an ankle-foot orthosis to stabilize the ankle and prevent foot drop.

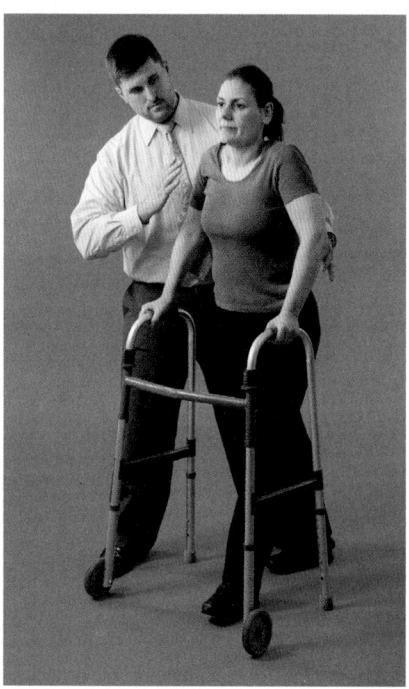

Figure 16.12 Locomotor training with a front-wheeled rolling walker.

walking" or "furniture walking." Devices also provide recognition to the community at large that patients are not staggering or losing their balance because they are "drunk," a frequent occurrence with many patients. The devices may be the difference between community

participation or remaining homebound because of fear of falling. Patients should be encouraged to try out different devices to determine which works best for them. For example, the patient with significant fatigue levels may benefit from a large-wheeled walker with locking hand brakes and a seat that allows for frequent rests. Recent technological advancements have brought a new breed of mechanical upright walking devices that have integrated computer chips, sensors, and motors to aid an individual in ambulation. Cosmesis is an important factor in promoting acceptance. There are many innovations in assistive technology that make the choices easier. For example, designer canes now come in many different colors and styles, including clear Lucite.

As the disease progresses, many patients benefit from a wheeled mobility device (powered scooter or wheelchair). The course and progression of the disease and presenting symptoms should be taken into consideration when deciding on a device. For patients with adequate trunk stability, UE function, and appropriate visual, perceptual, and cognitive skills, a scooter provides needed mobility while conserving energy. Scooters also do not carry the same negative stigma as wheelchairs. Both three- and four-wheeled scooters are available. Four-wheeled scooters have superior outdoor and uneven terrain performance but are not as easily transported. Features that should be recommended include a seat that rotates for easy mounting and dismounting, easy dismantling for loading into the car, and steering mechanisms that minimize the work of the UEs. One disadvantage of scooters is that seating cannot always be customized. They are often not designed for prolonged sitting or for patients with moderate to severe postural instability. Some new three-wheeled scooters are designed to turn in very small areas, while others have a wide turning radius and may not be suitable for in-home use. The individual with MS must be adequately educated on the safety precautions of a scooter, because the trunk strength and stability requirements are significantly higher than those of a power wheelchair.

A wheelchair should be considered when postural demands necessitate increased support. A standard wheelchair requires additional energy expenditure and coordination for propulsion. When prescribing a manual wheelchair to an individual with MS, it is important to include education on proper wheelchair propulsion for both preservation of shoulder strength and energy conservation. A power wheelchair should be considered when impairments prevent or limit manual propulsion or when fatigue is a major limiting factor in mobility (Fig. 16.13). However, they are costlier and require specialized transportation by a wheelchair-accessible van or bus. Most patients will navigate using a joystick. For patients with impaired hand strength and sensation, the joystick can be adjusted to increase

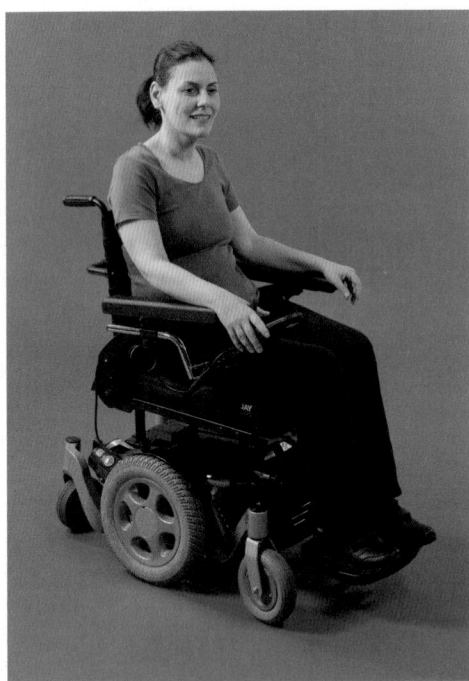

Figure 16.13 An individual with MS using a power wheelchair with joystick control for mobility. The correct power wheelchair prescription can encourage proper alignment of the pelvis, trunk, head, and limbs.

sensitivity. Wheelchair seating should ensure proper alignment of the pelvis, trunk and head, and limbs while enhancing function. Common malalignments include posterior tilting of the pelvis (sacral sitting) with kyphosis, typically the result of spasticity in the hamstring muscles. This can be improved with the addition of a seat cushion. Postural alignment can also be assisted by the addition of contoured seating (custom built). A solid back support and adjustable lateral trunk supports may be needed to enhance postural alignment and upright sitting. Footrests should be positioned to ensure that the thighs are parallel to the floor. If extensor spasms are strong, they can propel the patient out of the chair. A strong lap belt that secures firmly around the pelvis is necessary for safety. For patients with strong adductor spasticity, a medial knee block (pommel) may be necessary. Heel loops and straps may be required to maintain foot position on the footrests. Patients who no longer demonstrate adequate trunk and head stability require an alternate seating design. A tilt-in-space wheelchair with head/neck support is a better option than a reclining wheelchair with high back and elevating leg rests. The former maintains the normal hip sitting angle; the latter produces extension of the hips and may feed into strong extensor spasticity. Elevating leg rests tend to stretch hamstring muscles and may cause posterior pelvic tilting when spasticity is present. The reclining wheelchair with elevating leg rests also creates greater

environmental access problems. Motorized control of the seat back available in tilt-in-space wheelchairs will allow the patient to make easy adjustments in position, thus preventing skin breakdown. See Chapter 32, Seating and Wheeled Mobility, for additional discussion.

Patients should be instructed in transfer and wheelchair mobility/management skills. A transfer board or hydraulic lift may be necessary as UE function deteriorates. Attention to good sitting posture and pressure-relief techniques is essential to maintain alignment and prevent skin breakdown. Patients should be encouraged to balance time in the wheelchair with other activities, such as walking or exercising, and should be extra diligent in stretching muscles that tend to contract due to prolonged sitting (e.g., hip and knee flexors).

One of the constraints the therapist will have to deal with is financial reimbursement for the changing mobility needs of the patient with chronic MS. Private or public insurance organizations require a statement of medical necessity for payment. Because symptoms are not static in MS but rather typically exacerbate or remit, the therapist needs to provide clear and convincing documentation of need, stressing improved function and safety. Many third-party payers will not reimburse for new wheelchairs prescribed within specified time intervals or may be hesitant to finance expensive specialty wheelchairs such as the tilt-in-space chair or a second lightweight chair for traveling. The therapist will need to provide careful documentation of potential adverse outcomes to justify the cost of the new chair. For example, a likely deleterious outcome for a patient who is denied reimbursement for a tilt-in-space chair may be skin breakdown. The costs of nursing and surgical care for pressure injuries can then be compared with the cost of the new wheelchair, which can be justified as a preventive measure. It is equally important to anticipate future needs as they relate to rate of disease progression when ordering equipment.

Functional Training

Functional training should focus on problem-solving and the development of appropriate decision-making skills required to meet the challenges of being disabled. Skills should be adapted and practiced to ensure safe performance in both the home and community environments. Training in functional mobility skills (e.g., bed mobility, transfers, locomotion) is typically directed by the physical therapist, whereas ADL (e.g., dressing, personal hygiene, bathing, toileting, grooming, and feeding) and IADL (e.g., cooking, laundry, and bed making) training are directed by the occupational therapist, and training in communication skills is directed by the speech-language pathologist. Close communication and coordination among team members are necessary to ensure that training methods are applied consistently and successfully. Full participation of the patient in all phases of planning and training will increase personal involvement while decreasing dependency and passivity.

Many individuals with MS will use multiple adaptive devices. This requires careful attention to appropriate prescription of devices and environmental modifications to assist the patient in conserving energy and maintaining function. Assistive devices are discussed earlier in this chapter in *Orthotics and Assistive Devices*. Adaptive equipment can include bed or bathroom grab bars, overhead trapeze, raised seats, transfer board, or hydraulic lift. Appropriate positional and functional splints to facilitate writing or typing and plates and cups with lips to minimize spills are often helpful in assisting with hand function. Long-handled shoehorns, reachers, button hooks, sock aids, or Velcro closures can assist in dressing. Effective communication may require built-up writing utensils, a universal cuff for written communication, or more sophisticated computerized devices. Patients with severe speech problems may require voice amplification devices, electronic aids, or computer-assisted alternative communication systems. The team must recognize when a device is indicated and assist the patient in acceptance and in learning how to use the device *before* significant deterioration of function occurs.

Management of Speech and Swallowing

Impairments in communication and swallowing have been identified in individuals with MS.[220] Approximately 44% of patients with MS experience impairments of speech and voice early in the disease course, while 35% to 43% of MS patients can acquire voice, chewing, and swallowing disorders.[195] Respiratory deconditioning, characterized by reduced diaphragmatic support and shortening of the intercostal muscles, contributes to speech disorders and increases the likelihood of respiratory infections. Thus, collaborating with a speech-language pathologist to develop a *resistive breathing training* program paired with activities to improve trunk stability, head control, and sitting balance is an important component of the POC for patients with MS. Improved respiration can be facilitated through the implementation of prolonged phonation exercises, resistive breathing exercises, and incentive spirometry. The therapist should focus on diaphragmatic and segmental chest expansion, expiratory training, and volitional and effortful coughing.[221] Neuromuscular electrical stimulation (NMES) is more effective for the treatment of adult patients with dysphagia of variable etiologies than traditional treatment.[222]

When dysphagia or difficulty in swallowing occurs, physical therapists should work closely with speech-language pathologists to preserve safety of swallowing. Often a detailed examination is needed to investigate the deceptively complex swallowing mechanism. Diagnostic methods include *videofluoroscopic swallowing studies*

(VFSSs) and *fiberoptic endoscopic evaluation of swallowing*.[223] The role of the physical therapist is important in assisting with improving sitting position, body posture, and head control. An upright body posture with a slightly forward and downward-pointing chin position can be helpful in achieving a safe swallow and preventing aspiration.[224] Application of transcutaneous neuromuscular electric stimulation (NMES) to the submental muscles (suprahyoid triangle) to facilitate muscle reeducation was cleared by the FDA in late 2002, after the submission of data from over 800 patients (adults and children). NMES of the submental muscles paired with selected oral-motor exercises and swallowing maneuvers (e.g., Mendelsohn maneuver, effortful swallow, super-supraglottic swallow) can improve the strength, ROM, and coordination of the swallowing musculature.[221]

Thermal-tactile stimulation is a sensory technique whereby stimulation is provided to the anterior faucial pillars to improve swallowing reflexes and the pharyngeal phase of swallowing. Anecdotally, the use of cold and icy beverages such as shakes, fruit slushes, and ice chips provides heightened sensory input, which can improve the initiation of swallowing for many patients. Some patients also benefit from alternating small (teaspoon-sized) sips of liquids with their food during mealtime. Most patients should be discouraged from engaging in consecutive swallowing because it increases demand on the respiratory system and decreases airway protection. Resistive sucking through a straw can also be helpful, though therapists should use caution as use of straws can result in a larger amount of liquid compared with single sips. Thick liquids such as honey-thick and nectar-thick liquids can provide some resistance to facilitate muscle strengthening[225] and provide an alternate means of hydration when patients are unable to drink thin liquids due to aspiration risk. Moist foods (with sauces, broth, water, or milk) are easier to manage than dry ones. Semisolid and pureed foods are easier than regular solids. Foods that irritate the throat (e.g., vinegar) and crumbly or stringy foods (e.g., cake, cookies, potato chips, celery, cheeses) should be avoided. Patients also benefit when instructed to focus their effort on eating and never attempt to talk during active eating (mastication). Maintaining a quiet and peaceful environment during meals is helpful in improving attention and focus. Fatigue can also affect food intake. Many patients with MS benefit from reducing the size of their meals and eating smaller, more frequent meals or smaller, more nutrient-dense meals throughout the day. Percutaneous endoscopic gastrostomy feeding tubes and/or nasogastric tubes may become medically necessary for individuals with severe dysphagia.[226] For overall safety, it is important that family members, caregivers, and health-care providers are educated in the use of the Heimlich maneuver in the event of an emergency.[44] See Chapter 28, Neurogenic Disorders of Speech and Language, for further discussion.

Cognitive Training

Cognitive impairments can present major difficulties for the patient and for the rehabilitation team in general. Referral to a neuropsychologist may be indicated to determine the patient's strengths and weaknesses and to assist in the adaptive process. Compensatory strategies for memory deficits can be helpful. These include the use of memory aids, timing devices, and environmental strategies. Memory can be assisted by using a memory notebook to log daily events and reminders. With the increasing availability of mobile technologies, mobile devices, such as smartphones, have proven helpful for individuals with cognitive impairment related to memory and attention. A pill dispenser can assist the patient in maintaining a correct medication schedule. Cueing devices such as an alarm clock, bell timer, or watch alarm can help patients remember when to do certain tasks (e.g., taking medications, performing pressure relief). Structuring and labeling the environment are also effective strategies to assist memory (e.g., labeled drawers, cabinets). Directions for functional tasks (e.g., transfers, self-stretching techniques) should be carefully written down for both patients and caregivers. Complex tasks can be broken down with clear written directions provided for each step. Directions can be posted in different areas of the home (e.g., steps to follow for toilet or tub transfer posted in the bathroom). Additional cognitive strategies that may be helpful include mental rehearsal, requesting assistance, maximizing alertness, avoiding difficult situations, and mental exercises. Poor follow-through should be expected among patients with severe cognitive deficits, because often there is very little insight. In this situation, the efforts of family and caregivers must be fully maximized. As with healthy individuals, regular physical activity may have a positive effect on cognitive function, self-efficacy, and QOL.[88,227,228]

CBT for patients with MS can yield significant improvement in the ability to deal with distress, debilitating symptoms such as pain, fatigue and depression, impairment and disease exacerbation, and progression.[229] The goal of CBT is to change the way the individual thinks or feels about a particular impairment or problem. Significant improvements in QOL[230] and depressive symptoms result when CBT was applied in those with newly diagnosed MS.[231]

Cognitive rehabilitation conducted in both individual and group settings and through both in-person and computer-based methods is also useful for individuals with cognitive impairment[60,232–236] and has been shown to improve multiple domains of cognition including memory, attention, and information processing speed. Cognitive training may be more effective if the patient with MS is referred to a neuropsychologist for neuropsychological test assessment prior to treatment. This battery of tests can guide the focus of cognitive rehabilitation by identifying cognitive domains that are particularly impaired in the individual. See Chapter 27, Cognitive and Perceptual Dysfunction, for further discussion.

■ PSYCHOSOCIAL ISSUES

Individuals with MS and their families experience a variety of losses such as loss of social functioning, interpersonal relationships, employment status, independence, and functional skills. In contrast, these individuals are typically young adults who are normally engaged in establishing independence, careers, and social relationships. Disabilities emerge as the disease progresses over time. Various psychosocial adaptations can be seen, including anger, denial, and depression. The unique feature of a relapsing-remitting disease course is that it requires continual readjustment every time a new set of symptoms appears. Patients who appear well adjusted at one stage may regress as the disease worsens. The uncertainty of MS produces significant cognitive and emotional stress. Patients often feel out of control and unsure of themselves. Living with MS requires not only initial acceptance but also a tremendous flexibility to deal with this lack of closure. Patients also experience the cumulative effects of smaller, everyday stresses that are associated with fluctuating symptoms, inability to perform ADL, dependency on others, and architectural barriers. Many factors play a role in determining how an individual reacts to MS. These include the overall effect of the disease on daily life functioning, previous coping skills, perceived self-efficacy, extent of social support, and spiritual well-being. They may experience attitudes of "wait and see" or "nothing can be done." This may explain why many individuals with MS do not take medications to help control their MS despite medical guidelines recommending disease-modifying drugs. The longer they are influenced by these attitudes, the less likely they are to seek help. Learned helplessness, low self-efficacy, and lack of environmental mastery have been identified as major factors contributing to depression and fatigue.[237]

As mentioned, depression does not necessarily correlate to the severity of the disease. For example, a person with mild disease can be severely depressed, whereas the person with severe disability is not. The therapist must be alert to the signs of depression and intervene as appropriate. Chapter 26, Psychosocial Issues in Physical Rehabilitation, presents a complete discussion of this topic.

Despite the negative psychosocial effects of the disease, studies indicate that while initial diagnosis was met with negative reactions, over time positive changes in terms of values and outlook often occur. Interventions that target reexamination of the individual's role and identity result in an increased appreciation for life and can assist individuals with MS in better managing the disease and enjoying their lives.[238] *Self-efficacy* is the belief that an individual will be able to deal with particular situations that may contain novel, unpredictable, and stressful elements. Strategies that enhance self-efficacy and self-management (elements of CBT) empower the patient with MS.[239] Additional interventions include education, involvement in goal setting and treatment planning, wellness forums, and support or psychotherapy groups. The use of stress reduction techniques (e.g., relaxation techniques, meditation, and exercise) can also be helpful in promoting effective coping. Family and multidisciplinary support are key elements in effective psychosocial management.[240,241] Finally, referral for counseling or psychological services may be useful.

■ PATIENT AND FAMILY/ CAREGIVER EDUCATION

The primary roles of the clinician can be categorized as caring professional, expert teacher, and competent practitioner. A positive, affirming attitude can effectively influence patients' attitudes and assist them to view rehabilitation from a more positive perspective. The development of a strong collaborative relationship with the patient and family/caregivers in which there is respect, compassion, and effective communication is key to successful rehabilitation outcomes.[239] The overall focus should be on the maintenance of *hope* and *encouragement* tempered with *realism*.

As an educator, the therapist has an important role in assisting the patient and family/caregivers in providing information on the following:

- The disease process, clinical manifestations, and their significance in terms of management
- Prevention of secondary complications, indirect impairments, and activity limitations
- The rehabilitation process, the POC, and its specific interventions
- The HEP, including interventions that can be carried out independently
- Monitoring of the effects and possible adverse reactions of medications
- Use of assistive devices and adaptive equipment
- General health and stress management techniques
- Community resources
- Ongoing monitoring that includes wellness visits every 6 to 12 months to progress HEP and prevent decline as a result of deconditioning

- Referral to appropriate services including other health providers and community fitness and support services

Prompt referral to community resources including a support group can provide a necessary stabilizing base for patients and their families/caregivers. Within this environment individuals can gain accurate and useful information about the disease, discuss common problems and methods of coping, and share anxieties and resources. Thus, it provides a valuable forum to assist in the continual adjustment process. The NMSS (https://www.nationalmssociety.org) provides education, emotional support, and a variety of programs and services to individuals with MS and their families through their local chapters. Web-based resources are provided in Appendix 16.A (online).

A significant number of patients with MS (one out of every two patients) will require the assistance of another person at some point in the course of their disease. This places an extra burden on family members and on the financial resources of the patient if outside caregivers must be utilized. The majority of caregivers experience moderate levels of stress associated with their caregiving duties. As the level and duration of physical care increase, caregivers can experience a variety of signs and symptoms, including physical (e.g., fatigue, headache, sleep disturbances, appetite changes), psychological (e.g., anxiety, depression, frustration), social (e.g., family conflicts, decreasing social experiences or "lack of life"), and spiritual changes (e.g., hopeless and meaningless life and work).[242] This can also put stress on relationships, as the caregiver is often a spouse, and the dependency and degree of support needed to perform certain tasks can be a source of tension.[238] The therapist will need to be sensitive to these changes and to conflicts, problems, and tensions as they develop. Considerable time and energy will be devoted to counseling and educating caregivers and coordinating home management. Attention should also be paid to the children of patients with MS, because studies have indicated that parental MS has a negative impact on children's psychological well-being. This is due, in part, to lack of understanding about the disease, and education may help ameliorate some of the negative effects.[243]

SUMMARY

Timely referral to neurorehabilitation services is the key to successful management of activity limitations, disability, and QOL issues in patients with MS. Neurorehabilitation should be initiated early in the disease process, even at diagnosis, to discuss the importance of exercise, initiate a wellness HEP, and establish the therapist-patient relationship. Too often services are not begun until the individual becomes severely disabled. A comprehensive POC that addresses the needs of the whole patient and emphasizes meaningful functional activities, patient education, and self-management is ideal for such a complex neurodegenerative disorder. Activities that prove attainable and safe ensure patient success and build self-efficacy. Many patients with MS report that they lack the knowledge and skills needed to exercise safely. Promoting self-efficacy, self-management, and mastery can be achieved through supervised programs that focus on regular exercise, activity pacing, energy conservation, and overall healthy behaviors. Comprehensive efforts of the interdisciplinary team are needed to provide the coordinated and continuing care required with anticipated inpatient, outpatient, and home/community episodes of care.

Questions for Review

1. What are the pathophysiological processes involved in MS? What are the primary areas of CNS involvement?

2. Differentiate among the various disease courses (clinical subtypes) of MS.

3. How is the diagnosis of MS established? What tests and measures are used to confirm the diagnosis?

4. What is the role of disease-modifying drugs used in the medical management of MS? What are their indications and potential adverse effects?

5. Discuss the EDSS for patients with MS and indications for use.

6. Discuss the guidelines for an effective exercise prescription for the patient with MS to improve strength and conditioning.

7. Discuss the guidelines for an effective exercise prescription for the patient with MS to improve aerobic performance.

8. Discuss the problem of fatigue in MS and how it influences the design of an exercise program.

9. What strategies can be used to assist in the psychosocial adjustment of the patient with relapsing-remitting MS?

CASE STUDY

HISTORY

The patient is a 27-year-old graduate student who was admitted to an acute care facility with a chief complaint of double vision for 2 weeks. She reported that both lower extremities (LEs) seemed weaker recently. Four months earlier, she had noticed persistent tingling of her fingers on the left hand and some numbness on the left side of her face.

Neurological examination showed a scotoma in the upper field of the left eye, weakness of the left medial rectus muscle, horizontal nystagmus on left lateral gaze, and mild weakness of the left central facial muscles. All other muscles had normal strength. The DTRs were normal on the right and brisk on the left, and there was a left extensor plantar response. The sensory system was unremarkable. A diagnosis of suspected MS was made. The patient was discharged a few days later, seemingly improved after corticosteroid treatment.

The patient was readmitted to a neurological service 10 months later because she noticed increased difficulty in walking, and her speech had become thickened.

NEUROLOGIST REPORT

Patient presents with wide-based ataxic gait, minor slurring of speech, bilateral tremor in the finger-to-nose test, and dysdiadochokinesia. CT scan is within normal limits. MRI scan reveals numerous white areas indicative of lesions. LP shows 56 mg of protein with increased level of gamma-globulin. All other CSF findings are normal. Treatment with high doses of intravenous corticosteroids seemed to improve the neurological symptoms. Patient was discharged home with a referral for outpatient rehabilitation.

Two months later, the patient's symptoms worsened, and she is now admitted for intensive rehabilitation.

MEDICATIONS

Prednisone 20 mg po qid
Maalox 30 mL po qid
Valium 10 mg po qid
Copaxone 20 mg subcutaneously qid

CASE STUDY—cont'd

SOCIAL HISTORY

Patient has been living on her own for several years until her recent illness. She has taken a medical leave from graduate school and had returned home to live with her parents. They are both supportive and would like some advice as to how to modify their two-story home. There are five entry stairs with a handrail on both sides. There is a first-floor bathroom, and they plan to convert the first-floor study into a bedroom. The patient was driving but is currently relying on her parents for transportation. Patient does not have easy access to health care, having to travel close to an hour to therapy. Her parents are both in their early 60s and in good health. Both the patient and her parents are very anxious about their daughter's rapidly deteriorating condition. The patient is highly motivated to participate in therapy and to return to her prior level of function.

PHYSICAL THERAPY EXAMINATION FINDINGS

Mental Status

Alert, oriented

Memory: minimal impairment

At times lacks insight, seems unaware of the seriousness of her condition

Euphoric at times; other times she is depressed and cries easily

Communication

Speech is dysarthric, difficult to understand at times

Vision

Transient double vision

Gaze-evoked nystagmus to both left and right

Ocular dysmetria

Upper field defect of left eye

Endurance/Fatigue

Moderate impairment

Tolerance to activity is approximately 10 minutes before rest is required

Skin

WNL except for small bruise on right lateral malleolus

ROM

WNL except for 0° right dorsiflexion; 0° to 5° left dorsiflexion

Tone

Moderate extensor spasticity (2 on the modified Ashworth Scale) in both lower extremities (BLEs), left greater than right

Occasional BLE extensor spasms, which are a major safety risk when they occur during transfers

Sensation

Paresthesias in BLEs with moderate proprioceptive losses, ankle joints greater than proximal joints

Both upper extremities (BUEs): mild decrease in light touch, left greater than right

Strength

Moderate weakness in BLEs; generally functional muscle grades (able to move against gravity), with the greatest weakness noted at the hips

Standard MMT positions not used owing to spasticity

BUEs 3+/5 (fair+) to 4/5 (good) strength

Coordination

BUEs: Intention tremors with mild limb ataxia; voluntary movements are hypermetric; rapid alternating movements are moderately impaired

BLEs: Movements restricted by spasticity and spasms; unable to test

Gait

Ataxic

Wide BOS

Increased double support time

Decreased weight shift

Decreased gait speed

Increased pressure through UEs on walker

Forward flexion of trunk

(Continued)

CASE STUDY—cont'd

Decreased hip extension
Decreased heel strike bilaterally
Decreased hip and knee flexion bilaterally

Balance

Berg Balance Scale: 10
Sitting balance:
- *Static:* With eyes open (EO), able to maintain position independently up to 5 minutes with minimal postural tremor; with eyes closed (EC), truncal ataxia is pronounced
- *Dynamic:* With EO, able to weight shift to left and right to about 40% of LOS; with EC, experiences loss of balance with minimal weight shifts

Standing balance:
- *Static:* Able to maintain standing position in parallel bars with min assist × 1 for up to 3 minutes; during standing, patient is unable to maintain centered alignment; demonstrates moderate postural tremor; with EC, sway is increased dramatically, and patient quickly loses her balance
- Tends to keep her hips and knees stiff in extension/hyperextension
- *Dynamic:* Unable to weight shift or step without bilateral handhold

Expanded Disability Status Scale (EDSS) score: 6.5

PATIENT'S GOALS

She would like to regain ambulation skills and independent living status. She recognizes the need to live with her parents for the time being but sees this as only temporary.

GUIDING QUESTIONS

1. Using the ICF WHO model, identify/categorize body function and structure impairments, activity limitations, participation restrictions, and environmental and personal limiting factors.

2. Identify two outcome measures that will best address the patient's current functional level that represent the activity section of the ICF model. Provide a brief rationale for each.

3. Formulate four treatment interventions that could be used at the start of therapy to achieve the stated outcomes and goals. Provide a brief rationale for each.

4. What strategies can be used to develop self-management skills and promote self-efficacy and QOL?

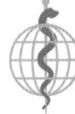

The reader is referred to Immersive Case D: A Patient With Multiple Sclerosis, an interactive case that guides users through the interview, examination, diagnosis, and writing of goals and the plan of care for a patient with multiple sclerosis, available online at **fadavis.com**.

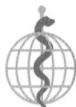

For additional resources, including answers to the questions for review, new immersive cases, case study guiding questions, references, and more, please visit **https://www.fadavis.com/product/physical -rehabilitation-fulk-8**. You may also quickly find the resources by entering this title's four-digit ISBN, 4691, in the search field at **http://fadavis.com** and logging in at the prompt.

Chapter 17

Amyotrophic Lateral Sclerosis

Vanina Dal Bello-Haas, PT, PhD

LEARNING OBJECTIVES

1. Describe the epidemiology, risk factors, etiology, pathogenesis, diagnosis, and general prognosis of amyotrophic lateral sclerosis (ALS).
2. Compare and contrast the Milano-Torino (MiToS) functional staging and King's clinical staging systems for staging disease progression.
3. Differentiate among impairments related to lower motor neuron, upper motor neuron, and bulbar pathology.
4. Discuss the medical and health-care management of individuals with ALS.
5. Outline a framework for rehabilitation for individuals with ALS.
6. Describe the components of the physical therapy examination for ALS.
7. Describe the role of the physical therapist in the management of individuals with ALS and the factors that influence intervention options.
8. Compare and contrast overwork damage and disuse atrophy as it relates to ALS.
9. Describe considerations that must be considered when designing an exercise program for an individual with ALS.
10. Describe common impairments associated with ALS and the physical therapy interventions to address these impairments.
11. Determine the goals and expected outcomes for an individual with ALS based on physical therapist examination findings.
12. Design a physical therapy plan of care for the individual with ALS.

CHAPTER OUTLINE

EPIDEMIOLOGY *636*
ETIOLOGY *637*
PATHOPHYSIOLOGY *638*
CLINICAL MANIFESTATIONS *640*
  Impairments Related to LMN Pathology *640*
  Impairments Related to UMN Pathology *642*
  Impairments Related to Bulbar Pathology *642*
  Respiratory Impairments *642*
  Cognitive Impairments *642*
  Other Impairments *643*
  Rare Impairments *643*
DIAGNOSIS *643*
DISEASE COURSE *644*
PROGNOSIS *645*
MANAGEMENT *645*
  Disease-Modifying Agents *646*
  Symptomatic Management *647*
  Sialorrhea and Pseudobulbar Affect *648*
  Dysphagia *648*
  Respiratory Impairments *649*
  Communication Impairments *649*
  Muscle Cramps, Spasticity, Fasciculations, and Pain *649*
  Fatigue *650*
  Anxiety and Depression *650*
FRAMEWORK FOR REHABILITATION *650*
PHYSICAL THERAPY EXAMINATION *658*
  Aerobic Capacity *659*
  Bulbar Function *659*
  Cranial Nerve Integrity *659*
  Cognition *660*
  Environmental Barriers *660*

Fatigue *660*
Functional Status *660*
Gait *660*
Integument *661*
Joint Integrity, Range of Motion, and Muscle Length *661*
Motor Function *661*
Muscle Performance *661*
Pain *661*
Postural Alignment, Control, and Balance *661*
Psychosocial Function *662*
Quality-of-Life *662*
Respiratory Function *662*
Sensation *663*
Tone and Reflexes *663*
PHYSICAL THERAPY INTERVENTIONS *663*
  Cervical Muscle Weakness *664*
  Dysarthria and Dysphagia *664*
  Pain *667*
  Upper Extremity Muscle Weakness *668*
  Respiratory Muscle Weakness *668*
  Lower Extremity Muscle Weakness and Gait Impairments *669*
  Activities of Daily Living *669*
  Decreased Mobility *669*
  Muscle Cramps and Spasticity *670*
  Psychosocial Issues *670*
EXERCISE AND ALS *671*
  Disuse Atrophy *671*
  Overuse Fatigue *671*
  Prescribing Exercise for People With ALS *671*
PATIENT/CLIENT-RELATED INSTRUCTION *672*
SUMMARY *674*

Motor neuron diseases (MNDs) include a heterogeneous spectrum of inherited and sporadic (no family history) clinical disorders of the upper motor neurons (UMNs), lower motor neurons (LMNs), or a combination of both[1] (Table 17.1).[1] Amyotrophic lateral sclerosis (ALS)*, also known as Lou Gehrig disease, is the most common and devastatingly fatal MND among adults. ALS is typically characterized by the degeneration and loss of motor neurons in the spinal cord, brainstem, and brain, resulting in a variety of UMN and LMN clinical signs and symptoms.[2] Clinical, genetic, postmortem, neuropathological, and imaging evidence supports that ALS should be regarded as a multisystem, heterogeneous disorder or syndrome rather than solely a motor disease, with variable involvement of extramotor networks and connections.

EPIDEMIOLOGY

The worldwide incidence of ALS has been reported to be 0.6 to 3.8 cases per 100,000 people per year,[3] with incidence differing based on ancestral origin; for example, the incidence rate for populations of European descent is about 2.1 to 3.8 cases per 100,000,[4–7] whereas the incidence rate in East and South Asia populations is lower, about 0.89 per 100,000 in East Asia populations and about 0.79 per 100,000 in South Asia populations.[8] Worldwide prevalence is about 4.1 to 8.4 cases per 100,000 people.[3] It is estimated that 30,000 individuals in the United States have ALS at any one time, and 15 cases are diagnosed every day, with decreased incidence in African-Americans and Asians compared to Americans of European descent, and decreased incidence in Hispanics compared to non-Hispanics.[9] Incidence in American Indian and Alaska Native populations has been reported as 0.63 cases per 100,000.[10] The prevalence of ALS is expected to increase by 69% by the year 2040, particularly in developing nations, due to an aging population globally.[11]

Studies have found ALS affects males slightly more than females, with a ratio of 1.2 to 1.5,[12–15] with male predominance decreasing after the fifth and sixth decades.[11] ALS can occur at any age; however, average age ranges from 51 years to 66 years,[4–7] with age of onset 10 years earlier in populations with mixed ancestral origins.[13,14] *Limb-onset (spinal) ALS,* with initial involvement in the extremities, is more prevalent than *bulbar-onset ALS,* with initial involvement in the bulbar muscles, with prevalence rates ranging between 60% to 80%;[2] Bulbar-onset ALS is more common in middle-aged women and individuals with associated cognitive impairments, and initial symptoms may include oro-motor dysfunction, with difficulty speaking, chewing,

Table 17.1	Motor Neuron Disorders
Subtype	Nervous System Pathology
Amyotrophic lateral sclerosis	Degeneration of the corticospinal tracts, neurons in the motor cortex and brainstem, and anterior horn cells in the spinal cord
Primary lateral sclerosis	Degeneration of UMNs
Progressive bulbar palsy	Degeneration of motor neurons of cranial nerves IX to XII
Progressive muscular atrophy	Loss or chromatolysis of motor neurons of the spinal cord and brainstem

Adapted in part from Rowland.[1]
UMN = upper motor neurons.

or swallowing.[3,16] About 5% of individuals present initially with trunk weakness or respiratory symptoms.[17]

The very large majority of adult individuals with ALS have no family history of the disease (referred to as *non-familial* or *sporadic* ALS), and about 5% to 10% of individuals have a family history of ALS (*familial ALS,* [FALS]).[3,16,17] Familial ALS is phenotypically and genetically heterogeneous, with intra- and interfamilial variability in age of onset and progression,[18] and is categorized by mode of inheritance and subcategorized by specific gene or chromosomal locus (Appendix 17.A [online]).[19–22] Numerous identified genes and chromosomal regions have been linked to ALS in the past three decades. The most common genes associated with ALS are: *C9orf72*, superoxide dismutase 1 (*SOD1*), TAR DNA-binding protein 43 (*TARDBP/TDP-43*), and fused in sarcoma (*FUS*).[23]

Of the hereditary adult ALS cases in people of European ancestry, about 25% to 40% are caused by a pathogenic defect (hexanucleotide repeat expansion, GGGGCC) in the *C9orf72* gene, which is responsible for making a protein found in cerebral cortex neurons and motor neurons.[24–26] *C9orf72* repeat expansion mutations cause frontotemporal lobar degeneration resulting in executive function, cognitive, language, and behavioral impairments. Frequency of the pathogenic repeat expansion in ALS varies greatly by ethnicity and geographic origin, with the lowest frequencies reported in Asian countries.[23] *C9orf72* mutations also cause frontotemporal dementia (FTD) in isolation or in combination with ALS, accounting for 25% of familial FTD cases[21] and 88% of combined ALS and FTD cases. Mean age of symptom onset in person(s) with ALS (PwALS) with *C90rf72* mutation is in the mid- to late-fifth decade, with about 40% bulbar onset and a median survival of 2.5 to 3 years.[27–29]

---

*The term *MND* is used to describe the disease in the United Kingdom, whereas the term *ALS* is used in North America and Europe. In Europe, ALS is also called Charcot disease.

Worldwide, approximately 20% of hereditary cases are a result of one of more than 100 mutations in *SOD1*,[16,30] a gene that encodes the copper-zinc superoxide dismutase enzyme. *Superoxide dismutases* are a group of enzymes that eliminate oxygen free radicals; although this group of enzymes are products of normal cell metabolism, they have been implicated in neurodegeneration. There are three isoforms of SOD in humans: cytosolic copper-zinc superoxide dismutase (CuZnSOD), mitochondrial manganese superoxide dismutase, and extracellular superoxide dismutase (ECSOD). *SOD1*, a gene on chromosome 21, encodes CuZnSOD. Mutations affect phenotype, disease severity, and disease progression.[31,32] In FALS, a vast majority of mutations change the amino acid sequence of the SOD1 protein at a single position, with that position different for most families. The most common *SOD1* mutation in North America is the alanine-to-valine mutation at codon 4, which accounts for 50% of *SOD1* mutations and causes an aggressive form of ALS with survival time of less than 2 years after onset.[31] The distribution of *SOD1* mutations differs markedly even within similar populations, and the same mutations in different populations may have highly variable clinical phenotypes (e.g., severity of symptoms and disease progression).[32] About 50% of individuals with a *SOD1* ALS variant are symptomatic by 46 years of age, and 90% are symptomatic by 70 years of age.[31]

■ ETIOLOGY

No single risk factor has been identified as the cause of ALS; rather, epidemiological and other evidence has identified several known and possible risk factors for ALS (Fig. 17.1), with both genetics and environment playing a role. The cause of FALS is genetic inheritance, with considerable and crucial progress having been made in unraveling the genetics of ALS.

The cause(s) of nonfamilial or sporadic ALS remain unclear and likely to be multifactorial,[33] with various cellular and molecular processes and multiple or cumulative or interacting mechanisms resulting in oxidative stress, aberrant RNA processing, exogenous neurotoxicity, excitotoxicity, impaired axonal transportation, axonal dysfunction, mitochondrial disruption, protein misfolding, protein aggregation, apoptosis (programmed cell death), and environmental factors thought to be responsible for ALS onset and progression.

1. *Genetics:* As noted, genetics play a role in the etiology of ALS. A very small percentage of individuals with nonfamilial/sporadic ALS have a mutation in *SOD1* (~2%) or *C9orf72* (6%–7%).[21,28] Monogenic factors (e.g., mutations in *SOD1* and *C9orf72*) account for the largest percentage of familial cases. *C9orf72*, *SOD1*, and other genes associated with ALS (e.g., *TARDBP* and *FUS*) are key to the normal functioning of motor neurons and other cells.

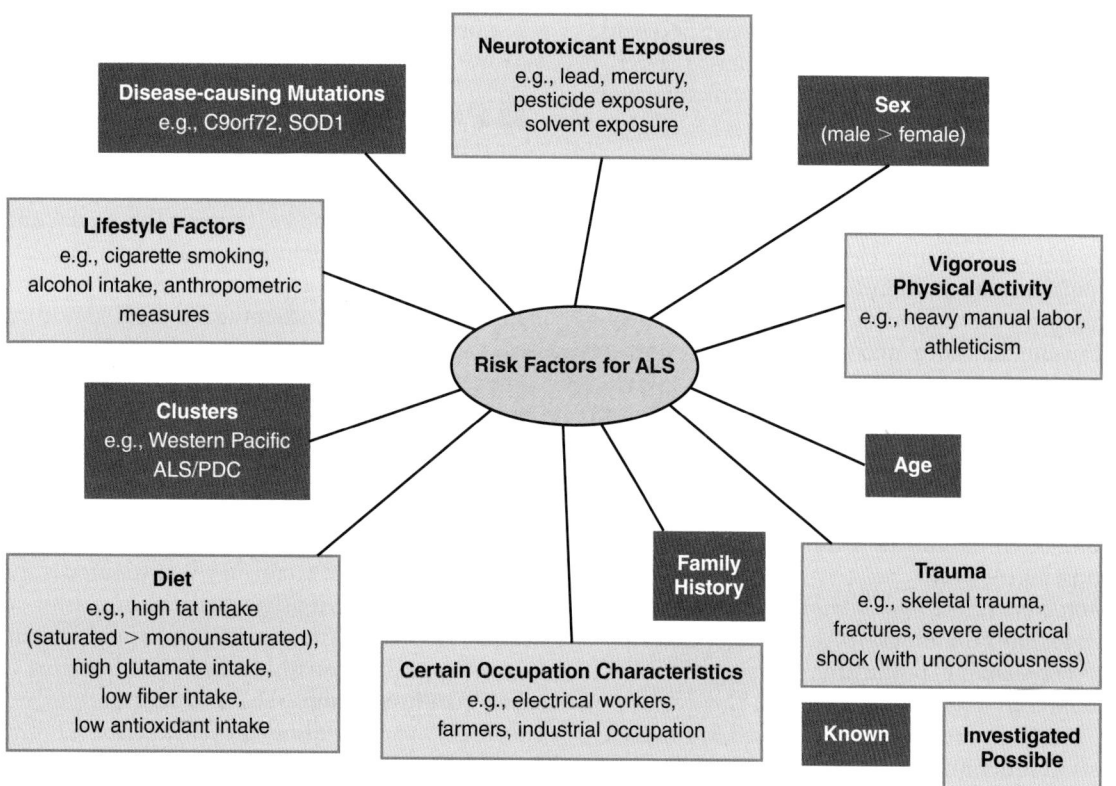

Figure 17.1 Known and possible risk factors for ALS.
ALS/PDC = amyotrophic lateral sclerosis and parkinsonism dementia complex.

Mutations identified in FALS have shown loss in SOD1 enzyme activity,[34,35] resulting in accumulation of free radicals causing toxicity and motor neuron death. Other mutations do not lead to reduced dismutase activity, supporting a toxic gain of function hypothesis.[28,36] Mutant *SOD1* is also more prone to adopt aberrant conformations that result in its aggregation in the intermembrane space of mitochondria, leading to mitochondrial dysfunction.[36]

TDP-43, a DNA/RNA-binding protein composed of 414 amino acids, is encoded by the *TARDBP* gene. TDP-43 is a regulator of gene expression and is involved in RNA regulation and multiple levels of RNA processing: RNA splicing, regulation of mRNA stability, mRNA transport, and translation. Both the loss, which affects expression of mRNAs and alters splicing events, and overexpression of TDP-43, will cause disruption of stress granules, which then aggregate and form protein inclusions and affect RNA metabolism, are thought to be causative of ALS.[37] FUS protein is structurally similar to TDP-43. FUS is also involved in RNA metabolism, and its depletion alters mRNA splicing, most of which is distinct from the mRNAs targeted by TDP-43.[37] FUS-positive inclusions have been found in PwALS with FUS mutations.[38,39]

2. *Glutamate,* an amino acid and excitatory neurotransmitter, has been implicated in neurodegeneration and is central to one hypothesis of ALS etiology. Motor neurons are particularly susceptible to glutamate, and excess glutamate triggers a cascade of events leading to cell death.[40,41] Increased levels of glutamate in the cerebrospinal fluid, plasma, and postmortem tissue of individuals with ALS have been reported.[41–43] A deficiency in excitatory amino acid transporter 2 (EAAT2), a specific glutamate transporter protein responsible for removal of glutamate from the synaptic cleft, in the motor cortex and spinal cord of postmortem ALS tissue has been reported lending support to the theory of excitotoxicity causing neurodegeneration.[44,45]

3. *Intraneuronal protein aggregates* (e.g., TDP-43, FUS, SOD1) have been identified in pathological studies of PwALS and animal models. Aggregates may disrupt normal protein homeostasis and induce cellular stress, bind to RNA and other proteins essential for normal cellular function, and impair axonal transport.[46]

4. *Neuroinflammation or an immune response* has been implicated in the etiology of ALS in several studies.[47,48] For example, proinflammatory cytokines interleukin-6 (IL-6), IL-1[beta], and TNF-[alpha] levels in the blood are increased in PwALS.[49] Defects in function or levels of T-regulatory lymphocytes (Tregs), important immunomodulatory cells that control the microglia and regulate the balance between activation and suppression of the immune response, have been found in PwALS, with lower levels of Tregs seen in more severe disease and poorer survival in those with Treg defects.[50,51]

5. *A lack of neurotrophic factors,* a group of growth factors essential for neuronal growth, maintenance and repair, has been thought to contribute to the development of ALS and other neurodegenerative disorders.[52] In vivo experiments and experiments with isolated motor neurons in cell culture have shown that neurotrophic factors are important in motor neuron survival.[53,54] However, factor deficits in ALS have not been conclusive and growth factor therapeutics have not been successful.

6. *Environmental factors,* specifically previous exposure to heavy metals including lead, previous exposure to pesticides, a history of physical trauma or injury, a history of electronic shock, and previous exposure to organic solvents, have been identified as having relatively strong associations with the onset of ALS.[55,56]

7. Other potential theories thought to contribute to neurodegeneration in ALS include apoptosis[48] and viral infections.[57] Mutations in *TP73,* an apoptosis regulator, have recently been identified in individuals with sporadic ALS, suggesting a role for apoptosis.[58] Viral exposure or infection has long been suspected as a causative pathogen for ALS. Enteroviruses, a family of positive-stranded RNA viruses that include poliovirus, coxsackievirus, echovirus, and enterovirus, can target motor neurons and both animal and human studies providing support for a possible link.[59]

■ PATHOPHYSIOLOGY

ALS is typically characterized by a progressive degeneration and loss of motor neurons in the spinal cord, brain stem, and motor cortex. The initial anatomical site of neurodegeneration is not known for certain (Fig. 17.2). The dying-forward hypothesis (corticomotoneuronal hypothesis, corticofugal axonal spread) proposes that ALS begins in the cortical motor neurons and progresses in an anterograde direction (Fig. 17.3).[60] The dying-back hypothesis proposes pathology begins with the muscles at the LMN level and advances into the central nervous system (CNS) in a retrograde direction from the neuromuscular junction.[60] A third hypothesis proposes upper and lower motor neurons degenerate independently.[60]

As noted previously, there is increasing evidence that ALS should be regarded as a multisystem health condition. Neuropathological and imaging findings have confirmed that ALS includes various nonmotor areas,[61–63] and the discovery of the *C9orf72* gene, which is linked to ALS-FTD, reinforces the concept that ALS comprises multiple, complex pathophysiological mechanisms.[64] Regions beyond the motor system affected by ALS include the autonomic nervous system; the basal

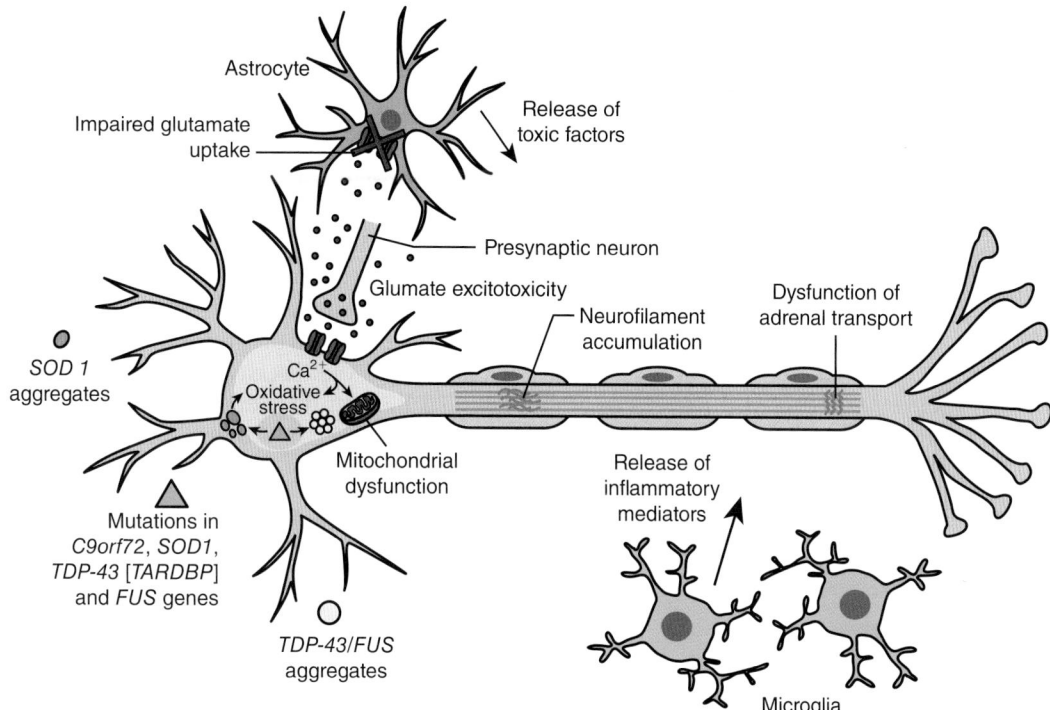

Figure 17.2 Causes of ALS are multifactorial. Causes include genetic mutations; various, multiple, cumulative, or interacting cellular and molecular processes; mechanisms that result in oxidative stress; aberrant RNA processing; exogenous neurotoxicity; glutamate excitotoxicity; impaired axonal transportation; axonal dysfunction; mitochondrial dysfunction; protein misfolding; protein aggregation; neuroinflammation; and apoptosis.

ganglia; and the cerebellar, frontotemporal, oculomotor, and sensory systems.[65,66]

UMNs in the cortex are affected, as are the corticospinal tracts. Brainstem nuclei for cranial nerves V (trigeminal), VII (facial), IX (glossopharyngeal), X (vagus), and XII (hypoglossal) and anterior horn cells in the spinal cord are also involved. Brainstem nuclei for cranial nerves controlling external ocular muscles (III: oculomotor; IV: trochlear; and VI: abducens) are usually spared; if degeneration occurs, it does so late in the course of the disease.[67] Motor neurons of the *Onufrowicz nucleus (Onuf nucleus)* are located in the ventral margin of the anterior horn in the second sacral spinal level and control striated muscles in the pelvic floor, including anal and external urethral sphincters. These neurons are also generally spared, and if they are affected, it is to a very limited extent.[68–70]

While ALS is thought to be mainly associated with motor and frontotemporal system degeneration, studies have reported degeneration of anatomical structures involved in somatosensory function and sensory pathways (e.g., medical lemniscus tract, visual, and auditory processing)[71] has been found in electrophysiology,[72,73] neuroimaging,[63,73] and neuropathology studies.[74–76] Sensory symptoms, such as numbness and mild parasthesia,[77,78] have been reported by some individuals, with increased prevalence of reporting in individuals with FALS.[79]

Regardless of the mechanism of ALS, the result is that as the motor neurons degenerate, they can no longer control the muscle fibers they innervate. Healthy, intact surrounding axons can sprout and reinnervate the partially denervated muscle[80,81] (Fig. 17.4), in essence assuming the role of the degenerated motor neuron and preserving strength and function early in the disease; however, the surviving motor units undergo enlargement.[80,82] Reinnervation can compensate for the progressive degeneration until motor unit loss is about 50%,[83] and electromyography (EMG) studies have found evidence of motor unit reinnervation in individuals with ALS. As the disease progresses, reinnervation cannot compensate for the rate of degeneration,[83] and a variety of impairments develop (Table 17.2).

The typical progression pattern of ALS spread is in a *contiguous* manner (e.g., within spinal cord segments [cervical segments to cervical segments]), before development of rostral or caudal symptoms,[84] with progression more likely and occurring more quickly to or from the region of onset to close spinal regions.[85] Although noncontiguous spread does occur,[86] signs and symptoms typically spread locally within a region (e.g., bulbar, cervical, thoracic, lumbosacral) before moving to other regions (see Figure 17.3). Rostral-to-caudal progression has been found to occur faster in PwALS with predominantly UMN signs. Caudal-to-rostral spread

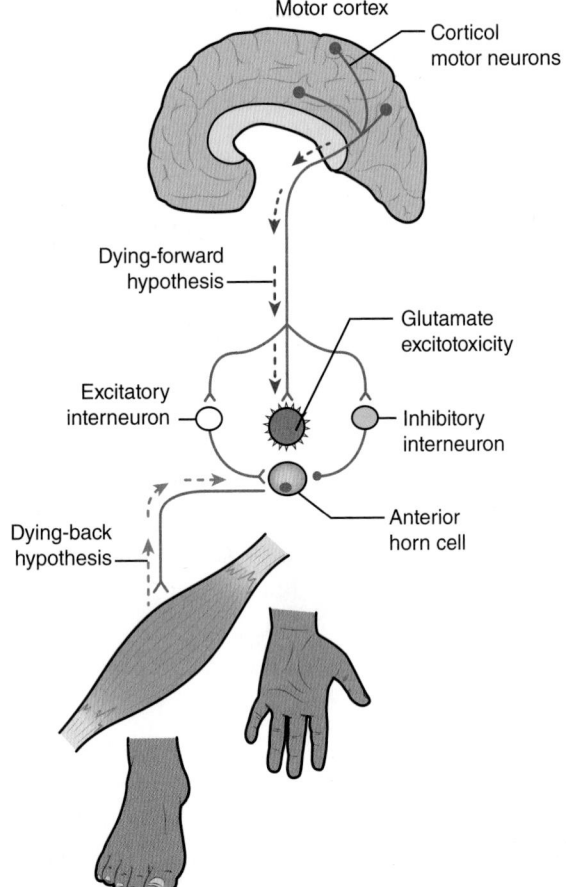

Figure 17.3 The dying-forward and dying-back hypotheses of ALS origin site. The dying-forward hypothesis proposes ALS begins in the pyramidal neurons of the motor and pre-motor cortices and via antegrade mechanisms causes dysfunction and death of the bulbar and spinal motor neurons (red dashed lines/arrows). The dying-back hypothesis proposes ALS begins at the muscle or neuromuscular junction level and progresses to motor neurons in the anterior horn of the spinal cord (anterior horn cells) via retrograde mechanisms (blue dashed line/arrow).

within the spinal cord and spread from the cervical to bulbar region appears to occur faster than rostral-to-caudal spread within the spinal cord.[84,86]

■ CLINICAL MANIFESTATIONS

The phenotypic expression of ALS is highly variable. Clinical manifestations of ALS vary depending on the localization and extent of motor neuron loss, the degree and combination of LMN and UMN loss, extrapyramidal areas affected and associated signs and symptoms, pattern of onset and progression, body region(s) affected, and stage of the disease. At onset, signs or symptoms are usually asymmetrical and focal,[2] although multifocal onset can occur. Progression of the disease leads to increasing numbers and severity of impairments.

Impairments Related to LMN Pathology

The most frequent presenting impairment, occurring in most people with ALS, is focal, asymmetrical muscle weakness beginning in the lower extremity (LE) or upper extremity (UE) or weakness of the bulbar muscles. For example, at onset an individual may notice difficulty with fine motor movements, such as buttoning, pinching, or writing, or may notice foot "slapping" or increased frequency of tripping while walking. Individuals with bulbar onset may notice changes in their voice, difficulty moving the tongue, or decreased ability to move the lips or open or close the mouth. Muscle weakness is considered the cardinal sign of ALS and may be caused by LMN or UMN loss. Initial muscle weakness is followed by progressive weakness and activity limitations.

In people with ALS, cervical extensor weakness is typical. Individuals may initially notice neck stiffness, feel "heavy-headed" after reading or writing, or may have difficulty stabilizing the head with unanticipated movements, such as in an accelerating car. Compared to age-matched, nonaffected individuals, neck movements in PwALS have been quantitatively characterized as having more "coupled movements"[87] (e.g., combinations of a prime movement together such as lateral flexion with one or more other secondary movements about [rotation] or along [translation] the axis, undesired

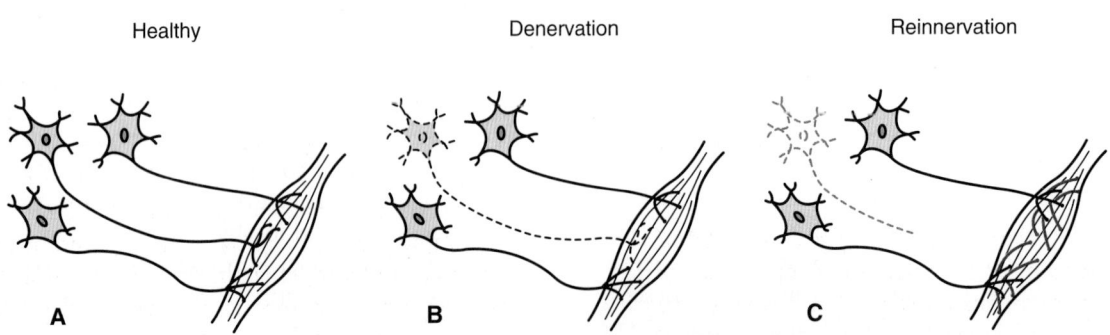

Figure 17.4 Sprouting: (A) normal motor neurons; (B) denervation; (C) reinnervation.

Table 17.2 Common Impairments Associated With Amyotrophic Lateral Sclerosis

Pathology/System Affected	Clinical Manifestations/Impairments
LMN pathology	Muscle weakness, hyporeflexia, hypotonicity, atrophy, muscle cramps, fasciculations
UMN pathology	Spasticity, pathologic reflexes, hyperreflexia, muscle weakness
Bulbar	Bulbar muscle weakness, dysphagia, dysarthria, sialorrhea, pseudobulbar affect
Respiratory	Respiratory muscle weakness (inspiratory and expiratory), dyspnea, exertional dyspnea, nocturnal respiratory difficulty, orthopnea, hypoventilation, secretion retention, ineffective cough
ALS-FTD, ALSci, ALSbi, ALScbi	Frontotemporal dementia-related impairments (e.g., loss of insight, emotional blunting), cognitive impairments (e.g., attention deficits, deficits in cognitive flexibility), behavioral impairments (e.g., irritability, social disinhibition)
Other	*Rare impairments:* sensory impairments, bowel and bladder dysfunction, ocular palsy *Indirect and composite impairments:* fatigue, weight loss, cachexia, decreased ROM, tendon shortening, joint contracture, joint subluxation, adhesive capsulitis, pain, balance and postural control impairments, gait disturbances, deconditioning, depression, anxiety

Adapted in part from van Es.[2]

ALS = amyotrophic lateral sclerosis; ALSbi = ALS with behavioral impairment; ALSci = ALS with cognitive impairment; ALScbi = ALS with cognitive and behavioral impairment; ALS-FTD = ALS with frontotemporal dementia; LMN = lower motor neuron; UMN = upper motor neuron.

out-of-plane movements, lower velocity movements, and movements that are less smooth).[88] As weakness progresses, the head may begin to fall forward, and in more advanced stages the neck becomes completely flexed with the head dropped forward, causing cervical pain and difficulties with ambulation, communicating. and feeding (Fig. 17.5).

Muscle weakness leads to secondary impairments, including decreased range of motion (ROM), predisposing the PwALS to joint subluxation (e.g., shoulder),

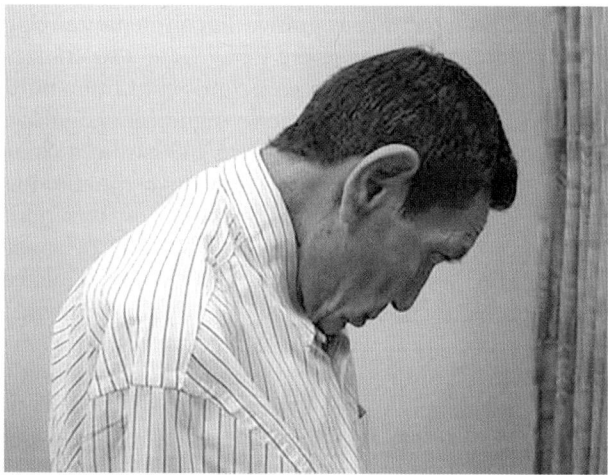

Figure 17.5 Marked head droop in a man with bulbar ALS. Weakness of the neck extensor muscles cause the head to droop resulting in chin-on-chest posture. *(Borrowed with permission from https://clinicalgate.com/motor-neuron-diseases/)*

tendon shortening (e.g., Achilles), joint contractures (commonly claw-hand deformity), and adhesive capsulitis. Weakness also results in ambulation difficulties, deconditioning, and impaired postural control and balance. Foot drop, secondary to distal weakness, and instability, secondary to proximal weakness, are common. The pattern and progression of LE weakness are characterized by greater losses of muscle force in distal muscles compared to proximal muscles.[89,90] A retrospective study found that decreases in walking ability from independent walking, to walking in the community with assistance, to walking only at home, to being unable to walk, were precipitated by relatively small changes in muscle force.[90] Falls are also common, reported to occur in 46% of individuals with ALS.[91]

As muscle fibers progressively denervate, their volume decreases, resulting in atrophy. *Fasciculations*, random spontaneous twitching of muscle fibers, often seen through the skin, are common in individuals with ALS, although they are rarely an initial symptom. The etiology of fasciculations remains unclear and is thought to be related to hyperexcitability of motor axons.[92]

Other LMN signs include hyporeflexia, decreased or absent reflexes, decreased muscle tone or flaccidity, and muscle cramping. The etiology of muscle cramping is not well understood and is also thought to be related to hyperexcitability of motor axons.[93] Muscle cramps are common in individuals with ALS and are usually movement-induced, short-lasting, and painful.[94] While common sites for cramps are the calf muscles, hand and finger muscles, and feet and toe muscles,[95] cramps can also occur in the tongue, jaw, neck, or abdomen.

Impairments Related to UMN Pathology

UMN loss is characterized by spasticity, hyperflexia, clonus, and pathological reflexes, such as a Babinski or Hoffmann sign, and may also cause muscle weakness. UMN signs may be less evident in the presence of muscle atrophy and weakness from LMN loss.[96]

Spasticity can eventually lead to contractures and deformities, as well as cause dys-synergic movement patterns, abnormal timing, loss of dexterity, and fatigue, all of which affect motor control and function.[97,98] For example, difficulties with the swing phase of gait secondary to distal spasticity and decreased balance owing to generalized spasticity are often seen in individuals with ALS.

Impairments Related to Bulbar Pathology

As bulbar UMNs and LMNs degenerate, *spastic bulbar palsy* or *flaccid bulbar palsy* (respectively) develops. In individuals with ALS, a mixed palsy that includes both flaccid and spastic components is common and may become more pronounced as the disease progresses.[99]

Dysarthria, impaired speech, can occur with either spastic or flaccid palsy, owing to weakness of the tongue and muscles of the lip, jaw, larynx, and pharynx. Initial symptoms include the inability to project the voice (e.g., shouting, singing) and problems with enunciation. With spastic dysarthria, the voice sounds forced, as more effort is needed to move air through the upper airway, whereas in flaccid dysarthria, the voice sounds hoarse or breathy. With pharyngeal weakness, air in the mouth leaks into the nose during enunciation, resulting in a nasal tone. As the disease progresses, speech becomes more difficult and unintelligible, and eventually the individual becomes *anarthric*.[99]

Dysphagia, impaired chewing or swallowing, is reported by all PwALS with bulbar-onset ALS and within 2 years of disease onset in about 60% of PwALS with spinal onset.[100] Dysphagia may also occur with either spastic or flaccid palsy. Manipulating food inside the mouth or moving food into the esophagus is difficult, and swallowing is impaired. With flaccid bulbar palsy, liquids may regurgitate into the nose because of pharyngeal weakness, and the cough reflex may be weak or absent, greatly increasing the risk of aspiration. Individuals with spastic bulbar palsy will have uncoordinated closure of the epiglottis, which may allow liquids or solids to pass to the larynx. Choking and slowed eating patterns are associated with dysphagia, placing the PwALS at risk for less than optimal fluid and caloric intake that results in weight loss and potentially cachexia.[99]

Individuals with ALS frequently experience *sialorrhea*, excessive saliva and drooling, owing to absence of automatic, spontaneous swallowing to clear excessive saliva, or because the lower facial muscles are too weak to close the lips tightly to prevent leakage.[2,101] Individuals with bulbar onset will experience this symptom relatively early. Initially, the individual may notice drooling at night (e.g., the pillow is wet in the morning); this eventually leads to needing to use a tissue repeatedly to wipe away the saliva.

Respiratory Impairments

Respiratory impairments in people with ALS are related to loss of respiratory muscle strength and a decrease in vital capacity (VC). Early signs and symptoms of respiratory muscle weakness may include fatigue, dyspnea on exertion, difficulty sleeping in supine, frequent awakening at night, recurrent sighing, excessive daytime sleepiness, and morning headaches due to hypoxia.[102,103] While some PwALS have evidence of respiratory function impairments at diagnosis,[104] others experiencing a gradual increase in respiratory muscle weakness may not report respiratory symptoms if they have decreased their overall level of physical activity because of muscle weakness in the extremities. The rate of decline of respiratory muscle strength differs among individuals, but it progresses at a linear rate.[105] As respiratory muscle weakness progresses, truncated speech, orthopnea, dyspnea at rest, paradoxical breathing, accessory muscle use, and a weak cough are typically evident. Respiratory muscle weakness is a significant predictor of impending respiratory failure and death.[105,106] If an individual does not receive ventilatory support, eventual CO_2 retention will lead to acidosis, coma, and respiratory failure.[107]

Cognitive Impairments

Neuropathological findings suggest that ALS affects the frontotemporal pathway and may be part of a wide clinicopathological spectrum of brain disorders known as TAR DNA-binding protein 43 (TDP-43) proteinopathies.[108,109] Although once considered rare outside the western Pacific region, cognitive impairments ranging from mild deficits[110] to severe FTD[111] are now considered part of the ALS disease spectrum.[112,113] Over a third of people with ALS have clinically significant cognitive impairment.[2,113,114] ALS-associated FTD has been characterized by cognitive decline; executive functioning impairments; difficulties with planning, organization, and concept abstraction; and personality and behavior changes.[115–118] Individuals with ALS, without FTD, have been reported to have a variety of cognitive impairments, including difficulties with verbal fluency, language comprehension, memory, abstract reasoning, and generalized impairments in intellectual function.[114,118,119] Risk factors for cognitive impairment include being female, having the C9orF72 repeat expansion, dysarthria, family history of ALS, predominantly UMN phenotype, and bulbar onset ALS.[120] It is important to know who may be at risk, as cognitive impairment (ALSci) and behavioral impairments (ALSbi) have important clinical implications, including increased caregiver burden and stress, as well implications related to effective communication, legal issues, and end-of-life decision-making.[121] Cognitive and behavioral impairments have also been linked with less adherence with management recommendations and decreased survival.[122,123] (Note: ALS with both cognitive and behavioral impairment is referred to as ALScbi.)

Other Impairments

Pseudobulbar affect is a term used to describe poor or pathological emotional control.[124] Spontaneous crying or laughter occurs in the absence of emotional triggers, or emotional responses are exaggerated and not related to the context.[125] This symptom is commonly seen in individuals with spastic bulbar palsy[126] and can occur in as many as 50% of individuals.[126]

Fatigue is highly prevalent in people with ALS.[127] Although ubiquitous, fatigue symptoms and characteristics vary between individuals, and the etiology of fatigue in ALS is not fully understood.[127] Fatigue in people with ALS has been reported as an inability to sustain motor function and as a "pervasive tiredness," often only partially relieved by rest.[128]

Fatigue is considered a composite impairment. Several factors may affect fatigue levels in PwALS, including central factors.[129] As motor neurons die, the remaining neurons or sprouted neurons are overburdened. Weak muscles must work at a higher percentage of their maximal strength to perform the same activity. This hastens muscle fatigue.[130] Fatigue may also be related to sleep disturbances, respiratory impairments, hypoxia, and depression. Sanjak et al.[131] demonstrated that individuals with ALS have abnormal physiological and metabolic responses to single bouts of exercise. Sharma et al.[132] found that in individuals with ALS, tetanic and maximal voluntary forces during sustained contraction were decreased compared to controls. No impairment was found in the muscular membrane or neuromuscular transmission, suggesting that muscle fatigue in ALS, in part, is due to impaired contraction activation.[132]

Many individuals with ALS report pain,[133] even though the disease does not typically affect pain pathways. Pain is typically a secondary impairment: musculoskeletal impairments, immobility, loss of ROM, decreased support from weakened muscles, positioning difficulty, dependent edema, and acute injuries (sprains, strains, and falls) can all cause pain.[134] Spasticity and cramps, especially if severe, and preexisting conditions can also cause pain. Pain is associated with decreased quality of life (QOL)[135] and may exacerbate depression and fatigue, both of which have been associated with decreased QOL in individuals with ALS.[136] (See the 2016 clinical guidelines on MND [https://www.mnd association.org/professionals/management-of-mnd/best-practice-guidelines-pathways] and Chiò et al.[28] for summaries of possible causes of pain in PwALS.)

Rare Impairments

As described above, sensory pathways can be affected. Some individuals may complain of vague, ill-defined sensory symptoms of paresthesia or focal pain in the limbs. External ocular muscles are usually spared in people with ALS; if degeneration occurs, it does so late in the course of the disease.[137] Individuals who have been maintained on ventilators for long periods of time may develop the inability to voluntarily close the eyes, or *ophthalmoplegia,* complete ocular paralysis.[137] Motor neurons controlling the anal and vesicourethral sphincter muscles and muscles of the pelvic floor are generally spared. Urinary symptoms such as urge incontinence, particularly in PwALS ages 60 years and older, those taking muscle relaxants and anticholinergics, and those with associated high symptom burden have been reported.[138] Incontinence of stool has low prevalence and constipation is more frequently reported.[138]

■ DIAGNOSIS

No definitive diagnostic test or diagnostic biological marker exists for ALS. For individuals with a clinical presentation of ALS, laboratory studies, EMG, nerve conduction velocity studies, muscle and nerve biopsies, and neuroimaging studies are used to support the diagnosis and to exclude other diagnoses. Studies have found that the time interval from symptom onset to diagnosis confirmation ranges from 8 to 16 months,[139-141] which may represent a significant proportion of disease duration. Individuals with bulbar-onset ALS have a shorter time to diagnosis.[141]

The diagnosis of ALS requires the *presence* of (1) LMN signs by clinical, electrophysiological, or neuropathological examination; (2) UMN signs by clinical examination; and (3) progression of the disease within a region or to other regions by clinical examination or via the medical history. The *absence* of (1) electrophysiological and pathological evidence of other diseases that may explain the UMN and LMN signs and (2) neuroimaging evidence of other disease processes that may explain the observed clinical and electrophysiologic signs are also evaluated.

The *World Federation of Neurology Research Group on Motor Neuron Diseases* established the *El Escorial criteria* in 1994, and revised criteria were published in 2000.[94] The El Escorial criteria have been considered standard for the diagnosis of ALS for clinical practice, therapeutic trials, and other research purposes for the past two decades. In the absence of pathological evidence, the diagnosis of ALS is classified into *clinically definite, clinically probable, clinically probable with laboratory support,* and *clinically possible* categories (Fig. 17.6).[142] A diagnosis of *clinically definite ALS* is defined as both UMN and LMN findings in at least three of four regions (bulbar, cervical, thoracic, or lumbosacral) or UMN and LMN signs in the bulbar region and at least

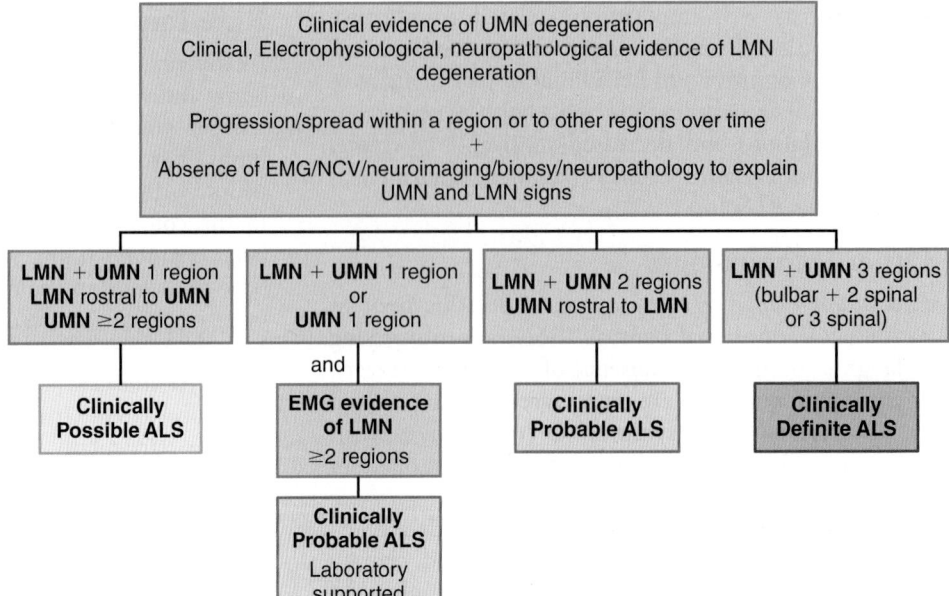

Figure 17.6 El Escorial Criteria for the Diagnosis of ALS.

two spinal regions. *Clinically probable* ALS is defined as UMN and LMN signs in two regions, with at least one UMN finding rostral to the LMN findings. *Clinically probable, laboratory-supported* ALS is defined as UMN and LMN clinical signs in one region only, or UMN signs alone present in one region and LMN signs defined by EMG criteria present in at least two regions. The EMG criteria include signs of active denervation, such as fibrillation potentials and positive sharp waves; and signs of chronic denervation, such as large motor unit potentials (increased duration, increased proportion of polyphasic potentials, increased amplitude) and unstable motor unit potentials. *Clinically possible* ALS is defined as UMN and LMN signs found together in only one region, or UMN signs found alone in two or more regions, or LMN signs found rostral to UMN signs and the inability to establish a diagnosis of clinically probable, laboratory-supported ALS.[142]

Awaji-Shima criteria were developed to increase diagnostic sensitivity for ALS, incorporating objective neurophysiological biomarkers of LMN dysfunction (e.g., chronic neurogenic changes, features of active denervation-presence of fasciculations).[143] The Awaji-Shima criteria are as follows: (1) *Clinically definite ALS*—clinical or electrophysiological evidence of LMN and UMN signs in the bulbar region and at least two spinal regions, or the presence of LMN and UMN in three spinal regions. (2) *Clinically probable ALS*—clinical or electrophysiological evidence of LMN and UMN in at least two regions, with some UMN signs necessarily rostral to the LMN signs. (3) *Clinically possible ALS*—clinical or electrophysiological signs of LMN and UMN signs in one region; or UMN signs found alone in two or more regions; or LMN signs found rostral to UMN signs.[143]

Because of the highly variable nature of ALS and clinical phenotypes, Al-Chalabi et al. proposed a comprehensive ALS classification system, combining current classification systems with the highly variable presentation of ALS. This system incorporates four components: disease stage (1 = early to 4 = late); phenotypic descriptors (e.g., site of onset, age of onset); diagnosis (e.g., LMN-dominant ALS or UMN-dominant ALS); El Escorial category; as well as diagnostic modifiers (FALS, FTD) and optional elements (specific mutation), thereby providing a more fulsome "picture" of the individual with ALS.[33]

Recently, a set of minimum diagnostic criteria, collapsing the criteria for possible, probable, and definite ALS, has been proposed and include: (1) progressive motor impairment as documented by history or repeated clinical assessment, preceded by normal motor function; (2) presence of UMN and LMN dysfunction in at least one body region (bulbar, cervical, thoracic, lumber), with UMN and LMN dysfunction noted in the same body region if only one body region is involved or LMN dysfunction in at least two body regions; and (3) investigations (e.g., nerve conduction studies and needle EMG, MRI or other imaging, blood or cerebral spinal fluid studies to exclude other disease processes).[144]

■ DISEASE COURSE

ALS has a progressive and deteriorating disease trajectory, and the progression from pathology to impairments to activity limitations to participation restrictions is inevitable. Although the disease course varies among individuals, with time from onset to death ranging from several months to 20 years, studies have found the average duration of ALS to be between 27 and 43 months, and the median duration to be between

Table 17.3	Comparison of ALS Milano-Torino and King's Disease Progression Staging	
	ALS Milano-Torino Staging[146]	King's Staging[147]

General Description	• Based on function as assessed by the ALSFRS/ALSFRS-R
	• Four domains:
	  • Movement (walking or self-care)–item 8 (Walking) OR 6 (Dressing and Hygiene)
	  • Swallowing–item #3
	  • Communicating–item #1 (Speech) AND item #4 (Handwriting)
	  • Breathing–item #10 (Dyspnea) OR #12 ALSFRS-R (Respiratory Insufficiency)
	• Each domain scored as 0 or 1
	• Stage score based on number of domains with loss of independence
		• Examines anatomical spread of ALS based on the number of affected regions, as per the El Escorial criteria–bulbar, upper limb, lower limb
		• Advanced stage defined by nutritional or respiratory failure

Stages	Stage 0 = functional involvement but no loss of independence in any domain Stage 1 = loss of independent function in one functional domain Stage 2 = loss of independent function in two functional domains Stage 3 = loss of independent function in three functional domains Stage 4 = loss of independent function in four functional domains Stage 5 = death	Stage 1 = involvement of first clinical region Stage 2 = involvement of second clinical region Stage 3 = involvement of third clinical region Stage 4 = late disease; need for gastrostomy (4A) or respiratory support (noninvasive ventilation, 4B) Stage 5 = death

ALSFRS/ALSFRS-R = ALS Functional Rating Scale/ALS Functional Rating Scale-Revised.

23 and 52 months.[145] Five-year and 10-year survival rates range from 9% to 40% and 8% to 16%, respectively. A 50% survival probability after the first symptom of ALS appears is slightly greater than 3 years unless mechanical ventilation is used to sustain breathing. In most PwALS, death occurs within 3 to 5 years after symptom onset and usually results from respiratory failure. However, about 10% of individuals have a much slower disease progression, living 10 years or longer.[145]

Disease progression staging systems have been developed to describe clinical milestones across the disease course that are reflective of disease severity, see Table 17.3 for a comparison of the Milano-Torino (MiToS)[146] and King's staging system.[147] The King's staging system has been found to differentiate early- to middle-stage disease well, whereas the MiToS staging system has been found to differentiate the late stages of ALS,[148] but neither system includes behavioral or cognitive impairments as components of the systems.

■ PROGNOSIS

Population- and clinical trial–based data sets have been used to identify prognostic factors. Specific individual characteristics have been reported to be associated with shorter or longer survival times.[145] Older age at symptom onset affects survival,[150] with PwALS ages 35 to 40 years of age or younger having better 5-year

survival rates than older individuals.[145] Individuals with limb-onset ALS have a better prognosis than do those with bulbar-onset ALS,[150] with 5-year survival rates reported to be 37% and 44%, compared to survival rates of 9% and 16% for individuals with bulbar-onset ALS.[151] Less severe involvement at the time of diagnosis, no symptoms of dyspnea at onset, and delayed time between symptom onset and diagnosis, which may be reflective of slower disease progression, have also been found to predict prognosis.[152] For example, individuals with ALS who had a delay of less than 6 months had a mortality rate of 45% compared to 6% mortality in those with longer delays (e.g., greater than 25 months). Psychological well-being has also been found to predict improved prognosis. Respiratory symptoms at onset, presence of FTD or *C9orf72* mutation, poor nutritional status, weight loss, poor respiratory function as evidenced by, for example, slow vital capacity (SVC) and other respiratory parameters, are associated with poorer prognosis.[151,153–156]

■ MANAGEMENT

Despite significant research efforts, there is no cure for ALS, and pharmaceutical options remain limited. Care is focused on managing symptoms and optimizing function, participation, and QOL.[2] People with ALS may receive care in a variety of health-care settings.

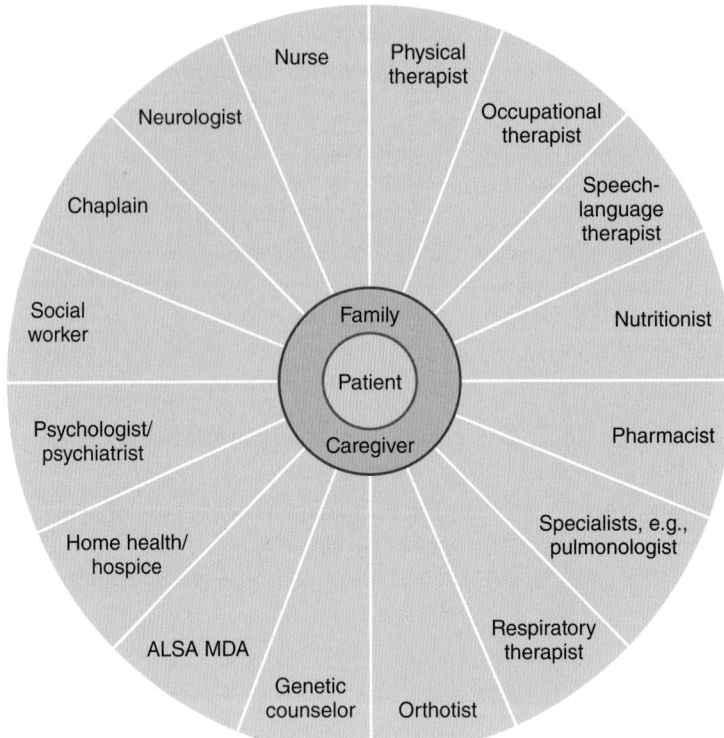

Figure 17.7 Multidisciplinary approach to the care of the individual with ALS. ALSA = Amyotrophic Lateral Sclerosis Foundation; MDA = Muscular Dystrophy Association.

Care via specialized centers or clinics with a team of health-care professionals that provide a comprehensive and multidisciplinary approach is considered the most advantageous owing to the complex and progressive nature of the disease and continually changing status (Fig. 17.7). A recent systematic review concluded that PwALS attending a multidisciplinary clinic had a significantly better survival, especially those individuals with bulbar onset, compared to PwALS attending a general neurology practice or other models of care.[157] Telemedicine and telehealth visits and monitoring via telehealth may be an alternative model or may augment multidisciplinary care clinics as these forms of care have been found to be acceptable, feasible, and satisfactory for PwALS and caregivers.[158–160]

The *Amyotrophic Lateral Sclerosis Association (ALSA)* and the *Muscular Dystrophy Association (MDA)*, both nonprofit voluntary health agencies, have developed standards for ALS clinics and centers. Clinics and centers that meet ALSA's clinical care and treatment standards regarding evidence-based multidisciplinary care, conduct ALS research, and pass a rigorous application and site visit are Certified Treatment Centers of Excellence. Clinics and centers that provide evidence-based, multidisciplinary care, similar to certified treatment centers, but that do not offer onsite research or opportunities for clinical trials participation are deemed ALS Association Recognized Treatment Centers. MDA centers that conduct ALS research and have staff with expertise in dealing with ALS earn special designations as MDA ALS Research and Clinical Centers.

Disease-Modifying Agents

Currently there are two U.S. Food and Drug Administration (FDA)-approved treatments for ALS. Riluzole (Rilutek), a glutamate inhibitor, has a standard dose of one 50 mg tablet two times a day. Although riluzole is generally well tolerated, regular monitoring of liver enzymes and blood counts and screening for nausea and fatigue are required.[161] Side effects include liver toxicity (which requires discontinuation), asthenia, nausea, vomiting, and dizziness. Evidence suggests the effects of riluzole to be modest, extending survival for 2 to 3 months.[162]

Radicava/Radicut (edaravone), a neuroprotective drug that has properties of a free radical scavenger, is delivered intravenously daily for 14 days, followed by no drug for the next 14 days. This initial course of treatment is then followed by another intravenous administration over 10 of the next 14 days, followed by another 14-day period without the drug. This cycle continues for as long as the treatment is to be administered.[163] Radicava seems to be more effective in the earlier stages of the disease, when people with ALS have less severe signs and symptoms and a greater forced vital capacity (FVC).[164] Results from two clinical trials found those who received Radicava had less decline compared to the placebo group, as measured by the ALS Functional Rating Scale-Revised (ALSFRS-R), over the short trial periods.[163,164] Reported side effects of Radicava seen in the clinical trials included contusion, gait disturbance, headache, dermatitis, eczema, respiratory issues (failure, disorder, hypoxia), glycosuria, and tinea infection.

Symptomatic Management

As noted previously, disease-modifying agents currently available are not curative and may extend survival for only a short time. Because the pathological process cannot be reversed and is progressive in nature, the context of medical management for individuals with ALS may be considered "palliative" by definition. As described by the World Health Organization, palliative care is an approach that improves the QOL of patients and their families who are facing problems associated with life-threatening illness through early identification; correct assessment and treatment of pain; and other physical, psychological, or spiritual problems.[165] Although there is no cure for ALS, it is still considered a "treatable disease." Medical and multidisciplinary health-care management and rehabilitation play an integral role in the overall comprehensive care of the PwALS.

Medical management is symptomatic and individualized and involves supportive care to address impairments as they arise. In order of decreasing prevalence, the following symptoms have been reported by individuals with ALS: fatigue (90%), muscle stiffness (84%), muscle cramps (74%), shortness of breath (66%), sleep difficulty (60%), pain (59%), anxiety (55%), depression (52%), increased saliva (52%), constipation (51%), pseudobulbar affect (38%), loss of appetite (37%), and weight loss (29%).[127]

In 2013, the American Academy of Neurology (AAN) Quality Measurement and Reporting Subcommittee undertook a literature review and evidence search of 378 recommendation statements from 20 guidelines and consensus papers,[166] available at https://www.ncbi.nlm.nih.gov/pmc/articles/PMC3863352/. Table 17.4 outlines the 11 final recommendation statements from the subcommittee. These statements were rated highest

---

Table 17.4   Amyotrophic Lateral Sclerosis Performance Measurement Set

Measure	Description
1. *Multidisciplinary Care Plan Development/Updating*	Multidisciplinary care plan should include a neurologist and at least four of the following: dentist, dietician, gastroenterologist, genetic counselor, occupational therapist, palliative care specialist, physiatrist, physical therapist, psychiatrist, psychologist, pulmonologist, respiratory therapist, social worker, specialized nurse, SLP. Plan should be updated at least once annually.
2. *Disease-Modifying Pharmacotherapy for ALS Discussion*	Riluzole should be offered.
3. *Cognitive and Behavioral Impairment Screening*	Screen for cognitive impairment at least once annually.
4. *Symptomatic Therapy Treatment Offering*	Symptomatic treatment should be offered for pseudobulbar affect, sialorrhea, and other ALS-related symptoms, if present.
5. *Respiratory Insufficiency Querying and Referral for Pulmonary Function Testing*	Query about symptoms of respiratory insufficiency (at each clinical visit). Test VC, maximum inspiratory pressure, SNP, or peak cough expiratory flow at least every 3 months.
6. *Noninvasive Ventilation Treatment for Respiratory Insufficiency Discussion*	Discuss treatment options of noninvasive respiratory support (e.g., noninvasive ventilation, assisted cough) at least once annually.
7. *Screening for Dysphagia, Weight Loss, and Impaired Nutrition*	Screen for dysphagia, weight loss, or impaired nutrition at least every 3 months.
8. *Nutritional Support Offering*	Dietary or enteral nutritional support via percutaneous endoscopy gastrostomy or radiographic-inserted gastrostomy at least once annually for those with dysphagia, weight loss, or impaired nutrition.
9. *Communication Support Referral*	Refer to a speech-language pathologist for augmentative/alternative communication evaluation at least once annually for those with dysarthria.
10. *End-of-Life Planning Assistance*	Assistance in planning for end-of-life issues, e.g., advanced directives, invasive ventilation, and hospice at least once annually.
11. *Falls Querying*	Query about falls within the past 12 months (at each clinical visit).

Data adapted from Miller 2013.[166]

ALS = amyotrophic lateral sclerosis; SLP = speech language pathologist; SNP = sniff nasal pressure.

on clinical importance, link to desired outcomes, evidence base, level of evidence, gaps in care associated with the recommendation, and validity and feasibility related to the implementation of the recommendation in practice in quality measure. They were approved by the subcommittee and other AAN committees. The report is currently being updated.

The recommendations related to symptom management, per the AAN Subcommittee and other guidelines, include the prescription of anti-cramping and anti-spasticity agents, drying agents for sialorrhea, and antidepressants; recommendations and referrals for *percutaneous endoscopic gastrostomy* tubes and ventilatory support (noninvasive ventilation, tracheostomy); and discussion of advanced care directives.[161,166] Unfortunately, evidence has determined low treatment prevalence for many ALS-related symptoms,[127] highlighting that more can and should be offered to individuals with ALS.

Sialorrhea and Pseudobulbar Affect

Management of *sialorrhea* in people with ALS and other diseases is often directed toward prescription of anticholinergic medications that decrease saliva production.[161,166] Examples include glycopyrrolate (Robinul), benztropine (Cogentin), transdermal hyoscine (scopolamine), atropine, and trihexyphenidyl hydrochloride (Artane). Side effects include constipation, difficulty urinating, dry eyes, and confusion. For individuals with associated thick mucus production, mucolytics or beta blockers, such as propranolol (Inderal) or metoprolol (Toprol), may be prescribed. Botulinum type injections into the parotid and submandibular glands and low-dose radiation have been found to be effective for PwALS with medically refractory sialorrhea.[167] Use of mechanical suction to remove oropharyngeal secretions and nonpharmacologic treatments that are used for clearing respiratory secretions (see section "Management of Respiratory Impairments") may also be useful.

For PwALS with pseudobulbar affect, tricyclic antidepressants, such as amitriptyline (Elavil), or selective serotonin reuptake inhibitors (SSRIs), such as fluvoxamine (Luvox), are often prescribed.[161,166] Nuedexta (DMQ), which contains both dextromethorphan hydrobromide (morphian family) and quinidine sulphate, is an FDA-approved medication for the treatment of labile emotionality associated with pseudobulbar affect. DMQ has been found to reduce the severity and frequency of crying and laughing behaviors and to improve bulbar function (e.g., speech, swallowing, and salivation).[167-169] Common side effects include fatigue, somnolence, dizziness, diarrhea, and nausea.

Dysphagia

Provisional Best Practices Guidelines for the Evaluation of Bulbar Dysfunction in ALS have been published.[170]

Early and aggressive nutrition intervention is recommended, as nutrition supplementation has been shown to promote weight stabilization or weight gain in PwALS, and nutrition status has been identified as a prognostic factor for survival and disease complications.[56,171] Dysphagia is addressed by a nutritionist or registered dietitian together with a speech-language pathologist (SLP). A nutritionist screens for and assesses nutritional and hydration status and needs and identifies malnutrition risk. To assist with the plan of care (POC), a nutrition-focused assessment includes oral nutritional intake and requirements; appetite, diet and weight history and change; barriers to adequate intake (e.g., ability to feed self and prepare foods, food access, chewing and swallowing function and difficulties); dietary supplement use; length of time to complete meals; and bowel changes (e.g., constipation).[172,173] The SLP's swallowing evaluation includes patient-reported outcomes, dietary intake, pulmonary function and airway defense physiological capacity, bulbar function, a dysphagia/aspiration screen, and a Videofluoroscopic Swallow Study for PwALS with dysfunction or failed screening.

Nutritionists provide counseling and diet management throughout the course of the disease. Regardless of whether poor nutritional status results from dysphagia, hypermetabolism, or inability to eat due to UE muscle weakness, there is a need for careful attention to nutritional and hydration status, in particular with individuals with impaired oral intake or arm or hand weakness limiting self-feeding.

Management of dysphagia is directed toward (1) dietary modifications, such as adapting foods textures and fluid consistencies for easier and safer swallowing; (2) compensatory strategies, maneuvers, and adaptations to promote swallowing such as tucking the chin down during swallowing or performing a clearing cough after each swallow; (3) addressing need for increased caloric requirements (e.g., recommendations for calorically dense foods or oral nutritional supplements); and (4) PwALS and caregiver education on the following topics: dietary strategies for maximizing calories and nutrients; maintaining adequate hydration; the role of proper oral hygiene, with emphasis on the association between poor oral hygiene and aspiration pneumonia in dysphagia; prescribed strategies and maneuvers, such as tucking the chin; importance of pulmonary hygiene and airway clearance; basic life-saving techniques; and the role of supplemental nutrition and hydration, including the role of percutaneous endoscopic gastrostomy (PEG).

As dysphagia and muscle weakness progress, the time required to consume a meal gradually increases owing to fatigue, increased difficulty chewing, and frequent choking. It is not uncommon for these difficulties to cause an accelerated weight loss. In these circumstances a PEG may be recommended. A PEG is a type of gastrostomy tube inserted via endoscopic surgery that creates a permanent opening into the stomach for the introduction of food. A PEG is useful for stabilizing body weight/mass and is typically offered to the PwALS and completed before the individual's VC falls below 50% of predicted at the time of the procedure.[174,175] A recent systematic review concluded that PEG is safe and probably prolongs survival in individuals who are not malnourished. Older age at onset, marked weight loss or reduced body mass index, and marked respiratory dysfunction were found to negatively influence the outcome after PEG insertion.[176] It is important for physical therapists to be aware that a PEG does not prevent the risk of aspiration.

Respiratory Impairments

Respiratory impairments place the PwALS at risk for respiratory tract infections. Important management considerations include (1) pneumococcal and yearly influenza vaccinations; (2) prevention of aspiration; and (3) effective oral and pulmonary secretion management. Supplemental oxygen is used with caution because it can suppress respiratory drive, exacerbate hypoventilation, and ultimately lead to hypercarbia and respiratory arrest.[161,166] Typically, supplemental oxygen is recommended only for individuals with concomitant pulmonary disease or as a comfort measure for those who decline ventilatory support.

Symptoms of respiratory insufficiency should be queried at each clinical visit, and VC, maximum inspiratory pressure, sniff nasal pressure (SNP), or peak cough expiratory flow testing should be conducted regularly.[166,177]

Positive-pressure noninvasive ventilation (NIV) typically is used for respiratory muscle support to decrease the work of breathing.[104,107] Guidance for optimal timing of the introduction of NIV varies, but early introduction is recommended.[178] Noninvasive ventilation has been shown to decrease symptoms of hypoventilation, decrease the rate of decline respiratory function decline, improve cognition, improve QOL, and increase survival time by several months.[179–181] Studies suggest that NIV for 4 or more hours a day has the greatest potential for long-term benefit.[179,181]

When NIV can no longer be tolerated or it is no longer effective, a decision must be made between invasive ventilation with tracheostomy via surgical intervention or hospice care to address late-stage respiratory symptoms. Owing to the emotional, social, and financial burden of invasive ventilation, PwALS and families must be carefully informed of the multiple direct and indirect costs and benefits of the intervention. Guidance for the withdrawal of ventilation at the request of the PwALS has been published by the Association for Palliative Medicine of Great Britain and Ireland.[182] Conditions for withdrawal of ventilation are discussed before or at the time of instituting invasive ventilation because the individual with ALS may become unable to communicate their wishes as the disease progresses.

Communication Impairments

Communication impairments are managed primarily by an SLP, with a focus on minimizing energy expenditure while maximizing collaborative engagement.[170] The time of diagnosis, regardless of whether speech impairments exist, is recommended for the initial SLP evaluation versus referral to an SLP as needs for augmentative and alternative communication (AAC) arise.

The SLP evaluation incudes review of relevant and related systems and functions, such as respiratory function (e.g., FVC or SVC), pseudobulbar affect, and cognition, and oral structural and motor studies, which may include video fluoroscopy to determine the degree and nature of the swallowing impairment and to assist in formulating a POC. Interventions for ALS-related speech changes may include back-up speech strategies; amplification strategies; environmental modifications (e.g., decreasing background noise); care partner training; use of a writing board for PwALS with adequate hand function; voice banking; message banking; use of a call system; and speech-generating devices.

A *palatal lift prosthesis* (partial lift, partial palatal augmentation prosthesis) may be prescribed for PwALS with hypernasality, articulation problems, a breathy voice quality or decreased loudness because of excessive air loss through the nose. The device, a dental appliance designed to attach to the existing teeth and to elevate the soft palate, is custom-made by a prosthodontist. It allows the soft palate to close around the surrounding structures such as the pharynx, making verbal communication more understandable by reducing or eliminating hypernasal speech and improving articulation.[183] The device also lowers the hard palate, which reduces tongue movement, allowing speech to be less fatiguing. Evidence related to palatal lift use for velopharangeal dysfunction in PwALS is limited to case reports and care series, with benefits including decreased hypernasality and improved articulation and intelligibility.[183]

Muscle Cramps, Spasticity, Fasciculations, and Pain

Anticonvulsant medication such as phenytoin (Dilantin) and carbamazepine (Atretol, Tegretol) may be prescribed for muscle cramps, if they are not relieved with a program of muscle stretching and adequate hydration and nutrition.[159,184] Both of these medications can cause gastrointestinal upset and rash, and carbamazepine can cause sedation. Benzodiazepines, such as diazepam (Valium), clonazepam (Klonopin), or lorazepam (Ativan) can also be prescribed for muscle cramps, and side effects may include sedation, dizziness, respiratory depression, and increased weakness. Benzodiazepines, especially diazepam, may be prescribed for spasticity, although baclofen (Lioresal) and tizanidine (Zanaflex) are more commonly used. Side effects include weakness, fatigue, sedation, and hypotension. Individuals with brisk, widespread fasciculations are generally instructed to avoid or minimize caffeine and nicotine. Lorazepam (Ativan) may be prescribed to decrease the intensity of the fasciculations.[185]

Depending on the etiology of pain, a variety of management strategies may be utilized, as, to our knowledge, there have been no pain medication trials conducted in individuals with ALS. Pain from muscle cramps or spasticity may benefit from stretching or ROM exercises. Mild pain or pain associated with joint discomfort is usually addressed with analgesics, such as acetaminophen or nonsteroidal anti-inflammatory drugs. For more severe refractory pain, opiates or opioids such as codeine, hydrocodone, or methadone may be prescribed. In the terminal stages of ALS, morphine may be administered to provide analgesia, sedation, and relief from respiratory distress.[121,161,166,185] See the Evidence Table (Table 17.5) for a recent systematic review of the prevalence of pain in people with ALS, and summary pathways for physical, psychological and spiritual pain management found at https://cdn2.assets-servd. host/mushy-parakeet/production/assets/resources/ mnd-pain-pathway-parkinsons.pdf.

Fatigue

Any reversible causes of fatigue (e.g., pain, depression, reduced caloric intake and weight loss, respiratory insufficiency, sleep disorders, a side effect of riluzole) are investigated and managed accordingly. A 2018 update of the 2014 systematic review update on the management of fatigue in ALS found four small studies each with a different intervention: (1) modafinil (a wakefulness promoting medication approved for the treatment of excessive sleepiness associated with narcolepsy); (2) inspiratory muscle training; (3) resistance exercise; and (4) repetitive transcranial magnetic stimulation (rTMS).[186] The three studies that found positive intervention effects (modafinil, inspiratory muscle training, rTMS) were of low quality. The positive effects of rTMS were short lived and no longer detected 2 weeks after cessation of treatment. The authors concluded that modafinil and inspiratory muscle training may play a role in the management of fatigue in ALS, but robust, high-quality studies of these and other interventions are needed.[186]

Anxiety and Depression

Anxiety and depression can greatly affect the QOL of PwALS and their families, as well as the ability to cope with and adapt to the progressive changes and losses of the disease. Additionally and more importantly, it has been reported that individuals with ALS are at a greater risk of suicidal behavior than the general population, in particular in the earliest stages of the disease, after diagnosis.[187] Thus, screening for mood disorders and

pharmacotherapy and psychological counseling are important management strategies for addressing the anxiety and depression that can develop. Individuals with depression may be prescribed an SSRI, such as fluoxetine (Prozac) or sertraline (Zoloft), or serotonin and norepinephrine reuptake inhibitor.[121,161,166] It is important to note that antidepressant effects may not occur for several weeks after initiation of the medications, and side effects may include agitation and insomnia. If the PwALS presents with depression and insomnia or agitation, a tricyclic antidepressant, such as amitriptyline (Elavil) or imipramine (Tofranil), is preferred.[166,185]

Benzodiazepines, such as chlordiazepoxide (Librium), clorazepate, diazepam, and flurazepam (Dalmane), may be prescribed for anxiety or for PwALS with depression and insomnia. For individuals whose respiratory status is affected, a non-benzodiazepine anxiolytic, such as buspirone (BuSpar), is preferred.[166,185]

■ FRAMEWORK FOR REHABILITATION

Interest in a rehabilitation approach for individuals with ALS has been increasing over the past decades, with an increasing number of articles published related to rehabilitation for PwALS or specific elements of physical therapy, such as exercise and falls. Physical therapy is perceived as important by people with ALS despite the functional deterioration that occurs over time.[188] As previously described, the course of ALS cannot be altered, and eventually PwALS will become dependent in essentially all aspects of mobility and self-care. However, rehabilitation programs comprised of appropriate physical therapy interventions should be designed and implemented to allow individuals to maintain independence and function for as long as possible, within the context of their goals and resources, throughout the disease and across health-care settings. Examples of general goals and outcomes for individuals with ALS can be found Box 17.1.

Consideration of the rehabilitation framework[189] elements will help guide the physical therapist in developing person-specific goals. Because of the progressive nature of ALS, it is imperative that the physical therapist not only addresses an individual's current problems but also plans ahead for future problems. A large body of evidence to help guide physical therapy decision-making is currently unavailable. As identified earlier, ALS has a progressive and deteriorating disease trajectory, with inevitable progression to disability. However, there is great variability among individuals across the disease trajectory. Staging ALS into *early,* *middle* (early-middle and late-middle), and *late* stages based on impairments, activity limitations, and participation restrictions may assist the therapist in designing appropriate and realistic interventions throughout the

Text continued on page 656

Table 17.5	Amyotrophic Lateral Sclerosis Evidence Summary

De Wit et al. (2018)[262]

Design	Systematic review of quantitative studies examining patient and informal caregiver factors related to caregiver burden. Databases used to identify relevant studies: PsycINFO, Medline (PubMed), CINAHL, EMBASE.
Level of Evidence	II
Subjects	People with ALS; informal caregivers
Intervention	*Not applicable*
Results	The review identified 25 articles that met the inclusion criteria: • High-quality evidence for relationship between caregiver burden and "behavioral impairments." • Moderate quality evidence for relationship between caregiver burden and "feelings of depression" of the caregiver and "physical functioning" of the patient. • Low-quality evidence for association between caregiver burden and caregiver factors ("feelings of anxiety," "distress," "social support," "family functioning," "age"); and patient factors ("bulbar function," "motor function," "respiratory function," "disease duration," "disinhibition," "executive functioning," "cognitive functioning," "feelings of depression," "age").
Comments	Only full-text articles; articles may have been missed. Peer-reviewed articles in English, Dutch, or German were reviewed. Quality of studies was assessed independently by two reviewers. Methodological quality scores ranged from 2–7 out of a maximum of 8 (high-quality) points, using Methodological Quality Assessment List. Grading of recommendations assessment, development, and evaluation approach used to assess overall quality of evidence for each factor (measured in at least three studies). Unable to perform meta-analysis due to heterogeneity of instruments and measures.

Hurwitz et al. (2021)[133]

Design	Systematic review of primary research studies or studies of secondary data analysis that included pain prevalence data to determine the pooled prevalence of pain in PwALS and explore the common evaluation characteristics of pain, e.g., location, intensity, type of pain. Databases used to identify relevant studies: MEDLINE, Embase (via OVID), Cochrane CENTRAL, CINAHL, AMED, PsycINFO, Scopus.
Level of Evidence	II
Subjects	People over the age of 18 years with a diagnosis of ALS.
Intervention	Not applicable
Results	Twenty-one eligible studies included 14 cross-sectional, 6 cohort, 1 case-control. • Pooled prevalence of pain across all studies was 60% (95% CI = 50%–69%), with a high degree of heterogeneity (I2 = 94%, p < .001). • 715 pain locations identified • Nine studies reporting pain location found location of pain was U/E including shoulders/extremities (41.5%); L/E including hips, groin, and extremities (33.7%); head/neck/trunk/back (24.8%). • Seven studies reporting pain intensity found that moderate ratings were reported most (78.8%, N = 1124), followed by severe ratings (17.5%, N = 250). Mild pain and very severe intensity pain were reported least (2.0%, N = 28 and 1.7%, N = 24). • Type of pain was commonly related to cramp or spasm, reported in seven studies.
Comments	Study quality assessed by one reviewer and moderated by an additional reviewer using either the Appraisal Tool for Cross-Sectional Studies or the Critical Appraisal Skills Programme Study checklist. Quality rated as adequate overall; specific issues with: sample size justification, measurement of confounders, use of valid, and standardized pain outcome measures, methodological clarity, and follow-up with participants. Variable and subjective reporting of pain characteristics between and within studies, resulting in merging of characteristics based on common elements.

(Continued)

Table 17.5	Amyotrophic Lateral Sclerosis Evidence Summary—cont'd
	Radunovic et al. (2017)[293]
Design	Systematic review (second update of a review first published in 2009) of randomized and quasi-randomized trials examining effects of mechanical ventilation on survival, functional measures of disease progression, and QOL with ALS, and adverse events related to the intervention. Databases were used to identify relevant studies: Cochrane Neuromuscular Disease Group Specialized Register, CENTRAL, EMBASE, CINAHL Plus, AMED, MEDLINE, and two registries to check for ongoing studies (ClinicalTrials.gov, World Health Organization International Clinical Trials Registry Platform). *Primary outcome: overall survival. Secondary outcomes: survival at 1 month and 6 months or longer; QOL using validated health status questionnaires, e.g., 36-Item Short Form Health Survey at 1 month and 6 months or longer; any validated functional rating scale, such as the ALSFRS or the ALSFRS-Revised or Appel scales at 1 month and 6 months or longer; the proportion of people experiencing adverse events related to mechanical ventilation.*
Level of Evidence	I
Subjects	People with a clinical diagnosis of ALS or MND, at any stage of disease and with any clinical pattern (e.g., bulbar and limb onset)
Intervention	Interventions included: • NIV • Tracheostomy-assisted ventilation Control group: no intervention or best standard care.

Results	• For the original *Cochrane Review*, review authors identified two RCTs involving 54 participants with ALS receiving NIV, but one trial published incomplete data. There were no new RCTs or quasi-RCTs at the first update. One new RCT was identified in the second update but was excluded.
	• Results were based on one study of 41 participants.
	• No adverse events reported.
	• Median survival was increased by an estimated 48 days, from 171–219 days. The survival benefit from NIV was much greater in people with ALS in whom the muscles used for speaking, chewing, and swallowing (bulbar muscles) were either unaffected or only moderately weak. Among these 20 participants, the median survival with NIV was increased by an estimated 205 days (216 days with NIV, compared to 11 days with standard care), although a sleep–related symptoms score improved.
	• Significant difference in median survival for NIV group, moderate quality evidence. Median survival was 219 days compared to 171 days with standard care.
	  • Survival benefit from NIV was significantly greater in PwALS with better bulbar function; median survival with NIV was 216 days with NIV compared to 11 days with standard care.
	  • Survival for PwALS with poor bulbar was 39 days less than the standard care group (222 vs 261 days).
	• Low-quality evidence that mechanical ventilation maintains or improves QOL.
	  • Significantly greater QOL scores in PwALS with better bulbar function, but not those PwALS with severe bulbar weakness.
	  • PwALS with poor bulbar function showed significant improvement in the Sleep Apnea Quality of Life Index, but not in the Short Form-36 Mental Component Summary score.

Comments	A thorough literature search was conducted that included: • Identification of unpublished theses • Inspection of reference lists of included studies Author(s) of included studies were contacted to obtain additional unpublished data. Quality of studies was assessed independently by four reviewers.

Table 17.5   Amyotrophic Lateral Sclerosis Evidence Summary—cont'd

Soofi et al. (2018)[294]

Design	Synthesis of qualitative evidence (qualitative metasynthesis) to answer the research question: how do PwALS perceive the potential of rehabilitation services in optimizing QOL? *Qualitative or mixed-methods studies that addressed domains or themes considered important to optimizing QOL for PwALS, published in English, were searched in seven databases: AMED, CINAHL, Embase, MEDLINE, OVID Health Star, PsycINFO, Global Health.*
Level of Evidence	II
Subjects	• Adult PwALS, 18 years and older • ALS diagnosis, any disease stage • PwALS had received rehabilitation
Intervention	• *PT, SLP, OT interventions or combination of PT, OT, SLP interventions*

Results	• Five studies included in the metasynthesis: four studies focused exclusively on PwALS, one focused on degenerative neurological conditions with specific identification of PwALS
	• Major themes identified from the studies:
	  • the concept of control
	  • adapting interventions to disease stage
	  • struggles with interventions
	  • barriers between health-care providers and patients
	• *Feeling in control was central to making life decisions related to accepting the disease, treatment options, and employment after diagnosis.*
	• *PwALS want their health-care providers to pay particular attention to their specific physical abilities and how these abilities change over the course of the disease.*
	• *A major issue identified by PwALS was the difficulty incorporating their assistive and AAC devices into their everyday lives because of access and accessibility issues, which negatively affected their QOL.*
	• PwALS and caregivers emphasized concerns regarding lack of knowledge and understanding of ALS by health-care professionals, which negatively impacted lives of PwALS.
	• *Rehabilitation interventions positively contributed to managing the goals of PwALS, especially in terms of independence and employment, which could optimize QOL.*

Comments	• None of the five included studies were conducted with the express purpose of examining rehabilitation and QOL. • Metasynthesis was guided by the ENTREQ guidelines; Sample, Phenomenon of Interest, Design, Evaluation, and Research type approach used for search strategy. • Quality of studies assessed using McMaster University's Guidelines for Qualitative Review Version 2.0 and the RF-QRA instrument. Four studies graded as RF-QRA Level 1 and one study as RF-QRA Level 2.

Jones et al. (2019)[295]

Design	Cross-sectional study. Survey tool, developed using the theory of planned behavior, examined health-care professionals' intention to provide exercise counsel to PwALS and the factors that contributed to that decision; whether mode of exercise (i.e., flexibility, strength, aerobic) influenced intentions; and differences between physicians and other health professional respondents.
Level of Evidence	III
Subjects	25 physicians and 53 non-physician health-care professional participants
Intervention	Not applicable

(Continued)

Table 17.5   Amyotrophic Lateral Sclerosis Evidence Summary—cont'd

Jones et al. (2019)[295]

Results	• Physicians (54%) and non-physician health-care professionals (64%) reported that exercise is discussed by more than 61% of PwALS. • Few reported moderate-to-strong familiarity with the ACSM guidelines for exercise with PwALS and ACSM guidelines were not typically during consultations regarding exercise. • Intentions of non-physician health professionals were strongly associated with their familiarity of the ACSM guidelines. • Clear preference for flexibility exercise for intentions over aerobic and strength training exercises, with strength training being the least preferred. • Most commonly cited potential barriers to providing exercise prescription of non-physician health-care professional participants were (1) patient tolerance, adherence, and interest and (2) lack of confidence or competence, another team member's responsibility.
Comments	• Of non-physician health-care professional participants, 23 of 53 indicated exercise prescription was within their scope of practice: physiotherapist (n = 10), occupational therapist (n = 6), nurse (n = 2), respiratory therapist (n = 2), speech language pathologist (n = 2), dietician (n = 1). • Convenience sample of voluntary respondents; response rate was 48%. • Study is subject to selection and response bias. • Generalizability to Canadian context only.

Plowman et al. (2019)[296]

Design	Randomized controlled trial. Patients were randomized to one of two groups: in-home, active EMST or Sham EMST. Primary outcome was change in MEP. Secondary outcomes: (1) voluntary cough spirometry using oral pneumotachograph; (2) swallowing function: physiological swallowing function first captured using videofluoroscopic swallowing study and evaluated as global swallowing function using Dynamic Imaging Grade of Swallowing Toxicity scale and airway safety using Penetration-Aspiration Scale (PAS); 3) daily oral intake using Functional Oral Intake Scale; 4) patient reported outcome of swallowing function using Eating Assessment Tool-10 (EAT-10); (4) FVC; 5) ALSFRS-R. Outcomes evaluated at baseline and immediately following 8 weeks of intervention.
Level of Evidence	II
Subjects	• Confirmed ALS diagnosis • FVC > 65% predicted • ALSFRS-R score > 30 • MMSE score >24 points • No allergies to barium • No tracheostomy or mechanical ventilation or diaphragmatic pacer
Intervention	*EMST group:* 8-week, at home EMST training using a handheld, one-way, spring-loaded valve trainer, set at 50% of participants' individual MEP. Training completed 5 days per week, with a single daily training session comprised of 25 targeted forced exhalations through the trainer, performed in five sets of five repetitions, with rests between each set; typical training session lasted about 20 minutes. *Sham EMST group:* Completed 8-week EMST training protocol with a trainer that looked identical to the high-physiological-load trainer, but with the internal spring removed.
Results	Main study findings: • EMST was well tolerated; adherence for completing prescribed exercises ranged between 95% and 100%. • Significantly higher increase in MEP in active EMST group compared to sham group. • Total DIGEST score and the DIGEST efficiency subscale score worsened in Sham group, but not active group. • Functional oral intake improved by 14.4% in the active group and worsened by 11.8% in the sham group. • PECF remained stable (0% change) for active EMST group and decreased in Sham group. • No significant group differences in DIGEST safety subscore, PAS score, EAT-10 score, cough spirometry, FVC, ALSFRS-R scores.

Table 17.5	Amyotrophic Lateral Sclerosis Evidence Summary—cont'd

Plowman et al. (2019)[296]

Comments	Prospective, single-center, double-blind, permuted block randomization; no formal sample size calculation. Limitations: • Small sample size from a single site

Kalron et al. (2021)[297]

Design	Randomized controlled trial. PwALS were randomized into one of two groups: combined aerobic-strengthening or flexibility training. Outcome measures included ALSFRS-R, SVC, FVC, MIP, MEP, 2-minute walk test, five-repetition sit-to-stand test, FSS, SF-36; assessed at 1 week before intervention, after 6 weeks of training, after 12 weeks of training.
Level of Evidence	II
Subjects	• Diagnosis of clinically probable, laboratory-supported probable, or definite ALS • Sporadic or familial ALS • Mild to moderate disabilities (Sinaki-Mulder stages I-II-III) • Percent predicted slow vital capacity > 40% • Ages ranging between 30 and 65 years
Intervention	Both interventions administered and supervised by a physical therapist and an exercise physiologist. *Combined aerobic and strength program* followed the ACSM Exercise Management Guidelines for Persons With Chronic Diseases and Disabilities and included 24 sessions over 12 weeks (two sessions per week), each session 50–60 minutes. Each session consisted of: (1) 20 to 30 minutes of aerobic training using recumbent cycling at 40%–60% of heart rate reserve, monitoring heart rate and oxygen saturation; (2) 10 minutes of stretching and passive ROM exercises; and (3) 20 minutes of strength training via functional exercises focusing on the large muscle groups of the trunk and U/E and L/E, e.g., squat, plank, lunge, "biceps curl, pelvic lift exercises. Aim was to perform one to two sets, 8 to 12 repetitions in each set, with rest periods as needed. *Stretching group:* provided with booklet with illustrations and brief text of basic stretching exercises of the UE and LE. Completed the stretching drill for 20 minutes, 5 times a week, for 12 weeks at home with the assistance of caregiver or family member. Adherence monitored by a self-report diary and contact by physical therapist every other week.
Results	Main study findings: • No adverse events occurred during the intervention period. • Significant differences in MEP, 2MWT, and ALSFRS-R in favor of the aerobic-strength group. • PwALS in aerobic-strength group maintained their scores, whereas a significant decrease was observed in the flexibility training group. • SF-36 subscales "physical functioning," "energy fatigue," and "well-being" were significantly higher following intervention in the aerobic-strength group compared with the stretching group.
Comments	Assessor blind, parallel group study. No formal sample size calculation; 1:1 randomization allocation, using sealed envelopes. Limitations: • Did not report adherence findings. • Small sample size (n = 28, 14 in each group) from a single site.

van Groenestijn et al. (2019)[298]

Design	Randomized controlled trial to explore the effectiveness of AET on disease-specific and HRQOL in ambulatory patients with ALS. Ambulatory PwALS were randomly assigned into one of two groups: AET + UC or UC. AET consisted of a 16-week aerobic cycling exercise program. Outcome measures included ALSAQ-40 and the MCS and PCS scores of the SF-36, with multiple secondary impairment, activity, and participation outcomes. Analysis was performed for those patients who attended ≥75% of the training sessions.

(Continued)

Table 17.5	Amyotrophic Lateral Sclerosis Evidence Summary—cont'd
	van Groenestijn et al. (2019)[298]
Level of Evidence	II
Subjects	• Age between 18 and 80 years • FVC of at least 80% • Possible, laboratory-supported probable, probable, or definite ALS (El Escorial criteria) • Life expectancy > 1 year • Ability to walk with or without walking aid (≥10 minutes) • Ability to cycle on a cycle ergometer (≥15 minutes)
Intervention	AET: Home-based training program with cycle ergometer and step board twice a week (time gradually increased from 20–35 minutes) and an individual training session once a week at a rehabilitation center or rehabilitation department of an academic hospital, supervised by specially trained intervention physiotherapists. The training session used stations including 5-minute warm-up, 30 minutes individually tailored aerobic exercises (cycle ergometer, step board, treadmill), 20 minutes muscle strengthening exercises (quadriceps, biceps, and triceps), and a 5-minute cool down. Heart rate–monitored training intensity was gradually increased from 50% (moderate) to 75% (vigorous) heart rate reserve during aerobic exercise. Training intensity for muscle strengthening gradually increased from 40%–50% of the maximum strength of different muscle groups (quadriceps, biceps, and triceps). Only muscle groups with a Medical Research Council score ≥3 were trained. Each exercise was repeated 10–15 times. Borg Ratings of Perceived Exertion Scale was also used to monitor training intensity.
Results	Main study findings: • No adverse events with AET. • No significant differences in ASLAQ-40, MCS, or PCS scores between groups.
Comments	Multicenter (five centers), assessor blinded, parallel group study. No a priori sample size calculation; 1:1 randomization allocation, using central randomization process. Limitations: • Only 10 participants completed or attended ≥75% of the training sessions.

2MWT = 2-minute walk test; ACSM = American College of Sports Medicine; AET = aerobic exercise therapy; ALS = amyotrophic lateral sclerosis; ALSFRS-R = Amyotrophic Lateral Sclerosis Functional Rating Scale—Revised; ASCM = American College of Sport Medicine; ASLAQ-40 = mental component summary; DIGEST = Dynamic Imaging Grade of Swallowing Toxicity; EAT-10 = Eating Assessment Tool-10; EMST = expiratory muscle strength training; FSS = Five Times Sit-to-Stand Test; FVC = forced vital capacity; HRQOL = generic health-related quality of life; MCS = mental component summary; MEP = maximum expiratory pressure; MIP = maximum inspiratory pressure; MMSE = Mini-Mental State Exam; MND = motor *neuron disease*; NIV = non-invasive ventilation; OT = occupational therapy; PAS = Penetration–Aspiration Scale; PCS = physical component summary; PT = physical therapy; PwALS = people with ALS; QOL = quality of life; RCT = randomized controlled trials; RF-QRA = Rosalind Franklin-Qualitative Research Appraisal; SLP = speech-language pathologist; UC = usual care; UE/LE = upper extremity/lower extremity; VC = vital capacity.

disease process, as well as anticipate the evolving needs of the individual[189] (Fig. 17.8).

In the *early* stage of the disease, ALS will manifest as a variety of signs and symptoms recognized by the individual as abnormal. The resultant impairments may or may not cause minor activity limitations and no participation restrictions are present. In the *middle* stage of ALS, the individual experiences increasing signs and symptoms, and develops an increase in the number of impairments and the severity of impairments. Minimal to moderate activity limitations will be noted and participation restrictions will develop. In the *late* stage of ALS, disease progression leads to numerous and increasingly more severe impairments. The individual becomes increasingly limited functionally owing to lack of voluntary motor control and numerous participation restrictions ensue. The individual becomes dependent in essentially all aspects of mobility and self-care, and may require mechanical ventilation to address respiratory compromise, if not already ventilated.[189]

Within this framework, impairments, activity limitations, and participation restrictions are managed through restorative, compensatory, or preventive physical therapy interventions.[138] These interventions should be tailored to the stage of the disease, keeping in mind individual variability throughout disease course (e.g., presence of cognitive impairments or respiratory signs and symptoms) and disease progression (e.g., slowly progressing

Box 17.1 Examples of General Goals and Outcomes for Individuals With ALS

Impact of Pathology/Pathophysiology Is Addressed

- Patient/client, family, and caregiver awareness and knowledge of the disease, prognosis, and POC are enhanced.
- Symptom management is addressed and enhanced.
- Changes associated with disease progression are monitored and addressed.
- Risk of secondary impairment(s) is reduced.
- Composite impairment(s) are addressed.
- Intensity of care is optimized.

Impact of Impairments Is Reduced

- Cognitive and psychosocial function are considered and addressed where possible.
- Pain is prevented, and if present, decreased.
- Respiratory impairment(s) are addressed and decreased to the extent possible.
- Dysarthria, dysphagia, and sialorrhea are considered and addressed.
- Joint integrity issues are prevented, and if present addressed.
- Motor function is addressed and enhanced to the extent possible.
- Muscle performance (strength, power, and endurance) issues are addressed and enhanced to the extent possible.
- Postural control and balance issues are addressed and enhanced to the extent possible.
- Mobility, gait, and locomotion are addressed and enhanced to the extent possible.
- Aerobic capacity is addressed and enhanced to the extent possible.
- Secondary and composite impairments are addressed and decreased to extent possible.

Ability to Perform Tasks and Activities Is Optimized and Enhanced Where Possible

- ADLs are addressed and optimized.
- Activity tolerance is addressed and optimized.
- Problem-solving and decision-making skills are enhanced.
- Safety of patient/client, family, and caregivers is increased.

Effects of Health Condition on Participation Are Addressed and Reduced to the Extent Possible

- Ability to engage in self-care and home management is optimized.
- Ability to engage in work (job/school), community, and leisure roles is optimized.
- Awareness and use of community and societal resources are improved.

Health Status Is Optimized and QOL of Patient/Client, Family, and Caregivers Is Enhanced

- Sense of well-being is enhanced.
- Stressors are reduced.
- Self-confidence and self-management skills are optimized and enhanced.
- Health, wellness, and fitness are optimized.

Patient/Client Satisfaction Is Enhanced

- Access and availability of services are acceptable to patient/client and family.
- Quality of rehabilitation services is acceptable to patient/client and family.
- Care is optimized.
- Care is coordinated with patient/client, family, caregivers, and other health-care professionals.
- Living arrangements are optimized.

QOL = quality of life.

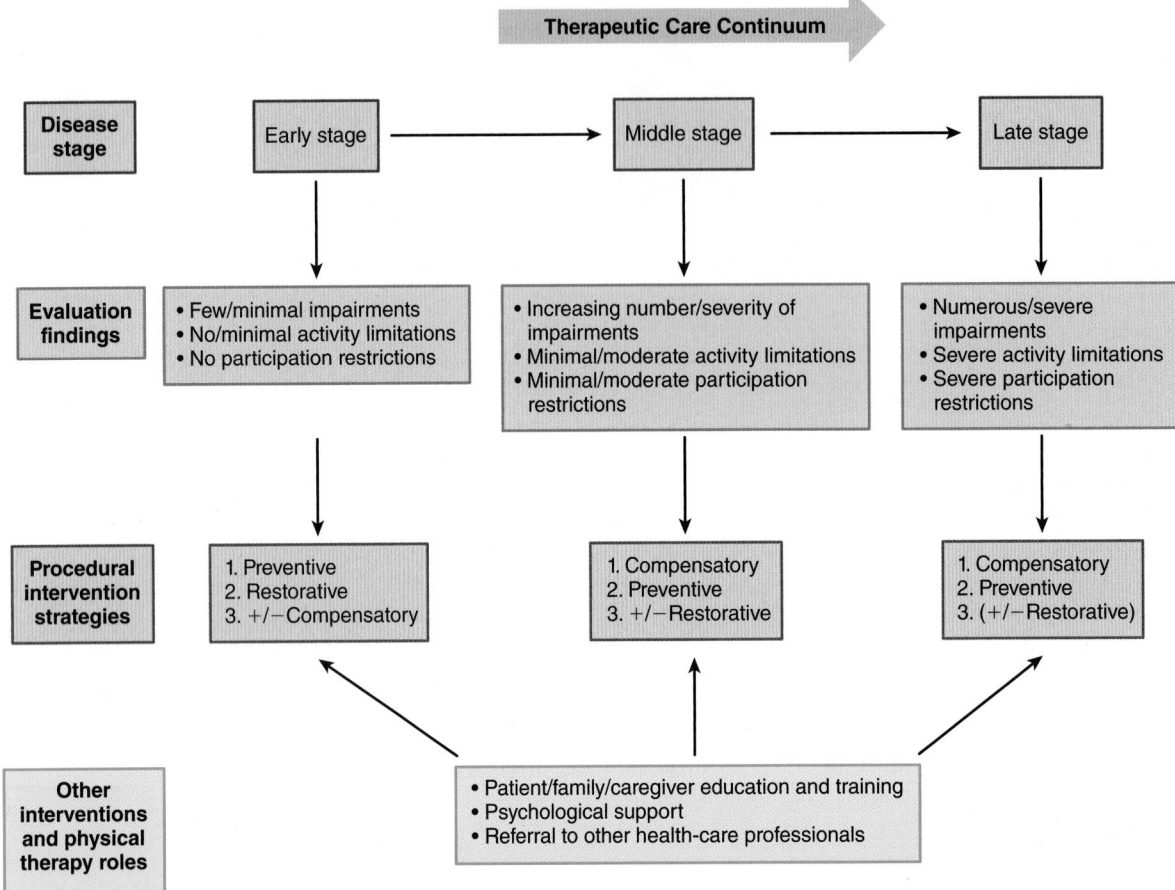

+ denotes may include; − denotes may not include

Figure 17.8 Framework for rehabilitation for individuals with ALS. *(Adapted from Dal Bello-Haas V,189 p. 116)*

versus fast progressing), and grounded in evidence-based research whenever possible. The individual's goals are paramount, and psychosocial factors that may influence decision-making, such as acceptance of the diagnosis, and social and financial resources must be considered.[189]

■ PHYSICAL THERAPY EXAMINATION

At any one time, a variety of body regions can be affected by ALS and in various combinations. Impairments may occur as a direct result of the pathology (*direct impairment*), as sequelae to the pathology (*indirect impairment*), or as the result of multiple underlying origins (*composite impairments*). Therefore, a careful and comprehensive examination is required to determine the extent of involvement as well as the impact of involvement on activity limitations and participation restrictions. With increasing evidence that ALS is a multisystem disease, the physical therapist needs to not only focus on subjective and objective assessment of the motor system, but also undertake evaluation of multiple systems (i.e., asking about pain and sensory

changes, testing for sensory system integrity, screening for cognitive impairments, and screening for extrapyramidal signs and symptoms).[134]

Elements of the examination for the individual with ALS are summarized in Box 17.2. Reexamination at regular intervals is necessary to determine the extent and rate of progression of the disease. However, at times it may be difficult to differentiate between the progressive course of the disease and the lack of impact of the interventions. In considering the tests and measures to include in a reexamination, the benefits should be carefully weighed against the psychological impact of repeating tests and measures when the PwALS is progressively deteriorating. This is especially true in the late-middle and late stage of the disease. It is important for the physical therapist to reexamine, monitor, and evaluate changes, because some medical decisions may be based on the physical therapist's findings, for example, percent predicted VC and the timing of PEG placement.

The PwALS' goals and individual psychosocial factors, rate of disease progression, extent and area of involvement, stage of the disease, and the extent of respiratory and bulbar involvement that may affect the

Box 17.2 Elements of the Examination for the Individual With Amyotrophic Lateral Sclerosis

Patient/Client History	Systems Review
• Age, sex/gender, race/ethnicity/cultural heritage, primary language, education level • Social history: cultural beliefs and behaviors, family, caregiver and other resources, social support systems • Occupation/employment/work, volunteer activities • Leisure, hobbies • Living environment: home/work barriers • Hand dominance • General health status: physical, psychological • Social/health and wellness habits (past, current) • Family history • Medical/surgical history • Current conditions/chief complaints • Medications • Medical/laboratory test results • Functional activity level, past, current • Role and social function(s), past, current	• Neurological • Musculoskeletal • Cardiovascular/pulmonary • Integumentary • Other, e.g., genitourinary, gastrointestinal, lymphatic Tests and Measures (see narrative) for: • Cognition and behavior • Psychosocial function • Pain • Muscle performance, strength, power, and endurance • Motor function • Tone and reflexes • Cranial nerve integrity • Sensation • Postural alignment and position symmetry • Postural control and balance • Gait and mobility • Respiratory function • Anthropometrics • Integument • Functional status • Environmental barriers • Fatigue

individual's ability to participate all need to be considered when structuring the initial examination. The types of data generated from the history and interview are presented in Chapter 1, Clinical Decision-Making. When collecting these data, determining what is important, relevant, and valued by the individual is key. By understanding what is most meaningful to a PwALS, the physical therapist can narrow the gap between an individual's expectations and hopes and actual experiences through realistic and appropriate interventions. For example, a young parent with ALS may inform the physical therapist their priority is caring for their children rather than maintaining employment. Thus, the initial examination would be structured around abilities and activities related to home, rather than work.

Many of the tests and measures described in this text are generally appropriate components of a comprehensive examination for an individual with ALS. However, selection is always based on specific individual need. The tests and measures frequently applicable to PwALS include examination of sensory function, muscle performance, motor function, coordination and balance, gait, functional status, the environment, respiratory function, and cognitive function (see Chapters 3 to 9, 12, and 27). The following section presents areas that typically warrant emphasis during the examination.

Aerobic Capacity

Aerobic capacity and cardiovascular–pulmonary endurance may be tested in the early stages of ALS using standardized, modified protocols to evaluate and monitor responses to aerobic conditioning.

Bulbar Function

The Center for Neurologic Study Bulbar Function Scale (CNS-BFS) is a self-administered questionnaire comprising 21 questions that assesses three domains of bulbar function: speech, swallowing, and salivation.[169,190] The CNS-BFS takes about 5 minutes to complete, and the recall period is 1 week. There are seven questions in each domain and each question is rated from 1 = does not apply to 5 = applies all the time. Internal consistency was found to be high, 0.97, test–retest reliability over a 2-week interval was 0.86, and the CNS-BFS total score was found to be highly and significantly correlated with the bulbar subscale of the ALSFRS-R ($r = -0.90$).[169,190]

Cranial Nerve Integrity

The cranial nerves commonly affected by ALS include V, VII, IX, X, and XII. Cranial nerves should be tested to determine the extent of bulbar involvement (see Chapter 5). Screening for oral motor function, phonation, and speech production can be accomplished through the interview and observation. Referral to an SLP is recommended.

Cognition

The ALS Cognitive Behavioral Screen (ALS-CBS) assesses executive function via two components: *cognitive*, which evaluates attention, concentration, working memory, fluency, and tracking using four subscales with a total score of 20; and *behavioral*, which evaluates changes in empathy, personality, judgment, language, and insight using 15 questions completed by the caregiver with scores ranging from 0 to 45.[191] Studies have found that the cognitive section differentiated individuals with cognitive impairments with 71% specificity and 85% sensitivity, and that the behavioral section predicted ALS-frontotemporal dementia (ALS-FTD) with 80% sensitivity and 88% specificity.[191,192] The utility of incorporating screening instruments into a busy ALS clinic has been documented, and it is recommended that PwALS be screened at least once annually for cognitive impairment (e.g., FTD screening, cognitive and behavioral impairment screening).[121,161,166] As cognitive impairment is often best identified through neuropsychological evaluation comprised of standardized measures and normative data, referral to a neuropsychologist may be warranted to identify specific cognitive impairments.

The Edinburgh Cognitive and Behavioural ALS Screen (ECAS) is an additional tool that incorporates short cognitive tests that have been shown to be sensitive to cognitive impairment in ALS. Executive functions, memory, language, visuospatial skills, and social cognition are assessed.[193–195] It also includes a short series of behavioral and psychosis interview questions for family or caregivers. The ECAS takes about 15 minutes to administer (score range from 0 to 136).

Environmental Barriers

The PwALS' home, work, and leisure environments should be examined for current and potential barriers, access, and safety.

Fatigue

Fatigue is very common in individuals with ALS. No ALS-specific measures exist; the *Fatigue Severity Scale*[196] has been used in clinical trials.

Functional Status

Functional mobility skills, safety, and energy expenditure are important considerations. Basic and instrumental activities of daily living and the need for adaptive equipment should be examined. The *Functional Independence Measure* (FIM)[197] and the *Schwab and England Activities of Daily Living Scale (SE)*[198] have been used

to document functional status in clinical trials. The SE is an 11-point global measure of functioning that asks the individual to report activities of daily living (ADL) function from 100% (normal) to 0% (vegetative functions only) and has been used to examine function in individuals with ALS. The ALS CNTF Treatment Study Group found the scale to have excellent test-retest reliability, to correlate well with qualitative and quantitative changes in function, and to be sensitive to changes over time.[199] See Chapter 18, Parkinson Disease.

The *ALS Functional Rating Scale (ALSFRS)*[199] and the revised version, ALSFRS-R[200] (Appendix 17.B [online]) examine the functional status of PwALS. The individual is asked to rate their function using a scale from 4 (normal function) to 0 (unable to attempt the task). The original scale, the ALSFRS, correlated positively with objective measures of UE and LE strength and was found to be valid and reliable for measuring the decline in function that results from loss of muscular strength. The ALSFRS-R was expanded to include additional respiratory items, and was found to have internal consistency and construct validity, and to have retained the properties of the original scale.[200] Telephone administration of the ALSFRS-R has also been found to be reliable.[201] Other disease-specific scales include the *Appel ALS Scale (AALS)*,[202] the *ALS Severity Scale (ALSSS)*,[203] and the *Norris Scale*.[204]

The *Rasch Overall ALS Disability Scale (ROADS)*[205] was developed using Rasch methodology, and methods in accordance with FDA 2009 Guidance for Patient Reported Outcomes (PRO). The ROADS is a 28-item, self-reported questionnaire of a broad range of disability levels. Each item is scored as 0 = unable to perform; 1 = abnormal, able to perform but with difficulty compared to before ALS symptoms; or 2 = normal, able to perform without difficulty as before ALS symptoms. Test–retest reliability for the ROADS was found to be very good (ICC = 0.97), as was construct validity. Variance of the measured construct was 58.2%, considered sufficient for unidimensionality. A 1-point change in the overall normed ROADS score was found to capture a measurable unit of disability consistent across the entire scale, and 2-point changes reflected twice the disability level compared with a 1-point change.[205]

Gait

Gait stability, safety, and endurance should be examined. Energy expenditure during gait; and alignment, fit, practicality, safety, and ease of use of orthotic and assistive devices should also be examined at regular intervals. No ALS-specific gait test or measure exists. Documentation of gait within a particular time period (e.g., within 15 seconds) or over a certain distance (e.g., 10 feet [3 meters]) has been measured in clinical trials. Gait speed, as measured during the 10-meter walk test was found to correlate with total ALSFRS-R score and ALSFRS-R gross motor subscale score in 50 consecutively enrolled people with ALS.[206] The 6-minute walk test (6MWT) has been found to demonstrate validity as a measure of walking capacity, defined as walking distance and speed, in a cross-sectional study of 186 consecutively enrolled ambulatory people with ALS—the 6MWT correlated with the 25-foot walk test, the Timed Up and Go (TUG) test, LE strength as measured by maximum voluntary isometric contraction (MVIC), total ALSFRS-R score and ALSFRS-R gross motor subscale score.[207]

Integument

In general, even in the late stage of ALS, skin integrity is rarely a problem. Skin inspection should be used to examine contact points between the body and assistive, adaptive, orthotic, protective, and supportive devices, mobility devices, and the sleeping surface. Such inspection is especially important when the PwALS' mobility becomes increasingly more dependent. If present, swelling should also be examined and monitored. Swelling of the distal limb may develop owing to lack of muscle-pumping action in a weakened extremity.

Joint Integrity, Range of Motion, and Muscle Length

Functional ROM, active, active-assisted, and passive range ROM, muscle length, and soft tissue flexibility and extensibility should be examined using standard methods.

Motor Function

Impairments in dexterity, coordination of large movement patterns, as well as gross and fine motor control, may be evident owing to spasticity and muscle weakness. Hand function and initiation, modification, and control of movement patterns should be examined.

Muscle Performance

Specific deficits of muscle strength, power and endurance, and muscle performance during functional activities should be determined. Specific deficits can be measured with manual muscle testing (MMT), isokinetic muscle strength testing, or handheld dynamometry.

In clinical trials, muscle strength has been examined as MVIC using a strain gauge tensiometer system.[208] This method eliminates muscle length and velocity as factors in testing and produces reliable, valid, interval data.[208] MVIC is considered the most direct technique for investigating motor unit loss and has been used extensively for examining muscle strength in individuals with ALS in the research context. Its range and sensitivity have been validated by natural history studies.[209] However, MVIC testing requires specialized equipment and training in its use. Test reliability of MMT and MVIC scores among uniformly trained physical therapists at several institutions has been examined.[210] Reproducibility between MMT and MVIC was found to be equivalent. Sensitivity to detect progressive muscle

strength changes in individuals with ALS favored MMT. However, six muscles were tested with MVIC and 34 muscles were tested with MMT; thus, the difference in detecting change was largely accounted for by the number of muscles sampled by MMT versus MVIC.[210]

Pain

Pain is common in individuals with ALS and should be examined subjectively and objectively, using a *visual analog scale* for example. Other outcome measures could be used, keeping in mind they have not been validated in the ALS population. For example, the Brief Pain Inventory (BPI)[211] has been utilized in studies. The BPI is comprised of pain intensity and interference of pain with daily functions questions, which are rated on a 0 to 10 scale using a recall period of 1 week. Pain location and quality descriptors are indicated on body drawings and there are questions about pain-relieving factors and the percentage of medication-related pain relief (scored on 0 to 100).[211] Pain is not necessarily a direct impairment of ALS, but rather an indirect (decreased ROM, adhesive capsulitis) or a composite impairment (joint malalignment secondary to spasticity and faulty posture). Further examination of underlying causes of pain is often required.

Postural Alignment, Control, and Balance

Static and dynamic postural alignment and body mechanics during self-care, functional mobility skills, functional activities, and work conditions and activities should be examined. Postural stability, reactive control, anticipatory control, and adaptive postural control should also be determined. See Chapter 6, Examination of Coordination and Balance for more information.

Falls in people with ALS lead to morbidity and mortality,[212] with fall-related deaths occurring in 1.7% of all PwALS.[212] Similar to other patient populations, PwALS should be queried about falls since the last visit and should be evaluated for known fall risk factors. Sanjak et al.[213] reported 37% of ambulatory individuals with ALS had decreased ability to use vestibular input and increased reliance on visual input for postural orientation to sustain equilibrium, despite relatively normal clinical balance and mobility test findings. The authors suggest these findings may be reflective of peripheral and central pathological abnormalities or ALS-related cerebellum pathology.[213]

No ALS-specific balance test or measure exists. A variety of balance status measures, originally designed for use with other patient populations, including the *Tinetti Performance Oriented Mobility Assessment* (POMA),[214] the *Berg Balance Scale*,[215] the *TUG test*,[216] and the *Functional Reach Test*,[217] can be used. Low total *Tinetti Balance Test* scores, indicating impaired balance, were found to be moderately to strongly related to LE muscle weakness and disability in individuals with

ALS.[218,219] Kloos et al.[219] suggest that the POMA is a reliable measure for individuals in the early or early-middle stages of ALS. A study of 31 individuals with ALS who underwent monthly TUG tests, Amyotrophic Lateral Sclerosis Functional Rating Scale—Revised (ALSFRS-R), FVC, MMT, and quality-of-life assessments for 6 months found that the TUG test was significantly associated with the risk of falling.[220]

Psychosocial Function

As depression and anxiety are common in individuals with ALS, screening is important and referral to a psychologist or psychiatrist for further evaluation may be indicated. The *Beck's Depression Inventory*,[221] the *Center of Epidemiologic Study Depression Scale*, the *Hospital Anxiety and Depression Scale* (HADS),[222] and the *State-Trait Anxiety Inventory*[223] have been used in clinical studies. The 12-item *Amyotrophic Lateral Sclerosis Depression Inventory* (ADI-12) is a short self-report screening questionnaire comprised of 12 items, rated on a 4-point scale, none of which refer to somatic or motor-related symptoms.[224] While the ADI-12 has been translated into Italian, the inventory has not undergone extensive or rigorous cross-cultural methodology or psychometric testing.

Quality-of-Life

QOL in individuals with ALS has been examined with generic measures, such as the *36-Item Short Form Health Survey* (SF-36),[225] the *Schedule for Evaluation of Individual Quality of Life—Direct Weighting* (SEIQoL-DW),[226] the *EuroQOL-5D* (EQ-5D),[227] and the *Sickness Impact Profile*.[228] The *World Health Organization Quality of Life BREF Scale* (WHOQOL-BREF), a shortened version of the generic 100-item WHOQOL, was recently validated in a large ALS/MND population. The WHOQOL-BREF is a self-report measure examining four domains: physical health and well-being (7 items), psychological health and well-being (6 items), social relationships (3 items), and environment (8 items).[229] Item responses are scored on a 5-point Likert scale, with higher scores indicating better QOL. A total score, and independent subscores for the Physical, Psychological, and Environmental domains can be calculated. Reliability across the domains was found to range from alpha values of 0.57 (Social) to 0.82 (Physical), and the WHOQOL-BREF domains (except social) were found to have adequate internal construct validity.[229]

A new ALS-specific preference-based (PB) health-related quality-of-life (HRQL) measure, the PB-ALS, was coproduced with PwALS and is currently available in English and French. PB HRQL measures summarize HRQL as a single score, developed using preferences to reflect a health status value and the value of that health status to the individual, along a continuum from 0.0 (death) to 1.0 (full health).[230] The PB-ALS followed the steps outlined by the FDA for the development of PRO

Measures and was developed in four phases: Phase 1, domain generation and development of item pool;[231] Phase 2, importance rating and refinement of items via cognitive debriefing;[232] Phase 3, translation into French using forward and back translation, expert committee review, and cognitive debriefing; and, Phase 4 (currently under way), development of a scoring algorithm based on the preferences of PwALS. The final version of the PB-ALS scale includes eight items: recreation and leisure, mobility, interpersonal interactions and relationships, eating and swallowing, handling objects, communicating, routine activities, and mood. The recall period is 2 weeks and there are four response options: I had no problems . . . ., I had some problems . . ., I had a lot of problems . . . ., I was unable to . . . .[232]

The *Amyotrophic Lateral Sclerosis Assessment Questionnaire (ALSAQ-40)*,[233] an ALS-specific QOL measure, contains 40 items that represent five distinct areas of health: mobility (10 items), ADL (10 items), eating and drinking (3 items), communication (7 items), and emotional functioning (10 items). The questions refer to the PwALS' condition during the past 2 weeks and responses are given on a 5-point Likert scale. The ALSAQ-40 measures health status in each domain using a summary score from 0 (best health status) to 100 (worst health status). The validity and reliability of this instrument have been examined and reported.[233,234] A 5-item subset of the ALSAQ-40, the ALSAQ-5,[235] was developed to minimize burden, with one item representing each domain of the ALSAQ-40.

The *ALS Specific Quality of Life-Short Form (ALSSQOL-SF)*,[236] is a 20-item short-form version of the original 50-item ALSSQOL-Revised questionnaire that measures overall QOL in individuals with ALS. The items address six domains and subscales: negative emotion, interaction with people and environment, intimacy, religiosity, physical symptoms, and bulbar function. Responses range from 0 = strongly disagree to 10 = strongly agree. The recall period is 1 week, and it takes only a few minutes to complete.[236]

Respiratory Function

Determination of respiratory status and function includes regular (at each clinical visit) querying about symptoms of respiratory insufficiency (dyspnea, orthopnea, excessive daytime sleepiness, insomnia, fatigue, morning headache), examination of respiratory symptoms and muscle function, breathing pattern, chest expansion, respiratory sounds, cough effectiveness, and regular pulmonary function testing. Peak cough expiratory flow is used to estimate cough effectiveness and airway clearance.[237] VC or FVC may be assessed using a handheld spirometer. Supine FVC may be a better indicator of diaphragm weakness than erect FVC, and if possible VC should be measured in standing, sitting, and lying.[155] Maximal inspiratory pressure may be useful in respiratory function monitoring because it can detect early respiratory insufficiency.[238] SNP may be effective in detecting hypercapnia and nocturnal hypoxemia; has been found to correlate well with transdiaphragmatic pressure and predict respiratory muscle function;[40,239] and, may be used for monitoring of inspiratory muscle strength, especially for those with bulbar involvement who cannot perform VC effectively because of bulbar weakness.

The Dyspnea ALS-15 (DALS-15) scale,[240] a 15-item ALS-specific self-reported questionnaire that detects and quantifies dyspena, was developed using Rasch methodology. Response options are 0 = never, 1 = occasionally, and 2 = often, and the recall period is the past 2 weeks. Individual item scores are summed to obtain an overall score ranging from 0 to 30 points. Cronbach alpha was reported as 0.88, test–retest reliability was 0.98 and minimally detectable change was 3.21 (10.87%) on the 0 to 30 scale.[240,241]

The Motor Neuron Disease Dyspnea Scale (MND-DS)[242] was developed in accordance with the FDA 2009 Guidance for Patient-Reported Outcomes. The MND-DS is comprised of three self-reported dyspnea symptoms, scored from 0 to 4: dyspnea while eating/talking, dyspnea while lying flat, and dyspnea during light activity. Total score ranges 0 = no dyspnea to 12 = severe dyspnea. While further validation studies are needed, reliability was found to be adequate, with ICC values ranging from 0.66 to 0.90, as was responsiveness to disease severity with higher MND-DS scores in individuals with more severe dyspnea.[242]

Sensation

If the PwALS complains of sensory symptoms or if sensory involvement is suspected, sensory testing should be completed, as described in Chapter 3, Examination of Sensory Function.

Tone and Reflexes

Muscle tone may be examined using the *Modified Ashworth Scale.*[243] Deep tendon and pathological reflexes should be tested to distinguish between UMN and LMN involvement. See Chapter 5: Examination of Motor Function: Motor Control and Motor Learning.

■ PHYSICAL THERAPY INTERVENTIONS

The role of the physical therapist in management of individuals with ALS and the extent of interventions provided vary depending on whether the therapist is working as a member of a team specialized in ALS care or as an independent or clinic-based therapist. Additional variables include the availability of other healthcare professionals in the practice setting and the reason the individual is seeking physical therapy (e.g., specific ALS-related issue versus a co-morbidity condition such as arthritis).

Restorative intervention is directed toward remediating or improving impairments and activity limitations. In the early and middle stages of ALS, restorative interventions are temporary at best because disease progression is expected, and permanent loss of function and disability is likely. Restorative interventions in the late stage of ALS are for the most part directed solely toward remediation of impairments that result from other systems pathology (e.g., pressure injuries, edema, pneumonia, atelectasis, adhesive capsulitis).[189]

Compensatory intervention is directed toward modifying activities, tasks, or the environment to minimize activity limitations and participation restrictions. In the early and middle stages of ALS, tasks or activities may be adapted to achieve function. As the disease progresses, increasing environmental adaptations will be necessary to maintain and promote function.[189]

In the early and early-middle stages of ALS, *preventive intervention* is directed toward minimizing potential impairments such as loss of ROM, aerobic capacity, or strength and preventing pneumonia or atelectasis, and reducing activity limitations. Beginning an early prevention program may alter impairments and maintain physical function temporarily, and may also improve well-being and decrease fatigue, as well as the secondary effects of immobility. In the late-middle and late stages, the pathology is more advanced, and mobility becomes progressively restricted. In these stages, it may be extremely difficult or impossible to prevent impairments and activity limitations that are directly related to the nervous system pathology. Thus, the role of prevention is *tertiary,* to mitigate the effects of the pathology that lead to impairments in other systems (e.g., educating caregivers about a passive ROM exercise program to prevent adhesive capsulitis in the shoulder).[189] In general, the role of the physical therapist includes the following:[134,189,244]

- Promoting independence and maximizing function throughout the stages of the disease, through restorative and compensatory interventions that address impairments, activity limitations, and participation restrictions
- Promoting health and wellness in the early and early-middle stages of the disease through restorative and preventive interventions
- Providing alternative means of carrying out functional activities with adaptive equipment and alternate methods for performing tasks and activities through compensatory interventions as the disease progresses
- Minimizing or preventing complications through preventive interventions throughout the course of the disease
- Providing education, psychological support, and recommendations for equipment and community and social resources to assist in adapting to the disease progression

Owing to the individual variability of the disease presentation, onset, course, and progression, PwALS will present with unique and different sets of problems; thus, interventions will vary. As described earlier, interventions are directed mainly toward addressing activity limitations and participation restrictions, because often the impairments causing the limitations and restrictions cannot be altered. However, in the early and early-middle stages of ALS, it may be possible to direct treatment toward the underlying CNS impairments, and perhaps postpone the onset of particular activity limitations. For example, a study of PwALS in the early stages of ALS (FVC ≥ 90% predicted and ALSFRS ≥ 30) who engaged in moderate load, moderate resistance exercises were found to have higher ALSFRS scores and SF-36 Physical Function scores compared to a matched control group who performed stretching exercises.[245] People with ALS and therapists must understand that any beneficial effects of an early prevention program will be short term and will not have an impact on the overall course of the disease. Much more research into the effectiveness of specific physical therapy and other interventions for individuals with ALS is needed.

In developing a POC, in addition to the PwALS' goals, the therapist must also consider the rate of disease progression, the extent and area of involvement, stage of the disease, respiratory and bulbar factors that may affect participation, timing of the intervention, acceptance and motivation, life support choices, availability of psychosocial support, and resources.

Some PwALS may view the need to use adaptive equipment, such as an ambulatory assistive device or wheelchair, as a definitive marker for disease progression and impending death. This may cause the PwALS to be hesitant to accept the recommended aid or device as a means of maintaining some aspect of control over the disease. The physical therapist will be required to maintain a balance between being realistic about what can be achieved and providing a sense of hope, not helplessness, when discussing intervention options. An overview of ALS disease stages and general intervention strategies is presented in Table 17.6. Common impairments and activity limitations associated with ALS and their respective interventions are described as follows.

Cervical Muscle Weakness

Progressive cervical extensor weakness will cause the head to fall forward, making eating, drinking, swallowing, seeing forward, and communicating difficult, and resulting in overstretching of the posterior musculature and soft tissues. This may cause acute pain or develop into anterior muscle tightness or chronic cervical syndrome. Some PwALS will compensate for the forward head position by increasing lordosis, as they attempt to maintain their posture during ambulation.

For mild cervical weakness, PwALS may prefer a soft foam or moldable collar to be worn during specific activities. Soft or moldable collars are lightweight, comfortable, and usually well tolerated. However, wear-induced compressibility requires that they be replaced frequently. For moderate to severe weakness, a semirigid or rigid collar are better options, as they provide firmer support. People with ALS may find these types of collars warm; may experience discomfort at points of body contact, such as the chin, mandible, sternum, or over clavicles; and may feel confined. A new cervical orthosis designed in collaboration with PwALS, the Head Up collar (previously known as the Sheffield Support Snood), is comprised of a stretchable fabric on a snood-like base on which various polypropylene supports can be attached in various configurations to adapt the support for tasks and limitations[246] (see Fig. 17.9). Several types of collars are presented in Figures 17.10 and 17.11, and the advantages and disadvantages of individual collar types are summarized in Table 17.7.

Neck weakness is often accompanied by shoulder girdle and thoracic extensor muscle weakness. Some PwALS with combined cervical and upper thoracic weakness may benefit from a cervical-thoracic orthosis. These devices provide greater support, but they are more expensive and heavier, and they may be difficult to don and doff. Some cervical collars (e.g., the Miami-J) have thoracic extensions available for when greater stability is needed. For severe or intractable neck weakness, referral to an orthotist for a custom-made device may be necessary.

In addition to wearing collars, individuals with cervical weakness may also benefit from taking frequent rest periods; using supportive seating, such as high-back chairs with neck support or recliners to allow a titled position for head, neck, and back support; using tilt-in-space or reclining wheelchairs; elevating reading material; and receiving education about good arm support for prolonged sitting, proper use of head rest when riding in a car, and ergonomic changes for workstations. It is important to note that when trunk weakness accompanies neck weakness, positioning for head support becomes more challenging.

Dysarthria and Dysphagia

In collaboration with the SLP and nutritionist, the physical therapist can play a role in managing dysarthria and dysphagia by addressing head and trunk control and sitting position. In addition, the physical therapist can reinforce the use of strategies for eating and swallowing (e.g., chin tuck), the use of prescribed communication devices, and the need for food consistency modifications. Because PwALS are at risk for aspiration, education of the individual, family, and caregiver is imperative (see section on "Respiratory Muscle Weakness").

Table 17.6 Amyotrophic Lateral Sclerosis Disease Stages and Common Intervention Strategies: Framework for Rehabilitation for Individuals With Amyotrophic Lateral Sclerosis Disease

Stage	Common Impairments and Activity Limitations§	Interventions
Early	Mild to moderate weakness in specific muscle groups Difficulty with ADL and mobility, especially toward the end of this stage [± *Pain*] [± *Dysarthria, dysphagia*] [± *Cognitive impairment*] [± *Respiratory compromise*]	**Restorative/Preventive** • Strengthening exercises* • Endurance, aerobic exercises • Active ROM, active-assisted ROM, stretching exercises • Address potential risk for secondary and composite impairment(s) • [± *Assess for VTE as needed*] **Compensatory** • Determine potential need for adaptive or assistive devices, supportive devices, orthoses • Determine potential need for ergonomic modifications of home/workplace • Energy conservation • Educate PwALS and caregiver about the disease process, energy conservation, community resources, support groups and resources
Middle	Progressive decrease in mobility throughout stage Wheelchair for long distances; increased wheelchair use toward end of stage Severe muscle weakness in some groups; mild to moderate weakness in other groups Progressive decrease in ADL abilities throughout stage ± Pain [± *Cognitive impairment*] ± *Dysarthria, dysphagia* ± *Respiratory compromise*	**Compensatory** • Support weak muscles via assistive and supportive devices, adaptive equipment, orthoses • Modifications to workplace/home, e.g., install ramp, move bedroom to first floor • Wheelchair prescription • Education of PwALS and caregivers regarding functional training **Preventive** • Active, active-assistive, and passive ROM, stretching exercises • Strengthening exercises (early middle) • Endurance, aerobic exercises (early middle) • Address potential risk for secondary and composite impairment(s) • Determine need for pressure-relieving devices (e.g., pressure-distributing mattress) • [± *Assess for VTE as needed.*]
Late	Wheelchair dependent or restricted to bed Complete dependence with ADL Severe weakness of UE, LE, neck and trunk muscles Dysarthria, dysphagia Respiratory compromise ± Pain [± *Cognitive impairment*]	**Preventive** • Passive ROM • Pulmonary care* • Hospital bed and pressure-relieving devices • Skin care, hygiene* • [± *Assess for VTE as needed*] **Compensatory** • Caregiver education regarding transfers, positioning, turning, skin care • Mechanical lift

Adapted from Dal Bello-Haas V.[189]
*May be restorative; §Amyotrophic lateral sclerosis is a heterogeneous, multisystem disease.
ADL = activities of daily living; LE = lower extremity; PwALS = person with amyotrophic lateral sclerosis; ROM = range of motion; UE = upper extremity; VTE = venous thromboembolism.

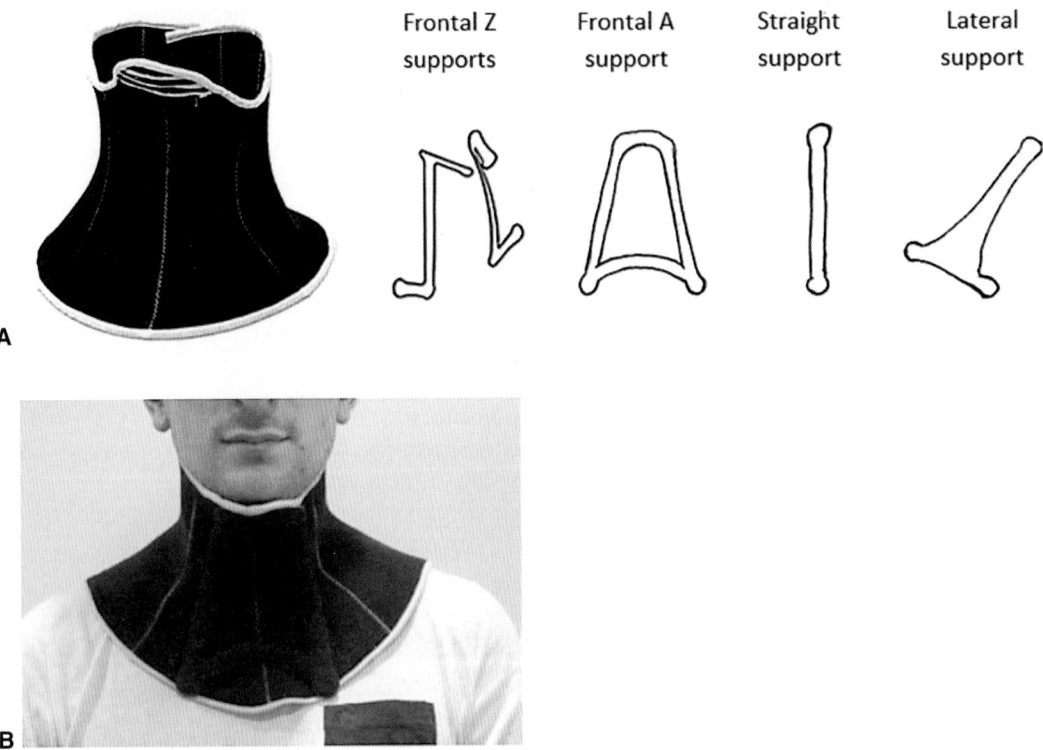

| Frontal Z supports | Frontal A support | Straight support | Lateral support |

A

B

Figure 17.9 The Head Up collar. From left to right: stretchable fabric snood, frontal Z-shape supports are placed under the jaw, frontal A-shape support is placed under the chin, straight support is placed on the back of the neck, lateral support is over the shoulder; ii. Frontal view, Head Up collar with an A-shape support. *(From Pancani S, Tindale W, Shaw PJ, Mazzà C, McDermott CJ. Efficacy of the Head Up collar in facilitating functional head movements in patients with Amyotrophic Lateral Sclerosis. Clin Biomech (Bristol, Avon). 2018; 57:114-120. doi: 10.1016/j.clinbiomech.2018.06.016; open access article distributed under the terms of the Creative Commons CC-BY license: https://creativecommons.org/licenses/by/4.0/). No changes to the original figure were made.*

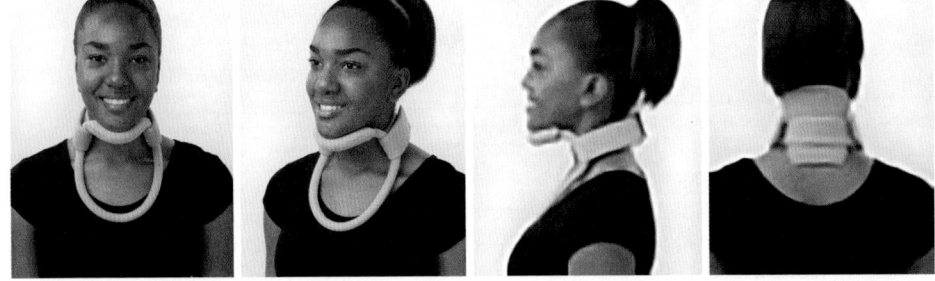

Figure 17.10 The Headmaster Collar. *(Courtesy of Symmetric Designs, Salt Spring Island, BC, Canada, V8K 2M4).*

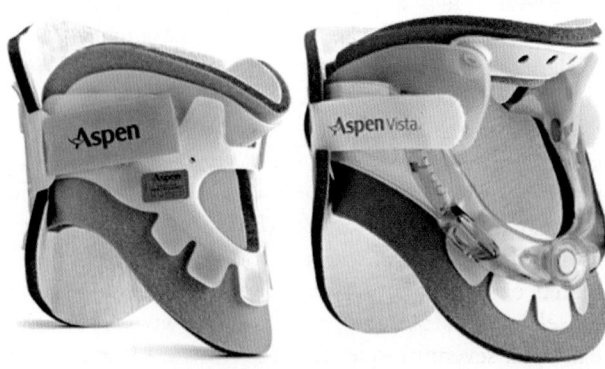

Figure 17.11 Types of anterior access collars. Aspen Vista Collar, Vista Cervical Collar. *(Courtesy of Aspen Medical Products Inc, Irvine, CA, USA, 92618).*

Table 17.7 Types of Semi-Rigid and Rigid Cervical Collars

Type	Examples	Advantages	Disadvantages
Collars without anterior neck access	Rigid plastic cervical collar	Supportive.	Stiff. Restrictive. PwALS may feel confined. May be uncomfortably warm. May increase pressure on chin, back of head, sternum. May cause difficulty with eating, drinking, swallowing.
	Head Up Collar[a]	*Provides support while allowing ROM. *Appearance and comfort acceptable to PwALS.	*May cause difficulty with eating and drinking for some PwALS. *Difficult to fit, requiring assistance to don.
Collars with anterior neck access (for tracheostomy)	Miami-J Select Collar[b] Aspen Vista Collar[c] Philadelphia Adjustable Tracheotomy Collar[d]	Padding absorbs and wicks moisture away from skin. Anterior cut away may make swallowing easier. Suitable for individuals with cervical weakness in all three planes.	PwALS may feel confined. May be uncomfortably warm.
	Headmaster Collar[e]	Open design allows for circulation of air. Lightweight. No pressure on trachea. Some PwALS consider collar more cosmetically appealing.	May put pressure on chin and sternum. Some models require custom cutting. Not adequate if rotation and lateral flexion weakness is also present.

[a]TalarMade Ltd, Derbyshire, UK.
[b]Össur, Reykjavik, Iceland.
[c]Aspen Medical Products Inc, Irvine, CA.
[d]Össur, Reykjavik, Iceland.
[e]Symmetric Designs Ltd., Salt Spring Island, BC, Canada.
PwALS = people with amyotrophic lateral sclerosis
*Sproson L, Lanfranchi V, Collins A, et al. Fit for purpose? A cross-sectional study to evaluate the acceptability and usability of HeadUp, a novel neck support collar for neurological neck weakness. *Amyotroph Lateral Scler Frontotemporal Degener* 2021;22:1-2:38-45. doi:10.1080/21678421.2020.1813308

Pain

Pain is common in people with ALS,[133,247] but it is not often addressed and is often poorly managed.[248] As noted earlier, pain is typically a secondary impairment resulting from decreased ROM, decreased mobility, and positioning issues. Shoulder, neck, and back pain are common.[249] It is imperative that pain be addressed, as pain can negatively affect QOL.[250] Pain intervention is dependent on what is causing the pain. Although the "best treatment" for pain is prevention, interventions may include modalities, ROM exercises, passive stretching, joint mobilizations, and education about proper positioning and joint support and protection. All that may be required are simple interventions such as asking individuals about comfort (pain) levels while seated or lying and making adjustments to the chair, wheelchair, or bed to provide adequate support. For example, severe muscle weakness in the LE may result in distal edema (and subsequent pain) due to lack of active muscle pump, and concomitant pain, when sitting in a wheelchair.

Shoulder Pain

Individuals with ALS may develop shoulder pain and present with capsular patterns of restriction. Pain may be caused by several factors: abnormal scapulohumeral rhythm secondary to spasticity or weakness causing imbalance that may lead to impingement, overuse of strong muscles, muscle strain, faulty resting position, glenohumeral subluxation secondary to weakness, or a fall.

A 20% incidence of adhesive capsulitis in individuals with ALS has been found.[251] Recommendations for managing the pain and decreased ROM include a protocol of an intra-articular analgesic and anti-inflammatory cocktail injection, followed by a course of aggressive ROM exercises. Some reported an acute resolution of pain, whereas others reported improvements over 2 to 3 weeks.[251]

UE Muscle Weakness

Weakness of the UEs greatly affects the PwALS' ability to carry out ADL. There is a large variety of adaptive equipment available that may help the individual prolong function for as long as possible (see section on "Activities of Daily Living").

Individuals with a painful shoulder due to subluxation may benefit from a sling, similar to those used with patients following stroke with decreased tone, although subluxation cannot be corrected completely. Splinting of the wrist or hand may be indicated to prevent contractures or to improve the PwALS' function, such as the ability to grasp.

Respiratory Muscle Weakness

Education is extremely important. People with ALS and caregivers must be taught how to balance activity and rest and educated about energy conservation techniques; and should also be educated about signs and symptoms of aspiration; positioning to avoid aspiration, such as upper cervical spine flexion during eating; causes and signs of respiratory infection; and strategies for managing oral secretions (use of oral suction device) or choking episodes (Heimlich maneuver). Specific breathing exercises and positioning to optimize ventilation/perfusion matching may also be incorporated, although their effectiveness in ALS has not been determined.

A 2019 systematic review found three studies comparing respiratory muscle training versus sham training in PwALS. The authors concluded the evidence did not demonstrate any clinically meaningful effect on physical functioning or QOL and there was uncertainty whether the intervention caused adverse effects.[252]

Clinical and research interest in cough augmentation techniques for individuals with ALS has been increasing. Airway clearance techniques may be necessary when conditions that cause secretion retention, such as pneumonia or atelectasis, arise. To compensate for a weakened cough, the PwALS and caregiver may be instructed in the use of manually assisted coughing techniques or the use of a mechanical insufflation–exsufflation (MI-E) device (cough assist device) to facilitate clearance of respiratory and oral secretions.

The MI-E device is designed to inflate the lung with positive pressure and assist cough with negative pressure through the flip of a switch. A positive-pressure breath of 30 to 50 cm H_2O over a 1- to 3-second period via an oral–nasal mask or tracheal airway is provided. The airway pressure is then reversed abruptly to −30 to −50 cm H_2O and maintained for 2 to 3 seconds. A peak expiratory cough flow (PECF) within normal range is achieved, thereby assisting with the clearance of secretions.[239] Studies of cough flows and pressures during cough augmentation have found that manual assistance increased flow 11% in those with bulbar ALS and 13% in those with nonbulbar ALS. MI-E increased flow by 26% in those with bulbar ALS and 28% in those with nonbulbar ALS. The greatest improvements were in those individuals with the weakest coughs.[239] The effectiveness of MI-E has not been demonstrated in people ALS, but case reports have described the benefits from regular use of a mechanical insufflation device.[253,254] A comparison study of MI-E versus breath-stacking found no statistically significant differences, which the authors attributed to under-powering and multiple confounders.[255]

The lung volume recruitment (LVR) technique (breath stacking, deep lung insufflation) may also be used to facilitate secretion clearance. LVR involves the administration of a series of stacked breaths using a resuscitator bag, which expands the lungs to a volume greater than spontaneous inspiratory capacity. LVR allows for the initiation of a cough from a higher lung volume. Thus, the greater respiratory system elastic recoil pressure generates a greater cough flow. LVR has been shown to increase peak cough flow in people with various NMDs and ALS.[256,257]

In people with NMD with respiratory muscle weakness, reduced tidal volumes, and decreased sighing and cough effectiveness leads to reduced compliance ("stiffening") of the lungs and chest wall over time, further contributing to respiratory insufficiency.[228] It has been proposed that in this context, the regular use of LVR can be viewed as an ROM exercise for the respiratory system to maintain normal compliance of the system and possibly delay the onset of ventilatory failure.[239]

Kaminska et al.[257] examined LVR in people with NMD, including eight individuals with ALS. The authors reported that after 3 months of regular LVR use, there was high acceptability and willingness to use LVR, and that there was a significant increase in lung inspiratory capacity-FVC difference, even though FVC declined (total subject analysis). Interestingly, adherence to LVR was highest in the participants with ALS.

High-frequency chest wall oscillation (HF-CWO) has garnered some interest in its applicability to the ALS population. HF-CWO is an external non-invasive modality that transmits high-frequency oscillatory pressures through the chest wall, thereby mobilizing secretions from the small peripheral airways and enhancing secretion clearance and gas exchange. HF-CWO has been effectively used in patient populations in which secretion retention and hypersecretion are issues (e.g., cystic fibrosis). A study comparing 19 PwALS who used HF-CWO to 16 who were not treated found that after 6 months, those using the device had significantly less breathlessness. In addition, those users with an FVC between 40% and 70% predicted had significantly less mean decrease in FVC and less breathlessness and fatigue.[258]

LE Muscle Weakness and Gait Impairments*

Orthoses may be recommended to improve function by offering support to weakened muscles and the joints they surround, decrease the stress on remaining functioning or compensatory muscles, conserve energy, or minimize local or general muscle fatigue. Controlling knee impairments can often be achieved through an ankle–foot orthosis (AFO); as such, addressing the ankle should be considered first. It is also important to consider the weight of the orthosis, as PwALS will have energy expenditure issues, and it may be more fatiguing to ambulate with a heavy orthosis than to ambulate without the impairment being corrected. For this reason, a knee-ankle-foot orthosis is not recommended.

Deciding between a commercially manufactured versus a custom-made orthosis is certainly dependent on the individual's resources, but the rate of disease progression should also be considered. For an individual with rapidly progressive ALS and who is likely to use the orthosis for a limited time, a commercially manufactured orthosis may suffice. Solid AFOs are a good choice for PwALS who have medial/lateral instability of the ankle with quadriceps weakness. The fixed-ankle position, combined with the quadriceps weakness, may make it difficult for sit-to-stand transfers, climbing stairs, and negotiating inclines. Hinged AFOs allow dorsiflexion and may be appropriate for the PwALS with adequate knee extensor strength and mild ankle strength loss. For more information on orthotics, see Chapter 30.

The type of ambulatory assistive device prescribed is dependent on the degree of proximal muscle strength or instability; function of the UEs; the pattern, extent, and rate of disease progression; acceptance by the PwALS; and financial constraints. Again, weight of the device is an important factor to consider in decision-making, while also considering which device will ensure optimal function and safety. Wheeled walkers, which do not require the individual to lift the device, are usually recommended. In general, PwALS are rarely prescribed crutches. If crutches are warranted, Loftstrand (Canadian) crutches are preferrable.

Activities of Daily Living*

A large variety of adaptive equipment is available to assist individuals with muscle weakness to perform everyday tasks. However, the benefits and effectiveness of adaptive equipment for people with ALS have not been evaluated systematically. No one type of device is suitable for every PwALS or for every stage of the disease. Reimbursement for the equipment is variable, and although a piece of adaptive equipment can help the individual maintain independence, limited financial resources may prevent recommending or purchasing the item. For example, in the early stages of ALS a universal cuff with a pocket for writing or feeding utensils may be beneficial. As the disease progresses and proximal shoulder weakness increases, a mobile arm support may be incorporated to allow the individual to maintain independence in eating. In the late stage of ALS when the individual is dependent on the caregiver for eating, a long straw and straw holder may be recommended to assist the caregiver with the activity. Examples of common adaptive equipment that may be beneficial for performing ADL are presented in Table 17.8.

Decreased Mobility*

Individuals with LE weakness may have difficulty with sit-to-stand or car transfers. Simple interventions include placing a firm cushion 2 to 3 in. (5 to 7.6 cm) thick under the buttocks in the chair or elevating the chair by placing the legs in prefabricated blocks. Self-powered lifting cushions are relatively inexpensive and

Table 17.8	Common Types of Adaptive Equipment
Feeding and eating	Foam tubing to increase the size of utensil handles; utensils and cups with modified handles or holders; long-levered jar opener; plate guard; serrated or rocker knife; wrist splint/adapted cuff (for holding tools and instruments); mobile arm support; Dycem
Self-care and bathing	Bathing benches; bathtub seats; shower commode; handheld shower head; grab bars; raised toilet seat; long-handled sponge; electric toothbrush or shaver; strap-fitted hairbrushes
Dressing	Zipper pulls or hooks; button hooks; long-handled shoehorn; hook and loop clothing closures; elastic shoelaces
Writing and reading	Foam tubing to increase the size of the pen or pencil; triangular pencil grip; pen holders; book holders; automatic page turner; adjustable angle table
Other	Key holders; doorknob adapters; lamp extension switch; personal alarm system; switch-operated environmental controls; speaker phone with automatic dialing; telephone holder; use of telecommunication devices for the deaf

*See https://www.youralsguide.com/ for photos of and videos about typical assistive, adaptative and other devices.

portable, but the individual needs adequate trunk control and balance to use the device safely. Upholstered reclining chairs with powered seat lifts may also be recommended but are more expensive. All these interventions increase the biomechanical advantage and make it easier for the PwALS to rise from a sitting position.

Caregivers will need to be educated regarding assisting the PwALS with transitional movements. Transfer boards may be used for transfers once the individual is unable to stand, either alone if the person has adequate arm strength and good sitting balance or the caregiver can be instructed in how to assist the individual. Other useful devices are transfer belts and swivel cushions or seats. Transfer belts ease the burden of the transfer for the caregiver and prevent potential pulling on the individual's UEs. Swivel cushions are lightweight, cushioned seats that swivel in both directions and make getting in and out of a car easier.

Once an individual cannot perform transfers, even with the assistance of a caregiver, a hydraulic or mechanical lift is required. Commonly recommended lifts devices include the Easy Pivot (Rand-Scot Inc., Fort Collins, CO), and the Hoyer Lift (Sunrise Medical, Longmont, CO). Use of an electric hospital bed may facilitate bed mobility and transfers both for the PwALS and caregiver, and, depending on resources, home modifications and automobile adaptations may also be considered.

Chair glides or stairway lifts can be suggested for those individuals who live in multilevel homes, but who cannot or should not climb stairs (see Chapter 9, Examination and Modification of the Environment). These lifts are measured and custom-made for individual staircases and are very expensive. Insurance companies usually do not reimburse for stairway lifts, but some medical supply companies offer "rent-to-own" options. In addition, local ALSA or MDA chapters may have lifts that have been recycled.

At some point as the disease progresses, the extent of muscle weakness or the energy requirements for ambulation will necessitate wheelchair use for mobility. In the early or early-middle stage of ALS a manual wheelchair, preferably lightweight, may be used for traveling long distances as an energy conservation technique. This wheelchair should be rented on a short-term basis or loaned from a local ALSA or MDA chapter or other source, because most insurance companies will reimburse for only one wheelchair purchase. As the disease progresses, a power wheelchair system tailored to the individual's current needs and potential future needs will be necessary. Numerous customized wheelchair features and options are available that can assist the individual in maintaining a maximum level of independence and comfort (see Chapter 32: Seating and Wheeled Mobility). A referral to a wheelchair and seating clinic may be the best option owing to the numerous, specialized, and evolving needs of the individual with ALS.

Trail et al.[259] surveyed 42 PwALS and moderate disability, as documented on the AALS, about the wheelchair features they found most beneficial. Sixty-one percent reported that their wheelchairs allowed them to maintain their previous activity levels. In order of priority, manual wheelchair users cited a lightweight frame, small turning radius, high reclining back, and supports for the head, trunk, and extremities as most desirable. Undesirable features included low, sling, nonreclining back; nonmotorized; static, nonadjustable leg rests; heaviness or large size; and nonremovable armrests. Desirable features for PwALS who used powered wheelchairs included independent mobility, maneuverability, overall comfort, and tilt-in-space/recline features. Undesirable features included low, nonreclining back, heaviness, or large size; uncomfortable seat; nonadjustable leg rests; and general discomfort.[259]

Although power scooters may be suitable for an individual with adequate UE and trunk strength in the earlier stages of ALS, the vehicle becomes limiting as the disease progresses and should not be prescribed. If the person with ALS has already been reimbursed for a scooter, most insurance companies will not pay for a power wheelchair, because the scooter is considered a power mobility device. If a scooter is to be recommended at all, the individual should rent or borrow the device for short-term use.

It is important for the physical therapist to recognize that PwALS with reduced mobility are at risk for venous thromboembolism (VTE). Leg-onset disease, increased age, LE muscle weakness, and progressive respiratory failure in PwALS are additional risk factors for VTE.[260] Physical therapists should consider VTE as a possible cause of new LE swelling and pain, as anticoagulation per standard VTE guidelines will be required.

Muscle Cramps and Spasticity

Muscle cramps may be alleviated with massage and a stretching program. Cold can temporarily decrease spasticity. Physical therapists can perform and instruct caregivers in slow prolonged stretches and passive ROM exercises to address spasticity. In addition, postural and positioning techniques can be incorporated to decrease spasticity and splinting may be necessary to prevent contractures. A published Cochrane review identified one randomized, controlled study that found PwALS who engaged in a 15-min, twice-daily, moderate intensity exercise had decreased spasticity, as measured by the *Modified Ashworth Scale,* compared to a control group who engaged in usual daily activities.[243]

Psychosocial Issues

A diagnosis of ALS is devastating for both the individual and family–caregiver unit. Because of the progressive nature of the disease, impairments readily lead to activity limitations and participation restrictions, which may affect QOL. The emotional responses of the person experiencing the disease, family members, and individuals caring for the individual are multifaceted and may fluctuate throughout the stages of the disease. Much is lost when living with a terminal, progressive disease: physical health and abilities, body image, work and family roles, identity, family and social networks, lifestyle, independence, control, hope, meaning, and the anticipated future.[261] The physical therapist must be able to recognize the PwALS' ability to cope and adapt, and their psychological reactions, level of acceptance, and willingness and ability to integrate therapeutic recommendations. It is also imperative that the physical therapist be able to differentiate between normal reactionary grief to losses or a change in physical function and the presence of clinical anxiety and depression, and refer the individual to the appropriate health-care team member, when necessary.[244]

When pervasive, anxiety and depressive symptoms need to be treated with pyschopharmacological medications, because left untreated these psychosocial impairments can adversely affect an individual's ability to adapt, cope, and participate in the POC. Depression may also lead to suicide. In addition, distress, anxiety and depression may also be prevalent among family members or caregivers.[262,263]

■ EXERCISE AND ALS

There is a high incidence of muscle weakness in PwALS and interest in the effects of exercise has significantly increased.[134] Often therapeutic exercise programs for PwALS comprise ROM and stretching exercises only. Despite the lack of research evidence, some discourage exercise because of fear of overuse weakness and believe that no exercise other than everyday activities is indicated. Systematic reviews of exercise in individuals with a variety of NMDs have found that exercise does provide benefits (e.g., improvements in aerobic and functional capacity, muscle strength, QOL, and well-being).[264–268] While some individuals with particular NMD's experienced musculoskeletal pain, swelling, and fatigue with exercise, overall tolerability of exercise training was high and serious adverse events were not reported.

When designing an exercise program for a PwALS, the physical therapist must consider the balance between overuse weakness and fatigue and disuse atrophy. Some animal studies have reported an inhibitory effect on sprouting in partially denervated muscle with neuromuscular activity,[269,270] whereas other studies have reported no effect[271,272] or promotion of sprouting or reinnervation with activity.[273,274] ALS animal model studies found that endurance exercise training at moderate intensities slowed disease progression;[275–277] while high-endurance exercise training had detrimental effects on male mice only.[278] Swimming-induced benefits including sustained motor function and increased the lifespan of ALS mice, and induced relative maintenance of the fast phenotype in fast-twitch muscles in the animals.[279]

Disuse Atrophy

A marked reduction in activity level secondary to ALS can lead to cardiovascular deconditioning and disuse weakness beyond the amount caused by the disease itself. Reduced physical activity, particularly if prolonged, reduces function of the neuromuscular system, in addition to the skeletal and other organ systems. With insufficient activity, disuse atrophy develops when muscle contractions are less than 20% of the total tension a muscle is capable of producing. As contractile proteins are lost, the muscle weakness progresses at a rate of 3% per day.[280] Strength loss through inactivity and disuse can significantly debilitate individuals with ALS, making them highly susceptible to deconditioning, and muscle and joint tightness leading to contractures and pain.

Overuse Damage

The potential for inducing overwork damage in individuals with ALS through excessive exercise is a common concern. Highly repetitive, high intensity, heavy resistance and eccentric exercise may cause muscle inflammation and damage, inability of skeletal muscle to repair itself, and prolonged loss of muscle strength in weakened, denervated muscle.[281–283] The effect of these types of exercises in PwALS has not been studied.

Sanjak et al.[131] found that individuals with ALS demonstrate abnormal physiologic and metabolic responses to single bouts of exercise. Oxygen consumption during submaximal exercise was increased in individuals with ALS compared to controls, and VO_{2max} and work capacity were decreased. In addition, it was found that several metabolic substrates of plasma and muscle compartments did not increase to the same level as untrained control subjects, indicating that the availability of substrate for energy production is affected.[131]

In individuals with ALS, the safe range for therapeutic exercise narrows, and the degree to which the range narrows is dependent on individual and disease heterogeneity, the extent of disease involvement and the rate of disease progression (Fig 17.12). It is important to note up to 50% of the motor neurons innervating a muscle may be lost prior to weakness or atrophy becoming clinically significant.[255] The remaining motor units will respond to training, and these motor units must work harder to handle a given amount of exercise stress.[271] A weak or denervated muscle may be more susceptible to overwork and ADL alone may cause impaired muscles to act as though in training. Exercise at intensities that would typically lead to improvements in "normal" muscles may actually cause overwork damage.

Prescribing Exercise for People With ALS

The physical therapist needs to be prepared for two common questions: *Can I exercise?* and *What exercises can I do?*

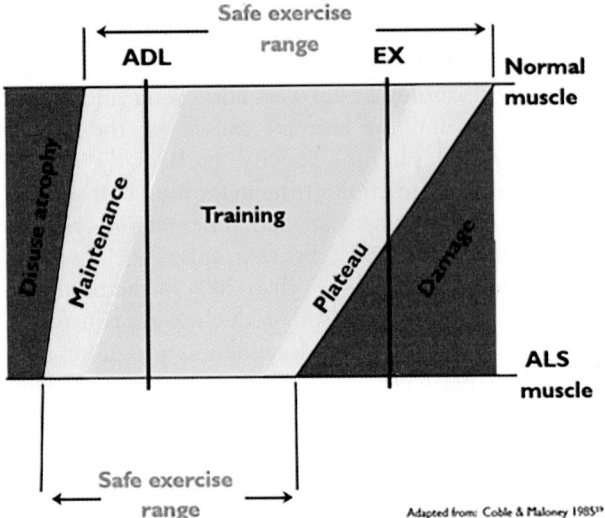

Figure 17.12 Exercise should be considered along a continuum: from disuse to maintenance and upper limit plateau, and if extreme, overwork (damage). With destroyed or lost motor units, the safe training range is decreased or narrowed depending on the extent of disease, the rate of progression, and individual and disease variability. The range continues to narrow as the disease progresses. Exercise is safe when the activity is sufficient to prevent disuse atrophy and less than the amount causing overwork damage. Within this window, effective training can occur. *Note*: As impaired muscles are already functioning close to maximal limits, activities of daily living alone may cause them to act as though in "training." As such, exercise that would result in improvement for normal muscles may actually cause overwork damage in impaired muscles. *Adapted from Coble, NO, and Mahoney, FP.280.*

When prescribed appropriately, exercise for PwALS may be beneficial, especially in the earlier stages of the disease or in those individuals with slowly progressive disease. Special attention should be paid to developing an exercise program for PwALS—physical therapists should err on the side of caution by prescribing exercise training at moderate to low intensities. Exercise may not improve the strength of muscles already weakened by ALS, particularly those below grade 3. Adverse events such as overuse weakness are less likely to occur in muscles with a MMT grade of 3 (fair) or greater out of 5 (normal). General active ROM and stretching of affected joints, resistive strengthening exercises with low to moderate weights, and aerobic activities, such as swimming, walking, and bicycling, at submaximal levels, may be prescribed to address therapeutic goals. See Box 17.3 for general considerations to assist in decision-making. The reader is referred to Dal Bello-Haas and Krivickas[284] for recommendations for prescribing exercise that consider physical therapy assessment findings,

the rehabilitation framework,[138] the nature and course of ALS, and the evidence.

The type and intensity of the exercise program should be carefully monitored and adjusted by the physical therapist to prevent excessive fatigue, while at the same time promoting optimal use of intact muscle groups. Individuals should be advised not to carry out any activities to the point of extreme fatigue, and should keep track of *symptoms of overuse*, such as the inability to perform daily activities following exercise due to exhaustion, increased weakness or pain, increased fasciculations, or increased muscle cramping. They may also be advised to exercise for several brief periods throughout the day, with sufficient rest in between.

While the evidence base related to exercise in individuals with ALS is increasing, studies are limited by: small samples sizes, high drop-out rates, variable study quality, lack of specific details on exercise interventions and training intensities, and heterogeneity of exercise interventions and outcomes.[285-287] Two early case studies demonstrated positive effects of specific strengthening and endurance exercises.[288,289] The effects of strengthening, aerobic, or combined strengthening and aerobic exercise in individuals with ALS have been evaluated with "larger samples." Studies have reported positive effects and adverse events in the exercise group were not evident across studies, suggesting safely and appropriately prescribed exercise may be beneficial and may not be harmful (e.g., no serious adverse events, does not hasten disease progression). However, definitive effectiveness of exercise for PwALS remains unclear and additional high-quality RCTs with larger sample sizes are needed. Some recent exercise studies for PwALS are presented in Table 17.5, the evidence summary table.

■ PATIENT/CLIENT-RELATED INSTRUCTION

A diagnosis of ALS is devastating for individuals and their families. They are faced with continual and multiple changes and losses, and eventual death. Assisting individuals and their family and caregivers to accept the impact of the disease is an important role for the physical therapist, and providing psychological support and opportunities for expression of feelings, frustrations, and concerns is imperative. Collaborating with and educating the PwALS, family, and caregivers in an open and encouraging environment may empower PwALS in their efforts to cope with their disease, foster a sense of purpose and self-efficacy, and enhance the overall effectiveness of the intervention by increasing adherence with recommendations.

Patient/client and family/caregiver education is integral throughout all stages of the disease. In addition to education topics discussed throughout this chapter, the

Box 17.3   Exercise Prescription for People With Amyotrophic Lateral Sclerosis: General Considerations and Principles

- An individualized approach is key.
- Decision-making considerations include:
  - disease stage
  - goals for PwALS
  - the wide variability in clinical presentation
  - disease progression overall and variability in disease progression
  - the type and amount of exercise that is warranted and safe to meet goals
  - balancing preventing disuse atrophy and causing overuse weakness
  - presence of cognitive and executive function impairments
  - extent of respiratory system involvement
- ROM and stretching exercises are typically accepted modes of exercise for PwALS.
- Aerobic/endurance and strengthening exercises can be effective only when a sufficient number of motor units are still functioning:
  - should be prescribed as soon as possible after diagnosis
  - more appropriate for PwALS in early or early-middle stage of ALS
  - more appropriate for PwALS with more slowly progressive disease
- Safe aerobic/endurance and strengthening exercise prescription may include:
  - Resistance exercises of unaffected muscles and possibly affected muscles with strength of at least grade 3, preferably above, using a low to moderate load and intensity
  - Aerobic activities, e.g., swimming, walking, and bicycling at submaximal levels, e.g., 50% and 65% of heart rate reserve
  - intermittent exercise with repetitive exercise–rest periods
- Educate PwALS about not engaging in exercise activities to the point of extreme fatigue and about signs and symptoms of overuse, e.g., inability to perform ADL post-exercise because of exhaustion or pain; decreased muscle force that gradually recovers; increased or excessive muscle cramping, soreness, fatigue, or fasciculations.
- Educate PwALS regarding self-monitoring and use of an exercise log to record the exercise sessions and adverse effects for the physical therapist to review.
- Principles apply to other modes of exercise, e.g., balance training.

ADL = activities of daily living; PwALS = Persons with amyotrophic lateral sclerosis; ROM = range of motion.

broad scope of education topics can include, but is not limited to, the following:

- Providing accurate, factual information about the disease process and clinical manifestations and their significance in overall medical and physical therapy management
  - Give only as much information as the PwALS, family, and caregivers need; information should be provided in a manner appropriate to their understanding.
- Instructing PwALS, family members, and caregivers regarding interventions that can be carried out independently such as monitoring the effects and side effects of medications, use of assistive devices and adaptive equipment, and preventing secondary impairments and complications. See https://www.youralsguide.com/overview.html for photographs and descriptions of the various types of assistive devices and adaptive equipment that may be prescribed and of benefit for people with ALS, as well as information about equipment funding.

- Advising the PwALS about methods to promote general health
  - Instruction regarding energy conservation, balancing rest and activity, and relaxation techniques may be beneficial in assisting the PwALS to cope with the daily constraints of the disease.
- Counseling regarding care and life decisions if the individual asks about these issues
- Referring PwALS to support groups or psychological counseling
- Providing information on health and available community, social, and support services

The ALSA and the MDA are two national voluntary organizations that provide many functions and programs for individuals with ALS and their families and caregivers, including the provision of written and video educational materials, local education programs, patient/client and caregiver support groups, equipment loan programs, respite programs, transportation programs, advocacy programs, and ALS Awareness Programs. Individuals and families can contact the ALSA and MDA for information and can explore available resources on the websites:

Amyotrophic Lateral Sclerosis Association (national office)
1300 Wilson Boulevard, Suite 600
Arlington, VA 22209
www.alsa.org
Care Services/Referral Resources: (800) 782-4747; alsinfo@alsa-national.org*
　　*Note: see https://www.als.org/contact-us for additional telephone numbers and emails depending on service required, as well as link to *Contact a Local Chapter*

Muscular Dystrophy Association—USA (national office)
161 N. Clark, Suite 3550
Chicago, Illinois 60601
800-572-1717
Email: ResourceCenter@mdausa.org
https://www.mda.org/

In addition, there are numerous international organizations whose websites provide various resources, including information about ALS, information about clinical trials, evidence-based reviews and practice guidelines, and publications about living with ALS. Appendix 17.C (online) includes web-based resources for clinicians, families, and PwALS.

SUMMARY

ALS, the most common and devastatingly fatal MND among adults, causes a progressive increase in the number and severity of impairments, activity limitations, and participation restrictions. Other than a small percentage of cases, etiology for the most part is unknown, and it is hypothesized that multiple mechanisms may be responsible for the disease. Although there is no cure for ALS and its course cannot be altered, it should be considered a "treatable disease." Medical management is primarily symptomatic, and a team approach to care is considered optimal. Rehabilitation management is focused on maximizing function and promoting independence to the highest level possible and ensuring optimal QOL throughout the course of the disease and across health-care settings.

The physical therapist plays an integral role in designing and implementing therapeutic interventions for individuals with ALS that will allow them to maintain independence and function for as long as possible. The selection of interventions, grounded in evidence-based research whenever possible, is based on the stage and progression of the disease and may be restorative, compensatory, or preventive. These interventions should take into consideration the individual's goals and psychosocial factors that may affect decision-making, such as the individual's acceptance of the diagnosis and the individual's social and financial resources. Because of the progressive nature of ALS, the physical therapist must not only address the PwALS' current problems but also plan for future needs.

Acknowledgments

Sincerest thanks to Katelyn Madigan, research assistant, for her editorial support, and Peggy Ingels-Allred for her thoughtful and critical review of earlier editions of this chapter.

Questions for Review

1. What are the differences between familial and nonfamilial ALS?

2. What genes are most commonly associated with ALS?

3. Why would it be important for physical therapists to know the results of genetic testing, e.g., the specific gene (mutation).

4. Compare and contrast the King's staging system and the MiToS staging system.

5. A) Describe the clinical manifestations of ALS. B) Differentiate among impairments associated with upper and lower motor neuron pathology, bulbar pathology, and respiratory system pathology. C) What cognitive, rare, indirect, composite, and other impairments might you see in an individual with ALS?

6. What medical examination procedures are used to help support the diagnosis of ALS?

7. A) Describe the disease course of ALS. B) What factors have a relationship to improved prognosis?

8. Considering the variety of impairments associated with ALS, what factors does a physical therapist need to consider when deciding on which tests and measures should be included in a comprehensive examination?

9. Differentiate *restorative, compensatory,* and *preventive* interventions.

10. When designing an exercise program for a PwALS, what factors need to be considered?

11. What information should be considered and included when developing a plan for a PwALS and family education following the diagnosis of ALS?

CASE STUDY

Mr. AB is 48-year-old male with ALS. Mr. AB has recently undergone genetic testing and is awaiting results. Mr. AB reports neck pain and fatigue that increases by the end of the workday. Pain is 1–2/10 in the morning and increases to 5–6/10 by the end of the day. About 8 months ago, Mr. AB noticed that his "balance seemed off" when walking quickly to cross the street. Mr. AB reports difficulty with opening packages for meal preparation, opening food containers he brings for lunch, and unwrapping sandwiches.

PAST MEDICAL HISTORY
Sprain R ankle 13 years ago playing rugby.

SOCIAL HISTORY
Mr. AB has been married for 20 years. Mrs. AB works full-time as a kindergarten teacher. The ABs have two daughters who are attending university in another state. Mr. AB lives in a two-bedroom condominium, with no stairs to access the building or his home.

Mr. AB takes the bus to work. The bus stop is across the street and about 300 meters from Mr. AB's office building. There are four steps, with a railing on the right, up to the front door of the building.

Mr. AB has a sedentary occupation and has not been physically active on a regular basis since he stopped playing rugby 13 years ago.

FAMILY HISTORY
Mr. AB's mother died of FTD at the age of 53 years.

OCCUPATION
Mr. AB is a data entry clerk for a school board.

MEDICATIONS
Riluzole two times a day.

DIAGNOSTIC TESTS
Electromyographic studies showed (1) low compound motor action potentials in all extremities; (2) normal sensory nerve conduction; (3) fibrillations and fasciculations in all extremities; and (4) widespread neurogenic changes in motor unit action potentials, abnormal recruitment patterns in the distal leg musculature, and mild changes in the UEs.

PHYSICAL EXAMINATION FINDINGS
- Height = 168 cm; Weight = 70 kg
- Observation: Mild wasting of the right calf muscles; moderate wasting of interossei muscle regions bilaterally.
- Posture: Slight forward head posture; Mr. AB sits slumped in the chair.
- Speech: Slow speech; mild hypernasality.
- ROM: Within normal limits for all joints, except the L ankle. He lacks 5° of L dorsiflexion.
- Strength: Bilateral L/E strength graded as 5/5, except for the hip flexor group, R and L = 4/5; and the L ankle dorsiflexors (3+/5). Shoulder muscle strength graded as 4+/5 R and L for all muscle groups; elbow muscle strength graded as 5/5 R and L for all groups. Neck muscle strength graded as flexion 4+/5, extension 4-/5, R and L rotation 4-/5, R and L side flexion 4+/5
- Hand strength: R = 92 lb; L = 84 lb (handheld dynamometer).

(Continued)

CASE STUDY—cont'd

- Pinch strength: R-tip = 13 lb; lateral = 18 lb; L-tip = 12 lb; lateral = 19 lb (see following for normative data on grip and pinch strength). *Note:* Tip pinch is thumb tip to index fingertip; Lateral pinch is pad of thumb to pad of second and third finger. Pinch strength measures obtained using a pinch gauge.

Grip and Pinch Strength Values (Pounds) for Men 45 to 49 (n = 28)

	Hand	Mean	SD	SE	Low	High
Grip	R	109.7	23.0	4.3	65	155
	L	100.8	21.7	4.3	58	160
Tip	R	18.7	4.9	0.92	12	30
	L	17.6	4.1	0.77	12	28
Palmar	R	24.0	3.3	0.63	19	33
	L	23.7	3.8	0.71	18	33
Lateral (Key)	R	25.8	3.9	0.73	19	35
	L	24.8	4.4	0.84	19	42

From Mathiowetz, V, et al. Grip and pinch strength: normative data for adults. *Arch Phys Med Rehabil.* 66:69,1984.

- Tone: 1+ for L calf (Modified Ashworth spasticity score).
- Reflexes: A clonic jaw reflex is evident; hyperreflexia in both UEs; hyporeflexia R L/E; hyperreflexia L L/E; positive Babinski reflex bilaterally.
- Gait: Independent of assistive devices; positive for slight L foot equinus during heel strike and hip hiking during swing phase; 6MWT distance = 499 m.

    Predicted distance equation:
    6MWT Distance = (7.57 * height) − (5.02 * age) − (1.76 * weight) − 309.

From: Enright PL, Sherrill DL. Reference equations for the six-minute walk in healthy adults. *Am J Respir Crit Care Med.* 1998;158:1384–1387.

- Balance: Tinetti Performance Oriented Mobility Assessment (POMA)[214] findings below

    1. **Sitting Balance**
        Leans or slides in chair   = 0
        Steady, safe   = 1
    2. **Arises**
        Unable without help   = 0
        Able, uses arms to help   = 1
        Able without using arms   = 2
    3. **Attempts to Arise**
        Unable without help   = 0
        Able, requires > one attempt   = 1
        Able to rise, one attempt   = 2
    4. **Immediate Standing Balance** (first 5 seconds)
        Unsteady (swaggers, moves feet, trunk sway)   = 0
        Steady but uses walker or other support   = 1
        Steady without walker or other support   = 2
    5. **Standing Balance**
        Unsteady   = 0
        Steady but wide stance (medial heels > 4 inches) apart and uses cane or
        other support   = 1
        Narrow stance without support   = 2

CASE STUDY—cont'd

6. **Nudged** (subject at maximum position with feet as close together as possible, examiner pushes lightly on subject's sternum with palm of hand three times)
   Begins to fall   = 0
   Staggers, grabs, catches self   = 1
   Steady   = 2
7. **Eyes Closed** (at maximum position of item 6)
   Unsteady   = 0
   Steady   = 1
8. **Turing 360 Degrees**
   Discontinuous steps   = 0
   Continuous steps   = 1
   Unsteady (grabs, staggers)   = 0
   Steady   = 1
9. **Sitting Down**
   Unsafe (misjudged distance, falls into chair)   = 0
   Uses arms or not a smooth motion   = 1
   Safe, smooth motion   = 2

   BALANCE SCORE: 13/16

10. **Initiation of Gait** (immediately after told to "go")
    Any hesitancy or multiple attempts to start   = 0
    No hesitancy   = 1
11. **Step Length and Height**
    Right swing foot
    Does not pass left stance foot with step   = 0
    Passes left stance foot   = 1
    Right foot does not clear floor completely   = 0
    Right foot completely clears floor   = 1
    Left swing foot
    Does not pass right stance foot with step   = 0
    Passes right stance foot   = 1
    Left foot does not clear floor completely   = 0
    Left foot completely clears floor   = 1
12. **Step Symmetry**
    Right and left step length not equal (estimate)   = 0
    Right and left step length appear equal   = 1
13. **Step Continuity**
    Stopping or discontinuity between steps   = 0
    Steps appear continuous   = 1
14. **Path** (estimated in relation to floor tiles, 12-inch diameter; observe excursion of 1 foot over about 10 ft. of the course)
    Marked deviation   = 0
    Mild/moderate deviation or uses walking aid   = 1
    Straight without walking aid   = 2
15. **Trunk**
    Marked sway or uses walking aid   = 0
    No sway but flexion of knees or back or spreads arms out while walking = 1
    No sway, no flexion, no use of arms, and no use of walking aid   = 2
16. **Walking Stance**
    Heels apart   = 0
    Heels almost touching while walking   = 1

    GAIT SCORE = 8/12

TOTAL SCORE (Gait + Balance) = 21/28
(<19, high fall risk; 19–24, medium fall risk; 25–28, low fall risk)

(Continued)

CASE STUDY—cont'd

- Respiratory: VC and SNiP are within normal limits.
- Functional status: ALSFRS-R (see Appendix 17.B [online]) scores below:

ALSFRS-R[200] Scores	
Item	Score
Speech	3
Salivation	4
Swallowing	4
Handwriting (pre-ALS dominant hand)	3
Cutting food and handling utensils (patients without gastrostomy)	3
Dressing and hygiene	3
Turning in bed; adjusting bed clothes	4
Walking	3
Climbing stairs	3
Dyspnea	4
Orthopnea	4
Respiratory insufficiency	4

GUIDING QUESTIONS FOR CASE STUDY

1. In what stage is Mr. AB, according to the framework for rehabilitation? MiToS staging? King's Staging?
2. What gene (mutation) would you not be surprised to see in Mr. AB's medical record once the genetic testing results have been finalized?
3. Identify Mr. AB's direct, indirect, or composite impairments.
4. What impact do the impairments have on Mr. AB's ability to function (i.e., activity limitations)?
5. Why was the Tinetti Performance Oriented Mobility Assessment chosen for balance testing?
6. What is the significance of the 6MWT distance and the POMA findings?
7. What additional tests, measurements, and assessments should be conducted? What consultations should be recommended?
8. At present, what are the initial key areas of education that should be addressed?
9. Identify the general elements of a physical therapy POC for Mr. AB.

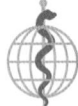 For additional resources, including answers to the questions for review, new immersive cases, case study guiding questions, references, and more, please visit **https://www.fadavis.com/product/physical -rehabilitation-fulk-8**. You may also quickly find the resources by entering this title's four-digit ISBN, 4691, in the search field at **http://fadavis.com** and logging in at the prompt.

Parkinson Disease

Tara L. McIsaac, PT, PhD
Edward W. Bezkor, PT, DPT, OCS, MTC, CAFS

Chapter 18

LEARNING OBJECTIVES

1. Describe the etiology, pathophysiology, clinical manifestations, and sequelae of Parkinson disease.

2. Identify and describe the examination procedures used to evaluate people with Parkinson disease to establish a diagnosis, prognosis, and plan of care.

3. Describe the role of the physical therapist in assisting a person with Parkinson disease in terms of direct interventions to maximize function, and in education to client, family/caregiver, community program instructors, and health-care team to optimize outcomes and participation.

4. Describe appropriate elements of the exercise prescription for individuals with Parkinson disease.

5. Identify the neuropsychological effects and social impact of Parkinson disease and describe appropriate interventions to maximize function, participation, and quality of life.

6. Analyze and interpret patient data, formulate realistic goals and outcomes, and develop a plan of care when presented with a clinical case study.

CHAPTER OUTLINE

INCIDENCE *679*
ETIOLOGY *680*
  Parkinson Disease *680*
  Secondary Parkinsonism *680*
  Parkinson-Plus Syndromes *681*
PATHOPHYSIOLOGY *681*
STAGES AND MODELS OF BRAIN PATHOLOGY *683*
DISEASE COURSE *683*
  Hoehn and Yahr Classification of Disability Scale *683*
  Movement Disorders Society Unified Parkinson Disease Rating Scale *683*
SYMPTOMS *684*
  Motor Symptoms *684*
  Nonmotor Symptoms *687*
MEDICAL DIAGNOSIS *691*
MEDICAL MANAGEMENT *691*
  Pharmacological Management *691*
  Nutritional Management *695*
  Deep Brain Stimulation *695*
FRAMEWORK FOR REHABILITATION *695*
  Rehabilitation Care Paths and Delivery *696*

PHYSICAL THERAPY EXAMINATION AND EVALUATION *697*
  Patient/Client History *697*
  Systems Review *698*
  Tests and Measures *698*
  Global Health Measures *698*
  Goals and Expected Outcomes *707*
PHYSICAL THERAPY INTERVENTION *708*
  Motor Learning Strategies *708*
  Exercise Training *709*
  Functional Training *711*
  Balance Training *712*
  Locomotor Training *715*
  Motor-Cognitive Dual-Task Training *716*
  Aerobic Exercise *719*
  Community-Based Exercise Prescription and Home Exercise Programs *719*
ADAPTIVE AND SUPPORTIVE DEVICES *720*
PSYCHOSOCIAL ISSUES *721*
PATIENT, FAMILY, AND CAREGIVER EDUCATION *721*
SUMMARY *722*

Parkinson disease (PD) is a progressive disorder of the central nervous system (CNS) with both motor and nonmotor symptoms. Motor symptoms include the *cardinal features* of *bradykinesia, tremor, rigidity,* and *postural instability.* Nonmotor symptoms (NMSs) may precede the onset of motor symptoms by an average of 10 years. These early premotor *(prodromal)* symptoms most commonly include constipation, rapid eye movement (REM) sleep behavior disorder, depression, anxiety, loss of sense of smell (anosmia), and orthostatic hypotension. Other NMSs include excessive daytime sleepiness, fatigue (a sense of exhaustion rather than sleepiness), pain, altered bladder function, erectile dysfunction, excessive saliva, integumentary changes, difficulty speaking and swallowing, apathy, and cognitive problems (reduced concentration and attention, slowed thinking, confusion, and in some cases dementia). Onset is insidious with a slow rate of progression. Disruptions in daily functions, roles, and activities are common in individuals with PD.[1]

■ INCIDENCE

PD is the second most common neurodegenerative disorder (the first is Alzheimer disease [AD]), and it affects an estimated 1 million Americans and 7 to 10 million people worldwide. The incidence increases by 5 to 10 times from the sixth to the ninth decades of life, ranging from 5 to over 35 in 100,000 new cases annually. The prevalence also increases from under 1% in people aged 45 to 54 years to 4% of men and 2% of women aged 85 years and older. Prevalence is expected to more than double by the year 2040. The average age of onset is 60 years with only 4% to 10% of patients diagnosed before the age of 50 years. This early-onset PD, often called young-onset PD (YOPD), is classified as beginning between 21 and 50 years of age, and juvenile-onset PD affects individuals less than 21 years of age. Men are affected 1.2 to 1.5 times more frequently than women, but this varies across the globe.[2,3]

■ ETIOLOGY

Parkinson disease, or *idiopathic parkinsonism,* is a generic term used to describe a group of neurologic disorders with PD-like movement problems (rigidity, slowness, tremor) and disturbances in the dopamine systems of basal ganglia (BG). Both genetic and environmental influences have been identified. Less common are *atypical parkinsonisms* (Parkinson-plus syndromes), which include other neurodegenerative disorders that mimic PD in some respects (multiple systems atrophy, progressive supranuclear palsy). *Secondary parkinsonism* results from a number of different identifiable causes, including viruses, toxins, drugs, and tumors (Box 18.1).[2]

Parkinson Disease

PD was first described as "the shaking palsy" by James Parkinson in 1817,[4] and the term refers to a clinical syndrome with a range of causes and clinical presentations. Two clinical subgroups (motor phenotypes) have been identified. One group includes individuals whose dominant symptoms include postural instability and gait disturbances *(postural instability gait disorder [PIGD] phenotype).* Another group includes individuals with tremor as the main feature *(tremor-dominant [TD] phenotype).* Patients who are tremor dominant typically demonstrate fewer problems with bradykinesia or postural instability, have lower prevalence of NMSs, including lower risk of developing dementia, and are less likely to have the known genetic mutations associated with PD.[5]

Genetic forms of PD represent less than 10% of cases overall. In a small number of families, several gene mutations have been identified (e.g., *SNCA, PRKN, PINK1, LRRK2, DJ-1,* and *GBA,* among others). Genes have been grouped into two categories: (1) causal genes, which actually produce the disease and (2) associated genes that do not cause PD but increase the risk of developing it.[1]

Secondary Parkinsonism
Postencephalitic Parkinsonism

The influenza epidemics of encephalitis lethargica that occurred from 1917 to 1926 affected large numbers of individuals. The onset of parkinsonian symptoms typically occurred after many years, giving rise to the theory that a slow virus infected the brain. Moving case histories are portrayed in the book *Awakenings* by Oliver Sacks.[6] With the 2019 onset of the global pandemic from

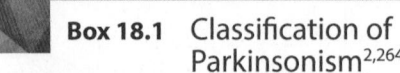

Box 18.1   Classification of Parkinsonism[2,264]

Idiopathic Parkinson Disease

Late-onset (older than 50 years; generally sporadic)
Early-onset (younger than 50 years; often familial)

• Young-onset (older than 21 years)
• Juvenile (younger than 21 years)

Parkinsonism Due to Identifiable Causes

Drug-induced: anti-dopaminergics used as neuroleptics and for gastrointestinal symptoms (e.g., aripiprazole, valproate, olanzapine, lithium, risperidone, quetiapine)
Hemiparkinsonism, hemiatrophy
Hydrocephalus (e.g., normal pressure hydrocephalus)
Hypoxia
Infectious (e.g., postencephalitic)
Metabolic
• Wilson disease
• Hepatocerebral degeneration
• Hallervorden-Spatz disease
• Hypoparathyroidism
Toxins (e.g., carbon monoxide, manganese, methylphenyltetrahydropyridine [MPTP])
Trauma
Tumors of basal ganglia
Vascular disease (multi-infarct)

Parkinsonism in Other Neurodegenerative Disorders

Cortical–basal ganglionic degeneration
Disorders with prominent and often early dementia:
• Diffuse cortical Lewy body disease
• Alzheimer disease with parkinsonism
• Frontotemporal dementia
Disorders with cerebellar/autonomic/pyramidal manifestation:
• Multiple-system atrophy
• Sporadic olivopontocerebellar atrophy
• Shy-Drager syndrome
• Striatonigral degeneration
• Machado-Joseph disease
Parkinsonism–dementia–amyotrophic lateral sclerosis complex of Guam
Progressive pallidal atrophy
Progressive supranuclear palsy

infection with the severe acute respiratory syndrome coronavirus (SARS-CoV)-2 and the resulting coronavirus disease 2019 (COVID-19), there are too few data as of this writing to know the long-term implications of COVID-19-related postencephalic parkinsonism.[7]

Toxic Parkinsonism

Parkinsonian symptoms can occur in individuals exposed to certain environmental toxins, including pesticides (e.g., paraquat, rotenone, permethrin, beta-HCH, maneb, Agent Orange) and industrial chemicals (e.g., manganese, carbon disulfide, carbon monoxide, cyanide, methanol). The most common of these toxins is manganese, which represents a serious occupational hazard to many miners from prolonged exposure.[8] Severe and permanent parkinsonism has been inadvertently produced in individuals who injected a synthetic heroin containing the chemical MPTP (1-methyl-4-phenyl-1,2,3,6- tetra/hydropyridine).[9] It is important to note that simple exposure is never enough to cause the disease.

Drug-Induced Parkinsonism

A variety of drugs can produce extrapyramidal dysfunction that mimics the signs of PD. These drugs are thought to interfere with dopaminergic modulation. They include (1) *typical neuroleptic drugs* such as chlorpromazine, haloperidol, and thioridazine; (2) *atypical neuroleptics* such as olanzapine and risperidone; (3) *anti-dopaminergics* such as reserpine and metoclopramide; (4) *calcium channel blockers* such as diltiazem and verapamil; and (5) *antiepileptics* such as valproate; among many others. High doses of these medications are particularly problematic in older adults. Withdrawal of these agents usually reverses the symptoms within a few weeks, although in some cases the effects can persist and may be related to subclinical PD.[10]

Parkinsonism can be caused in rare cases by metabolic conditions, including disorders of calcium metabolism that result in BG calcification. These include hypothyroidism, hyperparathyroidism, hypoparathyroidism, and Wilson disease.[2]

Parkinson-Plus Syndromes

Parkinson-plus syndromes are a group of neurodegenerative diseases that affect the substantia nigra and produce parkinsonian symptoms along with other neurological signs. These diseases include cortical–basal ganglionic degeneration (CBGD); progressive supranuclear palsy; multiple system atrophy syndromes (striatonigral degeneration [SND], Shy-Drager syndrome, sporadic olivopontocerebellar atrophy [OPCA], and motor neuron disease–parkinsonism). In addition, parkinsonian symptoms can be exhibited in patients with multi-infarct vascular disease; dementia syndromes (AD, diffuse Lewy body disease [DLBD], and frontotemporal dementia [FTD]); normal pressure hydrocephalus; Creutzfeldt-Jakob disease; Wilson disease (WD); and juvenile Huntington disease. Many of these conditions are rare and affect relatively small numbers of individuals. Early in their course, these diseases may present with rigidity and bradykinesia indistinguishable from PD. However, other diagnostic symptoms eventually appear (e.g., cognitive impairment in AD). Another diagnostic feature is that Parkinson-plus syndromes typically do not show measurable improvement from the administration of medications such as levodopa therapy (termed the *apomorphine test*).[11]

■ PATHOPHYSIOLOGY

The BG are a network of subcortical nuclei consisting of the *caudate nucleus,* the *putamen,* the *globus pallidus,* and the *subthalamic nucleus* along with the *substantia nigra.* The caudate and the putamen together are called the *striatum* (Fig. 18.1). The BG engages several parallel circuits or loops *(basal ganglia-thalamocortical loops),* including nonmotor loops. The *direct motor loop* through the BG consists of signals transmitted from the cortex to putamen to globus pallidus, to

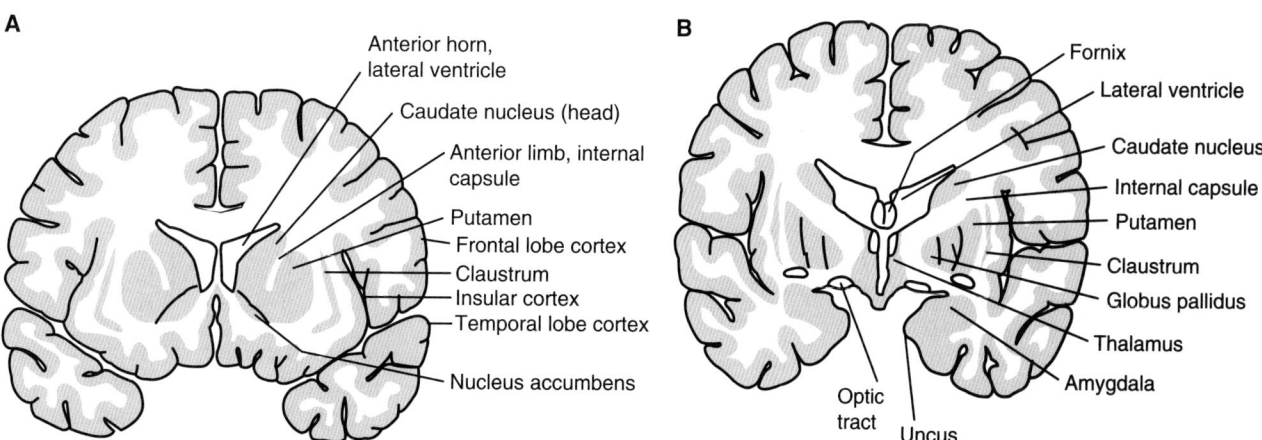

Figure 18.1 The major structures of the basal ganglia. (A) Coronal section through the rostral part of the frontal lobe showing the relation of the caudate nucleus, putamen, and nucleus accumbens to the surrounding telencephalic structures. (B) Coronal section through the caudal part of the front lobe showing the location of the lentiform nucleus lateral to, and the body of the caudate nucleus dorsal to, the diencephalon.

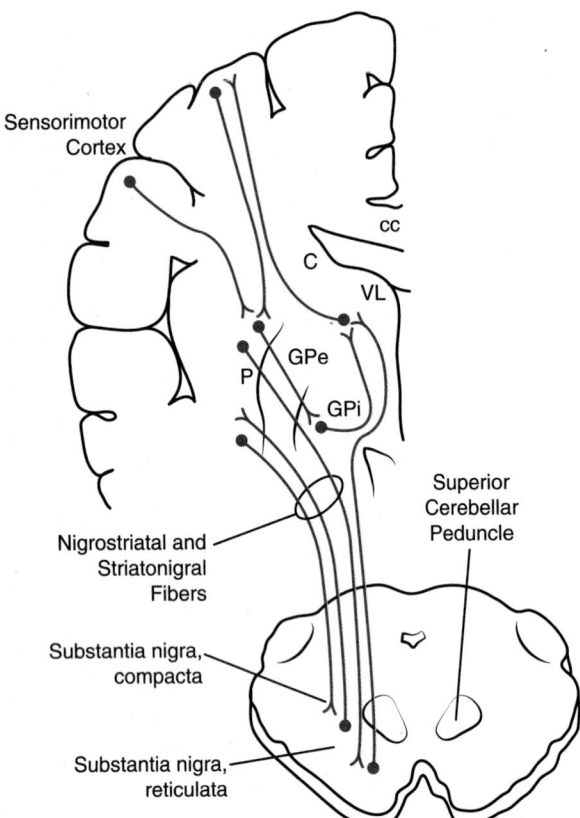

Figure 18.2 The direct loop through the putamen and the connections of the striatum with the substantia nigra pars compacta. The striatonigral fibers represented in this diagram arise in the putamen. However, most striatonigral fibers arise from the caudate. C = caudate nucleus; cc = corpus callosum; GPe = globus pallidus pars externa; GPi = glogus pallidus pars interna; P = putamen; VL = ventral lateral nucleus of the thalamus.

the substantia nigra that produce *dopamine* and (2) the presence of abnormal *alpha-synuclein,* cytoplasmic inclusions (misfolded proteins that clump) called *Lewy bodies,* that increase in quantity as the disease progresses and propagate from cell to cell through the *neural connectome.* Substantial neurodegeneration occurs from this spreading pathogenic alpha-synuclein in PD before the onset of motor symptoms and clinical signs (called *prodromal* period). Loss of the melanin-containing neurons produces characteristic changes in depigmentation in the substantia nigra with a characteristic pallor. Numerous other brain regions of people with PD show structural and functional changes, including impaired modulation of other neurotransmitters (acetylcholine, serotonin, noradrenaline, glutamate, and GABA).[13] Alpha-synuclein inclusions are seen very early in the disease in the *pedunculopontine nucleus* (PPN) and *nucleus basalis of Meynert* that release acetylcholine (ACh), and the *locus coeruleus* that releases noradrenaline.[14–16]

ventrolateral (VL) nucleus of the thalamus, and back to cortex (supplementary motor area [SMA]) (Fig. 18.2). This VL–SMA connection is excitatory and facilitates discharge of cells in the SMA. The BG thus serves to activate the cortex via a positive-feedback loop and assists in the initiation of voluntary movement. Inhibition of the thalamus by the BG is thought to underlie the hypokinesia seen in PD. An *indirect loop* through the BG involves the subthalamic nucleus, the globus pallidus interna, and substantia nigra pars reticulata to the superior colliculus and midbrain tegmentum (Fig. 18.3). This indirect loop serves to decrease thalamocortical activation. The BG projection to the superior colliculus assists in regulation of saccadic eye movements. The BG projection to the reticular formation assists in the regulation of trunk and limb musculature (via extrapyramidal pathways), sleep and wakefulness, and arousal. Other circuits in the BG are involved with memory and cognitive functions.[12]

PD is characterized by (1) degeneration of dopaminergic neurons in the BG in the pars compacta of

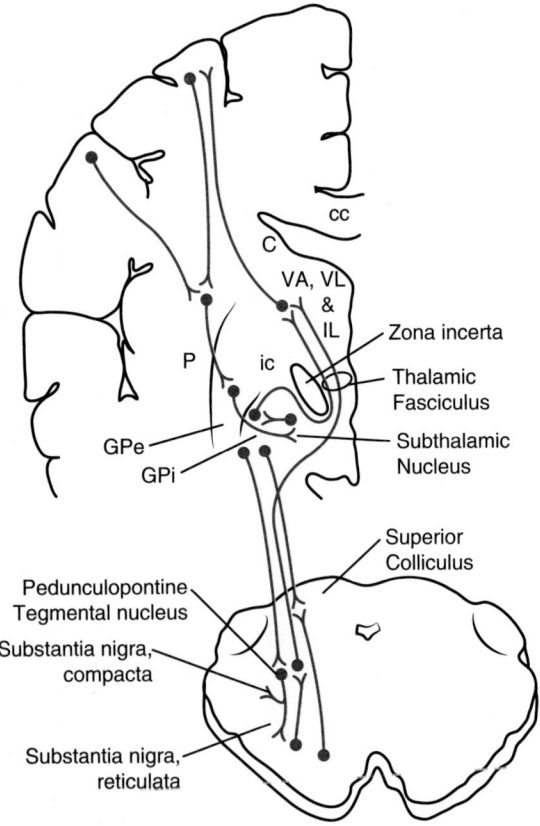

Figure 18.3 The indirect loop through the subthalamic nucleus; also represented are the efferents from the globus pallidus interna and substantia nigra pars reticulata to the superior colliculus and midbrain tegmentum. C = caudate nucleus; GPe = globus pallidus pars externa; GPi = globus pallidus pars interna; ic = internal capsule; IL = intralaminar nuclei of the thalamus; P = putamen; VA = ventral anterior nucleus of the thalamus; VL = ventral lateral nucleus of the thalamus.

■ STAGES AND MODELS OF BRAIN PATHOLOGY

Postmortem studies by Braak and colleagues have yielded evidence supporting the view that PD is a widely dispersed neurodegenerative disease that demonstrates a progression through different stages of brain pathology, *alpha-synucleinopathy*.[14–16] Early on *(stage 1)* lesions are found in the olfactory bulb, olfactory nucleus, and/or the dorsal IX/X nuclei in the brain stem. In *stage 2,* pathology is expanded to involve lesions in the pontine tegmentum (locus coeruleus, magnocellular nucleus of the reticular formation, and raphe nuclei). In *stage 3,* involvement of the nigrostriatal system is apparent (pars compacta of the substantia nigra). In *stage 4,* lesions are also found in the hypothalamus, parts of the thalamus, and cortex (temporal mesocortex and allocortex). In *stage 5,* pathology is extended to involve the sensory association areas of the neocortex and prefrontal neocortex. In *stage 6,* pathology is extended to involve the first-order association areas and primary areas of the neocortex.[14–17]

Recently, a model of PD pathogenesis has been proposed that aims to explain the motor asymmetry, the nonmotor phenotypes, and the cognitive decline. This alpha-synuclein origin and connectome model (SOC Model) proposes that in a brain-first subtype for some patients, the alpha-synuclein pathology first appears unilaterally within the CNS (e.g., in one amygdala), propagates to the ipsilateral (same side) substantial nigra and other structures, leading to asymmetric dopaminergic degeneration and motor signs. The model proposes that in a body-first subtype in other patients, the pathology begins in the peripheral enteric or autonomic nervous system (e.g., in the gut) and propagates along the vagus nerve to both right and left dorsal motor nuclei within the CNS, leading to more symmetric dopaminergic degeneration and motor signs.[18]

■ DISEASE COURSE

The disease is progressive, with a long preclinical/prodromal period estimated to be 5 to 25 years.[19,20] Mean PD duration is approximately 10 to 20 years with a life expectancy close to the general population. There is variability of the rate of progression. Patients with a young age at onset or who are tremor predominant typically demonstrate a slower progression. Patients with PD who present with postural instability and gait disturbances (the PIGD group) tend to have more pronounced deterioration with a more rapid disease progression. Neurobehavioral disturbances and dementia are also more common in this group.[21] With dopaminergic therapy, progression is generally slower with an overall improvement in mortality rates. The most common causes of death are cardiovascular disease and pneumonia.[22]

Hoehn and Yahr Classification of Disability Scale

An estimate of the stage and severity of the disease can be made using a staging scale. The most widely used in clinical practice and research trials is the *Hoehn and Yahr Classification of Disability Scale* (H&Y) (Table 18.1).[23] It provides a broad measure for charting the progression of the disease using motor signs and elements of functional status. H&Y stage I is used to indicate minimal disease involvement, whereas H&Y stage V is indicative of severe deterioration in which the patient is confined to bed or a wheelchair.

Movement Disorders Society Unified Parkinson's Disease Rating Scale

The *Unified Parkinson's Disease Rating Scale (UPDRS)* has been the "gold standard" for measuring the progression of PD since 1987.[24] Goetz and colleagues reported on a modification of this scale renamed the Movement Disorder Society–sponsored revision of the Unified Parkinson's Disease Rating Scale (MDS-UPDRS).[25,26] The goals of the revision were to improve ability to detect slower and smaller changes in mildly disabled patients and increase focus on nonmotor symptoms. Descriptors are added for each question. Parts I and II have been renamed: Part I is now *Non-motor Aspects of Experiences of Daily Living,* and Part II is now *Motor Experiences of Daily Living.* Part III is *Motor Examination* (same title), and Part IV is renamed *Motor Complications.*[26] The total time to administer the test is an estimated 30 minutes, with Parts I and II designed to be self-administered by the patient. This instrument can be found on the internet (http://www.movement disorders.org/MDS-Files1/PDFs/Rating-Scales/MDS-UPDRS_Vol23_Issue15_2008.pdf).

Table 18.1	Hoehn and Yahr Classification of Disability[23]
Stage	**Character of Disability**
I	Minimal or absent; unilateral if present.
II	Minimal bilateral or midline involvement. Balance not impaired.
III	Impaired righting reflexes. Unsteadiness when turning or rising from chair. Some activities are restricted, but patient can live independently and continue some forms of employment.
IV	All symptoms present and severe. Standing and walking possible only with assistance.
V	Confined to bed or wheelchair.

■ SYMPTOMS

The clinical presentation of PD is multifaceted, with many motor and nonmotor (including autonomic) signs and symptoms. The diagnosis is made based on the cardinal motor signs of *bradykinesia, tremor, rigidity,* and *postural instability* that often present many years (between 5 and 20) after the onset of nonmotor symptoms.

Motor Symptoms

Bradykinesia

Bradykinesia refers to slowness of movement and is the one cardinal feature common to all parkinsonian disorders, including PD. Weakness, tremor, and rigidity may contribute to bradykinesia but do not fully explain it. The principal deficit is the result of insufficient recruitment of muscle force during initiation of movement. Patients underscale movement commands in internally generated movements. The introduction of external cues (e.g., vision, sound) can partially ameliorate this and is used in treatment to guide movement. It is one of the most disabling symptoms of PD, with prolonged movement and reaction times resulting in increased time on task and dependence in daily activities. Slowness of thought, *bradyphrenia,* can contribute to bradykinesia.[27]

Akinesia refers to a poverty of spontaneous movement. For example, the patient with PD demonstrates *hypomimia* or masked facial expression, with significant social consequences. Other examples of akinesia include the absence of associated movements (e.g., arm swing during walking) or freezing (sudden, short, and transient inhibitions of movements while walking *[freezing of gait, FOG],* or during other movements such as writing, talking, or driving). Akinesia can be influenced by the degree of rigidity, as well as stage of disease, fluctuations in drug action, and disturbances in attention and depression.[28]

Hypokinesia refers to slowed and reduced movements and can also be seen in PD. For example, patients with moderate or severe PD typically present with handwriting that may start out strong but becomes smaller and smaller as writing proceeds *(micrographia).* During walking, rotational movements of the trunk with arm swing may also start out strong and decrease over time.

Tremor

Tremor, another cardinal feature of PD, involves involuntary shaking or oscillating movement of a part or parts of the body resulting from contractions of opposing muscles. In the early stages of the disease, about 70% of patients experience a slight tremor of the hand or foot on one side of the body, or less commonly in the jaw or tongue. It tends to be mild and occurs for only short periods. Tremor in PD tends to be of low frequency (4 to 6 Hz). The tremor is known as a *resting tremor* because it is present at rest, suppressed briefly by voluntary movement, and disappears with sleep. Tremor of the head, trunk, and limbs can be seen when muscles are used to maintain sustained postures against gravity, *postural tremor. Action tremor/kinetic tremor,* tremor that continues with movement, can occur in patients, but this occurs more often as the disease progresses. Tremor tends to be less severe when the patient is relaxed and unoccupied. It is aggravated by emotional stress or excitement. With disease progression, tremor can become severe, spread to the other side, and interfere with activities of daily living (ADL).[26,29]

Rigidity

Rigidity is one of the clinical hallmarks of PD and is defined as increased resistance to passive motion regardless of movement velocity. Patients frequently complain of "heaviness" and "stiffness." It is felt uniformly in both agonist and antagonist muscles and in movements in both directions and is often asymmetrical right to left. Spinal stretch reflexes are normal. Rigidity is constant regardless of the task, amplitude, or speed of movement. Two descriptive terms are sometimes used: cogwheel and lead pipe. *Cogwheel rigidity* is a jerky resistance to passive movement as muscles alternately tense and relax. It occurs when tremor is superimposed on a background of increased tone. *Lead pipe rigidity* is a sustained resistance to passive movement in all directions, with no fluctuations. Rigidity may initially be unilateral (limb rigidity), eventually spreading to involve the whole body, including the neck and trunk (truncal rigidity). As the disease progresses, rigidity becomes more severe, decreasing the ability to move easily. For example, loss of bed mobility or lack of reciprocal arm swing during gait, seen even early in the disease, is often related to the degree of truncal rigidity. Active movement, mental concentration, or emotional stress may all increase rigidity. Prolonged rigidity results in decreased range of motion (ROM) and serious secondary complications of contracture and postural deformity. Rigidity also has a direct impact on increasing resting energy expenditure and fatigue levels.[30]

Postural Instability

Achieving, maintaining, and regaining balance during posture and movement are all components of postural control that are impaired in individuals with PD, resulting in postural instability. Throughout the disease, several problems become evident across a broad spectrum of movement control. Patients demonstrate abnormal and inflexible postural responses controlling their center of mass (COM) within their base of support (BOS). They have smaller functional limits of stability (LOS) compared with healthy adults of the same age, reduced more anteriorly with forward lean than posteriorly with backward lean.[31] Narrowing of the BOS (tandem stance or single-limb stance) or competing attentional demands (alternating and divided attention situations) increases postural instability. Individuals with PD experience difficulty during dynamic destabilizing activities such as self-initiated movements (e.g., functional reach, walking, turning) and perform poorly under conditions of perturbed balance.[32] The response to instability is an abnormal pattern of coactivation, resulting in a rigid body and an inability to use normal postural synergies to recover balance.[32] Patients also demonstrate difficulty in regulating feedforward, anticipatory adjustments of postural muscles during voluntary movements. These anticipatory postural adjustments (APAs) are abnormally slow in people with PD (see the section "Gait"). Sensorimotor integration is impaired as evidenced by difficulty in adapting movement strategies to changing sensory conditions.[33] Visuospatial impairment has been identified in people with PD and correlates with lower scores in mobility, freezing episodes, and self-reported cognitive impairment.[28] Some patients are unable to perceive the upright or vertical position, which may indicate an abnormality in processing of vestibular, visual, and proprioceptive information contributing to balance. Contributing factors to postural instability include rigidity, decreased muscle torque production and weakness, loss of available ROM particularly of trunk motions, axial rigidity, and freezing. Medication side effects (e.g., postural hypotension and dyskinesias) also contribute.

Progressive development of postural deformity occurs. Weakness and force control deficits of antigravity muscles contribute to a flexed, stooped posture with increased flexion of the neck, trunk, hips, and knees.[34,35] This results in a change in the center-of-alignment position, placing the individual at the forward LOS. In the lower extremities (LEs), *contractures* develop in hip and knee flexors, hip rotators and adductors, and plantar flexors. In the spine, dorsal spine and neck flexors are involved, and in the upper extremities (UEs), shoulder adductors and internal rotators and elbow flexors are involved. Function becomes progressively more limited by these musculoskeletal constraints. Individuals with reduced activity levels and poor diet are likely to develop *osteoporosis*. Two involuntary and reversible postural abnormalities can occur in people with PD: (1) *Camptocormia*, flexion of the trunk when upright that resolves when supine of at least 30° at the lumbar fulcrum (L1-sacrum, hip flexion) and/or at least 45° at the thoracic fulcrum (C7 to T12-L1), and (2) *Pisa syndrome*, a lateral flexion of trunk over 10°. The pathophysiology is not well understood but likely involves abnormal central motor control that causes metabolic and structural changes in the paravertebral muscles.[36,37] Secondary contractures are a concern.

Frequent falls and fall injury are twice as likely to occur for individuals with PD as those without PD, and recurrent falls are nine times more likely in PD.[38] Falls can occur early in the disease, become increasingly prevalent during the middle portion of disease progression, and as the patient becomes progressively immobile, disappear during late disease. About 70% of patients with PD report experiencing falls within the past year, and 50% report recurrent falls. The rate of fall injury is about 40%. Although most injuries are not severe, some lead to hospitalization. Within 10 years of diagnosis, approximately 25% of patients will have developed a hip fracture. In a long-term study of over 3 million people in Sweden that explored fall risk *prior to* clinical diagnosis of PD (*prodromal/preclinical*), researchers found the risk of falls with injury was increased 10 years before diagnosis.[39] Disease severity, postural instability, and gait impairment including freezing are clearly linked to increased risk for falls.[32,40] Other risk factors include dementia, depression, postural hypotension, and involuntary movements associated with long-term use of antiparkinsonian medication (dyskinesias).[38,41] Falls can lead to "fear of falling" with increasing levels of immobility and dependency with a deteriorating quality of life (QOL).

Muscle Performance

A reduction in strength is evident in patients with PD. Torque production is decreased at all speeds resulting in activity limitations and muscle weakness.[42] Changes in strength may be dopamine related as patients on dopamine replacement ("on" state) demonstrate increases in strength when compared to testing the same muscles during an "off" state.[43] Electromyography (EMG) studies reveal that motor unit recruitment is delayed with under-recruitment of muscles and breakdown in the agonist–antagonist–agonist (triphasic) pattern of muscle activity. Once initiated, contraction is characterized by multiple bursts and *asynchronization,* that is, pauses and an inability to smoothly increase firing rate as contraction continues. These difficulties are compounded during the production of complex movements. As the disease progresses, disuse weakness evolves from inactivity and increases movement difficulties.

In patients with PD, *fatigue* is among the most common symptoms reported. The patient has difficulty in sustaining activity and experiences increasing weakness and lethargy as the day progresses. Performance decreases dramatically with great physical effort or stress. Rest or sleep may restore mobility. When levodopa therapy is initiated, the patient may notice a dramatic improvement initially and feel significantly less fatigued, but over time fatigue typically reappears. A common perception among patients is an increased sense of effort associated with movement that is manifested by difficulty activating and sustaining responses.[44]

Motor Function

The striatum of the BG (caudate nucleus, putamen, and nucleus accumbens) receive input from all cortical areas and project throughout the thalamus to frontal lobe areas (prefrontal, premotor, and supplementary motor areas) concerned with motor planning. In PD, motor planning deficits are evident, involving a loss of regulatory control of both automatic and voluntary movement responses directed through the pyramidal system.[45] Paucity of movement occurs with less accurate movements overall. This deficit in accuracy becomes more pronounced as the patient attempts to increase the speed of movement *(speed–accuracy trade-off)*. People with PD have difficulty performing complex, sequential, or simultaneous movements. The difficulties combining tasks or shifting attentional sets from one to another can also be seen with cognitive tasks or when combining cognitive and motor tasks *(dual-task control)*. Movement preparation (i.e., the when, where, and how to initiate movement) is significantly prolonged. This *start hesitation* is especially evident as the disease progresses. For example, the patient is delayed and slow in initiating movement during a transfer sequence.

Motor learning deficits can be seen in patients with PD.[46] Deficits in learning new motor skills, fine-tuning skills, and learning complex and sequential tasks have been demonstrated in all stages of disease. Healthy adults achieve better learning (determined by retention and transfer testing) with random order practice conditions and high levels of *contextual interference* (see Chapter 10, Strategies to Improve Motor Function). In contrast, for individuals with PD, learning is improved with lower levels of contextual interference through blocked practice conditions and with slower learning rates than healthy adults.[47] Learning deficits can be expected to be severe if multiple motor programs are required either simultaneously or sequentially (i.e., switching among tasks). For example, the patient may freeze when asked to carry out a second task while walking, when performing any two tasks that have separate task goals *(dual-tasking)*,[48] or when performing a complex task that requires increased cognitive processing.[49] Compounding variables that degrade learning include the severity of disease, dementia, and visual–perceptual deficits. Differences in learning can also be expected based on medication levels as motor learning is degraded when patients are in the "off" state of medication.[50,51]

Gait

More than 25% of patients present with gait disturbances and postural instability as their initial motor symptom and comprise a PIGD group.[52] The patient with PD demonstrates a number of significant gait changes that can generally be divided into continuous and episodic disturbances.[53] *Continuous gait control problems* have been characterized as three primary gait impairments that are relatively independent: (1) slowness (pace and rhythm), (2) increased variability and asymmetry, and (3) poor postural control.[32] Slowed walking is a hallmark characteristic of PD observed throughout the disease and primarily caused by bradykinesia (slower steps), hypokinesia (shorter steps), and rigidity

(increased tone). Reductions in arm swing and trunk rotation, also due to bradykinesia/hypokinesia, are seen throughout the disease. Axial rigidity (neck, trunk, and hips) contributes to an abnormal stooped posture, slowed gait, and an *en bloc* turning style with reduced speed and more steps to complete the turn. Variability of gait, seen as step width (mediolateral) and step length (anterior–posterior) fluctuations from stride to stride, is increased in people with PD and seen even early in the disease before the onset of shortened step length.[54] Asymmetry of arm swing (an early sign of abnormal gait in PD), step length, and time are increased in people with PD and may partially relate to the asymmetric onset of bradykinesia and rigidity.[55] All three components of postural control, achieving, maintaining, and restoring balance, are impaired in people with PD.[32] Postural sway is increased, particularly in the mediolateral direction, and LOS (peak displacement of COM without changing BOS) are decreased in standing, especially in the backward direction, which is seen even in very early disease.[56,57] In addition, people with PD have slow and small preparatory balance adjustments for an upcoming voluntary movement (APA). These reduced APAs contribute to the delayed step initiation and narrowed stance/step commonly seen in those with PD.[58] For example, in order to step with the right foot, one must first shift COM laterally toward that side in order to subsequently shift COM toward the stance side and allow right swing. The PD-related narrowed stance and slowed and small lateral-shifting APAs contribute to poorer gait initiation and balance during gait. Balance while walking is a complex temporal coupling of trunk control and stepping (posture and gait).[59]

Episodic gait disturbances refer to the intermittent, unpredictable and context-specific characteristics of *festination* (unintentionally rapid short steps) and *FOG* (trembling of the legs and transient inability to effectively step, or absence of leg movement/akinesia, described as being "stuck to the ground").[53] Gait can be *anteropulsive* (a forward festinating gait) or *retropulsive* (a backward festinating gait), typically seen when the individual is attempting to regain balance lost backward and is often unsuccessful.

Freezing episodes affect 38% of people with mild PD and 65% of those with severe PD.[60] FOG can be triggered by confrontation of competing stimuli. For example, the patient slows and stops walking when exposed to a narrowed space, an obstacle, or even a visual barrier such as a hallway, doorway, or change in flooring pattern. These freezing behaviors are consistent with findings from brain imaging studies in people with PD that indicate those with FOG have disruptions in the "executive-attention" and visual neural networks, compared with those who do not freeze.[61] The cognitive aspects that contribute to freezing are inhibition, attention, and visuospatial functions.[62] Stress and increased cognitive load, such as when dual-tasking, can exacerbate freezing episodes. Turning or changing direction is particularly difficult and typically accomplished by taking multiple small steps, which itself can elicit festination and freezing episodes.[63] In early disease, FOG is generally short in duration and rarely leads to falls. With disease progression, FOG becomes more frequent and disabling, often leading to falls.[64] Patients who are in the "off" medication state experience increased FOG and deterioration in gait performance, whereas gait patterns often improve with "on" medication levels. Most patients with mild gait deficits can compensate at least partially using external cues and attentional and self-cuing strategies.[64] Problems with controlling posture and balance limit independence, community ambulation, and safety.

Nonmotor Symptoms

Typically a person with PD will experience from 8 to 13 NMSs, regardless of the motor stage or duration of disease.[65,66] Seventeen NMSs are more common in early nonmedicated patients with PD than adults of the same age without PD. Fifteen of these NMSs are associated in four clusters: (1) REM sleep behavior disorder (RBD) symptoms (frequent nightmares, dream-enacting behaviors) and constipation, (2) cognition-related (memory complaints, fatigue, inattention, excessive daytime sleepiness), (3) mood-related (anhedonia, apathy, mood disturbance), and (4) sensory and dysautonomia (taste loss, chest pain, unexplained pain, excessive sweating, postprandial fullness). The most commonly reported early-onset NMSs (from 2 to greater than 10 years before motor symptoms) are smell loss, constipation, RBD symptoms, and mood disorders.[67]

Sensory Symptoms

Patients with PD do not suffer from primary sensory loss. However, 60% to 80% of patients with PD experience paresthesias and pain as early symptoms, including sensations of numbness, tingling, cold, aching pain, and burning.[68] Pain related to PD presents in five classifications: musculoskeletal, dystonic, neuropathic/radicular, central or primary, and *akathisia* (a feeling of inner restlessness and an inability to remain still).[68] The pathophysiology of PD-related pain is not clear but likely is complex and multifaceted. Central or primary pain may be due to abnormal modulation of pain caused by dopamine deficiency in the BG.[69] Pain is most commonly reported in the lower back and legs, and shoulders, but can also affect the face, head, mouth, pharynx, and internal/visceral regions.[68] Symptoms are typically intermittent and vary in intensity and location, often starting or being more severe on the side of the appearance of the first motor symptoms. Hypersensitivity to pain *(hyperalgesia)* is common and is linked to the motor fluctuations experienced during levodopa therapy (e.g., pain is more intense in an "off" state).[70] Pain may also be increased in patients experiencing depression.[66]

Proprioceptive regulation of voluntary movement and integration of somatosensory inputs may also be impaired. Patients with PD perform significantly worse than control subjects on tests of kinesthesia and proprioceptive position sense for the limbs and the trunk. Without visual guidance, patients demonstrate increased difficulty in accurately perceiving the extent of movement, consistently underscaling their movements.[71,72] Combined with the deficits in visuospatial skills that are common in PD, kinesthetic and proprioceptive impairments can contribute to balance and motor control problems. Patients demonstrate significantly more errors than normal on visual perception tasks involving spatial organization.

Olfactory Dysfunction

Olfactory dysfunction is common, with some studies showing up to 100% of patients affected. Most patients with PD report a decline or loss of sense of smell *(anosmia)*, often years before motor symptoms develop. Loss of smell therefore has important implications for diagnosis of early disease. It also increases the difficulty individuals have in maintaining a healthy diet and adequate nutrition.[66]

Visual and Visuospatial Perception

Visual and visuospatial perception disturbances are reported in over 70% of people with PD. These include visual hallucinations; misjudging objects and distances; impaired contrast sensitivity; abnormal color discrimination; peripheral visual disturbance; impaired face and emotion recognition; altered detection of visual motion, line orientation, pattern perception, and depth perception; and oculomotor changes, in particular with voluntary saccades.[73] Smooth pursuit movements may have a jerky quality, and saccades are hypometric. Decreased blinking can produce bloodshot, irritated eyes that burn and itch. Conventional drugs (e.g., anticholinergic drugs) used in PD can also cause visual disturbances (e.g., blurred vision and sensitivity to light [photophobia]). These drugs can worsen the normal visual changes associated with aging (presbyopia).

Vestibular Dysfunction

Vestibular dysfunction is common in individuals with PD. Dizziness that is unrelated to orthostatic hypotension is seen in up to 30% of those in early PD. There are too few studies of abnormalities of the vestibulo-ocular reflex in PD to draw reliable conclusions. However, substantial evidence shows patients have abnormal vestibulospinal reflexes measured by brain stem evoked potentials (vestibular-evoked myogenic potentials [VEMPs]). Balance and postural control involve the integration of somatosensory, visual, and vestibular information integration, and studies have shown impaired sensory integration with particular difficulty using vestibular information in people with PD.[74]

Auditory Dysfunction

Auditory dysfunction is a nonmotor feature of PD with impairments in a range of central auditory processes, including altered deviance detection of basic auditory features, auditory brain stem processing, auditory gating, and selective auditory attention. Brain stem auditory responses improve with dopaminergic medication (when patients are in the "on" phase). However, in clinical practice, little attention has been paid to hearing impairment.[75]

Dysphagia

Dysphagia, impaired swallowing, is present in as many as 95% of patients and is the result of rigidity, reduced mobility, and restricted range of movement. It is often an early symptom of the disease though it is present in all stages.[76] Individuals with PD experience problems in all four phases of swallowing: oral preparatory, oral, pharyngeal, and esophageal. Thus, the patient demonstrates abnormal tongue control and problems with chewing, bolus formation, delayed swallow response, and peristalsis. Dysphagia can lead to choking or aspiration pneumonia and impaired nutrition with significant weight loss. Nutritional inadequacy can contribute to the fatigue and exhaustion typically experienced by patients with PD. Patients also typically experience excessive drooling *(sialorrhea)* because of increased saliva production and decreased spontaneous swallowing. Drooling is particularly problematic while sleeping or initiating speech and in advanced cases increases the risk of aspiration. Excessive drooling has important negative social implications.[77]

Speech Disorders

Speech is impaired in 90% of people with PD and is the result of primary symptoms of PD (rigidity, bradykinesia, hypokinesia, and tremor).[78] People with PD experience *hypokinetic dysarthria,* which is characterized by decreased voice volume, monotone/monopitch speech, imprecise or distorted articulation, and uncontrolled speech rate. Vocal quality is degraded with speech described as hoarse, breathy, and harsh. In addition, patients experience timing difficulty of vocal onsets and offsets. Reduced mobility, restricted range, and uncontrolled rate of movement of muscles controlling respiration, phonation, resonation, and articulation are present. Reduced vital capacity results in reduced air expended during phonation. In advanced cases, the patient may speak in whispers or not at all, demonstrating *mutism.* Sensory problems may also contribute to speech difficulties. Patients who are instructed to upscale their speech sounds to produce increased volume consistently describe their speech as "too loud." Speech difficulties contribute to social isolation and impaired activity participation.[76,78]

Cognitive Impairment

Impairment in cognitive function is subtly present from the earliest stages of PD and prior to beginning medication *(de novo).*[79,80] Compared with similarly-aged healthy controls, most people with early-stage PD demonstrate problems with cognitive control (processing speed, attention, task switching, impulsivity, inhibition, apathetic motivation, verbal fluency, planning, and abstract reasoning), and almost half have visuospatial and verbal and visual memory deficits.[81–83] *Mild cognitive impairment (MCI)* is a state between normal cognition and early dementia. The frequency of MCI due to PD (PD-MCI) in those newly diagnosed is between 15% and 40% and predicts an increased risk of dementia within 5 years.[84] Although many people with PD-MCI during the first year after diagnosis went on to develop *PD dementia (PDD),* about 25% of patients with PD-MCI actually reverted to normal cognition by the fifth year.[84] The reasons for this are unclear but appear to be related to early diagnosis and treatment. The incidence of PD-MCI is 7% per year and increases to greater than 10% per year in patients diagnosed at 65 years and older. Older patients appear to be at greatest risk for progressing to dementia, with reported rates 4.4 times higher for individuals 80 years of age or older.[82,83] The conversion from PD-MCI to PDD is characterized by deterioration of previous impairments and development of language deficits (aphasia symptoms and confrontation naming/word-retrieval difficulties).[83] Psychosis can develop in up to 60% of patients, typically starting with visual illusions, progressing to visual hallucinations with then without insight, and ultimately delusions. Hallucinations are present in up to 70% of patients and can occur early in the disease before starting dopaminergic medication *(de novo),* with a lifetime risk of up to 50%.[85]

Depression, Anxiety, and Apathy

Depression is one of the first NMSs to appear in people with PD. Major depression is reported to occur in approximately 40% of patients and subclinical depression in nearly 55% of those in early-stage PD.[86] A significant number of patients develop depression before or just after onset of motor symptoms, suggesting an endogenous cause that may be related to genetic mutations associated with PD, underlying deficiencies of dopamine, serotonin, and norepinephrine. Patients demonstrate a variety of symptoms, including feelings of guilt, hopelessness, and worthlessness; loss of energy; poor concentration; deficits in short-term memory; loss of ambition or enthusiasm; and disturbances in appetite and sleep. Suicidal thoughts may also be present. Hypomimia, a reduction in facial expressiveness, can give the appearance of depression. Patients can also demonstrate *dysthymic disorder* characterized by chronic depression and dysphoric mood, resulting in poor appetite or overeating, insomnia or hypersomnia, low energy, low self-esteem, and poor concentration.

Anxiety is a common symptom in PD with a prevalence of 31%. Clinically, patients may present with symptoms of a panic attack (e.g., palpitations, sweating, trembling, shortness of breath) as well as social phobia (social withdrawal), agoraphobia, obsessive-compulsive disorder, or panic disorder. Anxiety symptoms may not be simply related to the psychological or social difficulties patients experience but due to specific neurobiological processes associated with the disease. Patients who are in the "off" medication state experience significant worsening of depression and anxiety.[86]

Apathy is characterized by decreased motivation, a reduction in goal-directed behavior, and includes affective, cognitive, and behavioral aspects. Apathy is found in 35% to 40% of people newly diagnosed with PD who have not begun medication treatment. The frequency appears to decrease with the onset of dopaminergic therapy and increases again after 5 to 10 years of disease to 40% in patients without dementia and to 60% in PDD.[86]

Autonomic Dysfunction

Autonomic dysfunction of both the sympathetic and parasympathetic limbs of the autonomic nervous system (ANS) occurs early in PD, is a direct manifestation of the disease, and is related to disease progression. Lewy bodies are found in neurons of the ANS. Thermoregulatory dysfunction includes *hyperhidrosis* (excessive sweating) and abnormal or uncomfortable sensations of warmth and coldness. Patients in the "off" state experience impaired peripheral vasodilation with difficulty dissipating body heat. *Seborrhea* (increased oil secretion of the sebaceous glands of the skin) and *seborrheic dermatitis* (oily, chafing, and reddened skin) are also common. Patients with PD exhibit abnormally slow pupillary responses to light and pain and reduced overall response to changes in light.[87]

Gastrointestinal disorders include poor motility (impaired gastric emptying occurs in up to 70% to 100%), changes in appetite, inadequate hydration, sialorrhea, and weight loss. *Constipation* is a common problem for most patients and typically occurs early in PD. *Urinary incontinence* occurs with associated symptoms of urinary frequency, urgency, and nocturia. Most individuals with PD report changes in libido, *erectile dysfunction* in males and *anorgasmia* in females, including impotence and reduced rates of sexual activity.[88]

Early and progressive sympathetic denervation of the heart occurs in most people with PD. This results in diminished heart function, which may be a contributory factor to the fatigue that most patients experience. People with mild to moderate PD exhibit blunted cardiovascular and metabolic responses to peak exercise (lower heart rate [HR], oxygen uptake [VO_2] and systolic blood pressure [SBP]) compared with their healthy peers. The motor limitations of PD may create a higher energy demand at the same absolute workload than for people without PD. Taking this into account, studies of submaximal exercise using ventilator thresholds as indicators of *relative* levels of intensity show that HR is lower and VO_2 and SBP are similar to healthy adults at this similar intensity. Thus, the blunted response to exercise in people with PD is present even at submaximal levels of exercise and worsens with increased intensity of exercise.[87,89]

Orthostatic hypotension (OH) is common in all stages of PD and is caused by a sharp drop in BP (20 mm Hg systolic and 10 mm Hg diastolic within 3 min) that occurs with position changes (e.g., supine to sit or sit to stand). Typical symptoms include light-headedness or dizziness. Patients can also experience pallor, diaphoresis, weakness, trembling, nausea, difficulty thinking, or syncope. The condition puts individuals at risk for loss of balance, falls, and fall injury. Medications (e.g., levodopa/carbidopa, bromocriptine) can contribute to OH.[89]

Patients with PD demonstrate respiratory impairments, reported in as many as 84% of patients, explained in part by dysfunction in the BG and other brain stem structures that control respiratory drive and muscles of respiration. *Airway obstruction* (e.g., air trapping, lung insufflation) is the most frequently reported pulmonary problem and has been linked to episodes of pulmonary failure. The etiology remains unknown but may be linked to bradykinetic disorganization of respiratory movements. *Restrictive lung dysfunction* is common and is linked to the decreased chest expansion that occurs because of rigidity of the trunk muscles, loss of musculoskeletal flexibility, and kyphotic posture. Patients with PD demonstrate lower forced vital capacity (FVC), lower forced expiratory volume in 1 sec (FEV$_1$), and higher residual volume (RV) and residual airway resistance (RAW) values when compared to age-matched controls. Daily function and activity participation are reduced in patients with pulmonary dysfunction. A sedentary lifestyle with decreased activity levels contributes to cardiopulmonary deconditioning.

Sleep Disorders

Individuals with PD can experience *excessive daytime somnolence* (sleepiness). At night, *insomnia* (disturbed sleep pattern) may occur. This includes problems falling asleep, staying asleep, and good quality of sleep. RBD occurs early in the prodromal phase of PD, affects as many as 50% to 60% of patients, and is the biomarker with the highest diagnostic strength potential. In people with RBD, the paralysis that normally occurs during REM sleep is incomplete or absent, allowing them to "act out" their dreams that are vivid, intense, and violent. Dream-enacting behaviors include agitation and physical activity during sleep (e.g., talking, yelling, punching, kicking, arm flailing, and grabbing).[90] Box 18.2 provides a summary of the cardinal features and clinical manifestations of PD.

Box 18.2 Cardinal Features and Clinical Manifestations of Parkinson Disease

Cardinal Features

- Rigidity
- Bradykinesia/akinesia
- Tremor
- Postural instability

Clinical Manifestations

Motor Performance

- Decreased torque production
- Fatigue
- Contractures and deformity common
- Masked face
- Micrographia
- Hypometria/undershooting target with limbs and with gaze

Motor Planning

- Start hesitation
- Freezing episodes
- Poverty of movement
- Visuomotor transformation difficulties

Motor Learning

- Slower learning rates, reduced efficiency
- Increased context-specificity of learning; impaired contextual flexibility
- Procedural learning deficits for complex and sequential tasks

Gait

- Reduced stride length; increased step-to-step variability
- Reduced step width
- Reduced speed of walking
- Cadence (steps per minute) typically intact; may be reduced in advanced Parkinson disease
- Increased time: double-limb support
- Insufficient hip, knee, and ankle flexion: shuffling steps
- Insufficient heel strike with increased forefoot loading
- Reduced trunk rotation: decreased or absent arm swing
- Festinating gait: anteropulsion common
- Freezing of gait
- Difficulty turning: increased steps per turn
- Difficulty stepping backward: retropulsion or decreased step initiation
- Difficulty sidestepping: decreased step initiation and narrowed steps
- Difficulty with dual-tasking: simultaneous motor and/or cognitive tasks
- Difficulty with attentional demands of complex environments

Posture

- Kyphosis with forward head and scapular protraction
- Leaning to one side with tonal asymmetries
- Increased fall risk

Sensory Systems

- Visual: blurring, decreased acuity, color discrimination, contrast detection, smooth pursuit, and age-related decreased adaptation to light, and sensitivity to light and glare
- Auditory: trouble detecting basic auditory features, reduced brain stem processing, auditory gating and selective auditory attention
- Vestibular: decreased ability to integrate vestibular information for postural control

Sensation

- Paresthesias
- Pain
- Akathisia
- Proprioceptive and kinesthetic deficits

Speech, Voice, and Swallowing Disorders

- Hypokinetic dysarthria
- Dysphagia

Cognition and Behavior

- Dementia
- Bradyphrenia
- Visuospatial deficits
- Depression
- Dysphoric mood
- Apathy
- Anxiety

Autonomic Nervous System

- Excessive sweating
- Abnormal sensations of heat and cold
- Seborrhea
- Sialorrhea
- Constipation
- Urinary bladder dysfunction
- Orthostatic hypotension

Cardiopulmonary Function

- Low resting blood pressure
- Compromised cardiovascular response to exercise
- Impaired respiratory function

■ MEDICAL DIAGNOSIS

Diagnosis at onset of PD is difficult with accurate diagnosis possible only with continued observation of evolving clinical motor and nonmotor signs and symptoms. The diagnosis is made based on history and clinical examination. The most widely accepted clinical criteria for diagnosis of PD, introduced in 1992 by the Parkinson Disease Society UK Brain Bank, focus on motor symptoms and exclude NMSs, which are now known to be central to PD.[91] To address this issue, in 2015 the Movement Disorder Society (MDS) proposed a revised set of criteria for PD diagnosis that retains the original motor criteria but also includes NMSs in determining the likelihood that the motor syndrome is specific to PD. The MDS Clinical Diagnostic Criteria for Parkinson Disease identify parkinsonism (bradykinesia plus rest tremor or rigidity) as the core feature of the disease.[92] Then, determining PD as the cause of parkinsonism relies on three categories of diagnostic features: (1) absolute exclusion criteria ruling out PD, (2) red flags that are potential signs that may rule out PD, and (3) supportive criteria that lend support to the diagnosis of PD, such as clear and dramatic benefit from dopaminergic therapy. Using these criteria, diagnosis can be made of either *clinically probable PD* or *clinically established PD*.[92] Exclusion of Parkinson-plus syndromes is necessary. The presence of extrapyramidal signs that are bilaterally symmetrical and do not respond to levodopa and dopamine agonists (apomorphine test) is suggestive of these syndromes, not PD. Imaging can be used to rule out other pathologies. In vivo functional imaging (MRI) using chemical markers to identify dopaminergic deficits in PD and related disorders identifies dopamine deficiency but does not discriminate between PD and other causes of parkinsonism. In the prodromal stage, nonmotor symptoms predominate. There is an increasing focus on use of questionnaires and tests (e.g., olfactory testing, imaging of cardiac sympathetic innervation) that focus on NMSs. Often symptoms of loss of smell, sleep disturbances, vivid dreams with REM alterations, foot dystonia and foot cramping, restless legs syndrome, OH, and constipation are symptoms that are present many years before a clinical diagnosis of PD is made.[93–96]

■ MEDICAL MANAGEMENT

Medical management is directed at slowing disease progression using neuroprotective strategies and symptomatic treatment of motor and nonmotor symptoms. Management becomes increasingly more challenging over time and progressing disease.

Pharmacological Management

Many agents are available as first-line neuroprotective and symptomatic therapy. Table 18.2 outlines the current pharmacological agents for treatment of PD, organized by type, mechanism of action, and potential side effects. (Updates on medications can be found at https://www.parkinson.org/blog/research/medication-treatment.) Selection is individualized according to the patient's characteristics with the benefits and risks of adverse side effects carefully weighed. Starting medication early has been shown to be beneficial in slowing the progression of the disease.[97,98] Drug delivery should be as close to constant as possible to avoid large peaks and valleys. The importance of taking the medication on a fixed schedule should be stressed to patients, family members, and caregivers. When patients with PD are hospitalized, it is important that they continue to receive their medication on schedule.[99] The *Aware in Care* kit from the National Parkinson Foundation can be helpful for these issues during hospital stays (https://www.parkinson.org/resources-support/hospital-safety-guide).

Carbidopa/Levodopa

Carbidopa/levodopa (Sinemet; Rytary) is the gold standard drug therapy for PD. Levodopa was first introduced in 1961 as an experimental drug and came into widespread clinical use in the late 1960s. It is a dopamine precursor that is metabolized to dopamine in the brain. Thus, administration of the drug represents an attempt to correct the essential neurochemical imbalance. Most of levodopa (almost 99%) is metabolized before reaching the brain, requiring administration of high doses that can produce numerous side effects. Today, levodopa is commonly administered with carbidopa, a decarboxylase inhibitor that allows a higher percentage of levodopa to enter the brain. Thus, lower doses of levodopa can be used with fewer adverse side effects. Levodopa remains the most effective drug for treating PD, but levels in the blood fluctuate throughout the day due to its short half-life and erratic absorption. Carbidopa/levodopa is available in immediate-release (IR) and controlled-release (CR) formulations. The IR form has a short half-life requiring multiple oral dosing throughout the day. The CR form is a long-acting, sustained-release preparation. Methods of drug administration are being explored that lead to a more sustained and consistent levodopa delivery, such as intestinal gel infusion, subcutaneous infusion, and inhaler.[100,101]

The primary benefits of dopamine replacement include controlling the PD motor symptoms of bradykinesia and rigidity. Increased movement velocity, initial burst of motor activity, and increased strength are all positive outcomes.[100] The effects on reduction of tremor are varied. Some individuals demonstrate little or no response to levodopa, whereas others demonstrate a positive reduction in tremor amplitude. The "on" state refers to the motor state when tremor, akinesia, or rigidity symptoms have improved with the medication, typically 20 to 60 minutes after dosing. The "off" state

Table 18.2   Pharmacological Agents for Treatment of Parkinson Disease[258]

Class/Type and Medication (available in United States)	Mechanism of Action	Potential Side Effects
Levodopa (carbidopa/levodopa in 1:4 ratio)		
• Carbidopa/levodopa (Sinemet) • controlled-release (Sinemet CR) • orally disintegrating tablet (Parcopa) • with entacapone (Stalevo) • extended-release capsules (Rytary) • enteral suspension (Duopa)	Replaces dopamine lost in PD. Carbidopa prevents levodopa from being converted to dopamine until after it crosses the blood-brain barrier.	• Low BP • Nausea • Dry mouth • Dizziness • Fluctuations and "wearing-off" of benefit between doses • Dyskinesias
Dopamine Agonists		
• Apomorphine (Apokyn) • bromocriptine (Parlodel) • pramipexole (Mirapex) • ropinirole (Requip) • rotigotine transdermal patch (Neupro)	Stimulates dopamine receptors in the basal ganglia.	• Low BP • Nausea • Leg swelling • Hallucinations • Sleepiness • Impulse control disorders • Dyskinesias
COMT Inhibitors		
• Entacapone (Comtan) • tolcapone (Tasmar)	Prolongs effects of levodopa by blocking its breakdown in the body. Used to alleviate "wearing-off," the return of PD symptoms between doses.	• Low BP • Nausea • Indigestion • Abdominal pain • Constipation • Back pain • Insomnia • Aggravation of dopaminergic side effects
MAO-B Inhibitors		
• Rasagiline (Azilect) • selegiline or deprenyl (Eldepryl) • Safinamide (Xadago)	Boosts the effects of levodopa by blocking enzyme in brain that breaks it down. Used early in PD as alternatives to levodopa and to control mild wearing-off phenomena. Low risk of inducing dyskinesias.	• Low BP • Nausea • Agitation • Insomnia • Dizziness • Headache • Back pain • Mouth sores • Indigestion • Dyskinesias • Hallucinations
Anticholinergics		
• Benztropine mesylate (Cogentin) • trihexyphenidyl (formerly Artane)	Reduces excessive acetylcholine influence caused by depleted dopamine. May reduce tremor and dystonias. Less commonly used due to many side effects. Central toxicity indicated by impaired memory, confusion, hallucinations, and delusions.	• Blurred vision • Dry mouth • Constipation • Urinary retention • Memory problems

Table 18.2 Pharmacological Agents for Treatment of Parkinson Disease[258]—cont'd		
Class/Type and Medication (available in United States)	**Mechanism of Action**	**Potential Side Effects**
Amantadine		
• (Symmetrel) • (Symadine)	An antiviral (influenza A) with unknown mechanism for PD, recently found to block effects of glutamate (excitatory amino acid). May reduce dyskinesias.[121]	• Dry mouth • Constipation • Urinary retention • Ankle swelling • Mottled skin rash • Aggravate hallucinations
Norepinephrine Precursors		
• Droxidopa (Northera)	Targets neurogenic orthostatic hypotension by increasing norepinephrine levels.	• Nausea • Headache • Confusion • High BP when lying down
Cholinesterase Inhibitors		
• Rivastigmine tartrate (Exelon)	Inhibits enzymes that break down acetylcholine. Used to improve memory function and gait stability.[123]	• Diarrhea • Dizziness • Weakness • Drowsiness • Insomnia • Increased sweating • Loss of appetite • Nausea
Atypical Antipsychotics		
• Pimavanserin (Nuplazid)	Blocks some effects from serotonin. Used to reduce hallucinations and psychosis from side effects of other PD medications.[124]	• Leg swelling • Nausea • Confusion • Constipation • Difficulty walking

BP = blood pressure; COMT = catechol-O-methyl transferase; MAO-B = monoamine oxidase-B; PD = Parkinson disease.

applies to the motor state when the patient experiences tremor, akinesia, or rigidity because no medication or not enough was taken, or because the medication taken is not effective.

Symptoms that are less or nonresponsive to dopaminergic therapy include postural instability, freezing, speech abnormalities, cognitive changes, dementia, depression, sensory abnormalities, and many autonomic dysfunctions.[100,102] However, these variations in responsiveness of different symptoms to levodopa may in fact be due to *relative* under- or overdosing.[82,102] Different regions of the BG–thalamocortical circuitry (the motor, cognitive, affective, and behavioral "loops" discussed in the "Pathophysiology" section) are thought to be affected by dopaminergic loss along a gradient of depletion. This *gradient of dopaminergic depletion* is thought to be greatest in the dorsal striatum involving the "motor loop" and weakest in the ventral striatum involving the "affective loop."[82] For example, freezing is a symptom that

abates at a higher dosage of levodopa than is typically given to alleviate bradykinesia or rigidity.[64] At the other end of the dopamine-depletion gradient for which there is not as much loss of dopamine are circuits for mood and behavioral symptoms (e.g., gambling, reversal learning). These symptoms are effectively "overdosed" at the therapeutic level for cardinal motor symptoms.[82] The decision about when to start levodopa/carbidopa is determined by the neurologist and is different for every person. Initial dosing improves low levels of levodopa often with dramatic improvements in functional status.

Complications of chronic dopamine replacement therapy include motor fluctuations, dyskinesias, and dystonias. As the disease progresses, the window becomes smaller between therapeutic benefit (4 to 6 years) and motor complications when the optimal benefit wears off (termed *wearing-off state*). Motor fluctuations include both the "on–off" phenomenon and wearing-off. The term *"on–off" phenomenon* refers to abrupt, random fluctuations in motor performance and responses. Production of movement errors is common. *Wearing-off* refers to *end-of-dose deterioration,* a worsening of symptoms toward the end of the expected time frame of medication effectiveness. The levodopa-related motor fluctuations are further complicated by disease severity and duration. Early in the disease, remaining dopaminergic neurons act to store the dopamine converted from the therapeutically administered levodopa. The neurons buffer the pulsatile aspect of taking levodopa medication and allow for gradual release of dopamine and a more stable motor response. As the disease progresses and more dopaminergic neurons have disappeared, there is less buffer storage capacity for the administered medication. As this happens, the effects of dopamine more directly follow the fluctuating (pulsatile) blood levels of levodopa medication, and more frequent dosing is needed to keep an adequate and constant level of dopamine. These unbuffered peaks of dopamine concentration in the BG lead to drug-induced hyperkinetic movements (levodopa-induced dyskinesia).[102,103]

Levodopa-induced dyskinesias (LIDs) are dynamic uncontrolled or involuntary movements that include choreic, athetotic, dystonic, and ballistic qualities. They are described based on their pattern of appearance within the "on–off" cycle of medication state. *Peak dose* or *"on"* state dyskinesia occurs with high plasma levels of levodopa when the patient has the maximum benefit of reducing akinesia and rigidity. These are often choreic in quality and are seen in the neck, face, trunk, and upper limbs. *Diphasic dyskinesia* appears when the patient is transitioning between "on" and "off" states when the plasma levels of levodopa are rising or falling. These dyskinetic movements are more repetitive, slow, and stereotyped, or resemble ballisms and can affect walking and balance. Risk factors for developing dyskinesias within 5 years of treatment include duration of levodopa therapy and younger age of onset of PD. LID occurs in 50% of those with age of onset of 40 to 59 years, 25% with age of onset of 60 to 69 years, and 16% after the age of 70 years.[104]

Dystonia, a prolonged involuntary contraction that causes twisting or torsion of body segments, can also occur. The patient typically complains of clawing of the toes or fingers, or cramping of the calf, neck, face, or paraspinal muscles. Dystonia is associated with pain and occurs typically during "off" periods. Patients may experience akathisia and significant disruptions in sleep and relaxation. This affects as many as 25% of patients and is relieved with movement (e.g., walking). *Akathisia* is associated with advanced PD and is more commonly seen in the "off" state.

Unsupervised reduction or sudden discontinuation of levodopa/carbidopa is contraindicated and may produce dangerous, life-threatening adverse effects. Adverse interactions can occur with several medications, including antacids, antiseizure drugs, antihypertensives, and antidepressants.[105]

Patients may also experience other changes that are dose related and may indicate the need for drug modification. These include (1) disabling psychiatric toxicity (visual hallucinations, delusions, and paranoia); (2) depression; (3) gastrointestinal changes (nausea, dry mouth); (4) cardiovascular changes (hypotension, dizziness, arrhythmias); (5) genitourinary changes (dysuria); and (6) sleep disturbances (insomnia, sleep fragmentation).[105]

Dopamine Agonists

Dopamine agonists (DAs) are a class of drugs designed to directly stimulate postsynaptic dopamine receptors. They are administered alone as a first-line monotherapy or along with levodopa/carbidopa, allowing lower doses to be administered with prolonged effectiveness. The greatest benefit of these drugs is reducing rigidity, bradykinesia, and motor fluctuations. Adverse effects are similar to those of levodopa with nausea, sedation, dizziness, constipation, and hallucinations being the most common. These medications have also been linked to an increased risk of impulse control disorders (see earlier for discussion of *relative overdosing;* e.g., pathological gambling, compulsive shopping, hypersexuality, overeating).[100,106]

Other Agents

The other categories of pharmacological agents that are used in the treatment of PD include catechol-O-methyltransferase (COMT) inhibitors, monoamine oxidase-B (MAO-B) inhibitors, anticholinergic agents, and amantadine. Norepinephrine precursors target OH, cholinesterase inhibitors target memory function and gait stability, and atypical antipsychotics are used to treat hallucinations and psychosis.[100] Refer to Table 18.2 for details.

Implications for the Physical Therapist

The therapist needs to be fully aware of each of the medications the patient is taking and potential adverse effects. It is important to remember that patients on dopamine replacement will develop motor complications at some point. Optimal performance can be expected at peak dosage, whereas worsening performance is associated with end-of-dose cycle and medication depletion.[100,102] Timing of physical therapy examination and intervention should be consistent and occur whenever possible during optimal dosing cycle. Therapists are involved in monitoring drug effectiveness on motor performance, activity levels, and participation. As the disease progresses, patients may develop an intolerance for a particular medication, necessitating a change in prescription. Often, the therapist first notices a change in functional status as the patient's system adapts to either the amount or type of drug prescribed. Accurate observation, examination, and reporting of these changes greatly assist the physician in modifying a drug prescription. Therapists may also be involved with clinical drug trials as new medications or combinations are developed.

Nutritional Management

A high-protein diet can block the effectiveness of levodopa. The dietary amino acids in protein compete with levodopa absorption. This is particularly problematic in patients with chronic disease who exhibit fluctuations in motor performance. Thus, patients are generally advised to follow a high-calorie, low-protein diet. Generally, no more than 15% of calories should come from protein. Dietary recommendations may also include shifting the intake of daily protein to the evening meal when patients are less active. These modifications minimize motor fluctuations and maximize responsiveness to levodopa therapy. Patients are also advised to increase their daily intake of water and dietary fiber to help control problems of constipation.[107,108]

Deep Brain Stimulation

Deep brain stimulation (DBS) involves the implantation of electrodes into the brain where stimulation of a relatively small area can result in network-wide changes that can improve symptoms of PD.[109] While the exact mechanisms of symptom improvement by DBS are unknown, it is believed that cell bodies close to the electrodes are inhibited, axons are excited, neurochemical changes are triggered, neurovascular and neurogenic changes are induced, and changes in the oscillatory behavior of certain groups of neurons of the BG appear to play important roles.[109] Brain electrodes are most often placed in the subthalamic nucleus (STN) or the globus pallidus internus (GPi) with the location being chosen according to individual patient needs. The GPi is considered if there are dyskinesias or cognitive or behavioral concerns, whereas the STN might be considered if medication reduction is the goal.[109] More recently, the pedunculopontine nucleus (PPN) and substantia nigra have been explored as targets for DBS to specifically improve gait and balance difficulties that are unresponsive to medication and DBS in the STN or GPi.[109] An impulse generator (IPG), similar to a pacemaker, is implanted in the subclavicular area, and a thin wire goes under the skin to connect to the brain electrodes. High-frequency stimulation is provided. The patient can control the pacemaker's "on–off" switch using a controller while the physician determines the amount of stimulation it delivers, tailoring it to the individual's needs.

DBS in either the STN or GPi has shown overall improvements in tremor and motor symptoms, particularly in the off periods and particularly in advanced stages of disease. Advantages of the STN target for DBS are greater medication reduction early after implantation and less frequent IPG battery changes. DBS of the GPi has the advantage of a more robust suppression of dyskinesias, greater flexibility of medication adjustments in the long term, and easier programming of DBS parameters to optimize effects. Other motor symptoms of akinesia, rigidity, weakness, and reduced walking speed may improve with DBS though the responses are more variable across individuals. Adverse effects can include confusion, depression, headache, speech problems, gait disturbances, and falling. Surgical risks (intracerebral hemorrhage, infection) and mechanical problems with the device (lead breakage, generator malfunction) are also possible. Newer adaptive DBS (aDBS) operates on a closed-loop feedback by adapting the stimulation parameters according to input signals from the brain representing symptoms and motor or other behavior activity.[109,110]

The most critical factor for successful DBS outcomes is selection of appropriate patients. Levodopa responsiveness is considered the single best predictor of DBS outcome. Symptoms that are under- or unresponsive to levodopa (gait, postural instability, speech, and posture) will likely not improve with DBS and may in fact worsen. A multidisciplinary evaluation is important for uncovering potential risks and benefits and to individualize alternative approaches. These teams include the neurologist, neurosurgeon, psychologist, psychiatrist, speech-language pathologists, and physical and occupational therapists. After separate evaluations by each team member, the decision to reject or to recommend DBS surgery is made.[109,110]

■ FRAMEWORK FOR REHABILITATION

Rehabilitation has an important role in early and long-term management to reduce activity limitations and disability and optimize function, activity participation, and independence. Disability is seen even early in the disease with nonmotor signs and symptoms being prevalent in the prodromal period and accumulated motor and nonmotor signs by the time of diagnosis. Growing evidence points to the importance of physical therapy, exercise, and physical activity for addressing motor and nonmotor symptoms, function, and disability.[111] Optimal management involves person-centered, team-based care with a coordinated interdisciplinary team to oversee a comprehensive plan of care to address individual clinical problems, concerns, needs, and goals as they change through every stage of the disease. The team begins with the patient and their family and care partners and typically includes the neurologist (ideally a movement disorders specialist), nurse, physical therapist, occupational therapist, speech-language pathologist, and social worker. The team may also include other specialists such as a psychologist, psychiatrist, nutritionist, gastroenterologist, urologist, pulmonologist, and others as needed.

The ideal rehabilitation program considers the patient's age of onset, disease history, course, and symptoms, together with impairments, activity limitations, and participation restrictions. Of equal importance are the patient's abilities (assets), priorities, and resources, including family, home, work, and community resources.

Eventual medication-induced fluctuations in performance and deterioration of condition should be expected, but early intervention with moderate to high physical activity can slow this deterioration. Depression and anxiety are common and should be carefully monitored. The overall focus is on improving level of physical activity and associated health behavior changes throughout all stages of the disease, followed by long-range planning and episodes of care including hospital-based, outpatient, and home-/community-based care. Interventions are restorative (aimed at improving impairments, activity limitations, and participation restrictions), preventive (aimed at minimizing potential complications and indirect impairments), and compensatory (aimed at modifying the task, activity, or environment to improve function) (see discussion in Chapter 1, Clinical Decision-Making). It is critical for the whole team to provide a supportive environment and promote active participation, health behavior change, shared decision-making, autonomy, and empowerment in living with a chronic and progressive disease. This approach and focus on the relief of symptoms, pain, and stress of a serious illness, called *palliative care,* is misunderstood as end-of-life care. However, palliative care is appropriate throughout *all* stages of the disease and can be provided in parallel with curative treatments with the goal of improved QOL for patients and families.[112,113]

Rehabilitation Care Paths and Delivery

Rafferty et al.[114] proposed a framework of care delivery that incorporates the different stages of PD: (1) a consultative, proactive rehabilitation approach in the early stage; (2) a traditional restorative approach addressing functional improvements in mid-stage; and (3) a skilled maintenance approach for long-term monitoring in advanced-stage PD. The newest model of care for people with PD recommends rehabilitation visits with clinicians having specialty training in PD for reevaluation every 6 to 12 months.[111,114,115] Early in the disease and at the time of diagnosis, the consultative, proactive approach can be considered secondary prevention. Individuals at this stage are functional and independent with minimal impairments. The numerous and mild motor and nonmotor symptoms can be measured, assessed, and addressed at this early stage, including changes in the person's voice, cognitive function, performance at work, and the more complex aspects of daily tasks. Traditionally, referral for physical therapy has been delayed at this stage. However, there is growing evidence that benefits could clearly be obtained in improving fitness levels and delaying or preventing indirect impairments. Studies of interdisciplinary intensive rehabilitation in newly diagnosed individuals with PD have suggested that early and intensive exercise might slow the progression of motor decline, delay the need for increasing drug treatment, and therefore have a neuroprotective

effect.[116,117] Patients in the early stage are typically seen on an outpatient basis, and the proactive, consultative rehabilitation can often be provided in four or fewer visits across a couple of months. Specific mobility strategies such as gait and balance practice, treadmill training, use of external cues, and large-amplitude movement can be introduced in this early stage to take advantage of intact or only mildly affected motor learning and cognition.[114]

During the *middle* stage of the disease, symptoms are more readily apparent, and activity limitations emerge. The patient may still be independent in gait and ADL, although performance is slowed and less efficient. Some assistance may be required. The patient may be seen as an outpatient, during home care, or during a brief inpatient admission. Rehabilitation goals in this stage are often achieved with visits two to four times a week for at least a month.[114] Exercise training programs have been shown to be effective for patients with mild to moderate PD in improving motor performance.[111] Perceived QOL and subjective well-being are also improved. Family and caregiver instruction is intensified to assist the patient in remaining as functionally independent as possible.

In the *late* stage, disease progression leads to increased and more severe impairments and complications. Patients are dependent in many or most of their daily functional mobility skills and ADL and are typically wheelchair bound or bedridden. Family and community resources are vital in maintaining the patient in the home. Some patients may require placement in a chronic care facility. These changes can be a source of great anxiety and frustration to the patient and family. Goals need to be restructured. The therapist needs to focus on preventive care to avoid secondary complications that may be life threatening (e.g., pneumonia, pressure injuries). Compensatory training focuses on maintaining function, including being upright and out of bed as much as possible. Safety for both the caregiver and the patient becomes a primary concern as maximal assist dependent transfers become the norm. Often, environmental adaptations may mean the difference between total dependence and modified dependence. The rehabilitation team should be supportive of the patient's efforts no matter how small they may be. Patients in late-stage PD demonstrate extremely limited skills to interact with their environment, with increasing social isolation and withdrawal. Families also suffer from the increasing demands of care, burnout, and social isolation. Therapists need to maximize psychosocial support and be readily available for consultation, with a visit every few months or so as needed, on an ongoing basis.

Maintenance therapy is defined as a series of occasional clinical, educational, and administrative services designed to maintain the patient's current level of function. Individuals with PD who benefit from maintenance therapy typically are in the late stages of the disease. Maintenance programs have historically not been well funded by insurance and require careful documentation. The Centers for Medicare and Medicaid Services (CMS), which cover services for older adults and those with disabilities, cover maintenance therapy if the *professional skills of a therapist* (specialized knowledge and judgment) are needed to prevent or slow deterioration of a person's condition and maintain the maximal predictable level of function. As the result of a legal settlement agreement on January 24, 2013, in the case of *Jimmo v. Sibelius,* CMS issued a clarification that the coverage of skilled services "does not turn on the presence or absence of a beneficiary's potential for improvement, but rather on the beneficiary's need for skilled care" (https://www.cms.gov/Center/Special-Topic/Jimmo-Center). For example, risk of secondary impairment and loss of functional capabilities is reduced, or safety of caregivers is enhanced. More information on the *Jimmo* settlements and implementation resources can be found on the Academy of Neurologic Physical Therapy (ANPT) website (http://neuropt.org/professional-resources/advocacy/jimmo-implementation-information). A variety of interventions are used to achieve goals and outcomes, including limited direct interventions, patient-/client-related instruction, and supportive counseling. The therapist tapers the frequency of the visits as the patient or family/caregivers are able to assume independent self-management of the care plan. Table 18.3 presents an overview of intervention strategies and rehabilitation goals across stages of PD, modified from Rafferty et al.[114]

■ PHYSICAL THERAPY EXAMINATION AND EVALUATION

A comprehensive examination is required to determine the level of impairments and extent of neurological and functional involvement. Subsequent reexamination at specified intervals is used to distinguish change in status as well as effects of treatment. Consider the patient's medication schedule and fatigue level when scheduling the examination, as function may fluctuate throughout the day. Physical therapy examination data are obtained from the history, systems review, and relevant tests and measures. The selection of examination procedures and instruments is determined by the patient's unique status and related to disease stage.

This section presents strategies for examination as well as relevant tests and measures. Complete descriptions of many of the tests and measures identified are provided in earlier chapters focusing on examination, including the Core Set of Outcome Measures for Adults with Neurologic Conditions recommended by the ANPT.[118]

Patient/Client History

A thorough interview with the patient/family/care partners and medical records review will provide information on demographics, social participation and employment history, family history, living and working environments, general health history, social and health habits, leisure and exercise/activity history, disease duration,

Table 18.3 Rehabilitation Care Path Framework for Parkinson Disease—Physical Therapy[114]		
Consultative and Proactive Rehabilitation in Early PD	**Restorative Rehabilitation for Functional Improvement (any stage)**	**Skilled Maintenance for Long-Term Monitoring in Advanced PD**
Assessment, education about the disease, and advice on recommended activities and self-management	Address impairments and function limitations that affect activities and participation through any stage of PD	Maintain vital functions, prevent complications (pressure sores, contractures), support care partners/nurses
• Assess baseline functional measures • Prevent inactivity through individually tailored exercise advice, prescription, and coaching • Address and prevent fear of movement or falling • Improve physical capacity • Address pain • Delay onset of activity limitations	• Assess functional measures • Prescribe exercise to address impairments • Address walking, balance, transfers, manual activities, and motor function problems • Train movement strategies	• Assess function as needed • Support exercise to minimize reduction in physical capacity • Correct body posture in bed/wheelchair • Support periodic changes in position • Involve and coach the care partners/nursing staff in the interventions • Maintain vital functions, prevent complications (pressure sores, contractures), support care partners/nurses

PD = Parkinson disease.

medication and medical procedures history, coexisting health problems, past and current falls, current/primary complaints, and current functional status.

Systems Review

Data obtained from the history and medical record will inform the systems review and help focus selection of appropriate tests and measures (Box 18.3). Review of the following systems is included: (1) cardiovascular/pulmonary; (2) cognitive, affective, and communication; (3) genitourinary; (4) integumentary; (5) musculoskeletal; and (6) neuromuscular.

Tests and Measures
Musculoskeletal Function
Joint Flexibility and Posture

An examination of musculoskeletal ROM and flexibility is important. The therapist can document specific active range of motion (AROM) and passive range of

---

 Box 18.3 Elements of the Examination for a Patient With Parkinson Disease

History

- Demographic information: age, sex, race/ethnicity, primary language, education
- Social history: cultural beliefs and behaviors, family and care partner resources, social support systems
- Occupation/employment/work information
- Living environment: home/work barriers
- Hand dominance
- General health status: physical, psychological, social, role function, and behavioral health risks
- Social and health habits (current and past)
- Family history
- Medical/surgical history
- Current conditions/chief complaints
- Medications
- Medical/laboratory/clinical test results
- Functional status and activity level: premorbid and current

Systems Review

- Cardiovascular/pulmonary
- Cognitive, affective, and communication
- Genitourinary
- Integumentary
- Musculoskeletal
- Neuromuscular

Tests and Measures

- Aerobic capacity and endurance: during functional activities and standardized exercise protocols including cardiovascular signs and symptoms in response to exercise and activity (see Autonomic); pulmonary signs and symptoms in response to exercise and activity
- Anthropometric characteristics: body mass index, girth, length; edema
- Assistive or adaptive devices: fit, alignment, function, use; safety
- Autonomic nervous system integrity: thermal responses, sweating; gastrointestinal signs and symptoms, constipation/bowel incontinence, urinary urgency/incontinence; salivation/drooling; orthostatic hypotension; cardiac sympathetic denervation
- Circulation: response to position change, degree of orthostatic hypotension (see Autonomic)

- Cognition: mental status, learning, memory, hesitation, slowness of thought processes, attention, visuospatial processing
- Communication
- Cranial and peripheral nerve integrity
- Environment, home, and work barriers
- Functional status and activity level: performance-based examination of functional skills, basic and instrumental activities of daily living; functional mobility skills; home management skills
- Gait and locomotion: gait pattern and speed, safety
- Integumentary integrity: skin condition, pressure-sensitive areas; activities, positioning, and postures to relieve pressure
- Joint integrity, alignment, and mobility: range of motion (active and passive); muscle length, and soft tissue extensibility
- Motor function: motor control and motor learning: tone, voluntary movement patterns; involuntary movements; hesitation, slowness, arrests of movements; poverty of movements
- Muscle performance: strength, power, and endurance
- Neuromotor control and sensory processing
- Oromotor function: communication (fluctuations, reduced volume), swallowing
- Pain: intensity, quality, behavior, and location
- Perceptual function: visuospatial skills
- Postural control and balance: degree of postural instability, balance strategies, safety
- Posture: alignment and position, symmetry (static and dynamic); ergonomics, and body mechanics
- Procedural learning for complex and sequential tasks
- Psychosocial function: motivation, apathy, self-efficacy, fear of falling, anxiety, and depression
- Range of motion (see Joint integrity)
- Reflex integrity
- Self-care and domestic life
- Sensory integrity and integration
- Skeletal integrity
- Ventilation and gas exchange
- Work, community, and leisure activities: ability to participate in activities, safety

motion (PROM) impairments using goniometric measurement. Patients with PD are likely to present with losses in hip and knee extension, dorsiflexion, shoulder flexion, elbow extension, dorsal spine and neck extension, and axial rotation.

It is particularly important to examine spinal ROM (ability to rotate, side-bend, flex, and extend the spine) because patients with PD have been shown to exhibit impairments in this area.[119] All segments of the spine should be examined, including cervical, thoracic, and lumbar segments. Spinal inclinometers such as the Back Range of Motion II (BROM II) and Cervical Range of Motion instruments have been shown to be valid and reliable in measuring spinal ROM and forward head posture.[120] The use of a head-mounted laser and wall measurements is a novel way to assess transverse plane spine ROM. Standing with feet stationary, the patient rotates as far as possible to one side. An objective measurement of full body (trunk) rotation is obtained by measuring the distance that the laser moves along the wall. This multisegmental measurement may be a better predictor of functional trunk mobility than isolated measurements of cervical and lumbar ROM. The mobility of the spine can also be examined using a series of functional movements, such as axial rotation (looking behind) in sitting and standing and walking. Hamstring length can be determined using a straight leg test.

An examination of resting posture and changes in posture that occur with movement is indicated. The therapist can use posture grids, plumb lines, still photography, or videotape to document changes. A flexible ruler contoured to the patient's spine in standing and then traced onto graph paper can be used to record static sagittal plane posture. This technique is affordable, with good intratester and intertester reliability, and was shown to have a high correlation to radiographic measurements of the lumbar and thoracic spine.[121] In standing, patients with PD typically assume a flexed, stooped posture (kyphosis with forward head) with the COM placed forward within the reduced LOS (Fig. 18.4). The Occiput to Wall test has been found to be a valid and reliable measurement of forward head posture in individuals with PD.[122] In supine, the flexed posture with forward head is still evident (shadow pillow posture) (Fig. 18.5).

Muscle Performance

An examination of strength and endurance is indicated. The therapist can measure strength using manual muscle testing. Handheld and isokinetic dynamometry can be used to quantify peak force (torque output). Patients with PD have been shown to exhibit impairments in the rate of force development and in maximum torque production capability. Isokinetic dynamometry can also be used to document muscle endurance and has been suggested for documenting tremor, using slow speeds of movement (25 mm/sec) and low torques.

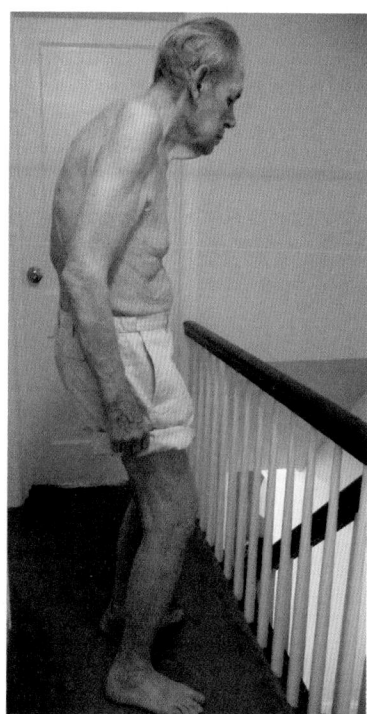

Figure 18.4 In standing, the patient with Parkinson disease demonstrates the typical flexed, stooped posture with kyphosis, forward head, and hip and knee flexion.

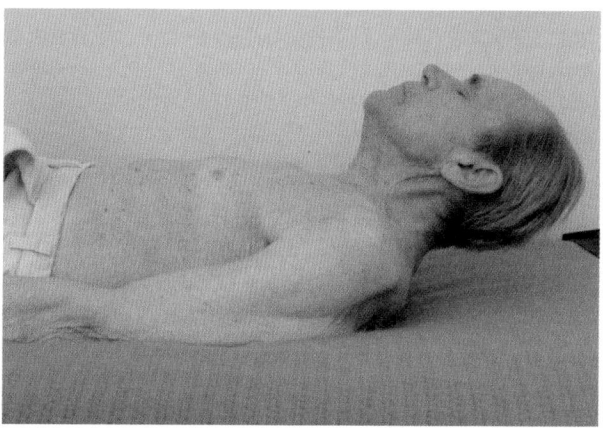

Figure 18.5 In supine, the patient with Parkinson disease demonstrates the typical flexed posture (shadow pillow posture).

Motor Function
Bradykinesia

Initially movements are slowed, then movements decrease in amplitude (hypokinesia); in later stages, movements become arrhythmic with frequent start hesitations and arrests (akinesia). A stopwatch can be used to quantify detectable slowing of movement *(movement time)* and start hesitancy or *reaction time* (elapsed time between the patient's desire to move and the actual movement response). The therapist should examine overall amplitude of movement and fluctuations in amplitude. For example, impaired coordination and asymmetry of arm swing during walking is a common finding in early PD. As the disease progresses, movements are characterized by marked slowness, poverty, and reduced amplitude. Timed tests for rapid alternating movements (RAM) can be used to determine the effects of bradykinesia. Examples of RAM include repeated opposition of the forefinger and thumb, alternating between pronation and supination, opening and closing of hands, and tapping (finger or foot tapping). Dexterity in complex motor tasks (e.g., writing, dressing, skilled object manipulation) can be expected to be impaired and should be examined. This is also true for motor tasks involving simultaneous use of both sides (e.g., bilateral RAM between pronation and supination). See items 3.4 to 3.8 and 3.14 in Part III of the MDS-UPDRS,[26] and Chapter 6, Examination of Coordination and Balance, for additional test examples.

Tremor

The location, persistence, and severity (amplitude) of tremor should be recorded. The therapist should determine if tremor is present at rest (initial typical pattern) or present with action and interferes with function. This latter pattern may occur in severe, long-standing disease. UE functional skills such as drinking from a cup, feeding, dressing, and writing can be used to test for the effects of tremor during movement. With severe tremor, the patient will be unable to complete the functional task. Stress can increase tremor. See items 3.15 to 3.18 in Part III of the MDS-UPDRS for test examples.[26]

Rigidity

Rigidity is usually equal in both agonist and antagonist muscle groups. As mentioned earlier, it can be sustained (lead pipe) or intermittent (cogwheel). Distribution of rigidity is often asymmetrical, especially in the early stages of the disease, and can vary throughout the day, at various points in the medication cycle, and with stress. It is therefore important to determine which body segments are affected and the severity of involvement. The patient should be seated or supine in a relaxed position. The therapist moves each extremity through full PROM. For head and neck and spinal PROM, the patient can be seated on a mat or at the edge of a chair, perch sitting, to allow for excursion of spinal motions (flexion, extension, rotation). A determination of severity of rigidity can be made based on the level of resistance to passive movement and availability of ROM. See item 3.3 in Part III of the MDS-UPDRS for test examples.[26] Deficits in functional mobility and postural reactions should be suspected in the presence of significant trunk rigidity.[123] The patient should also be examined for facial mobility (e.g., hypomimia or masked face) including ability to produce spontaneous expressions and part the lips; the ability to smile or use

the muscles of facial expression should also be examined. An inspection of voluntary repetitive movements should be performed to determine active limitations imposed by rigidity.

Dyskinesia

Drug-induced dyskinesias have a profound effect on physical and social functioning. Risk factors include high total dosage of dopaminergic drugs, young age at onset of PD, and extended duration of the disease process.[103,124] The *Rush Dyskinesia Scale* assesses functional disability by grading the subject walking, drinking from a cup, and putting on and buttoning a coat.[125] This scale has been used extensively in clinical trials and patient care and has undergone extensive clinimetric testing.[126] The *Unified Dyskinesia Rating Scale (UDysRS)* is a four-part comprehensive rating tool developed by the MDS to assess dyskinesias using the patient perspective, objective impairment, and objective disability approaches.[26] The therapist can explore the impact of motor fluctuations using questions that address changes in performance during the day.

Postural Control and Balance

A thorough examination of postural control and balance is indicated. The therapist should first observe the patient's resting posture in sitting and standing. The patient's perception of trunk rotation and of vertical may be impaired; some patients with advanced disease will perceive themselves as fully upright when they are actually leaning forward or to one side.[127]

Clinical measures of balance performance have been shown to be reliable and sensitive in the examination of functional performance and balance in patients with PD.[128] These include the *Berg Balance Scale* (BBS),[129] the *Functional Reach Test* (FRT),[130] the *Timed Up-and-Go test* (TUG),[131] the *Cognitive Timed Up-and-Go* (CTUG),[132] and the *Dynamic Gait Index* (DGI).[133] These tests are discussed in Chapter 6, Examination of Coordination and Balance. The BBS correlates well with the UPDRS and has been found to be a good overall measure of function in this population.[134,135] Dibble and Lange demonstrated that each of these tests has the ability to discriminate among people with PD who had a history of falls from those without a history of falls and suggested cutoff scores to maximize sensitivity and minimize false negatives.[136] False negatives can also be reduced when interpretation is based on the collective interpretation of multiple balance tests. A clinical decision-making algorithm that involves the serial use of clinical balance tests has been proposed.[137] Studies evaluating the BBS, the *Fullerton Advanced Balance Scale (FAB)*,[138] the *Functional Gait Assessment (FGA)*,[139] the *Balance Evaluation Systems Test (BESTest)*,[140] and the *Mini Balance Evaluation Systems Test (Mini-BESTest)*[141] have shown that all tests demonstrated high reliability scores.[142,143] The FAB, Mini-BESTest, and BBS showed similar accuracy in predicting falls, and the BESTest was most sensitive for identifying fallers.[142-144] The BBS, FGA, and DGI all have ceiling effects in early-stage PD.[128,144] Steffen and Seney found high reliability scores for the BBS, the 6-minute Walk Test (6MWT), and gait speed.[145] In contrast, the *Tinetti Gait Assessment* was not sensitive for detecting change in gait impairments in people with moderately disabling PD.[128] Strong stability of measurements on balance tests occurs during the "on" phase of the medication cycle, while stability of measurements is not maintained during the "off" period.[146] See Table 18.4 for descriptions, scoring, and minimal detectible change values.

Reduced postural control is evident during quiet standing (static control), with increased oscillations in both medial–lateral and anterior–posterior planes.[147]

During dynamic posturographic tests, postural restabilization strategies are often inadequate to maintain balance. Available postural strategies and reactions should be carefully documented (e.g., use of ankle, hip, and stepping strategies). Healthy individuals typically respond initially using an ankle strategy with small shifts in their COM, followed by hip and stepping strategies with larger shifts in the COM. Persons with PD and the older adult population in general typically respond to destabilizing forces with postural strategies involving more the hip joints than ankle joints. Start hesitation, abnormal coactivation patterns (rigid body) with an inability to recover a stable posture, is common. An absence of postural strategies (i.e., patient would fall if not for overhead body support harness) is also seen in advanced disease. During complex postural

Table 18.4 Selected Outcome Measures for Persons With Parkinson Disease by International Classification of Functioning, Disability, and Health Domain

Outcome Measure and ICF Category	Description	Scoring	MDC/MCID
MoCA[162] *Body Function and Structure*	16-item screen of multiple cognitive domains to detect mild cognitive impairment	Criteria are given for scoring each item for a total score (max 30 points). Cutoff scores: less than 26/30 mild cognitive impairment (PD-MCI); less than 22/30 dementia (PDD).	MDC: not established MCID: not established
Mini-BESTest[140] *Body Function and Structure Activity*	14-item clinical balance assessment in four domains, shortened version of the BESTest*	Items are scored on a three-point scale (0–2) for a total score (max 28).	MDC: 17.1% or 5.52 points (PD) MCID: four points (balance disorders)
PFS-16[175] *Body Function and Structure Activity*	16-item self-report measure for physical fatigue and its impact on daily function	Items are scored from 1–5 and summed for a total score (16–80).	MDC: not established MCID: not established
MDS-UPDRS[25] *Body Function and Structure Activity Participation*	Four-part comprehensive clinical rating scale for assessment of the extent and burden of PD	Items are scored from 0–4 and summed for each part. Parts I and II (13 questions each) rate nonmotor and motor experiences of daily living. Part III motor exam has 33 scores on 18 items. Part IV has six questions on motor complications.	MDC: not established MCID: not established
NMSQuest[73] *Activity Participation*	30-item self-report questionnaire covering 10 domains based on the previous month to screen the presence of NMS in PD and their impact of quality of life	Items scored as "yes," "no," or "don't know."	MDC: not established MCID: not established

(Continued)

Table 18.4   Selected Outcome Measures for Persons With Parkinson Disease by International Classification of Functioning, Disability, and Health Domain—cont'd

Outcome Measure and ICF Category	Description	Scoring	MDC/MCID
NMSS[161] *Body Function and Structure* *Activity* *Participation*	30-item scale covering nine dimensions based on the previous month for the assessment of frequency and severity of NMS in PD	Items scored on Severity (0–3) and on Frequency (1–4). Each item Severity and Frequency scores are multiplied, then summed within each domain. Total score is sum of domain scores.	MDC: not established MCID: not established
PDQ-39[259] or **PDQ-8** *Participation*	39-item self-report questionnaire based on previous month for assessment of PD-related health quality in eight dimensions Eight-item version of the PDQ-39	Items scored from 0–4 on previous month's experience. Scores are summed for each dimension, divided by max possible dimension score, and multiplied by 100. Overall summary index is sum of dimension total scores divided by 8.	MDC: 12–24 points across dimensions MCID: –11.4–1.3 points across dimensions
NFOG-Q[156] *Activity* *Participation*	Nine-item questionnaire in three parts based on previous month: Part I Distinction of freezer or nonfreezer; Part II Severity; Part III Impact on daily life	Criteria are given for scoring each item for a total score (max 29 points). High score indicates more severe freezing.	MDC: 9.95 (7.90–12.27) points MCID: 35.5%[157]
†**6MWT**[145] *Activity*	A measure of walking endurance	Utilize a marked course (33 meters) and measure wheel to obtain distance traveled in 6 minutes.	MDC: 82 meters or 269 feet (PD) MCID: 54–80 meters (COPD, geriatrics, stroke)
†**10MWT**[260] *Activity*	A measure of comfortable and fast walking speeds	Times are recorded to walk 10 m at the individual's (1) comfortable and (2) fastest safe speed.	MDC: 0.02–0.18 m/s comfortable speed; 0.09–0.25 m/s fastest speed (PD) MCID: 0.10–0.16 m/s (geriatrics, stroke)
Nine-Hole Peg Test[184] *Activity*	A measure of manual dexterity; the individual removes nine pegs from a pegboard to a well, one at a time, and then returns the pegs to the pegboard, one at a time	Time to complete this task is measured in seconds for both the dominant and nondominant hands.	MDC: 2.6 sec dominant, 1.3 sec nondominant hand (PD) MCID: not established
†*****Activities-Specific Balance Confidence Scale** *Activity* *Participation*	16-item self-report measure evaluating confidence performing home and community functional activities on a 0%–100% scale	Sum of the scores divided by 16 gives the final average score. Higher scores indicate better balance confidence.	MDC: 11.12–13 (PD) MCID: not established

Table 18.4 Selected Outcome Measures for Persons With Parkinson Disease by International Classification of Functioning, Disability, and Health Domain—cont'd

Outcome Measure and ICF Category	Description	Scoring	MDC/MCID
†*BBS *Activity*	14-item balance performance test	Items are scored 0–4 for a maximal score of 56. Scores ≤45 are associated with greater fall risk.	MDC: five points (PD) MCID: not established
*DGI *Activity*	Eight-item walking test examining changing task demands when walking (i.e., head turns, change in speed, obstacles, turns, stops, stairs)	Items are scored 0–3 for a maximal score of 24.	MDC: 2.9 points and 13.3% (PD)[152] MCID: four points (migraine and vestibular disorders)
*Functional Reach *Activity*	A measure of the maximal forward reach of an individual	A yardstick is secured to the walk at shoulder height; the individual flexes their arm forward 90° with the hand in a fist. After reaching as far forward as possible, the distance is recorded at the third metacarpal head.	MDC: 9 cm (PD) MCID: not established
†Functional Gait Assessment[139] *Activity*	10-item assessment of dynamic gait	Items scored from 0–3 for a maximum score of 30.	MDC: five points (stroke) MCID: not established
†Five Times Sit-to-Stand Test[186-188] *Activity*	A measure of functional leg strength	Time to stand up from and return to sitting in a chair five times consecutively is recorded. Cutoff score of 16 sec discriminates PD fallers from nonfallers.	MDC: 10 sec MCID: not established
*TUG *Activity*	A measure of dynamic balance	Time to stand from a chair, walk 3 meters, turn, and return to sitting in the chair is recorded.	MDC: 3.5–11 seconds (PD) MCID: not established
TUG Cognitive[132] *Activity*	A measure of dynamic balance with the addition of a secondary challenge	Time to perform the TUG with a cognitive task (subtract by 3's).	MDC: not established MCID: not established

Measures included in the Core Set of Outcome Measures for Adults with Neurologic Conditions recommended by the Academy of Neurologic Physical Therapy.[118]

*Please reference Chapter 6, Examination of Coordination and Balance, for additional information on these balance measures.

†Measures included in the Core Set of Outcome Measures for Adults with Neurologic Conditions recommended by the Academy of Neurologic Physical Therapy.[118]

All measures but the NMSQuest and NMSS are "highly recommended" or "recommended" by the *PD EDGE Task Force* for use across settings (acute, inpatient rehabilitation, home health, skilled nursing facility, and outpatient) *and* required at entry-level education (http://www.neuropt.org/docs/default-source/parkinson-edge/pdedge-all-documents-combined.pdf?sfvrsn=2).

BBS = Berg Balance Scale; COPD = chronic obstructive pulmonary disease; DGI = Dynamic Gait Index; ICF = International Classification of Functioning, Disability, and Health; MCID = minimal clinically important difference; MDC = minimally detectable change; MDS-UPDRS = Movement Disorders Society sponsored Unified Parkinson Disease Rating Scale; Mini-BESTest = Mini-Balance Evaluation Systems Test; MoCA = Montreal Cognitive Assessment; NFOG-Q = New Freezing of Gait Questionnaire; NMS = nonmotor symptom; NMSQuest = Nonmotor Symptoms Questionnaire; NMSS = Nonmotor Symptoms Scale; PDD = Parkinson disease dementia; PD-MCI = frequency of mild cognitive impairment due to Parkinson disease; PDQ-8 = Parkinson Disease Questionnaire-8; PDQ-39 = Parkinson Disease Questionnaire-39; PFS-16 = Parkinson Fatigue Scale-16; 6MWT = 6-minute Walk Test; 10MWT = 10-meter Walk Test; TUG = Timed Up and Go.

situations involving sensory conflict (e.g., the Sensory Organization Test), persons with advanced PD typically demonstrate reduced postural performance, suggesting inadequate sensory organization.[148] Balance control can also be expected to degrade under conditions of reduced cognitive monitoring. Patients with PD, especially in the early stages of the disease, may not demonstrate balance impairments in response to steady standing with normal BOS or self-initiated movements as long as their attention is fully directed to the task at hand. However, if competing attentional demands are instituted (i.e., *dual-task interference* such as talking while balancing), instability can be seen.[147] Balance confidence is also related to functional mobility and falls in people with PD.[149]

Gait

Parameters and characteristics of gait that should be examined during unobstructed walking on level surfaces include start time or gait initiation, speed of walking, stride length, cadence, stability, variability, and safety. The *10-meter Walk Test* can be used to determine speed, average stride, and cadence, or more sophisticated kinetic analysis can be obtained from embedded force plates, body markers, and computerized equipment (motion analysis systems typically seen in the laboratory setting). Persons with PD frequently demonstrate decreased step length and trunk rotation, difficulty initiating gait, and difficulty attaining increased walking speed. When instructed to walk as fast as possible, the movements produced are smaller and more variable when compared to healthy older adults.

Gait should be examined for kinematic or qualitative changes, including reductions in hip, knee, and ankle motions that result in a short-stepped, shuffling (festinating) gait pattern with reduced trunk rotation and arm swing. Postural abnormalities that contribute to the development of a festinating gait pattern should be documented (i.e., flexed, stooped posture). Gait should be examined in all movement directions: forward, backward, and sideways. A complex gait pattern such as cross-stepping or braiding can be used to examine deficits in motor planning. Patients with advanced PD typically have difficulty with adaptability and cannot easily vary walking or walk in complex confined areas such as narrow doorways or open environments. Walking should be examined in varied environments (e.g., community environment) or negotiating an obstacle course. Increased difficulty in walking is also experienced in response to varying attentional demands and dual-task interference. Changes in gait speed, stride length, and cadence can be observed while simultaneously performing a secondary cognitive task (e.g., talking while walking) or walking while simultaneously performing a secondary motor task (e.g., buttoning a coat). Gait performance in individuals with PD was significantly impaired when walking and talking on the cell phone.[150] The degree of change was similar with regard to type of dual-task interference.[151] Clinical measures of locomotor performance shown to be reliable and sensitive for people with PD include the DGI, FGA, and TUG (all previously discussed). Huang et al.[152] identified the minimal detectable change values for both the TUG and the DGI.

Freezing of Gait

FOG is an episodic inability to generate effective stepping in the absence of any known cause, and it has a dramatic effect on QOL and risk of falls for patients with PD.[153,154] Assessment is often difficult due to the unpredictable nature of the episodes. The therapist needs to document triggers or provoking factors. Common triggers for FOG include initiating gait, walking through narrow passages (e.g., doorway) or turning in tight spaces, a change in the environment or attentional demands, and walking under time pressure, anxiety, or stress. In the early stages of the disease, episodes are levodopa sensitive and more common in the "off" time. In advanced stages, FOG can occur during the "on" time.[155] The *New Freezing of Gait Questionnaire (NFOG-Q)* is a three-part questionnaire and short video to detect and rate FOG severity and impact but is only able to reliably detect changes above 35%.[156,157]

Falls and Fall Risk

A determination of fall history and fall injuries is an important component of the examination of balance and gait function. There is a strong association between duration and severity of PD with increased risk of falls. Of particular significance are balance and walking impairments including shortened stride length, decreased cadence, slower walking speed, FOG, anterior displacement of COM, decreased postural righting reactions, and the presence of dyskinesias.[40] Other linked factors include postural hypotension, dementia, depression, and prior history of falls.[158–160] A *fall diary* can be used to assist the patient and family/caregivers in accurately recording a fall event and the context of daily life in which the fall occurred. For example, activity at the time of the fall, relation to timing of medication and food intake, type of footwear, degree of fatigue and injury, and other risk factors all should be documented. The need for assisted gait and frequency of contact guarding from family members or caregivers during walking should also be documented.

Nonmotor Symptoms and Autonomic Function

The *Nonmotor Symptoms Questionnaire (NMSQuest)* was the first comprehensive self-report measure to assess the presence NMSs of PD and their impact on activities and QOL.[94] The *Nonmotor Symptom Scale (NMSS)* was developed in conjunction with the NMSQuest to assess the frequency and severity of NMSs in patients with PD across all stages.[161] The therapist should examine for problems with autonomic dysfunction.

Excessive drooling (salivation) or sweating, greasy skin, and abnormalities in thermoregulation should be noted. Excessive sweating and flushing during the "on" state are linked to the presence of dyskinesias.

Cognitive Function

Learning and memory, visuospatial processing, orientation, conceptual reasoning, problem-solving, and judgment should be examined. Speed of information processing, attention, and concentration are particularly important to determine if bradyphrenia is suspected. A brief screen of cognitive function across multiple cognitive domains (visuospatial and executive function, attention, orientation, naming, memory, language, abstraction) can be obtained using the *Montreal Cognitive Assessment (MoCA),* available with training and certification at https://www.mocatest.org/.[162]

Psychosocial Function

The therapist should determine overall levels of depression, stress and anxiety, and available coping strategies. It is important to ask the patient about the presence of symptoms such as sadness, apathy, passivity, insomnia, anorexia, weight loss, inactivity and dependency, inability to concentrate and impaired memory, or suicidal ideation. Instruments recommended for screening and measuring severity of depression in PD include the *Geriatric Depression Scales* (GDS-15 and GDS-30) and the *Hamilton Depression Rating Scale* (HAMD-17).[163–165] Anxiety is prevalent and disabling in this patient population. The *Geriatric Anxiety Inventory* and the *Parkinson Anxiety Scale* (PAS) are recommended for use in detecting and grading the severity of anxiety in PD without dementia.[166–168] The Emotional Well-Being index of the Parkinson Disease Questionnaire–39 (PDQ-39) has been found to be sensitive for detecting depression and anxiety.[169]

Sensory Function

A screening examination of sensation is indicated (superficial and deep sensations, combined cortical sensations). Sensory changes can be expected with aging, such as blunting of touch sensations and proprioception with greater losses in LEs than UEs, and distal more than proximal. Specific areas of sensory loss may be indicative of comorbid pathology, for example, stroke and diabetic neuropathy. The patient with PD should be asked about the presence of paresthesias (sensations of numbness or tingling) and pain. Mild aching and cramplike sensations are common and are often poorly localized. It is important to examine for musculoskeletal aches and pains linked to lack of movement, faulty movements or posture, and ligamentous strain.

An examination of vision should include a determination of acuity, peripheral vision, color discrimination, contrast sensitivity, tracking, accommodation, light and dark adaptation, and depth perception. Visual changes in PD include loss of visual acuity (both distance and near acuity), blurring of vision and difficulty reading not improved by corrective lenses, loss of color discrimination, difficulty detecting low contrast (shades of gray), problems with eye pursuit (cogwheeling), age-related decreased adaptation to light, and sensitivity to light and glare.[170] Medications may also produce impaired or fuzzy vision, for example, antidepressants and anticholinergics.

Vestibular function should be assessed with particular attention to examining sensory integration for balance. The processing of all three sensory systems is impacted by PD (somatosensory/proprioception, visual, vestibular), and identifying the relative contribution to postural control of each system is important for addressing balance and gait impairments. Vestibular rehabilitation has been shown to improve balance, eye tracking and gaze function, fatigue, and ADL, although the mechanism of action is unclear.[171] See Chapter 21, Vestibular Disorders, for more information on vestibular testing and rehabilitation.

Fatigue

Fatigue is a common impairment associated with PD. As the disease process progresses so does the prevalence of fatigue and its impact on QOL.[172] The International Parkinson and Movement Disorder Society (https://www.movementdisorders.org) created a task force to evaluate and make recommendations on available fatigue rating scales.[172] Following the systematic review, the task force recommended the *Multidimensional Fatigue Inventory (MFI),* the *Fatigue Severity Scale (FSS),* and the *Parkinson Fatigue Scale (PFS-16)* for assessment of fatigue in patients with PD. The MFI is a 20-item self-report scale that measures general fatigue, physical fatigue, mental fatigue, reduced motivation, and reduced activity.[173] The FSS is a self-administered nine-item rating scale that emphasizes the functional impact of fatigue.[174] The PFS-16 is a 16-item self-reported measure of physical fatigue and its impact on daily function,[175] described in Table 18.4.

Cardiorespiratory Function

Endurance may be reduced due to impaired cardiorespiratory function and long-standing inactivity, both common problems in PD. An examination of respiratory function should include inspection of rib cage compliance, chest wall mobility, and thoracic expansion. Visual inspection of breathing patterns and an examination of the influence of posture and activity on breathing should be performed. Objective measurements include respiratory rate (RR) and circumferential measurements of the chest. Specific ventilation parameters may be determined in patients with significant respiratory compromise. These can include FVC, FEV_1, maximal expiratory flow, maximal inspiratory flow, total lung capacity, RV, and RAW.

Individuals with mild PD (H&Y stages I and II) can demonstrate aerobic exercise capacities like healthy adults. Individuals with more advanced disease (H&Y stages III and IV) demonstrate greater variability and lower aerobic capacities compared to healthy adults. It is important to remember that many older adults are at high risk for latent cardiovascular disease. Exercise testing can be used to determine the patient's level of fitness before commencing an exercise program. Patients who have balance deficits or freezing episodes should not be tested on a treadmill without the use of a safety harness. Cycle ergometry (arm or leg) may be an acceptable alternative. A *6- or 12-min Walk Test* can be used to determine endurance capacity and walking velocity. The therapist should document vital signs (HR, RR, BP), exertional symptoms (dyspnea, dizziness or confusion, excessive fatigue, pallor, etc.), time, distance, and number of rest stops.[176] For patients with advanced PD (H&Y stages III and IV), the *2-minute Walk Test* to evaluate walking endurance is a sensitive and feasible test.[177] Perceived exertion can be documented using *Borg's Rating of Perceived Exertion Scale (RPE Scale)*.[178]

Orthostatic Hypotension

OH with positional change should be examined. Subjective signs and symptoms of OH on sitting up and standing up are documented (e.g., dizziness, lightheadedness, pallor, diaphoresis, or syncope). A drop in SBP of 20 mm Hg, or a drop of 10 mm Hg in diastolic blood pressure, *and* a 10% to 20% increase in pulse rate are diagnostic of the condition. The examination begins with the patient resting supine for 2 to 3 minutes. Resting BP and HR are taken. The patient is then asked to move from supine to sitting. After at least 1 minute, BP and HR are taken. If the patient is stable after at least 3 minutes (no symptoms), testing can be performed in the standing position. The patient is asked to move from sitting to standing with BP and HR again taken after at least 1 minute and repeated between 3 and 5 minutes. BP that continues to drop after at least 1 minute of standing is problematic and is evident in advanced PD.[89]

Integumentary Integrity

Sympathetic skin responses may be abnormal. For example, the skin may become oily (e.g., on the face). Seborrhea or seborrheic dermatitis occurs frequently in patients with PD. The therapist should examine the patient closely for areas of bruising and skin breakdown. Patients who are severely disabled (H&Y stage V) are restricted to bed, wheelchair, or both. Incontinence may occur during late-stage disease. The effect of these problems on skin integrity should be carefully documented. Use and effectiveness of pressure-relieving strategies and devices should also be documented.

Functional Status

An examination of functional status is indicated, including performance of functional mobility skills, basic ADL (BADL), and instrumental activities of daily living. A commonly used instrument for patients undergoing

active rehabilitation is the *Continuity Assessment Record and Evaluation (CARE) Item Set,* replacing the Functional Independence Measure (see Chapter 8, Examination of Function).[179] Need for and appropriate use of protective and supportive devices are an important component of the functional status examination. Close collaboration with the occupational therapist is essential.

Hand function is impacted by PD with dexterity problems being reported as one of the top contributors to disease burden.[180] For example, problems are common with ADL such as fastening clothes, tying shoes, using eating utensils, handling coins, turning pages, handwriting, using a cell phone, and typing on a touch screen tablet. Contributing factors include bradykinesia, tremor, dyskinesias, reduced coordination of the wrist and fingers, difficulty making sequential movements, impaired planning, and abnormal grip force adjustments.[181,182] There are few recommendations for outcome measures to assess hand function and its impact on QOL in people with PD.[183] The *Nine-Hole Peg Test* is commonly used, has shown high test–retest reliability, and its performance has been related to scores of bradykinesia and FOG.[184] The *Dexterity Questionnaire 24 (DextQ-24)* is a valid and reliable tool for evaluating dexterity in patients with PD.[185]

During functional performance tests, each skill should be analyzed to determine the impact of direct and indirect impairments on performance. For example, sit-to-stand transfers typically present a significant challenge for patients with moderate to severe PD as evidenced by increased time and increased falls. These changes have been attributed to hypokinesia, decreased rates of force production, and changes in distal muscle timing. The *Five Times Sit-to-Stand Test (FTSS)* is a timed test that has been used to determine performance in patients with PD at different disease stages and to discriminate between fallers and nonfallers with PD.[186,187] The average time for FTSS performance for community-dwelling individuals with PD was 20 seconds with a cutoff time of 16 seconds discriminating between fallers and nonfallers. Peterson et al. reported the minimal detectable change for the FTSS at 10 seconds.[188] Timed performance can also be used for other functional tasks such as rolling over in bed or moving from supine to sitting that are likely to prove difficult. These activities have a large rotational component of the trunk, typically lacking in many patients with PD.

Functional testing should be balanced with adequate rest to ensure that fatigue does not degrade performance with resultant fluctuations. Repeat testing should be undertaken at the same time of day and importantly at the same time in the medication cycle. Filming task activities can provide an objective record of functional performance. This is particularly useful to document motor fluctuations and dyskinesias. An examination of functional performance in the home (or work) environment is also indicated. The patient's physical environment is examined for barriers, access, and safety.

The *Profile of Function and Impairment Level Experience With Parkinson Disease* (*PROFILE PD*) was developed to assist the physical therapist's examination and evaluation of individuals with PD in the early and middle stages of disease. Half the test relates to deficits in body systems and cognitive/emotional factors. These include questions on tremor (with activity and at rest), rigidity, posture, postural stability, dyskinesia, dystonia, clinical fluctuations, falling, FOG, bradykinesia, speech, depression, memory, and involvement (routine daily/leisure/social activities). The other half of the test focuses on functional activities that are typically difficult for individuals with PD (e.g., dressing, hygiene, mealtime activities, transfers, bed mobility, chair rise, gait, fine and gross motor performance). Initial testing revealed it to be a reliable and valid scale with an estimated administration time of 15 minutes.[189]

Disease-Specific Measures

Disease-specific measures are designed to determine attributes unique to a specific disease entity. Items are included that provide information about the disease process and outcomes, and ideally document clinically meaningful change over time. Thus, these instruments have greater responsiveness or sensitivity to change than general health measures. The *Parkinson Disease Questionnaire (PDQ-39)* is a 39-item questionnaire developed from in-depth interviews with patients with PD.[190] It focuses on the subjective report of the impact of PD on daily life and addresses eight health-related quality-of-life dimensions (mobility, ADL, emotional well-being, stigma, social support, cognition, communication, and bodily discomfort). The PDQ-39 produces a profile of scores on the eight individual dimensions, and a summary score using the *Parkinson Disease Summary Index* can also be determined. It provides a useful indication of the global impact of PD on health status. Internal and test–retest reliability were moderate to high. Construct validity was good with significant and high correlations found between the PDQ-39 and the SF-36 and the H&Y staging score.[190]

The *Parkinson Database to Guide Effectiveness (PDEDGE)* task force of the ANPT compiled a list of measures for each relevant International Classification of Functioning, Disability, and Health (ICF) category together with instrument analysis, recommendations for use, and relevant references. The document can be found at http://www.neuropt.org/docs/default-source/parkinson-edge/pdedge-all-documents-combined.pdf?sfvrsn=2. Selected outcome measures are listed in Table 18.4.

Global Health Measures

Global health measures can be used to determine individual outcomes across a broad spectrum of populations. Instruments typically include items that examine ability to perform routine daily activities and QOL (e.g., physical and social function, general health and vitality, emotional well-being, bodily pain, and so forth).

General health measures have been used to study large populations and are most useful in determining long-term health outcomes. They lack the sensitivity needed to document short-term outcomes of treatment. Commonly used measures of general health status include the *Rand 36-Item Health Survey SF-36*[191] and the *Sickness Impact Profile.*[192]

Goals and Expected Outcomes

The general goals and expected outcomes for patients with progressive disorders of the CNS are presented in Box 18.4. These general goals will provide the basis for development of specific anticipated goals and expected outcomes for an individual patient.[114,193]

Box 18.4 Examples of General Goals and Expected Outcomes for Patients With Progressive Disorders of the Central Nervous System

Impact of pathology/pathophysiology is reduced.

- Decrease: risk of secondary impairment; intensity of care
- Improve: patient/client, family and care partner knowledge of disease, prognosis, and plan of care; symptom management

Impact of impairments is reduced.

- Decrease: pain
- Improve: cognitive function; joint integrity; mobility; sensory awareness; skin integrity; motor function; muscle performance; postural control and balance; gait and locomotion; management of fatigue; aerobic capacity

Ability to perform physical actions, tasks, or activities is improved.

- Improve: independence with activities of daily living; tolerance of positions and activities; activity pacing and energy conservation; problem-solving and decision-making skills; safety of patient, family, and care partners

Disability associated with chronic illness is reduced.

- Improve: ability to assume/resume self-care and home management; ability to assume work (job/school/play), community and leisure roles; patient/client and family knowledge and awareness of personal and environmental factors associated with condition worsening; awareness and use of community resources

Health status and quality of life are improved.

- Decrease: stressors
- Improve: sense of well-being; insight, self-confidence, and self-management skills; health, wellness, and fitness

Patient/client satisfaction is enhanced.

- Improve: acceptability of access and availability of services and quality of rehabilitation services to patient/client and family; coordination of care with patient/client, family, care partners, and other professionals

▪ PHYSICAL THERAPY INTERVENTION

A combined approach of physical therapy and pharmacological intervention is key in the management of the patient with PD. Despite best efforts, progressive disability develops and affects the patient's QOL. A variety of interventions to maximize functional ability and minimize secondary complications are used to achieve goals and outcomes, including direct interventions, supervision of assistive personnel, patient/family/caregiver instruction, environmental modification, and supportive counseling. Early intervention is critical in reducing the rate of decline and optimizing function and preventing secondary impairments. Interventions also focus on improvement of motor function, exercise capacity, functional performance, and activity participation. Education and support of patients, family members, and care partners at each stage of the disease are critical to attaining optimal outcomes. Strong evidence for evaluations and interventions by the rehabilitation team (PT, OT, SLP) has been summarized in clinical practice guidelines (see Table 18.3).[114,193]

Motor Learning Strategies

Patients with PD typically demonstrate motor learning deficits, including slower learning rates, reduced efficiency, and increased context-specificity of learning. Learning complex movement sequences and movements dependent on internally generated cues are more difficult than those dependent on external cues. In the early and middle stages of the disease, patients can improve their performance through practice and by using additional sensory information. The amount and persistence of learning are variable and can be expected to be lower than in healthy age-matched people. In more advanced stages and in the presence of pronounced cognitive deficits, training will likely be less successful.[46] The therapist needs to structure treatment sessions to optimize motor learning.

Critical elements of practice include many repetitions to develop procedural skills. The therapist should instruct the patient to deliberately focus their full attention on the desired movement, emphasizing self-awareness of the amplitude of movements. The environment should also be modified to reduce clutter and competing attentional demands that may trigger freezing episodes. The task should be modified to minimize competing cognitive demands (e.g., dual-tasking). Long and complex movement sequences should be limited initially or simplified, then progressed in complexity as the patient gains success. Initially, *random practice order* (i.e., practice in which the patient switches back and forth between tasks) should be avoided in favor of a *blocked practice order,* thereby reducing the effects of contextual interference. For example, walking patterns can be improved with focused instructions of "swing your arms," "walk

fast," or "take large steps." Self-controlled practice results in more effective skill learning than when the practice is determined by someone else.[194] For the patient with advanced disease and cognitive deficits, repetitive practice should be used together with an increased focus on caregiver training to ensure safety.

Cuing Strategies

External cues are effective in triggering sequential movements and improving movement characteristics in individuals with mild to moderate PD. *Visual cues* include stationary floor markings (e.g., brightly colored lines on the floor placed perpendicular to the gait path and spaced about one step length apart) and dynamic transportable cues (e.g., laser light signals). A laser light that projects a line onto the floor in front of the patient can be mounted on an assistive device (cane or walker) or on a subject's chest harness. Visual cues have been shown to improve stride length and velocity, while cadence was relatively unchanged.[195] Freezing episodes are also reduced. *Rhythmic auditory stimulation (RAS)* includes use of a metronome beat or a steady beat from a musical listening device. RAS has been shown to improve gait speed, cadence, and stride length, but for freezers a slight increase in frequency (10%) of the beat resulted in *reduced* step length compared to the *increased* step length for nonfreezers.[196] The beat is typically set 25% faster than the patient's preferred pace. Auditory cues such as "big step" have also been shown to improve gait. Cues should be consistent, not rushed, and have a rhythmical quality to them. Auditory cues appear to have a greater influence on the temporal components of movement (e.g., gait cadence, stride synchronization) rather than on spatial components. *Multisensory cuing* (use of both visual and auditory cuing) has been used for patients with PD. When sensory-enhanced therapy using multisensory cuing was compared with conventional therapy, significant improvements were found in the sensory training group.[197] However, the possible gait benefits of auditory cuing came at a cost in energy and poorer walking economy for patients walking on the treadmill at self-selected and slightly faster walking speed.[198]

External cues appear to facilitate movement by utilizing different brain areas. For example, the premotor cortex is active in the generation of movement in response to visual or auditory stimuli. Normally the SMA with inputs from the BG is involved in the initiation of self-generated movements and the performance of well-learned, repetitive movement sequences. External cues heighten patient attention through a common mode of action, that is, to bypass the diminished internal cuing of the BG. Thus, focus is shifted to less automatic movement using alternative, more conscious motor control pathways. This is supported by the finding that when patients were requested to carry out a secondary task while walking (dual-tasking), the beneficial effects of visual and attentional cues were reduced.[199]

Selection of the type of cue and successful use will depend on the individual patient with predicted long-term benefit of a particular type of cue linked to its initial success. Cues should be varied based on severity of the disease process and goals of treatment.[200] External cues are clearly not effective for all patients with PD. For patients with advanced disease and severe reductions in stride length, cuing is not effective. When cuing is withheld, performance can be expected to deteriorate. Focused attention with cuing requires constant vigilance and is cognitively demanding. Thus, cuing is not suitable for patients with dementia.

Amplitude-Scaling Strategies

Amplitude-based behavioral intervention is a concept that can be applied across all exercises and in different contexts in the treatment of PD.[201] These approaches are based on the concept that repetitive high-amplitude movements with high effort yield greater improvements in motor performance, following principles of neuroplasticity.[202–206] Patients are guided by a physical therapist to exercise at a high intensity (8/10 Borg's RPE Scale) with large amplitude, multiple repetitions, and whole-body movements that increase in complexity. These vigorous large movements of the trunk and extremities are counter to the akinesia/bradykinesia, the hallmark of PD, and relate to the role of scaling by the BG. Improvements in UPDRS motor scores, TUG, and timed 10-meter walking have been reported after 4 weeks of high-amplitude, high-effort training four times per week.[207] Hirsch et al.[208] reviewed studies of exercise-induced neuroplasticity in people with PD (N = 144), suggesting exercise elicits plasticity-related events including corticomotor excitation, changes in gray matter volume, and changes in brain-derived neurotrophic factor. The addition of high-intensity interval training was shown to improve hemodynamic variables and functional mobility in individuals with PD.[209] Moderate-intensity continuous exercise training had no impact on the same variables.

Exercise Training

Relaxation Exercises

Diaphragmatic breathing during exercise can promote relaxation of excessive muscle tension owing to rigidity. For example, yoga and Pilates movements and coordinated breathing with large-amplitude trunk and arm movements overhead can be used to expand the restricted chest and promote shoulder ROM (see Fig. 18.6 and the chair gate pose in Appendix 18.A [online]). The patient's attention can be focused on deep inspiration during arm elevation ("breathe in deeply") and on expiration ("breathe out deeply") while lowering the arms. Patients may also benefit from cognitive imaging, motor imagery, or meditation techniques.[210] Relaxation audiotapes can be used at home as part of

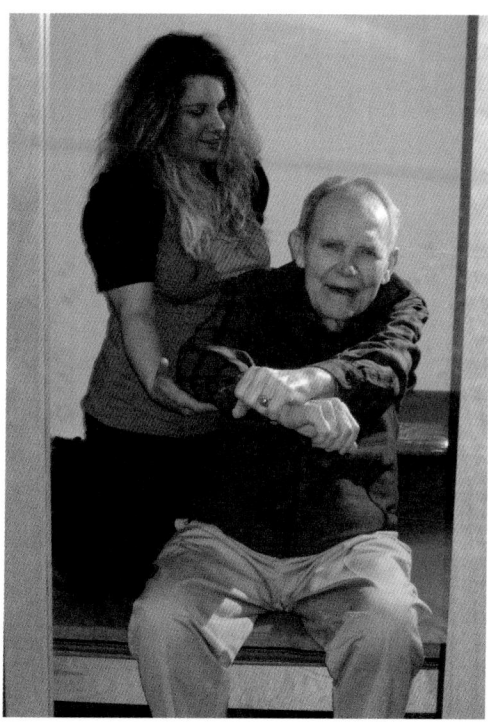

Figure 18.6 The patient with Parkinson disease performs bilateral arm raises while sitting (note the difficulty in achieving full shoulder flexion).

the home exercise program (HEP). Stress management techniques are an important adjunct to relaxation training. A daily schedule needs to be planned to accommodate the restrictions of the disease and the functional needs of the patient. Lifestyle modifications and time management strategies reduce anxiety associated with movement difficulties and prolonged times required to complete basic functional tasks.

Flexibility Exercises

The purpose of flexibility exercise (stretching) is to improve ROM and physical function. A combination of static (PROM) and dynamic (AROM) exercises is used to achieve maximum ROM. Flexibility exercises should be performed a minimum 2 to 3 days per week and ideally 5 to 7 days per week. A minimum of four repetitions per stretch held for 15 to 60 seconds is recommended.[176] Special consideration should be given to stretching common areas of limitation (Table 18.5) and dystonia (hands/fingers, feet/toes). Stretching can be combined with joint mobilization techniques to reduce tightness of the joint capsule or of ligaments around a joint (Fig. 18.7). By using selected grades of accessory movement, both improved ROM and decreased pain can be achieved. The stretching will be more effective if the muscles have been warmed with active exercise or with an external heating modality. Stretching exercises are an important component of the HEP. The patient and caregiver should be instructed in the appropriate

Table 18.5   Common Areas of Range of Motion Limitation and Suggested Stretching Exercises

Areas of ROM Limitation	Suggested Stretching Exercises
Cervical retraction	• Sitting, back against wall (or supine), head retractions (chin tuck position)
Cervical rotation	• Sit (or supine), with head retracted, head turns side to side
Shoulder flexion with trunk extension	• Sitting, hands clasped together, overhead arm lifts with thoracic extension • Supine, pillow under thoracic spine, hands clasp together, overhead arm lifts with thoracic extension
Elbow extension	• Sitting (or standing, modified plantigrade) weight-bearing with both UEs, elbows extended
Wrist and fingers extension	• Sitting or standing, palms together with fingers spread and pointing upward • Sitting or standing, roll tennis ball between fingers
Trunk extension	• Sitting, thoracic extension over the back of a chair with elbows bent and shoulders retracted • Prone lying, prone push-ups (press-ups) • Standing trunk extension, hands positioned on hips
Trunk rotation	• Supine, upper trunk rotation, hands clasped together (or holding a small ball), arms move with trunk rotation side to side • Hook-lying, lower trunk rotation, knees move with trunk rotation side to side • Sitting or standing, both arms out to one side (clasped together or holding a small ball), arms move with trunk rotation side to side
Hip extension	• Supine with one LE over edge of mat (hip extended, knee flexed), other knee held to chest • Supine, hips and knees extended • Hook-lying bridging • Standing, active hip extension or forward lunge • High-kneeling with hips extended
Hip abduction	• Supine, one LE extended and abducted, other LE in hook-lying
Knee extension	• Standing, forward lean with wall push-ups
Ankle dorsiflexion	• Standing, both forefeet on edge of step or block, heels off step, lower heels down with light touch-down support of both hands • Standing, forward lean with wall push-ups
Toe dorsiflexion/foot intrinsics	• Sitting, place foot on tennis ball, roll arch of foot back and forth over ball

LE = lower extremity; ROM = range of motion; UE = upper extremity.

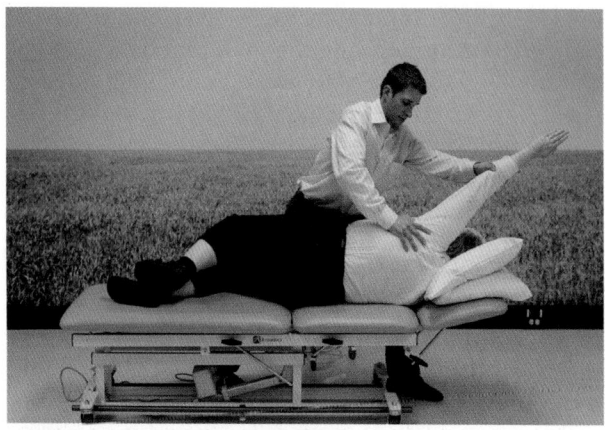

Figure 18.7 Shoulder range of motion with scapular mobilization performed in the side-lying position.

stretching exercises. A yoga sequence can be used effectively to focus attention on developmental postures, core stability, and stretching of structures that are traditionally restricted with PD, as well as to promote relaxation (see Appendix 18.A [online]).[211]

Patients with PD benefit from additional attention and cuing strategies during active stretching exercises. Patients are instructed to think of the end (goal) of the movement, and to "move BIG, with purpose and power" through the whole range with full focus and attention on the ending position for each repetition. Additional tactile or visual cuing can assist in maximizing range during active motions. For example, during active trunk rotation and reaching movements in sitting, the patient can be cued to touch an object or target. Ballistic stretches (high-intensity bouncing stretches) should be avoided because they are linked to increased injury. Muscle tears or ruptures of weakened tissues are especially prevalent in older, sedentary adults. Vigorous stretching can stimulate pain receptors and cause rebound muscle contraction. Older adult patients with PD who have long-standing disease must be considered at risk for osteoporosis and therefore must be stretched accordingly.

Positioning can also be used to stretch tight muscles and soft tissues. Patients in late-stage PD are likely to demonstrate severe flexion contractures of the trunk and limbs. Early on, the patient may benefit from daily positioning in prone-lying. As the disease progresses and significant postural deformity and cardiorespiratory impairments develop, the patient may not tolerate this position. The patient with a developing lateral curvature can be positioned in side-lying with a small pillow under the lateral trunk. Positional stretching is prolonged, with times typically ranging from 20 to 30 minutes.

Strength Training

Progressive resistance training to improve strength and power is indicated for patients with PD, due to primary muscle weakness with impaired motor unit recruitment and rate of force development and disuse weakness associated with prolonged inactivity. Specific areas of weakness are targeted, such as the antigravity extensor muscles. Weakness of these muscles is associated with poor posture (e.g., a flexed, stooped posture) and functional deficits (e.g., inability to get out of a chair, limitations in gait function). Weakness also contributes to postural instability, falls, and fall injury, as well as increased sense of effort. Strength training has been shown to improve muscle force, bradykinesia, functional mobility, balance, gait, fall risk, and QOL in patients with PD. Compared with resistance training alone, resistance training with instability (progressive increases in instability [e.g., balance pad, Dyna Discs, balance disks, BOSU and Swiss ball] along with the progressively increased resistance) and multimodal interventions that included resistance training showed the same or better improvements in strength/power, some nonmotor symptoms, and balance, and also reduced falls.[193]

Resistance training is based on the *progressive overload principle*. The amount of resistance is increased during training. Load can be applied using resistance machines, free weights, elastic resistance bands, or manually. With older adults, the recommendation is to begin at a lower intensity (e.g., using an RPE Scale of somewhat hard, 5 to 6 on a 10-point scale), ensuring that a set of 10 to 12 repetitions per set can be completed.[176] Research supports progressing the load by 2% when the patient successfully tolerates performing three sets of 15 repetitions.[193] Strength training can be performed 2 days per week on nonconsecutive days. Exercise machines may be safer than free weights for patients with more advanced disease because the movements are

more controlled, especially for the patient who demonstrates dyskinesia at peak dose or cognitive changes.[176] Because patients with PD already demonstrate too much stiffness and coactivation, isometric training is generally contraindicated. Functional training activities (see next section) can also be effective interventions to improve strength.

Corcos et al.[212] found a significant interaction between medication and strength. Withdrawal of levodopa during an "off" state period caused a decrease in strength and rate of force development. Exercise training should therefore optimally be timed for "on" periods when the patient is at their best (i.e., 45 minutes to 1 hour after medication has been taken). Exercising during an "off" period may not be possible or pose great difficulty for the patient. The patient should consistently exercise at the same time during a medication cycle.

Mobilizing facial muscles is another important component of the exercise program because the patient will have limited social interaction and poor feeding skills in the presence of marked facial rigidity and bradykinesia. These factors can greatly influence the patient's overall psychological state, motivation, and social participation. Massage, stretch, manual contacts, and verbal cuing can be used to enhance facial movements. The patient can be instructed to practice lip pursing, movements of the tongue, swallowing, and facial movements such as smiling, frowning, and so forth. A mirror can be used to provide visual feedback. In cases where eating is impaired by immobility, the movements of opening and closing the mouth and chewing should be combined with neck stabilization in a neutral position. Verbal skills should be practiced in association with breath control.

Functional Training

An exercise program should be based on focused practice of functional skills. The overall emphasis is on improving functional mobility with specific emphasis on improving mobility of axial structures, the head, trunk, hips, and shoulders. Progression to more difficult motor activities should be gradual. The more severely involved patient may benefit initially from assisted movements progressing to active movements to improve initial motor performance.

Bed Mobility

Bed mobility skills (i.e., rolling, bridging, supine-to-sit transitions) are essential skills that are often very difficult owing to truncal rigidity and bradykinesia. Side-lying rolling activities that emphasize segmental rotation patterns (i.e., isolated upper and lower trunk rotations) should be practiced rather than a log-rolling pattern. Patients with very stiff trunks may benefit from compensatory rolling strategies using the UE or LE to reach over and initiate the movement. Using large-amplitude and high-effort movements is particularly helpful for patients working on bed mobility and managing the

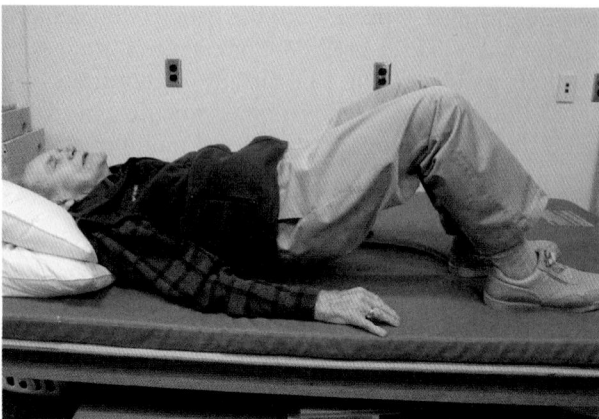

Figure 18.8 The patient with Parkinson disease practices bridging (note the difficulty in achieving full hip extension).

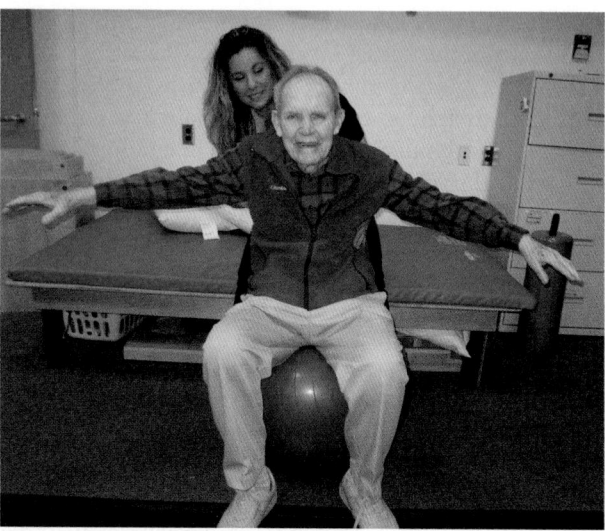

Figure 18.9 The patient with Parkinson disease practices sitting on a ball with upper extremities abducted to the sides, hands open.

bedsheets. For example, an overhead and cross-body reach with high and explosive effort can create trunk rotation and a momentum strategy of rolling. Rolling should be practiced on different surfaces progressing from firm to soft and finally simulating the patient's bed surface at home. Bridging is an important activity that improves scooting in bed as well as sit-to-stand transfers. Practicing large-amplitude, purposeful and effortful steps with each leg then trunk and shoulders facilitates bridging and scooting (Fig. 18.8).

Sit to Stand

Sit to stand (STS) is a difficult activity for many patients with PD, especially with moderate or advanced disease or when in the "off" state. Improving pelvic and hip mobility by stretching the tight hip flexors, adductors, and internal rotators will lead to improved STS. Anterior and posterior tilts, side-to-side tilts, and pelvic clock exercises with legs apart (hips in full abduction) can be practiced while sitting on a therapy ball, which enhances lumbopelvic and hip mobility (Fig. 18.9). Sitting activities should include weight shifting emphasizing large-amplitude upper trunk rotations and reaching. Patients demonstrate poor timing in controlling their COM forward velocity, which tends to be slower. Insufficient upward momentum (LE extension torques) in standing up is also problematic.[213] Other factors include level of agonist–antagonist coactivation and rigidity. STS training begins with the patient scooting to the edge of the mat and placing both feet under the knees and apart. Goal-directed forward trunk and hip flexion can be enhanced through reaching forward and toward the floor between widespread knees. Strengthening of the hip and knee extensors can be achieved through repeated sit-to-stand activity with emphasis on anterior pelvic tilt, and partial squats while standing at the sink or counter. Practice standing up from a firm *raised* seat decreases the total excursion and work of extensor muscles and promotes

ease of rise. Once control is achieved, progression is then to lower, standard height seats. Standing directly in front of the patient should be avoided, because this may block initial standing attempts. Instead, the therapist or caregiver should stand to the patient's side. If safety issues are apparent, a safety gait belt should be used.

Floor Transfers

Patients with PD typically experience a high number of falls and should be taught how to get up after a fall. To that end, scooting while seated on the floor, or transferring to hands and knees, should be practiced with the same large-amplitude movements mentioned previously, so the patient is able to move to a nearby stable chair or couch at home. The patient should also practice transitions moving from the floor to standing (supine to hands and knees to kneeling to half-kneeling and finally to standing) using UE support. Blocked, repetitive practice of powerful, rapid, and purposeful movements should be practiced. For example, during the transition from floor on hands and knees to one hip flexed, the patient steps that foot forward beside the hand, then pushes up and extends hips and trunk to upright with arms opened up and out to half-kneeling, then pushing up with UEs to standing.

Balance Training

There is high-quality and strong evidence recommending balance training programs to reduce impairments in postural control, and improve balance, gait, mobility, balance confidence, and QOL in individuals with PD.[193] It is important to recall that learning is task and context specific. Thus, a balance training program should include a variety of activities that alter task demands and expose the patient to varying environmental conditions.

Whenever possible, the therapist should try to duplicate the conditions the patient will encounter in everyday life. The level of challenge is important. A therapist should know the limitations of the patient and the specific demands of the task and environment to select and progress tasks accordingly and ensure patient safety. See Chapter 10, Strategies to Improve Motor Function, for a more complete discussion of balance training.

An important focus of balance training for the patient with PD is COM and LOS control training. Patients should be instructed in how COM influences balance and how to improve posture in sitting, in standing, and during dynamic movement tasks. Patients should be encouraged to explore their LOS and practice working toward expanding them in both sitting and standing. In standing, patients with PD typically demonstrate restricted LOS with forward displacement of center of foot pressure. Patients should be instructed in how to improve postural alignment and in ways to avoid postural disturbances and falls. The therapist should encourage the patient to self-assess and pay attention to their balance strategies, generating their own movement solutions, with feedback from the therapist. A standing platform training device (i.e., posturography system) can be valuable in providing COM position and LOS biofeedback. The patient is instructed in weight shifting that expands the LOS. The Nintendo Wii Balance Board is a widely available and economical force platform and biofeedback system. When compared to a laboratory-grade force platform, the Nintendo Wii Balance Board was valid in quantifying center of pressure, an important component of standing balance.[214] Subjects with poor positional awareness who trained on the Wii Balance Board with real-time visual biofeedback demonstrated significant improvements in weight-bearing symmetry.[215] Subjects with PD who trained with this device for 30 minutes three times a week, over a 4-week period improved on average 3.3 points on the BBS, 2.8 points of the DGI, and decreased their variability of postural sway by 31%.[216]

Balance training should emphasize practice of dynamic stability tasks (e.g., weight shifts, alternating unilateral weight-bearing, reaching, axial rotation of the head and trunk, axial rotation combined with reaching with and without added resistance bands [Fig. 18.10], stepping to reach in all directions). Seated activities can include sitting on a compliant surface (inflatable disk) or a therapy ball. To stabilize the floor-to-stand transfers in fall recovery skills, challenges to balance can be introduced in quadruped (Fig. 18.11), kneeling (Fig. 18.12), half-kneeling (Fig. 18.13), and standing on a disk (Figs. 18.14 and 18.15). Altering arm positions (e.g., arms out to side, arms folded across chest, reaching); altering foot/leg positions (e.g., feet apart, feet together); or adding voluntary movements (e.g., overhead arm clapping, head and trunk rotations, single leg raises, stepping or marching in place) can all

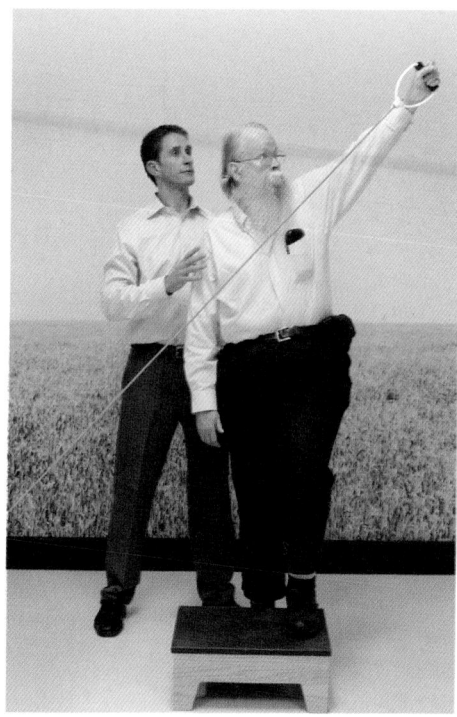

Figure 18.10 The patient with Parkinson disease practices maintaining a step-up position while performing resisted upper extremity shoulder abduction and flexion using elastic band resistance. The patient is encouraged to turn and look at the hand.

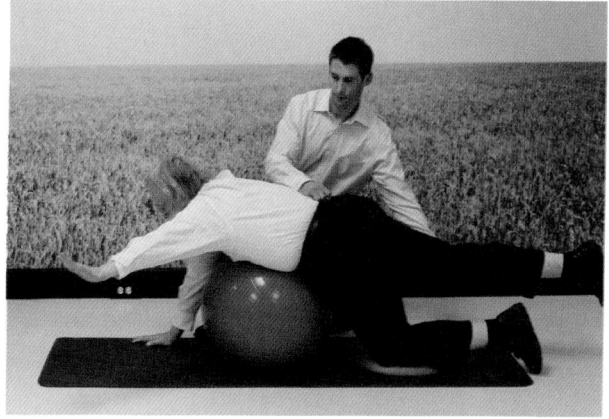

Figure 18.11 The patient with Parkinson disease practices contralateral upper extremity/lower extremity lifts in quadruped over a ball.

be used to increase difficulty of the activity. Training should focus on achieving faster initiation and execution movement times (i.e., large, fast, and powerful) supported by the use of appropriate cuing strategies. Strategies for varying environmental demands include altering the support surface (e.g., standing on foam), changing visual inputs (e.g., reduced lighting, eyes closed), or challenging the patient with a variable open environment (e.g., busy clinic setting).

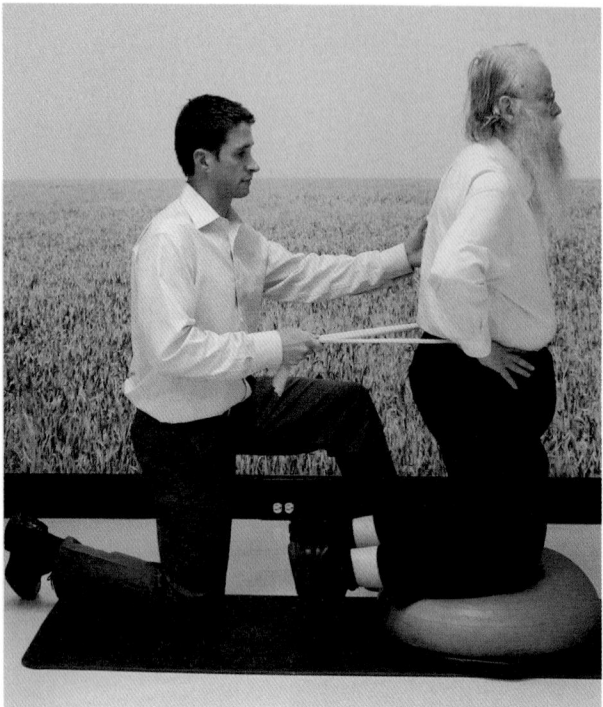

Figure 18.12 The patient with Parkinson disease practices kneeling on a BOSU disc. The therapist provides resistance using an elastic band to promote full hip extension.

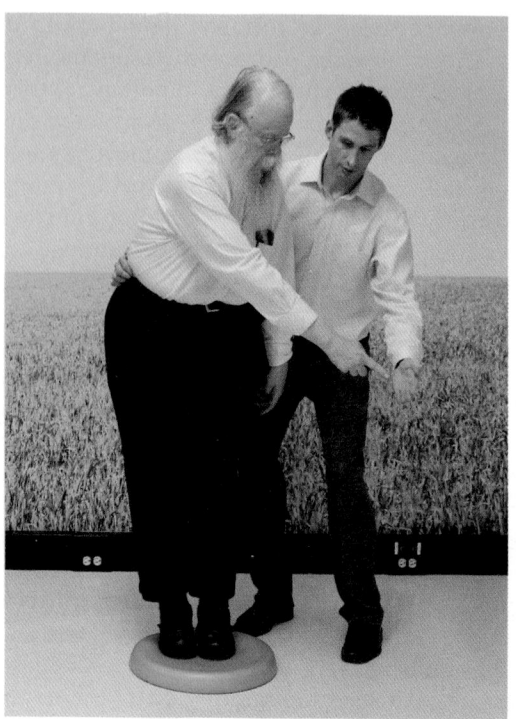

Figure 18.14 The patient with Parkinson disease practices standing on an inflated disc while reaching across, promoting upper trunk rotation.

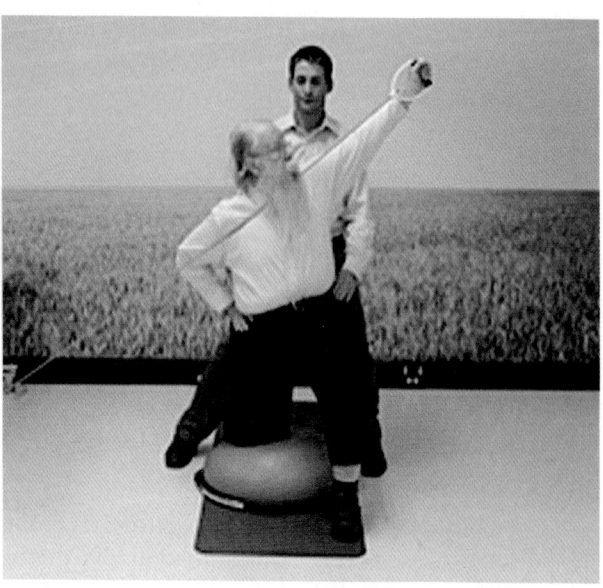

Figure 18.13 The patient with Parkinson disease practices half-kneeling on a BOSU disc while performing resisted upper extremity shoulder abduction and flexion using elastic band resistance.

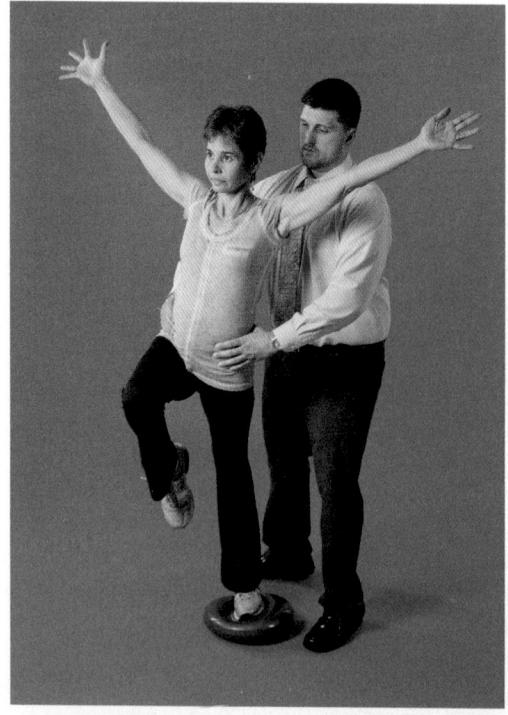

Figure 18.15 The patient with young-onset Parkinson disease practices standing with one foot on an inflated disc with bilateral "big arms" and hands open, palms up.

Adequate strength and ROM are important components needed to withstand the challenges of balance. The patient can be instructed in standing exercises to enhance balance, including heel-rises and toe-offs, partial squats and chair rises, single-limb stance with side-kicks or back-kicks, and marching in place. Collectively, these exercises are sometimes referred to as the "kitchen sink exercises" and are important components of the HEP for patients with balance deficiencies. The patient may require light touch-down support of the hands (e.g., on the kitchen sink) to start in order to stabilize yet keep COM over feet; progression should be to no support as soon as possible.

Locomotor Training

Locomotor training goals, whether overground or on a treadmill, focus on preventing falls, increasing safety of mobility, and improving agility by reducing the primary gait impairments of slowed speed, decreased stride length, lack of a heel–toe sequence with forward progression characterized by a shuffling (festinating) gait pattern, diminished contralateral trunk movement and arm swing, and an overall attitude of flexion while walking. Effective strategies for improving gait parameters and safety include having the patient walk with vertical poles overground (pole walking) (Fig. 18.16) or on a treadmill, and the use of *verbal instructional sets* (e.g., "Walk tall," "Walk fast," "Take large steps," "Swing both arms"). As previously discussed, visual (transverse more than parallel) and auditory cues are also effective in improving gait speed and step length. Strategies to

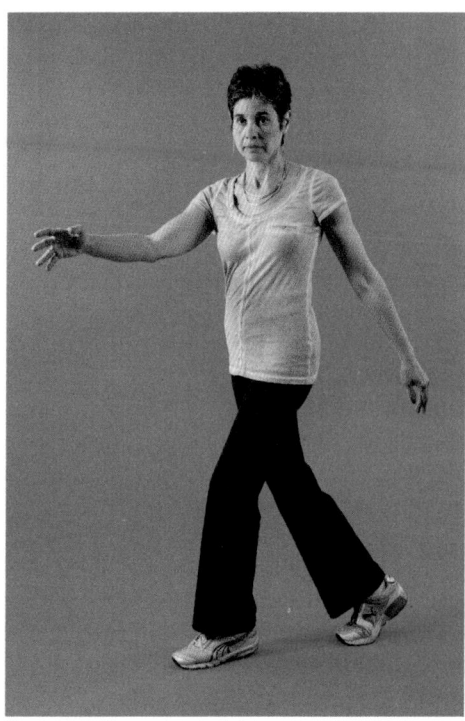

Figure 18.17 The patient with young-onset Parkinson disease practices cross-step walking.

improve step height include marching in place, walking using an exaggerated high stepping pattern, and stepping over obstacles. Advanced stepping and balancing that include large hip and pelvic movements can be achieved by having the patient practice juggling scarves or move through an agility course. Agility courses can include turns, cross-stepping (Fig. 18.17), crossing obstacles of different heights, changing surfaces, reaching, boxing, creeping through tunnels or under bars, crawling, floor-to-stand transitions, and more.[153] Reciprocal arm swing during gait can be enhanced by having the patient and therapist hold opposite ends of a set of two dowels (one in each hand). The therapist walks behind the patient and uses their arm swing to assist the patient's. Alternatively, from behind the therapist can lightly facilitate trunk rotation at the shoulders/upper trunk, thereby arm swing occurs passively due to the "natural" trunk rotation. With both of these strategies, the therapist must bring the patient's attention to how the cued movement feels, then the patient repeats the activity without cuing or assist.

Patients with PD who practiced locomotor training on a motorized treadmill, including robot-assisted gait training (RAGT),[217] downhill treadmill training,[218] circular/curved treadmill training,[219] and forward treadmill walking with virtual reality (VR),[220] demonstrated improvements in postural stability, gait (e.g., walking speed, step and stride length), motor function, and QOL. The treadmill may be acting as an external cue to enhance gait rhythmicity and reduce gait variability. The benefits of treadmill training, as with exercise training in general,

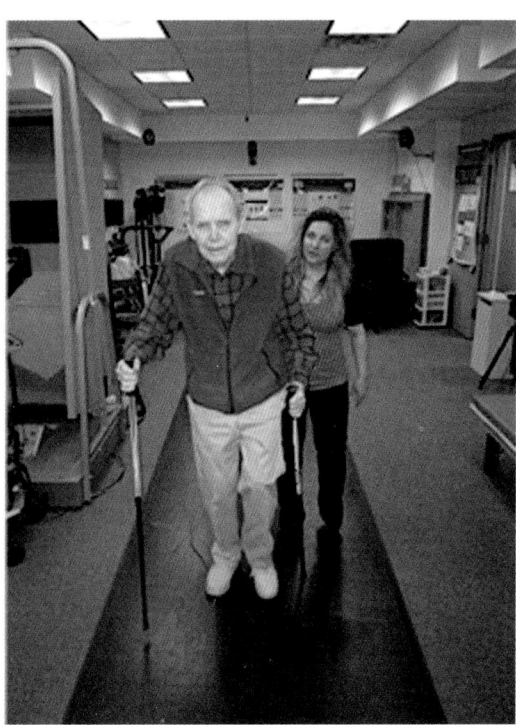

Figure 18.16 The patient with Parkinson disease practices walking using two vertical poles.

are dose dependent. More pronounced improvements are noted with high-intensity practice and incremental increases in treadmill speed.[221] High-intensity treadmill training has been shown to normalize corticomotor excitability in early PD and to increase neuroplasticity of dopaminergic signaling in the BG.[222] The treadmill can also be used for step training in people with PD. While supported in a safety harness, patients practice stepping in all four directions in response to suddenly turning the treadmill on and off [223] or by turning 90° or 180° to change direction of walking without pausing the treadmill, for patients in earlier stages of PD.

Locomotor training should also include task-specific training designed to promote full participation in social roles pertaining to family life, leisure, and community participation. This includes varying the walking task (e.g., walking on a tile floor, on carpet, outdoors on sidewalks and grassy terrain). Additional challenges include walking in the community (e.g., variable open environments), stair climbing, up and down curbs and ramps, over obstacles, and while also carrying out another task (e.g., buttoning a coat/shirt, talking on the phone, getting coins from a purse or pocket). Patients with PD often demonstrate difficulties in obstacle stepping due to deficits in cognitive and sensory-motor processing [224] and reduced foot clearance. Foot clearance can be improved with repeated practice of stepping over horizontal floor markers or laser light signals.

Patients in the advanced stage of the disease will be limited in terms of walking and variations that can be used. The overall goal at this stage is to promote regular walking while maintaining safety and preventing falls. Compensatory training strategies are indicated. Caregiver instruction regarding assisted walking and safety is imperative.

Freezing of Gait

FOG episodes are common and are often resistant to drug therapy. The therapist and patient should identify and practice strategies for unfreezing gait.[64] For example, some compensatory strategies include external cuing (visual cues, rhythmic auditory cuing, verbal cues, attentional cues) or "trick" movements such as dropping a tissue that the patient must step over. Having the patient focus extra attention to gait, making wide turns, walking and turning with wide and rocking steps, high-knees marching, and modifying the environment to reduce exposure to closed, tight spaces can also be successful strategies in reducing freezing.

Action observation training (AOT) is an approach that is based on the concept of the mirror neuron system in the frontal and parietal lobes.[225] Patients with freezing episodes watched video clips of strategies and movements that were helpful in reducing freezing, three times a week for 4 weeks. Each 60-minute session consisted of 24 minutes of observation and 36 minutes of imitation performed separately. The control group watched the same number and length of video clips of static landscapes followed by performance of the same movements/actions of the AOT group. After treatment, both groups showed reduced severity of freezing, but only the AOT group showed improved motor impairment (MDS-UPDRS scores), walking speed, balance, and QOL at 1 month post-training. These motor improvements were associated with functional MRI (fMRI) findings of increased recruitment of motor regions, and areas of the brain involved in attention, goal-directed processing, and the mirror neuron system.

FOG is associated with cognitive dysfunction, specifically in the areas of response inhibition, conflict resolution, visuospatial function, and switching or divided attention.[62,226] Cognitive training for people with PD has shown to be successful.[227] Considering the evidence that indicates an overlap of cognition and mobility, combining cognitive and physical exercise training for people with PD may reduce freezing from a restorative versus compensatory perspective.[153] Peterson et al.[153] suggest example activities that could be done with patients to specifically challenge the deficits in cognitive domains associated with freezing. Consider, for example, an agility course (divided attention) as described previously, the *Walking Trail-Making Test* in which the patient walks from a letter to a number alternating in ascending order (attention shifting),[228] the *Stroop* walking task (inhibition),[229] and the *Go-No-Go* boxing task with congruent and incongruent visual and verbal cues (inhibition, selection), among others.

Motor-Cognitive Dual-Task Training

Many ADL require doing two or more tasks at once such as driving, having a phone conversation while walking, and conversing while preparing dinner. Dual-tasking is the simultaneous execution of two tasks that can be performed independently, can be measured separately, and have distinct task goals.[48] *Dual-task interference* is a measure often used to represent the degree of performance deterioration from single-task (ST) to dual-task (DT) conditions. Successful DT performance relies on the cognitive ability to process and integrate the requirements of both tasks and to perform tasks automatically to some degree.[230] Individuals with PD have deficits in cognitive/executive functions, automaticity, and movement control, as discussed earlier in the chapter. These deficits influence dual-tasking which can lead to problems including imbalance and falls[231] and impaired driving and car accidents.[232] Most commonly, DT interference during walking is seen as decreased gait speed and stride length and increased variability and asymmetry. Drivers with PD and DT interference show decreased steering accuracy and speed adaptation and increased braking reaction time.[232]

Dual-task training (DTT) shows benefits on gait, balance, and motor symptoms in people with PD.[233] Table 18.6 presents a review of selected research in the area of motor-cognitive dual-task training for people with PD.

Table 18.6   Evidence Summary Motor-Cognitive Dual-Task Training for Individuals With Parkinson Disease

Fritz et al. (2015)[234]

Design	SR to determine the effectiveness of motor-cognitive dual-task training compared with usual care on mobility and cognition in individuals with neurologic disorders.
Level of Evidence	Level I
Subjects	Subjects with PD and AD (AD)
Intervention	Cued walking, cognitive tasks paired with gait, balance, and strength training and virtual reality or gaming.
Results	DTT improves single-task gait velocity and stride length in subjects with PD and AD, dual-task gait velocity and stride length in subjects with PD, AD, and brain injury, and may improve balance and cognition in those with PD and AD.
Comments	Improvement of dual-task ability in individuals with neurologic disorders holds potential for improving gait, balance, and cognition.

Killane et al. (2015)[235]

Design	RCT to examine the effect of dual motor-cognitive virtual reality training on dual-task performance in FOG in individuals with PD.
Level of Evidence	Level II
Subjects	Twenty community-dwelling participants with PD (13 with FOG, 7 without FOG).
Intervention	Eight 20-min intervention sessions consisting of a virtual reality maze through which participants navigated by stepping in place on a balance board combined with a cognitive task (Stroop test).
Results	Significant improvement in dual-task cognitive and motor parameters (stepping time and rhythmicity), dual-task effect for those with FOG and a noteworthy improvement in FOG episodes. Improvements were less significant for those without FOG.
Comments	A dual motor-cognitive approach to treatment improves dual-task performance and decreases FOG in subjects with PD.

Conradsson et al. (2015)[261]

Design	RCT to evaluate the short-term effects of the HiBalance program, a highly challenging balance-training regimen that incorporates both dual-tasking and PD-specific balance components.
Level of Evidence	Level II
Subjects	Ninety-one older adult participants with mild to moderate PD
Intervention	Participants randomized either into a 10-week program of highly challenging balance-training incorporating DTT or usual care for older adults with mild to moderate PD.
Results	Training group demonstrated significantly improved balance and gait performance. In addition, the training group improved their performance of the cognitive task while walking.
Comments	The HiBalance program showed promising transfer effects to everyday living.

Yitayeh, Teshome (2016)[262]

Design	SR to determine the effectiveness of conventional physiotherapy interventions in the management of balance dysfunction and postural instability in persons with idiopathic PD.
Level of Evidence	Level I
Subjects	248 participants with idiopathic PD
Intervention	Highly challenging balance training that incorporates both dual-tasking and PD-specific balance components in the form of stance and gait tasks which require feedforward and feedback postural control and in the form of technology-assisted balance training.

(Continued)

Table 18.6   Evidence Summary Motor-Cognitive Dual-Task Training for Individuals With Parkinson Disease—cont'd

Yitayeh, Teshome (2016)[262]

Results	Training that incorporates both dual-tasking and PD-specific balance components significantly benefited balance and gait abilities when compared with usual care. Repetitive exercises, highly challenging balance training, and incremental speed-dependent treadmill training improved ROM, endurance, gait parameters, functional reaching activities, and postural stability. In addition, it was demonstrated that these exercises help to decrease fall rate and fear of falling.
Comments	Results of study on high balance training can only be generalized to older adult, community-dwelling individuals with mild- to moderate-stage PD without cognitive impairments.

Ford et al. (2015)[263]

Design	SR to determine the effectiveness of DTGT on individuals with PD
Level of Evidence	Level I
Subjects	Subjects with PD
Intervention	DTGT
Results	DTGT improved gait speed, stride length, cadence, and balance. The addition of gait patterns and rhythmic music produced positive effects on dual-task walking.
Comments	DTGT can offset the negative effects of PD on patient's ability to dual-task while ambulating.

Strouwe et al. (2017)[230]

Design	RCT to evaluate and compare the efficacy and possible fall risk of two DTT interventions for improving gait delivered in the home for 6 weeks.
Level of Evidence	Level II
Subjects	One hundred twenty-one patients with PD, H&Y II–III
Intervention	Participants randomized into either (1) a CTT group that trained on gait and cognitive tasks separately, or (2) an IDT group that trained gait and cognitive tasks simultaneously. Post-tests occurred immediately after training and at 12-week follow-up.
Results	Both groups improved in dual-task gait velocity that was retained after 12 weeks. Fall risk was unchanged for both groups.
Comments	Gains in dual-task walking are likely due to *both* improved task automaticity from the CTT *and* more efficient integration of task-related neural networks from the IDT. DTT can be safe, even when delivered in the home.

Li et al. (2020)[233]

Design	SR and MA to determine the effectiveness of DTT on gait parameters, motor symptoms (disease rating scale), and balance in individuals with PD
Level of Evidence	Level I
Subjects	Three hundred twenty-two patients with PD, H&Y I–IV
Intervention	Cued walking, balance, tasks paired with gait: cognitive tasks, attentional focus, mindfulness breathing, complex daily tasks, tango, music, and virtual reality or gaming.
Results	DTT improved gait velocity, stride and step length, cadence, motor symptoms, and balance. Improved gait velocity was maintained at 3-week or 6-month follow-up testing.
Comments	DTT may improve attention during gait and improve gait performance, motor symptoms, and balance relative to other forms of training.

AD = Alzheimer disease; CTT = consecutive task training; DTGT = dual-task gait training; DTT = dual-task training; FOG = freezing of gait; H&Y = Hoehn and Yahr Classification of Disability Scale; IDT = integrated dual-task training; MA = meta-analysis; PD = Parkinson disease; RCT = randomized controlled trial; SR = systematic review.

In a systematic review to assess the effectiveness of motor-cognitive DTT compared with usual care in individuals with neurologic disorders, Fritz et al.[234] found that, regardless of the method used, motor-cognitive DTT interventions improved single- and DT walking (stride length and velocity). Furthermore, DTT resulted in more moderate improvements in balance and cognition. See Table 18.6 for details.

Specifically exploring the effects of DTT intervention for FOG using virtual reality, Killane et al.[235] found that the participants with FOG improved in dual-task cognitive and gait measures (reaction time, stepping time, and rhythmicity), whereas the non-FOG group only improved in stepping time. In addition, for the FOG group, the number of FOG episodes per trial was reduced after DTT intervention compared with before. The authors suggest that virtual reality DTT interventions such as these, that integrate cognitive and motor tasks together in training, could be used in the home and improve the QOL for patients who experience FOG.

FOG is a risk factor for falls, as discussed earlier in the chapter. Therefore, an intervention that uses cognitive functions known to contribute to falls in people with PD, and with FOG in particular, may pose a safety risk.[236] Strouwen et al.[236,237] addressed this issue and the efficacy of two different DTT programs for improving dual-task gait delivered in the home. One program was consecutive task training (CTT) in which gait training and cognitive exercises (verbal fluency, reciting switching and working memory tasks) were delivered separately to improve task *automaticity*. The other program was integrated dual-task training (IDT) consisting of gait practice and cognitive training simultaneously to improve DT *integration*. Results showed that DT gait improved after training, regardless of which method was used, and benefits were retained 12 weeks later. Importantly, the risk of falls did not increase with either of the two community-delivered interventions. The authors note that the improved DT performance gains are likely due to improved task automaticity after CTT *and* to better integration of task-related neural networks after IDT.

Aerobic Exercise

An individualized exercise prescription should be prescribed based on the American College of Sports Medicine guidelines for frequency, intensity, time (duration), and type of intervention (the FITT equation),[176] and on the Clinical Practice Guideline from the APTA.[193] Intensities should be moderate (60% to 75% of maximum HR) to high (75% to 85% of maximum HR) based on the patient's level of disease, fitness, and lifestyle. When lower intensities are used, longer-duration or more frequent exercise sessions are necessary to improve fitness. Careful monitoring is indicated because autonomic dysfunction is common. For example, long-term levodopa use can produce arrhythmias and OH and should

be considered. The therapist should monitor vital signs (HR, RR, BP), RPE, fatigue levels, and symptoms of exertional intolerance (e.g., significant dyspnea and hypotensive response). Endurance exercise training at a relatively high level improves cardiorespiratory capacity and endurance through increased VO_2max in mild and moderate PD.[238] Aerobic capacity and cognitive function improved in people with PD after a high-intensity aerobic exercise training program on a stationary recumbent bike, three times/week for 12 weeks, starting at 5 minutes/week up to 40 min/week.[239] These changes were correlated with functional changes measured with fMRI in brain areas involved in motor learning (increased activity in the hippocampus, striatum, and cerebellum).

Training modes can include leg and arm ergometry and walking. Selection will depend on the specific abilities of the patient; for example, postural instability and increased risk of falls may rule out use of a treadmill without an overhead harness. Recumbent or seated LE ergometry is a suitable alternative. A community-based indoor tandem cycling program, three times per week for 10 weeks, was designed to promote high cadence, consistency, and intensity of practice.[240] The authors found that most participants with PD achieved their training goals for target HR of 60% to 75% max, cadence of 80 to 90 revolutions per minute, and had 100% attendance. For most patients, a program of regular walking is recommended. The duration, speed, and terrain covered can be modified, based on individual ability. Accessibility to a supervised walking program using an indoor walking track is important for some to ensure safety. A shopping mall can provide an acceptable environment for community walkers in case of inclement or extremes of weather. A supervised aerobic pool program can also provide an acceptable mode of exercise for some patients. The warmth of the water may be relaxing, and the buoyancy may enhance stepping movements. The minimum recommended aerobic exercise frequency is three sessions per week. Daily walking with short multiple bouts (20 to 30 min) spaced throughout the day is recommended for individuals with lower functional capacity. Intermittent exercise with adequate rest intervals is indicated for older adult patients who are deconditioned, and those who present with restrictive pulmonary dysfunction. Aerobic training programs have been shown to be safe and effective for patients with PD in improving aerobic capacity.[238–240]

Community-Based Exercise Prescription and Home Exercise Programs

Community-based exercise is defined as (1) programs in which groups of individuals exercise together or (2) programs in which individuals follow a predetermined exercise program in a community setting either at home or in a community facility.[193] They do not need to be led by a physical therapist and are not part of the individualized physical therapy assessment.[193] Instead, they can be prescribed by the physical therapist as a result of their assessment and periodic reassessment. Community-based exercise should be recommended and prescribed as appropriate for the individual by the physical therapist, as there is high-quality and strong evidence for community-based exercise to reduce motor disease severity and improve nonmotor symptoms, functional outcomes, and QOL in individuals with PD.[193] Patients also benefit from the positive support, camaraderie, and communication the group situation offers.[241,242] Exercise groups and neuro-wellness fitness centers providing classes with an integrated focus on PD-related issues are beginning to appear. Careful evaluation of each patient before admission into a group or class is essential to ensure appropriate matching of the patient's fitness level with the class demands.[243,244] To this end, a two-part decision-making tool has been developed to help the physical therapist with prescription for and referral to the appropriate community-based group exercise classes.[243] Personal factors and clinical measures are used to appropriately match patients to multilevel group classes. Importantly, continued reassessment at regular intervals (every 6 months) by the physical therapist should include reassessment of the patient's involvement in their community-based exercise and updating of the prescription as needed.[111]

Patients should be able to perform the therapeutic core of the class. Selecting patients with similar levels of disability is often advisable because the sense of competition can frequently be a key factor in motivating groups. The ratio of staff to patients should be kept small (ideally 1:8 or 1:10), and extra staff should be added if patients are unable to work on their own. A variety of activities can be used, such as progressions from floor and seated exercises to standing and walking balance exercises. A combination of stretching, strengthening using body weight or bands, simple to complex movements using the whole body, and aerobic exercises are an appropriate focus for a group class. Music is used to provide necessary stimulation to movement and movement pacing. Exercise stations set up as a circuit class (e.g., stationary bicycle, mats, pulleys, and agility course) can also be used. Exercises done by the whole group together should focus on important exercise goals (e.g., improving ROM, mobility).

Recreational activities can be included such as dancing, partnered tango, ball activities, partnered boxing, and drumming. The activities selected should be interesting and varied. A relaxation segment should be incorporated into each class. Pole-striding groups (walking with trekking poles) are gaining in popularity, and this is another effective way to exercise at moderate to high intensity.[245-247] Yoga,[211] Pilates,[248] Alexander technique,[249] Tai Chi,[250] and dance[251,252] group classes effectively address multiple components of PD by improving posture,

flexibility, core stability, functional mobility, balance, relaxation, and socialization. King and Horak[253] recommend incorporating Tai Chi with other agility exercises (e.g., kayaking, boxing, lunges, agility training, Pilates exercises) to delay loss of mobility in people with PD.

The home-based exercises include exercises designed to improve relaxation, flexibility, strength, and cardiopulmonary function (all previously discussed). A key element is stressing the importance of regular daily exercise and avoiding prolonged periods of inactivity. The HEP should be realistic and of moderate duration and intensity. Early morning warm-up exercises and stretches are often helpful in reducing the increased stiffness patients may experience on arising. Stretching and strengthening exercises are performed in supine, sitting, and standing positions. Home ROM exercises can often be assisted by use of adaptive equipment. For example, to reduce the effects of forward head and kyphotic posture, the patient can be instructed to hang by the hands using an overhead bar. Standing, corner wall stretches can also be used to provide a maintained stretch on the upper trunk flexors. Use of a wand or cane can be effective in promoting overhead motions. In standing, a countertop or back of a sturdy chair can be used to assist in stabilization during standing calisthenics and balance activities. Home-based exercise programs have been found to be effective in improving postural control, mobility, functional status, and motor complications in people with PD.[254-257]

ADAPTIVE AND SUPPORTIVE DEVICES

Attention should be directed toward needs for adaptive and supportive devices that can improve function. To promote bed mobility, the patient can be helped to assume a sitting position by elevating the head of a powered hospital bed or with commercially available blocks approximately 4 in. (10 cm) high (furniture legs fit into a recess in the block). A simpler solution might include attaching a knotted rope or canvas "ladder" to the end of the bed to pull on. The bed should be stable and the mattress firm to facilitate mobility. Satin sheets and pajamas have sometimes been helpful to enhance bed mobility. Patients should be instructed to select firm chairs with armrests and avoid soft, low seats such as a low sofa. The chair can be raised (i.e., 4 in. [10 cm] and secured with blocks or tilted forward by elevating only the back legs about 2 in. [5 cm]). Some patients benefit from the use of a rocking chair to facilitate independent sit-to-stand transfers. Chairs that have spring-loaded seats that push the patient into standing are heavily marketed to older adults but should be used with caution. The patient is propelled into standing but may have difficulty stopping the movement and/or attaining balance within an appropriate time frame when first reaching the standing position. A raised toilet seat and toilet rails are also essential devices to facilitate ease of sit-to-stand transitions in the bathroom.

Loose-fitting clothing and sneakers with hook and loop closures can be used to facilitate dressing. If the patient demonstrates a shuffling gait, shoes should have leather or hard composition soles, because shoes with crepe or rubber soles will not slide easily and can result in falls. A festinating gait can sometimes be alleviated by the addition of modified heel or shoe wedges. A flat heel or toe wedge may slow down a propulsive gait. The use of assistive devices can be problematic owing to movement difficulties. A cane can be helpful for patients with mild to moderate disease to assist in balance or cue stepping (inverted walking stick). It is important that the height of the device not promote increased flexion of the trunk. Patients with more pronounced movement difficulties and poor balance are not likely to benefit from assistive devices. Walkers with wheels are particularly hazardous and are likely to increase a festinating gait; hand brakes are an essential requirement.

Adaptive devices can also assist with ADL. Reachers can be used to aid in dressing as well as for other activities. Eating can be facilitated in several ways. The patient should be seated properly, close to the table, with good posture. Specially adapted utensils, plate guards, and enlarged handles can aid the patient's efforts. Because eating time will be prolonged, heated plates or pads may help keep food warm and palatable. Drooling and/ or spills should be anticipated and clothing protected. Extra time should be planned, and the patient should not feel rushed.

■ PSYCHOSOCIAL ISSUES

The progressive nature of PD necessitates frequent personal and social adjustments and affects all aspects of life for both the patient and family. Disruptions in daily functions, roles, and activities are experienced. Some of the changes associated with PD are socially isolating (masked face, progressive immobility, and unintelligible speech), whereas other changes (increased salivation, perspiration, decreased sexual function) are distressing and can be socially embarrassing. The patient may feel increasingly isolated, and family relationships may suffer. The principal goal for team members is to assist the patient and family in their understanding of the disease and in developing insights and adjustments that lead to more effective self-management. Some individuals can successfully deal with the changes associated with the disease; others cannot. Coping skills can be facilitated. First and foremost, education is the key to assisting patients and family members in assuming responsibility. Feelings of hopelessness and dependency are reduced as the patient develops a sense of control over their own life. Self-management skills that should be promoted include advanced planning of activities, effective time management strategies, and stress management techniques. It is equally important to ensure that patients do not become isolated and that appropriate services are available. Team members must be vigilant regarding their assumptions and expectations. A condescending or pessimistic and limiting attitude can become a self-fulfilling prophecy. Patients and family members need reassurances and encouragement. An overall emphasis on what patients *can do* rather than what they cannot do helps to empower patients. Therapists need to provide a message of *hope tempered with realism.*

■ PATIENT, FAMILY, AND CARE PARTNER EDUCATION

The interdisciplinary team provides information about a variety of topics related to living with PD. These are presented in Box 18.5. Interventions can take the form of direct one-on-one instruction, group sessions, printed materials, and video or computer presentations. The therapist's overall approach needs to be positive and supportive.

Box 18.5 Elements of a Patient, Family, and Care Partner Education Program

• Parkinson disease: clinical presentation, strategies to manage symptoms
• Medications: purpose, dosage, possible adverse side effects, signs of either overmedication or undermedication
• Preventive measures to minimize the secondary complications and impairments
• Impact of Parkinson disease on movement and effective strategies to manage movement problems
• Barriers to exercise and effective solutions to regular exercise participation
• Impact of Parkinson disease on function and effective strategies to maintain independent function in home, community, or work environments
• Strategies for energy conservation and activity pacing
• Strategies for ensuring activity participation in valued leisure and family activities
• Community resources for patients: support groups, in-home interventions, community training programs, day programs
• Community resources for care partners: counseling, support groups, exercise programs, respite care

Community support groups are available for patients and their families. They disseminate information and offer a chance to discuss common issues, problems, and management tips. They also can provide a stabilizing influence, assisting patients and families to focus on healthy behaviors, coping skills, and effective self-management. For some patients in the early stages of the disease, participation in a support group may increase levels of anxiety as they observe more disabled patients. Groups particularly targeted to patients with early-stage disease and similar ages may be more helpful.

Educational pamphlets, newsletters, and location of support groups can be obtained through national PD associations. Web-based resources for clinicians and patients/families living with PD are presented in Appendix 18.B (online).

SUMMARY

PD is a chronic, progressive disorder of the BG characterized by the cardinal features of rigidity, bradykinesia, tremor, and postural instability. Additional impairments include the development of abnormal fixed postures, poverty of movement, fatigue, masked face, contractures, a festinating gait pattern, swallowing and communication difficulties, visual and sensorimotor disturbances, cognitive and behavioral dysfunction, autonomic dysfunction, and cardiopulmonary changes. Pharmacological interventions have become the mainstay of treatment and provide protective and symptomatic treatment. Effective rehabilitation focuses on the patient's stage of disease and symptoms, activity limitations and participation restriction, and residual abilities and assets. Interventions are restorative; that is, rehabilitation is focused on the improvement of strength, ROM, mobility, balance, functional skills, and endurance. Individuals with PD also benefit from functional maintenance programs designed to manage the effects of progressive disease. Strategies are developed to prevent or reduce indirect impairments and promote regular exercise, good health, and self-management skills. A comprehensive team approach including active involvement of patient and family provides optimal benefits. Team members need to be active during all stages of the disease, assisting the patient and family in maintenance of function and providing psychosocial support as needed.

Questions for Review

1. What are the major CNS structures involved in PD, and what are the pathophysiological changes associated with the disease?
2. Differentiate between cogwheel rigidity and lead pipe rigidity.
3. What impairments in postural stability are typically seen in patients with PD?
4. What are the nonmotor impairments in cognition associated with PD?
5. What are the major adverse effects associated with long-term use of levodopa/carbidopa?
6. How might the goals/outcomes and interventions vary by stage of disease?
7. OH is a common problem in patients with PD. How should it be examined?
8. Identify appropriate motor learning strategies for the patient with PD in terms of practice and feedback.
9. Describe the gait impairments common in patients with PD. What interventions can be used to improve locomotor function?
10. What guidelines for aerobic training are appropriate for the patient with early- to middle-stage PD?

CASE STUDY

Patient presented for physical therapy evaluation with his wife. The patient is a 63-year-old male with an 8-year history of PD. Patient reports a recent progression of decreased function, feelings of heaviness throughout his body. Wife reports that he has been moving more slowly with increased episodes of freezing and a new onset of hopelessness and depression. Patient referred to physical therapy to improve safety with ambulation and ability to perform ADL with improved independence.

HISTORY

The patient is a retired construction foreman/supervisor and a martial arts teacher/boxing trainer. He lives in a private house with his wife. The patient's initial onset of PD manifested with slight bilateral hand and lower extremity tremors right greater than left. He lived a very active life until recently when symptoms progressed to include freezing, shuffling gait pattern, decreased coordination of upper and lower body, rigidity, and decreased balance. Bed mobility has deteriorated including difficulty getting in and out of bed and freezing in bed. Speech volume has also deteriorated over time. Pt has a history of a fall out of a window and cervical trauma from a martial arts fight that has left him with chronic cervical and bilateral shoulder pain.

CURRENT STATUS

The patient is currently taking carbidopa-levodopa, ropinirole, and rasagiline. His chief complaints are:
- Difficulty walking, especially on uneven terrain, when getting up from office chair, and when moving in tight confined spaces
- Episodes of gait blocks (FOG) worse with dual-tasking, stopping–starting movement, and changing positions and directions with turns
- Increased bouts of uncontrolled or unsteady balance; experienced three falls in the past year
- Decreased endurance with ambulation; currently only able to walk 200 ft before requiring a break
- Increased difficulty rolling and getting into and out of bed
- Inability to dress independently
- Increased trunk rigidity
- Decreased speech volume
- Due to decreased hand coordination and respiratory tidal volume, patient frustrated that he is unable to play the harmonica anymore
- Bilateral shoulder pain left greater than right aggravated with movement and sleep postures

EXAMINATION FINDINGS

Cognition
Alert, oriented × 3

Psychosocial
Patient is showing signs of depression and frustration with progression of disease. He has always prided himself on how active he was with martial arts and ADL. Patient presents with a fear of falling in unfamiliar places.

Speech
Mild dysarthria, hypophonia

Sensation
Slightly decreased proprioception bilaterally in both ankles; otherwise intact

Tone
Rigidity (cogwheel type) moderate in all extremities R greater than L
Marked rigidity throughout neck and trunk
Masklike face

RANGE OF MOTION

Decreased due to moderate rigidity; with limitations in:
- Bilateral cervical rotation (0° to 30°)
- Bilateral shoulder abduction (0° to 130°)
- Bilateral elbow extension (10° to 140°)
- Bilateral hip extension (0° to 10°)
- Bilateral knee extension (10° to 115°)
- Bilateral ankle dorsiflexion (0° to 10°)

Strength
Generally fair (3/5) to good minus (4–/5)
Poor (2/5) bilateral shoulder abduction, bilateral ankle dorsiflexion

(Continued)

CASE STUDY—cont'd

MOTOR FUNCTION

Moderate to severe resting tremors, R hand greater than L hand
Bradykinesia: marked slowness, poverty of movement
Hesitation on initiation of movement

POSTURE

Forward head position; flexed; kyphotic spine
Stands with flexion of elbows and hips

BALANCE

Decreased LOS

The Lower Extremity Functional Scale Score: 40/80, LOB negotiating steps, freezing and hesitation of movement ambulating through doorways and elevators

Single Leg Stance: Right and Left 0 seconds. Ankle strategies used to maintain static standing on even surfaces

Berg Balance Measure: 43/56 requires increased time for turning 360° (10 sec), turns clockwise 10 steps and counterclockwise 9 steps, shuffling/freezing throughout, loss of balance with tandem stance

Sitting static control: good (able to maintain balance without handhold)
Sitting dynamic control: fair (accepts minimal challenge; able to lift both arms)
Standing static control: good (able to maintain balance without handhold)
Standing dynamic control: poor (unable to accept minimal challenge without handhold)

He has slowed reactions to loss of balance with decreased rotational movements of head/trunk and ineffective use of stepping strategies.

Timed Up and Go score is 38 seconds.

Functional Mobility

Generally decreased

Requires moderate assist: rolling in bed, supine-to-sit and sit-to-stand transfers. Retropulsion during sit-to-stand transfer, poor eccentric control with transfer to sofa with a low soft surface, poor posture and body mechanics and slowness of movement with car transfers.

Locomotion

Patient ambulates independently with a narrow BOS with narrow-based gait pattern evident with changes of directions and when negotiating around obstacles. Poor hip/trunk dissociation with minimal trunk rotation with no arm swing worse on the left. Poverty and slowness of movement with shuffling gait pattern more pronounced when negotiating small/confined spaces and through doorways. Difficulty negotiating busy environments, DT challenge gait deviations worsen with talking/carrying object.

Self-Care

Requires minimal assistance to supervision for feeding
Requires minimal to moderate assist for dressing/bathing

Cardiopulmonary Function/Endurance

Shallow (upper respiratory) breathing pattern

Generally decreased functional capacity (estimated functional work capacity is six metabolic equivalents [METs])

Fatigues easily and requires frequent rest periods

Skin

Intact, no areas of breakdown

GUIDING QUESTIONS

1. Identify/categorize this patient's problems in terms of:
   a. Direct impairments
   b. Indirect impairments
   c. Activity limitations
   d. Participation restrictions/disability

2. Identify two outcomes (the remediation of activity limitations and disability) and two goals (remediation of impairments) for this patient.

CASE STUDY—cont'd

3. Determine four interventions that could be used at the start of therapy to achieve the outcomes and goals provided for question 2. Provide a brief rationale for each.

4. What motor learning strategies will assist in improving his motor function?

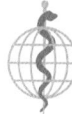

The reader is referred to the following interactive cases that guides users through the interview, examination, diagnosis, and writing of goals and the plan of care for Immersive Case E (mini-case): A Patient With Mild Parkinson Disease and Immersive Case F: A Patient With Freezing of Gait Due to Parkinson Disease. Both cases are available online at **fadavis.com**.

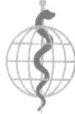

For additional resources, including answers to the questions for review, new immersive cases, case study guiding questions, references, and more, please visit **https://www.fadavis.com/product/physical -rehabilitation-fulk-8**. You may also quickly find the resources by entering this title's four-digit ISBN, 4691, in the search field at **http://fadavis.com** and logging in at the prompt.

Traumatic Brain Injury

Chapter 19

George D. Fulk, PT, PhD, FAPTA
Coby Nirider, PT, DPT
Gavin Williams, PT, PhD, FACP
Amy DeBlois, PT, DPT, NCS

LEARNING OBJECTIVES

1. Describe the pathophysiology of traumatic brain injury.
2. Analyze the impact of cognitive, neurobehavioral, and neuromuscular impairments, activity limitations, and participation restrictions on outcomes of people with traumatic brain injury.
3. Identify the different team members and settings in the management of the patient with traumatic brain injury.
4. Compare and contrast unresponsive wakefulness and minimally conscious state.
5. Identify key components of the physical therapy examination during the acute stage of recovery in patients with severe to moderate traumatic brain injury.
6. Create a plan of care for a patient with a severe to moderate traumatic brain injury that presents with disorder of consciousness in the acute stage of recovery.
7. Select evidence-based outcome measures to use during the physical therapy examination of a patient with moderate to severe traumatic brain injury during the active rehabilitation stage of recovery.
8. Explain the impact of cognitive and neurobehavioral impairments on the physical therapy plan of care in the active rehabilitation stage of recovery.
9. Create a plan of care for a patient with a severe to moderate traumatic brain injury in the active rehabilitation stage of recovery.
10. Select evidence-based outcome measures to use during the physical therapy examination of a patient with a mild traumatic brain injury.
11. Outline a return to play/activity timeline for a patient with a mild traumatic brain injury.
12. Create a plan of care for a patient with a mild traumatic brain injury.

CHAPTER OUTLINE

PREVALENCE 727
MECHANISM OF INJURY AND PATHOPHYSIOLOGY 727
  Primary Injury 727
  Secondary Injury 728
IMPACT OF TRAUMATIC BRAIN INJURY 728
  Body Structure/Function Impairments 728
  Activity Limitations 730
  Participation Restrictions 730
  Potential Long-Term Impact 730
DIAGNOSIS AND PROGNOSIS 731
CONTINUUM OF CARE AND INTERDISCIPLINARY TEAM 732
  Continuum of Care 732
  Interdisciplinary Team 732
EARLY MEDICAL MANAGEMENT 734
PHYSICAL THERAPY MANAGEMENT OF MODERATE TO SEVERE TRAUMATIC BRAIN INJURY EARLY AFTER INJURY 734
  Examination Early After Injury 734
  Goals and Outcomes 736
  Interventions 736
PHYSICAL THERAPY MANAGEMENT OF MODERATE TO SEVERE TRAUMATIC BRAIN INJURY DURING ACTIVE REHABILITATION 739
  Examination During Active Rehabilitation 739
  Goals and Outcomes 742
  Intervention Strategies 742
  Interventions 745
  Behavioral Factors 749
  Community Reentry 749
PHYSICAL THERAPY MANAGEMENT OF MILD TRAUMATIC BRAIN INJURY 751
  Mild Traumatic Brain Injury 751
  Physical Therapy Management 752
  Evidence-Based Care 755
SUMMARY 755

A traumatic brain injury (TBI) is defined as "an alteration in brain function, or other evidence of brain pathology, caused by an external force."[1] The population of patients with TBI is one of the most challenging and rewarding that a physical therapist is likely to encounter. Because of the multiple body systems affected by a brain injury and the strong likelihood of secondary impairments, a physical therapist must be proficient in a wide variety of examination procedures and intervention techniques. Owing to behavioral difficulties encountered during recovery, a physical therapist working with this population must also possess strong communication and interpersonal skills, must be able to react quickly and effectively to suddenly changing situations, and must have keen observation skills. These factors and others can make working with this population challenging. However, the rewards of assisting a patient with a severe brain injury to return to home, work, or school vastly outweigh the challenges of rehabilitation.

The patient with a brain injury is treated across a wide continuum of care, which includes the intensive care unit, acute hospital, in-patient rehabilitation center, skilled nursing facility (subacute rehabilitation), and long-term care facility. Additional services may include outpatient services, community reintegration program, comprehensive day treatment, and residential programs for assisted living and neurobehavioral services. Because of the wide variety of presenting impairments, activity limitations and participation restrictions, rehabilitation for the patient with TBI requires a strong interdisciplinary team. A physical therapist is an important member of this team. It is crucial that there be open communication between and among all team members to ensure safe, timely, and consistent treatment. Regardless of the setting, it is important to remember that the patient is the central member of the team.

■ PREVALENCE

Traumatic brain injury is the leading cause of injury-related death and disability in the United States. Globally, the incidence of TBI is approximately 200 cases per 100,000 people per year, which equates to roughly 15 million people. Of these, approximately 5.5 million experience a severe TBI.[2] In the United States, there are approximately 3 million hospital visits, 300,000 hospitalizations, and 57,000 deaths per year due to TBI.[3,4] Because of differences in definitions of TBI and underreporting of mild TBI, these numbers likely underrepresent its true incidence.

Falls are the leading cause of TBI, followed by struck by/against events and motor vehicle/traffic crashes. Older adults (>75 years) are at greatest risk of TBI, followed by infants (0 to 4 months) and older adolescents/young adults (l4 to 24 years).[5] Hospitalization and death as a result of TBI are most common in older adults (65 years old and over).[6,7] For individuals with moderate to severe TBI, motor vehicle crashes are the most common cause in younger adults and decreases with age. Falls are the most common cause in older adults.[8]

The long-term consequences of TBI on the healthcare system, society, and the individual and their family are high. There are approximately 3.2 to 5.3 million people living in the United States who are disabled as a result of TBI.[9–11] The annual economic burden is estimated to be $75 billion, including direct medical costs, injury-related disability and work loss, and lost income due to premature death.[2] One in five individuals who receive inpatient rehabilitation services post TBI are dead within 5 years, and of those that survive, 50% are readmitted to the hospital at least once.[12] Approximately 50% of people with moderate to severe TBI are able return to work after their injury, but only 33% return to their preinjury employment.[13] One quarter to one-third of people with severe to moderate TBI require assistance with activities of daily living (ADL) and approximately 20% to 30% report a full recovery.[12,14]

■ MECHANISM OF INJURY AND PATHOPHYSIOLOGY

Traumatic brain injury is a heterogenous injury, with a wide variety of pathophysiological mechanisms, but most typically occur as a result of a high-velocity or high-impact blow to the head.[15] The brain damage results from external forces that cause brain tissue to make direct contact with an object (bony skull or penetrating object), rapid acceleration or deceleration forces, or blast waves from an explosion.[16] Generally speaking, brain tissue damage can be categorized as either primary injury that is due to direct trauma to the parenchyma or secondary injury that results from a cascade of biochemical, cellular, and molecular events that evolve over time due to the initial injury and injury-related hypoxia, edema, and elevated intracranial pressure (ICP).[15,17]

Primary Injury

Primary TBI results from either brain tissue coming into contact with an object (e.g., bony skull or external object such as a bullet or sharp instrument, creating a penetrating injury) or rapid acceleration/deceleration or rotation of the brain creating cortical disruption. Contact injuries often result in contusions, lacerations, and intracerebral hematomas. This damage is generally focal in nature as the brain comes into contact with bony protuberances on the inside surface of the skull or damage from the penetrating object. Common areas of focal injury are the anterior temporal poles, frontal poles, lateral and inferior temporal cortices, and orbital frontal cortices.

Acceleration and deceleration cause shear, tensile, and compression forces within the brain, which causes *traumatic axonal injury* (TAI).[18] Traumatic axonal injury is a more recent term for *diffuse axonal injury* (DAI) as this type of injury may not always be diffuse. Traumatic axonal injury commonly occurs in the corpus callosum, internal capsule, cerebral peduncles, and brainstem.

The mechanism of TAI is microscopic, so there may be minimal initial findings on computed tomography (CT) and magnetic resonance imaging (MRI).

Secondary Injury

Secondary cell death occurs as a result of the cellular cascade that follows tissue damage in addition to the secondary effects of hypoxemia, hypotension, ischemia, edema, and elevated ICP. Secondary processes develop over hours and days and include glutamate neurotoxicity, influx of calcium and other ions, free radical release, cytokines, and inflammatory responses that can lead to cell death.[16,17] The release of glutamate and other excitatory neurotransmitters exacerbates ion-channel leakage and contributes to brain swelling and raised ICP.[16] Hypoxic-ischemic injury results from a lack of oxygenated blood flow to the brain tissue. It can be caused by systemic hypotension, anoxia, or damage to specific vascular territories of the brain. Because the rigid skull surrounds the brain, swelling, abnormal brain fluid dynamics, or hematoma can result in elevated ICP. Hematomas are usually classified according to their site (epidural, subdural, or intracerebral). Normal ICP is 5.9 to 8.3 mm HG in upright posture and 0.0 to 16.3 mm HG in supine.[19] Severely increased ICP may result in herniation of the brain, requiring prompt emergency treatment. Common types of herniations are uncal, central, and tonsillar.

It is important to keep in mind that both primary and secondary mechanisms of injury are not mutually exclusive and often do not occur in isolation. This is one reason that the impact of TBI is so widespread across the International Classification of Functioning, Disability, and Health (ICF) spectrum. Further, the nature of the mechanism of how a TBI may occur means that concurrent chest, spinal, abdominal, and limb injuries may occur.

■ IMPACT OF TRAUMATIC BRAIN INJURY

Traumatic brain injury is associated with a wide spectrum of body structure/function impairments, activity limitations and participation restrictions that can lead to diminished quality of life (QOL).[12,20–23] Box 19.1 identifies some of the prevalent body structure/function impairments, activity limitations and participation restrictions associated with TBI. Although physical therapy interventions primarily address physical limitations related to mobility, the cognitive and behavioral changes associated with TBI are often more disabling.

Body Structure/Function Impairments
Neuromuscular Impairments

Individuals with TBI commonly exhibit impaired motor function.[24] Upper extremity (UE) and lower extremity (LE) paresis,[24,25] impaired coordination,[24–26]

Box 19.1 Impairments, Limitations, and Restrictions Commonly Associated With Traumatic Brain Injury

Body Structure/Function Impairments
Neuromuscular

- Paresis
- Abnormal tone/spasticity
- Motor function
- Postural control

Cognitive
- Arousal level
- Attention
- Concentration
- Memory
- Learning
- Executive functions

Neurobehavioral
- Agitation/aggression
- Disinhibition
- Apathy
- Emotional lability
- Mental inflexibility
- Impulsivity
- Irritability
Communication impairments
Swallowing impairments
Activity limitations

- Walking/locomotion
- Basic mobility
- Basic ADL
- Instrumental ADL

Participation restrictions
- Vocational
- Family role
- Community/social role

impaired postural control,[27–31] abnormal muscle tone,[25] and abnormal gait[30,32,33] may be present as life-long impairments. Abnormal, involuntary movements such as tremor and choreiform and dystonic movements are less common.[24] Patients may also present with impaired somatosensory function, depending on the location of the lesion.

Abnormal tone may present as spasticity, hypertonicity, or spasms.[34] Primitive postures may include those associated with decorticate or decerebrate rigidity. In decorticate rigidity, the UEs are in a flexed posture and the LEs are extended. With decerebrate rigidity, both the UEs and LEs are positioned in extension. The distribution and severity of abnormal tone may vary considerably, ranging from spasticity that severely affects the entire body and greatly inhibits normal functional movement, to lesser levels of tone that affect individual muscle groups.

Cognitive Impairments

Cognition is the mental process of knowing and applying information. Owing to the complex nature of many cognitive processes it is difficult to localize the exact neuroanatomical structures responsible for many different cognitive functions. However, many cognitive functions are controlled in the frontal lobes. This makes people with TBI particularly susceptible to cognitive impairments. Cognition includes many complex neural processes, including arousal, attention, concentration, memory, learning, and executive functions.[35–37] Executive functions can be categorized into the following main areas: planning, cognitive flexibility, initiation and self-generation, response inhibition, and serial ordering and sequencing.[36] Chapter 27, Cognitive and Perceptual Dysfunction, provides an in-depth discussion.

Early after injury, patients often present with disorders of consciousness.[38,39] Coma, unresponsive wakefulness (referred to as vegetative state in earlier literature), and minimally conscious state are disordered arousal states seen after severe brain injury. It can be difficult to distinguish among these states.

Coma

Many severe injuries begin with coma. In a coma the arousal system is not functioning. Arousal and awareness are absent. The patient's eyes are closed, there are no sleep/wake cycles, and the patient is ventilator dependent. There is no auditory or visual function and no cognitive or communicative function.[39] Abnormal motor and postural reflexes may be present. A coma is usually not permanent, often lasting two to four weeks. Patients may become brain dead, enter an unresponsive wakefulness state, or minimally conscious state.

Brain death, or death by neurological criteria, is the "irreversible cessation of circulatory and respiratory functions, or irreversible cessation of all functions of the entire brain, including the brainstem. . . ." Despite this definition, clinical diagnosis of brain death remains controversial[40–42] and has clinical decision-making and legal implications. A neurological diagnosis that can lead to brain death is vital, and conditions that mimic it need to be excluded. Two key criteria related to brain death are the cessation of circulation and respiration; however, both can be masked by medications. Guidelines for pediatric brain death vary compared to adults, but in both cases there is no response to external stimuli, pupils are nonreactive and ocular reflexes absent, and gag and cough reflexes are absent.[42]

Unresponsive Wakefulness

In an unresponsive wakefulness state, there is disassociation between arousal and awareness. The higher central nervous system (CNS) centers are not integrated with the brainstem. Patients may be aroused to external stimuli, reflexive movement (chewing, crying, vocalizations) may be present, but patients are not aware of self or the environment. Eyes may open though awareness of surroundings is absent, and sleep/wake cycle is present. Patients may reflexively startle to visual or auditory stimuli and briefly orient to sound or visual stimuli. Although patients in an unresponsive wakefulness state may appear to have purposeful movement, these movements are nonpurposeful and reflexive in response to external stimuli. However, meaningful cognitive and communication function is absent.

Minimally Conscious State

In a minimally conscious state, there is evidence of self- or environmental awareness. Cognitively mediated behaviors occur inconsistently and are reproducible or sustained such that they can be differentiated from reflexive behaviors. Instead of withdrawing or posturing to stimuli, patients in a minimally conscious state will localize to stimuli and may inconsistently reach for objects. Patients may localize to sound location and demonstrate sustained visual fixation and visual pursuit, and inconsistently communicate through yes/no responses.

Commonly used terms to describe other altered levels of consciousness are *stupor* and *obtunded.* Stupor is an unresponsive state from which the patient can be aroused only briefly with vigorous, repeated sensory stimulation. The patient in an obtunded state sleeps often and when aroused exhibits decreased alertness and interest in the environment and delayed reactions.

Neurobehavioral Impairments

Patients can exhibit profound behavioral changes as they progress through recovery. These impairments can be closely linked to cognitive impairments and are often more debilitating in the long run than physical disability. Common behavioral sequelae include low frustration tolerance, agitation, disinhibition, apathy, emotional lability, mental inflexibility, physical and verbal aggression, impulsivity, and irritability.[43] The prevalence of aggression in the inpatient and rehabilitation settings for patients with TBI and posttraumatic amnesia (PTA) may be as high as 44%.[44] Factors related to this prevalence include premorbid substance use disorder and psychiatric conditions such as personality and affective disorders.

Communication Impairments

Language and communication deficits after brain injury are generally nonaphasic in nature[45] and are related to cognitive impairment. Common language and communication deficits include disorganized and tangential oral or written communication, imprecise language, word retrieval difficulties, and disinhibited and socially inappropriate language. Patients may also exhibit difficulties communicating in distracting environments, reading social cues, and adjusting communication to meet the demands of the situation.[46] These communication deficits can affect employability, social integration, and QOL.[47,48] Chapter 28, Neurogenic Disorders of Speech and Language, provides more detail on communication deficits and intervention strategies.

Paroxysmal Sympathetic Hyperactivity

Elevated sympathetic nervous system activity occurs as a normal response to trauma; following TBI, this response may become overactive. Paroxysmal sympathetic hyperactivity (PSH), also known as sympathetic storming, occurs early after injury (weeks). Increased sympathetic activity results in increased heart rate, respiratory rate, and blood pressure; diaphoresis; and hyperthermia. Other symptoms of dysautonomia include decerebrate and decorticate posturing, hypertonia, and teeth grinding. The incidence of PSH ranges from 8% to 33% in patients with TBI in the intensive care unit. The incidence of PSH is approximately 30%, and individuals with PSH often have longer hospital stays and poorer outcomes.[49]

Posttraumatic Seizures

Seizures after TBI can generally be categorized as immediate (<24 hours postinjury), early (1 to 7 days postinjury) or late (>7 days postinjury). Approximately 10% of people with TBI have an immediate seizure, 2% an early seizure, and 10% a late seizure.[50] Presence of seizures is associated with longer hospitalization and greater likelihood of discharge to a nursing facility rather than home.[51] Phenytoin, an antiseizure medication, is recommended for use to prevent early seizures. However, it is not recommended for prevention of late seizures.[51]

Disordered Sleep

Impaired sleep is common in people with TBI both in the early and chronic stages of recovery. Common sleep disorders include insomnia, hypersomnia, and sleep apnea. Disturbed sleep early after injury is particularly prevalent during PTA (see below).[52] In the later stages of recovery, disordered sleep is associated with poorer functional outcomes and lower QOL.[53] Cognitive-behavioral therapy for insomnia, sleep hygiene, exercise, and blue wavelength light therapy may help improve sleep, fatigue, and depression.[54,55]

Secondary Impairments and Medical Complications

Due to the high potential of prolonged immobility and concomitant injury, patients with TBI are at risk of developing a number of secondary impairments and other medical issues. Box 19.2 lists some of the more common secondary impairments and concomitant injuries associated with TBI.

Box 19.2 Secondary Impairments and Concomitant Injuries

- Deep vein thrombosis
- Heterotopic ossification
- Pressure ulcer
- Pneumonia
- Chronic pain
- Contractures
- Decreased endurance
- Muscle atrophy
- Fracture
- Peripheral nerve damage

ADL – activities of daily living.

Activity Limitations

The activity domain of functioning in the ICF is related to the execution of a task or action by an individual. Activity limitations involve difficulties with walking, carrying/handling objects, changing and maintaining body position, washing/bathing, dressing, eating, drinking, and other ADL. People with TBI are likely to have limitations in walking ability, high-level mobility, eating, dressing, bathing, grooming, and other ADL. Individuals with TBI are more likely to experience long-lasting limitations in cognitive-related activities such as problem-solving, memory, and cognitive comprehension, rather than motor-related activity limitations such as ADL and basic mobility.

Participation Restrictions

According to the ICF, the participation domain of functioning is related to a person's life situations, including but not limited to role in the home, vocation, and leisure and recreational involvement. Participation restrictions involve the difficulties a person may experience while attempting to engage in typical life situations due to the presence of disability related to their health condition. Although many people with TBI are able to return to some level of independence in relation to basic ADL,[56] given the potentially severe and widespread cognitive impairments, persons with TBI may experience significant, long-term participation restrictions.[12,23] Survivors are often challenged when attempting to return to their prior roles in workforce, family, or community. Approximately 50% of people with TBI are able to return to some type of work,[12] but only 33% return to their previous employment.[13] Age of onset, injury severity, severity of cognitive and behavioral impairments, preinjury employment, and length of hospital stay are predictors of return gainful employment post TBI.[57,58]

Potential Long-Term Impact

In addition to the immediate and near-term effects of TBI, there is also a correlation between TBI and the development of certain neurodegenerative and psychiatric diseases. In a review of the topic, Young and colleagues suggest that for those with TBI, as the brain ages, there is a long-term risk of developing Alzheimer disease, Parkinson disease, frontotemporal dementia, and chronic traumatic encephalopathy.[59] There also appears to be a relationship between the presence of a TBI and the development of depressive and anxiety disorders.[59]

■ DIAGNOSIS AND PROGNOSIS

Traumatic brain injury is generally categorized as severe, moderate, or mild using the *Glasgow Coma Scale* (GCS) (Fig. 19.1).[60] The GCS, developed by Teasdale and Jennett, is the most widely used clinical scale that helps define and classify the severity of brain injury. The GCS comprises three response scores: motor response, verbal response, and eye opening. The scores from the separate responses are summed to provide a score between 3 and 15. Scores of 8 or less are classified as severe, scores between 9 and 12 are defined as moderate, and scores of 13 to 15 are classified as mild brain injury. Table 19.1 provides an overview of some of the characteristics that distinguish mild, moderate, and severe brain injury. However, these terms can be somewhat misleading in that a mild TBI can have a profound impact across the ICF spectrum.

Owing to the wide range of cognitive, motor, and neurobehavioral impairments that accompany brain injury, it can be difficult to establish and predict long-term outcomes and set goals for these patients, even

Table 19.1 Characteristics of Mild, Moderate, and Severe Traumatic Brain Injury

Mild TBI	Moderate TBI	Severe TBI
LOC: 0–30 min	>30 min and <24 hr	>24 hr
AOC: <=24 hr	>24 hr	>24 hr
PTA: 0–1 day	>1 and <7 days	>7 days
GCS: 13–15	9–12	<9
Neuroimaging: normal	Normal or abnormal	Normal or abnormal

TBI = traumatic brain injury, LOC = loss of consciousness, AOC = alteration of consciousness, PTA = posttraumatic amnesia, GCS = Glasgow Coma Scale.

for an experienced clinician. However, researchers have identified some factors that are useful in predicting outcomes, commonly measured by the Glasgow Outcome Scale (GOS), which categorizes outcomes as good recovery (resumption of preinjury life with minor deficits), moderate disability (independent with ADL), severe disability (dependent with ADL), unresponsive, and death. Low initial scores on the GCS, particularly motor score and pupillary reactivity, age, CT showing mass lesions or signs of raised ICP are predictive of poorer outcomes.[61,62]

The *Medical Research Council* (MRC) CRASH (corticosteroid randomization after significant head injury) study provides a Web-based calculator (www.crash2.lshtm.ac.uk/Risk%20calculator/index.html) that allows clinicians to enter demographic and prognostic information (country, age, GCS score, pupil reactivity to light, presence of major extra cranial injury, and CT findings, if available); it calculates the 14-day mortality risk and unfavorable outcome at 6 months, along with the 95% confidence interval.[63] Unfavorable outcome is defined as dead, unresponsive state, or severe disability as measured by the GOS.

Duration of PTA, the length of time between the injury and the time at which the patient can consistently remember ongoing events, is also an important factor in predicting recovery. Brown et al.[64] found that duration of PTA as measured by the *Galveston Orientation and Amnesia Test* (GOAT), the revised GOAT, or the *Orientation Log* (O-Log) during inpatient rehabilitation is able to predict functional independence, employment, good overall recovery, and independent living 1 year after injury. Traditionally, it was believed that people in PTA may have reduced capacity to benefit from rehabilitation due to the inability to remember. However, recent studies have shown this not to be the case, and people in PTA can actively engage in physical therapy despite the presence of confusion, agitation and fatigue.[65–67]

Glasgow Coma Scale	
Activity	**Score**
Eye Opening	
Spontaneous	4
To speech	3
To pain	2
No response	1
Best Motor Response	
Follows motor commands	6
Localizes	5
Withdraws	4
Abnormal flexion	3
Extensor response	2
No response	1
Verbal Response	
Oriented	5
Confused conversation	4
Inappropriate words	3
Incomprehensible sounds	2
No response	1

Figure 19.1 Glasgow Coma Scale. *(From Teasdale and Jennett,[60] with permission.)*

■ CONTINUUM OF CARE AND THE INTERDISCIPLINARY TEAM

Continuum of Care

The rehabilitation of patients with TBI occurs across a continuum of care in a variety of settings (Fig. 19.2). Patients who are in an unresponsive wakefulness state may receive ongoing therapy in a nursing home or other long-term care facility once they are medically stable. Patients who are beginning to recover from coma with moderate to severe cognitive, behavioral, and physical impairments often continue rehabilitation in either an acute or subacute inpatient rehabilitation facility. As patients progress in recovery, they will be discharged to other community-based settings depending on the needs of the individual patient.

Interdisciplinary Team

The foundation for successful rehabilitation following TBI is an *interdisciplinary team*. Within the context of the team, it is vital to place the patient at the center, develop goals that are patient centered and focused on participation, and for team members to collaborate.[68] Communication and open mindedness are key to any team. The various members must share their skills and findings with the whole team and be willing to learn from other team members to promote optimal recovery. The physical therapist must be willing to share a unique knowledge of movement and motor control and be open to learning from other team members. Each team member should develop an approach to treatment that considers information obtained from all other participating disciplines. This will lead to a consistent and comprehensive approach to care. An interdisciplinary approach to rehabilitation for this population has been shown to be effective for improving activity levels and participation in society.[69]

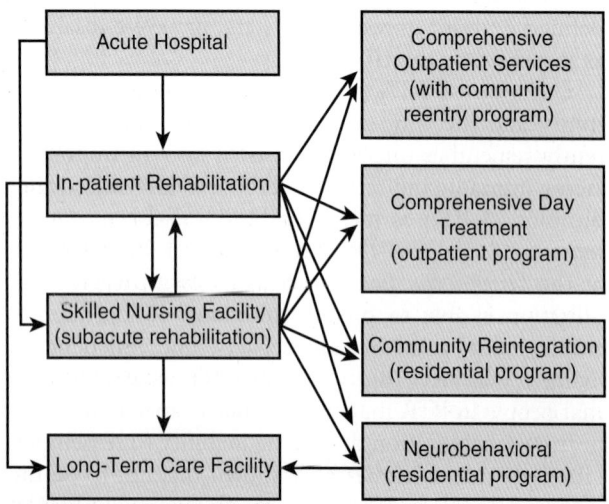

Figure 19.2 Rehabilitation settings for individuals with TBI across the continuum of care.

Some members may play more prominent roles depending on the setting and stage of recovery. For example, a recreational therapist will not likely be involved with a patient in the acute hospital but would play a vital role in a community reentry setting. The following subsections identify some of the team members involved in the care of individuals with brain injury and their roles in an acute rehabilitation hospital.

Patient and Family

The patient and their family are at the center of the team. The lives of both the patient and family members are likely to be dramatically changed as a result of the injury. Familial roles often change. The patient who previously took care of the children may now be on the receiving end of care. The team must garner information regarding the patient's work, school, financial status, and social history. Family members should be interviewed to obtain information about the patient's lifestyle (work/school/leisure), favorite social and recreational activities, and so forth. Information about the family dynamics should be ascertained. What is the patient's role in the family? Is the patient the primary wage earner? Is the patient responsible for taking care of children? Is the patient in school? Is the patient working? All of these and many other similar questions should be answered in order to develop a comprehensive plan of care (POC).

Physician

In the acute rehabilitation hospital, the physician overseeing the care of the patient with a brain injury is usually a physiatrist or neurologist. The physiatrist has expertise and training in physical medicine and rehabilitation. A neurologist's skills lie in the realm of the brain and nervous system. A neurologist will have particular knowledge related to how the brain may recover, and what impairments and activity limitations are likely to be seen given the location and the extent of the injury. Both a physiatrist and neurologist have vast knowledge in neuropharmacology, an extremely important part of management with this patient population. Certain medications may have harmful side effects that may not be readily apparent. For example, the physician may be able to prescribe a less-sedating drug than would normally be used to treat a certain clinical problem in other patient populations.

Speech-Language Pathologist

Owing to the nature of a brain injury, the speech-language pathologist (SLP) plays an important and diverse role in rehabilitation. The SLP examines, evaluates, and treats communication, swallowing, and cognitive impairments. As can be seen from the cognitive and communication impairments described above, this can be a challenging task. It is important for the physical therapist to be in close communication with the

SLP to provide consistency of care in relation to cognitive, swallowing, and communication impairments. With the guidance of the SLP, the team will be able to devise the most effective and consistent way to communicate with the patient. The SLP will also be able to instruct the team in how the patient's cognitive impairments may impede new learning, which in turn will affect everyone's interactions with the patient and their approach to treatment.

Occupational Therapist

The occupational therapist (OT) examines, evaluates, and treats the patient's diminished ability to perform ADL, visual/perceptual impairments, UE functional loss, and sensory integration problems, and will often work with the SLP in treating cognitive impairments. Basic ADL (BADL) includes dressing, self-feeding, bathing, and grooming. Instrumental ADL (IADL) includes home management, housekeeping, grocery shopping, driving, and telephone use. In the rehabilitation hospital, the occupational and physical therapists often work very closely together. A useful treatment approach is cotreatments with the OT. Having two trained professionals working at the same time with the patient can be very productive. This is especially true with patients who have severe motor control and cognitive deficits.

One example would be a scavenger hunt in the community with a higher functioning patient. The patient is given a list of tasks to do or items to find in a community setting such as a grocery store. During the scavenger hunt the PT might address specific mobility barriers or dual-task deficits in balance whereas OT might work toward improved problem-solving and social skills. The OT will also work closely with the nursing staff to educate them on the best ways to assist the patient with ADL. Following the subacute phase of rehabilitation, the OT may assist training and reintegration for a range of community-based activities such as driving, work or school, shopping, and money management.

Rehabilitation Nurse

In a rehabilitation hospital, the nurse is responsible for continually assessing the patient's medical status as well as the level of emotional and behavioral stability. Additional responsibilities include dispensing medications and closely monitoring their effects, and initiating and managing programs for bowel and bladder retraining to assist the patient in learning to become continent again. Bowel and bladder control is extremely important for self-esteem and is related to discharge placement. The nurse performs daily monitoring of vital signs to make sure the patient remains medically stable. The nurse will inspect the patient's skin daily to ensure there are no signs of skin breakdown. The nurse also has the difficult task of consistently following through with the team's treatment plan throughout the day. For example, each

shift of nursing staff must follow splinting schedules established by the physical and occupational therapists. The nurse often has the most interaction on a regular basis with the patient and family.

Neuropsychologist

The neuropsychologist plays an important role on the team. They will often perform neuropsychological testing when appropriate to determine the patient's baseline cognitive functioning. They also assist the team in developing a cognitive and behavioral management program. When the patient with a brain injury has severe behavioral impairments, the neuropsychologist may assume the role of the team leader and meet regularly with the patient and family for counseling sessions.

Case Manager/Team Coordinator

The case manager acts as the coordinator for the team. The case manager is often a nurse, social worker, or other health professional. The case manager will direct team meetings, schedule family conferences, and act as a liaison with third-party payers. The case manager must promote good communication among all team members to ensure that the rehabilitation care being provided is truly team oriented. The case manager will also be in constant communication with the patient and family to ensure that their needs are being met and that questions and concerns are adequately addressed. The case manager will coordinate payment and insurance benefit issues with the case manager from the patient's insurance company. In addition, the case manager is responsible for setting up follow-up and discharge services for the patient and family.

Social Worker

The social worker provides much needed support to both the patient and family. During the first few days after the initial injury, the family is often in a state of crisis. They are thrown into a world that they, most likely, never knew existed. The social worker can support the family with education and counseling. The social worker may also interface with insurance companies. As the patient progresses with recovery, the social worker will also provide counseling for the patient. This is particularly important as the patient begins to develop greater awareness and insight into their deficits. If the patient has behavioral impairments, the social worker can be pivotal in assisting both the patient and family. By providing counseling to both the patient and family, the social worker assists in the development of coping strategies for what may be a life-long disability.

Vocational Rehabilitation Counselor

The vocational rehabilitation counselor (VCR) plays a critical role when the patient is out of the hospital and beginning to integrate back into the work force. The

VCR provides support to secure employment and vocational counseling and training. In the United States, vocational counseling services are often provided by state agencies. The VCR, patient, and employer work together to develop an individualized plan to overcome barriers to work and provide coaching and skills training.[70]

Other Team Members

There are a variety of other health professionals that may also be a member of the interdisciplinary team supporting recovery. Patients with severe brain injury may require ventilatory support in the early stages of recovery. The respiratory therapist is a vital participant in the evaluation and treatment of respiratory impairments. In the rehabilitation hospital, the respiratory therapist contributes to monitoring the patient's pulmonary status and providing appropriate treatment. A registered dietician monitors patients' diet, which is critical during recovery.

In people with TBI with visual impairments, a neuro-ophthalmologist or neuro-optometrist may prescribe prism glasses to address visual field deficits or other interventions to improve vision. A recreational therapist assists the patient's return to activities enjoyed before the accident, or in helping identify new activities that the patient will find rewarding. Therapeutic recreation is an extremely important part of rehabilitation. Being able to participate in some type of leisure or recreational activities is a significant step in returning to a fulfilling lifestyle.

■ EARLY MEDICAL MANAGEMENT

Medical treatment following brain injury starts at the scene of the accident. Early resuscitation with the goal of stabilizing the cardiovascular and respiratory systems is important to maintain sufficient blood flow and oxygen to the brain. Once the patient arrives at the medical center, the primary goals are to minimize secondary brain injury by optimizing cerebral blood flow and oxygenation, stabilize vital signs, perform a complete examination, identify and treat any non-neurological injuries, and continuously monitor the patient.[71] Systolic blood pressure should be kept above 90 mm Hg and oxygen saturation above 90%.[72] Patients with severe injury and some with moderate injury will need to be intubated. The patient's neck should be stabilized with a collar and the head elevated 30°.[72] This is done to protect the spine in case of instability, as well as avoid an increase in ICP. Once the stability of the spine is confirmed through imaging, the protective collar can be removed. The GCS is used to determine the severity of the brain injury. A complete neurological examination is also done. Additional information about the extent of the injury is obtained through x-ray films and neuroimaging studies such as CT and MRI. This is done to determine if neurosurgery is warranted.

Intracranial hematomas or other mass lesions may need to be addressed surgically.

Cerebral perfusion pressure (CPP) and ICP are monitored.[73] For patients with a GCS of 8 or less, any acute abnormality on CT, a systolic pressure of less than 90 mm Hg, or age greater than 40 years, ICP monitoring is recommended.[72] However, some patients may not require continuous ICP monitoring.[74] External ventricular drains, a subdural bolt, and a fiberoptic catheter provide methods of monitoring ICP. Elevated ICP can be treated with sedating medications, moderate head-up positioning (head elevated to 30°), osmotherapy, hypothermia, and barbiturates.[72,75] Intracranial pressure should be less than 20 mm Hg and CPP greater than 60 mm Hg.[72] If ICP cannot be treated successfully, inducing a pharmacologic coma or surgical decompression may be necessary.

The remainder of this chapter is divided into three main sections: (1) physical therapy management of patients with severe to moderate TBI during the early stages of recovery focusing on patients with altered levels of consciousness, (2) physical therapy management of patients with severe to moderate TBI during active rehabilitation, and (3) physical therapy management of patients with mild TBI.

■ PHYSICAL THERAPY MANAGEMENT OF MODERATE TO SEVERE TRAUMATIC BRAIN INJURY EARLY AFTER INJURY

Patients in the early stage of recovery after severe to moderate TBI often demonstrate an altered level of consciousness as described earlier. The primary goals of physical therapy in this early stage of recovery are early mobilization, prevention of secondary complications due to the TBI and associated prolonged bedrest/immobilization, and initiation of family education.

Examination Early After Injury

The first step in beginning an examination at this early stage of recovery is to conduct a complete review of the medical record. Because the patient may not be medically stable and may have various contraindications, precautions, and complications that impact physical therapy interventions, it is important to obtain all critical information from the medical record, nursing staff, and physician before seeing the patient. The patient may be on a ventilator with ongoing monitoring. They may have weight-bearing restrictions owing to musculoskeletal injuries or open wounds. A thorough medical record review provides a comprehensive perspective about the patient's condition, as well as a complete understanding of the precautions and contraindications that must be observed during the examination and subsequent treatment. Because the patient's medical status may be dynamic, it is important to check with the patient's primary nurse before beginning any session. Team members should always observe universal precautions and may need to wear gowns, gloves, masks, and other personal protective equipment when treating the patient.

For patients with altered levels of consciousness, it is vital to perform a comprehensive and standardized examination to determine level of consciousness (coma vs. unresponsive wakefulness vs. minimally conscious state).[39,76] There are a variety of challenges associated with accurately determining the patient's level of consciousness. Limited motor function, communication impairments, sedating medications, impaired sensation, and impaired executive function can impact the patient's ability to respond to sensory stimuli and commands. The examination should be performed in a closed environment, in a structured manner, at multiple times, to capture the patient's response over time as the patient's response may not be consistent. The entire team should do the examination with all members carefully documenting the patient's response. The Coma Recovery Scale-Revised (CRC-R; see below for details on this test) is recommended for this purpose.[77,78] Identifying the patient's level of consciousness is critical as patients with disordered levels of consciousness are easily misdiagnosed. A misdiagnosis at this early stage of recovery can lead to a lack of appropriate rehabilitation services and poorer outcomes.

In addition to examining arousal, attention, and cognition other key areas to examine include the following:

- Integument integrity
- Sensory integrity
- Motor function
- Range of motion
- Reflex integrity
- Ventilation and respiration/gas exchange
- Mobility, including bed mobility, transfers, sitting and standing balance, and walking if the patient is able to participate in these activities

If not medically contraindicated, the examination should include early mobilization such as assisted bed mobility and sitting, and if possible, supported upright posture/standing. The therapist should monitor vital signs and observe for changes in arousal and motor function during assisted mobilization. A more upright posture may change the patient's level of arousal compared to when they are supine in bed. Care must be taken for those with prolonged disorder of consciousness (DOC) or polytrauma, as hypotension may result from early mobilization. For this reason, a tilt table that provides for a graduated vertical position may be preferable to a standing frame. When appropriate, the patient should be transferred into a wheelchair. The patient may require the assistance of two to three people to transfer at this stage. In most cases, a reclining or tilt-in-space wheelchair is the best option for positioning, with a pressure-reducing cushion. Often it may require several treatment sessions to complete the entire examination. Because early patient status is often dynamic, any signs of progress or regression should be carefully monitored and documented.

Outcome Measures

Arousal, Attention, and Cognition

The *Coma Recovery Scale–Revised* (CRS-R) is recommended to assess patients with disordered consciousness.[77,78] The CRS-R is a valid and reliable 23-item measure with six subscales: auditory, visual, motor, oromotor, communication, and arousal.[79] Scores range from 0 to 23. Data are useful in distinguishing between different states of consciousness (unresponsive wakefulness, minimally conscious state, and emerging), determining the prognosis, and informing treatment planning.[79]

The *Disorders of Consciousness Scale* (DOCS) is a valid and reliable scale designed to measure arousal and neurobehavioral recovery in patients with disorders of consciousness.[80,81] It consists of 23 items, which assess social knowledge, taste/swallowing, olfactory function, proprioception, tactile sensation, auditory function, and visual function. Scoring is based on patient response and includes no response, generalized response, or localized response. The DOCS can be used to differentiate states of consciousness (i.e., unresponsive wakefulness and minimally conscious state) and assist in determining prognosis for recovery. A training manual is available for the DOCS at https://www.sralab.org/sites/default/files/2017-06/manual_2011.pdf

The *Rancho Los Amigos Levels of Cognitive Functioning* (LOCF) scale is a descriptive scale used to examine cognitive and behavioral recovery in individuals with TBI (Box 19.3) as they emerge from coma.[82] This scale does not address specific cognitive deficits, but rather is useful for communicating general cognitive and/or behavioral status and for treatment planning. The eight categories describe typical cognitive and behavioral progress after a brain injury. Patients may plateau at any level. The LOCF has been shown to be a reliable and valid measure of cognitive and behavioral function for individuals with brain injury.[83] It can also be used to predict global outcome.[84]

Spasticity and Hypertonicity

Following TBI, spasticity and hypertonicity may be severe and challenging to treat. Numerous guidelines exist for spasticity management, but there is no consensus as to the best assessment tool.[85,86] The two most common clinical measures of spasticity are the modified Ashworth Scale[87] and the modified Tardieu Scale.[88] It has been suggested that although used interchangeably, spasticity and hypertonicity are different phenomena and should be assessed as such.[89] Consequently, the Modified Ashworth Scale (MAS) has been suggested for

Box 19.3   Rancho Los Amigos Levels of Cognitive Functioning[a]

I. No Response

Patient appears to be in a deep sleep and is completely unresponsive to any stimuli.

II. Generalized Response

Patient reacts to stimuli inconsistently, without purpose, and in a nonspecific manner. Responses are limited and often the same regardless of stimulus presented. Responses may be physiological changes, gross body movements, and/or vocalization.

III. Localized Response

Patient reacts specifically but inconsistently to stimuli. Responses are directly related to the type of stimulus presented. May follow simple commands such as closing eyes or squeezing hand in an inconsistent, delayed manner.

IV. Confused-Agitated

Patient is in a heightened state of activity. Behavior is bizarre and nonpurposeful relative to immediate environment. Does not discriminate among persons or objects; is unable to cooperate directly with treatment efforts. Verbalizations frequently are incoherent and/or inappropriate to the environment; confabulation may be present. Gross attention to environment is very brief; selective attention is often nonexistent. Patient lacks short- and long-term recall.

V. Confused-Inappropriate

Patient is able to respond to simple commands fairly consistently. However, with increased complexity of commands or lack of any external structure, responses are nonpurposeful, random, or fragmented. Demonstrates gross attention to the environment but is highly distractible and lacks ability to focus attention on a specific task. With structure, may be able to converse on a social automatic level for short periods of time. Verbalization is often inappropriate and confabulatory. Memory is severely impaired; often shows inappropriate use of objects; may perform previously learned tasks with structure but is unable to learn new information.

VI. Confused-Appropriate

Patient shows goal-directed behavior but is dependent on external input or direction. Follows simple directions consistently and shows carryover for relearned tasks such as self-care. Responses may be incorrect due to memory problems, but they are appropriate to the situation. Memories from long in the past show more depth and detail than do more recent memories.

VII. Automatic-Appropriate

Patient appears appropriate and oriented within the hospital and home settings; goes through daily routine automatically, but frequently robot-like. Patient shows minimal to no confusion and has shallow recall of activities. Shows carryover for new learning but at a decreased rate. With structure is able to initiate social or recreational activities; judgment remains impaired.

VIII. Purposeful-Appropriate

Patient is able to recall and integrate past and recent events and is aware of and responsive to environment. Shows carryover for new learning and needs no supervision once activities are learned. May continue to show a decreased ability relative to premorbid abilities, abstract reasoning, tolerance for stress, and judgment in emergencies or unusual circumstances.

[a]Condensed from Professional Staff Association, Ranchos Los Amigos Hospital, with permission.[108]

---

hypertonicity (the non-velocity-dependent resistance to passive movement) and the modified Tardieu Scale for spasticity (velocity-dependent resistance).

Goals and Outcomes

A list of general goals and outcomes anticipated for patients in Levels I, II, and III (LOCF) are presented in Box 19.4. These can be used to guide the development of specific anticipated goals and expected outcomes for an individual patient.

Interventions

Early Mobilization

Early physical therapy is beneficial for individuals with disorders of consciousness.[76,90–92] Patients with TBI who receive physical therapy early in the ICU and acute care hospital (<72 hours) are likely to have shorter lengths of stay and experience fewer secondary complications, such as pneumonia and skin breakdown.[93] Contraindications to early mobilization include unstable spine

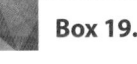

Box 19.4 General Goals and Outcomes Anticipated for Patients With Severe to Moderate Traumatic Brain Injury in the Acute Stage

Impact of impairment is reduced

- Risk of secondary impairments is reduced.
- Motor function is improved.
- Joint integrity and mobility are improved or remain functional.
- Level of arousal and alertness is increased.

Ability to improve physical actions, tasks, or activities is improved.

- Tolerance of upright postures and activities is improved.
- Functional mobility is improved.
- Safety of patient, family, and caregivers is improved.

Patient/client satisfaction is enhanced

- Family and caregivers are educated on patient's diagnosis, physical therapy interventions, goals, and outcomes.
- Care is coordinated among all team members.

and increased ICP. Precautions include weight-bearing restrictions, skin and joint integrity, autonomic instability, and cardiovascular status.

A tilt table, or specialized tilt table with a stepping system built in, can be used to safely assist the patient into an upright posture. Assumption of early upright posture (with or without a stepping system) is safe and may improve level of consciousness.[94-97] A harness system used either overground or over a treadmill can be used to safely assist the patient to a standing position and take assisted steps.[92] However, due to the limited research in this area and the lack of a control group in many of the studies, the benefits compared to other interventions and the optimal dosage of this early, assisted assumption of upright postures is not known.[98] When patients are assisted into an upright posture and during early mobilization, the physical therapist should closely monitor vital signs and observe for changes in level of arousal during the intervention session. A hard or soft cervical collar may be useful to assist with head control. Other interventions that can be done to promote early mobilization include passive seated bikes that use a powered system to pedal the bike, a functional electrical stimulation bike, and assisted sitting. Importantly, we should not automatically assume that patients with low levels of arousal cannot be mobilized. Early mobilization may be an important active ingredient to promote beneficial neuroplastic changes to improve outcomes.

Preventing Secondary Impairments

Because of the patient's inability to move at these levels, they are susceptible to secondary impairments such as

contractures, pressure injuries, pneumonia, and deep vein thrombosis. If prevention is not addressed early, these impairments are likely to impede future progress and can be life threatening. Proper positioning both in bed and in a wheelchair are essential. Appropriate positioning will assist in preventing skin breakdown and contractures, improve pulmonary hygiene and circulation, and may modify muscle tone. When the patient is in bed, the head should be kept in neutral. The hips and knees should be slightly flexed, but range of motion (ROM) should be monitored to ensure that contractures do not develop. Splints may be used to assist in positioning. Special boots can be used to position the foot to prevent foot drop and skin breakdown on the heel (Fig. 19.3). Turning will help prevent skin breakdown and pneumonia. Patients should be repositioned every 2 hours when in bed. Specialized air mattresses are another effective way to assist with the prevention of pressure injuries.

Serial casting may be used to maintain or improve ROM.[99,100] Serial casting is often used for plantarflexor or biceps contractures. With an elbow flexion contracture, the elbow is stretched into extension, and a short cast is applied (Fig. 19.4). In approximately 2 to 5 days, the cast is removed. The muscle is stretched again, and another cast is applied in an improved position. This procedure is repeated until satisfactory gains in ROM have been achieved, or no further progress is made. Because the individual with brain injury is likely to have impaired sensation and communication, as well as behavioral deficits, there is a risk of skin breakdown or the patient hurting themself or others with the cast. The decision to use casts should be made carefully and weigh the potential benefits of a prolonged stretch that the cast provides against a

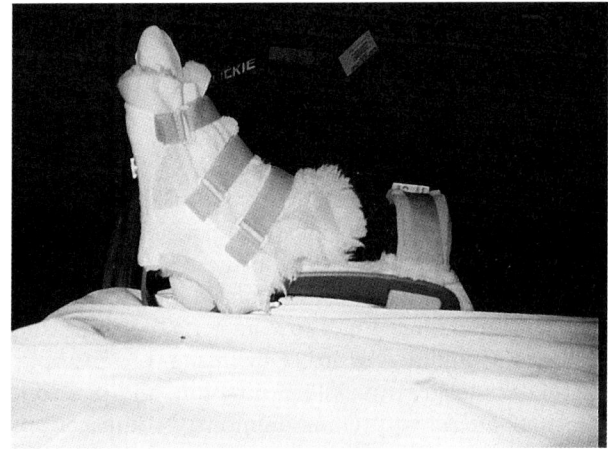

Figure 19.3 Multi-Podus boot used for ankle and foot positioning and to prevent skin breakdown on the heel. This type of positioning device may not be beneficial for the patient with moderate to severe tone at the ankle; it is not strong enough to prevent the ankle from plantarflexing.

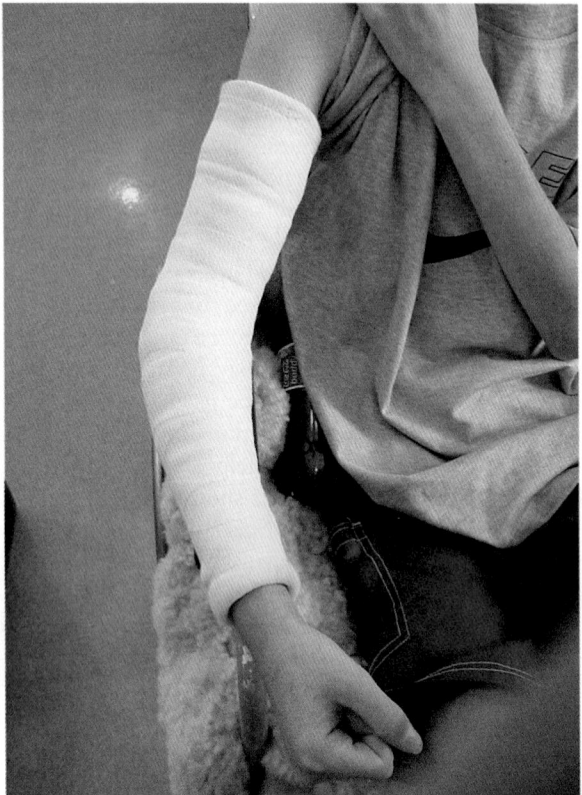

Figure 19.4 Serial casting applied to the elbow.

shorter but stronger stretch obtained on a tilt table. The benefits and possible side effects should be thoroughly discussed with input from appropriate team members. It is also important to monitor the patient's swelling, pain, and skin color after the cast is applied. In some instances, a splint may be able to be used in place of a serial cast. Hands-on experience under the supervision of a skilled clinician is recommended before attempting cast applications.

Proper wheelchair positioning is important. Because of a patient's reduced postural control, an individualized seating system—a reclining or tilt-in-space wheelchair—may be needed to promote optimal positioning and reduce pressure from prolonged sitting. Proper pelvic positioning and head positioning are key elements in promoting good posture in a wheelchair, preventing secondary contractures, and optimizing sensory stimulation. Refer to Chapter 32, Seating and Wheeled Mobility, for further discussion of this topic. Postural drainage, percussion, vibration, and positioning can be used to prevent pulmonary complications and improve pulmonary function.

Treating Spasticity and Hypertonicity

Many treatments are available for spasticity and hypertonicity, and they should align with the severity, chronicity, and distribution.[86] Focal or multifocal muscle spasticity affecting a localized group of muscles can be effectively treated with botulinum neurotoxin-A. When the distribution of spasticity and hypertonicity is more generalized, an oral systemic agent such as Baclofen may be the treatment of choice. In more severe generalized cases of spasticity, Baclofen can be administered via a pump inserted in the abdomen to deliver the medication directly to the spinal cord. Pumps that deliver Baclofen may be the preferred option if higher doses are required, as they have fewer side effects.[101] However, complication rates may be as high as 40%.[102] If severe, spasticity and hypertonicity are associated with established contractures, and musculotendinous surgery may be required.[103,104]

Sensory Stimulation

Sensory stimulation is an intervention used to increase the level of arousal and elicit movement in individuals with low levels of arousal. The theory is that by providing stimulation in a controlled, multisensory manner, with a balance of stimulation and rest, the reticular activating system may be stimulated, causing a general increase in arousal.[105] In general, multisensory stimulation involves the presentation of sensory stimulation in a highly structured and consistent manner while the patient is closely monitored to determine their behavioral response to the sensory stimulation. The following sensory systems can be systematically stimulated: auditory, olfactory, gustatory, visual, tactile, kinesthetic, and vestibular. The value of sensory stimulation for patients who are slow to recover is not clear. Two recent systematic reviews suggest that multimodal sensory stimulation improves arousal.[106,107] However, the designs of many of the included studies have a high potential for bias, the sample sizes are small, and the outcomes used may not be sensitive to change.

Family Education

Family education at this early stage after injury is critical. It is important to provide a realistic and consistent message to family members regarding prognosis. Family members should be included in decision-making when determining the POC and goals of physical therapy. Families should be educated on how patients with DOC present and the differences between reflexive and purposeful movements. Since family members may be with the patient often, they can be taught how to perform ROM exercises and learn how to position the patient to help prevent secondary complications. Family members can also assist with early mobilization interventions described above. Because some patients with TBI may not achieve full independence, family members should also be instructed in how to aid with basic ADL. Although family members value physical therapy, they may also view it negatively if they perceive it causes the patient pain or distress, so it is important to promote open communication with the patient's family.

■ PHYSICAL THERAPY MANAGEMENT OF MODERATE TO SEVERE TRAUMATIC BRAIN INJURY DURING ACTIVE REHABILITATION

As patients with severe to moderate TBI recover, they require extensive and protracted rehabilitation across a variety of settings throughout the continuum of care. This may include acute and subacute inpatient rehabilitation, postacute rehabilitation, day treatment program, and outpatient or home care. The many cognitive, physical, and behavioral impairments that impact activity levels and social participation often necessitate multiple episodes of physical therapy care over the patient's lifetime. Goals and interventions should be focused on the patient's abilities and personal goals regardless of setting and episode of care.

Examination During Active Rehabilitation

Irrespective of injury chronicity, patients with TBI may have cognitive and behavioral impairments that create challenges with the examination process. Disorientation, confusion, physical aggression, memory deficits, and limited attention span can make the examination challenging. It may be difficult to gather data using standardized tests, such as goniometry or the Berg Balance Scale, because the patient may be unable to understand the directions or cooperate. In these cases, the therapist must utilize observation skills as the patient moves to gain insight to the extent of the body structure/function impairments and activity restrictions. The physical therapist should assess the patient's cognition and communication because these will affect the ability to follow directions and relearn motor skills. Orientation, attention span, memory, insight, safety awareness, and alertness should all be assessed. Key initial questions that warrant consideration include the following:

- Is the patient able to follow commands: one-step, two-step, or multistep- commands?
- Is the patient oriented to person, place, and/or time?
- Does the patient recognize family members?
- Does the patient demonstrate insight into what has happened and the impact of the injury?

It is beneficial to consult with other team members, to obtain additional information about the patient's cognitive status. As the patient's cognitive and behavioral impairments become less obtrusive to the process, the physical therapy examination should include the elements and outcome measures found in Box 19.5.

Depending on the status of the individual patient, some of these areas may be screened, whereas others require more in-depth examination. Determination of the patient's functional abilities should be done in

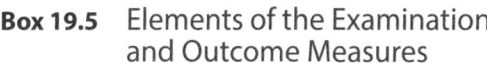

Box 19.5   Elements of the Examination and Outcome Measures

- Aerobic capacity/endurance
- Balance
  - *Berg Balance Scale, Community Balance and Mobility Scale*
- Behavioral status
  - *Supervision Rating Scale, Neurobehavioral Rating Scale–Revised, Agitated Behavior Scale*
- Community, Social and Civic Life
  - *Mayo-Portland Adaptability Inventory, Community Integration Questionnaire, Quality of Life After Brain Injury*
- Cranial nerve integrity
- Locomotion/Walking Ability
  - *10-meter Walk Test, 6-minute Walk Test, High-Level Mobility Assessment Tool, Modified Walking and Remembering Test*
- Integumentary integrity
- Joint integrity and mobility
- Mental Functions
  - *Coma Recovery Scale–Revised, Disorders of Consciousness Scale, Rancho Los Amigos Levels of Cognitive Functioning, Moss Attention Rating Scale, Test of Everyday Attention, Trail Making Test Part B, Galveston Orientation and Amnesia Test, Orientation Log*
- Mobility
  - *Continuity Assessment Record and Evaluation and GG Codes, Functional Independence Measure, Functional Assessment Measure*
- Motor function
- Muscle performance, including strength, power, and endurance
- Neuromotor development and sensory processing
- Pain
- Posture
- Range of Motion
- Reflex integrity
- Self-care and domestic life
  - *Functional Independence Measure, Functional Assessment Measure*
- Sensory integrity
- Ventilation and respiration
- Work life
  - *Mayo-Portland Adaptability Inventory, Community Integration Questionnaire, Quality of Life After Brain Injury*

a variety of environments because some patients may perform well in the closed environment of a private room, but performance may deteriorate in an open environment with multiple distractions. Section One of this book (Chapters 1 through 9 on clinical decision-making and examination) provides a detailed description of procedures, tests and measures, and specific outcome measures for examining the above-mentioned areas. A brief description of some of the more clinically useful outcome measures for individuals with TBI follows.

Outcome Measures: Body Structure/Function
Attention and Cognition

The Moss Attention Rating Scale (MARS) is an observational rating scale that provides a reliable and valid measure of attention-related behavior after TBI. The scale allows the therapist to rate a patient's behavior on a 5-point scale across 22 items that capture the effects of impaired attention on cognitive and motor performance.[108] Other measures of attention most often employed by neuropsychologists include the *Test of Everyday Attention*[109] and the *Trail Making Test Part B*.[110] Although all three of these measures capture attentional deficits and may serve as useful global outcome measures, they will be less helpful in measuring changes in attention behavior attributable to physical therapy interventions.

The GOAT is a measure of PTA.[111] The GOAT is administered by asking a series of standardized questions related to orientation and the ability to recall events before and after the injury. Scores between 100 and 76 are considered normal, and patients with scores below are considered to have PTA. The GOAT has high interrater reliability and is a valid measure of PTA.[111,112] The *Orientation Log* (O-Log) measures orientation to time, place, and circumstance.[113] The O-Log can be used for serial assessment of orientation to document improvements during rehabilitation.[114] It is reliable, is valid, and can be used to predict outcome.[113,115] Measures of dual-task performance (see later discussion) are more specific to physical therapy practice.

Behavior and Safety

Rehabilitation teams often use an outcome measure that captures the impact of behavior and safety on overall independence. The *Agitated Behavior Scale* measures the type and degree of agitation after TBI.[116] The *Supervision Rating Scale*[117] provides a one-step method for rating a patient's current level of supervision, ranging from independent to full-time direct supervision. The *Neurobehavioral Rating Scale–Revised* (NRS-R) is a 29-item multidimensional, clinician-based assessment instrument designed to measure neurobehavioral disturbances.[118] The items cover numerous cognitive and behavioral constructs such as memory, attention, communication, mood, and agitation.

Outcome Measures: Activity and Participation
Functional Balance

The Berg Balance Scale is a valid and clinically useful measure of balance in individuals with TBI and is recommended as a core outcome for people with neurological conditions.[119] However, as patients improve,

the Berg Balance Scale may exhibit a ceiling effect, and more challenging alternatives may be required.[120] The *Community Balance and Mobility Scale* (CB&M) by Howe et al.[121] is an instrument developed specifically for patients with persistent balance deficits following TBI. The CB&M is a reliable and valid tool that assesses higher level balance abilities typically associated with community mobility.

Locomotion

Gait deficits are common following TBI.[122] Classification systems of gait disorders can assist in clinical decision-making, selecting interventions, and prognosis. Williams and colleagues[33] developed a gait classification system for people with TBI that includes six categories: spastic hemiparesis, nonspastic hemiparesis, ataxia/dyspraxia unilateral, spastic bilateral paresis, nonspastic bilateral paresis, and ataxia/dyspraxia bilateral. These descriptors provide a common, clinically useful method when describing gait limitations and communicating findings.

Physical therapists use *observational gait analysis* (OGA) as a preferred method in the clinic to evaluate gait. One instrument used clinically is the *Rancho Los Amigos (RLA) OGA System*. Refer to Chapter 7, Examination of Gait, for further discussion of this instrument. However, caution should be used when interpreting OGA findings. Some gait abnormalities identified by quantitative gait analysis may not be detected by OGA.[122] Chapter 7 reviews instrumented walkways and other methods of more precisely and accurately measuring specific kinematics and kinetics associated with gait.

Gait speed is an important measure of walking ability. The *10-meter Walk Test* (10MWT) is a reliable measure of both fast-paced and self-paced gait speed in patients with TBI.[123] Caution should be used when interpreting gait because there is evidence suggesting that the gait speed may not fully reflect the many different demands of walking in the community (e.g., crossing a busy street, walking in a crowded mall, walking on uneven surfaces, and so forth).[123]

Higher levels of mobility are important for many people with TBI.[124] The *High-Level Mobility Assessment Tool* (HiMAT) is a unidimensional measure of higher-level motor performance for individuals with TBI. It was developed by Williams and colleagues to quantify higher level mobility required of physically demanding vocational and social roles, as well as sporting activities.[125,126] The HiMAT contains 11 items ranging from walking, walking on toes, walking over an obstacle (Fig. 19.5), running, bounding (Fig. 19.6A, B, C), and ascending/descending stairs. A revised version of the HiMAT has a minimal detectable change score of 2 points.[127]

Fatigue and deconditioning are common following TBI.[128,129] As such, measuring walking endurance is clinically useful. The *6-minute Walk Test* (6MWT) is a

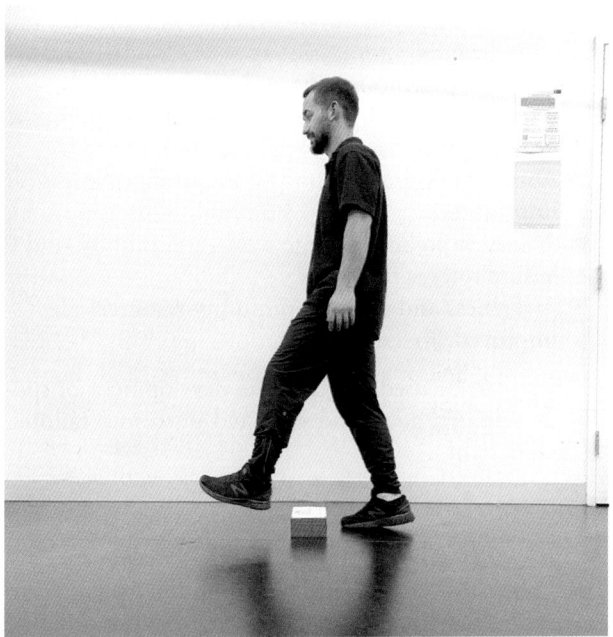

Figure 19.5 HiMAT: Walking over an obstacle.

common, reliable, and valid way to measure this aspect of walking ability.[119,130]

Several tests of dynamic balance (see above) and walking ability are appropriate for this population; however, they do not offer insight into how walking and balance are affected by the addition of a cognitive load. Measures of *dual-task performance* allow the therapist to examine the extent to which deficits in attention and memory affect gait speed and safety. These two cognitive abilities (attention and memory) are strongly associated with dual-task performance and are commonly impaired in persons with TBI.[131,132] There are a variety of clinical tests

of dual-task performance that can be used for clients with acquired brain injury. One such measure is the *Modified Walking and Remembering Test* (WART) developed by McCulloch et al.[131] The WART involves a single-task condition (simple walking task) and a dual-task condition (walking task and cognitive task).

Global Functioning

The *Functional Independence Measure (FIM)*[133] is a commonly used measure of functional mobility, ADL function, cognition, and communication. The FIM was designed to measure level of disability and burden of care in individuals undergoing inpatient rehabilitation and is useful for monitoring patient progress and evaluating outcomes. The *Functional Assessment Measure (FAM)*[134,135] was developed as an adjunct to the FIM. It includes functional areas not addressed in the FIM that are important for individuals with TBI and stroke. The other items include community access, reading, writing, safety, employability, and adjustment to limitations. The FIM, in combination with the FAM, is a valid and reliable measure of disability after TBI.[136] More recently the Centers for Medicare and Medicaid Services (CMS) has implemented the collection of Section GG codes in place of the FIM.[137] These codes are the self-care and mobility items from the *Continuity Assessment Record and Evaluation* item set.[138] In addition to measuring the amount of physical assistance required to perform a functional task, the therapist should also analyze how the patient performs the movement task.[139] A thorough movement analysis of how functional tasks (sit to/from stand, rolling, etc.) are performed will aid the therapist in identifying the motor function and other impairments that underlie specific activity limitations.

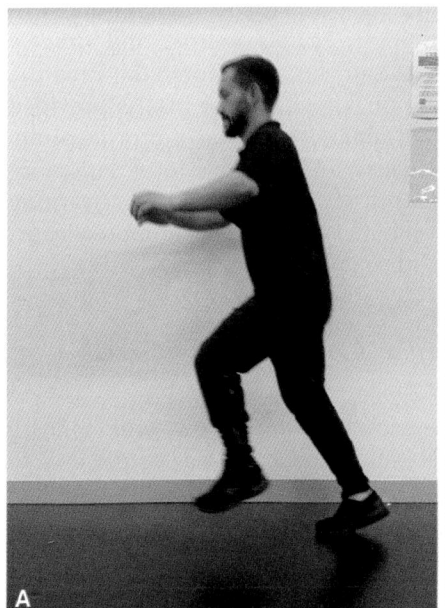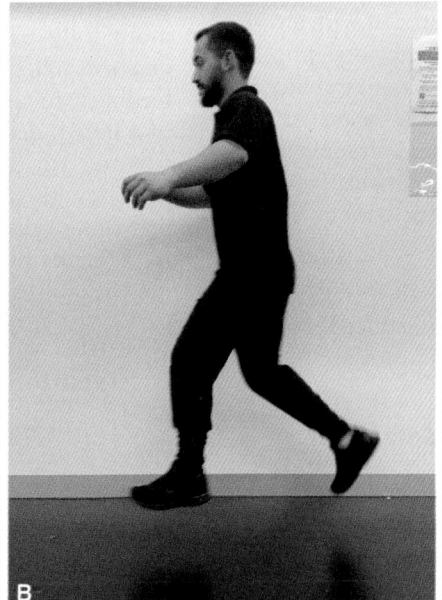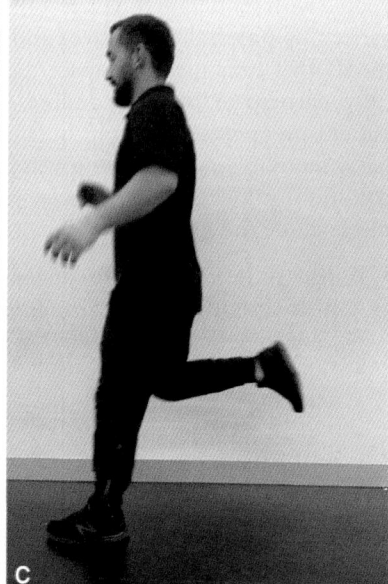

Figure 19.6A, B, C: HiMAT: Bounding.

Community Reintegration and Quality of Life

Rehabilitation teams commonly employ the use of a participation-level measure that quantifies the extent of reintegrate into social, familial, and vocational roles. One such measure is the *Mayo-Portland Adaptability Inventory*,[140] which is frequently used in postacute TBI rehabilitation. Another, similar measure is the *Community Integration Questionnaire* (CIQ).[141] The CIQ consists of 15 items relevant to home integration, social integration, and productive activities. Whiteneck and colleagues[142] developed the *Participation Assessment With Recombined Tools-Objective* (PART-O) that combines aspects of other participation level measures. The PART-O is a 24-item participation measure that is currently being used by the Traumatic Brain Injury Model System for use in clinical trials and outcome measure validation studies.[143] Another useful measure is the *Quality of Life After Brain Injury* tool.[144] This is a health-related QOL measure with 37 items and eight subscales addressing issues of thinking, feelings and emotion, autonomy in daily life, negative feelings, and perceived restrictions.

Further information on these and other outcome measures specifically used in TBI rehabilitation can be found at the *Center for Outcome Measurement in Brain Injury (COMBI)* website (www.tbims.org/combi/index.html, the Rehabilitation Measures Database at the Shirley Ryan Ability Lab (https://www.sralab.org/rehabilitation-measures), and at the Academy of Neurologic Physical Therapy Outcome Measures Recommendations webpage (http://www.neuropt.org/professional-resources/neurology-section-outcome-measures-recommendations/traumatic-brain-injury). Table 19.2 summarizes information on these outcome measures.

Goals and Outcomes

People with moderate to severe TBI present with a wide variety of physical, cognitive, and behavioral impairments that may greatly impact the patient's ability to fully participate in their desired social roles. As the patient progresses, goals and outcomes will move from basic mobility and self-care toward skills that facilitate community inclusion and social participation. Examples include the following:

- Impact of impairment is reduced.
  - Risk of secondary impairments is reduced.
  - Joint integrity and mobility are improved.
  - Motor function is improved.
  - Muscle performance is improved.
  - Cognition is improved.
  - Postural control is improved.
- Ability to improve physical actions, tasks, or activities is improved.
  - Walking ability is improved.
  - Independence in ADL is increased.

- Tolerance of upright postures and activities is increased.
- Safety of patient, family, and carepartners is improved.
- Ability to participate in social roles is enhanced.
  - Ability to assume/resume home management is improved.
  - Ability to assume/resume work, community, and leisure roles is improved.
  - Awareness and use of community resources are improved.

These can be used to guide the development of specific anticipated goals and expected outcomes tailored to each patient.

Intervention Strategies

Motor (Re)Learning Strategies

Treatment sessions should be thoughtfully planned to maximize the patient's motor-learning capabilities. The Optimizing Performance Through Intrinsic Motivation and Attention for Learning model outlines strategies to enhance motor learning. Intervention strategies that provide motivation (autonomy and enhanced expectations that influence effort) and with an external focus on the movement outcome enhance motor performance and learning.

Other motor learning factors that should be considered when designing the POC include the practice schedule and feedback. Initially, practice should be *distributed*, with frequent rest periods. Owing to cognitive impairments, patients may experience cognitive as well as physical fatigue during treatment sessions. Signs of cognitive fatigue may include increased irritability, decreased attention and concentration, deterioration in performance of physical skills, and delayed initiation. As the patient recovers and can more fully participate, *massed practice* and *random practice* schedules can be incorporated. Extrinsic feedback focusing on knowledge of results provided in a faded, delayed manner supports motor learning. Chapter 10, Strategies to Improve Motor Function, provides an in-depth discussion of motor learning principles. Unfortunately, there is little motor learning research literature that focuses specifically on people with TBI.

Restorative Versus Compensatory-Based Interventions

As discussed previously, an early, interdisciplinary approach to rehabilitation after TBI has been shown to be beneficial. There are many intervention approaches available to the physical therapist that can promote functional recovery following brain injury. Two basic treatment strategies are the *compensatory* and *restorative* (recovery) approaches. The compensatory approach

Table 19.2   Outcome Measures

Outcome, Measure, and ICF Category	Description	Scoring	MDC and MCID
6MWT ICF: 2	Performance-based test: assesses functional walking endurance.	Distance walked in 6 minutes when walking as fast as possible.	MDC = 61 meters, (estimated data based on data from Mossberg et al.)[130] MCID: NA
10MWT ICF = 2	Performance-based test: assesses walking capacity.	Time to walk middle 6 m of a 10-m walk; allows for a 2-m acceleration and deceleration phase.	MDC: 0.10 m/s MCID: NA
Berg Balance Scale ICF = 2	Performance-based test: assesses balance during 14 functional tasks.	14 items scored on a 5-point ordinal scale of 0–4, where 0 unable to perform/needs assistance to 4 = able to perform safely and independently	MDC = 4 MCID: NA
Community Balance and Mobility Scale ICF = 1, 2	Performance-based test: assess balance and mobility in ambulatory patients with TBI who have balance impairments that impact their ability to fully participate in normal social activities. Less of a ceiling effect than the Berg Balance Scale.	13 items scored on a 6-point ordinal scale of 0–5, where 0 = unable to perform or requires assistance to 5 = completes task independently, safely, in a coordinated manner, and in allotted time frame.	MDC: 8–10 points
Functional Assessment Measure ICF = 1, 2, 3	Performance-based test with 12 items that are added to the FIM that address functional areas that are not addressed in the FIM such as community functioning and behavior.	12 items added to 18 items of the FIM for a total of 30 items scored on a 7-point ordinal scale 1–7 where 1 = complete dependence to 7 = independent without assistive device.	MDC: NA MCID: NA
Quality of Life After Brain Injury ICF = 3	Self-report measure that assesses health-related quality of life. Contains six subscales: cognition, self, daily life and autonomy, social relationships, emotions, and physical problems.	Items scored on a 5-point ordinal scale 1–5. Scale means are converted to a 0–100 scale with a lowest possible value of 0 (worst possible quality of life) and a maximum value of 100 (best possible quality of life).	MDC: NA MCID: NA
Coma Recovery Scale Revised ICF = 1	Observational measure used to assist with differential diagnosis, prognostic assessment, and treatment planning in patients with disorders of consciousness. It has six subscales: auditory, visual, motor, oromotor, communication, and arousal functions.	Scores are based on the presence or absence of operationally defined behavioral responses to specific sensory stimuli.	MDC: NA MCID: NA
Agitated Behavior Scale ICF = 1, 2	Observation-based test: measures behavioral aspects of agitation during the early stages of recovery. In addition to total score, subscores for disinhibition, aggression, and lability can be calculated.	14 items, each item scored on an ordinal scale of 1–4 where 1 = behavior not present, to 4 = behavior is present to an extreme degree.	MDC: NA MCID: NA

ICF Category: 1 = Body Structure/Function; 2 = Activity; 3 = Participation
FIM = functional independence measure; ICF = World Health Organization International Classification of Functioning; MCID = minimal clinically important difference; MDC = minimal detectable change; NA = not available; 6MWT = 6-minute Walk Test; TBI = traumatic brain injury; 10MWT = 10-meter Walk Test.

seeks to improve functional skills by compensating for the lost ability. A simple example of this would be teaching one-handed dressing techniques to a patient with UE hemiparesis resulting from a TBI. A restorative approach seeks to restore the "normal" use of the affected UE. Both approaches seek to reinstitute functional independence.

Compensation is commonly defined as the resumption of the ability to complete a task using alternative motor patterns and strategies. The definition of recovery varies. Some feel that it refers to the resumption of the ability to complete a task using the same motor patterns and strategies as before the injury. Another, more liberal, definition is completing a task using similar strategies despite inferior efficiency, speed, and/or accuracy. Levin et al.[145] addressed this topic and proposed explicit definitions for recovery and compensation. The authors argue that the definitions of recovery and compensation will change based on whether performance or function is measured. To make this point clearer, the authors used the framework of the *World Health Organization's ICF Model.* Refer to Table 19.3 for more details.

In most cases involving moderate to severe TBI, clinical management will likely require a balance between both restorative and compensatory approaches. As an example, a therapist may determine that a restorative approach to gait training is indicated but may also choose to ensure that, for safety, the client and carepartner have adequate training in the use of an assistive device during the earlier stages of recovery, should it be needed. Current literature offers little guidance for the practitioner attempting to choose between approaches. Table 19.4 offers questions that can guide this aspect of clinical decision-making. After a thorough examination and consideration of the patient's unique personal and environmental barriers and facilitators, these questions can help lead the clinician and patient to a shared agreement about which approach will be used.

Translational and applied research in the areas of neural plasticity, motor learning, and neurological rehabilitation has heightened awareness that relearning is directly related to the rehabilitative experiences to which patients are exposed. Using the example above, interventions that seek compensation will result not only in learning how to use the less-affected UE but also in learning not to use the more affected UE. Alternatively, a restorative rehabilitative experience that allows the patient to practice using the affected arm for everyday tasks will result in greater functional independence and affected UE use. This knowledge is useful in clinical decision-making when developing the POC.

Table 19.3	Motor Recovery and Compensation Across Three Levels of the ICF	
Level	**Recovery**	**Compensation**
ICF: Health Condition (neuronal)	*Restoring function in neural tissue that was initially lost after injury. May be seen as reactivation in brain areas previously inactivated by the circulatory event. Although this is not expected to occur in the primary brain lesion, it may occur in areas surrounding the lesion (penumbra) and in the diaschisis.*	*Neural tissue acquires a function that it did not have prior to injury. May be seen as activation in alternative brain areas not normally observed in nondisabled individuals.*
ICF: Body Functions/ Structure (performance)	*Restoring the ability to perform a movement in the same manner as it was performed before injury. This may occur through the reappearance of premorbid movement patterns during task accomplishment (voluntary joint ROM, temporal and spatial interjoint coordination, etc.).*	*Performing an old movement in a new manner. May be seen as the appearance of alternative movement patterns (i.e., recruitment of additional or different degrees of freedom, changes in muscle activation patterns such as increased agonist/ antagonist coactivation, delays in timing between movements of adjacent joints, etc.) during the accomplishment of a task.*
ICF: Activity (functional)	*Successful task accomplishment using limbs or end effectors typically used by nondisabled individuals.[a]*	*Successful task accomplishment using alternate limbs or end effectors. For example, opening a package of chips using one hand and the mouth instead of two hands.*

ICF = World Health Organization International Classification of Functioning; ROM = range of motion.
[a]Note that task performance may be successful using compensatory motor strategies and movement patterns.
Levin, MF, Kleim, JA, and Wolf, SL. What do motor "recovery" and "compensation" mean in patients following stroke? *Neurorehabilitation and Neural Repair* 23(4):313–319, 2009. Reprinted by permission of SAGE Publications.

Table 19.4	Compensation Versus Restoration: Guiding Questions to Consider
Category	**Questions to Consider**
Injury Severity	• Are sensorimotor deficits so severe that restorative approaches are not possible or appropriate? • Do secondary complications or comorbidities exist that pose barriers to recovery (e.g., contractures, fractures)? • Is an appropriate motor recovery program (specificity, intensity, frequency, duration, difficulty) feasible? • How chronic is the injury?
Motor Learning	• What strengths and weaknesses does the patient have relative to their ability to learn motor tasks? • Are there significant cognitive, behavioral, or medical barriers?
Resources	• Does the patient have any financial or support barriers? • Will funding lapse before functional recovery occurs? • Do financial resources suggest that a more rapid approach be used? • What impact will discharge destination have on the prescribed treatment approach?

Restorative Interventions and Neural Plasticity

No studies to date have identified what types of restorative interventions are the most beneficial for persons with TBI. Current research has demonstrated that task-specific interventions with large amounts of practice at a moderate to high intensity can induce beneficial neuroplastic changes in the CNS and restore function.[146–149] Studies involving animal models of brain injury have demonstrated the importance of intensive, task-oriented training on neuroplastic changes in the motor cortex and functional recovery.[150,151] This line of research was extended to include human models with neurological deficits, and later the sum of these findings was translated into tangible principles of experience-dependent neural plasticity.[146,152] Table 19.5 provides examples of several of these principles. Current evidence suggests that treatment interventions that are most beneficial will be specific to the function/task being retrained, meaningful to the client, delivered at a moderate to high intensity level, and challenging to the cortical systems involved in the activity.

Task-Oriented Approach

Current theories of motor learning and research support a task-oriented approach to interventions for individuals with neurological deficits. Interventions should directly involve the task that is the primary goal. For example, if the goal is to improve walking ability, then the intervention should focus on the task of walking. Although walking requires dynamic balance control, an intervention that focuses on weight shifting and reaching in standing will not carry over to improved walking ability. Most of the research on the principles that underpin effective, task-oriented interventions for clients with neurological disorders has been done with persons with stroke. However, it is likely that these same principles will serve the physical therapist well in selecting and applying appropriate interventions for persons with TBI.[153]

Interventions

Locomotor Training/Walking Recovery

The current best evidence strongly recommends task-specific, moderate- to high-intensity training (targeting 60% to 80% of heart rate [HR] reserve or 70% to 85% of maximum HR) and virtual reality–based (VR-based) interventions, although most of the intensity and VR

Table 19.5	Principles of Experience-Dependent Neuroplasticity
Principle	**Description**
Use it or lose it	Failure to drive specific brain functions can lead to functional degradation.
Use it and improve it	Training that drives a specific brain function can lead to an enhancement of that function.
Specificity	The nature of the training experience dictates the nature of the plasticity.
Repetition matters	Induction of plasticity requires sufficient repetition.
Intensity matters	Induction of plasticity requires sufficient training intensity.
Time matters	Different forms of plasticity occur at different times during training.
Salience matters	The training experience must be sufficiently salient to induce plasticity.
Age matters	Training-induced plasticity occurs more readily in younger brains.
Transference	Plasticity in response to one training experience can enhance the acquisition of similar behaviors.
Interference	Plasticity in response to one experience can interfere with the acquisition of other behaviors.

From Kleim, JA, and Jones, TA. Principles of experience-dependent neural plasticity: Implications for rehabilitation after brain damage. *J Speech Lang Hear Res.* 51(1):S225–239, 2008, with permission.[152]

literature is in people with stroke.[149] A treadmill with a safety harness (without weight support) to reduce fall risk is used to provide an environment in which the task of walking can be repeated at a moderate to high intensity. Manual assistance to move the limbs and control the trunk is minimized. The speed of the treadmill gradually increased to achieve targeted intensity levels. The speed of the treadmill and the direction of walking (backward, sidestepping) can be varied. Overground walking training follows walking on the treadmill. For safety, an overhead harness can also be used for overground training. During overground training, the patient is encouraged to walk fast to achieve targeted intensity levels. Specific walking skills can also be performed, such as backward walking, sidestepping, stepping over obstacles, walking while carrying objects, and providing unexpected perturbations to the patient while walking.

The Academy of Neurologic Physical Therapy (ANPT) has developed online resources guided by the findings of the Clinical Practice Guideline to Improve Locomotor Function, following Chronic Stroke, Incomplete Spinal Cord Injury, and Brain Injury to support physical therapists as they implement walking interventions at a moderate to high intensity level. These are available at the ANPT website: https://www.neuropt.org/practice-resources/best-practice-initiatives-and-resources/intensity-matters. Additionally, ANPT has developed video cases that highlight different interventions delivered at a high to moderate intensity to people with various neurological health conditions, including spinal cord injury. These are available at the ANPT YouTube site: https://www.youtube.com/playlist?list=PLH8hBAd9u40lSIGbP9s3dz2BiveybZKW7.

Another task-oriented approach for improving walking and running was developed by Williams and Schache.[154] They used a conceptual framework based on the hierarchical ordering of high-level mobility tasks based on the HiMAT (see above) and biomechanical parameters[155] associated with normal walking and running as the basis for the specific interventions. Easier items on the HiMAT are set as goals and mastered before moving on to more difficult tasks. For example, once a patient can walk backward, the next, more difficult tasks (walking on toes and walking over obstacles) are set as goals. Important biomechanical aspects of walking and running, such as the generation of ankle and hip flexion power at push-off, are targeted through specific interventions.

Similarly, Peters and colleagues[156] utilized an intensive, task-oriented, mobility-training intervention to improve walking ability. Participants received gait training on a treadmill, overground gait training, sit to/from stand transfer training, standing balance activities, resistance training, coordination training, and ROM exercises for a total of 150 minutes per session for 20 sessions.

An important consideration for these and other task-oriented strategies is treatment dosing. Dosage entails more than just the number of physical therapy sessions/week and length of the individual session. When critically examining the treatment dosage, the following factors should be considered: sessions/week (or day), amount of practice time per task within a session, number of repetitions of the task performed within a session, and the intensity at which the task is being performed. However, it can be difficult to achieve the optimal dose in clinical practice due to varying constraints such as fatigue, cognitive and behavioral concerns, and insurance limitations. Although not well researched for persons with TBI, literature on UE rehabilitation and locomotor training after stroke suggests that these interventions are commonly underdosed[157,158] and that there is a dose-response relationship.[159]

Upper Extremity Function

Similar to walking, UE function may be compromised due to problems with contracture, spasticity, paresis, or reduced motor control. Each of these impairments may require individualized treatment, but task practice provides a method for training that may directly impact on the goal being targeted. UE task practice should be provided within the framework established for motor learning or skill acquisition (i.e., structured practice, movement specificity, feedback, knowledge of results) to improve performance (Fig. 19.7). The application of the principles of motor skill acquisition may require

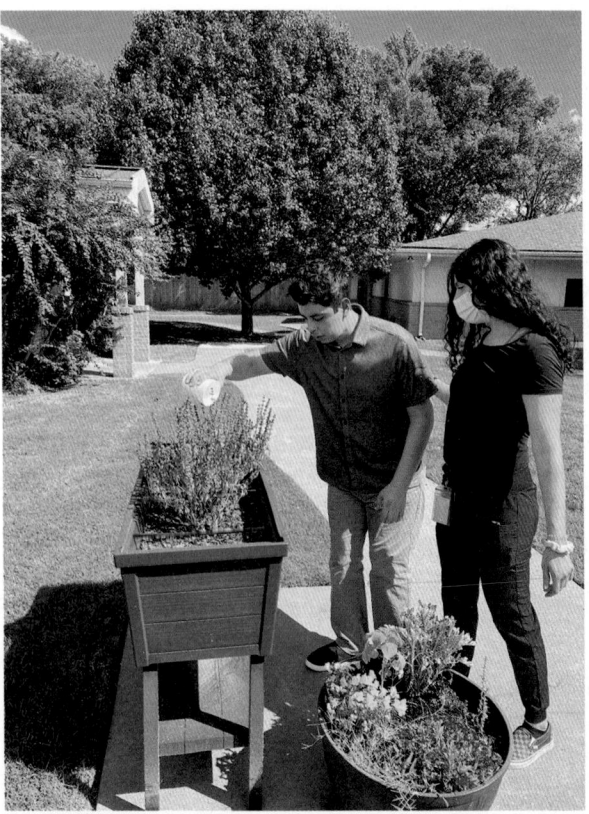

Figure 19.7 Upper extremity task practice.

modification (e.g., how many instructions are given, and how feedback is provided) in the presence of the cognitive impairment that is commonly associated with TBI.

Constraint-induced movement therapy is a method for intensive task practice and involves promoting the use of the more affected UE for up to 90% of waking hours and reducing compensatory use of the least-affected UE. Intensive, task-oriented training is provided for the affected UE for up to 6 hours per day over a 2- to 3-week period.[160] Most of the research published on CIMT has been done in people with stroke. However, this same intervention may also be useful for people with TBI.[161] Given the frequency of behavioral and cognitive impairments after TBI, patients undergoing CIMT may require greater structure and carepartner support outside of therapy to maximize their adherence to the protocol.

Balance

Reduced postural control and ability to balance is a major problem following TBI.[162] Ironically for some, poor balance may lead to falls and further TBI. Falls are the leading cause of TBI in older adults. The causes of reduced postural control and balance dysfunction following TBI may be complex and multifactorial. Somatosensory and proprioceptive changes, muscle paresis, spasticity and hypertonicity, visual problems and diplopia, dizziness, vestibular dysfunction, and benign paroxysmal positional vertigo (BPPV) may all contribute to problems with balance. The impact of balance dysfunction is broad, ranging from those who experience difficulty sitting to those who are deemed to be well recovered.[163]

It is important to differentially diagnose the factors contributing to reduced postural control and balance as they usually require different interventions. Vestibular rehabilitation and balance training are effective for improving balance, dizziness, and mobility for people with TBI.[164,165] Randomized clinical trials typically demonstrate significant improvements in intervention and control groups, but between-group differences are not always evident. Further investigations are required to identify the active ingredient of a treatment and the best platform (i.e., individual, group, home-based) for delivery.

Aerobic Conditioning

Fatigue and cardiopulmonary pathology are common after TBI.[128] The severity of deconditioning found in persons with TBI is significantly greater than that found in sedentary persons without disabilities.[129] Aerobic training is effective and should be prescribed for persons with TBI.[166,167] There are many options when developing an aerobic training program. The mode of training can vary from traditional exercises (e.g., walking, jogging, treadmill, elliptical machines, and ergometers)

to circuit training. The American College of Sports Medicine Guidelines for Exercise Testing and Prescription recommends a frequency of 3 to 5 days/week at an intensity of 40% to 70% of HR reserve (or a rate of perceived exertion of 11 to 14) for 20 to 60 minutes per session (multiple 10-minute sessions can be considered) for people with stroke.[168] They do not have specific guidelines for people with TBI. Aerobic exercise may also improve cognition[169,170] and sleep and reduce depression and fatigue.[171]

High-intensity interval training (HIIT) may be another safe and effective method to improve cardiovascular conditioning and other markers of health. However, it has not been specifically evaluated in people with TBI. A meta review of 33 systematic reviews of the topic concludes that HIIT has beneficial effects on cardiorespiratory fitness, glycemic control, exercise endurance, and muscle mass as well as reducing depression and anxiety.[172] They also noted that this form of training is not associated with adverse events such as acute injuries or cardiovascular compromise. Other authors have noted similar improvements when used by persons with stroke.[173,174] Acute bouts of HIIT training may also induce short-term improvements in executive functioning.[175]

Resistance Training

Interventions aimed at improving strength should also be a part of the POC.[176,177] As in aerobic training, there is little research on the effect of strength training specifically with people with TBI. ACMS guidelines for people with stroke recommend resistance training be performed at least 2 days/week on nonconsecutive days, 1 to 3 sets of 8 to 15 repetitions at 50% to 70% of 1-RM.[168] Postural and balance impairments may require modification of positions and equipment used. As with the general population, people with TBI benefit from regular exercise. Aerobic and resistance exercise should be a regular part of a healthy lifestyle after formal rehabilitation is complete.

Dual-Task Interventions

Patients with moderate to severe TBI may make significant improvements in physical function. However, although they may demonstrate independence with basic mobility skills such as walking, transferring, and stair climbing in a closed environment, residual motor and persistent cognitive deficits can severely impact community mobility. As discussed in the examination section, a dual-task paradigm can give valuable insight into how safely and efficiently patients will ambulate when also performing secondary, cognitive tasks. Research suggests that dual-task decrements, such as reduced walking speed and postural stability, are common after brain injury, even in those who are seemingly well recovered.[178]

Like many other interventions, improvements in dual-task performance are training specific. The dual-, multi-, and environmental tasks required for safe community mobility have been well documented.[179] This should be taken into consideration when designing and progressing a dual-task training regimen. The tasks and environments used in training should match those that the patient is anticipated to return to. Progressing this type of training can involve manipulation of the training environment, motor task (type and difficulty), and also the cognitive demands of the secondary task. A training program to improve dual-task performance can coincide with the achievement of independence in walking across different terrains. For example, once independent while walking down a corridor, progressively more challenging cognitive tasks such as serial subtraction or visual scanning tasks can be added. Furthering this example, the client might be asked to ambulate in a parking lot and scan for vehicles with certain characters in their license plate or walk the aisle of a busy grocery store and find specific items. Training speed can also be varied to add challenge. Walking while carrying a cup of water and maintaining a conversation is another example of a dual-task intervention (Fig. 19.8) as is reading out loud while walking on a treadmill (Fig. 19.9).

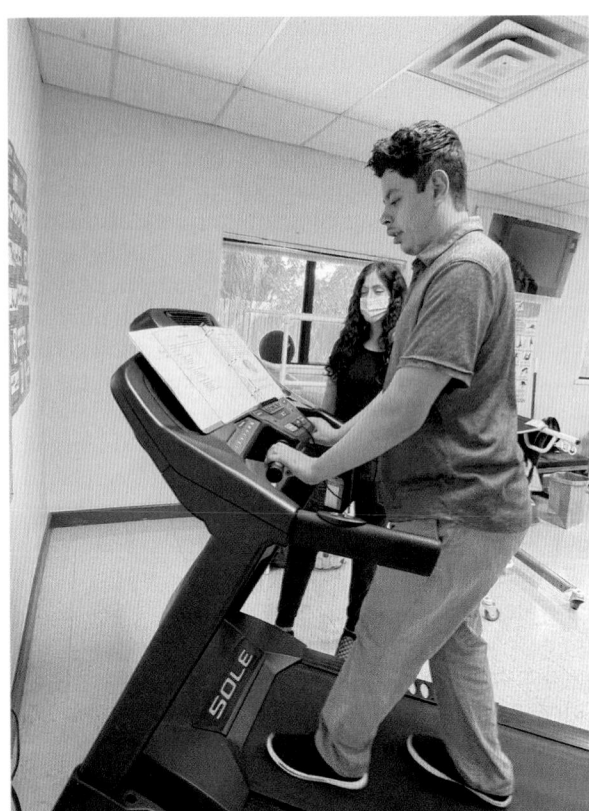

Figure 19.9 Dual-task training: walking on treadmill while reading out loud.

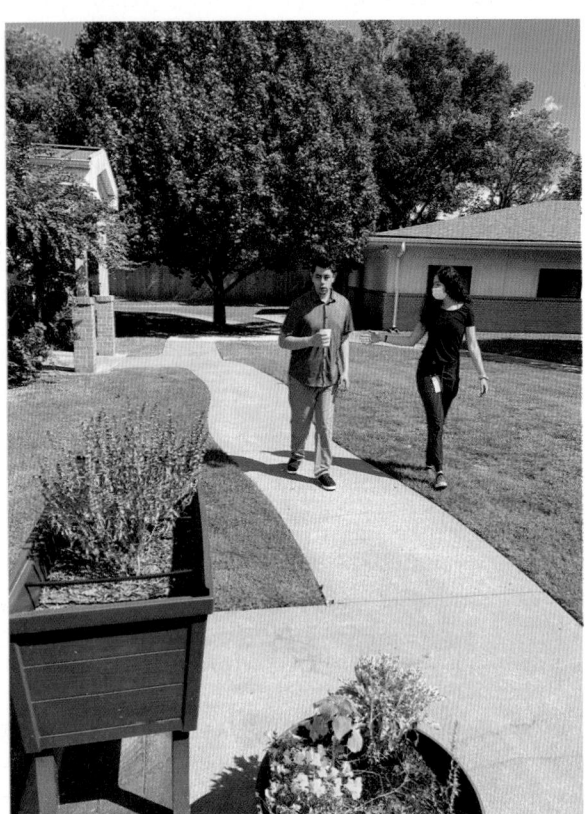

Figure 19.8 Dual-task training: walking in an open environment while carrying an object and talking.

Patient/Family/Carepartner Education

Patient/family/carepartner education and training is important across each level of rehabilitation. The goals of education and training will vary based on the cognitive and behavioral abilities of the patient. Clients in the early phase of recovery may go through a period where they are significantly confused and agitated. It is difficult to provide education for the patient at this level; the patient has very little, if any, ability for new learning. However, it is extremely important to provide education for the patient's family. Above all, the family should understand that the patient does not have control of their behavior. The patient is not striking out or cursing because of intent to hurt others, but because of agitation and confusion. Many times, families do not understand why a patient is exhibiting these behaviors. They should be educated that these behaviors are a symptom of the brain injury, just as is the patient's inability to walk or eat. It is important to educate the family that entering this level of recovery is a good sign because it indicates the patient is moving toward the next level of recovery. Aggressive behaviors are usually short lived, typically lasting only a few weeks at most. Family members should also be taught to use specific behavioral strategies (see below) when interacting with their loved one. Consistency is important for everyone, including family members. If a behavioral plan is being implemented, the family should be a part of devising it and carrying it out.

It is important to emphasize safety awareness education with the patient and carepartners. As the individual begins to exhibit improved mobility skills they may lack the insight to recognize that are not yet safe to ambulate or transfer independently. Family members and carepartners should learn how to safely assist the patient with functional mobility. This typically includes training in bed mobility, transfers, ambulation, and wheelchair mobility skills. Carepartners should be instructed in proper body mechanics and techniques when assisting with functional mobility, so as to avoid risking injury to the patient or themselves. Family members/ carepartners should be educated about how to assist the patient with strengthening exercises, passive ROM, and other elements of the exercise program. They should also be made aware of methods to enhance the patient's decision-making skills and safety awareness. Family members typically become the primary care partner for the patient upon discharge to home.

Behavioral Factors

Therapists may encounter a variety of behavioral barriers to examining and treating patients with moderate to severe TBI. As patients begin to emerge from coma, they often experience a period of acute posttraumatic agitation.[36] The confusion, amnesia, and disorientation during this phase of recovery often result in agitation, aggression, noncompliance, and combative behavior. However, patients exhibiting confusion and agitation can still participate in and benefit from structured interventions.[65,67] The therapist should incorporate creativity and flexibility when designing and providing interventions with individuals who are in the confused and agitated stage of recovery. At this stage, the therapist should work near the patient's physical level of function using familiar activities, rather than progress to more challenging skills, because the patient does not have the capacity for new learning. Interventions should be done in a closed environment in order to not overstimulate or distract the patient. The neuropsychologist can assist the team by providing insight into different ways to manage the patient's agitated behavior and may set up a behavioral modification program. Behavioral modification techniques such as positive reinforcement using a point or reward system, redirection, and compliance training are useful in managing these inappropriate behaviors and improving participation in therapy. Different medications may be effective in helping the patient manage behavior as well. These include propranolol, trazadone, selective serotonin reuptake inhibitors, Tegretol, and Seroquel.

Ativan should be used only with severe agitation. Table 19.6 summarizes special considerations for the management of patients who display significant cognitive and/or neurobehavioral impairments.

Professionals who frequently encounter aggressive and disruptive behaviors from patients with TBI may benefit from further training in managing these events. *Non-Violent Crisis Intervention Training* and *Brain Injury Specialist Training*, available through the Brain Injury Association of America, are two such training programs.

Community Reentry

Many clients will make significant progress in the early phase of rehabilitation. Before discharge from physical therapy, it is crucial to begin to wean the patient from the external structure provided by the hospital setting that is important in the early and middle stages of recovery. As the patient becomes better able to control themselves, external control provided by the environment should be lessened. Doing so will prepare the patient for the challenges of the next level of rehabilitation, postacute community reentry programming.

This level of therapy can be delivered in a comprehensive day treatment setting, residential setting, or community group home setting with an interdisciplinary emphasis on community reentry; return to work or school; and cognitive, behavioral, and psychosocial issues. The major goal of treatment at this level is to assist the patient in integrating the cognitive, physical, and emotional skills necessary to function in the community. Skills in judgment, problem-solving, planning, self-awareness, health and wellness, and social interaction are emphasized. For the demands of treatment to approximate the demands of the real world, treatment focuses on advanced activities such as community skills, social skills, and daily living skills. Examples of these skills are presented in Table 19.7. The interdisciplinary team emphasizes patient assumption of self-responsibility. Because the patient now has some insight into their own strengths and weaknesses, it is important to involve the individual in decision-making.

Independent as well as cooperative work with others is encouraged. Group treatment sessions are an important part of the POC. Feedback from the therapist and support group is crucial in order for the patient to learn how to function in society with their present abilities and limitations. Trial periods of independent living and supported work are important. The success and failures of these trials should be communicated to the interdisciplinary team so that clinical decisions regarding interventions modification or progression can be made. Adaptations are often required by the family, work, and school to accommodate to the needs of the individual.

Table 19.6   Special Considerations for Confused and Agitated Patients

Strategy	Rationale and Clinical Application
Consistency	• Consistency is important. All team members, including family members, should interact and address inappropriate behaviors in a consistent manner. • Remember that the patient is confused. To help decrease confusion, the patient should be seen by the same person at the same time and in the same location every day. • Establishing a daily routine is very important. It is calming and reassuring to have a sense of familiarity. Additionally, orientation (i.e., person, place, and time) should be provided frequently and in a nonthreatening manner. At this level, it is often better to provide orientation information than to challenge the patient to provide it, particularly if the patient is not expected to succeed.
Expect Limited Carryover	• Teaching new skills at this level is unrealistic. The patient may begin to perform a functional task, such as brushing teeth or ambulating. However, this does not indicate a general learning ability, because brushing one's teeth and especially walking are automatic skills with an ingrained neural network. • The use of charts or graphs may be useful to help the patient progress each day. Without the use of such aids, the patient is likely to have no recall of the previous day's performance.
Model Calm Behavior	• The patient is likely to perceive, and may reflect, the demeanor of the caregiver. Therefore, it is important for the therapist to assume a calm and focused affect. • The patient may not be able to control their behavior and may not feel safe. To help the patient feel safe, it is important for the therapist to be perceived as being in control of their emotions and behavior.
Expect Egocentricity	• At this level of recovery, the patient cannot be expected to see another's point of view. They will tend to think only of themselves, and at this point, it is unwise to stress the patient with attempts to do otherwise.
Flexibility/Options	• The patient will have a limited attention span and may not be able to concentrate on any given activity for a very long time. It is important to be prepared with numerous activities. If the patient cannot be redirected to the selected task, it is appropriate to attempt to engage him or her in another. For example, it may be difficult for a client to tolerate a full constraint-induced therapy protocol. You might, however, be able to engage the client in a variety of UE reaching tasks in various environments allowing the patient's level of attention and tolerance to dictate the duration of each. • Treat the patient at an appropriate age level. • Give control to the patient when it is safe and appropriate. Control can be given while maintaining focus on therapeutic goals by phrasing questions as "Would you rather play ball or go for a walk?" This prevents situations where the patient chooses an undesirable or unrealistic activity if asked, "What would you like to do?" or the case where the patient simply answers "No" when asked, "Would you like to . . . ?" • Provide safe choices for the patient. This allows the patient to feel that they have some control over the situation. This is important because the patient typically feels considerable loss of control during prolonged hospitalization.
Safety	• Owing to the patient's often unpredictable and inappropriate behaviors, it is important to keep the patient and those interacting with him or her safe. • In addition to utilizing some of the above-mentioned behavioral strategies, patients in this level of recovery may be kept on a locked unit of the hospital. Patients may require one-to-one staff supervision and assistance throughout the day.
Environment	• Initially, interventions should be performed in a closed environment with limited distractions. An open environment, such as a busy rehab gym, will likely have too many distractions and can lead to increased agitation and limited ability to participate in the intervention. • Progress to more open environment to challenge the patient as they improve.

UE, upper extremity.

Table 19.7	Components of Community Skills, Social Skills, and Daily Living Skills Programs	
Daily Living	Social Skills	Community Skills
Food preparation	Introductions	Shopping
Housekeeping	Nonverbal communication	Public transport
Money management	Assertiveness	Map reading
Meal planning	Listening skills	Leisure planning
Telephone use	Giving/receiving feedback	Community resources
Time management		

■ PHYSICAL THERAPY MANGEMENT OF MILD TRAUMATIC BRAIN INJURY

Mild Traumatic Brain Injury

It is estimated that between 1.6 and 3.8 million sports- and recreation-related mild TBIs (mTBIs) occur annually in the United States,[180] and a range of 8% to 23% of military personnel experience combat-related mTBI.[181] Other common causes of mTBI include falls, motor vehicle crashes, and assault. An mTBI is a type of TBI induced by biomechanical forces that disrupts physiological brain function.[182] It results from a direct blow to the head, face, or neck or an impulsive force elsewhere on the body that is transmitted to the head.[183] Mild TBI is primarily a functional disturbance of the CNS, which is thought to be due to neurometabolic dysfunction, neurotransmitter disturbances, and microstructural changes.[184–186] The impact of an mTBI is typically short, with most individuals with mTBI fully recovering in approximately 10 to 14 days for adults and up to 4 weeks for children.[182] There are risk factors that can increase the recovery time, such as previous history of concussions, presence of attention-deficit/hyperactivity disorder, female sex, history of migraines, delayed removal from play, and prolonged rest after injury. Prolonged recovery is more common in individuals who experience symptoms of dizziness, migraines, or depression after concussion injury.[183] It is estimated that up to 25% of people with mTBI experience persistent postconcussion symptoms and may have deficits months to years after the initial injury.[187–189]

As outlined in Table 19.1, the GCS defines mTBI as a score between 13 and 15. Individuals with mTBI may or may not experience a loss of consciousness (must be less than 30 minutes if loss of consciousness occurs) and if present, PTA and altered mental state would last less than 24 hours. Structural imaging in cases of mTBI is normal.

A diagnosis of mTBI is a clinical diagnosis and is made through an assessment of mechanism of injury and clinical symptoms. It is important to keep in mind that the appearance of symptoms may be delayed several hours. Declining consciousness, pupillary asymmetry, seizures, unrelenting vomiting, progressing neurological signs, or skull or cervical spine instability would warrant an emergency medical evaluation as they are indicative of more serious injury.[183,190] Common concussion symptoms can be divided into physical, cognitive, and behavioral domains as outlined in Table 19.8. If any of these elements are present, an mTBI should be suspected. Because an mTBI results in functional changes, neuroimaging is usually not indicated.[182] Recent studies have questioned the validity of neurocognitive testing, such as Immediate Post-Concussion and Cognitive Testing (ImPACT), and its role in diagnosis.[191–194] There is currently no diagnostic test for concussion although evolving research for fluid biomarkers (saliva, serum), HR variability, cerebral blood flow assessment, visual assessments, and advance neuroimaging may be useful to assist with the diagnosis in the future, but at this time there is insufficient evidence to support their use.[182,195,196]

Researchers have described distinct clinical trajectories of mTBI that may affect recovery and determine specific interventions. Identified clinical trajectories of mTBI include physiologic, cognitive/fatigue, vestibular, ocular, post-traumatic migraine, cervicogenic, and anxiety/mood.[197,198] Symptoms of mTBI are heterogeneous and as such require interventions that are

Table 19.8	Possible Postconcussion Symptoms	
Physical Symptoms	Cognitive Symptoms	Behavioral/ Emotional Symptoms
• Headache	Problems with:	• Depression
• Dizziness/Vertigo	• Attention	• Anxiety
• Balance problems	• Concentration	• Agitation
• Nausea	• Memory	• Irritability
• Fatigue	• Speed of processing	• Impulsivity
• Sleep disturbance	• Judgment	• Aggression
• Visual disturbance	• Executive functions	
• Sensitivity to light	• Speech and language	
• Hearing difficulties/loss	• Visual–spatial function	
• Tinnitus		
• Sensitivity to noise		

individualized for the patient depending on their presentation. Although physical therapists may play a role in the treatment of patients across all of these clinical trajectories, the physical therapist is most likely to play a prominent role in patients with vestibular (vestibular/balance rehabilitation), oculomotor (gaze stabilization exercises), cervical (musculoskeletal interventions), and physiologic trajectories (exercise interventions). Evidence supports an interdisciplinary approach to concussion management given the variation in symptom presentation with support from disciplines such as physical therapy, occupational therapy, speech therapy, psychology, and neuropsychology in addition to medical management.[199]

Physical Therapy Management

The Clinical Practice Guideline (CPG) specific to physical therapy published in 2020 provides an evidence-based guideline for rehabilitation after mTBI.[183] Other comprehensive resources include the U.S. Department of Veterans Affairs (VA) and U.S. Department of Defenses (DoD) clinical practice guideline for postacute mTBI management and rehabilitation (VA/DoD CPG) and the Consensus Statement from the Concussion in Sport Group.[182,190] These resources continue to be regularly updated based on new evidence. Current evidence for concussion management supports a period of rest for 24 to 48 hours, with a graded return to symptom-limited activities after the initial rest period.[182,183]

Return to Sport/Activity

Return to sport (RTS) or activity after an mTBI should follow a graduated, stepwise progression of increasing activity levels with an initial 24- to 48-hour relative physical and cognitive rest period.[182] Rest guidelines have changed with recent evidence showing that too much rest may actually be detrimental to recovery.[200,201] An initial period of 24 to 48 hours of relative physical and cognitive rest is now recommended compared to previous RTS versions in which rest was recommended if symptoms persisted. It is important to recognize that in addition to rest from physical activity, rest from activities that require cognitive skills such as attention and concentration (e.g., schoolwork, playing video games) is also recommended. There are six stages in the RTS strategy outlined as symptom-limited activity, light aerobic exercise, sport-specific exercise, noncontact training drills, full-contact practice, and return to sport.[182] There should be at least 24 hours spent in each step of the RTS progression, so that it will take approximately 1 week to return to full activities or full-contact sports activity. If any symptoms return during the progressive increase in activity, the athlete should return to the previous step.

The Progressive Return to Activity Following Mild TBI (PRA) guidelines for military service members was revised in 2021.[190,201] The stages of PRA recommends monitoring symptom severity as measured by the Neurobehavioral Symptom Inventory (NSI)[202] to guide progression of activity through six stages: relative rest (no longer than 72 hours), symptom-limited activity, light activity, moderate activity, intensive activity and return to full duty. Relative rest includes physical and cognitive activities that do not provoke symptoms. After an initial relative rest period, individuals can progress to the next activity level as long as symptom severity on the NSI does not exceed mild and there are no new symptoms. These PRA guidelines also provide more specific guidance related to environment, amount, and type of physical and cognitive/oculomotor activity. The 2021 full mTBI guidelines developed by the VA/DoD is available online at https://www.healthquality.va.gov/guidelines/Rehab/mtbi/VADoDmTBICPGProviderSummaryFinal508.pdf.

A similar individualized, balanced approach between rest and cognitive activity and graded increase in cognitive activity should be taken when students with concussion return to the classroom (return to school).[182] Return to school should be prioritized for children before RTS. Students who are removed from school should start with 5 to 15 minutes of cognitive load at a time and gradually build up as tolerated. Once the student can tolerate increased cognitive activity with minimally provoking symptoms, a gradual return to school or part-time attendance should be considered, with the goal to be able to return to full-time academics. Adjustments in the school such as frequent breaks, planned rest in a quiet area, reduced brightness levels on computer screens, use of sunglasses or hats, lunch in a quiet area, early dismissal from class to avoid noisy hallways during transitions, and extra time for tests may be helpful during the initial period of return to school/learning. Similar graded step-wise paradigms can be applied to return to work scenarios, depending on the job demands and safety at work.

Physical Therapy Examination

The physical therapy examination should proceed based on levels of irritability; tests that are least likely to provoke symptoms should be done first and progression to tests that are more likely to provoke symptoms.[183] Because the exam is likely to provoke symptoms, it may not be possible to perform all the desired tests during one session. Further testing is likely to be necessary to fully understand the patient's presentation. It is important to obtain thorough history prior to the physical examination, including past medical history, mental health history, mechanism of injury, symptom history, and management strategies.[183]

Symptoms

There are many self-report symptom scales to use in the concussion population that can help grade levels of irritability and track progress over time.[203] These scales ask patients to rate the severity of postconcussion symptoms such as headache, dizziness, vision difficulties, difficulty concentrating, fatigue, depression, sleep disturbance, and sensitivity to light and noise. The NSI (mentioned previously) asks the individual to rate 22 symptoms using a 5-point Likert scale (None to Very Severe). The NSI measures four different factors: somatosensory, affective, cognitive, and vestibular.[202] The Postconcussion Scale (revised) (PCS)[204] is a 22-item symptom list that the patient rates the severity of symptoms using a 7-point Likert scale (no symptom to severe). The Postconcussion Symptom Inventory (PCSI) was adapted from the Postconcussion scale for easier readability in adolescents and children and has been found to be valid and reliable to track using a 23-item symptom list and 7-point Likert scale, while also asking if the symptoms change with physical or mental activity.[205] The Rivermead Post-Concussion Symptom Questionnaire (RPQ) is a 16-item scale using a 5-point ordinal scale (no symptom to severe symptom) for a total sum ranging from 0 to 64.[205] There is no gold standard measure for symptom scales. They are useful to provide an initial impression of current symptoms and severity of symptoms.

The Sport Concussion Assessment Tool 5 (SCAT5) is a short test that can be completed on the sideline of a sports event within minutes of injury to assess mental status, symptom severity, balance, coordination, and cervical involvement.[182,206] The SCAT5 incorporates the Standardized Assessment of Concussion and the Maddocks questions and is designed for on-the-field/sideline assessment of acute concussion and should not replace more a comprehensive evaluation.

Cognition

Computerized tests have been developed to assess cognition after mTBI. One such test is the ImPACT. The ImPACT assesses attention span, working memory, sustained and selective attention time, response variability, nonverbal problem-solving, and reaction time. The ImPACT can be used to track recovery and assist in the return-to-play decision after mTBI and is often given for baseline testing during preseason.[207–209]

Four system domains have been identified as key areas for comprehensive physical therapy examination after concussion: cervical musculoskeletal, vestibulo-oculomotor, autonomic/exertional tolerance, and motor function.[183]

Cervical Musculoskeletal

Cervical injury can occur with a concussive event, and cervical dysfunction may contribute to the presence of headache, dizziness, and balance problems.[210] Tests and measures for cervical involvement should include passive and active ROM of the neck, muscle strength and endurance of cervical and thoracic muscles, palpation of musculature, joint mobility of the spine, and cervical

joint position error.[183,211,212] The cervical spine should be screened for involvement, even in individuals who do not report neck pain. If neck pain is a primary functional limitation, the Neck Disability Index (NDI) is a useful outcome measure to track progress over time.[213]

Vestibular-Oculomotor

Concussion injury may contribute to peripheral and/or central vestibular dysfunction as well as oculomotor dysfunction.[183,214] Examination should include ocular alignment, smooth pursuits, saccades, vergence and accommodation, gaze stability, dynamic visual acuity, visual motion sensitivity, and orthostatic hypotension.[183] Positional tests such as the Dix-Hallpike test and supine roll test for BPPV should also be performed.[215] Chapter 21, Vestibular Disorders, provides detailed information on these and other tests of vestibular and oculomotor function.

Mucha and colleagues[216] developed the Vestibular/Ocular Motor Screening (VOMS) tool, which examines five aspects of vestibular oculomotor function: smooth pursuit, horizontal and vertical saccades, near point convergence distance, horizontal vestibular ocular reflex, and visual motion sensitivity. Patients rate symptom provocation and severity while they undergo the vestibular/oculomotor tests. The VOMS was able to accurately distinguish between subjects who had a concussion and healthy controls.[216] It is recommended to use the VOMS as a screening tool but not as a replacement for a full vestibulo-oculomotor examination.[183]

The Dizziness Handicap Inventory is a valid and reliable self-report measure specific to the impact of dizziness on function.[217] Chapter 21, Vestibular Disorders, provides detailed information on these and other tests of vestibular and oculomotor function.

Autonomic/Exertional Tolerance

Autonomic dysfunction in response to exertional activities can contribute to functional deficits after concussion and exacerbate symptoms.[218,219] Exertional assessment is key to identify exertional intolerance and can help predict recovery.[220] The Buffalo Concussion Treadmill Test (BCTT) is a standardized, progressive exercise test that can diagnose physiological dysfunction after concussion and differentiate between factors other than exercise tolerance that may be impacting postconcussion symptoms.[221,222] The Buffalo Concussion Bike Test may be utilized for individuals with limited mobility or those not able to tolerate the treadmill test.[223] Exertional testing is safe, even within 1 week of injury, and can be useful to help to make return to play decisions and design targeted exercise programs.[183] A Dynamic Exertion Test has also been supported in the research, incorporating exertional challenge with more dynamic movements, such as quick changes in direction.[224]

Motor Function

Postural control deficits including divided attention and dual task motor functions may be impacted by concussion injury.[183,225] Examination of static and dynamic balance, motor control and coordination, and dual task assessment (cognitive or complex tasks) should be performed.[183,226]

The NeuroCom Sensory Organization Test (SOT) is a computerized, force plate–based, dynamic posturography test that assesses the ability to use and integrate sensory information from the visual, somatosensory, and vestibular systems to maintain balance.[227] The Balance Error Scoring System (BESS) is a clinical analog to the SOT. Both of these measures (SOT and BESS) have been used to demonstrate impaired postural control in people with sports-related mTBI.[228,229] Other measures of high-level balance activity such as the HiMAT,[125,126] Dynamic Gait Index,[230,231] Functional Gait Assessment,[232] and Balance Evaluation Systems Test[233]can also be used to assess balance. Sensor-based systems that utilize accelerometers and magnetometers to measure balance/postural control may be more sensitive than clinical measures but less expensive and more portable than force plate measures.[234–236] Self-report measures specific to perceived balance include the Activities-Specific Balance Confidence scale.[217] Table 19.9 summarizes some of the primary tests and measures and outcome measures.

Physical Therapy Interventions

Education

Education is a key component to concussion management. Patients should be provided with educational material regarding the symptoms of mTBI, expected recovery, and the importance of playing an active role in the rehabilitation process. Education regarding risk of further injury, such as second impact syndrome, may be warranted if individuals continue to participate in high-risk activities. Second impact syndrome is rare, but it can occur if the patient experiences a second mTBI after the initial one. The brain swells rapidly and can result in death. Concussion management strategies (sleep hygiene, rest breaks, and progressive physical activity) should be the focus of education. Refer to Box 19.6 for important educational topics. Appendix 19.A (online) contains Internet resources that may be beneficial for patients and their families.

Cervical Musculoskeletal

Identified cervical impairments from the examination should be addressed. Common interventions may include neck ROM, strength, motor control, proprioceptive or postural exercises.[183] Manual therapy for joint mobility in the cervical or thoracic spine may also be indicated. The neck pain CPG may be beneficial to guide specific cervical musculoskeletal

Table 19.9	Tests and Measures/Outcome Measures Commonly Used in Patients With Mild Traumatic Brain Injury
Concussion Symptom Self-Assessment	• Postconcussion Scale–Revised (PCS) • Rivermead Postconcussion Symptom Questionnaire (RPQ) • Neurobehavioral Symptom Inventory (NBI)
Cervical	• Neck Disability Index (NDI)
Vestibular-Ocular	• Dizziness Handicap Inventory (DHI) • Vestibular positional tests (Dix-Hallpike and Roll Test) • Vestibular Ocular Motor Screening (VOMS)
Motor/Balance	• Activities-Specific Balance Confidence scale (ABC) • Sensory Organization Test (SOT) • Balance Error Scoring System (BESS) • Dynamic Gait Index (DGI) • Functional Gait Assessment (FGA)
Autonomic/Exercise Tolerance	• Buffalo Concussion Treadmill Test (BCCT) • Buffalo Concussion Bike Test (BCBT)

Box 19.6   Education Topics

• Education on symptoms and expected recovery
• Reassurance about a positive recovery
• Prevention of further injury
• Empowerment for self-management
• Progression exercise or activity tolerance
• Sleep hygiene
• Rest breaks as needed

management.[183,237] There is some evidence that neck strength may be associated with concussion risk, so exercises to strengthen cervical and other postural musculature may be indicated.[238,239]

Vestibular-Oculomotor

Vestibular rehabilitation has been found to be an effective intervention after concussion injury.[240] If BPPV is encountered, repositioning techniques (canalith repositioning maneuvers) should be performed.[183] Other vestibular and oculomotor interventions include exercises for gaze stabilization (VOR x 1), habituation exercises, substitution exercises, and balance exercises with head movement.[183] See Chapter 21, Vestibular Disorders, for specifics on these interventions. The resources of the Vestibular Hypofunction CPG[241] and BPPV CPG[242] may also help to guide interventions.

Aerobic Exercise

Active rehabilitation with aerobic exercise has wide-ranging beneficial effects including improving neuronal function and faster symptom resolution.[243–245] While deconditioning with prolonged rest that may occur follow mTBI may have detrimental effects, progressive aerobic exercise has been shown to be safe and can result in a decrease in concussion symptoms.[183,221] Leddy and colleagues[221,222] recommend 20 minutes of aerobic training on the treadmill at 80% of threshold HR (established by the BCTT, level of exercise at which symptoms are exacerbated) five times a week, and progressively increasing the intensity by 5 to 10 beats per minute every 2 weeks as long as symptoms are not exaggerated. Other studies use ratings of perceived exertion or symptom ratings to guide exercise progression. In general, multiple modes of exercise progression are supported as long as the symptoms provoked are mild and resolve quickly.[183]

Motor

As described above in the section on interventions for persons with moderate to severe TBI, high-level, task-oriented balance and gait training can be performed, although evidence in the mTBI is more limited. Activities that are challenging to balance integration such as walking with head turns and on uneven, varied surfaces are recommended, as well as sport-specific skill training.[215] Balance training that incorporates the use of different sensory modalities such as standing on dense foam with eyes open and eyes closed can be performed. Balance training using computerized dynamic posturography can also be performed. Dual-task training and reactive balance training are another important intervention particularly linked to the functional needs of RTS or return to work.[217,225,246] See additional discussion in Chapter 10, Strategies to Improve Motor Function.

Evidence-Based Care

Mild TBI is an area of rapid research, and clinical guidelines are evolving quickly. Because of the evolving evidence related to the assessment and treatment of mTBI, it is important for the reader to employ evidence-based practice skills to remain up to date.

Although the term "mild" is used, a mild TBI can lead to debilitating impairments, limitations, and restrictions. In most cases the symptoms subside relatively quickly, and individuals are able to return to prior level of activity. However, for some individuals, symptoms can persist for long periods of time post-injury.[247] Patients with mTBI can be challenging to work with because it can be difficult to develop a targeted POC given the heterogeneity of the diagnosis. Just as with patients with severe to moderate TBI, because of the wide spectrum of signs and symptoms, it is important to consult and work with other health-care professionals in order to support the patient with mTBI to maximize their recovery.

SUMMARY

A TBI is a devastating and life-changing event for the individual and their family. The resulting complexity of impairments, activity limitations, and participation restrictions make working with a patient with brain injury extremely rewarding and challenging. There are a multitude of issues to consider. The physical therapist must adapt traditional physical therapy examination procedures and interventions to the unique motor function, cognitive, and behavioral challenges presented. The interdisciplinary team offers a unique opportunity for the physical therapist to learn and collaborate with experienced professionals. By working together with a team, the physical therapist is able to provide appropriate care that will help the individual with a TBI to maximize performance of activities and enhance social participation.

Questions for Review

1. List primary and secondary mechanisms of TBI.
2. Identify common neuromuscular, cognitive, and neurobehavioral impairments that result from TBI.
3. Contrast unresponsive wakefulness and minimally conscious state.
4. Identify key prognostic factors for individuals with TBI.
5. Identify and describe the roles of the interdisciplinary team members working with a patient with TBI.
6. Discuss the primary goals of physical therapy during the early stage of recovery in patients with severe to moderate TBI.

7. Select key outcome measures to use during the active rehabilitation stage in patients with severe to moderate TBI.

8. Describe strategies that should be considered when designing a POC for a patient with a severe to moderate TBI with cognitive and neurobehavioral deficits.

9. Contrast *restorative* versus *compensation-based interventions*. Give an example of each.

10. Develop a physical therapy POC for a patient with a severe to moderate TBI, which incorporates principles of experience-dependent neuroplasticity.

11. Outline a graduated return to play for a patient that has experienced a mild TBI.

12. Develop a physical therapy POC for a patient with a mild TBI.

CASE STUDY

The patient is a 22-year-old male who was involved in a motor vehicle crash. He was struck by another car as he exited his car. The patient suffered a severe closed brain injury, GCS score of seven at the emergency department, and both pupils were reactive to light. He was taken to a local hospital. CT scan revealed a left parietal subarachnoid hemorrhage. He also experienced a fracture of his right scapula. Two weeks after his injury, the patient is now transferred to an acute rehabilitation hospital.

Medications
Ritalin, Tegretol, Anaflex, and Ativan prn.

Social History
Patient is a graduate student in a computer science program at a local college. His parents live approximately 2 hours away. They are very supportive, and his mother has taken a leave of absence from her job to be with the patient and assist in his rehabilitation. He has private insurance through his parents, which covers inpatient and outpatient rehabilitation.

PHYSICAL THERAPY EXAMINATION

1. Screening: cardiopulmonary: HR 78, BP 110/76; integumentary: intact; musculoskeletal: see below; neuromuscular: see below.

2. Arousal, attention, and cognition: Rancho Los Amigos Levels of Cognitive Functioning: Level V. Easily distracted.
   a. Agitated behavior scale: 26/56
   b. GOAT: 66
   c. Moss Attention Rating Scale:
      1. Total Raw Score: 84
      2. Average MARS Item Score: 3.82
      3. Factor 1 (Restlessness/Distractibility) Score: 4.60
      4. Factor 2 (Initiation) Score: 4.00
      5. Factor 3 (Consistent/Sustained Attention) Score: 3.67

3. Assistive and adaptive devices: in the hospital environment, currently uses a standard wheelchair with gel cushion and solid back.

4. Balance
   a. Sitting balance: able to sit on edge of bed or mat with supervision
   b. Standing balance: able to stand with close supervision ×30 seconds, decreased weight bearing on right LE, Berg Balance Scale score: 36/56

5. Locomotion
   a. With minimal assistance able to ambulate with small-based quad cane for 150 feet using three-point step to/through pattern
   b. Gait speed: 0.34 m/s
   c. Observational gait assessment: difficulty clearing right foot in swing, right knee in extension throughout swing phase, circumducts and hip hikes right hip to clear foot, initial contact with midfoot on right.

6. Joint mobility: decreased posterior and inferior glide right glenohumeral joint.

7. Motor function, tone: increased extensor tone in right hip, knee, and ankle, 2 on Modified Ashworth Scale (MAS), increased flexor tone in right UE, 2 on MAS. Able to fractionate movement in left UE and LE but not able to fractionate movement in right UE or LE. However, patient exhibits active right dorsiflexion, wrist, and finger extension.

8. Orthotic, protective, and supportive devices:
   a. Has a bivalve cast at ankle and elbow from the acute care hospital for positioning ankle into dorsiflexion and elbow into extension

9. ROM: passive within normal limits, except:
   a. Right LE
      1. Dorsiflexion: has 5° plantar flexion contracture
      2. Knee extension: has 5° flexion contracture
   b. Right UE
      1. Shoulder flexion: 95°; abduction: 90°; external rotation: 65°; internal rotation: 80°; extension: 45°
      2. Elbow extension: has a 10° flexion contracture
      3. Wrist extension: 0°

10. Self-care and home management:
    a. FIM score:

Motor Items	Score	Cognitive Items	Score
Self-Care		*Communication*	
Eating	4	Comprehension	4
Grooming	4	Expression	4
Bathing	3	*Social Cognition*	
Dressing UE	3	Problem-solving	3
Dressing LE	2	Memory	2
Toileting	3	Social interaction	3
Sphincter control			
Bladder	4		
Bowel	4		
Transfer/Mobility			
Bed-Chair-Wheelchair	4		
Toilet	3		
Tub-Shower	3		
Locomotion			
Walk-Wheelchair	4		
Stairs	2		
Motor Score	43	***Cognitive Score***	16
Total Score	59		

11. Sensory integrity:
    a. Proprioception, light touch, and sharp/dull discrimination intact right and left extremities

CASE STUDY—cont'd

CASE STUDY GUIDING QUESTIONS

1. List factors that support a good prognosis for this patient, as well as factors that support a poor prognosis.

2. What factors make a restorative intervention approach appropriate for this patient? What factors make a compensatory approach appropriate for this patient?

3. List three long-term goals for this patient related to balance, walking ability, and transfer ability that are appropriate for discharge from the acute rehabilitation hospital.

4. Describe interventions to improve this patient's walking ability.

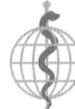

For topics related to dysautonomia, the reader is referred to Immersive Case A: A Patient With Long COVID/ Post-Acute Sequelae of COVID-19, an interactive case that guides users through the interview, examination, diagnosis, and writing of goals and the plan of care for a patient with dysautonomia due to long COVID/ post-acute sequelae of COVID-19, available online at **fadavis.com**.

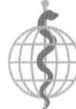

For additional resources, including answers to the questions for review, new immersive cases, case study guiding questions, references, and more, please visit **https://www.fadavis.com/product/physical -rehabilitation-fulk-8**. You may also quickly find the resources by entering this title's four-digit ISBN, 4691, in the search field at **http://fadavis.com** and logging in at the prompt.

Traumatic Spinal Cord Injury

Amy DeBlois, PT, DPT, NCS
Mark Bowden, PT, PhD
George D. Fulk, PT, PhD, FAPTA

Chapter 20

LEARNING OBJECTIVES

1. Identify the major etiologic factors associated with traumatic spinal cord injury.
2. Describe the clinical presentation following damage to the spinal cord.
3. Given a patient with a spinal cord injury, identify the motor and sensory level of injury and the American Spinal Injury Association Impairment Scale classification.
4. Analyze the impact of complications associated with spinal cord injury on the physical therapy plan of care and outcomes.
5. Identify the expected functional outcomes for patients with spinal cord injury at various lesion levels.
6. Explain how common precautions will affect physical therapy interventions.
7. Evaluate different outcome measures commonly used in people with spinal cord injury.
8. Analyze and interpret patient data, formulate goals and expected outcomes, and develop a plan of care when presented with a clinical case study.
9. Justify the selection of different interventions for the acute and active rehabilitation stages of recovery.
10. Discuss the use of neurotechnologies for people with spinal cord injury.

CHAPTER OUTLINE

DEMOGRAPHICS AND ETIOLOGY *760*
CLASSIFICATION OF SPINAL CORD INJURIES *760*
  Neuroanatomical Organization and Structure *760*
  Designation of Lesion Level *762*
  Complete Injuries, Incomplete Injuries, and Zone of Partial Preservation *763*
  ASIA Impairment Scale *763*
  Clinical Syndromes *764*
IMPACT OF SPINAL CORD INJURY ACROSS THE INTERNATIONAL CLASSIFICATION OF FUNCTIONING, DISABILITY, AND HEALTH *765*
  Body Structure/Function Impairments *765*
  Activity Limitations, Participation Restrictions, and Quality of Life *772*
ACUTE MEDICAL MANAGEMENT *773*
  Emergency Care *773*
  Fracture Stabilization *773*
  Immobilization *774*
PHYSICAL REHABILITATION *775*
  Physical Therapy Examination *776*

PROGNOSIS FOR RECOVERY OF MOTOR FUNCTION AND WALKING ABILITY *783*
OUTCOMES AND GOALS *783*
PHYSICAL THERAPY INTERVENTIONS *787*
  Strengthening *789*
  Respiratory *789*
  Skin Care *791*
  Cardiovascular/Endurance Training *792*
  Mobility Skills *793*
  Activity-Directed Upper Extremity Training *809*
WHEELCHAIR AND SEATING SYSTEM *809*
HEALTH, WELLNESS, AND PREVENTION *810*
  Exercise to Prevent Chronic Health Conditions and Treat Secondary Health Conditions *810*
SUMMARY *812*

Spinal cord injury (SCI) is a relatively low-incidence, high-cost injury that results in tremendous change in an individual's life. Paralysis or paresis of the muscles below the level of the injury can lead to limited and altered mobility, self-care, and ability to participate in valued social activities. In addition to the neuromuscular and musculoskeletal systems, many other body systems are impaired after an SCI, including the cardiopulmonary, integumentary, gastrointestinal, genitourinary, and sensory systems. The psychosocial impact of SCI can be just as great as the physical impact. Changes in body image and sexual function, incontinence, and having to rely on others to assist with the completion of everyday tasks that were previously done without thought or effort can profoundly influence a person's identity. Physical rehabilitation is an important component of the recovery process that helps people with SCI achieve a fulfilling and active life after their injury. Wellness and prevention strategies are critical so that individuals with an SCI can age successfully and lead meaningful lives. Physical therapists play a key role in supporting people with SCI during the rehabilitation process and afterward.

■ DEMOGRAPHICS AND ETIOLOGY

It is estimated that approximately 18,000 new cases of SCI occur in the United States annually,[1] while the global incidence of traumatic SCI is approximately 800,000.[2] The prevalence of SCI in the United States varies, with estimates ranging from 300,000[1] to over 2 million.[3] The average age at injury is 43 years.[1] Although the average age of a person who sustains a SCI has been increasing, approximately 50% of all SCIs occur in individuals between the ages of 16 and 30 years, with the most common age at injury being 19 years. The majority of persons with SCI are male (80% male versus 20% female)[1] Approximately 25% of SCIs occur in non-Hispanic blacks and 13% in individuals of Hispanic ethnicity.

SCIs can be grossly divided into two broad etiologic categories: *traumatic* injuries and *nontraumatic* damage. Trauma is the most frequent cause of injury in adult rehabilitation populations. Motor vehicle crashes (38%), falls (32%), and violence (14%) are the top three causes of traumatic SCIs.[1] Falls are the most common cause of SCI in older adults.[4] Nontraumatic SCI in adult populations generally results from disease or pathological influence. Conditions that may damage the spinal cord are vascular dysfunction (arteriovenous malformation [AVM], thrombosis, embolus, or hemorrhage), spinal stenosis and other degenerative processes, spinal neoplasms, and infection.[5–8] Nontraumatic etiologies account for approximately 38% of all SCIs[5] and are more common in older adults.[8] Although there is conflicting evidence on length of stay during inpatient rehabilitation between people with traumatic versus nontraumatic SCI,[7,9] outcomes after rehabilitation tend not to differ between people with traumatic and nontraumatic SCI.[10,11]

Incomplete tetraplegia (33%) is the most common neurological category, followed by complete paraplegia (24%), incomplete paraplegia (18%), and complete tetraplegia (18%).[1] The length of hospital stay, both in acute care and inpatient rehabilitation, has decreased considerably since the 1970s.[1,12] The median length of stay in the acute care hospital has decreased from 24 days in the 1970s to 11 days between 2015 and 2020. This trend is true for length of stay of inpatient rehabilitation as well, 98 days in the 1970s compared to 32 days between 2015 and 2020.[1] Individuals with complete tetraplegia have the longest length of stay, 59 days, while those with incomplete paraplegia stay in inpatient rehabilitation for approximately 33 days.

Life expectancy for people with SCI significantly improved in the middle of the 20th century, plateaued in the late 1900s and early 2000s, and slightly increased in the 2010s. However, it is still lower than people without SCI.[13] Factors that influence life expectancy are age at onset, level and extent of neurological injury, and ventilator dependency. Individuals with a functionally incomplete neurological SCI have a longer life expectancy than those with a complete injury, and individuals with more caudal injuries also have a longer life expectancy. A 20-year-old healthy individual without an SCI has a life expectancy of an additional 60 years (total life expectancy of 80 years). A person who experiences an SCI at age 20 years with a functionally incomplete injury has a life expectancy of an additional 52 years, with complete paraplegia an additional 45 years, with low tetraplegia (C5–C8) an additional 40 years, with high tetraplegia (C1–C4) an additional 34 years, and an individual who is dependent on a ventilator has a life expectancy of an additional 17 years.[1] These numbers are only estimates and vary based on the method of calculation.[14]

The financial impact of SCI for the individual and society is high. SCI is characterized by lengthy hospitalization, medical complications, extensive follow-up care, attendant care, and recurrent hospitalizations. It is estimated that the annual direct medical costs in the United States are over $2 billion.[3] Expenses during the first year post-injury vary based on level and type of injury from $1 million for high tetraplegia (C1–C4), $500,000 for paraplegia, and $350,000 for individuals with a functionally incomplete injury.[1,3] Average lifetime medical costs for an individual injured at 25 years of age are $3.5 million for high tetraplegia (C1–C4), $2.5 million for low tetraplegia (C5–C8), and $1.6 million for paraplegia.[15] Lifetime indirect costs for an individual with an SCI (lost wages and earnings) range from $0.5 million to $2.3 million.[16]

This brief presentation of demographic information provides some important general perspectives on characteristics of SCI. It is a relatively low-incidence disability affecting predominantly younger males and is associated with lengthy and costly care as well as a shorter life expectancy.

■ CLASSIFICATION OF SPINAL CORD INJURIES

SCIs typically are divided into two broad functional categories: tetraplegia and paraplegia. *Tetraplegia* refers to motor and/or sensory impairment of all four extremities and trunk, including the respiratory muscles, and results from lesions of the cervical cord. *Paraplegia* refers to motor and/or sensory impairment of all or part of the trunk and both lower extremities (LEs), resulting from lesions of the thoracic or lumbar spinal cord or cauda equina.[17]

Neuroanatomical Organization and Structure

Before considering designation of spinal cord lesions, it is useful to briefly review the anatomy of the spinal cord and its relationship with nerve roots to the vertebral bodies. The spinal cord exits the foramen magnum and extends to approximately the L1 vertebral level. It contains white matter, which consists mainly of ascending sensory tracts, descending motor tracts, and an H-shaped central area of gray matter. The primary ascending tracts are the dorsal column (conveys proprioception, vibratory sensation, deep touch, and discriminative touch); anterolateral system, consisting of the spinothalamic, spinoreticular, and spinotectal tracts (conveys pain, temperature, and crude touch); and the dorsal and ventral spinocerebellar tracts (conveys unconscious proprioception; Fig. 20.1). The primary descending tracts are the lateral corticospinal (voluntary movement); anterior corticospinal (voluntary movement of axial muscles, minimal functional significance due to small size); medial vestibulospinal (positioning of head and neck); lateral and medial vestibulospinal (posture and balance); lateral and medial reticulospinal (posture, balance, automatic gait-related movements); and rubrospinal (movement of limbs; Fig. 20.1). In addition to these long tracts, the white matter contains axons of interneurons, which convey information between spinal cord segments. The H-shaped gray matter is arranged such that the dorsal section in each half contains neurons involved in sensory function, the middle portion contains interneurons, and the ventral section contains neurons involved in motor function (anterior horn cells) that project to the peripheral muscles.

There are 31 pairs of spinal nerves: eight cervical, 12 thoracic, five lumbar, five sacral, and one coccygeal (Fig. 20.2). The cervical nerves are relatively horizontal as they exit the intervertebral foramina. The nerve roots for C1–C7 exit above the corresponding vertebrae. C8 exits below the C7 vertebrae. The remaining nerves exit in a downward direction and do not emerge at the corresponding vertebral level. During fetal development, the cord fills the entire length of the vertebral canal, and the spinal nerves run in a horizontal direction. As the vertebral column elongates with growth, the spinal

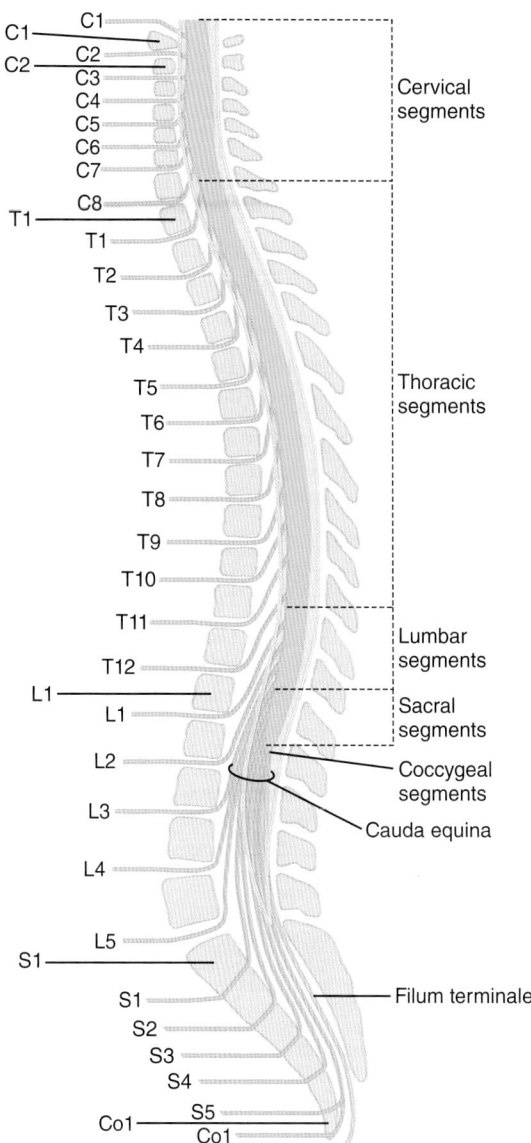

Figure 20.2 Relationship between spinal cord and nerve roots to vertebral bodies.

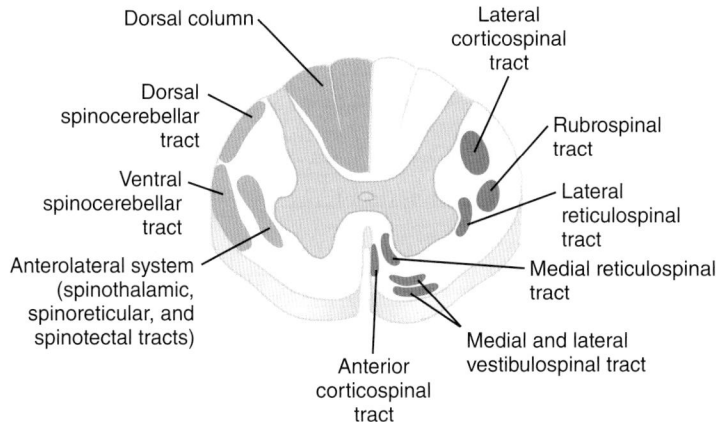

Figure 20.1 Main ascending sensor tracts: dorsal column, spinothalamic, spinoreticular, spinotectal, and dorsal and ventral spinocerebellar tracts. Main descending motor tracts: lateral corticospinal, anterior corticospinal, lateral and medial vestibulospinal, lateral and medial reticulospinal, and rubrospinal tracts.

cord, which does not elongate at the same rate or as much, is drawn upward. In adults the spinal cord ends in the conus medullaris at the L1 vertebral level. The nerve roots assume an increasingly oblique and downward direction, running in an almost vertical direction in the lumbar area, giving the appearance of a "horse's tail" (cauda equina) (Fig. 20.2). Because of this, in more caudal injuries, the vertebral level of injury does not correspond directly to the spinal cord segment level of injury.

Designation of Lesion Level

It is extremely important for clinicians and researchers to be able to accurately determine the extent of neurological impairment in terms of motor and sensory loss when working with individuals with SCI. The extent of motor and sensory function after injury has a large impact on the medical and rehabilitation needs of the individual. In an effort to standardize the way in which severity of injury is determined and documented, the American Spinal Injury Association (ASIA) created the *International Standards for Neurological Classification*

of Spinal Cord Injury (ISNCSCI)[17] (Fig. 20.3). The ISNCSCI provides a standardized examination method to determine the extent of motor and sensory function loss after an SCI. It promotes better communication between and among professionals, provides guidance for establishing the prognosis, and is an important tool for clinical research trials.

The *neurological level of injury* is defined as the most caudal level of the spinal cord with normal motor and sensory function on both the left and right sides of the body. *Motor level* is determined testing the strength of 10 key muscles on the right and left sides of the body. (See Fig. 20.3 for key muscles.) Key muscle strength is scored using the six-point ordinal scale commonly used for manual muscle testing (MMT). The motor level is the lowest myotome with a key muscle that has a grade of at least 3, provided that the muscle functions in the key muscles above this level are normal (MMT = 5). *Sensory level* is determined by testing the patient's sensitivity to light touch and pinprick on the left and right sides of the body at key dermatomes. (See Fig. 20.3 for key sensory points.) Scoring of sensation is based

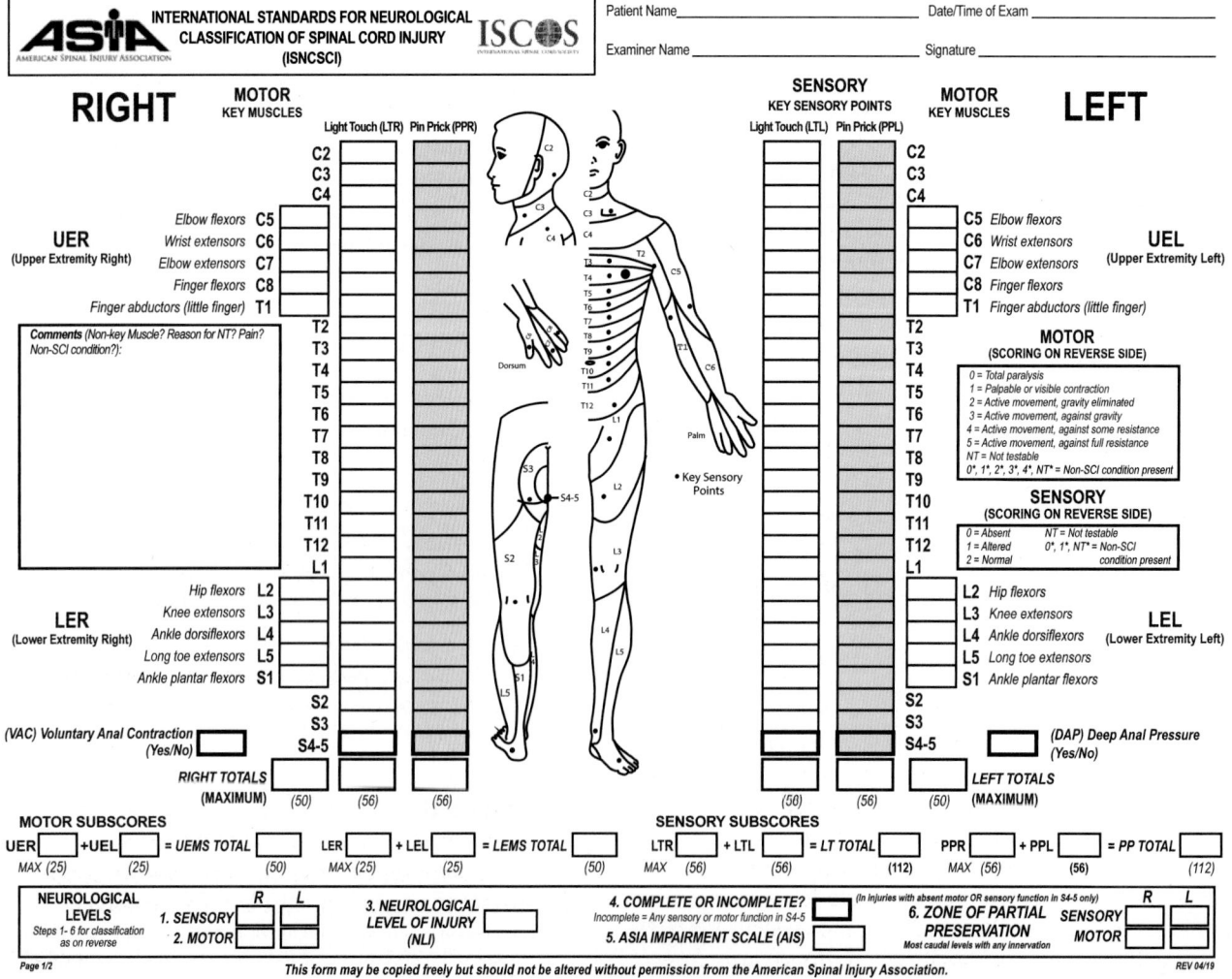

Figure 20.3 American Spinal Injury Association: *International Standards for Neurological Classification of Spinal Cord Injury*, revised 2019; Richmond, VA. With permission.

on a three-point ordinal scale, where 0 is absent, 1 is impaired, and 2 is normal. The sensory level is the most caudal level with normal light touch and pinprick sensation. For an individual patient, the motor and sensory levels may differ and may be different between the left and right sides of the body.[17]

Assigning a single muscle to represent one myotome is a generalization. Most muscles are innervated by more than one segmental nerve root; usually two nerve roots innervate each muscle. For example, the extensor carpi radialis longus receives innervation from the C6 and C7 spinal nerve roots. The ISNCSCI key muscles have two levels of innervation, adding to the validity of the scoring. For the purpose of determining motor and neurological level, the key muscle is defined as having intact innervation if it has an MMT score of at least 3/5 (fair), and the rostral key muscles exhibit 5/5 (normal) strength. If the rostral key muscle does not demonstrate 5/5 strength but the therapist feels that the muscle would test normally except for factors that would impede normal testing (e.g., pain with testing or difficulty with positioning), then this information should be carefully documented. For myotomes that are not clinically testable (i.e., C1–C4, T2–L1, and S2–S5), the motor level is defined as the same as the sensory level.

As mentioned, when determining neurological level, there may be differences in the level of sensory and motor function and between the left and right sides of the body. For example, a patient's sensory level may be at C5 on the left and C8 on the right, and the motor level may be C5 on the left and T1 on the right. In these cases, it is still necessary to assign a neurological level so that ASIA Impairment Scale (AIS) classification can be assigned by determining the number of key muscles intact below the neurological level (see "AIS Impairment" section later). However, it should be noted that in some cases the neurological level assignment can be misleading in that the patient may have a mixed presentation of intact motor and/or sensory function below that level.

Complete Injuries, Incomplete Injuries, and Zone of Partial Preservation

A complete anatomical transection of the spinal cord is rare. However, even if the injury is not anatomically complete, it may present as neurologically complete. The ISNCSCI defines a *complete injury* as having no sensory or motor function in the lowest sacral segments (S4 and S5), with no sacral sparing. Sacral sparing is determined by preserved sensory or motor function at the S4–S5 level: ability to feel deep anal pressure, or voluntary anal sphincter contraction. An *incomplete injury* is classified as having motor and/or sensory function below the neurological level that includes sensory and/or motor function at S4 and S5, with presence of sacral sparing. If an individual has motor and/or sensory function below the neurological level without having sacral sparing, then the areas of intact motor and/or sensory function below the neurological level are termed *zones*

of partial preservation (ZPPs).[17] ZPPs were previously only recorded with complete injuries but more recently were expanded to include incomplete injuries, to give a more precise clinical picture.[17,18] If individuals present with motor or sensory loss due to preexisting or non–spinal-cord-injury-related conditions, grading for those motor or sensory scores are denoted with an asterisk (*). Examples of these non–spinal-cord conditions include musculoskeletal injury, amputation, and burns.[17,18]

ASIA Impairment Scale

The AIS (Box 20.1) was created to distinguish among different types of SCI—complete, sensory incomplete, and motor incomplete. Physical therapists may play a role in performing the testing to determine AIS levels.

Box 20.1 ASIA Impairment Scale (AIS)

A = Complete. No sensory or motor function is preserved in the sacral segments S4–5.

B = Sensory Incomplete. Sensory but not motor function is preserved below the neurological level and includes the sacral segments S4–5 (light touch or pin prick at S4–5 or deep anal pressure) AND no motor function is preserved more than three levels below the motor level on either side of the body.

C = Motor Incomplete. Motor function is preserved at the most caudal sacral segments for voluntary anal contraction (VAC) OR the patient meets the criteria for sensory incomplete status (sensory function preserved at the most caudal sacral segments S4–5 by LT, PP or DAP), and has some sparing of motor function more than three levels below the ipsilateral motor level on either side of the body.
(This includes key or non-key muscle functions to determine motor incomplete status.) For AIS C—less than half of key muscle functions below the single NLI have a muscle grade ≥3.

D = Motor Incomplete. Motor incomplete status as defined above, with at least half (half or more) of key muscle functions below the single NLI having a muscle grade ≥3.

E = Normal. If sensation and motor function as tested with the ISNCSCI are graded as normal in all segments, and the patient had prior deficits, then the AIS grade is E. Someone without an initial SCI does not receive an AIS grade.

Using ND: To document the sensory, motor and NLI levels, the ASIA Impairment Scale grade, and/or the zone of partial preservation (ZPP) when they are unable to be determined based on the examination results.

LT = light touch; PP = pin prick; DAP = deep anal pressure; NLI = neurologic level of injury.
From American Spinal Injury Association, with permission. American Spinal Injury Association: International Standards for Neurological Classification of Spinal Cord Injury, revised 2011; Atlanta, GA, Revised 2011, Updated 2015.

Certifications in the ISNCSCI testing are available on their website. Individuals with incomplete injuries may have variable clinical presentations in terms of motor and/or sensory function below the neurological level. For example, one patient may have close to normal sensory and motor function below the level of the lesion, whereas another with the same lesion level may have impaired sensation and no motor function below the neurological level. AIS grades may change over time, with the highest rates of conversion from complete to incomplete for tetraplegic levels of injury.[19] It is important to note that changes in AIS grades may not directly correlate with changes in function.

Clinical Syndromes

Despite the disparity associated with incomplete lesions, several syndromes have emerged with consistent clinical features. Approximately one-fifth of all SCIs result in an injury pattern similar to clinical SCI syndromes.[15] Information related to the anticipated sensory and motor functions of these syndromes is useful in establishing anticipated goals, expected outcomes, and plan of care (POC). The approximate area of cord damage of each syndrome is presented in Figure 20.4. The corresponding clinical features of the different syndromes are explained by the anatomical organization of the motor and sensory pathways described earlier. Patients who are identified as having one of these syndromes should still receive a neurological, motor, and sensory-level designation and be assigned an AIS classification.

Brown-Séquard Syndrome

Brown-Séquard syndrome occurs from hemisection of the spinal cord (damage to one side) and is typically caused by penetration wounds (i.e., gunshot or stab). Partial lesions (termed *Brown-Séquard plus syndrome*) occur more frequently; true hemisections are rare. The clinical features of this syndrome are asymmetrical. On the *ipsilateral* (same) side as the lesion, there is paralysis and sensory loss. The ipsilateral loss of proprioception, light touch, and vibratory sense is due to damage to the dorsal column, paralysis results from damage to the lateral corticospinal tract. Damage to the spinothalamic tracts results in loss of sense of pain and temperature on the side *contralateral* (opposite) to the lesion. This loss begins several dermatome segments below the level of injury. This discrepancy in levels and impairment on sides of the body occurs because the lateral spinothalamic tracts ascend two to four segments on the same side before crossing and the descending motor tract decussating in the medulla. Individuals with Brown-Séquard syndrome typically achieve good functional gains during inpatient rehabilitation.[20]

Anterior Cord Syndrome

Anterior cord syndrome is frequently related to flexion injuries of the cervical region with resultant damage to the anterior portion of the cord and/or its vascular supply from the anterior spinal artery. There is typically compression of the anterior cord from fracture, dislocation, or cervical disk protrusion. This syndrome is characterized by loss of motor function (corticospinal tract damage) and loss of the sense of pain and temperature (spinothalamic tract damage) below the level of the lesion. Proprioception, light touch, and vibratory sense are generally preserved, because they are mediated by the dorsal columns with a separate vascular supply from the posterior spinal arteries.[21] Individuals with anterior cord syndrome often require a longer length of stay during inpatient rehabilitation compared to people with other types of SCI clinical syndromes.[20]

Central Cord Syndrome

Central cord syndrome is the most common SCI syndrome.[20] It generally occurs from hyperextension injuries to the cervical region.[22] It also has been associated with congenital or degenerative narrowing of the spinal canal. The resultant compressive forces give rise to hemorrhage and edema, producing damage to the most central aspects of the cord. There is characteristically more severe neurological involvement of the upper extremities (UEs) (cervical tracts are more centrally located) than of the LEs (lumbar and sacral tracts are located more peripherally). Varying degrees of sensory impairment occur but tend to be less severe than motor deficits. With complete preservation of sacral tracts, normal sexual, bowel, and bladder function may be retained. Patients with central cord syndrome typically recover the ability to ambulate. Some distal UE weakness and loss of fine motor control remain, which can result in moderate to severe limitations in the ability to perform functional tasks.

Cauda Equina Injuries

The spinal cord tapers distally to form the conus medullaris at the lower border of the first lumbar vertebra.

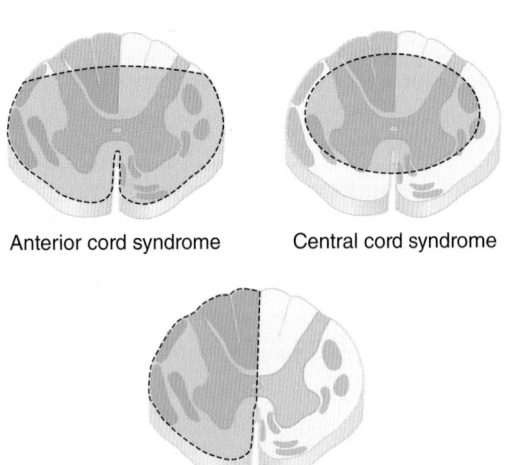

Anterior cord syndrome   Central cord syndrome

Brown-Sequard syndrome

Figure 20.4 Areas of spinal cord damage in clinical syndromes.

Although some anatomical variations exist, this is the typical termination point of the spinal cord. Below this level is the collection of long nerve roots known as the *cauda equina*. Complete transections in this area are rare. Cauda equina lesions are frequently anatomically incomplete owing to the great number of nerve roots involved and the comparatively large surface area they encompass (i.e., it would be unlikely that an injury to this region would involve the entire surface area and all the nerve roots).

Individuals with cauda equina injuries exhibit areflexic bowel and bladder and saddle anesthesia. Lower extremity paralysis and paresis are variable, depending on the extent of the injury to the cauda equina. Cauda equina lesions are peripheral nerve (*lower motor neuron* [LMN]) injuries. As such, they have the same potential to regenerate as peripheral nerves elsewhere in the body. However, full return of innervation is not common because (1) there is a large distance between the lesion and the point of innervation, (2) axonal regeneration may not occur along the original distribution of the nerve, (3) axonal regeneration may be blocked by glial-collagen scarring, (4) the end organ may no longer be functioning once reinnervation occurs, and (5) the rate of regeneration slows and finally stops after about 1 year.

Conus medullaris syndrome occurs when the very distal portion of the spinal cord is damaged. This type of injury often results in a mixture of LMN and *upper motor neuron* (UMN) damage. ASIA's website provides educational materials with more details on the ISNCSCI (http://asia-spinalinjury.org).

■ IMPACT OF SPINAL CORD INJURY ACROSS THE INTERNATIONAL CLASSIFICATION OF FUNCTIONING, DISABILITY, AND HEALTH

SCI results in a disruption of communication from higher centers in the central nervous system (CNS) to the periphery. This disruption results in many different body structure/function impairments, activity limitations, and participation restrictions.

Body Structure/Function Impairments
Spinal Shock

Immediately following SCI there is a period of areflexia that is part of *spinal shock*. This period of transient reflex depression is not clearly understood.[23] It is believed to result from the very abrupt withdrawal of connections between higher centers and the spinal cord. It is characterized initially by an absence of all reflex activity, impairment of autonomic regulation resulting in hypotension and loss of control of sweating and piloerection. In addition to the loss of deep tendon reflexes, there is

a loss of the bulbocavernosus reflex, cremasteric reflex, and Babinski response, and a delayed plantar response.

Spinal shock evolves over time. The initial period of total areflexia lasts approximately 24 hr. This is followed by a gradual return of reflexes 1 to 3 days after injury and a period of increasing hyperreflexia lasting 1 to 4 weeks.[23] Spinal shock should not be confused with neurogenic shock, which is changes in autonomic blood pressure (BP) control that occur in the acute stage of injury and result in severe bradycardia and hypotension.[24]

Motor and Sensory Impairments

Following SCI, there will be either complete (*paralysis*) or partial (*paresis*) loss of muscle function below the level of the lesion. Disruption of the ascending sensory fibers following SCI results in impaired or absent sensation below the level of the lesion.

The clinical presentation of motor and sensory impairments depends on the specific features of the lesion. These include the neurological level and the completeness of the lesion. See previous section on Classifications of SCI.

Autonomic Dysreflexia

Autonomic dysreflexia (AD) is an abnormal autonomic reflex that can be life threatening. Typically, AD occurs in lesions above T6 (above sympathetic splanchnic outflow). However, it has been reported in patients with lower injuries. The incidence of AD is approximately 48% to 70%. Although AD is more common in the chronic stage of recovery (usually first occurring between 3 and 6 months after injury), it may also occur in the early stages after SCI. It is more common with complete injury, but it may also occur with an incomplete SCI (iSCI).[25]

AD is a result of disruption of the autonomic control of the cardiovascular system. After SCI, supraspinal regulation of the sympathetic preganglionic neurons is disrupted. Initially, this results in reduced BP and sympathetic reflexes. Over time the spinal circuitry reorganizes, becoming hyperexcitable. This hyperexcitability of the sympathetic reflexes when combined with the loss of descending control results in abnormal reflex activation of the sympathetic system below the level of the injury when there is a noxious stimulus below the level of the lesion.[26] Noxious afferent reach the spinal cord below the level of the injury and initiate a mass sympathetic reflex response resulting in elevation of BP. Normally, the impulses stimulate the receptors in the carotid sinus and aorta, which signal the vasomotor center to readjust peripheral resistance. Following SCI, however, impulses from the vasomotor center cannot pass the site of the lesion to counteract the hypertension by vasodilation.[26] Owing to the lack of inhibition from higher centers, hypertension will persist if not treated promptly. Hypertension triggered by AD can result in seizures, cardiac arrest, subarachnoid hemorrhage, stroke, or even death.[26,27]

Initiating Stimuli

Although there are a variety of potential causes of AD, the most common cause is bladder issues, followed by bowel irritation (constipation, impacted feces, and obstruction). Common bladder issues that may trigger AD are distended bladder, blocked catheter, urinary tract infection (UTI), kidney stones, and irritation of bladder or urethra during catheterization or other procedures. Other precipitating stimuli include skin pressure injuries, heterotopic ossification, fracture, trauma, sexual activity, childbirth/labor, and other noxious stimuli below the level of the lesion.[25] Table 20.1 summarizes stimuli that may trigger an onset of AD, as well as common associated signs and symptoms.

Signs and Symptoms

The symptoms of AD include hypertension, bradycardia, headache (often severe and pounding), profuse sweating, increased spasticity, restlessness, vasoconstriction below the level of the lesion, vasodilation (flushing) above the level of the lesion, constricted pupils, nasal congestion, piloerection (goose bumps), and blurred vision. Less commonly, AD may also present as asymptomatic. A rise in systolic BP 20 mm Hg above baseline is diagnostic of an episode of AD. People with SCI typically have lower than normal resting BP; systolic may be in the range of 90 to 110 mm Hg for those with neurological level above T6. During an episode of AD, systolic BP may rise to 250 to 300 mm Hg and diastolic to 200 to 220 mm Hg.[25,26,28]

Intervention

The onset of symptoms should be treated as a medical emergency. If lying flat, the patient should be brought to an upright position, inasmuch as BP will be lowered in this position, and any tight clothing or restrictive devices should be loosened. BP and pulse should be monitored. Possible triggers should be identified, starting with bladder and bowel. If the patient is using an indwelling catheter, it should be checked to make sure it is not blocked. If any type of blockage is found, it should be removed immediately. If the patient catheterizes intermittently, a catheter should be placed and the bladder drained. The patient should then be questioned about when the last bowel movement occurred and checked for an impaction. The patient's body should be examined for other triggering stimuli such as tight clothing, restricting catheter straps, abdominal binders, or anything that may be a noxious stimulus.[25,26,28]

If hypertension and other symptoms do not subside with the identification and elimination of specific triggers, medical and/or nursing assistance should be sought emergently. Antihypertensive medications, nitrates, and nifedipine are used acutely,[25,26] and clonidine may be used in recurrent cases of AD.[29]

People with SCI who are at risk of experiencing AD should be educated on initiating stimuli, symptoms, and management of AD. In many cases, AD does not manifest itself until after the patient is discharged from

Table 20.1 Initiating Stimuli and Signs and Symptoms of Autonomic Dysreflexia	
Initiating Stimuli	Signs and Symptoms
Bladder distention/irritation/infection*	Hypertension (rise in systolic BP 20–30 mm Hg above baseline, individuals with SCI above T6 tend to have systolic blood pressure between 90 and 100 mm Hg)
Bowel distention/irritation*	Bradycardia, but may instead present with tachycardia
Stimuli that would normally be painful below level of lesion	Severe headache
Pressure injuries	Feeling of anxiety
Sexual activity	Constricted pupils
Childbirth/labor	Blurred vision and/or spots in visual field
Skeletal fracture/trauma	Flushing of skin and sweating above level of injury
Gastrointestinal irritation	Cool skin and pallor
Restrictive clothing or shoes	Piloerection may be above or below level of lesion
	Nasal congestion
	Increased spasticity
	May be asymptomatic

*Most common triggers of autonomic dysreflexia.

the hospital and rehabilitation, so the patient may no longer be able to rely on their health-care team for support in case they experience an episode of AD. Approximately 40% of people with SCI above T6 reported never having heard about AD, and 22% of those who did know about it did not know how to respond to an episode of AD.[30] Additionally, up to 40% of emergency department personnel may not have adequate knowledge or training related to AD.[31]

Spastic Hypertonia

Individuals with SCI and other CNS disorders such as traumatic brain injury, multiple sclerosis, and stroke often present with altered muscle tone, termed *spastic hypertonia*. Specifically, hypertonia refers to resistance to passive motion, while spasticity (a form of hypertonia) is defined as "a motor disorder characterized by a velocity-dependent increase in tonic stretch reflexes (muscle tone) with exaggerated tendon jerks, resulting from hyperexcitability of the stretch reflex, as one component of the upper motor neuron syndrome."[32] Hypertonia and spasticity are sometimes used interchangeably in the literature but should be distinguished due to hypothesized differences in neurophysiology. Spastic hypertonia is part of UMN syndrome, which encompasses a range of conditions including spasticity, muscle spasms, abnormally high muscle tone, hyperactive stretch reflexes, and clonus.[33] Approximately 65% of people with SCI have spasticity, and it is more common in people with cervical-level injuries.[34] Spastic hypertonia is thought to be a result of altered input at the spinal segmental level, which causes an imbalance between excitation and inhibition of the spinal motor neurons. Descending, suprasegmental signals are altered or eliminated following SCI, the anterior horn cell may become hyperexcitable, and there are changes in afferent input.[33]

Spastic hypertonia typically emerges below the level of the lesion after spinal shock evolves. There is a gradual increase in spastic hypertonia during the first 6 months, and a plateau is usually reached 1 year after injury. Various stimuli including positional changes, cutaneous stimuli, environmental temperatures, tight clothing, bladder or kidney stones, fecal impactions, catheter blockage, UTIs, pressure injuries, and emotional stress may trigger or increase spasticity and muscle spasms.

Spasticity varies in the degree of severity. Approximately 50% of people with SCI report that their spasticity is problematic and negatively impacts their function.[34-36] Spasticity is also associated with poorer health,[37] including pain, insomnia, pressure injuries, and contractures.[38] Patients with minimal to moderate involvement may learn to trigger the spasticity or muscle spasm at appropriate times to assist in functional activities. However, strong spasticity can be a deterrent to independent function. For example, severe spasms during transfers may cause loss of balance and a fall.

The management of spasticity must balance the potential benefits against the negative effects.

Spasticity is generally managed through a variety of methods including stretch, exercise, electrotherapy, heat, massage, and medications.[38] Although stretch and other modalities are commonly used in the clinic, systematic reviews have found that effects of physical therapy interventions and stretch are inconclusive or had no clinically important impact on spasticity.[38,39] However, one 2019 review evaluated 18 systematic reviews and found low-quality evidence for short-term benefits of vibration therapy.[40] This review found that focal vibration resulted in short-term spasticity decrease (lasting 24 hr), and whole-body vibration reduced spasticity for 6 to 8 days.[40] However, no evidence currently exists for long-term management rehabilitation of spasticity.

Medications typically used include muscle relaxants and spasmolytic agents such as baclofen,[30,32] tizanidine,[33] diazepam,[34] and dantrolene sodium.[34] Intrathecal baclofen (where an implanted pump delivers small amounts of baclofen directly at the spinal cord level to minimize side effects) can be used in cases of severe spasticity when individuals do not respond well to oral administration.[35] Intramuscular injection of botulinum neurotoxin can be used to manage focal spasticity.[36] Pharmacological management is often not successful in alleviating spasticity,[41] and its limited benefits must be weighed against potentially adverse side effects (e.g., weakness, dizziness, drowsiness). There is also some evidence that the use of antispasmodic medications may actually be associated with reduced recovery during inpatient rehabilitation.[42]

Cardiovascular Impairment

In healthy individuals with an intact spinal cord, cardiovascular function is regulated by the brain stem and hypothalamus via the sympathetic and parasympathetic nervous systems of the autonomic nervous system. Parasympathetic signals to the heart arise from the vagus nerve, decreasing heart rate and contractility. Sympathetic outflow comes from spinal segments T1 to L2 through the sympathetic trunk, increasing heart rate and heart contractility and peripheral vasoconstriction. More specifically, sympathetic outflow to the heart and blood vessels of the upper body comes from the cervical and upper thoracic region (above T6), while sympathetic outflow to blood vessels of the lower body comes from below T5 (T6–L2). Thus, a higher SCI (above T6) will result in loss of sympathetic control to the heart and blood vessels below the level of the injury and intact parasympathetic input to the heart. An SCI at T6 and below has intact sympathetic and parasympathetic control to the heart but loss of sympathetic control to the blood vessels below the level of the injury. The resulting imbalance between sympathetic and parasympathetic control of the cardiovascular system can result in a variety of cardiovascular impairments. These include AD (discussed earlier), neurogenic shock, bradyarrhythmias, hypotension, orthostatic hypotension, and impaired cardiovascular reflexes.[24,43,44]

A rostral SCI (above T6) may result in neurogenic shock because sympathetic output to the heart is lacking, and vagal (parasympathetic) input is unopposed. *Neurogenic shock* is defined as systolic BP ≤90 mm Hg and heart rate ≤50 bpm. Neurogenic shock results in bradyarrhythmias, atrioventricular conduction block, and hypotension. Neurogenic shock may resolve in weeks postinjury and is more likely in individuals with injuries at the cervical and upper thoracic levels.[43–45]

Because of the disrupted balance between sympathetic and parasympathetic input, as well as a lack of or decrease in active muscle contraction and prolonged time in bed, *orthostatic hypotension* (decrease in systolic BP of at least 20 mm Hg or decrease in diastolic BP of at least 10 mm Hg when assuming upright posture from supine) is often experienced early after injury. Approximately 75% of individuals with SCI experience orthostatic hypotension in the acute stage, and 50% of those with a cervical injury still experience it in the chronic stage. Symptoms of orthostatic hypotension include blurred vision, dizziness, ringing in the ears, light-headedness, nausea, dyspnea, and fainting.[24,46] Orthostatic hypotension is more common in people with SCI above T6, but it may also occur in those with a lower-level injury. Although the exact mechanism is not clearly understood, the cardiovascular system, over time, gradually reestablishes sufficient vasomotor tone to allow assumption of the vertical position.[39,47]

To minimize these effects when mobilizing patients early after SCI, the cardiovascular system should be allowed to adapt gradually by a slow progression to the vertical position. This frequently begins with incremental elevation of the head of the bed and progresses to a reclining wheelchair with elevating leg rests and use of a standing frame or tilt table. Vital signs should be monitored carefully. Use of compressive stockings, ACE wraps on the LEs, and an abdominal binder may further minimize these effects.[46,48,49] Medications such as midodrine, nitro-L-arginine methyl ester, fludrocortisone, ergotamine, and ephedrine may be used.[46,50,51]

Past the acute stage of injury, people with SCI below or within the thoracolumbar sympathetic output will exhibit a reduced exercise tolerance, lower stroke volume, and reduced cardiac output.[52,53] Individuals with cervical SCI are likely to demonstrate a lower peak heart rate, postexercise hypotension, and other abnormal cardiovascular responses to exercise.[54,55] In the long term, individuals with SCI are at risk for developing cardiovascular disease due to physical inactivity, impaired glycemic control, chronic inflammation, and abnormal cholesterol profiles.[24] A regular exercise program after rehabilitation should be developed and implemented (see later section on Health, Wellness, and Prevention).

Impaired Thermoregulation

Due to loss of peripheral sensory input to the thermoregulation centers of the brain and impaired vasomotor and sudomotor control below the level of the lesion, people with SCI experience impaired thermoregulation that is worse in those with injuries above T6. This autonomic (sympathetic) dysfunction results in impaired thermoregulatory responses. Individuals with cervical-level injuries may present with *poikilothermia,* a condition in which the environmental temperature dictates body temperature. During exercise or when in ambient high temperature, individuals with SCI have limited ability to vasodilate peripheral blood vessels and excrete body heat through sweat. This results in hyperthermia. Conversely, in cold ambient temperatures, the lack of ability to vasoconstrict peripheral blood vessels and shiver results in hypothermia. Thus, core body temperature fluctuates with the temperature of the environment.[56]

People with SCI also may present with hyperhidrosis (excessive sweating), anhidrosis (lack of sweating), or hypohidrosis (limited sweating). The most common presentation is hyperhidrosis above the level of the lesion and hypohidrosis below the level of the lesion.

Pulmonary Impairment

Ventilatory and respiratory function vary considerably, depending on the level of lesion. As with other impairments following SCI, the more rostral the injury, the greater is the impact on function. Pulmonary complications are a leading cause of death in both the early and late stages of recovery.[1,57]

The primary muscle of inspiration is the diaphragm. The scalenes and intercostals also play important roles by stabilizing and elevating the ribs. Other important accessory and stabilizing muscles of inspiration are the sternocleidomastoid, serratus anterior, pectoralis major and minor, serratus posterior superior, trapezius, levator scapulae, and abdominals. The primary muscles of expiration are the abdominals and internal intercostals. Normally, relaxed expiration is essentially a passive process that occurs through elastic recoil of the lungs and thorax. However, the abdominals and internal intercostals contribute several important functions related to movement of air out of the lungs. Loss of these muscles significantly decreases expiratory efficiency. Control of the abdominal muscles originates from T6 to T12. When fully innervated, they play an important role in maintaining intrathoracic pressure for effective respiration. They support the abdominal viscera and assist in maintaining the position of the diaphragm. They also function to push the diaphragm upward during forced expiration. With paralysis of the abdominal musculature, this support is lost, causing the diaphragm to assume an unusually low position. This lowered position and lack of abdominal pressure to move the diaphragm upward during forced expiration result in a decreased expiratory reserve volume. This subsequently decreases cough effectiveness and the ability to expel secretions. Table 20.2 presents the level of innervation of inspiratory and expiratory muscles in relation to level of SCI and the likely respiratory support a patient with an SCI at that level requires.[21,58-61]

With high spinal cord lesions at C1 and C2, phrenic nerve innervation and spontaneous respiration are lost. The only muscles of respiration that are intact are accessory muscles of inspiration: sternocleidomastoid and upper trapezius. An artificial ventilator or phrenic nerve stimulator is required to sustain life. Expiration is passive; as a result, individuals with SCI at these levels require assistance for airway clearance. C3- and C4-level injuries have partial diaphragm innervation, as well as scalenes and levator scapulae function. In the acute stage of recovery, individuals with an injury at these levels will require mechanical ventilation. With recovery and training they will likely be able to breathe on their own.[62] However, they may need part-time ventilatory support, especially individuals with C3-level injury. These individuals do not have innervation to muscles

of expiration (abdominals or intercostals), so they will need assistance for airway clearance.

Patients with mid to lower cervical-level injuries have better pulmonary function than those with higher cervical-level injuries. Injuries at C5–C8 have a fully innervated diaphragm, as well as many accessory muscles of inspiration. They are not likely to require ventilator support. However, forced expiration is severely impaired. Although some cough ability is preserved, it is usually weak.

Although individuals with paraplegia have better respiratory function than people with tetraplegia, they still have impaired respiratory function compared to healthy individuals without an SCI.[63] Individuals with weak or absent abdominal and intercostal musculature will have impaired airway clearance ability and be at a greater risk for developing pneumonia and atelectasis.

Other factors may further impair respiratory status. Additional trauma sustained at the time of injury, premorbid respiratory problems, age, weight, and smoking history can all further compromise respiratory function.[63,64]

Table 20.2   Innervation of Muscles of Inspiration and Expiration

Level of Spinal Cord Injury	Inspiratory Muscles* (Innervation)	Forced Expiratory Muscles* (Innervation)	Respiratory Support
C1–C2	Sternocleidomastoid and upper trapezius (accessory cranial nerve)		Requires mechanical ventilation or phrenic nerve stimulation.
C3–C4	Partial diaphragm (C3–C5), levator scapulae (C3–C5), scalenes (C3–C8)		Require mechanical ventilation early in recovery but likely able to breathe independently in long run. Will need assistance with airway clearance, not able to cough.
C5	Diaphragm (C3–C5)	Pectoralis major—clavicular (C5–C6)	Able to breathe independently. Will need assistance with airway clearance, not able to cough.
C6–8	Pectoralis major—sternal (C7–T1), pectoralis minor (C6–T1), serratus anterior (C5–C7)		Able to breathe independently. Will need assistance with airway clearance, may have weak cough.
T1–T5	Intercostals (T1–T11), serratus posterior superior (T1–T3)	Intercostals (T1–T11)	Able to breathe independently. May need assistance with airway clearance, have a weak cough.
T6–T10	Abdominals (T6–L1)	Abdominals (T6–L1), serratus posterior inferior (T9–T12)	Able to breathe independently. May need assistance with airway clearance, weak to strong cough.
T11 and below	All of the above	All of the above, quadratus lumborum (T12–L4)	Able to breathe independently. Independent with airway clearance, strong cough.

*Lower-level spinal cord injuries have intact innervation to muscles above the level of the injury. There are slight differences among sources in regard to muscle innervation levels.

Bladder and Bowel Impairment

Bladder Dysfunction

The effects of bladder dysfunction following SCI pose serious medical complications requiring consistent and long-term management. Urinary tract infections are a major cause of rehospitalization in people with SCI. Approximately 40% of people with SCI report having a UTI 1 year after injury.[65] SCI alters the complex reflexive and voluntary control of *micturition*. As a result, people with SCI often require a catheter to drain the bladder.

Spinal control for micturition originates from the sacral segments of S2, S3, and S4.[21] The level of the SCI dictates the type of bladder dysfunction. Patients with lesions that occur above the conus medullaris and sacral segments develop a *spastic* or *hyperreflexic bladder*.[21] This is also termed a *UMN bladder*. Following a lesion of the sacral segments or conus medullaris, a *flaccid* or *areflexic bladder* develops.[21] This is also termed a *LMN bladder*.

A spastic or hyperreflexic bladder (UMN lesion) contracts and reflexively empties in response to a certain level of filling pressure.[66] The reflex arc is intact with this type of injury. The detrusor muscle is generally hyperreflexive. There can be increased tone of the sphincter, contraction of the detrusor with small urine volumes, and lack of coordination between detrusor and sphincters (dyssynergia). A flaccid or areflexive bladder (LMN lesion) is essentially flaccid because there is no reflex action of the detrusor muscle.

There are generally two types of bladder dysfunction: failure to store urine and failure to empty urine.[66] These can be due to detrusor muscle or sphincter impairment. Inability to store urine may be due to an areflexive sphincter or spastic detrusor muscle. Inability to empty the bladder sufficiently may be due to an areflexive bladder or a sphincter that is unable to relax. Dyssynergia between the detrusor and sphincter can also cause incomplete drainage of the bladder.[66]

Bladder Management

The primary goal of bladder management is to prevent or minimize urinary tract complications. These include UTIs, *hydronephrosis* (swelling of kidney due to backup of urine), renal calculi, bladder calculi, and *vesicoureteral reflux* (backward flow of urine up the ureter).[66] Because urinary incontinence has very strong psychosocial implications for the patient, a coordinated approach to bladder management is particularly important. Knowledge of and participation in the bladder management program is an important consideration for the physical therapist.

In the early stage of recovery, while the patient is still in spinal shock, the bladder is flaccid, and an indwelling catheter is used. After the patient is stable during rehabilitation, the most frequently used method of bladder management is *intermittent catheterization*.[66,67]

Briefly stated, the program involves establishing a fluid intake pattern of approximately 2,000 mL/day. Intake is stopped late in the day to reduce the need for catheterization during the night. Initially, the patient is catheterized every 4 hours. A record is maintained of voided and residual urine. While in the hospital, sterile intermittent catheterization should be done; after discharge, a clean technique can be used.

Although intermittent catheterization is the most common method of bladder management after discharge from the rehabilitation hospital, many males switch to the use of an external, condom catheter.[67] Other methods of bladder management include suprapubic tapping and the Valsalva maneuver. *Suprapubic tapping* involves tapping directly over the bladder with fingertips, causing a reflexive emptying of the bladder. This technique only works for individuals with an UMN bladder without dyssynergia between the detrusor and sphincter, because the sphincter must open for the bladder to reflexively drain.[66,67] Individuals with an areflexive bladder can use the *Valsalva maneuver,* which is done by straining.[66,67] Some individuals may elect to use an indwelling, suprapubic catheter.[68] Use of intermittent catheterization is associated with lower incidence of UTI.[69]

The exact method or combination of methods used for bladder management will depend on a variety of factors: type of bladder dysfunction, level of injury, functional ability, and personal preference. Whichever method(s) is used, the goal is for the patient to avoid development of UTIs and other bladder complications, be catheter free, have low postvoid residual volume of urine in the bladder, and be without high bladder pressure during voiding.[70] Urodynamic testing is done after spinal shock resolves, approximately 3 months after injury, to help diagnose the specific type of bladder dysfunction and guide the selection of management strategies.

Symptoms of UTI include AD, increased spasticity, incontinence, fever, abdominal discomfort, and general discomfort.[71] Urinary system complications linked to chronic UTIs are development of bladder and kidney stones and kidney dysfunction.

Bowel Dysfunction

As with bladder dysfunction, bowel dysfunction is a major concern after SCI. Over 98% of people with SCI report problems with bowel care, and 34% require some level of assistance with bowel care.[72] People with SCI report that bowel function has a greater impact on daily life than many other impairments after SCI, including sexual function, bladder function, pain, spasticity, and skin integrity.[72–74] Bowel function also has a large impact on social activities and quality of life (QOL).[73] Neurogenic bowel conditions that develop after spinal shock subsides are of two main types. In spinal cord lesions above S2 there is a *spastic* or *reflex bowel* (UMN lesion).

Because the parasympathetic and internal sphincter connections from S2 to S4 are intact, reflex defecation can occur when the rectum fills with stool. In S2–S4 or cauda equina (peripheral nerves) lesions, a *flaccid* or *areflexive bowel* (LMN lesion) develops. With an areflexive bowel, the parasympathetic connections from S2 to S4 are not intact, so the bowel will not reflexively empty. This can cause feces to become impacted, and because the external sphincter is flaccid, incontinence can occur.[66] Common symptoms associated with impaired bowel function include constipation, incontinence, abdominal pain, difficulty with bowel movement, and urgency.[75]

Bowel Management

Safety and an appropriate, well-timed bowel care routine are common goals for bowel management.[75] Safety includes continence in order to maintain intact and healthy skin, prevent damage to colorectal structures, and prevent AD due to bowel dysfunction.[70] In addition to type of neurogenic bowel (UMN or LMN), the bowel care program also depends on the presence of other health conditions that may affect gastrointestinal function, medications, dietary habits, fluid intake, and functional ability.[66] A typical bowel program involves establishing a daily (or every other day) pattern of eliciting a bowel movement. The exact time of day is chosen by the patient based on lifestyle needs and should be consistent at the same time of day. This is usually in the morning or late evening. People with a reflex bowel may require the use of suppositories and digital stimulation techniques to cause a reflex defecation. Digital stimulation involves manual stretch of the anal sphincter, either with a lubricated gloved finger or an orthotic digital stimulator. This stretch stimulates peristalsis of the colon and evacuation of the rectum (mediated by S2, S3, and S4).[66] Valsalva maneuver and abdominal massage may also be performed. Transanal irrigation is also an effective technique, which can reduce incontinence and UTIs and improve QOL.[75] Nonreflex bowel management relies on manual evacuation techniques and gentle Valsalva.[66] Other factors that can play a role in maintaining a consistent, safe bowel program include eating a diet with appropriate amount of fiber, fluid intake, physical activity, stool softeners, laxatives, and bulking agents. Because many people with SCI will require assistance with their bowel program, it is important to support the patient/carepartner relationship with this important task.

Sexual Dysfunction

Sexuality encompasses much more than just the physical ability to have sexual intercourse. It is an important part of an individual's makeup and sense of self-esteem. SCI affects not only the physiological ability to have intercourse but also the psychosocial aspect of sexuality as well. Degree of sexual ability is an important

component of QOL.[76] People with paraplegia report that improved sexual function is the primary factor that would improve their QOL. For people with tetraplegia, it is the second most important after regaining hand function.[74] Education so that the patient can fully understand the impact of SCI on sexual function and psychosocial support so the patient can become confident in their new sexuality are important parts of rehabilitation.

Male Response

Sexual response is directly related to level and completeness of injury. As with bowel and bladder function, sexual capabilities are broadly divided between UMN (damage to the cord above S2–S4) and LMN lesions. There are two types of erections: reflexogenic and psychogenic. *Reflexogenic erections* occur in response to external physical stimulation of the genitals or perineum.[77] An intact reflex arc is required (mediated through S2, S3, and S4). *Psychogenic erections* occur through cognitive activity such as erotic fantasy.[77] Individuals with complete SCI above T10 will usually have reflexogenic erection capability, while those with a complete lesion that interrupts the sacral reflexes will have psychogenic erection capability.[77]

Generally speaking, erectile capacity is greater in UMN lesions than in LMN lesions and greater in incomplete lesions than in complete lesions. Although almost 75% of men with SCI report the ability to obtain an erection, the majority of them report that their erection is not reliable and of short duration.[78] Phosphodiesterase type 5 inhibitors (PDE5i) such as sildenafil, vardenafil, tadalafil (longer duration), and avanafil as well as intracavernosal injections can be used to treat erectile dysfunction in men with SCI.[79]

Men with SCI also have impaired ability to ejaculate. There is a higher incidence of ability to ejaculate with LMN lesions than with UMN lesions and incomplete as compared with complete lesions.[66] Penile vibrostimulation can be used to assist with ejaculation.[77,79] Men with SCI have adequate numbers of spermatozoa but abnormally low sperm motility and viability, which also negatively impacts fertility. Approximately 50% of men with SCI report being able to have an orgasm.[78]

Female Response

Female sexual responses also follow a pattern related to location of lesion. In patients with UMN lesions, the reflex arc remains intact. Therefore, components of sexual arousal (vaginal lubrication, engorgement of the labia, and clitoral erection) will likely occur through reflexogenic stimulation, but psychogenic response will be lost. Conversely, with LMN lesions, psychogenic responses will most likely be preserved and reflex responses lost.[77] Woman with SCI report lower sexual activity, lower sexual desire, and reduced ability to achieve orgasm.[80]

Fertility is not affected as severely in women as men with SCI. The menstrual cycle typically is interrupted for a period of 3 to 24 months following injury. After this time, normal menses return, and the potential for conception remains unimpaired.[77,79] Women with SCI who want to bear children should be closely supervised during pregnancy. They are more likely to encounter complications during pregnancy and childbirth than woman without SCI. Problems include UTIs, anemia, and venous thrombosis. Labor and delivery must be monitored. Depending on the neurological level of injury, the woman may not feel labor. There is a risk of AD during labor.[81] See guidelines by Bertschy and colleagues[81] for an overview of pre-, intra-, and postpartum care for women with SCI.

A major consideration for the physical therapist regarding sexual dysfunction is that a patient will often direct questions to the individuals with whom they feel most comfortable. It is not uncommon for such a discussion to arise during a physical therapy session. These questions or issues should be addressed openly and honestly. In addition, the therapist must anticipate and be prepared for these situations by (1) obtaining accurate information about the patient's physiological state and anticipated sexual function and (2) having knowledge of referral options and support services available to the patient for appropriate examination and counseling.

Pain

Pain is a common occurrence following SCI in both the acute and chronic stages of recovery. Approximately 68% of individuals with SCI experience chronic pain.[82] Pain can limit the performance of activities of daily living (ADL), affect sleep, and contribute to a lower QOL.[83,84] Pain can be grossly divided into two broad categories: *nociceptive pain* and *neuropathic pain.* Nociceptive pain can be musculoskeletal or visceral in origin. Neuropathic pain can be central or peripheral. The prevalence of chronic neuropathic pain and chronic musculoskeletal pain is approximately 58% and 56%, respectively, in people with SCI.[82] See Chapter 25, Chronic Pain, for an in-depth discussion of different types of pain.

Nociceptive Pain

Because of paralysis or paresis of the LEs, people with SCI rely heavily on their UEs for a variety of functional tasks (wheelchair propulsion, transfers, bed mobility, and self-care). This overreliance on the UEs places them at a high risk for developing overuse injuries of the UEs.[82,85] Musculoskeletal pain in the UEs is a common type of nociceptive pain in people with SCI. Overuse musculoskeletal injuries may be due to a variety of factors: repetitive stress from propelling a wheelchair while in a biomechanically poor position, increased weight-bearing on the UEs in a biomechanically compromised position while transferring or using pressure relief techniques, excessive weight-bearing on the UEs while using assistive device(s) for ambulation, muscular imbalances in the shoulder girdle, poor seated posture in a wheelchair, decreased flexibility, and poor positioning in bed.[85] Older age and higher body mass index (BMI) can also contribute to shoulder pain.[86] Specific musculoskeletal injuries that may occur are biceps tendonitis, lateral epicondylitis, shoulder impingement, rotator cuff tears, carpal tunnel syndrome, and wrist tendonitis.[87]

Neuropathic Pain

Neuropathic pain is caused by injury to the central or peripheral nervous system. Neuropathic pain can occur below, at, or above the level of the spinal cord lesion and can be spontaneous or evoked. Spontaneous neuropathic pain can be continuous, which presents as burning, cold, or squeezing; or intermittent, which presents as shooting, stabbing, or electric. Evoked neuropathic pain can present as hyperalgesia (increased sensitivity to pain) or allodynia (pain in response to a normal nonpainful stimulation).[88]

Neuropathic pain is particularly challenging to treat, and no single intervention option has established efficacy.[89,90] Nonpharmacological options include transcutaneous electrical nerve stimulation, massage, acupuncture, and mental imagery.[91] Pharmacological interventions commonly used are anticonvulsants such as gabapentin (Neurontin), pregabalin (Lyrica), and valproic acid (Depakote, Valparin); the antidepressant amitriptyline (Elavil, Vanatrip); and analgesics such as tramadol (Rybix, Ultram).[88,89] Only partial relief from pain can be expected, and self-management and behavioral interventions should be employed as well.[88] Exercise and activity can also improve QOL in people with SCI with chronic pain.[92] Chapter 25, Chronic Pain, provides an in-depth discussion on interventions for pain management.

Secondary and Other Impairments

Individuals with SCI are at great risk for secondary impairments throughout their life because of prolonged immobilization during the initial recovery period after injury and the wide-ranging effects of the SCI on multiple body systems. Common secondary complications include pressure injuries, UTI, pulmonary infection, heterotopic ossification, deep vein thrombosis, and musculoskeletal injuries (contractures, osteoporosis, fracture, heterotopic ossification [HO]).[65,93,94]

Activity Limitations, Participation Restrictions, and Quality of Life

As discussed later in the section on outcomes and goals, the neurological level of injury and whether the injury is complete or incomplete play a major role in determining an individual's independence with functional mobility tasks and ADL. While SCI-related impairments play a role, it is the interplay and relationship between impairments, activities, and participation which ultimately influence QOL after SCI. Personal factors such as education levels, financial status, social/emotional support, and motivation contribute, as well as environmental factors such as home setup, equipment, and community access. For example, participating in physical activity after injury is associated with higher QOL,[95] while higher levels of pain and spasticity and impaired bladder and bowel function are associated with lower QOL.[96,97]

Physical therapists play a collaborative role in enhancing patient motivation and influencing strategies to access role models and peer support to improve activity and participation.[96] Education specific to coping strategies and problem-solving can impact participation levels in physical activities. Physical therapists should measure participation outcome measures using measures such as World Health Orgnization Quality of Life BREF (WHO QOL-BREF), Needs Assessment Checklist (NAC), Life Satisfaction 9 (LISAT-9), Craig Hospital Assessment and Reporting Technique (CHART).[96]

SCI has a large impact on ability to be employed. At 1 year post-SCI, 18% of people with SCI were employed. By 20 years postinjury, this increased to 32%.[1] Individuals who had a college degree prior to injury or were injured at a younger age are more likely to be employed after their injury.[98,99] Reported barriers to employment are transportation; health and physical limitations; lack of experience, education, or training; environmental barriers; discrimination; and loss of benefits.[99] Vocational rehabilitation services, peer support groups, skills training, and early delivery of these interventions have been shown to be favorable for employment outcomes.[100]

■ ACUTE MEDICAL MANAGEMENT
Emergency Care

Management of SCI begins at the location of the accident. Techniques used in stabilizing, moving, and managing the patient immediately following the trauma can influence prognosis and recovery of motor function. Rescue personnel must be adept at questioning and examining for signs of SCI before moving the individual. Signs of SCI after a traumatic event include paresthesias, lack of or impaired movement or sensation in the extremities, spinal pain, and altered cognitive status or level of alertness. When an SCI is suspected, efforts should be made to avoid both active and passive movements of the spine. If the injury caused a displaced fracture, further damage to the spinal cord can occur. Movement of the spine is minimized by strapping the patient to a spinal backboard or a full-body adjustable backboard, using a supporting cervical collar, immobilizing the head, and obtaining assistance from multiple personnel in moving the patient to safety.[101] These measures assist in maintaining the spine in a neutral,

anatomical position and may prevent further neurological damage.

On arrival at the emergency department, initial attention is focused on stabilizing the patient medically with a primary emphasis on ventilation and circulation. Cardiac, hemodynamic, and respiratory status are closely monitored.[101,102] Diagnosis of SCI is based on the physical examination, neurological assessment, and imaging.[102] A complete neurological examination is performed once the patient is stabilized. Imaging studies assist in determining the extent of damage and plans for medical management. Attention is directed toward preventing progression of neurological impairment by restoration of vertebral alignment and early immobilization of the fracture site. A urinary catheter typically is inserted, and secondary injuries are addressed.

High doses of methylprednisolone had previously been used early after injury with the intention of reducing edema and improving motor recovery.[103–106] More recent studies find that the use of steroids early after injury does not lead to improved motor or functional outcomes.[107,108] Also, there may be serious complications associated with taking high doses of steroids over a prolonged time.[109,110] Current guidelines do not advocate for routine use of steroids.[107,108,111,112] Local and systemic hypothermia have also been studied as an intervention to reduce secondary damage and provide neuroprotection to the spinal cord early after injury and improve outcomes.[113,114] The evidence suggests that local and systemic hypothermia is safe; however, further research is needed to establish the effectiveness and optimal dosage.[115] Researchers continue to conduct clinical trials to identify therapeutic interventions to limit damage to the spinal cord and improve tissue healing with methods of neuroprotection, regeneration, and cell transplantation.[116]

Fracture Stabilization

The goal of fracture/spinal injury site management is to stabilize the spinal column to prevent further damage to the cord. Reduction and immobilization of spinal injuries can be achieved via conservative or operative methods. Indications for surgical stabilization are unstable fracture site, gross malalignment, cord compression, and deteriorating neurological status. In people with acute, traumatic SCI, early (within 8 hours) surgical decompression and stabilization are recommended.[117] Approximately 60% of patients with SCI admitted to model SCI system centers underwent surgical stabilization.[118] Closed reduction is indicated for patients with cervical subluxation or fracture dislocation injuries. It is achieved with the use of traction devices typically followed by use of spinal orthotics to maintain alignment through immobilization. Patients with thoracic or lumbar injuries that are managed conservatively without surgery require immobilization by positioning in a regular or rotating bed and use of spinal orthotics.

Immobilization

Following reduction of the fracture site, through either conservative or surgical means, the spine is immobilized for a period of time through the use of spinal orthoses and recumbent positioning.

Cervical Orthoses

Halos are used commonly to immobilize cervical fractures after both open and closed reduction. This spinal orthosis (Fig. 20.5) consists of a halo ring with four titanium alloy skull pins that attach directly to the outer skull. The halo is attached to a body jacket or vest by four vertical steel posts. A halo is extremely effective at limiting cervical motion in all planes. The most common complication of a halo orthosis is loosening of the pin site. This can create instability at the injury site in the vertebral column and/or be a sign of infection. Skin breakdown may also occur under the vest portion of the halo.

Although a halo is an effective means of immobilizing and protecting the injury site, it can make learning mobility skills challenging. The orthosis limits shoulder motion and changes the user's center of gravity. This may cause patients to feel unstable. It can also make bed and wheelchair positioning difficult and walking and stair negotiation challenging.

The *Minerva* is another type of cervical orthosis (CO) that also effectively limits motion in all planes. Like the halo, because it provides excellent cervical stability, the Minerva allows for early mobility and rehabilitation after SCI. The sterno–occipital–mandibular immobilizer (SOMI) is another type of CO. It is less effective in limiting cervical range of motion (ROM) than either the halo or Minerva. There are also a variety of cervical collars that can be used. Generally, these are constructed of semirigid foam and plastic and consist of two halves, which are held together with hook-and-loop closures. They do not effectively immobilize the spine.

However, they may be used as transitional support following removal of a more rigid device (e.g., halo). Common types of collars include Philadelphia collar, Miami J collar, Aspen collar, and foam soft collar.

Thoracolumbosacral Orthoses

A thoracolumbosacral orthosis (TLSO; Fig. 20.6) is commonly used to immobilize the spine in patients

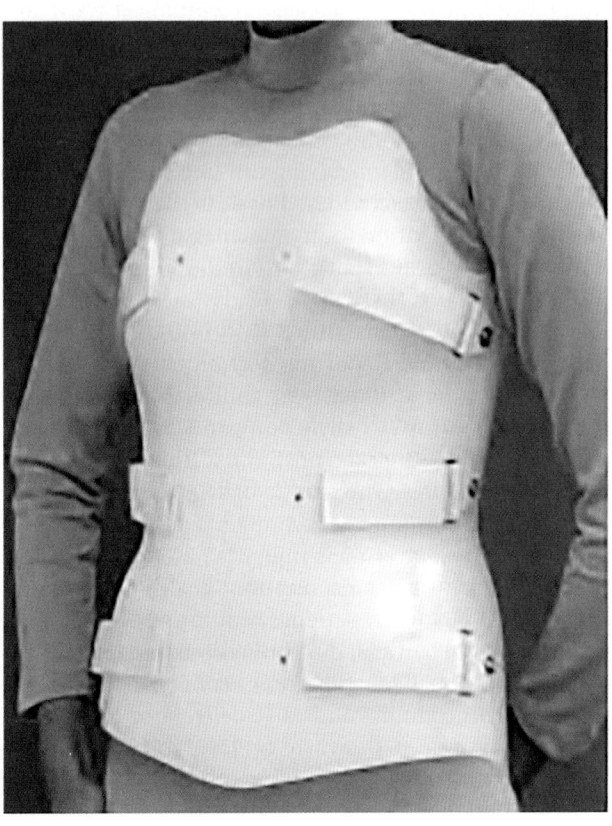

Figure 20.6 Thoracolumbosacral orthosis. *(Courtesy of Spinal Technology, Inc., West Yarmouth, MA 02673)*

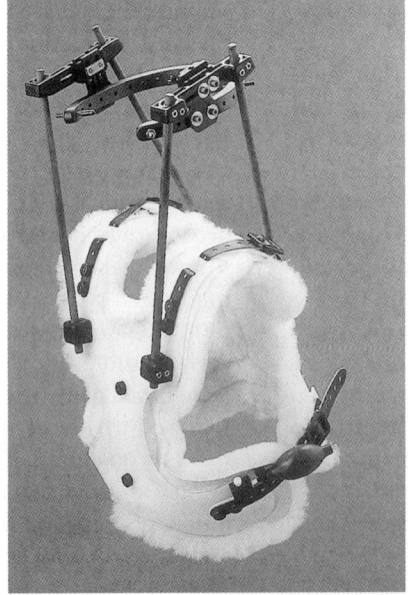

Figure 20.5 Halo orthosis.
(Courtesy of PMT Corp.)

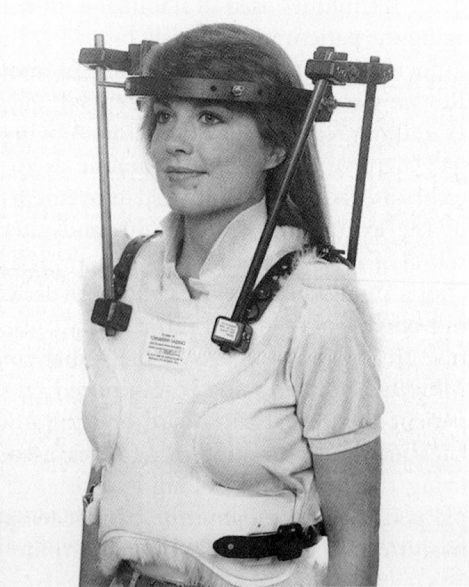

with thoracic or lumbar injuries. A TLSO is made by an orthotist who takes a cast of the patient's trunk and makes the molded body jacket from the impression. Body jackets are typically bivalved and connected by hook-and-loop closures, which allows for removal during bathing and skin inspection. An extension is necessary with high thoracic injuries and low lumbar injuries in order to provide effective immobilization of the spine in these areas. See Chapter 30, Orthotics, for a more in-depth discussion of spinal orthotics and physical therapy considerations for mobilizing patients with orthotics, including safely donning/doffing, if appropriate.

■ PHYSICAL REHABILITATION

The overarching goal of rehabilitation is to support the patient to become as independent as possible and to achieve the functional mobility necessary for everyday life, work, and recreation. Goals should be developed in collaboration with the patient to optimize function and health and meet the desires of the patient. Independent mobility can be achieved in a way that (1) either uses new movement strategies to compensate for neuromuscular impairments or (2) uses the neuromuscular system to accomplish the task with a movement pattern similar to that before the injury.[119,120] *Compensation* refers to use of an alternative or new movement strategy, or technology to compensate for neuromuscular deficits to accomplish a daily task.[121] *Recovery of function* refers to the restoration of the neuromuscular system so that the motor task is performed in a similar manner as it was before the SCI.[120,121]

For instance, if a patient cannot actively flex the fingers to grasp a bottle owing to weakness or paralysis of finger flexor muscles, use of wrist "tenodesis" is often taught as a compensatory strategy (Fig. 20.7). Active wrist extension simultaneously produces passive finger flexion and can be used to achieve a functional grasp. Knee-ankle-foot orthoses (KAFOs) may help a

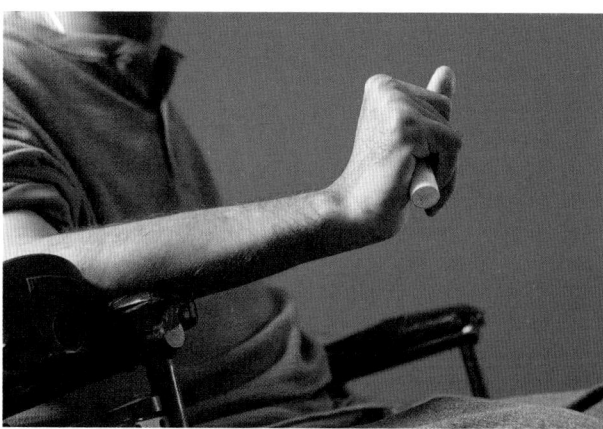

Figure 20.7 Tenodesis grasp. Patient extends the wrist, which causes the shortened long finger flexors to passively flex allowing a grasp.

patient achieve the goal of standing but do not have a therapeutic effect on retraining the neuromuscular system in the once familiar task of standing. Once the KAFOs are removed, the LEs cannot perform the task of standing. The braces compensate for the inability to activate antigravity LE muscles due to weakness or paralysis. The task of moving from sitting to standing with KAFOs entails the use of assistive devices and weight-bearing through the arms, further altering the preinjury movement pattern to accomplish the task. Transfers from a wheelchair to a bed that also incorporate weight-bearing through the arms and a *head–hips* movement strategy (the head moves in one direction to move the hips in the opposite direction; see below) is another example of a compensatory behavior using a biomechanical advantage to achieve a functional mobility task in a new way. Focusing on recovery of the once familiar task of sit-to-stand would require a movement pattern including weight shift from the buttocks forward over the feet, a powerful activation of antigravity muscles to lift the body off of the chair, the head moving up and forward, and then full extension of the limbs and trunk to achieve standing without the arms weight-bearing.

How a functional mobility task is achieved (or expected to be achieved) is thus important in treatment planning and goal setting. Historically, rehabilitation for persons after SCI has employed compensation strategies using muscles spared above the level of the lesion, substitution, novel movement patterns, and assistive devices/braces as the primary means for achieving independent functional mobility skills. Recent advances in our understanding of the neurobiological control of walking and in activity-dependent plasticity have provided the basis for new, alternative therapies that generate activity below the level of the lesion with the goal of recovery.[120] Our assumption that the spinal cord was simply a conduit for neural signals from the brain was incorrect. In fact, the spinal cord is quite responsive to the ensemble of sensorimotor information provided during task execution to generate a motor output. Activity elicited through such therapies (e.g., locomotor training, task-specific practice) is used to retrain the neuromuscular control required for function, then used in everyday activities, and finally integrated into daily use.[122–124]

Although both compensation and recovery-based approaches (activity-based therapies) are used in rehabilitation for SCI, compensation dominates current clinical practice. However, a large and expanding body of literature is providing new insights about integration of activity-based therapies into the POC,[125,126] their potential for improving outcomes with combinatorial approaches,[125,127,128] and the impact of these therapies on functional outcomes to advance recovery and QOL.

If independence cannot be achieved, whether using compensation or recovery-based strategies, then the patient may be interdependent on others for assistance in accomplishing certain tasks of daily life (e.g., the patient with a complete high cervical lesion). The patient, family, friends, and carepartners receive thorough instructions and training in the knowledge and skills required to address the individual's daily needs. For example, patients with a C4 complete SCI will need to learn how to self-direct aspects of their care that they cannot perform themselves, such as dressing, bed positioning, transfers using a lift, etc.

Physical Therapy Examination

The examination is the first step in the patient/client management process and includes identifying body structure/function impairments, activity limitations, participation restrictions, and personal and environmental factors and resources in order to develop an appropriate POC. The examination consists of history, systems review, and tests and measures.

History

The history should be gathered from the patient, family members, and medical record. It is important to take a patient-centered approach in order to understand the primary concerns of the patient and their goals for physical therapy. Key information to gather includes the patient's goals and concerns, level of knowledge the patient has regarding the injury, emotional state of the patient, preexisting health conditions that may impact the prognosis and POC, amount of social support from family members or others, current living or planned discharge arrangement (lives alone or with family), accessibility of the home environment for a wheelchair, preinjury employment and work environment, and hobbies. The following information should be obtained from the medical record: date and extent of injury, lesion level, AIS impairment scale designation, complications that may have developed, concomitant injuries, and rehabilitation services received previously. It is vital to find out any precautions or contraindications and what is the patient's understanding of these. For example, a patient with a thoracic complete SCI may have to wear a TLSO to protect the spine as it heals after the injury and surgery to stabilize the fracture site, or the injury may have occurred during a motor vehicle crash, and the patient also fractured their femur and there are weight-bearing restrictions.

Examination

There are a variety of standardized outcome measures and tests available to the physical therapist (Table 20.3). Using a modified Delphi process, the SCI Special Interest Group of the Academy of Neurologic Physical Therapy developed recommendations for use of outcome measures in clinical practice, research, and entry-level physical therapy education. These recommendations and psychometric properties of the recommended

outcome measures are available online (http://www.neuropt.org/professional-resources/neurology-section-outcome-measures-recommendations/spinal-cord-injury). The Rehabilitation Measures Database at the Shirley Ryan Ability Lab (https://www.sralab.org/rehabilitation-measures) and the SCI Research Evidence (https://scireproject.com) websites are also useful resources for information on outcome measures.

Which specific outcome measure to use or which areas to examine will depend on a variety of factors including the patient's presentation, acuity of injury, precautions/contraindications, level of injury, AIS classification, and patient goals. For example, early after injury the patient may not be stable enough to get out of bed so the exam may focus on muscle strength, sensation, respiratory status, integument, and ROM. However, later in the recovery process a more in-depth examination should be performed that examines mobility skills such as bed mobility, transfers, and wheelchair propulsion. Some of the more frequently used and recommended tests and measures are discussed here.

Body Structure/Function

MOTOR FUNCTION/MUSCLE PERFORMANCE/SENSORY INTEGRITY

Motor and sensory function should be assessed using the ISNCSCI described earlier to determine the level of neurological injury (see Fig. 20.3).[129] Care should be taken when performing MMT, particularly if the spine is not yet stabilized or fully healed after surgery. Forceful contraction of muscles that originate from the spine may cause instability at the fracture site. Discretion should be used in applying resistance around the shoulders in tetraplegia and around the lower trunk and hips in paraplegia. However, if the surgeon has indicated that the fracture site is stable after surgery, then these precautions are not likely needed.

In addition to testing the strength of the AIS key muscles, MMT should be performed for all muscle groups that are innervated based on findings from the ASIA ISNCSCI. For example, if the biceps are intact, then other muscles innervated by C5 such as the deltoids and rotator cuff muscles should also be tested. Although not included as key muscles in the ISNCSCI, examination of other functionally important muscles such as deltoids, scapular musculature, pronators/supinators, gluteals, and hamstrings will assist in establishing goals and expected outcomes. Handheld dynamometry can also be used to examine muscle strength, including trunk strength.[130]

There are several unique considerations when performing MMT for people with SCI. Patients often learn to functionally move joints by substituting intact muscle contraction for weak or paralyzed muscles. For example, supination of the forearm allows gravity to extend the wrist, and lower abdominal muscles can substitute for hip flexion by causing the pelvis to tilt posteriorly.

Table 20.3 Outcome Measures

Outcome Measure and ICF Category	Description	Scoring	MDC and MCID
International Standards for Neurological Classification of Spinal Injury, AIS ICF: 1	Test of capacity: assesses and classifies the current level of motor and sensory deficits.	Ability to sense and differentiate sharp and dull sensation as well as ability to resist the examiner at varying muscles. Classified between AIS A (complete) to AIS E (no) deficits.	MDC: 3.87 (total sensory), 1.87 (total motor) (all AIS classifications) MCID: 5.19 (total sensory), 4.48 (total motor) (all AIS classifications)
Handheld Dynamometry ICF: 1	Test of capacity: assesses muscular strength during grip task.	Force production (kg, N, or lb) during maximal isometric contraction for 3– seconds ("make") or examiner applies force to overcome patient ("break").	MDC: 5.1–8.2 lb (biceps), 6.0–6.7 lb (triceps), 0.7–4.8 lb (wrist extensors) (estimated based on data from Aufsesser et al.) MCID: NA
WUSPI ICF: 1	Self-reported measure: assesses shoulder pain in wheelchair users during functional activities and tasks that include transfers, wheelchair mobility, self-care, and general activities.	15 items across the four domains each have a 10-cm VAS that is anchored from "no pain" at 0 cm to "worst pain ever experienced" at 10 cm.	MDC: NA MCID: NA
6MWT ICF: 2	Test of capacity: assesses functional walking endurance.	Distance walked in 6 minutes when walking as fast as possible.	MDC: 45.8 m (150 ft) (incomplete SCI) (estimated based on data from van Hedel et al.) MCID: NA
10MWT ICF: 2	Test of capacity: assesses walking speed over a short distance.	Time to walk middle 6 meters of a 10-meter walk to allow for a 2-meter acceleration and deceleration phase.	MDC: 0.13 m/sec (incomplete SCI) MCID: 0.15
BBS ICF: 2	Test of capacity: assesses both static and dynamic balance during 14 functional tasks.	14 items scored on a five-point ordinal scale of 0–4 where 0 = unable to perform/needs assistance to 4 = able to perform safely and independently.	MDC: NA MCID: NA
WISCI ICF: 2	Test of capacity: assesses the need for physical assistance and/or assistive devices for ambulation.	Amount of assistance needed over 10-meter walk ranked on 20-point ordinal scale where 0 = unable to stand or participate to 20 = ambulates with no assistance.	MDC: 0.78 (self-selected level), 0.16 (maximum level) (estimated based on data from Burns et al.) (both paraplegia and tetraplegia) MCID: NA
CUEI ICF: 2	Self-reported measure: assesses impact of tetraplegia on UE motor function.	32 items scored on a seven-point ordinal scale of 1 to 7 where 1 = totally limited and cannot do at all to 7 = not at all limited.	MDC: 33.8 (estimated based on data from Marino et al.) (tetraplegia, mostly AIS A) MCID: NA

(Continued)

Table 20.3 Outcome Measures—cont'd

Outcome Measure and ICF Category	Description	Scoring	MDC and MCID
SCIM ICF: 2	Observation-based test of capacity with interview component: assesses ability to self-care, bladder/bowel management and general mobility.	19 items are scored over three domains that together in total range from 0–100 with greater scores indicating increased independence.	MDC: NA MCID: for total score: range of 26–62 depending on level of injury and complete versus incomplete injury; for mobility subscore range of 10–17 depending on level of injury and complete versus incomplete injury.[174]
GRASSP ICF: 2	Test of capacity: assesses hand (L/R) function, neurological recovery, and sensation in those with tetraplegia from cervical SCIs.	Five total subtests over three domains that measure sensory function (six locations) from 0–4, strength (10 locations) from 0–5, prehension (three grasps) from 0–4, and prehension performance (six tasks) from 0–5.	MDC: 5.1 (R), 5.3 (L) (strength), 1.8 (R), 1.7 (L) (prehension ability), 7.0 (R), 4.9 (L) (prehension performance) (estimated based on data from Kalsi-Ryan et al.)[169] (tetraplegia) MCID: NA
Wheelchair Skills Test ICF: 2	Test of capacity: assesses ability to navigate and utilize wheelchair for necessary tasks and activities.	32 items of increasing difficulty from indoor, outdoor, and community environment scored as "pass, safe" to "fail, unsafe" or "no part" for indicated skills.	MDC: NA MCID: NA
World Health Organization QOL-BREF ICF: 3	Self-reported measure: assesses impact of injury on domains in physical health, psychological health, social relationships, and one's environment in the past 4 weeks.	25 items across four domains scored on a 5-point Likert scale from 1–5 with scores indicating various meanings. Greater scores in total indicate greater QOL.	MDC: 6.6–21.5 (estimated based on data from Lin et al.)[189] MCID: NA
LISAT-9 ICF: 3	Self-reported measure: assesses self-care ability and relationships.	Nine domains; scores a single item for life satisfaction and eight additional items for each domain using a 6-point Likert scale with 1 = very dissatisfied to 6 = very satisfied.	MDC: 0.14–0.19 (estimated based on data from Geyh et al.)[185] MCID: NA
CHART ICF: 3	Self-reported measure: assesses degree of handicap within physical, social, and cognitive aspects in the community.	Six domains with 32 total items with each subscale ranging from 0–100 for a total score of 0–600, with greater scores indicating lesser handicap.	MDC: 53.3 (total score)[183] MCID: NA

ICF CATEGORY: 1 = Body Structure/Function; 2 = Activity; 3 = Participation.
AIS = American Spinal Injury Association Impairment Scale; BBS = Berg Balance Scale; CHART = Craig Handicap Assessment and Reporting Technique; CUEI = Capabilities of UE functioning Instrument; GRASSP = Graded and Redefined Assessment of Sensibility Strength and Prehension; ICF = International Classification of Functioning, Disability, and Health; LISAT-9 = Life Satisfaction Questionnaire; MCID = minimal clinically important difference; MDC = minimal detectable change; NA = not available; QOL = quality of life; 6MWT = 6-minute Walk Test; SCI = spinal cord injury; SCIM = Spinal Cord Independence Measure; 10MWT = 10-meter Walk Test; UE = upper extremity; US = upper extremity; VAS = visual analog scale; WISCI = Walking Index for Spinal Cord Injury; WUSPI = Wheelchair Users Shoulder Pain Index.

The physical therapist should carefully stabilize proximal areas to reduce substitution and palpate to ensure that the test muscle is contracting. Abnormal muscle tone and spasms can cause involuntary muscle contractions or a weak muscle to appear stronger. Orthoses and spinal precautions may preclude the patient from assuming a recommended test position or forcefully contract certain muscles. The use of alternate (nonstandard) test positions should be documented. See Chapter 3, Examination of Sensory Function, for details on a full sensory exam.

The presence of spastic hypertonia should be assessed as part of the motor function examination. The *Modified Ashworth Scale (MAS)* is commonly used to assess tone. The MAS is a six-point ordinal scale that rates the amount of resistance to passive movement of the joint and is valid and reliable for use in people with SCI.[131,132] (See Chapter 5, Examination of Motor Function: Motor Control and Motor Learning, for a description of the MAS.) The *Penn Spasm Frequency Scale* is a valid and reliable two-part self-report measure that assesses the frequency and severity of spasms.[132,133]

RESPIRATORY

The physical therapist should assess the strength of the diaphragm and intercostal muscles through observation while the patient is breathing. Normally, the epigastric region should rise and the chest wall expands during inhalation while in supine. Contractions of the sternocleidomastoids and scalenes or paradoxical breathing patterns indicate weakness or lack of innervation of the diaphragm or intercostal muscles. Respiratory rate should be assessed while the patient is unaware that it is being done. Normal respiratory rate is between 12 and 20 breathes per minute. To compensate for a weak diaphragm, the respiratory rate will typically increase.

Maximal chest excursion can be assessed using a tape measure with the patient supine. At both the level of the axilla and xiphoid process, the physical therapist should measure the chest's diameter at maximal exhalation and inhalation. Chest expansion measurements are the difference between chest measurements at maximal exhalation and at maximal inhalation. Normal chest expansion ranges from 2.5 to 3 in (6.35 to 7.62 cm), and negative values are an indication of paradoxical chest motions.

Vital capacity (VC) should be measured during the early stages of recovery. VC can be measured with a handheld spirometer and is strongly related to other measures of pulmonary function.[134] Forced vital capacity and volume of pulmonary secretion and gas exchange are predictive of airway management.[135] Typically, VC is approximately less than 25% of normal in individuals with high cervical lesions (above C3), 25% to 50% in midcervical lesions, 50% to 75% in lower cervical and upper thoracic lesions, and 70% to 80% in mid- to lower thoracic lesions.[64,136,137]

Owing to lack of full abdominal musculature innervation in many people with SCI, respiratory capability changes when the patient is sitting compared to supine. In sitting, the lack of abdominal muscle innervation causes abdominal contents to fall forward and pull down on the central tendon. This changes the motion of the diaphragm when it contracts during inspiration resulting in an inefficient breathing pattern.

The lack of full abdominal muscle function also impairs the ability to cough and clear the airway. The ability to effectively cough is vital for the removal of secretions. The abdominal muscles are the major contributors to generating enough force to expel secretions or foreign objects. Cough function can be categorized into three types: functional cough, weak functional cough, and nonfunctional cough.[138] A *functional cough* is loud and forceful, and the patient is able to generate two or more coughs with one exhalation. In this case, the patient is able to clear all respiratory secretions. A *weak functional cough* is soft, and the patient is only able to generate one per exhalation. The patient can clear small amounts of secretions and clear the throat. A *nonfunctional cough* is not a true cough; it is a clearing of the throat and has no expulsive force. In this case, assistance is needed to clear secretions from the airway.

INTEGUMENT

During the acute phase, meticulous and regular skin inspection is a shared responsibility of the patient and the entire medical/rehabilitative team. As management progresses into the active rehabilitation phase and throughout the patient's life, the patient will gradually assume greater responsibility for this activity. Patient education related to skin care is crucial and should be initiated early. The patient may view frequent position changes and skin inspection as bothersome or distracting from sleep if there is not adequate awareness of the importance and purpose of these activities.

Assessment for pressure injuries should combine both direct skin inspection, which combines both visual observation and palpation, with assessment of risk factors. The patient's entire body should be observed regularly with particular attention to areas most susceptible to pressure (Table 20.4). Palpation is useful for identifying skin temperature changes that may be indicative of a hyperemic reaction. This is particularly important in examining individuals with dark pigmented skin because early skin responses to pressure may not be readily apparent. Skin reactions to excess pressure include redness, local warmth, local edema, and small open or cracked skin areas. If the patient is wearing a halo, vest, or other orthotic device, contact points between the body and the orthosis must also be inspected.

In addition to skin inspection, factors that increase the risk for pressure injuries should be considered. Spasticity, bladder or bowel incontinence, and nutritional deficiencies can increase the risk of developing pressure

Table 20.4	Areas Most Susceptible to Pressure in Recumbent Positions	
Supine	**Prone**	**Side-Lying**
• Occiput	• Ears (head rotated)	• Ears
• Scapulae	• Shoulders (anterior aspect)	• Shoulders (lateral aspect)
• Vertebrae	• Iliac crest	• Greater trochanter
• Elbows	• Male genital region	• Head of fibula
• Sacrum	• Patella	• Knees (medial aspect from contact between knees)
• Coccyx	• Dorsum of feet	• Lateral malleolus
• Heels		• Medial malleolus (contact between malleoli)

injuries. A number of specific scales can be used to assess the risk of developing a pressure injury in people with SCI.[139] The Braden Scale is commonly used for a variety of patient groups who are at risk for developing pressure injuries, including people with SCI.[139] The Braden Scale is more sensitive (75%) than specific (57%) and is easy to administer and has adequate validity.[139] The SCI Pressure Ulcer Scale (SCIPUS) and SCIPUS-Acute were designed specifically for people with SCI in acute care and in active rehabilitation.[139] The SCIPUS is more specific (84%) than sensitive (37%), whereas the SCIPUS-Acute is more sensitive (88%) than specific (59%).[139] Both of these scales have adequate validity and are easy to administer.

If a patient develops a pressure injury, there are a variety of tools that can be used to examine and document the extent of the wound. The location, shape, size, and stage of the wound should be documented. A photograph of the wound on a grid is also an effective method of documenting the wound. Chapter 14, Vascular, Lymphatic, and Integumentary Disorders, provides more detailed information on wound examination.

RANGE OF MOTION

Goniometry can be used to assess joint ROM. Shoulder ROM is particularly important for patients with tetraplegia. Depending on the motor level of injury, people with tetraplegia may require more than normal ROM to perform certain mobility skills,[138] and decreased shoulder ROM is associated with shoulder pain.[140] Hamstring length, hip extension, and ankle dorsiflexion are important to measure as well, owing to the potential for contractures in these joints and the need for ROM in these joints for mobility skills.

AEROBIC CAPACITY/ENDURANCE

The *6-minute Arm Test (6MAT)* can be used to assess aerobic capacity and cardiovascular endurance.[141] The 6MAT requires the patient to perform 6 minutes of submaximal cycling on an arm ergometer at a single, steady-state power output. It is a valid and reliable measure for people with either tetraplegia or paraplegia. Steady-state power output for clients with tetraplegia should be set between 10 and 30 W based on use of a manual versus power wheelchair and activity level. For clients with paraplegia, the power output should be set between 30 and 60 W depending on gender, AIS motor score, and activity level. Heart rate is continuously recorded, and the final steady-state heart rate averaged over the last 30 seconds. Ratings of perceived exertion should also be documented.[141]

MENTAL FUNCTION

Because the majority of injuries are traumatic in nature, it is particularly important to screen patients for cognitive impairment.[142] Up to 60% of people who experience a traumatic SCI may also have a concomitant traumatic brain injury (TBI).[143] Motor vehicle crashes and falls are common causes of SCI that may also result in a TBI. In some cases, the impact of the TBI be subtle and not easily recognized. A concomitant TBI, whether mild or severe, can have a profound impact on recovery and the rehabilitation POC. Although they have not been validated in people with SCI, the *Mini-Mental State Examination* and the *Montreal Cognitive Assessment* are useful tools to screen for cognitive impairment.[144,145] If it is suspected that a patient has a TBI, a referral should be made to a neuropsychologist or psychiatrist.

Approximately 25% to 30% of people with SCI experience depression and anxiety,[146,147] and as such, it is important to screen patients for these and other mental health conditions. The Depression Anxiety Stress Scales[148] is a valid tool to screen for depression, stress, and anxiety in people with SCI.[149] It has 21 items and takes approximately 10 minutes to complete. Higher scores indicate greater distress. The Patient Health Questionnaire 9 (PHQ-9) is another valid screening tool that can be used to screen for depression in people with SCI.[150] A score of 10 or greater is an indication that the patient has moderate depression, although this cutoff score was determined from the general population, not people with SCI.[151]

PAIN

Pain should be examined continually. A *numeric pain rating scale* can be used to identify the intensity of pain. The patient rates pain on a scale from 0 to 10, where 0 is no pain and 10 is severe, disabling pain. There are also self-report measures of pain designed specifically for people with SCI. The *Wheelchair User's Shoulder Pain Index* measures the impact of shoulder pain on transfers, self-care, wheelchair mobility, and general activities.[152,153] Wheelchair users rate the amount of pain experienced while performing various activities on a scale from 0 to 10. Total score ranges from 0 to 150, with higher scores indicating a greater impact of pain. The *Classification System for Chronic Pain in SCI* can be used to classify type of pain (musculoskeletal or neuropathic) by location (below, at, or above the lesion level) and the effects of activity, position, and light touch.[154]

REFLEX INTEGRITY

Deep tendon reflexes, graded on a 0 to 4+ scale, with 2+ being normal, should be tested. Reflex testing assists in determining the resolution of spinal shock and distinguishing between UMN and LMN injuries. See Chapter 5, Examination of Motor Function: Motor Control and Motor Learning.

Activity/Participation
FUNCTIONAL BALANCE

Surprisingly, there are a limited number of clinical tests that measure functional sitting balance that have been validated in people with SCI.[155,156] The modified Functional Reach Test[156,157] has adequate reliability, validity, clinical utility, and responsiveness for patients with complete SCI. For patients with iSCI and the capability to stand and walk, functional balance can be assessed using the Berg Balance Scale (BBS). The BBS demonstrates adequate reliability, validity, clinical utility, and responsiveness in patients with iSCI.[156] The Mini-Balance Evaluation Systems Test (mini-BESTest) shows promise due to its ability to comprehensively assess balance; however, further research is needed in people with iSCI. See Chapter 6, Examination of Coordination and Balance, for more detailed information on these and other measures of balance.

LOCOMOTION

Wheelchair Propulsion. Most individuals with SCI will rely on a wheelchair as their primary means of mobility in the home and community. As such, it is important to examine the patient's ability to perform wheelchair skills. This includes setting and releasing the wheel locks, removing footrests and armrests, propelling the wheelchair on level surfaces, performing wheelies, ascending and descending curbs, and various other wheelchair skills necessary for independent mobility in the community. The *Wheelchair Skills Test* examines a wheelchair user's skills in performing 32 representative wheelchair skills (29 for power wheelchair use).[158–160] The skills are categorized according to three levels that reflect difficulty and setting in which they will be performed: indoor, community, and advanced. There are separate tests for manual and power wheelchair users.

The Wheelchair Skills Test can be used as a diagnostic tool to determine which wheelchair skills need to be addressed in therapy and to document improvement during rehabilitation.

Gait/Walking Ability. Gait and walking ability should also be examined in patients who maintain some ability to stand and walk. An observational gait analysis tool such as the *Rancho Los Amigos Observational Gait Analysis*[161] can be used to identify gait deviations. See Chapter 7, Examination of Gait, for a description of this instrument. Identifying abnormal gait patterns will inform selection of additional tests and measures needed to determine the underlying impairments that may be causing the abnormal movements as well as guide development of the POC.

The *Walking Index for Spinal Cord Injury (WISCI)* examines level of physical assistance, type of assistive device, and amount of bracing required to ambulate 10 meters.[162,163] Scores range from 0 (unable to stand or walk with assistance) to 20 (ambulates with no assistance, no braces, and no assistive device). The *Spinal Cord Injury Functional Ambulation Inventory (SCI-FAI)* is another outcome measure used to assess walking ability in people with iSCI.[164] It involves a 2-minute observational gait analysis performed using the patient's usual assistive device. Documentation includes the frequency and distances the patient typically walks in the home and community.

The *10-meter Walk Test*[165] and *6-minute Walk Test (6MWT)*[165] are reliable, valid, and responsive to change in people with iSCI. A change of 0.13 m/sec in gait speed is an indication that significant clinical change has occurred.[165] Gait speed can also be used as a predictor of functional walking ability. People with iSCI who walk at 0.09 m/sec are likely to be supervised ambulators. Walking speed of 0.15 m/sec is an indication that the person can likely walk indoors but use a wheelchair outside the home. Walking speed of 0.44 m/sec is an indication that the person will likely use an assistive device or orthosis to walk in and outside the home. Finally, a walking speed of 0.70 m/sec indicates the person can walk in and outside the home without an assistive device or orthotic.[166] The minimal detectable change of the 6MWT is 46 meters.[165] See Chapter 7, Examination of Gait, for more detail on measures of functional walking capacity.

UPPER EXTREMITY FUNCTION

The *Capabilities of Upper Extremity Instrument (CUEI)* is a self-report measure that assesses the ability to unilaterally and bilaterally grasp, release, and lift as well as assesses wrist and finger actions.[167] Each item is scored on a seven-point ordinal scale where 1 is totally limited, cannot do at all and 7 is not at all limited. Total scores range from 32 to 224, where higher scores indicate better UE function. The CUEI is reliable, valid, and responsive.[167,168] The minimal detectable change

(MDC) is estimated to be 34 points.[167] The *Graded and Redefined Assessment of Sensibility, Strength, and Prehension* (GRASSP) is a performance-based measure that assesses hand function, neurological recovery, and sensation in people with tetraplegia.[169]

SELF-CARE AND DOMESTIC LIFE

Among the main goals of rehabilitation is to promote independence in functional mobility skills and self-care. In addition to wheelchair propulsion skills and gait (if appropriate), it is important to carefully examine the patient's ability to perform other mobility skills such as transfers and bed mobility and also pressure relief. The amount of physical assistance, method of performing the task, verbal cues required, use of adaptive/assistive devices, characteristics of environment, and degree of safety should all be carefully documented. To be truly independent, the patient must be able to complete the task safely, without assistance, in a timely manner, without undue effort, in an open environment, in different environments, and consistently. It may be tempting to provide a small amount of assistance such as stabilizing the wheelchair while the patient transfers (to prevent sliding) and still document that the patient was independent with the bed-to-wheelchair transfer. However, in this case the patient was not truly independent with the task. The patient must be able to complete the task without assistance the physical therapist presents. The physical therapist must actually observe the patient performing the task because patients may overestimate their own ability (e.g., self-report).

The *Functional Independence Measure (FIM)*[170] scores task completion based on the amount of assistance required based on the percentage of active patient participation. The amount of assistance is scored on a seven-point ordinal scale that ranges from 1 = total assistance (patient performs less than 25% of the effort) to 7 = independent. The FIM assesses burden of care across 18 basic ADL; 13 motor tasks such as dressing, bathing, and transfers; and five cognitive tasks such as comprehension, problem-solving, and memory. In 2018, the Centers for Medicare and Medicaid Services (CMS) implemented the collection of GG codes in place of the FIM.[171] These codes are the self-care and mobility items from the Continuity Assessment Record and Evaluation (CARE) item set.[172] Each item is scored on a six-point scale from 01 (dependent) to 06 (independent). There are differences between the rating scale of the FIM and GG codes in how the amount of assistance is defined. For example, on the GG code scale there is no score for minimal assistance. The scoring is either partial/moderate or supervision or touching assistance. Additional information on the FIM and GG codes is provided in Chapter 8, Examination of Function.

Several SCI-specific outcome measures are available to examine self-care and domestic life. The *Spinal Cord Injury Independence Measure (SCIM)* was specifically created to assess function in people with SCI. It includes 19 items divided into three subcategories: self-care, respiration and sphincter management, and mobility. Total scores range from 0 to 100, where higher scores indicate greater independence. The SCIM is valid and reliable, with a minimal clinically important difference (MCID) between 10 and 17 on the mobility section depending on the level and completeness of the injury.[173,174]

The *Neuromuscular Recovery Scale (NRS)* is an outcome measure used to examine the ability to perform a functional movement in the manner used by the intact neuromuscular system before injury and without compensation.[175-178] In comparison, the FIM examines performance of functional tasks based on level of assistance required (i.e., burden of care). The FIM allows compensation as a movement strategy and addresses whether a goal is achieved but not how it is accomplished. The NRS uniquely examines how a goal is attempted (or achieved) and does not allow the use of compensation strategies during task performance. Thus, the standard for recovery is not only whether a goal is achieved but whether it is accomplished in the manner (i.e., behavioral pattern) used before injury. This scale is particularly relevant because newer interventions for rehabilitation after SCI are now beginning to target recovery to preinjury status as opposed to compensation for injury-related impairments. The NRS consists of 11 items ranging from sitting to sit-to-stand to walking.

ASSISTIVE TECHNOLOGY

Individuals with SCI benefit from a variety of assistive technologies to increase independence with mobility and ADL and to enhance participation in desired social roles and activities. These range from high-tech devices such as exoskeletons, power wheelchairs, environmental control units, and speech recognition software to lower-tech devices such as adaptive writing devices, a trapeze over the bed, and reaching devices. The *Psychosocial Impact of Assistive Devices* is a self-report tool that can be used to assess the impact of assistive technology on independence, well-being, and QOL.[179] The *Quebec User Evaluation of Satisfaction With Assistive Technology (QUEST)* is another self-report/interview scale that is designed to assess the patient's satisfaction with assistive technology.[180] Scores on the QUEST are moderately associated with QOL.[181]

COMMUNITY, SOCIAL, AND CIVIC LIFE

The ultimate goal of rehabilitation is to allow the individual to return to their normal roles and fully participate in society. Measures of participation provide insight into how the individual is functioning in the home and community. Some commonly used outcome measures are the *Craig Handicap Assessment and Reporting Technique*,[182,183] *Life Satisfaction Questionnaire*,[184,185] *Short Form 36*,[186,187] *Satisfaction With Life Scale*,[188] *Reintegration to Normal Living Index*,[189] and *World Health Organization QOL*.[190]

Contextual Factors

ENVIRONMENTAL FACTORS

It is also essential that the physical therapist examine the patient's home, community, and work environments to determine accessibility. Because structural modifications and/or additions to the home may be required to ensure patient safety and access, the rehabilitation team should perform an examination of the home environment early in the rehabilitation process (see Chapter 9, Examination and Modification of the Environment).

■ PROGNOSIS FOR RECOVERY OF MOTOR FUNCTION AND WALKING ABILITY

One of the most common questions that patients and families have after a SCI is how much recovery of motor function will occur and will the individual be able to walk again. The potential for recovery from SCI is directly related to the neurological level of lesion and completeness of the injury.[191] An incomplete lesion (AIS B, C, or D) is a good prognostic indicator of greater likelihood of recovery of motor function.[192,193] Approximately 67% of individuals with AIS A injuries will gain one level of motor recovery, 16% will gain two levels, and only 3% gain three or more levels.[194] Approximately 20% to 30% of individuals will convert from AIS A to B, C, or D, with high thoracic injuries having the lowest percentage (10%) and lumbar injuries the highest (10%).[195] If the injury is still assessed as motor and sensory complete at 1-month postinjury, the likelihood of converting to an incomplete injury drops to less than 10%.[196] In addition to level of injury and degree of completeness, many coexisting factors contribute to the degree of expected recovery. Age (particularly if older than 65 years), spasticity, decreased balance, impaired proprioception, decreased trunk control, and decreased cognition all have negative effects on expected recovery.[195] Recovery of motor function generally plateaus around 12 to 18 months after injury.[193,197]

Specific to walking, patients with an AIS impairment A are unlikely to regain the ability to walk; approximately 33% of patients with AIS B, 65% of patients with AIS C, and almost 100% of patients with AIS D regain some ability to walk.[191,198] However, even with complete lesions (AIS A), 70% patients with cervical-level injuries are likely to experience one level of motor recovery below the original neurological level.[199]

Preservation of pinprick sensation after injury in the LEs or sacral region is associated with a good prognosis for motor recovery and walking ability at 1 year after injury.[200,201] Lower extremity AIS motor score, quadriceps and gastrocnemius strength in particular, can be a useful predictor of functional walking ability in people with motor incomplete injuries. The *European Multicenter Study on Human Spinal Cord Injury* has published a clinical prediction rule for predicting ambulation after SCI.[202] In a cohort of almost 500 patients, findings indicated that age, motor scores of quadriceps and gastrocnemius, and light touch sensory scores at L3 and S1 were able to accurately distinguish between independent home ambulators and those who require assistance or cannot ambulate. The clinical prediction rule was 96% accurate. These findings corroborate findings from Hussey and Stauffer's landmark 1973 study.[203]

Prediction for recovery of walking based on SCI clinical syndromes is also fairly well established. Independent walking is highly likely after central cord injury but decreases from 97% likelihood to 41% when the patient is older than 50 years. Similarly, Brown-Séquard syndrome is associated with high degrees of recovery ranging from 75%[204] to 100%.[205] Lastly, while transcranial magnetic stimulation (TMS) assessments of motor-evoked potentials and MRI evaluations do not contribute to the predictive models, increased spinal cord edema is associated with poorer outcomes, particularly if the edema crosses multiple levels.[206]

As with any clinical prediction guide, it is important to keep in mind that these factors should only be used as a *guide* to assist in the development of goals and the POC. Other factors such as psychosocial support, insurance coverage, and patient psychological status and motivation can affect outcomes. Additionally, new therapies may be developed that improve neurological recovery.

■ OUTCOMES AND GOALS

Functional outcome after SCI is dependent on many factors; primary among these, especially for individuals with complete injuries, is level of motor function. With complete lower-level lesions (i.e., more musculature intact), there is greater potential for independence in mobility tasks and ADL. With incomplete lesions (AIS A, B, C, or D), there is greater functional potential as compared to AIS A injuries; AIS D injuries represent greater functional independence than those of AIS B or C injuries. Other factors that may affect functional outcomes include age, concomitant injury, preexisting health conditions, secondary complications (pneumonia, UTIs, pressure injuries), BMI, and psychosocial factors. Table 20.5 provides a guide to expected functional outcomes for people with complete SCI based on level of injury. The physical therapist, rehabilitation team, and patient can use these expected outcomes to establish goals and outcomes. However, as mentioned earlier, factors other than motor level may affect functional recovery.

Goals should reflect what is important and meaningful to the patient. This will increase motivation, promote achievement of goals, and enhance patient autonomy. Early after injury, patients are not likely to fully understand the consequences of a SCI and are still in the process of adjusting to the injury. It is important to educate patients on the impact of SCI and review the findings of the initial examination and all reexaminations. Potential functional goals should be discussed, and patients should be encouraged to participate in their own goal formation as well. While short-term goals may focus on body structure and function impairments, long-term goals should focus on activity and social participation. Goals should be specific by stating what the patient will achieve. The level of assistance, the environment/conditions,

and the length of time to achieve the goal should all be documented.

Examples of general goals and outcomes for patients with SCI as adapted from the *Guide to Physical Therapist Practice* are presented in Box 20.2.

For patients with high cervical SCI who may not be able to physically perform certain functional mobility tasks, goals should be directed toward patient ability to

Table 20.5	Functional Expectations for Patients With Spinal Cord Injury by Level of Injury*	

C1, C2, C3, C4

KM: Face/neck muscles, cranial nerves, diaphragm (partial innervation at C3 and C4)
A: Talking, mastication, sipping, blowing, scapular elevation

Mobility Expectations	ADL Expectations	Equipment Needs
Bed mobility: Dependent Transfers: Dependent, Aides use mechanical lift Wheelchair mobility: Power: Independent Manual: Unable Pressure relief: Dependent with positioning, use of tilt in space Standing: Dependent with tilt table Ambulation: Unable	Feeding: Dependent Grooming: Dependent Dressing: Dependent Bathing: Dependent Bowel and bladder: Dependent Home management: Dependent Driving: Unable Independently directs care when assist is needed	Power-adjustable bed with pressure-reducing mattress Mechanical Lift Power wheelchair with adaptive controls: head, chin, tongue, or sip-and-puff controls Wheelchair cushion and head support Portable ventilator, suctioning equipment Hand splints Shower/commode chair Environmental control unit: smart technology for electronics Brain–computer interface

C5

KM: Biceps, brachialis, brachioradialis, deltoid, infraspinatus, rhomboid (major/minor), supinator
A: Elbow flexion and supination, shoulder external rotation, shoulder abduction and flexion to 90°

Mobility Expectations	ADL Expectations	Equipment Needs
Bed mobility: Assistance to dependent Transfers: If dependent use mechanical lift, may be able to use transfer board with assist Wheelchair mobility: Power: Independent Manual: Independent to some assist on level surfaces; assist for outdoors Pressure relief: Independent in power wheelchair Standing: Some assist needed with tilt table/standing frame Ambulation: Unable	Feeding: Some assistance/setup Grooming: Some assistance/setup Dressing: Some assistance/setup Bathing: Some assistance/setup Bowel and bladder: Dependent Home management: Some assistance/setup Driving: May be independent with van with adaptive controls Independently directs care when assist is needed	Power-adjustable bed with pressure-reducing mattress; bedrails and loops Mechanical lift Transfer board Power wheelchair with joystick and powered tilt/recline Wheelchair cushion Manual wheelchair with power assist wheels or rims/extensions Adapted utensils and splinting Mobile arm supports, deltoid aid Adapted bathing equipment Hand splints Shower/commode chair Accessible van with adaptive controls

Table 20.5   Functional Expectations for Patients With Spinal Cord Injury by Level of Injury*—cont'd

C6

KM: Extensor carpi radialis, infraspinatus, latissimus dorsi, pectoral major (clavicular portion), pronator teres, serratus anterior, teres minor
A: Shoulder flexion, extension, internal rotation, and adduction; scapular abduction, protraction, and upward rotation; forearm pronation; wrist extension (tenodesis grasp)

Mobility Expectations	ADL Expectations	Equipment Needs
Bed mobility: Independent to some assistance Transfers: Independent to some assist for level, assistance needed for uneven surfaces Wheelchair mobility: Power: Independent for community Manual: Independent to some assist on level surfaces; some assist for outdoors Pressure relief: Independent Standing: Tilt table or standing frame Ambulation: Unable	Feeding: Assistance to independent with set up or equipment Grooming: Assistance to independent with setup or equipment Dressing: Assistance to independent with setup or equipment, assist for LE dressing Bathing: Assistance to independent with set up or equipment Bowel and bladder: Assistance typically needed, may be independent with adaptive equipment Home management: Assistance, may be independent with light household tasks and adaptive equipment Driving: Independent with van with adaptive controls Independently directs care when assist is needed	Power-adjustable bed with pressure-reducing mattress; bedrails and loops Transfer board Power wheelchair for community Manual wheelchair with coated rims/extensions, power assist wheel option Wheelchair cushion Universal cuff and adaptive utensils for feeding/grooming Adaptive equipment for dressing, bathing Hand splints Shower/commode chair Accessible van with adaptive controls

C7

KM: Extensor pollicis longus and brevis, extrinsic finger extensors, flexor carpi radialis, triceps
A: Elbow extension, wrist flexion, finger extension

Mobility Expectations	ADL Expectations	Equipment Needs
Bed mobility: Independent with adaptive equipment Transfers: Independent, may need assist on unevens Wheelchair mobility: Manual: independent in home and community, may need assist with ramps, curbs, unevens Pressure relief: Independent Standing: Standing frame Ambulation: Unable	Feeding: Independent with adaptive equipment Grooming: Independent with adaptive equipment Dressing: Independent with adaptive equipment Bathing: Independent with adaptive equipment Bowel and bladder: Independent with adaptive equipment Home management: Assistance for heavy household tasks Driving: Independent with adaptive controls	Bedrails and loops if needed Transfer board for uneven surfaces Manual wheelchair with coated rims Wheelchair cushion ADL adaptive equipment Hand splints Shower/commode chair Van/car with adaptive controls

(Continued)

Table 20.5   Functional Expectations for Patients With Spinal Cord Injury by Level of Injury*—cont'd

C8

KM: Extrinsic finger flexors, flexor carpi ulnaris, flexor pollicus longus and brevis, intrinsic finger flexors
A: Finger flexion

Mobility Expectations	ADL Expectations	Equipment Needs
Bed mobility: Independent Transfers: Independent, may need assist on unevens; may be able to do floor transfers Wheelchair mobility: independent in home and community, less assist needed with ramps, curbs, unevens than C7 Pressure relief: Independent Standing: Standing frame Ambulation: Unable	Feeding: Independent with adaptive equipment Grooming: Independent with adaptive equipment Dressing: Independent with adaptive equipment Bathing: Independent with adaptive equipment Bowel and bladder: Independent with adaptive equipment Home management: Assistance for heavy household tasks Driving: Independent with adaptive controls	Bedrails and loops if needed Transfer board for uneven surfaces Manual wheelchair with coated rims or power assist wheels Wheelchair cushion ADL adaptive equipment Hand splints Shower/commode chair Van/car with adaptive controls Less need for adaptive equipment due to increased hand function compared to C7

T1–T12

KM: Intercostals, long muscles of back (sacrospinalis and semispinalis), abdominal muscles (T7 and below)
A: Improved trunk control with more caudal SCI, increased respiratory reserve, pectoral girdle stabilization for lifting objects

Mobility Expectations	ADL Expectations	Equipment Needs
Bed mobility: Independent transfers: Independent, including floor transfers Wheelchair mobility: Independent in home and community with manual wheelchair, including ramps, curbs, unevens Pressure relief: Independent Standing: Independent standing with assistive device and orthotics Ambulation: Independent to some assist for household distances with assistive device and orthotics More caudal thoracic injuries will need less assistance for ambulation	Feeding: Independent Grooming: Independent Dressing: Independent Bathing: Independent Bowel and bladder: Independent with adaptive equipment Home management: Assistance for heavy household tasks Driving: Independent with adaptive controls	Manual wheelchair, lightweight Wheelchair cushion Assistive device for ambulation walker or loftstrands Orthotics for ambulation: HKAFO,KAFO Adaptive equipment Shower/commode chair Vehicle with adaptive controls

L1, L2, L3

KM: Gracilis, iliopsoas, quadratus lumborum, rectus femoris, sartorius
A: Hip flexion, hip adduction, knee extension

Mobility Expectations	ADL Expectations	Equipment Needs
Bed mobility: Independent Transfers: Independent Wheelchair mobility: may use wheelchair for long distances Pressure relief: Independent Standing: Independent with assistive device and orthotics Ambulation: Independent with assistive device and orthotics	Feeding: Independent Grooming: Independent Dressing: Independent Bathing: Independent Bowel and bladder: Independent Home management: Independent Driving: Independent with adaptive controls	Manual wheelchair for community distances Wheelchair cushion Assistive device for ambulation (walker, loftstrands, canes) Orthoses: HKAFO, KAFO, AFO depending on motor function

Table 20.5	Functional Expectations for Patients With Spinal Cord Injury by Level of Injury*—cont'd

L4, L5, S1

KM: Quadriceps (L4), anterior tibialis (L5), hamstrings (L5–S1), gastrocnemius (S1), gluteus medius and maximus (L5–S1), extensor digitorum, posterior tibialis, peroneals, flexor digitorum (L5, S1)

A: Strong hip flexion, strong knee extension, knee flexion, ankle dorsiflexion, ankle plantarflexion, ankle eversion, toe extension

Mobility Expectations	ADL Expectations	Equipment Needs
Bed mobility: Independent	Feeding: Independent	Manual wheelchair for community distances
Transfers: Independent	Grooming: Independent	Wheelchair cushion
Wheelchair mobility: may use wheelchair for long distances	Dressing: Independent	Assistive device for ambulation (lofts-trands, canes)
Pressure relief: Independent	Bathing: Independent	Orthoses: AFO, SMO, or foot orthotic insert
Standing: Independent with assistive device and orthotics	Bowel and bladder: Independent	
Ambulation: Independent with assistive device and orthotics	Home management: Independent	
	Driving: Independent with adaptive controls	

A = available movements; ADL = activities of daily living; AFO = ankle-foot orthoses; HKAFO = hip-knee-ankle-foot orthoses; KAFO = knee-ankle-foot orthoses; KM = key muscles; LE = lower extremity.

*This table presents general functional expectations at various lesion levels. Each progressively lower motor includes the muscles from the previous levels. Although the key muscles listed frequently receive innervation from several spinal levels, they are listed here at the key neurological levels where they add to functional outcomes. Although intact musculature plays a main role in determining functional capability, many other factors influence function, including concomitant injuries, premorbid health status, age, body type, and psychosocial factors. Individuals with an incomplete injury will likely have greater functional abilities.

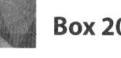

Box 20.2   Examples of General Goals and Outcomes for Patients With Spinal Cord Injury

- Impact of pathology/pathophysiology is reduced
  - Decrease risk of secondary impairment (i.e., pressure injury)
  - Educate patient/client, family/care partner regarding health condition, prognosis, and plan of care
- Impact of body structure/function impairments is reduced
  - Airway clearance is improved
  - Muscle performance is increased
  - Aerobic capacity is increased
  - Joint mobility and integrity are improved or remain functional
- Ability to perform physical actions, tasks, or activities is improved
  - Tolerates upright sitting posture
  - Independence with bed mobility tasks
  - Independence with wheelchair mobility
  - Independence with transfers
  - Independence with self-directing care
  - Independence with pressure relief
- Disability associated with chronic health condition is reduced
  - Independence with self-care and home management
  - Resume work, community, and leisure roles
  - Education on community resources

independently direct an attendant carepartner to perform the task appropriately and include specific equipment that may be necessary to accomplish the goal.

■ PHYSICAL THERAPY INTERVENTIONS

Improvements in body structure/function impairments, the ability to perform activities that are important to the individual, and a return to participating in normal, desired social roles can be achieved through interventions that are based on compensatory strategies, restorative strategies, or a combination of the two. The intervention strategy selected is largely based on the amount of preserved motor function. Independence in functional skills in patients with complete motor SCI (AIS A and B) is largely achieved through compensatory mechanisms, and interventions are developed accordingly. For example, a person with a C6 injury (AIS A) is taught to transfer from bed to wheelchair using a sit-pivot method. Patients with AIS C or D, depending on the degree of motor return, may relearn how to perform functional tasks using more normal movement strategies. For example, a person with an AIS C or D may relearn to walk through locomotor training using a body weight support (BWS) and treadmill (TM) system, an intervention that promotes normal movement patterns during gait training. This restorative approach attempts to minimize compensatory movement strategies and promote normal movement patterns to drive beneficial neuroplastic changes within the CNS.

Because SCI affects many different body systems, certain precautions (Box 20.3) and general principles must be considered when performing interventions. Common principles used across compensatory intervention strategies to promote functional independence in mobility tasks are momentum, head–hips relationship, and muscle substitution. These compensatory strategies allow performance of functional mobility by substituting for lost motor function and strength below the lesion level. For example, a patient with a T1 AIS A will use momentum by swinging the arms across the body multiple times to roll from supine to side-lying as a compensation for lost trunk or LE muscles that would normally assist in performing the task.

For compensatory training, the overarching goal is to teach techniques to move the body using available musculature and motor control. These techniques will vary from individual to individual based on multiple factors, among them preexisting health conditions, body type, and ability to incorporate motor learning. Even individuals with the same level of injury may adapt seemingly very different techniques to maximize independence with function. There are, however, several principles that can be applied to all compensatory strategies, and examples of how these may be incorporated are covered in later sections:

- *Head–hips relationship:* this compensatory strategy is applicable to a variety of functional tasks. It involves moving the head in one direction to cause movement of the hips in the opposite direction. For example, a compensatory strategy for sit-pivot transfers or wheelchair positioning is to lead with the hips while the head leans in the opposite direction (see Figure 20.8).
- *Momentum:* body segments with available motor function can be used to generate momentum (force × velocity) to facilitate movement of denervated body segments.
- *Muscle substitution:* to improve function, individuals with SCI typically become very adept at using intact muscles to substitute for those that are lost. If deemed safe and effective, these substitutions should be incorporated into movement training.

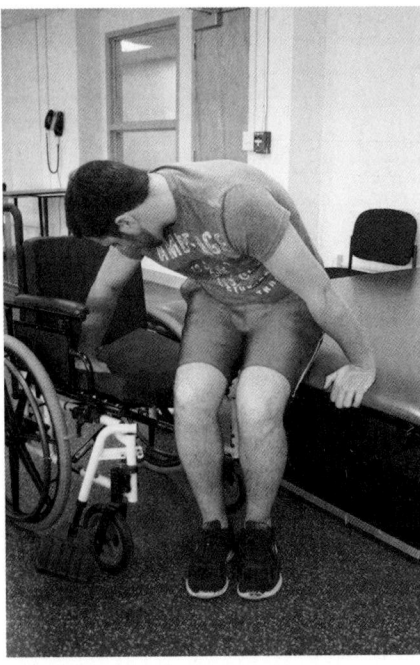

Figure 20.8 Head–hips relationship during transfer.

- *Task modification:* modifying the task to make it easier allows for a progression and builds confidence and self-efficacy for the patient. Examples include placing a wedge behind the back to assist with early rolling activities, modifying the height for uneven transfers, or using adaptive equipment (trapeze system over the bed to promote independence with bed mobility).
- *Working in and out of the task:* failure to complete a functional task might be due to a lack of skill or a lack of required components (flexibility, strength, stability). Patients benefit from both task-specific skill training as well as out-of-task impairment-focused training (e.g., muscle strengthening and stretching).

Motor learning concepts should be incorporated into the POC. In the early stages of motor learning, when the patient is not skillful and cannot perform the task independently, extrinsic feedback regarding task performance may be useful. For example, the physical therapist may provide tactile and verbal cues on correct hand placement on the hand rim when the patient is practicing and learning how to perform wheelies. Extrinsic feedback provided on a faded schedule promotes motor learning. In later stages of motor learning, it is beneficial to have the patient use intrinsic feedback and rely less on extrinsic feedback. The practice schedule and environment can also be set up to promote motor learning. A random practice schedule is more beneficial to learning than a blocked practice schedule. The environment should be varied as the patient develops more skill in performing the task. For example, the patient should practice transferring to and from a variety of different surfaces (e.g., wheelchair to/from mat, bed, chair, car, sofa) once basic competence in the skill has been achieved.

For mobility tasks, it is often beneficial to break down the task into component parts for practice followed closely by practice of the integrated whole (parts-to-whole practice). For example, when learning to move from supine to long-sitting, practice first focuses on a component part such as transitioning to supine-on-elbows. See Chapter 10, Strategies to Improve Motor Function, for a discussion of motor learning strategies.

Strengthening

Strengthening all remaining innervated musculature is an important component of the POC. Key UE muscles to strengthen include serratus anterior, latissimus dorsi, pectoralis major, rotator cuff, and triceps brachii.[207,208] These muscles are particularly important for independent transfers. Initially, strengthening exercises may be done daily during early rehabilitation. A variety of methods can be used to implement strengthening exercises such as pulley systems, free weights, manual resistance, elastic bands, and weight cuffs. With very weak muscles (grade ≤2), strengthening can be performed in gravity-reduced positions on a powder board or with active assistive ROM. Strengthening can be done in functional postures as well. For example, push-ups can be performed in prone-on-elbows and supine-on-elbows. Regardless of the strengthening modality or baseline level of strength, it is important to exercise at an appropriate intensity level; 60% to 80% of the 1RM or 100% of the 10RM, the intensity required to complete 10 repetitions before fatigue.

Respiratory

Respiratory care will vary according to the level of injury and individual respiratory status. Primary goals of management include improved ventilation, increased effectiveness of cough, and prevention of chest tightness and ineffective substitute breathing patterns.

Individuals with cervical injuries at and above C5 often require ventilatory support using an intermittent positive pressure ventilator. Invasive mechanical ventilation (MV) is often done through a tracheostomy and can be provided through a stationary or portable ventilator. Noninvasive positive pressure ventilation provides an alternative to invasive MV.[61] Intubation may impair the function of the airway cilia, leading to chronic bacterial colonization and chronic inflammatory changes of the airway. Patients may also prefer noninvasive ventilation.

Diaphragm pacing (DP) uses intramuscular diaphragm stimulation to improve respiratory function and helps wean from MV if long-term ventilation assistance is necessary, minimizing long-term complications from MV.[209] Newer respiratory rehabilitation models advocate for earlier consideration of DP and use of task-specific respiratory training models to enhance functional gains.[209] More evidence is needed to determine long-term outcomes with DP, including QOL measures, although DP has been shown to decrease hospital-related costs and decrease time to wean off MV.[210]

Respiratory Muscle Training

Similar to other muscles, strength training can improve respiratory muscle strength and endurance. Two systematic reviews concluded that respiratory muscle training is effective for improving respiratory muscle strength, VC, maximal inspiratory pressure, maximal expiratory pressure, and residual volume.[211,212] Diaphragmatic breathing should be encouraged. To facilitate diaphragmatic movement and increase VC, the therapist can apply light pressure during both inspiration and expiration. Manual contacts can be made just below the sternum. This will assist the patient in concentrating on deep-breathing patterns even in the absence of thoracic and abdominal sensation.

Inspiratory muscles can be trained using relatively inexpensive handheld devices, which increase the resistive or threshold inspiratory load on muscles of inspiration (Fig. 20.9). There are two general categories of handheld inspiratory muscle training devices: resistive or threshold trainers. Breathing through these devices increases the resistive or threshold inspiratory load on the muscles. The load can be progressively increased as the patient progresses. Inspiratory muscle training can improve pulmonary function, reduce dyspnea, and improve cough function.[213] Another method of strengthening inspiratory muscles is to provide manual resistance (and progress to weighted resistance) to the epigastric area as the patient breathes.

Expiratory muscle training can assist in improving pulmonary function.[211,214] Similar to inspiratory muscle training, expiratory muscle training can be done by breathing through a device with a small diameter that

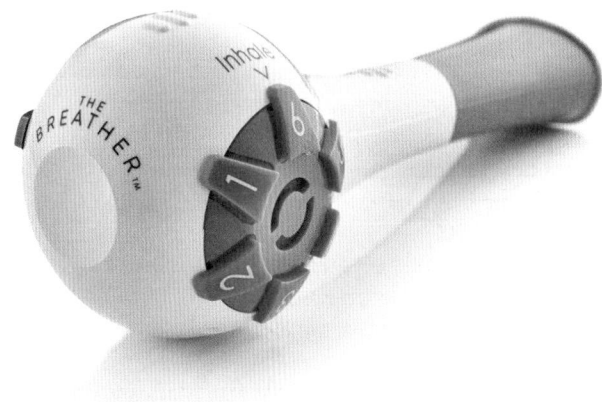

Figure 20.9 Respiratory muscle trainer. *(The Breather, Courtesy of PN Medical, Inc.)*

limits the airflow, increasing the resistance to expiration (resistive training); or breathing with enough force to overcome a valve and allow airflow (threshold training). Expiratory muscle training can also be accomplished with functional activities such as blowing into an instrument to produce sound, into a straw to move light objects, or singing.[215] The impacts of respiratory muscle strengthening on functional outcomes and QOL are not clear, with decreased risk of pulmonary infection and decreased mortality being most evident.[216] Also, the most effective dosage of strength training has not been established although training intensity seems more relevant than training volume.[217]

Patients who are not able to produce a functional cough should be taught to perform a self-assisted cough. This can be accomplished in a seated position (Fig. 20.10) or supine. Those who cannot perform a self-assisted cough may benefit from a manually assisted cough to help remove secretions (Fig. 20.11).[218] To assist with coughing and movement of secretions, manual contacts are placed over the epigastric area. The therapist pushes quickly in an inward and upward direction as the patient attempts to cough.

Glossopharyngeal Breathing

Glossopharyngeal breathing may be appropriate for patients with high-level cervical lesions who are

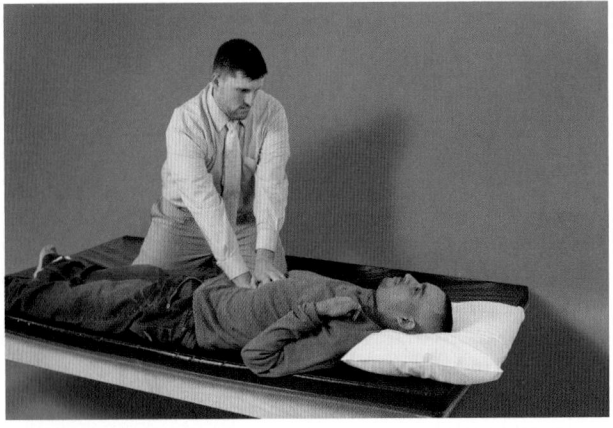

Figure 20.11 Assisted cough in supine using abdominal thrust maneuver to clear secretions.

dependent on a mechanical ventilator for ventilation, as well as for patients with mid- to high cervical-level injuries who are not dependent on MV. Glossopharyngeal breathing utilizes the lips, pharyngeal muscles, and tongue to inhale air.[219,220] The patient is instructed to take in small amounts of air, using a "gulping" pattern, thus utilizing available facial and pharyngeal muscles. The patient repeats these 6 to 10 times. By using this technique, enough air is gradually inspired. Exhalation occurs owing to the elastic recoil of the lungs. Glossopharyngeal breathing provides a method for individuals with high cervical lesions who are dependent on MV to breathe independently for a period of time in emergency situations[219] and as a way to increase VC in people with cervical lesions who are not dependent on a mechanical ventilator. Teaching a patient to perform glossopharyngeal breathing requires specialized skills and experience beyond entry level.[138]

Abdominal Binder

An abdominal binder may improve respiratory function,[221] cough ability,[222] and speech[221] in patients with high thoracic and cervical lesions. An abdominal binder may improve respiratory mechanics by compensating for nonfunctioning abdominal muscles. The binder compresses abdominal contents to increase intraabdominal pressure and elevates the diaphragm into a more optimal position for breathing. In addition, abdominal binders may provide secondary benefits of maintaining intrathoracic pressure and decreasing postural hypotension.

Manual Stretching

Mobility and compliance of the thoracic wall can be facilitated by manual stretching chest wall muscles in supine. This is done by placing one hand around the side of the chest wall with the fingertips on the transverse processes and the other on top of the chest with the base of the hand on the edge of the sternum. The

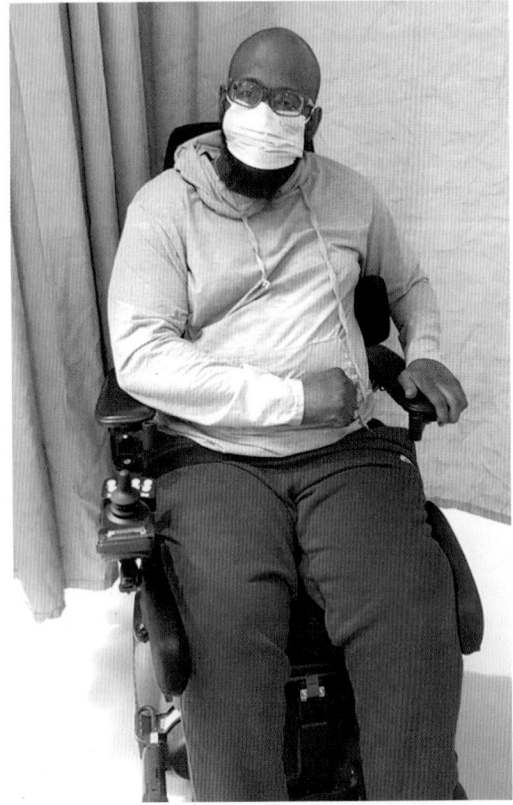

Figure 20.10 Individual with spinal cord injury performing self-assisted cough in sitting.

hands are moved in a wringing motion. Pressure should be distributed across the surface of the hands. Wetzel[220] provides an in-depth discussion of interventions to enhance respiratory function.

Skin Care

Prevention is the most effective intervention for skin care; this entails positioning, consistent and effective pressure relief, skin inspection, and education. Areas that are susceptible to skin pressure injury (see Table 20.3) should be adequately protected when the patient is in bed by using pillows, foam, and positioning devices (Fig. 20.12). Positioning should also be used to prevent development of joint contractures and secondary pulmonary complications. Specific positioning of the extremities to prevent contractures will depend on the level of the SCI. Certain joints may be more prone to contracture depending on which muscles surrounding the joint are innervated. For example, a patient with a C5-level injury may tend to position the shoulder in adduction and the elbow in flexion. When positioning this patient, the shoulders should be abducted and elbows extended when possible.

When in bed, patients should be repositioned at least every 2 hours.[223] Increased and consistent pressure over bony prominences, shear forces, heat, and moisture should be minimized. A variety of beds and rotating beds with foam, air, low air loss, and air fluidized mattresses and overlays can assist in the prevention of pressure injuries and aid with healing (Fig. 20.13).

The wheelchair and seating system should also assist in promoting optimal positioning for reducing pressure and shear forces on susceptible areas. The pelvis should be positioned in a neutral position or slightly tilted anteriorly and be symmetrical (i.e., left anterior-superior iliac spine [ASIS] even with the right ASIS). A variety

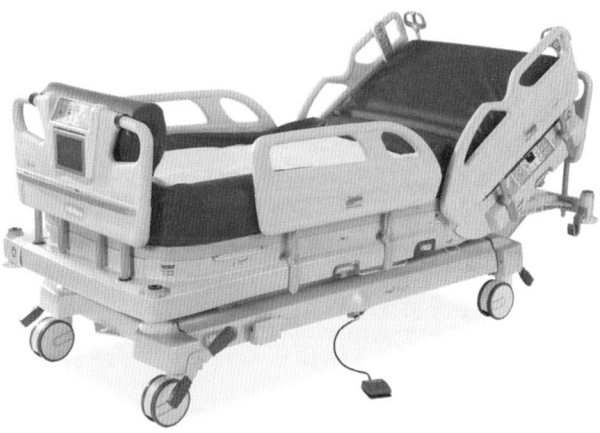

Figure 20.13 Envella air fluidized bed. (© Hill-Rom Services, Inc. Reprinted with Permission. All Rights Reserved.)

of wheelchair cushion types are designed to assist with positioning and redistribution of pressure. Positioning should optimize weight-bearing on the ischial tuberosities while minimizing pressure on the greater trochanters and sacrum/coccyx, which are able to accommodate much less pressure without the breakdown of skin tissue. The main types of cushions are foam, gel, air, and flexible matrix and differ in the balance between support and pressure compensation. Cushions are often contoured to further assist in the redistribution of pressure and to reduce shear. No one type of cushion is the most effective, although air-based cushions have been shown to be more consistently effective in interface pressure reduction than gel- and foam-based cushions.[224] The exact type of cushion selected should be based on the individual patient and should consider both pressure relief and seated postural control. Chapter 32, Seating and Wheeled Mobility, provides more detail about wheelchairs and seating systems as well as their advantages and indications for use.

Patients should perform a pressure relief maneuver every 15 minutes when in the wheelchair, either with assistance or independently.[225] From the seated position, this can be done by using a push-up maneuver, leaning to the side, or leaning forward (Fig. 20.14). If using a forward lean, the lean should be greater than 45°.[226] Patients who are not able to perform these maneuvers initially can be assisted or their wheelchair can be tilted back. If tilting the entire wheelchair back, it should be tilted to at least 65° in order to adequately shift the pressure off of the ischial tuberosities. All pressure relief maneuvers should be maintained for at least 2 minutes to be effective.[227] A tilt-in-space or reclining wheelchair can also be used to redistribute pressure.

The patient's skin should be routinely inspected to ensure there are no developing pressure injuries. Enhanced education on prevention and management with consistent follow-up can reduce the development and recurrence of pressure injuries.[228] As the

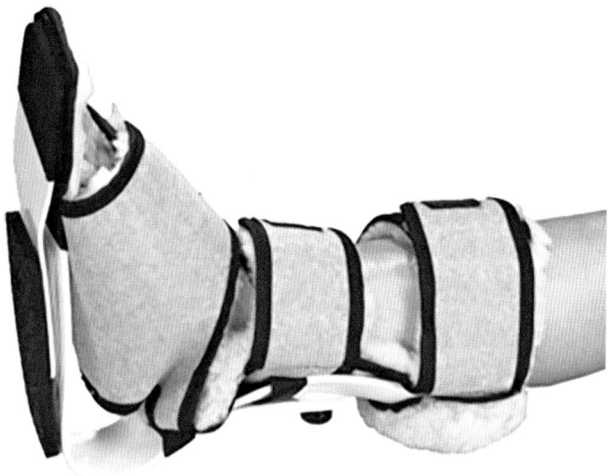

Figure 20.12 Ankle/foot positioning to prevent skin breakdown and contracture. (Roylan Podus Boot, Courtesy of © Performance Health.)

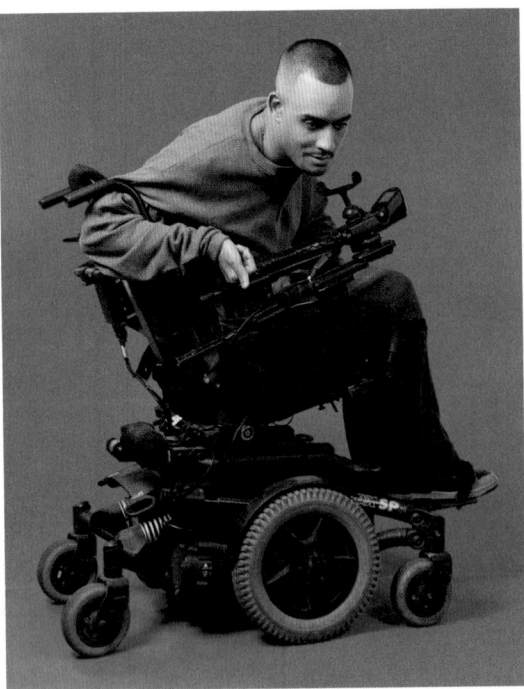

Figure 20.14 Lateral lean in wheelchair for pressure relief.

rehabilitation program progresses, the patient gradually assumes responsibility for skin care. Preparation for assumption of this responsibility will include patient education about the potential risks of pressure sores, the importance of hygiene, instruction in skin inspection techniques, the use of pressure relief equipment and procedures, and what to do if a pressure injury develops.

If the patient develops a skin pressure injury, the preventive measures described earlier should continue to be employed. Various therapies directed at wound healing should be initiated. Chapter 14, Vascular, Lymphatic, and Integumentary Disorders, provides a comprehensive perspective on these and other specific wound healing interventions.

Cardiovascular/Endurance Training

As with able-bodied people, cardiovascular training has important health benefits for people with SCI. A number of studies have shown that endurance training can improve aerobic fitness.[229–231] Upper extremity–based exercises such as arm ergometry, wheelchair propulsion, and swimming are the most common methods of aerobic training. In people with iSCI with sufficient walking capacity, locomotor training on a TM with or without BWS is another method of endurance training.[232] Walking training in various forms has been shown to decrease cardiovascular risk factors in individuals with chronic SCI.[233] For cardiovascular benefit, adults with SCI should perform 30 minutes of moderate- to vigorous-intensity exercise three times per week.[234] The American College of Sports Medicine (ACSM) recommends

aerobic training 3 to 5 days a week, with a total duration per day of 20 to 60 minutes at 40% to 90% of oxygen consumption reserve (VO_2R).[235] There is no evidence to show adverse effects of cardiovascular exercise if safety guidelines are followed, including monitoring for osteoporosis, autonomic dysfunction, and overuse injuries.[236] SCI adversely affects exercise response, including decreased cardiac output, decreased BP response, and impaired thermoregulation.[237] Peak heart rate for individuals with tetraplegic level of injuries is typically 100 to 120 beats/min due to sympathetic impairment.[237] If individuals are not capable of increasing heart rate (HR), a rating of perceived exertion (RPE) of 13 to 17 may be substituted for maximum HR percentage.[238] The duration and intensity of the training should be gradually increased for those not able to initially tolerate these training levels. Modifications of using gloves or hand/leg wrappings to improve ability to grasp exercise equipment or maintain foot placement may be necessary. Surface functional electrical stimulation (FES)–induced cycling or walking is also an effective means of improving cardiovascular fitness.[239] Surface electrodes are attached bilaterally to the hamstrings, quadriceps, and gluteal muscles; a computer controls the intensity of the muscle stimulation and cadence based on the position of the pedals (Fig. 20.15). Any activity, including functional training and strength training, that keeps the HR or RPE in the target zone for 20 to 60 minutes constitutes cardiovascular training and may be an

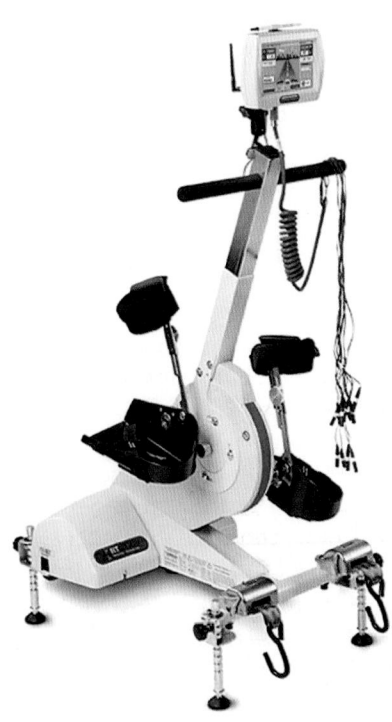

Figure 20.15 Functional electrical stimulation–powered lower extremity ergometer. *(Courtesy of Restorative Therapies, Baltimore, MD 21224.)*

appropriate substitution for those who are not capable of utilizing traditional endurance training techniques or equipment.

Mobility Skills

Once the patient is physician-cleared to assume an upright posture, functional mobility skills can be initiated. The patient typically will experience symptoms of orthostatic hypotension (e.g., dizziness, nausea, ringing in ears, loss of vision, or loss of consciousness) when first assuming sitting and/or standing (if able). A gradual acclimation to upright postures is necessary. The use of an abdominal binder and elastic stockings may reduce venous pooling and prevent orthostatic hypotension. During early upright positioning, elastic wraps may also be used in combination with (placed over) the elastic stockings.

Initially, upright activities can be initiated by slowly elevating the head of the bed and progressing to a reclining or tilt-in-space wheelchair with elevating leg rests. Use of a standing frame provides another option for orienting the patient to a vertical position. A tilt table can also be used. Vital signs should be monitored carefully and documented during this acclimation period to ensure that systolic and diastolic BP values do not fall below a safe range. If the patient experiences any of the signs or symptoms of orthostatic hypotension during sitting or standing activities, the patient should be brought safely to a supine position (or trunk reclined) with the legs elevated.

When the patient is acclimated to upright postures (sitting and standing), specific training can begin on basic mobility skills. Interventions designed to teach bed mobility skills such as rolling and transitioning supine to/from long- and short-sitting and transfer skills can be initiated. These and other functional mobility skills become the focus of rehabilitation once the patient is stable. Specific intervention techniques on these and other functional mobility skills are discussed next.

Bed Mobility

Bed mobility skills are necessary to promote independence in functional mobility. Bed mobility skills include rolling, transitioning supine to/from sitting on the edge of the bed, and LE management. Independence in these skills is also necessary for dressing, positioning in bed, and skin inspection. The degree to which these skills can be performed independently varies depending on the individual's level of injury and other factors. The exact method of performing the task will vary with the individual. The skills and intervention techniques described later provide a general guide; however, these may need to be adapted depending on the unique presentation of the patient. Also, as mentioned earlier, certain precautions need to be observed when teaching patients these techniques. For example, excessive friction on the elbows while weight shifting in prone-on-elbows may result in skin breakdown. Patients may begin training wearing protective elbow pads.

At first, bed mobility skills are learned and practiced on an exercise mat, which is firmer and larger than a typical bed. However, as skill improves, they should be practiced on a bed similar to that used at home. A patient may be independent performing these skills on a mat but still require more practice to become independent performing the same task on a bed due to the softer and smaller surface.

Individuals with complete SCI will need to use compensatory movement strategies (e.g., momentum, muscle substitution, and head–hips principle) to move the entire body. For example, a patient with a T1 AIS A injury will use momentum by swinging the arms up and across the body to generate momentum that will cause the trunk and legs to roll to the side-lying position from supine. A patient with a T10 AIS A injury will use muscle substitution by using the UEs to lift the legs up onto the mat from a short-sitting position when transitioning to supine from sitting. Individuals with iSCI may be able to use more normal movement strategies to perform these tasks, depending on the extent of motor recovery. Regardless of whether the injury is complete or incomplete, the recovery of normal movement patterns should be attempted and assessed.

Rolling

Rolling is a basic foundational skill required for functional bed mobility, progressing to sitting on the edge of bed, turning in bed for pressure relief, and performing daily activities such as dressing. It requires the patient to learn to use the head, neck, and UEs, as well as momentum, to move the trunk and/or LEs. It is usually easiest to begin rolling activities from the supine position, working toward the prone position. If asymmetric involvement exists, rolling should be initiated with movement toward the weaker side. While rolling is a prerequisite skill for many other functional tasks, it is also very difficult and may require an extended period of time to master.

To develop maximum independence, adaptive devices such as bedrails, ropes, canvas loop "ladders," or overhead devices such as trapezes should be avoided, if possible. However, if these adaptive devices allow more efficient or independent task performance or when the task cannot be otherwise accomplished, they should be incorporated into the overall POC. In addition, the patient should work toward achieving independent rolling when covered by sheets and blankets. To begin training and facilitate rolling, several strategies can be used:

- Flexion of the head and neck with rotation may be used to assist movement from supine to prone positions.
- Extension of the head and neck with rotation may be used to assist movement from prone to supine positions.

- Bilateral, symmetrical UE rocking with outstretched arms produces a pendular motion when moving from supine to prone positions. The patient rhythmically rocks the outstretched arms and head from side to side and then forcefully "tosses" them to the side to which the patient is rolling. The trunk and hips will follow (Fig. 20.16). The head and arms should be synchronized and may be facilitated by the therapist. Use of wrist cuff weights (2 to 3 lb) may be used initially to increase kinesthetic awareness and momentum. The number of rocking motions necessary will depend on the patient's skill, level of SCI, and body type.
- Crossing the ankles will also facilitate rolling initially (see Fig. 20.16). The therapist crosses the patient's ankles so that the upper limb is toward the direction of the roll (e.g., the right ankle would be crossed over the left when rolling toward the left). When first learning, flexing the hip and knee of the top LE and placing it over the opposite limb (e.g., the hip and knee of the right LE would be flexed and placed over the left when rolling toward the left) can assist.
- In moving from the supine position to the prone position, pillows may be placed under one side of the pelvis (or scapula, if needed) to create initial rotation in the direction of the roll (Fig. 20.17). The activity can be started with two pillows, progress to one, and then to rolling without the use of pillows. If difficulty is encountered in initiating the roll, the activity can be started from a side-lying position. To facilitate movement from prone to supine positions, pillows may be placed under one side of the chest and/or pelvis. Again, the number and height of pillows should be reduced gradually and eventually eliminated.

Transitioning Supine To/From Sitting

The ability to transition from supine in bed to sitting on the edge of the bed is a critical skill necessary for

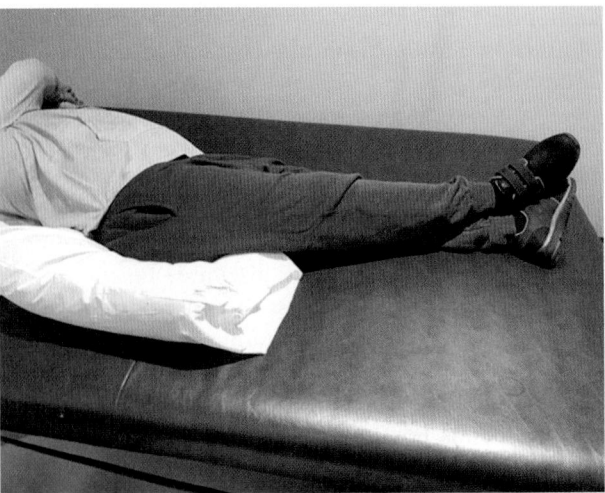

Figure 20.17 Pillows may be placed under one side of the pelvis to initially assist with rolling.

independent mobility. Before a person can transfer out of bed to a wheelchair, the ability to sit up on the edge of the bed must first be achieved. There are two basic methods (with variations) to transition from supine to sitting: (1) "walking" onto elbows from prone or side-lying and (2) coming straight up from supine. Both of these methods transition the patient from supine to long-sitting. The patient then must learn to manage the LEs to move into short-sitting on the edge of the bed. In addition to rolling, two important prerequisite skills/postures that are necessary to come to long-sitting from supine are the ability to assume and move within prone-on-elbows and supine-on-elbows. Long-sitting requires at least 90° of hamstring length bilaterally, and it may be assisted by having the patient long-sit with external rotation of the hips with the knees slightly flexed.

Prone-on-Elbows

The prone-on-elbows position can be assumed from either prone or side-lying. In prone, the shoulders can be either abducted (elbows out away from the body) or adducted (elbows at the side of the trunk), and the patient weight shifts from side to side while moving the unweighted arm to eventually position both elbows directly underneath the shoulder joints (Fig. 20.18A and B). From side-lying, the patient pushes the elbow that is on the mat down into the mat by extending the shoulder, then swings the top arm forward while rolling to prone so the elbow comes onto the mat in the prone-on-elbows position.

Transitioning into prone-on-elbows position is a challenging skill, particularly for individuals without functioning triceps. The patient can be assisted into the position and practice stability and controlled mobility interventions initially.

- Weight-bearing in the prone-on-elbows position will improve stability and strength at the upper trunk, neck, and shoulders.

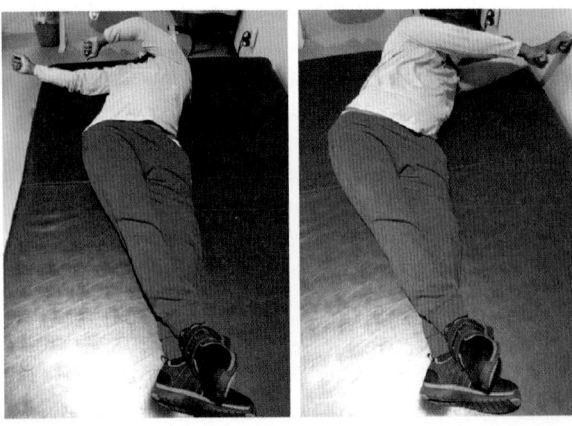

Figure 20.16 Rolling from supine to side-lying using upper extremity momentum and crossing the ankles.

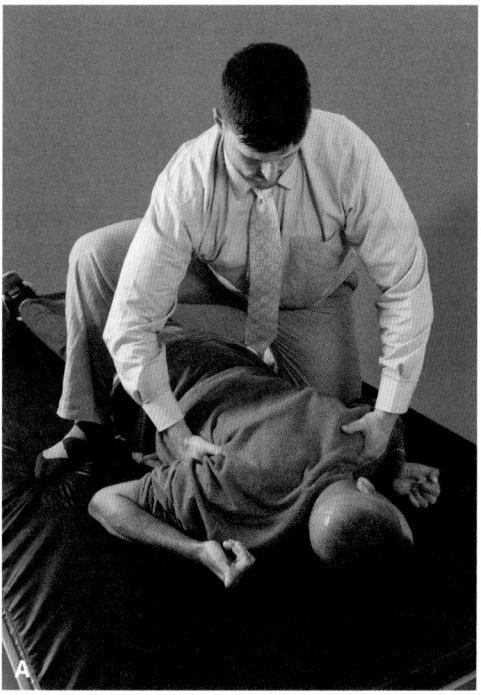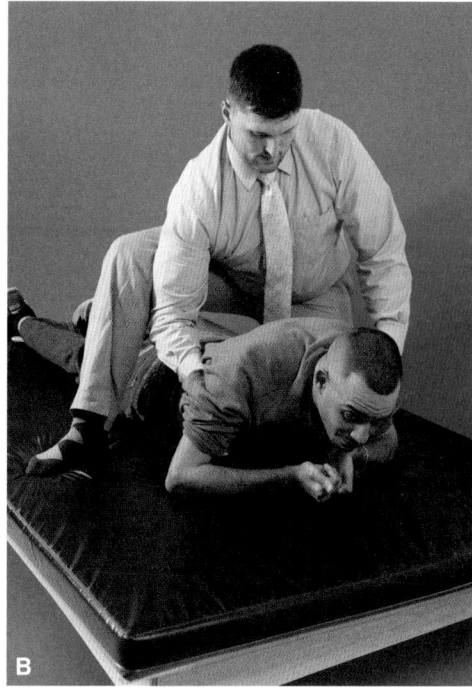

Figure 20.18 Transitioning from prone (A) to prone-on-elbows (B) with shoulders initially abducted and weight shifting.

- Weight shifting assists with development of controlled mobility and is usually easiest in a lateral direction with a progression to anterior or posterior movements.
- Unilateral weight-bearing on one elbow can be achieved in the prone-on-elbows position by having the patient lift one arm. This further facilitates co-contraction in the weight-bearing limb.
- Movement within this posture can be achieved by walking on elbows to both sides, up toward the head of the mat, and backward toward the foot of the mat.
- Strengthening of the serratus anterior and other scapular muscles can be achieved with prone-on-elbows push-ups. This is accomplished by having the patient push the elbows down into the mat and tuck in the chin while lifting and rounding out the shoulders and upper thorax. This is similar to the "cat/camel" maneuver used in the quadruped position. The patient lowers the upper chest to the mat again by allowing the scapula to adduct.

Supine-on-Elbows

There are several approaches to assuming the supine-on-elbows position. If control of abdominal muscles is present, the patient may have sufficient strength to achieve the position by pushing the elbows into the mat and lifting into the position. A common technique is for the patient to "wedge" the hands under the hips or to hook the thumbs into pants pockets or belt loops. By contracting the biceps and/or wrist extensors, the patient can pull up partially into the posture. By shifting weight

from side to side, the elbows can then be positioned under the shoulders (Fig. 20.19A, B, and C).

Some patients may find it easiest to assume this position from side-lying. The lower elbow is first positioned and pushed into the mat. The patient then rolls toward the supine position and quickly extends the upper arm, landing on the elbow as close to the shoulder as possible. By weight shifting, placement of the elbows can then be adjusted.

Much of the inherent benefit of this activity is achieved in learning to assume the posture and then move into long-sitting. In addition to its direct functional significance, this activity is also an important strengthening exercise for shoulder extensors and scapular adductors.

- Lateral weight shifting can be practiced in this position.
- Side-to-side movement in this posture will enhance the patient's ability to align the trunk with the LEs when in bed or in preparation for positional changes.
- Precautions should be taken with this posture because it may cause increased shoulder pain due to the pressure exerted on the anterior shoulder joint capsule.

Walking on Elbows to Assume Long-Sitting Position

From prone the patient walks on elbows toward one side into a "C" position. The patient then unweights

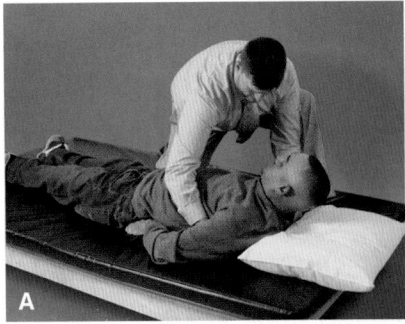
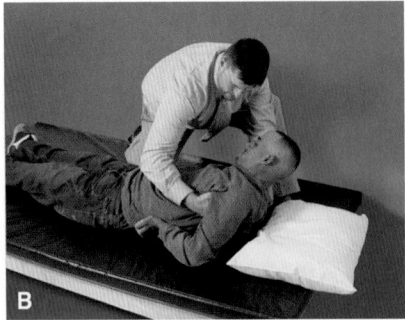
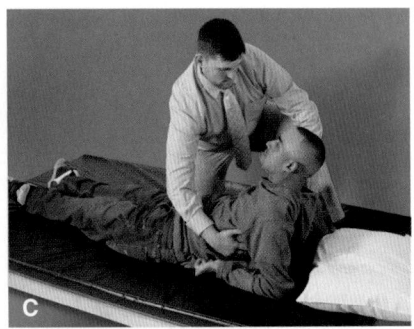

Figure 20.19 Patient transitioning from supine (A) to supine-on-elbows position (B) by stabilizing hands under the pelvis, forcefully pulling up by contracting the biceps, weight shifting side to side, and placing elbows farther underneath the shoulder joints (C).

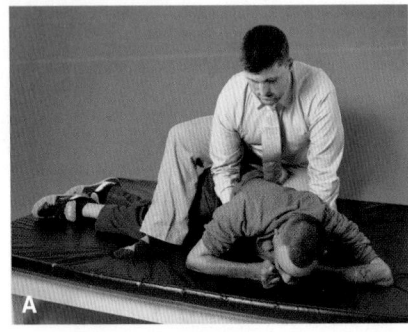
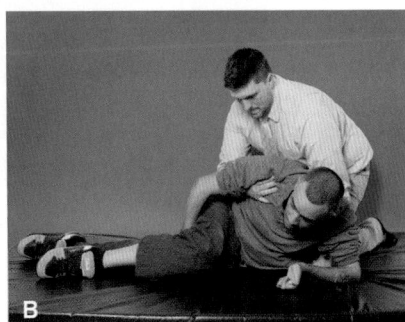
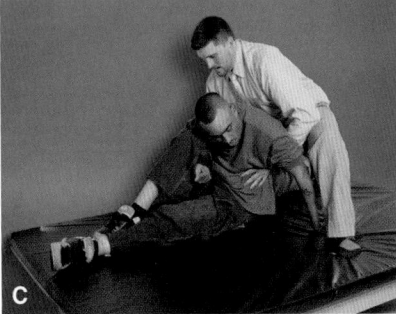
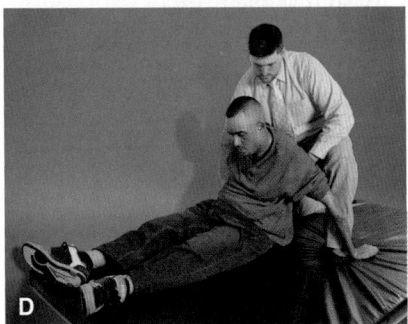

Figure 20.20 Patient transitioning from prone-on-elbows (A) to long-sitting position (B); walks into a "C" position (C), pulls trunk up to long-sitting position (D).

the elbow closest to the legs and hooks it around the knees and pulls the trunk toward the legs. At a certain point the patient can then shift weight off the weight-bearing elbow to the palm and push with one arm while pulling with the other up to a long-sitting position (Fig. 20.20A, B, C, and D).

This method of coming to long-sitting does not require as much ROM in the shoulders as coming to sitting straight up from supine (see later). Practicing component parts of the task (e.g., walking on elbows or pulling up with one arm once in the "C" position) followed closely by practicing the whole task can be used to facilitate learning.

Coming Straight to Long-Sitting Position From Supine

To come to long-sitting from supine requires a more than normal amount of shoulder extension and strong

elbow flexors and wrist extensors. From supine, the patient should assume the supine-on-elbows position as described earlier. From this position, the patient unweights one elbow by shifting onto the opposite elbow. For the patient with a midlevel cervical SCI, the unweighted UE is thrown back into hyperextension and external rotation with the elbow extended so that the palm is on the mat. The patient then rotates the upper trunk onto the UE that was just thrown back in order to unweight the other UE. The unweighted UE is now thrown back in a similar manner so that the patient is now weight-bearing on both hands, then weight shifts side to side and walks the hands up to assume a long-sitting position (Fig. 20.21A, B, and C). Again, it is useful to practice parts of the task to assist in learning how to perform the entire skill.

Patients without sufficient strength or ROM, or due to other factors, may use adaptive equipment such as

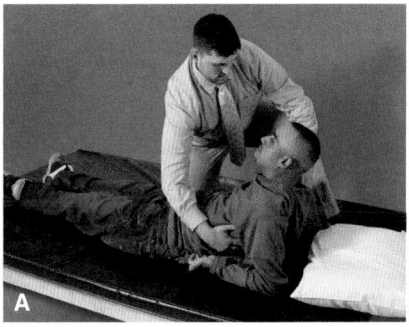
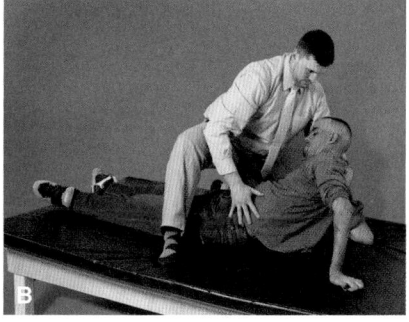
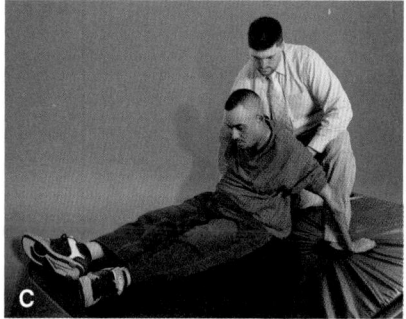

Figure 20.21 Patient transitioning to long-sitting from supine-on-elbows (A). Bears weight on one elbow while the other upper extremity is thrown back into shoulder extension with the elbow extended to bear weight on the other upper extremity (B), then weight shifts onto the other upper extremity and throws the other upper extremity back into shoulder extension with elbow extended to come into long-sitting (C).

bed rails, loop ladder, suspended trapeze, or suspended loops to assist in coming to long-sitting (Fig. 20.22).

Once in long-sitting position, patients must learn to move the LEs off the edge of the bed to come to short-sitting, back onto the bed when moving from short-sitting to supine, and to position themselves in bed using their UEs. Patients without full finger and hand musculature innervation can slide the wrist under a leg so that the palm of the hand is facing the mat and extend the wrist to help move the legs. Alternatively, leg loops can be placed around the thighs to slide the hand in and extend the wrist to lift the leg (Fig. 20.23).

Sitting Balance

Independent sitting balance, both in short-sitting and long-sitting positions, is an important skill for many different functional tasks such as transfers, dressing, and wheelchair mobility. Sitting posture will vary considerably with lesion level. Patients with low thoracic lesions can be expected to sit with a relatively erect trunk. Individuals with low cervical and high thoracic lesions maintain sitting balance by forward head displacement and trunk flexion (Figs. 20.24 and 20.25).

Owing to sensory and motor impairments, patients need to relearn their center of balance and limits of stability as well as how to maintain postural control. The following are some suggestions that can be incorporated to improve sitting balance, both in long- and short-sitting positions.

- Sitting balance training is initially done by assisting the patient into a balanced short- or long-sitting position. In short-sitting, the patient should initially be positioned with the feet firmly supported on the floor and the hips and knees flexed to 90°. In long-sitting, patients should have approximately 90° to 100° of straight leg raise ROM to avoid overstretching the low back muscles. Initially, it is easier to maintain balance in long-sitting due to the larger base of support. The LEs can be placed with the hips

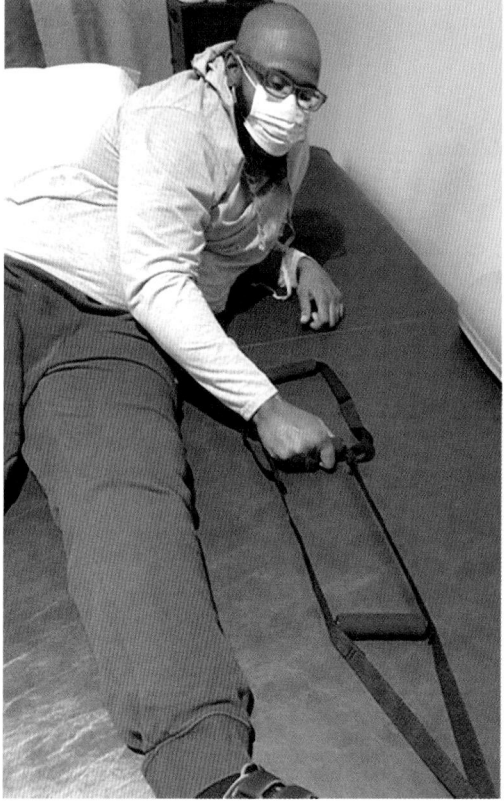

Figure 20.22 Individual with spinal cord injury using loop ladder to assist with bed mobility.

in external rotation and slight abduction to allow knee flexion to avoid overstretching the low back muscles if there is insufficient hamstring flexibility.
- Patients may initially need to bear weight through the UEs to maintain the sitting position. For patients with cervical-level lesions who utilize a tenodesis grasp to hold and manipulate objects, the fingers should be flexed at the proximal and distal interphalangeal joints when the wrist is in full extension to prevent overstretching the finger flexor

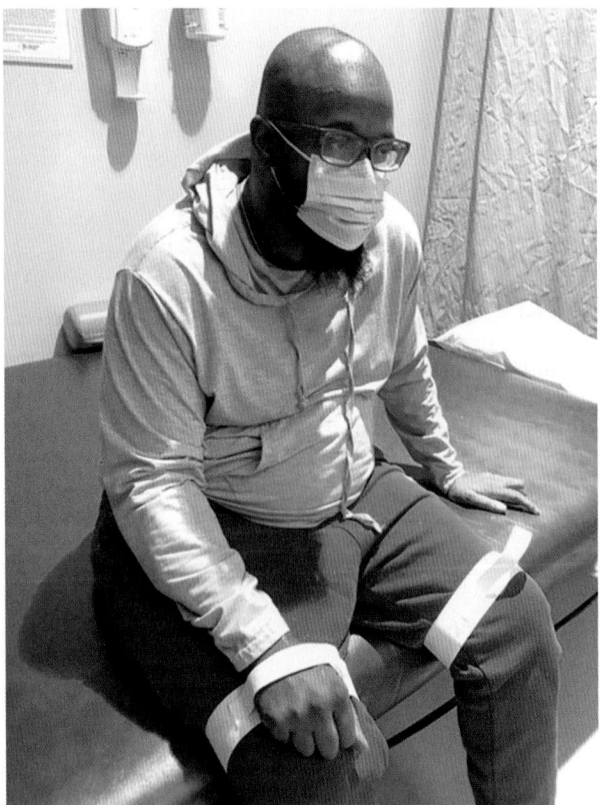

Figure 20.23 Individual with spinal cord injury using leg loops to assist with managing lower extremities during bed mobility.

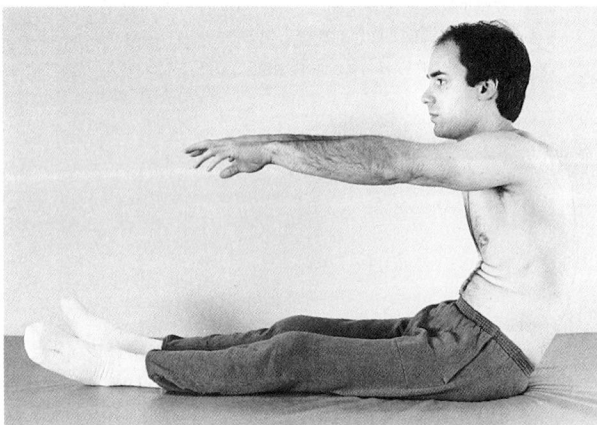

Figure 20.24 Individual with a T4 AIS A injury in long-sitting position.

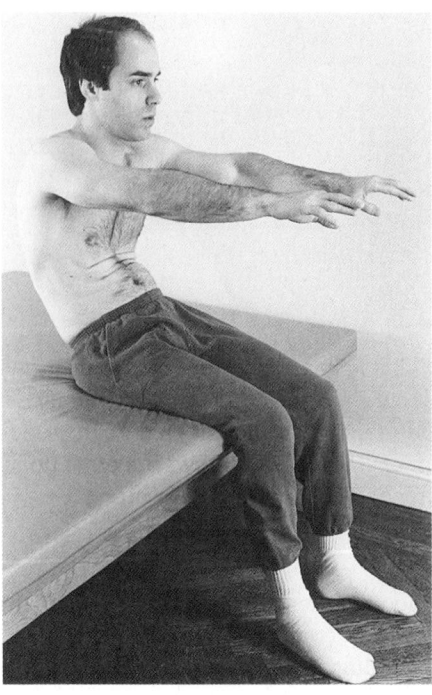

Figure 20.25 Individual with a T4 AIS A injury in short-sitting position.

tendons. Patients who do not have triceps innervation need to learn to keep the elbows extended through muscle substitution. In a closed-chain position, extended elbows combined with shoulder external rotation will assist in maintaining the tripod position. The patient throws back the shoulder into full extension while externally rotating the shoulder and supinating the forearm. When the UE is weight-bearing in this position, the patient can contract the anterior deltoids to flex the shoulder in a closed chain, which will extend the elbow.

- Stability in sitting can be enhanced by providing manual resistance to the upper or lower trunk. Sitting practice should include altering UE support (bilateral, unilateral, with progression to no support). Reaching for objects with one and both UEs can improve anticipatory balance reactions. Patients should also practice maintaining postural control while manipulating objects and performing ADL in sitting.
- Patients should safely learn their new limits of stability. This can be accomplished by weight shifting until the point is reached where balance can no longer be maintained; close supervision/assistance is warranted.
- Unexpected perturbations can be provided in a safe manner to practice reactive postural control.
- Balance interventions should be practiced on a variety of surfaces: firm mat, bed, dense foam, sofa cushion, and so forth. Balance interventions should also be practiced while sitting in the patient's wheelchair.

Transfers
Sit-Pivot Transfers

There are three components to the sit-pivot transfer (e.g., bed to/from wheelchair in a seated position): preparatory phase, lift phase, and descent phase.[240] During the *preparatory phase,* the trunk flexes forward, leans laterally, and rotates toward the trailing arm in order to lead with the hips (see description of head–hips relationship below) (Fig. 20.26A). The *lift phase* starts when the buttocks lift off the sitting surface and continues while the trunk is lifted halfway between the two surfaces (Fig. 20.26B). The *descent phase* denotes the period when the trunk is lowered to the other seating surface, from the halfway point until the buttocks are on the other surface (Fig. 20.26C).

The following are key components and intervention strategies that can be used to improve transfer ability:

- Provide support and assistance so the patient feels safe and comfortable while learning transfers.
- Confidence and skill in maintaining sitting balance is critical (see previously discussed strategies).
- The head–hips relationship is important. Moving the head and upper trunk in one direction causes the lower trunk and buttocks to move in the opposite direction. For example, if the patient wants to transfer from bed to the wheelchair, which is positioned to the patient's right, the patient rocks the head and upper trunk forward/downward and to the left. In combination with protracting the scapulae to lift the buttocks, this will cause the lower trunk and buttocks to lift upward and swing to the right into the wheelchair.
- For patients without innervated triceps, the strategies described can be used to place and maintain the elbows in extension. For patients without full finger function, overstretching the finger flexors as described should be avoided.
- Hand position is important. The hands should be positioned forward of the hips to form a tripod with the buttocks. Greater force is generated in the trailing UE[240,241] (UE farthest from the surface transferring to); if one UE is weaker or more painful, it should be the lead UE. The lead UE should be farther from the trunk/buttocks and the trailing UE closer to the trunk/buttocks.
- Part to whole task training, protracting the scapulae while leaning head and upper trunk forward and down (head–hips relationship) should be practiced to lift the buttocks off the sitting surface. The physical therapist can assist by placing their hands under the patient's hips and assisting the lift or by placing one hand on the front of the chest and the other between the scapulae to guide and assist the forward/downward lean and lift. Practicing the push-up is a key task that may be made easier utilizing push-up blocks to get more clearance, especially for individuals with shorter arm-to-trunk ratios (Fig. 20.27). Part to whole task training should also include lifting the buttocks and shifting laterally to the left and right on the sitting surface. The patient should lean the head/upper trunk forward and downward, then twist to left or right to lift and shift the hips in the opposite direction. Patients may initially lift the hips and then twist the upper trunk to shift the lower trunk and buttocks in the opposite direction in two motions. As the patient improves, these two movements should be performed as a single motion.
- LEs should be positioned with the feet supported and the hips and knees at approximately 90° of flexion or slightly more at the hips. The legs should be midway between the two surfaces so they do not block the movement of the trunk and body toward the transfer surface. A stable position of the

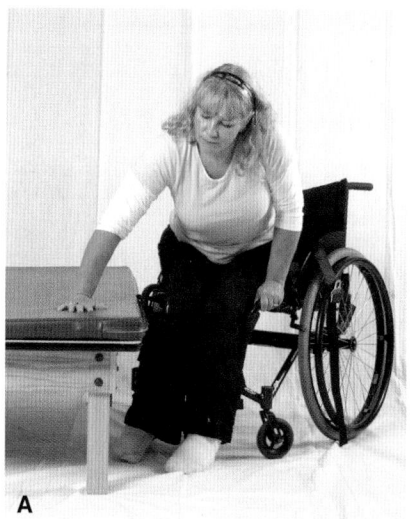 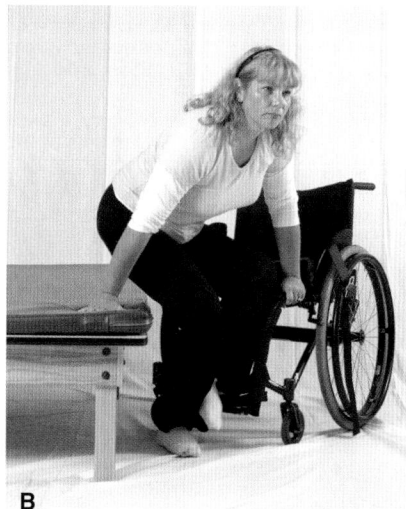 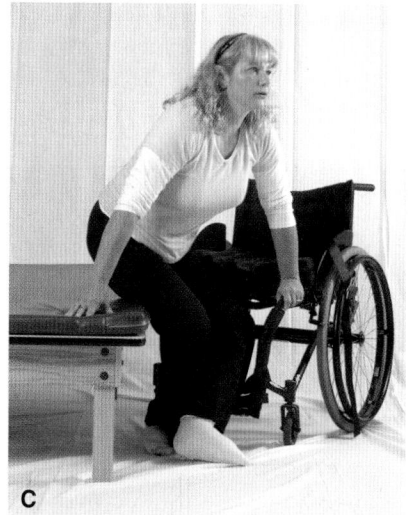

Figure 20.26 (A) Preparatory phase of the transfer; trunk is flexed forward and laterally away from surface transferring to. (B) Lift phase; buttocks are lifted off the seating surface as the trunk rotates. (C) End of the descent phase when the buttocks are on the other sitting surface. *(From O'Sullivan S, Schmitz T. Improving Functional Outcomes in Physical Rehabilitation. F.A. Davis: 2010. With permission.)*

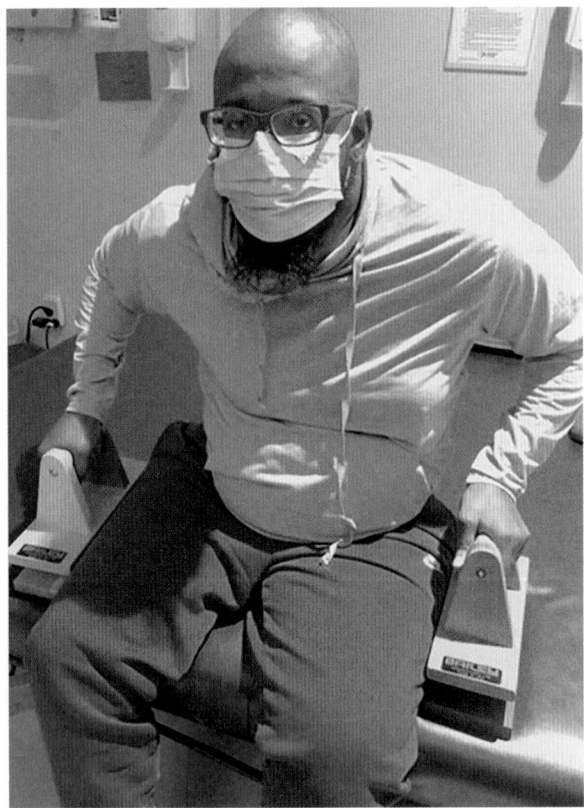

Figure 20.27 Individual with spinal cord injury using push-up blocks while practicing transfers.

feet, even in those without LE motor control, will provide a pivot point and increase stability during the transfer.

- Emphasis should be placed on lifting and shifting laterally instead of sliding/scooting to the side to avoid shearing of the skin. Control of movement should be promoted during the descent phase to avoid trauma to the skin. A transfer board may be used initially until the patient gains more skill with the task. Some patients with midcervical SCI may always require a transfer board.
- Transfer training should include a variety of surfaces from the wheelchair (bed, sofa, toilet, car, and so forth) and to varying heights (higher and lower than the wheelchair surface).

In addition to the task of transferring from one surface to another, there are important complementary skills that patients need to be able to perform to be fully independent with transfers. These include positioning the wheelchair, setting wheel locks, removing and replacing armrests on the wheelchair, removing and replacing leg rests on the wheelchair, managing LEs, and managing body position in the wheelchair.

Floor-to-Wheelchair Transfers

There are several basic floor-to-wheelchair techniques including forward and sideways approaches (Figs. 20.28 A–D, and 20.29 A–C). *Improving Functional Outcomes*

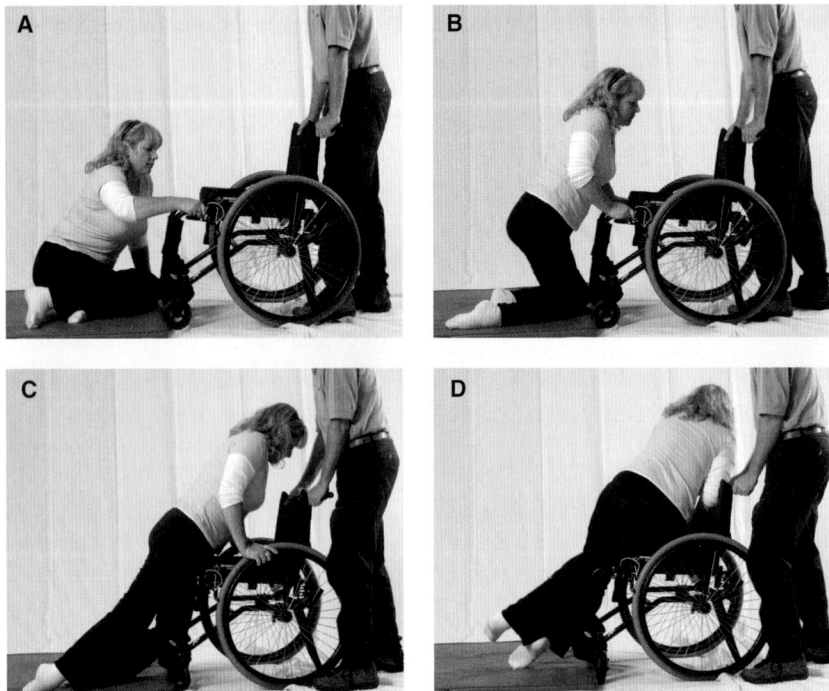

Figure 20.28 (A–D) Floor-to-wheelchair transfer using a frontward approach. *(From O'Sullivan S, Schmitz T. Improving Functional Outcomes in Physical Rehabilitation. F.A. Davis; 2016. With permission.)*

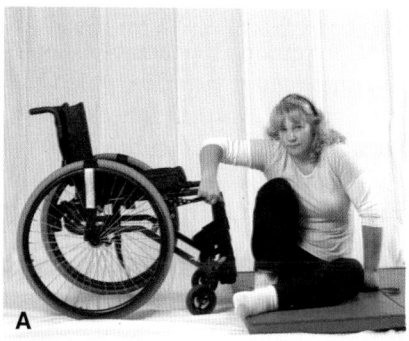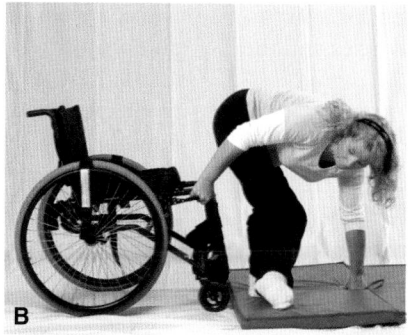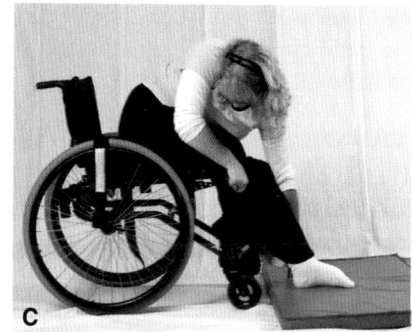

Figure 20.29 (A–C) Floor-to-wheelchair transfer using a sideways approach. *(From O'Sullivan S, Schmitz T.* Improving Functional Outcomes in Physical Rehabilitation. *F.A. Davis; 2016. With permission.)*

in Physical Rehabilitation[242] and *Spinal Cord Injury: Functional Rehabilitation*[138] provide more detail on how to perform these transfers and other interventions to improve transfer ability.

Locomotor Rehabilitation
Wheelchair Skills

For individuals who use a manual wheelchair, the ability to propel and maneuver over and around various obstacles and terrains in their home and community is essential for functional independence. In order to propel a manual wheelchair independently in the home and community environments, patients must be able to perform certain basic wheelchair mobility skills: propelling forward and backward, turning, ascending and descending inclines, assuming and maintaining a wheelie, and propelling on uneven terrain.

PROPULSION ON EVEN SURFACES

To propel the wheelchair forward, the patient reaches back and grasps the wheelchair hand rims (Fig. 20.30), then pushes forward, releasing the hand rims after the hands have passed in front of the hips. Patients should practice reaching far back on the hand rims to initiate the stroke and pushing far forward before releasing the hand rims. A longer pushing stroke is more efficient. Patients who do not have the ability to grasp the hand rims propel the wheelchair by pressing their palms against the lateral aspect of the hand rims and then pushing forward. These patients will often use hand rim projections or have plastic-coated hand rims.

The technique used to turn depends on how quickly the patient needs to turn, as well as the size of the turning radius. To make a large radius or slow turn, the patient just pushes harder with one arm (e.g., if turning to the right, the patient pushes harder with the left arm). To make a tight and/or quick turn, the patient pushes forward with one hand while pulling back with the other (e.g., if turning to the right quickly, the patient pushes forward with the left arm while pulling back with the right arm).

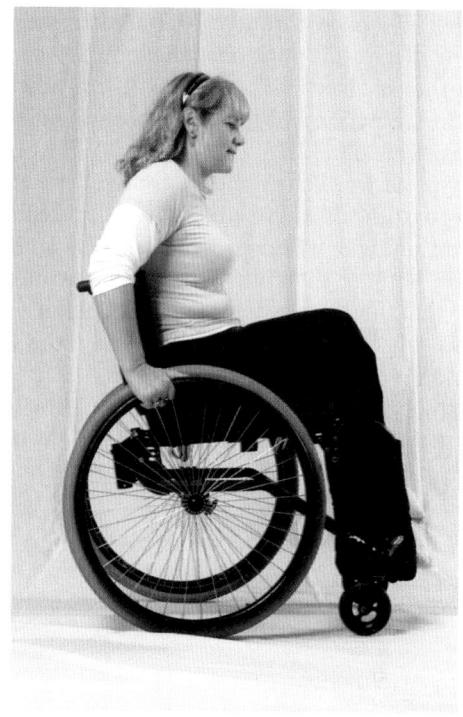

Figure 20.30 Propelling wheelchair forward. *(From O'Sullivan S, Schmitz T.* Improving Functional Outcomes in Physical Rehabilitation. *F.A. Davis; 2016. With permission.)*

ASCENDING AND DESCENDING INCLINES

There are a variety of surfaces with inclines that wheelchair users need to negotiate to be independent in their home and community. These include ramps, curbs, slopes, and hills. The basic techniques used to ascend and descend these inclines are the same. To ascend an incline, the patient takes shorter and quicker strokes and pushes on the hand rims more forcefully. If possible, the patient should lean forward with the head and trunk while pushing forward to prevent the chair from tipping backward.

To control or slow the descent of the wheelchair, grip the hand rim, and slowly release the grip in a controlled manner. Patients without full hand function control the descent of the wheelchair by applying pressure to the hand rims with the palms and slowly releasing the pressure.

ATTAINING AND MAINTAINING WHEELIES

The ability to perform a wheelie (Fig. 20.31) is an essential skill to negotiate curbs, steep declines, uneven terrain, and other areas of the community. To attain a wheelie, the patient reaches back on the hand rim and forcefully pushes forward to lift the front casters off the ground (as if attempting to tip the wheelchair over backward). When first learning any skill that involves a wheelie or if there is a risk of the wheelchair tipping over, the patient should always be closely supervised and guarded. To ensure safety while practicing wheelies, a gait belt is looped through the frame of the wheelchair. The therapist is positioned behind the wheelchair, holding the gait belt in one hand with the other hand placed on the patient's shoulder or push handle of the wheelchair (Fig. 20.32).

The type of wheelchair and its configuration impact how easy or difficult it is to attain a wheelie. Achieving a wheelie in a heavier wheelchair and one with a posterior axle plate is more difficult. An axle that is more forward, so that the user's center of mass is behind the axle, causes the wheelchair to be less stable and more "tippy." This makes it easier to assume a wheelie.

The ability to maintain a wheelie should be learned in conjunction with attaining a wheelie. Both of these skills are important lead-up activities to more advanced wheelie skills such as ascending and descending curbs and propelling over uneven terrain. The therapist should assist the patient into the *balance point* in which the front casters are off the ground with the wheelchair in equilibrium. The patient's hands should lightly grip the hand rim in a position near the hips. Pushing forward on the hand rims causes the chair to tip backward and pulling backward causes the wheelchair to tip forward onto the casters and back into a stable position. The patient should practice lightly pushing and pulling on the hand rim to learn the balance point; the hand rim should slide through the patient's grip as they do this. The patient should not keep the hand firmly grasped at the same point on the hand rim.

When propelling a wheelchair on uneven surfaces (e.g., gravel, grass), there is a possibility of the front casters catching, causing the wheelchair to tip over in a forward direction. Being able to propel the wheelchair forward while maintaining a wheelie can minimize this risk and allow the patient to propel the wheelchair independently over a variety of terrains. When learning to propel the wheelchair forward and backward and while turning in a wheelie position, the patient should be instructed again not to use a firm grip but to allow the hand rims to slide within their grip.

On some uneven surfaces, it may be easier to "pop up" into a wheelie for only a brief time (not maintain the wheelie) and push forward. The patient then crosses

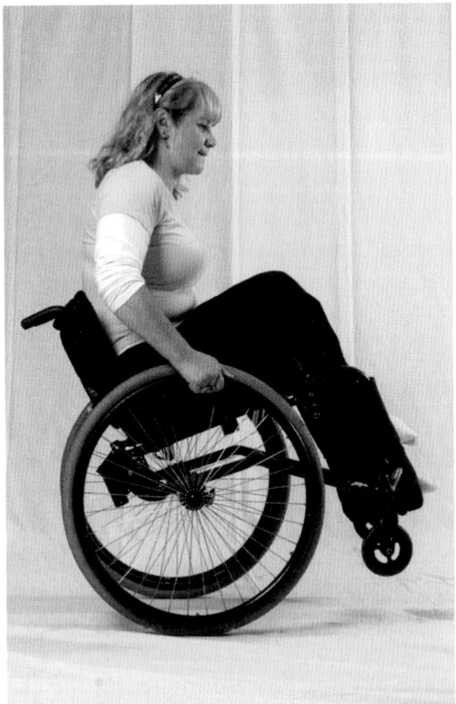

Figure 20.31 Performing a wheelie. *(From O'Sullivan S, Schmitz T. Improving Functional Outcomes in Physical Rehabilitation. F.A. Davis; 2016. With permission.)*

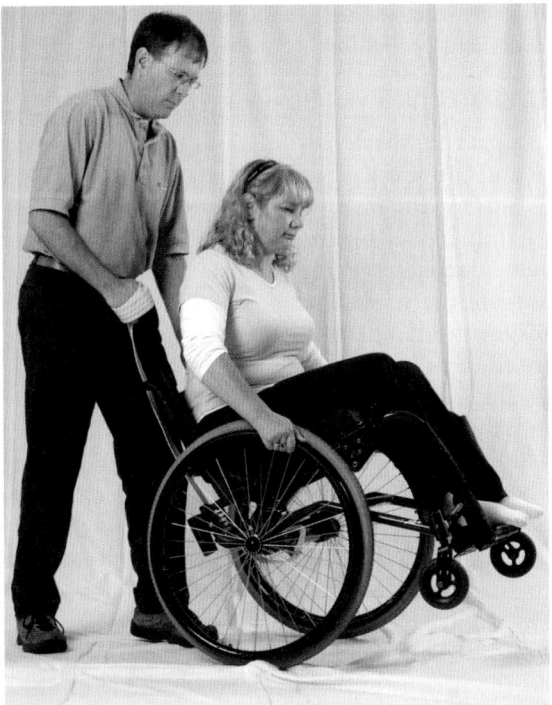

Figure 20.32 Technique to safely spot a patient while practicing performing wheelies. *(From O'Sullivan S, Schmitz T. Improving Functional Outcomes in Physical Rehabilitation. F.A. Davis; 2016. With permission.)*

the surface in a series of short wheelies while pushing forward.

Wheelies are also used to ascend and descend curbs. To ascend a curb while moving, the patient pops a wheelie while moving forward just before reaching the curb. This lifts the front casters so they are up on top of the curb. As the wheels make contact with the curb, the patient pushes forward on the hand rims and leans the head and trunk forward (Fig. 20.33A–C). To descend a curb, the patient pushes the wheelchair forward, and just as the casters approach the edge of the curb, the patient pops a wheelie. The wheelie is maintained as momentum carries the back wheels off the curb. The patient maintains the wheelie so the back wheels land first; then the casters land (Fig. 20.34A–C).

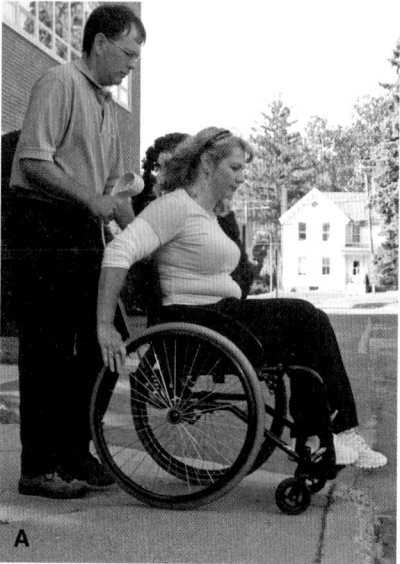

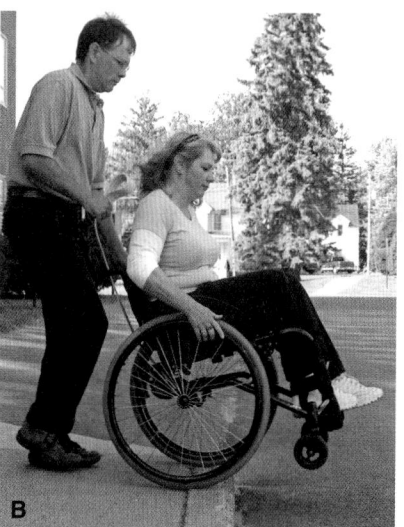

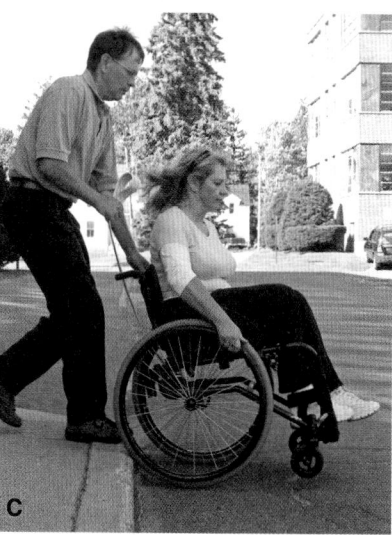

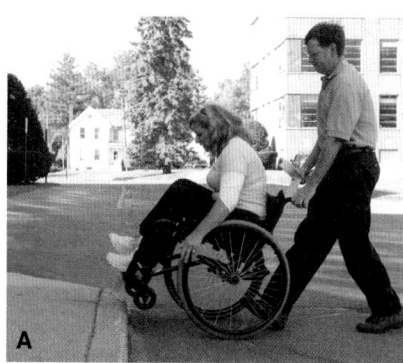

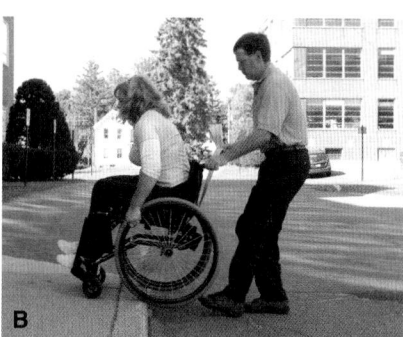

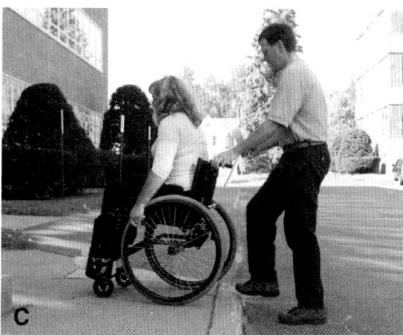

Figure 20.33 (A–C) Ascending a curb in a wheelie. *(From O'Sullivan S, Schmitz T. Improving Functional Outcomes in Physical Rehabilitation. F.A. Davis; 2016. With permission.)*

Figure 20.34 (A–C) Descending a curb in a wheelie. *(From O'Sullivan S, Schmitz T. Improving Functional Outcomes in Physical Rehabilitation. F.A. Davis; 2010. With permission.)*

Other wheelchair skills that patients should learn include turning in place, turning while moving, falling from a wheelchair, picking up objects off the floor, opening and closing doors, and negotiating obstacles. Patients should also learn how to manage the parts of the wheelchair: putting wheel locks on and off, removing and returning leg rests, folding the wheelchair, removing the cushion, moving armrests, and removing and putting the wheels back on.

POWER WHEELCHAIR DRIVING TASKS

Individuals who require a power wheelchair for their mobility needs also will need training in specific mobility skills using a power wheelchair. In addition to learning how to perform some of the skills listed earlier such as moving forward and backward, negotiating inclines and obstacles, turning in place and while moving, and maneuvering on uneven/soft surfaces, individuals that use a power wheelchair will also need to learn how to operate the controller and the ability of the seating system to position the body (i.e., pressure relief using a tilt-in-space seating system).

In addition to the Wheelchair Skills Test described earlier, Kirby and colleagues developed the *Wheelchair Skills Training Program*. Based on the skills of the Wheelchair Skills Test and principles of motor learning, the Wheelchair Skills Training Program was designed to improve manual wheelchair user performance and safety, and it is a safe and effective training method for new wheelchair users, community-based wheelchair users, and care partners. The Wheelchair Skills Test and Wheelchair Skills Training Program are available at https://wheelchairskillsprogram.ca. This website provides details on how to perform the Wheelchair Skills Test and has videos demonstrating how to perform the different skills. *Spinal Cord Injury: Functional Rehabilitation*[138] and *Improving Functional Outcomes in Physical Rehabilitation*[243] are other resources that provide more detail on interventions to improve the previously mentioned and other wheelchair skills.

Gait/Walking Skills

Regaining the ability to walk is a common goal for most individuals following SCI. Several factors will influence the success or failure in attaining this goal. Patients must possess adequate muscle strength, postural alignment, postural control, ROM, and sufficient cardiovascular endurance to become functional ambulators. Becoming a functional ambulator following a complete SCI is very difficult. Walking with orthoses and assistive devices is slower and requires considerably more energy than walking before the injury. Many individuals with motor complete SCI who learn to walk with these devices may not continue walking once they stop rehabilitation. Patients with motor iSCI (AIS C and D) are more likely to regain functional ambulation skills than those with complete or sensory incomplete injuries.

This section on strategies to improve walking function is divided into two sections. The first deals with gait retraining using a compensatory-based approach for people with motor complete SCI. This compensatory approach utilizes bracing, assistive devices, and new strategies to achieve walking, and relying exclusively on compensatory strategies often does not result in functional locomotion. The second section highlights a recovery and activity-based approach for people with motor iSCI that aims to recruit multiple aspects of the neuromotor system to promote functional recovery of walking.

COMPENSATORY-BASED APPROACH

When initiating a program to improve locomotor function for individuals with complete SCI, therapists should be realistic and provide a clear picture of the costs and potential benefits. Patients who wish to relearn to ambulate following SCI should be given this option even if their potential for functional ambulation is limited. Although some patients may not become functional ambulators, standing alone may provide other important benefits such as improved circulation, skin integrity, bowel and bladder function, sleep, and a sense of well-being.[244]

Individuals with complete SCI rely on orthotic and assistive devices, adequate ROM, and maximizing strength of neurologically intact musculature for standing and walking. Full ROM in hip extension is essential in attaining balance in the upright position. The patient learns to lean into the anterior ligaments of the hip with the trunk extended to stabilize the trunk and pelvis (often referred to as the "parastance" position). The absence of knee flexion and plantarflexion contractures is also important in attaining upright standing balance.

Adequate cardiovascular endurance also is a criterion for functional ambulation. Because the energy cost of ambulation for a patient with complete paraplegia is higher than it is for people without SCI, endurance becomes an important factor in determining success or failure and continued ambulation once rehabilitation is complete. In addition, the energetic cost (oxygen utilization per unit distance) of walking with braces and compensatory strategies is very high compared to normal ambulation.[245]

Other factors that may restrict ambulation include severe spasticity, loss of proprioception (particularly at the hips and knees), pain, obesity, and the presence of secondary complications such as pressure injuries, heterotopic bone formation at the hips, or deformity. In addition, the patient's motivation plays a key role in determining success or failure in ambulation. A highly motivated patient can learn to walk using hip-knee-ankle-foot orthoses (HKAFOs) or knee-ankle-foot orthoses (KAFOs) and assistive devices. However, these patients often find that the energy cost of ambulation is too great.

Follow-up studies of long-term continuation of ambulation have not been extensive. Mikelberg and Reid[246] surveyed 60 individuals with SCI for whom orthotics had been prescribed. From this group, 60% used their wheelchairs as the primary means of mobility. Thirty-one percent completely discarded their orthoses. Those who did use their orthoses reserved them primarily for standing and exercise activities. It was reported as early as 1973 that functional ambulation required knee control in at least one leg,[203] and there are little data to suggest that individuals with SCI become long-term functional ambulators using bilateral HKAFOs or KAFOs.

For patients with complete SCI, training emphasis is on strengthening available musculature; using assistive devices and orthoses to support weak or denervated muscles; and learning new, compensatory methods of walking. Forearm crutches are most often selected for patients with paraplegia. These crutches provide several advantages. They are lightweight; they allow use of the hand without the crutch becoming disengaged; they fit more easily into an automobile; and, most important, they improve function in ambulation and stair climbing by allowing full hip extension and unrestricted movement at the shoulders. See Chapter 30, Orthotics, which provides a detailed discussion of different types of orthoses.

Swing-through (Fig. 20.35) and four-point gait patterns are two common walking patterns learned by patients with complete SCI using HKAFOs and KAFOs. Initial standing balance and gait training should be done in the parallel bars and then progressed to the appropriate assistive device when the patient is ready. Relevant training activities include those described next.

Performed in Sitting or Supine

- *Putting on and removing orthoses.* The patient is first taught the correct way to don and doff the orthoses. The patient must be cautioned to continuously monitor skin for pressure areas, particularly after brace removal.

Performed in Parallel Bars

- *Sit-to-stand activities.* These activities should be practiced using a wheelchair, then progressed to using the forearm crutches. The patient must learn to slide to the edge of the chair and unlock and lock the orthoses. Initially the patient is taught to pull to standing, using the parallel bars. A progression is made to using the wheelchair armrests to push to standing. This progression should be accomplished as quickly as possible to avoid dependence on the pulling mechanism. Once in an upright position, the patient pushes down on the hands and tilts the pelvis forward in front of the shoulders. Return to sitting is a reversal of this procedure. To begin this activity with crutches, the patient first places the crutches behind the chair, leaning against the push handle(s). To assume a standing position with crutches, the patient moves forward in the chair, locks both knee joints, crosses one leg over the other, and then rotates the trunk and pelvis (Fig. 20.36). Hand placements on the armrest are reversed, and the patient pushes to standing by pivoting around to face the chair. The reverse of this technique is used to return to the chair.
- *Static standing balance.* The patient learns to balance in standing with the hips in hyperextension and the upper trunk, head, feet, and arms behind the pelvis. The feet are approximately 6 in. apart. The patient should first practice maintaining this position with both hands on the parallel bars then progress to balancing with one hand off the parallel bars and finally with both hands off the bars. The greater the amount of dorsiflexion at the ankle, the more anterior the pelvis can be.
- *Weight shifting in standing.* This entails controlling the pelvic position using UE support and positioning the head and shoulders forward ahead of the pelvis. The head–hips relationship applied in transfers

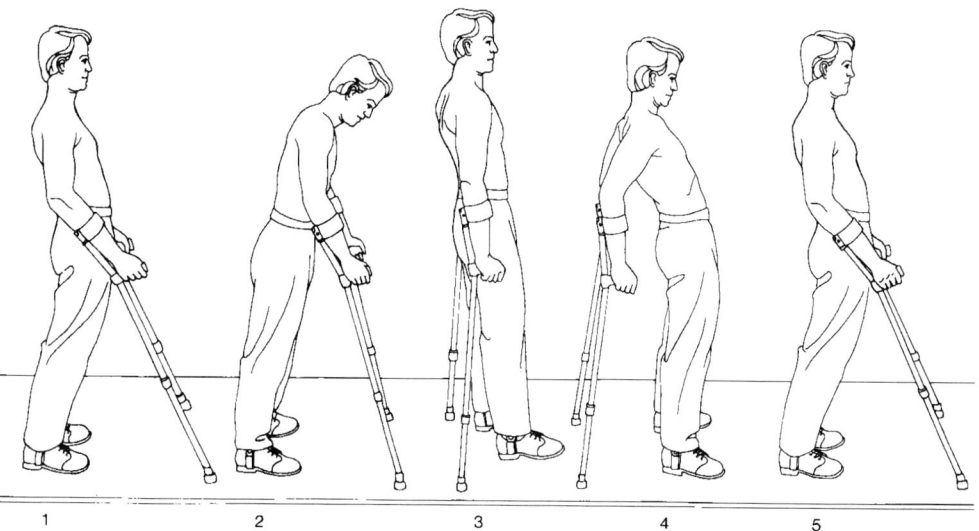

Figure 20.35 Swing-through gait pattern.

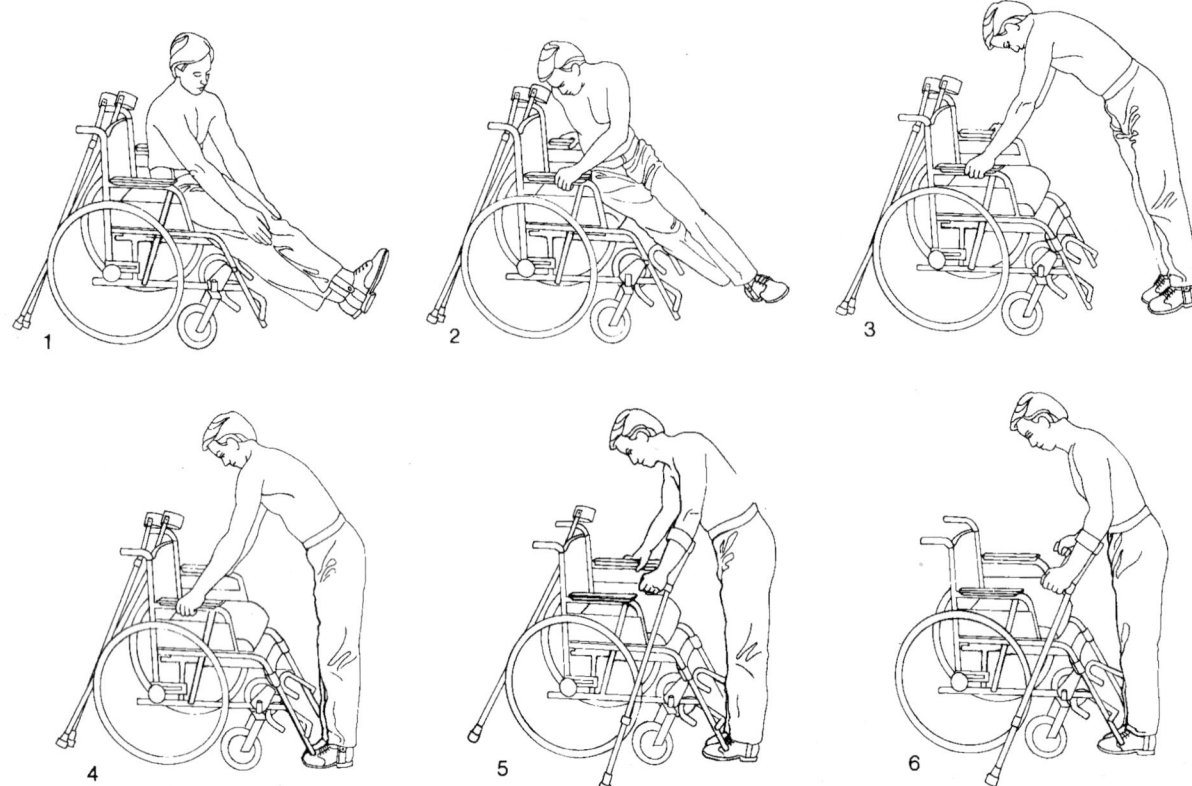

Figure 20.36 Standing from wheelchair using forearm crutches and knee-ankle-foot orthoses. The reverse sequence is used to return to sitting in the wheelchair.

also applies in standing. The patient must be taught recovery to overcome and/or to prevent jackknifing from happening during ambulation. Jackknifing occurs when the patient's COM falls anterior to the hips causing the patient to flex forward suddenly.

- *Push-ups.* This includes lifting the body off the floor using elbow extension and scapulae depression and protraction, tucking the head to gain added height, and controlled lowering of the body.

Performed in Parallel Bars Progressed to Overground

- *Swing-through pattern.* From a balanced standing position with the hands posterior to the pelvis, the patient moves the hands forward causing the trunk to flex. Then the patient lifts by extending the elbows and protracting/depressing the scapula and tucking the head. Gravity will cause the trunk and legs to swing forward. When the heels strike the ground, the patient quickly extends the upper trunk and head and pushes the pelvis forward to come back to the starting position (see Fig. 20.35).
- *Four-point pattern.* This gait pattern is slower but safer than a swing-through pattern; three points are always in contact with the ground, as opposed to a swing-through pattern, in which there are times when only two points are in contact with the ground. From a standing position with the

pelvis forward, both feet on the ground, and hands posterior to the pelvis, one hand/crutch is lifted and placed forward. Weight is shifted away from the contralateral LE so it can swing forward as the hip is hiked and the head is moved down and away from the swing leg. This unweighting and hip hiking allows gravity to assist the forward swing. This process is repeated on the opposite side.

FUNCTIONAL, RECOVERY-BASED APPROACH

The past several decades have seen a huge rise in the number and types of interventions geared toward the promotion of recovery of walking function. This functional, recovery-based approach is a product of translational research that emerged from animal models of the neural control of locomotion. This approach minimizes the use of orthotic and/or assistive devices while utilizing the neuromotor system's ability to interpret sensory input in order to modulate motor output. Knowledge gained by basic science researchers concerning the neurobiological control of walking laid the foundation for developing therapeutic interventions with application to human, clinical populations. Principles that emerged from this literature to promote the intrinsic ability of the nervous system to control rhythmical movement patterns and modulate sensory input into task-specific motor output include the following:

- The legs are maximally loaded for weight-bearing, minimizing, or eliminating loading of the arms.
- Sensory cues provided are consistent with the task of walking (e.g., treadmill speed, manual cues to facilitate flexor or extensor muscle activation).
- The posture, trunk, pelvis, and limb kinematics are coordinated and specific to the task of walking.
- Compensatory strategies for movement (i.e., hip hiking) are minimized or eliminated with recovery of preinjury movement patterns as the goal.[123,247]

The utilization of these principles should not in any way imply that compensatory strategies are to be avoided: in fact, many of the examples of recovery-based strategies utilize assistive devices in the least restrictive fashion.[248,249] As demonstrated in Figure 20.37, the goal is not to eliminate compensatory strategies from the recovery continuum but rather to facilitate potential recovery before "filling in the gap" between functional capacity and functional requirements for independent walking.

Given the interest in functional, recovery-based approaches and the developing research in this area, a relative paucity of randomized clinical trials is available to help guide clinical decision-making. In a recent Clinical Practice Guideline for improving walking speed and timed walking distances after chronic neurological injury (greater than 6 months after SCI, stroke, and TBI), the primary findings were strong recommendations for moderate- to high-intensity training (targeting 60% to 80% of HR reserve or 70% to 85% of maximum HR)[250] and virtual reality (VR)–based interventions (although most of the VR literature involves stroke recovery and not SCI).[251] Weaker evidence exists for utilizing strengthening interventions for the purpose of increasing speed and endurance.[251–253] The guidelines further demonstrate strong evidence against BWS treadmill training, robotic training, or sitting/standing balance training without virtual reality for the purposes of increased walking speed or timed distances.[251] However, as noted earlier, many of these interventions aim to improve motor control, cardiac conditioning, effector strength, or additional mechanisms of impaired walking other than speed or endurance limitations.[254] Additionally, the majority of evidence supporting these recommendations are from studies with people with chronic stroke.

The Academy of Neurologic Physical Therapy (ANPT) has developed online resources guided by the findings of the Clinical Practice Guideline to Improve Locomotor Function following Chronic Stroke, Incomplete Spinal Cord Injury and Brain Injury to support physical therapists as they implement walking interventions at a moderate- to high-intensity level. These are available at the ANPT website (https://www.neuropt.org/practice-resources/best-practice-initiatives-and-resources/intensity_matters). Additionally, ANPT developed video cases that highlight different interventions delivered at a high to moderate intensity with people with various neurological health conditions, including SCI. These are available at the ANPT YouTube site (https://www.youtube.com/playlist?list=PLH8hBAd9u40lSIGbP9s3dz2BiveybZKW7).

Even less evidence exists in the subacute populations (less than 6 months post-SCI). The majority of these investigations assess robot-assisted gait training (RAGT) either with stationary devices (such as the Lokomat) or with mobile devices such as robotic exoskeletons[255–260] with no clear evidence of superiority of RAGT over traditional walking rehabilitation or manually assisted BWS treadmill training. High-intensity training is sparse in the acute population due to the difficulty in delivery with early reports showing no difference when compared to moderated-intensity training and conventional rehabilitation.[261]

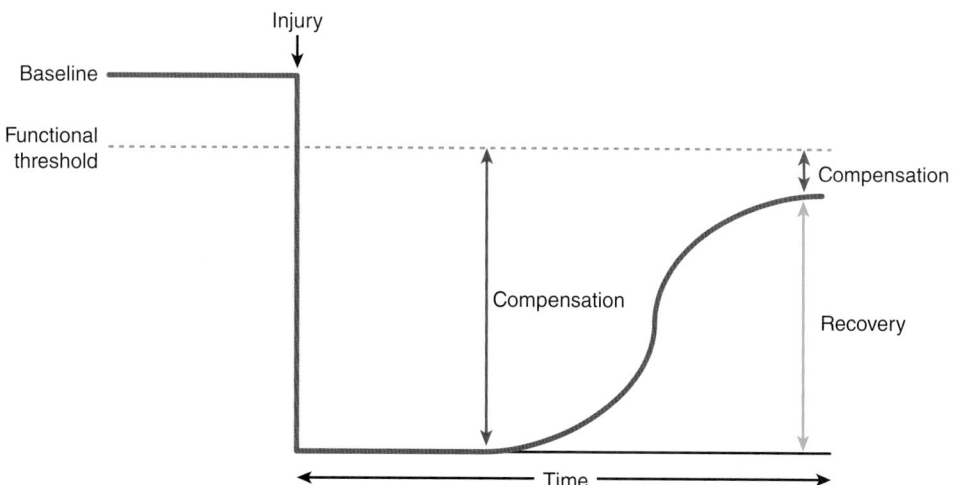

Figure 20.37 The relationship between recovery, compensation, time, and functional threshold.

TECHNOLOGIES TO ENHANCE WALKING RECOVERY

Robotic devices are a form of neuroprosthetic devices that can be used during walking training to move the LEs in a stepping pattern to promote recovery of walking ability.[262] Exoskeleton robots allow people with complete SCI to walk overground with assistance from the robot.[263] In 2014, the U.S. Food and Drug Administration approved the use of robotic exoskeletons for use in the home and community. These devices range from those that provide full movement support at the hip and knee (e.g., ReWalk, Berkley Bionics eLEGS, and Indego) to those that require at least some movement to engage locking and unlocking mechanisms at the knee (OttoBock E-MAG). The devices range in weight from approximately 20 lb to over 200 lb and may be used by individuals up to 6 ft 4 in. in height. While the devices are expensive and are currently not covered by most third-party payers, the technology is progressing rapidly and may provide more full-time walking assistance for some individuals with SCI.

Neurostimulation techniques when combined with activity-based walking interventions may also hold promise to improve walking function in people with SCI. Harkema and colleagues[125] combined epidural spinal electrical stimulation with locomotor training on a TM with BWS and stand training in an individual with a chronic AIS B C7 injury. After training, the individual was able to stand with full LE weight-bearing requiring assistance only for balance and voluntarily activate some LE muscles when the stimulator was on. The authors speculate that this combination therapy (epidural electrical stimulation with task-specific locomotor and stand training) may be a viable method to improve function after SCI. Research is currently under way to translate these invasive stimulation techniques to non-invasive direct current stimulation, both at the level of the brain and directly to the spinal cord.[264,265]

FES to cause the contraction of paralyzed or weak muscles below the level of the lesion for exercise, walking, and functional use of the UEs can also be used. As discussed earlier, surface FES can be used with an LE ergometer as a method of cardiovascular training.[239,266] Surface FES can also be applied to LEs to allow standing and walking in people with SCI.[267] Surface electromyography (EMG) has been paired with FES to provide patients with a method of triggering the FES to produce a more normal walking pattern than FES alone.[268] Implanted FES systems allow people with SCI to stand and walk[269] as well as those with high cervical SCI to use their hand to grasp and manipulate objects.[270] Implanted FES systems can also be used for phrenic nerve stimulation to allow patients with high cervical SCI to breathe without a ventilator[271] and to provide patients with bladder control.[272,273]

In the absence of clear evidence for interventions with proven efficacy to improve walking function, therapists often must define their own treatment protocols based on the best available evidence and the presentation/goals of the patient. The functional, recovery-based training principles presented earlier are not dependent on clinical modalities (i.e., TM and/or BWS system) but should be utilized overground in the clinic, home, and community. When possible, these principles should be incorporated with high-intensity training that is dosed on either HR or RPE. Adaptations can be made for advancing skills in any environment and should be consistent with training principles. For example, a rolling walker may permit a faster walking speed initially; however, training with the earlier principles may facilitate improved activation of leg muscles in an activity-dependent manner, even while temporarily decreasing speed. The long-term goal of this strategy is to maximize walking outcomes with a less restrictive device allowing for more independence in complex environments such as stairs and uneven terrain. Certainly, use of clinical modalities such as BWS and/or treadmills has advantages (such as optimizing posture, limiting falls during training, and increasing the number of steps taken during a treatment session) and may be the optimal environment for consistent practice and retraining the neuromuscular system, but the transition and application to community ambulation are critical. Modifying the parameters of training in both permissive (training-specific) and overground community environments will challenge the use of new skills, reinforce new patterns and independence, and inform goal setting across environments.

Engaging the client in each aspect of goal setting and understanding of the therapy principles empowers the client to extend "training" beyond the time in the clinic to the rest of the day. The choices that the therapist and client make daily may significantly affect the rate and magnitude of the client's recovery and achievement of goals. For instance, a client's choice to walk using a grocery cart instead of shopping from a wheelchair reinforces the principle of maximizing weight-bearing through the LE and provides greater opportunity to practice walking. Similarly, setting the assistive device higher than normally prescribed will decrease the ability to bear excessive weight through the UEs and promote a more upright posture. If the individual walks with an upright posture, the goal is further enhanced with increased load bearing on the LE versus the arms and achievement of hip extension during loading. This simple choice will advance the individual's recovery. Many more choices can be made by the client to support recovery regardless of where one is on a continuum of recovery.

An important area for future research is the benefits of walking rehabilitation to a person's health after SCI, whether an incomplete or a complete injury. Additional questions that need to be answered include the following: Does walking rehabilitation decrease the risk of pressure injuries or bladder infections; reduce bone loss or muscle atrophy? Do benefits for health warrant increased access to walking rehabilitation? Can robotic devices provide an avenue to cost-effectively provide this service? What is the impact of walking outcomes on the QOL of the person with SCI and the impact on the family or care partner(s)?

Guidance for walking rehabilitation after SCI and for safe and effective use of therapeutic equipment is essential to the practice of evidence-based physical therapy following SCI. As research findings are published, clinicians should seek information to guide their decision-making and practice. Such future research may identify the following:

- When is the best time after injury to provide an intervention for optimal recovery of walking—in the acute stage of rehabilitation, after discharge from rehabilitation, or at some other point after SCI (and if so, what is the appropriate time after injury)?
- Will early engagement of recovery-based walking limit the onset of maladaptive plasticity observed in the chronic phases of other neurological conditions?[274]
- What is the optimal dose of therapy (i.e., intensity, frequency, and duration of the training)?
- How is a patient trained and progressed? How is new training equipment examined as it reaches the market (e.g., suspension systems, robotic devices)? How are the trainers' body ergonomics monitored during training?
- Are there any medical precautions and safety issues for persons with SCI, and what are their effects on walking rehabilitation (e.g., AD, skin, bowel and bladder, falling, osteoporosis, spasticity, cardiovascular health)?
- What therapies may augment recovery, or what combined therapies enhance the recovery of walking (e.g., strengthening, FES)?[126]

Activity-Directed Upper Extremity Training

For people with a cervical SCI, the recovery of UE function is a primary goal.[275] Interventions aimed at improving functional use of the UE have primarily been compensatory in nature. For example, patients with active wrist extension are taught how to manipulate and pick up objects using a tenodesis grasp, use the hand as a hook, and use different types of orthoses to feed themselves. Some patients with cervical SCI may choose surgical interventions such as nerve or tendon transfer or implanted neuroprosthetics, although the focus after surgery remains activity-based training to improve function. Surgery options require prolonged immobilization and limit extremity use postsurgery which may not be feasible for individuals.[276,277] Researchers continue to explore interventions to promote UE functional recovery and corticomotor and spinal

reorganization.[278–281] Evidence suggests both unimanual and bimanual massed practice may help improve upper limb function, especially when combined with electric stimulation.[282] Improvements in hand function have been shown both with repetitive transcranial magnetic stimulation (rTMS) to corticomotor areas with repetitive task practice[283] and with transcutaneous spinal cord stimulation.[284] Optimal dosing of UE interventions has not been determined, and compared to extensive research for high-intensity task-specific training for the UE with stroke, evidence is limited with SCI.[285]

Activity-directed interventions for both gross motor function (dressing, washing, bathing, wheelchair propulsion) and fine motor function (grooming, feeding, buttoning, zipping) target improvements in performance of functional activities.[286] Robotic-assisted UE rehabilitation has been shown to be safe and feasible, but effectiveness has been inconclusive compared to conventional rehabilitation.[287] Current evidence for VR interventions directed at UE motor function is limited, but early research showed comparative results to conventional therapy, with improved motivation and adherence with VR.[288]

Preservation of UE function is critical. Education regarding overuse and mechanics for transfers and wheelchair propulsion may help to reduce the risk.[289] Particular exercises to maintain strength in all major shoulder muscle groups and overall glenohumeral and pectoral muscle flexibility are important long-term concepts to counteract common mechanical imbalances that may occur.[289]

■ WHEELCHAIR AND SEATING SYSTEM

Many people with SCI will use a wheelchair as their primary means of mobility. A wheelchair acts as a mobility base and serves to provide postural support. Because patients with SCI will have varying degrees of trunk, hip, and shoulder girdle paralysis, the wheelchair and accompanying seating system provide postural support to keep the pelvis, spine, and extremities in optimal alignment. Postural alignment affects a variety of areas, including respiration, bowel and bladder function, skin integrity, and mobility. Poor posture in the wheelchair can negatively affect all these areas. Because most patients will be using a wheelchair exclusively, it should be custom ordered (prescribed) for each individual. When prescribing a wheelchair, consideration should be given to the patient's goals and characteristics as well as the activities and environment in which it will be used.

The first choice is between a power and manual wheelchair. Generally, individuals with intact triceps function can independently propel a manual wheelchair. Individuals with a C6- or C5-level injury may also be able to independently propel a manual wheelchair but may not have the endurance or strength for community wheelchair mobility. The selection of a manual or power wheelchair in these cases should be done on an individual basis. Individuals with higher cervical injuries generally rely on a power wheelchair for their mobility needs (see Table 20.5). Before prescribing a wheelchair, a series of trials with different types of chairs with different components will assist with making an informed decision on what specific type of wheelchair to obtain.

There are two basic frames for manual wheelchairs—a *folding* or a *rigid* frame—and three weights (standard, lightweight, and ultralight). Folding chairs are an important consideration for patients who plan to transfer into a car because they can be folded compactly for storage without having to remove as many parts as possible. Folding frames typically incorporate a below-seat crossbar and generally provide a smoother ride on uneven surfaces. Potential drawbacks include heavier and more moveable parts, causing it to be less energy efficient during propulsion than rigid frames.

A rigid frame is generally lighter, is more energy efficient, and often has an adjustable seat-to-back angle. This type of frame may be more difficult to store in a car. Both wheels must be removed for storage. A rigid frame is often more durable than a folding frame.

A variety of different components and options can be selected for a manual wheelchair. There are benefits and drawbacks to the different options. For example, the wheel locks can be mounted high or low on some wheelchair frames. High-mounted wheel locks are easier to access but can be an obstacle to transfers. Conversely, low-mounted wheel locks are more difficult to access but are not in the way of transfers or during propulsion.

Power wheelchairs are indicated for all patients with C4 lesions and above. Patients with C5-level lesions may also elect to use power wheelchairs, particularly for community mobility. A tilt-in-space or reclining seating system provides improved postural control and allows the user to independently perform pressure relief. There are various types of controls, ranging from a hand-operated joystick to a sip-and-puff control.

Some patients may require more than one wheelchair. Many lightweight "everyday" chairs are not suitable for sport and recreational activities. Depending on the interests of the patient, a second chair specifically designed for a particular sport such as tennis or racing may be desired. Chapter 32, Seating and Wheeled Mobility, provides detail on the wheelchair and seating evaluation, drawbacks, and benefits of different wheelchair components, seating systems, and a variety of other issues associated with selecting a wheelchair and seating system.

■ HEALTH, WELLNESS, AND PREVENTION

Individuals with SCI experience a number of long-term consequences, including changes in activities, participation, and QOL (as mentioned previously), health, and longevity. These outcomes are interrelated and are associated with numerous protective and risk factors, including demographic, injury, socioenvironmental characteristics, psychological, and behavioral factors. One long-term goal of health and rehabilitation research and practice is to optimize the health and well-being of those living with chronic SCI and ultimately promote longevity by targeting these potentially preventable or modifiable factors.

High incidence and prevalence of secondary health conditions (SHCs) and chronic health conditions (CHCs) are observed among those with long-standing SCI.[290–293] SHCs are generally defined as physical and psychological health conditions that are causally related to the disability.[294] Though the conceptualization of SHC varies,[291,295] they include pathologies, impairments, and functional limitations that arise *after* the disability (either directly or indirectly), and they may be acute, recurrent, or persistent. Common SHCs include pain, spasticity, neurogenic bladder, pressure injuries, infections (including UTIs and septicemia), and fractures. CHCs in comparison are characterized as progressing slowly and lasting for an extended period (greater than 12 months); they may include preexisting conditions. Although CHCs are not specific to a disability, having an SCI increases the risk of experiencing conditions that are generally associated with the aging process, including heart disease, hypertension, diabetes, and cancer.[296–299] SHCs and CHCs may limit daily activities and participation and decrease QOL.[300] Additionally, the presence of these conditions may hinder rehabilitation progress or outcomes, necessitate continued medical management and increase health-care utilization (including hospitalizations and emergency department utilization),[301–306] and increase the risk of mortality.[301,307–309]

Exercise to Prevent Chronic Health Conditions and Treat Secondary Health Conditions

Aerobic exercise training is an established treatment approach for combating many of the CHCs common following SCI (e.g., cardiovascular disease, hypertension, diabetes, obesity). In addition, aerobic exercise is effective for treating conditions less commonly recognized as responsive to exercise therapy but frequent in individuals following SCI (i.e., depression, cognitive decline, and certain cancers). Importantly, properly designed aerobic exercise training in individuals following SCI can also significantly improve functional performance and QOL. Although the goals for and prescription of aerobic exercise training do not differ substantially for individuals following SCI (versus able-bodied individuals), exercise options can be limited as is access to facilities and appropriate support personnel. For example, LE aerobic exercises such as treadmill walking/running or cycling are not easily accomplished after SCI, even in those with motor incomplete injuries (e.g., AIS C or D). UE cycling (arm or wheelchair ergometry) is common in individuals with SCI to achieve requisite intensities of exercise known to result in benefits to health and function. Other modes of aerobic exercise include FES-assisted cycling or rowing or walking on a treadmill (with or without the use of robotics), though these forms of exercise require specialized equipment and may not be readily available to all individuals with SCI. Whatever the type of exercise performed, recommendations are for 20 to 40 minutes of moderate to vigorous activity performed at least two to three times per week. Although the benefits of regular aerobic exercise are substantial, it should be noted that exercise in individuals with SCI comes with some unique risks such as the potential for AD, joint contractures, as well as limited thermoregulatory function in those with higher levels of injury. However, with proper attention given to risk mitigation, the benefits of aerobic exercise in individuals following SCI are substantial, and aerobic exercise should be a primary component of daily life.

One model developed by Krause et al.,[310,311] the Theoretical Risk and Prevention Model, was developed to categorize and order multiple sets of risk and protective factors for health outcomes, and the ultimate health outcome—mortality (Fig. 20.38). The model presents a sequence of factors and, importantly, identifies points for intervention or prevention strategies (represented as arrows), with earlier points in the model preferred for prevention rather than treatment. Consider pressure injuries as an example. They are related to sensory and motor impairments as well as mobility limitations.

However, they are also related to a number of behavioral risk (e.g., smoking, medication use and misuse) and protective factors (e.g., healthy lifestyle, exercise, diet, fitness level, increased hours out of bed, and days out of house).[312–316] With appropriate attention and prevention efforts, including focus on health maintenance behaviors and proper equipment, pressure injuries may be avoided.[317–323] Prevention is highly important due to their high cost[324] and effect on overall health, QOL, health-care utilization, and longevity.[309,325–328]

Related to the management of SHCs and/or CHCs (and often multimorbidity), individuals with chronic SCI are at increased risk of treatment with high-risk medications (e.g., opioids, benzodiazepines)[329–331] and polypharmacy (using multiple medications), posing a unique risk for medication errors and misuse[332–336] and adverse health outcomes including overdose, hospitalization, and death.[337–339] Furthermore, polypharmacy and high-risk medication use may impact rehabilitation goals, community participation, and employment outcomes.[340] Interventions or therapies to address conditions such as pain and spasticity that are often treated with high-risk medications may ultimately prove beneficial in reducing the risks related to medication use.

As mentioned, health conditions increase the risk of costly hospitalizations and emergency department visits. Many of the leading causes of utilization (SHC and CHC) are potentially preventable,[301,306] and many risk factors are modifiable,[303,305,341,342] presenting unique opportunities for intervention. Interestingly, differences in utilization are observed by ambulatory ability, and walking independently is associated with fewer hospitalizations, suggesting a valuable role for rehabilitation professionals.

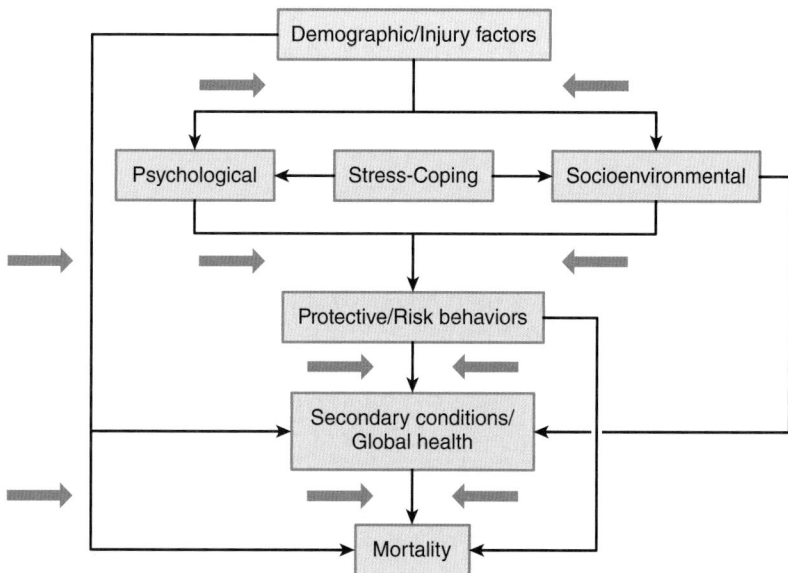

Figure 20.38 Theoretical Risk and Prevention Model. *(Courtesy of J. Krause.)*[311]

SUMMARY

SCI has a profound impact on many different body systems, which can greatly affect a person's ability to move, perform everyday tasks, and participate in expected social roles. This chapter reviewed the impact of SCI on different body systems, common impairments that result from SCI, classification of different types of SCI, and secondary complications associated with SCI. Physical therapists play a role across the continuum of care from the acute care hospital through rehabilitation to community reintegration. Standardized outcome measures are an important element of the examination process. The POC should be individually tailored to the patient's presentation, concerns, and goals. Interventions may be compensatory or recovery based depending on the presentation of the patient. Patient education is a critical component of the POC. Patients unable to perform certain activities should be educated to direct others about their care. People with SCI, no matter at what level, can lead a productive, healthy, and high-quality life. See Appendix 20.A (online).

Questions for Review

1. Identify the clinical features of Brown-Séquard, anterior, central, and posterior cord syndromes.

2. Define *spinal shock.*

3. Describe complications associated with SCI.

4. What is AD? Describe the initiating stimuli and symptoms of this syndrome. What action would you take if a patient experienced an onset of symptoms during a physical therapy treatment?

5. Identify two primary factors affecting prognosis following SCI.

6. What is included in a physical therapy examination during the acute phase of recovery? How might some of the standard examination techniques need to be modified?

7. Describe potential goals and interventions to improve respiratory function during the acute phase of management.

8. Identify tests and measures and outcome measures used during the active rehabilitation phase of management.

9. List factors that will have an impact on the prognosis for recovery of walking ability.

10. Outline interventions to improve transfers for a patient with C6 and AIS A tetraplegia. Describe the specific activities you would include. What type of progressive strengthening and endurance training activities would you suggest for each patient as an adjunct to the mat program?

11. What are key training parameters to consider when developing a POC to improve walking ability with an individual with an incomplete SCI?

CASE STUDY

HISTORY

The patient is a 21-year-old male who was transferred to a rehabilitation hospital yesterday. He suffered a traumatic cervical SCI 8 days ago. He was given methylprednisolone in the emergency department. He had surgery to stabilize the fracture site, internal fixation, and decompression using a right iliac bone graft. He was discharged to your facility yesterday and is currently wearing a Philadelphia collar. He is able to extend his elbows but cannot flex his fingers in either hand. He is a senior at college, computer science major. Lives in on-campus apartment, not wheelchair accessible. His parents live in the next state.

MEDICATIONS

Lovenox, midodrine, amitriptyline, OxyContin, and Dulcolax.

CASE STUDY—cont'd

PHYSICAL THERAPY EXAMINATION

Cardiopulmonary
HR: 75

BP: supine: 110/72; sitting: 100/66 (only able to tolerate sitting for about 10 minutes, then blood pressure drops due to orthostatic hypotension)

Forced VC: 2.2 L

Weak functional cough

Communication/Cognition
Alert, oriented ×3, able to follow multistep commands; MMSE: 30/30

Muscle Performance
Bilateral: biceps: 5/5, wrist extensors: 5/5, triceps: 4/5, no active contraction below C7

Sensory Integrity
Intact pinprick and light touch bilaterally C2–T4, absent below T4

Intact anal sensation

Functional Mobility
Bed mobility: moderate assistance to roll to the left and right

Supine ↔ short sit: maximal assistance

Supine ↔ long-sit: maximal assistance

Transfer wheelchair ↔ bed: FIM score 2 (requires maximal assistance with transfer board)

Transfer wheelchair ↔ toilet: FIM score 2 (requires maximal assistance with transfer board)

Locomotion
Unable to ambulate.

Able to propel wheelchair 150 ft on level surface with minimal assistance

Wheelchair Skills
Requires assistance with locking wheel locks, removing foot rests and armrests, and to perform pressure relief. Wheelchair Skills Test score: 4%

Currently uses a lightweight, folding wheelchair with hand rim projections

Gel cushion

Tolerates sitting in wheelchair for 20 to 30 minutes.

Balance
Long-sitting: able to maintain balance on mat for 1 minute with UEs in weight-bearing position with supervision

Short-sitting: able to maintain balance on edge of mat for 1 minute with UEs in weight-bearing position with minimal assistance, 0 in. for modified functional reach

Motor Function
Increased spasticity in bilateral hip flexors, 1+ on MAS

Passive ROM
WNL except bilateral ankle dorsiflexion is 5° from neutral

Skin Integrity
Stage 1 wound on right heel

Self-Care
Dressing upper body: FIM score 2 (requires maximal assistance)

Dressing lower body: FIM score 1 (dependent)

Bathing: FIM score 1 (dependent using shower chair)

Feeding: FIM score 3 (moderate assistance with adapted utensils)

Grooming: FIM score 3 (moderate assistance with adapted utensils)

Toileting: FIM score 2 (maximal assistance)

Bowel and Bladder
Bladder: FIM score 1 (just began intermittent catheterization program and requires total assist to manage)

Bowel: FIM score 1 (just began bowel training program with nursing, has been incontinent of bowel during the past day)

(Continued)

CASE STUDY—cont'd

CASE STUDY GUIDING QUESTIONS

1. What is the patient's neurological level of injury, motor level of injury, and sensory level of injury? What is the patient's AIS classification?

2. Identify/categorize this patient's problems in terms of
   a. Body structure/function impairments
   b. Activity limitations
   c. Restrictions in social participation

3. Identify three anticipated goals and three expected outcomes for this patient.

4. Formulate three interventions with one progression that could be used during the first 3 weeks of therapy to improve bed mobility skills.

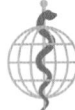

For additional resources, including answers to the questions for review, new immersive cases, case study guiding questions, references, and more, please visit **https://www.fadavis.com/product/physical -rehabilitation-fulk-8**. You may also quickly find the resources by entering this title's four-digit ISBN, 4691, in the search field at **http://fadavis.com** and logging in at the prompt.

Vestibular Disorders

Wagner H. Souza PT, PhD
Michael C. Schubert, PT, PhD, FAPTA

Chapter **21**

LEARNING OBJECTIVES

1. Differentiate vestibular symptom pathology from other manifestations of vertigo, dizziness, and disequilibrium.
2. Identify the examination procedures used to evaluate patients with vestibular dysfunction to establish a diagnosis, prognosis, and plan of care.
3. When presented with a clinical case study, analyze and interpret examination data and determine appropriate interventions for the clinical problems presented.
4. Determine appropriate elements of the rehabilitation program for patients with vestibular dysfunction.

CHAPTER OUTLINE

ANATOMY *816*
  Peripheral Vestibular System *816*
  Semicircular Canals *816*
  Otolith Organs *817*
  Central Vestibular System *817*
PHYSIOLOGY AND MOTOR CONTROL *818*
  Tonic Firing Rate *818*
  Vestibulo-Ocular Reflex *818*
  Push–Pull Mechanism *819*
  Inhibitory Cutoff *819*
  Velocity Storage System *820*
EXAMINATION *820*
  History and Systems Review *820*
  Tests and Measures *821*
VESTIBULAR SYSTEM DYSFUNCTION *828*
  Peripheral Pathology *828*
  Central Nervous System Pathology *830*
  Discerning Peripheral Vestibular Pathology From Central Vestibular Pathology *830*
INTERVENTIONS *831*
  Benign Paroxysmal Positional Vertigo *831*

Unilateral Vestibular Hypofunction *833*
Bilateral Vestibular Hypofunction *837*
Abnormal Central Vestibular Function *838*
Patient Education *838*
DIAGNOSES INVOLVING THE VESTIBULAR SYSTEM *843*
  Ménière Disease *843*
  Perilymphatic Fistula *844*
  Vestibular Schwannoma *844*
  Vestibular Atelectasis *844*
  Vestibular Paroxysmia *845*
  Mal de Debarquement *845*
  Vestibular Migraine *845*
  Multiple Sclerosis *845*
  Multiple System Atrophy *845*
  Cervicogenic Dizziness *846*
  Superior Canal Dehiscence Syndrome *846*
CONTRAINDICATIONS TO VESTIBULAR REHABILITATION *846*
SUMMARY *846*

Physical therapists are likely to encounter patients with vestibular disorders in a variety of clinical settings, including the emergency department. At an incidence of 5.5%, dizziness in the United States affects more than 15 million people each year.[1] The reported prevalence of dizziness as a medical symptom in community-dwelling adults varies based on subjects' age, sex, and definition of the complaint (1% to 35%).[2] Dizziness is among the most common complaints adults report to their health-care providers, and prevalence increases with age.[3] A cross-sectional study of emergency department visits for dizziness found that otologic/vestibular pathology was the number one cause (32%).[4] Among community-dwelling adults, it has been suggested that nearly one-third of the U.S. population

has a vestibular disorder.[5,6] Patients who experience dizziness report a significant disability that reduces their quality of life.[7,9] Furthermore, it has been reported that greater than 70% of patients with initial complaints of dizziness will not have a resolution of symptoms at a 2-week follow-up. Of patients with persistent dizziness, 63% reported recurrent symptoms continuing beyond 3 months.[10]

Cawthorne[11] and Cooksey[12] were the first clinicians to advocate exercises for persons suffering from dizziness and vertigo. It has been only within the last three decades, however, that our knowledge of vestibular function and related disorders has profoundly changed rehabilitation approaches. Once an accurate diagnosis involving the vestibular pathways has been made, activity limitations are minimized and progression toward disability can be prevented. Evidence suggests that an individualized approach to vestibular rehabilitation is important for a better outcome.

The peripheral vestibular system serves as the primary focus of this chapter because it is the most common origin of patient signs and symptoms. The physical therapist, however, must recognize patterns of signs and symptoms from a central pathology as well. With an appreciation of the complexity of the vestibular system coupled with an understanding of tests to measure its function, the reader will be able to discern anomalies of the system and begin to formulate effective rehabilitation strategies.

■ ANATOMY
Peripheral Vestibular System

The three primary functions of the peripheral vestibular system are (1) stabilizing visual images on the fovea of the retina during head movement to allow clear vision; (2) maintaining postural stability, especially during movement of the head; and (3) providing information used for spatial orientation.

Semicircular Canals

Within the petrous portion of each temporal bone (base of the skull between the sphenoid and occipital bones) lies the membranous vestibular labyrinth. Each labyrinth contains five neural structures that detect head acceleration: three *semicircular canals* and two *otolith* organs (Fig. 21.1). The three semicircular canals (SCCs)

(*horizontal, posterior* [inferior], and *superior*[anterior]) respond to angular acceleration and are orthogonal (at right angles) with respect to one another. Alignment of the SCCs in the temporal bone is such that each canal has a contralateral coplanar mate. The horizontal canals form a coplanar pair while the posterior and contralateral anterior SCCs form coplanar pairs. The anterior aspect of the horizontal SCC is inclined 30° upward from a plane connecting the external auditory canal to the lateral canthus. The posterior and anterior SCCs are inclined about 92° and 90°, respectively, from the plane of the horizontal SCC.[13] Angular head rotation stimulates each canal to varying degrees.[14]

The SCCs are filled with *endolymph* (fluid) that has a density slightly greater than water.[15] Endolymph moves freely within each canal in response to the direction of the angular head rotation. The SCCs enlarge at one end to form the *ampulla*. Within the ampulla lies the *cupula*, a gelatinous barrier that contains the sensory hair cells (Fig. 21.2). The *kinocilia* (mechanosensing cilia involved in the sense of movement) and *stereocilia* (mechanosensing organelles) of the hair cells are seated in the *crista ampullaris* (sensory organ of angular rotation). Deflection of the stereocilia caused by motion of the endolymph results in an opening (or closing) of the transduction channels of hair cells, which results

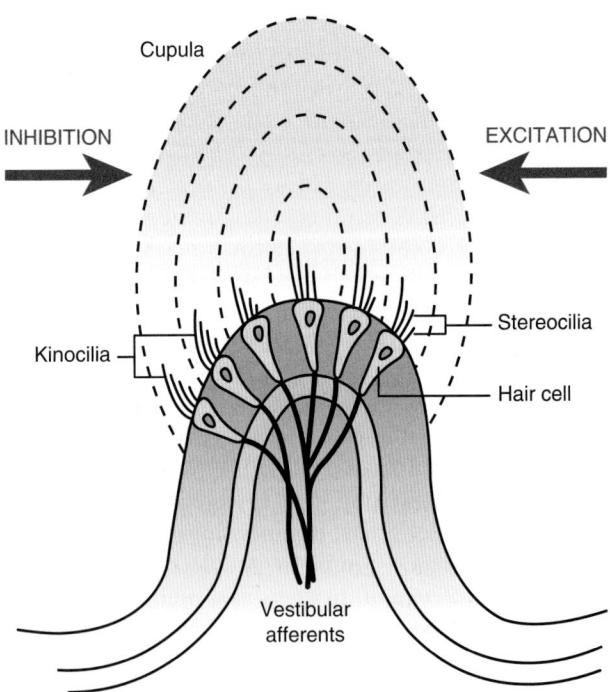

Figure 21.2 The cupula of the ampulla is a flexible, gelatinous barrier that partitions the canal. The crista ampullaris contains the kinocilia and stereocilia sensory hair cells. The hair cells generate action potentials in response to cupular deflection. Deflection of the stereocilia toward the kinocilia causes excitation; deflection in the opposite direction causes inhibition.

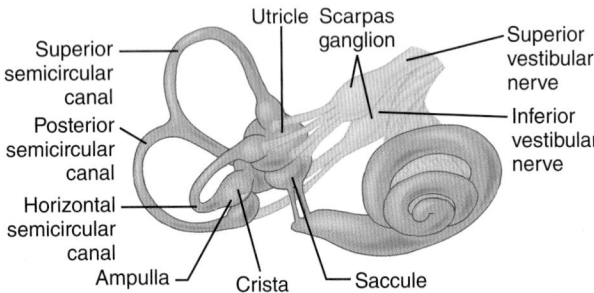

Figure 21.1 Anatomy of the vestibular labyrinth. Structures include the utricle, sacculus, superior semicircular canal, posterior semicircular canal, and the horizontal semicircular canal. The three semicircular canals (SCCs) are orthogonal with each other. Note the superior vestibular nerve innervating the superior (anterior) and horizontal semicircular canals as well as the utricle. The inferior vestibular nerve innervates the posterior semicircular canal and the saccule. The cell bodies of the vestibular nerves are located in Scarpa ganglion (Gangl. Scarpae). Also note that the semicircular canals enlarge at one end to form the ampulla.

in changes in the membrane potential of the hair cells. Deflection of the stereocilia toward the kinocilia in each hair cell leads to excitation (*depolarization*), and deflection of the stereocilia away from the kinocilia leads to inhibition (*hyperpolarization*).

Each of the SCCs responds best to motion in its own plane with coplanar pairs exhibiting a *push–pull dynamic*. For example, as the head is turned to the right, the hair cells in the right horizontal SCC are excited, while hair cells in the left horizontal SCC are inhibited. The brain detects the direction of head movement by comparing input from the coplanar labyrinthine mates.

Otolith Organs

The saccule and utricle make up the otolith organs of the membranous labyrinth and respond to linear acceleration and static head tilt. Sensory hair cells project into a gelatinous material that has calcium carbonate crystalline-structure material (otoconia) embedded in it, which provides the otolith organs with an inertial mass (Fig. 21.3). Similar to the SCCs, motion toward the kinocilia causes excitation, while motion away leads to inhibition. Utricular excitation occurs during horizontal linear acceleration and/or static head tilt, and saccular excitation occurs during vertical linear acceleration.

Central Vestibular System

Brain stem processes provide primary control of many vestibular reflexes. Tracing techniques used to follow axonal projections from their source to point of termination have identified extensive connections between the vestibular nuclei and the reticular formation, thalamus, and cerebellum[16–18] (Fig. 21.4). In addition, vestibular pathways appear to terminate in a unique cortical area. Primate studies have identified the junction of the parietal and insular lobes as the location for a vestibular cortex.[19–21] Evidence in human studies using functional magnetic resonance imaging (fMRI) appears to confirm the parietal and insular regions as the cortical location for processing vestibular information.[22] Connections with the vestibular cortex, thalamus, and reticular formation enable the vestibular system to contribute to the integration of arousal and conscious awareness of the body, as well as to discriminate between movement of self and the environment.[23,24] The cerebellar connections help maintain calibration of the vestibulo-ocular reflex (VOR), which stabilizes images on the retina during head movements, contributes to posture during static and dynamic activities, and influences the coordination of limb movements.

Vestibular connections with the autonomic nervous system contribute to cardiovascular function (i.e., blood pressure), validated in astronauts who, upon returning to Earth's gravitational field (and the return of vestibular afference of gravity), suffer orthostatic intolerance after long-duration space exposure.[25]

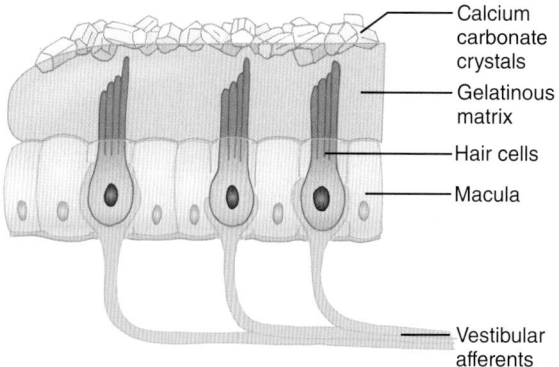

Figure 21.3 Otoconia are calcium carbonate crystals that are embedded in a gelatinous matrix that provides an inertial mass. Linear acceleration shifts the gelatinous matrix and excites or inhibits the vestibular afferents depending on the direction in which the stereocilia are deflected.

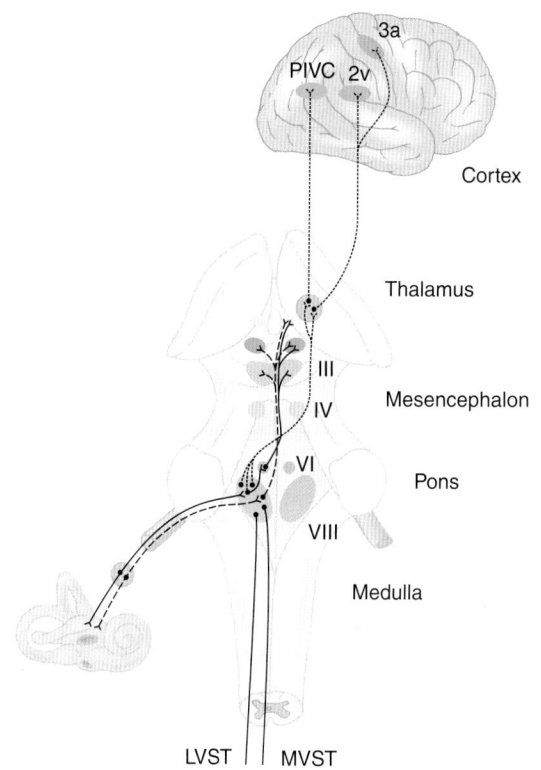

Figure 21.4 The semicircular canal (angular) and otolith (linear) input is sent to the vestibular nuclei. From the vestibular nuclei, the input travels to the ocular motor nuclei (III, IV, VI) for mediation of the vestibulo-ocular reflex. For arousal and conscious awareness of the head and body in space, information proceeds further to the thalamus and cortex. For maintenance of postural control, the peripheral vestibular input is sent distally as the medial and lateral vestibulo-spinal tracts (MVST, LVST). PIVC = Parieto-insular vestibular cortex.

■ PHYSIOLOGY AND MOTOR CONTROL

Foundational knowledge of vestibular neurophysiology is important for understanding the signs and symptoms of vestibular dysfunction. Important principles of the vestibular system include the *tonic-firing rate, VOR, push–pull mechanism, inhibitory cutoff,* and *velocity storage system.*

Tonic Firing Rate

In primates, primary vestibular afferents of the healthy vestibular system have a resting firing rate that is typically 70 to 100 spikes/sec.[26-27] The presence of the high tonic firing rate means each vestibular system can detect head motion through excitation or inhibition. During angular head rotations, ipsilateral vestibular afferents and ipsilateral central vestibular neurons are excited.[28] Such head movements also result in inhibition of peripheral afferents and of many central vestibular neurons receiving innervation from the contralateral labyrinth.

Vestibulo-Ocular Reflex

The VOR is responsible for maintaining stability of an image on the fovea of the retina during rapid head movements. To do this, the VOR must generate rapid compensatory eye movements in the direction opposite the head rotation. The VOR achieves this with relatively simple patterns of connectivity in the central vestibular pathways. In its most basic form, the pathways controlling the VOR can be described as a three-neuron arc:

- Primary vestibular afferents from the anterior SCC synapse in the ipsilateral vestibular nuclei.
- Secondary ipsilateral vestibular neurons receiving innervation from the ipsilateral labyrinth decussate and synapse in the contralateral oculomotor nucleus.
- Motor neurons from the contralateral oculomotor nucleus then synapse at the neuromuscular junction of the ipsilateral superior rectus and the contralateral inferior oblique muscles, respectively (Fig. 21.5).

Similar patterns of connectivity exist for each SCC and the eye muscles that receive innervations from them (Table 21.1). See Figure 21.6 for insertions of the ocular muscles.

Vor Gain and Phase

Normally, as the head moves in one direction, the eyes move in the opposite direction with equal velocity. This relationship of eye velocity to head velocity is expressed as the gain (*VOR gain*) of the vestibular system (eye velocity/head velocity = −1). For example, when the head is moved down, the anterior SCCs are stimulated. Excitation of the anterior SCC afferents rotates both eyes in the direction opposite the angular head movement, or up (see Fig. 21.5). *VOR phase* is a second useful measure of the vestibular system and represents the

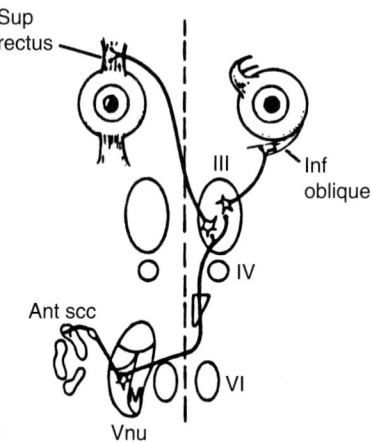

Figure 21.5 From the anterior semicircular canal (Ant scc), afferent input travels to the vestibular nuclei (Vnu). The signal continues to the contralateral oculomotor nuclei (III). From there, motoneurons synapse with the superior rectus muscle that moves the eye upward, and the inferior oblique muscle that moves the eye upward and torsionally. Also shown are the oculomotor nuclei IV and VI. *(Adapted from Baloh and Honrubia,[33, p. 52] with permission.)*

Table 21.1	Innervation Pattern of Excitatory Input From the Semicircular Canals		
Primary Afferent	**Secondary Neuron**[a]	**Extraocular Motor Neuron**	**Muscle**
Horizontal (left)	Medial vestibular nucleus	Left oculomotor nucleus[b] Right abducens nucleus	Left medial rectus Right lateral rectus
Posterior (left)	Medial vestibular nucleus	Right trochlear nucleus Right oculomotor nucleus	Left superior oblique Right inferior rectus
Anterior/Superior (left)	Lateral vestibular nucleus	Right oculomotor nucleus	Left superior rectus Right inferior oblique

[a]Ascending secondary neurons travel in the medial longitudinal fasciculus.
[b]In the horizontal semicircular canal, secondary neurons also travel in the ascending tract of Dieters.

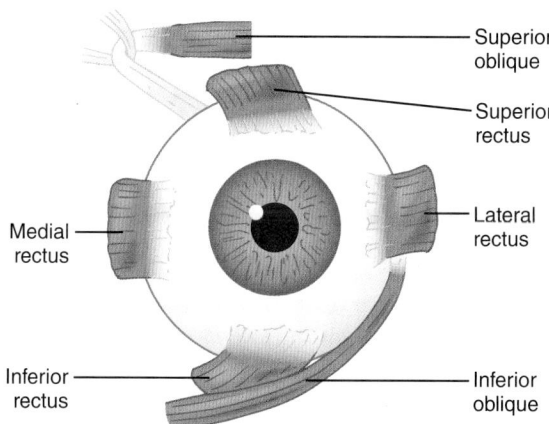

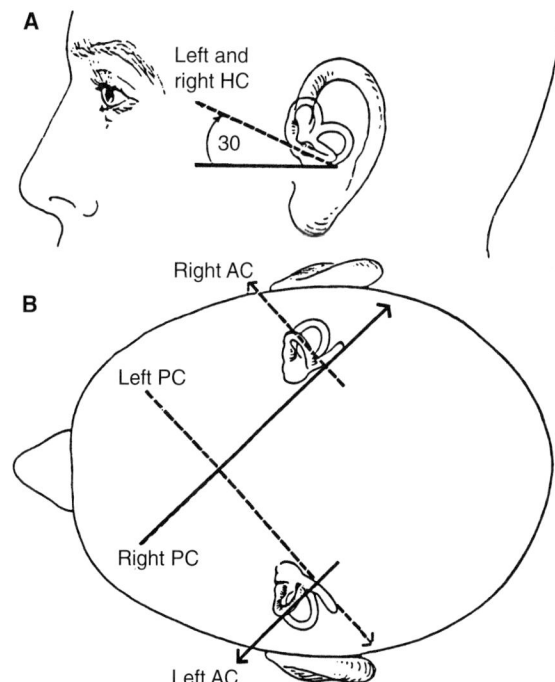

Figure 21.6 Muscle insertions of the left eye. Six extraocular muscles insert into the sclera and can be considered as complementary pairs. The medial and lateral rectus muscles rotate the eyes horizontally, the superior and inferior rectus muscles rotate the eyes vertically, and the superior and inferior oblique muscles rotate the eyes torsionally with some vertical component. By convention, the torsional rotation is noted as it relates to the superior poles of the eyes. The superior oblique muscle rotates the eye downward and toward the nose, whereas the inferior oblique muscle rotates the eye upward and away from the nose. The superior oblique muscle travels through the fibrous trochlea, which attaches to the anteromedial superior wall of the orbit.

Figure 21.7 (A) Orientation of the horizontal semicircular canals (HC) in situ, with the head neutrally aligned. (B) The semicircular canals (ipsilateral anterior and contralateral posterior, and each horizontal) work in pairs, as a push–pull mechanism. The arrows indicate the angular pitch direction of individual SCC stimulation. The dashed and continuous lines illustrate each SCC has an equally opposing SCC, sensitive to the opposite angular pitch direction of the head. For example, the left anterior canal (left AC) is paired with the right posterior canal (right PC) and collectively recognized as the left anterior right posterior (LARP) plane.

amplitude relationship between the eye and head. VOR phase should represent an equal but opposite head and eye position relationship. Therefore, if the head moves 10° to the right, the eyes should be positioned 10° to the left. When the head and eyes are equally positioned but oppositely directed, this is described as a zero phase shift. *Note*: VOR phase is not equivalent to VOR gain, which examines the difference between head and eye velocity.

In individuals with healthy oculomotor function, for head velocities below 60°/sec, *gaze stability* can be maintained fairly well using *smooth pursuit* (the ability to move the eyes with smooth, continuous motions in order to follow the movement of a target of interest and maintain the moving image on the fovea).[29] In situations where head velocity is greater than 60°/sec, the vestibular system is primarily responsible for generating eye movement (in the direction opposite the head movement) to maintain *gaze* on the target.[30] The VOR operates at head velocities as great as 350° to 400°/sec.[28]

Push–Pull Mechanism

The brain detects head movement and direction through comparison of inputs between the two vestibular systems. The SCCs each work in coplanar fashion as mentioned earlier; as the head is turned to the right, the

right horizontal SCC will have an increased firing rate while the left horizontal SCC has a decreased firing rate. This is called the *push–pull mechanism* (Fig. 21.7). The brain is then responsible for recognizing the difference and interpreting movement. A faulty interpretation will lead to difficulties with gaze stabilization, postural stability, and motion perception.

Inhibitory Cutoff

Recall that during angular head rotations (rotations about an axis) ipsilateral vestibular afferents can be excited up to 400 spikes/sec.[28] A simultaneous hyperpolarization (reduction of the spontaneous firing rate) of the opposite labyrinth also occurs. However, the inhibition of the hair cells in the opposite labyrinth can only reduce the firing rate to zero, at which point the inhibition is cut off (*inhibitory cutoff*). Thus, for ipsilateral rapid head rotations, the contralateral vestibular afferents cannot detect head rotation when the ipsilateral head velocity is greater than the inhibitory cutoff of those contralateral afferents. The response to head movements that hyperpolarize the hair cells is therefore limited to a velocity range up to 70° to 100°/sec. For example, if the tonic firing rates of the vestibular afferents are 80 spikes/sec, with a rotation to the right of 120°/sec, the vestibular afferents increase their firing rate from 80 to 200 spikes/sec (tonic firing rate + rotational velocity). In contrast, the left ear will decrease from 80 to 0, not to negative 40 (−40), which limits the afferents from the left ear from adequately detecting the head velocity. (It is generally accepted that a 1:1 ratio exists between head velocity and spikes per second neuronal firing rate.) Because the resting discharge rate of these afferents and central vestibular neurons averages 70 to 100 spikes/sec, inhibitory cutoff is more likely to occur than is excitation saturation.

Velocity Storage System

The signal generated by movement of the cupula is brief, lasting only as long as the cupula is deflected (~6 sec).[31] The response is sustained, however, by a circuit of neurons involving the medial vestibular nucleus and the cerebellum, extending the duration of nystagmus beyond 10 seconds in people with normal vestibular function. It is generally believed that the purpose of sustaining vestibular input is to assist the brain in detecting low-frequency head rotation.

■ EXAMINATION
History and Systems Review

Physical therapists examining people who report dizziness and imbalance have the difficult task of sorting through potential causes. Capturing a thorough history and performing a systems review are critical components of the process. Key elements of taking the history are identification of symptoms, as well as their duration and the circumstances under which the symptoms occur.

Identification of Symptoms

Many patients use the imprecise term *dizziness* to describe a vague sensation of light-headedness or a feeling that they may fall. The imprecision of the term can entangle clinical management decisions. It is essential to determine what the patient is experiencing when the term *dizziness* is used. Most complaints of being "dizzy" can be categorized as vertigo, light-headedness, dysequilibrium, or oscillopsia (targets in visual field appear to move during head motion). Generally, dizziness is vaguely defined as the sensation of whirling or feeling a tendency to fall. Ideally, patients should be directed away from using the word dizziness and to instead use more precise terms that will help the clinician develop more direct treatment approaches.

Vertigo is defined as an illusion of movement. Many patients use the term *vertigo* incorrectly, and thus the clinician must be certain to inform patients of the true definition, as well as identify their unique experience. Patients may describe that they sense their environment is moving or that they see the environment moving (spinning). Vertigo tends to be episodic and to indicate pathology at one or more locations along the vestibular pathways. It is most common during the acute stage of unilateral vestibular hypofunction (UVH) but may also manifest itself via displaced otoconia (benign paroxysmal positional vertigo) or an acute unilateral brainstem lesion affecting the root entry zone of the peripheral vestibular neurons or the vestibular nuclei.

Light-headedness is often defined as a feeling that fainting is about to occur and can be caused by nonvestibular factors such as hypotension, hypoglycemia, or anxiety.[32] Light-headedness is vague and less localizing than vertigo.

Dysequilibrium is defined as the sensation of being off balance. Typically, acute and chronic vestibular lesions will produce dysequilibrium. Often, however, this symptom is associated with nonvestibular problems such as decreased somatosensation or weakness in the lower extremities (LEs; Table 21.2).

Oscillopsia is the subjective experience of motion of objects in the visual environment that are known to be stationary. Oscillopsia can occur with head movements in patients with vestibular hypofunction since the vestibular system is not generating an adequate compensatory eye velocity during the head motion. Such a deficit in the VOR results in motion of images on the fovea and in a decline in visual acuity. The severity of gaze instability, however, varies across individuals with vestibular hypofunction.[33–36]

Table 21.2   Symptoms and Possible Causes

Symptom	Possible Cause
Vertigo	BPPV, UVH, unilateral central lesion affecting the vestibular nuclei, migraine affecting the central vestibular pathways
Light-headedness	Orthostatic hypotension, hypoglycemia, anxiety, panic disorder
Dysequilibrium	BVH, chronic UVH, lower extremity somatosensation loss, upper brainstem/vestibular cortex lesion, cerebellar and motor pathway lesions

BPPV = benign paroxysmal positional vertigo; BVH = bilateral vestibular hypofunction; UVH = unilateral vestibular hypofunction.

Duration and Circumstances of Symptoms

The physical therapist must determine how recently the patient has had an acute attack of vertigo, lightheadedness, dysequilibruim, or oscillopsia and whether the symptom is constant or episodic. If the symptom is episodic, the clinician must attempt to determine the average duration of the episodes in seconds, minutes, or hours. For example, vertigo lasting seconds to minutes commonly suggests benign paroxysmal positional vertigo. In contrast, vertigo lasting minutes to hours suggests Ménière disease (see "Diagnoses Involving the Vestibular System"), and vertigo lasting for days implies vestibular neuronitis or migraine-associated dizziness.

The physical therapist must also determine under what circumstances the patient experiences symptoms. It is important to discern whether the patient experiences symptoms with particular movements, positions, or at rest. For example, is the patient sensitive to motion as the passenger in a moving car? Or does the patient experience a vigorous vertigo when the head is moved into certain positions?

Tests and Measures
Visual Analogue Scale

Use of a *visual analogue scale* (VAS) is an effective tool to obtain subjective intensity ratings of vertigo, lightheadedness, dysequilibrium, and oscillopsia.[37,38] The patient is asked to answer a question (e.g., *How intense are your symptoms?*) and mark on a 10-cm line (on a continuum from "none" to "worst possible intensity") where the symptoms exist at that moment. The clinician then measures the line and obtains a quantified value.

Dizziness Handicap Inventory

The *Dizziness Handicap Inventory* (DHI) is a popular tool used to measure a patient's self-perceived handicap as a result of vestibular disorders (Table 21.3).[39] The DHI has excellent test–retest reliability ($r = 0.97$) and good internal consistency reliability ($r = 0.89$). Patients respond to 25 questions, subgrouped into functional, emotional, and physical components. The DHI provides quantification of the patient's perception of dysequilibrium and its impact on daily activities. It is useful to establish subjective improvement. Measures of subjective impairment and physiological improvement are often not correlated;[40,41] therefore, it is likely that factors other than organic recovery of vestibular function are responsible for subjective impairment.

Vestibular Rehabilitation Benefit Questionnaire

The *Vestibular Rehabilitation Benefit Questionnaire* (VRBQ) was developed to specify the benefit from vestibular physical therapy and includes questions that address avoidance behavior, which is often absent in similar measures.[42] The VRBQ is a 22-item questionnaire that uses seven unique choices (word descriptors) to answer questions from one of four subscales: Dizziness, Anxiety, Motion-Provoked Dizziness, and Quality of Life. The VRBQ has excellent test–retest reliability ($r = 0.92$) and is moderately correlated with the DHI (0.59).

Table 21.3 Sample of the Types of Questions Included in the Dizziness Handicap Inventory, Based on the Three Subcomponents

Domain	Questions
Physical domain	Does looking up increase your problem? Does walking down the aisle of a supermarket increase your problem? Does performing more ambitious activities like sports, dancing, or household chores (such as sweeping or putting dishes away) increase your problem? Does bending over increase your problem?
Emotional domain	Because of your problem, do you feel frustrated? Because of your problem, are you afraid to leave your home without having someone accompany you? Has your problem placed stress on your relationships with members of your family or friends? Because of your problem, are you afraid to stay home alone?
Functional domain	Because of your problem, do you restrict your travel for business or recreation? Because of your problem, do you have difficulty getting into or out of bed? Does your problem significantly restrict your participation in social activities such as going out to dinner, going to the movies, dancing, or going to parties? Because of your problem, is it difficult for you to walk around the house in the dark?

The patient instructions are as follows: The purpose of these questions is to identify difficulties that you may be experiencing because of your dizziness. Please answer "yes," "no," or "sometimes" to each question. Answer each question as it pertains to your dizziness or balance problem only.

Motion Sensitivity Quotient

The *Motion Sensitivity Quotient* (MSQ) was developed to provide a subjective score of an individual's sensitivity to motion.[43] The test involves placing patients into positions incorporating head or entire body motion to determine whether the movement reproduces dizziness (Fig. 21.8). If the patient reports an increased symptom intensity moving into a provoking position, the intensity is assigned a point, graded by the patient between 1 (mild) and 5 (severe). The duration of symptoms is also assigned points from 0 to 3 (0 to 4 seconds = 0; 5 to 10 seconds = 1; 11 to 30 seconds = 2; greater than 30 seconds = 3). The symptom intensity and duration values are then added together for a score. The MSQ is calculated by multiplying the number of positions that provoked symptoms by the score. This number is then divided by 2,048. An MSQ score of 0 indicates no symptoms, whereas a score of 100 means severe dizziness in all positions.

Examination of Eye Movements

Owing to the direct relationship between vestibular receptors in the inner ear and eye movements produced by the VOR, the examination of eye movements is critical for defining and localizing vestibular pathology. The key tests include observation for nystagmus, the Head Impulse Test (examination of the VOR at high acceleration), the Head-Shaking Induced Nystagmus (HSN) test, positional testing, and the Dynamic Visual Acuity (DVA) test.

Observation for Nystagmus

Nystagmus is the primary diagnostic indicator used in identifying most peripheral and central vestibular

Name: _____ Age: _____ Gender: _____ Date: _____

Baseline Symptoms	INTENSITY	DURATION	SCORE
1. Sitting-to-supine			
2. Supine-to-left side			
3. Supine-to-right side			
4. Supine-to-sit			
5. Left Dix-Hallpike test			
6. Return from Dix-Hallpike test			
7. Right Dix-Hallpike test			
8. Return from Dix-Hallpike test			
9. Sitting: nose toward left knee			
10. Return to sitting			
11. Sitting: nose toward right knee			
12. Return to sitting			
13. Sitting: head rotation 5×			
14. Sitting: head flexion and extension 5×			
15. Standing: turn right (180°)			
16. Standing: turn left (180°)			
Intensity: rated from 0 to 5 (0 = no symptoms; 5 = severe symptoms)			
Duration: rated from 0 to 3 (5-10 sec = 1 point, 11-30 sec = 2 points, ≥30 sec = 3 points)			

Figure 21.8 Motion sensitivity quotient. *(Adapted from Smith-Wheelock et al.,48, p. 221 with permission.)*

Motion sensitivity quotient: $\dfrac{\text{\#Provoking positions} \times \text{score} \times 100}{2048}$ = _____ Total

Note: An MSQ score of zero means no symptoms, and 100 means severe dizziness in all positions.

lesions. An involuntary eye movement, nystagmus due to a *peripheral vestibular lesion* is composed of both slow and fast components. The direction of the nystagmus is named by the direction of the fast component. For individuals with a unilateral vestibular lesion, the slow component is due to relative excitation of one side of the vestibular system. The fast component is generated from the parapontine reticular formation in the brainstem and repositions the eye to the center of the orbit. For example, in left-beating nystagmus, the eyes move slowly to the right (VOR), and the resetting eye movement is to the left (fast component). Therefore, the direction opposite the quick component of the nystagmus localizes the side of the vestibular reduced firing rate (possible hypofunction).

Nystagmus due to a vestibular lesion is most commonly seen after an acute unilateral insult, *spontaneous* (at rest) *nystagmus*. This type of nystagmus occurs in the absence of motion because of the asymmetry between the healthy functioning and reduced/absent functioning vestibular systems. The brain perceives the asymmetry as active stimulation from the more neutrally active (i.e., healthy) ear. Resolution of spontaneous nystagmus in the light typically occurs within 3 to 7 days, but may vary, and it can last as long as 2 months.[44,45] Spontaneous nystagmus may always be present in the dark after a unilateral loss of vestibular function. Regardless, resolution of spontaneous nystagmus in the light or dark occurs when symmetry between the resting firing rates of both vestibular systems is reestablished.[46]

Vestibular nystagmus can be suppressed in light and when a person visually fixates on a target.[47] As a result, the observation of nystagmus should be performed under conditions in which the person cannot see. This can be achieved with Frenzel lenses or an infrared camera system. Frenzel lenses look like large goggles with magnifying lenses that enable the clinician to observe for nystagmus while preventing the patient from fixating on a target (Fig 21.9). An infrared camera uses infrared light to illuminate the eyes while the patient remains in complete darkness.

Head Impulse Test (Examination of the VOR at High Acceleration)

The HIT is a widely accepted clinical tool used to examine semicircular canal function.[48–52] Cervical range of motion (ROM) should be determined before performing the head impulse test and the physical therapist should explain why the head must be moved quickly. The head impulse test is performed by having the patient first fixate on a near target (e.g., the clinician's nose). Patients are asked to keep their eyes focused on a target while their head is manually rotated in an unpredictable direction using a small-amplitude (5° to 15°), moderate-velocity (approximately 200°/sec), and high-acceleration (3,000° to 4,000°/sec²) angular impulse

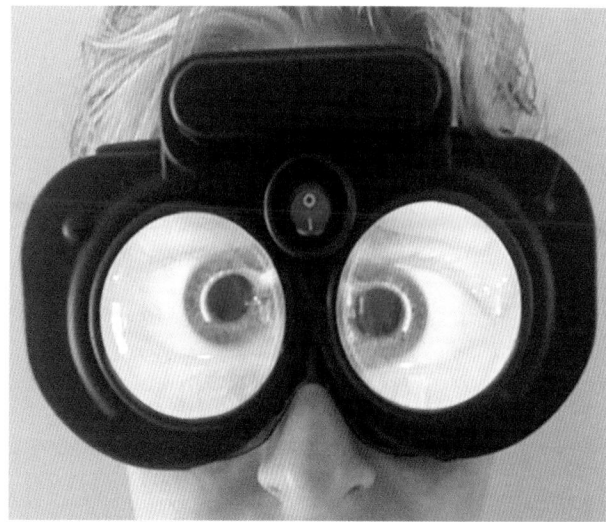

Figure 21.9 Frenzel lenses placed over a subject. The lenses both enlarge the eyes and block the subject's ability to fixate on a target, enabling proper assessment for nystagmus.

(Figs. 21.10 and 21.11). When the VOR is functioning normally, the eyes move in the direction opposite to the head movement, and gaze will remain on the target. In a patient with a loss of vestibular function, the VOR will not move the eyes as quickly as the head rotation, and the eyes move off the target. The patient will then make a corrective saccade (a rapid eye movement used to reposition the eyes to the target of interest) to reposition the eyes (fovea) on the target. The appearance of corrective saccade indicates vestibular hypofunction as determined by the HIT and occurs because inhibition of vestibular afferents and central vestibular neurons on the intact side (persons with UVH) are less effective in encoding the amplitude of a head movement than excitation. A patient who has a unilateral peripheral lesion or pathology of the central vestibular neurons will not be able to maintain a gaze when the head is rotated quickly toward the side of the lesion. A patient with a bilateral loss of vestibular function will make corrective saccades after a head impulse to either side. The HIT provides a sensitive indication of vestibular hypofunction in patients with complete loss of function in the affected labyrinth that occurs following ablative surgical procedures such as labyrinthectomy.[48,51–53] The test is less sensitive in detecting hypofunction in patients with incomplete loss of function.[54–57]

A video oculographic version of the HIT (vHIT) has been available since 2012, and it has become the preferred test to use in patients with a suspected vestibular disorder,[58] though the caloric exam is still useful.[59] The vHIT not only provides a measure of the VOR gain, but it also enables the identification of compensatory saccades that may occur during the head rotation (covert) or

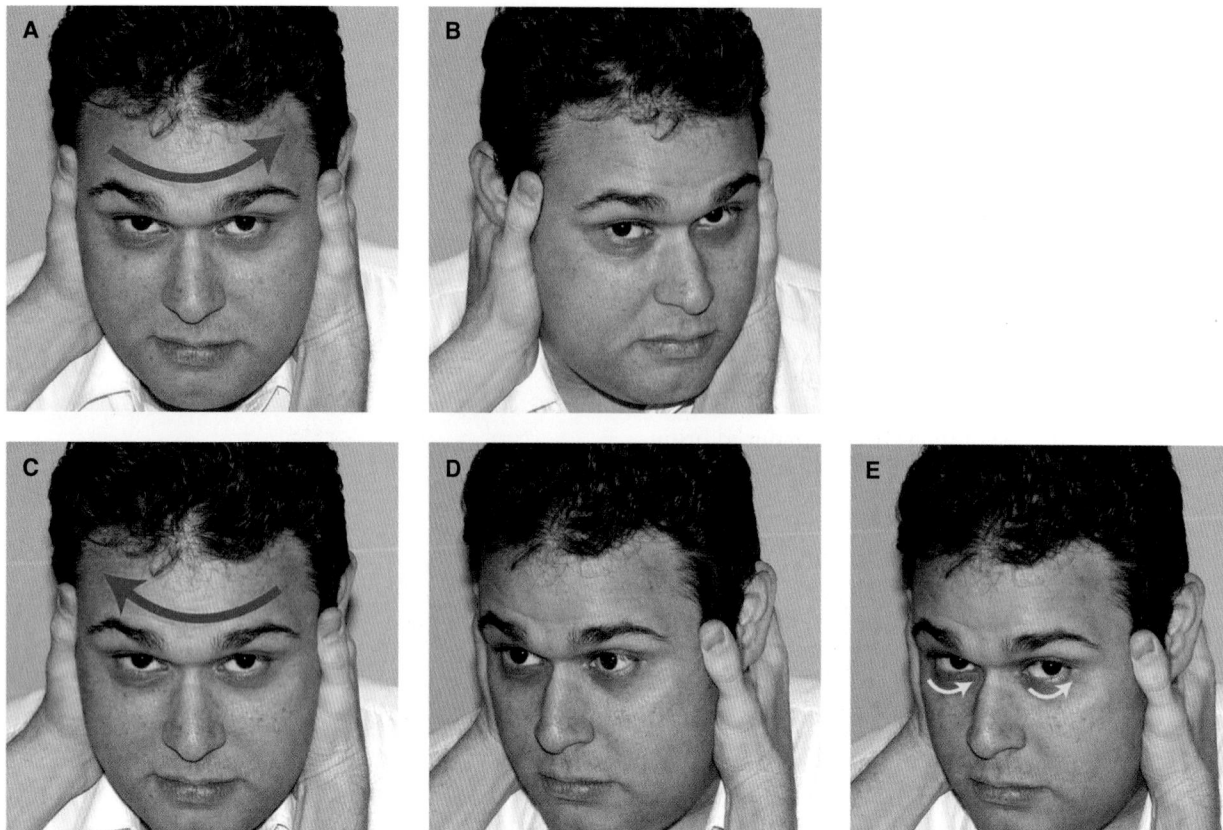

Figure 21.10 Normal horizontal canal head impulse test to the left (A, B), abnormal to the right (C–E). The examiner applies the head impulse test (HIT) to the patient. Large arrow denotes direction the head will be turned. (A) Initial starting position places subject's head into cervical flexion; eyes are focused on the target. (B) On stopping the head turn, the eyes are still on target and no corrective saccade is observed. In photographs A and B, the subject's eyes stay fixed on the examiner's nose throughout the test. (C) Initial starting position places subject's head into cervical flexion; eyes are focused on the target. (D) As the head is turned rapidly to the right, the eyes fall off the target and move with the head. (E) The subject must make a corrective saccade (small arrows) to bring the eyes back to the target of interest. For patients with cervical spine pathology, the clinician may choose to perform the horizontal canal HIT by first positioning the head in 15° of rotation and then returning the head to center. *(From Schubert et al.[62, p.153] with permission of the American Physical Therapy Association.)*

after the head stops moving (overt). The vHIT software includes data to compare using age-matched controls. Clinicians using the HIT test should consider that VOR gains decline with older age on both the horizontal canal (over 70 years of age) and the vertical canal (over 80 years of age).[60]

Head-Shaking–Induced Nystagmus Test

The head-shaking–induced nystagmus (HSN) test is a useful aid in the diagnosis of a unilateral peripheral vestibular defect. During this test, vision is occluded. The patient is instructed to close their eyes. The clinician flexes the head 30° before oscillating horizontally for 20 cycles at a frequency of two repetitions per second (2 Hz). A metronome can be used to ensure the frequency of

oscillations. When the oscillation stops, the patient opens their eyes and the clinician checks for nystagmus. In subjects with normal vestibular function, nystagmus will not be present. An asymmetry between the peripheral vestibular inputs to central vestibular nuclei, however, may result in HSN. Typically, a person with a UVH will manifest a horizontal HSN, with the quick phases of the nystagmus directed toward the healthy ear and the slow phases directed toward the lesioned ear.[61] Not all patients with a UVH will have HSN. Patients with a complete loss of vestibular function bilaterally will not have HSN because neither system is functioning. As a result, there is no asymmetry between the tonic firing rates. The presence of vertical nystagmus after either horizontal or vertical head shaking suggests a central lesion.

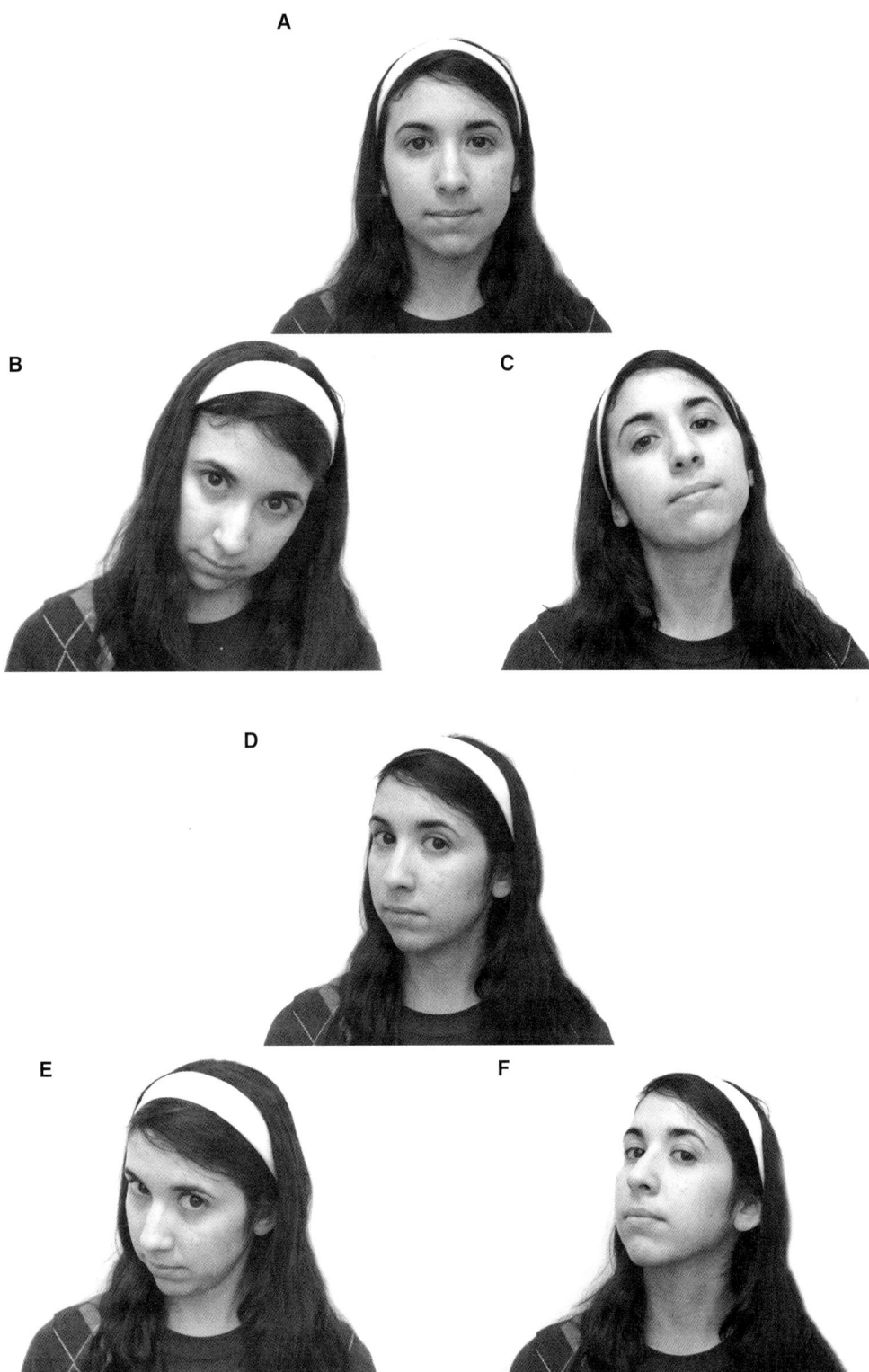

Figure 21.11 Vertical semicircular canal HIT, examiner's hands not shown here. There are two ways to investigate the VOR from each coplanar pair; methods A–C and D–F illustrate the two methods for the LARP VOR. (A) The head is placed in a neck neutral position. Next, the head is rapidly moved pitch down while being rolled to the left, (B) as if the head were moving diagonally. This examines the VOR from the left anterior SCC. From here, the clinician should return to (A) before rapidly moving the head pitch up and rolled to the right (C). This examines the VOR from the right posterior canal. Alternatively, the head is rotated 45° to the right (D). From this static position, the head is rapidly pitched down (E), examining the left anterior SCC. The head should be returned to the start position (D) and then the head rapidly moved pitch up to examine the right posterior SCC (F). In this figure, the HIT is normal for the LARP plane since the eyes remain gazing straight ahead.

Positional Testing

Positional testing is commonly used to identify whether otoconia have been displaced into the SCC, causing a condition referred to as *benign paroxysmal positional vertigo* (BPPV). The addition of the otoconia into the endolymph makes the semicircular canals sensitive to changes in head position. The Dix-Hallpike test is the most common positional test used to examine for BPPV.[62] The patient is moved from a long-sitting position with the head rotated 45° to one side, to a supine position with the head extended 30° beyond horizontal, head still rotated 45° (Fig. 21.12). The maneuver places each of the SCCs in a gravity-dependent position and the physical therapist should observe the eyes for nystagmus. The direction of the nystagmus is unique to the involved SCC. The direction and duration of the resultant nystagmus can help determine whether the patient has BPPV or a central lesion. An alternative form of the Dix-Hallpike test asks the patient to move into a side-lying position (Fig. 21.13). In both versions illustrated, the ear toward the ground is the labyrinth being tested. If horizontal SCC BPPV is suspected, the roll test can be used instead (Fig. 21.14). In this test, the patient is positioned supine with the head flexed 20°. Rapid rotations to the sides are done separately and the clinician observes for nystagmus and vertigo. To prevent neck injury, patients may perform their own head rotation.

Dynamic Visual Acuity Test

Dynamic visual acuity (DVA) is the measurement of visual acuity during horizontal motion of the head. A "bedside" and computerized form of the test can be used to identify the functional significance of the vestibular hypofunction.[63,64] Head velocities need to be greater than 100°/sec at the time DVA is measured to ensure that the vestibular afferents from the contralateral side are driven into inhibition and the letters (acuity chart) are not identified with a smooth pursuit eye movement. To perform the test, static visual acuity is determined first. The patient is asked to "Read the lowest line you can see" on a wall-mounted acuity chart. Lighthouse ETDRS (Early Treatment Diabetic Retinopathy Study) wall charts are recommended because they provide uniform light luminance for each of the letters. The patient then attempts to read the chart while the clinician horizontally oscillates the patient's head at a frequency of 2 Hz. A metronome can be useful to ensure correct frequency of the oscillation. For patients with loss of vestibular function, the eyes will not be stable in space during head movements. This causes a decrement in DVA compared with visual acuity when the head is still. Using the acuity chart, a three-line or more decrement in visual acuity during head movement is suggestive of vestibular hypofunction.[61] For people with normal vestibular function, head movement results in little or no change of visual

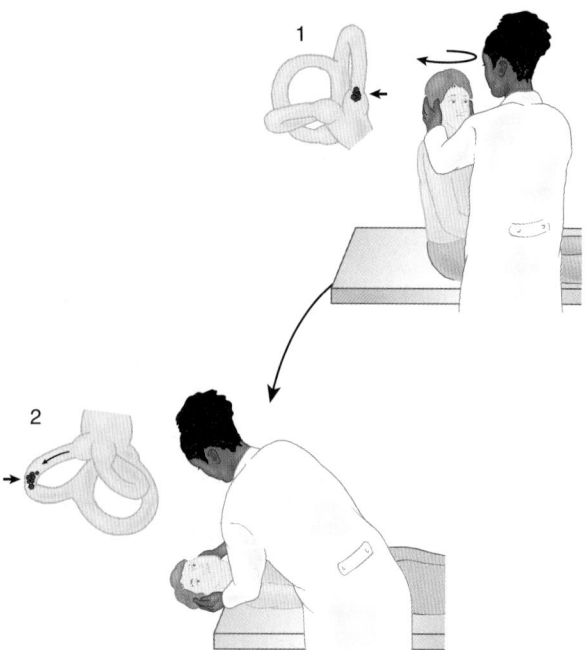

Figure 21.12 The Dix-Hallpike test. (1) The patient sits on the examination table, and the clinician turns the head horizontally 45°. (2) As the examiner maintains the 45° rotation, the patient is quickly brought to a supine position with the neck extended 30° beyond the horizontal. The examiner must look for nystagmus and ask the patient if vertigo is being experienced. The patient is then slowly brought back to the starting position, and the other side is tested. The side that reproduces nystagmus and vertigo is the side that has the BPPV. Shown here for testing right posterior or right anterior semicircular canal BPPV.

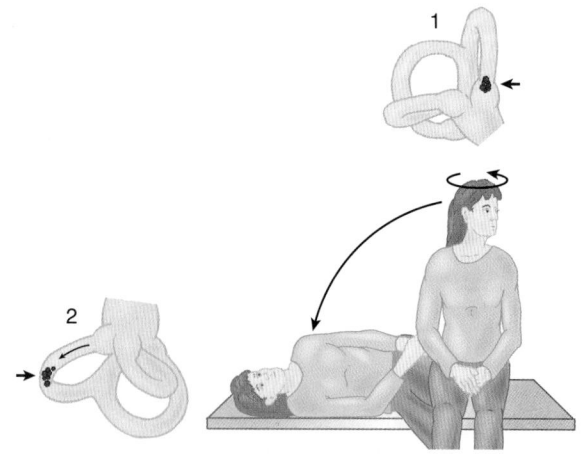

Figure 21.13 The Dix-Hallpike test (side-lying). (1) The patient sits on the edge of the examination table. The clinician turns the head horizontally 45°. (2) As the examiner maintains the 45° rotation, the patient is quickly brought down to the side opposite the head rotation (pictured here as the right side). The examiner checks for nystagmus and vertigo, then slowly brings the patient to the starting position. The other side is then tested.

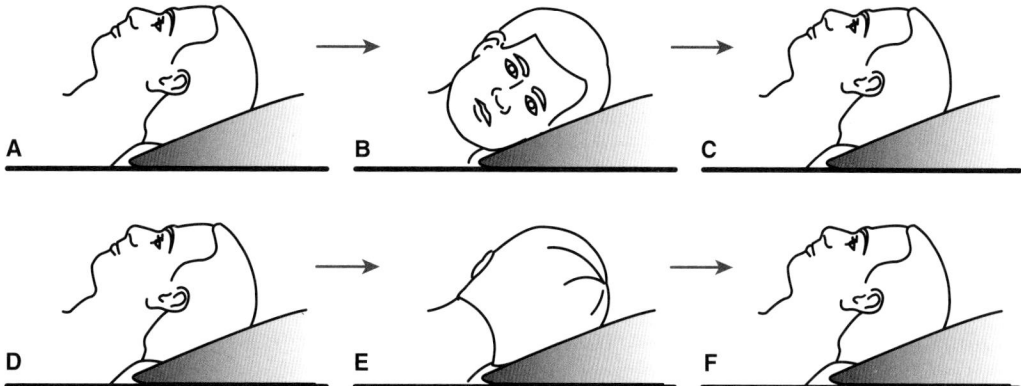

Figure 21.14 Roll test for horizontal semicircular canal BPPV. The patient is positioned in supine. (A) Initially, the patient's head should be placed in 20° cervical flexion. (B) The head is quickly turned 90° to the left side. The clinician then checks for nystagmus and vertigo. (C) The head is then gently returned to the neutral starting position. (D–F) The test is repeated to the other side (head is quickly turned 90° to the right side). The therapist again must check for nystagmus and vertigo. The head is then returned to the neutral starting position.

acuity compared with the head still (less than one line difference). Computerized DVA has been found to correctly identify the side of lesion in patients with unilateral hypofunction for self-generated and unpredictable head motion[64,65] and can be used to identify single SCC lesions.[66]

Examination of Gait and Balance

Examination of gait and balance problems is important for determining a patient's functional status. Testing should address both static and dynamic balance (e.g., weight shifting, automatic postural responses, and ambulation). Gait and balance tests *cannot* uniquely identify pathology within the vestibular system. Table 21.4 includes common balance tests and expected results.

Vestibular Function Tests
Semicircular Canal Tests

The more common SCC tests include *electronystagmography* (ENG) or *videonystagmography* (VNG) testing and *rotational chair tests* and are often performed in a clinical vestibular function test laboratory. ENG includes a battery of tests that measure central and vestibular *oculomotor* function. The test also examines for nystagmus in different head positions. The ENG oculomotor tests typically examine saccadic and smooth pursuit including velocity, latency, and gain. The vestibular component includes the *caloric test* and infuses the external auditory canal with separate cold and warm air or water. This stimulus introduces

Table 21.4   Common Balance Tests and Expected Results Related to Specific Diagnosis

Test	BPPV	UVH	BVH	Central Lesion
Romberg	Negative	Acute: positive Chronic: negative	Acute: positive Chronic: negative	Often negative
Tandem Romberg	Negative	Positive, eyes closed	Positive	Positive
Single-legged stance	Negative	May be positive	Acute: positive Chronic: negative	May be unable to perform
Gait	Normal	Acute: wide-based, slow, decreased arm swing and trunk rotation Compensated: normal	Acute: wide-based, slow, decreased arm swing and trunk rotation Compensated: mild gait deviation	May have pronounced ataxia
Turn head while walking	May produce slight unsteadiness	Acute: may not keep balance Compensated: normal	May not keep balance or slows cadence	May not keep balance, increased ataxia

BPPV = benign paroxysmal postural vertigo; BVH = bilateral vestibular hypofunction; UVH = unilateral vestibular hypofunction.

a temperature gradient. In the presence of gravity, this temperature gradient results in the convective flow of endolymph that deflects the cupula and generates nystagmus from the horizontal SCC. This test is particularly useful for determining the side of the deficit because each labyrinth is stimulated separately. A variation with ice water is useful to determine whether minimal function exists in the vestibular system for patients with severe loss. However, the caloric test provides limited information since only the horizontal SCCs can be stimulated and that stimulation corresponds to a frequency (0.025 Hz) that is much lower than the natural frequencies of head movement (1 to 20 Hz).[67]

The rotational chair test stimulates each horizontal SCC by rotating subjects in the dark. In subjects with normal vestibular function, nystagmus should be generated by the rotation. In the presence of a vestibular disorder, the extent of pathology can be determined by comparing VOR gain and phase from rotations toward one ear with rotations toward the opposite ear. In addition, VOR gain and phase of people with normal vestibular function can be compared with that of people with suspected vestibular hypofunction. The rotational chair test is considered the standard test for bilateral vestibular hypofunction. Rotational chair testing is limited because only the horizontal SCCs are routinely tested to determine extent of pathology.

Otolith Tests

Advances in vestibular diagnostic testing have extended the region of identifiable pathology to include the otolith organs.[68–70] The *vestibular-evoked myogenic potential* (VEMP) test is a laboratory test that has gained broad clinical use and includes two subtypes: *cervical* and *ocular* VEMP. Both types use the threshold and amplitude of a muscle contraction (electromyography [EMG]) to classify pathology. The cervical VEMP test exposes patients to aural stimuli in the form of a series of ipsilateral loud (95-decibel [dB]) clicks. During the sound application, the ipsilateral sternocleidomastoid (SCM) muscle is tested for myogenic potentials. In people with healthy vestibular function, an initial inhibitory potential (occurring at a latency of 13 milliseconds [msec] after the click) is followed by an excitatory potential (occurring at a latency of 21 msec after the click). For patients with vestibular hypofunction, the VEMPs are absent on the side of the lesion. The saccule has been implicated as the site of afferent stimulation during cervical VEMP testing because saccular afferents provide ipsilateral inhibitory disynaptic input to the SCM muscle,[71] are responsive to click noise,[72–74] and are positioned close to the footplate of the stapes (inner most auditory ossicle) and therefore are subject to mechanical stimulation.[69,72]

The ocular VEMP exposes subjects to loud clicks (aural stimuli) or bone vibration applied to the forehead at Fz at midline at the hairline. During the stimulus, EMG is measured from the inferior oblique muscle while subjects look upward to bring the muscle belly closer to the surface electrode. The ocular VEMP is a crossed, excitatory otolith-oculomotor response and in patients with UVH will be absent from the contralateral superior oblique.[75] The ocular VEMP is considered a test of the utricle and the superior vestibular nerve based on its absence in patients with abnormal caloric but preserved cervical VEMP.[75]

The *subjective visual vertical* (SVV) and *subjective visual horizontal* (SVH) tests are used to examine otolith function, though they cannot be used to uniquely detect saccular or utricular pathology. During the SVV test, patients are asked to align a dimly lit luminous bar (in an otherwise darkened room) with what they perceive as being vertical. The SVH test asks patients to align a bar with what they perceive as being horizontal. In the absence of vestibular problems, subjects typically align the bar within 1.5° of true horizontal. Patients with UVH generally align the bar more than 2° from true vertical or horizontal with the bar tilted toward the lesioned side.[70,76]

The *video ocular counter roll* (vOCR) test is sensitive enough to identify dysfunction in the pathway carrying otolith afference, though it cannot localize the side of the vestibular loss.[77] The vOCR test is done with video-oculography (VOG) goggles worn over the eyes to enable measuring the amount of ocular counter roll (in degrees) during a simple bedside maneuver that tilts the patient's head.[78] It has been shown that vOCR testing can detect loss of vestibular function with validity similar to the VEMP, with the best threshold for abnormality being less than 3° ocular counter roll.[77]

■ VESTIBULAR SYSTEM DYSFUNCTION

Peripheral Pathology

Mechanical

The most common cause of vertigo, BPPV, is a biomechanical disorder. Symptoms of BPPV include nystagmus and vertigo with change in head position, occasionally nausea with or without vomiting, and dysequilibrium. In the most common form, latency to onset of the vertigo and nystagmus occurs within 15 seconds once the head is in the provoking position. The duration is usually less than 60 seconds. The vertigo and nystagmus are direct impairments caused by the misplaced otoconia. BPPV is believed to occur via one of two mechanisms: *cupulolithiasis* and *canalithiasis*. Both of the theories involve the otoliths becoming dislodged from the utricle and falling into the SCCs. Schuknecht[79] first theorized that fragments of otoconia break away and adhere to the cupula of one of the SCCs (cupulolithiasis). When the head is moved into certain positions, the weighted cupula is deflected by the pull of gravity. This abnormal signal results in vertigo and nystagmus, which persists as long as the patient is in the provoking position. Cupulolithiasis, therefore, does not explain the brief duration of the vertigo common in BPPV.[80] A second theory was proposed, canalithiasis, in which the otoconia are floating freely in one of the SCCs.[81] When a patient changes head position, the pull of gravity causes the freely floating otoconia to move inside the SCC, resulting in endolymph movement and deflection of the cupula. Figure 21.15 illustrates BPPV occurring from cupulolithiasis or canalithiasis.

Decreased Receptor Input

The most common causes of UVH leading to decreased or eliminated receptor input are viral insults, trauma, and vascular events.[82,83] Patients who sustain a UVH will experience direct impairments of vertigo, spontaneous nystagmus, oscillopsia during head movements, postural instability, and dysequilibrium. Initially, the patient will experience vertigo and nystagmus impairments due to the asymmetry created when one vestibular system is no longer functioning. This resolves within 3 to 7 days, assuming the patient is exposed to common daylight conditions.[84] Spontaneous nystagmus in room light, beyond this time period, should alert the clinician to a possible central lesion or an unstable peripheral vestibular lesion. The direct impairments of visual blurring, postural instability, and dysequilibrium respond to physical therapy intervention. Because vertigo caused by asymmetry typically resolves within 7 days, persistent symptoms of vertigo beyond 2 weeks should be considered chronic, also necessitating vestibular rehabilitation.[80]

The most common cause of bilateral vestibular hypofunction (BVH) is ototoxicity. Certain classes of antibiotics such as aminoglycosides (e.g., gentamicin, streptomycin) are readily taken up by the hair cells of the vestibular apparatus and continue to build in this system even after the person has stopped using the antibiotic. Less common causes of BVH include meningitis, autoimmune disorders, head trauma, tumors on each eighth cranial nerve (including bilateral vestibular schwannoma), transient ischemic episodes of vessels supplying the vestibular system, and sequential unilateral vestibular neuronitis.[85–87] The primary complaint is dysequilibrium, though oscillopsia and gait ataxia are common clinical signs with a BVH diagnosis, all direct impairments. Unless the BVH is asymmetrical, the patient will not experience nausea, vertigo, or nystagmus because there is no asymmetry in the tonic firing rate of the vestibular neurons. Halmagyi et al.[88] reported that patients with gentamicin ototoxicity have

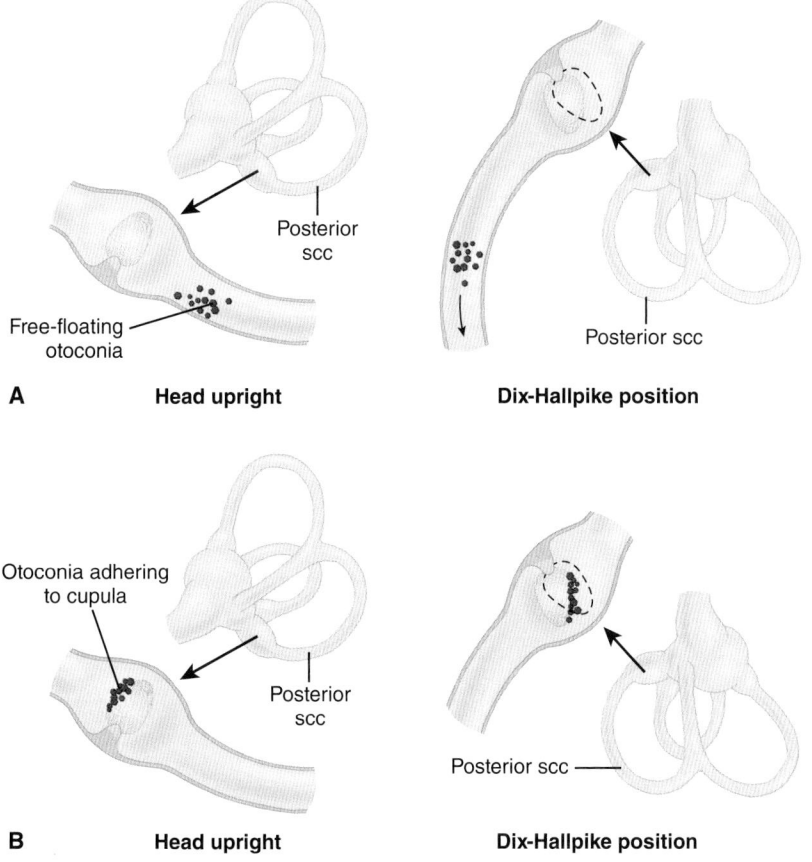

A Head upright — Posterior scc / Free-floating otoconia

Dix-Hallpike position — Posterior scc

B Head upright — Otoconia adhering to cupula / Posterior scc

Dix-Hallpike position — Posterior scc

Figure 21.15 Illustrated is BPPV of the posterior SCC. (A) Canalithiasis indicates free-floating otoconia within the SCC. When the head is moved into a position that places the SCC parallel to the pull of gravity (e.g., Dix-Hallpike position), the free-floating otoconia move to the dependent position within the canal. The movement of the free-floating otoconia results in deflection of the cupula. (B) Cupulolithiasis indicates otoconia adhering to the cupula. When the head is moved to a position placing one of the SCCs parallel to the pull of gravity (e.g., Dix–Hallpike position), the cupula is continually displaced. Illustrated is BPPV of the posterior SCC; also note the cupular deflection. Note that the cupula is drawn with the superior aspect detached from the ampulla.

posture and gait abnormalities, decreased visual acuity with head movement, and reduced VOR gains resulting in a positive head impulse test. These impairments are likely permanent, though patients with BVH can return to high levels of activity.

Central Nervous System Pathology

Various central nervous system (CNS) injuries can affect the vestibular system.[89] Cerebrovascular insults involving the *anterior-inferior cerebellar artery (AICA)*, *posterior-inferior cerebellar artery (PICA)*, and *vertebral artery* may cause vertigo, though other signs associated with these infarcts are present and help clarify the site of pathology. Signs and symptoms between an AICA and PICA infarct can be difficult to distinguish, though hearing loss is usually more common with AICA infarcts. Lesions of the vertebral artery may affect the cerebellum only and can mimic a peripheral vestibular hypofunction in its clinical presentation. Most patients with cerebellar lesions, however, will have associated signs such as dysdiadochokinesia or past pointing.[90] Individuals with transient ischemic attacks (TIAs) may present with sudden vertigo that lasts minutes, and they may also report hearing loss. For more thorough reading discerning types of central vestibular pathology, see Brandt and Dieterich[89] and Delaney.[90]

Signs and symptoms associated with *vertebrobasilar insufficiency* (VBI) typically do not involve the classic signs and symptoms of vestibular pathology. The most common cause of VBI is motor vehicle crash.[91] Purvin et al.[92] identified the most common symptoms of VBI as visual field cuts, whereas an older study reported visual dysfunction, drop attacks (sudden, spontaneous falls), and unsteadiness/incoordination as the three most common symptoms.[93] Another cause of VBI is cervical spondylosis. In these patients, vertigo and decreased blood flow velocity through vertebral arteries after head rotation have been reported.[94]

Patients who have sustained a traumatic brain injury (TBI) due to labyrinthine or skull fractures may complain of vertigo.[95] As many as 78% of patients sustaining a mild head injury reported acute vertigo, and 20% to 37% still experienced the vertigo 6 months to 5 years later.[96,97] Abnormal central processing as well as reduced receptor input may cause the perseveration of the vertigo reported in patients with TBI.

Demyelinating diseases such as multiple sclerosis (MS) can affect cranial nerve VIII where it enters the brainstem. In such a case, signs and symptoms may be identical to a UVH. An MRI scan will need to be performed to ensure an accurate diagnosis of MS.

Discerning Peripheral Vestibular Pathology From Central Vestibular Pathology

Observation of nystagmus is a useful tool for assisting in determining a diagnosis of CNS pathology. Nystagmus from a cerebellar lesion may be in a pure vertical direction.[98] The nystagmus may not have a slow component, and the eyes therefore oscillate at equal speeds called *pendular nystagmus*. Pendular nystagmus is often indicative of congenital disorders, such as the absence of central vision (cortical visual processing). Another clue to discern a central versus a peripheral vestibular pathology is the recovery time. Unlike nystagmus following a peripheral vestibular lesion, nystagmus from a central vestibular lesion often never resolves.

Vertigo can be a symptom with central pathology, but that is rare and if present, is often much less intense than with a peripheral vestibular lesion.[99] Patients with lesions of the vestibular nuclei can present with vertigo, nystagmus, and dysequilibrium similar to patients with a peripheral vestibular lesion. However, central lesions above the level of the vestibular nuclei will manifest lateropulsion, head tilt, and visual perceptual difficulties, as well as oculomotor signs. *Lateropulsion* refers to the person's tendency to fall to one side.

Brandt et al.[100] classify central vestibular syndromes from a clinical consensus of establishing perceptual, oculomotor, and postural signs. They report that the most sensitive signs of unilateral brainstem infarct are tilt of the patient's SVV and ocular torsion. *Ocular torsion* refers to the superior pole of the eyes moving together in a roll direction.

Ocular torsion combined with head tilting and skew deviation encompass a triad of signs termed a complete *ocular tilt reaction* (OTR; Fig. 21.16).[101] Skew deviation of the eyes appears as one eye being superiorly displaced in comparison with the other eye. Kattah et al.[102] examined 101 subjects with symptoms that may have been due to a central pathology (acute vertigo, nystagmus, nausea/vomiting, head-motion intolerance, unsteady gait). Each subject underwent neuroimaging at admission (generally 72 hours after symptom onset). CVAs were diagnosed by MRI or CT. The initial MRI diffusion-weighted imaging was falsely negative in 12% (48 hours after symptom onset) of subjects. However, the presence of normal horizontal head impulse test, direction-changing nystagmus in eccentric gaze, or skew deviation was 100% sensitive and 96% specific for stroke. Furthermore, the presence of skew deviation correctly predicted lateral pontine stroke in two of three cases in which an abnormal horizontal head impulse test erroneously suggested peripheral localization. In conclusion, skew is an important predictor of brainstem involvement and can identify CVA when an abnormal horizontal head impulse test may falsely suggest a peripheral lesion. The study recommended a three-step bedside oculomotor examination (HINTS: Head-Impulse, Nystagmus, Test-of-Skew) as a more sensitive measure for stroke than early MRI.[102]

Red flags that should alert the physical therapist to a central vestibular etiology include horizontal or vertical diplopia lasting longer than 2 weeks after the onset of signs or symptoms thought to be due to UVH, persistent pure vertical *positional nystagmus* (anterior canal cupulolithiasis should be ruled out), a spontaneous upbeating nystagmus (rare), and a positive test for skew deviation. The therapist should refer a patient with these manifestations to a neurologist.

It is not within the scope of this chapter to expand on the differential diagnosis within the CNS, identifying the site of lesion. However, the physical therapist must recognize the difference between central and peripheral vestibular dysfunction because this guides the treatment strategy. The symptoms presented in Table 21.5 can be used to discern central vestibular pathology from peripheral vestibular pathology.

■ INTERVENTIONS
Benign Paroxysmal Positional Vertigo
The development of specific goals and outcomes for the individual patient with BPPV is based on the following general goals:

- The otoconia will be returned in to the vestibule.
- The patient will demonstrate reduced vertigo associated with head motion.
- The patient will demonstrate reduced or absent nystagmus associated with head motion.
- The patient will demonstrate improved balance.
- The patient will demonstrate independence in daily activity (basic activities of daily living [BADL] and instrumental activities of daily living [IADL]) involving head motion.

Because BPPV is the most common peripheral vestibular pathology, physical therapists should be familiar with treating this disorder. The type of nystagmus generated as result of placing the SCCs in gravity-dependent positions indicates which SCC is involved (Table 21.6) and directs the clinician to choose an appropriate treatment approach. Three different treatment approaches have been developed, each based on pathophysiological theories of this disorder. The techniques include the canalith repositioning maneuver, the Liberatory (Semont) maneuver, and Brandt–Daroff exercises.

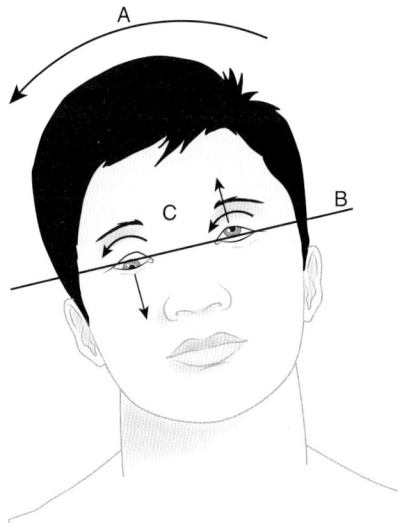

Figure 21.16 The OTR consists of a triad of signs: (A) Head tilting to the right, indicated with the large arrow. (B) Skew deviation of the eyes (right eye is down, left eye is up), indicated with the bisecting line and straight arrows. (C) Torsion of the eyes to the right, indicated with the two smaller rounded arrows.

Table 21.5 Common Symptoms Associated With Central Versus Peripheral Vestibular Pathology	
Central Vestibular Pathology	**Peripheral Vestibular Pathology**
Ataxia often severe.	Ataxia mild.
Abnormal smooth pursuit and abnormal saccadic eye movement tests.	Smooth pursuit and saccades usually normal; positional testing may reproduce nystagmus.
SX usually do not include hearing loss; if so, it is often sudden and permanent.	SX may include hearing loss (insidious—may recover), fullness in ears, tinnitus.
SX might include diplopia, altered conscious, lateropulsion.	SX of acute vertigo usually suppressed by visual fixation.
SX of acute vertigo not usually suppressed by visual fixation.	SX of acute vertigo usually intense (more than central vestibular pathology).
Pendular nystagmus (eyes oscillate at equal speeds).	Nystagmus will incorporate slow and fast phases (jerk nystagmus).
Pure persistent vertical nystagmus persists regardless of positional testing (persistent downbeat nystagmus in Dix–Hallpike test may indicate anterior canal BPPV).	Spontaneous horizontal nystagmus usually resolves within 7 days in a patient with UVH.

BPPV = benign paroxysmal postural vertigo; SX = symptoms; UVH = unilateral vestibular hypofunction.

Table 21.6   Type of Nystagmus Based on Semicircular Canals Location and Mechanism of Benign Paroxysmal Postural Vertigo

SCC[a]	Mechanism	Nystagmus[b]	Incidence (%)[12]
Right posterior	Cupulolithiasis	Persistent UBN and right torsion[d]	62
	Canalithiasis	Transient UBN and right torsion	
Left posterior	Cupulolithiasis	Persistent UBN and left torsion	
	Canalithiasis	Transient UBN and left torsion	
Horizontal[e]	Cupulolithiasis	Persistent ageotropic[f]	35
	Canalithiasis	Transient geotropic[g]	
Right superior	Cupulolithiasis	Persistent DBN and right torsion	3
	Canalithiasis	Persistent DBN and right torsion	
Left superior	Cupulolithiasis	Persistent DBN and left torsion	
	Canalithiasis	Persistent DBN and left torsion	

BPPV = benign paroxysmal positional vertigo; DBN = downbeat nystagmus; SCC = semicircular canals; UBN = upbeat nystagmus
[a]Testing for BPPV in the SCC assumes the patient is in the appropriate positional test.
[b]Nystagmus is labeled by the direction of the fast component. UBN means the fast component of the nystagmus is beating upward.
[c]The incidence of BPPV refers to the affected semicircular canal, not the type of BPPV.
[d]Torsional rotation is noted as it relates to the superior poles of the eyes from the perspective of the examiner.
[e]When BPPV occurs in the horizontal SCC, nystagmus will be present when the head is positioned to either side.
[f]Ageotropic nystagmus = fast component beats away from the ground.
[g]Geotropic nystagmus = fast component beats toward the ground.

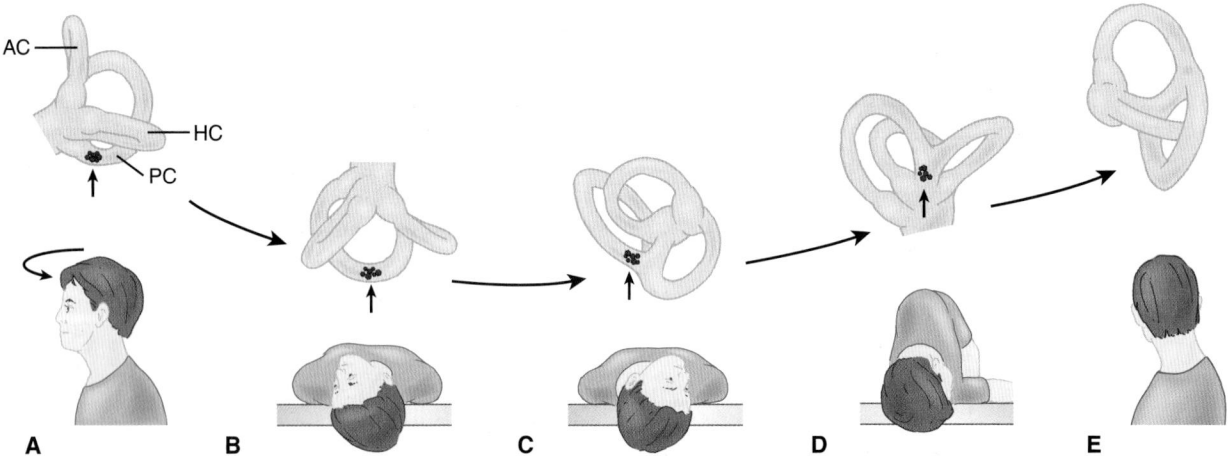

Figure 21.17 CRM for posterior or anterior semicircular canal BPPV. (A) The patient's head is first rotated 45° toward the involved side, pictured here at the left. (B) The patient is then moved into the Dix-Hallpike position with the affected left ear toward the ground. (C) Next, the head is rotated 90° to the right. It is important to maintain the 30° neck extension during this step. The head should now be positioned 45° to the right. (D) The patient is rolled onto the right shoulder and (E) slowly brought up to sitting position, head still rotated 45° to the right. The patient may then be fitted with a soft collar. Note the orientation of the labyrinth for each stage. The arrow points to the free-floating debris and shows its movement through the canal into the common crus (D). AC = anterior SCC; PC = posterior SCC; HC = horizontal SCC. Between each step, the clinician should wait 1 to 2 minutes or until the vertigo and nystagmus have stopped to ensure otoconia flow through the canal.

The *canalith repositioning maneuver* (CRM) is based on the canalithiasis theory of free-floating debris in the SCC.[103] The patient's head is moved into different positions in a sequence that will move the debris out of the involved SCC and into the vestibule (general term for the location of the utricle and saccule; see Fig. 21.1). Once the debris is in the vestibule, the signs and symptoms should resolve. The positions used in the treatment of posterior and anterior SCC canalithiasis can be the same. Figure 21.17 illustrates the CRM as applied to either the left posterior or left anterior SCC. It is important to instruct the patient that horizontal movement of the head is not contraindicated and should be performed to prevent stiff neck muscles. Patients may wish to limit vertical head motion. CRM has also been adapted for application to the horizontal SCC (Fig. 21.18), although BPPV is less common in either the horizontal or anterior SCC.[104] The original post-CRM instructions asked patients to remain upright for one to two nights (sleep in a recliner chair) and then to avoid sleeping on the involved side for five additional nights. There is no evidence to support sleeping upright after CRM.[105] Recurrence of BPPV varies depending on the study involved.[106,107] There is no evidence that prophylactic CRM prevents recurrence.[108]

The *Liberatory (Semont) maneuver* was first offered as a treatment for posterior SCC BPPV based on the

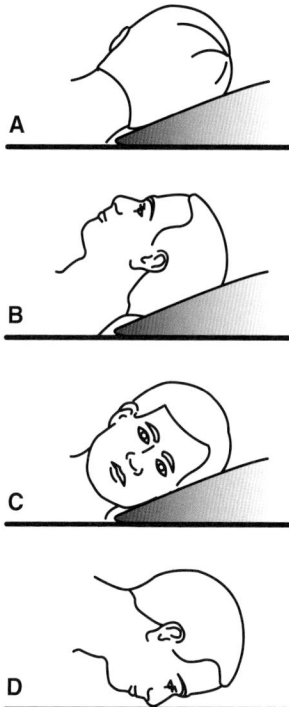

Figure 21.18 CRM for right horizontal semicircular canal BPPV. Initially, the patient's head should be placed in 20° cervical flexion. (A) For treating a right-sided horizontal canal BPPV, the patient's head is initially placed 90° to the right. (B) Next, the head is rotated 90° to the left. The therapist should wait in this position for 15 seconds or until the vertigo and nystagmus stops. (C) The head should then be rotated another 90° to the left; again, the therapist must wait for 15 seconds or until the vertigo and nystagmus stops. (D) The patient must then roll into prone position and await the signs or symptoms to stop. The therapist must attempt to keep the head in 20° flexion during the transition from C to D. If the CRT has been successful, nystagmus and vertigo should resolve once the patient is in the prone position. The patient may need assistance to sit up from the prone position.

cupulolithiasis theory.[109] It involves rapidly moving the patient through positions designed to dislodge the debris from the cupula (Fig. 21.19). Data suggest it is effective as an alternative treatment for canalithiasis, though it may be more difficult for the patient to tolerate.[110,111]

Brandt–Daroff exercises were originally designed to habituate the CNS to the provoking position.[112] Evidence now suggests that Brandt–Daroff exercises are not effective to remove displaced otoconia.[113] They may still be useful to treat motion-induced dizziness that is not caused by BPPV, or perhaps to habituation dizziness sensations once BPPV has been resolved. Figure 21.20 illustrates the exercises. The exercise should be performed for 5 to 10 repetitions, three times a day until the patient has no vertigo for 2 consecutive days. If the patient has severe vertigo or complaints of nausea, decreasing the number of repetitions to three, performed three times a day, may render the exercises more tolerable. It is important to explain to the patient that the movements must be performed rapidly and that this will probably provoke vertigo. Education should also include informing the patient that it is normal to have some residual symptoms of dysequilibrium and nausea on completing the exercises. The residual symptoms are usually temporary, and patients need to continue the exercises.

The goal of performing CRM and liberatory procedures is to replace the otoconia into the vestibule, where the calcium crystals can be reabsorbed or perhaps dissolved. The Brandt–Daroff exercises, although originally designed to habituate the peripheral vestibular response, have also led to a complete remission of symptoms, sometimes after the first exercise session.[112] Physical therapy outcomes should also include teaching the patient how to use the appropriate techniques at home, in the case of recurrence. See Table 21.7 for suggested guidelines for use of the CRM, the Liberatory (Semont) maneuver, and Brandt–Daroff exercises.

Unilateral Vestibular Hypofunction

The development of specific goals and expected outcomes for the individual patient with UVH is based on the following general goals:

- The patient will demonstrate improved stability of gaze during head movement.
- The patient will demonstrate diminished sensitivity to motion.
- The patient will demonstrate improved static and dynamic postural stability.
- The patient will be independent in a home exercise program (HEP) that includes walking.

Patients with UVH should be informed that recovery time after initiating vestibular rehabilitation averages 5 to 7 weeks. To ensure adherence with the vestibular rehabilitation exercises, patients should be encouraged

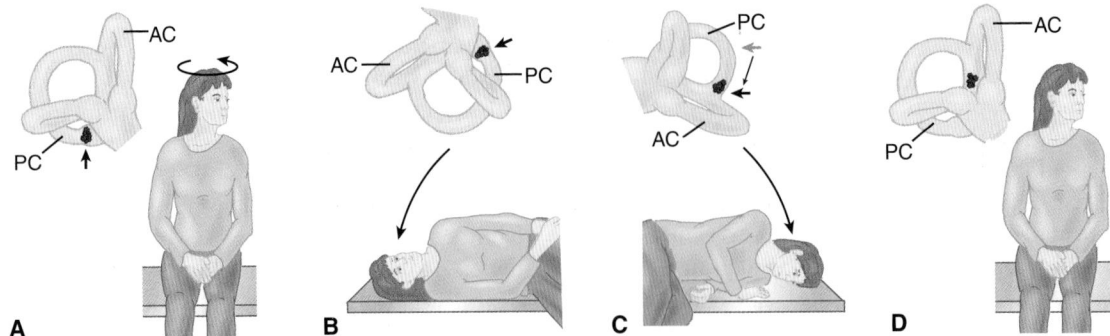

Figure 21.19 Liberatory (Semont) maneuver for right posterior SCC BPPV. The physical therapist should assist the patient through this positioning procedure. Note the otoconia adherent to the cupula in A and B. (A) The head is rotated 45° to the left side. (B) With assistance, the patient is then moved from sitting to right side-lying and stays in this position for 1 minute. (C) The patient is then rapidly moved 180°, from right side-lying to left side-lying. The head should be in the original starting position, left rotated (nose down in final position) in this example. Note that the otoconia have been dislodged from the cupula. After 1 minute in this position, (D) the patient returns to sitting. AC = anterior SCC; PC = posterior SCC.

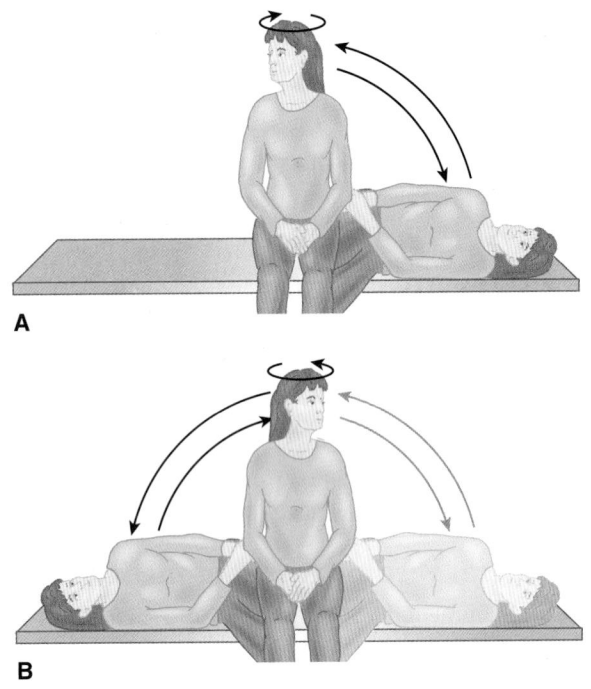

Figure 21.20 Brandt–Daroff exercises for posterior SCC BPPV. (A) The patient starts in a sitting position and turns the head 45° to one side (*right*), then quickly lies down on the opposite shoulder (*left*). The patient should be instructed to remain in this position for 30 seconds or until the vertigo stops. The patient then slowly returns to the starting position (A), maintaining the head rotation (*right*) until sitting upright. (B) Next, the patient turns the head to the opposite direction (*left*) and lies down on the other shoulder (*right*), observing the similar 30-second time guidelines. The exercise should be done 10 to 20 times, three times per day until the patient is without vertigo for 2 consecutive days.

Table 21.7	Benign Paroxysmal Positional Vertigo Treatment Techniques	
Treatment Procedure		**Diagnosis/Symptoms**
CRM		BPPV due to canalithiasis Posterior SCC canalithiasis the most common
Liberatory maneuver		BPPV due to canalithiasis or cupulolithiasis
Brandt–Daroff exercises		Persistent/residual or mild vertigo (even after CRM) For the patient who may not tolerate CRM

BPPV = benign paroxysmal positional vertigo; CRM = canalith repositioning maneuver; SCC = semicircular canal.
Note: This table presents an overview of the treatment procedures for
 BPPV. For more in-depth content on the many different CRM for each
 semicircular canal, please see Gold et al. in Supplemental Reading.

frequently, and mutually agreed on goals and outcomes should be regularly reinforced. According to the 2021 clinical practice guideline for rehabilitation of vestibular hypofunction,[114] clinicians should not include voluntary saccadic or smooth-pursuit eye movements alone to improve gaze stability in vestibular hypofunction. Therapists may target activity limitations and participation restrictions by offering specific exercise techniques, such as virtual reality or augmented sensory feedback. It is recommended that vestibular rehabilitation be done under the supervision of a specialty trained clinician, who can prescribe weekly clinic visits in addition to a home exercise program of gaze stabilization exercises.

Gaze Stability Exercises

The purpose of these gaze stability exercises (GSE) is to improve the VOR and other systems that are used to assist gaze stability with head motion. There is some evidence suggesting VOR gain does change after performing GSEs.[115] Vestibular adaptation exercises are designed to expose patients to retinal slip. *Retinal slip* occurs when the image of an object moves off the fovea of the retina, resulting in visual blurring. Retinal slip is necessary as this is the signal used to drive vestibular adaptation within the brain. Because the brain can tolerate small amounts of retinal slip yet see a target clearly, the patient must try to keep the target in focus. Otherwise, head motion that is too rapid will result in excessive retinal slip. The two primary paradigms of vestibular adaptation are ×1 (times 1) and ×2 (times 2) exercises.[37] In the ×1 exercise, the patient is asked to move the head horizontally (and vertically if appropriate) as quickly as possible while maintaining focus on a stable target. The patient must learn to slow the head movement if the target becomes blurred. A good target to use is a business card, asking the patient to focus on a word or a

letter within a word. The starting target distance should be an arm's length away. The ×2 paradigm requires the patient to move the head and target in opposite directions (Fig. 21.21). Both paradigms should be made increasingly more difficult as the patient improves. Examples of increasing difficulty include the use of a distracting background while the patient attempts to focus on the letter or word (checkerboard, Venetian blinds), varying the distance from which the patient performs the exercises, moving the head more rapidly, and performing the exercise while standing or walking. GSE programs should be performed at a minimum of three times a day for at least 12 minutes in individuals diagnosed with acute/subacute UVH. For individuals with chronic UVH, these exercises should be performed between 3 to 5 times per day for a minimum of 20 minutes daily over 4 to 6 weeks. The *computerized DVA* test is a useful measure of improved gaze stability for individuals with UVH and TBI.[64,116] Additionally, clinicians may prescribe static and dynamic balance exercises for a minimum of 20 minutes daily for at least 4 to 6 weeks for chronic unilateral vestibular hypofunction.

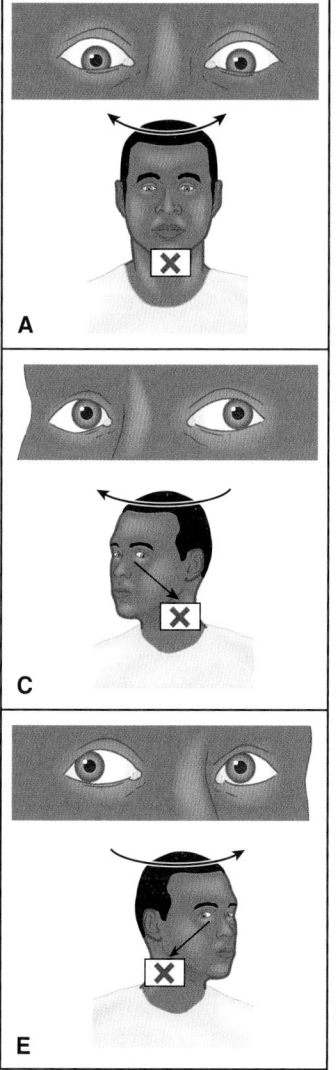
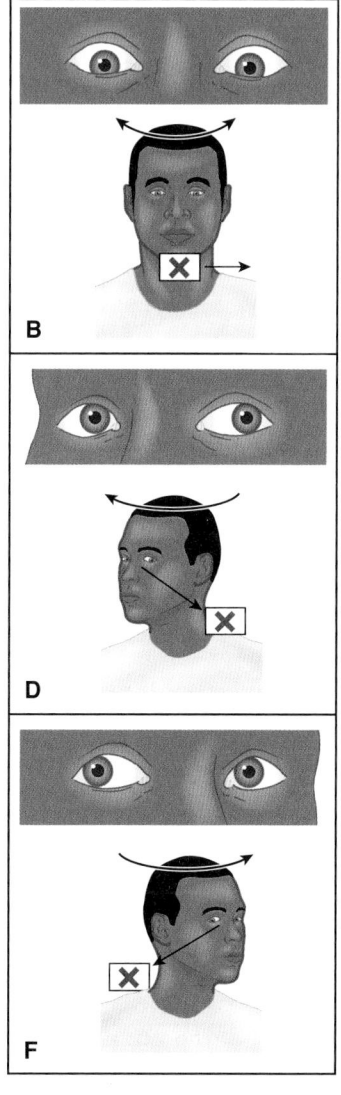

Figure 21.21 Gaze stability exercises. (A, C, E) ×1 paradigm: The patient is instructed to focus the eyes on a near target. While maintaining focus on the target, the patient horizontally rotates the head, keeping the target still. (B, D, F) ×2 paradigm: The patient is instructed to focus the eyes on a near target. While the focus is maintained, the patient horizontally rotates the head and the target in *opposite* directions. Both ×1 and ×2 paradigms require vigilance of the patient to ensure clear vision during the motions. Both exercises are typically performed for 1 to 2 minutes, five times a day. It can be repeated using vertical head movements.

Postural Stability Exercises

The purpose of postural stability exercises is to improve balance by encouraging the development of balance strategies within the patient's limitations, be they somatosensory, visual, or vestibular. The exercises should challenge the patient and be safe enough to perform independently (Table 21.8). Exercises must be updated and progressed to incorporate more challenges (Fig. 21.22). In addition, it is important to incorporate head movement into the exercises because many patients with vestibular loss tend to decrease their head movement.

Habituation Exercises (Motion Sensitivity)

Habituation exercises are warranted when a patient with a UVH has continual complaints of dizziness. *Habituation* is defined as the reduction in response to a repeatedly performed movement. These exercises were the first successful methods used to treat persons with vestibular disorders. Various investigators[43,117] have developed versions of positional tests based on the original exercises and studies by Cawthorne,[11] Cooksey,[12] Norre and DeWeerdt,[118] and Dix.[119,120] As our knowledge of the vestibular system improves, however, we are able to provide more specific exercises than what habituation offers. Clinicians should not use habituation exercises to treat all patients with vestibular disorders.

To determine which habituation exercises to prescribe, the physical therapist first must determine the provoking positions (see Fig. 21.8). When a position elicits a mild to moderate dizziness, the patient remains in the provoking position for 30 seconds or until the symptoms abate, whichever comes first.[43] The patient is provided with an HEP based on the results of the positional test.[43,112] The provoking exercises are performed from three to five times each, two to three times a day.

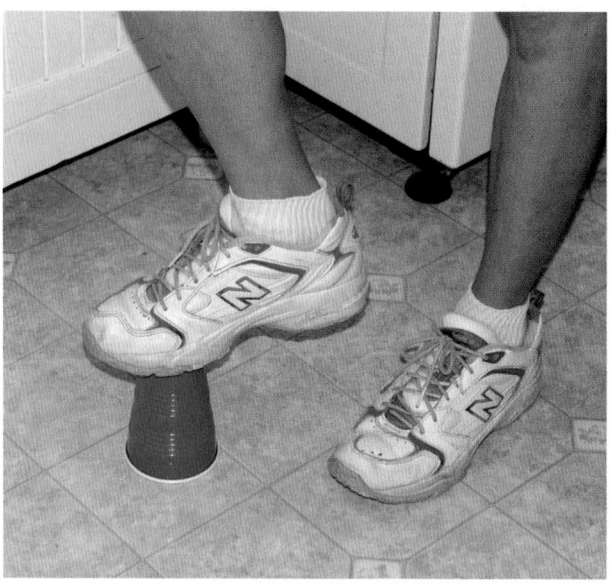

Figure 21.22 Example of a more difficult balance exercise. Instruct the patient to gently place his or her foot on a plastic cup and maintain his or her balance without crushing the cup. Initially, the patient should be advised to use a handhold. The exercise can be progressed to eyes closed, no handhold, or stepping while alternating foot placement on the cup.

Table 21.8   Balance Exercises and Progressions

Begin With	Progress To	Purpose
1. Stand with feet shoulder-width apart, arms across the chest.	Bringing feet closer together. Close eyes. Stand on a sofa cushion or foam.	Enhances the use of vestibular cues for balance by decreasing base of support. Eyes closed increases reliance on vestibular cues for balance.
2. Practice ankle sways: medial-lateral and anterior-posterior.	Doing circle sways. Close eyes.	Teaches the patient to use a correct ankle strategy.
3. Attempt to walk with heel touching toe on firm surface.	Doing the same exercise on carpet.	Enhances the use of vestibular cues for balance by decreasing base of support. Doing the exercise on carpet alters proprioceptive input, increasing difficulty.
4. Practice walking five steps and turning 180° (left and right).	Making smaller turns. Close eyes.	Turning provides a greater challenge to the vestibular system.
5. Walk and move the head side to side, up and down.	Counting backward from 100 by threes.	Uses distracting cognitive or motor demands to challenge balance.

Note: This table presents a limited number of exercises that are effective at improving functional balance. Each of the balance exercises should be performed three times a day for 1 to 2 minutes each repetition.

Figure 21.23 provides an example of an HEP using vestibular habituation training. An activity diary can be a useful method to monitor response to training. The exercises are designed to reproduce the dizziness the patient experiences, and the patient should be encouraged that the symptoms normally decrease within 2 weeks. If after 2 weeks the symptoms are no better, first the habituation exercises should be changed. If this is not helpful, the patient should be referred to either a physical therapist with special training in vestibular rehabilitation or a physician for further evaluation.

Bilateral Vestibular Hypofunction

The development of specific goals and expected outcomes for the individual patient with BVH is based on the following general goals:

- The patient will demonstrate improved stability of gaze during head movement.
- The patient will demonstrate reduced subjective complaints of gaze instability.
- The patient will demonstrate improved static and dynamic balance.
- The patient will be independent in an HEP that includes walking.
- The patient will demonstrate enhanced decision-making skills during performance of basic and IADL.

Treatment of patients with a BVH is designed to address the primary complaints of gaze instability during head motion, dysequilibrium, and gait ataxia. Gaze stability exercises can be similar to the ×1 paradigm described in treatment for UVH. GSE programs should be carried three to five times a day for a total minimum of 20 to 40 minutes daily over 5 to 7 weeks.[114,121] Use of the ×2 paradigm is generally not recommended for a patient with a BVH because this exercise may cause excessive retinal slip. However, many patients have an asymmetrical BVH, in which the ×2 exercise may be useful. Instead, exercises that incorporate sequenced eye and head movements and the use of imaginary targets may improve gaze stability by enhancing central preprogramming of eye movements (Table 21.9).

Additionally, clinicians may prescribe static and dynamic balance exercises for a minimum of 20 minutes daily for at least 6 to 9 weeks.[114,121] Patients with BVH depend on somatosensation and/or vision to maintain postural stability. Balance exercises should enhance the use of these cues. Care must be taken that the exercises are performed safely because people with BVH are likely to fall.[122] It is imperative to begin the patient on a walking program, daily if tolerated. This can be progressed to ambulating on different surfaces (grass, gravel, sand) and in different environments (grocery store, mall). Recovery from a lesion involving both vestibular systems takes much longer than a unilateral lesion. Patients should be informed that as long as 2 years may be necessary to ensure as complete a recovery as possible. For this reason, patient education emphasizing daily activity is a high priority. Daily activity must continue beyond the course of vestibular rehabilitation. Other recommended activities include exercises in a pool and Tai Chi. A pool provides an environment of buoyancy, allowing the patient to move safely without the risk of falling quickly to the ground. Tai chi incorporates slow, controlled motions used to improve balance, flexibility, and increase strength. In most cases, a person with a BVH will incur an activity limitation or disability. Certain activities may always be limited, such as walking in the dark, night driving, or

Instructions for the Patient:
Once in the provoking position, wait for 10 seconds to determine if the dizziness will occur. If you experience symptoms of dizziness, remain in the position for an additional 20 seconds (30 seconds total) or until the dizziness abates, whichever comes first. If you do not experience any symptoms you may return to your starting position. Now that you have returned to your starting position, remain here for 10 seconds to monitor your dizziness. If you are dizzy, remain in the return position for an additional 20 seconds (30 seconds total) or until the symptoms abate, whichever comes first. Repeat five times.

Example of Exercises:
1.) Quickly move from sitting upright to bending at the trunk as if to touch your nose to your knee.
2.) Quickly move from sitting at the edge of the bed to lying flat.
3.) In supine, roll onto your left then right side.

Guidelines for the Therapist:
Often, the patient may complain of a certain movement that provokes the symptoms that the examination does not incorporate. This movement can be adapted to be a part of the patient's home exercise program.

	Mon	Tues	Wed	Thur	Fri	Sat	Sun
Duration (0–30 seconds)							
Intensity (0–5)							

Figure 21.23 Example of a home exercise program using habituation therapy. Intensity refers to symptoms (or dizziness) on a 5-point scale (0 = none; 5 = most severe).

Table 21.9 Bilateral Vestibular Lesion Exercises to Improve Gaze Stability	
Begin With	**Progress To**
1. In sitting, hold two targets at arm's length from your head (i.e., X and Y). Look with your eyes first to one of the targets (X) and make sure your nose is pointed to the "X" as well. Now look at the "Y" with your eyes only, followed by turning your head horizontally to point your nose to the "Y." Repeat this sequence of alternating between the two targets. Attempt to do this for 60 seconds. The patient should be instructed to always first make an eye rotation followed by a head rotation.	Progress to increasing the distance used to see the target. Use a busy background (checkerboard, venetian blinds). Progress to doing this standing.
2. In sitting perform exercise 1 above using vertical head turns.	Same as above.
3. In sitting, hold one target at arm's length from your head. Close your eyes and turn your head horizontally away from the target, attempting to keep your eyes focused on the target. Open your eyes only after having turned your head.	Progress to doing this standing. Progress to decreasing base of support.

sports involving quick movements of the head.[123] Older patients may have to use an assistive device such as a cane for safe ambulation at night or on uneven surfaces. Habituation exercises do not work for the patient with a bilateral vestibular loss.[43]

Vestibular adaptation exercises are an excellent starting point for rehabilitation of patients with vestibular hypofunction (UVH and BVH). Research supports the beneficial effects of vestibular adaptation exercises on gait, posture, and DVA.[37,115,124–132] For a thorough report on the beneficial effects of vestibular rehabilitation, see the systematic review of literature by Hall and colleagues.[133] The Evidence Summary in Table 21.10 presents outcome studies using GSEs for vestibular hypofunction. Resolution of symptoms or the achievement of normalized balance and vestibular function could be used as reasons for stopping therapy in both unilateral and BVH.

Abnormal Central Vestibular Function

The development of specific goals and expected outcomes for the individual patient with a central vestibular lesion is based on the following general goals:

- The patient will demonstrate enhanced decision-making skill regarding fall prevention strategies and necessary safety precautions to allow safe functioning within the home and community.
- The patient will demonstrate enhanced decision-making skills regarding use of compensatory strategies to assist in gaze stability.
- The patient will be independent in performance of an HEP that includes walking.

Once an accurate diagnosis of central vestibular pathology is made, expectations for recovery should be described initially to the patient. Generally, the time to recover will be 6 months or more, and full recovery may not be achieved.[134] Many of the adaptive mechanisms thought responsible for recovery of the vestibular system are central processes that may have been damaged in the initial central lesion. Physical therapists treating patients with TBI must be cautious not to be too aggressive, which will greatly exacerbate the patient's symptoms. Though vestibular rehabilitation offers promise for treating persons with TBI,[134] it may not always be the treatment of choice owing to its irritative nature.

The physical therapy intervention for a central vestibular lesion at the level of the brainstem (vestibular nuclei) likely will be similar to a UVH, with the same expectations for recovery. Vestibular cortical lesions may also recover, similar to the process in which recovery from a CVA might occur.

Because many patients with central vestibular lesions complain of dizziness, a good treatment approach is to start with habituation exercises. However, the exercises should not be too aggressive, thereby aggravating the patient's condition. In addition, gait and balance exercises designed to incorporate somatosensory, visual, and vestibular contributions are also effective with this patient population.

Patient Education

The vestibular system requires movement to recover from most lesions. This basic tenet should be thoroughly discussed when educating patients about returning to daily activity, exercising independently at home, and as a general guideline for their recovery. Appendix 21.A (online) includes Web-based resources for clinicians, families, and patients with vestibular disorders. The vestibular system will not improve to its greatest extent without head motion. The challenge for both outpatient and inpatient management is determining the amount of exertion the patient can tolerate and creating an effective vestibular rehabilitation strategy without causing deleterious effects.

Text continued on page 843

Table 21.10 Evidence Summary Outcome Studies Using GSEs to Improve Gait, Balance, and Dynamic Visual Acuity in Subjects With Vestibular Hypofunction

Reference Citation	Subjects	Design	Intervention	Results	Comments
Cole et al., 2022[121]	138 trials in the review	Scoping review on gaze stabilization exercises used to address vestibular dysfunction or gaze instability whether vestibular dysfunction was present or not. Databases searched included PubMed, CINAHL, Scopus, and Cochrane.	Examined and quantified the parameters of dose (duration, speed, head excursion) and dosage (daily and weekly frequency, duration) of gaze stabilization exercises used to improve gaze-related performance in peripheral vestibular dysfunction (50), bilateral and/or unilateral peripheral vestibular hypofunction (53), other peripheral diagnoses (e.g., dehiscence and cervicogenic dizziness) (5), central dysfunctions (e.g., stroke, MS) (16), TBI (11),and vestibular hypofunction in healthy vestibular populations (7).	Only 13 studies reported all six dose and dosage parameters of GSE prescription. Nine of the studies, however, were based on very short interventions. Most studies reviewed only reported three out of six parameters. Dosage parameters (duration, daily frequency and weekly frequency) were more frequently reported than dose parameters (repetition duration, speed and excursion). 12.3% of studies omitted information on both dose and dosage. 113 of the investigated studies used GSE as an adjunct to other rehabilitation interventions.	Very recent review on GSE ability to improve gaze performance in patients with/without vestibular dysfunction. It suggests that to date, there is still a lack of consensus or well-structured guidelines for the standardized use of GSE in neurorehabilitation.
Wang et al., 2021[183]	18 participants. E: Nine patients with vestibular schwannoma at pre- and 6-weeks postsurgery stages. Mean age 56.1 ± 15.7 years. C: Nine age-matched healthy controls. Mean age 49.3 ± 15 years.	Cross-sectional study with follow-up at 6 weeks on head kinematics performance during GSE following vestibular schwannoma resection.	Angular head velocity was collected with a wearable sensor attached to the participant's head during 12 GSE (six continuous and six transient) performed before surgery, 1 week after surgery and 6 weeks after surgery.	Head movement in both continuous and transient GSE paralleled that of natural head movement; however, only continuous exercises yielded kinematic patterns that could differentiate patients from healthy controls. Specifically, coupling of kinematic measures present in control subjects was absent in patients during continuous but not transient head rotations.	This study relied on objective kinematic measures to determine that continuous head motion, unlike transient head motion, could be used to distinguish vestibular hypofunction from healthy vestibular behavior during GSE.

(Continued)

Table 21.10	Evidence Summary Outcome Studies Using GSEs to Improve Gait, Balance, and Dynamic Visual Acuity in Subjects With Vestibular Hypofunction—cont'd				
Reference Citation	Subjects	Design	Intervention	Results	Comments
Wang et al., 2021[184]	18 participants. E: nine patients with vestibular schwannoma at pre- and six-weeks postsurgery stages. Mean age 56.1 ± 15.7 years. C: Nine age-matched healthy controls. Mean age 49.3 ± 15 years.	Cross-sectional study with follow-up at 6 weeks on head kinematics performance during GSE following vestibular schwannoma resection.	Angular head velocity was collected with a wearable sensor attached to the participant's head during performance of six continuous GSE before surgery, one week after surgery, and 6 weeks after surgery.	Kinematic measures were significantly abnormal in patients compared to age-matched healthy controls, both pre- and postsurgery, with patients taking longer time to move their heads regardless of movement direction.	The assessment and prescription of GSE are often subjective. This study used inertial measurement units to objectively show for the first time that head kinematic measures during GSE are altered in patients with vestibular hypofunction due to schwannoma, even before tumor resection.
Rinaudo, et al., 2021[185]	20 participants. E: 10 UVH patients. Mean age 62 years (35–72). C: 10 sex-matched healthy controls. Mean age 49 years (24–69).	Cross-sectional study based on a two-session exposure to GSE.	Training was classified as ×1 and ×2. During ×1 training, patients actively moved their head sinusoidally while viewing a stationary target. For ×2 training, patients moved their outstretched hand antiphase with their head rotation while attempting to view a handheld target. GSE incrementally increased head rotation from 0.5–2 Hz over 20 minutes. Active and passive sinusoidal and head impulse VOR gains were measured.	Patients showed an increase in impulse but not sinusoidal VOR response after a single session of manual ×2 training. Patients had more variability in VOR demand during manual ×2 training compared to controls.	This study suggests that the clinical ×1 gaze-stabilizing exercise used was a weak stimulus for VOR adaptation in UVH.

Table 21.10 Evidence Summary Outcome Studies Using GSEs to Improve Gait, Balance, and Dynamic Visual Acuity in Subjects With Vestibular Hypofunction—cont'd

Reference Citation	Subjects	Design	Intervention	Results	Comments
Millar et al., 2020[186]	43 patients with UVD surgery were recruited. Mean age 52 ± 13 years. E: N = 19 patients with completed protocol. C: N = 38 age-matched healthy controls for DVA test (mean age 46.9 ± 15.9 years); and N = 28 healthy controls for video-head impulse testing (mean age 45 ± 17 years).	Cross-sectional study on a 5-week GSE protocol implemented with static and dynamic postural stability tasks.	Patients were assigned an exercise group. Each exercise group (A, B, C) completed six exercises including two active gaze stability, two static balance, and two dynamic balance exercises. Each exercise was performed in three repetitions of 1.5 minutes for a total of 27 minutes, 7 days a week, for 5 weeks.	Subjective and fall risk measures showed clinically meaningful improvement. DVA during active head rotation improved. As a group, passive yaw VOR gain did not change after rehabilitation. The velocity of the overt compensatory saccades during ipsilesional head impulses were reduced after rehabilitation. Preserved utricular function was correlated with improved yaw DVA and preserved saccular function was correlated with improved pitch DVA.	This study showed that combining gaze and gait stability exercises improved subjective and behavioral performance in UVD despite absent change in VOR gain in most patients, which could be associated to residual otolith function.
Lacour et al., 2020[187]	28 patients with UVH in three experimental groups. E: First (early) group, N = 10; mean age 66.1 ± 8.7 years. Second (late 1) group, N = 9; mean age 63.1 ± 9.3 years. Third (late 2) group, N = 9; mean age 60.2 ± 9.1 years. EC: central vestibular or ocular motor dysfunctions, positional vertigo.	Prospective study with between-groups comparison.	Patients were tested under passive conditions before (pretests) and after (post-tests) a protocol that consisted in active gaze stabilization exercises with two training sessions per week, each lasting 30 minutes, for 4 weeks.	Early rehabilitation improved dynamic visual acuity score by increasing passive aVOR gain and decreasing compensatory saccades. The late one and late two groups showed less DVA improvement, with no change in the aVOR gain and an increase in compensatory saccades. All groups showed significant reduction in DHI score, with higher improvement in subjective perception of dizziness handicap in the patients receiving early rehabilitation.	This study shows evidence that earlier GSE-based rehabilitation is better to improve DVA and passive aVOR gains.

Table 21.10   Evidence Summary Outcome Studies Using GSEs to Improve Gait, Balance, and Dynamic Visual Acuity in Subjects With Vestibular Hypofunction—cont'd

Reference Citation	Subjects	Design	Intervention	Results	Comments
Meldrum and Jahn, 2019[188]	Nonsystematic literature review	Review of evidence-based clinical advances	Included studies addressing the effects of GSE on vestibular rehabilitation compared to habituation exercises, and how performance in GSE could serve as measures of vestibular function.	Active vestibulo-ocular reflex improves with short periods of GSE, but passive VOR gains do not improve to the same degree. GSE seem to have a modifying effect on compensatory saccade organization and could improve dynamic visual acuity.	This study summarizes important findings on GSE and highlights the current paradigm shift from delivering GSE via traditional pen and paper toward technology-based methods with more objective outcome measures.
Schubert et al., 2008[115]	E: $n = 4$ UVH and one BVH; mean age 54.4 ± 8.9 years; C: $n = 5$ age-matched healthy controls, mean 54 ± 12.8 years EC: patients with dizziness not confirmed as true vestibular hypofunction, BPPV.	Age-matched control intervention study E: VOR adaptation and balance exercises 4–5×/day for 20–30 minutes C: No intervention	Mean 5.0 ± 1.4 visits; over 66 ± 24 days Outcome measures: a VOR gain and DVA	DVA improved (mean, 51% ± 25%, range 21%–81%) AVOR gain during the head rotation increased in each patient mean range, 0.7 ± 0.2 to 0.9 ± 0.2 (35%) For control subjects, a VOR gain during DVA was always near one. Patients also increased use of compensatory saccades.	First study to show mechanistic effect of exercises explaining improved DVA Saccade system also modifiable with GSE.
Hillier and McDonnell., 2007[131]	21 trials in the review.	Cochrane review of RCT on vestibular rehabilitation in adults living in the community, diagnosed with symptomatic unilateral peripheral vestibular hypofunction.	Included studies addressing the effectiveness of vestibular rehabilitation against control/sham interventions, nonvestibular rehabilitation interventions, by comparing the subjects in each group who had significant resolution of symptoms and/or improved function.	Individual and pooled data showed a statistically significant effect in favor of the vestibular rehabilitation over control or no intervention; there were no reported adverse effects.	Moderate to strong evidence that vestibular rehabilitation is a safe, effective management for UVH.

Table 21.10 Evidence Summary Outcome Studies Using GSEs to Improve Gait, Balance, and Dynamic Visual Acuity in Subjects With Vestibular Hypofunction—cont'd

Reference Citation	Subjects	Design	Intervention	Results	Comments
Herdman et al., 2007[124]	13 Patients with BVH E: N = 8; mean age 63.6 ± 9.4 C: N = 8; mean age 63.6 ± 10.8 EC: presence of nystagmus in room light, static visual acuity with the worse than logMAR 0.500, minors/people incapable of understanding the purpose.	RCT; double blind; repeated measures with control E: VOR adaptation exercises and balance retraining C: smooth pursuit and balance exercises; DVA measured weekly for 6 weeks; VAS-O measured.	E and C groups exercised 4–5xxday for 20–30 minutes in addition to 20 minutes of balance exercises	Seven of eight individuals in E group had improvement only in DVA; those in C group did not. Change in VAS-O did not correlate with change in DVA.	Only type of exercise was correlated with change in DVA, not age, time from onset, initial DVA, or complaints of oscillopsia and disequilibrium.
Herdman et al., 2003[37]	21 patients with UVH E: N = 13; mean age 65.1 ± 16.5 C: N = 8; mean age 64.9 ± 16.2. EC: normal DVA, BVH.	RCT; double blind; repeated measures with control E: VOR adaptation exercises and balance retraining C: smooth pursuit and balance exercises; DVA measured weekly for 4 weeks.	E and C groups exercised 4–5x/day for 20–30 minutes in addition to 20 minutes of balance exercises.	12 of 13 individuals in the E group demonstrated DVA that returned to age-matched normal values; no change in DVA for control group; only the type of exercise contributed to change in DVA.	Important first study showing the beneficial effect of VOR adaptation exercises to improve gaze stability in persons with UVH as measured by the DVA.

aVOR = angular vestibulo-ocular reflex; BVH = bilateral vestibular hypofunction; C = control group; CINAHL = Cumulative Index to Nursing and Allied Health Literature; DHI = Dizziness Handicap Inventory; DVA = dynamic visual acuity; E = experimental group; EC = exclusion criteria; GSE = gaze stabilization exercise; HZ = hertz; MS = multiple sclerosis; RCT = randomized controlled trial; UVD = unilateral vestibular deafferentation; UVH = unilateral vestibular hypofunction; VAS-O = visual analogue scale oscillopsia; VOR = vestibulo-ocular reflex.

■ DIAGNOSES INVOLVING THE VESTIBULAR SYSTEM

Ménière Disease

Ménière disease is confirmed by a documented low-frequency hearing loss and episodic vertigo.[135] The patient may also complain of a sense of fullness in the ear and tinnitus. According to a clinical practice guideline revised by the Barany Society and published in 2020,[136] the diagnosis of Ménière disease as *definite* or *probable* includes the following criteria: two or more spontaneous attacks of vertigo, each lasting 20 minutes to 12 hours, are reported; audiometrically documented fluctuating low- to midfrequency sensorineural hearing loss (SNHL) in the affected ear on at least one occasion before, during, or after one of the episodes of vertigo; fluctuating aural symptoms (hearing loss, tinnitus, or fullness) in the affected ear and possible causes are excluded by specific tests. Probable Ménière disease is assigned when the following criteria are met: at least two episodes of vertigo or dizziness lasting 20 minutes to 24 hours; fluctuating aural symptoms (hearing loss, tinnitus, or fullness) in the affected ear; and other possible causes are excluded by specific tests.

Vestibular rehabilitation, including GSE, is recommended as one of the noninvasive therapies available to address Ménière disease symptoms, although evidence is limited. It should be highlighted that Ménière disease symptoms gradually increase in severity and that vestibular exercises are not recommended during an episode.

Chronic Ménière disease, however, can result in UVH, for which rehabilitation is appropriate. The pathophysiology of Ménière disease, in part, probably involves an increase in endolymphatic fluid causing distention of the membranous tissues.[137] Medical treatment is therefore directed toward reducing or preventing fluid buildup. Many patients can manage the symptoms well with a controlled diet. Patients with Ménière disease are often placed on a 2 g/day or less sodium diet. This is the most important dietary restriction to follow. Other substances to be avoided are caffeine and alcohol. Sometimes medical management includes use of a diuretic to control the amount of water in the body. Surgery to either prevent the fluid buildup in the inner ear (endolymphatic shunt placement) or to stop the abnormal vestibular signal (vestibular nerve section or chemical ablation using transtympanic gentamicin injection) may be indicated if the episodes are frequent enough to disturb daily function. Although physical therapy is beneficial in treating the effects of a UVH owing to chronic Ménière disease, the therapy will not stop the episodes of vertigo. Combining gaze and postural stability exercises may be appropriate. Physical therapy is also useful in the treatment of dysequilibrium occurring after a vestibular neurectomy or chemical ablation.

Perilymphatic Fistula

Perilymphatic fistula (PLF) is most commonly caused by a rupture of the oval or round windows, the membranes that separate the middle and inner ear. A rupture of these membranes results in leakage of the perilymph into the middle ear. The result is vertigo and hearing loss. Normally, perilymph bathes the SCCs and serves as a protective barrier between the bony and membranous labyrinth. PLF usually is caused from a traumatic event, such as excessive pressure changes as in deepwater diving, blunt head trauma without skull fracture, or extremely loud noise.[138] This diagnosis is much debated, and the treatment for PLF is similarly ambiguous. Patients often are treated first with bedrest in hopes of allowing the membrane to heal. Surgical patches of the fistula are also performed. Physical therapy is contraindicated for most patients with PLF; however, it can be beneficial for those who experience continual dysequilibrium or develop a vestibular hypofunction postoperatively. Medical management will likely include strict limitations on activities, warranting good communication between physical therapist and the health care provider.

Vestibular Schwannoma

Vestibular schwannomas (VSs), historically known as *acoustic neuromas,* are benign tumors arising from the Schwann cell of the eighth cranial nerve, often in the internal auditory canal (IAC). The IAC also contains the facial nerve (cranial nerve VII) and the internal auditory artery, along with the vestibulocochlear nerve.

Symptom presentation is usually related to where the tumor arises. If the tumor arises in the IAC, then tinnitus and hearing loss are often the first symptoms. However, if the growth occurs in the cerebellar-pontine angle, the tumor may become quite large before symptoms of hearing loss are revealed. Thus, although unilateral hearing loss is often the initial sign of VS, the pathogenesis of the associated structures within the space can sometimes result in vestibular (i.e., vertigo, imbalance), facial, or even vascular symptoms. Generally, VS tumors grow slowly. As a result, the extent of impaired vestibular or facial nerve function is often not appreciated until the tumor is removed. This is because the tumor gradually compresses the cranial nerves, and in the case of vestibular function, allows the brain to compensate. However, as the VS enlarges, symptoms of hearing loss, tinnitus, and vestibular hypofunction worsen, resulting in the primary deficits. Treatment usually involves surgical excision of the tumor, though gamma knife radiation is also an option. On tumor removal, most unilateral vestibular afference is lost and the brain now perceives asymmetrical vestibular input. Optimally, physical therapy is initiated during the early postoperative period to help the patient resolve symptoms of dysequilibrium and oscillopsia.[126] Outpatient treatment should be considered similar to the treatment for a UVH.

Vestibular Atelectasis

Atelectasis commonly refers to the collapse of a lung. However, previously described histologic studies suggest that the peripheral vestibular labyrinth, too, might suffer from a collapse of the endolymph-containing portions of the labyrinth.[139] In a retrospective case series, Wenzel et al.[140] described four patients with BVH, sound and/or pressure-evoked nystagmus, and normal hearing thresholds. None of these patients presented with a history suggestive of damage to the end-organ (i.e., exposure to toxins, aminoglycosides, head trauma). More recently, Eliezer et al.[141] presented evidence that an MRI can be used to capture unilateral collapse of the utricle and the ampullas of the semicircular canals in patients with vestibular atelectasis. In fact, additional evidence from the same research team showed that MRI technology could also identify bilateral atelectasis in a patient who described unsteadiness and dizziness when exposed to loud sound (Tullio phenomenon).[142] In that case, CT imaging was also used to differentiate vestibular atelectasis from labyrinthine dehiscence syndrome, which also presents sound-induced symptomatology. The latter, however, is caused by a defect in the bone enclosing the vestibular semicircular canals of the inner ear and can be often repaired through surgery.[143] The physical therapist may be one of the clinicians treating patients with vestibular atelectasis; therefore, familiarity with the clinical vestibular examination remains critical when treating patients with symptoms of dizziness.

Vestibular Paroxysmia

Vestibular paroxysmia refers to a vascular compression of the eighth cranial nerve. Compression of cranial nerves is thought to cause their demyelination, affecting firing rate and perhaps making the nerve susceptible to aberrant excitation.[144] Patients with putative vestibular paroxysmia typically report frequent, spontaneous, brief attacks of vertigo or dizziness that generally last less than 1 minute. MRI has revealed the neurovascular compression of the eighth nerve,[145] with recent evidence presenting 3D Constructive Interference in Steady-State (CISS) MRI sequence as the superior approach to image the neurovascular contact.[146] However, contact of the eighth cranial nerve can be detected by MRI in up to 45% of normal individuals, which makes MRI indication in this condition mostly an alternative to rule out other etiologies.[147] Treatment includes surgical decompression or antiepileptic medication. While physical therapy would not be expected to help, understanding paroxysmia expression could be important to diagnosis differentiation. This remains critical considering other conditions such as lower brainstem tumors (e.g., melanocytoma) can masquerade as vestibular paroxysmia through the presentation of paroxysmal vertigo and tinnitus.[148]

Mal de Debarquement

Mal de Debarquement (MdD) means feeling sick upon disembarkment, as when exiting from a water or airborne vessel. Thus, MdD generally occurs after exposure to continuous motion as experienced from sea voyages or turbulent long-duration air travel, although it can also occur spontaneously.[149] Patients with MdD report a persistent rhythmic motion (sense of rocking, swaying) while at rest that typically resolves when they start moving. The diagnosis should be made when the history includes a phantom self-motion perception that occurs after exposure to passive motion (e.g., boat, plane).[150] The neurophysiology behind MdD is not precisely known, although postulates drawn from experiments in subhuman primates[149] suggest that MdD is produced at the velocity storage integrator[151] by activation of vestibular-only neurons, driven by signals from the Purkinje cells in the cerebellar nodulus. Long exposure to movement in the roll axis (e.g., sea, air travel) putatively conditions nodulus neurons to realign their orientation vector away from a vertical or gravity alignment to a new alignment that is tilted in the roll plane. MdD is not to be confused with the commonly felt "sea legs," which occurs after return to land and resolves within 24 hours. Instead, MdD usually persists longer than a month following the triggering exposure.[152] Treatment options are limited and include mediation[150] and cross-axis habituation techniques.[153] There is limited indication that physical therapy offers much benefit.[154] Recent evidence, however, suggests that successful treatment would include rolling of the head at the frequency of the perceived motion (e.g., rocking, swaying, bobbing) under a full-field optokinetic stimulus rotating around the spatial vertical countering the direction of the vestibular imbalance.[149]

Vestibular Migraine

Vestibular migraine can be deceptively similar to a peripheral vestibular lesion, whether it is BPPV or UVH. Vestibular migraine symptoms include vertigo, dizziness, imbalance, and motion sickness. A recent study reported 100% of patients with vestibular migraine had abnormal nystagmus during a migraine episode if they were positionally tested as part of an oculomotor examination.[155] The prevalence of migraine is significant, affecting 6% of men and 15% to 18% of women between the ages of 25 and 55.[156] The clinical examination will often provide the differential diagnosis between vestibular pathology and migraine. The history is crucial, and important questions for patients in whom migraine is suspected include asking if symptoms worsen when barometric pressure changes and whether headache or eating certain foods is associated with any of the symptoms. If the therapist suspects migraine, the patient should be referred to a neurologist, preferably one with a special interest in headache. Vestibular migraine is often well controlled with medication and diet. Migraine that is not controlled may become worse with exercises such as vestibular rehabilitation, which stimulate the peripheral vestibular end organ and central VOR pathways.[157] Vestibular rehabilitation in patients with vestibular migraine can be very helpful, but patients with both vestibular hypofunction and migraine do not respond as well.[158] Strupp et al.[159] provide a thorough discussion of this topic.

Multiple Sclerosis

Multiple sclerosis (MS) can affect cranial nerve VIII where it enters the brainstem, potentially causing symptoms identical to a unilateral vestibular pathology, including a disabling oscillopsia.[160] Patients with MS may also present with impaired saccadic eye movements.[161] MRI scans add to a more accurate diagnosis of MS. However, imaging outcomes should be critically assessed to avoid misdiagnosis given that vestibular migraine can lead to white matter scaring (hyperintensities) similar to those caused by MS.[162,163] Conversely, MS can initially present with migraine symptoms and hence be mistaken for a more benign diagnosis, hindering early care.[164,165]

Multiple System Atrophy

Multiple system atrophy (MSA) is a progressive degenerative disease of the nervous system involving four clinical domains: *cerebellar ataxia, autonomic dysfunction, Parkinson disease–like symptoms,* and *corticospinal dysfunction.* MSA has been found to be a cause of dizziness and imbalance.[166] The effect of physical therapy for persons with MSA has not been thoroughly investigated and is mostly limited to case reports.[167] The scarce information on rehabilitation strategies specific to MSA is likely associated with poor diagnostic tools. In addition, lack of a diagnosis during the early stages of the disease likely hinders participation in potentially disease-modifying trials,[168] thus missing opportunities to know about treatment options. Nevertheless, a few studies in specific groups (e.g., Parkinson variant of MSA) are emerging with promising evidence that physical therapy can improve motor function.[169]

Cervicogenic Dizziness

Cervicogenic dizziness is a term meant to imply that the cause of symptoms such as dizziness or imbalance arise from pathology affecting the cervical spine or related soft tissue. Unfortunately, the term *cervical vertigo* is still often used, which implies true vertigo due to cervical pathology, which is not documented in humans. The mechanisms of involvement are believed to be from at least two sources. First, the upper cervical spine sends proprioceptive input to the contralateral vestibular nucleus.[170] Soft tissue injury and joint dysfunction might alter the afferent input contributing to spatial orientation. Indeed, a recent case report showed that cervicogenic dizziness can be associated with craniocervical instability.[171] While vestibular rehabilitation appears to be warranted for these individuals,[172] manual therapy[173] and upper cervical traction[174] have also been reported as alternatives to appease cervicogenic dizziness. Second, a patient might have VBI (see earlier section on "Central Nervous System Pathology"). If VBI is suspected, vascular compromise must first be ruled out as a cause of the patient's symptoms. The VBI test can be performed while the subject is seated, though little evidence exists for the sensitivity and specificity of this test. The patient leans forward and extends the neck. The neck is then rotated 45° to the suspicious side. Persons suspected of having VBI should be referred to a neurologist immediately. Repeated episodes of vertigo without the associated VBI symptoms usually suggest a peripheral vestibular diagnosis.

Superior Canal Dehiscence Syndrome

Superior canal dehiscence syndrome (SCDS) is characterized by an absence or thinning of the bony encasement over the superior semicircular canal, thereby creating a third mobile window (in addition to the oval and round windows) in the inner ear. This must be confirmed using CT or MRI.[175] SCDS is the most common subtype of the third mobile window syndromes. It often manifests through recurrent attacks of vertigo in response to changes in intracranial or middle-ear pressure, loud noises, autophony, increased bone conductions, or pulsatile tinnitus.[147] Although imaging remains the gold standard for the identifying SCDS, a bony defect does not always result in signs and symptoms, and a consensus in SCDS characterization has recently been proposed.[176,177] Imaging, audiometry, and VEMPs are usually combined as a strategy for diagnosing SCDS. Surgery to plug the affected superior semicircular canal is often recommended.[178] Physical therapy (e.g., vestibular rehabilitation) is recommended at the postsurgical stage[179,180] when about 40% of patients present transient vestibular hypofunction,[181] while many patients experience symptoms of BPPV, likely treated with canalith repositioning maneuvers.[182]

■ CONTRAINDICATIONS TO VESTIBULAR REHABILITATION

Physical therapy is not appropriate for unstable vestibular disorders such as Méniere disease (with the exception mentioned above), uncontrolled migraine, PLF, or an unrepaired superior semicircular canal dehiscence. Other contraindications the physical therapist should be alert to include sudden loss of hearing, increased feeling of pressure or fullness to the point of discomfort in one or both ears, and severe ringing in one or both ears. When treating patients who have had a surgical procedure, the clinician must be observant for discharge of fluid from the ears or nose, which may indicate cerebrospinal fluid leak. Patients with acute neck injuries may not be able to tolerate some components of the physical examination, the CRM, or some of the GSEs.

SUMMARY

High incidence and prevalence rates of vestibular disorders oblige the physical therapist to recognize signs and symptoms associated with inner ear disorders. It is essential to differentiate a peripheral pathology from a central one. Peripheral and central lesions have separate manifestations and may require different intervention strategies. In addition, all vestibular disorders should not be treated similarly. The most common form of vertigo, BPPV, is a biomechanical problem readily treated, often with a single maneuver. This is in stark contrast to a patient with a BVH, which requires a greater rehabilitation effort. Evidence supports the use of vestibular adaptation exercises for patients with vestibular hypofunction.

Research in vestibular rehabilitation is ongoing, and it remains imperative to answer important questions related to dosing, recruitment of compensatory strategies to assist gaze stability, recurrence prevention for BPPV, and more. Exciting future treatments may involve instrumentation to improve the VOR, virtual reality, vibrotactors to alert patients of abnormal posture, and the inclusion of computer gaming platforms. Currently, humans are being implanted with a vestibular prosthesis as part of an early efficacy and safety trial. Within the next 5 years, we will have good evidence realizing the utility of such prosthetics to improve quality of life for those suffering from BVH. Regardless of technological advances, rehabilitation will still be important for these patients.

The *Vestibular Disorders Association* (VEDA) has a list of physical therapists in each state who are interested in treating patients with vestibular disorders. VEDA can be contacted via phone (800-837-8428; 24-hour voice mail) or through the "contact us" link on their website (www.vestibular.org). The supplemental reading list contains other excellent literature for the reader interested in pursuing a greater depth of knowledge in vestibular rehabilitation.

Questions for Review

1. Why is it important to perform the head impulse test using rapid velocity?
2. What is the name of the linear accelerometers within the vestibular labyrinth?
3. Why does the patient with an acute unilateral vestibular lesion experience spontaneous nystagmus?
4. How will cupulolithiasis present differently from canalithiasis of the posterior semicircular canal?
5. What are the key elements in taking a history for a patient with a suspected vestibular disorder?
6. Explain inhibitory cutoff.
7. Differentiate the ×1 exercise paradigm from the ×2 exercise paradigm.
8. In a patient with vestibular nystagmus, which part of the eye movement (slow or fast) is from the vestibular system? Why?
9. Describe how the Dix-Hallpike test would elicit nystagmus for posterior SCC BPPV.
10. Differentiate between adaptation and habituation training for patients with vestibular dysfunction.

CASE STUDY

CASE STUDY 1
You are performing an initial examination of a patient with new onset of complaints of imbalance and dizziness. In a sitting position, at rest, the patient is observed to have purely torsional and vertical nystagmus. You also notice that the patient's head is tilting to the left. The nystagmus is not altered with any change in head position, and the head-shaking induced nystagmus test is negative.
Guiding Questions
1. Do you suspect a central or peripheral pathology as a cause of the imbalance and dizziness?
2. Is physical therapy appropriate at this time?

CASE STUDY 2
On your patient's return to sitting up after you have performed the CRM for a left posterior canalithiasis, you notice left beating nystagmus that stops after 15 seconds. The patient is complaining of vertigo.
Guiding Questions
1. Where do you suspect the otoconia is now located?
2. What positional test might you use to confirm where the otoconia are located?
3. How will you treat for BPPV the second time?
4. Following the second treatment for BPPV, the patient complains of dizziness and neck pain. The vertigo and nystagmus are gone. Can you prescribe any other forms of exercise for the remaining dizziness? What about the neck pain?

CASE STUDY 3
A patient with UVH complains of feeling worse after 7 days of starting a vestibular rehabilitation program. The patient has had no falls. The complaints consist of increased dizziness with head motion, nausea, and fatigue.

(Continued)

CASE STUDY—cont'd

Guiding Questions

1. Is your rehabilitation program making the patient worse?

2. How can you modify the program?

3. What information will you tell your patient with an UVH regarding time to recover? What will you tell patients with BPPV, BVH, or CNS pathology regarding times to recover?

CASE STUDY 4

A patient presents transient downbeat nystagmus that was initially treated as a peripheral benign paroxysmal position vertigo with no significant change in symptoms. Additional positional testing done with the patient in upright position (non–gravity dependent) revealed a downbeat nystagmus. Static angiography and imaging studies showed normal results.

Guiding Questions

1. Which semicircular canal may be causing the short-duration downbeat nystagmus?

2. What other non-peripheral vestibular conditions lead to positional downbeat nystagmus?

3. What should the physical therapist do in face of normal results for static angiography and traditional imaging (e.g., MRI, CT)?

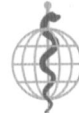

For additional resources, including answers to the questions for review, new immersive cases, case study guiding questions, references, and more, please visit **https://www.fadavis.com/product/physical -rehabilitation-fulk-8**. You may also quickly find the resources by entering this title's four-digit ISBN, 4691, in the search field at **http://fadavis.com** and logging in at the prompt.

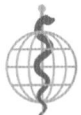

The reader is referred to video Case Study 13: Patient With Vestibular Disorder for additional review and study. The full written case study, including tables, figures, charts, and three video segments (examination, intervention, and outcome), appears online at FADavis.com. The case study poses questions for the reader's consideration with suggested answers to the case study questions, also posted online at **FADavis.com**.

Amputation

Tzurei Chen, PT, PhD, GCS
Kevin K. Chui, PT, DPT, PhD, GCS, OCS, CEEAA, FAAOMPT
Sheng-Che Yen, PT, PhD
Kevin M. Parcetich, Jr. PT, DPT, NCS
Margery A. Lockard, PT, PhD

Chapter **22**

LEARNING OBJECTIVES

1. Discuss the role of the physical therapist in the care of any individual following lower extremity amputation.
2. Describe the major etiological factors leading to lower extremity amputation.
3. Explain the major concepts involved in lower extremity amputation surgery.
4. Develop an evaluation plan for any individual following lower extremity amputation.
   a. Prioritize data gathering for the acute postsurgical period and the preprosthetic phase.
5. Design an effective plan of care for the acute postsurgical period.
   a. Explain the rationale for, and teach patient and caregiver, proper positioning.
   b. Teach sitting and standing balance to enhance transfers and mobility.
   c. Ensure continuity of care following discharge from acute care.
6. Design an effective plan of care for the preprosthetic period.
   a. Teach proper residual limb care, including bandaging as indicated.
   b. Teach standing balance to help the patient attain the highest functional level of mobility with appropriate ancillary support.
   c. Teach residual limb strengthening exercises to facilitate eventual prosthetic fitting.
   d. Teach range of motion exercises to prevent/alleviate secondary contractures.
7. Respond appropriately to patient/family from an awareness of the psychological impact of lower extremity amputation.
8. Analyze and interpret patient data, formulate realistic goals and expected outcomes, and develop a plan of care when presented with a clinical case study.

CHAPTER OUTLINE

CAUSES OF AMPUTATION 850
LEVELS OF AMPUTATION 851
AMPUTATION SURGERY 852
HEALING PROCESS 854
POSTSURGICAL DRESSINGS 855
   Rigid Dressings 855
   Semirigid Dressings 856
   Soft Dressings 856
PHASES OF CARE 857
   Preoperative Phase 857
   Postsurgical Phase 857
   Preprosthetic Phase 861

   Preparatory and Definitive Prostheses 873
   Patient Education 874
   Bilateral Amputation 874
PREDICTING PROSTHETIC POTENTIAL 874
PROSTHETIC TRAINING 876
   Gait Training 876
   Advanced Training 880
FUNCTIONAL OUTCOME MEASUREMENTS 883
SUMMARY 885

There are more than 2 million people living with limb loss in the United States today with an estimated 185,000 new amputations per year.[1] This number of individuals with limb loss is expected to increase, and it has been projected that by 2050 the prevalence of amputation will reach 3.6 million Americans (with an estimated 2.27 million due to dysvascular disease and 1.33 million due to trauma).[2] The most common causes of amputation are peripheral vascular disease (about 54%), trauma (about 45%), malignancy (< 1%), and congenital limb deficiency (< 1%).[3]

■ CAUSES OF AMPUTATION

The primary cause of lower extremity (LE) amputation continues to be peripheral vascular disease (PVD), particularly with associated diabetes. The Centers for Disease Control and Prevention (CDC) reports that 10.5% of the U.S. population (34.2 million people in 2018) has diabetes.[4] There are approximately 130,000 LE amputations each year due to diabetes (5.6 per 1,000 adults with diabetes in 2016).[4] Stated another way, an adult with diabetes is 10 times more likely to have an amputation than an adult who does not have diabetes.[5] Among those with diabetes, some are disproportionally affected by amputation. Amputation has its highest incidence in those who are in the oldest age groups, male, and Black.[6] It is also interesting to note that foot and leg ulcers were the most commonly found comorbidity or precipitating factor in people with diabetes who undergo LE amputation.[7] Overall, in the U.S. Medicare population, the incidence of diabetic foot ulcers is approximately 6 per 100 individuals with diabetes per year, and the incidence of LE amputation is about 4.9 per 1,000 persons with diabetes per year.[8] Despite these data, the rate of amputation as a complication of diabetes has been decreasing in the United States,[9] which is consistent with global trends.[10] A recent clinical practice guideline summarizes and grades the evidence using a multidisciplinary management approach to prevent diabetic foot ulceration, off-loading diabetic foot ulcers, and wound care for diabetic foot ulcers.[11]

Major amputation (level of amputation above the ankle or wrist), which is considered a treatment of last resort for conditions, including infected diabetic foot ulcers and critical limb ischemia, like all major surgeries carries mortality risk. Perioperative (30-day) mortality has been reported between 7% and 13%. Thirty-day mortality (4.6%) was predicted in patients after major LE amputation by eight easily obtainable clinical metrics: do not resuscitate orders, congestive heart failure, age greater than 80 years, creatine greater than 1.5 g/dL, above-knee amputation (vs. below-knee amputation), dependent living status, coronary artery disease, and chronic obstructive pulmonary disease.[12]

The overall 5-year mortality rate for patients with diabetes and PVD after major amputation is very high: 40% to 82% after transtibial amputation and 40% to 90% after transfemoral amputation.[13] In a meta-analysis examining the same patient population, the long-term mortality associated with amputation was reported at follow-up to be 48% at 1 year, 61.3% at 2 years, 70.6% at 3 years, and 62.2% at 5 years.[14] This is higher than the 5-year mortality rate for breast cancer, colon cancer, and prostate cancer together.[15] When planning rehabilitation programs for patients with amputation, it is also important to be aware of the status of the contralateral or remaining lower limb. Five years after a major amputation in persons with PVD, 52% had undergone a major amputation of the contralateral lower limb.[16] An independent risk factor for contralateral limb amputation is atherosclerosis with or without diabetic neuropathy.[16] Additionally, 41% had a revision or additional amputation to the originally amputated lower limb in the same time frame.[16] Stated in a simpler but dramatic way: about 50% of patients with amputation owing to poor vascular status will die in the 5 years following surgery; of those who live, 50% will have a contralateral limb amputation. Many of the patients that therapists treat in all types of settings have diabetes and/or peripheral arterial disease (PAD). Therapists can be more effective by being knowledgeable about diabetes and PAD and by making patient education for prevention of amputation an integral part of the plan of care (POC). Resources report positive outcomes associated with early/continuous patient education on the prevention of foot ulcers, including proper foot care, and reduction in amputations.[17–19]

The second leading cause of amputation is trauma, usually from motor vehicle crashes, accidents with machines, war, or gunshot injury. Individuals with traumatic amputations are often young adults, more frequently men, and have often been involved in an active lifestyle before amputation. The incidence of civilian trauma-related amputation has been declining over the past several decades, with the majority of amputations involving the upper limb (approximately 67%).[20] Civilian trauma-related amputations of the lower limb have a high incidence of postsurgical complications, including pneumonia, acute kidney injury, deep-vein thrombosis/thrombophlebitis, and revision amputation. Significant predictors of need for revision amputation include injury severity, crush fracture, and compartment syndrome.[21] The presence of these complications may extend hospital stays and delay prosthetic fitting. Combat-related amputations during the wars in Afghanistan and Iraq have increased the numbers of service members with amputation returning to civilian life due to higher survival rates in the war zones.[22] During these wars, the mean amputation rate was 5.29 per 100,000 deployed troops: 41.8% transtibial amputation (TTA), 34.5% transfemoral amputation (TFA), 6.7% transradial, 5.5% through knee, and

5% transhumeral.[22] Thirty percent of service members with amputations have multiple amputations, which is significantly greater than in any other American wars. The most common combinations are TFA/TFA (27%), TTA/TTA (20%), TFA/TTA (16%), and TTA or TFA/knee disarticulation (10%).[22]

The incidence of amputation from malignancy, primarily osteogenic sarcoma, has been reduced owing to improved imaging techniques, more effective chemotherapy, and better limb salvage procedures. Osteogenic sarcoma is most prevalent in adolescents and young adults. Amputation may be necessary if the tumor is large and cannot be resected without substantial removal of bone and tissue. However, the surgeon may choose to remove the tumor and incorporate one of several limb salvage procedures. Many factors go into this decision, including the age of the patient, the size of the tumor and bone, social concerns, and, if the patient is young, the potential for future growth.[23] Limb salvage with adjunctive chemotherapy, however, is now the treatment of choice in 80% to 95% of patients with extremity osteosarcoma, and their 5-year survival rate is 60% to 75%.[24]

Congenital limb deficiency may be caused by genetic factors, exposure to teratogens or environmental agents, and infection.[25,26] The incidence of congenital deficiencies is quite small (2 to 7 per 10,000 live births or 0.8% of all limb losses) and has been stable over 10 years.[3] However, when limb deficiencies do occur, they are most common in the upper limb.

Regardless of the cause of amputation, physical therapists have a major role in rehabilitation. Early initiation of rehabilitation influences the eventual outcome of the episode of care. It is critically important, especially for the older individual, for the therapist in the acute care setting to ensure continuity of care once the patient is discharged from the hospital. Too often, the patient is sent home and is not seen again for several weeks or months. By that time, the patient may have become debilitated and developed contractures that interfere with prosthetic use and function.

■ LEVELS OF AMPUTATION

Traditionally, levels of amputation have been identified by anatomical considerations such as below knee and above knee. In 1974, the Task Force on Standardization of Prosthetic-Orthotic Terminology developed an international classification system to define amputation levels.[27] Table 22.1 describes the major terms in common use today.

Amputations following trauma may be performed at any level. The surgeon tries to maintain the greatest

Table 22.1 Levels of Amputation

Level	Description
Partial toe	Excision of any part of one or more toes.
Toe disarticulation	Disarticulation at the metatarsal phalangeal joint.
Partial foot/ray resection	Resection of the third, fourth, fifth metatarsals and digits (a ray is a metatarsal and its associated phalanges).
Transmetatarsal	Amputation through the midsection of all metatarsals.
Tarsometatarsal (Lisfranc)	Amputation through the tarsometatarsal joint (the distal bones in the foot are the cuneiforms and the cuboid).
Ankle disarticulation (Syme's)	Ankle disarticulation with attachment of heel pad to distal end of tibia; may include removal of malleoli and distal tibial/fibular flares.
Long transtibial (below knee)	More than 50% of tibial length.
Transtibial (below knee)	Between 20% and 50% of tibial length.
Short transtibial (below knee)	Less than 20% of tibial length.
Knee disarticulation	Amputation through the knee joint; femur intact.
Long transfemoral (above knee)	More than 60% of femoral length.
Transfemoral (above knee)	Between 35% and 60% of femoral length.
Short transfemoral (above knee)	Less than 35% of femoral length.
Hip disarticulation	Amputation through hip joint; pelvis intact.
Transpelvectomy or Hemipelvectomy	Resection of part of the pelvis.
Hemicorporectomy	Amputation of both lower limbs and pelvis below L4–L5 level.

bone length and save all possible joints, while providing adequate soft tissue coverage to produce a *residual limb* (RL) that will be comfortable and functional in a prosthetic socket. A variety of surgical techniques may be necessary to create a functional RL. Guillotine amputations (skin, muscle, and bone all transected at approximately the same level) may precede secondary closure with skin flaps; occasionally, free tissue flaps, taken from some other area of the body, may be used to cover the wound. Amputations for vascular diseases are generally performed at partial foot (transmetatarsal), transtibial, or transfemoral levels.

Patients with unilateral transtibial amputations, regardless of age, are quite likely to become functional prosthetic users; many individuals with bilateral transtibial amputations also become functional ambulators with a prosthesis. An updated systematic review identified the following variables as the strongest predictive factors of prosthetic candidacy: amputation level, age, physical fitness, and comorbidities.[28] Patients with bilateral transfemoral amputations may become prosthetic users with microprocessor-controlled and externally powered prosthetic components. However, this is a difficult task and requires good balance, strength, endurance, and coordination. Hip disarticulations, transpelvectomies, and hemicorporectomies are generally performed either for tumors or for severe trauma and represent a small percentage of the population of individuals with amputations. An important factor in determining the prosthetic potential of an individual is their level of activity prior to amputation.[29] Hip extension strength and balance (single limb stance) are also predictive of the ability to ambulate functionally with a prosthesis.[30] Furthermore, strong evidence supports the relationship between balance and walking ability after lower limb amputation.[31] Comorbidities and the extent of injuries from war and trauma must be considered, but individuals who led an active life before amputation—even those with diabetes and related comorbidities—are likely to become functional prosthetic users if they can demonstrate good balance, hip strength, and coordination.[28–31]

■ AMPUTATION SURGERY

The specific type of surgery is determined by the surgeon, whose decision depends on the status of the extremity at the time of amputation.[32] The surgeon must allow for primary or secondary wound healing and construct an RL for optimal prosthetic fitting and function. Numerous factors affect the selection of level of amputation. Conservation of RL length, uncomplicated wound healing, and the creation of a pain-free limb that can be fitted with a prosthesis that maximizes the individual's functional mobility are all important considerations. Tools have been created to predict the probability of achieving independent mobility at each major LE amputation level[28,33–35] as well as individual

risk of death and reamputation.[34,36] Although a description of each type of surgical procedure is beyond the scope of this chapter, an understanding of the basic principles of amputation surgery is important.[32,37]

Skin flaps are as broad as possible, and the residual scar should be pliable, painless, and nonadherent to optimize comfort and mobility outcomes. For most transfemoral and some transtibial amputations without vascular impairment, equal length anterior and posterior flaps are used, placing the scar at the distal end of the bone (Fig. 22.1). Long posterior flaps are often used in transtibial amputations with compromised circulation because the posterior tissues have better blood supply than the anterior skin (Fig 22.2).[38] Additionally, the calf muscles provide better distal cushioning for the tibia and fibula. A long posterior flap places the scar anteriorly over the distal end of the tibia; care must be taken to ensure that the scar does not become adherent to the bone (Fig. 22.3). Some surgeons believe the skew flap, developed in England, is a better approach for individuals with severely compromised distal circulation, ulceration, or gangrene, and may offer the benefit of improved prosthetic fit[39] as the skew flap naturally gives a more cylindrical RL shape.[40] The skew flap is an angular medial–lateral incision that places the scar away from bony prominences. While an updated systematic review on the use of different skin flaps for below-knee amputations did not find evidence of a benefit of one type of incision over another,[41] a recent retrospective observational cohort study reported better functional outcomes for patients who received a long posterior flap when compared to a skew flap.[42]

Stabilization of the major muscles that are cut during surgery allows retention of muscle tension and maximum muscle function. Muscle stabilization may be achieved by myofascial closure, myoplasty, myodesis, or tenodesis. In most transtibial and transfemoral amputations, a combination of *myoplasty* (muscle-to-muscle closure) and *myofascial* (muscle-to-fascia) closure is used to ensure that the muscles are properly stabilized and do not slide over the end of the bone. *Myodesis* (muscle attached to periosteum or bone) may also be used to provide a very stable muscle attachment. More rarely, a *tenodesis* (tendon attached to bone) may be used for muscle stabilization, particularly in partial foot amputations where extrinsic muscle tendons are cut. Regardless of the technique, muscle stabilization under some tension is desirable to ensure that the transected muscles can contract to maintain muscle bulk and function.

Severed peripheral nerves can form *neuromas* (a collection of nerve cell ends) in the RL. The neuroma must be well surrounded by soft tissue so as not to cause pain and interfere with prosthetic wear. Surgeons identify the major nerves, pull them down under some tension, and then cut them cleanly and sharply, allowing them to retract into the soft tissue of the RL. Neuromas that form close to scar tissue or bone generally cause pain

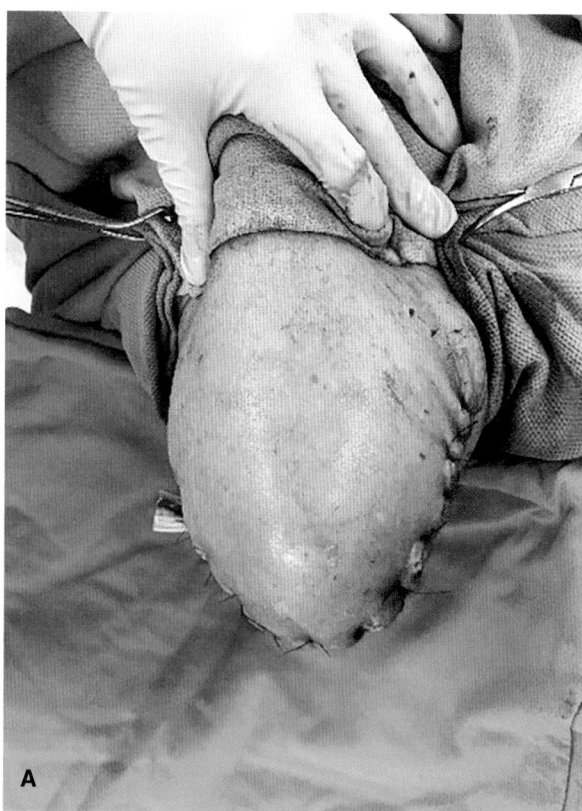
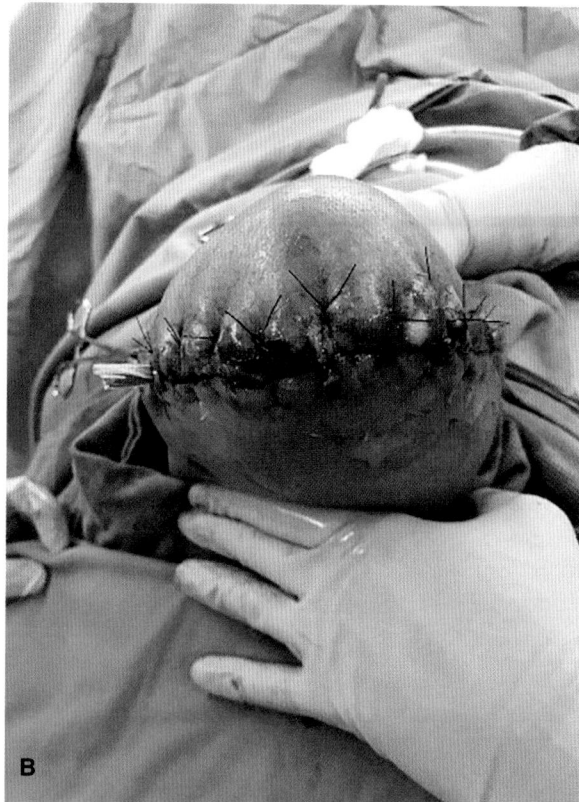

Figure 22.1 (A) Anterior view. (B) Superior view of a transfemoral RL with incision from equal-length flaps. *(Photos courtesy of Dr. Chin Ping Lin.)*

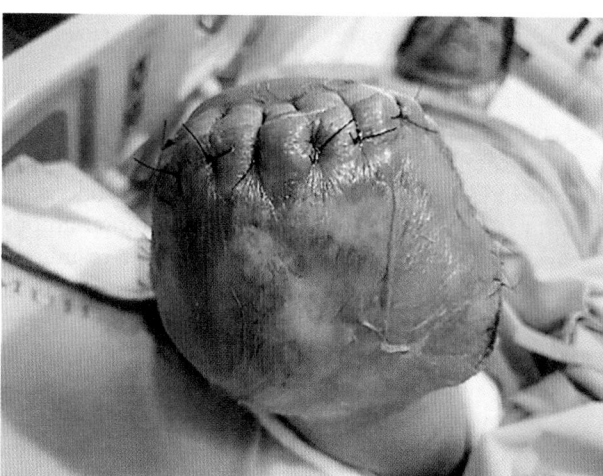

Figure 22.2 Transtibial RL with anterior incision from a long posterior flap. *(Photo courtesy of Dr. Chin Ping Lin.)*

and may require later resection or revision. *Hemostasis* is achieved by ligating major veins and arteries; *cauterization* is used only for small bleeders. Care is taken not to compromise circulation to distal tissues, particularly the skin flaps, which are important for uncomplicated wound healing.

Bones are sectioned at a length to allow wound closure without excessive redundant tissue at the end of

the RL and without placing the incision under great tension that might impair healing. Sharp bone ends are smoothed and rounded without disturbing or stripping the periosteum; disruption of the periosteum from the bone may cause development of *osteophytes* (bone spicules) and RL pain during prosthetic use. In transtibial amputations, the anterior portion of the distal tibia is *beveled*, and the fibula is cut slightly shorter than the tibia (approximately 1 cm) to reduce pressure between the end of the bones and the prosthetic socket. Alternatively, an Ertl, or *osteoplasty*, procedure may be performed during transtibial amputation. In this procedure, an autologous piece of bone (often from the amputated fibula) is placed between the ends of the tibia and fibula, secured, and allowed to solidly fuse in place. This results in a more cylindrically shaped RL, which may permit better fitting with a prosthetic socket and increase the ability to take direct end-pressure on the RL to dissipate force.[43–45] Whatever procedure is used, care is taken to ensure that the bone is physiologically prepared for the pressures of prosthetic wear. Tissue layers are approximated under normal physiological tension and the incision is closed, usually with regular sutures. A drainage tube may be inserted as necessary.

In a traumatic amputation, the surgeon attempts to save as much bone length and viable skin as possible and preserve proximal joints while providing for appropriate

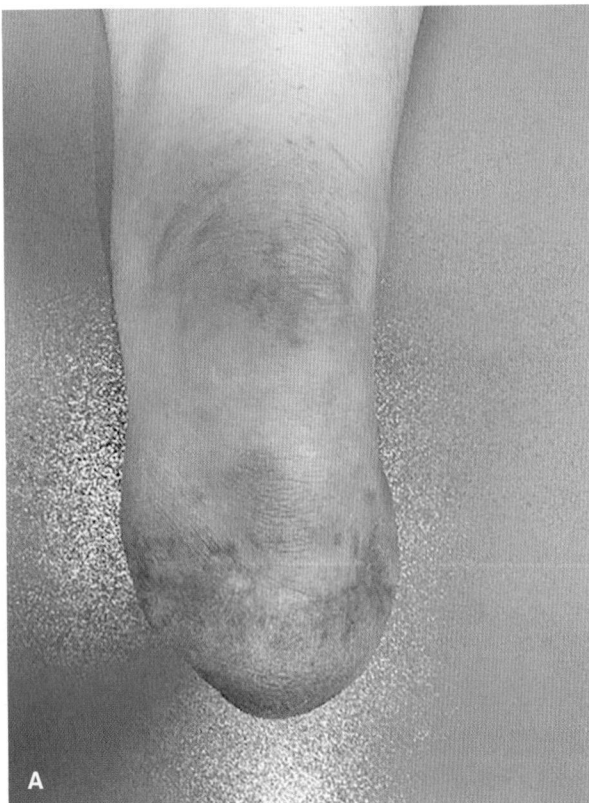
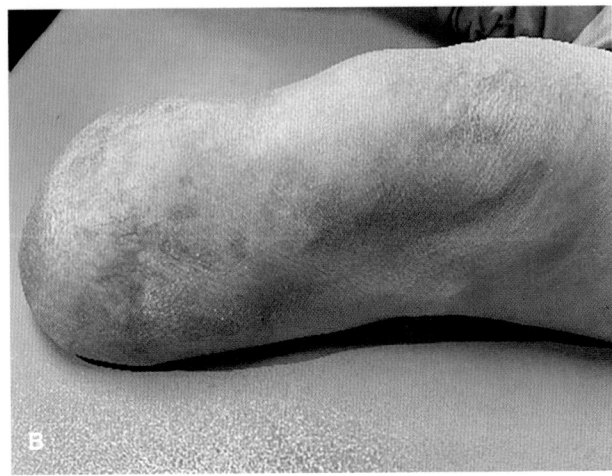

Figure 22.3 (A) Anterior view and (B) lateral view of the scar of a transtibial RL with anterior incision from a long posterior flap.

healing of tissues without secondary complications such as infection.[46] In potentially "dirty" (involving foreign substances) amputations, the incision may be left open with the proximal joint immobilized in a functional position for 5 to 9 days to prevent invasive infection. Secondary closure also allows the surgeon to shape the RL appropriately for prosthetic wear and function.

Osseointegration is a newer technique that has developed over the last few decades as a solution for individuals who are unable to successfully use a conventional prosthesis that attaches to the RL with a socket and suspension system.[47] This is often the case in individuals who have very short or atypically shaped transfemoral or transhumeral RLs due to trauma or tumor resection amputations. In osseointegration, the prosthesis is surgically connected into the residual bone, in a method similar to dental implants or the insertion of a prosthesis in a total hip arthroplasty.[37] The basic components include a fixture that is inserted into the intramedullary canal of the bone and a percutaneous abutment that is attached to the fixture and connects the prosthesis directly to the bone. Benefits of this approach include improvements in pain due to socket-RL fit issues, sensory feedback owing to direct connection of the prosthesis into the skeleton, mobility, and quality of life.[48–51] Despite these benefits, problems can arise due to superficial skin and bone infection, bone fracture, implant

breakage or loosening, revision surgical procedures, soft tissue refashioning, and mechanical complications In the United States, this procedure received FDA (Food and Drug Administration) approval in 2015;[52] however, research on this technique and the rehabilitation of individuals who have had the procedure supports its use.[53–56]

Amputation for vascular disease is generally considered an elective procedure; the surgeon determines the level of amputation by examining tissue viability through a variety of measures. Segmental limb blood pressures can be determined by Doppler systolic blood pressure measurement.[57] Transcutaneous oxygen measurement and skin blood flow by radioisotope or plethysmography are also determined. Doppler systolic blood pressure measures have been reported to be quite accurate in predicting viable level of amputation.[58] Improvements in noninvasive examination techniques have greatly reduced the use of arteriography to determine amputation level.[59,60]

■ HEALING PROCESS

Numerous factors influence the course of the healing process in each patient.[61] One of the greatest postoperative concerns is infection, whether from external or internal sources. Individuals with contaminated wounds from injury, infected foot ulcers, or other causes are at greater risk of infection. Research indicates that smoking is a major deterrent to wound healing; one systematic review found that smoking significantly increases the risk of foot amputation in diabetic patients.[62] Other factors affecting wound healing are the severity of the vascular problems, diabetes, renal disease, and other physiological problems such as cardiac disease.[38] The physical therapist can influence optimal wound healing by teaching proper bed mobility, avoiding pressure on the newly amputated limb, and facilitating mobilization as soon as it is medically approved.[63]

POSTSURGICAL DRESSINGS

Surgeons have several options regarding the postoperative dressing, including (1) rigid dressing, (2) semirigid dressing, or (3) soft dressing. It is important for some type of edema control to be used because excessive edema in the RL can compromise healing and cause pain. Table 22.2 outlines the major postsurgical dressings in use today with their advantages and disadvantages.

Rigid Dressings

Rigid dressings, developed in the early 1960s, can be applied as a removable rigid dressing or as an *immediate*

postoperative prosthesis (IPOP).[64,65] In either case, the socket may be custom- or handmade from plaster or fiberglass casting materials or purchased as a prefabricated device made from plastic or other materials in various sizes. The IPOP socket is applied by the surgeon or a prosthetist in the operating room over wound dressings and padding to protect the wound, skin, and bony prominences. The IPOP cast, most commonly used with transtibial amputations, extends to midthigh and immobilizes the knee in extension.[66,67] A removable pylon (pipe that replaces the missing tibia) and prosthetic foot is added to the cast so that the patient is able to walk with very limited weight-bearing on the first day following surgery. In about 2 weeks, the cast is removed to inspect the incision and remove sutures. The cast and pylon are reapplied, and the patient continues with this process until fitted with a temporary or definitive prosthesis. Prefabricated IPOP devices that use pneumatic compression have also been used. As healing progresses the patient is able to increase the amount of weight-bearing on the device. Advantages of this system include early mobilization, decreased RL edema and pain, improved balance and safety during transfers, protection of the wound from trauma,

Table 22.2 Postsurgical Dressings

Type of Dressing	Advantages	Disadvantages
Elastic roller bandage	Readily available, accessible Inexpensive Easy access to incision	Can be difficult for patients and family members to learn to apply correctly with appropriate pressure. May produce areas of high pressure that may impair healing. Minimal RL protection. Requires frequent rewrapping. Increased likelihood of developing knee flexion contracture with transtibial amputation.
Shrinker	Easy to apply, particularly for transfemoral level Can effectively control edema with even pressure	Not used until sutures are removed. Requires changing as RL shrinks. Can be expensive to replace. Increased likelihood of knee flexion contracture with transtibial amputation.
Semirigid dressing	Better edema control than soft dressing RL protection	Needs frequent changing. Cannot be applied by patient. No access to incision.
Removable rigid dressing	Effective edema control RL protection Access to incision	Requires skilled practitioner to fabricate or may be expensive to purchase.
IPOP	Excellent edema control Excellent RL protection Control of RL pain Decreased time to fitting with prosthesis	No access to incision. More expensive than other dressings. Requires proper training for use. Requires skilled practitioner for frequent reapplications and fittings. Patient must carefully adhere to all procedures.

IPOP = immediate postoperative prosthesis; RL = residual limb.

prevention of knee flexion contracture, decreased time to fitting with a prosthesis, and the psychological benefit of early prosthetic fitting. Not all patients, however, are good candidates for this method. Patients must be free of infection, have been ambulatory prior to surgery, and able and willing to follow all directions carefully.[66] *Removable rigid dressings* (RRDs), whether handmade from plaster or fiberglass casting materials or prefabricated, are applied over dressings, a RL sock, stockinette, or a silicone gel liner.[65,68] Prefabricated RRDs are adjustable as the limb shape and volume changes and may be removed as needed for wound inspection. RRDs used with transtibial amputations can extend over the knee to maintain knee extension or end below the knee to permit active knee flexion.

Use of immediate postoperative rigid dressings varies greatly and is more prevalent in some areas of the country than others. Rigid postsurgical dressings, whether used immediately after surgery or in the early postoperative period, have been found to be successful in reducing postoperative edema and pain, knee flexion contractures, healing time, injury due to falls, and the time to fitting with a prosthesis.[65–67]

Semirigid Dressings

Semirigid dressings provide better control of edema than soft dressings. *Unna's dressing* (Unna boot), gauze impregnated with a compound of zinc oxide, gelatin, glycerin, and calamine, may be applied in the operating room. Its major disadvantage is that it may loosen easily and is not as rigid as the plaster of Paris dressing. However, it has been shown to be superior to the soft dressing in enhancing healing and reducing edema.[69,70]

Soft Dressings

The soft dressing is the oldest method of postsurgical management of the RL and probably the one that most physical therapists in acute care hospitals will encounter. A soft postoperative dressing typically includes a nonadherent dressing over the incision, gauze pads and fluff placed over the distal and anterior aspect of the RL secured with roll-over gauze. Typically, but not always, an elastic bandage is applied over the dressing to control edema. After the fluff gauze is no longer needed, edema is managed with an elastic bandage or an elastic or silicone shrinker.[67,71]

Elastic Wraps

With care taken to ensure proper compression, an elastic bandage, 4 inches wide or more, may be applied over the postsurgical dressing. The elastic bandage must apply even pressure without areas of excessive pressure that might impair circulation and healing. The patient or a family member should learn to apply the wrap using effective technique as soon as possible after wound care is no longer necessary. Many older individuals with transfemoral amputations may not have the necessary balance and coordination to wrap effectively.

Some surgeons prefer delaying elastic wrapping until the incision has healed and the sutures have been removed. Leaving the RL without any compression allows for full development of postoperative edema, which may increase pain and interfere with circulation in the small vessels in the skin and soft tissue, thereby potentially compromising healing. The therapist can discuss the benefits of early wrapping with the surgeon if no other form of rigid dressing is used. There is strong evidence in the literature of the benefits of either the IPOP or the RRD.[65,70,71]

One of the major drawbacks of the elastic wrap is that it needs frequent rewrapping. Movement of the RL against the bedclothes, bending and extending the proximal joints, and general body movements cause slippage and changes in pressure. Covering the finished wrap with stockinet helps to reduce some of the slippage; however, careful and frequent rewrapping is the only effective way to prevent complications. Nursing staff, family members, and the patient, as well as the physical therapist or physical therapist assistant, need to assume responsibility for frequent inspection and rewrapping of the RL. Residual limb wrapping is described in detail later in this chapter.

Elastic Shrinkers

Shrinkers are sock-like garments manufactured from an elastic material; they are conical in shape and come in a variety of sizes (Fig. 22.4). Shrinkers are difficult to use in the early postoperative period because the process of pulling the shrinker onto the RL may put undesirable stress on the unhealed incision. Silicone liners are applied with a "roll-on" process that is less traumatic to the incision. Another potential disadvantage of a shrinker is that as the RL shrinks in volume, new smaller shrinkers must be purchased several times before limb volume stabilizes. However, shrinkers have

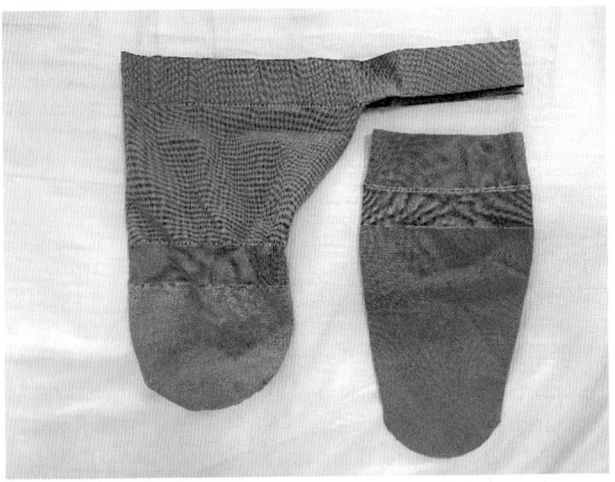

Figure 22.4 (Right) Transtibial shrinker. (Left) Transfemoral shrinker.

several advantages over elastic bandages. Unlike elastic bandages, shrinkers do not require frequent reapplication or extensive training. Therefore, in many clinical settings, the shrinker has replaced the elastic bandage for RL shrinking and shaping during the preprosthetic phase.

■ PHASES OF CARE

Early onset of rehabilitation produces greater potential for success. A long delay is likely to result in the development of complications such as joint contractures, general debilitation, and depressed psychological state. The rehabilitation process includes several stages of varying duration: preoperative phase; postsurgical phase; preprosthetic phase; and, if applicable, prosthetic training. The desired expected outcome of the episode of care is to help the patient regain the presurgical level of function. For some, it will mean return to gainful employment with an active recreational life. For others, it will mean independence in the home and community. For still others, it may mean living in an assisted living environment or nursing home. If the amputation resulted from long-standing chronic disease, the rehabilitation approach may be to help the person function at a higher level than that immediately before surgery.

Preoperative Phase

In the case of traumatic amputation, there is no option for a preoperative phase of rehabilitation. However, when amputation is presented as a likely intervention for patients with PVD and critical limb ischemia, optimal rehabilitation care begins before the amputation with multidisciplinary medical, physical, and functional assessments, including assessment of the contralateral limb and psychosocial and cognitive factors that can affect functional prognosis.[70,72,73] Patient education, including discussions with the patient and family members about phantom and RL pain and realistic short- and long-term goals, is also important at this stage. Patients whose pain expectations are realistic for the postamputation year are more satisfied with their rehabilitation outcomes, regardless of their actual reported pain levels.[74] When possible, patients should also begin a cardiorespiratory conditioning program prior to surgery.[75] Learning about prosthetic rehabilitation, seeing a prosthesis, and even meeting or talking with a successful prosthesis user helps individuals be less fearful of amputation as a treatment option.

Postsurgical Phase

The postsurgical phase is the time between surgery and discharge from the acute care hospital. The primary goal of this phase of care is to prepare the patient for discharge to the appropriate placement site for continued rehabilitation. Box 22.1 presents the general goals of the postsurgical phase of care.

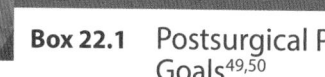

Box 22.1 Postsurgical Phase General Goals[49,50]

- Promote RL wound healing
- Residual limb pain management and control
- Phantom limb pain/sensation management
- Optimize ROM of both lower and upper limbs, without impairing RL healing
- Optimize strength of both lower and upper limbs, without impairing RL healing
- Protect remaining limb (if dysvascular)
- Demonstrate functional sitting and standing balance
- Perform independent transfers and bed mobility
- Ambulate with appropriate assistive device
- Demonstrate proper sitting and bed positioning
- Begin psychological adjustment
- Understand the process of prosthetic rehabilitation

RL = residual limb; ROM = range of motion.

Box 22.2 outlines the data necessary for the therapist to develop a physical therapy POC for the hospitalized patient following amputation. This data is collected from review of the medical record and patient interview and examination. Data gathering must be prioritized according to the person's physiological status and cause of amputation; however, the information obtained on initial and subsequent examinations will influence discharge planning and future care. Thus, it is important that the therapist include evidence of the patient's physical capabilities required to qualify for various post-hospitalization levels of care. For example, to qualify for some inpatient rehabilitation facilities, patients must be able to tolerate 3 hours of therapy per day. Patients may be discharged to home with home services (including physical and occupational therapy) or outpatient services. Other options include discharge to an inpatient rehabilitation facility or a subacute/skilled rehabilitation facility.

Physical therapists must advocate for their patients to ensure appropriate continuation of rehabilitation services following hospital discharge. Studies show that persons with amputation who receive rehabilitation at comprehensive inpatient rehabilitation facilities achieve a higher level of mobility success with their prostheses and are more satisfied with their mobility when compared to those who went home or to subacute/skilled facilities.[76–78]

For all patients, current cardiovascular status, physiological response to surgery, presence of infection, pain level, and medication will influence to what extent the patient will be able to actively participate in the therapy program. Individuals with amputations secondary to severe trauma, blast injuries in war, and similar problems will require a somewhat different approach from individuals with vascular disease. The type of postsurgical dressing will also influence both data gathering and

Box 22.2   Postsurgical Phase Examination[50]

- Medical Record Review
- Onset and duration of symptoms and reason for admission
- Height, weight, BMI
- Tobacco use
- Comorbid chronic conditions (e.g., diabetes, PAD, CAD, MI, COPD, CHF)
- Medications and relevant laboratory results
- Previous or ongoing medical or surgical treatments
- Type and level of amputation; relevant specifics of amputation surgery
- Status of RL incision healing, infection
- Social history, including prior functional level and use of mobility aids, home environment, social support, and patient goals and expectations
- Out-of-bed status; orders that affect mobility
- Physical examination
- Observation
- Lines and tubes
- Residual limb position and dressings; presence of devices (e.g., knee immobilizer)
- Mental status, cognition, communication
- Affect and psychological considerations (e.g., fear, anxiety, emotional lability)
- Systems review
- Vital signs, SpO_2—at rest and following activity
- Cardiovascular (e.g., pulses, edema, pitting edema)
- Respiratory (signs of respiratory distress; effort of breathing, dyspnea)
- Integumentary (e.g., skin integrity, wounds, scars); remaining intact foot
- Neuromuscular (e.g., sensation, protective sensation in intact foot)
- Pain
- RL pain; incisional pain
- PLP or sensation
- Other
- Musculoskeletal
- ROM of residual limb joints and intact UEs and LEs
- Gross functional muscle performance, UEs and intact LE (e.g., strength, coordination)
- Balance (sitting, standing, response to perturbation)
- Functional status
- Bed mobility, transfers, sitting, standing
- Ambulation with ambulatory aid (distance, assistance required)
- Safety awareness during functional activities

BMI = body mass index; CAD = coronary artery disease; CHF = congestive heart failure; COPD = chronic obstructive pulmonary disease; LE = lower extremity; MI = myocardial infarction; PAD = peripheral vascular disease; ROM = range of motion; SpO_2 = oxygen saturation; UE = upper extremity.

interventions. A person with a rigid dressing may be able to move more easily in bed than someone with a soft dressing. Typically, an individual in the early postsurgical phase will have limited mobility and functional capabilities. They may also have compromised endurance, RL postoperative pain and phantom limb pain/sensation that may interfere with participation in the program. The specific POC is developed to achieve patient goals based on critical examination findings.

Intervention: Postsurgical Phase

The therapist treating a patient in the hospital has only limited time in which to achieve the goals because hospital lengths of stay are typically short. Interventions must be aimed at preparing the patient for discharge from acute care to appropriate continuing rehabilitation care. Box 22.3 outlines interventions included in the postsurgical rehabilitation POC.

Positioning

Persons with amputation are at risk for developing RL joint contractures that make it difficult to comfortably wear and use a prosthesis. The development of contractures

Box 22.3   Postsurgical Phase Interventions

- Interventions to prevent development of RL joint contractures
- Positioning (e.g., prone lying; for transtibial amputations, devices to maintain full knee extension of RL)
- Active ROM exercise; caution to prevent unwanted stress to the incision
- Functional training
- Bed mobility (rolling, supine to and from sitting, supine to and from prone)
- Transfers (bed, chair, wheelchair, toilet)
- Standing and sitting balance training
- Ambulation training with crutches or a walker; stairs, if appropriate
- Exercises for intact extremities (upper limbs and remaining lower extremity)
- Active exercise to maintain joint ROM and muscle function
- Exercise to maintain cardiorespiratory endurance necessary for functional activities
- RL care and protection; edema management (when appropriate, elastic bandage, rigid dressing, shrinker)
- Care of the remaining lower extremity (if circulation compromised)
- Patient and caregiver education
- Education on amputation rehabilitation and prosthetics
- Safety awareness during all functional activities

RL = residual limb; ROM = range of motion.

also delays fitting with a definitive prosthesis. The most common type of contracture that develops in a transtibial amputation is a knee flexion contracture. Frequently seen with transfemoral amputations are hip flexion and abduction contractures owing to muscle imbalance. For example, the hamstrings are cut and secured, but the iliopsoas is unaffected by the amputation; the long adductor muscles are cut and secured, but the abductor muscles are intact. Additionally, persons with lower limb amputations tend to spend much of their time sitting, which can predispose to development of flexion contractures. Persons with partial foot amputations may develop plantarflexion contractures, particularly if weight-bearing is restricted for a long period of time. When a tarsometatarsal amputation is performed, the foot may assume an inverted position because of loss of the attachment of peroneus longus, resulting in eversion weakness.

Figure 22.5 illustrates the positioning strategies appropriate for a patient with either a transtibial or transfemoral amputation. Although the figure represents someone with a transtibial amputation, the general principles are the same. It is critical in both instances to prevent hip flexion contractures, and the patient should be encouraged to spend at least 30 minutes in the prone position each day, if at all possible. A pillow under the RL while the patient is supine is never recommended, nor is prolonged sitting. In the early days, the patient

will want to avoid side-lying on the amputated side and the RL should be kept in extension at both hip and knee. Some facilities use a knee immobilizer or a posterior splint to maintain knee extension following a transtibial amputation. If a knee immobilizer is used, care must be taken to avoid excessive pressure to the RL. It is also most likely not safe to use the knee immobilizer during ambulation. A rigid dressing usually extends to midthigh and maintains knee extension. Patients can also perform active range of motion (ROM) of the joints of the RL; however, prior to healing, care must be taken to avoid movements that place excessive tension on the incision.

Functional Training

The loss of part of a limb shifts the body's center of mass (COM) and alters weight distribution among the limbs and trunk. As a result, some patients may have difficulty turning in bed or moving from a supine to sitting position. Usual procedures for teaching functional mobility are typically effective in helping patients to achieve independence in bed mobility. Transfers require the patient to demonstrate good sitting and standing balance. The shift in COM owing to the amputation will require the patient to adjust his or her balance responses accordingly. Persons with intact vision, vestibular function, and proprioception accommodate quickly. Those with impairments in these functions may require more time

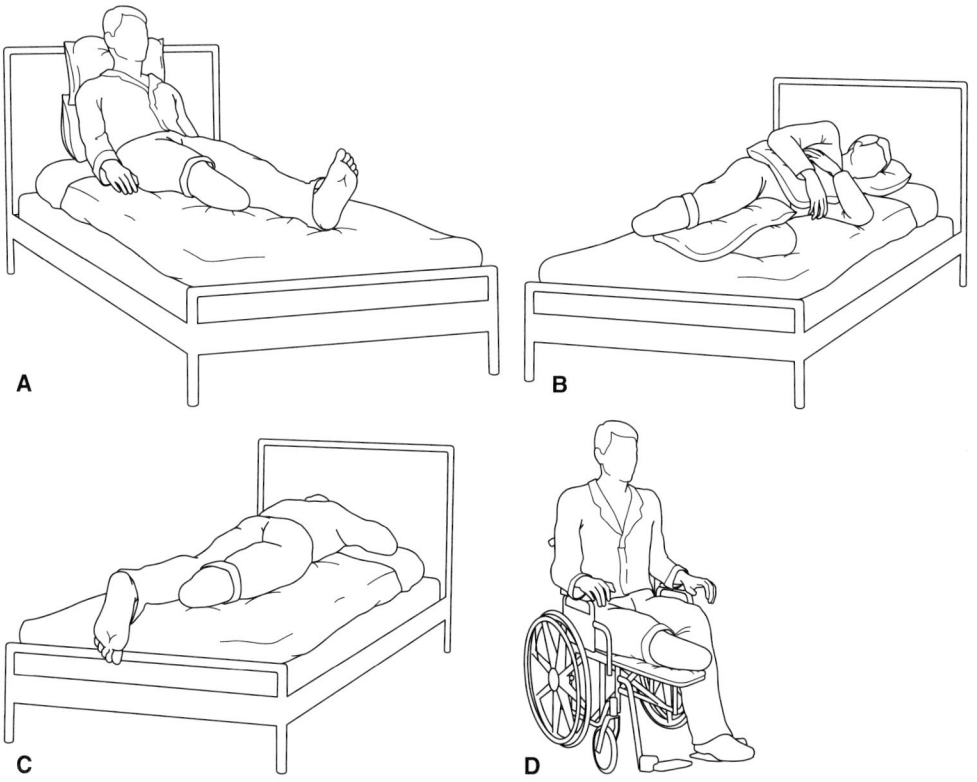

Figure 22.5 Proper transtibial position: (A) Supine. (B) Side-lying. (C) Prone. (D) Sitting. *(From May and Lockard, 46, p. 67 with permission.)*

and training. It is important to include safety awareness during transfer training, since at this point postamputation, most patients have phantom sensations (nonpainful sensations in the part of the limb that has been amputated and removed) and may default to learned motor patterns that include the now-absent limb. Patients will need to learn new motor patterns for functional activities and transfers. During transfer training in the early postsurgical period, the person should stand and transfer leading with the unamputated limb to protect the RL from possible injury against the chair or bed.

Balance Training

Sitting balance is usually not a problem with unilateral amputations; however, persons with a transfemoral amputation may have difficulty in unsupported sitting, if pushed in a posterior direction. Individuals with bilateral amputations may require more specific training in sitting balance. For persons with unilateral amputation, standing balance exercises on the remaining extremity are helpful to regain appropriate balance responses. The better the person can balance on the remaining extremity the more likely they will be to use crutches and lead an active life during the period before prosthetic fitting. A variety of balance exercises may be used, including balancing on a compliant surface.

Ambulation and Gait Training

Many physical therapists fit patients with a walker for ambulation. Although this is appropriate for some individuals, teaching the patient safe and independent mobility with crutches is more beneficial because the crutch gait pattern is similar to the pattern that will be used when walking with a prosthesis. While there is more stability in a walker, there is greater flexibility in accomplishing activities of daily living (ADL) with crutches, particularly when forearm (Loftstrand) crutches are used. The added balance needed for crutches will also serve the individual well when it is time for prosthetic fitting.

If the patient has been fitted with an IPOP rigid dressing and has good control of weight-bearing, a pylon and prosthetic foot may be added to the rigid dressing, making partial weight-bearing gait possible. In this instance, the patient must be fitted with crutches because the walker will inhibit the natural function of the prosthetic components.

When teaching mobility to someone with diabetes or any vascular compromise, it is important that the patient wear a shoe on the remaining foot. The remaining foot must be protected from injury, and hospital-provided slippers, or any slippers, do not provide the necessary protection. The family should bring in an appropriate shoe (low heel, cushion sole, good heel support, and laces to firmly secure the shoe to the foot). If the patient has lost protective sensation or has deformity in the unamputated foot, consider fitting the foot with an accommodative shoe to prevent trauma.[79]

Residual Limb Care

The physical therapist should discuss volume containment for edema management with the patient and family and provide instruction in how to properly implement the technique. If the patient has been fitted with an IPOP or RRD, the physical therapist must be alert to excessive bleeding or drainage through the cast. A primary focus at this point is to teach the patient how to protect the RL while moving in bed, coming to sitting, and transferring. Patients should not put pressure on the limb or drag it on the bed. Slightly raising the RL and moving it to the side while rolling to the unamputated side is the best way to come to sitting. Careful monitoring of RL healing status is important during postsurgical rehabilitation. The patient should be encouraged to move the limb gently within a pain-free range both at the knee (transtibial) and at the hip (both levels). Gentle hip extension performed several times a day (for transtibial amputations, with the knee straight) is an excellent exercise to teach the patient while lying prone or on the unamputated side. Resistive exercises for the RL are contraindicated at this time.

Care of the Remaining Lower Extremity

Since the majority of individuals undergoing amputation do so as a result of poor circulation, it is important to evaluate the status of the remaining extremity and teach the patient and family proper care, as presented in Chapter 14, Vascular, Lymphatic, and Integumentary Disorders. A proper shoe must be obtained before standing and mobility activities.[79] ROM and strengthening exercises can be implemented as appropriate for the status of the remaining limb.

Patient Education

Patient education is an important element throughout all phases of amputation rehabilitation.[70] Effective patient education can positively influence the patient's outcome and promote healthy behaviors.[70] Throughout the examination and implementation of the POC, the physical therapist continuously involves the patient and caregivers, answering questions and providing information at a level and rate commensurate with the capabilities of the individuals. The goals are to have the patient and caregivers assume responsibility for care and safety awareness during functional activities, understand the need for continued care, and become active participants in the rehabilitation program.[80] Regardless of the specific discharge placement, the patient should be given a home program and encouraged to be as mobile as possible.

Discharge Planning

Physical therapists, as part of the multidisciplinary team caring for the patient, should actively participate in discharge planning and placement discussions. As mentioned, evidence shows that persons with amputation who receive rehabilitation at comprehensive inpatient rehabilitation facilities achieve a higher level of mobility success with their prostheses and are more satisfied with their mobility when compared to those who went home or to subacute/skilled facilities.[76–78,81] Furthermore, greater prosthetic use and satisfaction were found for those who were admitted to an inpatient rehabilitation facility versus a skilled nursing facility or home.[78] When discharge to home is planned, physical therapists must coordinate with the occupational therapist and social services to ensure that appropriate equipment, an ambulatory aid, home evaluation and modification, and continued rehabilitation services are arranged for safety and continuity of care.[82]

Preprosthetic Phase

The preprosthetic phase is the time between discharge from the acute care hospital and fitting with a preparatory (temporary) or definitive prosthesis, or the decision not to fit the patient with an artificial limb. Regrettably, for many individuals this period lasts too long and does not include a regular program of physical therapy, resulting in poor outcomes. The general goals for the prosthetic phase of care are presented in Box 22.4. Box 22.5 provides a guide for preprosthetic examination.

Examination
Residual Limb

Approximately 7 to 12 days after surgery, depending on the condition of the RL, the amount of healing, and the postsurgical dressing, specific data about the RL and adjacent joint(s) can be gathered. Residual limb girth and length measurements are taken after initial postsurgical edema has diminished. Circumferential measurements are then taken regularly throughout the preprosthetic phase to document RL shaping and shrinkage. Measurements are made at regular intervals over the length of the limb to reflect the specific limb shape. Circumferential measurements of the transtibial RL are started at the medial tibial plateau (medial joint line of the knee) and taken every 2 to 3 in. (5 to 8 cm), depending on the length of the limb. Length of the RL is measured from the medial tibial plateau to the end of the bone, then to the end of the skin. Circumferential measurements of the transfemoral RL are started at the ischial tuberosity, greater trochanter, or the insertion of the adductor longus tendon onto the pubic ramus, whichever is most reliably palpable, and are taken every 3 to 4 in. (8 to 10 cm). Length is measured from the same proximal landmark to the end of the bone, then to the end of the skin. For accuracy of repeat measurements, exact landmarks are carefully noted. If the ischial tuberosity is used in transfemoral measurements, hip joint position is noted as well. Other information gathered about the RL includes a description of its shape (conical, bulbous, or cylindrical; presence of redundant tissue), skin condition, sensation, and joint proprioception.

Box 22.4   Preprosthetic Phase General Goals

- Independent in RL care
- Volume containment and edema management: elastic bandage, shrinker, or removable rigid dressing application; IPOP care
- Skin care and desensitization
- Positioning
- Independent in mobility, transfers, and functional activities
- If fitted with IPOP, partial weight-bearing crutch walking; full weight-bearing when tolerated
- Single-leg ambulation with crutches/walker if fitted with soft dressing or removable rigid dressing; demonstration of a gait pattern that will allow easy transition to prosthetic gait
- Ability to ambulate safely on level surfaces, uneven surfaces, inclines and steps, as appropriate for the ability of the patient
- Ability to perform all transfers, including in the bathroom, car transfers, and to and from the floor, as appropriate for the ability of the patient
- Perform an exercise program accurately and with good form
- ROM and resisted exercises for all parts of residual LE
- ROM and strengthening exercises for the unamputated LE and trunk
- Muscle strengthening and endurance exercises for UEs to support functional needs
- Perform appropriate care of the remaining lower extremity if amputation was for vascular reasons
- Demonstrate cardiorespiratory endurance necessary for prosthetic use and community mobility

BMI = body mass index; IPOP = immediate postoperative prosthesis; LE = lower extremity; ORIF = open reduction internal fixation; ROM = range of motion; UE = upper extremity.

Range of Motion

Gross ROM estimations are generally adequate for examination of the uninvolved extremity unless there are specific limitations or contractures. Specific goniometric measurements are necessary for the amputated side, bilateral hip extension, and ankle dorsiflexion of the unamputated side. Functional balance requires good ankle motion, and many older individuals have developed limited range in ankle dorsiflexion leading to catching the toes during swing, stumbling, or falling. Hip and knee measurements are taken following transtibial amputation. Hip flexion, extension, abduction, and adduction measurements are taken following transfemoral amputation. Measurement of internal and external hip rotation is difficult to obtain and unnecessary if no gross abnormality or pathology is evident. Hip flexion contractures are particularly important to note because the patient

Box 22.5   Preprosthetic Phase Examination Guide

General and Social History

- Patient demographics (age, sex, body weight, BMI)
- Family and social data
- Living arrangements, home architectural challenges or hazards
- Social support/caregivers
- Preamputation status (work, physical activity level, avocation, independence, community mobility)
- Insurance status, relative to coverage for prosthesis, durable medical equipment, and continued rehabilitation
- Psychological and emotional status (adjustment to and acceptance of amputation; body image)
- Other as relevant

History of Present Illness and Past Medical History

- Amputation history
- Cause of amputation (disease, tumor, trauma, congenital)
- Date of surgery, hospital, surgeon; any surgical/medical complications
- Associated diseases/symptoms (e.g., diabetes, neuropathy, visual disturbances, cardiopulmonary disease, cardiovascular disease, renal disease, stroke, arthritis, congenital anomalies, history of depression/anxiety)
- Other relevant surgeries (e.g., total joint replacements, fracture repairs with ORIF)
- Medications

Systems Review

- Cardiopulmonary
- Vital signs and SpO$_2$ measured with pulse oximeter, at rest and after activity
- Observation for signs of respiratory distress, dyspnea at rest and after activity
- Auscultation of heart and lungs, if required
- Integumentary
- Lesions (location, size, shape, open, scar tissue)
- Skin condition, turgor, and texture (moist, dry, scaly, cracked, callous)
- Trophic changes (changes due to neuropathy, such as dryness, loss of hair, nail thickening)
- Grafts (location, type, healing)
- Dermatological lesions (psoriasis, eczema, rashes, maceration, cysts)
- Neuromuscular
- Mental status, cognition and communication
- Pain (location, intensity, nature, frequency, duration)
- RL pain
- Phantom limb sensation and PLP
- Other locations
- Sensation (absent, diminished, hyperesthesia; protective sensation in intact foot)
- Balance (sitting, standing, with perturbation)
- Coordination (quality of movements)
- Vascular (both lower limbs)
- Pulses (femoral, popliteal, dorsalis pedis, posterior tibial)
- Color (red, pallor, cyanosis)
- Temperature (glove-stocking presentation)
- Edema (location, type [pitting or nonpitting]; girth measurements)
- Intermittent claudication in intact lower extremity
- Musculoskeletal (all four extremities and trunk)
- ROM (patients are vulnerable to insidious development of joint contractures during this phase; therapists must monitor and carefully measure and remeasure)
- Muscle strength and endurance (core trunk strength is very important to prosthetic control and should be assessed in addition to the extremities)

Box 22.5 Preprosthetic Phase Examination Guide—cont'd

Residual Limb

- Length
- Bone length (transtibial limbs measured from MTP; transfemoral limbs measured from ischial tuberosity or greater trochanter)
- Soft tissue length (note distal redundant tissue)
- Shape
- Cylindrical (desirable), conical, bulbous end, and so forth
- Abnormalities ("dog ears," adductor roll)
- Incision (healed, adherent, invaginated, flat, dehiscence, signs of necrotic flap)
- Skin condition

Functional Status

- Transfers
- Bed-to-chair, to toilet and tub/shower, to car
- Assistance required; safety awareness
- Mobility and ambulation
- Wheelchair or type of ambulatory aid
- Required assistance or supervision; safety awareness, balance and recovery from balance loss
- Distance and cardiorespiratory response to sustained mobility
- Basic ADL (bathing, dressing)
- Instrumental ADL (cooking, cleaning)
- Functional outcome measures (choose instrument to measure progress or regression)
- Performance-based measurement
- Quality of life measurement

ADL = activities of daily living; BMI = body mass index; MTP = medial tibial plateau; ORIF = open reduction internal fixation; PLP = phantom limb pain; RL = residual limb; ROM = range of motion; SpO_2 = oxygen saturation.

will not be able to stand and bear weight properly using a prosthesis without adequate hip extension (Fig. 22.6). Additionally, hip extension participates in prosthetic knee control for some transfemoral prostheses.

Muscle Strength

Manual muscle testing (MMT) of functional muscle groups in the upper extremities (UEs) and uninvolved LE is performed as part of the initial examination. MMT of the involved LE must usually wait until most healing has occurred. With a transtibial amputation, good strength in the hip extensors and abductors, as well as the knee extensors and flexors, is needed for satisfactory prosthetic ambulation. For the patient with a transfemoral amputation, good strength of the hip extensors and abductors is a requirement. Hip abductor strength should also be monitored as it is important for pelvic stability during gait. The POC should include monitoring and strengthening of these muscles throughout the preprosthetic phase. Hip extensor strength has been identified as a predictor of successful prosthetic use[30,33] and running ability.[83] Strength of the muscles that stabilize the trunk must also be assessed. Side-to-side trunk muscle asymmetries were found in people with lower

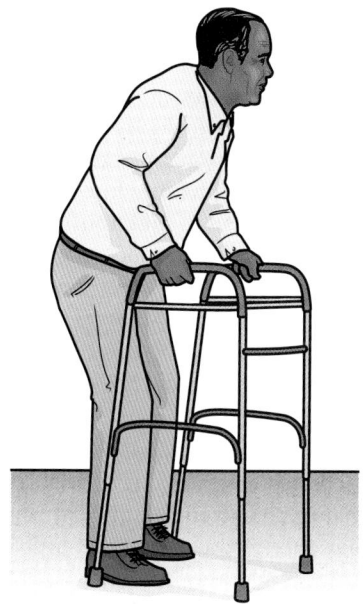

Figure 22.6 Hip flexion contractures alter upright postural alignment and lower extremity weight-bearing.

limb loss.[84] In addition, core strengthening exercises were found to be beneficial for functional mobility and walking speed.[85]

Status of the Uninvolved Limb

The vascular status of the uninvolved LE is determined and documented. Data gathered include condition of the skin, presence of pulses, sensation, temperature, edema, pain on exercise or at rest, presence of wounds, ulceration, or other abnormalities. Chapter 14, Vascular, Lymphatic, and Integumentary Disorders, presents further information on examination and evaluation of peripheral vascular status. In addition to examination of the remaining lower limb's vascular status, ROM, and strength, the presence of deformities and other orthopedic problems should also be identified. Contralateral knee pain, which affects quality of life, is a common complaint after amputation.[86] The presence of preexisting conditions, such as arthritis, should be noted early so that accommodations can be made to prevent them from limiting function in the future.

Functional Status

Activities of daily living and functional mobility skills, including transfer and ambulatory status, are examined, measured, and documented. Sitting balance and standing balance on the remaining extremity are important and should be examined. Data regarding presurgical activity level are obtained through interview and are often indicative of potential functional prosthetic use.[87] An individual who had an active lifestyle before the amputation, regardless of age, is more likely to be able to learn to use a prosthesis well. Individuals with a long history of a sedentary lifestyle may encounter more difficulty, particularly if the amputation is at the transfemoral level.[35,87] A performance-based functional outcome measure should be included in the examination and used as a baseline for subsequent assessment of function.[88] Functional outcome measures are discussed at the end of this chapter.

Phantom Limb

The majority of individuals will encounter *phantom limb sensations* following amputation.[89] Phantom sensation is the perception that the part of the limb that has been amputated is still present. The phantom, which may occur initially immediately after surgery, is variably described as feeling normal in character, feeling warmth or tingling, or feeling that part of the amputated limb is held in a particular position. Occasionally the person may feel the whole extremity. The phantom is more often described as "telescoping" in which the patient perceives the distal part of the limb without sensation from the midportion of the limb.[89] Phantom pain occurs when the phantom sensations are noxious, often interfering with prosthetic use and function. It is most commonly described as burning, aching, or cramping. The lifetime prevalence of phantom limb pain (PLP) is high (76% to 87%).[89]

PLP may be localized or diffuse, continuous or intermittent, or may be triggered by some external stimuli. PLP often improves over time. Most people experience a reduction in PLP frequency and duration during the first 6 months, but many continue to experience some level of PLP for years.[90] However, despite its commonality among individuals with amputation, a specific etiology for PLP has not been determined. A leading theory suggests that phantom phenomena are due to maladaptive neuroplasticity (changes to the cerebral cortex, particularly the motor and sensory cortex) driven by the deafferentation that occurs with amputation.[91]

During examination, it is important to document the presence of phantom sensation and pain. Patients should be asked to describe their sensation, rate its intensity using a numerical rating scale, and describe the frequency of occurrence and the duration of the episodes.[92] In some patients, PLP can be evoked by applying pressure.[91] Therefore, palpation and physical exam may be helpful in understanding PLP in these patients. In addition, patients should be asked to qualify or quantify the effect of their phantom on ADL and quality of life. The effects of phantom limb sensation/pain should be noted in functional outcome measurements. Baseline data documenting the status of phantom limb sensations during the preprosthetic phase should be recorded as a basis for evaluating the effects of time or interventions.

Emotional and Psychological Status

Initial reaction to the traumatic loss of a limb may be grief and depression. The person may experience insomnia and restlessness and have difficulty concentrating. Some individuals may mourn the possible loss of a job or the ability to participate in a favorite sport or other activities rather than the lost limb per se. In the early stages, the person's grief may alternate with feelings of hopelessness, despondency, bitterness, and anger. Socially, the patient may feel lonely, isolated, and the object of pity. Concerns about the future, about body image and sexual function, about the responses of family and friends, and about employment all affect the individual's reactions.[93,94] If the amputation is the result of vascular disease or other long-term problem, the amputation may actually come as a relief. The fight to save the limb, sometimes long and painful, is finally over. However, regardless of the cause of amputation, the prevalence of psychiatric disorders among people with limb loss is high and ranges from 32% to 84%, including rates of depression ranging from 10.4% to 63%, and rates of post-traumatic stress disorder ranging from 3.3% to 56.3%.[95] In addition, people with limb loss experience higher levels of anxiety and depression than do the general population.[96]

During examination, therapists should encourage patients to express personal feelings about their limb loss and address concerns with patient education or referral for counseling. Although it is difficult to predict long-range adjustment initially, there is some evidence that early counseling before the surgery and the opportunity to explore the feelings associated with amputation and rehabilitation may be beneficial for individuals in all age groups.[97] Often seeing others in the treatment area with similar problems, particularly if involved in prosthetic training, may help the patient with a new amputation realize what can be achieved.

Social integration is another important factor to evaluate. Social integration refers to the contacts and interactions between the person with amputation and his or her social network. Increased social interaction is associated with both improved function and quality of life.[98] Therapists should identify and facilitate patients' participation in important social relationships.

Cognition

Rehabilitation following amputation requires learning new methods of performing functional mobility and ADL, which may prove challenging for persons with a vascular amputation and impaired cognition.[99] Although there is no evidence that those with cognitive impairment should be excluded from consideration for prosthetic fitting and rehabilitation, therapists must be aware of their patients' cognitive abilities when planning and implementing rehabilitation plans of care. Effective learning styles for each patient should be identified and alternative or supplemental methods to facilitate learning and remembering safe procedures should be included.[100] Evaluation of cognitive abilities in persons with a vascular amputation should be performed at intervals in the postamputation period. Overall, cognitive performance appears poorest before surgery, but improves after amputation. Cognitive improvement generally stabilizes between 6 and 12 weeks postsurgery.[101] Higher cognitive function has been reported to be associated with better functional mobility outcomes and increased prosthesis use.[99]

Clinical Note (The Older Adult With Amputation). Older individuals are subject to considerable stress from concerns about financial limitations, loss of control over their lives, and fear of becoming dependent. An older adult who requires an amputation must often cope with multiple physical problems. Loss is a part of normal aging—loss of physiological capabilities, loss of a spouse or friends, loss of the self-esteem related to one's career or job, and now loss of function. It is helpful to give the client as much control over decision-making as possible to provide opportunities to be involved in goal setting and sequencing of activities. As with any client during examination, physical therapists need to learn about the stressors affecting the individual and assist with coping by being reflective listeners and enablers.

It is a myth that older individuals cannot learn a new skill, have difficulty remembering, and cannot achieve functional independence.[102] A longitudinal study revealed that older adults with lower limb amputation can improve their functional independence after rehabilitation.[103] Some older adults may have difficulty learning a new skill, but many are able to adapt successfully to a disability such as an amputation and lead a full and normal life. Although some suffer from dementia, others who are labeled as having dementia because of confusion in the acute care setting may actually only be responding to medications, metabolic imbalances, infection toxicity, insecurity in a strange environment, or the sequelae of anesthesia. It is important to reassess cognition in postacute care rehabilitation settings because cognition typically improves postsurgery.[101] Understanding the client's cognitive capabilities is necessary to structure learning experiences appropriately. Goal-oriented statements may be clearer than step-by-step instructions. For example, asking the patient to "stand up" may be more successful than instructions involving multiple steps. We do many activities almost automatically—getting up from a chair, turning in bed, and walking. Most of us have developed particular patterns of movements over the years. The physical therapist can draw on such patterns while focusing on the movement goals.

Intervention: Preprosthetic Phase
Residual Limb Care and Edema/Volume Management

Changes in RL volume occur due to postoperative edema and overall body weight. The limb should be healed and postoperative edema minimized to be ready for prosthetic fitting. The RL is subjected to considerable and varied pressures during prosthetic walking and is generally not fully healed and prepared for these stresses for 8 to 12 weeks after surgery. Although using the IPOP method enables partial weight-bearing with a prosthesis earlier than this time frame, it is only variably used in the United States.[66,67] Individuals not fitted with an IPOP or rigid dressing use elastic bandages or shrinkers to reduce the size of the RL. The patient, family member, or professional staff member applies the bandage, which is worn 23 hours a day (full time, except when bathing). Using an elastic wrap or a shrinker to reduce edema is a slow process. Edema may be difficult to control in individuals with diabetes, particularly if they have renal disease or congestive heart failure.

Body weight also contributes to the size of the RL. After amputation, some individuals gain weight because their appetite returns or they become less active. Others lose weight because they become more active. Body weight must be monitored by regular weighing, just as RL girth measurements must be taken to monitor edema reduction. Patients require education regarding the importance of maintaining a stable body weight because fluctuations in body weight will make prosthetic socket fit difficult.

Residual Limb Wrapping

The basic principles of wrapping are presented in Box 22.6. When the wrap is complete, all skin of the RL should be covered with a smooth (wrinkle-free), snug wrap. The shape of the RL should be cylindrical. All wraps will slip and move, regardless of how well they are applied; rewrapping should be performed about every 4 hours. Whenever possible, patients should be able to independently wrap their own RL using good technique; a family member or caregiver should also be able to apply a good wrap. This usually requires considerable practice and should be a treatment goal.

Figure 22.7 and Box 22.7 illustrate and describe the wrapping technique for the transtibial amputation. Figure 22.8 and Box 22.8 illustrate and describe the wrapping technique for a transfemoral amputation. An alternate view of the wrapping techniques from the patient's perspective is available online.[104]

Shrinkers

The transtibial elastic shrinker is rolled onto the RL to midthigh and is designed to be self-suspending. Individuals with heavy thighs may need additional suspension with a waist belt to prevent distal slippage. Transfemoral shrinkers typically incorporate a hip spica (encircles the pelvis), which provides good suspension except with obese individuals (see Fig. 22.4). Care must be taken that the patient understands the importance of proper suspension; any rolling of the edges or slipping of the shrinker can create a tourniquet around the proximal part of the RL and form an adductor roll. Shrinkers are not used until the incision is healed and the sutures removed; distraction forces that may occur during donning can cause wound dehiscence (splitting open). Shrinkers are more expensive to use than elastic wrap; the initial cost is greater, and new shrinkers of smaller sizes must be purchased as the limb volume decreases. However, shrinkers are easier to apply than elastic bandages and are a viable option for individuals who are not able to properly wrap the limb due to cognitive impairment, poor vision, or limited mobility.[105] As mentioned, the shrinker has replaced the elastic bandage for RL shrinking and shaping in many clinical settings due to this advantage. When comparing the effectiveness of shrinkers and elastic bandages in RL management, current literature provides limited evidence that can be used to guide clinical decision-making. Therefore, the selection of compression method should be individualized for the patient.[105]

Skin Care

Proper hygiene and skin care are important. The RL is treated as any other part of the body; it is kept clean and dry. The application of lotions is usually not

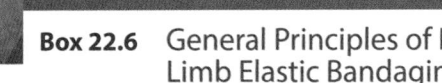

Box 22.6 General Principles of Residual Limb Elastic Bandaging

- The general direction of wrapping should be from distal to proximal.
- Use figure-eight wrapping pattern, with diagonal turns—NOT circular turns that can constrict or choke.
- Diagonal turns should be about 45° from horizontal and should form an X pattern as the diagonal turns cross each other.
- Each turn should partially overlap previous turns so there are no gaps in the wrap, and pressure is even throughout the wrap.
- Apply the wrap diagonally over the distal "corners" of the RL to prevent "dog ears" or a bulbous shape. After the RL is wrapped, the shape should be cylindrical.
- Pressure should be even throughout the wrap, with a slight gradient from more distally to less proximally.
- The elastic in the wrap should be stretched about half of its available elasticity for a snug wrap.
- There should be about three layers of wrap evenly applied over the RL; more layers in one area will cause localized higher pressure.
- Secure with tape applied wrap to wrap. Do not apply tape to skin or secure the wrap with clips or pins.
- When the wrap is complete, the RL should be totally covered with no gaps between turns.
- There should be no wrinkles or folds in the wrap; wrinkles cause increased pressure.
- In the TT RL, the patella may be covered or left open; the full wrap should cover the supracondylar region of the thigh.
- Wrapping the TF RL requires a hip spica (about two wraps around the waist to prevent the wrap from sliding down).
- While applying the TF wrap, make sure that the wrapping does not pull the RL into hip flexion or abduction by moving the RL into good position while wrapping.
- While applying the TT wrap, ensure that the wrapping does not pull the RL into knee flexion by maintaining the knee in extension during wrapping.
- Two elastic bandages are usually required, but the number is determined by the size of the RL.
- TT usually use two 4-inch wraps.
- TF usually use one 4-inch and one 6-inch wrap; a large TF may require three wraps.
- Wraps should be removed and reapplied about every 4 hours or whenever slippage occurs.

BMI = body mass index; ORIF = open reduction internal fixation; RL = residual limb; SpO$_2$ = oxygen saturation; TF = transfemoral; TT = transtibial.

recommended, unless there is a specific reason; however, if a lotion is used, it should be non-alcohol-based, hypoallergenic, and fragrance free. Care must be taken to avoid abrasions, cuts, and other skin problems.

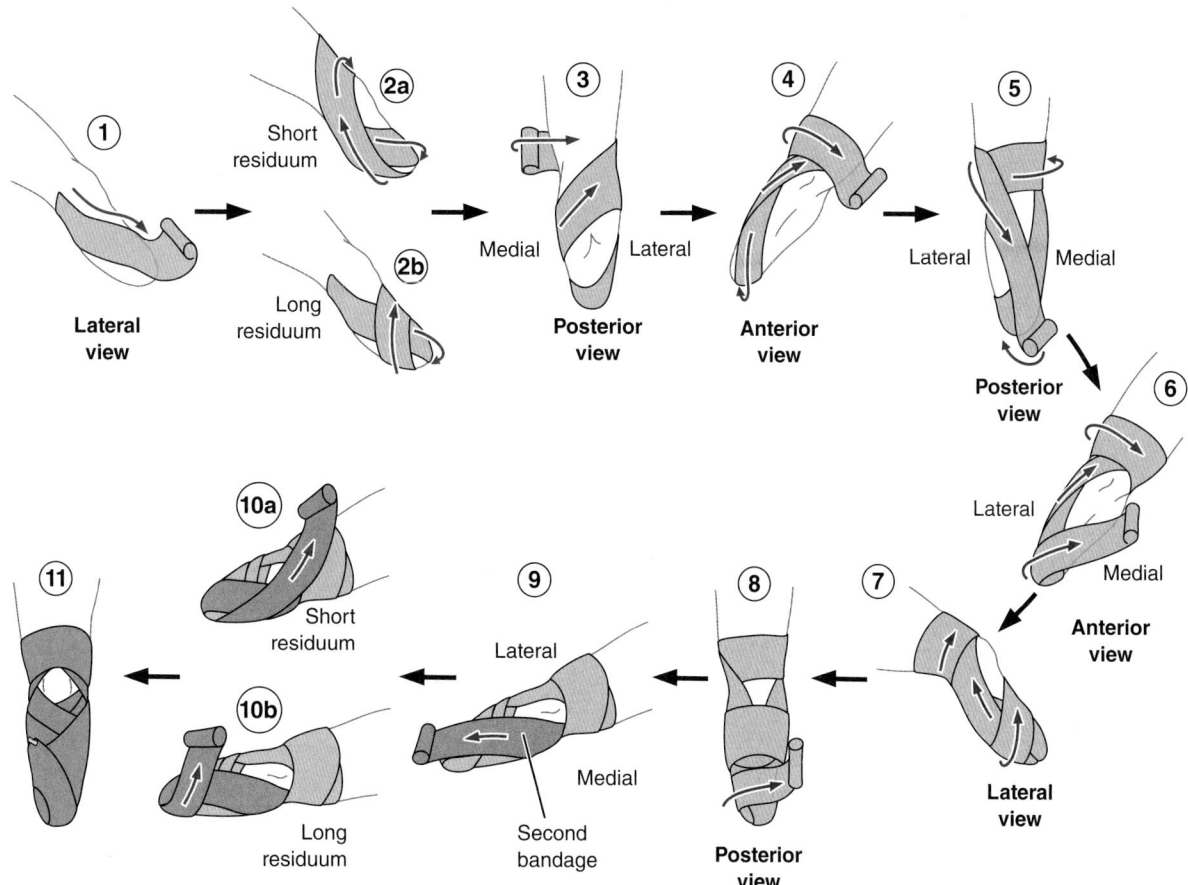

Figure 22.7 Transtibial RL bandaging. *(From May and Lockard, 46, p. 75 with permission.)*

Box 22.7   Transtibial Residual Limb Bandaging Technique*

- **Step 1:** Start the wrap at the medial or lateral tibial condyle and wrap diagonally over the anterior surface of the RL to the distal end, covering the midline of the incision. Continue diagonally over the posterior RL, to the beginning turn as an anchor. If the incision is anterior, wrap from posterior to anterior over the distal end to pull the soft tissue forward over the bone to facilitate a distal muscle cushion under the bone at the end of the RL.
- **Step 2:** The wrap may be brought directly over the beginning point (step 2a) or across the front of the residual limb in an X design (step 2b). The latter is useful with long RLs and aids in bandage suspension. Anchoring turns over the distal thigh suspend the wrap and shape the supracondylar region of the thigh for prosthetic fitting.
- **Steps 3–5:** After anchoring above the knee, the bandage is brought back around the opposite tibial condyle and down to the distal end of the RL. The bandage should overlap the midline of the incision and the other wrap by one-half inch to ensure adequate distal support.
- **Steps 6–8:** The figure-eight pattern is continued until all the bandage is used, making sure to distribute the turns so the wrap is not too thick in any area from the distal end of the RL to the supracondylar region of the thigh. The patella may be covered or left open, depending on the specific needs of the individual.
- **Steps 9–11:** The second bandage is wrapped like the first, except that it is started at the opposite tibial condyle from the first wrap. Bringing the weave of each bandage in contraposition exerts a more even pressure. Effort is made to bring the angular turns across each other rather than in the same direction.
- After completing the wrap, check for and correct any gaps or wrinkles. Check to make sure that the knee has not been pulled into flexion by the wrap.

*Step numbers refer to Figure 22.7.
RL = residual limb.

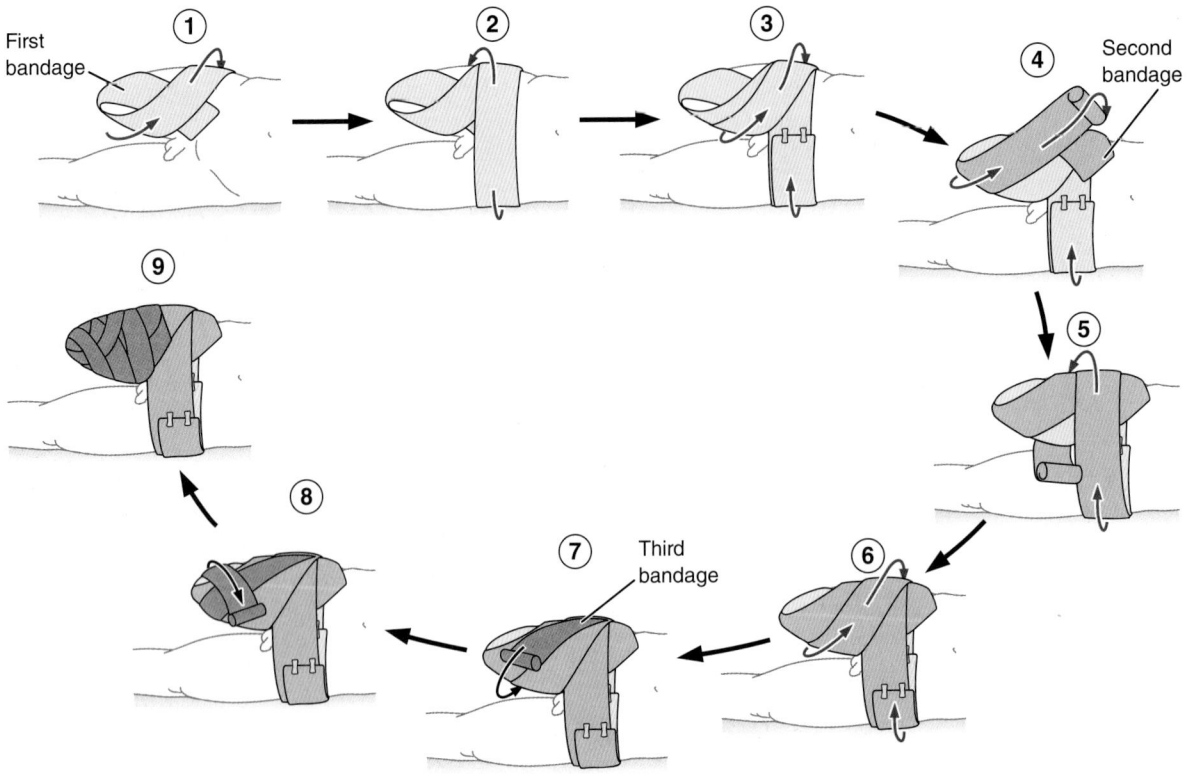

Figure 22.8 Transfemoral RL bandaging. *(From May and Lockard, 46, p. 76 with permission.)*

Box 22.8   Transfemoral Residual Limb Bandaging Technique*

- Positioning in side-lying or standing is preferred. Wrapping in sitting or supine can result in pulling the RL into flexion or abduction.
- A combination of 6- and 4-inch elastic bandages are used depending on RL size. Double-length wraps can be purchased. Two or three wraps may be used.
1. **Step 1:** Start the first bandage in the groin; wrap diagonally over the anterior surface to the distal lateral corner, covering at least half of the distal end of the RL. Continue diagonally up the posterior RL and cross and anchor the beginning of the wrap high in the groin. Continue around the iliac crest to form a hip spica. Move the hip into extension to prevent a flexion and abduction pull by the wrap.
2. **Steps 2 and 3:** Continue figure-eight wraps with diagonal turns. The wrap must be high in the groin (to the pubic ramus) to prevent an adductor roll (proximal soft tissue that is not contained within the wrap). An adductor roll makes prosthetic socket fitting difficult and socket wear painful.
3. **Steps 4–6:** The second bandage is wrapped like the first but is started more laterally; it is anchored in a hip spica after the first figure eight. Prevention of an adductor roll is important but be careful not to create a proximal tourniquet effect.
4. **Steps 7–9:** If a third 4-inch bandage is used, it should exert greater pressure over middle and distal areas of the RL without a spica. Start laterally to bring the wrap across the previous wraps.
- After completing the wrap, check for and correct any gaps or wrinkles. Check to make sure that the hip has not been pulled into flexion or abduction by the wrap.

*Step numbers refer to Figure 22.8.
RL = residual limb.

Appropriate scar massage techniques can be used to prevent or mobilize adherent scar tissue. The massage is done gently, after the wound is healed and when no infection is present. Properly performed gentle friction massage to mobilize the scar and RL tissues may help decrease hypersensitivity to touch and pressure. Early handling of the RL by the patient is an aid to acceptance and is encouraged, particularly for individuals who may be repulsed by the limb. For individuals with hypersensitivity, desensitization techniques can be used, including gently brushing the RL with a soft material, progressing to rougher materials or tapping.[106]

The patient is taught to inspect the limb with a mirror each night to ensure there are no sores or impending problems, especially in areas not readily visible. If the person has diminished sensation, careful inspection is particularly important. Because the RL tends to become edematous after bathing, nightly bathing is recommended, particularly once a prosthesis has been fitted. The elastic bandage, shrinker, or removable rigid dressing is reapplied after bathing. If the person has been fitted with a prosthesis, a shrinker or elastic bandages should be used at night and any time the prosthesis is not worn until it is fully mature (i.e., does not develop edema when not wearing a prosthesis).

The skin of the RL may be affected by a variety of dermatological problems such as eczema, psoriasis, contact dermatitis, or other rashes. Specific care is prescribed and coordinated among the physician, therapist, and prosthetist.

Range of Motion Exercise

An important deterrent to successful and comfortable use of a prosthesis is contractures of the hip or knee. In fact, contractures have been shown to predict poor prosthetic functional mobility.[107] The most common and functionally limiting contractures in the transfemoral RL are flexion and abduction; in the transtibial RL, hip and knee flexion contractures are most common and limiting. These contractures make prosthetic fitting difficult and walking with a prosthesis painful, slow, or inefficient. Joint contractures in the intact limb also affect gait and must be identified and reduced. The best treatment for contractures is prevention. Patients should understand the importance of proper positioning and regular exercise in preparing for eventual prosthetic fit and ambulation. For all levels of lower limb amputation, full hip ROM, especially hip extension, is critical in allowing the individual to assume a balanced upright posture and is found to significantly influence basic prosthetic moblity.[108]

With the transtibial amputation, full ROM in both hips and the knee, particularly in extension, is needed. While sitting, the patient can keep the knee extended by using a posterior splint or an extension board attached to the wheelchair; some facilities recommend using a knee immobilizer during sitting or lying. The patient with a transfemoral amputation needs full ROM in the hip, particularly in extension and adduction. Prolonged sitting should be avoided by all. At least 30 minutes each day should be spent in the prone position.

Some individuals, however, will develop hip or knee flexion contractures. Mild contractures may respond to various stretching techniques, including active and passive exercises and neurophysiological techniques, such as contract-relax[109] and hold-relax methods.[110] Although low-load prolonged stretching exercises are effective for

improving ROM, they are often difficult to administer in the presence of amputation because the RL lever arm length may be too short to effectively position and load the shortened tissues. It is very difficult to reduce moderate to severe contractures by manual stretching, especially hip flexion contractures. A systematic review found that the effect of passive stretching on contracture prevention or treatment is unclear.[111] An alternative method to reduce a transtibial knee flexion contracture for an individual who is ready for prosthetic fitting is to provide a prosthesis that is aligned to place the hamstrings on stretch with each step.[112] If this "stretch during walking" technique is used, therapists must carefully instruct and monitor the patient while walking to ensure that stretching occurs without excessive abnormal socket pressure on the RL. This technique requires careful monitoring and frequent alignment adjustments to produce a good outcome. Hip flexion contractures are frequently found in persons with transfemoral amputations. It is difficult to "walk out" a hip flexion contracture with the transfemoral prosthesis because prosthetic knee instability and falls may result. Alternatively, pelvic and spinal compensation may occur that lead to lower back pain. In some instances, depending on the severity of the contracture and the length of the RL, the contracture can be accommodated in the alignment of the prosthesis. A knee flexion contracture of less than 15° is not usually a problem. A recent systematic review found that fitting a prosthesis in a person with a flexion contracture ≥25° is possible.[113] Prevention, however, continues to be the best treatment for contractures.

Exercises to Improve Muscle Function

Current literature indicates that exercise programs have positive effect on muscular fitness and functional mobility for persons with amputation.[114-116] In addition, there is evidence that mobility level is a factor that predicts prosthetic success.[87] Thus, exercise programs to improve muscle function are included in preprosthetic rehabilitation.[114] Exercises to improve muscle strength and endurance are prescribed for the RL as well as the intact lower limb and UEs. The type of postsurgical dressing, volume containment, degree of postoperative pain, and healing of the incision will determine when resistive exercises for the involved extremity can be started. The exercise program can take many forms and must include exercises that the patient performs independently when not in therapy. The hip extensors and abductors, core trunk stabilizer muscles, and knee extensors are particularly important for effective prosthetic ambulation.[117,118] Figures 22.9 and 22.10 depict examples of exercises to strengthen key muscles around the hip and knee. Exercises in which the patient pushes the RL against a towel roll or bolster to lift the trunk using hip extensors (Fig 22.9F) and resistive hip abduction exercises (Fig 22.10E) performed in supine and side-lying are important because they simulate activity

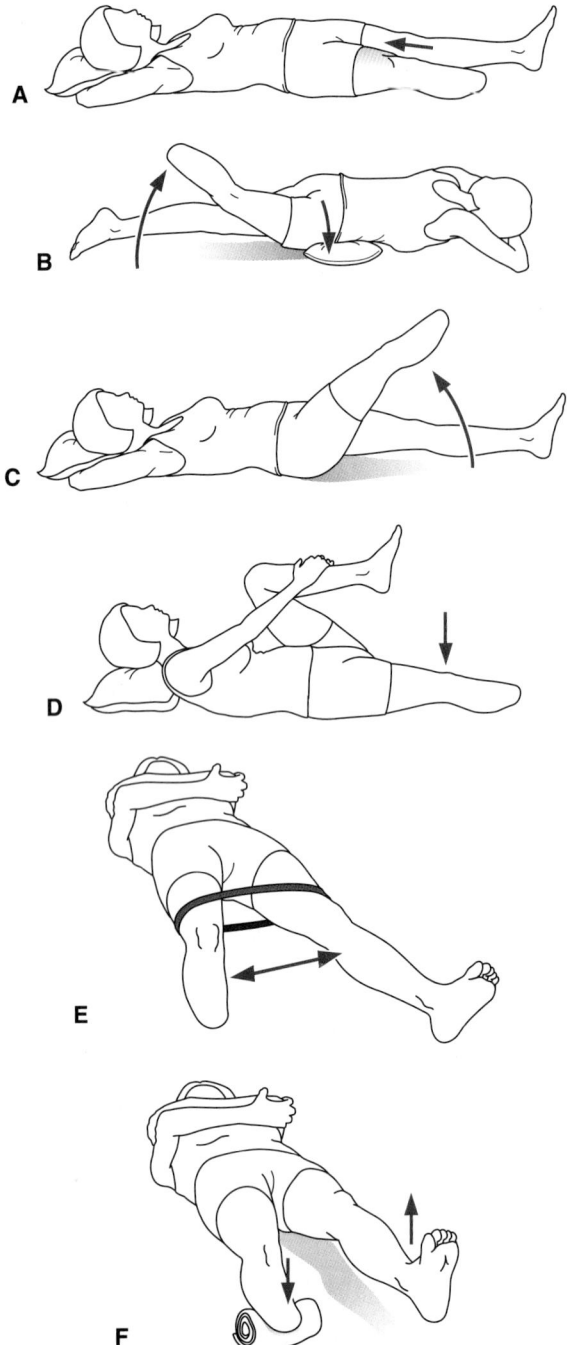

Figure 22.9 Transtibial exercises: (A) quadriceps sets. (B) Hip extension with knee straight. (C) Straight leg raises. (D) Hip and knee extension of the RL with opposite knee against chest. (E) Hip abduction against resistance (also performed in side-lying). (F) Hip extension against a towel roll "bridging." *(From May and Lockard, 46, p. 77 with permission.)*

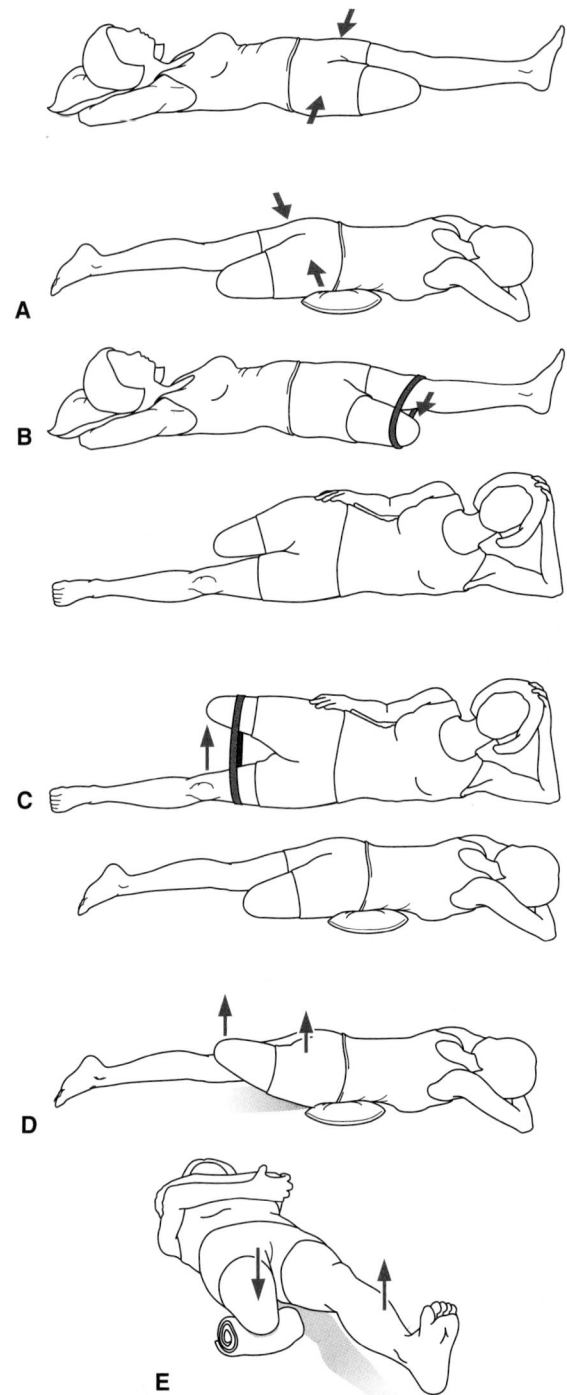

Figure 22.10 Transfemoral exercises: (A) Gluteal sets. (B) Hip abduction supine against resistance. (C) Hip abduction side-lying active and resistive. (D) Hip extension prone. (E) Hip extension against a towel roll "bridging." *(From May and Lockard, 46, p. 78 with permission.)*

of important muscles used during gait. These exercises also expose the RL to contact pressures, simulating the pressure imposed by the prosthetic socket while walking. Exercises to strengthen trunk and spine stabilizer muscles are also important for all persons with amputation.[85] Exercises must be progressed with increased resistance or modifications to increase the challenge when appropriate and to remain relevant.

Balance and Mobility Activities

Early mobility and independence in functional activities are important to physiological and psychological recovery following amputation. Balance is a key element to safe and effective mobility. Poor balance and fear of falling have been found to negatively affect walking ability and community participation in people with lower limb loss.[119,120] Although individuals with unilateral amputation usually do not have a problem with unperturbed sitting balance, it is important for the individual to develop good standing balance on the remaining limb. Poor balance and increased fall risk are reported in all stages of recovery after amputation.[121] Even after prosthetic fitting, many prosthesis users continue to report that they modify their participation because of the potential for falls.[122] Patients with amputation have lost some of the proprioceptive input and response strategies used for balance. In addition, recent systematic review found that excess confidence in balance and walking ability and less cautious stair climbing impose an elevated risk of falling. Efforts should be made to access and educate patients about their balance confidence and performance.[121] Activities to help patients develop balance skills and confidence must begin early in rehabilitation. Single leg balance exercises can be designed by progressively introducing balance challenges with compliant surfaces, upper limb movements, and distracting activities, such as throwing/catching a ball. Figure 22.11 illustrates one type of standing balance exercise on a compliant surface. Weight-bearing through the RL is also beneficial to future prosthetic training. This can only be safely achieved in patients with transtibial amputations. Figure 22.12 depicts a person kneeling on a chair of appropriate height, shifting weight on and off the amputated side. Weight-bearing and shifting activities can also be performed kneeling on a mat table with progression to "stepping" forward and backward with alternate knees.

Walking is excellent exercise and necessary for independence in daily life. Gait training can start early, and the person with a unilateral LE amputation can become quite independent using a three-point gait pattern on crutches. Many older individuals have difficulty learning to walk on crutches. Some are afraid, some lack the necessary balance and coordination, and others lack endurance. It is of importance to note that walking with crutches without a prosthesis requires a greater expenditure of energy than walking with a prosthesis in adults with transtibial amputation.[123]

Independence in crutch walking is an outcome worthy of therapy time. The individual who can ambulate with crutches will develop a greater degree of general fitness than the person who spends most of the time in a wheelchair. Crutch walking is good preparation for prosthetic ambulation, and the person who can learn to use crutches generally will not have difficulty learning to use a prosthesis. However, the individual who cannot learn to walk with crutches independently may be independent using a walker.

A walker is more stable than crutches but cannot be used safely on stairs and curbs. It is sometimes difficult

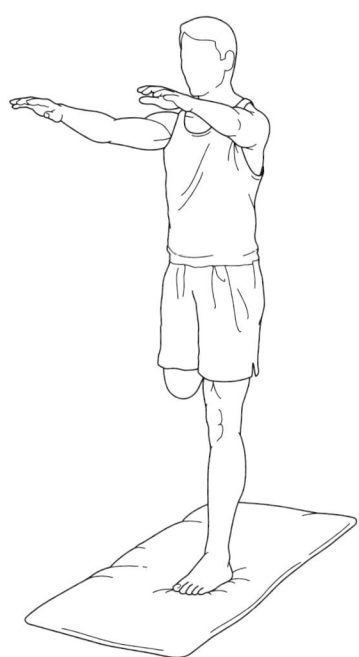

Figure 22.11 Standing balance exercise on a compliant surface. *(From May and Lockard, 46, p. 73 with permission.)*

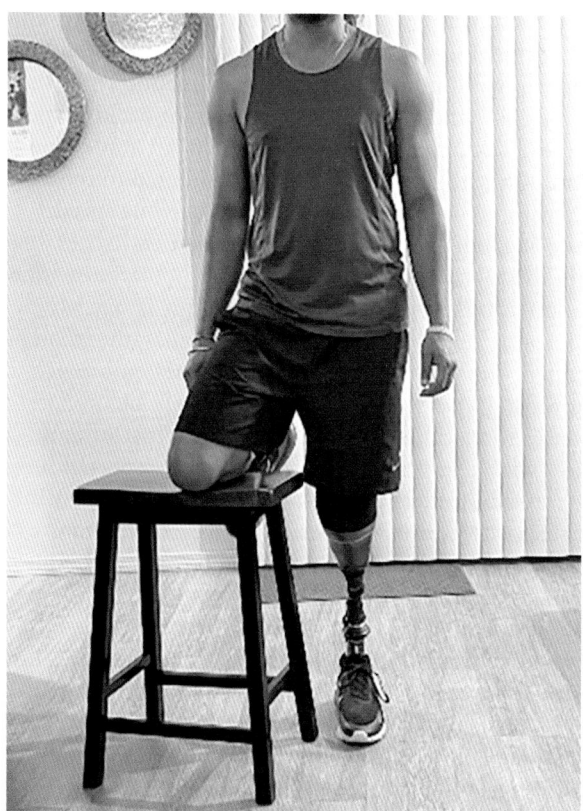

Figure 22.12 Kneeling on a chair provides an opportunity for some weight-bearing. *(Photo courtesy of Vamshi Krishna.)*

for the person who has used a walker following the amputation to switch to crutches or a cane when fitted with a prosthesis. The gait pattern used with a walker is not appropriate with a prosthesis and should not be used for prosthetic training. A walker encourages a flexed posture and a step-to gait pattern, whereas efficient prosthetic use requires an erect, extended posture and a step-through gait pattern. However, all individuals with an amputation need to learn some form of safe mobility without a prosthesis for use at night or when the prosthesis cannot be worn. For some individuals, this may need to be a walker.

Exercise for Cardiopulmonary Endurance

Ambulation and functional activity require energy expenditure. At rest in healthy individuals, the rate of metabolic energy expenditure (oxygen consumption or VO_2) is 3.5 mL/kg per minute. As the rate of ambulation or functional activity increases, oxygen consumption and heart rate response increase linearly, using aerobic metabolism. When the intensity of the activity requires an individual to consume oxygen ≥50% of his or her maximum capacity (VO_2max), the anaerobic threshold (AT) is reached, and a portion of the metabolism becomes anaerobic. Continued higher intensity activity will be limited by the accumulation of metabolites and muscle fatigue. The relationship between energy expenditure and ambulation speed with an amputation is also linear, but the slope is greater than in normal individuals. Thus, at any walking speed, individuals with an amputation use metabolic energy at a higher rate and will reach AT at a slower walking speed. In addition, they exhibit a greater heart rate response and increased cardiac work load compared to individuals without amputation walking at the same speed.[124,125] Another important variable to consider when evaluating the metabolic consequences of ambulation with an amputation is energy cost. Energy cost is oxygen consumption relative to the distance walked, rather than per unit of time. Thus, this variable defines endurance, or how long a person can continue to walk before fatigue causes him or her to stop. The energy cost of ambulation with a prosthesis has been variably reported but is increased at all levels of lower limb amputation.[124] A systematic review and meta-analysis revealed that oxygen consumption and heart rate increased with a more proximal amputation.

As mentioned, ambulation without a prosthesis using crutches is more energy expensive than walking with a prosthesis.[123] Additionally, walking with a prosthesis and crutches shows increased energy expenditure compared to walking with a prosthesis alone.[126] Many additional factors may affect the energy cost of walking, including prosthetic componentry, gait pattern and symmetry, the level of walking skill or efficiency, and balance confidence. Although the reason for amputation is not a predictor for oxygen consumption,[127] some studies report older persons with high-level vascular amputations have a higher energy cost of walking and walk at slower, less efficient speeds, resulting in poorer walking endurance.[128,129] Prosthesis users may be able to walk at the same speed as peers without amputation, but they are working at a higher percentage of their maximum aerobic capacity; thus, they use more energy and may not be able to sustain the speed (Box 22.9).[129] Therefore, peak aerobic capacity is an important determinant for walking ability, and appropriately prescribed aerobic exercise training must be included in rehabilitation programs at all levels.[129]

Various types of exercise can be used to increase aerobic capacity, walking distance, and speed, but it is important to define the aerobic-training stimulus with a specific target heart rate and duration and frequency of the exercise. Some examples include LE ergometry using the intact leg alone, and UE ergometry and treadmill training, with or without body weight support.[114] It important to note that military personnel with traumatic amputations who were provided with a comprehensive, intensive rehabilitation program achieved metabolic energy expenditure with their prostheses that was equivalent to their able-bodied peers.[130]

Management of Phantom Limb Pain

Postoperative RL pain usually improves as healing progresses, edema is reduced, and mobility restored. PLP, however, can become persistent and debilitating. A systematic review found that the prevalence of PLP is high among individuals with amputations, with the highest prevalence reported in upper limb amputees.[89,131] In a cross-sectional study of 71 adults with lower limb loss, 90.1% reported PLP and the average intensity reported was 5.9 (1 = extremely mild pain; 10 = extremely intense pain).[132] In the same study, 38% of the those with PLP experience the pain at least once daily. Thus, PLP must be identified and addressed early. There is some evidence that preemptive epidural anesthesia and immediate postoperative regional analgesia may prevent the development of PLP, but firm evidence is lacking equivocal.[133]

There are many and varied treatments for PLP because its specific cause is still undetermined. Treatments are classified as pharmacological and nonpharmacological. Usual analgesics, such as acetaminophen and

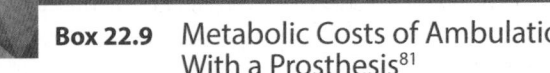

Box 22.9   Metabolic Costs of Ambulation With a Prosthesis[81]

- Partial foot: increased approximately 15%
- Traumatic transtibial: increased approximately 25%
- Vascular transtibial: increased approximately 40%
- Traumatic transfemoral: increased approximately 68%
- Vascular transfemoral: increased approximately 100%

NSAIDs, may mildly reduce pain intensity.[134] Opioids, such as morphine, and ketamine, offer some short-term pain relief but have some adverse effects, which interfere with usual functional activity.[135,136] Gabapentin may also be effective in decreasing pain intensity with limited adverse effects.[136] The effects of medications, such as tricyclic antidepressants and anticonvulsants, used to treat chronic neuropathic pain, are variable, and it is unclear when to use them to treat PLP.[134,135] Botulinum toxin A and calcitonin did not appear to be effective.[135] Owing to the lack of evidence for the effectiveness of pharmacological treatments for PLP and the relatively high occurrence of adverse effects, there is a greater focus on nonpharmacological interventions.

Nonpharmacological treatments for PLP include invasive and noninvasive interventions.[134,136] Invasive neuromodulation interventions include deep brain stimulation, spinal cord or dorsal root ganglion stimulation, and prophylactic regenerative peripheral nerve interfaces.[134,137,138] In some small studies, dorsal root ganglion stimulation has shown some success, without significant negative side effects.[137] Regenerative peripheral nerve interfaces are surgical constructs made of a transected peripheral nerve implanted into an autogenous free muscle graft. Prophylactic regenerative peripheral nerve interfaces in major limb amputees reduce the incidences of phantom limb pain compared with control patients undergoing amputation without regenerative peripheral nerve interfaces.[138] Noninvasive techniques that have shown some efficacy in small trials include transcranial direct current stimulation of the motor cortex, transcutaneous electric nerve stimulation, acupuncture, and hypnosis.[136,139–142]

A current theory for the cause of PLP is neuroplastic changes in the brain due to deafferentation caused by amputation.[143] Based on this theory, treatments have been developed that target neuroplastic mechanisms to restore neural representation of the missing limb through motor imagery.[144] Therapies in this domain include the use of visual feedback via mirrors or virtual reality, whereby the patient observes movements executed by their intact limb, viewed in a mirror or a virtual environment, and then couple the observed movement with movement of the phantom limb.[145,146] A recent systematic review concluded mirror therapy is a simple, inexpensive method that seems to be effective in reducing the intensity and duration of PLP. However, authors of the systematic review noted that most publications in this field have low to moderate methodological quality, and more high-quality studies are needed.[146] In augmented virtual reality, myoelectric signals from activation of the muscles of the RL are used to create a virtual body part that executes motor tasks in a virtual environment. Using a conventional webcam and monitor, patients observe themselves with a virtual limb (replacing their phantom) that they can actively move to accomplish virtual tasks by activating their RL muscles.

Because the virtual limb images are created from myoelectric signals from the RL, unlike mirror therapy, this treatment can be used by persons with bilateral amputations. Early results have been quite favorable.[147,148] However, all of the studies were small-scale case reports. Further research with higher quality studies are need to fully explore the benefits of augmented virtual reality for PLP management.[145]

Psychological Support

The patient needs to receive reassurance and understanding from the entire rehabilitation team. Team members should create an open and receptive environment and be willing to listen to the patient's questions and concerns. The patient should know what to expect during the entire process. The physician and therapists should carefully explain the steps and expectations of rehabilitation, using methods that are compatible with the patient's preferred learning style. The Amputee Coalition of America (ACA) is a national, nonprofit consumer education and advocacy organization representing people who have experienced amputation or were born with limb differences (www.amputee-coalition.org). The ACA provides training for peer visitors, individuals with amputations who are trained to provide emotional support and motivation by visiting individuals with recent amputations. Therapists should be cognizant of local ACA chapters and make use of the organization to support and educate their patients. A peer visitation program can also be developed from previous successful patients.

Patients have various attitudes and goals regarding a prosthesis. Some are most concerned with regaining the greatest level of function possible; others are more concerned about its appearance and cosmesis. Therapists must be sensitive to the specific concerns of each patient and advocate for their individual goals in prosthetic prescription and training. Good predictors for adjustment to the prosthesis are active involvement in the rehabilitation program and consistent attempts to return to an active lifestyle and social interaction. Therapists must foster and develop active participation by the patient.

Preparatory and Definitive Prostheses

Many individuals are not fitted with a prosthetic appliance until the RL is healed and free from edema. During this 6- to 12-week period, the patient is limited to mobility using a wheelchair or ambulation with crutches or a walker. The first prosthesis may be a temporary or preparatory prosthesis, made with simple components. A definitive prosthesis is one that is permanent. Since definitive prosthetic componentry is modular (parts can be changed out or replaced without affecting the rest of the prosthesis), if the RL continues to shrink and the socket is too large, a new socket can be manufactured to replace the original one without replacing the rest of the prosthesis. Once fitted with a first prosthesis, the RL may continue to change in size, and a second socket is often required within the first 2 years. Many third-party payers (insurers) will not fund a temporary prosthesis, so early permanent fitting is advocated, even though the socket may become too big quite quickly and require replacement.

Early bipedal ambulation is a desired goal for most individuals following amputation. The longer the delay in fitting with a prosthesis, the lower the potential for effective rehabilitation. Care should be taken that the patient is fitted with optimum components for his or her expected level of function. Too often, older individuals are fitted with low-cost, low-function components when they probably could achieve a higher level of function with more functional components.[149] Therapists must clearly and objectively document functional performance and potential and justify the prescription of an appropriate prosthesis that will maximize function and ambulation.

Patient Education

Patient education is an integral and ongoing part of the rehabilitation program.[70,150] Information on the care of the RL—proper care of the uninvolved extremity, positioning, exercises, and diet (if the patient has diabetes or is overweight)—is necessary for the patient to be a full participant in the rehabilitation program. Discussions should also be held regarding patient goals, projected activity levels, funding, and prosthetic components. If the patient underwent the amputation for vascular problems, the education program should include information on proper footwear.

Care must be taken not to overwhelm the patient with too much information at one time; information overload leads to forgetfulness. It is more effective to prioritize the information and ask the person to remember one new thing each session rather than try to teach a complex program at one time. Visual materials using media compatible with the client's preferred learning style are necessary to supplement the teaching and help the patient remember what is required. It is also important for the program to be tailored to the individual's way of life. Involving the patient in establishing priorities enhances adherence. Appendix 22.A (online) includes Web-based resources for clinicians, families, and patients with amputation.

Bilateral Amputation

Intervention for the person with bilateral LE amputations is similar to the program developed for someone with a unilateral amputation. If the individual was previously fitted with a prosthesis and ambulated after unilateral amputation, the prosthesis is useful for transfer activities and limited ambulation. Some individuals may be able to use the prosthesis with external support to get around more easily, particularly for bathroom activities.

Most individuals with bilateral amputations need a wheelchair on a permanent basis, even if they use prostheses for ambulation, because there will always be times when the prostheses cannot be worn. The chair should be as narrow as possible (for the size of the patient with prostheses, if worn) and lightweight to facilitate community mobility. Removable desk arms and removable leg rests are necessary. Elevating armrests are useful to assist in sit-to-stand transfers. Amputee wheelchairs with offset rear wheels and no leg rests are not recommended unless the therapist is sure that the person will never be fitted with prostheses. It is easier to add antitipping devices to the rear of the wheelchair or attach small weights to the front uprights (counterbalance) for use when the footrests are removed, and no prostheses are worn.

The exercise program includes mat activities designed to help the person regain a sense of body position and balance; balance is usually more challenging for individuals with bilateral lower limb amputations. Upper extremity and RL strengthening and ROM exercises are also important. Functional mobility training should stress independence in bed mobility, transfers, and wheelchair use. With bilateral amputations, individuals spend considerable time sitting and are therefore more prone to develop flexion contractures, particularly around the hip joints. The patient should be encouraged to sleep prone if possible, or at least spend time in the prone position each day. With the variety of prosthetic componentry options available today, many persons with bilateral lower limb amputations can walk functionally with prostheses.[151] Thus, rehabilitation for persons with bilateral amputations should be similar to, and as intensive as, rehabilitation for individuals with unilateral amputations. Energy expenditure during functional activities with or without prostheses is quite high. Thus, all programs for persons with bilateral amputations must include cardiopulmonary exercise training to maximize functional potential.

■ PREDICTING PROSTHETIC POTENTIAL

The ability to accurately predict prosthetic functional mobility from pre- and postamputation patient characteristics has been pursued for many years. Recognition of characteristics that predict prosthetic use and positive functional outcomes at different levels of amputation would help the patient with poor vascular status and critical limb ischemia and the patient's surgeon to decide on the best surgical approach to disease management.[33] Evidence that certain patient characteristics are strongly associated with successful prosthetic mobility would also help therapists and physicians advocate for patients with third-party payors to provide for prostheses and prosthetic rehabilitation.

To this end, researchers developed and validated the AMPREDICT, an instrument that can be used by clinicians to predict mobility outcome after LE amputation at different levels secondary to vascular compromise.[33] This instrument utilizes the presence or absence of patient characteristics that were identified as important to predict the probability of achieving independent basic or advanced functional mobility with a prosthesis.[33] A recent systematic literature review identified characteristics of all types of patients (not just those with dysvascular amputation) that predict prosthetic walking ability following lower limb amputation.[152] The most strongly supported factors for considering prosthetic candidacy were amputation level (lower), age (younger), physical fitness (cardiorespiratory endurance/aerobic capacity), and no or few comorbidities. Moderately supported factors for prosthetic candidacy included cognition/mood disturbance, etiology, ability to stand on one leg, and preamputation living status. Another research group identified clinical assessments administered to patients after amputation, but before the decision to fit with a prosthesis, that yield predictors of prosthetic use.[107] The report indicated that age (younger), level of amputation (lower), absence of contractures, ability to stand on one leg for 10 seconds or more (a proxy for balance and strength), and cognitive function (as measured by the Trail Making Test) were predictive of successful functional mobility with a prosthesis.[107] Another study identified balance on the remaining leg and RL hip extensor strength as predictive of successful prosthetic use.[30] A recent 15-year retrospective cohort study also indicated that female gender could be an important predictor for successful functional mobility with a prosthesis.[35] However, this result needs to be carefully verified as the study was unbalanced in male (82.8% of the sample) and female participants. AMPREDICT has been incorporated into a clinical support tool (DST), and a recent mixed methods found strong usability characteristics and clinical relevance in AMPREDICT DST.[34]

Although recognition of the factors associated with successful prosthetic use is helpful, it still leaves unanswered questions regarding the decision to fit a particular patient with a prosthesis. For example, there is evidence that being older and having a higher level of amputation makes it less likely that a patient will become an independent prosthetic user, but in fact, some older individuals with transfemoral amputations do become independent in ambulation with a prosthesis. Thus, an instrument that predicts the likelihood that a particular individual with an amputation will be able to ambulate successfully with a prosthesis based on his or her current performance is most desirable.

Medicare developed a functional classification system for persons with amputation. It is used to classify individuals according to their potential to achieve independent functional mobility with a prosthesis at home and in the community, as well as to achieve advanced sports or work-related activities. The classification

levels are described in Box 22.10. These levels are used to determine the medical necessity of a prosthesis and to determine the types of prosthetic components (e.g., types of prosthetic knees and feet) available to patients in each category. Although the classification system is promulgated by Medicare, it is used by many insurers to determine coverage for a prosthesis for an individual. Thus, it is important for therapists to be able to objectively measure individual patient functional capabilities. However, substantiating and justifying a prosthetic prescription require an instrument that measures current physical performance without a prosthesis to predict ability to ambulate with a prosthesis. The Amputee Mobility Predictor (AMP) is a reliable instrument that has been validated to make this prediction.[153] For patients with unilateral amputation, versions are available for those with a prosthesis (AMPPRO) as well as for those without a prosthesis (AMPnoPRO). It is a 20-item assessment of a patient's ability to perform functional tasks required for successful prosthetic ambulation. It can be administered and scored in about 15 minutes.[153] To make the instrument usable for individuals with bilateral amputations (AMP-B), five items were modified and the scoring system adjusted.[154] All instruments have been shown to predict performance on the 6-minute Walk Test.[153,154]

Box 22.10   Medicare Functional Classification Levels

- **Functional level 0 (K0):** The patient does not have the ability or potential to ambulate or transfer safely with or without assistance, and a prosthesis does not enhance his or her quality of life or mobility.
- **Functional level 1 (K1):** The patient has the ability or potential to use a prosthesis for transfers or ambulation on level surfaces at fixed cadence. Typical of the limited and unlimited household ambulator.
- **Functional level 2 (K2):** The patient has the ability or potential for ambulation with the ability to traverse low-level environmental barriers such as curbs, stairs, or uneven surfaces. Typical of the limited community ambulator.
- **Functional level 3 (K3):** The patient has the ability or potential for ambulation with variable cadence. Typical of the community ambulator who has the ability to traverse most environmental barriers and may have vocational, therapeutic, or exercise activity that demands prosthetic utilization beyond simple locomotion.
- **Functional level 4 (K4):** The patient has the ability or potential for prosthetic ambulation that exceeds basic ambulation skills, exhibiting high-impact, stress, or energy levels. Typical of the prosthetic demands of the child, active adult, or athlete.

■ PROSTHETIC TRAINING

The major goal of prosthetic rehabilitation is to attain a smooth, energy-efficient gait that allows the individual to perform ADL and participate in desired social, employment, and recreational activities. Prosthetic ambulation is a skilled psychomotor activity, and the person must learn to adapt well-developed patterns of movement to new situations. Box 22.11 outlines general motor skills required to achieve an effective prosthetic gait. In general, gait training must guide the individual to integrate the prosthesis into all mobility activities. Table 22.3 presents basic prosthetic training elements, starting with basic balance and progressing to ambulation.[155] Although the table depicts training with a transfemoral prosthesis, the sequence is equally appropriate for transtibial prosthetic training other than the knee control step.

Some gait or prosthetic control skills are specific for certain prosthetic components. For example, certain types of microprocessor-controlled knees and power knees require specific techniques to operative their control features.[156,157] Walking with a microprocessor knee is different from walking with a prosthesis with a conventionally controlled knee. The therapist must be knowledgeable of the requirements of each type of componentry and teach the appropriate gait skills. To use energy storing and releasing (ESAR) prosthetic feet effectively, users must shift weight onto the foot at initial contact and advance the pelvis over the foot through late stance phase to ensure deflection of the toe and optimal use of foot features. Box 22.12 provides examples of specific exercises that can be used in prosthetic gait training with an ESAR prosthetic foot.[158]

It is important to accomplish as much training as possible without the use of external support, as walking is more efficient without it. If found necessary, a cane may be added for safety once there is good control of weight shifting on and off the prosthesis and a step-through progression has been achieved. Therapists should not plan to begin prosthetic training with a walker and progress to a cane or less restrictive device because this will most likely not be successful. In addition, it is very difficult to use an appropriate prosthetic gait pattern with a walker. Leaning on a walker makes it almost impossible to advance the pelvis in the transverse plane to achieve proper weight-bearing through the prosthesis. A walker should be reserved for situations where the individual is so limited that it is the only safe option.

Gait Training

Gait training is a key component of successful rehabilitation of lower limb amputation. Abnormal gait patterns, particularly gait asymmetries and over-dependence on the intact lower limb, can lead to musculoskeletal overuse injuries and arthritis. Knee pain in the intact lower limb and back pain are common problems reported by prosthesis users.[159,160] People with limb loss commonly complain of back pain, which may be associated with a variety of possible causes, including poor posture, abnormal movements during gait, leg length discrepancy, poor prosthetic fit or alignment, or general deconditioning.[159] Knee pain and osteoarthritis in the intact leg are common and may be caused by increased stress and loading of the intact lower limb during walking and functional activities.[159] Physical therapy should include gait training to improve spaciotemporal and kinematic symmetry and the bioenergetics or efficiency of gait. A variety of traditional gait training techniques are used, but few large or randomized controlled trials are published. A recent systematic literature review identified studies that reported on prosthetic gait training.[161] They classified studies as overground or treadmill training and reported with high confidence that gait training under skilled supervision is effective in improving spaciotemporal gait parameters in patients with LE amputations.[161] Table 22.4, the Evidence Summary Table, presents studies that investigated a variety of traditional approaches to improve gait and gait symmetry in persons with amputation.

In addition to traditional gait-training techniques, novel neural rehabilitation and bioengineering approaches have been developed and preliminarily tested to improve the training outcome. A recent study shows that it is feasible to use game-based exercises (e.g., Wii Fit) in the clinic or at home as a gait-training strategy.[162,163] The incorporation of virtual reality shows promising results in enhancing the outcome of balance and gait training.[164-166] Adding task-oriented mental practice (motor imagery) in a training program

---

Box 22.11 Skills Required for Efficient Prosthetic Gait

- Accept and support body weight on each leg at the instant of initial contact.
- Balance on one foot in single-limb support without excessive sway.
- Symmetrical stance time on prosthetic and intact lower limb.
- Maintain erect trunk and spine stability in stance and swing; minimize pelvic tilt and excessive frontal plane trunk compensatory movements.
- Execute anterior transverse pelvic rotation (on the prosthetic side) during stance to advance pressure on the prosthetic foot all the way to the toe.
- Advance each limb with symmetrical step lengths.
- Adapt to environmental demands, such as uneven terrain, obstacle avoidance, inclines, and steps without stumble.

Table 22.3	Prosthetic Training Elements	
Element	Activity	Details
Stability—both legs (TT/TF)	Secure standing without hand support; reaching for objects.	Hold an object a reachable distance; patient reaches and touches objects with either hand looking at object. Objects placed high/low/right/left encouraging goal-oriented weight shifting.
Knee control (TF)	Secure standing without hand support; slightly bend and straighten prosthetic knee to varying degrees.	Encourage patient to develop kinesthetic feel of knee position by socket pressures.
Stability on prosthesis (TT/TF)	Secure standing without hand support; place 6–8-in. stool directly in front of patient.	In a controlled manner, patient places unamputated foot on stool and back on the floor.

(Continued)

Table 22.3   Prosthetic Training Elements—cont'd

Element	Activity	Details
Stability on prosthesis (TT/TF)	Secure standing without hand support; place soccer ball in front of unamputated leg.	In a controlled manner, patient kicks the ball with the unamputated foot.
Prosthetic control (TT/TF)	Secure standing without hand support; place soccer ball in front of prosthesis.	In a controlled manner, patient kicks the ball with the prosthetic leg.
Proprioception (TT/TF)	Secure standing both legs on a piece of paper with a clock face drawn and without hand support.	On command, patient shifts weight to 12, 3, 6, and 9 o'clock in random order. Learns to recognize where prosthetic foot is in relation to weight-bearing.

Table 22.3 Prosthetic Training Elements—cont'd

Element	Activity	Details
Pelvic control (TT/TF) 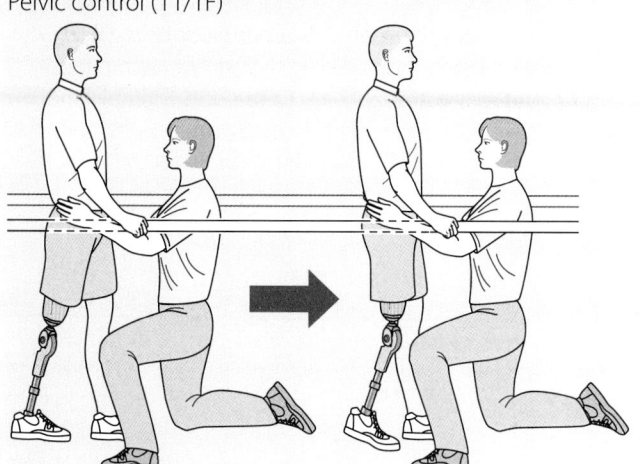	Secure standing without hand support, prosthetic leg behind unamputated leg. Provide resistance to forward pelvic progression at initial contact to foot flat.	Encourage patient to transfer weight smoothly with forward and slight lateral pelvic motion by providing resistance as patient brings prosthesis forward.
Stepping with prosthesis (TT/TF) 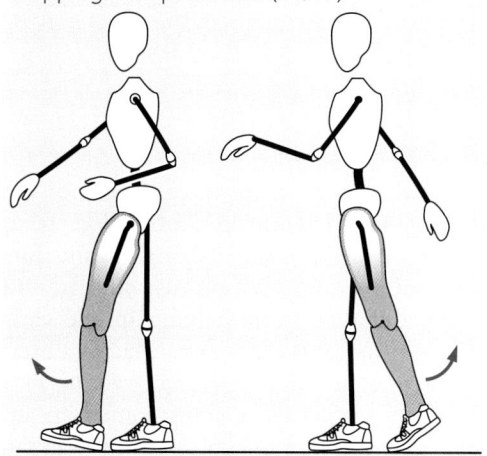	Secure standing without hand support, step forward and back with prosthesis.	Start with double leg stance, shift weight to unamputated leg and steps forward with prosthesis. Returns prosthesis to position behind sound leg. Emphasize knee control with TF.
Stepping with sound leg (TT/TF) 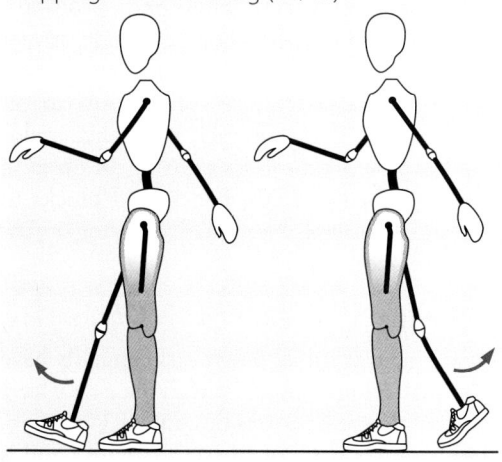	Secure standing without hand support, step forward and back with unamputated leg	As above but with unamputated leg. Make sure patient brings weight to forward part of foot before stepping on unamputated leg. Emphasize toe-off on TF to activate swing initiation.

(Continued)

Table 22.3	Prosthetic Training Elements—cont'd		
Element		**Activity**	**Details**
Sidestepping; backward stepping (TT/TF) 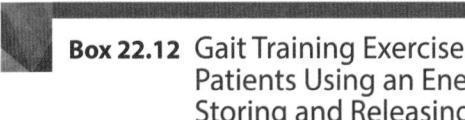		Consecutive steps to the right, then to the left without hand support. Stepping backward several steps.	Sidestepping, emphasize picking up the leg and placing it several inches to the side, then picking up the other leg to the first leg. TF backward stepping generally requires a larger prosthetic step than the unamputated for knee control.

From May and Lockard,[46, pp. 136–141] with permission.
TF = patient with transfemoral prosthesis; TT = patient with transtibial prosthesis

---

Box 22.12 Gait Training Exercises for Patients Using an Energy Storing and Releasing (ESAR) Prosthetic Foot[109]

- Stool stepping to improve single limb standing balance on the prosthetic foot
- Resistive gait training to enhance transverse pelvic rotation, pelvic advancement, and symmetry of movement during ambulation
- Resistive ambulation to promote dynamic balance and proper prosthetic toe-loading during late stance
- Ball rolls (with the intact foot) in three planes to increase the speed of hip muscle contraction to maintain prosthetic single limb balance during stance
- Trunk rotation to assist with balance and symmetry of movement
- Change of direction and turning skills; agility skills

---

also shows beneficial effects on improving gait performance.[167] Robotic technology such as exoskeletal has been developed and tested to assist in prosthetic gait training.[168] Initial evidence shows that lower limb amputees can adapt to split-belt treadmill walking and improve gait symmetry, and it may be a useful tool to be applied in clinical settings.[169] Mobile health technology, such as using a custom application (app) to deliver a home exercise program (HEP), shows promising ability to improve functional mobility in individuals with lower limb amputation.[170]

Advanced Training

Changing the environment is an integral part of the gait-training program. Functional ambulation takes place in complex environments. Walking around furniture, through narrow doorways, on rugs, and around obstacles is very different from walking in the clear open space of the physical therapy gym. Placing obstacles on the floor to step around or over, walking in a busy hallway or on a sidewalk, picking something up from the floor, and carrying an object while walking are all advanced activities that require balance, coordination, and the ability to shift one's weight on and off the prosthesis smoothly in different body positions. During advanced training, the client is taught to get up and down from chairs of different heights and seat resilience, including toilet seats, as well as how to get up and down from the floor. Obstacle avoidance is also important and can be practiced by creating an obstacle course using chairs, single steps, cones, and blocks to walk around, and should also be practiced using a variety of walking surfaces.

Steps and Ramps

Individuals wearing transtibial prostheses generally have little difficulty mastering steps and ramps once they have achieved good balance and prosthetic control. Going up, step over step, requires good quadriceps strength and is easier for individuals with medium to long RL length. Descending steps requires accommodating for lack of prosthetic ankle dorsiflexion by placing it over the edge of the step. Safely descending steps is important; those with poor balance should use a step-to pattern, placing

Table 22.4   Evidence Summary Prosthetic Gait Training

Schafer et al. (2021)[192]

Personalized 12-week exercise program for individuals with lower limb amputation

Design	Randomized controlled trial
Level of Evidence	II
Subjects	Individuals with transfemoral and transtibial amputations; seven subjects in the experimental group and seven in the control group.
Intervention	Experimental group: a personalized home-based exercise program consisting of balance, endurance, strength, and flexibility training. Control group: Normal daily activities
Results	The personalized exercise program improved postural control, reduced reliance on visual input, and enhanced somatosensory interpretation in lower limb amputees.
Comments	A personalized home-based exercise program is effective.

Miller et al. (2017)[115]

Balance, balance confidence, and gait

Design	Repeated Measures
Level of Evidence	III
Subjects	16 individuals with transfemoral or transtibial amputations.
Intervention	A 6-week supervised exercise program focusing on stretching, core and lower extremity strength and flexibility, and static and dynamic balance and gait activities.
Results	The exercise program improved dynamic balance and self-selected walking speed.
Comments	A supervised exercise program consisting of strengthening, stretching, dynamic balance and gait activities is effective.

Highsmith et al. (2016)[161]

Gait training interventions

Design	Systematic review
Level of Evidence	I
Subjects	Individuals with transfemoral and transtibial amputations.
Intervention	Prosthetic gait training.
Results	Thirteen studies using over-ground training and five studies using treadmill training met the inclusion criteria. Eight evidence statements were synthesized: three with moderate evidence, five with low evidence.
Comments	Therapeutic gait training under supervision with appropriate prosthetic component prescription is effective.

Agrawal et al. (2013)[193]

Influence of gait training and prosthetic foot category

Design	Randomized repeated measures trial
Level of Evidence	III
Subjects	Five subjects with transtibial amputations, K-level 2; five subjects with transtibial amputations, K-level 3
Intervention	Each subject was tested with four different prosthetic feet on the same socket: SACH, SAFE, Talux, Proprio, and standardized gait training.

(Continued)

Table 22.4	Evidence Summary Prosthetic Gait Training—cont'd
Results	The Talux (J-ankle, heel-to-toe footplate) provided the best symmetry of work for K-level 2 subjects.
Comments	Gait training can influence gait symmetry; K-level 2 subjects achieved greater work symmetry with K-3 feet (Talux, J-foot).

Kaufman K, et al. (2014)[194]
Fall prevention training

Design	Prospective cohort study
Level of Evidence	III
Subjects	Eleven males with traumatic transtibial amputations, ages 18–40; all experienced prosthesis users.
Intervention	Trip-specific fall prevention training program with a microprocessor-controlled treadmill to provide bidirectional trip stimulus; six 30-min training sessions over 2 weeks.
Results	Post-tests were at completion of training, 3 months, and 6 months. All subjects decreased trunk flexion angle (indicator of decreased falls risk on perturbation) and increased stepping ability on both legs and improved in balance confidence.
Comments	Results were maintained at 3 and 6 months.

Darter BJ, et al. (2013)[195]
Home-based treadmill training

Design	Repeated measures cohort
Level of Evidence	IV
Subjects	Eight subjects with transfemoral amputations who had lost their limbs due to trauma or cancer at least 3 years ago.
Intervention	Home-based treadmill walking for 30 min/day, 3 days/week for 8 weeks. Each session involved walking at three speeds.
Results	Improvement in all outcome measures: stance phase duration and step length, energy expenditure, and energy cost; self-selected walking speed and maximum walking speed; and 2-minute Walk Test.
Comments	Home-based treadmill walking is an effective method to improve gait in patients with transfemoral amputations, even beyond the traditional rehabilitation period.

SACH = solid ankle cushion heel; SAFE = stationary attachment flexible endoskeleton

the prosthesis down first until balance has improved. Some gait adaption may be needed for steep ramps or hills, depending on the type of prosthetic foot used. The more limitation of dorsiflexion, the harder it is to go up a steep hill step over step. Going down a steep hill requires good quadriceps strength and prosthetic control but can be accomplished by most individuals.

The technique for going up and down stairs and ramps will vary for an individual wearing a transfemoral prosthesis based on the type of knee component. Generally, the person will ascend stairs one step at a time leading with the unamputated leg, unless the prosthesis has a powered knee. A power knee joint permits ascending stairs using a foot-over-foot pattern, although it is quite energy expensive. Individuals fitted with a microprocessor-controlled knee with stance phase control can descend steps using a foot-over-foot pattern. The patient should be carefully instructed to operate the features of the prosthetic knee correctly. For descending stairs with many fluid/hydraulic prostheses, it is necessary to place the prosthetic heel only on the step and to "sit back" to create a flexion moment at the knee, thereby allowing the knee to flex. Table 22.5 presents examples of advanced training activities for individuals

Table 22.5	Advanced Activities (Transfemoral)
Activity	Procedure
Sitting on the floor	Place the prosthesis about half a step behind the sound foot, keeping the weight on the sound foot. Bend from the waist and flex at the knees and hips, reaching for the floor with both arms outstretched and pivoting to the sound side. Then gradually lower the body to the floor. This activity is one continuous movement.
Getting up from the floor	Get on the hands and knees; place the sound leg forward, well under the trunk, with the foot flat on the floor while balancing on the hands and the prosthetic knee. Then extend the sound knee while maintaining the weight over the sound leg. Move to an erect position by pushing strongly with the sound leg and the arms bringing the prosthesis forward when almost erect.
Kneeling	Place the sound foot ahead of the prosthetic foot keeping the weight on the sound leg. Slowly flex the trunk, hip, and knee until the prosthetic knee can be gently placed on the floor. Clients with transfemoral limbs usually kneel on the prosthetic leg. Getting up from a kneeling position is like getting up from the floor.
Picking up an object from the floor	Place the sound foot ahead of the prosthetic foot with the body weight remaining on the sound leg. Bend forward at the waist flexing the hips and knees until the object can be reached. Care must be taken to maintain the weight on the sound leg if wearing a mechanical knee. Some individuals like to bend sideways rather than forward, whereas others find it easier to keep the prosthetic knee straight and bend the sound leg until the object can be picked up.

Adapted from May and Lockard.[155, p. 147]

with a transfemoral prosthesis. Once good balance, prosthetic control, and gait have been achieved, many individuals develop their own method of doing each of these activities.

■ FUNCTIONAL OUTCOME MEASUREMENTS

Use of standardized functional outcome measures is an important strategy to monitor change in patients over time, identify effective interventions, and enhance the quality of the care provided. Since 2013, the Centers for Medicare and Medicaid Services (CMS) requires therapy providers to document patients' initial function and their achieved outcomes during and after treatment by including G codes (and modifiers) on requests for reimbursement.[171] These codes are used to document functional activity limitations and participation restrictions, as defined by the International Classification of Functioning, Disability and Health (ICF). Thus, it is important for clinicians to include appropriate measurements of functional status in all patient examinations, including clients with amputation. Several studies have assessed or reviewed the psychometric properties of some commonly used functional outcome measurements in rehabilitation of lower limb amputation.[172–174]

Functional status measures can be grouped into two general categories: self-report or performance-based assessments. Instrument selection should be based on available data addressing reliability as well as its validity for use with the patient population. Other important psychometric information about the instrument include its responsiveness to change and how much change must occur to be real or clinically important (minimally detectable change [MDC]; minimal clinically important difference [MCID]). Additional factors considered when selecting an instrument include ease of completion, time required to administer, and space or specialized equipment requirements. It is important to note whether it can be used with individuals with or without a prosthesis or if the instrument is limited to current prosthesis users only. Table 22.6 presents examples of commonly used outcome measures that are valid, reliable, responsive to change, and relatively easy to administer. Assessment of functional status is an important component of determining effectiveness of physical therapy treatment and justifying reimbursement. Interventions used for patients with amputation, whether an exercise or a prosthetic component, should have a measurable effect on function. If interventions are not effective, they should be abandoned and an alternative approach pursued.

Table 22.6   Outcome Measures: Self-Report and Performance-Based Functional Status Measures for Persons With Amputation

Outcome Measure and ICF Category	Description	Scoring	MDC and MCID
Self-Report Functional Status Measures			
PEQ[175] **ICF: 2**	82 questions divided into 4 domains; 12-item mobility subscale (PEQ-MS) assesses prosthetic ambulation and transfers	Linear analog scale response for met	MDC (PEQ-MS): 5.5[176] MCID (PEQ-MS): 8[176]
LCI-5[177–179] **ICF: 2**	14 questions about ambulation in various circumstances and performing activities while walking	5-level ordinal scale (0–4); higher scores indicate better locomotor capabilities using prosthesis	MDC: 5.66[180] MCID: 7[180] Large Improvement: 12[180]
PLUS-M[181] **ICF: 2**	Version 1 is designed for clinical practice; includes 44 mobility items; 2 short forms (12 and 7 items)	5-point rating of difficulty in walking and performing activities; raw score is converted to T-score and percentile. Available online at https://plus-m.org/	MDC: 5.59 (7-item); 5.36 (12-item)[173]
ABC[182,183] **ICF: 2**	16-item scale; patients rate level of balance confidence while performing functional mobility activities	5-level ordinal rating scale (no, low, moderate, high, and complete confidence). Score is average of all ratings.	MDC: 0.49[173]
PROMIS-29[184] **ICF: 2, 3**	Measures eight symptoms and QOL constructs: physical function, anxiety, depression, fatigue, sleep disturbance, social role satisfaction, pain interference, pain intensity.	T-score and percentiles	MDC: Physical function subscore 7.3; others range from 2.3 (pain intensity) to 9.2 (fatigue)[173]
Performance-Based Measures			
TUG[185] **ICF: 2**	Patient rises from a chair, walks 3 meters, turns, returns to chair and sits.	Time in seconds from buttocks off chair to buttocks back on chair. Can be used with all patient populations but has been validated for use with patients with LE amputations.	MDC: (90% confidence): 0.96 seconds for lower limb amputees;[186] may have ceiling effect for more active patients.
L Test[187] **ICF: 2**	Modification of the TUG for more active patients with amputation; arise from armless chair, walk 3 meters, make right-angle turn, continue walking 7 meters and turn 180° and walk back along same path and sit down (20 meters total)	Time in seconds from buttocks off chair to buttocks back on chair.	MCID: 4.5 sec[188]
6MWT[189] **ICF: 2**	Patient walks on a smooth, level surface 100-foot path. Instructions: Walk as far as possible for 6 minutes, but don't run or jog; patient may stop and rest, but clock continues.	Total distance walked in meters in 6 minutes.	MDC (90% confidence): 45 m[174]

Table 22.6	Outcome Measures: Self-Report and Performance-Based Functional Status Measures for Persons With Amputation—cont'd			
Outcome Measure and ICF Category	**Description**	**Scoring**	**MDC and MCID**
2MWT[190] ICF: 2	The same as the 6MWT, but patient walks for only 2 minutes.	Total meters walked in 2 minutes.	MDC (90% confidence): 34.3 m[174]
Amputee Mobility Predictor[153] ICF: 2	Patient is asked to perform 21 tasks in four categories (static and dynamic sitting activities, static and dynamic standing activities, transfer skills, and gait skills).	Based on quality of performance; score is sum of ratings for all items; scoring adjustments made for those with unilateral amputations who do not have a prosthesis and for those with bilateral amputations, for whom some tasks will be difficult, even for very able individuals.	MDC: 3.4[174]
CHAMP[186,191] ICF: 2	Developed for military service-members who demonstrate proficient strength, balance, postural stability, prosthetic control and endurance; designed to test speed, power and agility.	Scores for each item are added to produce a composite score, with 40 the highest level of performance.	MDC: 3.74 for total CHAMP score[186]

ICF CATEGORY: 1 = body structure/function; 2 = activity; 3 = participation
ABC = Activities Balance Confidence Scale; CHAMP = Comprehensive High-Level Activity Mobility Predictor; LCI-5 = Locomotor Capabilities Index; LE = lower extremity; MCID = minimal clinically important difference; MDC = minimal detectable change; PEQ = Prosthetic Evaluation Questionnaire; PEQ-MS = Prosthetic Evaluation Questionnaire-mobility subscale; PLUS-M = Prosthetic Limb Users Survey of Mobility; PROMIS-29 = Patient-Reported Outcomes Measurement Information System (29-Item); QOL = quality of life; TUG = Timed Up and Go Test.

SUMMARY

Most individuals with lower limb amputations can return to a full and useful life following the loss of a limb. A program of postoperative care that includes consideration of physical and emotional needs will enable most patients to become functional prosthetic users. Many prosthetic problems can be avoided by properly preparing the individual for prosthetic wear. In this chapter, concepts related to the postoperative and pre-prosthetic management of the individual with LE amputation have been presented. Through a process of careful evaluation and open communication, a comprehensive program designed to meet the needs of an individual patient can be achieved.

Questions for Review

1. Describe the advantages and disadvantages of the following postoperative dressings: (a) compressible soft dressing, (b) semirigid dressing, (c) removable rigid dressing, and (d) immediate postoperative prosthesis.

2. What are the general goals of the postsurgical phase of amputation care?

3. What critical information would you provide a family member about patient positioning following a transtibial amputation?

4. A 72-year-old man with a history of diabetes, cardiovascular disease, and PVD has been referred for physical therapy 24 hours post–right transtibial amputation performed due to an infected foot ulcer. What examination data are needed to plan an appropriate treatment program? Which are the most critical to obtain on the first visit?

5. Describe the patient data that you would gather to justify prescribing a prosthesis for a patient.

6. Plan three gait-training activities that could be used to improve stability during weight-bearing on the prosthesis.

CASE STUDY

REFERRAL

The patient is a 68-year-old female status post–right transtibial amputation yesterday secondary to an infected nonhealing plantar pressure ulcer on the foot.

CURRENT MEDICAL HISTORY

Type 2 diabetes since age 48 controlled by insulin 20 units bid. Arteriosclerosis; hypertension controlled by medication; treated for a pressure ulcer on the plantar surface of right first metatarsal area for past 4 months. Ulcer did not heal, leading to amputation. Body mass index (BMI) is 29.

PAST MEDICAL HISTORY

Hysterectomy at age 42; otherwise unremarkable.

SOCIAL HISTORY

Widow who lives alone. Three grown children and six grandchildren in the area.

Retired school teacher; enjoys gardening, and until her foot ulcer, she was active in volunteer activities, including teaching in an English as a second language (ESL) program.

She does not smoke; drinks wine occasionally; does not use drugs.

Physical activity was moderate: she took a yoga class twice per week. She had decreased physical activity during wound treatments and has been sedentary for the last 4 months.

PHYSICAL THERAPY EXAMINATION (INITIAL)

Chart Review

Patient alert and awake in no apparent distress. Right residual limb wrapped in soft gauze dressing covered with an elastic wrap. Drain in place. Incision clean on dressing change.

BP: 142/70, pulse 66, respiration normal.

Respiratory therapist reports patient using spirometer properly, normal cough, and no evidence of respiratory problems; SpO$_2$ is 97%.

Patient complains of some pain in residual limb (pain medication prescribed). Reports some uncomfortable phantom limb sensation, but denies pain.

Patient has been sitting at the side of the bed twice/day.

Examination Data

Gross muscle strength of left LE and both UEs grossly within functional limits (WFL). Muscle strength of right hip flexion, abduction, and adduction grossly WFL; hip extension tested side-lying and graded 3+/5. Demonstrates active motion of right knee flexion and extension with no resistance given at this time.

Residual limb measurements deferred until initial healing has taken place.

Gross ROM of left LE and both UEs WFL. Left hip extension measurements deferred until patient can lie prone or on right side. Gross ROM of the right hip WFL except hip extension to 0° measured side-lying. Right knee flexion and extension grossly WFL. Specific measurement deferred until dressing can be removed.

Left LE is hairless below the ankle. Skin is warm to touch. Dorsalis pedis pulse not palpable. Toes are warm to touch. Proprioceptive sensation at the ankle and toes is intact. She is unable to detect the 5.07 Semmes Weinstein monofilament under metatarsal heads on the left. Diminished sensation over plantar surface of left foot and dorsum of first metatarsal. No evidence of edema in left LE. Sensation testing of right residual limb (RL) deferred owing to presence of dressing.

FUNCTIONAL STATUS

Bed Mobility

Rolling to left: independent; rolling to right and prone: not tested.

Supine-to-sit and return: modified independent using side rail of bed.

Sitting Balance

Independent

Standing Balance

Single leg balance (without hand support): 5 seconds

Transfers

Sit-to-stand with walker: moderate assistance. No orthostatic hypotension.

Stand-to-sit in chair or bed: moderate assistance.

Locomotion
Ambulation with walker: moderate assistance for 5 feet. Complains of increased RL pain when her right leg is dependent.
Vital signs (post-ambulation): HR, 82; BP, 150/72; RL pain rated: 7/10
Expected outcomes of physical therapy episode of care (achieved before discharge from hospital):

1. The patient will be independent in all transfers and bed mobility.

2. The patient will be independent in ambulation with crutches or walker for 40 feet.

3. The patient will demonstrate knowledge of proper residual limb positioning, bandaging, and care.

4. The patient will demonstrate knowledge of basic RL exercises.

5. The patient will demonstrate knowledge of proper care of the left LE.

PREPROSTHETIC HOME CARE PHYSICAL THERAPY
The patient is discharged on day 5 to the home of one of her daughters. She is referred to home care physical therapy.

Examination Data
Examination data obtained following discharge from hospital by home care physical therapist:
Residual limb: Sutures in place, incision healing well, no drainage; length 5.4 in. (13.6 cm) from medial tibial plateau (MTP) to end of RL.
Circumferential measurements from MTP:
- 2 in. (5 cm) below MTP = 14 in. (35 cm)
- 4 in. (10 cm) below MTP = 15 in. (38 cm)
- 5 in. (12 cm) below MTP = 14.5 in. (37 cm)

RL sensation intact. She continues to have phantom limb sensation (throbbing, like the wound she had before the amputation), but denies PLP. She rates her RL pain: 5/10.
Psychosocial. She is somewhat anxious because she doesn't want to be a burden to her daughter. She is able to look at and touch her RL and is anxious to get moving. She acknowledges that she is worried because she has never known anyone with an amputation and is not sure she can learn to use a prosthesis. She also is fearful that she will fall, so she stays in her chair unless someone is with her.
ROM right knee: WFL.
ROM right hip: extension to 0° (all other motions WFL).
The patient's daughter is present and tells you that she is worried because her mother seems more forgetful now than she was before the surgery. The daughter is concerned that her mother will forget safe procedures and fall or not be able to learn to use a prosthesis.

Expected Outcomes
Expected outcomes for physical therapy episode of care during preprosthetic home care intervention:

1. The patient will be independent in care of RL, including bandaging or using a shrinker.

2. The patient will be independent in crutch (or walker) ambulation in and around the home and community.

3. The patient will be independent in HEP.

4. The patient will be independent in self-care and functional activities in the home.

Ten weeks after surgery the patient is fitted with a transtibial prosthesis (total surface-bearing socket with seal-in liner, suction suspension, and ESAR prosthetic foot). When she receives the prosthesis, she will be admitted to an acute rehabilitation hospital for 10 days of prosthetic training. Her goal is to return to her own home when discharged from rehabilitation.

GUIDING QUESTIONS

1. The patient's RL was wrapped in a soft dressing after amputation. Discuss the advantages and disadvantages of the volume containment options (rigid, semirigid, and soft dressings) for this patient.

2. Review the initial examination data given for the patient. What data would be important to obtain on the first postoperative visit and what can be deferred? What other data would you obtain and when?

(Continued)

CASE STUDY—cont'd

3. As the home health therapist:

   a. What additional examination data do you need to develop an appropriate POC?
   b. Describe your initial plan of interventions.
   c. Describe your mobility program.
   d. How will you address your patient's anxiety regarding falling and her ability to be successful with a prosthesis?
   e. Describe possible causes for your patient's cognitive issues and how you will address her daughter's concerns.

4. When the patient receives her prosthesis and is admitted to the acute rehabilitation hospital, what will be the focus of her prosthetic training program? Outline your program.

   a. Describe your initial balance training program.
   b. How will you teach her to use her ESAR prosthetic foot effectively? What gait training techniques will you include to ensure that she develops a symmetrical gait pattern?
   c. How would you teach this person to get down to and up from the floor?

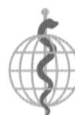 The reader is referred to Immersive Case G: A Patient With Limb Loss Following Amputation, an interactive case that guides users through the interview, examination, diagnosis, and writing of goals and the plan of care for a patient with limb loss following amputation, available online at **fadavis.com**.

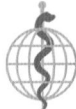 For additional resources, including answers to the questions for review, new immersive cases, case study guiding questions, references, and more, please visit **https://www.fadavis.com/product/physical -rehabilitation-fulk-8**. You may also quickly find the resources by entering this title's four-digit ISBN, 4691, in the search field at **http://fadavis.com** and logging in at the prompt.

Arthritis

Maura Daly Iversen, PT, DPT, SD, MPH, FNAP, FAPTA
Michelle Wormley, PT, MPT, PhD, CLT

Chapter 23

LEARNING OBJECTIVES

1. Discriminate between the epidemiology, pathophysiology, disease course, and clinical manifestations of two common rheumatic diseases: rheumatoid arthritis and osteoarthritis.

2. Identify the medical (clinical) diagnostic procedures commonly used in the examination of patients with arthritis, including laboratory tests and imaging.

3. Apply common principles of medical and rehabilitation management to the plan of care for individuals with rheumatoid arthritis and osteoarthritis.

4. Identify and understand when, why, and how to apply and interpret clinical examination and outcome measures commonly used in assessing individuals with rheumatoid arthritis or osteoarthritis.

5. Describe environmental, psychosocial, and other personal factors associated with arthritis that affect participation, intervention adherence, achievement of anticipated goals, and expected outcomes.

6. Explain the importance of a team-based chronic disease management approach for persons with arthritis.

7. Analyze, synthesize, and interpret patient data, formulate realistic intervention goals and outcomes, and develop a plan of care when presented with a clinical case study.

CHAPTER OUTLINE

RHEUMATOID ARTHRITIS 889
  Epidemiology 890
  Etiology 890
  Pathophysiology 890
  Laboratory Tests 891
  Radiography/Diagnostic Imaging 892
  Classification and Diagnostic Criteria 892
  Disease Onset and Course 893
  Clinical Presentation 893
  Prognosis 901
  Remission Criteria 901
OSTEOARTHRITIS 901
  Epidemiology 901
  Etiology 902
  Pathophysiology 902
  Disease Onset and Course 904

  Classification and Diagnostic Criteria 904
  Radiography/Diagnostic Imaging 905
  Clinical Presentation 905
  Prognosis 910
MEDICAL MANAGEMENT 910
  Pharmacological Therapy in Rheumatoid Arthritis 910
  Pharmacological Therapy in Osteoarthritis 912
REHABILITATIVE MANAGEMENT 914
  Physical Therapy Examination 914
  Physical Therapy Intervention 923
  Physical Activity 932
  Education and Self-Management 935
  Telehealth/Telerehabilitation 935
SUMMARY 935

The terms *arthritis, rheumatism,* and *rheumatic disease* are generic references to an array of more than 100 diseases that are divided into 10 classification categories. Two major forms of arthritis are considered in this chapter: *rheumatoid arthritis (RA),* a systemic inflammatory disease, and *osteoarthritis (OA),* a more localized process known previously as *degenerative joint disease.* RA and osteoarthritis account for most arthritis cases treated by physical therapists.

■ RHEUMATOID ARTHRITIS

RA is a major subclassification within the category of diffuse inflammatory connective tissue diseases that also includes juvenile idiopathic arthritis, systemic lupus erythematosus, progressive systemic sclerosis or scleroderma, polymyositis, and dermatomyositis. RA is primarily a disease of the *synovium.* The first clinical description of RA is attributed to A. J. Landré-Beauvais in 1800, although analysis of pictorial art of the late Renaissance suggests the existence of RA in earlier times. Early descriptions of patient symptomatology were complicated by the lack of uniform agreement about the distinguishing disease characteristics, given its wide spectrum of clinical presentations. The term *RA* was first used by Sir Alfred Baring Garrod in 1858 but was not accepted by the American Rheumatism Association as the official terminology until 1941.[1] Diagnostic criteria and terminology have been developed and, in some cases, revised based on current data.[2,3]

Epidemiology

The estimated prevalence of RA among adults in the United States is approximately 1.3 million, and its prevalence increases with age.[4] Women are affected two to four times more often than men. Differences in prevalence exist among certain subpopulations, which suggests a possible role for genetic or environmental factors in disease etiology. For example, Black Americans have a lower prevalence of RA than White Americans, whereas several Native American groups demonstrate higher prevalence rates. There also is a lower prevalence of RA in native Japanese and native Chinese peoples compared to those of European descent.[4,5] A diagnosis of RA is associated with premature mortality, specifically, an average reduced life expectancy of 3 to 10 years.[6]

Etiology

RA is an autoimmune disease of unknown complex etiology. RA has a substantial genetic basis and a heritability estimate of 60%, demonstrated by the increased disease risk and clustering in families.[7,8] Among the genetic factors associated with RA risk, human leukocyte antigen–DR isotype (*HLA–DRB1*) positivity is the strongest genetic risk factor, increasing disease risk by roughly threefold.[9,10]

Briefly, an *antigen* is a substance, usually foreign to the host, that provokes the immune system into action. The immune system may respond to the antigen directly (cellular immunity) or by the production of *antibodies* that circulate in the serum (humoral immunity). These responses involve two general types of lymphocytes: T cells, which are responsible for cellular immunity, and B cells, which produce circulating antibodies specific to the antigen. Antibodies are immunoglobulins, a type of serum protein.[1]

Given that individuals with RA produce antibodies to their own immunoglobulins, such as rheumatoid factor (RF) and anticitrullinated protein antibody, and these antibodies precede the clinical presentation of RA by years,[11,12] RA is considered an autoimmune disease.[12] It is not clear, however, whether this antibody production is a primary event or results as a response to a specific antigen from an external stimulus. Current theory and research on the cellular basis of autoimmunity suggest that aberrant functioning of cell-mediated immunity and defective T lymphocytes may trigger the autoimmune response that underlies RA.[12] A specific etiologic agent for RA has not been identified. However, external agents may trigger disease expression through various and differing mechanisms. Behavioral risk factors, such as low fish intake, obesity, poor dental health, and smoking are associated with an increased risk of developing RA.[13–17] Bacterial organisms, including streptococcus, clostridia, diphtheroids, and mycoplasmas, have been suggested as triggers, but no connections have been definitively proven. There has also been discussion of a viral etiology for RA. A recent systematic review of studies suggests an increased risk of RA incidence following parvo B19 and hepatitis C viral exposure. As with other investigations seeking to identify an etiology for RA, research remains speculative.[18]

Rheumatoid factors are antibodies specific to immunoglobulin G (IgG) and are found in the sera of approximately 70% of all patients with RA. Current theory suggests that RFs arise as antibodies to "altered" autologous (the patient's own) IgG. Some modification of IgG changes its configuration and renders it an autoimmunogen, stimulating the production of RF. IgM is the first class of immunoglobulins formed after contact with an antigen, and most RFs are of this class, although RFs may be of any immunoglobulin class.[1] The exact biological role of RF is unknown. Although RF has been implicated in the pathogenesis of RA, the disease occurs in the absence of RF in a substantial number of individuals.[19] Research indicates that the presence of RF affects disease severity, because those who have RF, or seropositive disease, have increased frequency of subcutaneous nodules, vasculitis, and polyarticular involvement and worse health outcomes.[1]

Worthington and Eyre examined the literature investigating a genetic predisposition to the development of RA.[7] HLAs found on the surface of most human cells are capable of generating *an immune response* when genetically incompatible tissues are grafted to each other, for example, during organ transplants. Genes controlling these HLAs are found on the sixth chromosome. Four loci have been described: HLA-A, HLA-B, HLA-C, and HLA-D. RA has been associated with increased HLA-D and HLA-DR (D-related) antigens, suggesting that certain genes determine whether a host is more or less at risk for an immunologic response that leads to RA.[7] A *rheumatoid epitope* has been identified through DNA typing of HLA-DR4 as a particular sequence of amino acids common among patients with RA.[20] A national case-control study conducted in Sweden focused on citrulline-modified proteins, proteins not normally present in healthy adults but found in about two-thirds of patients with RA, to determine if smoking and the presence of shared epitope HLA genes triggered RA. The investigators concluded that the interaction of smoking and carrying two copies of the SE gene increases the risk of developing RA by 21-fold.[21,22] Further studies of genomic organization of the HLA-D region specifically implicate a short sequence on the *HLA-DRB1* gene and suggest that HLA-DRB1 alleles (alternate forms of a gene) modify disease expression and progression.[1] Various studies of different ethnic groups have also shown that particular variations of the HLA-DRB1 allele are overrepresented in people with RA.[1]

Pathophysiology

In early RA, synovial inflammation leads to pain, stiffness, and restricted range of motion (ROM). Inflammation typically begins as low-grade, protracted responses to pathogens or certain endogenous or exogenous substances.[23] As the disease progresses, the joint capsule becomes inflamed, and immune cells degrade the cartilage. With long-standing RA, the synovium appears grossly edematous with slender villous or hair-like projections into the joint cavity (Fig. 23.1). Distinctive vascular changes, including venous distention, capillary obstruction, neutrophilic infiltration of the arterial walls, and areas of thrombosis and hemorrhage, may be evident. Synovial proliferation of vascular granulation tissue, known as *pannus,* dissolves collagen as it extends over the joint cartilage. Eventually, with disease progression, the granulation tissue leads to adhesions, fibrosis, or bony ankylosis of the joint. Chronic inflammation associated with RA weakens the joint capsule and supporting ligamentous structures, altering joint structure and function. Tendon rupture and fraying tendon sheaths produce imbalanced muscle pull on pathologically altered joints resulting in the characteristic musculoskeletal deformities seen in advanced RA.[24]

Following alterations in blood flow, rapid changes in the cellular content and volume of the synovial fluid may result, owing to low pressure in the joint space and the lack of a limiting membrane between the joint space and synovial blood vessels. High molecular weight substances such as macroglobulins and fibrinogens can pass through the synovial capillaries during periods of inflammation and are not easily cleared.[1] Antigen–antibody complexes may be isolated within the joint cavity and stimulate phagocytosis and further development of pannus. Although sustained inflammation requires the proliferation of new blood vessels, the exact mechanism of capillary growth is not understood. One hypothesis suggests that activated macrophages, responding to antigen–antibody complexes, may stimulate this development. With established synovitis, polymorphonuclear (PMN) leukocytes are drawn into the joint cavity and coupled with lysosomal enzyme activity contribute to destruction of synovial tissues.[19]

Laboratory Tests

Elevated *erythrocyte sedimentation rate (ESR)* and *C-reactive protein (CRP)* are acute-phase reactants that indicate the presence of active inflammation. Although patients with RA characteristically have active inflammation, up to 40% may have normal values for these tests despite clinical evidence of inflammation. Normal ESR and CRP values are nonspecific and alone cannot confirm or refute a diagnosis of RA. RF is found in approximately 80% of patients with RA in time but in as few as 30% at onset.[12] The presence or absence of RF alone neither confirms nor rules out a diagnosis of RA. Nearly 25% of people with RA do not have a positive RF (seronegative RA), whereas a positive RF is seen in a number of other immunologic conditions (e.g., leprosy, tuberculosis, chronic hepatitis) and occasionally in individuals with no disease.[12] In recent years, the anticyclic citrullinated peptide antibody (anti-CCP) has been researched and included as one of the most important serological biomarkers for diagnosing RA. A positive RF and anti-CCP in combination with clinical criteria may help to confirm a clinical impression.[20]

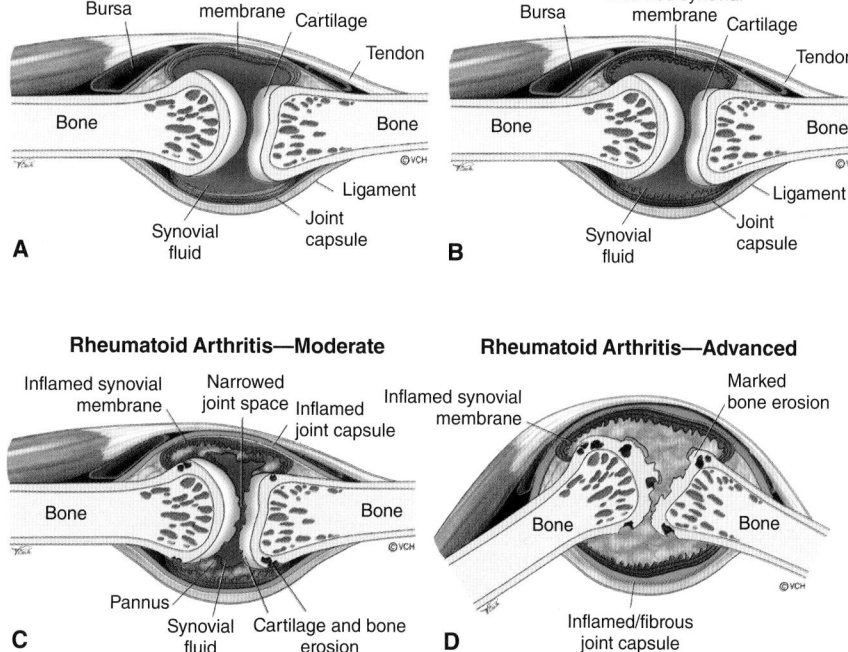

Figure 23.1 Progression of joint changes due to rheumatoid arthritis inflammation: early to advanced disease.

A *complete blood count (CBC)* is routinely ordered because many findings are commonly associated with RA. Red blood cell counts are often decreased, indicating the anemia of chronic disease found in approximately 20% of individuals with RA.[25] By comparison, the white blood cell count is generally normal. *Thrombocytosis,* a high platelet count, is not uncommon in active RA.

Synovial fluid analysis can greatly enhance the process of differential diagnosis. Normal synovial fluid is transparent, yellowish, viscous, and without clots. Synovial fluid from inflamed joints is cloudy, less viscous owing to a change in hyaluronate proteins, and will clot. Significant inflammation also increases the number of fluid proteins. A culture can be performed to identify potential bacterial agents as the cause of joint inflammation. If the joint is inflamed, white blood cells will be elevated in the fluid. Crystals are not common. If present, they may confirm the diagnosis of gout (urate crystals) or *pseudogout* (calcium pyrophosphate crystals). A mucin clot test (a measure of viscosity) of the synovial fluid can be used to discriminate between acute infectious arthritis and inflammatory arthritis, such as RA. Poor clotting accompanies acute infectious arthritis, whereas RA produces fair mucin clotting.[1]

Radiography/Diagnostic Imaging

Radiographic study is essential in a diagnostic workup for RA.[24] Physical therapists practicing in rheumatology should develop a basic proficiency in identifying abnormalities in joint structure and the surrounding soft tissues as these abnormalities influence the course and outcome of rehabilitation. To identify radiographic abnormalities, the therapist must be able to describe how a normal joint appears on a radiograph. Therapists can orient themselves to a radiograph by considering several parameters: alignment, bone density and surface, and cartilaginous spacing. Normal alignment is present when the long axes of the proximal and distal bones of the joint are in their normal spatial relationships and the convex surface of one bone fits well with the concavity of the other. Bone density, in the absence of *osteoporosis,* should be somewhat opaque and milky and appear evenly distributed throughout. The cortices of each bone should be distinct, appropriately thick, and well defined. The joint soft tissues should conform to known anatomical shape. A normal joint surface should be smooth and should conform to known anatomical shape without bony formations or outgrowths around the end of a joint (osteophytes). Soft tissue swelling and evidence of uneven spacing between joint surfaces on radiograph may suggest activity limitations. Uneven, reduced, or absent spacing suggests joint cartilage loss or joint surface erosion (see Fig. 23.1). RA progression can be characterized in four sequential stages using periodic radiographic examination. Radiographic changes evident in early RA are nonspecific and usually limited to soft tissue swelling, joint effusion, and periarticular demineralization. Diagnostic confirmation is made when the disease process leads to bilateral joint space narrowing and erosions in the hands and feet.[1]

Ultrasound and MRI may also be used to assess RA-associated changes and to monitor disease activity. Both are more sensitive to use than physical examination of the joints.[26] A systematic review comparing MRI and ultrasound to assess joint inflammation indicates that ultrasound is a valid technique for identifying synovitis in the hand and wrist joints and is easier and more practical to implement than MRI.[27] In addition to detecting synovitis, ultrasound can be applied to almost all synovial joints to examine for the presence of erosion, cartilage loss, or tendon damage. A recent systematic review found ultrasound to be more sensitive than conventional radiography identifying the prevalence of erosions, particularly in small joints of the hands and feet, when validated definitions and scoring systems were used.

Classification and Diagnostic Criteria

The differential diagnosis of RA is predicated on the history, clinical examination of signs and symptoms, and careful exclusion of other disorders. The *American College of Rheumatology* (ACR) classification criteria,[2] developed using data from patients in outpatient clinics, are commonly used to confirm whether an individual's clinical presentation is, in fact, a case of RA. In 2010, the ACR and the *European League Against Rheumatism* (EULAR; in 2021 renamed the *European Alliance of Associations for Rheumatology*) revised the original 1987 classification criteria for RA[2] to help identify early RA. These criteria are based on a combination of signs, symptoms, and laboratory findings that have persisted for a specified period of time, and a full explanation can be found at the following link: https://rheumatology.org.[3] A diagnosis of definite RA is now established on the confirmed presence of synovitis in at least one joint, absence of an alternative diagnosis that better explains the synovitis, and a total score of 6 or greater (out of a possible 10) from four domains. The domains are (a) *Joint Involvement,* designating the number and site of involved joints (score range 0 to 5); (b) *Serology,* indicating serological abnormalities (score range 0 to 3); (3) *Acute-Phase Reactants,* describing elevated acute-phase response (score range 0 to 1); and (4) *Duration of Symptom* (two levels; range 0 to 1).[3] The inclusion of criteria for early RA may help rheumatologists to target treatment at earlier stages of the disease and decrease RA progression.

Patients with RA can also be classified based on global functional status criteria.[28] There are four functional classifications based on a person's ability to complete functional and self-care activities. Class I is defined as the complete ability to perform usual activities of daily living (ADL) (such as dressing, bathing) and vocational activities (school, work) and avocational activities (recreation and leisure). Class II is defined as the ability to perform usual ADL and vocational activities but with limited avocational activities. Class III is considered when a patient is limited in the ability to perform usual ADL and vocational and avocational activities. Class IV is full dependence.[28] In addition to their clinical relevance, these functional classifications enable clinicians and researchers to classify subjects in clinical trials and inform evidence-based clinical recommendations for therapies.

Disease Onset and Course

RA is characterized by an exacerbating and remitting disease course. Disease onset is accompanied by complaints of generalized joint pain and stiffness, usually in multiple small joints *(polyarthritis)* though it may be localized to a single joint. Symptoms may appear spontaneously or over a prolonged time period. Disease progression is highly variable. High RF titers indicate a more severe disease course. Spontaneous remissions can occur. Some patients experience an intermittent course characterized by partial to complete remissions longer than the periods of exacerbations. A third group experiences the full unremitting destructive process of progressive RA.[1] Comparisons of late-onset RA with early-onset RA revealed that abrupt onset and large joint involvement, particularly of the shoulder girdle, were more common in older adults. The late-onset group demonstrated clinical features more commonly associated with *polymyalgia rheumatica,* a separate and distinct disease affecting the shoulder and pelvic musculature leading to muscle inflammation.[29]

Clinical Presentation

Systemic

Systemic features of RA include weight loss, fever, and extreme fatigue. Fatigue greatly affects function and participation in daily life and is often underappreciated on physical examination. Fatigue may result from chronic pain and is associated with cerebral inflammation and physical inactivity.[20] A hallmark clinical feature is *morning stiffness* in and around the joints lasting at least 1 hr before maximal improvement.[3] In contrast, OA-induced stiffness results from inactivity. Morning stiffness can be qualified in its severity and duration, both of which are directly related to the degree of disease activity.

Joint Impairments (Articular and Nonarticular)

RA is characterized by bilateral and symmetrical synovial joint involvement. Clinically, patients present with limited mobility and signs of inflammation including pain, redness, swelling, and warm joints. The most common joints involved are the hands, feet, and cervical spine (Fig. 23.2). The hands are generally affected early in the disease course, and severity of hand involvement is indicative of severity of disease.[30] The term *arthralgia* refers to joint pain. The joint examination may reveal *crepitus,* an audible or palpable grating or crunching evident as the joint is moved through its ROM. Crepitus is the result of uneven degeneration of the joint surface.

Cervical Spine and Temporomandibular Joint

The cervical spine is often involved in RA, and on examination, ROM may be limited in all planes. The occipitoatlantal (occiput–C1) and atlantoaxial (C1–C2) joints are frequently affected due to their extensive synovial tissue. The midcervical region is also a common site of inflammation, leading to decreased ROM, particularly in rotation, accompanied by instability. Chronic inflammation in the cervical region can lead to ossification of the anterior and posterior longitudinal and transverse ligament, the major stabilizers of movement in the C1–C2 region. Three patterns of cervical spine involvement are described: atlantoaxial subluxation aka dislocation (65%), atlantoaxial impaction (20% to 25%), and subaxial subluxation (10% to 15%).[31] Atlantoaxial subluxation is defined as a malalignment and excess movement of the body of C1 and the odontoid process of C2 with neck flexion, leading to impairments in cervical rotation and cervical radiculopathy consistent with the degree of spinal cord impingement (Fig. 23.3A–C). Involvement of the C1 and C2 vertebrae may produce life-threatening situations if the transverse ligament of the atlas should rupture or if the odontoid process should fracture or herniate through the foramen magnum, compressing the upper cervical cord. Patients presenting with cervical radiculopathy and neurological signs should be immediately referred to a physician. MRI is the most effective tool to visualize both the spinal column and the cord.[31] *Ankylosing* (i.e., fusion) of one or more vertebrae of the spine may accompany RA and can lead to loss of ROM and function of the involved joints.

The temporomandibular joint (TMJ) is usually among the last joints involved. Inflammation of the TMJ results in pain, swelling, and limited movement and eventually to ankylosis. With early disease, TMJ x-rays are usually negative but with time and chronic inflammation can demonstrate bone destruction. The use of cone-beam computed tomography has been helpful in early identification of degenerative TMJ changes, which may affect the ability to open the mouth fully (approximately 2 in. [5.08 cm]) with normal side-to-side gliding and protrusion.[32] In resting position, the normal approximation of the upper and lower teeth may be altered following persistent inflammation.

Shoulders and Elbows

Shoulder involvement may be evident in the glenohumeral, sternoclavicular, or acromioclavicular joints leading to joint surface degeneration, pain, and loss of ROM. Shoulder pain is often referred to the deltoid region. The scapulothoracic articulation may

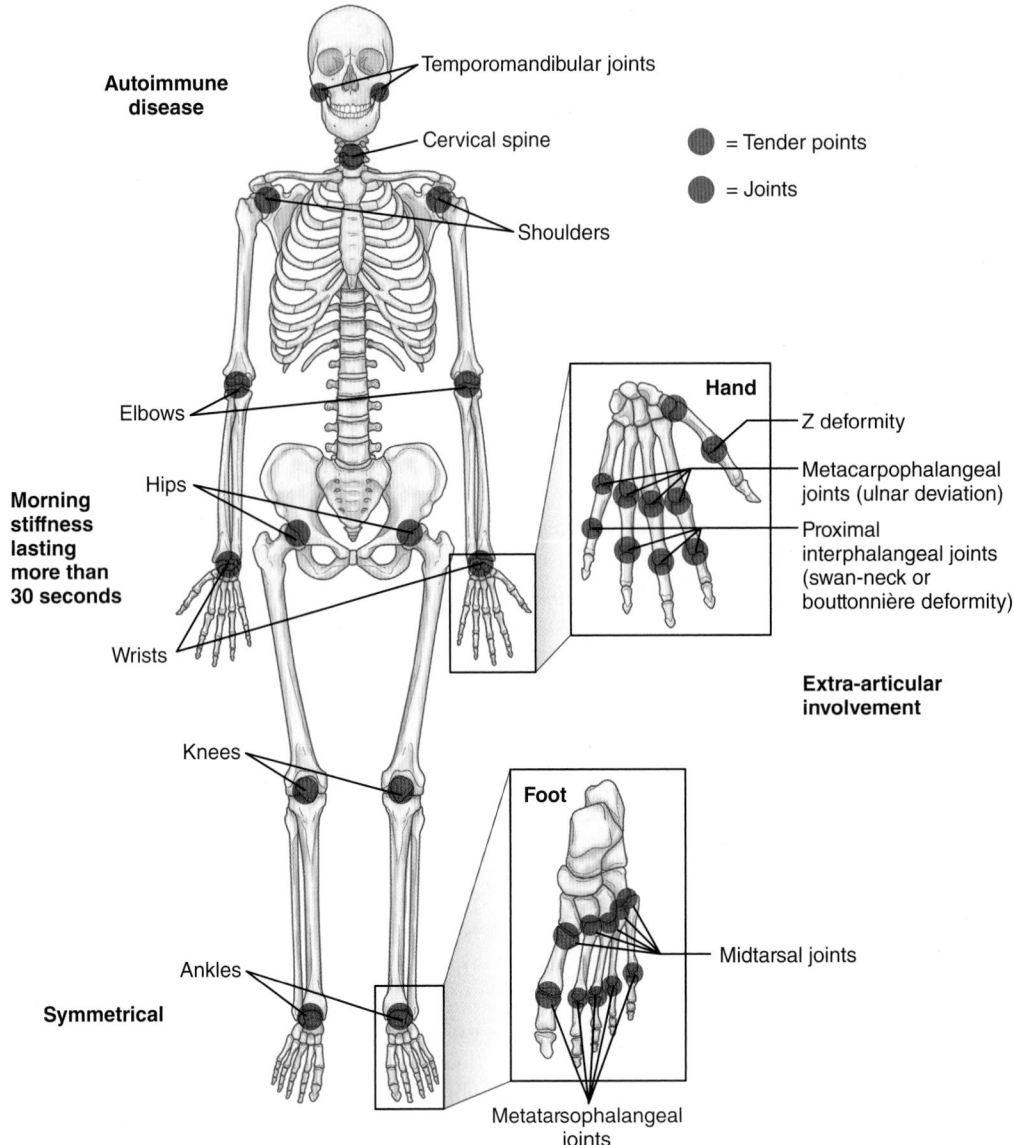

Figure 23.2 Homunculus showing common joints affected by rheumatoid arthritis.

secondarily exhibit a loss of ROM. Chronic shoulder inflammation causes the capsule and the ligaments to become distended and thinned. As joint surfaces erode, the shoulder eventually becomes unstable. In addition, tendinitis and bursitis may complicate management. Typical elbow joint findings include effusions between the lateral epicondyle and olecranon prominence, bilateral swelling of the olecranon bursa (more prevalent with severe disease), and rheumatoid nodules on the olecranon or extensor surface of the proximal ulna.[31] Inflammation, capsular and ligamentous distention, and joint erosion may lead to instability and irregular or catching movements. Flexion contractures frequently develop due to patient posturing to reduce pain and persistent spasm.

Wrists

The ulnar styloid may be tender on examination, suggesting inflammatory synovitis. Early synovitis among the carpal bones and the ulna leads to a fairly rapid development of a flexion contracture, which ultimately diminishes the ability to grasp. Additionally, *carpal tunnel syndrome* may occur due to compression of the median nerve in the carpal tunnel. Chronic inflammation around the ulnar styloid coupled with laxity of the radioulnar ligament produces the *piano key sign* on examination. The piano key sign is defined as an up and down movement of the styloid in response to point pressure from the examiner. Over time ulnar deviation or drift may occur from chronic inflammation causing movement of the wrist toward the ulna (Fig. 23.4).

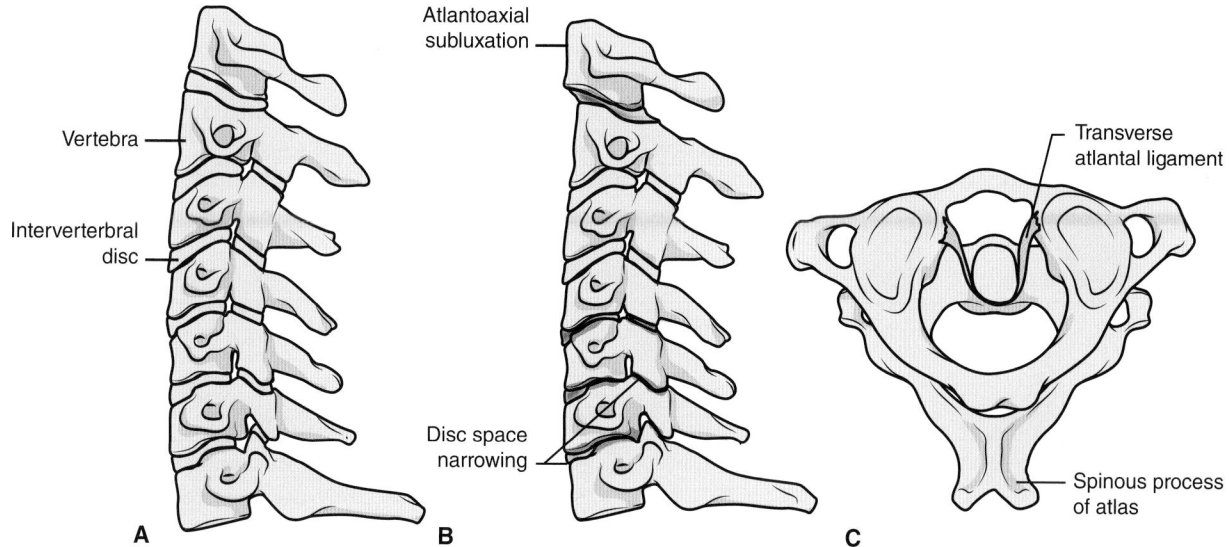

Figure 23.3 Rheumatoid arthritis cervical spine involvement including atlantoaxial subluxation and atlantoaxial impaction.

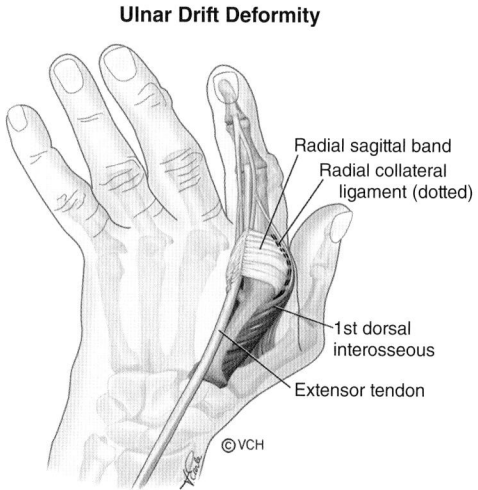

Ulnar Drift Deformity

Radial sagittal band
Radial collateral ligament (dotted)
1st dorsal interosseous
Extensor tendon
©VCH

Figure 23.4 Ulnar drift (deviation) of the fingers. This drawing depicts the impact of metacarpophalangeal joint swelling, soft tissue laxity due to synovitis, which leads to ulnar deviation of the fingers in rheumatoid arthritis.

Chronic inflammation of the proximal row of carpals can lead to a volar *subluxation* of the wrist and hand on the radius, accentuating the normal 10° to 15° of volar inclination of the carpus on the distal radius (Fig. 23.5). In addition, radial deviation of the distal carpals can occur due to loss of radial ligamentous support, destruction of the extensor carpi ulnaris and the fibrocartilage on the distal ulna. This allows the proximal carpals to slide down the distal radius toward the ulna, contributing to radial deviation of the distal row of carpals relative to the two bones of the forearm, where normally there is 5° to 10° of ulnar deviation.[33] Stenosing tenosynovitis of the first dorsal compartment of the wrist

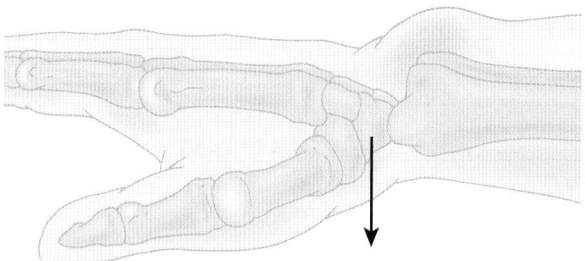

Figure 23.5 Volar subluxation of the wrist seen with rheumatoid arthritis. Chronic inflammation of the proximal carpals can eventually lead to a volar subluxation of the wrist and hand on the radius, accentuating the normal 10° to 15° of volar inclination of the carpus on the distal radius.

(*de Quervain disease*) may also occur leading to pain and swelling at the base of the thumb and difficulty moving the thumb and wrist when picking up objects or grasping. Some patients experience a stiffness in movement or stop-and-go movement phenomenon.

Hand Joints

METACARPOPHALANGEAL

Soft tissue swelling around the metacarpophalangeal (MCP) joints, especially the index and long fingers, is common (Fig. 23.6). Volar subluxation and ulnar drift of the MCPs frequently seen in RA results from exaggeration of the joints' normal structural shape that tilts the proximal phalanges in an ulnar direction. Ulnar "drift" is a feature of gripping, and repeated gripping can further lead to this deformity. The anatomical placement and length of the collateral ligaments, which are most stretched during MCP flexion, and the insertions of the intrinsics, which also pull from an ulnar direction, contribute to ulnar drift at the MCPs during hand motion. Weakened ligaments cannot resist a pull toward volar subluxation during power pinch or grasp when flexor tendons bowstring across MCPs through frayed tendon sheaths damaged by long-term synovitis. The *bowstring effect* results from moving the fulcrum of the flexor

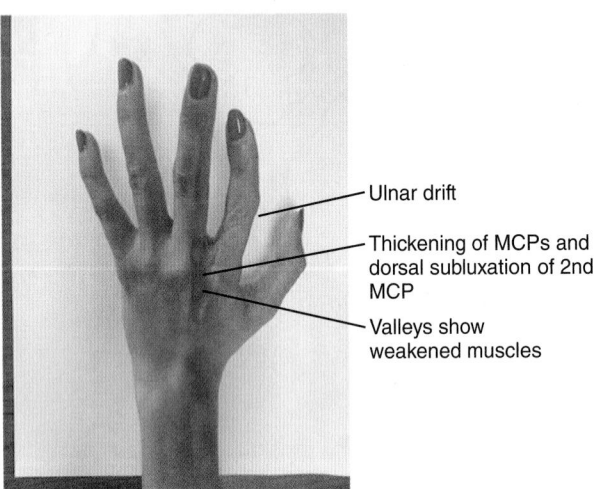

— Ulnar drift

— Thickening of MCPs and dorsal subluxation of 2nd MCP

— Valleys show weakened muscles

Figure 23.6 Hand with rheumatoid arthritis illustrating thickening of the metacarpals, ulnar deviation of the phalanges, and muscle wasting.

tendons distally, placing an ulnar and volar pull on the proximal phalanges. Radial deviation of the carpals further enhances MCP ulnar drift as the phalanges try to compensate for the loss of normal ulnar deviation at the wrist. This is known as the *zigzag effect,* where forces in the hand try to move the index finger back into its normal functional position in line with the radius. A *trigger finger* may be evident whereby a snapping sensation is felt when flexing or extending the finger due to flexor tenosynovitis and resultant slippage of the tendon, friction with movement, or presence of tendon nodules[31,34] (Fig. 23.7).

PROXIMAL INTERPHALANGEAL

Swelling of the proximal interphalangeal (PIP) joints is common and is easily appreciated with lateral joint palpation. There are two characteristic irreversible deformities (if not surgically repaired early) seen at the PIPs in individuals with severe RA. The first of these is known as *swan neck deformity* and consists of PIP hyperextension and distal interphalangeal (DIP) flexion (Fig. 23.8). Swan neck deformities arise in three distinct ways, depending on the site of initial involvement. Most commonly, swan neck deformity follows from initial synovitis of the MCP, where the pain of chronic synovitis leads to reflex muscle spasm of the intrinsics. The biomechanical force of the intrinsics then combines with the hypermobility found in the chronically

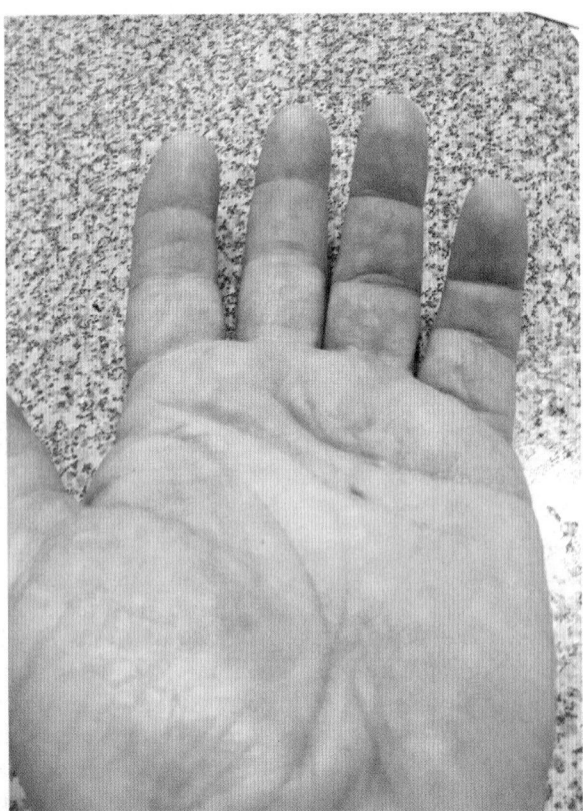

Figure 23.7 A patient with a trigger finger.

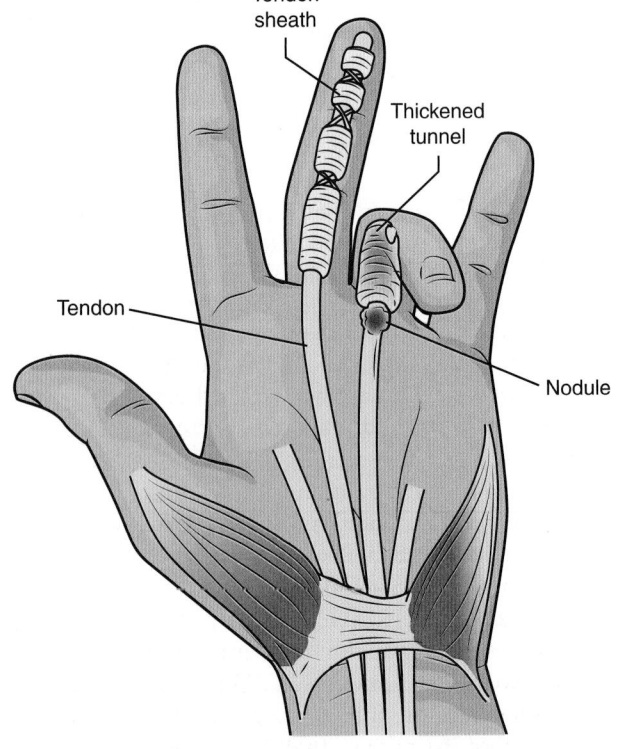

Tendon sheath

Thickened tunnel

Tendon

Nodule

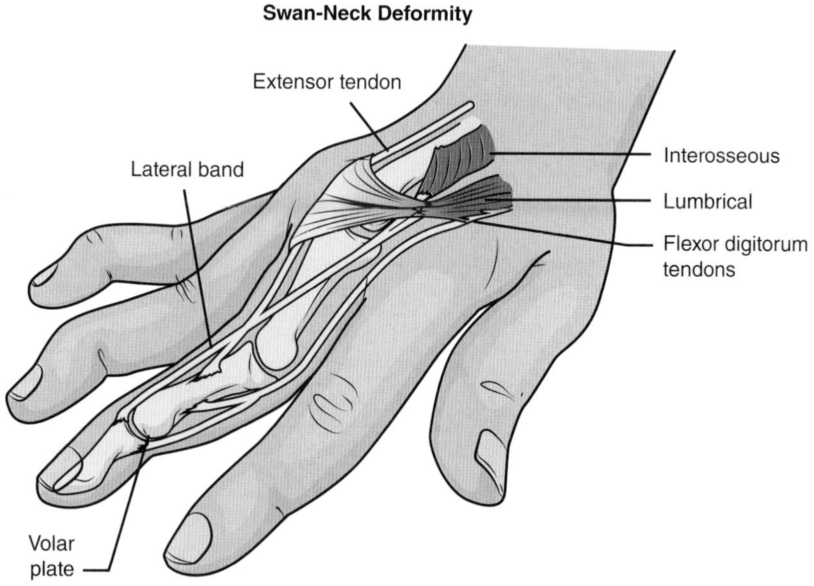

Swan-Neck Deformity

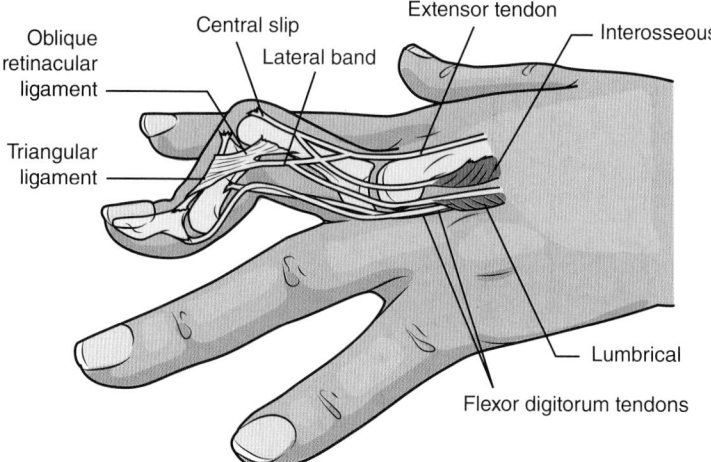

Figure 23.8 Swan neck deformity is characterized by PIP hyperextension and DIP flexion.

Figure 23.9 Features of a boutonnière deformity include DIP extension with PIP flexion.

inflamed and structurally changed PIP, resulting in volar subluxation and PIP hyperextension. Swan neck deformity may also result when the volar capsule of the PIP is stretched, the lateral bands move dorsally, and tension is placed on the flexor digitorum profundus by the PIP which flexes the DIP. In these instances, a rupture of the flexor digitorum sublimis further predisposes an individual to swan neck deformity. A third mechanism for developing swan neck deformity involves a rupture of the extensor digitorum communis at its insertion on the DIP resulting in DIP flexion and PIP hyperextension owing to unrestrained pull by the flexor digitorum profundus.[31,33]

The other characteristic deformity of the PIP is known as a *boutonnière deformity* and consists of DIP extension with PIP flexion (Fig. 23.9). As a result of chronic synovitis, the insertion of extensor digitorum communis into the middle phalanx (known as the central slip) lengthens, and the lateral bands slide volarly to force the PIP into flexion. Osteophytes found at the PIP

are known as *Bouchard nodes* and may be seen in OA. They are unrelated to RA, although an individual may have both kinds of arthritis at the same time.[31,34]

DISTAL INTERPHALANGEAL

The DIP joints are rarely affected in RA. Occasionally, a *mallet finger* deformity will result from rupture of the extensor digitorum communis tendon, pulling the DIP into flexion as force from the flexor digitorum profundus is unopposed.[34]

THUMB

Synovitis can lead to many deformities in the thumb. The most prevalent is a *flail IP* in which the patient loses the ability to flex the interphalangeal (IP) joint. The structures particularly affected include the fibers of the dorsal hood mechanism over the MCP, the joint capsule, collateral ligaments, and the tendons of extensor pollicis brevis and extensor pollicis longus. The exact mechanism of thumb deformities depends on the particular combination of affected structures. Similar to other hand deformities, the actual presentation depends on the site of initial synovitis, the direction of imbalanced muscle forces, and the integrity of the surrounding joint structures. A *type I deformity*, consisting of MCP flexion with IP hyperextension without involvement of the carpometacarpal (CMC) joint, is most seen. *Type II deformity* occurs when the CMC is subluxed and the IP is held in hyperextension. CMC subluxation and MCP hyperextension is classified as a *type III deformity* and is more common in RA than a type II deformity.[31,33,34]

MUTILANS DEFORMITY (OPERA-GLASS HAND)

Grossly unstable thumbs and severely deformed phalanges are indicative of *mutilans-type deformity*. Also known as *opera-glass hand,* the transverse folds of the skin of the thumb and fingers resemble a folded telescope. Radiographic study of the bones of the hand reveals severe bone resorption, erosion, and shortening of the MCP, PIP, radiocarpal, and radioulnar joints especially. The negative impact of this deformity on hand function and ADL is significant.[34]

Hips and Knees

Hip synovitis is less frequent in early RA. Hip synovitis often presents as pain in the groin or lower buttock. Pain over the greater trochanter may be secondary to trochanteric bursitis though recent MRI and ultrasound studies indicate that may not be the case. In a small prospective case-controlled study with researchers blinded to histological data, MRI and ultrasound studies combined with histology suggest no etiologic role of bursal inflammation in RA trochanteric pain syndrome.[35] Radiographic hip disease is evident in approximately half of all patients with RA.[34] Severe inflammatory destruction of the femoral head and the acetabulum may push the acetabulum into the pelvic cavity, a condition known as *protrusio acetabuli*. With progressive hip disease, patients may require a total hip *arthroplasty*.[31]

The clinical presentation of the knee joint frequently includes synovitis, causing accumulation of relatively large amounts of fluid. Special tests can be used to assess these symptoms. The knee ballottement test is used to examine for knee effusion. The examiner presses on the patella with the index finger, resulting in a downward motion of the patella; a sensation of bogginess indicates effusion of the knee. Posterior accumulation of fluid in the knee produces a *Baker cyst* (Fig. 23.10). If a Baker cyst ruptures, it produces pain, swelling, and heat in the posterior calf like symptoms of a deep vein thrombosis. To assess for the presence of anterior synovitis, a bulge test can be performed. With this procedure, the examiner strokes the medial aspect of the knee in an upward motion and then presses on the lateral aspect of the knee. A positive sign is a *wavelike* movement of fluid medially. Chronic synovitis results in distention of the joint capsule, attenuation of the collateral and cruciate

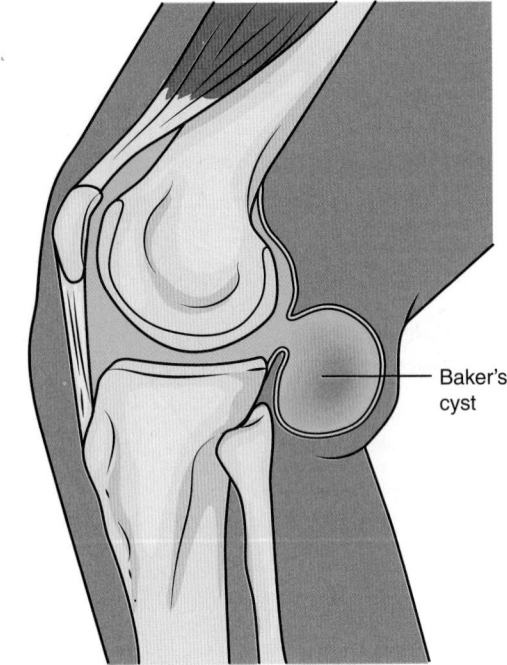

Figure 23.10 Baker cyst.

ligaments, and destruction of the joint surfaces. Painful knees may be held in slightly flexed positions, ultimately resulting in joint tightness or flexion contractures.[31]

Ankles and Feet

Early inflammation of the feet is often evident in the forefoot. On examination, patients often note pain with forefoot compression. Chronic synovitis accentuates the natural tendency of the talus to glide medially and plantarward, resulting in pressure on the calcaneus and leading to hindfoot pronation. The spring ligament is also stretched by these occurrences, flattening the medial longitudinal arch. The calcaneus may erode or develop bony *exostoses* known as spurs. As synovitis weakens the transverse arch, the metatarsals spread, and a splayed forefoot (*splayfoot*) may develop. Instability of the talocalcaneal joint, if severe, can lead to the need for surgical fusion. Synovitis of the metatarsophalangeal (MTP) joints is extremely common, and *metatarsalgia* (pain over the metatarsal heads) may develop. A *hallux valgus* and *bunion* (a painful bursitis over the medial aspect of the first MTP joint) may also be present. When volar subluxation of the MTP combines with flexion of the PIP and hyperextension of the DIP joints, this condition is commonly referred to as *hammer toes*. The MTPs may also exhibit volar subluxation of the metatarsal head with flexion of the PIP and DIP joints, known as *cock-up* or *claw toes*. As the capsule and intertarsal ligaments are weakened and stretched, the proximal phalanges move dorsally on the metatarsal head. Similar to conditions observed in the hand, the long toe extensors "bowstring" over the PIP joints while the flexors are displaced into the intertarsal spaces.[31] Figure 23.11 illustrates the typical changes seen in the foot with RA.

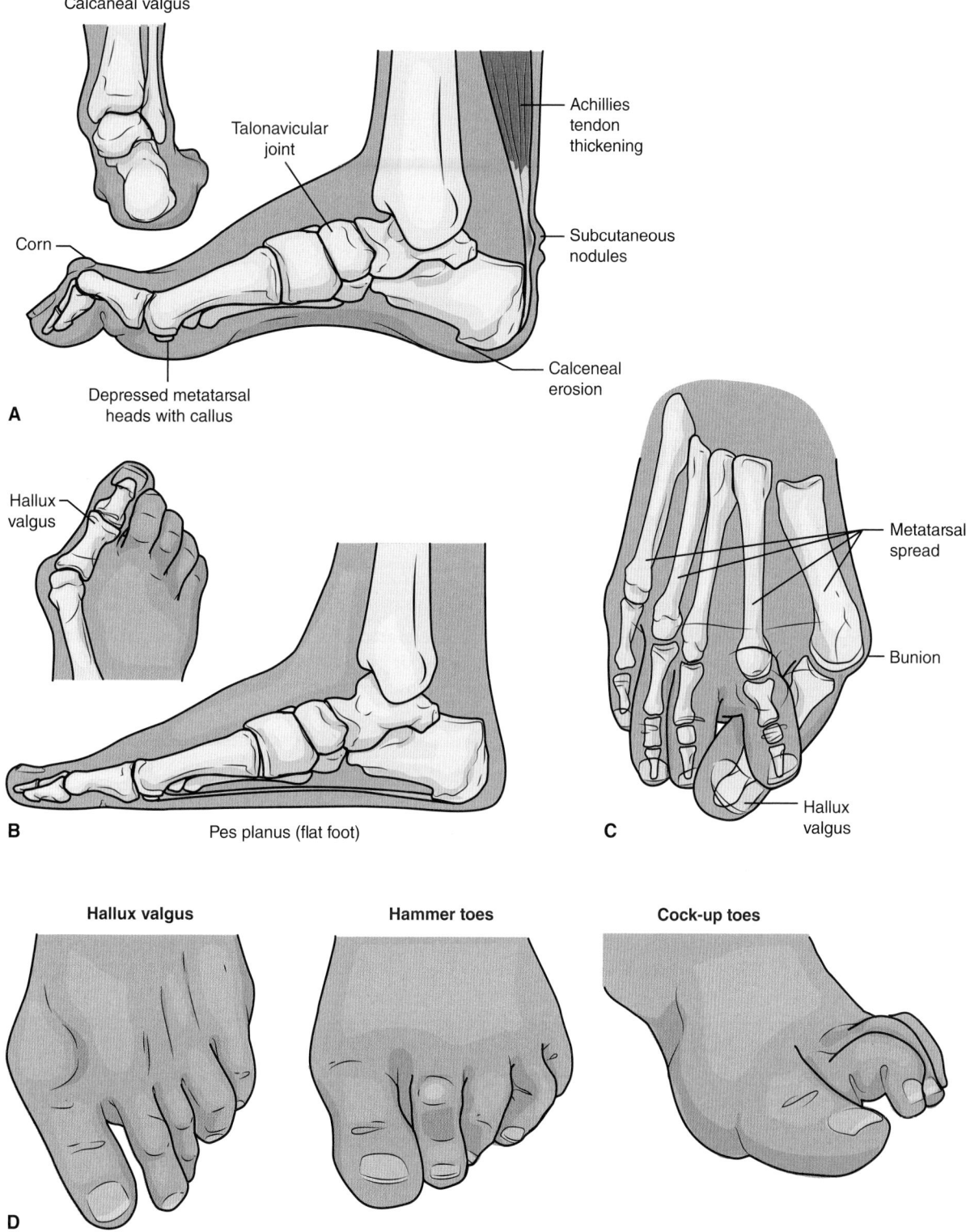

Figure 23.11 Foot involvement with rheumatoid arthritis.

Muscle Involvement

Muscle atrophy around affected joints may be present early. Roughly 50% of patients with RA will develop *rheumatoid cachexia,* a loss of muscle with concurrent increase in fat mass and in body mass index.[36] It is not definitively known, however, whether this atrophy results from disuse or selective attrition of muscles owing to some unspecified mechanism related to the disease process. It appears that individuals with RA who have rheumatoid cachexia experience selective attrition of type II (phasic) muscle fibers through some unknown mechanism.[36,37] Evidence suggests that elevated production of *cytokines* (i.e., TNF-α and IL-1β) may contribute to rheumatoid cachexia by triggering cell death by nuclear apoptosis in skeletal muscle[36] perhaps leading to muscle loss.[38] There is also some evidence that type I (tonic) muscle fibers of the quadriceps will undergo selective atrophy following anterior cruciate ligament damage.[37] Loss of muscle bulk may also be attributed to peripheral neuropathy or steroid-induced myopathy. Muscle weakness may result from either reflex inhibition secondary to pain or atrophy.[36-38] With long-standing disease, hand intrinsics and quadriceps atrophy are particularly evident although the mechanisms for these changes may not be the same.

Tendon Involvement

Tenosynovitis, inflammation of the tendon sheath lining, may occur with active disease and interferes with the smooth gliding of the tendon through the sheath. Inflammation may directly damage the tendon, eventually leading to a tendon rupture. Common sites of tenosynovitis are wrist flexors, thumb flexors, patella, and Achilles tendons. Trigger finger and *de Quervain tenosynovitis* may occur. A patient with tendon damage or muscle weakness may exhibit a *lag phenomenon,* a nonspecific finding that refers to a substantial difference in passive versus active ROM. Thus, therapists need to examine a lag carefully to determine its cause and design appropriate treatment.[34]

Deconditioning

Research indicates deconditioning is a significant clinical feature of RA. Persons with RA have diminished cardiorespiratory status, muscular strength and endurance, flexibility, and altered body composition when compared with healthy individuals of the same age and gender without arthritis. Deconditioning results from both direct and indirect impairments.[36-38] Direct impairments of RA include loss of type II muscle fibers, systemic fatigue, cachexia (wasting of lean body mass),[30-32] and shortening of contractile tissues. Indirect impairments include deconditioning secondary to inactivity and elevated resting energy expenditure (calories required by the body during a 24-hour period under resting conditions). Immune system activity and inflammation, even in individuals with well-controlled disease, create an increased metabolism with subsequent loss of lean body tissue.[37,39]

Rheumatoid Nodules

Rheumatoid nodules occur in approximately 20% to 25% of patients and are associated with a positive serological RF test and greater disease severity. Nodules are generally tender. Nodules are found in the subcutaneous or deeper connective tissues in areas subjected to repeated mechanical pressure such as the olecranon bursae, the extensor surfaces of the forearms, and the Achilles tendons. The presence of nodules on tendon mechanisms may lead to mechanical breakdown and tenosynovitis. Nodules present in early RA are suggestive for a greater likelihood of severe *extra-articular* manifestations.[31,34]

Vascular and Neurological Complications

Vasculitis, or inflammation of the blood vessels, is found in 25% to 30% of individuals with RA on autopsy.[34] Most forms of RA-associated vascular lesions are silent and difficult to diagnose due to variability in the size of the blood vessels affected. Skin vasculitis is the easiest to observe and can present as discoloration of the nail beds, purpura (red or purple discoloration), and petechiae (red or purple spots). The fulminant form of *rheumatoid arteritis* (arterial inflammation associated with a rheumatoid disorder) can be life threatening and accompanied by malnutrition, infection, congestive heart failure, and gastrointestinal bleeding. Vasculitis of the vessels supplying nerves can lead to peripheral neuropathies such as foot or wrist drop.[1] Peripheral neuropathies may also occur secondary to mechanical compression of nerves such as carpal tunnel or tarsal tunnel syndrome. Cervical spine inflammation can produce spinal cord compression (see section on cervical spine and TMJ). If clinical signs of cord compression are present, this requires immediate medical attention.[1]

Cardiovascular and Pulmonary Complications

Morbidity and mortality from cardiovascular disease are elevated in persons with RA due to a greater prevalence of ischemic heart disease, secondary to accelerated atherosclerosis. In fact, patients with RA have nearly a twofold increased risk of developing coronary artery disease (CAD), a risk similar to adults with diabetes.[39] Although the exact etiology of accelerated atherosclerosis is unclear, it is hypothesized that metabolic and vascular effects of chronic inflammation may be the causative factor.[39,40] Subclinical pericarditis may be present and has been found at autopsy. Heart failure is also more prevalent among adults with RA, especially among RF-positive patients as compared to those who are RF negative. However, patients with RA who have heart failure have an atypical presentation making it harder to detect and resulting in less aggressive management. Some evidence suggests patients with RA have heart failure related to diastolic dysfunction.[41]

Pulmonary involvement, such as *pleuritis* and pulmonary nodules, is frequent. Pulmonary involvement is more prevalent in men than women and among those with high rheumatoid titers. Nodes are more commonly found in the periphery of the upper and middle regions of the lung. Pulmonary nodules are found among seropositive patients with profuse synovitis and associated with the presence of nodules elsewhere in the body. Nodules may be 0.40 to 3 in. (1 to 8 cm) in size and affect gas exchange.[31]

Ocular Complications

Keratoconjunctivitis, inflammation of the cornea and conjunctiva, is the most common ocular complication in RA, impacting about 10% of all patients. The severity of this condition, however, is not proportional to the severity of RA. *Uveitis,* inflammation of the uvea located between the sclera and retina when present in RA, leads to blurred vision, dark, floating spots, eye pain, redness, and light sensitivity. *Episcleritis* is a benign and self-limiting process, affecting the episcleral tissues located between the conjunctiva and sclera, which typically correlates with RA disease activity.[42] Patients present with red and painful eyes with a diffuse or nodular distribution. *Scleritis,* inflammation of the sclera, is associated with long-standing disease and leads to eye pain, redness, blurred vision, tearing, and sensitivity to light. Untreated scleritis may lead to *scleromalacia,* a thinning of the sclera, and eventual blindness. The difference between episcleritis and scleritis is difficult to detect clinically. Therefore, patients with RA should undergo annual eye examinations and may require referral to an ophthalmologist.[34]

Activity Limitation and Participation Restriction

Patients with milder forms of RA suffer from activity limitations and decreased participation in ADL due to joint destruction. Almost 50% of individuals with RA will eventually have marked restrictions in ADL.[1,4] Late-onset RA is generally associated with better functional outcomes and less activity limitations and participation restrictions, though the cause of these findings is unclear. Loss of income is a major consequence of RA and is directly attributable to work disability. In a large international comparison study, work disability rates were high in persons with RA, and disability was associated with disease factors as well as societal factors.[43]

Prognosis

RA causes increased morbidity and reduces life span by as much as 3 to 10 years.[44] The question of mortality associated with RA is controversial. Previously, it was believed that RA itself was not usually a cause of death, although conditions such as systemic vasculitis and atlantoaxial subluxation could be fatal. There is presently a growing body of evidence that individuals with RA have decreased survival compared to their siblings and may not live as long as their counterparts without disease, especially if the early years of RA are marked by aggressive disease and poor functional status. Causes of death occurring more frequently in patients with RA as compared to the general population are infections; ischemic heart disease; and renal, respiratory, and gastrointestinal disease.[31,34,45]

Although numerous potential prognostic factors have been identified, there is no firm consensus regarding specific prognostic factors. Research suggests that individuals with a positive RF are more likely to progress to severe disease, as are those with high ESR and CRP at baseline. Baseline CRP is also associated with radiographic changes later in life.[46,47] Similarly, baseline radiographic tests are strongly associated with the

pattern of progression. Genetic research suggests that a shared epitope in the hypervariable region of the HLA-DR is associated with disease severity in a dose-dependent manner.[48]

Remission Criteria

Remission is the state of little to no active RA disease. In 2011, in response to the increasing ability to achieve remission with appropriate medical management, the ACR, EULAR, and the ACR Outcomes Measures in Rheumatology Initiatives developed a rigorous set of remission criteria, as new medications increased the chance patients could achieve remission and help researchers uniformly define remission as a therapeutic target for clinical practice and research. RA remission can be operationally confirmed based on one of two definitions: (a) when scores on the tender joint count, swollen joint count, CRP (in mg/dL), and the *Patient Global Assessment* (0–10 scale rating how patient feels overall) are all less than or equal to 1, or (b) when the score on the *Simplified Disease Activity Index* (numerical sum of all of the above plus the score on the Physician Global Assessment) is less than or equal to 3.3.[49]

■ OSTEOARTHRITIS

Osteoarthritis (OA) is primarily confined to one or more synovial joints and their surrounding soft tissues. Two predominant pathological features once defined OA: the progressive destruction of articular cartilage and the formation of bone at joint margins.[1] OA is now recognized as a disease involving the entire joint including the periarticular musculature.[50] Studies confirm that synovitis is an important pathological feature of OA, and synovial involvement (thickening and edema) may occur earlier than cartilage involvement.[51,52] Impairments, activity limitations, and participation restrictions related to OA extend far beyond the boundaries of the synovial joint. Data on the personal and societal impact of OA increasingly demonstrates its importance as an individual and public health issue.

Epidemiology

Osteoarthritis is the most common form of arthritis and extremely prevalent among individuals over 40 years of age. Based on data from A National Public Health Agenda for Osteoarthritis 2020, it is estimated that 32.5 million adults in the United States (1 in 7) are living with OA.[53] It is widespread in adults older than 65 years and affects men more than women before age 50 years, but distribution reverses after age 50 years.[1] Studies concerning racial predisposition to OA have yielded conflicting data, depending on the joint studied. Several longitudinal studies revealed the prevalence of radiographic and symptomatic knee OA was highest in non-Hispanic Black Americans compared to non-Hispanic White Americans or Mexican Americans, who had similar prevalence rates.[54] Chinese women were found to have a higher prevalence of radiographic and symptomatic knee OA compared with White females of the same age. Conversely, radiographic hip OA is lower among Chinese women, whereas similar rates of hip OA are reported when comparing Americans of African and European descent.[54]

Etiology

Similar to RA, no single factor has been identified that predisposes an individual to OA. Although aging is indeed strongly associated with OA, it must be emphasized that aging in itself does not cause OA, nor should OA be considered synonymous with the "normal" aging process.[1,55] In fact, many OA-related changes seen at both a cellular and tissue level are opposite those seen with normal aging.[56] Several factors related to aging may, however, contribute to its development. Genetic factors account for between 39% and 65% of radiographic OA of the hand, hip, and knee in women and as much as 70% of OA cases of the spine.[57] Recent data suggest the biomarkers, immunoglobulin lambda constant 1 (*IGLC1*) and immunoglobulin lambda variable 1-44 (*IGLV1–44*), both protein coding genes, may potentially play an important role in development of OA.[58]

Trauma before adulthood may initiate bone remodeling that alters joint mechanics and nutrition in a way that becomes problematic only later in life. Repetitive *microtrauma* has been implicated in the etiology of OA.[1] Specifically, occupational tasks involving heavy lifting are associated with the development of hip OA,[59] and those involving kneeling and heavy lifting are related to the development of knee OA.[59,60] Malalignment, including *varus* and *valgus* deformities, and leg length discrepancy are associated with greater prevalence of knee and hip OA, respectively[60,61] (Fig. 23.12). The strongest predictor of knee OA disease progression is varus malalignment.[62] *Femoroacetabular impingement* (FAI), a mechanical mismatch between the femoral head and acetabulum, plays a role in development of hip OA.[63] Obesity has been identified as a risk factor for the development of OA in later life, most evident in the knee OA and to a lesser extent for OA in the hip and hands.[1,61] Obesity is also associated with greater functional decline in knee OA.[64] The relationship between obesity and incidence of OA is stronger in women than in men. Risk factors for OA can be classified as systemic or local (Box 23.1), and OA most likely results from the combined effect of multiple factors acting on a vulnerable joint that leads to disease.[61,65] An important aspect of physical therapy management is the role the physical therapist plays in educating and counseling patients regarding modifiable factors for OA that are amenable to therapeutic interventions.

Pathophysiology
Normal Cartilage

Healthy articular cartilage is composed of an extracellular matrix and *chondrocytes*. By weight, the matrix consists

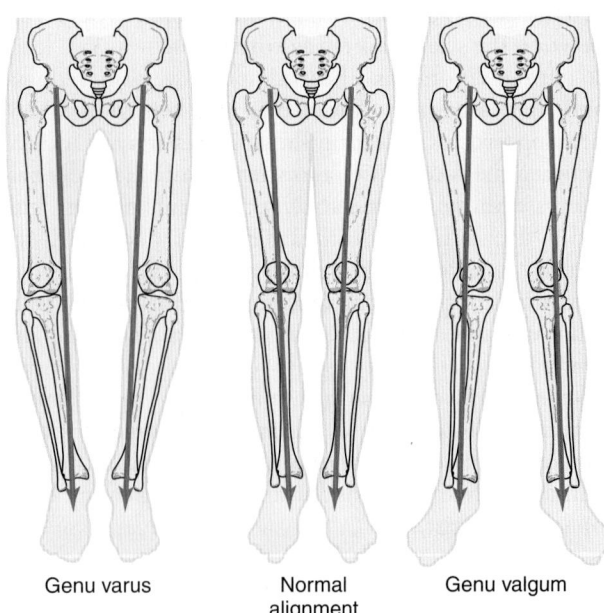

Genu varus   Normal alignment   Genu valgum

Figure 23.12 Varus and valgus knee alignment.

Box 23.1 Risk Factors for Osteoarthritis[61]

Systemic Factors
- Age
- Gender
- Race
- Genetics
- Metabolic/endocrine
- High bone density
- Nutritional status (e.g., vitamin D deficiency)
- Congenital/developmental
- Obesity

Local Factors
- Obesity
- Major joint trauma (e.g., anterior cruciate ligament rupture)
- Repetitive stress (occupation)
- Muscle weakness/imbalance
- Altered joint biomechanics
- Joint malalignment
- Proprioceptive impairments

of between 65% and 80% water, approximately 10% of mostly type II collagen, and the remainder consists of *proteoglycans* (molecules found in articular cartilage), noncollagenous proteins, and glycoproteins.[60,65] The matrix protects the chondrocytes from damage during normal joint use. Chondrocytes, the only cells in articular cartilage, secrete the matrix, yet make up only 1% of the total volume of adult human articular cartilage.[60]

Chondrocytes are dispersed throughout the extracellular matrix but are most concentrated in the deep layer. The superficial layer has the highest concentration of water and collagen fibers giving this zone the greatest tensile stiffness and strength to resist shearing forces.[60] Proteoglycans consist of a protein core and one or more glycosaminoglycans (GAGs), including hyaluronic acid (HA) and chondroitin sulfate. Proteoglycan concentration is highest in the middle and deep zones.[60]

Articular cartilage contains no nerves, blood vessels, or lymphatic vessels. It receives its nutrition and eliminates waste via diffusion through synovial fluid and by facilitated *imbibition* (absorption of fluid by a solid body).[60] The multiple roles of articular cartilage include decreasing friction between articulating joint surfaces, distributing static and dynamic joint forces to the underlying bone, and absorbing shock.[60,66] Cartilage's shock-absorbing function is minimal (1% to 3% of load forces), however, compared to that of subchondral bone (30%)[60] and periarticular muscles (which requires timely and coordinated muscle contraction). These joint structures together with ligaments, menisci, capsule, synovium, and synovial fluid serve to protect the joint from regular wear and tear and damaging forces. Regular forces acting on the articular cartilage include body weight, muscle contractions, and ground reaction forces that vary with the rate and duration of loading and the available load-bearing surface.[60,65] Extremes of joint loading in either direction can lead to detrimental morphological and metabolic changes in the cartilage, whereas moderate, cyclic loading enhances proteoglycan synthesis and concentration.[50,60]

Joint Pathology

Although traditionally viewed as a noninflammatory disease, improved detection methods suggest that inflammation does play a role and that inflammatory pathways are upregulated (increased responsiveness) with an increased production of cytokines.[1,55,60,66] Further inflammatory reactions occur in response to cartilage fragments in the synovial cavity and resultant low-grade synovitis.[60]

The first osteoarthritic change in articular cartilage confirmed in humans is an increase in water content. The increase in water suggests that the proteoglycans have become swollen far beyond normal. This process, combined with disruption of other components of the extracellular matrix, decreases matrix stiffness and leads to further mechanical damage.[60,65]

In later stages of disease progression, proteoglycans are lost. The loss of proteoglycans diminishes the water content of cartilage, and the articular cartilage loses its compressive stiffness and elasticity, which, in turn, results in the transmission of compressive forces to underlying bone. While collagen synthesis is increased initially, there is a shift from type II collagen fibers to a larger proportion of type I collagen, the kind found in skin and fibrous tissue. In response to early tissue damage, chondrocytes

synthesize new matrix molecules, proliferate, and form cell clusters.[60,66] As the articular cartilage is destroyed, the joint space narrows.[50] In summary, the early phases of cartilage degeneration are characterized by biosynthesis and repair as the chondrocytes attempt to restore the damaged matrix, while the later phase is degradative in nature as catabolic enzyme activity digests the matrix and erodes the cartilage. Age-related oxidative stress and *cell senescence* (reduced proliferation of cells) can further contribute to increased production of inflammatory *cytokines* and catabolic matrix metalloproteinases.[55,60,66]

One of the first noticeable changes in cartilage is the mild fraying or "flaking" of superficial collagen fibers. Deeper fraying, or "fibrillation," of the upper third of the cartilage follows in areas of greater weight-bearing and may progress to full-thickness fissures (Fig. 23.13). As the cartilage degenerates, there is evidence of increased density of subchondral bone (also called *subchondral sclerosis*), creation of cyst-like bone cavities, and formation of marginal *osteophytes*.[1,60,67] Cartilage degeneration may progress to the point where exposed subchondral bone becomes necrotic and *eburnated* (polished or ivorylike). The stiffer than normal subchondral bone further reduces the shock-absorbing properties of the joint and results in greater impact loading.[60] The traditional view of OA is that the disease process begins with an unrepaired articular cartilage injury; however, evidence suggests that reduced compliance in subchondral bone and periarticular structures may initiate degenerative processes.[60,66]

Osteophytes may be fibrous, cartilaginous, or bony in composition, and marginal prominences are palpable and often tender in more superficial joints.[1,60,67] The process of osteophyte formation in OA is not well understood. Current hypotheses have implicated increased vascularity in the deepest layers of the degenerated cartilage, venous congestion from subchondral cysts and thickened subchondral trabeculae, and continued sloughing of articular cartilage.[67] Each of these hypotheses may explain how bony growth contributes to the pain and motion loss that accompany OA. Subchondral cysts containing myxoid, fibrous, or cartilaginous tissue along with bone marrow lesions identified through MRI are associated with painful knee OA.[66,68]

Osteoarthritis Phenotypes and Endotypes

Given the heterogeneity of OA, *phenotypes* (observable characteristics of individuals including genetic and environmental factors) have been identified to better detect OA in early stages and identify those at risk of disease progression. These factors include the presentation of joint involvement, radiographic severity, depression, body mass index (BMI), muscle strength, and pain.[66] Greater recognition of those at risk of progression can, in turn, be used to guide clinical decision-making and lead to phenotype-specific therapeutic interventions.[65,69] Six different phenotypes have been described and include a chronic pain phenotype with central

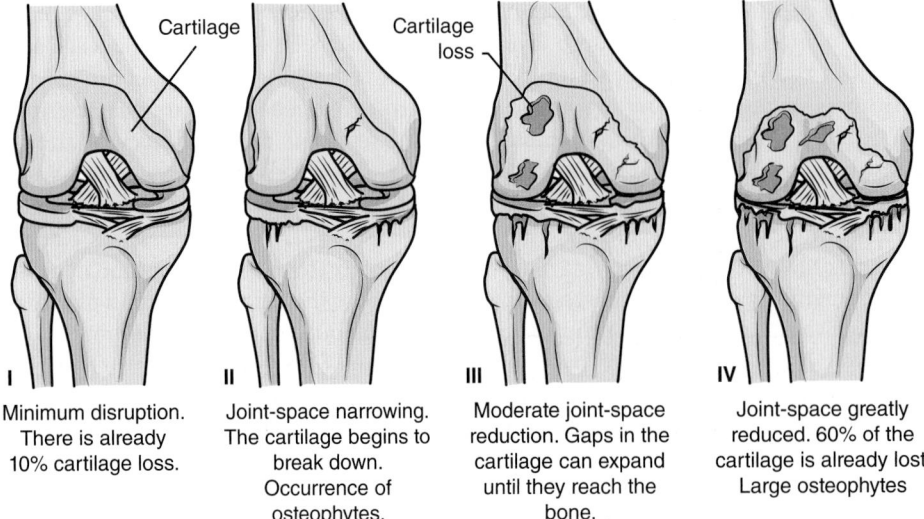

I	II	III	IV
Minimum disruption. There is already 10% cartilage loss.	Joint-space narrowing. The cartilage begins to break down. Occurrence of osteophytes.	Moderate joint-space reduction. Gaps in the cartilage can expand until they reach the bone.	Joint-space greatly reduced. 60% of the cartilage is already lost. Large osteophytes

Figure 23.13 Early to advanced osteoarthritis joint changes. Early joint changes are characterized by superficial damage to articular cartilage and mild inflammation (cartilage, clefts, and fibrillation). Progression to moderate joint changes includes joint space narrowing with full-thickness damage to cartilage and thickening of the subchondral bone. Advanced joint changes are marked by bony hypertrophy (marginal osteophytes), significant joint space narrowing, and possible angulation (deformity).

sensitization, an inflammatory phenotype, a metabolic syndrome phenotype, a bone and cartilage metabolism phenotype, a mechanical (malalignment) phenotype, and a minimal joint disease phenotype.

More recently, *endotypes* have received attention, and the discussion surrounding endotypes continues to evolve. *Endotypes* are another stratification of OA disease based on a functional or pathological molecular mechanism. For example, an inflammatory endotype can be related to a specific cytokine. Thus, an endotype can be helpful in developing a targeted intervention in OA.

Disease Onset and Course

Osteoarthritis usually starts in an insidious fashion and may progress undetected in some individuals when early, aneural articular cartilage is the only involved tissue. Pain is initially episodic and triggered by specific activity. In later disease, pain becomes a chronic, dull ache accentuated with episodic severe pain.[50] It is pain that leads an individual to seek medical help. Unlike RA, there are no systemic features such as fatigue, fever, or malaise with OA onset.

OA is typically a slowly progressive condition; however, most people with radiographic evidence of joint damage in their hips or knees stabilize and do not require joint replacement surgery[1] (see Fig. 23.13 and Fig. 23.14). The pathological process involved in OA appears to be cyclical with active periods of increased matrix protein turnover interspersed with inactive phases.[70] Prognosis is variable and not necessarily bad. However, comorbidities increase with normal aging,

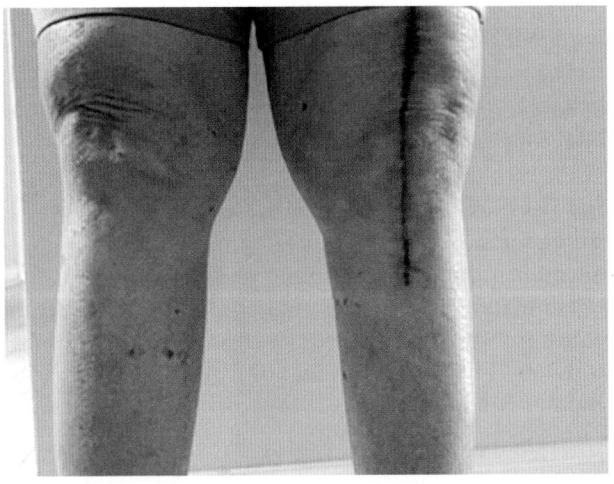

Figure 23.14 Patient with knee osteoarthritis who has had a total knee arthroplasty.

leading to greater risk of physical inactivity which can contribute to increasing disability.[1]

Classification and Diagnostic Criteria

OA is typically differentiated in two ways: *primary* (*idiopathic*) and *secondary* disease.[1] When the disease etiology is unknown with no known prior event, it is termed *primary* or *idiopathic* OA. This category can be further divided into *localized* (one or two joints affected) or *generalized* OA (affecting three or more joints).[1] Generalized OA typically involves the hands in a more symmetrical fashion not unlike inflammatory forms of arthritis and has a stronger genetic association.[1] Secondary OA is defined as known etiology (e.g., trauma, biomechanical factors, congenital malformation, or other musculoskeletal disease). As our ability to detect subtle and early biochemical, histological, morphological, and biomechanical factors improves, the evidence suggests many cases categorized as idiopathic are more appropriately recognized as secondary disease.

Most researchers have used Kellgren and Lawrence's *radiographic classification system* and their grade 2 definition (the presence of definite osteophytes) as the criterion for identifying disease, although a few others have required evidence of joint space narrowing (grade 3 corresponding to clinically identified disease) to designate OA.[71] This five-point system remains the most widely used criteria for grading radiographic changes both clinically and for purposes of research.[71]

- Grade 0: normal radiograph
- Grade 1: doubtful narrowing of the joint space and possible osteophytes
- Grade 2: definite osteophytes and absent or questionable narrowing of the joint space
- Grade 3: moderate osteophytes and joint space narrowing, some sclerosis, and possible deformity
- Grade 4: large osteophytes, marked narrowing of joint space, severe sclerosis, and definite deformity

It is widely recognized, however, that radiographic findings are not strongly correlated to clinical symptoms and pain severity[61] and add little to the accuracy of the clinical diagnosis. In knee OA, muscle strength and pain are more explanatory of functional loss than radiographic findings.[72] Radiographs are frequently used to confirm the extent of joint damage and disease progression and continue to be a component of the ACR diagnostic criteria.[50] The clinical criteria for hip,[73] knee,[74] and hand[75] OA are described primarily in terms of pain and limitation of motion (Box 23.2).

Radiography/Diagnostic Imaging

Newer imaging techniques including high-resolution MRI are able to detect early structural changes and pathology in pain-sensitive structures well before changes are observable on radiographs.[50,76] Real-time ultrasound allows visualization of both bony and soft tissue structures and is more sensitive than clinical examination in detecting effusion, synovitis, and early osteophytes in OA.[76] Ultrasound imaging has greater potential for routine use in clinical practice than MRI.

Clinical Presentation

Signs and Symptoms (Impairments)

As noted already, the clinical diagnosis is often made based on signs and symptoms (e.g., pain and swelling, loss of ROM, and bony deformity). Not all joints are equally affected by OA. In the upper extremity (UE),

Box 23.2 Clinical Classification Criteria for Knee, Hip, and Hand Osteoarthritis

Knee Osteoarthritis[74]

- Persistent knee pain
- Limited morning stiffness ≤30 minutes
- Reduced function
- Crepitus
- Bony enlargement
- Restricted movement

Hip Osteoarthritis[b73]

Pain present in combination with either

- Hip internal rotation ≥15°; morning stiffness ≤60 minutes; and age older than 50 years, and pain on internal rotation, *or*
- Hip internal rotation less than 15° and hip flexion less than 115°

Hand Osteoarthritis[c75]

- Presence of Heberden nodes
- Age older than 40 years
- Family history of nodes
- Joint space narrowing in any finger joint

[a]Correctly diagnoses 99% of knee osteoarthritis when all six criteria are met.[74]
[b]86% sensitivity, 75% specificity.[73]
[c]Correctly diagnoses 88% of patients when all four criteria are met.[75]

the finger DIP and PIP joints and CMC of the thumb are commonly involved. The cervical and lumbar spine, hips, knees, and MTP of the great toe are also sites for OA. The MCP joints, wrists, elbows, and shoulders are usually spared in primary OA.[1] Unlike RA, OA does not have a bilateral, symmetrical presentation (with the exception of generalized OA)[1]. A single joint or any combination of joints may be affected and may be of differing etiologic origins. OA is not a systemic disease; however, severe fatigue is reported by nearly half of patients with hip and knee OA and is associated with factors such as greater pain, less physical activity, and depression.[77] Individuals with OA may experience some stiffness in particular joints on awakening that is similar to the stiffness felt when moving the same joints after inactivity during the day, but this stiffness (articular gelling) typically does not last more than 30 minutes, nor is it generalized to the entire body.[1,50] Crepitus is a common clinical finding in OA and may progress from a painless grating sensation to an extremely painful, high-pitched sound as a result of bone-on-bone articulation.

Although cartilage degeneration is the primary manifestation of OA, cartilage is aneural and therefore not the cause of a person's pain. Pain in OA can arise from any innervated tissue and may be attributed to incongruent articulations of joint surfaces, periosteal elevation secondary to osteophytes, vasocongestion in subchondral bone, trabecular microfractures, distention of the joint capsule and ligaments, and muscle spasm or strain.[50,66,68] Many patients with knee OA will also experience a secondary synovitis and effusion.[66,68]

As noted earlier, symptoms do not always match disease severity on radiographs. Further, some patients with OA may have an amplified pain experience and central pain sensitization at the spinal or cortical level.[66] Unlike individuals with RA who often report more pain and stiffness at rest, the pain associated with OA is likely to occur or worsen with motion, except in the later stages of the disease when it is present at rest and with activity.[1,50]

Joints

OA may present differently and result in varied levels of impairment depending on the joints involved.

The most affected joints are described and noted on the homunculus (Fig. 23.15).

HANDS AND FINGERS

In the hand, DIP and PIP involvement may result in reduced ROM, poor grip strength, bony nodes, and joint angulation because of stretched collateral ligaments or bone erosion. *Bouchard nodes* at the PIP joints and *Heberden nodes* at the DIP joints are often tender in the early stages and can lead to marked restrictions in finger ROM and fine motor skills as the disease advances (Fig. 23.16). Osteoarthritic damage in the first CMC joint results in pain or aching at the base of the thumb and can lead to decreased pinch strength and squaring of the thumb (thickening and prominence of CMC due to subluxation of first metacarpal) as a result of weakness and contracture of the thenar muscles.[78] This in turn affects abduction, extension, and opposition ROM

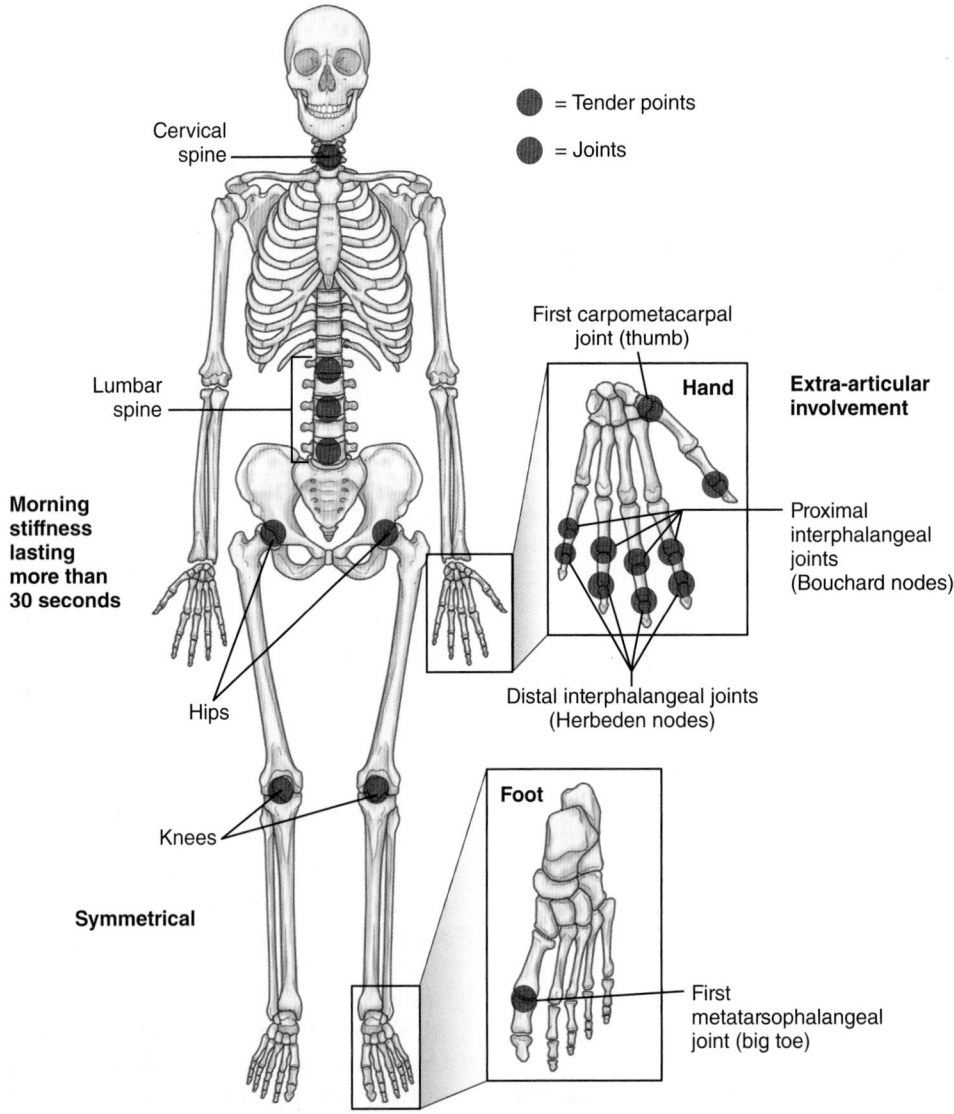

Figure 23.15 Homunculus showing common joints affected by osteoarthritis.

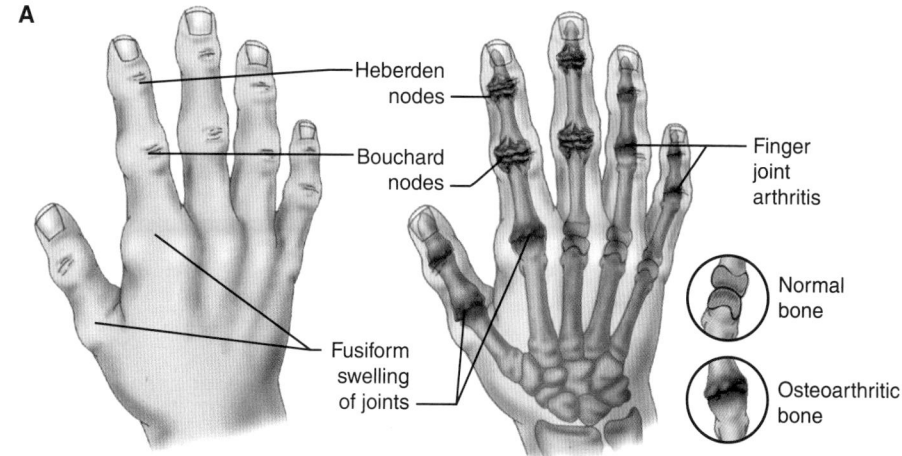

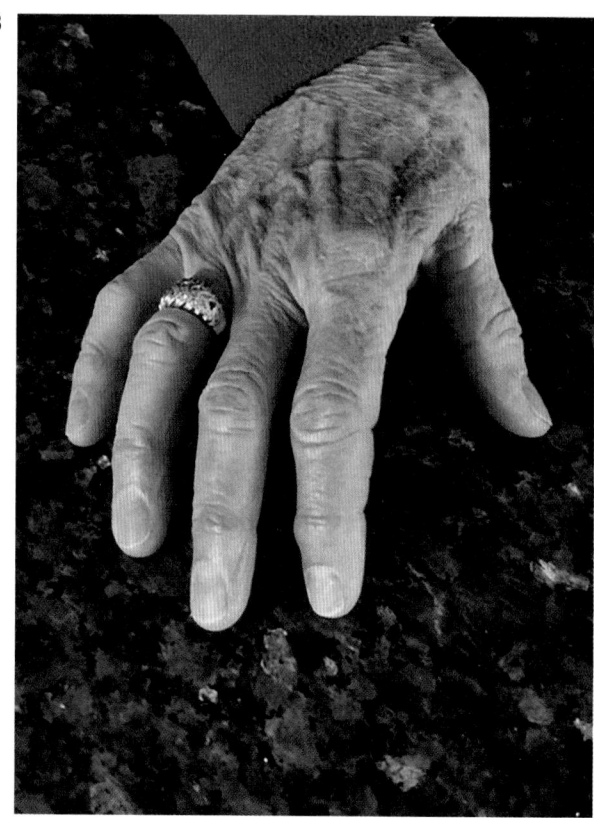

Figure 23.16 (A) Osteoarthritis (OA) of the hand showing Heberden and Bouchard nodes and OA changes at the carpal metacarpal joint involvement. (B) OA in the hand illustrating patient with Heberden nodes at the index finger.

of the thumb and greatly affects grip strength and hand function.[79] In cases of generalized OA, the hands are always affected and in a more symmetrical pattern.[1] Painful inflammation with synovitis, erosive changes, cystic swellings, and osteophytes are present in this less common form of OA and may lead to ankylosis of the DIP and PIP joints.[1,78]

Hips

Symptoms of hip OA are usually insidious in onset and may include antalgic gait and decreased ROM with a tendency for the hip to be held in a somewhat flexed,

abducted, and externally rotated position. Internal rotation is usually restricted and painful.[80] Pain arising from the hip joint is commonly experienced in the groin but can also be felt in the buttock, trochanteric, or knee region.[80,81] Lateral hip pain is most often associated with gluteus medius and minimus tendinopathy and often misdiagnosed as trochanteric bursitis.[82] Decreased hip ROM and proximal hip weakness, most notably the gluteal muscles, and soft tissue shortening, especially in the rectus femoris, are common.[83] Hip OA is associated with decreased walking speed, decreased stride length, poor balance, and increased energy leading to an increased risk of falls.[81] Even early hip OA is associated with a 52% increased risk of falls.[84]

KNEES

Early presentation of knee OA includes pain with weight-bearing activities such as climbing stairs and squatting. In later stages, both pain and stiffness are reported after prolonged sitting. Symptoms of joint locking and buckling (giving way) may occur with damage to stabilizing menisci and ligaments[80] and lead to increased risk of falls.[50] Knee OA more commonly affects the medial joint due to the higher weight-bearing load placed on this compartment. As a result, medial joint space narrowing often results in *pseudolaxity* of the medial collateral ligament (the ligament no longer covers the same distance as before joint changes occur), stretching of the lateral collateral counterpart, and genu varus deformity (see Fig. 23.12). Genu valgus due to greater lateral compartment involvement is less common. A *flexion deformity* of several degrees can develop quickly in the painful knee and contribute to a functional leg length discrepancy, decreased step length, and quadriceps muscular fatigue or strain. Patellofemoral compartment OA, with its hallmark anterior knee pain, can occur in isolation as a result of patella malalignment, abnormal tracking and loading, and direct trauma to the patella.[80]

FEET AND TOES

Two distinct phenotypes of foot OA are suggested. Isolated first MTP joint OA is the most common and may result in hallux rigidus or hallux valgus deformities, first interphalangeal joint hyperextension, and hindfoot eversion. Polyarticular foot OA with changes in the other MTP joints, toes, and medial tarsal joints can lead to shortening of the long extensors, hammer toes, reduced MTP flexion, and flattened sagittal arch[85,86] (Fig. 23.17). Forefoot involvement contributes to painful and limited push-off in the terminal stance phase of gait, slower walking speed, and balance issues.[85,86]

SPINE

The lower cervical and mid to lower lumbar regions are most susceptible to OA. All spinal articulations can experience degenerative changes; however, the facet (zygapophyseal) joints are the only true synovial joints in the spine.[87] Degeneration of the intervertebral disks may precede facet joint involvement by many years and lead to increased compressive loads and degenerative changes. Facet joint osteophytes can contribute to lateral and central lumbar stenosis and subsequent nerve root impingement[87] (Fig. 23.18). Pain from lumbar facet joint OA can originate from the joint itself and affected nerve roots (radicular pain) in the lumbar area, and typically increases with spinal extension, rotary motions, and prolonged standing or sitting.[87]

Consequences of Osteoarthritis

Although not a systemic illness, OA has been linked to an increased risk of cardiovascular disease (CVD) and all-cause mortality. In a large Canadian cohort of older adults with hip/knee OA followed over 10 years, greater self-reported functional disability, walking disability, and use of a walking aid were associated with all-cause mortality and risk for a serious CVD event even after controlling for comorbidities such as obesity, diabetes, and hypertension.[88] Physical therapy interventions to reduce walking disability may have an important protective effect.

Osteoarthritis dramatically affects quality of life, leading to a higher incidence and prevalence of depression and anxiety. Indeed, roughly 20% of patients with knee OA suffer from depression and anxiety.[89] Anxiety and depression are significantly correlated with one another and with pain experience and are key influencers of outcomes. The variability of depression and anxiety cannot be explained by pathology alone. In fact, depression and anxiety are better predictors of disability than radiographic evidence of OA. Thus, physical therapists

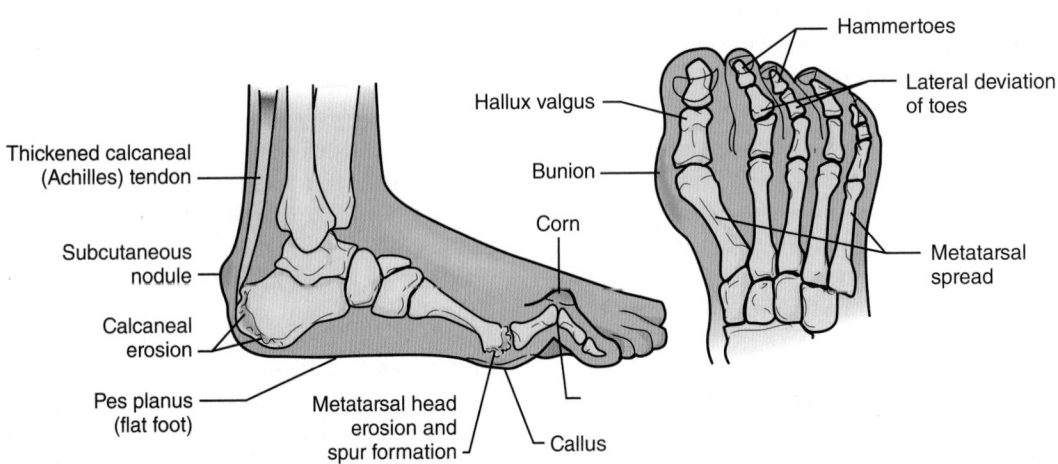

Figure 23.17 Osteoarthritic foot.

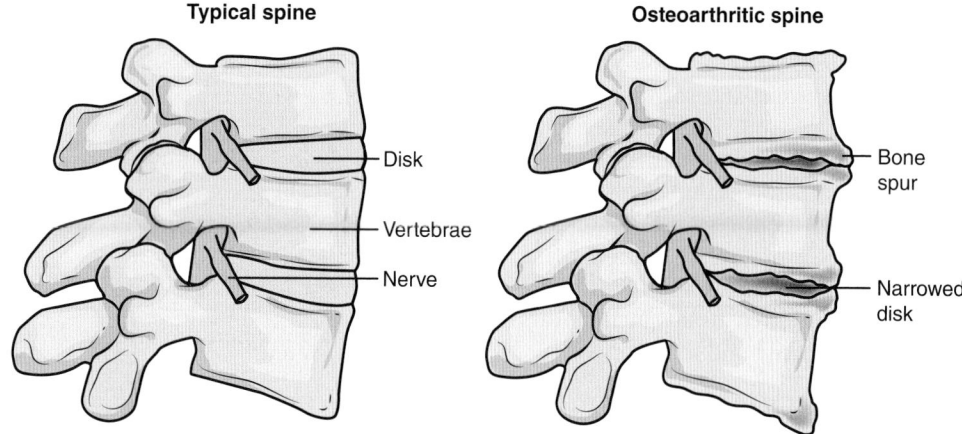

Figure 23.18 Osteoarthritis of the spine.

should incorporate a simple depression and anxiety screen for patients with OA in their comprehensive physical examination (Box 23.3).

Activity Limitations and Participation Restrictions

Overall, OA of the knee can impose functional limitations to a degree equivalent to heart disease, congestive heart failure, and chronic obstructive pulmonary disease and accounts for a substantial proportion of the burden of disability among community-living older adults.[90]

Patients with the most severe disease may not move their joints as often or in the ways that exacerbate their symptoms. Therefore, pain, disease severity, and functional disability in individuals with OA are interrelated. Among older adults, it has been shown that the functional loss associated with severe radiographic OA without pain is more likely than the loss associated with symptomatic but milder disease.[91] One explanation for this finding is that individuals with OA limit their functional activities to avoid movements that are painful. Given that individuals with OA may reduce or eliminate their symptoms by avoiding certain activities, clinicians should explore activity limitations and physical inactivity–related symptoms in patients with OA separately from the evaluation of symptoms.

OA is a leading cause of disability and major contributor to work-related disability, reduced productivity, and absenteeism.[92] In a study of Finnish adults ages 60 to 80 years with advanced knee OA, greater self-reported disability was associated with pain, joint laxity, age, and BMI, while performance-based functioning was related to the self-reported function using the *Western Ontario and McMaster Universities Osteoarthritis Index* (WOMAC) function score, pain, and obesity.[72] Of interest, the authors found no association between radiographic severity of knee OA and self-reported and performance-based function.[72] The comprehensive *International Classification of Functioning, Disability,*

 Box 23.3   Depression and Anxiety Screening Questions and Tools

Patient Health Questionnaire

Screening Questions for Depression
- During the past 2 weeks have you been bothered by feeling down, hopeless, or depressed?
- During the past 2 weeks have you been bothered by little interest in doing things?

RESPONSES: not at all (0) several days (1) more than half of the days (2) nearly every day (3). The score ranges from 0–6. A cut point of 3 is used to identify possible depressive disorder. Patients should be further screened with the Patient Health Questionnaire-9 and referred to the appropriate licensed mental health provider.

Screening Questions for Generalized Anxiety Disorder (GAD-2)
- Over the last 2 weeks how often have you felt nervous, anxious, or on edge?
- Over the last 2 weeks how often have you not been able to stop or control worrying?

RESPONSES: not at all (0) several days (1) more than half of the days (2) nearly every day (3). Thus, the score range is 0–6. To determine risk score, sum the points allocated to the two items based on the patient's response. A cut point of 3 is the threshold indicating a need for further follow-up by a licensed mental health provider.

Source: Adapted from Mental Health Disorder Screening available at https://www.hiv.uw.edu/page/mental-health-screening/gad-2

and Health (ICF) *Core Set* of impairments, activity limitations, and participation restrictions was established by an international team of researchers, clinicians, and patients to identify areas of functioning that are affected by OA, with the shorter Brief ICF Core Set created for clinical purposes.[93,94]

Prognosis

OA is a slow-progressing disease that can be self-limiting or can progress to advanced joint and soft tissue damage and complete joint failure. In such a case, joint surgery including *arthrodesis* of some joints in the foot, or *arthroplasty* (replacement), for example, of the hip or knee is used to help the patient regain function and reduce pain. However, rapidly progressive joint damage is uncommon; in most cases, patients stabilize.[1] Increasing disability may be more related to advancing years and comorbidities such as obesity and inactivity.

■ MEDICAL MANAGEMENT

Pharmacological Therapy in Rheumatoid Arthritis

Current medical management is based on the implementation of an early, aggressive, treat-to-target approach. The treat-to-target approach to disease management is an aggressive pharmacological approach with regular clinical monitoring, designed to help the patient reach remission or low disease activity and eventually to halt disease or decrease progression.[95] Medical therapies also focus on decreasing pain and inflammation. Early aggressive pharmacological therapy is associated with diminished joint damage and long-term maintenance of function. The major classifications of drugs used in RA management include nonsteroidal anti-inflammatory drugs (NSAIDs), corticosteroids, and disease-modifying antirheumatic drugs (DMARDs), which include the biological response modifiers (BRMs) and Janus kinase (JAK) inhibitors.[95]

Nonsteroidal Anti-Inflammatory Drugs

NSAIDs are generally given in combination with other DMARDs. NSAIDs provide both *analgesic* and *anti-inflammatory* effects depending on the dose prescribed; however, they do not alter disease progression. Discontinuance of NSAIDs quickly leads to exacerbation of symptoms. At lower doses, the NSAID effect is analgesic through the peripheral inhibition of pro-inflammatory prostaglandin synthesis. At higher doses, the effect is anti-inflammatory, probably through both prostaglandin inhibition and alterations in macrophage and neutrophil function. Due to the mechanism of action of these medications, adverse effects include gastrointestinal (GI) complaints and renal effects. Mild GI adverse effects include distress and nausea. However, approximately 2% to 4% of patients experience serious adverse effects including GI bleeding, ulcers, and perforation. Patients are encouraged to take these medications with food, to monitor GI signs, and are given prophylactic therapy to decrease GI damage. Renal and other adverse effects associated with continued use and high doses of NSAIDs include dizziness, drowsiness, headache, tinnitus (ringing in the ears), kidney dysfunction, and elevation of liver enzymes. CBCs and stool guaiac analyses for occult blood should be conducted every 3 to 4 months to monitor for potential adverse effects.[95]

There are two primary categories of NSAIDs, based on whether they inhibit COX-1 and COX-2 enzymes or COX-2 enzymes alone. These enzymes are responsible for synthesis of prostaglandins. Traditional NSAIDs block both COX-1 and COX-2 enzymes. The main function of the COX-1 enzyme is synthesis of prostaglandins in the endothelium and gastric mucosa, tissues present in the stomach lining and kidneys. Caution should be taken when prescribing NSAIDs to specific groups of patients at risk for GI complications such as older adults, smokers, those taking corticosteroids, and those with severe arthritis, comorbidities, and history of GI symptoms. The selective COX-2 inhibitors were designed to decrease the risk of GI toxicity by inhibiting only the COX-2 enzyme, which is responsible for the pain and swelling associated with inflammation. Early studies of short-duration exposure supported the reduced risk of GI side effects and increased tolerability of COX-2 inhibitors.[96] However, studies of longer selective COX-2 exposure and systematic evaluation of the data from numerous trials indicate that patients on selective COX-2 inhibitors are at greater risk of acute myocardial infarction and other cardiovascular events.[97–99]

NSAIDs are an accessible and relatively inexpensive drug to manage inflammation; however, the decision to prescribe an NSAID must be based on risk factors, known toxicities, and dosing preferences. Individual response to an NSAID is extremely variable in effectiveness and tolerance. Therefore, it often requires several month-long trials to find the best product. Taking more than one NSAID increases the risk of toxicity with no increase in benefit. NSAIDs are prescribed for patients with RA at the onset of symptoms to provide rapid pain relief and control of inflammation while waiting for the slower-acting DMARD to become effective.

Disease-Modifying Antirheumatic Drugs

DMARDs are the primary class of drugs for managing disease progression in RA. These include an array of drugs with varying chemical structures, modes of actions, clinical indications, and toxicities. There are three classifications of DMARDs: conventional DMARDs (cDMARDs), BRMs, and *Janus kinase (JAK) inhibitors*. Each class is discussed in the following sections.

Conventional Disease-Modifying Antirheumatic Drugs

Conventional DMARDs used to manage RA include antimalarials, methotrexate (MTX), sulfasalazine, and leflunomide. Although DMARDs are effective in reducing disease progression, these medications do not provide an analgesic effect and are slow acting, taking from 3 weeks to 3 months to take effect. A drug that is classified as a DMARD must show evidence of affecting the course of RA for at least 1 year (improved function, reduced inflammation, and slowing or prevention of structural damage). Given its relative low cost and safety profile, oral MTX is the most widely used conventional cDMARD[100] and is also considered the drug of choice for DMARD-naive patients with moderate to high disease activity.[101]

DMARDs may be given alone or in combination for best effectiveness.[101] DMARDs are most often used to treat adult-onset RA, and individuals taking them should be monitored regularly for the toxicities accompanying the specific drug.[34] Advances in medical management and the treat-to-target approach have led to a recognition of the importance of initiating conventional synthetic (csDMARD) therapy in combination with low-dose glucocorticoids. Additionally, it is well noted that MTX given in proper doses and in conjunction with folate is the major player in the management of RA.[100] The ACR provides specific recommendations regarding the types of DMARDs given to patients who have comorbidities such as heart failure, hepatitis B infection, or pulmonary disease.[101]

Biological Response Modifiers

BRMs are a class of disease-modifying agents used since 1998. These medications are biologically engineered to mimic the activities of targeted immune cells to reduce or block the inflammatory process. These drugs are approved to treat moderate to severe RA that is nonresponsive to traditional therapy. Unlike other RA medications, these drugs are engineered to target specific components of the immune system. The mechanism of action of BRMs varies and inhibition of cytokine activity, by blocking tumor necrosis factor–alpha (a pro-inflammatory cytokine) or interleukin-1 to their receptors. Some biologics are immunoglobulin isotypes, such as IgG1, fusion proteins that block the costimulatory signal required for T-cell activation (T cells or T lymphocytes are a subtype of white blood cells), a central component of the RA inflammatory response. Thus, the drug will work "upstream" in the inflammatory cascade compared with other biologic agents. Another form of biologic therapy is a monoclonal antibody (MAb) that binds to CD20, a cell marker expressed on mature B cells (B lymphocytes) and pre-B cells, leading to selective depletion of CD20+ B cells via several mechanisms.[102] The half-life and dosing of these drugs are important considerations as they impact the frequency, cost, and mode of drug delivery (e.g., IV). Research demonstrates these drugs result in inhibition of the progression of structural damage and improvement of physical function in RA. Biologics represent a significant advancement in the treatment of RA. Patients who begin BRMs usually continue with their NSAIDs, corticosteroids, or other RA medication. These medications can be given by injection or infusion. In fewer than 30% of patients, there may be a rash and an injection site reaction. Severe allergic reaction is also a potential outcome, so patients are routinely monitored during infusion of the medication. Adverse effects of these medications can be quite serious, and patients must be monitored for signs of infection, including colds and flus, which can rapidly progress during immunosuppression. Those with a history of tuberculosis (TB) are at risk for reactivation of TB and may be excluded from this form of therapy. The number of diseases in which these agents are useful continues to expand as do the number and types of agents available.[102]

Janus Kinase (JAK) inhibitors

In recent years, a third category of DMARDs, *Janus kinase (JAK) inhibitors,* have been introduced in the treatment of individuals with RA who experienced an inadequate response to conventional DMARDs. JAK inhibitors are small-molecule oral treatments that block the four Janus kinase enzymes: JAK1, JAK2, JAK3, and tyrosine kinase 2 (TYK2), that play a role in the cell-signaling processes leading to inflammation and immune responses observed in RA.[103] They are cytoplasmic tyrosine kinases that mediate the intracellular signaling by association with type 1 and type II cytokine receptors. JAK activation leads to activation of their downstream substrates, the signal transducer and activator of transcription (STAT) proteins, followed by their nuclear translocation and subsequent activity of target genes. JAK activation stimulates cell proliferation, differentiation, migration, and apoptosis.[104,105] Since many type I and II cytokines that are involved in RA pathogenesis exert their function through the JAK-STAT pathway, JAK targeting may cause immunosuppression. Their rapid clinical efficacy, the lack of immunogenicity, oral administration, and their short half-life are important advantages, though medication costs are high. Their safety profile is in line with other DMARDs, and adverse reactions include an increased risk of herpes zoster infection and thromboembolic events that need further evaluation. JAK inhibitors may be prescribed on their own or in conjunction with other DMARDs in the treatment of RA.[101]

Corticosteroids

Corticosteroids are powerful anti-inflammatory drugs creating rapid and potent suppression of inflammation. Corticosteroids are generally not given alone and may be administered orally, intravenously, or via intra-articular or periarticular injection. Often, they are prescribed in the presence of unremitting disease and severe extra-articular inflammation and given in combination with other RA medications (e.g., a slower-acting DMARD) until the DMARD has reached therapeutic levels. Unfortunately, these potent inflammatory medications also produce serious adverse effects when used long term or in high doses. Potential adverse effects include thinning of the skin, osteoporosis, muscle wasting, adrenal suppression, increased susceptibility to infections, impaired wound healing, cataracts, glaucoma, hyperlipidemia, and aseptic bone necrosis. Resistance exercise or heavy physical activity in the presence of high-dose steroids can lead to tendon rupture.[106]

Corticosteroids are often prescribed in *pulse doses* (low tapering doses over a specific time period) to reduce the risk of side effects. Patients on corticosteroids should have their blood counts, serum potassium, and glucose levels monitored and be observed for potential side effects.[34] When inflammation is confined to a specific location, steroid injections into a joint, bursa, tendon, or tendon sheath may be administered. However, use of steroid injections is commonly limited to no more than two to four per year to reduce the risk of osteonecrosis and soft tissue damage.

Immunization

Patients with RA are at risk of infection due to the nature of the disease pathology (autoimmune) as well as the immunosuppressive agents used to treat the disease. The influenza and herpes zoster (if over 50 years old) vaccine should be given annually, diphtheria-polio-tetanus every 10 years, and the pneumococcal vaccine every 5 years, in accordance with the vaccines recommended for the general population. With regard to the COVID-19 vaccine, the Centers for Disease Control and Prevention (CDC) recommends those who are immunocompromised receive a COVD-19 vaccine primary series as well as a booster shot. Those who are moderately or severely immunocompromised may receive an additional primary shot in lieu of the booster. It is necessary for patients with RA to discuss vaccine type and timing with rheumatologists or primary care doctors to ensure safe administration.[107,108]

Pharmacological Therapy in Osteoarthritis

To date, drug therapy in OA has no effect on disease progression and is ancillary to nonpharmacological approaches to pain management including patient education and self-management, weight loss, joint protection, and exercise.[62,74,109–112] The goals of drug therapy in patients with OA are to relieve pain and decrease inflammation when it is present. Oral and topical NSAIDs and corticosteroid injections are the primary medications used in OA management.[1,109,110,112]

Nonsteroidal Anti-Inflammatory Agents

NSAIDs are the primary medications in the management of persons with OA and are strongly recommended for use in managing OA. NSAIDs should be kept to the lowest effective dose and for the shortest durations needed to minimize GI toxicity. The COX-2 NSAIDs, described for RA management, had been prescribed for people who are at increased risk for GI problems until longer-term trials called their safety into question.

Topical Analgesics and Anti-Inflammatory Preparations

Topical agents include analgesics and anti-inflammatory preparations. Topical analgesics may be rubefacients, which contain methyl salicylate, chemical compounds that produce a counterirritant effect, or capsaicin compounds, which reduce pain through depletion of the neurotransmitter substance P in peripheral nerves. To date, the only topical analgesic to show consistent efficacy in controlled clinical trials is capsaicin, and this is the only topical agent recommended in the 2019 ACR clinical practice guidelines.[110] Capsaicin is an alkaloid derived from red chili peppers and is available in topical analgesic creams in varying concentrations (Zostrix, Capsaicin-P, Dolorac). It has been shown to decrease pain approximately 33% when applied to specific joints four times daily.[109] The initial stinging or burning sensation disappears after several days of use; however, the need for frequent daily applications may limit the acceptability of this therapy for some patients. Topical NSAIDs (diclofenac sodium) are recommended as alternative or adjunctive therapy in symptomatic peripheral joint OA and are conditionally recommended for use by the ACR.[110] Topical preparations delivered through gel, liquid, or patch formulations are absorbed through the skin with the help of an absorption enhancer and are slightly less or equally effective as oral NSAIDs with fewer adverse events.[50,109,113]

Corticosteroid Injections

Intra-articular corticosteroid injections are strongly recommended for adults with hip or knee OA and conditionally recommended for those with hand OA. Intra-articular corticosteroid injections are often used for acute episodes with a moderate effect for pain relief, irrespective of the number of injections.[109] The knee is the most common site; however, soft tissue injections for subacromial, anserine, and trochanteric bursitis also may be effective. The use of ultrasound guidance of injection is recommended when available.

Viscosupplementation

Viscosupplementation or intra-articular knee injections using a form of HA is conditionally recommended in some guidelines.[109,114] A number of synthetic forms are available (Synvisc, Hyalgan, Artzal). HA is a naturally occurring polysaccharide that contributes to the thickness and viscosity of joint fluid in the healthy joint. In a knee with OA, the levels of HA are lower and the joint fluid is thinner and less dense, reducing the ability of the fluid to lubricate and attenuate shock. Viscosupplementation therapy consists of a series of weekly injections. The reported effects of treatment are reduced pain and stiffness and improved function in people with mild to moderate knee OA, which may last for several months.[109] It is not clear if HA injections are more effective than corticosteroid injections, NSAIDs, or placebo injections. The injected HA does not replace normal joint fluid to achieve its effect as most is absorbed and cleared from the joint within a week. The risk of adverse effects is low. The most serious reported adverse event is an allergic reaction, and less serious effects are injection site reactions and joint swelling. There is no evidence that supports increased efficacy of one product over another; however, high molecular weight hylan (Synvisc) may have greater efficacy.[109]

Glucosamine Sulfate and Glucosamine Hydrochloride

Despite its widespread use by patients, recent clinical practice guidelines published by the ACR strongly recommend against the use of glucosamine sulfate (GS) and glucosamine hydrochloride (GH) in the management of hip and knee OA. Glucosamine, naturally produced by the body, is a structural component of cartilage. Many synthetic versions are available commercially as dietary supplements. The recent recommendation against GS and GH is due to conflicting results in clinical trials and little to no benefit over placebo.[110]

Acetaminophen

Acetaminophen, an oral analgesic, is conditionally recommended for adults with hip, knee and hand OA due to the limited impact on pain in randomized controlled trials of acetaminophen for this population.[110] Acetaminophen-containing compounds (Tylenol, Panadol, Anacin-3) have been cited as having almost no toxicity in recommended doses (up to 4 g/day) and little or no GI side effects. Since acetaminophen has no anti-inflammatory effect, it cannot be substituted for NSAIDs in this regard. Acetaminophen also has no significant effect on stiffness or physical function in patients with symptomatic knee OA.[74] Further, acetaminophen use can lead to liver and, less commonly, kidney toxicity, especially in individuals who drink excessive amounts of alcohol. There is increasing evidence of an increased incidence of hospitalization due to GI perforation, peptic ulceration, and bleeding with acetaminophen use of greater than 3 g/day compared to lower doses (less than 3 g/day).[74] In individuals where NSAIDs are contraindicated, acetaminophen may be appropriate.

Antidepressants

Due to the high prevalence of depression and anxiety experienced in persons with hip and knee OA, the 2019 ACR practice guideline conditionally recommends duloxetine, an antidepressant, for the management of OA. Among the variety of centrally acting medications used to manage chronic pain, only duloxetine has sufficient evidence of benefit. However, the use of antidepressants involves discussion and shared decision-making with the patient and provider.[110]

Opioids

Prescription opioids are medications that may be used in the treatment of acute and chronic pain; however, a lack of evidence exists of their long-term effectiveness for individuals with arthritis.[115] Data demonstrate that between 4% and 40% of patients with RA use opioids on a long-term basis. Similarly, long-term opioid use is reported for 8% to 26% of Medicare patients with OA.[116] Over the last two decades there has been an increase in the prescription of opioids; however, opioids may cause significant side effects in addition to the risk of misuse, addiction, overdose, and death. Opioids were involved in 49,860 overdose deaths in 2019.[117] A study of adults with knee and hip OA suggested that a year of taking over-the-counter medications resulted in a greater reduction in pain than among those taking opioids. The ACR conditionally recommends tramadol, an opioid, only for those patients who have contraindications for NSAIDs use or are not candidates for surgery. Physicians must carefully evaluate and consider the risk of addiction when prescribing tramadol.[110] In alignment with the American Physical Therapy Association's stance on pain management, pain should be patient-centered with attention to functional status, comorbid disease, severity of pain, and expected outcome goals. Physical therapy can reduce the symptoms of chronic disease which may help to avoid surgery and prescription drug use while maximizing mobility and improving physical function and quality of life.

Medical Marijuana (Cannabis)

Cannabis has been used for thousands of years to treat a multitude of medical conditions including chronic pain.[118] The *Cannabis* plant affects the human body through its chemically active substances or compounds termed cannabinoids. Of those identified, tetrahydrocannabinol (THC) and cannabidiol (CBD) are most well studied and used as medications. Tetrahydrocannabinol has the more psychoactive component in cannabis (i.e., the "high"), while CBD is the major nonpsychoactive component. The Food and Drug Administration has approved several drugs containing the cannabinoids to treat conditions such as severe childhood epilepsy, nausea, and decreased appetite, and others are being researched in clinical trials. A recent meta-analysis found that one in six patients suffering from rheumatologic disease actively consume cannabis, resulting in pain reduction.[119] While legalization and utilization of medical marijuana continues to expand, it is likely that physical therapists may encounter patients with RA or OA who use marijuana to treat their symptoms, although systematic studies regarding efficacy are lacking.[119]

Physical therapists should monitor the patient's pain using a valid and reliable pain scale, along with vital signs to assess any potential side effects related to the patient's cardiovascular status. Side effects may include increased heart rate, blood pressure, chest pain, palpitations, or dizziness. Other side effects may include decreased balance, safety, and changes in mood or cognition that may impede participation in personal or work-related obligations. Patient education regarding possible adverse effects is recommended as well as a consultation with a physician before patients administer this medication in any form.[118]

■ REHABILITATIVE MANAGEMENT

The chronic progressive nature of arthritis dictates a plan of care (POC) that includes patient education and self-management beyond the initial presentation. Although RA is systemic and OA is a more localized condition, both diseases can significantly affect health, function, participation, and quality of life. The rehabilitation of persons with arthritis requires comprehensive and coordinated efforts of a health professional team, including physical therapists, and ensures that the patient is first in treatment planning. The patient's ability to self-manage successfully is a major predictor of better health outcomes.[120] The physical therapist plays a pivotal role in helping the patient to minimize disability and gain confidence and experience in using self-management skills to deal with the condition. The general goals and outcomes for persons with RA and OA are similar.

The remainder of this chapter discusses physical therapist examination and interventions for people with RA and OA of the hip and knee. Although OA also presents at other joints, these two joints are the most common and disabling sites for OA, and patients with hip and knee OA are most frequently seen by a physical therapist.

Physical Therapy Examination

A comprehensive history and multisystem examination are essential components of physical therapy management. Whether the patient is a direct access client or seen in a system-based clinical setting, collaboration and communication with other care providers working with the patient are imperative. As with all patient-centered care, the patient is the primary stakeholder and should be actively engaged in goal setting and in the development of the POC.

Careful observation of the patient during the initial meeting and a thorough history can help inform the POC process. For example, observation of the patient's gait, ability to remove outerwear, and transfer into a chair for the history will provide the therapist with a quick assessment of functional ability.

History

The medical and social history will direct and inform the examination and provide insight into the development of a POC and need for potential resources. Ascertaining the patient's understanding of the disease and the disease impact on daily life is an important component of the interview process. History taking should focus on the patient's current health status, past medical history, family history of disease, RA/OA disease course, and past medications. The therapist should be concerned with identifying "red flag" signs and symptoms that indicate the need for immediate medical follow-up (Table 23.1) as well as "yellow flags" (Table 23.2) that represent psychosocial and behavioral risks that may exacerbate RA or OA symptoms.[121]

Pain assessment questions should include location, duration, pattern, quality, and intensity. Specific details regarding joint inflammation such as joint heat, swelling, and erythema should be recorded and confirmed during the physical examination.[122] A determination of joint stiffness (morning versus after prolonged static posture), previous activity level, pattern and degree of fatigue, presence of comorbidities, and current medication is also essential. The physical therapist should ascertain the patient's prior use of nonpharmacological interventions and their perceived effectiveness and how these experiences influence the patient's expectations, attitudes, and beliefs about physical therapy interventions. Although many physical therapy tests and measures are used during the examination, specific adaptations may be made to tailor the examination to the person with RA or OA. At the end of the examination after synthesizing all the data, patients can be classified into three types: (a) those who will require education for self-management and an independent exercise program, (b) those who require education and exercise plus brief physical therapist intervention, and (c) those who require information, education, and longer-term physical therapy intervention.

Observation, Joint Tenderness, and Sensory Integrity

Clinical examination of the patient begins with careful observation of posture, gait, and functional transfers. A general guideline for clinical observation of any RA joint begins with a careful joint inspection. Examine the joint and surrounding tissues for swelling, muscle wasting, thinning and bruising of the skin (an indication of long-term steroid use), joint deformity, and the presence of nodules, rashes, and scars. Especially in RA, the tender and swollen joint count appears to be a sensitive measure of systemic disease activity and guides the exercise prescription.[29] A comprehensive physical therapist examination includes examination of the nails of the hands and feet for pitting or nail fold vasculitis and comparison of the joint on one side of the body with the other to determine whether changes are symmetric or asymmetric. To assess joint inflammation, it is recommended to place the dorsal side of your hand over the joint surface.

Palpate soft tissue to determine whether there is tendon thickening or joint pain. To assess joint pain, gently compress the joint (e.g., squeeze MCPs using a

Table 23.1 "Red Flags" Suggesting the Need for Urgent Evaluation and Management

Red Flag	Differential Diagnosis
History of significant trauma	Soft tissue injury, internal derangement, or fracture
Hot, swollen joint	Infection, systemic rheumatic disease, gout, pseudogout
Constitutional signs (e.g., fever, weight loss, malaise, malnutrition, congestive heart failure)	Infection, sepsis, systemic rheumatic disease, fulminant form of rheumatoid arteritis
Weakness	Peripheral or central nerve impingement
Focal	Focal nerve lesion (compartment syndrome, entrapment neuropathy, mononeuritis multiplex, motor neuron disease, radiculopathy[a])
Diffuse	Myositis, metabolic myopathy, paraneoplastic syndrome, degenerative neuromuscular disorder, toxin, myelopathy,[a] transverse myelitis
Neurogenic pain (burning, numbness, paresthesia): Asymmetrical	Radiculopathy,[a] reflex sympathetic dystrophy, entrapment neuropathy myelopathy,[a] peripheral neuropathy
Neurogenic pain: Symmetrical	Soft tissue injury, internal derangement, or fracture
History of significant trauma	Peripheral vascular disease, giant cell arteritis (jaw pain), lumbar spinal stenosis
Claudication pain pattern	Vascular versus spinal stenosis
Fever, severe cold symptoms in patients with rheumatoid arthritis on biologic therapy	Risk of rapid progression and serious infection due to immunosuppression, triggering of inactive tuberculosis
Body rash in patients with rheumatoid arthritis on sulfasalazine	Adverse reaction to drug, liver toxicity

[a]Radiculopathy and myelopathy may be due to infectious, neoplastic, or mechanical processes.

Table 23.2 "Yellow Flags" Suggesting the Patient Is At Risk for Exacerbation of Symptoms[121]

Yellow Flag	At-Risk Indicator	Action to Be Taken
Exhibiting symptoms of anxiety	Answers yes to two screening questions	Relay information to primary care physician and monitor closely; integrate relaxation activities into intervention
Exhibiting symptoms of depression	Answers yes to two screening questions	Relay information to primary care physician and monitor closely; integrate social activities into intervention plan
Fear-avoidance behaviors	At risk for deconditioning	Assess level of fear with a self-reported measure such as the Fear-Avoidance Beliefs Questionnaire and address in intervention plan

medial–lateral pressure). Check peripheral pulses. In patients with RA, alterations in sensation may be evident with the presence of *Raynaud disease* or with nerve compression due to inflammation or joint derangement. Any indication of peripheral neuropathy or nerve involvement should be investigated using standard examination procedures (see Chapter 3, Examination of Sensory Function). Sensory changes resulting from other comorbidities or from the normal aging process should be considered.

Range of Motion

Tenderness and subjective reports of pain with passive range of motion (PROM) are highly indicative of inflammation; thus, gentle pressure and appropriate hand position are paramount during examination.

Following a total body gross joint screening, goniometric measurement of PROM is indicated to assist in monitoring treatment effectiveness. Standardized procedures (e.g., testing positions) are essential for reliable and valid measures.[123] Otherwise, potential variations in intrarater and interrater reliability will reduce the accuracy of data comparison throughout the disease course. If joint pain or poor activity tolerance prohibits PROM measurement, the therapist may consider substituting a functional ROM test by asking the patient to touch various body parts (e.g., the top of the head and small of the back) to determine the available ROM for performing self-care activities. The therapist should note any tenderness, crepitus, or pain during examination of ROM.

Regardless of whether the patient has OA and monoarticular involvement or RA with polyarticular involvement, the impact of an involved joint on the kinematic chain or on the contralateral side should be considered. When there is OA in a hip or knee, active motion in functional positions should be examined in all joints of both lower extremities (LEs). It is also important to observe motion for symmetry and smoothness during gait, stair climbing, and rising from a chair. Research indicates that 50° hip flexion and 90° knee flexion are required to recover balance from a stumble during walking[124] and that decreased ROM at the hip and knee increases the risk for injury and falls. In patients with RA, changes in the ankle and feet are associated with a greater fall risk.[125] Ascending stairs requires the greatest amount and velocity of knee flexion and may be one of the best activities to determine knee function.

Strength

Pain and joint effusions impede muscle contraction and may limit the examination of muscular force. A patient may be able to generate force in the pain-free range but unable to completely contract in the painful range secondary to reflex inhibition. Traditional strength tests (e.g., manual muscle tests) are not appropriate in the presence of severely deformed or deranged joints. In that case, functional strength assessments will provide sufficient data to formulate treatment goals. Individuals who demonstrate a *lag phenomenon* will have limited active range and will not be candidates for traditional grading systems, because these grading systems are not sensitive to changes in the quality and quantity of muscle contraction. It is important to note that the severity of knee pain, obesity, and perceived helplessness to manage OA have been identified as important determinants of disability.[126] Thus, pain experience will influence the strength assessment and may create a sense of helplessness or fear of movement.

When documenting strength, the therapist should include information on the modifications made to standardized testing positions, the grade of strength exhibited in that arc of motion, and the method of strength testing used (e.g., break test, isometric holding at the end of range, or resistance throughout the ROM). Modifying the test protocol to include an isometric break test at midrange or most comfortable joint position generally yields higher grades than would be received if full range testing were done (see Chapter 4, Musculoskeletal Examination). In addition to modifications, it is important to document the time of day the patient was tested as well as the use and timing of medications that might alter performance or exercise tolerance.

The functional threshold for LE strength has yet to be determined. However, data from studies examining knee strength as a percentage of body weight suggest that isokinetic strength measured at velocities between 60° and 180° per second should be 20% to 30% body weight for knee extension and 20% to 25% for knee flexion.[127] It is also important to perform strength testing of the muscle groups proximal to the affected joints to detect deficits that can affect function and contribute to abnormal biomechanics.

Joint Stability

Joint stability is essential for normal biomechanics, function, and independence. Inflammatory aspects of RA can lead to joint instability and eventual deformity. Intra-articular ligaments are highly susceptible to inflammatory and erosive changes in RA. Thus, ligamentous laxity of any affected joint should be fully investigated. More RA-specific tests for joint stability of the wrist and hand are described in the literature.[128,129] *Pseudolaxity*, often detected in unicompartmental knee OA, should be differentiated from *true ligamentous laxity*. Standard ligamentous integrity tests including those for the anterior and posterior cruciate and collateral ligaments of the knee are appropriate for both knee OA and knee involvement from RA.

Cardiovascular Status

Fatigue is one of the systemic manifestations of RA and is frequently underappreciated.[20] Individuals with OA also report fatigue.[77] To best ascertain the impact of fatigue on patient functioning and independence, assessments should be made over the course of a single day and over several days. The increased incidence of asymptomatic cardiovascular disease, elevated risk for ischemic heart disease, and decreased cardiovascular fitness of individuals with RA[39–41] demand specific attention. It is also important to determine cardiovascular fitness in individuals with OA, because cardiovascular deficits and increased risk for coronary artery disease are clearly associated with long-standing or severe disease, inactivity, and walking disability.[88] Assessment of heart rate, respiratory rate, blood pressure, and ratings of perceived exertion (RPE) should all be measured during a functional activity that is reasonably stressful for the patient's current level of fitness. Excessive increases in RPE may indicate the presence of inflammation or impairment of pulmonary and cardiac function that requires more extensive and formal evaluation.

Standardized Outcome Measures

Standardized outcome measures provide a rich and patient-centered approach to assessment. Measures may include *patient-reported outcome measures*, physician-reported data that may merge laboratory findings with the physician's judgment of the patient's function, or performance-based measures (see Chapter 8, Examination of Function). The selection of a functional measure is based on the patient's demographic features (e.g., age, gender), the depth of information required, the measure's sensitivity and responsiveness in gauging the efficacy of treatment, and clinical feasibility (e.g., available resources, space). As with goniometric measurement, reliability and validity of tests are important for individual and comparative purposes.

In the management of patients with arthritis, generic and disease-specific patient-reported outcome measures are incorporated as part of a core set of measures. The revised *Arthritis Impact Measurement Scales 2* (AIMS2) include physical function and performance in psychological and social domains and have been used in persons with RA, OA, psoriatic arthritis, ankylosing spondylitis, and fibromyalgia.[130,131] The AIMS2 also measures the patient's satisfaction with current functional status and individual preferences for outcome. The AIMS2 is not well suited for program evaluation or clinical purposes due to its complicated scoring algorithm and associated costs (Table 23.3).

The *Health Assessment Questionnaire* (HAQ)[132] is one of the RA core measures and assesses the impact

Table 23.3 Outcome Measures for Rheumatoid Arthritis and Osteoarthritis Organized by International Classification of Functioning, Disability, and Health Categories			
Outcome Measure (ICF Category)	Description of Measure and Link to Measure (if available)	Scoring	Clinically Important Change Values
Arthritis—many forms			
AIMS2[130,131] (body structure and function, activity, and participation)	A PRO that measures physical, social, and emotional well-being using a series of items that ask about the level of disability the person is experiencing for each item. The AIMS2 also includes a measure of satisfaction with health. The AIMS2 has been proven a valid and reliable measure in many forms of arthritis. http://www.aqol.com.au/documents/MIC/OSTEO ARTHRITIS_MIC_qnr_180711.pdf	The response format for each item is a 5-point scale. Items are scored separately without weights. Greater disability = higher score. Total health score is calculated by summing the standardized scores for mobility, physical and household activities, dexterity, pain, and depression.	SRMs for changes in AIMS2-SF scores over 3-month range from 0.36 (small) to 0.8 (high).
Rheumatoid Arthritis			
CDAI[132,133] (body structure and function)	This is a provider and patient assessment measure. The CDAI includes the provider's assessment of 28 joints as either swollen (SJC-28) or tender (TJC-28) and the patient's self-assessment of overall RA disease activity (scale 1–10, where 10 is maximal activity) and the provider's global disease activity (scale 1–10; 10 is maximal activity).	Total score created by summing the four components of the measure. Interpretation as follows: Disease in remission CDAI ≤2.8 Low disease activity CDAI >2.8 and ≤10 Moderately active disease CDAI >10 and ≤22 Highly active disease CDAI >22	In general, MID is five points. MID cut points for improvement in adults with high disease activity, reduction of more than 11 units; patients with moderate disease reduction of 6 units; low disease activity, reduction greater than 2 units.

(Continued)

Table 23.3 Outcome Measures for Rheumatoid Arthritis and Osteoarthritis Organized by International Classification of Functioning, Disability, and Health Categories—cont'd

Outcome Measure (ICF Category)	Description of Measure and Link to Measure (if available)	Scoring	Clinically Important Change Values
	Rheumatoid Arthritis		
DAS[134] (body structure and function)	This measure includes the provider assessment and laboratory data. It is a four-item tool to assess RA disease activity in patients by counting tender joints and painful joints calculated by the RAI, a 44 swollen joint count, ESR, and a PtGA or General Health using a VAS. Validated for patients with RA.	Scores for each item are calculated as follows: the RAI ranges from 0–78, the 44SJC ranges from 0–44, the GH/PtGA VAS ranges from 0–100, and the ESR ranges from 0 to 100 mm/hr. The DAS ranges from 0–10. The level of disease activity is classified as follows: in remission, low, moderate, or high if the scores are between 0 and 1.6, 1.6 and 2.4, 2.4 and 3.7, and 3.7 and 10, respectively.	A change in the DAS greater than 1.2 is a significant change. Change is classified as good, nonresponsive, or moderate if scores and follow-up scores are greater than 1.2 and less than 2.4, greater than 0.6, or improvement between 0.6 and 1.2 and a follow-up greater than 3.7. All other responses are classified as moderate.
DAS28[135] (body structure and function)	Provider assessment plus laboratory data. This four-item tool is a modified version of the DAS. It is used to assess rheumatic disease activity in patients using a 28 swollen joint count, a 28 tender joint count, ESR, and a PtGA or GH using a VAS. Validated for patients with RA.	Scores for each item are calculated as follows: the 28TJC and 28SJC range from 0–28, the GH/PtGA VAS ranges from 0–00, and the ESR ranges from 0–100 mm/hr. The DAS28 ranges from 0–9.4. The level of disease activity is classified as in remission, low, moderate, or high if the scores are 0–1.6, 1.6–2.4, 2.4–3.7, and 3.7–10, respectively.	A change in the DAS28 greater than 1.2 is a significant change. Change is classified as good, nonresponsive, or moderate if scores and follow-up scores are greater than 1.2 and less than 2.4, greater than 0.6, or improvement between 0.6 and 1.2 and a follow-up greater than 3.7. All other responses are classified as moderate.
HAQ[136] **HAQ-DI**[136,137] (body structure and function and activity)	20-item–reported tool assessing physical function in daily living and the use of aids or help from others. Validated for patients with a variety of rheumatic conditions. http://www.rheumatoid-arthritis-decisions.com/HAQ.html HAQ-DI has 41 items (20 for daily activities, 13 for assistive devices, 8 for help from others).	HAQ scores are calculated for each subcategory on a scale from 0 (no difficulty) to 3 (unable to do) in 0.125 increments. Scores are adjusted upward by 1 for each category if aids/assistance are used and the score for that category was reported at 0 or 1. Scores process similar. The eight scores of the eight sections are summed and divided by 8.	MCID for scores is ~0.22, although the value can range from 0.07–0.87. MCID for HAQ-DI is a change of 0.22–0.25. A recent study suggests the MCII is a decrease of 0.375.

Table 23.3	Outcome Measures for Rheumatoid Arthritis and Osteoarthritis Organized by International Classification of Functioning, Disability, and Health Categories—cont'd		
Outcome Measure (ICF Category)	**Description of Measure and Link to Measure (if available)**	**Scoring**	**Clinically Important Change Values**
	**Rheumatoid Arthritis**		
MDHAQ[138] (body structure and function, activity, participation)	Patient reported 10-item tool assessing physical function in daily living and use of assistive devices or aid from others. Includes more difficult activities such as playing sports and walking more than 2 miles. Validated for patients with a variety of rheumatic diseases. A short-form MDHAQ is recommended for routine clinical use.	Scores calculated for each item on a scale from 0 (no difficulty) to 3 (unable to do). If at least 9/10 questions were answered, the scores are summed and then divided by the number of questions answered to reach a final score of 0–3 and rounded to the nearest 0.1.	MDHAQ scores are found to be significantly associated with amount of morning stiffness as compared to pain, fatigue, joint counts, and patient global and independently predict 10-year mortality.
PAS and PAS-II (body structure and function)[138,139]	Patient-reported outcome that includes three primary components: patient pain score (pain VAS) and PtGA via health assessment questionnaire (PAS) or using the health assessment questionnaire II (PAS II).	Take the mean of the sum of the three subscales (but in the process of summing a weighting applied to the HAQ score, multiply HAQ × 0.33). Similar process for PAS-II. Scores range from 0–10. Disease activity cutoffs (both): Remission (0–0.25) Low disease (0.26–3.7) Moderate (3.71 less than 8.0) High (≥8.0)	As this is a composite of three known measures treated with equal weighting, ability to detect change is moderate to good.
PROMIS[140–142] (body structure and function, activity, and participation)	Patient-reported physical function and disability measure is one component of the PROMIS set. These measures are part of a series of generic measures available for free from the National Institutes of Health. PROMIS also measures pain, fatigue, depression, anxiety, and social function. **Website:** https://www.healthmeasures.net/explore-measurement-systems/promis	For best information on scoring, see http://www.healthmeasures.net/promis-scoring-manuals	MCID for physical function from a longitudinal cohort study in RA was 0.2 SD.
RAPID-3[142]	Patient-reported outcome with three primary components: patient pain score, pain VAS and the Multidimensional HAQ (MDHAQ).	(MDHAQ × 3.33 + pain VAS + patient global assessment VAS)/3.	As this is a composite of three known measures treated with equal weighting, ability to detect change is moderate to good.

(Continued)

Table 23.3   Outcome Measures for Rheumatoid Arthritis and Osteoarthritis Organized by International Classification of Functioning, Disability, and Health Categories—cont'd

Outcome Measure (ICF Category)	Description of Measure and Link to Measure (if available)	Scoring	Clinically Important Change Values
Rheumatoid Arthritis			
SDAI[136,138] (body structure and function)	This measure combines physician assessment and laboratory data to determine disease activity. It includes a physician global assessment, patient global assessment, 28 total tender joint count, and 28 total swollen joint count plus CRP level.	The score is calculated by taking the total of the 28 tender joint count score + 28 swollen joint count score + provider global assessment + patient global assessment + CRP.	As this is a composite of three known measures treated with equal weighting, ability to detect change is moderate to good.
Osteoarthritis			
DASH (body structure and function, activity)[142]	A 30-item self-report questionnaire designed to assess musculoskeletal disorders of the upper limbs. It has two shortened versions, the QuickDASH and the QuickDASH-9. https://www.sralab.org/rehabilitation-measures/disabilities-arm-shoulder-and-hand-questionnaire	Each item scored 1 (no difficulty, not at all, not limited, none, strongly disagree) to 5 (unable, extremely, unable, strongly agree). Online version and scoring at: http://www.orthopaedicscore.com/scorepages/disabilities_of_arm_shoulder_hand_score_dash.html	MDC = 12.75 in adults with upper extremity musculoskeletal problems.
HOOS (body structure and function, activity, and participation)	A 40-item survey that assesses pain, symptoms, function in daily living, function in sports and recreation, and quality of life over the past week. Validated for hip OA and THR patients. A short-form HOOS-PS is recommended for routine clinical use[142] (http://www.koos.nu).	Scores calculated for each subscale with 0 being lowest score and 100 being highest.	MCII 1 year after THA is 24 points for pain subscale and 17 for QOL subscale.
KOOS[142,143] (body structure and function, activity, and participation)	A 42-item tool that assesses pain, symptoms, function in daily living, function in sports and recreation, and QOL over the past week. Validated for knee injury (e.g., ACL), OA, and TKR. A short-form KOOS-PS is recommended for routine clinical use (https://www.sralab.org/rehabilitation-measures/knee-injury-and-osteoarthritis-outcome-score).	Scores calculated for each subscale with 0 being lowest score and 100 being highest.	MDC for knee OA ranges from 13.4 points for pain subscale to 21.1 for QOL subscale.
LEFS[144] (activity)	A 20-item tool that assesses current (i.e., today) ability to undertake activities at home, work, school, recreation, and sport. Validated for hip and knee OA and TJR[144] (https://www.sralab.org/rehabilitation-measures/lower-extremity-functional-scale).	Scored 9–80 with higher score representing better function.	MDC and MCID is 9 points.

Table 23.3 Outcome Measures for Rheumatoid Arthritis and Osteoarthritis Organized by International Classification of Functioning, Disability, and Health Categories—cont'd

Outcome Measure (ICF Category)	Description of Measure and Link to Measure (if available)	Scoring	Clinically Important Change Values
	Osteoarthritis		
Oswestry Disability Index[145] (body structure and function, activity, participation)	A 10-item tool that assesses pain intensity, personal care, lifting, walking, sitting, standing, sleeping, sex (if applicable), social, and travel. https://www.sralab.org/rehabilitation-measures/oswestry-disability-index	Each item scored 0 (least disability) to 5 (greatest disability) for total score of 0–50. Online version and scoring at: http://www.orthopaedicscore.com/scorepages/oswestry_low_back_pain.html	MDC = 12.72 for population with chronic back pain.
PSFS[145] (activity and participation)	Patients select activities important to them and rate their current ability to complete each on an 11-point scale. https://www.sralab.org/rehabilitation-measures/patient-specific-functional-scale	Each item rated 0 (unable to perform) to 10 (able to perform at prior level).	MDC = 1.4 for low back pain. MCID = 1.34 for spinal stenosis.
ABC[216]	A 16-item self-report measure of balance confidence in performing various activities without losing balance or experiencing a sense of unsteadiness. https://www.sralab.org/rehabilitation-measures/activities-specific-balance-confidence-scale#non-specific-patient-population	Items are scored on a 0–100 rating scale. Score of 0 represents no confidence, a score of 100 represents complete confidence.	MDC = 15 points for older adults seeking outpatient therapy.

ABC = Activities Specific Balance Confidence Scale; ACL = anterior cruciate ligament; AIMS2 = Arthritis Impact Measurement Scales 2; CDAI = Clinical Disease Activity Index; CRP = C-reactive protein; DAS = Disease Activity Score; DASH = Disabilities of the Arm, Shoulder, and Hand; ESR = erythrocyte sedimentation rate; GH/PtGA = General Health - Patient Global Assessment; HAQ = Health Assessment Disability Questionnaire; HAQ-DI = Health Assessment Disability Questionnaire—Disability Index; HOOS = Hip Disability and Osteoarthritis Outcome Score; ICF = International Classification of Functioning, Disability, and Health; KOOS = Knee Injury and Osteoarthritis Outcome Score; LEFS = Lower Extremity Functional Scale; MCID = minimal clinically important difference; MCII = minimum clinically important improvement; MDC = minimal detectable change; MDHAQ = Multidimensional Health Assessment Questionnaire; MID = minimal important difference; OA = osteoarthritis; PAS = Patient Activity Scale; PRO = patient-reported outcome measures; PROMIS = Patient-Reported Outcomes Measurement Information System; PSFS = Patient-Specific Functional Scale; PtGA = patient global assessment of disease activity; QOL = quality of life; RA = rheumatoid arthritis; RAI = Ritchie Articular Index; RAPID-3 = Routine Assessment of Patient Index Data 3; SDAI = Simplified Disease Activity Index; SRM: standardized response mean; THR = total hip replacement; TKR = total knee replacement; VAS = Visual Analog Scale.

of disease activity on function and disability. The HAQ consists of five domains or subscales—disability, discomfort, pain, drug side effects (toxicity), and costs of care—and has been shown to correlate highly with measures of disease progression in RA (x-ray changes). There are numerous versions of the HAQ available.[132–134] The *Modified HAQ*, an abbreviated version of the HAQ, is quick and easy to complete and score. The *Multidimensional HAQ* includes a sports item and an item that assesses the ability to walk more than 2 miles,

in order to reduce the floor effects typically found with the HAQ.[134] Online versions are available for free.

Although there are numerous (more than 60) disease activity measures in RA, the six most highly recommended include the *Disease Activity Score* (DAS) with 28-joint counts (ESR or CRP),[135] the *Clinical Disease Activity Index* (CDAI),[136] the *Patient Activity Scale* (PAS), PAS-II,[137] the *Routine Assessment of Patient Index Data with 3 measures* (RAPID-3),[134] and the *Simplified Disease Activity Index* (SDAI).[138] These measures were recommended due to their accuracy; sensitivity to change; and ability to discriminate adults with low, moderate, and high disease activity states following a systematic literature review combined with input from an expert panel of clinician researchers.[139] All measures have criteria to establish remission and are easy to use in the clinic. As an example, both the DAS28[135] and the Rheumatoid Arthritis Disease Activity Index (RADAI)[140] combine data from the physician's physical examination of the patient with clinical laboratory biomarkers of inflammation. These measures are used frequently to assess and monitor disease activity in RA and determine whether the patient has achieved either remission or low disease activity in response to medical therapy (see Table 23.3).

For patients with OA, the WOMAC is a widely used, valid, and reliable self-report instrument of 24 items that address three categories specific to hip and knee OA (pain, stiffness, and function).[141] The WOMAC, however, requires a licensing fee to use making it less appropriate for routine clinical use.[142] The *Knee Injury and Osteoarthritis Outcome Score* (KOOS)[143] was developed based off the WOMAC and includes sports, recreation, and quality of life items. This measure is readily accessible; is relatively easy to score; and demonstrates strong validity, reliability, and responsiveness in adults.[141] A modified version of the KOOS was developed for persons with hip OA, the *Hip Disability and Osteoarthritis Outcome Score* (HOOS).[143] Short forms of both tools are recommended for routine clinical use.[142] The *Lower Extremity Functional Scale* (LEFS) is another short (20-item) tool that has been validated in the OA population, is feasible for clinical use, and enables comparison of disability across a variety of LE conditions[144] (see Table 23.3).

The Osteoarthritis Research Society International (OARSI) has suggested the use of five performance tests thought to be the most valuable for patients over age 40 years with knee and hip OA or who are undergoing joint arthroplasty surgery.[145] The selected tests encompass different aspects of functional mobility and aerobic capacity. The *30-second Chair Stand Test* (30CST) evaluates sit-to-stand ability, the 4-by-10 meter fast-paced walk test is a test of walking activity and speed over short distances with changing directions. The *Timed Up and Go* evaluates functional mobility and gait speed, the timed stair climb test assesses stair negotiation, and the 6-minute Walk Test (6MWT) acquires information regarding aerobic capacity and walking longer distances. These tests were chosen to be complementary to established patient-reported outcome measures and are considered the best available clinometric evidence. However, OARSI acknowledges the need for further evidence.

Mobility, Gait, and Balance

A complete and detailed gait examination by the physical therapist is one of the most important contributions to the rehabilitation team's understanding of a patient's functional abilities and serves to identify additional areas for examination and intervention. (See Chapter 7, Examination of Gait, for a complete discussion.) Substantial differences in fall risks, knee ROM, and gait velocity between patients with either OA or RA and their peers without arthritis have been demonstrated. Persons with RA demonstrate alterations in joint kinematics and kinetics as a result of chronic synovitis, in some instances joint derangement, and a high prevalence of significant foot and ankle involvement. Studies of three-dimensional gait analysis indicate that persons with arthritis develop an antalgic gait pattern characterized by reduced walking speed, stride length, and cadence. These individuals also demonstrate reduced joint motions, prolonged weight-bearing periods, and diminished joint power. At the foot, there is decreased plantarflexion, reduced and often delayed heel rise in early stance, and diminished power.[146]

During ambulation, adults with knee OA and medial compartment involvement tend to outwardly rotate their leg and walk at a slower speed with a reduced knee extensor moment. Ligamentous instability further alters normal knee biomechanics during level ground walking and stair negotiation. Gait patterns in individuals with hip OA tend to be altered to accommodate reduced hip ROM, hip pain, and lateral muscle weakness. Typically, these individuals demonstrate increased cadence and ankle power generation, maintenance of anterior pelvic tilt throughout the gait cycle, decreased step width, reduced hip extension, and a dropped pelvis (Trendelenburg gait) during stance. These deviations are quite different from comparisons with age- and gender-matched healthy controls.[146]

Psychosocial Status

Individuals with chronic arthritis experience years of functional and social loss that would stress any person's ability to cope and adapt.[147] The overall psychological status of the individual with RA is generally similar to individuals with other chronic diseases that threaten a severe change in body image and disruption of social integration (see Chapter 26, Psychosocial Issues in Physical Rehabilitation). Individuals respond to these threats with various coping strategies to maintain psychological well-being. No single strategy can be deemed definitely better than another, although for some individuals, different strategies will lead to better coping and more positive outcomes than others. Exploration of the patient's attitude toward rehabilitation and readiness to make health behavior changes as well as the availability of social support can assist the therapist and patient in mutual goal setting and identifying realistic expectations of future functional ability. Persons with RA face the additional challenges of living with a chronic disease that is characterized by a fluctuating disease course and must learn to adapt their lifestyle, activity level, medications, and sleep schedule according to their disease activity. As the physical therapist works collaboratively with the patient to establish realistic, achievable goals, patient education regarding the warning signs of flares is needed to help patients self-manage.

Due to the chronic nature of OA and RA pain, fear avoidance behaviors are prevalent.[148,149] Avoidance of physical activity results in physical consequences such as loss of muscle strength, impaired mobility, and falls and psychological changes, such as depression and anxiety. Given the adverse consequences of falls, fear of falling is also common among these patients with RA and OA. A simple self-report measure, the Activities-Specific Balance Confidence (ABC) Scale can be used to assess a patient's confidence in performing various activities and to identify balance impairments and fall risk. Fear of falling can lead to activity restriction, reduced quality of life, and increased medication use. On the contrary, not participating in physical activities may lead to feelings of confinement and isolation. Chronic pain, fatigue, loss of function, and reduced activity levels can all contribute to emotional distress. Studies indicate anxiety and depression are common in patients with OA and RA and may alter their pain experience, function, and response to treatment interventions.[150] Participation in the *Arthritis Self-Management Program* has been shown to improve coping.[151,152]

Environmental and Socioeconomic Factors

Therapists should be aware of environmental factors in the home, work, and leisure environments that might serve as facilitators or barriers to functioning and warrant specific identification, examination, and recommendations (see Chapter 9, Examination and Modification of the Environment). A discussion about the home and work environments may reveal conditions that threaten independence that can be addressed through ergonomic and environmental modifications and school or workplace accommodations. The cost of such changes may be a limiting factor for implementing these recommendations. The work environment affects employment and disability in more ways than the physical setting and task requirements.[153] Acceptance and understanding by supervisors and coworkers of the disease and self-management requirements of the worker with arthritis are important determinants of maintaining employment and income. In the event adults with OA or RA experience career disruption or reduced work productivity, this may lead to financial impact on employment wages, inability to afford the costs of clinical care, and burden on personal and family financial situations. As a result, patients may experience considerable distress, anxiety, and possible depression.[154]

Other environmental factors common to both the RA and OA ICF Core Sets include technology and assistive devices for ADL, mobility, transportation, and employment; design and access to buildings; climate;

and attitudes of family, friends, and health professionals.[155–157] Considering the psychosocial, environmental, and socioeconomic factors associated with RA and OA and assessing quality of life, with standardized measures, is an important component in evaluating well-being, disease progression, and intervention efficacy. Effective communication with the patient, family, and members of the multidisciplinary team is necessary to ensure that individuals with OA and RA receive effective care and support.

Physical Therapy Intervention

The development of specific goals and expected outcomes for the individual with arthritis is based on the following general goals and expected outcomes developed in conjunction with the patient (Box 23.4).

The specific goals and outcomes identified for each patient will depend on the type of arthritis, disease activity level, clinical presentation, and patient preferences. Mutual goal setting promotes patient participation in treatment. It is the physical therapist's responsibility to document the POC, implement that plan safely and effectively, and delegate responsibility appropriately to ensure that the patient's goals can be reached.

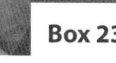 **Box 23.4** Examples of General Goals and Outcomes for Patients With Arthritis

Reduce Impact of Impairments of Body Functions and Structures

- Decreased pain
- Maximized range of motion of all joints sufficient for functional activities
- Maximized muscle performance (strength, power, endurance) sufficient for functional activities
- Maximized joint stability and decreased biomechanical stress on all affected joints to prevent deformity
- Increased endurance for all functional activities and desired leisure activities
- Improved ability to perform physical actions, tasks, or activities
- Greater independence in activities of daily living, including dressing, transfers, and self-care
- Enhanced efficiency and safety of gait pattern and balance with reduced fall risk
- Established adequate physical activity or exercise patterns to maintain or improve musculoskeletal and cardiovascular fitness and general health

Improve Health Status and Quality of Life

- Improved capacity for self-management, including joint protection, through education of patient, family, and caregivers

Source: Adapted from *APTA Guide to Physical Therapist Practice 3.0,* 2014.

All intervention goals need to be SMART goals (i.e., goals that are specific, measurable, attainable, relevant, and time bound) and documented with specific time frames. For example, an intervention goal may be to increase left shoulder flexion ROM by 10° in 2 weeks, or the patient should be able to ambulate independently on level surfaces for at least 250 ft using platform crutches without complaints of fatigue within 1 month. Failure to achieve goals within the stated time frame indicates the need for reevaluation and reformulation of goals. Goals and outcomes should be revised to reflect changes owing to both personal and environmental factors that may affect progress or alter the proposed time frames (see Chapter 1, Clinical Decision-Making).

Modalities for Pain Relief

A variety of therapeutic modalities are available to relieve pain and prepare the patient for passive and dynamic stretching and other exercise interventions. The most common form is thermotherapy. Many thermal modalities have limited scientific evidence of benefit. Thermotherapy is conditionally recommended by the ACR.[110]

Heat

Superficial heat is heat that penetrates only a few millimeters, produces localized analgesia, and increases circulation in the vicinity where it is applied. Types of superficial heat include moist hot packs, dry heating pads, lamps, paraffin wax, and hydrotherapy. The evidence supporting the effectiveness of these modalities is weak, but patients often report they gain comfort from moist heat. Paraffin is particularly useful in delivering superficial heat to irregularly shaped joints or to individuals who cannot tolerate the weight of a moist hot pack. Paraffin combined with exercises can provide beneficial short-term effects for arthritic hands. Hydrotherapy or aquatic therapy allows the therapist to combine tissue heating with exercise.[158] Systematic reviews of heat and cold therapy in arthritis suggest little to no effect on objective measures of disease activity.[159]

Deep heating modalities, such as ultrasound, may affect the viscoelastic properties of collagen and increase the plastic stretch of ligaments, providing modest improvements in pain and function in individuals with knee OA.[160] However, their efficacy in RA is not demonstrated. The use of deep heating modalities for individuals with RA is contraindicated during an acute stage of inflammation as it may stimulate collagenase activity within the joint, furthering joint destruction.[161] Additionally, modalities that do not readily translate to home use may foster a dependency on clinical care.

Cold

Local applications of cold will produce local analgesia, decrease intra-articular temperature, and improve superficial circulation at the site of application following an initial period of vasoconstriction.[161] Cold is particularly useful around joints that are inflamed and swollen, a condition that usually worsens with the application of superficial heat modalities. Therapists may use either wet or dry cold application techniques. In patients with OA, ice massage had a statistically beneficial effect on ROM, function, and knee strength, and cold packs were shown to decrease edema. Contrast baths, where the hand or foot is alternately immersed in hot and cold water for a specified ratio of time, have been used to decrease swelling, joint stiffness, and pain; however, there is no common approach or consistent findings.[162] Superficial cold is contraindicated in patients with Raynaud phenomenon or *cryoglobulinemia,* linked to an abnormal protein (cryoglobulins) in the blood that gels at low temperatures. Both may be associated with RA.

Electrotherapy Modalities

Transcutaneous electrical nerve stimulation (TENS) has been used for patients with RA and OA, although the reported value of TENS in the literature is inconsistent, and TENS is not recommended based on a recent RA clinical practice guideline.[121] A meta-analysis of studies investigating TENS for knee OA pain concluded that the mode of TENS applied did affect results, repeated use was more effective than a single application, and use for at least 4 weeks was the most effective.[163] Another meta-analysis reported high-frequency TENS provided moderate pain relief, while interferential current (IFC) resulted in even greater pain reduction when compared to control or sham interventions.[159] International guidelines are uncertain or provide conditional recommendations regarding the use of TENS,[110] and none include IFC in their recommendations for OA.[110]

Rest and Energy Conservation

Complete bedrest is rarely recommended. An adequate night of sleep (roughly 8 to 10 hr) is recommended combined with periodic rest periods during the day. Daily rest breaks from 15 to 60 minutes with joints properly supported can alleviate joint pain coupled with small breaks during tasks to reduce joint fatigue. Proper rest also helps reduce pain and minimize joint stress, allowing the body to heal and address inflammation.

An important component of patient education is instruction in the principles of energy conservation. Energy conservation does not mean patients should spend all day resting, rather it is the process of simplifying activities, employing pacing, and using adaptive devices. Any activity that results in pain for 1 to 2 hr after completion of the activity is an activity that requires modification and pacing. Patients should be encouraged to rest before they feel fatigue. General principles of energy conservation include planning the task to eliminate extra unnecessary movement, using proper body mechanics and posture, and using adaptive equipment.

Joint Protection, Splints, Orthoses, and Braces

JOINT PROTECTION

Joint protection is a key component of arthritis management as overuse can lead to progressive joint destruction and soft tissue inflammation. Joints in persons with RA or OA can be mechanically weak and lack stabilization during movement, leading to overstretching and damage to tendons, ligaments, and cartilage, and ultimately pain. The focus of joint protection strategies is to minimize joint strain during daily use through good posture, modifications to activities to reduce repetitive motions, or pacing of ADL. Joint protection interventions should focus on the joints most involved. Joint protection techniques for patients include instruction on sharing weight across many joints versus one (e.g., carrying items with two arms and using built-up handles), maintaining good postural alignment with all activities when possible, and avoiding flexed static positions of joints and maximizing extension. For patients with RA, the hands are generally the first to be involved. Positions and activities to avoid include putting pressure on the bent knuckles, putting pressure on the outside of the hand, twisting the wrist toward the thumb, carrying objects with fingers versus forearm, maintaining any position for long periods of time, and tapping or putting pressure on the inside of the wrist (as with typing on a keyboard). Patients need to learn to avoid activities if their pain persists for more than 1 to 2 hr after stopping the activity or if their body is exceptionally stiff the next day.

There are numerous adaptive items available for purchase for work and home to assist with ADL, such as long-handled reachers, modified grips and door handles, modified gardening tools, and assistive and safety devices for the bathroom (shower seat, safety bars, etc.). Patient education for joint protection also includes teaching the basics of body mechanics such as bringing an object close when lifting, bending with the knees not the back, avoiding twisting the back and moving the feet when lifting from one surface to another, carrying items in a backpack instead of a handbag to reduce strain on fingers and wrists, and limiting the weight of loads.

A randomized controlled trial compared the effects of a 3-month educational–behavioral joint protection program for adults with hand OA to standard education. Each session consisted of a 20-minute session and provision of a piece of Dycem nonslip matting to use when opening jars. This single-blinded study demonstrated that patients in the joint protection and exercise group increased grip strength by 25%, and both groups reported better hand function with the joint protection information.[164] Physical therapists should encourage patients to incorporate joint care into all ADL to minimize pain and conserve energy.

With RA, hand and wrist orthoses are used to immobilize specific joints and help reduce pain and swelling by providing local rest and support.[165] There are three primary types of splints: resting (used to maintain joint alignment and reduce pain), functional (used to restore or improve function), and corrective (used to improve alignment). Resting splints are worn at night or periodically during the day to reduce synovitis and tenosynovitis or in patients with end-stage disease to reduce contractures of the hand intrinsic and extrinsic muscles. When volar subluxation at the metacarpophalangeal (MCP) joint is present, the splint design should apply a gentle force on the volar aspect of the proximal phalange to reduce volar subluxation.[129] While frequently prescribed, there is little to no evidence that resting splints are effective in reducing pain and inflammation.[166–168]

For patients with RA who have moderate synovitis or early-to-moderate soft tissue changes, a functional MCP splint, which provides support to MCP joints in slight flexion and neutral deviation, is used to reduce pain, decrease flexion forces during grip, and help maintain good joint alignment. To optimize hand function, functional splints should only be prescribed for involved joints. MCP splints are contraindicated in patients with significant proximal phalangeal synovitis, as the splint may increase joint forces and may be too restrictive for daily function and gripping. Data indicate functional hand splints provide small benefits for pain reduction and increased function including grip and pincher strength. There is evidence that wearing a functional wrist splint decreases grip strength and does not affect quality of life with regular wear.[169] A study investigating the effects of functional wrist splint wear on task performance reported that wearing a commercially available elastic wrist orthosis resulted in some decrement in performance speed on a number of common tasks, though pain was significantly reduced for all tasks.[170] To enhance patient adherence to splint wear, patients need to be educated on how to properly wear the splint and understand the use of the splint and any restrictions associated with the splint.[171] In OA management, hand orthoses are strongly recommended for first CMC involvement as the scientific evidence for benefits in pain reduction and function is substantial.[110]

ORTHOSES

In addition to reducing pain and improving function, orthoses also may provide support and protection for vulnerable and painful joints. Foot orthotics or specially designed shoes can serve the dual purpose of relieving biomechanical stresses and enhancing function for the person with RA foot involvement.[172] A good shoe will provide support and eliminate unnecessary joint motion in the talocalcaneal joint with a firm and wide heel counter. A good shoe should also help to maintain normal bony alignment and accommodate all existing foot deformities within a toe box of adequate dimensions. Pressure should be evenly distributed along the plantar surface of the foot during weight-bearing. If the cost of special shoes is not reimbursable under insurance programs, commercially available gel inserts may be helpful and are inexpensive. However, with more advanced biomechanical changes in the foot, the fabrication of orthoses may be required. A *rocker sole* (shoe sole that is curved at the toe) can be used to facilitate push-off with limited ankle motion. A controlled trial examining the effect of off-the-shelf extra-depth orthopedic footwear for people with RA who had at least 1 year of foot pain found patients wearing extra-depth shoes improved significantly on self-reported disability, weight-bearing and non-weight-bearing pain, and gait. In addition to extra depth in the shoe toe box, the shoes provided greater rear foot stability, an arch support, a stiff shank, and a padded heel collar above the counter for improved fit. This study reported that walking pain accounted for 75% of the variability in physical function level of the subjects.[173] A systematic review on this topic found inconclusive results regarding the long-term effects of different footwear on knee and hip OA pain.[174] The authors did suggest, however, that there was increasing evidence that shock-absorbing insoles, subtalar taping, and avoidance of high heels and sandals early in life may prevent LE joint pain later in life.

In patients with RA, foot orthoses are a conservative treatment option used to optimize foot biomechanics and function or for providing cushioning and off-loading of foot structures.[175] Variations of foot orthoses exist based on the materials used (rigid versus soft), the shoe type (custom made or off-the-shelf), and type of modifications (metatarsal bars, shock-absorbing pads). The target of treatment for individuals with RA is typically reduction of forefoot plantar pressure or forefoot pain. A systematic review indicates a medium effect for the immediate reduction of forefoot plantar pressure in favor of treatment with soft foot orthosis compared to semirigid orthosis.[175]

In patients with knee OA, foot orthoses are used to alleviate pain through biomechanical support or correction for individuals with knee OA. Data indicate a lateral wedge insole designed to reduce medial compartment stress compared to no insole appears to reduce pain and NSAID use in some individuals with knee OA. There is evidence to support a conditional recommendation for the use of lateral wedge insoles to manage knee OA but not for foot orthoses.[110]

Knee OA clinical practice guidelines published by the American Academy of Orthopaedic Surgeons include moderate to strong recommendations for bracing treatment in early pain management.[176] Unloader braces include those that adjust alignment appropriately to unload the articular compartment that is the source of pain. For example, a lateral unloader knee brace applies a varus moment for lateral component OA and is recommended for mild to severe unicompartmental OA. Unloader braces have been reported to improve quality

of life and have the potential to delay or avoid the need for a total knee arthroplasty. Patellofemoral knee braces may decrease knee OA pain perhaps because of the adjustment of patellar tracking that distributes forces more evenly, unloading the extensor mechanism of the knee and improving the Q angle. Because of the uncertainty on the exact mechanism of action of these braces, their efficacy is unclear. Knee sleeves can be used for patients with knee OA during a symptomatic exacerbation; although they do not provide structural support, they may reduce swelling and pain and improve proprioceptive feedback.[176] There is strong evidence for the benefits of tibiofemoral braces and some support for the use of patellofemoral braces in the management of knee OA. It is important to note that all orthotic interventions require professional evaluation, selection, education, and monitoring of use.[177]

KINESIO TAPING

Kinesio Taping (KT) is a technique that uses waterproof, hypoallergenic, elastic tape capable of stretching up to 130% to 140% of its resting static length, ensuring free mobility of the applied muscle or joint.[178] Kinesio Tape can be applied directly to the skin and can be left for several days with good adherence. The ACR conditionally recommends KT for patients with knee and/or first CMC joint OA. The protocol for application varies; however, a common application is single, double, or triple Y-shape along the quadriceps femoris muscle and wrapping the tape end medially and laterally around the patella. Systematic reviews indicate patients experience a reduction in pain, improvements in knee ROM, and isokinetic strength.[178,179] Studies also support KT as an adjunct to a program of closed- and open-chain exercises with individuals with knee OA to reduce pain and improve function, ROM, and quality of life compared to a program of closed- and open-chain exercises alone. KT is not recommended for use in patients with RA.[121]

Complementary and Alternative Medicine

The use of complementary and alternative therapies is increasing.[180] About 30% to 69% of adults over 65 years reported using complementary and alternative therapies to improve various health conditions, with arthritis being the most cited reason.[181,182] Complementary and alternative medicine therapies used for arthritis include meditative movement therapies (yoga and Tai Chi), acupuncture, diet and nutritional supplements, herbal medicine, massage therapy, and dry needling.

The practice of yoga offers a holistic approach combining physical and breathing exercises with relaxation and meditation, intended to promote physical, mental, and spiritual well-being. A recent randomized controlled trial found that individuals with RA completing a yoga program (90 minutes, twice a week for 12 weeks) demonstrated improvements in fatigue and mood compared to the control group; however, this was not associated with change in quality of life. More studies with large sample sizes are required to determine duration, intensity, and frequency for implementing yoga as part of a POC to promote physical activity for individuals with RA. Within the management of knee OA, there is strong evidence for the use of yoga. Benefits may be gleaned from a combination of physical effects and psychological effects of treatment.[110]

Tai Chi, a Chinese martial art, includes slow, smooth, rhythmic movements that reproduce postures inspired by nature. This activity has been used to improve postural control, strength, and flexibility, and reduce risk of falls in addition to promoting interaction between body and mind. The evidence is limited regarding this treatment approach for individuals with RA. A systematic review included three studies with only one presenting high-quality methodology and reported improvements in disability, quality of life, depression, and mood, but no clear benefits to pain.[183,184] However, the evidence for the benefits of Tai Chi for both knee and hip OA is sufficient to warrant a strong recommendation by the ACR for the use of Tai Chi for adults with hip and knee OA.[110]

Dry needling techniques (DNTs) are used in the management of various neuromusculoskeletal pain syndromes by inserting fine monofilament needles through the skin, most commonly involving needling the myofascial trigger points (MTrPs).[185] Other DNTs include periosteal stimulation (PST) and intramuscular electrical stimulation (IMES). Physical therapists performing DNTs must do so within state regulations and with appropriate educational training. A recent systematic review investigating DNTs in knee OA indicated a lack of good quality studies on MTrP DNT. The PST technique was found to have moderate-quality evidence on the short-term effect of PST on pain and function, but long-term effects could not be confirmed. IMES demonstrated potential for a significant effect on pain in knee OA; however, due to heterogeneity of the studies and limited number, further research is required.[186] DNTs are also not recommended for patients with RA in a recently published clinical practice guideline due to lack of evidence of effectiveness.[121]

Rest

Complete bedrest is rarely recommended. Adequate quality and quantity of sleep at night and short rests during the day are preferred. General recommendations include 8 to 10 hr of sleep per night and brief 30-minute rest periods during the day. Inactivity is a common problem for people with arthritis and may lead to deconditioning, depression, lower pain thresholds, diminished bone and soft tissue health, and increased risk for other serious health conditions. Thus, a major goal of therapy is to assist patients to maintain or regain adequate levels of physical activity and avoid the unnecessary consequences of inactivity.[29,187]

Range of Motion and Flexibility Exercise

A major factor affecting joint mobility in individuals with RA is the level of inflammation and the resting position in which specific joints are maintained. For example, intra-articular pressure is reduced when joints are in flexion. Although helpful in reducing joint pain, this flexed position may lead to capsular and musculotendinous shortening and eventual contracture. Patients should be taught proper positioning when resting and should be encouraged to perform daily, active ROM as tolerated to maintain motion. Active-assisted, passive, and proprioceptive neuromuscular facilitation techniques may also be applied to shortened muscles. Pain should be respected at all times and should be minimal during and after exercise. Evoking a pain response during stretching may lead to a reflex contraction of the agonist muscle as opposed to creating a relaxation response. Patients should be taught to stretch muscles slowly, to hold the position for 20 to 30 seconds and perform stretching exercises 2 to 3 days a week or more often if indicated. Patients should avoid stretching inflamed, swollen joints because they are at risk for capsular stretching and rupture.[29,187] Common wisdom recommends that *exercise-induced pain should subside within 1 hr.* If patients report discomfort lasting longer than 1 hr, it may indicate that the technique, intensity, or duration of the exercise was too great and should be reduced or modified at the next exercise session. Encourage patients to exercise on their own during periods of the day when they feel best. Local pain-relieving modalities before or immediately after exercise may be useful and increase exercise adherence.

In hip and knee OA, manual therapy offers some additional benefit within a comprehensive treatment program that includes exercise.[188] In a systematic review of manual therapy techniques including passive physiological and accessory movements, muscle stretching, and soft tissue mobilization, moderate to large effects for pain and self-reported function were found when compared to alternate interventions and exercise alone.[188] The ACR clinical practice guidelines recommend manual therapy combined with exercise for knee OA management.[110] Manual therapy is not generally recommended for individuals with RA who have joint inflammation or resultant laxity. According to a recent RA clinical practice guideline, short-term passive mobilization is conditionally recommended only when provided to support exercise therapy in patients without active inflammation.[121]

Strengthening Exercise

Decreased muscle function (strength, endurance, power) arises from both direct and indirect effects of the disease. These include intra-articular and extra-articular inflammatory disease elements, side effects of medication, disuse, reflex inhibition in response to pain and joint effusion, impaired proprioception, and loss of mechanical integrity around the joint. A variety of conditioning programs can be effective for improving strength, endurance, and function without exacerbation of pain or disease activity. Exercise has also been shown to reduce RA-related cachexia with concurrent increases in fat-free body mass.[189]

Initially, isometric exercise may be indicated to improve muscle tone, strength, and static endurance; to recruit or activate specific muscles; and to prepare joints for more vigorous activity. Although isometric exercise does avoid dynamic joint stress and mechanical irritation, it can produce other unwanted effects. Isometric exercise performed at more than 50% of maximal voluntary contraction constricts blood flow through the exercising muscle, leading to postexercise muscle soreness, and the increased peripheral vascular resistance produces increased blood pressure.[187] In the knee and hip, high-intensity isometric contractions are associated with significant increases in intra-articular pressure and reductions in synovial circulation.[190–192] Patients with cardiovascular disease should perform these exercises with caution and be sure to breathe during the contraction as holding one's breath can increase intra-abdominal pressure (*Valsalva maneuver*). Patient instructions for isometric exercise should include the cautions to (a) maintain the contraction for no more than 6 seconds, (b) avoid maximal effort because it is neither necessary nor desirable, (c) exhale during the contraction and inhale during a similar time period of relaxation, and (d) not contract more than two muscle groups at a time.

Dynamic exercise includes both shortening (concentric) and lengthening (eccentric) contractions. Strength and endurance may be improved through resistance (physiological overload) supplied by weight of the body part or external resistance in the form of free weights, elastic bands, or a variety of resistive exercise equipment. A cautious approach to resistance training is recommended to protect unstable or inflamed joints from damage. Strengthening exercise should be performed within the pain-free range. Maximum benefit and maintenance can be achieved by incorporating functional movements and body positions in the recommended exercise routine. The use of well-controlled smooth movement toward the end of the movement range is advised, and modifications to resistance, repetitions, or frequency are recommended as needed. Assessment of strength via a one-repetition maximum (1RM) test is recommended to establish the proper exercise intensity. A warm-up and cooldown should precede any exercise session. Longer cooldown periods are recommended for those who are deconditioned and older adults. Gradual progression of resistance and repetition over a 2- to 3-week period is recommended. Reduce exercise intensity, frequency, or motion if increased joint swelling or pain occurs (local inflammatory response).[29]

Individuals with RA benefit from maintaining or restoring muscular fitness. Several systematic reviews and meta-analyses of the literature illustrate that there is moderate-level evidence for the benefits of both short- (8 to 12 weeks) and long-term progressive land-based and aquatic resistance exercise (a year or more) of up to 70% of one repetition of maximal contraction (1RM) for muscle strength and functional performance. Loads of up to 70% 1RM used in a circuit training resistance program for persons with controlled RA demonstrated no exacerbation in joint symptoms and significant improvements in strength and function. Studies of higher intensity tended to yield greater improvements. Data are presented in Table 23.4 Evidence Summary.[121,193–195]

Designing exercise interventions for individuals with RA requires careful consideration of the patient's disease activity, disease severity, and systemic disease features. Persons with RA in an active flare-up should limit their exercise to daily ROM exercises incorporated into ADL to promote adherence to active joint movement and isometric exercises to promote strength. It is also important to use caution with resistance exercise in individuals on high doses of corticosteroids to reduce the risk of tendon rupture and osteoporosis-related fractures. Walking as tolerated is encouraged together with daily periods of rest and a full night of sleep to manage fatigue. When the disease activity subsides, the exercise program can be progressed by adding dynamic strengthening exercises, with caution to avoid stress on deranged joints or cysts, and greater repetitions of isometric exercises as well as greater engagement in physical activity. When the disease is in remission, aerobic exercises and dynamic exercises with resistance should be considered to promote cardiovascular health and improve strength and conditioning. When RA affects the large weight-bearing joints, patients should be cautious with high-intensity impact exercise especially in the presence of established joint changes.[196] For patients with RA who are deconditioned or not sure if they should to exercise, it is recommended to begin a strengthening program at 50% to 60% of 1RM and a perceived exertion rating (PRE) score of roughly 12 to 13. Those accustomed to exercise may begin at 60% to 80% of 1 1RM and PRE score 14 to 16, with two to four sets of 8 to 15 repetitions incorporating 30- to 60-seconds rest periods between sets.[121] Exercises should focus on large muscle groups and be performed bilaterally.

In persons with knee OA, the evidence is strong and consistent indicating LE exercise that includes neuromuscular and functional training reduces pain and improves function. Interventions have included isometric, isotonic, functional, and aquatic exercise, as well as proprioceptive and balance training. Interventions have been tested in both clinically supervised and self-directed settings with positive results and acceptable adherence.[197] Evidence supporting the use of exercise

Table 23.4 Evidence Summary Systematic Reviews and Clinical Practice Guidelines of Interventions for Adults With Rheumatoid Arthritis

Subjects	Methods	Duration/Dosage	Results/Comments
Hammond et al. (2016)[193]			
665 adults with mean age of 59 years (one study had adults with early RA)	Seven RCTs of supervised home hand exercise therapy: ROM and resistance exercise (three RCTs with low risk of bias and four with moderate risk of bias assessed with PEDro scale)	Duration ranged from 4–52 weeks. Frequency ranged from one individualized session with home exercise follow-up to daily, supervised sessions.	Data indicated significant short-term gains in hand function, pain, and grip strength. Long-term improvements found for hand and upper extremity function and pinch strength. Data suggest high-intensity home hand exercise programs led to better short-term outcomes than low-intensity programs, and these programs are cost-effective.
Wen and Chai (2021)[194]			
512 in. resistance exercise group and 498 in. control group; all female participants	17 RCTs included in the meta-analysis, mean quality score of 3.83/5	Duration ranged from 3 weeks–24 months; Frequency 1–7 times per week; time ranged from 20–80 min; intensity ranged from max load 40%–80%	Resistance exercise significantly decreased DAS-28 scores, reduced ESR and shortened the time of 50-ft walking. No significant difference was observed in VAS scores and HAQ scores.
Ye et al. (2022)[195]			
967 adults with RA, of varying degrees of functional status, age range 45–70.11 years	13 RCTs with aerobic exercise interventions; low to moderate quality evidence	Duration was from 15 to 90 minutes; frequency two to five times a week, intensity 30%–90% of max heart rate.	Moderate-quality evidence for significant gains in functional capacity and pain; low-quality evidence for increase in aerobic capacity.
Peter et al. (2021)[121]			
Clinical Practice Guideline	Patients with varying clinical presentations of RA	Refer to article for detailed parameters.	Exercise therapy—conditional to strong recommendation. Avoid using passive modalities—conditional recommendation. Patient education—conditional recommendation.

DAS-28 = disease activity score in 28 joints; ESR = erythrocyte sedimentation rate; HAQ = health assessment questionnaire; PEDro = Physiotherapy Evidence Database; RA = rheumatoid arthritis; RCT = randomized controlled trial; ROM = range of motion; VAS = visual analog scale.

in the management of knee and hip OA is presented in Table 23.5 Evidence Summary.[110,183,198-202] Exercises should be performed bilaterally for hip and knee OA, and exercises with high mechanical load should be avoided in patients with knee OA. To enhance adherence to exercise, physical therapists should routinely incorporate strategies including exercise booster sessions (periodic follow-up appointments), goal setting, and other self-efficacy enhancing practices.[187,203]

Cardiovascular Training

Individuals with RA or OA are usually deconditioned compared to their age-matched peers. A number of systematic reviews have reported significant improvements in aerobic capacity and activity levels through regular cardiovascular conditioning without aggravating joints and other disease symptoms. If weight-bearing is a barrier to exercise, low- or non-weight-bearing activities such as stationary cycling, pool-based aerobics, or deep water running may be options.[19,157,203] For most people, walking and stationary bicycles are safe and effective means of aerobic exercise.[19,204] Furthermore, patients who have engaged in such a program often report improved self-esteem and emotional status.[19] Medical screening as appropriate for age and medical condition (e.g., *Revised Physical Activity Readiness Questionnaire* [PAR-Q]) (http://eparmedx.com) should be completed before beginning an aerobic exercise program. The use

Table 23.5	Evidence Summary: Systematic Reviews and Clinical Practice Guidelines of Therapeutic Exercise in the Management of Knee and Hip Osteoarthritis		
Subjects	**Methods**	**Duration/Dosage**	**Results/Comments**
Brosseau et al. (2017)[198]			
Adults with clinical diagnosis of knee OA. Total of 36 (yoga) and 196 (Tai Chi) participants. No mean age or demographics provided.	Guidelines with systematic review of four RCTs up to May 2016 examining effects of mind–body exercise programs (e.g., yoga, Tai Chi). Expert consensus panel assigned Grades A to D based on statistical significance and clinical importance (≥5% improvement).	Interventions ranged from 8–12 weeks. No details on frequency or intensity provided.	Significant improvement with Hatha yoga for pain relief (Grade B) and physical function (Grade C+). Tai Chi Qigong resulted in significant improvement for quality of life (Grade B), pain relief (Grade C+) and physical function (Grade C+). Sun-style Tai Chi gave significant improvement for pain relief (Grade B) and physical function (Grade B).
Brosseau et al. (2017)[199]			
Adults with clinical diagnosis of knee OA. Total of 3,621 participants with mean age ranging from 55–70 years (reported for nine studies only).	Guidelines with systematic review of 26 RCTs examining effects of strengthening exercises. Expert consensus panel assigned Grades A to D based on statistical significance and clinical importance (≥5% improvement).	Interventions ranged from 4–52 weeks. No details on frequency or intensity provided.	Significant improvement for pain relief and physical function (Grade A) and quality of life (Grade B). Strengthening in combination with exercise (e.g., balance, functional) also showed a significant improvement in these outcomes (Grade A).
Brosseau et al. (2017)[200]			
Adults with clinical diagnosis of knee OA. Total of 650 participants with mean age ranging from 58–68 years.	Guidelines with systematic review of five RCTs examining effects of aerobic exercise. Expert consensus panel assigned Grades A to D based on statistical significance and clinical importance (≥5% improvement).	Included trials ranged from 4–12 weeks with varied interventions including walking, running, and cycling. Most included a strengthening component.	Significant improvement for pain relief (Grade B), physical function (Grade B), and quality of life (Grade C+). Aerobic exercise in combination with strengthening exercises also showed significant improvement for pain relief (Grade A) and physical function (Grade A).

Table 23.5 Evidence Summary: Systematic Reviews and Clinical Practice Guidelines of Therapeutic Exercise in the Management of Knee and Hip Osteoarthritis—cont'd

Subjects	Methods	Duration/Dosage	Results/Comments
		Hu et al. (2021)[183]	
Patients with knee OA were included. Total of 986 subjects; mean age of 59.9–78.9 years.	Systematic review of 16 RCTs examining the effects of Tai Chi on the physical and mental health of individuals with knee OA.	Duration was between 5 and 52 weeks.	Moderate-quality evidence for improvements in pain and stiffness, physical function, dynamic balance, physiological and psychological health.
		Luan et al. (2022)[201]	
Patients with knee OA were included. Age range 35–91 years old.	A systematic review and meta-analysis of 18 RCTs evaluated the effectiveness of stretching exercises for pain relief in individuals with OA.	Duration was between 6 and 16 weeks.	Stretching exercises alone may be sufficient to improve pain in individuals with KOA. Quality of evidence was low to moderate as several items had low-quality scores due to heterogeneity and small sample size.
		Turner et al. (2020)[202]	
1,428 participants with KOA were included with mean age range 51.9–71.2 years to determine if resistance training affects pain and physical function.	12 RCTs, mean CONSORT quality score 20.3 (range 17–24.5).	30–60-minute session of two to three sets of 8–12 repetitions with an initial resistance of 50% to 60% of maximum resistance that progressed over three sessions per week for 24 weeks.	Quadriceps muscle strengthening has positive effects on pain and function, whether with open- or closed-chain techniques.
		Kolasinski (2019)[110]	
ACR/Arthritis Foundation Guideline for the Management of Osteoarthritis of the Hand, Hip, and Knee.	Patients with hip, knee, and hand OA.	Refer to article for details regarding specific parameters.	Aerobic exercise, strengthening, neuromuscular training, aquatic exercise are strongly recommended; balance exercises are conditionally recommended; weight loss is strongly recommended for patients who are overweight or obese; self-efficacy and self-management programs are strongly recommended; Tai Chi is strongly recommended; Yoga is conditionally recommended; thermal interventions are conditionally recommended.

KOA = knee osteoarthritis; OA = osteoarthritis; RCT = randomized controlled trial.

of performance-based standardized outcome measures (as well as vital signs, pain, and RPE) are important to assess, monitor, and modify the patient's individualized POC. For patients with RA who are not accustomed to aerobic exercise, a general guideline is to initiate aerobic conditioning exercises at 40% to 60% of maximum heart rate and a PRE of 12 to 13. Ensure a gradual buildup in intensity to greater than 60% of maximum HR and a PRE of 14 to 17 and follow the training principles.[121]

Physical Activity

Patients with RA and OA are less physically active than their healthy counterparts despite the benefits of physical activity in reducing disease activity and improving health status.[205] The U.S. Department of Health and Human Services has established *Physical Activity Guidelines*. These guidelines recommend accumulating 150 to 300 min/week of moderate-intensity or 75 to 150 min/week of vigorous-intensity aerobic physical activity for adults with chronic health conditions.[206] Additionally, muscle-strengthening activities of moderate or greater intensity that involve all major muscle groups on 2 or more days a week is recommended. In a study by Lee et al., 42% of patients with RA accumulated no moderate/vigorous physical activity over a 1-week period.[207] In a longitudinal study of a large cohort of adults, those with knee OA spent two-thirds of their daily time in sedentary behavior (e.g., watching TV, using computer, reading).[208] Sedentary behavior is an independent risk factor for increased morbidity and mortality; therefore, it is vital that physical therapists counsel and support patients to "move more and sit less" throughout the day. Fortunately, there are many technologies (mobile apps used with smartphones, wearable devices, Internet tracking programs, etc.) that can help motivate patients to be physically active, enable them to track their progress, and serve as a coaching tool for physical therapists (Table 23.6).

Functional Training

Functional training for the individual with arthritis proceeds in the same fashion as for other individuals with similar deficits. Therapists may choose to reduce the functional demands of an activity either temporarily, due to acute inflammation, or permanently by incorporating a variety of adaptive equipment into ADLs that substitute for lost ROM and strength. To ensure patients with RA can engage in functional training activities, modifications can be made to handles of devices for easier grasp. Occupational therapists may be involved to recommend aids for dressing and grooming as well as personal hygiene. By breaking functional tasks, such as rising from a chair or climbing stairs, into smaller movements and incorporating these into a therapeutic exercise program, the therapist can help the patient identify faulty movement patterns and address specific movement components that are causing

difficulty. Functional exercises aim to replicate daily activities including house, yard, work, and leisure activities that are important to the patient. Such exercises often incorporate body weight for resistance and the use of actual tools/equipment or movements that make up that activity.

Rearranging the home or work environment also can improve a person's functional abilities. Raising beds or chairs can reduce the effort needed to stand up. Railings placed around the bed, bath, and along stairways also can help increase an individual's independence.

Gait and Balance Training

Specific deviations will be evident throughout the gait cycle in both RA and OA. These may include gait asymmetries, decreased velocity, cadence and stride length, prolonged period of double support, inadequate initial contact and push-off, and diminished joint excursion through both swing and stance phases. Gait deviations in the patient with RA, specifically owing to foot pain or deformities, may also be evident (Table 23.7).[146,209] Interventions should target underlying joint and muscle impairments that contribute to these deviations for individuals with any type of arthritis.

The degree to which a patient's gait should, or can, approximate normal is one of the most difficult questions in designing a therapeutic program. Some "abnormalities" such as antalgic limping may in fact reduce joint loading. Joint destruction may necessitate the introduction of assistive devices as simple as a standard cane or walking poles. UE involvement in RA, particularly of the wrist and hands, may complicate the choice of an ambulatory assistive device by precluding any weightbearing on these affected joints. In these instances, platform attachments can be added to crutches or walkers to transform the forearm into a weight-bearing surface. Use of a properly fitted, standard cane in the contralateral hand is associated with decreased joint loading and pain in individuals with both hip and knee OA. The gait of the individual with RA or OA should be safe, functional, and cosmetically acceptable to the patient rather than an unattainable idealized version of the norm.

Decreased gait speed in arthritis is common, and there is general agreement that increased speed is a meaningful measure of functional capacity and improvement.[210] For example, a person's ability to walk fast enough to cross the street with the timing of the traffic light is important for functional and safe community locomotion. However, increased gait speed without attention to joint biomechanics may be undesirable. In a clinical trial of a nonsteroidal drug for persons with knee OA, all with a varus deformity, gait variables were included as outcome measures. The researchers found that self-reported pain diminished and walking speed increased in the active therapy group. At the same time, kinetic analysis of joint forces showed the increased speed was accompanied by increased adductor movement at the

Table 23.6 Mobile and Internet Applications for Tracking and Promoting Physical Activity

Application	Description and Link
ArthritisPower	Mobile application where you can enter exercise as well as data on fatigue, sleep, and medications, and you can track your disease symptoms. https://arthritispower.creakyjoints.org
Health Log	This mobile app for smartphones helps a patient record and track exercise, weight, hours of sleep, mood, and other useful functions. https://play.google.com/store/apps/details?id=andrew.arproductions.healthlog&hl=en
MyRA Touch	This RA symptom tracking app allows you to record information about your joint pain, fatigue, and other RA-related symptoms in your phone. You can also print out the information to share with your rheumatologist or rheumatology health professional. Available for iPhones and Androids.
RheumaTrack	This mobile app allows you to track your RA symptoms as well as physical activity. It includes a personal lock system to keep health information safe.
Track+React	Developed by the Arthritis Foundation, this app enables people with RA to track their fitness, nutrition, sleep, and self-management activities to see what impact it has on their symptoms. http://www.arthritis.org/living-with-arthritis/tools-resources/track-and-react/track-and-react-app.php
tRAppen	This mobile Internet service was designed specifically to help adults with RA self-manage their disease. A recent study of its use suggests tRAppen may support a physically active lifestyle. http://rmdopen.bmj.com/content/rmdopen/2/1/e000214.full.pdf
Walk With Ease	This Internet-based and mobile app allows you to track your steps. The application is based on the Arthritis Foundation's Walk With Ease 6-week program. http://www.arthritis.org/living-with-arthritis/tools-resources/walk-with-ease/about.php
Wokamon	A simple gamification of walking in which the Wokamon gets more food and grows larger the more you walk.
Stepz	This free app uses cell phone sensors to count steps, flights climbed, mileage covered, and calories burned. You can set your own goals or use an automatic goal. https://apps.apple.com/us/app/stepz-step-counter-tracker/id839671656
Raise	This free app was developed by or in conjunction with people with RA and knee pain. Provides suggestions for exercises to relieve arthritis symptoms. https://appadvice.com/app/raise-rheumatoid-arthritis/1035627318
5-min yoga	This free app provides a new yoga sequence each day including a photo of the pose and a description of the movement. Then, a countdown clock for how long to hold the pose or position. Not designed specifically for patients with RA or OA. https://apps.apple.com/us/app/5-minute-yoga-workouts/id362093404

OA = osteoarthritis; RA = rheumatoid arthritis.

knee and greater loading of the medial compartment.[211] This additional joint loading and increased stress on lateral supporting tissues may not be worth the gains of increased speed. Careful attention to biomechanical factors is necessary in comprehensive management, even when drug therapy decreases pain and improves gait speed.

Decreased proprioceptive input, impaired neuromuscular reflexes, altered joint biomechanics, pain, and muscle weakness contribute to static and dynamic balance problems in adults with LE arthritis. Balance training may include progression from static postures, moving from double- to single-limb support, transitioning from stable to unstable surfaces, and adding

perturbations, when safe. Dynamic balance activities include maintaining postural alignment while shifting weight from one limb to the other in various directions and walking on different surfaces to challenge the vestibular and proprioceptive systems. A systematic review of 17 randomized controlled trials and clinical controlled trials found no studies that separately evaluated balance training, rather exercise programs were comprehensive in nature including muscle strengthening, endurance, and functional activities.[212] Published clinical practice guidelines recommend the incorporation of balance and coordination training in the management of adults with OA and RA[110,121] (see Chapter 10, Strategies to Improve Motor Function).

Table 23.7   Analysis of Gait Deviations, Physical Examination Findings, and Intervention Goals

Gait Deviations	Physical Examination Findings	Intervention Goals
Pronated Foot		
Shuffled progression Decreased step length Initial contact with medial border of foot Decreased single-limb balance Prolonged double-support phase Late heel rise Plantarflexion of ipsilateral ankle in swing Genu valgus with weight-bearing	Tenderness over subtalar midtarsal area Limited inversion range Weak and painful posterior tibialis muscle Pronated weight-bearing posture of foot Lax medial collateral ligament of knee	Relieve subtalar and midtarsal joint stresses Increase ankle inversion Strengthen posterior tibialis muscle Stabilize hypermobile joints with rigid orthosis Maintain neutral alignment in stance by foot positioning
Hallux Valgus		
Lateral and posterior weight shift Late heel rise Decreased single-limb balance	Lateral deviation of great toe Swelling of first MTP joint Shortening of flexor hallucis brevis muscle Tenderness of great toe Weakness of great toe abduction	Accommodate foot with wide toe box shoe Increase extension of great toe Relieve weight-bearing stresses
Metatarsophalangeal Joint Subluxation		
Diminished roll-off Decreased single-limb stance Apropulsive progression Decreased single-limb balance	Painful MTP heads with weight-bearing Callus formation over MTP heads Ulcerations over MTP heads Limited MTP flexion Prominent MTP heads	Redistribute pressure with metatarsal bar Relieve pressure with soft cutout shoe insert Increase flexion mobility of MTP joints Accommodate foot with extra-depth shoe
Hammer or Claw Toes		
Diminished roll-off Decreased single-limb stance Apropulsive progression Decreased single-limb balance	Posture of MTP joint hyperextension with proximal and distal interphalangeal joint flexion Posture of MTP and distal interphalangeal joint hyperextension with proximal interphalangeal flexion Callus formation at plantar tips and dorsum of proximal interphalangeal joint Limited MTP flexion	Improve toe alignment with metatarsal bar Accommodate foot with extra-depth shoe Diminish pressure with soft insert Increase toe mobility
Painful Heel		
Toe-heel pattern No heel contact in stance Decreased stride length Decreased velocity Plantarflexion of ankle in swing Increased hip flexion in swing Decreased step length of contralateral limb	Painful active plantarflexion Painful passive and active dorsiflexion Swelling and pain at Achilles insertion Tenderness over spur Decreased ankle dorsiflexion range	Decrease inflammation with steroid injection or modalities Relieve weight-bearing stress Decrease pressure over spur with soft shoe insert Maintain ankle mobility

From Dimonte and Light[209] with permission.
MTP = metatarsophalangeal.

Education and Self-Management

Patient education in rheumatic diseases yields positive changes in knowledge, health behavior, beliefs, and attitudes that affect health status, quality of life, and health care utilization. In a review of the literature, researchers documented the well-established benefits of self-management programs on mental health.[120] As in any chronic illness, education should include information needed to deal with the condition (taking medications, exercise), self-management skills necessary to carry out important social and vocational roles, and resources to deal with the emotional consequences of chronic illness such as depression, fear, and frustration. The evidence was overwhelming that education designed to teach self-management skills and increase client self-efficacy for these tasks is the most effective.[120,213] Referral by physical therapists to local counseling services, peer support groups, or web-based resources is essential for the holistic approach to patient care. The *Arthritis Foundation* (https://www.arthritis.org) can supply the clinician or the individual with a variety of resources and self-help courses that will increase cognitive understanding of the disease process and self-management skills. (See Appendix 23.A [online].) Local chapters of the Arthritis Foundation hold individual and family support groups to increase psychosocial adaptation as well as conduct aquatic and land exercise programs in public facilities. The *Association of Rheumatology Health Professionals*, a division of the ACR (https://rheumatology.org), can provide the therapist with scientific and clinical resources for enhanced practice, as well as a network of professional colleagues who work in rheumatology. (See Appendix 23.B [online].)

Telehealth/Telerehabilitation

The World Health Organization (WHO), EULAR, and the American Physical Therapy Association (APTA) acknowledge the potential benefit of telehealth, the use of electronic information and telecommunication technologies to remotely provide health care information and services, when access to clinical practice is not possible. Approaches such as videoconferencing, phone conversations, text messaging, and online support groups have led to positive outcomes for individuals with OA and RA, specifically in the areas of pain reduction, self-management, and improved adherence. Additionally, with the expansion of telehealth/telerehabilitation, observation of gait can be accomplished with a family member or other individual present to record a patient's gait for the therapist in real time or for later evaluation. Smart phone mobile applications also exist which can record and provide some interpretation of the gait pattern to be incorporated in the physical therapists' gait and balance assessment.[214,215] These applications are relatively new, and their psychometric properties are consistently being evaluated. Further high-quality research regarding prescription and long-term effectiveness is required to evaluate optimal care delivery. It is recommended to regularly review telehealth state guidelines as variability of laws and regulations between states exist and telehealth practices are continuously evolving.

SUMMARY

RA and OA are the two most common forms of arthritis in adults. Both exact a high toll with respect to physical functioning and limitations in participation and quality of life. RA, due to its exacerbating and remitting course and systemic features, also impacts mental well-being. Advances in medical therapies for both conditions combined with physical therapy and physical activity allow patients to achieve maximum functioning. Physical therapy for these patients covers a broad array of interventions, from modalities and orthotics to exercise and self-management strategies. Exercise has the strongest evidence for benefits, equivalent to the effects of nonsteroidal medications, whereas the evidence for other interventions is less strong. Overall, data have shown that maintaining a physically active lifestyle is important for both joint and cardiovascular health and should be a component of all counseling discussions with patients.

Questions for Review

1. What epidemiological factors are associated with a diagnosis of RA?
2. What are the major pathological changes seen in RA?
3. State two hypotheses concerning the pathogenesis of RA.
4. Describe four modifiable risk factors that may predispose an individual to OA.
5. Describe two changes in articular cartilage associated with OA that differ from normal aging.
6. Name at least two laboratory tests used in the diagnosis of RA and state their purposes.
7. Describe the parameters used in examining radiographs of arthritic joints.

8. Describe the typical joint changes seen with RA for the following joints: occipitoatlantal, atlantoaxial, temporomandibular, carpals, knees, and talocalcaneal.

9. Define the following deformities: ulnar drift, swan neck, boutonnière, hammer toes, claw toes, and hallux valgus.

10. Describe the typical radiographic joint changes seen in advanced OA.

11. Describe the overall goals of medical management for RA and OA.

12. What are the primary indications for surgery in RA?

13. Describe the key points in taking a history for the individual with arthritis.

14. What adaptations of standard tests and measures might be required in examining the individual with RA?

15. What are the general physical therapy goals for individuals with RA or OA?

16. Explain the goals, modifications, and progression of a typical strengthening program.

17. Discuss treatment strategies for increasing ROM.

18. Design a cardiovascular conditioning program for an individual with LE arthritic joint involvement.

19. Describe strategies to enhance patients' adherence to therapeutic exercise programs.

20. State at least four principles of joint protection and give a practical application of each.

21. What criteria guide the selection of shoes for the individual with RA?

22. What are the purposes of splints?

23. Name two yellow flags and two red flags in adults with RA and OA.

24. What changes in gait are commonly associated with RA? What impairments contribute to static and dynamic balance problems in the individual with LE arthritis?

CASE STUDY

Two case studies are presented: Case 1, a patient with RA; and Case 2, a patient with OA.

CASE 1: RHEUMATOID ARTHRITIS
History
The patient is a 52-year-old woman who has two children in high school. She is a nurse and works about 40 hr/week. She has had symptoms of joint swelling and pain, fatigue, and increasing weakness for 2 years. During the initial onset of symptoms, a primary care physician diagnosed her with carpal tunnel syndrome, knee OA, and eventually, fibromyalgia. Her symptoms continued to worsen on NSAIDs. She was also prescribed antidepressants, and she was referred to a rheumatologist 3 months ago. Based on her history, physical examination, laboratory values (DAS = 3.2; RF = 12.30; ESR = 26), and radiographic evidence, the rheumatologist confirmed a diagnosis of seropositive RA. She began a course of methotrexate and has been referred to physical therapy.

Physical Therapy Examination
At the initial outpatient physical therapy examination, she reports her morning stiffness is now less than 30 minutes (previous high of 3 hr). The pain and swelling in her hands, feet, and elbows is markedly decreased, and she is feeling more energetic. Systems review of the integumentary system is unremarkable except for slight edema and redness of the distal finger joints and wrist right greater than left. Her blood pressure and respiratory rate are within normal limits. Her resting heart rate is 72 bpm but increases to 96 bpm with modest exertion.

ROM is limited at the shoulders, elbows, wrists, and MCPs. She lacks 10° of knee extension and has no ankle dorsiflexion or hip extension beyond neutral. Bilateral strength is grossly 4-/5. She exhibits a forward head, rounded shoulder posture, with the beginning of a marked kyphosis. Her pain is most prominent in her wrists, elbows, and ankles (4/10 visual analog scale [VAS]) and indicates general fatigue. She has pronated feet and moderate swelling of the metatarsal heads. She is relieved that she has been diagnosed with a condition for which there is effective treatment, and she trusts her rheumatologist. Her immediate goals are to regain comfortable motion, strength, and stamina and to avoid deformity.

Guiding Questions

1. Identify the general anticipated goals and expected outcomes of physical therapy for this patient.

2. What self-management strategies would you recommend and/or instruct the patient to use?

3. Describe the types of community resources you would recommend the patient explore.

4. What supportive devices might be used to decrease symptoms and increase function?

5. How would her physical therapist optimally schedule her return visits to the outpatient clinic?

CASE 2: OSTEOARTHRITIS

History

The patient is a 58-year-old woman with low back and bilateral knee pain that has increased over the past year. She is 5-ft 7 in. tall and weighs 195 lb. She has a past medical history of hypertension and chronic renal insufficiency for which she takes prescribed medication. She works part time as a teacher's assistant in a local elementary school and lives alone in a third-floor walk-up apartment. On weekends, she serves as the assistant building manager, which includes both cleaning and minimal maintenance duties. She has difficulty using stairs, getting up and down from sitting, getting on and off the bus, and walking for more than 15 minutes at a time. She has had progressively greater knee pain and stiffness for the past 3 years and has recently experienced episodes of "giving way" in the right knee. Her low back pain is worse after prolonged sitting, vacuuming, and at the end of the day. She avoids over-the-counter medications due to her underlying kidney disease but reports moderate pain relief with topical diclofenac gel applied to both knees three times a day. The patient recently joined an aquafit class at a local pool but admits to rarely attending classes.

On a recent visit to her primary care physician, she underwent radiographs of both knees that revealed bilateral joint space narrowing, with the right knee more affected than the left and greater lateral compartment involvement than medial. There is evidence of bony sclerosis, osteophytes, and mild malalignment (genu valgum) greater on the right. Her physician has suggested continued use of the topical NSAID, use of a cane, weight loss, and referred her to a physical therapist for evaluation and exercise advice. The patient and her doctor have agreed to discuss surgical options for the knee if she is not satisfied with her condition in 3 to 6 months.

Physical Therapy Examination

During the initial history and systems review, the patient reports that she is finding both of her part-time jobs difficult, in particular, her cleaning responsibilities in the apartment building. She is divorced with one grown son who lives out of town. She is frequently tired and lacks the energy to go to the pool classes despite enjoying the session she last attended 2 months ago. The patient admits to not sleeping well and having to take occasional sick days from her school-based job. She is concerned about finances and feels that she needs to avoid knee surgery and continue working for at least another 3 years. Her pain is intermittent during the day but wakes her up frequently during the night. Her heart rate is 82, her blood pressure is 140/85, and her respiratory rate is 16. Her skin and circulation in the LEs are unremarkable, and sensory integrity and reflexes are intact.

Selected tests and measures reveal weakness and loss of motion in hips and knees bilaterally and an antalgic and slow gait. Her spinal ROM is restricted in extension and rotation. Anterior–posterior knee stability is good, but there is moderate pseudolaxity of the lateral collateral ligaments bilaterally. She rates her left knee pain on the VAS as 7/10 while walking and 8/10 while climbing stairs. Right knee pain is at 6/10 for all activities. She is wearing unsupportive slip-on shoes and shows marked ankle pronation on the right and bilateral hallux valgus. Her static dynamic and balance are poor in both legs. She is unable to perform unilateral stance testing greater than 5 seconds secondary to pain, and her score on the Timed Up and Go Test was 11 seconds, indicating a fall risk. Her fast-paced walking speed is 0.94 m/sec.

Guiding Questions

1. What anticipated goals should the physical therapist discuss with the patient for the POC?

2. Formulate a home exercise program for this patient and determine an optimal schedule for follow-up by the physical therapist.

(Continued)

CASE STUDY—cont'd

3. What kind of orthotic device(s) or equipment would reduce this patient's symptoms and increase her function?

4. What should be included in patient-related instruction to maximize this patient's function?

5. What strategies would maximize this patient's adherence to a home exercise program and regular physical activity?

6. What other health professional(s) and or community resources would you recommend for this patient?

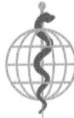

For additional resources, including answers to the questions for review, new immersive cases, case study guiding questions, references, and more, please visit **https://www.fadavis.com/product/physical-rehabilitation-fulk-8**. You may also quickly find the resources by entering this title's four-digit ISBN, 4691, in the search field at **http://fadavis.com** and logging in at the prompt.

Burns

R. Scott Ward, PT, PhD, FAPTA, BT-C Certified Burn Therapist
Ingrid S. Parry, MS, PT, BT-C

Chapter 24

LEARNING OBJECTIVES

1. Describe the anatomy and physiology of the skin as an organ in the healthy state and the damaged condition that occurs with a burn injury.
2. Discuss the pathology, symptoms, and sequelae of burn injuries.
3. Compare the treatment for various depths and extent of burn injury in relation to medical, surgical, and physical therapy management.
4. Identify the consequences of contracture formation after burn injury and the treatment of this condition.
5. Differentiate the options for management of hypertrophic scars.
6. Determine the type of skin care necessary after burn wound healing.
7. Design a physical therapy plan of care that appropriately incorporates positioning, splinting, and exercise.
8. Analyze and interpret patient data, formulate realistic goals and outcomes, and develop a plan of care when presented with a clinical case study.

CHAPTER OUTLINE

EPIDEMIOLOGY OF BURN INJURIES 939
SKIN ANATOMY AND BURN WOUND PATHOLOGY 940
CLASSIFICATIONS OF BURN INJURY 941
  Epidermal Burn 942
  Superficial Partial-Thickness Burn 942
  Deep Partial-Thickness Burn 943
  Full-Thickness Burn 944
  Subdermal Burn 945
  Electrical Burn 945
  Burn Wound Zones 945
  Extent of Burned Area 946
COMPLICATIONS OF BURN INJURY 946
  Infection 946
  Pulmonary Complications 946
  Metabolic Complications 946

Cardiovascular Complications 948
Heterotopic Ossification 948
Neuropathy 948
Pathological Scars 948
BURN WOUND HEALING 948
  Epidermal Healing 948
  Dermal Healing 949
MEDICAL MANAGEMENT 950
  Initial Treatment 950
  Surgical Management 951
PHYSICAL THERAPY MANAGEMENT 953
  Examination 954
  Goals and Expected Outcomes 954
  Intervention 954
COMMUNITY PROGRAMS 000
SUMMARY 964

B urn injuries are a major health problem of the industrial world. In the United States, 450,000 to 500,000 burn injuries require medical treatment each year, with an estimated 3,300 related deaths.[1] In addition, it has been estimated that burn injuries account for 40,000 hospitalizations per year, with about 30,000 patients being admitted to specialized burn treatment centers and the balance to other types of medical facilities.

Although these data report the extent of the health care problem caused by burn injury, recent medical advances have significantly reduced the number of deaths from burn injuries and have improved the prognosis and functional abilities of surviving patients.[1–3] The survival rate has improved annually owing to improved resuscitation techniques, the acute medical and surgical care now practiced, and continued research into the management and care of the patient with burns. The American Burn Association (ABA) reported an overall survival rate of 96.8% from 2005 to 2014.[1] As a result of improvements

in care, treatment, and survival of patients with burns, more physical therapists will become responsible for treating these patients for a significant portion of their rehabilitation in settings other than a hospital burn center (e.g., outpatient clinics, community hospitals).

This chapter introduces the clinical presentation of different depths of burn injury and the complications that can result from thermal destruction of the skin. Current techniques used in the medical, surgical, and rehabilitative management of the patient who has been burned will be described. For more in-depth information regarding the examination and treatment of the patient with a burn injury, the reader is referred to additional sources.[4–8]

■ EPIDEMIOLOGY OF BURN INJURIES

Although the morbidity and mortality rate of patients with burns has dramatically decreased in recent years, the epidemiology of burns remains basically the same.

The most common cause of burn injury in children 1 to 5 years of age is from scalds from hot liquids.[9–12] Fires are the most common cause of burn injury in other age groups. Men are twice as likely as women to suffer a burn injury.[1,9] Fire and flame burns make up 43% of the admissions to burn centers, with scald injuries contributing 34% of admissions, then contact burns (9%), electrical injury (4%), and chemical burns (3%), followed by a collection of other causes (7%).[1] The majority of burn injuries occur in the home (73%), followed distantly by occupational sites (8%), motor vehicles (5%), and recreation/sport activities (5%), with 9% of injuries occurring in other settings.[1] The chances of dying from a fire or smoke inhalation is about 1 in 1,442. The number of burn-related accidents has decreased, presumably because of better preventive measures such as smoke detectors, education, and more stringent fire codes.[13]

A major reason for the improved prognosis and survival of patients with severe burn injury is the availability of specialized burn centers.[2] The advent of the burn center and the concentrated team care and focused research that has been generated by these facilities have improved the outcome of the most severely burned patient, as well as reduced the average hospital stay in most cases. The ABA[14] has established criteria for admission to a designated burn center as follows:

- Partial-thickness burns greater than 10% of total body surface area (TBSA)
- Burns that involve the face, hands, feet, genitalia, perineum, or major joints
- Third degree burns in any age group
- Electrical burns, including lightning injury
- Chemical burns
- Inhalation injury
- Burn injury in patients with preexisting medical disorders that could complicate management, prolong recovery, or affect mortality
- Any patient with burns and concomitant trauma (such as fractures) in which the burn injury poses the greatest risk of morbidity or mortality. In such cases, if the trauma poses the greater immediate risk, the patient may be initially stabilized in a trauma center before being transferred to a burn unit. Physician judgment will be necessary in such situations and should be in concert with the regional medical control plan and triage protocols.
- Children with burns who are in hospitals that are without qualified personnel or equipment for the care of children; burn injury in patients who will require special social, emotional, or rehabilitative intervention.

Thirty-five years ago, there were only 12 specialized burn centers in the United States. Today there are over 125 specialized centers for the care of patients with burn injuries and other skin disorders.[15] This accounts for approximately 1,700 beds. Burn centers now have the opportunity to undergo a process of verification (voluntary quality assurance review) through the ABA.[16] Currently, over half of the burn centers in the United States are verified.

A burn center is staffed by specialists from multiple disciplines—physicians, nurses, physical therapists, occupational therapists, dietitians, psychiatrists, psychologists, social workers, child life therapists, chaplains, pharmacists, vocational rehabilitation specialists, and other support personnel—who direct their professional expertise toward the care, treatment, and rehabilitation of the patient with a burn injury. Each member is an integral part of the team, and the most effective burn centers are successful because of their team approach to the care of each patient.[2] It is historically noteworthy that burn personnel, with the founding and establishment of the ABA in 1967, initiated the interdisciplinary "team" approach to patient care.

SKIN ANATOMY AND BURN WOUND PATHOLOGY

The skin is the largest organ of the body, comprising approximately 15% of total body weight. Anatomically, the skin consists of two distinct layers of tissue: the **epidermis**, which is the outermost layer exposed to the environment, and the deeper layer, termed the **dermis** (subdivided into the *papillary* and *reticular* dermis).[17] Although not part of the skin per se, a third layer involved in the anatomical consideration of the skin is the subcutaneous fat cell layer directly under the dermis and above muscle fascial layers. These layers are illustrated in Figure 24.1.

The epidermis is avascular. Notwithstanding, it performs several vital functions. The *stratum corneum* gives the skin its waterproof characteristic and serves the role of protection from infection. The *stratum granulosum* is the layer responsible for water retention. The *stratum spinosum* adds a layer of protection to the underlying stratum basale layer. Cells in the *stratum*

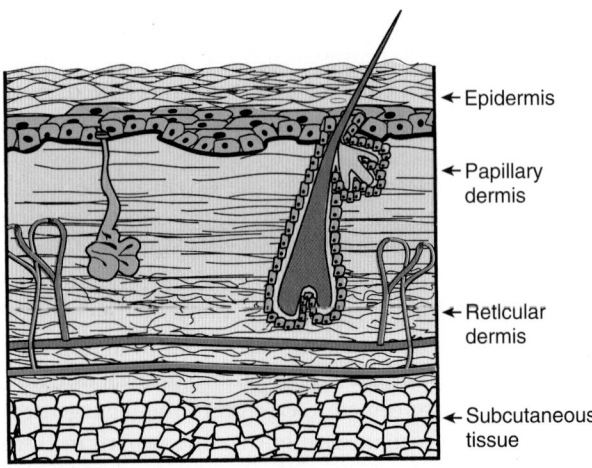

Figure 24.1 Cross-section of skin.

basale layer enable the epidermis to regenerate. This layer also contains melanocytes, the cells that determine skin pigmentation. The interface between the epidermis and the dermis is termed the *rete peg region*. This area consists of an extensive series of epidermal-dermal ridges and valleys that serve to increase the surface area between the epidermis and the dermis. These ridges act as a reservoir of skin and are needed to overcome frictional forces that skin is exposed to in daily activity. The lack of these ridges in the healed burn wound will result in blisters from abrasion and poor adherence of the new epidermal tissue when it comes in contact with clothing or other surfaces.

In earlier literature, the dermis is often referred to as the *corium*, or "true skin," because it contains blood vessels, lymphatics, nerves, collagen, and elastic fibers. It also encloses the epidermal appendages (sweat ducts, sebaceous glands, and hair follicles), which provide a deep source of epidermal cells for wound healing. The dermis is 20 to 30 times thicker than the epidermis. It is comprised primarily of interwoven collagen and elastic fibers, which provide the skin with its tensile strength and elasticity to resist deformation. The predominantly parallel orientation of normal collagen in the dermis is different from the whorls of collagen typically seen in scar tissue that result from burn injury.[18] The tiered location of sensory receptors in the skin is an important consideration in determining depth of burn injury (Table 24.1). The dermis is subdivided into two layers: the superficial *papillary* layer and the deep *reticular* layer.[17] The papillae of the papillary layer project upward and interlock with the epidermis. The papillae are vascular plexuses that serve, in part, to nourish the epidermis through osmosis. Morphologically, this layer is composed of a loose basket-weave network of collagen fibers. The reticular dermis lies below the papillary dermis and is composed of densely interwoven collagen fibers. The reticular dermis attaches to the subcutaneous tissue by an irregular interlacing network of fibrous connective tissue.

In addition to the functions mentioned already, the skin is important in temperature regulation through the emission of sweat and electrolytes, secretion of oils from the sebaceous glands to lubricate the skin, vitamin D synthesis, and it contributes to cosmetic appearance and identity. As the result of a burn injury, some or all of these functions may be impaired and/or lost, and a patient's protective barrier defense mechanisms will be compromised.

It is worth noting that, mechanically, skin elongates to accommodate joint motion, and this pliability is compromised following a burn injury.[19] Another basic pathophysiological consideration in a burn injury is the alteration of vascular integrity, which results in the formation of edema in the interstitial spaces. Edema formation occurs in the area of burn as well as in adjacent tissues. An initial concern of the physical therapist on the burn team is a decrease in joint range of motion (ROM) due to swelling.

The amount of skin destruction is based on temperature and length of time the tissue is exposed to heat.[20] The type of insult (i.e., flame, liquid, chemical, or electrical) also will affect the amount of tissue destruction. A tremendous amount of heat is not required to cause damage. At temperatures below 111°F (44°C), local tissue damage will not occur unless the exposure is for prolonged periods. In the temperature range between 111°F and 124°F (44°C and 51°C), the rate of cellular death doubles with each degree rise in temperature, and short exposures will lead to cell destruction.[20,21] At temperatures in excess of 124°F (51°C), exposure time needed to damage tissue is extremely brief.

■ CLASSIFICATIONS OF BURN INJURY

In the past, burn injury depth was categorized as *first*, *second*, and *third* degree. Although the lay public may use these classifications, most medical literature now classifies burn injuries by the depth of skin tissue destroyed (Table 24.2).[21] The *APTA Guide to Physical Therapist Practice* includes classification of wounds based on etiology and depth of tissue destruction.[22] The depth to which a burn injury causes damage depends on many factors, including the duration and intensity of heat, skin thickness of area, the distance of the area from the source of heat, the extent (percentage) of body area exposed, vascularity, and age.

The different classifications of burn wounds will present different clinical pictures, and each can change dramatically during the course of treatment. In addition

Table 24.1	Sensory Receptors, Location by Layer of Skin, and Sensation Mediated	
Sensory Receptor	Location	Sensation Mediated
Free nerve ending	Epidermis	Pain, itch
Free nerve ending	Dermis	Pain
Merkel's disks	Stratum spinosum	Touch
Meissner's corpuscle	Papillary dermis	Touch
Ruffini's corpuscle	Papillary dermis	Warmth
Krause's end bulb	Papillary dermis	Cold
Pacinian corpuscle	Reticular dermis	Pressure, vibration

Table 24.2	Burn Wound Classification: Differential Diagnosis		
Depth of Burn	Color and Vascularity	Surface Appearance/Pain	Swelling/Healing/Scarring
Epidermal	Erythematous, pink or red; irritated dermis	• No blisters, dry surface • Delayed pain, tender	• Minimal edema • Spontaneous healing • No scars
Superficial partial thickness	Bright pink or red, mottled red; inflamed dermis; erythematous with blanching and brisk capillary refill	• Intact blisters, moist weeping, or glistening surface when blisters removed • Very painful, sensitive to changes in temperature, exposure to air currents, light touch	• Moderate edema • Spontaneous healing • Minimal scarring, discoloration
Deep partial thickness	Mixed red, waxy white; blanching with slow capillary refill	• Broken blisters, wet surface • Sensitive to pressure but insensitive to light touch or soft pinprick	• VSS • Marked edema • Slow healing • Excessive scarring
Full thickness	White (ischemic), charred, tan, fawn, mahogany, black, red (hemoglobin fixation); no blanching; thrombosed vessels; poor distal circulation	• Parchment-like, leathery, rigid, dry • Anesthetic; body hairs pull out easily	• Area depressed • Heals with skin grafting • Scarring
Subdermal	Charred	• Subcutaneous tissue evident • Anesthetic; muscle damage; neurological involvement	• Tissue defects • Heals with skin graft or flap • Scarring

VSS = Vancouver Scar Scale.

Epidermal Burn

An epidermal burn, as the name implies, causes cell damage only to the epidermis (Fig. 24.2). The classic "sunburn" is the best example of an epidermal burn. Clinically, the skin appears red or erythematous.[23] The erythema is a result of epidermal damage and dermal irritation, but there is no injury to the dermal tissue. There is diffusion of inflammatory mediators from sites of epidermal damage and release of vasoactive substances from mast cells. The surface of an epidermal burn is dry. Blisters will be absent, but slight edema may be apparent. After an epidermal burn, there is usually a delay in the development of pain, at which point the area becomes tender to the touch. Following epidermal damage, the injured epidermal layers will peel off or desquamate in 3 to 4 days. Epidermal healing is spontaneous; that is, the skin will heal by itself, and no scar tissue will form.

to the amount of direct tissue damage from a burn, a patient's metabolic, physiological, and psychological condition can greatly affect clinical status. This section presents general clinical signs and symptoms seen in each of the burn wound classifications (see Table 24.2).

Superficial Partial-Thickness Burn

With a **superficial partial-thickness burn** (Fig. 24.3), damage occurs through the epidermis and into the papillary layer of the dermis. The epidermal layer is destroyed completely, but the papillary dermal layer sustains only

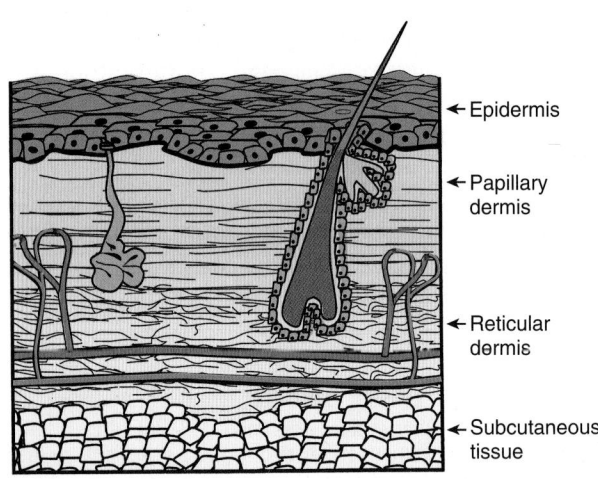

Figure 24.2 Red shading represents depth of skin involved in an epidermal burn.

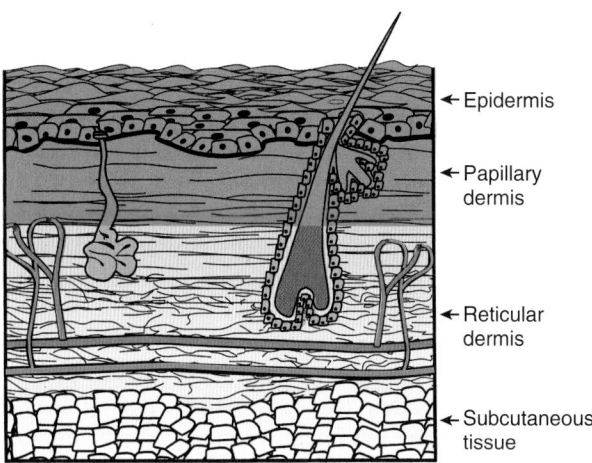

Figure 24.3 Red shading represents depth of skin involved in a superficial partial-thickness burn.

mild to moderate damage. The most common sign of a superficial partial-thickness burn is the presence of intact blisters over the area that has been injured.

Although the internal environment of a blister is considered sterile, it has been shown that blister fluid contains substances that increase the inflammatory response and retard the healing process, and it is recommended that blisters be evacuated.[24–28] Healing will occur more rapidly if the damaged skin is removed and an appropriate topical agent and wound dressing applied.[29] Once blisters have been removed, the surface appearance of the burn area will be moist. The wound will be bright red because the dermis is inflamed. The wound will **blanch**, which means if pressure is exerted against the tissue with a finger, a white spot appears as a result of displacement of blood in the capillaries under pressure. On release of pressure, the white area will demonstrate brisk capillary refill. Edema can be moderate.

This type of burn is extremely painful secondary to irritation of the nerve endings contained in the dermis. When the wound is open, the patient will be highly sensitive to temperature changes, exposure to air, and light touch. In addition to pain, fever may be present if areas become infected.

Some topical antimicrobial creams will cause the wound to develop a gelatin-like film that eventually will peel off, similar to the desquamation that occurs with sunburn. This exudate is a coagulum of the topical antibiotic used to prevent infection and serum that seeps from the wound as a result of the insult to capillary integrity.

Superficial partial-thickness burns heal without surgical intervention, by means of epithelial cell production and migration from the wound's periphery and surviving skin appendages. Coverage by new epithelium resumes the barrier function of the skin, and complete healing should occur in 7 to 10 days. There may be some residual skin color change owing to destruction of melanocytes, but scarring is minimal.

Deep Partial-Thickness Burn

A **deep partial-thickness burn** (Fig. 24.4) involves destruction of the epidermis and papillary dermis with damage down into the reticular dermal layer. Although as mentioned below, as this burn nears the deepest dermis it begins to resemble a full-thickness burn. Most of the nerve endings, hair follicles, and sweat ducts will be injured because most of the dermis is destroyed.

Deep partial-thickness burns appear as a mixed red or waxy white color. The deeper the injury, the whiter it will appear. Capillary refill will be sluggish after the application of pressure on the wound. The surface usually is wet from broken blisters and alteration of the dermal vascular network, which leaks plasma fluid. Marked edema is a hallmark sign of this burn depth. There is a large amount of evaporative water loss (15 to 20 times normal) because of tissue and vascular destruction.[20,26,30] An area of deep partial-thickness burn has diminished sensation to light touch but retains the sense of deep pressure due to the location of the Pacinian corpuscle deep in the reticular dermis. Healing occurs through scar formation and reepithelialization. By definition, the dermis is only partially destroyed; therefore, some viable epidermal cells may remain within the surviving epidermal appendages and serve as a source for new skin growth.

The depth of a deep partial-thickness injury is sometimes difficult to determine, so allowing the wound to demarcate (between normal and damaged tissue) during the first few days is necessary. Demarcation becomes evident after several days as the dead tissue begins to slough. Hair follicles that penetrate into the deeper dermal regions below the burn level remain viable. Preservation of hair follicles and new hair growth will

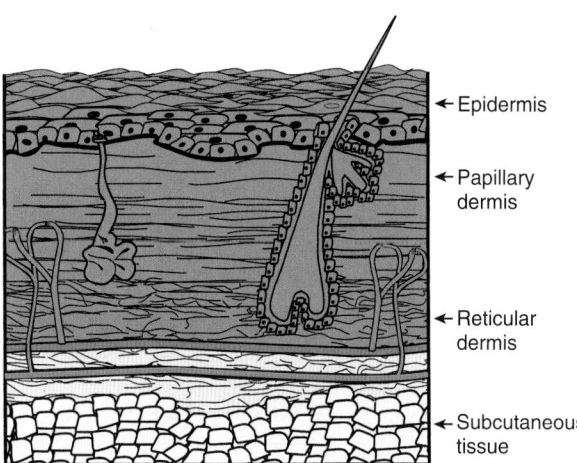

Figure 24.4 Red shading represents depth of skin involved in a deep partial-thickness burn.

indicate a deep partial-thickness burn rather than a full-thickness injury, and there is a corresponding greater potential for spontaneous healing. Factors that determine which epidermal structures survive and which die include the thickness of the skin in a particular location and/or the distance of the area from the source of heat.

Deep partial-thickness burns that are allowed to heal spontaneously will have a thin epithelium and may lack the usual number of sebaceous glands to keep the skin lubricated. New tissue usually appears dry and scaly, itchy, and is easily abraded. Creams are necessary to artificially lubricate the new surface. Sensation and the number of active sweat ducts will be diminished.

A deep partial-thickness burn generally will heal in 3 to 5 weeks if it does not become infected. It is critical to keep the wound free of infection, because infection can convert a deep partial-thickness burn into a deeper injury. The development of hypertrophic and keloid scars is a frequent consequence of a deep partial-thickness burn. **Hypertrophic scars** are typically raised, red, and sometimes pruritic but do not extend beyond the margin of the original wound, whereas **keloid scars** move beyond the original wound and rarely regress.[31] There are also histological differences such as the presence of collagen bundles laid in wavy and parallel to the epithelial surface in hypertrophic scars which are absent in keloid where the collagen is more loosely arranged in random orientation.

Full-Thickness Burn

In a **full-thickness burn** (Fig. 24.5), all of the epidermal and dermal layers are destroyed completely. In addition, the subcutaneous fat layer may be damaged to some extent.

A full-thickness burn is characterized by a hard, parchment-like eschar covering the area. **Eschar** is devitalized tissue consisting of desiccated coagulum of plasma and necrotic cells. Eschar feels dry, leathery, and rigid. The color of eschar can vary from black to deep red to white; the latter indicates total ischemia of the area. Frequently, thrombosis of superficial blood vessels is apparent, and no blanching of the tissue is observed. The deep red color of the tissue results from hemoglobin fixation liberated from destroyed red blood cells.

Hair follicles are completely destroyed, so body hairs pull out easily. All nerve endings in the dermal tissue are destroyed so the wound will be *insensate* (without feeling); however, a patient still may experience a significant amount of pain because adjacent areas of partial-thickness burn usually surround a full-thickness injury and the presence of inflammatory pain.

A major problem that arises from deep burns is the damage to the peripheral vascular system. Because large amounts of fluid leak into the interstitial space beneath unyielding eschar, the pressure in the extravascular space increases, potentially constricting the deep circulation to the point of occlusion (see discussion of cardiovascular complications in the section "Complications of Burn Injury"). Because eschar does not have the elastic quality of normal skin, edema that forms in an area of a circumferential burn can cause compression of the underlying vasculature. If this compression is not relieved, it may lead to eventual occlusion with possible necrosis of tissue distal to the site of injury. To maintain vascular flow, an **escharotomy** may be necessary. An escharotomy is a midline lateral incision of the eschar the length of an extremity or chest wall.[32,33] Figure 24.6 shows an escharotomy and the result of pressure that forces the incision to gap. Following an escharotomy, pulses are frequently examined to monitor restoration of circulation. If the escharotomy is successful, there will be an immediate improvement in the peripheral blood flow, demonstrated by normal pulses distal to the wound and by return of normal temperature and capillary refill of the distal extremity.

Although at times it may be difficult to differentiate a deep-partial from a full-thickness burn in the early postburn period, the differences will become evident after

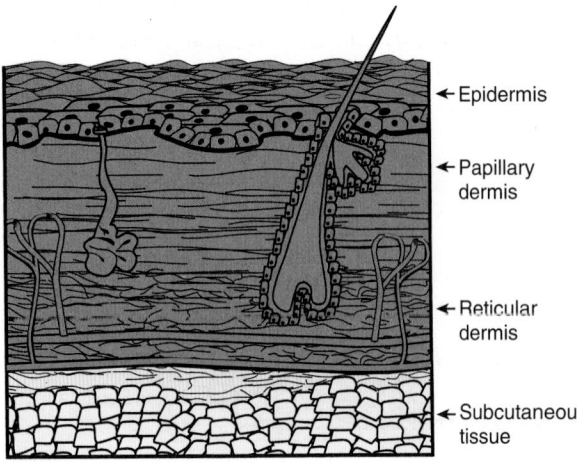

Figure 24.5 Red shading represents depth of skin involved in a full-thickness burn.

- ← Epidermis
- ← Papillary dermis
- ← Reticular dermis
- ← Subcutaneous tissue

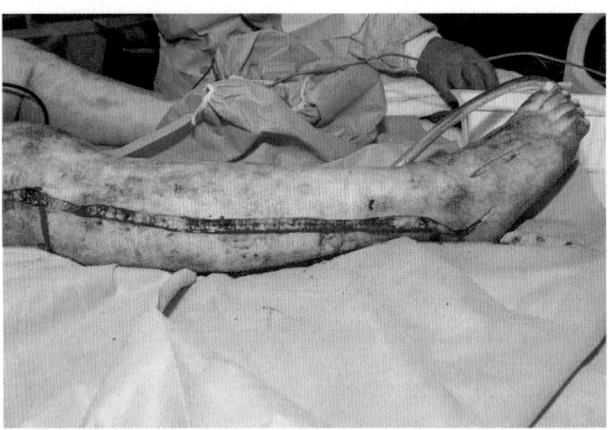

Figure 24.6 Escharotomy of the right lower extremity.

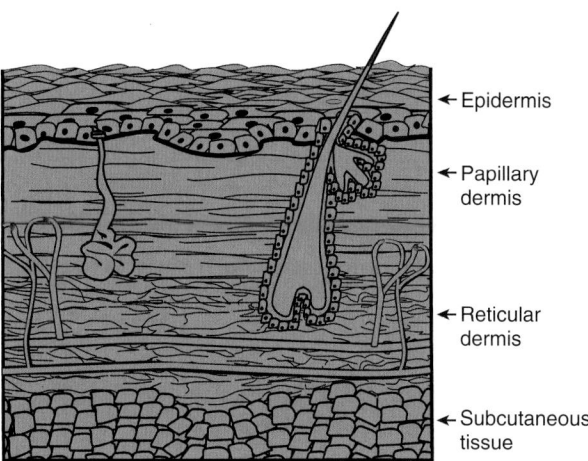

Figure 24.7 Red shading represents depth of skin involved in a subdermal burn.

several days. With a full-thickness burn, there are no sites available for reepithelialization of the wound. All epithelial cells have been destroyed, and skin grafting will be necessary. Grafting is discussed in detail in the section on "Surgical Management of the Burn Wound."

Subdermal Burn

An additional category of burn, the **subdermal burn**, involves complete destruction of all tissue from the epidermis down to and through the subcutaneous tissue (Fig. 24.7). Muscle and bone are subject to necrosis when burned. This type of burn occurs with prolonged contact with a heat source and routinely occurs as a result of contact with electricity. Extensive surgical and therapeutic management is necessary to return a patient to some degree of function.

Electrical Burn

The signs and symptoms of an **electrical burn** may vary according to the type of current, intensity of the current, and the area of the body the electric current passes through.[34] A burn results from the passage of an electric current through the body after the skin makes contact with an electrical source. Electric current follows the course of least resistance offered by various tissues. Nerves, followed by blood vessels, offer the least resistance. Bone offers the most resistance. Tissue damage results from tissue resistance to the passage of the current or by direct electrical current.[34-36]

Typically, contact sites will exist where the patient first came into contact with the electricity and a second site where the patient was grounded. The wound where initial contact was made (sometimes referred to as the *entrance wound*) will appear charred and depressed, and many times is smaller than the ground site. The skin appears yellow and ischemic. The ground site (sometimes referred to as the *exit wound*) often appears as though there was an explosion out of the tissue at the

site. It is dry in appearance. Tissues along the pathway of the current may be damaged owing to heat that developed as a result of tissue resistance to current passage. An extremity or area that appears viable after an injury may become necrotic and gangrenous in a few days. Arteries may undergo spasm, and there may be necrosis of the vascular wall. The blood supply to the surrounding tissues, including muscle, may be altered. Damaged muscle will feel soft. Because the course of tissue destruction is unpredictable, there may be unequal and uneven muscle damage. Time will be required to determine which tissues will remain viable and which will not.

There can be other consequences of electricity passing through the body, such as cardiac arrhythmias and acute renal failure secondary to fluid and electrolyte imbalances and release of myoglobin (protein present in muscle) into the blood. One of the most severe complications of electrical current damage is acute spinal cord damage or vertebral fracture. Clinically, these patients will have spastic paresis but may or may not have any sensory pathway changes over concomitant areas of spasticity. Possible causes of death from electrical burns are ventricular fibrillation and respiratory arrest.

Burn Wound Zones

A burn wound typically consists of three zones (Fig. 24.8).[21,37] In the **zone of coagulation**, cells are irreversibly damaged and skin death occurs. This area is equivalent to a full-thickness burn and will require a skin graft to heal. Because of the lack of viable tissue and the amount of eschar, the risk of infection is increased. This potential complication emphasizes the need for careful monitoring, the use of antibiotics, and the treatment of a burned patient in a specialized burn center. The **zone of stasis** contains injured cells that may die within 24 to 48 hours without diligent treatment. This is the area in which infection, drying, and/or inadequate perfusion of the wound will result in conversion of potentially salvageable tissue to completely necrotic tissue and enlargement of the zone of coagulation. Splints or compression bandages, if applied too tightly, can compromise the zone of stasis. Finally, the **zone of hyperemia** is a site

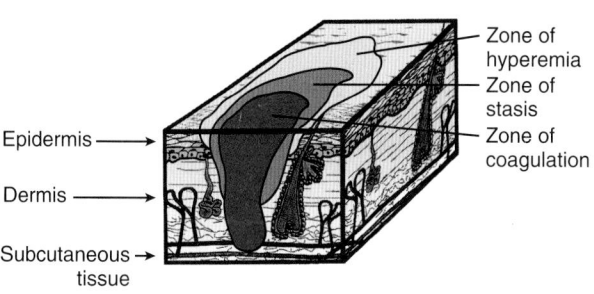

Figure 24.8 Zones of tissue damage as the result of a burn injury.

of minimal cell damage, and the tissue should recover within several days with no lasting effects.[38]

Extent of Burned Area

A major consideration when determining the severity of a burn is the extent of body burn. The **Rule of Nines** was developed by Pulaski and Tennison[39] to rapidly calculate an estimate of the percentage of total body surface area burned and was formally published by Wallace in 1951.[40] The Rule of Nines divides the body surface into areas of 9%, or multiples of 9%, of the TBSA. Figure 24.9 shows the percentages using the Rule of Nines for adults and children. Lund and Browder[41] modified the percentages of body surface area to account for a continuum of age and to accommodate for growth of different body segments. This method is the more accurate means of the two methods to determine the extent of burn injury. Figure 24.10 shows the relative percentages of burned area for children and adults according to the Lund and Browder formula. Although this formula provides an accurate assessment of TBSA, the use of the Rule of Nines is more practical in the emergent triage of a patient with a burn injury.

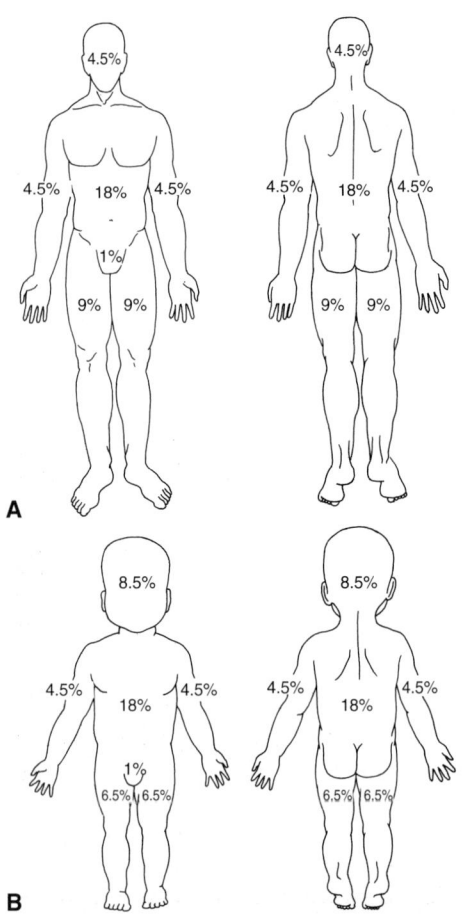

Figure 24.9 Rule of nines to determine percentage of body surface area burn in adults (A) and children (B).

■ COMPLICATIONS OF BURN INJURY

Depending on the extent of burn injury, the depth of the burn, and the type of burn, there may be secondary systemic complications.[42] In addition, the health, age, and psychological status of a patient who is burned will affect these complications. This section addresses selected systemic complications a patient may experience after a significant burn injury.

Infection

Infection, in conjunction with organ system failure, is a leading cause of mortality from burns.[43] Some virulent strains of *Pseudomonas aeruginosa* and *Staphylococcus aureus* are resistant to antibiotics and have been responsible for epidemic infections in burn centers.[1,43] Microbial invasion from the burn wounds to other healthy tissue can create sepsis.[43,44]

Systemic antibiotics are used to treat both burn and general system infections once they have been documented.[42-44] A bacterial count in excess of 10^5 per gram of tissue constitutes burn wound infection, and levels of 10^7 to 10^9 are usually associated with lethal burns. Most wounds are treated with topical antibiotics, discussed in the section on medical management.

Pulmonary Complications

Any patient who has been burned in a closed space should be suspected of having an **inhalation injury.**[45] Among patients with burns, the incidence of smoke inhalation may be in excess of 33%,[46] and this rises to 66% in patients with facial burns.[47] The incidence of pulmonary complications is extremely high after severe burns, and death due to pneumonia alone is attributed to a majority of the deaths following burn injury.[48] Direct trauma to the upper airways can also occur from the inhalation of hot gases.[49]

Signs of an inhalation injury include facial burns, singed nasal hairs, harsh cough, hoarseness, abnormal breath sounds, respiratory distress, and carbonaceous sputum and/or hypoxemia.[49]

The primary complications associated with this injury are carbon monoxide poisoning, tracheal damage, upper airway obstruction, pulmonary edema, and pneumonia. Lung damage from inhaling noxious gases and smoke may be lethal. To determine the extent of inhalation injury, several diagnostic procedures can be performed. The most helpful diagnostic procedure is bronchoscopy.[48]

Metabolic Complications

Thermal injury involving greater than 40% of the TBSA causes a great metabolic and catabolic challenge to the body. Severe burn injury is associated with a hypermetabolic state and prolonged catabolism resulting in associated protein loss and reduction of lean body mass.[50,51]

**Burn Estimate and Diagram
Age vs. Area**

Initial Examination

Cause of Burn_____

Date of Burn_____

Time of Burn_____

Age _____

Gender_____

Weight _____

Date of Admission _____

Signature _____

Date _____

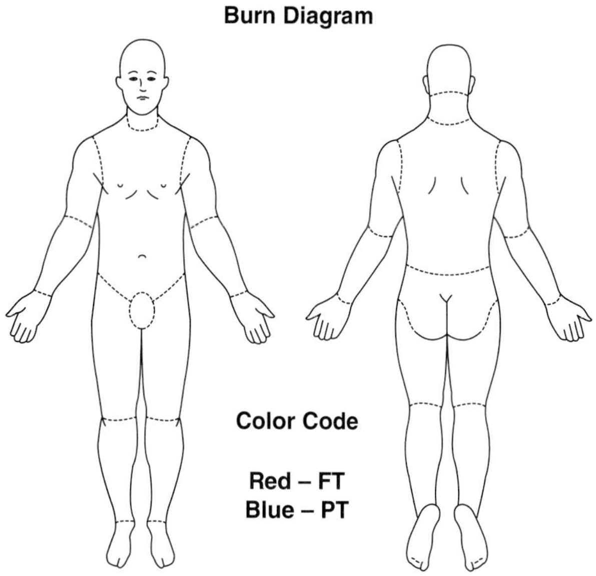

Burn Diagram

Color Code

Red – FT
Blue – PT

Area	Birth yr.	1–4 yrs.	5–9 yrs.	10–14 yrs.	15 yrs.	Adult	PT	FT	Total	Donor Areas
Head	19	17	13	11	9	7				
Neck	2	2	2	2	2	2				
Anterior Trunk	13	13	13	13	13	13				
Posterior Trunk	13	13	13	13	13	13				
Right Buttock	2¹/₂	2¹/₂	2¹/₂	2¹/₂	2¹/₂	2¹/₂				
Left Buttock	2¹/₂	2¹/₂	2¹/₂	2¹/₂	2¹/₂	2¹/₂				
Genitalia	1	1	1	1	1	1				
Right Upper Arm	4	4	4	4	4	4				
Left Upper Arm	4	4	4	4	4	4				
Right Lower Arm	3	3	3	3	3	3				
Left Lower Arm	3	3	3	3	3	3				
Right Hand	2¹/₂	2¹/₂	2¹/₂	2¹/₂	2¹/₂	2¹/₂				
Left Hand	2¹/₂	2¹/₂	2¹/₂	2¹/₂	2¹/₂	2¹/₂				
Right Thigh	5¹/₂	6¹/₂	8	8¹/₂	9	9¹/₂				
Left Thigh	5¹/₂	6¹/₂	8	8¹/₂	9	9¹/₂				
Right Leg	5	5	5¹/₂	6	6¹/₂	7				
Left Leg	5	5	5¹/₂	6	6¹/₂	7				
Right Foot	3¹/₂	3¹/₂	3¹/₂	3¹/₂	3¹/₂	3¹/₂				
Left Foot	3¹/₂	3¹/₂	3¹/₂	3¹/₂	3¹/₂	3¹/₂				
Total										

Key: FT – Full Thickness
PT – Part Thickness

Figure 24.10 Modified Lund and Browder chart for determination of percentage of body surface area burn for various ages. Values represent percentages of burned body area. *Courtesy Shriners Burns Hospital, Cincinnati, OH.*

A number of anabolic agents have effectively been used to mitigate muscle catabolism after severe burn injury and minimize the loss of lean body mass.[52,53] In addition, early enteral feeding has been shown to improve outcomes after burn injury, reducing the degree and extent of catabolism.[50,54] Understanding the metabolic demands of a burn injury and how to improve the patient's nutritional status to meet these demands has led to substantial improvements in burn care.[50,55]

As a result of the increased metabolic activity, there will be an increase of 1.8°F to 2.6°F (1°C to 2°C) in core temperature that seems to be due to a resetting of the hypothalamic temperature centers in the brain.[1] Wilmore et al.[56] hypothesized that there is a significant relationship between the increased evaporative heat loss from the impaired skin barrier over a burn and the hypermetabolic state. In any event, if individuals with burns are placed in a room with normal ambient temperature, excessive heat loss will be exhibited, and this will further exaggerate the stress response seen in these patients.[1,56] Therefore, it is recommended that room temperature be kept at 86°F (30°C), which will significantly reduce the metabolic rate.

As part of the patient's altered metabolism, protein from muscle tissue is preferentially used as a source of energy. This situation, coupled with the effects of bedrest, causes muscles to atrophy and renders patients weak.

Much of the improved management of burns has been attributed to the greater focus of research on the nutritional needs of patients. It is beyond the scope of this chapter to detail nutritional supplementation, and the interested reader is referred to several excellent reviews of advances in burn nutrition.[55,57–60]

Cardiovascular Complications

Hemodynamic changes result from a shift in fluid to the interstitium, which subsequently reduces the plasma and intravascular fluid volume in a patient with a burn.[61,62] The fluid shifts occur as a result of local and temporary systemic changes in capillary dynamics. This shift of fluid to the interstitium can result in significant edema. Capillary permeability returns to normal after about 24 hours. Also, with these fluid shifts, there will be a tremendous initial decrease in cardiac output, which may reach as low as 15% of normal within the first hour after injury.[63,64] Fluid replacement therapy is utilized initially to manage the loss of circulatory fluid. This additional fluid allows perfusion of vital organs but also increases the amount of tissue edema.[61,65]

Hematological changes also occur after a severe burn injury. These changes include alterations in platelet concentration and function, clotting factors, and white blood cell components; red blood cell dysfunction; and decreases in hemoglobin and hematocrit.[66] These physiological alterations, coupled with cardiac changes and injured vascular beds, will significantly affect initial resuscitation efforts and, if the patient survives, how rapidly they will recover. Additionally, patients will exhibit decompensation from an endurance standpoint resulting in functional deterioration.

Heterotopic Ossification

Heterotopic ossification (HO) is the abnormal development of bone in areas of soft tissue. It is relatively uncommon following burn injury, but when it occurs it often leads to pain and functional limitation.[67] The number of cases that progress to become clinically problematic ranges from less than 1% to nearly 6%.[68–70] The etiology of HO is unclear. Burn-induced inflammatory response may stimulate abnormal osteogenic differentiation of stem cells; other suspected causes include immobilization, microtrauma, high protein intake, and sepsis.[67,71] Physiologically, HO can appear anywhere in the body. Some case reports suggest the elbows are most commonly affected. Schneider et al. found that grafts to the arm, head/neck, and trunk are significant predictors

of developing HO.[72] The TBSA is also a predictor of risk for HO. The risk of HO increases as TBSA increases, especially if the burn size is beyond 30% TBSA.[68] Usually, HO occurs in areas of full-thickness injury or sites that remain unhealed for a prolonged time. Symptoms appear late in a patient's course of recovery and include decreased ROM and point-specific pain (i.e., pain location that differs from the generalized pain typically experienced).

Neuropathy

Peripheral neuropathy in patients with burns can take two forms: polyneuropathy (damage to multiple peripheral nerves, usually with a distal bias) or local neuropathy.[73] The cause of polyneuropathy is unknown; however, direct thermal injury, vascular occlusion, compressive nerve entrapment, and edema are suggested causes.[74] Similar to those with HO, patients with peripheral neuropathy generally have a large TBSA burn, and the condition may be more commonly associated with electrical injury.[74] Fortunately, most neuropathies resolve over time, but some may be long-term.

Local neuropathies can be caused by several burn treatment issues such as compression bandages applied too tightly, poorly fitted splints, or prolonged and inappropriate positioning.[73] The most common sites of involvement are the brachial plexus, ulnar nerve, and common peroneal nerve.

Pathological Scars

Burn scars occur in areas of deep partial-thickness burns that are allowed to heal spontaneously and in full-thickness burns that have been skin grafted, but graft coverage is incomplete. If maturing tissue demonstrates a greater rate of collagen production than degradation, a scar becomes raised and thick.[75,76] Scars become pathological when they take on the form of **hypertrophy**, contracture, or both. Each of these scar conditions is unique and should not be viewed as synonymous. A patient can have a hypertrophic scar that does not interfere with movement or a scar contracture band that is not hypertrophied. However, both conditions can exist simultaneously, and specific treatment for each is discussed later in this chapter.

The burn wound has been described, and the causes and complications of burn injury have been presented. The following sections address wound healing[77] and medical, surgical, and physical therapy management of the patient with a burn.

■ BURN WOUND HEALING

The two layers of the skin—the epidermis and dermis—differ morphologically and heal by separate mechanisms.

Epidermal Healing

If a burn injury is isolated to the epidermis, or if there are viable cells lining the skin appendages, **epithelial healing** can occur on the surface of a wound.

The stimulus for epithelial growth is the presence of an open wound exposing subepithelial tissue to the environment. The intact epithelium attempts to cover an exposed wound through mitosis and the ameboid movement of cells from the basal layer of the surrounding epidermis into the wound. The epithelial cells stop migration when they are completely in contact with other epithelial cells. Following this **contact inhibition**, cells begin to differentiate to form the various epithelial layers. While epidermal cells move about the wound site, they maintain a connection with the normal epithelium at the wound margin. To continue migration and proliferation, a suitable base for the epithelial cells must be provided by adequate nutrition and blood supply, or the new cells will die.

The process of epithelialization is most evident clinically in the partial-thickness wound that has intact hair follicles and glands. The skin appendages provide a source of epithelial cells from which the wound may heal. The cells migrate outwardly from the appendages and appear as epidermal islands from which they spread peripherally across the wound. Skin growth and coverage from these epithelial islands actually can be visualized over time.

Damage to sebaceous glands may cause dryness and itching of a healing wound. Lubrication can be a problem, and newly healed skin is characteristically dry and may split. Dryness may continue for a long time because many of the sebaceous glands do not return to their normal function after a wound is epithelialized. Therapists need to educate patients about the type, frequency, and techniques of moisturizing cream application to lubricate newly healed tissue.

Dermal Healing

When an injury involves tissue deeper than the epidermis, **dermal healing**, or scar formation, occurs. Scar formation can be divided into three phases: *inflammatory, proliferative,* and *maturation*. Although these phases will be described separately, they occur on a continuum, and one phase often overlaps another.

Inflammatory Phase

The primary reaction of viable tissue to a burn wound is inflammation, which prepares the wound for healing through hemostatic, vascular, and cellular events. Inflammation begins at the time of injury, ends in about 3 to 5 days, and is characterized by redness, edema, warmth, pain, and decreased ROM. Initially, when a blood vessel is ruptured, the wall of the vessel contracts to decrease blood flow. Platelets aggregate, and fibrin is deposited to form a clot over the area. Fibrin serves a threefold function: (1) to partially retain body fluids; (2) to protect the underlying cells from desiccation; and (3) to provide a firm coagulum substance from which cells can infiltrate. Therefore, fibrin can be thought of as forming a lattice network, from which cells can climb and work themselves into the healing structure.

After a transient vasoconstriction of the vasculature, which lasts about 5 to 10 minutes, vessels vasodilate to increase blood flow to the area. There is increased permeability of the blood vessels, with leaking of plasma into the interstitial space and subsequent edema formation. Leukocytes infiltrate the area and begin to rid the site of contamination. Of particular importance is the presence of macrophage cells, which are responsible for attracting fibroblasts into the area.

Proliferative Phase

During this phase, reepithelialization is occurring at the surface of the wound, while deep within the wound, fibroblasts are migrating and proliferating. **Fibroblasts** are the cells that synthesize scar tissue, which is composed of collagen and protein polysaccharides in the form of a viscous ground substance that surrounds the collagen strands. The collagen is deposited with a random alignment and no true architectural arrangement of fibers. Stress (e.g., a force intended to elongate the scar) applied to the developing tissue during this time causes the fibers to align along the direction of force.[78] During this period of fibroplasia, the tensile strength of the wound increases at a rate proportional to the rate of collagen synthesis.

In conjunction with collagen deposition, granulation tissue is formed during this phase. Granulation tissue consists of macrophages, fibroblasts, collagen, and blood vessels.[77] Newly formed blood vessels bring a rich blood supply to the area and encourage further wound healing. However, granulation tissue formation is not necessary for skin graft adherence, and excess granulation tissue may lead to an increase in hypertrophic scarring.

During the proliferative phase, **wound contraction** occurs. Wound contraction is an active process in which the body attempts to close a wound where a loss of tissue has occurred. The amount of contraction is determined by the amount of available surrounding mobile skin. It involves movement of existing tissue at the wound edge toward the center, not formation of new tissue. Wound contraction ceases when (1) the edges of the wound meet, or (2) tension in the surrounding skin equals or exceeds the force of contraction. Skin grafting may decrease contraction, with thick grafts causing less contraction.

Maturation Phase

A wound is considered closed at the time epithelium covers the surface; however, wound healing involves remodeling of the scar tissue. During the maturation phase, there is a reduction in the number of fibroblasts, a decrease in vascularity owing to a lesser metabolic demand, and remodeling of collagen, which becomes more parallel in arrangement and forms stronger bonds. The ratio of collagen breakdown to production determines the type of scar that forms. If the rate of breakdown equals or slightly *exceeds the rate of production*, maturation results in a pale, flat, and pliable scar.

If the rate of collagen production *exceeds breakdown*, then a hypertrophic scar may result. This scar is characterized by a red and raised appearance with rigid texture; it stays within the boundary of the original wound. A *keloid* is a large, firm scar that overflows the boundaries of the original wound; it is more common in darkly pigmented individuals. Both of these scars take a prolonged period of time to mature. The presence and contraction of the scar can lead to both functional and cosmetic deformities. The active process of scar contraction during both this maturation phase and the proliferative phase creates a risk of contracture formation. A contracture over a joint will limit ROM and affect joint function.[79]

MEDICAL MANAGEMENT

Advances in the medical management of patients with burn injury have resulted in the survival of thousands of patients who 25 or 35 years ago would have died from their injuries.[3] Research findings and current techniques available at modern burn centers have enabled patients to receive better care through use of more sophisticated interventions. This section addresses the initial treatment of burn injuries and surgical management, including primary excision, skin grafts, and correction of scar contracture.

Initial Treatment

The goals of initial medical treatment of a patient with a burn are to address critical life-threatening problems and stabilize the patient through procedures designed to (1) establish and maintain an airway; (2) prevent cyanosis, shock, and hemorrhage; (3) establish baseline data, such as extent and depth of burn injury; (4) prevent or reduce fluid losses; (5) clean the patient and wounds; (6) examine injuries; and (7) prevent pulmonary and cardiac complications. Triage (assigning degree of urgency and order of treatment) using these procedures applies to major burn trauma.

Initially, a patient must be transported from the site of injury to a treatment facility. If possible, transportation will be directly to a burn center, rather than to a hospital emergency department. The goals of treatment in transit are to stabilize the patient and maintain an airway. During the initial transportation phase, patient history and personal data are gathered when possible. The type of agent causing the burn is noted, and initial examination of the burn injury takes place. Emergency medical personnel may use the Rule of Nines to estimate the percentage of burn injury. In addition, they prepare the individual for triage at the burn center by removing all burned clothing and jewelry and initiating administration of fluid through an intravenous line.

One of the major advances in burn care has been in fluid volume replacement initially and throughout a patient's treatment. Research has led to an improved understanding of the physiological changes that occur

in a patient after a burn injury and of the fluid volumes necessary to optimize the chance for survival.[64] Information about the physiological changes responsible for shifts in body fluids and protein has led to the use of intravenous solutions in an amount necessary to replace vital fluids and electrolytes.[80]

After a patient arrives at a burn center and adequate fluid resuscitation (replacement) has been initiated, the burn team determines the extent and depth of injury and begins initial wound cleansing. Burn units typically use showers, spraying over a tub, or "bed baths" for the removal of dressings and daily cleaning of wounds. The use of hydrotherapy tubs for wound cleansing is no longer recommended.[81,82] The initial wound care session allows the team to determine body weight, fully examine the patient, remove hair where necessary, and start the **debridement** process by removing any loose skin. The goals of wound cleansing and debridement are to remove dead tissue, prevent infection, and promote revascularization and/or epithelialization of the area. Depending on the facility, physical therapists may be involved in the wound-cleaning procedures.[83]

The wound should be inspected carefully. The appearance, depth, location, and size are determined, and the presence of exudate or odor is noted. *Infection* is characterized by thick, purulent drainage, odor, fever, a brownish-black discoloration, rapid separation of eschar, boils in adjacent tissue, or conversion of a deep partial-thickness burn to a full-thickness injury.

Wound care is carried out using sterile technique and instruments. If **sharp debridement** (the use of surgical scissors or scalpel and forceps to remove eschar) is performed, sloughed epidermis and loose eschar are removed, and pockets of pus are drained. The procedure needs to be performed carefully so that bleeding is minimal.

After the wounds have been cleaned, the patient should be kept warm to reduce any further metabolic demand due to additional heat loss. Topical medications and/or dressings are then applied. Table 24.3 presents common topical medications used in the treatment of burns. The technique of applying a topical cream or ointment without dressings is called the **open technique** and allows for ongoing inspection of the wound and examination of the healing process. With this technique, the topical medication must be reapplied throughout the day.

The **closed technique** consists of applying dressings over a topical agent. Dressings serve several purposes: (1) they hold topical antimicrobial agents on the wound, (2) they reduce fluid loss from the wound, and (3) they protect the wound. Dressings are changed once or twice a day, depending on the size and type of wound and the type of topical antimicrobial used.

Dressings consist of several layers. The first layer is nonadherent to protect the fragile healing surface from disruption. This may be followed by cotton padding to

Table 24.3 Common Topical Medications Used in Treatment of Burns

Medication	Description	Method of Application
Silver sulfadiazine	Most commonly used topical antibacterial agent; effective against *Pseudomonas* infections.	White cream applied with sterile glove 2–4-mm thick directly to wound or impregnated into fine mesh gauze.
Mafenide acetate (Sulfamylon)	Topical antibacterial agent; effective against gram-negative or gram-positive organisms; diffuses easily through eschar.	White cream applied directly to wound with thin 1–2-mm layer twice daily; may be left undressed or covered with thin layer of gauze.
Mafenide acetate solution (Sulfamylon 5% solution), silver nitrate	Topical solution with antimicrobial function against gram-positive and gram-negative organisms. Maintains moist environment. Antiseptic germicide and astringent; will penetrate only 1–2 mm of eschar; useful for surface bacteria; stains black.	50-g packet of white powder that is mixed with either 1,000 mL sterile water or 0.9% sodium chloride–soaked gauze. Dressings or soaks used every 2 hours; also available as small sticks to cauterize small open areas.
Bacitracin/Polysporin	Bland ointment; effective against gram-positive organisms.	Thin layer of ointment applied directly to wound and left open.
Collagenase, Accuzyme	Enzymatic débriding agent selectively débrides necrotic tissue; no antibacterial action.	Ointment applied to eschar and covered with moist occlusive dressing with or without an antimicrobial agent.

absorb wound drainage. The final layer consists of roll gauze or elastic bandages, which hold the other layers in place but allow movement.

Surgical Management

Primary Excision

Primary excision is the surgical removal of eschar. The excision generally includes removal of peripheral layers of eschar until vascular, viable tissue is exposed as the site for skin graft placement.[84] Much of the increased survival rate of patients with extensive burns is associated with early primary excision of burn wounds.[85] Typically, a patient is taken to surgery after successful resuscitation, usually within 1 week of the injury. As much of the eschar is removed at one time as possible. Proponents of early primary excision believe that this approach is easier on the patient than repeated debridement and that it promotes more rapid healing, reduces infection and scarring, and is more economical in terms of staff and hospital time.[84]

Skin Grafts

In many burn centers, a wound is closed with a skin graft at the time of primary excision. Many types of grafts can be used to close a wound. An **autograft** is a patient's own skin, taken from an unburned area and transplanted to cover a burned area. Autografts are desirable because they provide permanent coverage of the wound. An **allograft** (or **homograft**) is skin taken from an individual of the same species, usually cadaver skin. The skin can be kept frozen in skin banks for

prolonged periods. Allografts are temporary grafts used to cover large burns when there is insufficient autograft available. **Xenograft** (or **heterograft**) is skin from another species, usually a pig. Allografts or xenografts are used until there is sufficient normal skin available for an autograft.

Perhaps the most progressive advancement in the care of patients with burns in recent years is the use of **skin substitutes** for coverage of an excised wound.[86–93] Skin substitutes consist of cultured autologous skin, which is grown in a laboratory from a biopsy of a patient's own tissue, the use of altered cadaver skin, or other biologically engineered tissues. Skin substitutes are used when large areas of burn exist and coverage is necessary for a patient's survival. Cultured autologous skin takes several weeks to grow and is highly susceptible to infection. Other biologically engineered tissues are more readily available and have demonstrated more reliable adherence than in the past. With the use of most skin substitutes, ROM exercises may be delayed, and shearing forces must be avoided. Although skin substitutes are an expensive intervention for wound coverage, they are useful and have proved effective in managing patients with large burn wounds. Examples of skin substitutes include the following:

- *Cultured epidermal autografts (CEAs):* A skin biopsy is obtained from a patient, and only the epidermal cells are cultured.[86,87]
- *Cultured autologous composite grafts:* A skin biopsy is obtained from a patient, and both epidermal and dermal cells are cultured. This forms a bilayer structure.

- *Autologous skin cell spray:* The autologous skin cell spray technique uses a suspension of isolated progenitor cells from the patient and solution sprayed back onto the patient's wound bed to facilitate reepithelialization. This treatment is often used for partial and deep partial thickness wounds.[94]
- *Allogenic skin substitute:* The epidermal layer of skin and all immune cells are removed from cadaver skin. This tissue is applied to the graft bed, and once adhered, a thin epidermal autograft or CEA is applied.[95]
- *Cultured dermis (temporary):* Cultured dermal matrix is seeded with human neonatal fibroblasts and used as a temporary covering in place of cadaver skin. This substitute eventually is removed and replaced with an autograft.[91,92]
- *Cultured dermis (definitive):* This skin substitute is composed of cultured bovine collagen with a silicone outer layer. Pores in the material allow for controlled growth of a neodermis. After approximately 14 days, the silicone layer is removed, and a very thin skin graft or CEA is applied.[93]
- *Artificial dermal template (partially temporary):* This is a fully synthetic dermal template in the form of a biodegradable polyurethane foam and a temporary nonbiodegradable polyurethane seal.[96] The polymers have minimal cytotoxicity allowing human keratinocytes, dermal fibroblasts, and microvascular endothelial cells to grow within the polyurethane matrix, leaving a vascularized dermis when the sealing membrane is removed. These are used to promote dermal growth prior to wound closure.[91,97]

The removal of skin to graft onto a burn wound is done surgically under anesthesia. The skin used for a graft usually is removed with a **dermatome**. This instrument not only allows the surgeon to obtain a large amount of skin, but a more consistent thickness of skin can be obtained. The dermatome is adjusted to remove a predetermined thickness of skin for a **split-thickness skin graft**. A split-thickness skin graft contains epidermis and a variable amount of dermis, as opposed to a **full-thickness skin graft**, which consists of the full dermal thickness.

The site from which a skin graft is taken is called a **donor site**. Common donor sites include the thighs, buttocks, and back. These wounds heal by reepithelialization, like a partial-thickness burn, and require appropriate care to prevent additional dermal damage with resultant scar formation. A full-thickness skin graft has the disadvantage of leaving a full thickness wound at the donor site that will require either primary closure or grafting with a split-thickness skin graft.

Generally, the thinner the skin graft, the better the adherence, and the thicker the graft, the better the cosmetic result. Additionally, a thin graft will contract more than a thick skin graft once it has adhered to the wound bed. Selection of depth depends on many factors,

including whether the donor site needs to be used again for another skin graft. Taking a thicker graft adversely affects the possibility of taking another graft from the same site for a prolonged period of time. Harvesting from split-thickness skin graft sites may be repeated in 10 to 14 days, depending on the amount of time the donor site takes to heal.

A **sheet graft** is a skin graft applied to a recipient bed without alteration following harvesting from a donor site (Fig. 24.11). The face, neck, and hands are covered with this type of graft for optimal cosmesis and function. When limited donor skin is available, most areas are covered with a **mesh graft** (Fig. 24.12). The meshing of a graft consists of processing the sheet graft through a device that makes tiny parallel incisions in a linear arrangement. This process permits the skin graft to be expanded before it is applied to the wound bed.[98] This technique allows coverage of a larger area, and once the graft adheres, the interstices heal through reepithelialization.

A skin graft usually is held in place with sutures, staples, or Steri-Strip skin closures. Once a graft is fixed in position, any blood or serum that might have collected between the graft and the recipient site should be

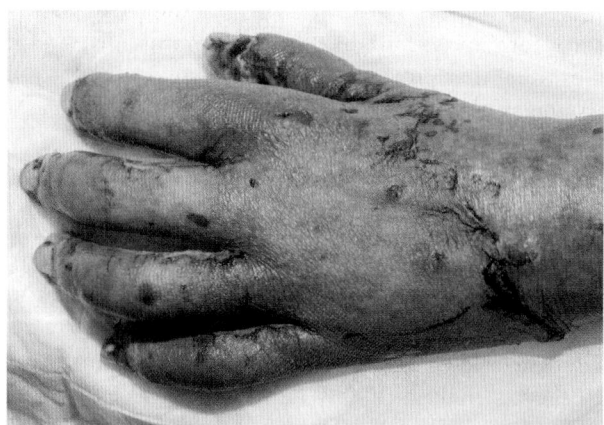

Figure 24.11 Sheet graft on dorsum of left hand.

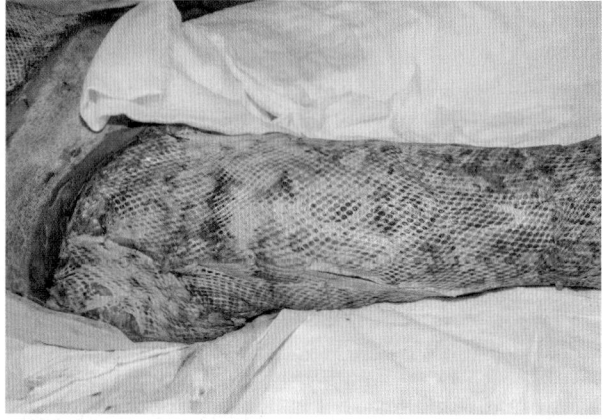

Figure 24.12 Meshed split-thickness skin graft applied to freshly excised wound on right lower extremity.

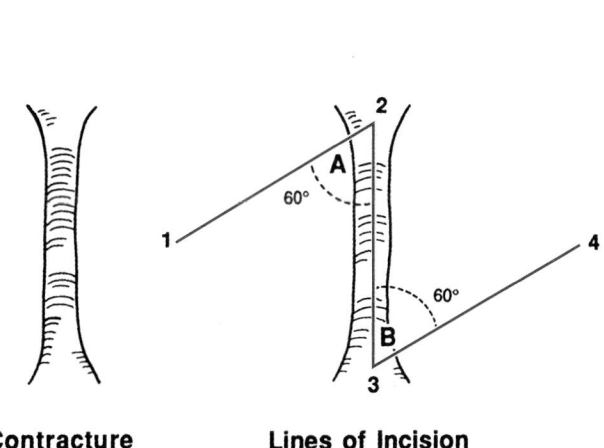

Contracture   **Lines of Incision**

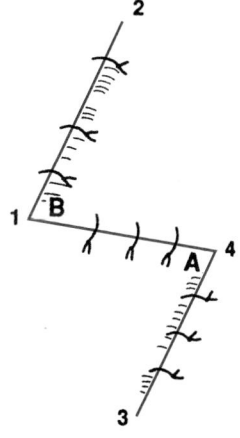

Result of Z-plasty

Figure 24.13 Schematic diagram of Z-plasty procedure. *From Richard and Staley,*[4(p192)] *with permission.*

removed. Application of a pressure dressing facilitates contact between the graft and recipient site.

A basic necessity for successful adherence of a graft is sufficient vascularity within the wound bed. Grafts will not adhere to poorly vascularized areas, such as tendon. Once a skin graft has been applied, separation of a graft from its bed must be prevented. Separation may result from shear force, mechanical trauma, or hematoma formation. Initially, the area is immobilized with a dressing that provides firm, even compression on the wound. Other reasons for graft failure include inadequate excision of necrotic tissue and infection.

Survival of a skin graft depends on several factors: (1) circulation, which provides a nutritive supply to the graft; (2) inosculation, or the process by which a direct connection is established between a graft and the host vessels; and (3) penetration of the host vessels into a graft site. Except in darkly pigmented skin, grafts are white in color at the time of transplantation and begin to show a pinkish hue within a matter of hours after their placement on an adequate vascular bed.

The reestablishment of circulation in a skin graft will take place through the formation of direct anastomosis between respective vessels, invasion from the host bed forming new channels, or both. Twenty-four hours after grafting, numerous host vessels will have penetrated the graft.[77] The invasion of new capillaries seems to be the most important consideration in vascularization. Normally, within 72 hours, inosculation has proceeded to the point where the skin graft is secure. Initially, structural connections are fibrous. Collagen is then laid down to secure attachment of the graft.

Correction of Scar Contracture

If physical therapy interventions are unsuccessful in averting scar contracture formation, and limitations are noted in ROM and function, surgery may be required. In the past, reconstructive surgery usually was postponed while a burn wound was in the active, immature phase of scar formation.[99] Successful release of scar contractures before scar maturation has been documented.[100] Each patient's scar will require an individualized evaluation and treatment. Many surgical treatment options are available to eliminate scar contractures; among the more common procedures are skin grafts and Z-plasties.[101]

A schematic diagram of a Z-plasty is shown in Figure 24.13. The Z-plasty serves to lengthen a scar by interposing normal tissue in the line of the scar. Skin grafts are used after surgical release for more severe contractures.

■ PHYSICAL THERAPY MANAGEMENT

Concurrent with skin healing is the initiation of the physical therapy plan of care (POC). Commonly, physical therapy interventions are directed toward prevention of scar contracture, preservation of normal ROM, prevention or minimization of hypertrophic scar formation and cosmetic deformity, maintenance or improvement in muscular strength and cardiovascular endurance, return to preburn function, and performance of activities of daily living (ADL).[4] The POC for a patient with burns is an evolving process that may require daily modification.[5–7,102]

Rehabilitation is a continuum of care through the entire course of recovery and will vary in intensity and interventions required, with each individual and each phase of recovery.[103] The overall focus of rehabilitation is to restore the patient's preinjury function and lifestyle. The physical therapist collaborates with other team members to obtain these outcomes. With adherence to a well-designed treatment plan, a patient can expect to return to a normal, productive life. For many patients, the most difficult phase of rehabilitation occurs after the wounds have healed and the scar tissue begins to contract. At this point, patient education about adherence to strategies designed to prevent or minimize contractures is particularly important. The remainder of this chapter will address the physical therapist's role in the rehabilitation of a patient who has sustained a burn injury.

Examination

After the initial examination for depth of burn and percent of TBSA involved, the physical therapist then examines the patient to determine the presence of impairments and activity limitations.[104] The therapist needs to obtain an accurate history from the patient and family members regarding any preexisting limitations or previous injuries that may affect rehabilitation potential. The therapist must also anticipate the potential for development of indirect impairments as the burn wounds heal and mature. For example, active or passive ROM may be limited as a result of edema, restrictive eschar, or pain, and an initial baseline measure should be obtained. The physical therapy evaluation and subsequent treatment plan can be guided by the World Health Organization's International Classification of Functioning, Disability and Health, which describes health outcome in terms of body function and structure, activity and participation.[104]

Other tests and measures discussed in this text are appropriate for inclusion in the initial examination and reexamination of a patient following burn injury (e.g., gait, balance, mobility, reaching, and functional status). See discussion of outcomes measures in Chapter 6, Examination of Coordination and Balance (also Table 6.7), and Chapter 8, Examination of Function. Because healing of a burn wound is a dynamic process and changes may occur daily, the physical therapist needs to examine and monitor patients routinely for changes in skin integrity, ROM, and functional mobility. Frequent evaluation will keep the physical therapist and other members of the burn care team abreast of potential problems so that intervention can occur before a potential problem becomes a real one. Studies addressing assessment of burn scars are presented in Table 24.4, Evidence Summary.

In addition to the physical damage imposed by a burn, there also may be an enormous psychological impact.[105-107] The physical therapist should be cognizant of a potential problem during ongoing evaluations because psychological trauma may affect the patient's motivation, progress, outlook, and compliance with the POC. Referral to an appropriate professional for intervention may be necessary, which is discussed in Chapter 26, Psychosocial Issues in Physical Rehabilitation.

Goals and Expected Outcomes

Based on evaluation of examination data with consideration to the severity of burn, and the patient's current health status, age, and physical and psychological condition, the patient's prognosis can be estimated. Development of goals and expected outcomes are informed by the prognosis and current medical status. It is difficult to identify specific goals and outcomes owing to the varied nature of each burn injury. Suggestions for formulating goals and outcomes include:[22]

- Peripheral edema is minimized.
- Joint integrity and mobility are improved.
- Muscle performance (strength, power, and endurance) is improved.
- Range of motion is improved.
- Caregivers are independent in safe patient handling.
- Physical function is improved.
- Utilization of rehabilitation services is optimized.
- Self-management of symptoms is improved.
- Access, availability, and services provided are acceptable to the patient or client.
- Coordination of care is acceptable to the patient or client.

The optimal outcome of rehabilitation is the return of a patient to normal, preinjury function and lifestyle.

Intervention

Patients with burns usually begin physical therapy on the day of admission. The initial examination will determine which areas need to be addressed first. Control and resolution of edema and preserving ROM usually are the first priorities of intervention. Edema can be minimized through elevation of the extremities and active movement, especially of the hands and ankles. Prevention of scar contractures can be accomplished through positioning, splinting, exercise, and ambulation. Exercise and ambulation also will help to minimize deconditioning and other deleterious effects of bedrest.[108] Following wound closure, massage and compression therapy will assist with minimizing contracture formation and management of burn scars.

The scar that forms across a joint skin crease while a burn wound is healing is composed of immature collagen. A scar will shorten as a result of the contractile or pulling forces in scar tissue.[109-112] This scar contraction remains a major potential cause of burn morbidity in the United States as it leads to about one-third of patients with a severe burn injury developing some level of contracture.[113] Scar contracture may be more common in areas where access to expert care is absent or limited.[114] Scar contraction can limit ROM and function unless interventions are taken against this process. Although measures to prevent a contracture are undertaken in expectation of the best result, the risk of scar contracture development must be acknowledged and countered with an appropriate plan of care. There are several interventions available to address prevention and/or treatment of scar contracture.

As stated, positioning, splinting, exercise, and ambulation are interventions utilized in opposing the scar contracture process. Active exercise and patient participation in functional activities are important strategies to prevent or minimize contractures. However, owing

Table 24.4   Evidence Summary Studies Addressing the Assessment of Burn Scar

Sullivan et al. (1990)[192]

Design	Observational rating
Level of Evidence	II
Subjects	73
Intervention	Burn scars less than 1 year old were observed and rated on the following characteristics and scale scores: Pigmentation (normal = 0, hypopigmentation = 1, hyperpigmentation = 2); vascularity (normal = 0; 1–3 = signs of increased vascularity); pliability (normal = 0, 1–5 = signs of decreased pliability); and height (0 = normal or flat, 1 = <2 mm, 2 = <5 mm, 3 = >5 mm).
Results	Moderate interrater reliability was reported. No data related to intrarater reliability or validity were reported.
Comments	The study suggested that the VSS may have potential as a clinical rating of burn scars. Although the strength of this study is low and despite some published modifications to this scale, the VSS remains the current standard for assessing burn scar.

Crowe et al. (1990)[193]

Design	Observational
Level of Evidence	II
Subjects	Four (two therapists with scar care experience and two without scar care experience)
Intervention	Four-color photographs (slides), each of 10 patient's scars were rated using the VSS and two other assessment scales.
Results	Interrater reliability ranged from 0.66 (vascularity assessment) to 0.90 (color assessment). Test-retest reliability ranged from 0.73 (vascularity assessment) to 0.89 (proportion of irregular scar assessment). Novice therapists were generally as reliable as expert therapists in assessment of the scars.
Comments	Findings suggested that the use of photographs with application to a scar assessment scale holds potential for evaluation of scar surface, thickness, border height, and color. Subject and evaluator numbers were low.

Martin (2003)[194]

Design	Observational
Level of Evidence	II
Subjects	Scars (37 scars on 20 subjects) were assessed. Follow-up reassessment of scars included 17 scars on eight subjects.
Intervention	A modified VSS and a VAS were used for both the initial and follow-up assessments. Scar assessment by the clinicians included pigmentation, vascularity, and height of the scar. The VAS was used to obtain subject responses to two questions: 1. *How would you rate your scar?* (Best possible, most attractive = 0 and worst possible, least attractive = 10); and 2. *I feel this scar is unattractive to other people.* (Completely disagree = 0, completely agree = 10). Scars less than 6 months old were initially rated, and some of these same scars were reassessed approximately 1.5 years after the burn injury.
Results	There was significant improvement of the scar from early to late assessment ($p \leq 0.001$) and with VAS question 2 ($p \leq 0.006$). There was no correlation between VSS scores and the patient's responses to the VAS questions.
Comments	This study included not only clinician assessment of scars, but also involved feedback provided by the patients about their perception of the appearance of the scar. Findings suggested that while subjects might feel their scars improve with time, their feelings (1) may not match the clinician's assessment of improvement and (2) be different regarding acceptance of the scar by others.

(Continued)

Table 24.4 Evidence Summary Studies Addressing the Assessment of Burn Scar—cont'd

Draaijers et al. (2004)[195]

Design	Observational
Level of Evidence	II
Subjects	Four independent observers used the observer score of the POSAS and the VSS on 49 scars on 20 patients.
Intervention	The observer portion of the POSAS includes assessment of the variables of vascularization, pigmentation, thickness, relief, and pliability on a 1–10 scale (1 = normal, 10 = worst scar possible). Patients also completed the patient response portion of the POSAS. The questions for the patient include the level of pain and itching, respectively (rated on a 1–10 VAS with 1 = no complaints and 10 = worst imaginable); and color of the scar, stiffness of the scar, thickness of the scar, and irregularity of the scar (rated on a VAS scale with 1 = like normal skin, and 10 = very different from normal). Independent observers also completed the VSS on each of the same scars assessed using the POSAS.
Results	Internal consistency of the patient and observer scales were acceptable. Reliability of POSAS completed by a single observer was acceptable (ICC = 0.73), better than VSS. The observer scale shows less variability than the VSS between repeated measures. The observer scale had significant correlation with the VSS (Spearman's rho = 0.89, $p < 0.001$). Significant influences from the patient's point of view were pain and itching.
Comments	The authors conclude the observer scale is feasible because a single observer can use the scale reliably. The POSAS scar assessment tool is suitable for clinical studies because the opinion of the patient is incorporated.

Nedelec et al. (2008a)[196]

Design	Observational
Level of Evidence	II
Subjects	Four skin areas evaluated (three scar sites; one normal skin area) on each of 30 subjects. The four sites included: • The most severe scar • A less severe scar • A donor skin site • A normal skin site
Intervention	Modified VSS used to assess scar height, pliability, and vascularity. Other measures included the following: • Cutometer used to assess skin elasticity. • Mexameter used to further assess scar erythema and melanin. • Dermascan used to assess scar thickness. Each site was evaluated by the same observer using a modified VSS, a cutometer, mexameter, and dermascan. Each site was assessed on three different days within a 2-week period. The observer was blinded to any previous measurement results.
Results	The ICC for the modified VSS for height, pliability, and vascularity subscales was adequate (0.81). The cutometer did not discriminate between normal skin and scar. The mexameter was acceptable for erythema (>0.75) and melanin index (>0.89), as was the dermascan for thickness (>0.82). *Note:* Thresholds were described for some of these measurements.
Comments	Variable sensitivity and specificity noted with some measures. Questions raised about intrarater reliability of the modified VSS with hypertrophic scar. The interrater reliabilities for the mexameter and the dermascan were acceptable, allowing consideration of these instruments for measuring the relevant scar.

Table 24.4 Evidence Summary Studies Addressing the Assessment of Burn Scar—cont'd

Nedelec et al. (2008b)[197]

Design	Observational
Level of Evidence	II
Subjects	As with the previous study also by Nedelec et al., four skin areas were evaluated (three scar sites; one normal skin area) on each of 30 subjects. The four sites included the following: • The most severe scar • A less severe scar • A donor skin site • A normal skin site
Intervention	Modified VSS used to assess scar height, pliability, and vascularity. Other measures included the following: • Cutometer used to assess skin elasticity. • Mexameter used to further assess scar erythema and melanin. • Dermascan used to assess scar thickness. Each site was evaluated by the same observer by using a modified VSS, a cutometer, mexameter, and dermascan. Each site was assessed on three different days within a 2-week period. The observer was blinded to any previous measurements results.
Results	Interrater reliabilities of all subscales of the modified VSS were not acceptable (≈0.50). Acceptable reliability was reported for the cutometer (>0.89), the mexameter, and the dermascan (0.82). Concurrent validity was significant with the VSS in every case except with the pliability subscale and the cutometer in cases of severe scar.
Comments	The interrater reliabilities of the cutometer, mexameter, and dermascan and their concurrent validity with the modified VSS suggest they are objectively measuring the same scar characteristics as the modified VSS.

Simons, Tyack (2011)[198]

Design	Observational
Level of Evidence	II
Subjects	Three-phase assessment of rating burn scars from photographs included the following: • Opinions from 38 health professionals about current practice in scar assessment • Opinions from 36 therapists (PTs and OTs) about what should be included in a photographic scar scale • Opinions of 10 health-care consumers about scar evaluation
Intervention	Each site was evaluated by the same observer by using a modified VSS, a cutometer, mexameter, and dermascan. Each site was assessed on three different days within a 2-week period. The observer was blinded to any previous measurement results. Responses and answers to open-ended questions were linked for similarity. Linked responses and answers were converted to percentages for descriptive purposes and then analyzed for significance using chi-square analysis.
Results	Some agreement was reached that vascularity, color, contour, height, and overall opinion of the burn scar were parameters that could be assessed using color photography.
Comments	The authors suggest that a categorical scale with clear descriptors and strategies may improve photographic evaluation of burn scar.

OT = occupational therapy; POSAS = Observer Scar Assessment Scale; PT = physical therapy; VAS = visual analogue scale; VSS = Vancouver Scar Scale.

to the relentless forces of scar tissue and pain associated with exercising a burned area, additional interventions may be necessary (e.g., skin grafts and Z-plasty). Early and ongoing patient and/or family education is needed to help these individuals understand the necessity of the burn rehabilitation process.

Clinical Note. A Burn Rehabilitation Therapist Competency Tool (BRTCT) has been developed to define the core knowledge and skills central to the role of physical and occupational therapists in burn management.[115] The BRTCT provides standards of care for patients with burn injuries throughout the full spectrum of rehabilitation.[116]

Positioning and Splinting

A positioning program should begin on the day of admission to counteract contraction of damaged and scarring tissue.[6,7,83,117] The goals of a positioning program are to (1) minimize edema; (2) prevent tissue destruction; (3) maintain soft tissues in an elongated state; and (4) preserve function.[118] Positioning strategies for common deformities are presented in Table 24.5. To mitigate the development of scar contracture and joint limitation, a positioning program must be designed based on the distribution of the burn injury relative to adjacent joints. Joint position should be opposite the anticipated contracture based on evaluation of

the wound distribution and depth. Examples of proper positioning of different body segments are provided in Figures 24.14 through 24.17. Burned areas should be positioned in an elongated state or neutral position of function.[119,120]

Splinting can be viewed as an extension of a positioning program. There are certain "anti-deformity" positions in which patients generally are splinted; however, positioning is individualized based on the location of the burn and which movements are difficult for the patient to achieve. With the exception of splints designed to immobilize a skin graft after surgery, splints should be fabricated for patients only if ROM or function would be lost without them. General indications for the use of splints include (1) prevention of contractures, (2) maintenance of ROM achieved during an exercise session or surgical release, (3) reduction of developing contractures, (4) protection of a joint or tendon, and (5) reduction of the overall pain experience.[121,122] Splint design should be kept simple so that it is easy to apply, remove, and clean.[123] Splints are usually worn at night, when a patient is resting, or continuously for several days following skin grafting. Splints should conform to the body part, and care must be taken to ensure that there are no pressure points that may cause a breakdown in healing or normal skin. Splints should be checked routinely for proper fit and revised if necessary. Active motion is important, and splints and positioning are intended to serve as adjuncts to the therapy program

Table 24.5	Positioning Strategies for Common Deformities		
Joint	Common Deformity	Motions to Be Stressed	Suggested Approaches
Anterior neck	Flexion	Hyperextension	Use double mattress; position neck in extension (Fig. 24.14); with healing, use rigid cervical orthosis
Shoulder-axilla	Adduction and internal rotation	Abduction, flexion, and external rotation	Position with shoulder flexed and abducted (airplane splint)
Elbow	Flexion and pronation	Extension and supination	Splint in extension
Hand	Claw hand (also called intrinsic minus position)	Wrist extension; metacarpophalangeal flexion, proximal interphalangeal and distal interphalangeal extension; thumb abduction	Wrap fingers separately. Elevate to decrease edema. Position in *intrinsic plus* position, wrist in extension, metacarpophalangeal in flexion, proximal interphalangeal and distal interphalangeal in extension, thumb in abduction with large web space
Hip and groin	Flexion and adduction	All motions, especially hip extension and abduction	Hip neutral (zero degrees of flexion/extension), with slight abduction
Knee	Flexion	Extension	Posterior knee splint
Ankle	Plantarflexion	All motions (especially dorsiflexion)	Plastic ankle-foot orthosis with cutout at Achilles tendon and ankle positioned in neutral

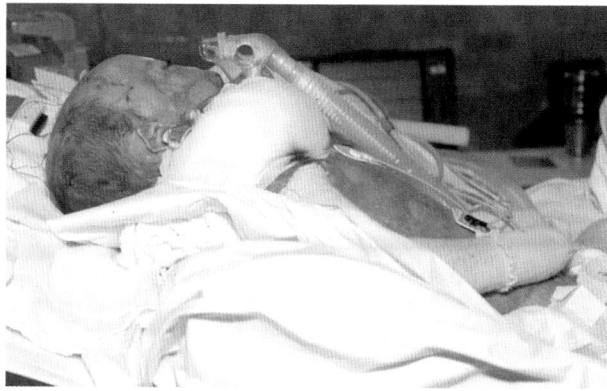

Figure 24.14 Positioning in bed of patient with burns of the anterior neck. *From Richard and Staley,[4(p225)] with permission.*

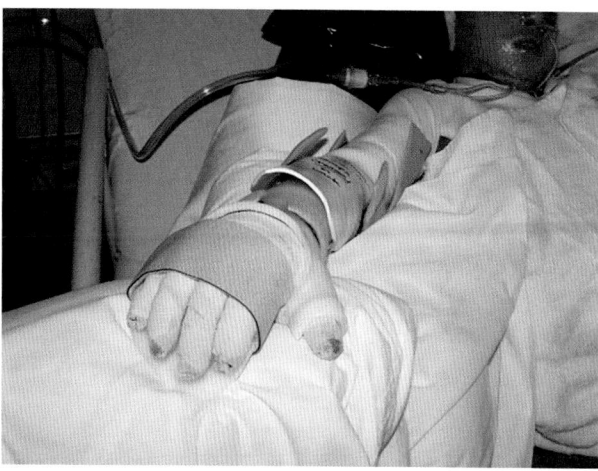

Figure 24.15 Positioning in bed of patient with burns of the axilla. *From Richard and Staley,[4(p228)] with permission.*

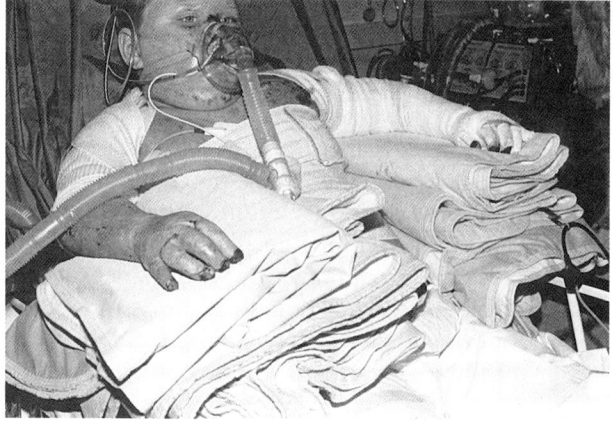

Figure 24.16 Proper positioning of upper extremities to reduce edema while seated. *From Richard and Staley[4(p231)] with permission.*

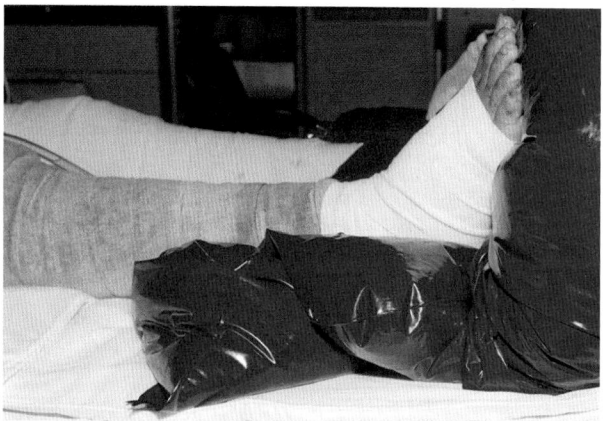

Figure 24.17 Positioning of feet with gel pads that help distribute pressure on the heels.

until full active motion can be achieved. Recent practice guidelines highlight the mixed evidence supporting orthotic use but recommend consideration of orthoses for improving ROM or reducing contracture in adults after burn injury and provide recommendations for use based on expert opinion.[124]

Most splints used for burn injuries are static. This type of splint has no moveable parts and maintains a position or immobilizes an area following skin grafting (Fig. 24.18). Static splints may be made from rigid materials with adjustable parts that allow modification to accommodate increases in ROM, termed static progressive splints. Dynamic splints also have been used successfully in the care of patients with a burn injury (Fig. 24.19).[125–128] These splints have moveable parts that allow joint movement. At the same time, dynamic splints apply a low-load, prolonged stress that can be adjusted to a patient's tolerance. They offer great potential for correcting a developing contracture and the early return of active function in areas of extensive burn and grafting.[128]

Therapeutic Exercise
Active and Passive Exercise

Active exercise begins on the day of admission.[5–7,83,129] Any patient who is alert and able to follow commands is encouraged to perform active exercises of involved body parts frequently throughout the day. A patient should perform active exercise of all extremities and trunk, including unburned areas. Dressing changes are an opportune time for exercise because the burn wound is visible, and the therapist can monitor the wound during movement. In the presence of a recent skin graft, the timing of reintroduction of active and passive exercise of the area is variable, depending on surgeon protocol. However, initiating movement of the area as soon as possible is desirable. Once it is determined to be safe to begin exercise again, gentle ROM—first active and then passive, if needed—is reinstituted.[120,130,131]

Active-assistive and passive exercise should be initiated if a patient cannot fully achieve active ROM. To

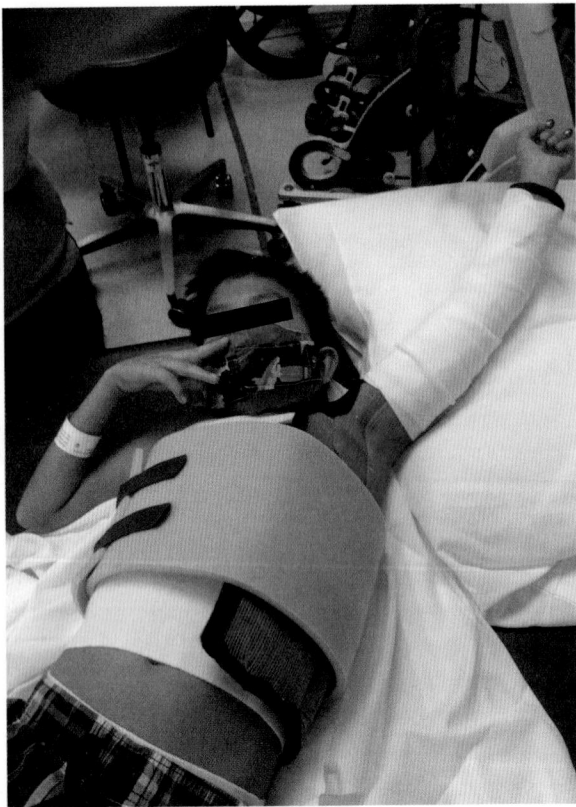

Figure 24.18 Splint that helps prevent neck flexion contracture and contours the anatomy of the neck.

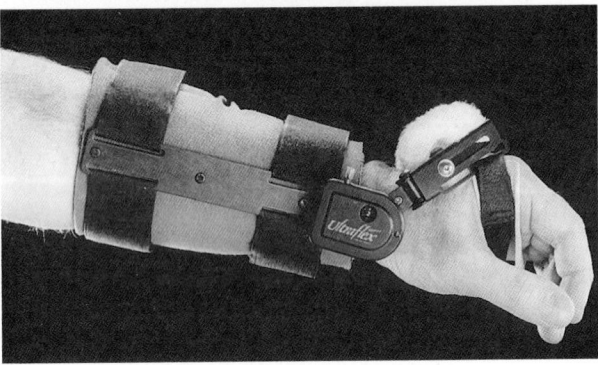

Figure 24.19 Dynamic splint used to provide a low-load, prolonged stress to scar tissue on volar aspect of forearm to gain wrist extension.

keep the healed burned area moist, it should be lubricated before exercise is initiated. Care should be taken around areas of skin grafts, and stress should be applied in a gentle, prolonged, and gradual fashion. If the burn wounds are well healed, heating modalities (e.g., paraffin, ultrasound) may be used to increase the pliability of the tissue before exercise therapy.[132,133]

Range of motion in the area of unhealed burns can be extremely painful, and patients may voice that they would rather lose their motion than be subjected to the

additional pain that occurs with movement. It usually is difficult and mentally draining for the physical therapist to push patients to exercise in and through pain, but it is critical that the therapist be persistent. Coordinating exercise activities with the administration of pain medication can lessen the painful experience for the patient.[100,129] Physical therapists should elicit the assistance of the family and caregivers in keeping the patient motivated and mobile as much as possible.

Because limited range of motion due to scarring is one of the most common impairment findings for a burn survivor, it is helpful for the therapist to understand how skin or scar affects motion of adjacent joints. The concept of *cutaneous functional units* (CFUs)[134,135] that describes fields of skin that functionally contribute to ROM of an associated joint contributes to the comprehension of mobility limitations caused by skin contraction (Figure 24.20). For example, the identified CFU area for the motion of neck extension is the skin on the anterior torso. As the neck extends, skin is recruited as distal as the skin covering the pubis bone in some individuals. Therefore, the concept that CFUs are associated with movement of a joint and those CFUs may extend some distance from the joint crease itself is helpful when designing treatment programs or evaluating the source of range of motion limitation. Beyond the CFU area involved in a burn injury, percentage of the CFU area scarred, proximity of the scars to joint skin creases and associated burn depth are also considerations of burn scar contracture development. Research using CFUs has reported that CFUs are a better method

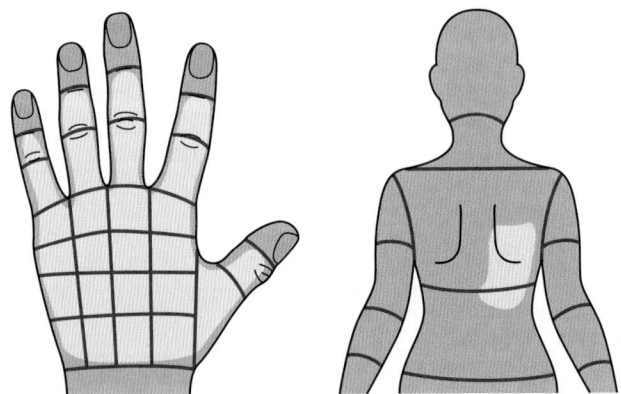

Figure 24.20 Comparison of the number of affected cutaneous functional units (CFUs) in burn injuries to the dorsal hand (left) and the posterior trunk (right). The area of the burn injury is highlighted. The overlaid red skin mapping lines demarcate individual CFUs. Note that the burn injury to the hand involves multiple CFUs compared with only two CFUs on the posterior trunk. The more CFUs involved, the relative proximity of skin creases in the burned area, as well as the depth of injury, are all associated with increased risk for development of burn scar contracture.

than TBSA for determining patient outcome from a rehabilitation perspective.[136,137] The percentage of the CFU burned has been shown to be a factor related to moderate limitations in ROM.[138] A computerized body mapping system has been developed using CFUs to quantify the number of potential burn scar contracture (BSC) sites a patient has and thereby provide the beginnings of an acuity determination of a patient's extent of burn involvement. In addition, adequate burn rehabilitation based on treatment time per CFU was found to be associated with preventing the development of BSC.[139,140]

Resistive and Conditioning Exercise

Patients show a decline in physical fitness after burn injury, which is linked to multiple factors including hypermetabolism, skeletal catabolism, and prolonged bedrest.[52,141] When compared to healthy individuals, those with a burn injury show decreased aerobic capacity,[142] lean body mass,[143] pulmonary function,[144] and strength.[145,146] As a patient continues to recover, the rehabilitation program should include strengthening and cardiovascular exercises.[5,83,147,148] Exercise may consist of isokinetic, isotonic, or other resistive training devices. General principles of exercise training and strength improvement should be followed, but they may need to be modified based on the patient's condition and stage of wound healing. Resistive devices such as free weights and pulleys can be used to prevent loss of strength in areas not burned.

When a patient initially begins strengthening or conditioning (endurance) exercises, the physical therapist should monitor vital signs to assess cardiovascular and respiratory responses to treatment.[149] Overexertion may occur. Monitoring of pulse, blood pressure, and respiratory rate before, during, and after exercise, particularly in the recovery period after exercise, will yield valuable information about the status of the cardiovascular and pulmonary systems (see Chapter 2, Examination of Vital Signs).

Patients should be encouraged to participate in exercises that will stress the cardiovascular system, such as walking from the burn unit to the physical therapy department. Cycling or rowing ergometry, treadmill walking, stair climbing, and other forms of aerobic exercise should be encouraged and progressed throughout the stages of recovery. These activities will not only increase cardiovascular endurance, but also have the added benefit of improving strength and ROM of the extremities. Interactive video games have been used in the rehabilitation of patients with burns as a means to increase activity, improve participation, and distract patients from pain.[150,151] In addition, such activities introduce variety into the rehabilitation program. The physical therapist needs to be creative and innovative to motivate patients to increase their exercise capacity.

Ambulation

Ambulation activities should be initiated as soon as possible after burn injury and/or skin graft surgery.[152–154] When ambulation is initiated after a skin graft, the lower extremities (LEs) should be wrapped in elastic bandages in a figure-eight pattern to support the new grafts and promote venous return. If the upright position cannot be tolerated owing to orthostatic intolerance or LE pain from being in a dependent position, gradual increases in time and duration on a tilt-table will assist in preparation for standing.[155–157] Initially, a patient may require an assistive device to ambulate. However, independent ambulation without a device should be achieved as soon as possible.

The physical therapist will spend a great deal of time with an individual patient during each treatment session. The rewards of a successful POC are tremendous when a patient who has suffered a life-threatening burn is able to walk out of the hospital and return to productive community involvement.

Scar Management

Following wound closure, a skin graft or healed burn wound is vascular, flat, and soft. During the following 3 to 6 months, dramatic changes may occur. The newly healed areas may become raised and firm. Pressure has been used successfully to hasten scar maturation, minimize hypertrophic scar formation, and improve scar appearance.[158] Studies have shown that pressure can decrease scar thickness,[159] hardness,[160] height,[161] and erythema.[162] However, no one study validates the mechanism by which pressure alters scar tissue. Pressure may exert control over hypertrophic scarring by (1) thinning the dermis, (2) altering the biochemical structure of scar tissue, (3) decreasing blood flow to the area, (4) reorganizing collagen bundles, or (5) decreasing tissue water content. Constant pressure dressings or garments exerting pressure exceeding 25 mm Hg will decrease the vascularity, decrease the amount of mucopolysaccharides, decrease collagen deposition, and significantly lessen localized edema.[5,158,162] The early hypertrophic scar is readily influenced by compressive forces and thus will respond to pressure therapy. The earlier the scar tissue is exposed to pressure, the better the result.[163,164] Usually, if the scar is less than 6 months old, it will respond to pressure therapy by conforming to the pressure, remaining flat on the surface, and not developing into a hypertrophic scar.[143] If the scar is still active or shows evidence of vascularity (red color), pressure therapy may be successful, even if the scar is as much as 1 year old.

Practice guidelines for use of compression recommend pressure therapy be used prophylactically with wounds that take longer than 14 to 21 days to heal or those that have undergone grafting. Pressure should be applied (1) as soon as tolerated by the healing skin;

(2) be worn 23 hours per day through scar maturation (removed for bathing); (3) be fitted by a trained professional; and (4) modified or replaced every 2 to 3 months or as needed.[165]

Pressure Dressings

Elastic wraps can be used to provide vascular support of skin grafts and donor sites, as well as to control edema and scarring. Elastic wraps should be used until a patient's skin or scars can tolerate the shearing force of pressure garment application, and open areas are minimal. Elastic wraps are applied in a figure-eight pattern on the LEs. A spiral wrap can be used on the upper extremities (UEs) and a circular wrap on the trunk.[158]

A self-adherent elastic bandage can be used for the hand and toes.[158,166,167] This bandage adheres only to itself and can be used over dressings before the wounds have healed. It helps to minimize edema and control scar formation. It may be used before application of a customized pressure glove or as definitive pressure on an infant's hand.

Tubular support bandages come in various circumferences and garment styles. They provide moderate compression and may be used as interim garments before a custom-made garment is fitted.[158,168] The tubular support bandage is especially useful for small children who grow rapidly and require frequent alterations in garment size.

Several companies manufacture pressure garments. Some are ready made and come in several sizes to fit most patients; others are custom made for the individual patient. For custom-made garments, the physical therapist uses a tape measure to determine the periodic circumference and linear length of each limb and trunk or face so fit of the garment is exact to apply proper pressure. Garments are measured when a patient has only a few remaining open areas. The garments are very tight, and difficult to apply, but the pressure is necessary to prevent scar hypertrophy. Garments can be ordered for any or all body parts, including the face and head, and they come in many styles, options, and colors (Fig. 24.21).[158] As mentioned, garments can be worn when the skin or scars can tolerate the shearing force of application. Pantyhose may be used under waist-height pressure garments to assist with donning. Garments should be washed daily to prevent buildup of perspiration and moisturizing cream, which may lead to scar maceration. The patient usually receives two sets of garments, one to wear and one to wash.

Adequate pressure may not be obtained with elastic wraps or pressure garments over concave surfaces, such as the sternum or axilla. In these instances, an insert may be necessary.[168,169] Inserts can be made of many materials, including foam, silicone elastomer, elastomer putty, and gel pads.[158,169–173] These items also need to be removed and cleaned regularly to prevent maceration of the underlying tissue.

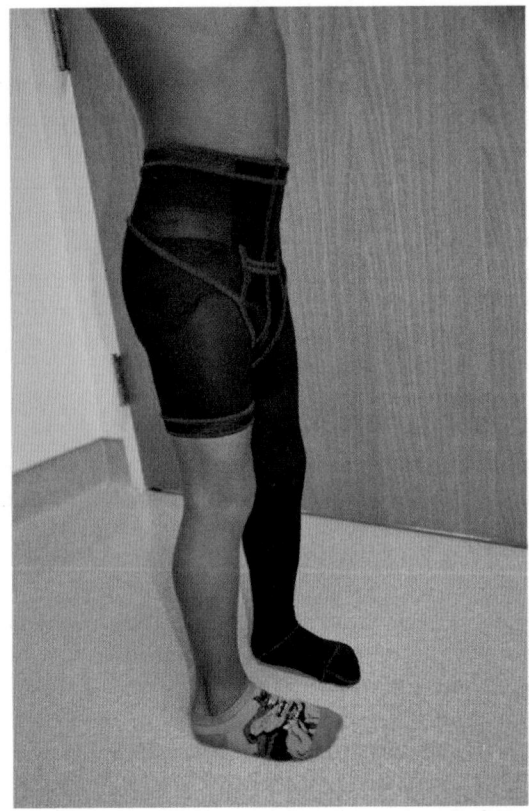

Figure 24.21 Pressure garments are worn to minimize hypertrophic scar formation. In this figure, the patient is wearing pressure garments for scars on the left lower extremity and upper hip. Pressure garments are customized for individual patents and their needs and can be custom fit for all extremities (including gloves for the hands), torso, and face.

Early, consistent use of pressure will result in flat, pliable scars, desensitization and protection of scars, and relief of itching. Pressure is necessary until scar maturation when the scars are pale, flat, and soft.

Silicone Gel

Silicone gel has demonstrated effectiveness in managing hypertrophic scars.[174-176] Available in a variety of sizes, application of silicone gels or gel sheets is recommended for immature burn scars at risk for hypertrophy (i.e., wounds that heal in more than 21 days). Silicone gel sheets may be applied directly over an actively maturing scar.[177] The mechanism of action of this intervention is not well understood.[178] The only reported complication with silicone gel sheet use is a local rash with the potential for, though rare, skin breakdown. Rashes that develop are readily reversible by temporarily deferring the use of the gel sheet. Once the site is clear of the rash, the gel sheet can be reapplied.

Massage

Scar massage is used quite readily in the rehabilitation of patients after burn injury.[179] It requires relatively very few resources and can be used in a variety of settings. Deep friction massage is thought to loosen scar tissue by mobilizing cutaneous tissue from underlying tissue and acting to break up adhesions.[5,180] When massage is used in conjunction with ROM exercise, the immature scar can be elongated more easily, and a developing contracture can be corrected. Although short-term benefits of massage to scar pliability, thickness, and texture have been shown, evidence for long-term changes of scar characteristics as a result of massage has not been proven.[181] However, studies have shown other benefits of massage for burn management, such as decreased pain, itching, and anxiety.[182–184] Firm scars that are routinely massaged tend to soften.[185] The edges or seams of grafts or any area that is raised and firm may benefit from massage. A video presentation of specific massage techniques for the individual with a burn is available online.[186]

Camouflage Makeup

For scars of the face, neck, and hands, camouflage make-up can be used.[7,158] This type of make-up may be useful when a person has either hyperpigmentation or hypopigmentation of the skin due to the burn injury. In addition, make-up can be used before scar maturation, when the scar is still red, and a patient wants to go out in public without their pressure garments for short periods of time. The cosmetics are opaque, color-correct for burn scars, and are available in multiple shades to accommodate various skin colors. They also are waterproof and can be worn during all activities. These products can be purchased in larger department stores or where theatrical products are sold.

Follow-Up Care

Well before patients are discharged from the hospital, the therapist should provide information regarding a home exercise program (HEP), a splinting and positioning program, and skin care.

An HEP should continue to stress frequent ROM exercises in combination with massaging areas involved in the burn injury. In addition, patients should be encouraged to perform as many ADL skills as possible independently. Therapists can film the patient's exercise program to provide the patient, family, and outpatient therapist with a visual of the actual ROM and movement patterns used in each exercise. Instructional programs facilitate education of those involved in the patient's rehabilitation program and will help to ensure consistency of treatment after discharge.[187]

The splinting schedule and pressure program that was followed in the hospital just before the patient's discharge should be continued at home. Before discharge, the patient and/or family members should be able to apply and remove all splints and pressure appliances independently.

Proper skin care requires specifying the type of soap and cream a patient is to use. In general, soap should be mild without perfumes or other irritants. A moisturizing soap can be used after all open areas are healed. Moisturizing creams should be applied two to three times daily and should not contain perfumes or have a significant alcohol content. Patients should be instructed to massage the cream completely into their skin to avoid buildup on the surface. If a patient will be unavoidably exposed to the sun, a sunscreen with a skin protection factor of at least 30 should be used and reapplied frequently.[188] Patients should be cautioned to avoid the sun if at all possible and to use hats or clothing to help protect their skin against the sun's rays.

Small, superficial open areas may plague a patient for many months after wound closure because of the fragility of a healed burn wound. The patient should be instructed to wash these areas twice daily, apply a small amount of antibiotic ointment, and cover the areas with a nonadherent dressing. To help prevent further irritation or maceration, the patient should be cautioned to avoid shearing forces, improper fit of clothing, brisk cleansing, soaking in water too long, or application of too much cream.

Itching may intensify when wounds have healed. A patient should be instructed to pat, rather than scratch, the irritated areas. Application of cream may help decrease itching; however, some patients may require oral antihistamine medication to help control this problem.

Some patients with burn injury may require outpatient therapy to supplement the HEP and monitor and adjust their splinting and pressure program. Frequency of outpatient therapy is based on each patient's needs. Regardless of whether patients receive outpatient therapy, they should be monitored at regular intervals through an outpatient clinic. This will allow burn team members to evaluate adjustment back into society and alter the HEP or other management strategies according to each patient's physical abilities and extent of scar maturation. When an adult patient's burns have matured and full ROM is achieved, further follow-up care is unnecessary. However, children need to be monitored until they are fully grown, because burn scars may not keep pace with a child's growth. In these cases, surgical release of scar tissue may be necessary.[189]

Community Programs

There are various community programs available to individuals who have sustained a burn injury. The therapist should be aware of those in the patient's home community so an appropriate referral can be made. If programs are not available, someone in the hospital or community may consider initiating a program. Examples of community resources include the following:

• The American Burn Association (www.ameriburn. org) provides access to a large variety of resources (e.g., educational materials, facts sheets, newsletters, meeting announcements).

- School Reentry Programs are provided by the hospital staff for the students and staff in the child's school.[7,188]
- Burn Camps (https://resources.phoenix-society.org/resource-marketplace/international-association-of-burn-camps) are weekend- to week-long camps that provide an opportunity for children to interact in a controlled, outdoor environment with peers who have sustained a similar injury.[187] The American Burn Association has a Burn Camp Special Interest Group with readily available information about camps throughout the United States and Canada.

- Adult Support Groups provide an opportunity for individuals with or without their families to share experiences and gain support from others who have had similar injuries.[187]
- Phoenix Society for Burn Survivors (www.phoenix-society.org) is a nonprofit organization dedicated to supporting burn survivors and families in recovery. The Phoenix Society offers many programs and resources that promote return to a meaningful life.[190]

Appendix 24.A (online) includes web-based resources for patients, families, and clinicians.

SUMMARY

Specific impairments and complications from a burn injury vary based on the extent and depth of thermal destruction of the skin. The classification of burn injuries is based on the depth of tissue destroyed and includes epidermal burn, superficial partial-thickness burn, deep partial-thickness burn, full-thickness burn, and subdermal burn. The Rule of Nines[39] and the Lund and Browder[41] formula were developed to assist with the initial determination of the extent of burn injury. The specific clinical signs and symptoms vary based on burn classification. Indirect impairments can include infection, pulmonary, metabolic, skeletal, muscular, neurological, and cardiovascular and pulmonary complications. Medical management addresses life-threatening problems and stabilization of the patient. Dressings with topical medications, debridement, surgical excision, and skin grafting are primary treatment measures. Skin substitutes are slowly becoming a practical alternative to skin grafting.

Rehabilitation is an essential component of recovery for the patient with a burn.[191] Physical therapy management focuses on the prevention of scar contracture, maintenance of normal ROM, development of muscular strength and endurance, improvement of cardiovascular conditioning, independence in functional activities, and prevention of hypertrophic scarring. Although burn trauma and subsequent recovery can be a devastating life occurrence, there are treatment facilities and medical professional teams to assist patients with burn injuries and their families return to as normal a lifestyle as possible.

Questions for Review

1. Identify the two primary layers of skin and two functions of each.
2. Discuss the initial management of a patient with an acute burn injury.
3. Describe the differences between epidermal, superficial partial-thickness, deep partial-thickness, and full-thickness burns.
4. Explain how a deep partial-thickness burn can convert to a full-thickness burn.
5. Compare the treatments for deep partial-thickness and full-thickness burns.
6. Describe the primary involvement of the pulmonary system associated with extensive burns.
7. What is the primary metabolic complication associated with burns, and how is it treated?
8. Identify and describe the three phases that occur in dermal healing of a burn wound.
9. Differentiate (1) between a split-thickness and full-thickness skin graft and (2) between a sheet and a meshed skin graft.
10. Identify three essential factors for successful skin graft adherence.
11. For the patient with a burn injury, identify five general goals and outcomes that may be included in the physical therapy plan of care.
12. What interventions can be used to prevent (1) burn scar contractures and (2) hypertrophic scar formation?

CASE STUDY

A 29-year-old male sustained a 30% total body surface area burn 6 weeks before this outpatient examination and evaluation. The patient was burned at home while he was refueling a lawnmower with gasoline, which ignited. Areas of the body affected by the burn include the right upper extremity, portions of the posterior and anterior trunk, lateral neck, right side of face, and thigh. Areas skin grafted included the right dorsal hand, forearm, and arm up to the axillary crease. The remaining wounds healed secondarily. The neck, face, and thigh burns were superficial. The patient was initially treated at a regional burn center and now is referred to the local hospital for follow-up outpatient physical therapy owing to decreased right elbow extension, decreased shoulder flexion, and inability to reach overhead. The right upper extremity lacks 15° of elbow extension (i.e., 15° to 120°) and flexion of the shoulder is limited to 0° to 155°. Scar contracture bands are noted at both locations at the end of available range with movement. The patient states that he has some difficulty donning shirts and his jacket. All other movements are within functional limits. The patient's strength overall is within functional limits. His wounds are all closed. The patient lives with his girlfriend and has medical benefits through his employer.

One week after his discharge from the hospital, the patient presented for his initial outpatient examination wearing interim pressure garments, as instructed. He also brought the static elbow splint that had been issued to him during his acute hospitalization, but which "doesn't fit right anymore." The expected outcome for this patient is to regain full right upper extremity range of motion and function.

GUIDING QUESTIONS

1. Describe how you would approach the clinical problems presented. Your answer should address positioning, splinting, exercise, and scar-management interventions.

2. Identify the impairments and activity limitations you will address in determining the prognosis and the plan of care.

3. Establish *general* goals (short term) and outcomes (long term) for this case. Develop one goal/outcome that will affect each of the following areas: *impairments, muscle performance, activity limitations,* and *risk reduction/prevention.*

4. Determine the prognosis.

5. Develop a plan of care. Your response should include specific interventions, patient instruction, and required coordination, communication, and/or documentation.

6. Describe the discharge plan.

7. What is the anticipated rehabilitation potential for this patient? Your thought process should include time from burn injury and stage of healing.

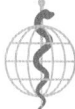 For additional resources, including answers to the questions for review, new immersive cases, case study guiding questions, references, and more, please visit **https://www.fadavis.com/product/physical-rehabilitation-fulk-8**. You may also quickly find the resources by entering this title's four-digit ISBN, 4691, in the search field at **http://fadavis.com** and logging in at the prompt.

Chronic Pain

Chapter **25**

Leslie N. Russek, PT, DPT, PhD, OCS

LEARNING OBJECTIVES

1. Assess the impact of chronic pain on individuals and society.
2. Clarify terminology associated with nociception, pain, and chronic pain.
3. Compare and contrast nociceptive, neuropathic pain, and nociplastic pain.
4. Apply the International Classification of Functioning, Disability, and Health (ICF) model to chronic pain.
5. Explain the pathophysiological processes underlying chronic pain, including peripheral and central sensitization, as well as immune, endocrine, and autonomic system involvement.
6. Propose risk factors associated with chronic pain.
7. Describe methods for obtaining a thorough, biopsychosocial history from patients.
8. Contrast various outcome measures for examining chronic pain and its impact on activity and participation.
9. Describe tests and measures appropriate for examining individuals with chronic pain.
10. Relate examination findings to evaluation and prognosis for individuals with chronic pain.
11. Describe appropriate physical therapy interventions for individuals with chronic pain.
12. Summarize medical management of chronic pain.
13. Discuss complementary and alternative medicine approaches to managing chronic pain.

CHAPTER OUTLINE

PAIN TERMINOLOGY AND BASIC CONCEPTS 967
  Evolution of the Biopsychosocial Model of Pain 971
PATHOPHYSIOLOGICAL PROCESSES UNDERLYING CHRONIC PAIN 971
  Changes in Neural Processing Associated With Chronic Pain 972
  Chronification of Neuropathic Pain 976
RISK FACTORS ASSOCIATED WITH CHRONIC PAIN 977
  Genetic Risk Factors 978
  Psychosocial Risk Factors 978
  Pain Beliefs and Behaviors 979
EXAMINATION OF PATIENTS WITH CHRONIC PAIN 980
  Impact of Pain on Physical and Psychosocial Function 981
  Pain Characteristics 982
  Identification of Psychosocial Factors Impacting Pain 984
  Challenges in the Subjective Examination 986
  Systems Review and Review of Systems 987
  Physical Therapy Tests and Measures 987

PHYSICAL THERAPY EVALUATION, DIAGNOSIS, AND PROGNOSIS 990
  Evaluation and Diagnosis 990
  Prognosis 992
PHYSICAL THERAPY MANAGEMENT OF CHRONIC PAIN 993
  The Multidisciplinary Pain Management Team 993
  Therapeutic Alliance 995
  Patient-/Client-Related Instruction 995
  Cognitive Behavioral Therapy, Cognitive Functional Therapy, and Pain Coping Skills 999
  Physical Self-Care Strategies 1002
  Neuromuscular Reeducation 1003
  Exercise 1004
  Manual Therapy 1005
  Assistive Devices 1006
  Biophysical and Other Modalities 1006
MEDICAL MANAGEMENT OF CHRONIC PAIN 1007
  Medical Diagnostic Testing 1007
  Pharmacological Management 1007
  Other Medical Management 1007
COMPLEMENTARY AND ALTERNATIVE APPROACHES 1008
SUMMARY 1008

Pain is the most common reason people visit health-care providers and physical therapists. According to the 2019 National Health Interview Survey, *chronic pain* affects more than 50 million adult Americans—more than 20% of the U.S. adult population.[1] Chronic pain is the leading cause of long-term disability in the United States, affecting more people than diabetes, heart disease, and cancer combined.[2] Chronic pain is more prevalent among women, minorities, military veterans, and rural and marginalized populations.[3]

Chronic pain exacts a huge toll in medical care, lost workdays, and compromised quality of life. In the United States, the national economic cost of chronic pain in 2010 was estimated at $560 billion to $635 billion per year, with $261 billion to $386 billion per year of that due to direct medical costs. Lost productivity due to pain costs $297 billion to $336 billion per year.

Quality of life is severely compromised for people with chronic pain.[4]

This chapter focuses on individuals with chronic pain who are most likely to present for PT intervention. It is not the goal of this chapter to address cancer or visceral pain, even though they are growing specialty areas within PT. Recent advances in pain physiology are presented as a foundation for understanding common chronic pain conditions and the appropriate management for those conditions.

■ PAIN TERMINOLOGY AND BASIC CONCEPTS

Pain is defined as "An unpleasant sensory and emotional experience associated with, or resembling that associated with, actual or potential tissue damage"; the International Association for the Study of Pain (IASP) has added "six key notes" to further qualify the definition (Box 25.1).[5] Pain is not just the firing of nociceptive neurons, it is an interaction among internal and external stimuli, context, and emotional and social factors. An analogy would be that some people perceive spicy food as unpleasant or even painful, while others perceive it as delicious; interpretation depends in part on internal stimuli (physical sensations, cognitive and emotional factors) and external stimuli (e.g., social factors and context). The experience of pain reflects a perception of danger and the need for protection. Tissue threat/damage and nociception, while sometimes associated with pain, are

---

Box 25.1   IASP Pain Definition and Six Key Notes Terminology [5]

Pain: An unpleasant sensory and emotional experience associated with, or resembling that associated with, actual or potential tissue damage.

Six key notes:

1. Pain is always a personal experience that is influenced to varying degrees by biological, psychological, and social factors.
2. Pain and nociception are different phenomena. Pain cannot be inferred solely from activity in sensory neurons.
3. Through their life experiences, individuals learn the concept of pain.
4. A person's report of an experience as pain should be respected.
5. Although pain usually serves an adaptive role, it may have adverse effects on function and social and psychological well-being.
6. Verbal description is only one of several behaviors to express pain; inability to communicate does not negate the possibility that a human or a nonhuman animal experiences pain.

---

neither necessary nor sufficient for an individual to experience pain.[2,6-9]

Additional pain terminology relates to ways in which pain is classified or described. This section briefly presents terminology related to pain mechanisms, and the physiology is explained in later sections. See Box 25.2 for terminology,[2,5,9] and Table 25.1 for a description of different types of pain.[9-12] Pain may be nociceptive, neuropathic, or nociplastic. *Central sensitization (CS)* now refers to a mechanism underlying nociplastic pain and amplifying nociceptive and neuropathic pain. Clinical states usually involve a combination of several types of pain.

Nociceptive pain is associated with activation of primary nociceptors through noxious stimulation (mechanical, thermal, or chemical/inflammatory) or through non-noxious stimuli in the presence of inflammation; nociceptive pain typically signals impending tissue damage or danger. Nociceptive pain typically leads to a protective withdrawal response and is therefore beneficial. Nociceptive pain may be transient, recurrent, or persistent. For example, transient pain may occur after a shoulder subluxation, while recurrent pain may occur after repeated subluxations, and persistent pain may occur in the case of osteoarthritis (OA).[9,13,14] Because neural connective tissue is innervated by nociceptors (nervi nervorum), neural connective tissue may also generate nociceptive pain, which tends to be deep, aching, and localized with discomfort generally proportional to stimulus.[15] Deep tissues may present with more diffuse and vague pain. What used to be considered deep muscle pain, including delayed-onset muscle soreness, is now thought to be associated with richly innervated deep fascia.[11,16,17] Fascial pain is included in discussions of nociceptive pain, inflammation, and sensitization.

Visceral pain is sometimes considered separate from musculoskeletal pain,[6] though both are forms of nociceptive pain. While some visceral pathology refers pain to somatic tissues, much of the vagal afferent information projects to pre-emotional processing regions of the brain, such as the solitary tract projecting to the anterior cingulate. This results in the distress often associated with visceral pain. This chapter does not address visceral pain, though it is a common source of chronic pain and can present as musculoskeletal pain and can produce CS. Readers are referred to Pacheco-Carroza for further information about how visceral pain may contribute to musculoskeletal conditions.[10]

Some sources also distinguish *inflammatory pain* as different from other nociceptive pain because nociceptors are not only activated but may be sensitized by local or systemic inflammatory mediators, and low-threshold stimuli that are normally not painful may become painful.[6] There is growing evidence that some chronic pain conditions (e.g., fibromyalgia, long COVID, hypermobile Ehlers-Danlos syndrome) are associated with mast

Box 25.2   Pain Terminology[2,5,9]

- **Acute pain:** Pain associated with tissue damage or the threat of such damage and typically resolves once the tissue heals or the threat resolves; often nociceptive dominant.
- **Adjuvant medication:** Medications whose primary indication is a condition other than pain but which have demonstrated benefit in pain management.
- **Allodynia:** Pain due to a stimulus that does not normally provoke pain.
- **Analgesia:** Absence of pain in response to stimulation that would normally be painful.
- **Causalgia:** A syndrome of sustained burning pain, allodynia, and hyperpathia after a traumatic nerve lesion, often combined with vasomotor and sudomotor dysfunction and later trophic changes.
- **Central neuropathic pain:** Pain initiated or caused by a primary lesion or dysfunction in the central nervous system.
- **Central sensitization:** Amplification of neural signaling within the central nervous system, resulting in pain hypersensitivity.
- **Chronic pain:** Pain lasting more than 3 or 6 months.
- **Chronic pain syndrome:** Pain that exists when individuals have developed extensive pain behaviors such as preoccupation with pain, passive approach to health care, significant life disruption, feelings of isolation, being demanding, being angry, or doctor shopping.
- **Chronic primary pain:** *International Classification of Diseases, 11th revision*, classification for pain with no clear underlying cause, or in which the emotional distress and/or functional disability is not better accounted for by another condition.
- **Chronic secondary pain:** Pain secondary to an underlying disease.
- **Dysesthesia:** An unpleasant abnormal sensation, whether spontaneous or evoked.
- **High-impact chronic pain:** Chronic pain associated with substantial reduction in work, social, and self-care activities.
- **Hyperalgesia:** Increased pain from a stimulus that normally provokes pain.
- **Hyperesthesia:** Increased sensitivity to stimulation, excluding the special senses.
- **Hyperpathia:** A painful syndrome characterized by an abnormally painful reaction to a stimulus, especially a repetitive stimulus, as well as an increased threshold.
- **Malignant pain:** Pain associated with cancer.
- **Neurogenic inflammation:** The process of nociceptive afferents releasing inflammatory molecules at the peripheral terminal, causing a localized inflammatory response in the peripheral tissues.
- **Neurogenic pain:** A term previously used for neuropathic but now only indicates that pain comes from the nervous system, such as "neurogenic inflammation."
- **Neuromatrix:** A complex network of synaptic links within the central nervous system, initially determined by genetics but modified by psychological and sensory inputs. Because the neuromatrix that processes pain is not dedicated to only process pain, the term "pain neuromatrix" is not ideal, though it is often used.
- **Neuropathic pain:** Pain caused by a lesion or disease of the somatosensory nervous system.
- **Nocebo (nocebo effect):** The opposite of a placebo or the placebo effect. A nocebo is an inert treatment or event that increases symptoms because the patient believes it will increase symptoms. The expectation of pain can result in both increased pain from painful stimuli and allodynia, pain from a normally nonpainful stimulus.
- **Nociceptive pain:** Pain that arises from actual or threatened damage to non-neural tissue and is due to the activation of nociceptors. Nociceptive pain occurs only when the somatosensory nervous system is normal.
- **Nociplastic pain:** Pain that arises from altered nociception despite no clear evidence of actual or threatened tissue damage causing nociceptor activation, nor lesion of the somatosensory system causing pain.
- **Paresthesia:** An abnormal sensation, whether spontaneous or evoked.
- **Peripheral neuropathic pain:** Pain caused by a lesion or disease of the peripheral somatosensory nervous system.
- **Peripheral sensitization:** Increased responsiveness and reduced threshold of nociceptors to stimulation of their receptive fields.
- **Persistent pain:** Pain related to tissue damage or the threat of such damage that persists because the causative factors persist.
- **Placebo (placebo effect):** An inert treatment such as a sugar pill or fake treatment that is beneficial because the patient believes it will be beneficial.
- **Psychogenic pain:** An older term for pain believed to be caused by psychological factors when organic factors were absent or not severe enough to explain the pain complaint.
- **Referred pain:** Spontaneous pain outside the area of injury or source of pain.
- **Sensitization:** Increased responsiveness of nociceptive neurons to their normal input, and/or recruitment of a response to normally subthreshold inputs.
- **Suffering:** The multidimensional experience of severe stress that occurs when there is a significant threat to the whole person, and processes that would normally enable adaptation are insufficient.

Table 25.1   Subjective and Objective Characteristics Associated With Different Pain Mechanisms[9-12]

Type of Pain	Tissue Source	Subjective Characteristics	Objective Characteristics
Nociceptive: Cutaneous or superficial	Skin and subcutaneous tissues (A-delta and C fibers). History of damage or potential tissue damage.	Usually intermittent, well-localized, stabbing, sharp; may be constant dull ache or throb at rest. Varies relative to tissue damage or potential damage.	Clear, consistent, proportional pain reproduced through movement or mechanical testing of target tissues. Localized or with somatic referral. No sensory loss.
Nociceptive: Deep somatic	Fascia and other connective tissues, bone, muscle, blood vessels (greater predominance of C fibers over A-delta)	Vague, tearing, cramping, pressing, aching. Often referred to other locations.	Vague, sometimes referred pain reproduced through movement or mechanical testing of deeper tissues; spasm, trigger points common. No sensory loss.
Nociceptive: Visceral	Organs and the linings of the body cavities (more C fibers than A-delta). Spinal and vagal pathways.	Often referred to other locations; poorly localized, diffuse, deep cramping or splitting, sharp, stabbing. Poorly correlated to tissue damage.	Vague pain reproduction on movement or mechanical testing of visceral tissues, sometimes autonomic dysfunction. No sensory loss.
Peripheral neuropathic	Nerve fibers (A-delta and C fibers, but may involve A-delta and autonomic). History of lesion or disease to peripheral nerve.	Pain variously described as burning, shooting, pricking, stabbing, or "electric shock." Paresthesias: tingling, pricking. Pain and sensory dysfunction neuro-anatomically logical (dermatomal or peripheral nerve patterns). May have allodynia.	Sensory or motor/strength deficits depending on nerve. Pain or symptom provocation with movement or mechanical tests that move, load, or compress neural tissues; pain may be spontaneous (no external stimulus).
Central: Central neuropathic	Spinal cord and brain. History of lesion or disease to spinal cord or brain.	Pain neuro-anatomically logical. Continuous or paroxysmal; evoked by mechanical stimuli or spontaneous; unpredictable. May have allodynia.	Evidence of CNS damage or disease such as spasticity, dystonia. Pain and sensory abnormalities are neuro-anatomically logical. Pain may be triggered by mechanical stimuli or spontaneous.
Nociplastic	Neuroplasticity in spinal cord and brain but no injury or disease. Peripheral and/or central sensitization. Not consistent with tissue damage.	Pain is typically vague and dull, widespread, and not neuro-anatomically logical. Disproportionate, nonmechanical, unpredictable pattern of pain in response to multiple, nonspecific aggravating or easing factors. Often has visceral and autonomic pain or nonpain complaints. May have maladaptive beliefs and pain behaviors. Fatigue; may have weakness due to deconditioning.	Disproportionate, inconsistent, or nonanatomical pattern of sensory abnormalities and pain provocation in response to movement or mechanical testing. Autonomic dysfunction. Wind-up (temporal summation), allodynia, and decreased conditioned pain modulation.

CNS = central nervous system.

cell activation that sensitizes both the peripheral and central nervous systems.[18-20] Inflammation may therefore be both a source of nociceptive pain and a modulator of nociception, neuropathic and nociplastic pain, and CS.

Peripheral neuropathic pain is defined as pain caused by a lesion or disease of somatosensory nerves. Peripheral neuropathic pain can occur in response to diseases (e.g., diabetes, herpes zoster, HIV infection), medical interventions (e.g., chemotherapy, surgery), or traumatic or overuse injuries (e.g., carpal tunnel, brachial plexus avulsion, herniated disc). It can also occur spontaneously (i.e., with no known peripheral tissue damage or threat) or in response to normally innocuous stimuli. When axons are involved, symptoms can also include hypoesthesia, anesthesia, paresthesia, or dysesthesia such as burning, prickling, tingling, searing, or crawling sensations in the innervation pattern of the nerve.[5,12,21-23] Although the terms *neurogenic* and *neuropathic* are often used interchangeably, the IASP nomenclature uses the term *neuropathic* for pain associated with neural injury or disease.[5] The IASP does not formally define *neurogenic*, but it is generally used to more broadly refer to pain caused by the nervous system, which includes inflammation in or caused by nerves.

Central neuropathic pain is defined as pain caused by a lesion or disease of the central nervous system (CNS).[5] It can exist in the absence of peripheral nociceptive input and can, in fact, be generated in body regions that are denervated, such as spinal cord injury (SCI). Other common conditions include stroke, traumatic brain injury, multiple sclerosis (MS), brain tumors, epilepsy, or Parkinson disease (PD). Central neuropathic pain may be burning, cold, stabbing, shooting, lancinating, pricking, pressing, or squeezing, and both hyperalgesia and allodynia may exist. Peripheral and central neuropathic pain may become chronic because changes in the neural system cannot be reversed or due to neuroplasticity.[5,12,21-23]

Nociplastic pain was defined by the IASP in 2017 as the third mechanism for pain which results from altered nociception, in the absence of evidence for tissue or neural injury or disease.[5] These include functional pain syndromes, such as fibromyalgia, irritable bowel syndrome (IBS), and complex regional pain syndrome. Nociplastic pain may contribute to nociceptive or neuropathic pain if the pain and disability exceed what can be justified by tissue or neural injury or disease. CS still refers to a process by which the CNS amplifies neural signals associated with pain, can occur in the absence of observed neural lesions or disease, and is a primary mechanism for nociplastic pain. However, CS can occur in the presence of any type of pain.[13,14] Neuropathic pain can be considered a "hardware problem," while nociplastic pain would be a "software problem."

Pain is often described as acute or chronic based on the duration of pain. However, pain physiology is distinct from acute, subacute, remodeling, or chronic stages of tissue healing. The term *acute pain* is generally used to refer to transient, nociceptive-dominant pain—that is, acute pain is often associated with nociceptor activation due to tissue damage or the threat of such damage and typically resolves as the threat resolves or during the healing process as tissue heals. Acute, nociceptive-dominant pain is often associated with physiological signs of distress, such as sweating, pallor, nausea, and heart rate (HR) changes. However, acute/recent pain is not simply nociceptor activation; cognitive and emotional factors have a powerful effect on the pain experience. Also, nociceptive-dominant pain is not always recent, acute, or transient; nociceptive-dominant pain can be of long duration if recurrent or persistent,

as in the case of osteoarthritis. So, while the term *acute pain* is commonly used to contrast with chronic pain, the term does not quite correspond to a single aspect of pain physiology. Patients may also have *acute-on-chronic pain* with acute, nociceptive-dominant pain superimposed on chronic pain.

Chronic pain has been defined in a variety of ways. The simplest and most common is to define it as any recurrent or persistent pain lasting more than 3 months.[2,6,8,24] This is the definition adopted by the *International Classification of Diseases, 11th revision (ICD-11)*, because it is simple and clearly defined.[25] Although this definition is simple to apply, it does not reflect the significant physiological and psychosocial changes that occur in "chronic pain."[26] The *ICD-11* defines *chronic primary pain* as pain with no clear underlying cause or in which the emotional distress and/or functional disability is out of proportion to the underlying cause; pain due to another condition is defined as *secondary chronic pain*. This new definition is controversial, as there may be underlying causes that have not yet been identified; patients with poorly understood or underdiagnosed conditions could be mislabeled as primary chronic pain.[27] The *ICD-11* classification for chronic pain is given in Box 25.3.[28]

Box 25.3 ICD-11 Classification for Chronic Pain: MG30.0[44]

- MG30 **Chronic pain:** Any persistent or recurrent pain lasting longer than 3 months.

Subclassification of Chronic Pain:

- **MG30.0 Chronic primary pain:** Chronic primary pain is chronic pain in one or more anatomical regions that is characterized by significant emotional distress (anxiety, anger/frustration or depressed mood) or functional disability (interference in daily life activities and reduced participation in social roles). Chronic primary pain is multifactorial: biological, psychological, and social factors contribute to the pain syndrome. The diagnosis is appropriate independently of identified biological or psychological contributors unless another diagnosis would better account for the presenting symptoms. Subclassification includes chronic primary visceral pain, widespread pain, musculoskeletal pain, headache or orofacial pain, complex regional pain syndrome, and unspecified primary pain.

Chronic Secondary Pain
- **MG30.1 Chronic cancer related pain**
- **MG30.2 Chronic postsurgical or posttraumatic pain**
- **MG30.3 Chronic secondary musculoskeletal pain**
- **MG30.4 Chronic secondary visceral pain**
- **MG30.5 Chronic neuropathic pain**
- **MG30.6 Chronic secondary headache and orofacial pain**

Clinical Implications. While chronic pain is typically defined as pain persisting for more than 3 months, chronic pain is often physiologically different from acute pain. Consequently, treatments that work for acute pain do not always work for chronic pain.

Pain research frequently uses thermal, mechanical, or chemical stimuli that stress but do not damage tissues. This *experimental pain* is typically acute, short-duration, nociceptive-dominant pain. Experimental pain is often studied in healthy individuals, in contrast to *clinical pain,* which is observed in people experiencing pain due to clinical conditions. Clinical pain can be any combination of nociceptive, peripheral, or central neuropathic. The difference between experimental and clinical pain is important because neuroanatomy and neurophysiology related to pain may not be the same in these two situations. This chapter addresses clinical pain.

Many terms have been used in the past to describe medically unexplained pain: *maladaptive, pathological, psychogenic, affective,* and *nonorganic pain.* Altered neural processing due to neural plasticity is now called "nociplastic" pain, which may be due to peripheral or CS. Terms such as *psychogenic, affective,* and *nonorganic pain,* once commonly used for medically unexplained pain, are no longer consistent with understanding of pain physiology and should not be used. Other definitions related to pain are presented in Box 25.2.[5,29]

Evolution of the Biopsychosocial Model of Pain

In the 17th century, Descartes set the groundwork for the *specificity model,* where pain was believed to travel along dedicated nerve fibers to a pain center in the brain. This mechanistic view provided the foundation for the *biomedical model* of pain, in which pain was directly correlated to tissue damage or threat of damage. According to the biomedical model, pain should resolve once tissue damage heals. The biomedical model works reasonably well for many types of acute, nociceptive pain; however, it is unable to explain many other examples of pain where the pain experience is inconsistent with tissue damage or healing. The failure of the biomedical model to explain many instances of pain led to the adoption of the *biopsychosocial model* of pain, which recognizes that biological factors interact with personal and environmental factors to influence body function and structure, activity, and participation in life activities.[30-32] Some have also proposed a *biopsychosocial-spiritual model.*[33] The IASP definition of pain includes "6 key notes" that clearly define pain as a biopsychosocial phenomenon.[5] The biopsychosocial model is more effective than the biomedical model in explaining and managing chronic pain.[30-32]

Clinical Implications. The biomedical model often works well for patients with acute, nociceptive-dominant pain. However, it does not work well for patients with chronic pain. Patient examination and management strategies for patients with chronic pain must include understanding and addressing a wide range of emotional, cognitive, social, and environmental factors as well as biological contributors to the pain.[2,6-8]

Although the concept is still controversial,[25] the Institute of Medicine has proposed that chronic pain be considered a disease, rather than just a symptom, because chronic pain results in pathological changes in the nervous system that can progress over time, independent of the initial cause of pain. Just as a myocardial infarction may have many contributing factors but ultimately results in some common outcomes, chronic pain has multiple contributing factors that result in some common outcomes, and it needs to be managed if it cannot be cured.[34] The *ICD-11* classifies primary chronic pain as a disease and secondary chronic pain as a symptom/body function impairment.

The World Health Organization's (WHO's) ICF model treats pain as an abnormal body function classified under the designation *Sensory Function and Pain.* The physiological changes observed in chronic pain may also be associated with changes in the *Structure of the Nervous System* at the level of body structure.[35] The multidirectional nature of the ICF model is particularly pertinent to chronic pain where personal factors, structure, function, activity, participation, and environmental factors are interrelated and can all affect one another. This complex interaction is discussed further in the Risk Factors section, later in this chapter.

■ PATHOPHYSIOLOGICAL PROCESSES UNDERLYING CHRONIC PAIN

A detailed discussion of the neuroanatomy and neurophysiology involved in the pain experience is beyond the scope of this chapter. Therefore, the current discussion focuses on ways in which anatomical or physiological changes associated with chronic pain may impact interventions. Readers can find more extensive coverage of pain physiology in one of the textbooks on pain: *Mechanisms and Management of Pain for the Physical Therapist,*[36] *Pain Neuroscience Education: Teaching People About Pain,*[37] and *Explain Pain Supercharged.*[38]

There are several models describing pain neurophysiology. The *neuromatrix model* describes pain as a neuromatrix comprising a widespread network of neurons initially determined by genetics but modified by psychological and sensory inputs both before and during the pain experience.[39,40] The initial neuromatrix theory identified three components of the pain phenomenon, with each component potentially contributing to and an output of the pain experience. The *sensory-discriminative dimension* refers to localization, intensity, duration, and the nature of the pain (burning, sharp, etc.). The *motivational-affective dimension* refers to the emotional component, including stress. The *cognitive-evaluative dimension* relates to how pain is interpreted in the context of past and present experience, culture, and so forth.[29,40] Although it is often referred to as the "pain neuromatrix," these pathways are more accurately described as a *dynamic neural representation of pain* or *salience network*. The involved pathways also serve a variety of other, non–pain-related neural processes responsible for maintaining homeostasis, and activity in these regions is not proportional to pain intensity, and the pain experience is not proportional to activity in any single brain network, as was once believed.[41]

The *triple network model of pain* identifies three neural networks associated with pain: one ascending pathway includes the lateral pain pathway for localization, the medial pain pathway processes affective and emotional aspects of pain, and a descending modulatory pathway can inhibit or facilitate pain processing. Functional MRI studies suggest that chronic pain develops when the descending modulatory becomes inactive and fails to inhibit pain. The triple network model also proposes that suffering (mediated by the medial pathway) includes cognitive, emotional, and autonomic components.[42] The autonomic component may involve decreased activation of the vagus nerve, whose descending fibers contribute to both analgesia and anti-inflammatory effects, and whose ascending fibers contribute to the emotional experience of pain.[10,43] The *allostasis model of pain* proposes that autonomic system activation, hypothalamic–pituitary–adrenal (HPA) axis dysfunction, and neuroplastic adaptations interact to increase inflammation, sympathetic arousal, fear conditioning, and a hyperalgesic state and vulnerability to chronic pain.[44]

While CS appears to be the primary underlying mechanism for nociplastic pain, it may also result from peripheral sensitization, changes in descending inhibition, immune system activation, and other neuroplastic changes.[9,14,45] Therefore, any of the following pathophysiological processes may contribute to nociplastic pain except for frank nerve damage or disease, which result in neuropathic pain.

> **Clinical Implications.** Chronic pain is a complex, multisystem phenomenon that involves multiple regions of the brain. The neuromatrix reflects both genetic and experiential influences (sensory, emotional, and cognitive activity). Over time, certain pathways become well worn, the connections become stronger, and activity in these networks is more easily reproduced in response to non-nociceptive stimuli as well as nociceptive stimuli. The neuromatrix becomes more "skilled" at perceiving pain.[46]

Changes in Neural Processing Associated With Chronic Pain

Peripheral Sensitization

Peripheral sensitization exists when nociceptor activity is increased, resulting in primary *hyperalgesia* or *allodynia*. Increased nociceptor sensitivity in the presence of acute inflammation normally leads to resting the injured tissues; ideally, nociceptors return to their normal state once local tissues have healed. However, in peripheral sensitization associated with chronic pain, nociceptors either become too sensitive or remain sensitized for too long. Repeated or persistent noxious stimulation of muscle nociceptors can lead to changes in the size, number, threshold, and receptive field of dorsal horn neurons[47] and coupling between autonomic and nociceptive nerves.[9] Peripheral sensitization differs from neuropathic pain that, by definition, involves nerve injury or disease. The mechanism of sensitization can be through tissue damage, neurogenic inflammation, abnormal sympathetic activity, or systemic inflammation. Tissue damage (including prolonged muscle spasm or trigger point activity) releases a multitude of chemicals or ions that can increase nociceptor sensitivity by decreasing activation threshold or by activating "silent nociceptors" (mechanically insensitive C fibers that develop mechanical sensitivity in response to chemical stimuli such as inflammation, hence acquiring a lower mechanical threshold). Tissue damage also activates the sympathetic nervous system, which can lead to autonomic imbalance.[48]

Nociceptor activity can be modified through several cellular mechanisms, such as activation of ion channels, increased receptor density or type, decreased firing threshold, increased conduction velocity, increased sensitivity to circulating catecholamines, activation of intracellular messengers, or increased receptive field.[49,50] Changes at the periphery can propagate to the nociceptor cell body, where modifications to ion channels can produce ectopic activity, and increased transcription can lead to sprouting of additional peripheral terminals. When multiple factors are present (e.g., inflammation and low pH), nociceptor firing intensity and duration can both be increased. Silent nociceptors may also be chemically activated by tissue damage or inflammation.[51] Overall, the mechanisms of peripheral sensitization contribute to hyperalgesia, where pain threshold is decreased, and allodynia, where non-painful stimuli such as movement or light touch can activate nociceptors. Peripheral sensitization also provides increased input into the CNS, leading to CS.[50]

> **Clinical Implications.** Joint nociceptors are normally responsive to noxious pressure or extreme joint movement, but silent nociceptors, once activated by tissue damage or inflammation, respond to any mechanical stimulus. Consequently, when peripheral sensitization is present, motion that would not normally activate nociceptors now does.[49]

Immune Involvement in Chronic Pain

The immune system modulates nociception through systemic, local, and neuroinflammation. Mast cells, neutrophils, macrophages, dendritic cells, and T cells are all involved in local or systemic inflammatory effects on pain. Inflammation activates silent nociceptors, which remain active by producing sustained discharge long after removal of the stimulus. Cytokines can increase or decrease neural excitability and modify neural growth or interconnections. Neuroimmune interactions from tissue damage contribute to peripheral sensitization in chronic pain.[52-54] The role of inflammation in CS is discussed in the section on Central Sensitization.

Neurogenic inflammation is another mechanism for increasing nociceptor sensitivity. Nociceptors generally act as afferent neurons, responding to environmental stimuli such as heat, cold, mechanical, or chemical triggers. However, they are actually pseudo-unipolar, where the central and peripheral stalks of the axon can both receive and transmit signals. Injured nerves may also respond at the site of injury. *Neurogenic inflammation* refers to the process where afferent nerves activate in an antidromic direction, stimulating inflammatory processes in peripheral tissues by releasing calcitonin gene-related peptide, substance P, neuropeptides, glutamate, neurokinins, vasoactive peptides, nitric oxide, and cytokines at the peripheral terminal.[55,56] This *dorsal root reflex* in nociceptive neurons can therefore stimulate chemotaxis of neutrophils, macrophages, and lymphocytes to the peripheral terminal; cause vasodilation, vascular leakage, and edema; and prime the differentiation of T helper cells. Neurogenic inflammation thus facilitates tissue healing and immune defense in acute conditions when danger is perceived, but it contributes to peripheral and CS when persistent.[55,57-59]

> **Clinical Implications.** Nociceptors can transmit antidromic signals to peripheral tissues leading to vasodilation, increased capillary permeability, plasma extravasation, and edema associated with neurogenic inflammation even if there was no local tissue damage. Consequently, tissue inflammation might be generated by the CNS and not tissue damage.[55]

Fascia normally serves as a lymphatic drainage system to remove inflammatory mediators from tissues. If fascia is unable to perform this function, inflammatory mediators can accumulate in a variety of tissues, both previously injured and previously healthy. Since fascia is highly innervated with nociceptors, this inflammation can trigger pain; pain and inflammation can increase contractile activity in myofibroblasts, increasing fascial restrictions that compromise both physiological and mechanical function. Chronic, widespread fascial inflammation can sensitize peripheral nerves, trigger excess autonomic activity, and contribute to CS.[16,17,60,61]

which in turn increases neurogenic inflammation that perpetuates the cycle.

Autonomic Dysfunction in Chronic Pain

The autonomic system is involved in many chronic conditions involving chronic pain and/or inflammation: fibromyalgia, chronic headache, rheumatoid arthritis (RA), osteoarthritis (OA), IBS, interstitial cystitis, and chronic fatigue syndrome. Vagus nerve efferent activity both inhibits systemic inflammation via the cholinergic anti-inflammatory pathway and provides analgesic effects via afferent input into brain structures processing pain.[43,48,62] The vagus nerve provides the primary afferent input to the solitary tract nucleus and anterior cingulate, which contribute to pre-emotional processing, leading to affective and emotional components of chronic pain.[10] The true picture is likely more complex, with polyvagal theory proposing that the dorsal and ventral vagus nerves serve different functions and may be activated or inhibited separately.[63]

Acute pain normally activates the sympathetic nervous system and inhibits the parasympathetic system as part of the response to perceived danger. Sympathetically maintained pain *(causalgia)* typically presents as neuropathic pain (burning pain and allodynia) accompanied by edema, changes in skin blood flow and temperature, and trophic changes. There are several mechanisms by which the autonomic nervous system can alter pain. First, epinephrine can increase sensitivity of nociceptors through peripheral sensitization, as discussed already. Second, after peripheral nerve injury, nociceptors can express catecholamine receptors that then respond to sympathetic activity, causing stress to directly activate nociceptors. Third, nerve injury results in sympathetic nerves sprouting postganglionic basketlike structures around injured neuronal cell bodies. Activation of these sympathetic fibers may result in increased activity in the injured neurons.[64,65] Decreased parasympathetic activation has also been associated with chronic pain.[43,66] The autonomic system involvement in chronic pain helps explain (a) trauma and psychosocial stress as risk factors; (b) prevalence of signs, symptoms, and comorbidities associated with autonomic dysfunction; and (c) the benefits of aerobic exercise, relaxation, and stress management as interventions for chronic pain.[43,48,62] Furthermore, decreased parasympathetic function, measured using HR variability, results in maladaptive responses to both physical and psychological health problems, perpetuating both.[43,66]

> **Clinical Implications.** Sympathetic nervous system activation can both sensitize and directly activate nociceptors to amplify pain. In contrast, an active parasympathetic nervous system has analgesic and anti-inflammatory effects. This provides physiological justification for stress management and relaxation as essential components of physiological pain management.

Central Sensitization

Both central neuropathic pain and CS are associated with changes to the CNS. Changes in CNS processing can lead to secondary hyperalgesia and allodynia in areas adjacent to or remote from actual tissue injury.[67] Some conditions may generate pain without any nociceptive input, whereas others appear to be mediated by centrally amplified and perpetuated peripheral nociceptive pain.[68] *Placebo* and *nocebo* (the reverse of placebo), while not unique to chronic pain, involve some of the same CNS pathways.[69]

Chronic pain is associated with widespread neuroplasticity, including changes in CNS structure, function, and chemistry, affecting both neurons and glia in the peripheral and central nervous systems.[70] That is, chronic pain is not simply ongoing nociception. Figure 25.1 shows changes observed in the brain with chronic pain.[50,71] Changes include decreased gray matter volume in some areas, increased gray matter in other areas, and both increased and decreased connectivity among regions of the brain. Furthermore, CNS changes observed vary across different pain syndromes.

CS presents as increased sensitivity to sensory input, which may include nociceptive, non-nociceptive, visceral, and special senses; multisystem hypersensitivity is key to identification of CS.[72,73] CS can result in increased

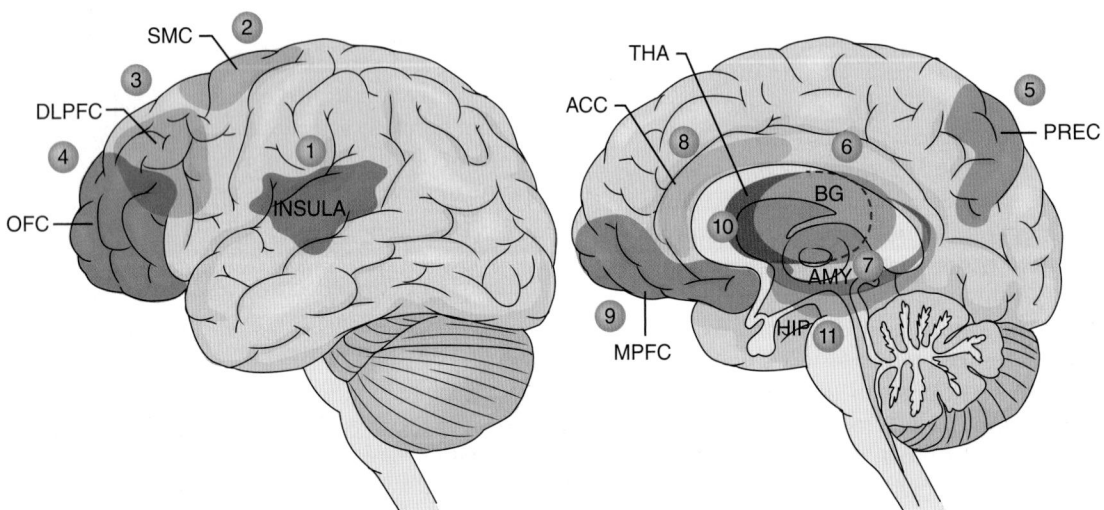

Figure 25.1 Brain regions that change in patients with chronic pain.[50,71,75,341]
Diagram shows regions of the brain that are believed to change in patients with chronic pain:

1. Insular cortex: Involved in consciousness, body awareness/perception, motor control, and some emotional processing. Decreased gray matter volume observed in patients with chronic pain.
2. Supplemental motor cortex: Primarily controls movement and posture.
3. Dorsolateral prefrontal cortex: Executive function and motor planning. Decreased gray matter in chronic low back pain.
4. Orbitofrontal cortex: Associated with decision-making, expectations, emotional processing of reward/punishment.
5. Precuneus: Associated with self-awareness, memory processing, visuospatial perception. Reduced cortical gray matter volume observed in patients with chronic back pain.
6. Basal ganglia: Associated with movement, motor planning, learning. Increased gray matter volume in chronic back pain, fibromyalgia, temporomandibular disorder.
   - Thalamus: Relays sensory and motor inputs to other brain areas and regulates consciousness. Reduced gray matter density in patients with chronic back pain.
7. Amygdala: Part of the limbic system, strong modulators of fear, associated with memory, decision-making, and emotional processing. Increased gray matter observed in patients with back pain.
   - Hippocampus: Part of the limbic system, functions in memory formation and consolidation. Altered hippocampal–cortical connectivity observed in patients with chronic back pain.
8. Anterior cingulate cortex: Participates in consciousness, autonomic functioning, decision-making, emotional processing of pain, reward-based learning. Descending projections link to autonomic responses to stimuli. Reduced gray matter density correlated to neurocognitive deficits in chronic tension-type headache and fibromyalgia.
9. Medial prefrontal cortex: Decision-making, including risk/reward. Decreased gray matter density in patients with chronic back pain.

or prolonged response to noxious stimulation (hyperalgesia), pain in response to normally innocuous input (allodynia), increased responsiveness in regions surrounding the initial area of injury (secondary hyperalgesia), increased response over time (temporal summation or wind-up), and pain lasting beyond the duration of the initial stimulus.[72,74] *Wind-up* or *temporal summation* is a normal process whereby firing of a postsynaptic neuron increases after the stimulus has been present for a few seconds; however, wind-up can be enhanced or its threshold decreased in the presence of CS.[67,75,76] Wind-up can result in long-term potentiation, in which the neural response is strengthened through increased neurogenic inflammation and altered gene expression resulting in altered nerve phenotype, with different receptors and transmitters.[67]

> **Clinical Implications.** Wind-up, or temporal summation, reflects CS. Wind-up can easily be measured as a part of the clinical examination to document CS.[77] Instructions are given later in this chapter, in the section on Examination.

CS is common in chronic pain conditions, but the abnormal sensory processing may begin early after trauma and may contribute to transition of acute into chronic pain. Both *central neuropathic pain* (CNP) and CS involve dysfunction of neurons and glial cells in the CNS; however, CS can occur in the absence of CNS lesion or disease.[74] CS is associated with increased activity in some brain areas involved in acute pain as well as regions not typically associated with acute pain and descending facilitatory pathways, and is associated with decreased activity in descending inhibitory pathways.[72-74] CS appears to be a neuroinflammatory process involving activation of glial cells (microglia, astrocytes, and oligodendrocytes), increased production of cytokines and chemokines, and increased vascular permeability and leukocyte infiltration. The neuro-immune interactions are bidirectional: glia perpetuate sensitization by releasing neuroactive signaling molecules that perpetuate an immune response. Once CS is initiated, nociplastic pain can occur in the absence of further peripheral nociceptor input.[50,58,74,75,78]

> **Clinical Implications.** The structure, physiology, and function of nociceptors change in CS. These sensitized nociceptors do not behave as in acute, nociceptive-dominant pain. Patients can therefore experience excessive pain (hyperalgesia) or pain as a result of movement or sensory stimuli that would not normally be painful (allodynia). Hyperalgesia and allodynia are therefore the result of physiological and functional changes in the nervous system. The terms *psychogenic, affective, nonorganic,* and *medically unexplained* are not appropriate. While we do not yet fully understand "primary pain," it is real, and it reflects real physiological and neuroplastic changes.

Endocrine Roles in Chronic Pain

The endocrine system also modulates the pain experience, and the hypothalamic–pituitary–adrenal (HPA) axis plays a central role in mediating stress-related chronic pain syndromes, such as fibromyalgia, whiplash-associated disorder, chronic fatigue syndrome, pelvic pain, IBS, posttraumatic stress disorder (PTSD), and burnout. Several brain regions are involved: hypothalamus, amygdala, prefrontal cortex, and hippocampus.[79,80] The locus coeruleus (LC) appears to be integrally involved in the link between stress and emotional-cognitive components of pain; that is, the LC amplifies aversion to painful experiences, a component of the emotional response to pain, without necessarily altering the sensory dimension. Stress also triggers multiple mediators that impact chronic pain.[81] Ultimately, physical or emotional stress activates the HPA axis, leading to a self-perpetuating cascade of events resulting in chronic sympathetic activation, which increases or perpetuates chronic pain.[44,82,83] Although the research is currently inconsistent, chronic pain appears to be associated with a blunted cortisol response; since cortisol is a strongly anti-inflammatory hormone, this stunted response could contribute to both peripheral and CS.[79,84] These physiological changes compound the psychological impact of stress and chronic pain on one another, which is discussed more later in this chapter. So, while the stress response is adaptive for acute pain, it becomes maladaptive when pain persists and contributes to chronification.[79,80]

The endocrine system also contributes to both peripheral and CNS changes seen in chronic pain. Chronic stress can be caused by either external circumstances (psychosocial or physical, including pain) or inappropriate responses such as negative cognitions, rumination, worry, catastrophization, or helplessness. When stress or pain is present for a prolonged period, the endocrine response becomes maladaptive with dysregulation of the HPA axis contributing to dysregulation of the corticolimbic system (including the amygdala, prefrontal cortex, and hippocampus), which can lead to increased inflammation, morning fatigue, muscle atrophy, compromised tissue growth and repair, autonomic dysfunction, cognitive changes, and pain.[44,83] Ultimately, chronic activation of the stress response appears to exhaust the HPA axis, as shown in Figure 25.2.[79,85] Hypocortisolism associated with chronic stress has been shown in fibromyalgia, chronic fatigue syndrome, temporomandibular disorder, and chronic pelvic pain. Cortisol is a potent anti-inflammatory hormone, and the decreased levels seen in chronic stress contribute to systemic inflammation and increased pain-related cytokines, which then lead to both peripheral and CS.[79] The exact mechanisms are not clear, but they are believed to be a combination of genetic vulnerability with a neurotoxic effect of hormones, such as glucocorticoids, secreted from the HPA axis during chronic

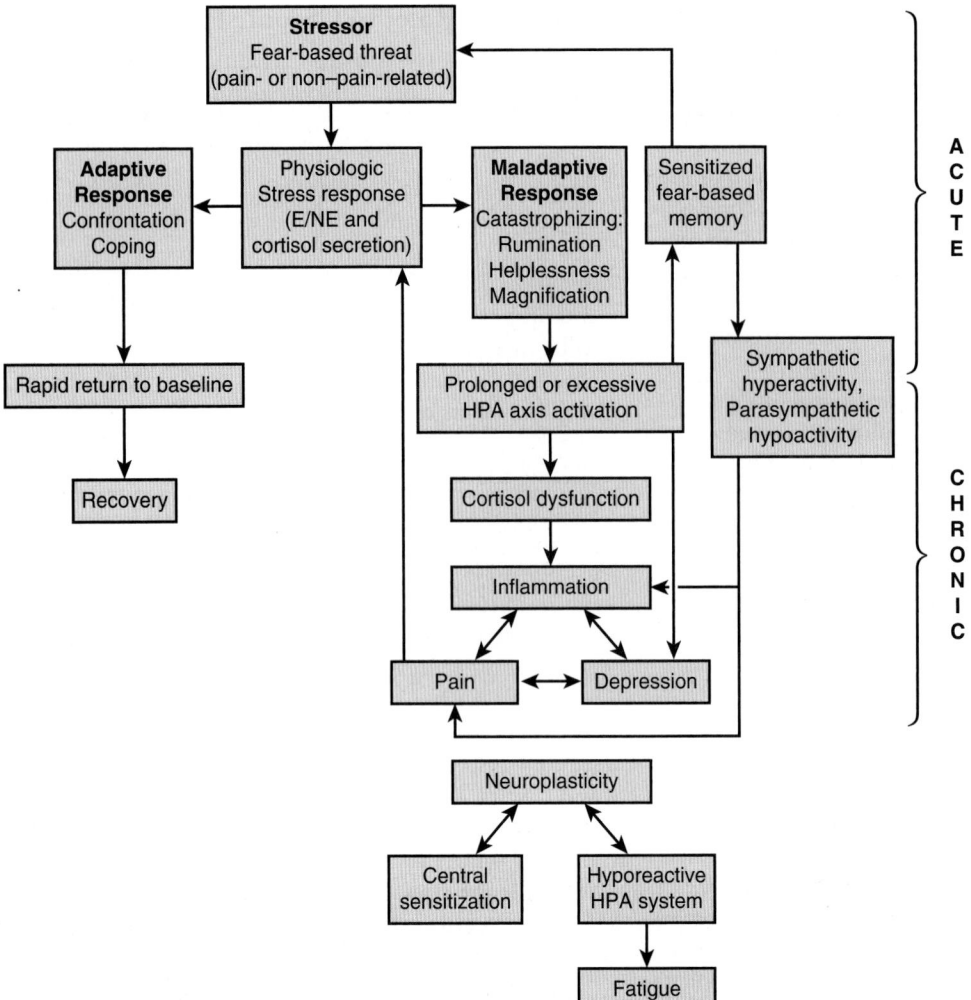

Figure 25.2 Relationship between stress and chronic pain. A physical or psychological stressor causes a stress response. Healthy individuals have an adaptive response and return to baseline. People who have a maladaptive response may have a prolonged or excessive hypothalamic–pituitary–adrenal (HPA) response and excessive sympathetic response that exacerbate the fear response and contribute to neuroplasticity associated with neuropathic pain or CS. A prolonged stress response can also lead to a hypoactive HPA system, which can lead to the fatigue often seen in chronic pain, and decreased parasympathetic function, which can lead to visceral symptoms.[79,342,343]

stress. The endocrine link helps to explain the interrelationships seen between cognitive, emotional, and physical components of the pain experience.[44,79,80]

Clinical Implications. Physical and emotional stress activate neuroendocrine processes that contribute to the transition from acute to chronic pain, and to the perpetuation of chronic pain. Stress compromises immune function, tissue growth and repair, as well as autonomic function. Stress also leads to cognitive changes and structural changes in the brain. A biopsychosocial management approach should address both pain- and non–pain-related stressors in patients.[44,79,83]

Chronification of Neuropathic Pain

While chronic pain is often musculoskeletal, up to 40% is neuropathic, due to conditions such as stroke, SCI, diabetes, MS, HIV/AIDS, amputation, PD, cancer, and chemotherapy or radiation for cancer.[23] Furthermore, neuropathic chronic pain may be particularly disabling.[21,86] Nerve injury sensitizes peripheral nerves through direct compromise to the axons or immune reaction of glial cells. The pathological changes observed in peripheral neuropathic pain develop as a result of normal healing processes, a complex interaction among the peripheral nerve, glial cells, and inflammatory mediators. However, neurotrophic factors and cytokines travel retrograde to the cell body where they modulate gene expression, sensitizing nociceptors at the dorsal root ganglion, and to the spinal cord where they stimulate CS and epigenetic changes. Microglia in the dorsal and ventral horns release neurotrophic factors that decrease descending inhibitory activity.[12,74,79,80,87-89]

Ultimately, prolonged peripheral neuropathic pain results in maladaptive neural plasticity, leading to decreased stimulation threshold, increased sensitivity, ectopic impulses, altered or eliminated axonal conduction, abnormal growth, reduced inhibition, and glial scarring. As a consequence of demyelination, uninjured fibers may be activated by adjacent fibers, a process called *crosstalk*. Also, innocuous input can trigger pain when A-beta fibers form synapses in the dorsal horn with neurons that normally transmit nociceptive information. What appears to be spontaneous activity may actually be due to sensitized nerves now activated by normal body temperature or innocuous motion.[12]

CNP may be chronic either because the underlying lesion/disease is chronic or because of the development of CS and nociplastic changes. Up to 73% of people with SCI, 86% of those with MS, 50% of those with stroke, and many people with PD develop chronic CNP.[12,21,90] Pain may occur when the balance between descending inhibition and descending facilitation is lost. Imbalance may be mediated by glia and astrocytes, leading to synaptic remodeling and synaptic connections forming between general sensory afferents and nociceptive fibers (allodynia) and resulting in descending facilitation.[70,74,91] For example, pain in SCI may be generated by ectopic activity in spinal cord nociceptive pathways, either from microglial activation or decreased descending inhibition. Pain due to stroke may be due to disinhibition; for example, lesions in the lateral thalamus can disinhibit the medial thalamus, allowing increased activity. Changes at the site of CNS injury can generate CNS changes in remote regions; for example, SCI can lead to microglial activation in the thalamus. The progression of neuropathic pain into nociplastic pain is from ectopic activity to peripheral and CS, impaired inhibitory modulation, and finally changes in microglia.[12,70,92,93] Nociceptive pain due to musculoskeletal dysfunctions secondary to CNS pathology is not considered CNP; for example, spasticity due to SCI, stroke, or PD is nociceptive pain and not CNP.[92] Additional neuroanatomical changes associated with chronification of CNP are described in the literature.[12,70,93]

Clinical Implications. Peripheral and central neuropathic conditions can trigger peripheral and CS and nociplastic changes through both neuroinflammatory processes and decreased descending inhibition. Patients with neuropathic pain should always be assessed for sensitization and nociplastic pain.

RISK FACTORS ASSOCIATED WITH CHRONIC PAIN

While injury or disease often triggers the development of pain, additional risk factors influence the likelihood that acute pain will transition into chronic pain, and that chronic pain will persist. Figure 25.3 shows a "Bucket Model" of pain, with a variety of risk factors and contributing factors as inputs into the pain "bucket." Risk factors contributing to chronic pain act cumulatively to trigger or amplify pain. The model may also help patients understand that the apparent cause of injury (e.g., lifting a box at work) was probably only one of many contributing factors. Contributing factors are cumulative, and the apparent cause of injury might have been a minor event on top of many other inputs into the bucket (see Box 25.4). This model can also be helpful in explaining to patients why addressing a variety of lifestyle issues, such as sleep, stress, and nutrition, may

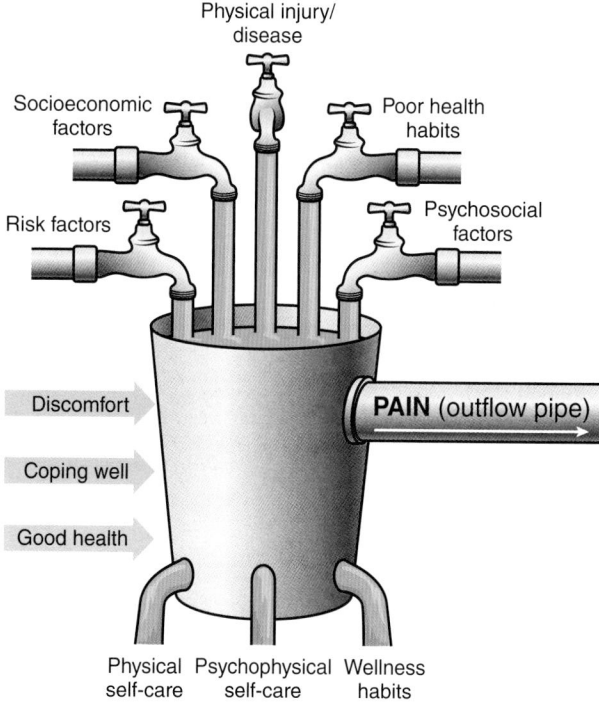

The Bucket Model of Pain

Figure 25.3 The "Bucket Model" of pain, showing that many factors contribute to activating the neuromatrix. The more or stronger the input into the neuromatrix, the higher the water level in the bucket and the more likely the brain is to interpret the experience as discomfort or pain. At the bottom of the bucket are self-care methods to drain the bucket, so neuromatrix activation is decreased, and less likely to result in discomfort or pain. Sensitization can be visualized as the water levels leading to coping well, discomfort, and pain moving down on the bucket, so lower levels of stimulus (water) trigger pain earlier and with fewer inputs.

Box 25.4 Filling and Emptying the Pain "Bucket"

Filling the Pain "Bucket"

Physical injury/disease
- Mechanical tissue stress
- Local inflammatory/chemical stress from tissue damage
- Neural damage/disease
- Systemic inflammation
- Comorbidities

Poor health habits
- Poor diet/nutrition
- Sedentary lifestyle
- Insufficient sleep
- Smoking
- Obesity

Psychosocial factors
- Psychosocial stress
- Negative thinking, anxiety, catastrophizing
- Fear, fear of movement or reinjury

Socioeconomic and environmental factors
- Limited access to health care
- Work demands
- Environmental toxins
- Stressful home/family

Risk factors
- Genetic
- Adverse childhood events
- Prior physical or emotional trauma
- Gender

Emptying the Pain "Bucket"

Wellness habits
- Healthy diet, nutraceuticals
- Good sleep
- Regular activity, healthy weight

Physical self-care
- Joint/tissue protection
- Appropriate exercise/activity
- Pain-relieving exercises
- Self-care (topicals, transcutaneous electrical nerve stimulation, ice, etc.)
- Medications

Psychophysical self-care
- Pain neuroscience education
- Diaphragmatic/slow breathing
- Relaxation strategies, meditation

decrease pain. For example, stress or sleep disturbance might not be the primary cause of pain, but managing them may decrease the overall input into the pain neuromatrix. These risk factors are profoundly interrelated, so cause and effect can sometimes be impossible to distinguish.[94-97] Denk et al.[95] explain the neurophysiological mechanisms of factors impacting pain vulnerability.

The discussion in this chapter highlights factors likely to be most relevant to physical therapists.

Genetic Risk Factors

Up to 50% of the variability in prevalence and severity of pain appears to be due to genetic factors; the catechol-O-methyltransferase (*COMT*) gene was identified early on, but many other genes may be involved.[74,85,98,99] Epigenetic mechanisms can enhance or suppress gene expression due to interaction between the individual and the environment, contributing to synaptic plasticity, learning, and memory.[79,80,100,101] Traumatic personal history affects epigenetics in ways that amplify and perpetuate chronic pain through changes in the CNS, immune and endocrine systems, as well as contributing to psychological distress and maladaptive behaviors that exacerbate pain.[102,103]

A sedentary lifestyle is separately associated with increased back pain and joint degeneration, independent of weight; inactivity also exacerbates fear of movement, which further limits activity.[96,104] Smoking also increases the likelihood of chronic pain.[105] Sleep disorders are highly correlated to chronic pain, increased disability, and suffering due to pain, and increased health-care utilization. Furthermore, sleep disorders may be aggravated by a sedentary lifestyle.[106-109]

Evidence suggests that nutrition and gut microbiota can contribute to pain through their influence on the neurochemical and behavioral responses to stress, anxiety, and depression via the HPA axis, neurotransmitters, cytokines, bacterial metabolites, immune response, and the vagus nerve. Nutrition has been linked to CS, and physical therapists are encouraged to recognize the role of nutrition as a risk factor for chronic pain.[110-112]

> **Clinical Implications.** Sleep dysfunction and chronic pain create a self-perpetuating cycle, where pain makes it difficult to sleep, and lack of sleep amplifies pain. Assessment and management of sleep are an important part of pain management.[109,113]

Psychosocial Risk Factors

Psychosocial factors can sometimes have stronger correlations with chronic pain than imaging or neurological test results.[114] The term *negative affect* encompasses negative emotions, thoughts, and behaviors, such as depression, anxiety, distress, and catastrophizing. Research shows that negative affect is the primary determinant of chronic pain severity across all types of chronic pain.[115] Neurobiological pathways that link psychological factors with chronic pain include epigenetics; autonomic dysfunction; cellular priming; altered brain pathways associated with reward, motivation, and learning; immune response; diurnal cortisol patterns; hypothalamic–pituitary regulation; and descending modulation leading to somatosensory amplification and CS. Psychosocial stress contributes to increased sympathetic and decreased parasympathetic tone associated with chronic pain and inflammation.[43] Pain can become a physiologically conditioned response from trauma-related cues.[116] Socioeconomic status influences prevalence of chronic pain through impaired descending inhibition, demonstrating a physical link between psychosocial factors and pain physiology.[117,118] Several good resources review the interaction between psychological factors and chronic pain.[85,97,119]

Yellow flags have been defined as psychosocial factors that increase the likelihood that acute pain will progress into chronic pain and disability.[24,94] Table 25.2 outlines terminology for flags proposed by Nicholas et al.[94] In this terminology, *yellow flags* include beliefs, emotional responses, and pain behavior; *orange flags* represent frank psychiatric symptoms; and *blue flags* reflect the interaction between work and health perceptions. The yellow flags with greatest impact appear to be (a) the belief that pain and activity are harmful, (b) a depressed mood and social withdrawal, (c) the expectation that passive treatment will help more than active treatment, and (d) low self-efficacy.[120] Other important factors include sickness behavior (e.g., excessive rest), history of pain or disability, poor job satisfaction, overprotective family or lack of support, and problems with claims or compensation.

> **Clinical Implications.** Psychosocial "yellow flags" should be considered for each patient, because interventions addressing specific psychosocial factors are more successful than interventions that do not.[2,6-8,24]

Pain Beliefs and Behaviors

Pain-related beliefs include people's understanding about what is causing their pain, the meaning of their pain, and expectations regarding the impact pain has on their present and future lives. Beliefs associated with better outcomes include having control over pain, global self-efficacy, pain self-efficacy, control over life, and internal pain control. Beliefs associated with poor outcomes include believing pain indicates injury/damage and should be avoided, pain will be constant, pain is disabling, emotions influence pain, and that other people should be solicitous because of the pain, helplessness, and external locus of control (the belief that pain is controlled by someone other than the individual in pain).[121] Beneficial coping responses include activities to distract oneself from the pain, task persistence, exercise, ignoring pain, coping self-statements, and acceptance of the condition. Detrimental coping responses include guarding, resting, venting emotions, passive coping (avoidance), and asking for assistance.[121]

Pain behaviors can be grouped in different ways. Table 25.3 contrasts *fear avoidance* with *pain persistence* and provides an evidence-based classification into four pain behavior clusters.[122-124] It is important to note that pain behavior and pain behavior clusters can change over time, so these factors need to be reassessed periodically. The impact of social responses to pain behaviors depends on the nature of the behavior and whether the response is supportive, solicitous, or punishing. Social reinforcers for wellness behavior tend to be beneficial.[121] Solicitous behaviors such as sympathy, encouragement to avoid pain and do less, and allowing people to avoid tasks due to pain lead to altered neural processing in the brain, increased pain, and decreased function.[121,125] Punishing or negative responses to pain behaviors lead

Table 25.2	Alert Flags for Chronic Pain[94]	
Flag Color	Type of Problem	Examples
Red	Serious physical pathology	Cauda equina syndrome, fracture, tumor
Orange	Psychiatric symptoms	Clinical depression, posttraumatic stress disorder, personality disorder
Yellow	Beliefs, appraisals, and judgments	Negative pain beliefs Expectation of poor outcome
	Emotional responses	Fear, anxiety, catastrophization, distress
	Pain behavior, including pain coping strategies	Fear avoidance behavior, dependence on passive interventions
Blue	Perceptions about relationship between work and pain	Belief that work will cause further injury and pain Belief that supervisor and coworkers are unsupportive
Black	System or contextual obstacles	No modified duty options at work Legislation restricting return to work options Lack of insurance coverage Overly solicitous family or health providers

Table 25.3   Pain Behavior Clusters[122-124]*

Classification	Characteristics	Recommended Approaches
Fear Avoidance Versus Pain Persistence		
Fear avoidance[†]	Pain-avoidant behavior, fear of pain, catastrophizing, hypervigilance, social reinforcement for pain behaviors	Decrease focus on symptoms, set functional goals, gradual increase in activity despite symptoms, reinforce healthy behaviors, ignore pain behaviors, graded exposure, movement visualization
Pain persistence[†]	Ignore or deny pain, continue activity in spite of pain, set unrealistic goals, ignore physical limits, low social support	Realistic goal setting, pacing, alternating activity and inactivity, cognitive restructuring, gradually progressed conditioning exercises, gradual increase in activity, assertiveness training
Pain Behavior Clusters		
Well adapted[‡]	Low levels of pain, distress and interference with life; high self-efficacy and activity	Pain education and pain coping skills, cognitive behavioral therapy
Dysfunctional[‡]	High pain intensity, interference with activity, pain behavior, social support and solicitousness; negative pain self-talk	Operant restructuring (reinforce healthy behaviors and do not reinforce pain behaviors), cognitive behavioral therapy
Distressed with little social support[‡]	Low self-efficacy, social support, solicitousness of others; "punished" rather than rewarded for pain behavior; high affective distress and perceived daily stress	Cognitive behavioral therapy including stress and pain management, help managing dysfunctional relationships
Psychophysiologically highly reactive[‡]	High stress reactivity, muscle tension, daily stress; low social support, little reinforcement for pain behavior, low activity due to pain	Relaxation, biofeedback, cognitive behavioral therapy

*Reproduced from Russek L, McManus C. A practical guide to integrating behavioral and psychologically informed approaches into physical therapist management of patients with chronic pain. *Orthopaedic Physical Therapy Practice.* 2015;27(1:15):8–16 with permission from the Orthopaedic Section, APTA, Inc.

to increased pain and depression. Table 25.3 also relates social support and behavior.[122-124]

Clinical Implications. While fear avoidance is well recognized, some patients use a pain persistence behavior that is equally dysfunctional. Customizing pain management to the patient's pain behavior pattern is likely to result in improved patient adherence and better outcomes.[94,121,122,126]

The *Fear-Avoidance Model* of pain proposes that some people have amplified fear that movement will cause reinjury and/or increase pain. Fear of pain can even become more disabling than the actual pain. Figure 25.4 shows how these factors lead to maladaptive hypervigilance, inaccurate predictions about pain, misinterpretation of body sensations, muscular reactivity, and physical deconditioning.[127,128] On the other hand, *pain persistence* can be equally dysfunctional. In pain persistence, the individual denies or ignores the pain, often due to reluctance to rely on others or lack of social

support. Individuals with pain persistence tended to have high levels of activity, overcommitment to work, and perfectionist behaviors before developing chronic pain; they can be inflexible and often do not accept functional limitations or want to be labeled as lazy.[124,129] Pain persistence is associated with cycles of overactivity, severe pain, forced rest, decreased function, and overactivity as shown in Figure 25.4.

■ EXAMINATION OF PATIENTS WITH CHRONC PAIN

The goals of the subjective portion of the chronic pain examination include listening to the patient's narrative, developing a rapport, assessing both the pain and the patient's experience of the pain, understanding the patient as a person, and engaging in shared decision-making.[6-8,24] In addition to obtaining standard medical history, the subjective component should address (a) the impact of pain on physical and psychosocial function, (b) pain characteristics to identify biological contributing factors, and (c) identification of psychosocial factors

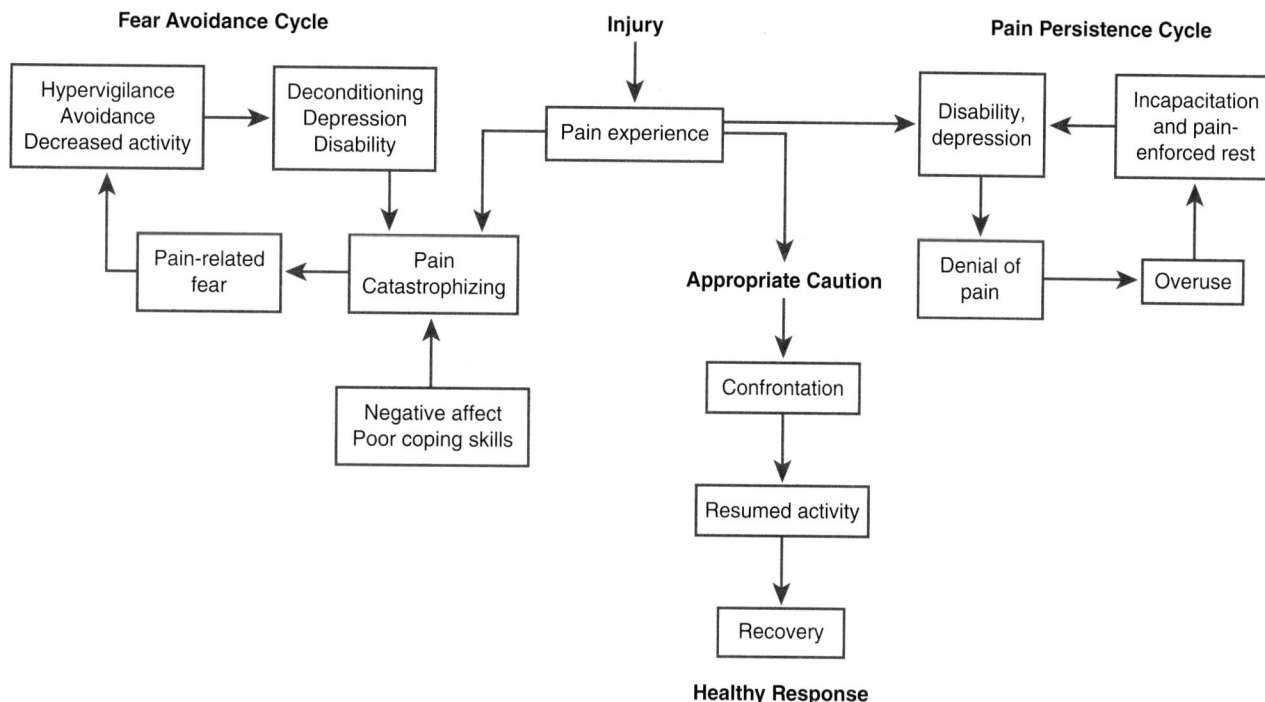

Figure 25.4 Fear avoidance and pain persistence. The Fear-Avoidance Model shows how the pain experience can resolve in the absence of fear or become a vicious cycle in the presence of either pain-related fear or pain persistence. The healthy response to pain is appropriate caution, which leads to confrontation and resumed activity. In fear avoidance, negative affect and poor coping skills cause the pain experience to be perceived as a threat; pain catastrophizing increases pain-related fear, hypervigilance, and avoidance. In the pain-persistence cycle, individuals ignore or deny pain and are overactive until they crash due to the pain; they are then forced to rest. These individuals may demonstrate catastrophization, or depression when not in denial about limitations. In both fear avoidance and pain persistence, inactivity leads to secondary problems such as deconditioning, depression, and additional disability, which further exacerbate the negative aspects of the pain experience.

impacting pain so they can be addressed. Figure 25.5 shows a general flow for the physical therapist's examination, which may need to be distributed over several visits.

Impact of Pain on Physical and Psychosocial Function

Unidimensional measures of pain intensity, such as the *Numeric Rating Scale* (NRS), *Verbal Rating Scale, Visual Analog Scale, Facial Pain Scale,* or pain thermometer, are inadequate for measuring chronic pain. The move, in the 1990s, to consider pain rating "the fifth vital sign" is no longer endorsed by medical organizations as it did not improve patient outcomes and is believed to have contributed to the opioid epidemic by overemphasizing lower numeric pain rating as a clinical goal.[130] The Functional Pain Scale is a unidimensional measure that strives to make patient reporting more objective by linking pain rating to specific functional deficits,[131] but research does not show whether it avoids the pitfalls of other unidimensional measures.

Ideally, a comprehensive outcome measure of the impact of pain on physical and psychosocial function

should examine each of the domains within the ICF: body structure or function, activity, and participation. A multitude of pain questionnaires and outcome measures exist to measure both nonspecific and disease-specific severity and impact of pain; the choice of tool depends on the purpose for which the information will be used.[132,133] Several measures are specifically to identify or quantify neuropathic pain.[88] Table 25.4 provides a short list of outcome measures appropriate for assessing severity and impact of chronic pain and yellow flags, and where many of these tools can be found online.[134-144]

Tools to measure pain severity in the clinic should be convenient to use and score, and they should have good measurement properties (see https://www.sralab.org/rehabilitation-measures). Examples of multidimensional pain-specific tools include the *Pain Disability Index, Global Pain Scale,* and *Brief Pain Inventory* (BPI). Overall health-related quality-of-life tools and condition-specific tools have been developed to examine specific conditions. The *Patient-Specific Functional Scale* allows patients to identify specific functional

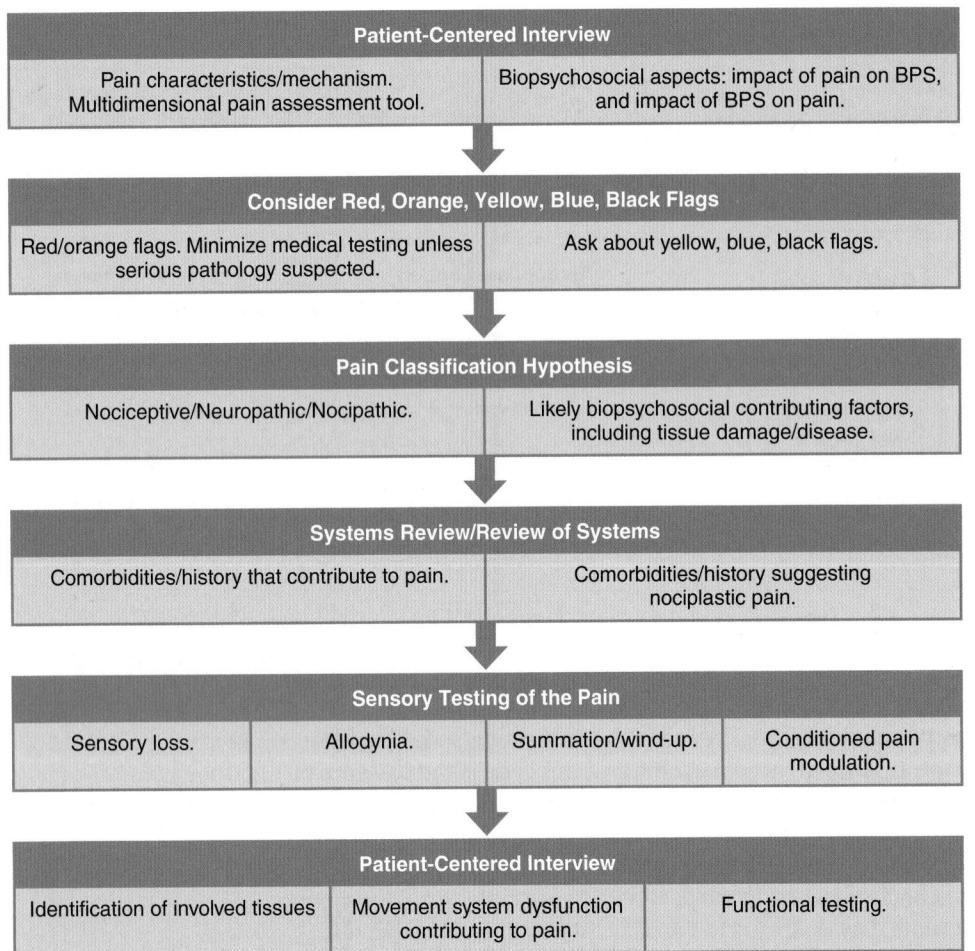

Figure 24.5 A general flow for the physical therapist's examination of people with chronic pain. The order may change based on each individual patient's needs, but each step should be addressed. Often, this cannot all be accomplished in a single visit so may be distributed over several visits.

activities of personal importance affected by their pain condition, which can be helpful in identifying a few key functional goals for a patient whose presentation may otherwise be somewhat overwhelming to the clinician.[145] Postexertional malaise, common in several chronic pain conditions, can also be assessed using the *DePaul Symptom Questionnaire—Post-Exertional Malaise short form* (DSQ-PEM).[146] Therapists should be cautious about interpreting restrictions as due solely to physical limitations, as some functional limitations may be due in part to difficulty focusing attention, difficulty handling stress, fear of movement or fear of pain, and other psychological factors.

Pain Characteristics

Pain can be classified as nociceptive, neuropathic, or nociplastic; peripheral and CS can amplify each of these mechanisms.[9,14,76] (See Table 25.1 for characteristics of different types of pain.) Chronic pain may be mixed, with variable contribution from nociceptive, neuropathic, and nociplastic input that may change from day to day. For example, a patient may have acute nociceptive-dominant or neuropathic conditions superimposed on nociplastic pain: that is, a person with fibromyalgia may still have rotator cuff impingement, myofascial trigger points, lumbar instability, or

a urinary tract infection. Neuropathic pain may also be associated with nociceptive or nociplastic pain. For example, a person with neuropathic pain due to a stroke may also have shoulder instability or pain from muscle spasticity. Moreover, one source of pain can trigger or amplify another: nociception can increase sensitization, and sensitization can amplify neuropathic pain.

Characterization of pain begins with understanding *somatic dimensions* of the pain such as intensity, location, duration, nature, temporal variation, and other signs and symptoms. Recognizing different characteristics of superficial, deep somatic, and visceral nociceptive pain can help in identifying tissues involved. Standard mnemonics for pain assessment can be helpful for asking about somatic characteristics of chronic pain (see Box 25.5).

Body diagrams provide information about pain location, radiation, and character. Pain and symptom location can be assessed using a body map. Traditional pen and paper pain diagrams required more patient instruction, were difficult to interpret, and hence were more time-consuming to administer. However, technology allows for much easier collection and interpretation of information.[147] Patients can distinguish between aching, burning, stabbing, pins and needles, and numbness, and sometimes sensations such as heaviness,

Table 25.4   Pain Severity and Functional Assessment Tools for Chronic Pain

Pain Scale	Properties	Items	References/Websites
Pain Interference and Function			
Brief Pain Inventory (long and short forms)	Multidimensional scale includes pain ratings, body function, activity, and participation	Long form has 32 items; short form has nine items	Atkinson et al., 2011[147] https://www.mdanderson.org/ research/departments-labs-institutes/ departments-divisions/symptom -research/symptom-assessment-tools .html (fee for use)
GPM (regular and short forms)	Multidimensional scale includes body function, activity, and participation	GPM has 24 items; GPM-SF has 12 items	Ferrell et al., 2000[148]; Blozik et al., 2007[149] http://www.palliativecareswo.ca/docs/ Geriatric%20Pain%20Measure%20GPM .pdf [online access]
Global Pain Scale	Subscales: pain, emotions, clinical outcomes, activities	33 items for full version, 20 items on short form	Gentile, 2011[144] https://www.paindoctor.com/globa l-pain-scale [online access]
Graded Chronic Pain Scale Revised	Assesses domains of impairment, activity, and participation restriction	Six items	Von Korff, 2020[135] https://www.ncbi.nlm .nih.gov/pmc/articles/PMC7097879/ [online access]
Pain Disability Index	Impact of pain on home responsibilities, recreation, social and sexual activities, occupation, activities of daily living	Seven items	Tait, 1990[146] https://www.oregon.gov/oha/HPA/ dsi-pmc/PainCareToolbox/Pain%20 Disability%20Index.pdf
Pain Disability Questionnaire	Subscales: functional and psychosocial	15 items	Anagnostis et al., 2004[150] https://coa.org/docs/Pain-Disability -Questionnaire.pdf [online access]
PEG	Subscales: average pain, enjoyment of life, general activity	Three items	Krebs, 2009[151] https://health.gov/hcq/trainings/ pathways/assets/pdfs/PEG_scale.pdf
PROMIS-Global	Measures physical, mental, and social health, fatigue, and pain; can compute physical and mental health subscales	10 items asking about biopsychosocial function	Cook, 2016[142] https://www.healthmeasures.net/ explore-measurement-systems/promis/ obtain-administer-measures
DePaul Symptom Questionnaire–Post-Exertional Malaise	Measures frequency and severity of physical and mental fatigue in response to physical and mental activity	10 items	Cotler, 2018[143] https://www.researchgate.net/ publication/358281945_DePaul _Symptom_Questionnaire_-_Post -Exertional_Malaise_short_form _DSQ-PEM
OSPRO-YF	Assesses yellow-flag psychosocial concerns including mood, fear avoidance, and positive affect/coping	10 or 17 items	Butera, 2020[144] https://www.orthopt.org/yf/OSPRO_ YF_Tool_questions.pdf

GPM = Geriatric Pain Measure; PEG = Pain, Enjoyment, General activity.

swelling, or other autonomic symptoms. Information about the location and nature of the pain can be used to hypothesize about the source of the pain: sclerotomes, referred pain, dermatomes, and peripheral nerve patterns all implicate specific structures, whereas other patterns implicate neuropathic involvement.[148] A recent study used computer analysis to identify patient clusters using body diagram markings, and those clusters were correlated with psychosocial factors and response to intervention.[149]

Box 25.5 Mnemonics for Assessing Somatic Characteristics of Pain

PQRST

- **P**rovoking/precipitating factors
- **Q**uality of pain
- **R**egion and radiation
- **S**everity or associated symptoms
- **T**emporal factors/timing

SOCRATES

- **S**ite: Where is the pain?
- **O**nset: When and how did it start? Sudden or gradual? Trauma, illness, or other possible cause?
- **C**haracter: How does the pain feel? Sharp? Stabbing? Burning? Aching? Other?
- **R**adiation: Does the pain radiate? Where? What causes radiation?
- **A**ssociations: Other symptoms, such as numbness, paresthesias, heaviness, other?
- **T**ime course: How does the pain vary over the day?
- **E**xacerbating/relieving: What aggravates or relieves the pain?
- **S**everity: Intensity rating

Several questionnaires can help identify the primary mechanism of pain, with most distinguishing neuropathic from either non-neuropathic or nociceptive pain. (Balzani et al. present a comparison of neuropathic assessment tools.)[88] For example, the *Neuropathic Pain Scale, Neuropathic Diagnostic Questionnaire* (DN4), *Leeds Assessment of Neuropathic Symptoms and Signs* (LANSS), and *PainDETECT* attempt to distinguish between neuropathic and non-neuropathic pain (some sensitivities and specificities are given in Table 25.5).[150-170] The *McGill Pain Questionnaire* (MPQ) and the *Short Form MPQ* (SF-MPQ) examine sensory, affective-emotional, evaluative, and temporal aspects of pain.[150,151] The SF-MPQ includes fewer verbal descriptors, and the SF-MPQ-2 is said to have better differentiation of pain type.[152] The *Central Sensitivity Index (CSI)* and the shorter *CSI-9* measure CS.[153,154]

Clinical Implications. Many people with chronic pain have a mix of pain mechanisms (nociceptive, neuropathic, nociplastic), and the proportion of one mechanism over another may change over time based on contributing factors. Assessment of pain mechanism is therefore an ongoing process, not a one-time decision.

Interpretation of findings to classify pain is discussed in the section on Evaluation. Note that classifying the pain is *not* the same as seeking a biological source of pain; there might or might not be damaged or diseased tissues, or the extent of tissue damage might not correlate to the impact of pain. If damaged or diseased tissues are identified, the examination can seek to determine the specific pathophysiology through standard PT tests and measures.

Identification of Psychosocial Factors Impacting Pain

Research suggests that physical therapists are good at collecting information about the somatic components of pain, as described already, but are not as good at collecting information about cognitive, emotional, behavioral, and social domains.[155] Focusing the interview on somatic characteristics of the pain limits the evaluation to a biomedical, rather than biopsychosocial, view of pain. There are several models that can help physical therapists collect a broad spectrum of biopsychosocial information. Oostendorp et al.[155] developed a list of 51 questions spanning the biopsychosocial spectrum of chronic pain. They summarized their findings as the SCEBS model, which addresses somatic/biological, psychological (cognitive, emotional, and behavioral), and social domains. Wijma et al.[32] modified the SCEBS model to include type/mechanism of pain and motivation, ending up with the PSCEBSM model of patient examination (see Box 25.6). This approach strives to first classify the mechanism(s) of pain (nociceptive, neuropathic, CS/nociplastic). "Somatic and medical factors" addresses the biological contributions to pain, including current medical management and medications. Cognitive, emotional, behavioral, and social factors are similar to the SCEBS model, though not identical.

The last component of PSCEBSM is motivation, or the patient's perceptions about the source of pain, expectations, and readiness to change. Motivation is a critical issue for patients with chronic pain, as patients need to be active participants in their pain management program. Patients with a passive approach to health care, or with low pain-related self-efficacy, are less likely to be successful in pain management. Since patients with chronic pain have typically failed several treatment attempts before, the approach of *Motivational Interviewing* is recommended by clinical practice guidelines to determine what obstacles could be interfering with patients' adherence to self-management.[6,156]

Evidence shows that physical therapists are not accurate in determining the presence of yellow flags such as depression or fear avoidance based on observation; consequently, screening tools for psychological factors may be appropriate. *The Optimal Screening for Prediction of Referral and Outcome Yellow Flag tool (OSPRO-YF)* is an example of a multidimensional tool that assesses multiple yellow flag dimensions, such as catastrophizing, negative mood, fear avoidance, and positive affect/coping.[144] Stearns et al.[157] propose a process for integrating yellow flag screening into standard outpatient

Table 25.5	Pain Classification Tools		
Pain Scale	Properties	Items	References/Websites
Pain Quality and Location			
Central Sensitivity Inventory-9	Score indicates the presence of central sensitivity. Score≥20 indicates CSS	9 health-related symptoms	Nishgami, 2018[154] https://journals.plos.org/plosone/article?id=10.1371/journal.pone.0200152#sec034 [online access]
Chronic Pain Questions	Distinguishes nociceptive, neuropathic, and CS pain	14 items about symptoms and pain interference. Includes ID pain.	Coyne, 2017[332] https://eprovide.mapi-trust.org [online access]
ID Pain	Score distinguishes neuropathic from non-neuropathic pain. Score ≥3 Sn = 78%, Sp = 74% (Padua, 2013)	Six items	Portenoy, 2006[333] https://eprovide.mapi-trust.org [online access]
LANSS	Score distinguishes between neuropathic and non-neuropathic pain; includes self-report and objective testing. Sn = 82%–91%, Sp = 80%–94%[†]	Seven self-report and two sensory testing items for allodynia and hyperalgesia	Bennett, 2001[334] https://eprovide.mapi-trust.org [online access]
MPQ	Assesses pain intensity, sensory, affective, evaluative, and miscellaneous pain	78 items: 20 pain descriptors (sensory [1–10], affective [11–15], evaluative [16], and miscellaneous [17–20]), one pain intensity item	Melzack, 1975[151] https://eprovide.mapi-trust.org [online access]
SF-MPQ and SF-MPQ-2	Assesses pain intensity, sensory, and affective pain	17 items: 11 sensory descriptors, four affective descriptors, two pain intensity	Melzack, 1987[150] https://eprovide.mapi-trust.org [online access]
DN4	Distinguishes between neuropathic and non-neuropathic pain. Score ≥4/10: Sn = 83%, Sp = 90%[†]	10 pain descriptor items	Bouhassira, 2005[335] https://eprovide.mapi-trust.org [online access]
Neuropathic Pain Symptom Inventory	Identifies subgroups of neuropathic pain	10 pain descriptor items and two temporal	Bouhassira, 2004[336] https://eprovide.mapi-trust.org [online access]
Neuropathic Pain Scale	Distinguishes neuropathic from non-neuropathic pain. Sn = 66%, Sp = 74%[†]	10 items: seven sensory descriptors, one temporal, one unpleasantness, one intensity	Fishbain et al., 2008[159][337] https://eprovide.mapi-trust.org [online access]
PainDETECT	Distinguishes nociceptive from neuropathic. Sn = 85%, Sp = 80%[†]	Seven sensory descriptors, one temporal, one about radiation	Freynhagen, 2006[338] https://eprovide.mapi-trust.org [online access]
PQAS	Distinguishing types of pain and is an outcome measure	20 pain descriptor items and one temporal pattern; differentiates between nociceptive and neurogenic pain	Victor, 2008[339] https://eprovide.mapi-trust.org [online access]
S-LANSS	Distinguishes neuropathic from non-neuropathic pain; S-LANSS is the LANSS without the two objective testing items	Seven self-report questions	Bennett, 2005[340] https://bpac.org.nz/BPJ/2016/May/docs/s-lanss.pdf [online access]

CS = Central Sensitization; CSS = Central Sensitivity Syndrome; DN4 = Neuropathic Pain Diagnostic Questionnaire; MPQ = McGill Pain Questionnaire; LANSS = Leeds Assessment of Neuropathic Symptoms and Signs; PQAS = Pain Quality Assessment Scale; SF-MPQ = McGill Pain Questionnaire Short Form; S-LANSS = Self-report Leeds Assessment of Neuropathic Symptoms and Signs.

Box 25.6   PSCEBSM Model for Taking a Biopsychosocial History[32]*

1. **Pain type:** Distinguish between nociceptive, neuropathic, and central sensitization.
2. **Somatic and medical factors:** Comorbidities, changed movement patterns, exercise capacity, strength: medications.
3. **Cognitive factors:** Cognitions and perceptions about the physical and mental aspects of pain, expectations regarding care, prognosis, and emotional representation of pain. Catastrophizing, perceived injustice or harm.
4. **Emotional factors:** Anxiety, anger, fear, depression, and posttraumatic stress. Fear of movement, avoidance behaviors, psychological issues related to work, family, finances, or social issues.
5. **Behavioral factors:** Behavioral adaptations to pain: (a) healthy response, (b) fear avoidance, (c) pain persistence.
6. **Social factors:** Housing/living situation, social environment, work, relationships. Prior treatments and attitudes toward prior/other health-care providers. Social support.
7. **Motivation:** Readiness to change, perceptions about the cause of pain and treatment expectations. Psychological flexibility, stage of change.

*Wijma et al.[32] provide additional detail, along with suggested assessment tools.

PT. Questionnaires can also help assess the patient's knowledge and beliefs about pain. The *Multidimensional Pain Inventory* classifies patients into one of three pain-behavior clusters: adaptive copers, dysfunctional, and interpersonally stressed[118] (corresponding to "well-adapted," "dysfunctional," and "distressed with little social support" in Table 25.3).[122-124] Several sources discuss other useful tools for assessing psychosocial factors relevant to disability and chronic pain.[158-160] The *Physical Therapy Healthy Lifestyle Appraisal* asks about lifestyle habits that contribute to chronic pain, and readiness to change.[161]

Since a high proportion of people with chronic pain have experienced some form of abuse, physical therapists need to be sensitive to the needs of this population, especially given the importance of touch to PT.[162] Polyvagal theory proposes that trauma survivors may present with either agitation caused by excess sympathetic activation, or with a "freeze" state driven by activation of the dorsal vagal complex. Consequently, a patient's appearance of calm may actually be a "freeze" state demonstrating high levels of distress.[43,163] Survivors of abuse may have difficulty distinguishing fatigue from distress or pain, or distinguishing physical from emotional pain. Physical therapists working with this population should know how to ask about and respond to revelations of past or present abuse. The physical therapist's response to a revelation is critical to developing a trusting relationship.[164]

The current emphasis on factual data collection should not overshadow the importance of a compassionate, patient-centered approach to examining patients with chronic pain. It is important to listen to the patient's story, illness experience, beliefs, fears, and expectations rather than to simply quantify or objectify pain.[7,24]

Clinical Implications. Trauma and abuse can sensitize the CNS, autonomic, and endocrine systems in ways that amplify nociplastic pain throughout life. One of the mechanisms for this sensitization appears to be epigenetic changes and not just psychological state. It is therefore important to help patients feel safe in PT.[97,103]

Challenges in the Subjective Examination

Psychological or socioeconomic issues can compound difficulties for patients who have chronic pain. Patients who believe in a purely biomedical model may arrive wanting a purely physical problem to be identified and fixed; such patients may deny that psychosocial factors are relevant. Patients with a history of frequent treatment failures may be frustrated, angry, demanding, or hopeless. Patients may have financial or family stressors associated with being unable to work outside or in the home or having frequent medical appointments. CS, anxiety, or catastrophization lead patients to overreact, appearing to "symptom magnify." Most patients are doing the best they can, but some may appear angry, abusive, demanding, deceitful, nonadherent, or engaging in doctor-shopping.[165,166]

Understanding the source of these patient behaviors helps clinicians empathize and improves communication. For example, patients may be defensive or hostile because of previous negative interactions with unsupportive medical professionals.[165] Since chronic pain can lack objective findings of a physical cause for the pain, many patients have struggled with not being believed by health-care providers[166] and have been treated as malingerers, liars, hysterics, or drug seekers. Because psychosocial factors often exacerbate chronic pain, prior health-care providers may have treated patients as though the pain was not real or was due to a purely psychiatric problem.[74] Accepting that the patient's pain experience is real can accomplish a great deal in establishing rapport. Strategies to diffuse anger, relieve anxiety, eliminate ambiguity, and maintain appropriate professional boundaries are as important to clinical practice as the skillful application of any treatment technique.[165,166]

Interviewing patients with chronic pain can also be overwhelming simply because of their complexity and the need to address such a range of psychosocial factors. Histories of adverse childhood events can be emotionally draining to hear. Chronic pain is difficult to treat, often leaving both patients and providers unsatisfied with the results. Clinicians may feel frustrated and inadequate, leading to stress and burnout.[166] Even when patient–provider interactions are constructive, the emotional needs of patients with chronic pain can lead to *empathy fatigue* for the clinician, a state of emotional, mental, and physical exhaustion. Health-care providers need to take care of their own emotional well-being. Stebnicki et al.[167] offer strategies for avoiding empathy fatigue: provide a support system within the facility where clinicians can discuss the stress of working with difficult patients, provide mentoring for new clinicians, encourage support networks outside the workplace, avoid having one clinician treat many difficult patients at one time, and promote education and wellness programs within the clinic or organization.

Since the prevalence of abuse is very high among people with chronic pain,[162] the physical examination should be performed carefully. Survivors of abuse often become stressed by physical contact needed in the examination and may demonstrate hypervigilance, anxiety, disempowerment, distrust, somatization, transference, or dissociative reactions. Strategies to build trust include the following: ensure two-way communication, observe body language, establish positive rapport and a trusting therapeutic relationship, give the patient control and respect boundaries, obtain consent frequently, keep the patient an active participant, pay attention to physical stressors, recognize and respond to triggers, check in with the patient, and try alternative examination/treatment approaches if the patient is uncomfortable.[164]

Systems Review and Review of Systems

The complex nature of chronic pain means that the systems review component of the patient examination is extremely important. Systems review in the *Guide to Physical Therapist Practice*[168] includes cardiovascular/pulmonary, integumentary, musculoskeletal, neuromuscular, and communication components. The goals of systems review are to identify areas that will require further testing and to identify body structure/function deficits that might impact rehabilitation or that might require referral. For patients (especially women) presenting with widespread chronic pain, musculoskeletal systems review should include the *Beighton Score* for generalized joint laxity, and individuals who score ≥5/9 should be assessed for hypermobility spectrum disorders (i.e., hypermobile Ehlers-Danlos syndrome [hEDS]). Patients with hEDS may present with diagnoses of fibromyalgia, myofascial pain syndrome, chronic headaches, or spinal pain; if the underlying hypermobility is not identified and addressed, treatment is more

likely to fail.[169] Cardiovascular screening of vital signs may indicate whether there are cardiovascular restrictions to aerobic exercise. While measuring respiratory rate, clinicians should observe the breathing pattern, because overuse of accessory breathing muscles can aggravate pain. The integumentary system should be examined, particularly for old injuries or surgeries that could compromise fascial mobility or lymphatic flow. Neuromuscular screening should include balance, locomotion, and transfers. Testing for clonus, hyperreflexia, and hypertonicity may be important if there is any suspicion of *serotonin syndrome* (see section "Pharmacological Management").[170] The communication, affect, cognition, and learning style component of the systems review is particularly important given the psychosocial aspects of chronic pain.

A review of systems is important because visceral and musculoskeletal pain referral is bidirectional, and chronic pain often involves multiple body systems.[10] For example, symptoms of pruritis, abdominal pain, vague "allergies," interstitial cystitis, and brain fog suggest mast cell activation, which can exacerbate chronic pain by amplifying neurogenic inflammation both in peripheral tissues and the CNS.[171] Gastrointestinal (GI) issues such as IBS are associated with increased CS.[172] Therapists should be looking for not only "red flag" systemic conditions that require urgent medical care but also milder visceral functional disorders that contribute to CS, inflammation, and distress[10] by filling the biopsychosocial pain "bucket" (see Figure 25.3). Several outcome measures can assess sleep quality.[173] Fatigue is common in chronic pain,[174] so assessment of fatigue may include the *Fatigue Severity Scale,* which measures physical aspects of fatigue, and *Fatigue Assessment Scale,* which measures both physical and cognitive fatigue. If cognitive fatigue is most disabling, referral to an occupational therapist or psychologist may be appropriate. Goodman and Snyder[175] provide a comprehensive discussion of review of systems.

Physical Therapy Tests and Measures

PT tests and measures for patients with chronic pain provide information about the type of pain or abnormal sensory function (e.g., neuropathic versus nociceptive pain); irritability of the condition; underlying tissue pathology, if there is any (e.g., OA, nerve compression, fascial restrictions); body structure/function deficits due to injury/disease, if present; body structure/function deficits resulting from the chronic pain, either secondary to pain (e.g., trigger points) or disuse (e.g., weakness or balance deficits); and initial functional status. Some tests can identify underlying conditions that might not have been diagnosed. If the patient has reported severe fatigue and autonomic symptoms, a Stand/Lean Test can assess *postural orthostatic tachycardia syndrome* (POTS).[176] The specific body structure and function measures needed will be determined by how the patient presents, because each patient with chronic pain has different structural and functional involvement. If the clinician hypothesizes that a specific neuromusculoskeletal condition may be contributing to nociceptive, inflammatory, or peripheral neurogenic pain, the examination should include specific tests and measures for those conditions. For example, a patient with stroke-related pain may have shoulder instability, a patient with diabetic neuropathy may have carpal tunnel syndrome, or a patient with postconcussion headaches may have cervical instability. Patients with systemic pain conditions, such as MS, could have an acute musculoskeletal injury superimposed on the underlying chronic pain. Therefore, standard musculoskeletal and neurological tests may be appropriate.

Patients with CS may have a positive response to many or all pain provocation tests due to hyperalgesia and allodynia, even in the absence of local tissue pathology. Provocation tests may therefore produce false-positive results due to sensitization. Sometimes, several weeks of treatment to reduce CS are necessary before standard provocation tests are helpful for identifying tissue injury. Furthermore, signs of inflammation, such as edema, warmth, and rubor, may be due to neurogenic inflammation in the absence of local tissue damage. The following discussion addresses some tests and measures that may be useful in examination of patients with chronic pain.

> **Clinical Implications.** When patients have peripheral and central sensitization, all provocative tests may be positive, even when there is no corresponding tissue pathology. Therefore, it is sometimes necessary to spend a few weeks of treatment decreasing sensitization before performing provocative tests to identify specific tissue involvement.

Sensory Integrity

Since many types of chronic pain are associated with abnormal activity in sensory nerves, sensory integrity is important. *Quantitative sensory testing* (QST) refers to a set of psychophysical measurements to assess neuropathic changes, peripheral and CS. While QST is a powerful research tool, it is not practical for clinical use. Several "bedside-QST" or "clinical sensory test" batteries of 5 to 13 tests have been proposed that use equipment easily available in the clinic and take 5 to 15 minutes.[77,177,178] While each battery is standardized, protocols differ so there is currently no single standard technique. One version of a Clinical Sensory Test is given in Table 25.6.[179]

The specific tests used depend on whether the goal is to distinguish neuropathic pain from nociceptive[177] or nociplastic from nociceptive and neuropathic.[178] Sensory loss to cold, touch, and vibration is typical in neuropathic pain. Static allodynia can be assessed with light pressure from 5.46 (26 g) Semmes-Weinstein filament or pencil eraser pressure held 10 seconds. Dynamic mechanical allodynia can be tested using a brush, Q-tip, or cotton wisp four to five times. Any report of pain in the dynamic tests is considered allodynia. Although CS cannot be directly measured,[180] *wind-up*, or *temporal summation*, is a key finding in CS.[76] Wind-up can be measured by comparing pain reported after a single touch with a 6.67 (300 g) Semmes-Weinstein monofilament (or toothpick) with pain after 10 repetitions at one per second. It can be reported as a ratio of NRS after multiple repetitions divided by a single repetition, or as the difference between final pain and single repetition pain.[77] *Conditioned pain modulation* (CPM) measures descending inhibition by comparing pain threshold (e.g., using Semmes-Weinstein monofilament) before and after a conditioning noxious stimulus (e.g., immersing a nonpainful body part into ice water); decreased inhibition is present if the pain threshold does not increase.[76,181] Test clusters may be most helpful for identifying characteristics of peripheral sensitization (thermal allodynia) and CS (mechanical allodynia and wind-up).[77]

Proprioception deficits due to either underlying pathology or as a result of the pain[97,182] may perpetuate microtrauma, macrotrauma, and pain. For example, poststroke shoulder pain is associated with impaired proprioception,[183] and cervical joint position sense is compromised in patients with chronic neck pain.[184] Joint position sense can be examined using traditional tests for proprioceptive awareness (see Chapter 3, Examination of Sensory Function), a goniometer, or a laser pointer.

Cranial and Peripheral Nerve Integrity

Standard tests for sensory or motor nerve function are indicated based on suspected pathology. Neurodynamic assessment can assess nerve mobility, including a proposed neurodynamic test for the vagus nerve.[185] Function of the vagus nerve and autonomic function can be tested using heart rate variability (HRV).[186]

Palpation

Palpation for tenderness may be useful for identifying tissue damage, muscle spasm, trigger points, or hyperalgesia and allodynia. Palpation can be quantified through use of an *algometer,* which measures palpation pressure, or standardized using techniques from clinical sensory testing, as described earlier. *Pressure pain threshold (PPT)* is the point at which pressure changes from comfortable pressure to slightly unpleasant pain. Decreased PPT may be noted in areas of primary or secondary hyperalgesia or may be widespread and observed at remote sites, providing evidence of CS.[181] Because patients may present with widespread hyperalgesia and allodynia, palpation for tenderness might not be useful

Table 25.6 Clinical Sensory Test

Subjects tested on unaffected, symptom-free location first, then at location of pain. See Zhu, 2019,[179] for pictures and detailed instructions.

Item	Tool/Test	Interpretation
Loss of Function		
1. Cold detection	Large coin at room temperature	Is stimulus at affected site less than at symptom-free location?
2. Warm detection	Large coin kept in pocket for 30 min	Is stimulus at affected site less than at symptom-free location?
3. Mechanical detection	Light stroke with cotton wool or Sensitivity to 16 mN von Frey filament	Is stimulus at affected site less than at symptom-free location?
4. Vibration detection	128 Hz tuning fork	Is stimulus at affected site less than at symptom-free location?
5. Mechanical pain threshold	Toothpick or von Frey 256 mN	Is stimulus at affected site less than at symptom-free location?
Gain of Function		
6. Cold pain threshold	Ice cubes in plastic bag, held on skin for 10 seconds	Pain rating 0–10. Is pain greater at affected site than at symptom-free location?
7. Hot pain threshold	Glass vial filled with hot tap water (40°C) held on skin 10 seconds	Pain rating 0–10. Is pain greater at affected site than at symptom-free location?
8. Mechanical pain threshold	Toothpick or von Frey 256 mN (same test as for loss of function)	Pain rating 0–10. Is pain greater at affected site than at symptom-free location?
9. Pressure pain threshold	Pencil eraser (7-mm diameter) pressure for 10 seconds to indent tissues and cause blanching or finger pressure	Pain rating 0–10. Is pain greater at affected site than at symptom-free location?
10. Wind-up ratio	Toothpick pressure once followed by series of 10 stimuli	Wind-up ratio = Final pain/single stimulus pain
11. Dynamic mechanical allodynia	Brush stroked five times	Patient rates 0/100 Allodynia is any pain rating above 0

for identifying involved tissues as uninjured tissues may be tender. Palpation may also be helpful for assessing fascial restrictions, which may both compromise lymphatic flow and contribute to peripheral and CS.[61]

Muscle Performance

Standard muscle strength testing and functional tests such as a 30-second Sit to Stand can be helpful to assess the effects of deconditioning. Many widespread pain complaints are associated with myofascial trigger points. Palpation may elicit local tenderness or referral along the pattern specific for that muscle. To elicit the referred pain pattern associated with trigger points, pressure needs to be maintained for at least 10 seconds or only local tenderness will be detected.[187] Palpation of a trigger point may elicit a local twitch response, a transient contraction of the muscle fiber, or a *jump response,* which is patient vocalization or withdrawal from the palpation. Trigger points can cause a variety of

symptoms other than pain, such as tinnitus, dizziness, tachycardia, shortness of breath, nausea, constipation, diarrhea, and so forth.

Motor Control

Many patients with neurological conditions have chronic musculoskeletal pain due to abnormal motor control or muscle performance.[92] Chronic low back pain (CLBP) and whiplash also appear to be associated with motor control deficits.[184,188] Testing for spinal pain may include use of the Stabilizer for lumbar or cervical motor control.[189] Patients with underlying neurological disorders may be tested as described in Chapter 5, Examination of Motor Function: Motor Control and Motor Learning.

Balance

An examination of balance is often indicated because the primary injury or disease, deconditioning, and/or fear of movement may compromise balance.[190] Chronic pain has been associated with balance impairments and increased risk of falls among older adults, and even near-falls can exacerbate pain conditions by straining muscles. The specific choice of balance test depends on the patient (see Chapter 6, Examination of Coordination and Balance, for a discussion of balance tests). Some patients will have difficulty with a basic *Romberg test*, whereas others will have no difficulty completing the *Berg Balance Scale*. The *Activity-Specific Balance Confidence Scale (ABC)* is a self-report tool for balance confidence, which may reflect imitations due to kinesiophobia as well as to physical balance deficits.[191]

Activity and Participation Measures

Activities commonly affected by chronic pain include physical functions such as walking, mobility, changing or maintaining body position, toileting, preparing meals, doing housework, parenting, or completing job tasks (see Chapter 8, Examination of Function). Quantification of activity and participation restrictions can be examined through either self-report or performance measures. Self-report assessment tools were discussed in the Subjective Examination section, and summarized in Table 25.4. Note, however, that some of these outcome measures are designed to assess pain rather than physical function. The *Oswestry Low Back Pain Disability Questionnaire,* for example, asks how much each activity is restricted by pain; this depends on psychosocial context as much as patient's physical ability.

For patients with widespread pain, physical performance measures can assess multiple body regions with one test. For example, the *30-second Sit to Stand Test, Timed Up and Go,* and *10-meter Walk Test* are efficient ways to assess functional lower extremity strength and balance. Combined performance tests such as the *Short Physical Performance Battery* (SPPB), which combines sit-to-stand transitions, balance, and walking velocity, reflect activity and predict participation restrictions.[192] Although the SPPB was designed for older adults, it provides an appropriate level of challenge for many adults with chronic pain who have very limited function. Chronic pain is often associated with deconditioning, which exacerbates activity and participation restrictions.[190] A *2- or 6-minute Walk Test* can provide valuable information about endurance and willingness to exercise, as well as activity tolerance.[193] Formal functional capacity evaluations can be useful for establishing a person's physical work capability. These standardized test batteries can last from 3 hr to 2 days and may include any aspect of physical job requirement, such as fine motor control, cardiovascular fitness, postural tolerance, and lifting strength.

Fatigue and cognitive fatigue can also be functionally limiting in people with chronic pain, especially in myalgic encephalomyelitis/chronic fatigue syndrome (ME/CFS) and long COVID. ME/CFS and long COVID may also present with postexertional malaise (persistent and disabling fatigue after even minor physical or mental effort). Postexertional malaise may limit physical performance testing and function even more than pain but might not be evident until after the patient has left the clinic.[194,195]

Clinical Implications. Physical and cognitive fatigue are very common in people with chronic pain. Fatigue may compromise both quality of life and patients' ability to engage with exercise and self-care. The PT plan should consider fatigue when developing the management plan.[196]

■ PHYSICAL THERAPY EVALUATION, DIAGNOSIS, AND PROGNOSIS

Evaluation and Diagnosis

The PT evaluation and diagnosis of patients with chronic pain builds on the examination to (a) classify the pain mechanism(s) to guide treatment, (b) identify physical and psychosocial factors impacting pain so they can be addressed, (c) assess the impact of pain on physical and psychosocial function to select appropriate goals, and (d) determine whether the patient requires referral to other health-care providers.[132]

Therapists can use several approaches to classify mechanisms/types of pain. They may use the descriptions provided in Table 25.1, a decision flowchart as shown in Figure 25.6,[13,14] pain classification tools as described in Table 25.5, or the Clinical Sensory Test as described in Table 25.6.

The following description is vastly oversimplified, but in general, pain that is localized and responds appropriately to mechanical stressors is likely to be nociceptive. Localized pain that responds excessively to mechanical stressors may involve peripheral sensitization.[49] Pain corresponding to peripheral nerve injury or disease that follows a dermatomal or peripheral nerve pattern and includes paresthesias, burning/electrical sensations and/or numbness, hyperalgesia and/or allodynia, and can be mechanically provoked or spontaneous is likely to be peripheral neuropathic.[12,88] Neuropathic pain corresponding to CNS injury or disease with a neuroanatomically consistent distribution is likely to be central neuropathic.[92] Widespread pain and hypersensitivity that are disproportionate to peripheral tissue threat or damage; present in the absence of identifiable tissue damage or has spread beyond the initial damage; that may include multiple senses (light, sound, smell, as well as touch); includes summation, hyperalgesia, and/or allodynia, and multiple system sensitivity (e.g., GI, urogenital, skin) is likely to be nociplastic and involve CS.[72,73] Visceral pain tends to be diffuse, may be referred, and can be associated with autonomic changes.[10,47] Patients may have multiple pain mechanisms that may

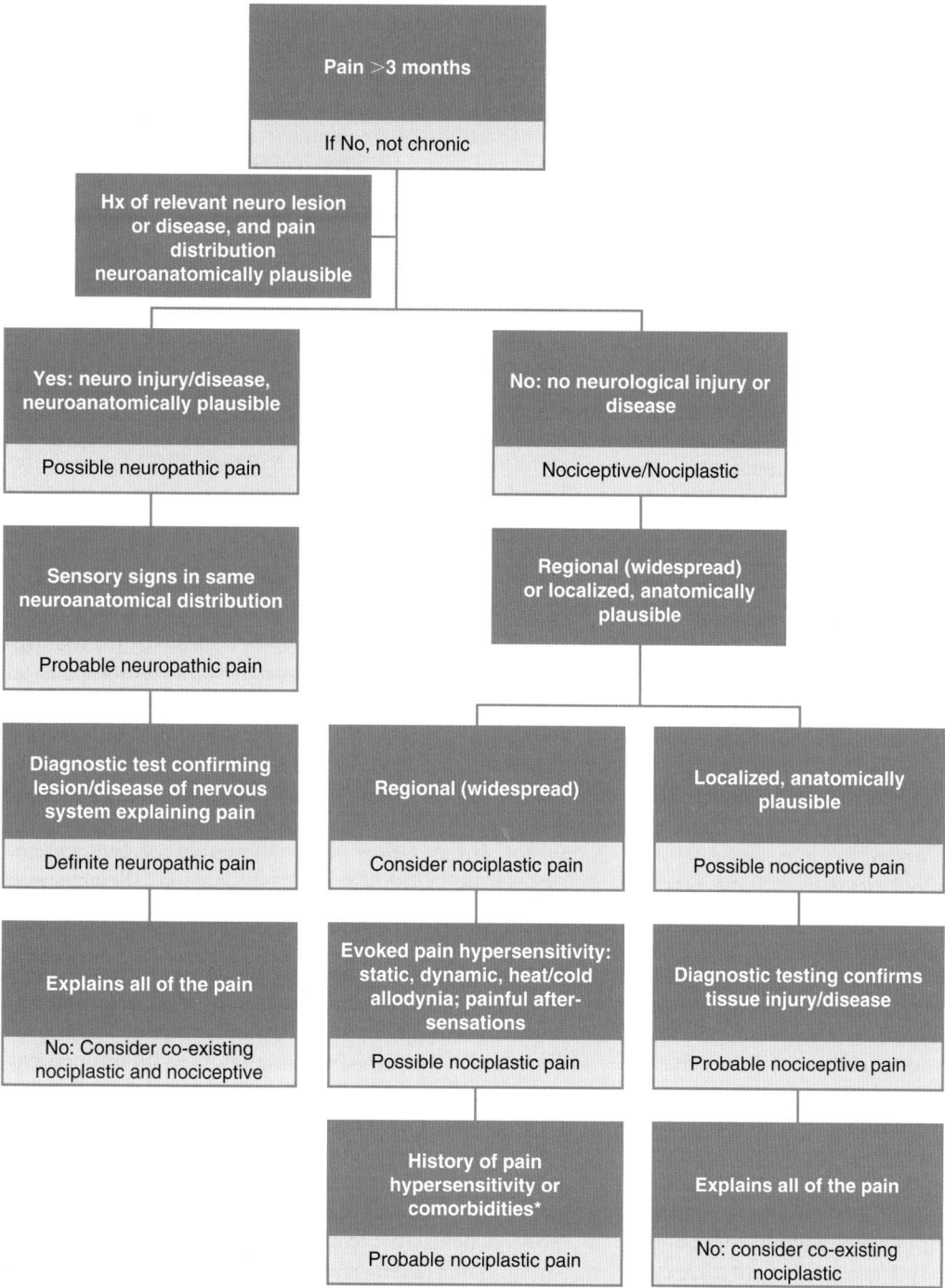

Figure 25.6 Flowchart for distinguishing pain mechanisms. This flowchart shows a decision-making process for identifying the dominant mechanism of pain. If there is a neurological lesion or disease, evaluation continues through the left branch to confirm neuropathic pain and determine whether it is peripheral or central. In the absence of a known neurological lesion, evaluation passes through the right branches to determine whether pain is due to nociplastic changes or normal nociception. Note that most pain is often a mix of more than one pain mechanism, so the presence of nociceptive or neuropathic pain does not rule out nociplastic pain.[13,14]

* Pain hypersensitivity includes any one: touch, pressure, movement, heat/cold. Comorbidities included here include any one: increased sensitivity to sound and/or light and/or odors; sleep disturbance with frequent awakenings; fatigue; cognitive problems with brain fog such as difficulty with focus, attention, memory.[13,14]

vary over time. Furthermore, the Bucket Model reflects how different contributing factors combine to result in pain, and it is sometimes impossible to identify a single source of pain.

Clinical Implications. Convergence between somatic and visceral structures means that activation of visceral nociceptors can result in pain, sensitization, and hyperalgesia in the tissues at the somatic referral site. Similarly, activation of somatic nociceptors can result in pain, sensitization, and hyperalgesia in visceral tissues.[10,47]

If the pain has a nociceptive component, evaluation should identify the movement system impairment and aggravating factors that persistently irritate the tissues.[197] For example, someone with drooping shoulders may have persistent trigger points due to overstretched trapezius muscles or thoracic outlet pain due to stretched peripheral nerves; if the underlying postural dysfunction is not addressed, treatment of the irritated tissues is likely to fail. A person with hEDS may have mechanical pain due to overstretched joints or instability due to poor proprioception; if the underlying proprioceptive and motor control deficits are not identified and addressed, treatment is more likely to fail.[169] A person with PD or SCI may have muscle pain due to spasticity. Some peripheral neuropathic pain has mechanical causes that can be identified and addressed, such as abnormal neural tension in carpal tunnel syndrome. Some of these nociceptive and peripheral neurogenic sources of pain can be addressed through standard, movement system PT approaches. Furthermore, patients with sensitization or CNP may have musculoskeletal factors, such as poor posture, muscle imbalance, or poor motor control that fuels sensitization and exacerbates other sources of chronic pain.

Identification of contributing and perpetuating factors is also essential in managing chronic pain. The ICF model identifies personal and environmental contextual factors that can affect body function or structure, activity, or participation. Personal factors contributing to chronic pain include age, gender, heredity, past and present experience, occupation, education, personality, coping strategies, and social or cultural background. Personal factors include such traits as anxiety, fear avoidance, catastrophizing, depression, and low patient motivation. These traits may also be characterized as body function involvement (global psychosocial functions) in the ICF model.

The evaluation process should address the patient's knowledge and beliefs about chronic pain (and sometimes also the beliefs of family members or caregivers) and factors that might interfere with the patient's willingness or ability to actively participate in PT.[94] Active participation in self-management can be compromised if the patient strongly holds to a biomedical model and is convinced that the only solution is to find and fix the tissue pathology causing pain.[198] The patient's pain behavior (Table 25.3) can influence optimal treatment approach; for example, patients with high fear avoidance need to be encouraged to become more active, while patients with high pain persistence need to learn how to pace their activities.[122-124]

Possible outcomes of the evaluation process include referral to or consultation with another practitioner either instead of or in combination with PT intervention. Yellow flags suggesting psychosocial factors (Table 25.2) may require referral or may be addressed through psychologically informed PT management.[123,157] Examples of red flags suggesting systemic involvement include personal or family history of cancer, recent infection, significant weight change without effort, pain unrelieved by rest or change in position, inability to relieve or provoke symptoms during the examination, night pain, pain in a visceral referral pattern, and certain associated signs and symptoms. Readers are referred to Goodman and Snyder's *Differential Diagnosis for Physical Therapists* for an extensive discussion of how to screen for red flags and how to determine whether referral should occur at the same time as or instead of PT intervention.[175] Each patient's situation should be examined individually because many people with chronic pain have multiple red or yellow flags that may be readily explained, do not require referral, and do not preclude PT. When in doubt, the referring physician should be contacted to discuss these findings.

Prognosis

Prognosis predicts the level of optimal improvement that may be attained through intervention and the required amount of time required to reach that level. Prognosis depends on personal and environmental factors identified in the evaluation process. Again, the alert flags (Table 25.2) highlight biological, psychosocial, and contextual factors that may enhance or compromise prognosis. For example, medical comorbidities, anxiety, or a history of sexual abuse compromise prognosis, whereas a record of regular exercise, adequate stress management strategies, good social support, or good emotional function improve prognosis.

Pain readiness to change is a personal characteristic that may also influence prognosis. As with other forms of readiness to change based on the *Transtheoretical Model of Behavior Change*, individuals who are ready to change are more likely to incorporate pain management strategies into their lives; hence, their prognosis is better. Patients resistant to change are unlikely to be compliant with rehabilitation and are less likely to improve.[199] Environmental factors such as having a support system, attitudes of friends and family, or access to comprehensive health care all affect prognosis.

In the 20th century, the biomedical model strove to eliminate chronic pain by fixing the pathology causing pain; that often did not work. Focus on pain and pain reduction may lead individuals to become hypervigilant and fear avoidant; patients, families, and health-care providers often need to deemphasize pain severity as a measure of status or treatment effectiveness. Patients should focus on functional goals that emphasize active coping skills and wellness behavior rather than pain-based goals.[122] Activity and participation restrictions can be related more to fear avoidance and deconditioning than to pain. The American Chronic Pain Association now proposes that management minimize suffering and maximize return to a productive life even if chronic pain cannot be eliminated.[2]

Functional restoration aims to empower patients to optimize their physical and emotional well-being, activities of daily living, and return to vocational and avocational activities.[43] Rehabilitation strives to enable the patient to take primary responsibility for their physical and emotional well-being. Clinical practice guidelines recommend five components to the goals: increased function, increased physical activity, stress management, improved sleep, and decreased pain.[2,6,7]

■ PHYSICAL THERAPY MANAGEMENT OF CHRONIC PAIN

There are many clinical practice guidelines (CPGs) outlining recommended management approaches. Ernstzen et al. reviewed and consolidated recommendations from six high-quality CPGs for chronic musculoskeletal pain. Their findings are summarized in Table 25.7. Table 25.8 shows how treatment decisions should be based, in part, on the pain mechanism(s).[12,43,45,61,76,90,190,200-203] When referring to Table 25.8, recognize that different conditions within any given mechanism may respond very differently to one treatment or another.

Nociceptive and peripheral neuropathic pain are often driven by movement impairments creating persistent stress to tissues. In these cases, treatment must address the underlying movement impairment rather than just symptomatic tissues (i.e., nerve compression, inflammation, muscle spasm, fascia, trigger points).[197] Failure to identify and address the underlying movement impairment can lead to chronic, nociceptive pain. Nonpharmacological approaches should be emphasized in nociplastic pain, as medications typically provide inadequate benefit.[45]

The Multidisciplinary Pain Management Team

The principles of chronic pain management include a range of physical, psychological, vocational, and medical objectives. The physical therapist's role in management of chronic pain depends on both the patient and the environment in which the therapist practices. Figure 25.7 shows an overview of holistic, conservative

chronic pain management approaches. The four quadrants of the circle represent areas that often need to be addressed: comorbidities contributing to the pain, physical and psychosocial aggravating factors, healthy lifestyle, and pain sensitization. For example, sometimes managing comorbidities can decrease nociceptive and inflammatory input, making it easier to identify aggravating factors. Sometimes pain sensitization must be managed before patients have the emotional energy to make lifestyle changes. The order in which these issues are addressed will vary based on patient presentation and preference. These components of patient care may progress quickly: for some patients, progress is made in a few educational sessions that coincide with more traditional PT intervention; for others, it may take months for physiological and lifestyle changes to occur. The physical therapist may facilitate referral in areas outside their expertise. Once these foundational issues are sufficiently addressed, specific interventions addressing movement system impairments are more likely to be successful. Failure of standard PT intervention may be because patients do not have the physiological or psychological foundation to build upon.

A multidisciplinary pain management team may include any of the following health professionals: primary care physician, pain specialist, physiatrist, anesthesiologist, psychiatrist, psychologist, pharmacist, social worker, caseworker, physical therapist, occupational therapist, sleep specialist, nutritionist/dietician, or nurse. Although multidisciplinary care has been shown to be more effective than monotherapy or standard medical care, the optimal components of multidisciplinary care have not been identified, and the cost-effectiveness has been questioned.[204] Coordination of care and communication with other providers are essential to a comprehensive, patient-centered approach. It is especially important that the patient receive consistent information from providers regarding such things as the fact that there might not be current tissue damage other than that due to deconditioning and the need to maintain activity despite pain. All providers should be consistent about encouraging functional goals rather than using pain ratings as a guide of treatment success.[2,6-8]

A physical therapist working within a multidisciplinary pain clinic may be able to refer psychological issues to the team psychologist and coping skills to the occupational therapist. However, a therapist working in an isolated outpatient clinic might not have access to such collaborations and may need to integrate a broader range of components into the plan of care (POC) while remaining within the physical therapist's scope of practice. The following discussion emphasizes what may benefit patients with chronic pain; who provides a given service will depend on the context. In cases when multidisciplinary or specialist care is not available or practical, motivated patients may be able to pursue some aspects

Table 25.7   Merged Clinical Practice Guideline Recommendations for Chronic Musculoskeletal Pain

Shading groups clusters of recommendations with similar content.

Topic	Strength	Recommendation
Holistic assessment	A	Holistic patient evaluation includes history, physical examination, functional status, psychosocial risk factors, and contextual factors.
Assessment tools	A	Use appropriate, validated assessment tools to establish functional and psychological status and quality of life.
Reassessment	B	Regular reassessment to determine patient's response to Rx.
Special investigations	A	Caution when requesting imaging or special evaluations, and provide appropriate information about results to avoid increased fear, activity restriction, or maladaptive behavior in response to imaging results.
Classification of pain	B	Classification of chronic pain (neuropathic, inflammatory, mechanical, nociceptive) to guide management.
Patient centered	A	Patient-centered, compassionate, explores patient's beliefs, knowledge, and understanding.
Shared decisions	A	Collaborative decision-making, including patient goals and developing a patient-specific, comprehensive pain management program.
Interprofessional collaboration	A	Interprofessional collaboration to develop a plan based on a biopsychosocial approach.
Address patient concerns	A	Address patient's concerns and beliefs; teach the patient and family about pain management strategies.
Advice to stay active	B	Patients should stay active in addition to exercise therapy. Advice, alone, is insufficient.
Brief education	A	Brief education to help patients continue to work.
Self-management	A	Self-management strategies and resources to ensure active patient participation in early and long-term management.
Exercise	A	Exercise and exercise therapy.
Delivery of exercise	A	Supervised exercise, individualized exercise in group settings, home exercise, home exercise instructions.
Manual therapy	A	Manual therapy for relief of chronic pain.
Electrotherapy	B	TENS (low or high frequency).
Low-level laser	B	Low-level laser.
Cognitive behavioral therapies	A	Cognitive behavioral therapy for functional restoration and reduction of pain.
Respondent behavioral therapies	A	Progressive relaxation or EMG biofeedback.
Identification of psychological disorders	B	Identification and management of comorbid psychological conditions such as depression.
Operant behavioral therapies	B	Clinician awareness that their behaviors and the clinic environment can impact reinforcement of unhelpful patient responses.
Referral to psychologist	E	Explaining that referral to psychologist is to increase coping skills and improve quality of life with chronic pain.

Topic	Strength	Recommendation
Table 25.7		**Merged Clinical Practice Guideline Recommendations for Chronic Musculoskeletal Pain—cont'd**
Complementary medicine	A	Acupuncture can be considered for short-term pain relief in some patients.
Multidisciplinary management	A	Referral to a multidisciplinary pain management program.
Pain specialist referral	B	If nonspecialist management is failing, chronic pain is poorly controlled, there is significant distress, or specific specialist approaches are considered.

A = evidence; B = some evidence; C = conflicting evidence; D = limited evidence; E = expert consensus; F = insufficient/no evidence. Recommendations graded as C, D, and F were not included in the table.
Data from Ernstzen, 2022.[7]

of their care independently. (See Appendices 25.B [online] and 25.C [online] for a list of patient resources.)

Therapeutic Alliance

Perhaps the most important component of any PT intervention for chronic pain is the therapeutic alliance or relationship, as it is likely to modulate the effectiveness of other interventions provided. Therapeutic alliance is working rapport, harmony, or positive psychosocial connection between the patient and therapist. It relies on a combination of empathy, collaboration, communication, and technical skills. Research has demonstrated that therapeutic alliance impacts outcomes including pain, physical function, activities of daily living (ADL), depression, global health assessment, treatment adherence, and satisfaction. In some cases, therapeutic alliance with sham treatment can be more effective than real interventions with minimal patient–provider rapport.[205,206]

Patient and therapist expectations and the therapist's expression of confidence in the interventions also influence effectiveness. Therefore, the physical therapist should choose words with positive connotations and avoid negative or threatening words.[207] Finding out what treatments the patient believes have been effective or not effective in the past and the patient's treatment preferences can help the therapist select, from appropriate options, those that the patient believes will be most effective. Adherence and benefits are generally greater with treatments patients prefer. Instructions and explanations also impact outcomes, as patients are likely to perceive what they are told to expect. This overall approach is consistent with evidence-based practice, which is the integration of best available evidence with clinician experience and patient preference.

Expectation and therapeutic alliance appear to tap into the powerful placebo response, which is mediated by descending pain modulation pathways. While placebo is sometimes believed to be a psychological response, placebo analgesia has been shown to operate through physiological changes in several components of the neuromatrix, including enhancing descending

modulation of nociception[208] and modifying brain activity related to pain.[209,210] Consequently, positive thinking on the part of both the clinician and patient can have concrete physiological benefits that may specifically address neurological abnormalities associated with nociplastic pain. The placebo response has been demonstrated to occur even when the patient is aware that the placebo effect is involved.[211]

> **Clinical Implications.** Treatment for pain can be more effective when the patient feels the treatment is being given by a supportive healthcare provider who uses positive language. Words matter.[209,210]

Patient-/Client-Related Instruction

Ongoing patient self-care is key to effective management of chronic pain, and PT is ideally positioned to provide patients the education and skills for active self-care.[2,6-8,24] For the current discussion, the *Guide to Physical Therapist Practice* categories of Functional Training in Self-Care and Domestic, Education, Work, Community, Social, and Civic Life are combined with Patient-Related Instruction because so much of the content overlaps. The family may also require education about chronic pain to both recognize chronic pain as a real disease and to avoid fostering illness behavior in the patient. Patient instruction/education includes pain neuroscience education and self-management through both psychosocial (e.g., cognitive behavioral therapy) and physical means. Goals of the educational component of intervention are given in Box 25.7.[2,6-8,24]

Studies have shown that there is better patient adherence and effectiveness of pain self-management that is matched to a patient's pain behavior.[32,122,126] For example, patients who demonstrate fear avoidance require encouragement to be active despite pain, while patients demonstrating pain persistence need to pace themselves. Table 25.3[123] shows the educational approaches most likely to be effective for specific pain behavior clusters.[122,126] For example, patients who are

Table 25.8 Chronic Pain Interventions by Mechanism[12,43,45,61,76,90,109,190,200-203]				
Interventions	Potential Mechanisms	Noci	Neur	Plast
Therapeutic alliance, shared decision-making	Positive patient attitude, buy-in into treatment decisions	XX	xx	XXX
Functional approach: Treatment focus on function and quality of life in addition to decreasing pain	Functional improvements	XX	XX	xxx
Education				
Biopsychosocial/spiritual model of pain	Appropriate expectations	X	x	xxx
Pain neuroscience and "explain pain" to encourage self-management	Increased active engagement in self-care, altered central pain processing; decreases negative cognitions that contribute to dysfunctional neuroplasticity; may alter pain cognitions more than pain	xx	x	XXX
Self-care principles: posture, body mechanics, etc.	Decreased stress on tissues	xxx	XX	xxx
CBT skills such as coping, pacing, avoiding negative thinking	Decreased stress on tissues; increased active engagement in self-care; improved coping skills	XX	X	XX
Mindfulness or acceptance-based approaches	Autonomic stabilization (decreased sympathetic, increased parasympathetic activation); decreased inflammation; decreased pain	X	x	xxx
Importance of physical activity	Enhanced descending inhibition	XX	XX	XX
Weight management	Decreased systemic inflammation, decreased tissue stress	X		X
Sleep health promotion	Decreased neuroinflammation and CS	XX	XX	XX
Nutrition	Improved gut microbiome decreases inflammation; decreased central and/or peripheral sensitization	X	X	XX
Neuromuscular reeducation				
Physiological quieting, such as diaphragmatic breathing, slow breathing; HRV biofeedback, autonomic stabilization, meditation	Autonomic stabilization (decreased sympathetic, increased parasympathetic activation); decreased inflammation; decreased pain; decreased muscle spasm	xx	xx	XXX
Specific motor control training to address movement system dysfunctions	Decreased stress on tissues (including peripheral nerves); decreased kinesiophobia	XX	XX	X
Yoga, qigong, Tai Chi	Increased parasympathetic activation; flushing of inflammatory mediators from fascia and interstitial tissues	xx	x	xx
Exercise				
Condition-specific strengthening, stretching, stabilization	Decreased stress on tissues by minimizing contributing factors; improved neural function; improved fascial function, enhance/restore EIA, endorphin release	XXX	XX	XX

Table 25.8 Chronic Pain Interventions by Mechanism[12,43,45,61,76,90,109,190,200-203]—cont'd				
Exercise				
Nonspecific exercise	Enhance/restore EIA; endorphin and serotonin release; decrease systemic inflammation; reduces glial cell activation; increase muscular strength; improve cardiovascular condition and function; decreases central excitability in spinal cord, brain stem and cortex; improves learning, memory, and neurogenesis; improves mood; decreases negative cognitions, parasympathetic activation	XX	XX	XX
Aerobic exercise	Stimulates healing at sites of nerve injury; stimulates nerve fiber growth	XX	XX	XX
Graded exposure exercise	Decrease kinesiophobia	X	x	xx
Manual therapy				
Joint manipulation	Peripheral inhibition, release of mediators that reduce inflammation, spinal cord–level inhibition; decreased glial cell activation in spinal cord decreased central excitability; normalizes muscle function (decreases spasm of some muscles, increases strength of others)	XX		xx
Massage	Epigenetic changes that reduce inflammation, stimulates tissue repair, restores normal joint movement to decrease tissue stress; enhances descending inhibition via oxytocin; decreases psychological distress; decreases cortisol levels	XX	X	XX
Nerve mobilization (manual or exercise)	Improves myelin sheath; hypothesized to improve intraneural fluid mobility	xx	xx	xx
Fascial mobilization (manual or exercise)	Flushing of inflammatory mediators from fascia and interstitial tissues	xxx	xx	xxx
Trigger point management (manual or exercise)	Decreases trigger point pain, improves normal mobility	xx		xx
TENS	Alters sympathetic activity, activates peripheral endorphin release, decreases nociceptive neurotransmitter release; decreases peripheral and CS; increases central inhibition and reduces central excitability at spinal cord, brain stem, and cortical levels; endorphin and GABA release; decreases glial cell activity; decreases inflammation at spinal cord level; decreases muscle spasm	XX	X	XX
Other neurostimulation: vagus nerve, transcranial	Increased parasympathetic activity, vagus-nerve induced anti-inflammatory action	X	x	XX

CS = Central Sensitization; EIA = Exercise-induced analgesia; GABA = Gamma-aminobutyric acid; HRV = Heart rate variability. This table has been compiled from multiple sources using nonquantitative methods. The number of X's reflects the relative benefit with one x representing some potential benefit and three x's substantial benefit. The quality of evidence is reflected in lowercase versus capital Xs, with capital X reflecting stronger evidence, though evidence is generally weak for all interventions because of the difficulty in doing high-quality research on these interventions.

psychophysiologically highly reactive benefit from initial treatment focusing on relaxation, biofeedback, and cognitive behavioral therapy. Since patients can transition from one behavior cluster to another over time, educational approaches may need to be modified over time.[122]

Pain education should adapt based on the patient's readiness to change.[212] For example, patients in the precontemplation stage may benefit from the physical therapist taking on a "nurturing parent" role to overcome patient resistance and defensiveness, while patients in the action/maintenance phase might benefit most from

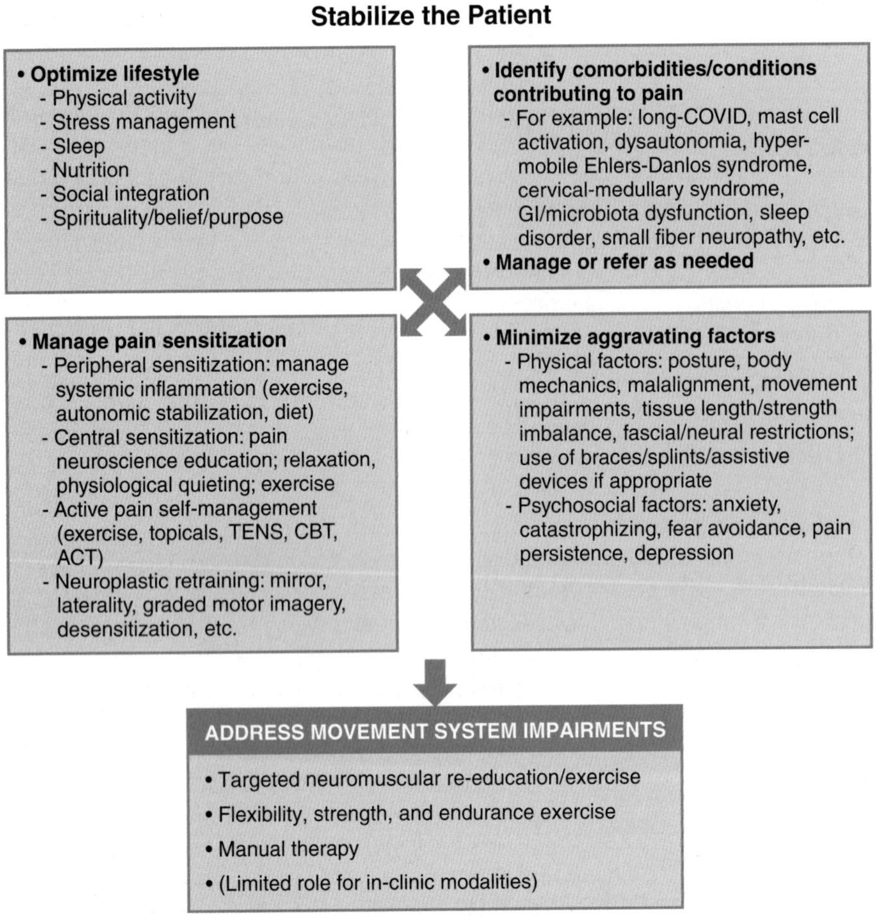

Stabilize the Patient

- **Optimize lifestyle**
  - Physical activity
  - Stress management
  - Sleep
  - Nutrition
  - Social integration
  - Spirituality/belief/purpose

- **Identify comorbidities/conditions contributing to pain**
  - For example: long-COVID, mast cell activation, dysautonomia, hypermobile Ehlers-Danlos syndrome, cervical-medullary syndrome, GI/microbiota dysfunction, sleep disorder, small fiber neuropathy, etc.
- **Manage or refer as needed**

- **Manage pain sensitization**
  - Peripheral sensitization: manage systemic inflammation (exercise, autonomic stabilization, diet)
  - Central sensitization: pain neuroscience education; relaxation, physiological quieting; exercise
  - Active pain self-management (exercise, topicals, TENS, CBT, ACT)
  - Neuroplastic retraining: mirror, laterality, graded motor imagery, desensitization, etc.

- **Minimize aggravating factors**
  - Physical factors: posture, body mechanics, malalignment, movement impairments, tissue length/strength imbalance, fascial/neural restrictions; use of braces/splints/assistive devices if appropriate
  - Psychosocial factors: anxiety, catastrophizing, fear avoidance, pain persistence, depression

ADDRESS MOVEMENT SYSTEM IMPAIRMENTS

- Targeted neuromuscular re-education/exercise
- Flexibility, strength, and endurance exercise
- Manual therapy
- (Limited role for in-clinic modalities)

Figure 25.7 Conservative chronic pain management overview. This patient management approach starts by stabilizing the patient through a combination of patient education and empowerment to implement self-care and decrease pain sensitization. These components can be provided in any order that is appropriate for the patient. Patients with chronic pain have often already failed the more traditional physical therapy approach beginning with neuromuscular reeducation, exercise, or manual therapy. Sometimes their pain has even been aggravated by traditional exercise and manual therapy approaches because of neurosensitization, inflammation, and autonomic dysregulation. Beginning with education and self-care training can often stabilize the patient, who is then more likely to succeed with direct interventions such as neuromuscular reeducation, exercise, or manual therapy. Direct interventions should take a movement system approach, identifying how inappropriate movement patterns may perpetuate pain.[44,72,197]

the therapist as a "consultant."[32] The physical therapist should identify potential learning barriers such as difficulty concentrating (including "brain fog" and cognitive fatigue), depression, refusal to accept a biopsychosocial model of pain, or lack of social support. People at all educational levels may have difficulty learning when they are experiencing chronic pain.

Patient education about pain and pain management can be provided in a variety of formats, and there are many excellent educational resources available. Education is often provided one-on-one in the clinic but may also be provided in small or large group settings, using computer resources or books.[38,198,213] Web- and phone-app–based resources for clinicians, families, and patients with chronic pain can be found in Appendix

25.B (online); Appendix 25.C (online) provides a selected list of books to educate patients about pain.

Pain Neuroscience Education and Explain Pain

Pain neuroscience education (PNE) includes the neurophysiology of pain, including the nociceptive pathways (including synapses and action potentials), as well as the processing systems (spinal modulation, peripheral and CS), neuroplasticity, and role of psychosocial factors in pain. Excellent PNE resources for both clinicians include *Pain Neuroscience Education: Teaching People About Pain*,[37] *Integrating Manual Therapy and Pain Neuroscience: Twelve Principles for Treating the Body and the Brain*,[214] and *Explain Pain Supercharged*.[38] One of the

Box 25.7   Goals of Educational Components of Chronic Pain Management[2,6-8,24]

The goals of patient education are for the patient to:

- Acknowledge that chronic pain is real.
- Recognize the complex, biopsychosocial nature of pain, and the need for a multifaceted management program in which the patient is an active participant.
- Understand the impact of pain on sleep, mood, energy, fitness, ability to work, family life, and stress.
- Avoid letting pain guide activity or medication use because pain-based treatment encourages pain behavior.
- Recognize and utilize wellness behaviors.
- Recognize the role of poor posture and body mechanics in perpetuating pain.
- Overcome fear of movement through gradual exposure to feared activities.
- Learn relaxation strategies.
- Actively participate in own management program.
- Enlist family support and participation in management program.
- Participate in an exercise program, either through physical therapy, independently, or using community resources.
- Minimize fear of movement and activity reduction due to fear of movement.

objectives of PNE is to "de-educate" patients prior to reeducation. Patients have often been given a biomedical explanation for their pain using pathoanatomical terms such as "deterioration," "herniation," "bone on bone," or "wear and tear"; use of these images can be counterproductive because they increase fear and anxiety, creating perceived danger that contributes to the pain experience. Once patients understand the different pain mechanisms and that most chronic pain is mixed, they can better understand the biopsychosocial contributing factors that need to be managed. PNE is intended to be provided with other PT interventions, especially neuromusculature reeducation and exercise; it is not intended to be a solitary intervention.[215-217]

Explain Pain, developed by Butler and Moseley, builds on PNE with an effort to shift the patient's conceptualization of pain away from believing that pain is necessarily an indicator of tissue damage or disease to the understanding that pain indicates the brain's perception that it needs to protect the body.[38,198] Table 25.9 lists the 10 key objectives of *Explain Pain,* which strive to help patients understand the biopsychosocial nature of pain.[38,218] *Explain Pain* is distinct from *cognitive behavioral therapy* (CBT) in that *Explain Pain* focuses on the neurophysiology (why CBT methods are helpful) rather than pain coping skills (e.g., how to implement CBT).

Patients should be told that this educational component is not just to make them more knowledgeable about their pathology (chronic pain), but that a shift in their understanding of the relationship between perception and pain can actually change the neurophysiology of pain. That is, pain results from the brain's perception of danger and, if education can modify patients' perceptions (i.e., help them realize that hurt does not always mean harm), it can potentially modify the actual pain experience.[38,198]

Key objectives of patient education about the nature of chronic pain are that (a) hurt does not always mean harm; and (b) there may be no tissue damage that surgery or medication can fix. Also, patients should understand what pain mechanisms they have to identify strategies that can most effectively manage the pain. For example, nociceptive-dominant pain due to RA may benefit from joint protection strategies, whereas patients with CS may benefit more from calming the CNS. Furthermore, patients who appreciate that the biopsychosocial nature of pain links mind and body are less likely to become defensive about suggestions of psychological management approaches.[213,219]

Evidence indicates that PNE can decrease disability, catastrophization, fear avoidance, pain behaviors, and health-care utilization while increasing pain knowledge, health behaviors, and physical movement.[213,219] The goal of PNE and *Explain Pain* is not just to get patients thinking about pain differently but to actually normalize neurological processes that have become maladaptive. Evidence shows that these interventions enhance neural processing and descending inhibition of pain; because of these neurological processing changes, pain education can be considered a form of neuromuscular reeducation.[216,220,221]

Physical therapists may also provide some education regarding nutrition and sleep, which both have significant impact on chronic pain. Diet and nutrition are likely to contribute to chronic pain in multiple ways, but particularly in the context of nociplastic pain through peripheral and CS via neuroinflammation, gut microbiota, and vagal mechanisms. The literature provides guidance regarding the role of PT in nutrition and specific educational recommendations.[112,222] Similarly, sleep dysfunction plays an important role in perpetuating chronic pain, and CBT approaches to sleep health are recommended over medication. Knowledgeable physical therapists should therefore provide education regarding healthy sleep habits as part of comprehensive chronic pain management.[109,113]

Cognitive Behavioral Therapy, Cognitive Functional Therapy, and Pain Coping Skills

Patients may benefit from CBT and pain coping skills in which beliefs, attitudes, and behaviors are modified to alter the experience of pain, overcome dysfunctional

Table 25.9	Explain Pain Concepts[38]
Target Concept	**Explanation**
Pain is normal, personal, and always real.	All pain experiences are normal and are an excellent, though unpleasant, response to what your brain judges to be a threatening situation. All pain is real.
There are danger sensors, not pain sensors.	The danger alarm system is just that—there are no pain sensors, pain pathways, or pain endings.
Pain and tissue damage rarely relate.	Pain is an unreliable indicator of the presence or extent of tissue damage—either can exist without the other.
Pain depends on the balance of danger and safety.	You will have pain when your brain concludes that there is more credible evidence of danger than safety related to your body and thus infers the need to protect.
Pain involves distributed brain activity.	There is no single "pain center" in the brain. Pain is a conscious experience that necessarily involves many brain areas across time.
Pain relies on context.	Pain can be influenced by the things you see, hear, smell, taste, and touch; things you say; things you think and believe; things you do; places you go; people in your life; and things happening in your body.
Pain is one of many protective outputs.	When threatened, the body is capable of activating multiple protective systems including immune, endocrine, motor, autonomic, respiratory, cognitive, and emotional pain. Any or all of these systems can become overprotective.
We are bioplastic.	While all protective systems can become turned up and edgy, the notion of bioplasticity suggests that they can change back, through the life span. It is biologically implausible to suggest that pain cannot change.
Learning about pain can help the individual and society.	Learning about pain is therapy. When you understand why you hurt, you hurt less. If you have a pain problem, you are not alone—millions of others do too. But there are many researchers and clinicians working to find ways to help.
Active treatment strategies promote recovery.	Once you understand pain, you can begin to make plans, explore different ways to move, improve your fitness, eat better, sleep better, demolish DIMs,* find SIMs,* and gradually do more.

*DIMs and SIMs are terms used in *Explain Pain Supercharged*[38] and *The Explain Pain Handbook: Protectometer.*[249] DIMs refers to "Danger in Me" factors that can increase pain; SIMs refers to "Safety in Me" factors that can decrease pain (https://noijam.com/2017/03/03/supercharging-explain-pain/ used with permission).

behaviors, improve function, and minimize disability.[2,6-8,24,122,223] CBT provides the "how to" as follow-up of PNE "why to." Evidence suggests that CBT strategies can modify several yellow flags associated with disability in chronic pain such as pain beliefs, self-efficacy, and psychological distress.[94,120] Research demonstrates that CBT can be effective in decreasing chronic pain, improving quality of life, and improved physical function, quality of life, sleep, fatigue, depression, and anxiety.[223,224] Cognitive functional therapy is similar but specifically focuses on functional goals. Acceptance and commitment therapy encompass CBT with more emphasis on decreasing suffering while implementing behavioral change.[225,226]

It is increasingly accepted for physical therapists to integrate psychologically informed content into patient care because therapists already educate patients about relaxation strategies, graded activity, pacing, problem-solving, and functional restoration.[82,94,123,227-229] For physical therapists unfamiliar with psychologically informed practices, guides are available in the literature.[123,228,229]

For therapists working with children, behavioral approaches (and phone apps) are available specifically for working with children.[230] Although patients benefit from guidance from a health-care professional, they may also learn many strategies independently using one of the self-help resources listed in Appendixes 25.B (online) and 25.C (online). Components of CBT and pain coping skills are listed in Box 25.8.[2,6,82,122,123,229] Some examples are described here.

Clinical Implications. PT is an ideal opportunity to apply cognitive behavioral approaches. Physical therapists already spend time educating patients and teaching them functional and problem-solving skills, graded exposure, and self-care.

Patients should set realistic activity goals that are meaningful to them, including pleasurable activities. Some patients feel that they hurt too much to participate in leisure activity or that they should not indulge in

Box 25.8 Cognitive Behavioral Strategies and Pain Coping Skills[2,6,82,122,123,229]

Cognitive Behavioral Strategies

- Pain education
- Importance of active self-management
- Demonstrating wellness behaviors rather than illness behaviors
- Goal setting
- Problem-solving
- Identifying and challenging negative thoughts (cognitive restructuring)
- Pleasant activity scheduling
- Elimination of fear avoidance or pain persistence
- Progressive activity/exercise
- Time-based rather than task-based pacing
- Not using pain as a guide
- Relaxation (through diaphragmatic breathing, mindfulness meditation, pleasant imagery, biofeedback, progressive muscle relaxation)
- Calming self-statements
- Distraction
- Flare management using self-care strategies

pleasurable activities if they cannot meet work, family, or household responsibilities. Losing pleasurable activities, however, aggravates depression, leads to loss of social life associated with those activities, and contributes to deconditioning.[123,228,229]

Patients should be encouraged to identify and challenge negative thinking using techniques of cognitive restructuring. Negative self-talk can increase pain.[207] Often, people with chronic pain will catastrophize, ruminate, or dwell on negative aspects of their lives.[94,231] Restructuring can be particularly helpful for highly reactive patients, such as those with PTSD.[232]

Patients may need to be taught effective problem-solving strategies. For example, if a patient is unable to schedule 30 min/day for exercise, help them identify 5-minute blocks or integrate exercise with other activities, such as including children in the exercise by using a DVD focused on yoga for children. If the patient is unable to garden due to knee pain, encourage them to use raised flower beds, take rest breaks, or use adapted tools. Problem-solving can help address fear-avoidant behavior by identifying and modifying aspects of an activity that cause anxiety.[123,228,229]

Pacing should generally be time based rather than task or pain based and should alternate activity and rest to avoid bursts of activity.[228] Pacing is particularly important for patients with postexertional malaise, who may be too physically and mentally exhausted to fully engage in PT exercises.[146,233] Patients who use task-based pacing (i.e., continuing until a task is done) often push themselves for too long and cause a flare, causing "yo-yo"

patterns of activity and rest commonly seen with pain persistent behavior.[124] If they stopped part way through the task and rested or did alternate activities, they might be able to go back to the original task and finish it without a flare. Patients often need to be reminded that "hurt does not equal harm" and that some pain with activity is okay; in fact, muscular soreness during or after exercise is a normal response.[123,228,229] Progressive or graded activity refers to patients gradually increasing their activity level not using pain as a guide, and is discussed further with exercise, as follows.

Since sleep disturbance is a common occurrence in chronic pain, patients should be educated in proper sleep management, which includes sleep education, sleep hygiene, CBT for insomnia, relaxation, and behavioral changes. The literature describes specific strategies physical therapists can use to address sleep disturbance, and many are similar to CBT for pain. There are also phone apps with good CBT for insomnia resources. Gentle exercises such as stretching, yoga, qigong, or Tai Chi may be particularly helpful at bedtime to improve quality of sleep due to their relaxing effects.[83,109,228,229,234]

Patients should learn that stress contributes directly to pain via sympathetic efferents connecting directly to nociceptive afferents. Although many people believe that activities such as watching television and playing video games are relaxing, these forms of passive relaxation are not as physiologically effective as active relaxation techniques discussed here. "Physiological quieting" is therefore a form of neuromuscular reeducation to decrease pain through reducing nervous system tone, muscle activity, and sympathetic and neuroendocrine reactivity.[82,83] A list of relaxation techniques is given in Box 25.9.[2,6,123,235] Slow, diaphragmatic breathing, which can decrease pain and sympathetic nervous system activity, is one of the simplest to teach patients and

Box 25.9 Relaxation Strategies[2,6,123,235]

- Diaphragmatic breathing: Slow diaphragmatic breathing
- Progressive relaxation: Selectively tensing and relaxing major muscle groups
- Visualization: Imagining a safe and relaxing environment, including sounds, smells, feel
- Autogenic training: Imagining your hands feeling warm and heavy
- Mindfulness meditation: Training the mind to be in the present moment, to be calm, kind, and curious
- Biofeedback using heart rate variability, electromyogram for muscle tension, or galvanic skin response, electroencephalogram, or skin temperature
- Body awareness activities such as yoga, qigong, or Tai Chi
- Virtual reality relaxation and calming programs

easiest for them to do.[236-238] Some evidence suggests that vagus nerve activation may be particularly helpful for chronic pain, especially if associated with high levels of distress or history of trauma.[43,48] Mindfulness meditation has been successful for managing stress-related diseases such as heart disease and chronic pain. Mindfulness and acceptance-based meditation teach people to focus on the present moment, attending to thoughts, emotions, sensations, and perceptions without judgment.[2,6-8,24,239-241] The acceptance aspect of mindfulness meditation helps patients differentiate between pain sensations and suffering and hence improves coping. Resources for many of these physiological quieting approaches are given in Appendixes 25.B (online) and 25.C (online).

Family and/or caregiver education can be just as important as patient education. Chronic pain affects the whole family through changes in family roles due to the patient's activity and participation restrictions. The family may reinforce the patient's "sick role" in an attempt to be supportive. Both the patient and the family need to understand the importance of maintaining normal activities and participation to minimize disability; patients must not perceive lack of physical assistance as lack of support or concern from family. In contrast, the family may be completely unsupportive, often owing to lack of objective evidence that the pain is real. Family members may be angry with the individual with pain and may blame that individual for financial, personal, or family problems.[2,7,8]

Personal intimacy is often very difficult with chronic pain, just as it is for other chronic injuries or diseases. Problems may be due to the pain, deconditioning and fatigue, depression, decreased sense of self-worth, or adverse reactions of medications. Distress is often greater for survivors of childhood sexual abuse.[242] It is important that both partners learn about chronic pain so that they understand the reasons for challenges faced. Both partners need to accept that the nature of the intimate relationship can change and not harbor anger, frustration, blame, or guilt. Individuals with chronic pain can improve their self-image through daily exercise, grooming, and cognitive strategies of CBT. Communication is critical so that both partners can contribute suggestions for problem-solving. For example, select a time of day with the least amount of pain and fatigue and find positions that minimize stress to the body. Appendix 25.C (online) includes several patient resources for working through the challenges of intimacy with chronic pain.

Physical Self-Care Strategies

Physical self-care strategies may include a variety of self-applied techniques such as exercise, heat, ice, massage, topical rubs, or transcutaneous electrical nerve stimulation (TENS). Although many can be considered passive treatments when provided by the physical therapists, they can all be components of active patient self-management. The effects of exercise are discussed later in this chapter.

While the popularity of TENS has waxed and waned over the years, current evidence suggests that it can indeed be helpful for pain management, especially when used as a self-management tool.[243-246] TENS operates through both peripheral (gate-control) and CNS mechanisms, including activation of descending inhibition, which is often deficient in patients with chronic pain.[247] High-frequency (greater than 50 Hz) and low-frequency (1 to 10 Hz) TENS operate through different physiological mechanisms, with the important consequence that low-frequency TENS will not reduce pain in people who are opioid tolerant. Hence, people with chronic pain who are taking opioid medications are likely to benefit more from high-frequency than low-frequency TENS. TENS has a strong dose-response curve and is most effective when the strongest nonpainful stimulus is used; the recommended method for setting intensity is not to increase to "strong but comfortable" but to instead increase until the stimulus is painful, then to back down slightly. TENS may be helpful in managing certain types of CNP, including MS and some types of SCI, but not for poststroke pain.[248] Finally, evidence suggests that TENS might be most effective in reducing motion-related pain compared to pain at rest; patients should therefore be encouraged to use TENS during activity or exercise when possible.[243,244]

Patients with chronic pain often develop myofascial trigger points that act as nociceptive triggers for peripheral and CS.[249] Although evidence for sustained improvements with manual trigger point treatments is weak, self-care using trigger point cane, tennis balls, or other pressure devices can provide a low-risk tool for patients who report benefits. All patients should recognize the role of poor posture and body mechanics in perpetuating pain syndromes. Several books listed in Appendix 25.C (online) can be helpful for patients managing multiple and variable trigger points. There is some evidence that use of self-acupressure can be helpful for musculoskeletal chronic pain.[250] These are all safe tools to include in the pain management toolbox.

Topical medications provide another self-care option for patients who want to minimize oral pain medication.[2,6,7,8,24,251] Topical rubs fall into three broad categories: those creating cooling sensations, those creating warmth sensations, and those with bioactive agents such as anti-inflammatories, anaesthetics, and cannabinoids. A variety of over-the-counter medications can be administered via topical rubs, especially if involved structures are superficial, as medication can be absorbed through the skin into muscle, synovium, and joint tissue.[252] Those that create a cooling sensation, generally menthol-based, work as a counterirritant, probably via the gate-control mechanism. Those creating the sensation of warmth are generally capsaicin-based. An important aspect of capsaicin-based topical medications is that the counterirritant effect begins immediately after application but the neurogenic effect requires daily use for 6 weeks to deplete nerve endings of substance P.[253] Lidocaine cream or patch can be beneficial for peripheral neurogenic pain.[6] While evidence for most topicals is weak, they are relatively safe and improve patient self-efficacy.[6]

Other self-care devices may include home lumbar or cervical traction units, paraffin, home massage devices, topical rubs, and hot tubs. Self-care training in all environments is critical to effective management of chronic pain (see Figure 25.7). Therapists can help patients create a sample personal care plan (for an example, see Appendix 25.A [online]). This personal care plan combines patient goals with patient responsibilities for self-care, including PT, independent exercise, stress management, and sleep hygiene; medications may be included as part of the self-care program. Patients should understand the importance of increasing activity and function; patients should not focus only on reducing pain.

Neuromuscular Reeducation

Several forms of neuromuscular reeducation (NMR) have already been discussed: diaphragmatic or slow breathing, physiological quieting with relaxation techniques, and even PNE, which works in part by changing neural processing of pain cognitions. Cognitive functional training (discussed earlier with CBT) includes motor control training and functional integration through increasing body awareness, relaxation, and control during specific functional movements. The goal is to recontextualize painful movements through motor learning and to integrate functional movement patterns into ADL that caused pain.[2,227]

One of the primary mechanisms by which NMR may benefit chronic pain is through addressing movement system dysfunctions[197] that contribute to persistent nociceptive pain.

Proprioceptive and motor control impairments throughout the body can affect the ability of people with chronic pain to perform exercises correctly, so repeated feedback during exercise instruction can maximize safety and success. External feedback, which is helpful in retraining motor control, can be achieved through a variety of approaches: laser pointer–guided exercise, virtual reality, and biofeedback.[254] Research suggests that laser pointer–guided exercise may improve proprioception and motor control, but more research is needed to determine whether currently available laser-pointer training programs are more effective than standard exercise.[255] Similarly, virtual reality–based rehabilitation appears promising, but more research is needed.[256,257] Kinesiophobia (fear of movement) can be reduced if early efforts at exercise are successful.[258]

NMR may utilize biofeedback for both motor control and to stimulate a relaxation response, decrease muscle spasm, and decrease autonomic function associated with stress and pain. HRV is probably the most widely available biofeedback tool, as patients can now implement HRV biofeedback at home using smartphone apps. Physical therapists may train patients in using HRV biofeedback as part of NMR. HRV is a measure of parasympathetic activity, with higher HRV indicating improved vagal tone, and increasing vagal activity associated with decreased pain and inflammation.[259-261] Electromyography (EMG), which measures intensity of muscle activation, can teach patients to relax overactive muscles and isolate functional muscles without widespread over-recruitment.[223,262] Galvanic skin response provides feedback about the autonomic nervous system for decreasing the stress response. Electroencephalographic neurofeedback shows benefit for SCI[263] and migraine.[264] Respiration rate and HR can also be used as low-technology biofeedback measures to evoke a relaxation response. Temperature biofeedback can be helpful for migraines. For back and neck pain, pressure biofeedback can be used for proprioceptive and motor control training.[262,265]

> **Clinical Implications.** Neuromuscular reeducation for chronic pain is more than just retraining motor function. Since nociplastic pain is a problem with neural processing, NMR can potentially retrain the peripheral, central, and autonomic nervous systems. Activities such as biofeedback may help increase vagus nerve function to decrease both pain and inflammation.

Certain chronic pain conditions respond to specific types of exercise or neuromuscular reeducation. For example, phantom limb, complex regional pain syndrome (CRPS), dystonia, and stroke are typically associated with changes in sensory and motor mapping in the sensorimotor cortex.[182] In these cases, sensory input through use of a myoelectric prosthesis, virtual reality or mirror training, or sensory discrimination training stimulates cortical reorganization that is generally associated with decreased pain.[266,267] Two-point discrimination training might be a simple strategy for restoring tactile acuity and decreasing nociplastic pain.[182] Graded motor imagery and mirror therapy have been shown effective for CRPS and chronic musculoskeletal pain, and visual imagery has been shown beneficial for CNP associated with SCI and Parkinson disease.[2] Overall, a systematic review of bodily illusions on clinical pain found mixed results but concluded that mirror therapy, bodily resizing, and functional prostheses show promise.[2] Overall, a systematic review of bodily illusions on clinical pain found mixed results but concluded that mirror therapy, bodily resizing, and functional prostheses show promise.[248,268-275] Finally, desensitization is a form of sensory retraining that may decrease neuropathic pain.[2]

NMR can address kinesiophobia. Graded motor imagery can help people overcome fear of movement through a gradual progression from left/right judgment, visualization, and mirror feedback. For patients who are extremely fearful of specific movements or activities, graded exposure can allow patients to be successful at lower levels of stimulus as they transition to progressively more stressful activities.[274] Patients can start with simple visualization of a position or movement and progress through simplified versions of the activity and then to the activity itself.[94,258] However, overall evidence for effectiveness of imagery in managing chronic pain remains weak.[269,270]

Yoga, Tai Chi, or qigong are alternative forms of NMR that work through a relaxation effect, proprioceptive training, alleviation of fear-avoidance behavior, sleep enhancement, and alleviation of depression and anxiety.[2,83,276-280] While previously considered with "complementary approaches," more PT clinics are integrating these into practice. Virtual reality–based motor control training is becoming more common, but research is not yet conclusive.[281,282]

Exercise

Therapeutic exercise is a key part of chronic pain management. Exercise addresses chronic pain in several ways: (a) It provides nonspecific exercise-induced hypoalgesia; (b) decreases inflammation; (c) stimulates regeneration of some neural tissues; (d) reduces deconditioning and functional limitations; (e) improves psychological function, sleep, and quality of life; (f) corrects movement system dysfunctions contributing to the pain; (g) decreases comorbidities such as deconditioning, obesity, diabetes, cardiovascular disease, autonomic and immune dysfunction; and (h) decreases chance of falls and further injury.[2,6-8,24,76,190,202,283,284] Graded exercise can decrease fear avoidance.[258]

Multiple CPGs recommend various forms of exercise for managing chronic pain, including aerobic, strength, flexibility, range of motion (ROM), core, balance training, yoga, Pilates, and Tai Chi.[2,6-8,190] In general, there is limited evidence that any one type of exercise is superior to others, though some conditions seem to benefit from specific types of exercise. For example, diabetic neuropathy responds best to aerobic exercise, while chemotherapy-induced neuropathy responds better to sensorimotor training.[285] Exercise can counteract aerobic deconditioning and muscle weakness that limit function, decrease inflammation, and stimulate peripheral nerve healing.[76,90,276,285,286] The selection of exercises will often depend on the patient's goals, body structure/function impairments, and preferences. Any type of exercise may also exacerbate pain, so it is critical to customize exercise programs developed in collaboration with patients.[203,287]

Exercise-induced hypoalgesia (EIH) is well documented in people without chronic pain, but research indicates that it may not occur consistently in people with chronic widespread pain, including neuropathies.[200,288,289] EIH appears to use the same descending inhibition pathways active in CPM. People with localized pain may show decreased EIH at the site of injury but normal EIH at remote sites. In addition to some variation between diagnoses, some of the variability in EIH appears due to the extent of underlying sensitization. People with high levels of widespread pain and those with decreased CPM (both indicators of CS) tend to have decreased EIH. Although EIH has traditionally been attributed to endorphin release, endocannabinoids and serotonergic mechanisms may also be involved. The role of the immune system in EIH is unclear, as some studies show increased inflammation after exercise, which could increase peripheral and CS. People with chronic pain have an abnormal sympathetic response to exercise and may have abnormal parasympathetic recovery after exercise, both of which may contribute to abnormal oxidative stress response.[84,101,233] Consequently, exercise prescription parameters used for healthy individuals might not be appropriate in some people with chronic pain, and more gradual progression of exercise may be appropriate. PNE may improve EIH if graded exercise is perceived as less of a threat.[200,290,291]

Clinical Implications. Exercise-induced hypoalgesia is often recommended for chronic pain, but the physiological process might not work normally in people with chronic pain. Physical therapists need to monitor patients for their response to exercise and modify the program if the desired response is not achieved.[200,288,289]

Exercise also decreases the systemic inflammation that is often associated with chronic pain, with increased frequency of exercise showing improved responses.[292-295] The mechanism is mediated by the autonomic nervous system and hypothalamic–pituitary–adrenal axis, which can stabilize the immune-neuroendocrine system in people with dysregulation. Activation of the vagus nerve may be particularly important.[294,295] Exercise reduces stress hormones and inflammatory cytokines and stimulates anti-inflammatory and "anti-stress" responses, which are opposite those seen in healthy individuals.[293]

As with NMR, exercise may help address movement system dysfunctions that contribute persistent nociceptive and peripheral neuropathic input; readers are referred to textbooks on exercise prescription for guidance on this group of exercises. Two special cases will be noted here, as recent research has changed our understanding regarding chronic pain. Fascial restrictions and adhesions can compromise tissue mobility and lymphatic flow, resulting in widespread interstitial inflammation and hence peripheral and CS. Exercises that mobilize fascial tissues may therefore be beneficial.[17,60,61] Since fascial entrapment is the most common cause of peripheral neuropathies,[296] fascial release can benefit patients with peripheral neuropathies. Neurodynamic exercises that enhance neural gliding may benefit patients with both nociceptive and neuropathic chronic pain, including peripheral neuropathies and MS.[297-299] Neurodynamic exercises and mobilization appear to work by improving flow of intraneural fluid, nerve conduction, and blood supply, and decreasing neural edema. Neurodynamic mobility may also produce changes in the CNS, improving descending inhibition in nociplastic pain.[297]

Patients are more likely to implement exercise plans that have been developed collaboratively with their input.[287] Exercise intensity should start conservatively and progress gradually. One systematic review recommends aerobic exercise start as low as 40% of the HR maximum but progressing up to 80%.[300] Strengthening could begin at 40% of 1-rep maximum and increase to 60%. Exercise two to three times per week for 20 to 60 minutes is beneficial. However, many patients with chronic pain cannot start exercising at this intensity and may need to break up their daily exercise into short units, even starting at 1 to 2 minutes at a time, if necessary. Exercise should be continued for at least 7 weeks for nociceptive conditions but 10 to 13 weeks for nociplastic pain.[203,300,301] People who have chronic pain associated with ME/CFS and long COVID have decreased parasympathetic reactivation after exercise[233] and are particularly likely to demonstrate exercise intolerance and postexertional malaise; exercise interventions with these individuals must therefore be carefully implemented, monitored, and modified if patients respond poorly.[146] Overall, most people with chronic pain need to "start low, go slow" to avoid flares that will discourage them or prevent them from continuing.[90,203,302-304]

Patients with nociplastic pain should not use pain as a guide in progressing exercise, and they should be reminded that hurt does not always indicate harm or tissue damage and that some discomfort is to be expected when beginning an exercise program. People with chronic pain may have trouble distinguishing psychological distress from physical pain, so they sometimes need guidance distinguishing fear of movement from actual pain. Specific performance-based targets can prevent overly enthusiastic patients from overdoing their exercise and triggering a yo-yo response of activity and inactivity. For example, exercises could progress a set amount determined by the therapist, such as 10% per week, allowing for an occasional easy day if the patient has a flare. Patients should be discouraged from omitting exercises entirely on flare days as this perpetuates cycles of inactivity; they should decrease exercise by, perhaps, 50% then return to prior targets once the flare has passed. Several resources[203,302-304] provide detailed charts of recommendations for exercise prescription and progression for patients with chronic pain.

Adherence to an exercise program can be challenging for people with chronic pain. People with chronic pain may report short-term increases in pain in response to exercise even though regular exercise can decrease pain. A Cochrane review of systematic reviews concluded that the studies show no long-term increases in pain in response to appropriately prescribed and progressed exercise, only expected transient increases in muscle soreness due to unaccustomed activity.[190] Patients should therefore be given specific guidelines about how to begin and progress using principles of pacing and gradual progression.[190,288,303] Patients should also be informed that temporary, "normal" soreness may occur but should subside with continued exercise, and that pain during exercise does not prevent pain relief from occurring after exercise.[190,283] The prevalence of obesity is high among patients with chronic pain, and exercise may be more difficult and uncomfortable for this population. Strategies for improving compliance for people who are obese include breaking exercise up into multiple shorter bouts, decreasing joint range during exercise, and replacing impact with nonimpact activity.[305]

Other barriers to adherence include the belief that pain is chronic and doubt about the effectiveness of the recommended exercises, lack of a clear rationale for the exercises, low self-efficacy, fatigue, forgetting, perceived lack of time, and symptoms associated with comorbidities. Table 25.10 lists common barriers to exercise and potential solutions.[190,306]

Patients will be most motivated if exercises relate directly to functional goals. For example, a patient who wants to go to the movies with his wife could follow an exercise program designed to overcome his specific obstacles, such as walking from the car to the movie theater and sitting comfortably throughout the movie. Exercises with a social component help address isolation often experienced by people with chronic pain; for example, group exercise programs, active family involvement, or dancing can make exercise more enjoyable.

Manual Therapy

Manual therapy may be beneficial in the case of persistent pain with ongoing nociceptive or inflammatory input or in cases where CS is perpetuated by peripheral nociceptive/inflammatory input. Manual therapy may reduce tissue inflammation, but lasting benefits are unlikely unless contributing factors are addressed. It may temporarily reduce CS and thus decrease other symptoms of CS such as hyperalgesia and anxiety or may improve movement or alignment to allow exercise.[2,6-8,24,307-311] Manual therapy may enhance patient expectations and improve participation in more active components of therapy, such as PNE, neuromuscular reeducation, and exercise.[308] The potential benefits of fascial and neurodynamic mobilization are similar to those with fascial and neurodynamic exercise, discussed earlier.[296,297] Fascial and neurodynamic mobilization may therefore address nociceptive contributing factors,

Table 25.10 Barriers and Potential Solutions for Exercise Adherence[190,306]

Perceived Barrier	Potential Solutions
Increased pain with exercise, symptoms due to comorbidities	• Appropriately selected exercises (e.g., using low-impact or decreased weight-bearing exercises, breaking exercise into shorter bouts) • Appropriately progressed exercises: using principles of pacing and graded progression • Patient education that some increase in pain due to exercise is normal and should decrease over time
Belief that pain is chronic and inevitable	• Patient education that exercise is an effective method for not only reducing pain but increasing function, psychological wellness, overall wellness, and quality of life
Doubt that the exercises will be effective, lack of clear rationale for exercises selected	• Patient education about exercise-induced hypoalgesia/pain relief, with explanation of physiological mechanisms • Patient education about the purpose of exercises selected, beyond exercise-induced hypoalgesia
Low self-efficacy	• Patient empowerment and reassurance
Fatigue	• Dividing exercise into smaller units • Reassuring the patient that fatigue decreases with regular exercise
Forgetting	• Helping the patient establish a routine including exercise • Encouraging family members to remind or encourage the patient
Lack of time, low prioritization	• Patient education regarding the importance of exercise for pain management and for decreasing future chronic pain • Encouraging patient to integrate social activities with exercise • Encouraging patient to problem-solve, for example, watching TV while exercising, exercising by walking more to and from work or shopping, etc.
Lack of resources	• Providing patient with low-resource options, such as walking, body-weight resisted exercises, etc.

including those that contribute to peripheral and CS. Because manual therapies seldom resolve pain permanently, there is a risk of patients becoming dependent on them. Interventions based solely on passive manual therapy modalities should therefore be limited to managing acute flares, addressing nociceptive contributing factors, and decreasing CS so that the patient can engage in active interventions such as exercise rather than an isolated intervention.[2,6-8] Patients may use fascial release and trigger point management as part of their self-care program.

Clinical Implications. Although manual therapy seldom entirely resolves chronic pain, it can be an important component of a comprehensive pain management program. Manual therapy can decrease both inflammation and CS so that patients are better able to engage in active self-management. Manual therapy can also strengthen the therapeutic alliance and increase patient motivation.[312] Improved understanding of the role of fascia in chronic pain and inflammation may lead to better understanding of the physical benefits for people with chronic pain.[11,16]

Assistive Devices

Patients with persistent activity limitations due to defined physical impairments may benefit from assistive devices to improve function. Patients with joint disorders, such as OA, RA, or hEDS (i.e., joint hypermobility) should consider devices that decrease stress to affected joints. For example, shoe orthotics and knee braces have strong evidence for modest improvements for OA of the knee.[313] Other devices that decrease stress to joints include items such as jar openers and carts for transporting groceries. Conditions associated with focal weakness, such as stroke, MS, or joint hypermobility, may benefit from braces or splints to support weakened structures and decrease muscle length and strength imbalances. Each patient's specific situation needs to be examined and evaluated, because overreliance on splints and appliances to protect painful regions in the absence of specific pathology can be counterproductive if it reinforces pain and illness behavior.[2,6]

Biophysical and Other Modalities

TENS, heat, and ice are helpful as self-management strategies; see section on self-management, aforementioned.[2,24,243,244,314] Some new noninvasive electrical modalities are promising, especially if they, like TENS, can become self-care tools for patients. Transcutanous vagus nerve stimulation at the neck or ear shows promise for a variety of systemic inflammatory and pain conditions, including CNS inflammation.[315,316] Transcranial direct current stimulation has strong evidence for nociplastic pain and is inconsistent for neuropathic pain.[317] Deep brain stimulation may be effective for chronic neuropathic pain associated with SCI and phantom limb.[248] Evidence for other biophysical modalities such as ultrasound, laser, and shockwave is generally weak, and prolonged use of these modalities is discouraged because they instill a passive approach to pain management.[2,6,36,307] Evidence for cervical or lumbar traction is also weak.

MEDICAL MANAGEMENT OF CHRONIC PAIN
Medical Diagnostic Testing

There is currently no clinically useful imaging or laboratory test diagnostic to measure chronic pain. Furthermore, abnormalities observed in imaging tests do not prove that the identified pathology is related to the patient's pain, as indicated in multiple studies showing positive lumbar imaging findings in people without LBP[7,318,319] and the mismatch between radiographic findings of OA and pain.[320] In fact, studies show that doing MRI imaging early in an episode of acute back pain is associated with poorer health outcomes and increased likelihood of disability.[321,322] CPGs recommend against extensive medical testing unless serious pathology is suspected.[7,230] Ultimately, repeated diagnostic testing to search for an undefined physical abnormality is generally not indicated because it fosters patients' obsession with obtaining a pathophysiological diagnosis that might not exist and thus fosters overadherence to a biomedical model rather than looking for strategies to identify contributing factors and manage the pain using a biopsychosocial model.[2,6-8]

Laboratory tests, such as thyroid hormone levels, sedimentation rates, Lyme titers, or general blood screening, can be appropriate to rule out conditions that are treatable. Electrodiagnostic testing, such as needle electromyography, is not indicated unless there is suggestion of specific neuropathy. Diagnostic nerve blocks (peripheral or sympathetic), joint blocks (facet or sacroiliac), and provocative discography can help determine whether a given structure is involved; see any of the clinical guidelines on chronic pain for more information on interventional testing.[2,6-8] Skin biopsy is becoming a more common diagnostic tool for small fiber neuropathy, which is often difficult to diagnose through other means. Neuroimaging using functional MRI (fMRI), positron emission tomography, and proton magnetic resonance spectroscopy (H-MRS) is currently used in research to observe neurophysiological or neuroanatomical abnormalities, but these techniques are not yet useful for making diagnoses other than frank neuropathy.[323]

Pharmacological Management

Medications used for chronic pain are rapidly evolving and beyond the scope of this chapter; readers are referred to current CPGs for recommendations[2,6-8,24] and explanation of physiological mechanisms.[324] Medications are typically staged, starting with those least likely to cause adverse side effects to those with greatest risk. Medications should ideally be selected based on the mechanism of pain (e.g., nociceptive, neuropathic, and nociplastic), and when possible, they should address underlying pathology rather than just pain as a symptom. For example, standard NSAIDs may be helpful for reducing both inflammation and pain, while medications that address neurogenic inflammation may be helpful for neuroinflammation associated with peripheral and CS.[57] *Adjuvant medications* (medications whose primary indication is a condition other than pain but which have demonstrated benefit in pain management) are typically added next. Muscle relaxants and weak opioids are added if prior medications, PT, and cognitive therapy are unsuccessful. Low-dose naltrexone appears to have benefits for nociplastic pain and may become more widely used as it appears to be much safer than opiates.[325] Given the current opiate epidemic, opiates are avoided if possible. If opioids are used, their risk/benefit should be reevaluated regularly, and they should be discontinued if not providing effective pain relief and improved function.[2,6-8] Goals for medication should include both pain and function. A large, WHO-led systematic review on management of pain in children found that although medication decreased pain, it did not improve physical function, whereas physical and psychological interventions did improve function.[326]

Serotonin syndrome (serotonin toxicity) is a potentially dangerous consequence of polypharmacy (use of multiple drugs to treat the same condition) with medications often used to manage chronic pain. The most likely medications involved are SSRIs, SNRIs, TCAs, some opioids, and triptans (used as an abortive medication for migraines). Because the condition is potentially lethal, the physical therapist should remain alert for symptoms of serotonin syndrome: confusion, hypomania, agitation, myoclonus, hyperreflexia, diaphoresis, shivering, tremor, diarrhea, incoordination, and fever.[327]

Other Medical Management

In a progression of interventions for patients with chronic pain, invasive procedures and opioid medications are to be avoided, if possible. Interventional management approaches are beyond the scope of this chapter, and readers are referred to current CPGs for more about medical management.[2,6-8]

■ COMPLEMENTARY AND ALTERNATIVE APPROACHES

"Complementary" treatments are used alongside standard medical care, while "alternative" treatments are used instead of standard medical care. Since 35% to 63% of people with chronic pain use these approaches,[83,277] physical therapists should be familiar with how they may be integrated into a comprehensive POC. Approaches such as yoga, Tai Chi, qigong, biofeedback, and mindfulness meditation are now sometimes integrated into PT care, though patients may pursue these outside the clinic. Movement therapies such as yoga, Tai Chi, and qigong now have substantial support as forms of exercise for improving flexibility, strength, balance, and proprioception, and decreasing fear of movement.[83,276-278,280,328] Mind–body movement and mindfulness meditation also decrease sensitization as well as foster relaxation and independence, which are all important components of self-management. Furthermore, many mind–body movement activities are practiced in a community-based group setting, which addresses issues of isolation and loss of recreational activities. Mindfulness meditation has the longest history of research supporting its beneficial effects for a variety of chronic health conditions.[222,277]

Other complementary approaches include chiropractic, acupuncture, hypnosis, reiki, magnets, and herbal and nutritional supplements. Magnets, herbal medicines, and supplements are beyond the scope of this chapter. Acupuncture, chiropractic, and osteopathy have inconsistent evidence for effectiveness, depending on the type of chronic pain condition, but benefits are typically not permanent. While they may be viable alternatives to medication, they are all passive interventions, making patients reliant on ongoing care. It is likely that patients experience a relaxation response with most manual therapy approaches; while promoting relaxation is beneficial during flare states, active self-directed methods of relaxation are preferable to passive approaches in which patients depend on health-care providers.[2,6-8] Hypnosis has been found to be at least as effective as other cognitive and physical interventions for pain; patients are often taught self-hypnosis to facilitate self-management.[329] In summary, several complementary and alternative approaches have documented benefit for patients with chronic pain while others do not. In general, side effects are minimal, especially compared to some of the pharmacological and surgical interventions.

SUMMARY

Chronic pain is a complex biopsychosocial phenomenon: the nervous system integrates physiological, psychological, and social factors to create the experience of pain. Chronic pain is often modulated by plasticity or dysfunction of the central and/or peripheral nervous systems, autonomic, endocrine, and immune systems. Pain may be classified as nociceptive, peripheral or central neuropathic, or nociplastic, with many patients experiencing a mix of pain mechanisms that may vary over time. Peripheral and CS can amplify pain, cause it to spread to previously uninvolved regions, and cause it to persist in the absence of noxious stimulus, injury, or disease. The psychological and social context of pain must be assessed and addressed for effective pain management.

Effective management of chronic pain needs to address the whole patient and often also the patient's family. The most powerful tools in patient management appear to be an effective patient–therapist alliance, patient education about the nature of chronic pain, exercise, and self-management using cognitive and physical means. Physical therapists are well positioned to provide these interventions and to be a key member of the pain management team to restore optimal function and quality of life to patients with chronic pain. The scientific understanding of chronic pain has changed substantially in recent decades. With better understanding of the biopsychosocial nature of pain and neuroplasticity, in time it may be possible to rehabilitate (i.e., reverse) chronic pain through retraining the brain.[14,37,38,330]

Questions for Review

1. Which of the following is NOT an accepted pain type or mechanism?
   a. Nociceptive
   b. Neuropathic
   c. Psychogenic
   d. Nociplastic

2. Pain associated with *neurogenic inflammation* is MOST likely associated with which of the following physiological processes?
   a. A systemic inflammatory condition
   b. Antidromic neural activity
   c. Non-neural tissue injury
   d. Injury of neural connective tissue

3. Contrast the physiology and presentation of acute, nociceptive-dominant pain versus chronic pain.

4. Contrast the biomedical and biopsychosocial models applied to pain.

5. List and propose the mechanism for five risk factors associated with chronic pain.

6. Explain central sensitization.

7. Which of the following components of a patient examination is MOST important with patients who have chronic pain? Why?
   a. MRI or CT scan of the brain
   b. Thorough medical testing for every possible condition
   c. A biopsychosocial interview
   d. Tests and measures for each area of pain

8. Outline the components of a PT evaluation for a patient with chronic pain.

9. Describe several educational and behavioral principles that physical therapists can integrate into the POC for patients with chronic pain.

10. Explain three reasons why neuromuscular reeducation and exercise are important for patients with chronic pain.

CASE STUDY

CHRONIC PAIN

The following case is based on a published case report.[331] Students are encouraged to read the full case report for additional detail.

HISTORY

The patient is a 64-year-old female attending an outpatient clinic complaining of a 3-year history of CLBP. She reported no traumatic onset. She progressively decreased activity and ultimately stopped working as a nurse 1.5 years previously due to the CLBP. Her pain diagram showed pain throughout her middle and lower back, as well as her entire legs (anterior and posterior). She rated her pain 9/10. Activity increased pain: for example, vacuuming more than half of a room led to a flare that required medication, rest, and no further housework. Taking medication, frequent resting, and lying down decreased pain. She had previously been treated by a number of health-care providers and received various types of exercise, manipulations, massage, physical modalities, relaxation training, and multiple medications. She had also received several epidural steroid injections and nerve ablations, with no sustained improvement in her pain.

PAST MEDICAL HISTORY

There were no other orthopedic or medical complaints. MRI revealed "bulging" discs at L2/3, L4/5, and L5/S1, and degenerative disc disease throughout the lumbar spine.

MEDICATIONS

Hydrocodone, OxyContin, Skelaxin, and Celebrex
Tests and Measures:
Self-Care and Domestic Life:
Oswestry Disability Index score: 54% (higher scores indicate greater disability). She reported being unable to stand to cook a meal and unable to sit at a desk for more than 30 minutes.
Mental Functions
Zung Depression Scale: 58/80 (scores greater than 55 indicate depression)
Fear Avoidance Behavior Questionnaire: FABQ-W: 25/42, FABQ-PA: 20/24 (higher scores indicate greater fear avoidance)

(Continued)

Pain
Diffuse tenderness in a nonanatomic pattern

Range of Motion
Screening motions for hip, knee, cervical, and thoracic ranges were normal.
Lumbar flexion: 10°, limited by fear that further motion would trigger her pain complaint. Further ROM testing was discontinued due to the patient's apprehension about moving.

Cranial and Peripheral Nerve Integrity
Lower-quarter neurological screening examination showed no abnormalities in myotomes, dermatomes, or stretch reflexes.
Straight leg raise: 70° B with "pulling" sensation that did not reproduce pain complaint.
Modified slump: decreased knee extension −30° B with "pulling" in low back and leg, with reproduction of primary pain complaint.

GUIDING QUESTIONS
1. Is the primary type of this patient's pain nociceptive, neuropathic, or nociplastic?
2. What findings support your answer to question 1?
3. What are the implications of the MRI findings?
4. Why were more physical tests and measures not performed?
5. What should be the emphasis of initial PT management for this patient?
6. What type of exercises (including NMR) would be most appropriate and why?

Answers to Guiding Questions

1. Is the primary type of this patient's pain nociceptive, neuropathic, or nociplastic?
   a. The primary pain mechanism is nociplastic pain driven by central sensitization. While there may have been some nociceptive and neuropathic components to her pain, those were likely less important for perpetuating her pain.

2. What findings support your answer to question 1?
   a. She had a high Fear Avoidance Behavior Questionnaire score, the pain diagram showed vague and widespread pain, spontaneous pain, pain was associated with emotional distress and maladaptive cognitions, and she had a history of failed treatments. The physical examination also showed diffuse and nonspecific findings.

3. What are the implications of the MRI findings?
   a. MRI findings for CLBP have been shown to have poor correlation to pain complaints. The MRI results would encourage a biomedical approach to managing her pain, which had been ineffective in the past. The patient's continued focus on a biomedical explanation of bulging and degenerative discs could interfere with her engagement in a biopsychosocial approach.

4. Why were more physical tests and measures not performed?
   a. Once it is apparent that nociplastic pain dominates, it is important to take a comprehensive biopsychosocial approach. Extensive physical tests and measures would perpetuate a biomedical perspective in the patient. Furthermore, with her initial pain complaint of 9/10, she would likely experience increased pain with most physical tests and measures; if everything is painful, the tests contribute less useful information. In patients with CS, it is often helpful to initially work toward decreasing CS, then consider whether further physical examination would be helpful. Sometimes nociceptive pain generators and movement system dysfunctions are more apparent once CS is decreased.

5. What should be the emphasis of initial PT management for this patient?
   a. Both manual therapy and exercise-focused interventions have previously failed for this patient, suggesting an alternative approach might be more effective. Initial PT management should focus on PNE to help decrease CS. A better understanding of pain can decrease fear associated with exercise and hence improve adherence. Prior PT had attempted a variety of exercise programs, which had not been successful for this patient; the patient would have expected failure again if PT started with an exercise approach without first understanding pain and CS. Patients with CS can sometimes respond well and sometimes poorly to manual therapy. Manual therapy

CASE STUDY—cont'd

can be combined with PNE, but manual therapy alone does not address the driving factors for CS, typically provides temporary benefit, and reinforces a biomedical model of pain. Since prior manual therapy was not successful, it should not be the focus of current treatment.

6. What type of exercises (including NMR) would be most appropriate and why?
   a. Gentle aerobic exercise can provide benefits through EIH; selecting forms of exercise that do not directly stress the low back will be better tolerated as the patient is less likely to be fearful. Aerobic exercise can also improve mood, sleep, and energy levels, which can provide positive reinforcement. Walking and aquatic exercise are good options for aerobic exercises as they would not significantly stress the low back, but any low-impact exercise that the patient enjoys and would perform could be considered. Neurodynamic mobilization exercises, such as slump sliders, could improve the health and mobility of neural structures. General strengthening exercises can provide both EIH as well as trunk strengthening through stabilizing the trunk while performing resistance exercises. Specific core strengthening could be used, but specific exercises are often no more effective than general exercise in nociplastic pain; furthermore, the patient might have a negative attitude toward "back" exercises that had been part of prior unsuccessful treatment episodes.

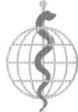

For additional resources, including answers to the questions for review, new immersive cases, case study guiding questions, references and more, please visit **https://www.fadavis.com/product/physical -rehabilitation-fulk-8**. You may also quickly find the resources by entering this title's four-digit ISBN, 4691, in the search field at **http://fadavis.com** and logging in at the prompt.

Psychosocial Issues in Physical Rehabilitation

Pat Precin, PhD, PsyaD, NCPsyA, LP, OTR/L, FAOTA

LEARNING OBJECTIVES

1. Discuss the psychosocial factors that influence rehabilitation.
2. Explain the impact of psychological functioning and social interaction on health, disease, accident proneness, and adjustment to illness and physical trauma.
3. Recognize the psychological impact of disability on the patient.
4. Differentiate the various professionals (and their roles) to which physical therapists can refer patients with psychosocial issues.
5. Apply the interventions used to handle challenging behavior—how to deescalate an agitated patient, manage violent patients, and identify signs of hypersexuality.
6. Describe the stages of psychosocial adaptation to loss and disability and apply them to treatment.
7. Differentiate between psychosocial adaptation and psychosocial adjustment.
8. Analyze different coping strategies that have been found to be important in psychosocial adaptation and adjustment to chronic disability and illness.
9. Analyze common defensive reactions to disability.
10. Understand how body image may be affected by disability and what a physical therapist can do to address body image issues.
11. Recognize the warning signs of possible post-traumatic stress disorder.
12. Describe the general adaptation syndrome, its aims, uses, and potentially dangerous outcomes.
13. Determine crisis points in the rehabilitation process and use clinical reasoning to problem-solve solutions.
14. Apply psychosocial techniques to facilitate patient-/client-centered intervention.
15. Compare strategies and resources for prevention, wellness, and psychosocial education.

CHAPTER OUTLINE

PSYCHOSOCIAL ADAPTATION *1015*
  Grief, Mourning, and Sorrow *1015*
  Phase Models of Psychosocial Adaptation *1016*
  Chronic Illness and Disability: Differences in Adaptation *1018*
  Post-traumatic Rehabilitation *1018*
PERSONALITY AND COPING STYLES *1019*
  Personality Types *1019*
  Personality Disorders *1020*
  Coping Styles *1021*
COMMON DEFENSE REACTIONS TO DISABILITY *1022*
COMMON PSYCHOSOCIAL ISSUES *1025*
  Anxiety *1025*
  Acute Stress Disorder and Post-Traumatic Stress Disorder *1029*
  Depression *1032*
  Substance Use *1037*
  Substance Use and Rehabilitation *1037*

Treating Patients Who Abuse Substances *1038*
Education on Substance Use *1038*
When to Make a Referral for Substance Use *1038*
Agitation and Violence *1038*
Hypersexuality *1040*
PSYCHOSOCIAL WELLNESS *1041*
  Barriers to Wellness for People With Disabilities *1041*
  Social Support *1041*
WELLNESS IN REHABILITATION *1041*
INTEGRATING PSYCHOSOCIAL FACTORS INTO REHABILITATION: CASE EXAMPLE *1042*
SUGGESTIONS FOR REHABILITATIVE INTERVENTION *1042*
  Patient Education *1043*
  Use of Jargon and Labels *1045*
  Trauma-Informed Care *1045*
  Rehabilitation Team Members' Self-Awareness *1051*
SUMMARY *1051*

Psychosocial factors pertain to the psychological development of individuals in relation to their social environment.[1] Psychosocial factors are numerous, as a person's psyche is affected by countless events in the internal and external environments. This chapter focuses on the psychosocial factors that may influence the direction of physical therapy intervention. Some examples of psychosocial factors include premorbid status or mental illnesses, personality styles, coping strategies, defense mechanisms, and emotional reactions to disability. Others include spirituality, values, environment, adjustment, cognitive abilities, motivation, family, social supports, life roles, and educational level. All these factors can affect patients and treatment outcomes.

This chapter identifies and describes how psychosocial factors can influence rehabilitation, demonstrates how to address such factors during physical therapy intervention, and provides indications for referral to psychosocial rehabilitation specialists. Psychosocial factors profoundly affect a patient's ability to recover. Patients who are emotionally upset will have difficulty concentrating on physical therapy goals until emotional issues are addressed. If a patient is motivated to participate in rehabilitation, but their family members do not support the patient's rehabilitation goals, the patient will be unlikely to progress on returning home. Mental health status has been shown to be one of the most important predictors of physical health.[2] Wickramasekera et al.[3] found that more than 50% of all visits to primary care doctors involved somatic complaints resulting from psychosocial problems. Patients with physical disabilities may fail to respond to treatment if a prominent psychosocial issue is affecting them as well.

Treatment outcomes will be influenced by patients' perceptions of their role in the rehabilitation process. Patients who believe that they possess control regarding their treatment and feel respected by staff tend to experience better health outcomes.[4,5] Empowerment, education, inclusion in goal setting, and a high level of engagement are important factors that positively influence recovery.

The mind and the body are highly connected.[6-8] Because of their reciprocal influence, psychosocial and physical issues should be addressed simultaneously to best facilitate recovery. A slow recovery may cause or prolong depression, which may in turn further delay the rehabilitation period. Watts[9] believes that mental health interventions should be provided to all rehabilitation patients because health outcomes tend to be poor and prolonged when psychosocial problems remain unaddressed.

Physical therapists regularly encounter patients who have psychiatric illnesses. Psychiatric conditions occur with some frequency in the general population (Table 26.1), but they occur at an even higher rate in rehabilitation settings.[10] For instance, panic disorder occurs in 10% to 30% of patients treated in cardiovascular, respiratory, and neurological rehabilitation units and in 60% of those treated in cardiology clinics

Table 26.1 Lifetime Prevalence of the Most Common Psychiatric and Personality Disorders in the United States[11]

Major Psychiatric or Personality Disorder	Incidence/Prevalence %
Alcohol abuse or dependence	12.4 adult men 8.5 for people ages 18+ 4.9 adult women 4.6 for people ages 12–17
Major depression	7
Schizotypal personality disorder	4.6
Post-traumatic stress disorder	3.5
Paranoid personality disorder	2.3
Obsessive-compulsive disorder	2.1–7.9
Panic disorder	2–3
Histrionic personality disorder	1.84
Borderline personality disorder	1.6–5.9
Autism spectrum disorder	1
Bipolar II	0.8
Bipolar I	0.6
Dependent personality disorder	0.49
Schizophrenia	0.3–0.7
Antisocial personality disorder	0.2–3.3
Gender dysphoria	0.005–0.014 Natal adult males 0.002–0.003 Natal adult females

(compared with 1% to 2% in the general population).[11] Conversion disorder has been reported to occur at a rate of up to 14% in general medical or surgical inpatient units (compared with 0.5% in the general population).[12] Friedland and McColl[13] found the prevalence of depression and substance use to be significantly higher among people with disabilities than in the general population, as did Turner and Beiser,[14] who documented the rate to be three times higher regardless of gender and age. Vulnerable populations such as older adults with disabilities are at higher risk for a diagnosis of major depression that interferes with daily activities.[15] Thirty-three percent of patients with stroke were found to be depressed and 20% were diagnosed with anxiety—findings that correlated with poorer rehabilitation outcomes.[16] Patients with traumatic brain injury (TBI), spinal cord injury (SCI), and Parkinson disease also reported higher levels of depression compared with the general public.[17,18]

Patients who do not have a preexisting psychosocial illness are more likely to develop one after the onset of physical illness. Anxiety disorders can result from many conditions: endocrine (e.g., hyperthyroidism and hypothyroidism, pheochromocytoma, hypoglycemia, and hyperadrenocorticism), cardiovascular (e.g., congestive heart failure, pulmonary embolism, and arrhythmia), respiratory (e.g., chronic obstructive pulmonary disease, pneumonia, and hyperventilation), metabolic (e.g., vitamin B_{12} deficiency and porphyria), and neurological (e.g., vestibular dysfunctions, encephalitis, and neoplasm).[11] The onset of depression has also been linked to the presence of an existing physical disability.[13,14] There is evidence for the converse as well; the longer a person has some form of mental health concern, the greater their risk for developing a physical illness. Depression is a risk factor for heart disease and poststroke mortality.[19,20] Heinemann et al.[21] found that alcohol-related automobile accidents are responsible for a significant number of SCIs, and Zegans[22] reported that psychological problems could be exacerbated by physical illness or injuries. Anxiety can also increase the risk of cardiovascular disease and hypertension.[23]

Although the co-occurrence of physical disabilities and mental illness is high, the rate of treatment for mental illness among people with disabilities is low. According to the World Health Organization's Comprehensive mental health action plan 2013–2030, 35% to 55% of individuals with serious mental illness in high-income countries receive no treatment, and up to 85% of individuals in low- and moderate-income countries receive no treatment.[15]

A thorough examination of the patient's psychological and social functioning can contribute significantly to a better understanding of needs, fears, anxieties, and capabilities, as well as furnish essential information about the patient's emotional adjustment to disability, assets and liabilities, personality structure, and cognitive functioning. These can then be used to better understand the patient's emotional barriers and behavioral difficulties that can impede recovery. Although not inclusive, Box 26.1 highlights the major areas of consideration in a mental health examination.

Whether physical therapists should address psychosocial issues during treatment or refer psychologically impaired patients to other professionals depends on several variables: (1) the severity of the patient's psychosocial issue; (2) the level of comfort with which the physical therapist can address psychosocial problems; and (3) the patient's ability to progress in rehabilitation if existing psychosocial issues are not addressed. Professionals to whom referrals may be made for additional psychosocial intervention include but are not limited to

Box 26.1　Elements of a Mental Health Examination

Client Demographics

- Gender, age, culture, ethnicity, education, economic status, primary (and secondary) language(s)
- Living environment (past, present, and projected future) and environmental supports
- Family history of psychiatric diagnoses/interventions
- Current complaints
- Psychiatric medication (past and current)
- Roles (past, present, and projected future)
- Occupation (past, present, and projected future)
- Social supports (past, present, and projected future)
- Leisure interests (past, present, and projected future)
- Goals (past, present, and projected future)
- Values (past, present, and projected future)
- History of psychiatric hospitalizations, substance use detoxifications, and/or rehabilitation stays
- Current use of time

Systems Review

- Psychosocial

Examination

Chosen to measure or identify the following:

- **Cognitive status** (orientation, memory [short-term, long-term, working memory], executive functioning, judgment, calculations, attention, processing, meta-cognition, use of cognitive strategies), volition, self-awareness, mental status, degree of organicity and cognitive disability and its relationship to the patient's rehabilitative capacity. *Primary impairments:* disorientation, amnesia, word-finding difficulty, impaired memory, poor judgment, executive functioning deficits, thought blocking, poor use of cognitive strategies and/or meta-cognition, lack of motivation, impaired self-awareness of limitations, impairments in mental status.[141]

| Box 26.1 | Elements of a Mental Health Examination—cont'd |

Examination

- **Emotional status**. *Primary impairments:* anxiety, depression, mania, hypomania, grief, mourning, shock, anger, suicidal ideation, emotional numbness, overwhelmed, paranoia, agitated, low self-esteem, regression, delusions, poor reality testing, inappropriate affect, blunted affect, hypervigilance or hypovigilance, anhedonia (inability to experience pleasure), mood swings.
- **Defense mechanisms.** *Primary impairments:* The use of predominantly primitive defense mechanisms (such as splitting, acting out, denial, devaluation, dissociation, idealization, isolation of affect, projection) as opposed to more mature defenses (sublimation, humor, rationalization, omnipotence, altruism, autistic fantasy). Defense mechanisms are rigid enough to impair ego functioning.
- **Personality types.** *Primary impairments:* personality disorders (paranoid, antisocial, dependent, borderline, histrionic, narcissistic, avoidant, obsessive-compulsive, schizoid, schizotypal).
- **Coping styles.** *Primary impairments:* external locus of control, self-blame, substance use, and nondirect passive and escape/avoidance modes of coping.
- **Determination of suicidal tendencies, decompensation, and other risks.** *Primary impairments:* history of suicide attempts in self or family members, current suicidal ideation, suicide note, plan for suicide, emotional and/or behavioral regression, substance use, feelings of hopelessness and/or helplessness, birthdays or anniversaries of deaths of loved ones, holidays, anniversaries of traumatic events.
- **Symbolic meaning of the disability and loss, and the compensatory reserves that can be elicited.** *Primary impairments:* Poor compensatory reserves or use of compensatory strategies. The meaning of the disability is both negative and fixed/rigid (e.g., the disability is karmic or a curse that is deserved).
- **Levels of pain, stress, tolerance, and secondary gain.** *Primary impairments:* Low frustration tolerance coupled with high levels of pain and/or stress. The secondary gain of the impairment is high (important) enough to cause a fixation at a lower than expected level of functioning, result in malingering, or interfere with rehabilitation.
- **Sexual practices.** *Primary impairments:* sexual dysfunction, impotence secondary to psychiatric medication, unprotected sex, impulsive sexual behavior, sexual abuse, perversions, hypersexuality, sexual addictions.
- **Current functional capacities.** *Primary impairments:* Problems with basic ADL or instrumental ADL, inability to perform in current roles and occupations, decreased community mobility, inability to live independently.

ADL = activities of daily living.

psychiatrists, psychologists, psychiatric nurses, occupational therapists, social workers, creative arts therapists, vocational counselor, rehabilitation counselor, substance use professionals, and pastoral counselor.

■ PSYCHOSOCIAL ADAPTATION

The combination of intense psychological stress, uncertain prognosis, prolonged treatment, and interference with daily activities can greatly affect the rehabilitation of patients with disabilities and chronic illnesses. Disability is loss of or diminished ability to perform specific social roles normally expected of the patient. Psychosocial adaptation to disability and chronic illness is an ongoing, dynamic, evolving process through which a patient strives to attain an optimal state of function within their environment.[24] Successful psychosocial adaptation may be characterized by (1) a sense of personal mastery; (2) participation in social, recreational, or vocational pursuits; (3) successful negotiation of the environment; and (4) a realistic awareness of one's current strengths, deficits, and functional capacities.[25] Adjustment is the final phase in adaptation and includes striving to achieve life goals, feeling self-confident and having positive self-esteem, possessing a positive attitude toward one's disability, forming emotional connections to others, and establishing a community member role.[26]

The processes of adaptation and adjustment are influenced by whether a chronic illness or disability is congenital or adventitious, of sudden onset or gradually progressive, and stable or unstable. Patients born with a physical disability and those who acquire them as a result of accident or disease later in life have substantial psychological differences.[27] Children born with a physical disability have only experienced life with their impairment; the development of their self-identity commonly mirrors that of children without disabilities.

In contrast, patients with adventitious disabilities often experience acute loss and grief. Patients with gradually progressive diseases or disabilities of sudden onset often experience anxiety and shock when first becoming aware of their condition. Such anxiety and shock are often followed by anger and depression, as patients realize the magnitude and consequences of their diagnosis.[24] Disabilities of sudden onset (e.g., injuries or accidents) are usually experienced as crises that will change the lives of patients and their families for all time.

Grief, Mourning, and Sorrow

Grief is a psychological state of distress resulting from a significant loss. In reaction to a disability, grief may emerge from lost function, broken relationships, the loss of one's familiar self-identity, and disrupted roles. Grief is characterized by preoccupation with loss and feelings of worthlessness or helplessness. Specific symptoms include feelings of tightness of the throat, muscular weakness, emptiness in the abdomen, anxiety that is described as painful, shortness of breath and choking, and periodic waves of physical distress lasting up to an hour. Other symptoms may include forgetfulness, poor concentration, dissociation, insomnia, loss of appetite, compulsive behavior, an inability to manage time in a productive manner, disorganized cognitive functioning, social withdrawal, guilt, decreased ability to make decisions, excessive speech, and hostility.[28] Severe, prolonged cases of grief can compromise the immune system.[29] The grief–mourning period is unpredictable, lasting anywhere from 6 months to 2 years or more. According to Donatelle and Davis, the grieving process consists of 10 stages: (1) frozen feelings; (2) emotional release; (3) loneliness; (4) physical symptoms; (5) guilt; (6) panic; (7) hostility; (8) selective memory; (9) struggle for a new life pattern; and (10) a sense that life is okay.[28] It is important to note that such stages do not always occur in a progressive, linear fashion, and some stages may occur simultaneously.

Grief is a natural experience necessary to regain or adapt to one's losses and construct a new self-concept. New coping skills are learned as patients adjust to unfamiliar challenges. There may be a difference between people grieving over loss from a disability and those grieving over other types of losses.[29] When grief occurs as a result of disability, it may become prolonged, as the patient must continuously strive to accept the disability and his or her altered self. Burke et al.[30] described the grief of people with disabilities as "chronic sorrow," or a grief regarding the loss of normality. Lindgren et al.[31] defined chronic sorrow as (1) progressive sadness that often increases after the initial loss; (2) prolonged periods of sorrow with no predictable end; and (3) recurrent or cyclic in nature as the sadness is continuously triggered by internal or external events that reawaken loss. Patients with chronic sorrow can eventually experience adaptation to their losses if they are highly motivated to rebuild their lives and find meaning in their experience. Conversely, patients with prolonged grief disorder often experience prolonged feelings of guilt, anger, and sadness that inhibit function and adaptation.

It is important to recognize that grief can be an all-encompassing experience that can take time and energy away from rehabilitation, thereby affecting the process of rehabilitation and its outcomes. Physical therapists must understand grieving, mourning, and sorrow so that a patient's lack of progress or motivation is not misinterpreted as malingering.

Phase Models of Psychosocial Adaptation

The literature regarding psychosocial adaptation to chronic disability and illness falls into two opposing theories of adaptation—one in which adaptation occurs as a set of nonsequential and independent patterns of behavior, and the other in which adaptation occurs progressively through a series of phases.

Phase models suggest that a patient's reaction to chronic disability or illness follows a stable sequence of phases, or stages, that are hierarchically and temporally ordered. This progression is gradual, linear, and involves the psychological assimilation of changes to one's body image and self-concept. The most frequently identified phases in the adaptation to chronic disability and disease are shock, anxiety, denial, depression, internalized anger, externalized hostility, acknowledgment, and final adjustment.[24]

Shock

Shock usually occurs as the initial reaction to a psychological trauma or severe and sudden physical injury. It results from an overwhelming experience and may include the inability to move or speak, psychic numbness, decreased cognitive skills, disorganization, and depersonalization.

During a traumatic event, an individual will respond primarily at the physiological level; emotional reactions are commonly delayed until the event is over, and the individual is medically stable. Likewise, the medical emergency team will first implement immediate lifesaving attempts before addressing accompanying psychological issues.

During a perceived or real catastrophic event, an organism would most likely respond with what Selye termed the general adaptation syndrome (GAS).[32] Selye described GAS as an organism's defensive adaptation attempt, which expresses itself through physiological and emotional responses aimed at dealing with such emergencies. During GAS, there is a physiochemical chain reaction, whereby a peptide called corticotropin-releasing factor (CRF) is secreted to stimulate the release of adrenocorticotropic hormone (ACTH). ACTH sets into motion an increase of specific physiological activity designed to maximize the body's defense capacity while minimizing the utilization of nonessential physiological activities. Although an increase in CRF serves the person's self-defensive strategies, its inhibitory effect on other body functions—such as the production of insulin and calcium—is undesirable in the long run.

Studies have shown that injection of a CRF antagonist reduces anxiety in stressful situations.[33] When the inhibitory effects of CRF are prolonged, however, the additional undesirable effects of hypertension, digestive problems, and interference with the immune system result. Selye[32] documented the devastating effect that a prolonged GAS response has on human mental and physical functioning.[32] Theorell et al.[34] documented the occurrence of resultant illnesses long after the stress-producing event had ended.

Anxiety

Once the magnitude of the traumatic event is comprehended, anxiety in the form of a panic-stricken reaction commonly occurs and is marked by compulsive activity, confusion, elevated pulse rate, difficulty breathing, and cognitive flooding (e.g., when emotions such as anxiety preclude logical thought). Situations that activate the sympathetic nervous system through repeated alarm or chronic stress may alter synaptic transmission and lead to depression and malfunction of normal body systems.

It should be noted that the physiological and psychological reactions to stress are not limited to catastrophic conditions. An extensive body of research shows stress reactions to be present in individuals under conditions that may not be traumatic but nevertheless persistent and disruptive. Everyday life frustrations, internal and external conflicts, and changes in life conditions are major causes of the stress reaction that, over time, have a deleterious effect on a person's function and health. Physical therapists should be cognizant that even though a patient's emergency is over, a stress reaction may continue to be present.

Denial

Denial is often used as a defense mechanism to alleviate the anxiety and pain associated with a disability or illness.[35] Denial occurs as a specific phase early in the adaptation process and protects the person from having to confront the overwhelming implications of illness or injury all at once. Instead, denial allows a gradual assimilation of one's altered reality. Breznitz[36] identified seven types of denial:

1. Denial of threatening information (using selective inattention and partial awareness)
2. Denial of vulnerability (exerting control and maximizing personal strengths)
3. Denial of urgency (using methods to see the situation as less pressing than it is)
4. Denial of affect (reduction of emotional impact)
5. Denial of affect relevance (diverting attention to other issues and believing that an emotion is coming from an unrelated cause)
6. Denial of personal relevance (attributing difficulties to a benign cause and blaming others when involvement was one's own)
7. Denial of all information (creating a barrier between external reality and one's psyche, resulting in total disbelief of having an illness or disability)

Patients in the stage of denial may selectively attend to the environment, choose facts that support their beliefs about themselves and their condition, and ignore facts that remind them of their new challenges. They may have unrealistic and wishful goals for recovery and may appear indifferent and aloof.

Depression

The phase of depression occurs as denial lessens, allowing a greater awareness of one's losses. Depression is a reactive response of bereavement for impending death, suffering, or the loss of body function. Neurochemical and biological changes resulting from disability or disease, premorbid personality and family history, and reactions to stress have all been identified as risk factors for depression.[37,38]

Internalized Anger

Anger occurs in reaction to anxiety, misperception, threats of abandonment, feelings of helplessness, or fear of losing control. Characteristics of anger include hostility, resentment, or hatred. Anger is a response to loss and if not expressed, is termed *internalized anger*. Internalized anger is associated with self-blame and is a manifestation of self-directed bitterness and resentment. Signs of internalized anger include manipulation, sabotage, and passive-aggressive behavior. Sometimes anger emerges when a patient attributes their own behaviors to the onset of disability or disease. In such cases, internalized anger can result in depression, suicidal tendencies, or psychosomatic complaints—particularly in people who have a chronic condition.[39]

There are many reasons why patients may not express anger: fear of losing loved ones or social isolation, cultural restraints, lack of awareness, fear of losing control, or belief that expressing anger is inappropriate or dangerous. Repressed anger not only affects a patient's psychological well-being but may also slow rehabilitation. It is important for physical therapists to encourage expression of angry feelings by providing a safe environment for patients to verbalize their anger in appropriate ways. Therapists might state that anger is a normal emotion—especially under the patient's circumstances; offer reasons why it is important to express anger; and provide anger management techniques (e.g., effective coping strategies). It is equally important for therapists to understand that although a patient's anger may be directed at the therapist, such anger more often reflects the patient's own projected feelings regarding their disability.

Externalized Hostility

Externalized hostility is anger directed toward other people or objects in the environment and is an attempt to retaliate against activity limitations. Challenges encountered during rehabilitation may trigger externalized hostility. As time from the onset of the disability passes, externalized hostility tends to become more apparent.[40] Signs include passive-aggressive behaviors that obstruct rehabilitation, aggressive acts, hypercriticism, demanding or antagonistic behaviors, falsely blaming others, and abusive accusations. Patients who express anger aggressively through physical or verbal abuse, sarcasm, or controlling behaviors need the help of the entire team to redirect their anger into productive therapeutic activities that further their rehabilitation goals.

Acknowledgment

Acknowledgment is the first sign that the patient has accepted or recognized the permanency of the condition and its future implications. The patient begins to integrate activity limitations into their self-concept. During this phase, the patient accepts themself as a person with a disability, develops a new self-concept, reassesses values, and searches for new goals and meaning.

Adjustment

Adjustment is the final phase in adaptation and involves the development of new ways of interacting successfully with others and one's environment. The person is now adjusted to the outside world after having fully assimilated their activity limitations from disability into a new, cohesive self. In this phase, the person regains self-worth, understands that new potentials are possible, pursues vocational[41,42] and social goals, and overcomes obstacles that arise in the attainment of goals.[43]

There is evidence that the phase model of adjustment to chronic disability or illness is nonlinear, multidimensional, and progressive. Phase models tend to have 10 common assumptions:[24]

1. People may skip one or more phases or may regress to an earlier phase, but adaptation is not usually reversible.
2. The pace and structure of adaptation can be influenced by external events or interventions (e.g., environmental changes or counseling) yet are mainly determined by internal processes.
3. Not everyone achieves adjustment; some fixate at earlier phases.
4. Adaptation is an unfolding, dynamic process that gradually shifts from initial experiences of distress to assimilation of loss and reconciliation.
5. The adaptation process is initiated by significant and permanent changes in the body's functional capacities and appearance, which are usually followed by alteration of self-concept and body image.
6. The amount of time spent in each phase varies and may be determined by a combination of the following factors: social support, financial and human resources, past exposure to crises, age at onset, severity, nature of the disability or illness, and premorbid personality.
7. Psychological maturity and growth occur as the patient progresses through the phases.
8. Psychological re-equilibrium occurs through gradual adaptation and integration of the perceived misfortune.
9. Human variability and uniqueness have a strong influence on the temporal ordering of phases—the sequence of phases is not universal.
10. Occasionally, phases may overlap, be nondiscrete, or fluctuate, causing patients to experience more than one reaction at a time.

Chronic Illness and Disability: Differences in Adaptation

There are marked differences in the way that people adapt psychosocially to a disability associated with a traumatic event, such as TBI, versus a chronic illness, such as multiple sclerosis (MS). The onset of disability in a traumatic event is sudden, and medical stability may be achieved shortly after. The onset of a chronic illness is usually insidious and gradual; its course is often uncertain and marked by states of remission and deterioration.[44] In chronic illness, each onset of symptoms can be experienced as a new illness.

Shock may not be experienced by people with gradually deteriorating medical conditions (e.g., Parkinson disease, rheumatoid arthritis, or diabetes mellitus), but is usually experienced following a trauma (e.g., TBI, myocardial infarction, amputation, or SCI). The phases of anxiety and depression relate more to the past, such as grieving over the loss of premorbid functioning. Shock may be present but is not as strong in people with life-threatening or end-stage diseases (e.g., AIDS, cancer, or amyotrophic lateral sclerosis). In a chronic illness, anxiety and depression relate more to the future (e.g., fear of death, feelings of hopelessness, and fear of the unknown).[45] The acknowledgment and adjustment phases may be more difficult to achieve in chronic, life-threatening conditions that require the internalization of and acceptance that the condition may worsen and result in death.

Post-traumatic Rehabilitation

The post-traumatic period may include phases of anxiety, depression, denial, internalized anger, and externalized hostility mentioned earlier, and is usually the time during which much, if not most, of the rehabilitative intervention takes place. It is also the period during which the psychological effects of the traumatic experience are more strongly felt by the patient. It seems as if the psychological defenses and reactions that became secondary during the initial traumatic period (shock phase) begin emerging as the physical injury is dealt with. These repressed reactions seem to interact with a growing awareness of the effects of the disability creating fears, anxieties, and behaviors that the rehabilitation team must address.

Regardless of which phase the patient is in, physical therapists need to be aware of each patient's psychological needs. During the initial phases of adaptation, patients may experience an awareness of their injuries that facilitates panic and fear of total dependence. Patients may also experience anxiety as a result of anticipating painful medical treatment. Some patients react to these feelings by desperately seeking control over their rehabilitation. Others experience shock regarding their losses and become overly dependent. Patients may idealize the past and have unrealistic expectations about the duration of their recovery.

During these early stages, physical therapists should praise small gains and work with caregivers so they can offer hope and support to the patient. Therapists should be supportive but careful not to make unrealistic predictions about the expected degree of recovery, because this may lead to disappointment, resentment, and depression.[46] One of the first approaches physical therapists can use to help patients regain self-control is diaphragmatic breathing, which may decrease pain and anxiety through the relaxation response.[47]

During the middle stages, physical therapists may need to educate patients about medical precautions, contraindicated movements or activities, how the patient's body has adapted to disability, and how to reformulate expectations. Psychosocial instruction should be integrated with information about activities of daily living (ADL),[48] mobility, strengthening, and endurance. The transition from the patient role to an independent adult member of society is a difficult adjustment and can result in anxiety, depression, and poor social integration.[24,49] Physical therapists should help patients prepare psychologically for discharge and reintegration into society. Some of the issues that patients may fear include negative reactions to their disability, feelings of inadequacy, having to identify new social supports, receiving help in the home environment, and adjusting to a new body image.

Body image includes judgment about one's appearance, an awareness of boundaries and personal space, judgment about one's bodily responses, perception of one's body parts and their movement, and an awareness of physical pleasure and pain. Body image is intimately related to self-concept and self-esteem. It affects a person's functional abilities, cognition, perceptions, attitudes, and emotions, as well as the reactions of others to oneself. Because body image changes throughout life, it is thought to be both dynamic and developmentally based. Difficulties brought on by a disability—such as activity limitations and pain and disfigurement—alter body image and threaten its stability. Patients must then reconstruct their body image and self-perception to adapt to this physical change.[24]

Biordi[50] has identified the following patterns in patients who experienced shifts in body image after disability: (1) denying the existence of one's body; (2) fantasizing about a lost or damaged body part being magically replaced or healthy; (3) concentrating solely on noninjured body parts to deny impairment of the affected area; and (4) experiencing a period of defensiveness followed by gradual acceptance and assimilation of their altered body. The physical therapist's comfort level with the patient's physical disability and the therapist's attention to the affected body part may help the patient feel less ashamed about body changes.

■ PERSONALITY AND COPING STYLES

The more patients have evolved socially and psychologically, the better they will be at using adaptive methods to deal with crises. Hence, a patient with a healthy premorbid personality but a severe physical disability may do better in rehabilitation than one with a less severe disability and a pathological premorbid personality.[51] When aware of their patients' personality styles, physical therapists will be more adept at strategizing interventions, developing a plan of care, and motivating and guiding patients through rehabilitation.

Personality Types

Although each personality is unique, personalities have been categorized into different types, such as *type A, perfectionistic, authoritative,* and *passive-aggressive.* These personality types are nonpathological and develop in response to one's environment when young.

Individuals with type A personalities have a compulsive need to be achievers in all aspects of life. They are extremely independent and productive. These qualities also serve as defenses against low self-esteem and interpersonal conflicts. These people usually derive satisfaction from being strong individuals who can help others. If they can no longer participate in this role, they may become depressed because of a perceived inability to confirm their worth through altruistic activities. Physical therapists can use these qualities in patients with type A personalities to motivate their interest in rehabilitation. Because they are often self-starters and take initiative for their own learning, they can usually be depended on to independently practice home exercise programs.

Individuals with perfectionistic personalities uphold high standards to maintain self-esteem. These individuals judge themselves by inflexible and possibly unachievable criteria and may not be able to tolerate slow progress during rehabilitation. Physical therapists may aid these patients by helping them derive pleasure from simple things, such as a meal, a sunset, a new shirt, or interesting information. Helping them discover value in these things offers them sources of self-esteem other than meeting impossibly high standards.

Individuals with authoritative personalities need to be in control and need things to be done in a particular way because of rigid perceptions regarding values, rules, and the manner in which others should behave. They are often concerned with status, tend to be judgmental, and have difficulty empathizing with others. During rehabilitation, these patients may try to dictate their treatment and engage in a power struggle with their physical therapists. Patients with authoritative personalities have difficulty adapting to disability, which often requires acceptance and compromise. They may require alternative strategies to solve what may have been perceived as an unsolvable problem. Physical therapists should engage patients in problem-solving to generate strategies to meet their goals.

Individuals with passive-aggressive personalities express hostility by using passive techniques such as procrastination, resistance, stubbornness, and intentional inefficiency. These personalities react to authority negatively and have difficulty working with others. Physical therapists may work more efficiently with passive-aggressive patients by placing the responsibility for progress on them. Patients can be instructed to make decisions about their treatment whenever possible and then summarize their progress after each session. This deemphasizes the physical therapist's role as an authority figure and therefore the need for a passive-aggressive response.

Personality Disorders

When an individual's personality style deviates from cultural norms over a long period of time, is inflexible or pervasive, causes distress to oneself and others, and leads to activity limitations, that personality style is considered dysfunctional.[11] Personality disorders have been thoroughly classified. They include paranoid, antisocial (also referred to as sociopath or psychopath), borderline, histrionic, narcissistic, avoidant, dependent, obsessive-compulsive, schizoid, and schizotypal personalities. Freidman and Booth-Kewley[52] state that disability exacerbates preexisting pathology, meaning that the stress of dealing with a physical illness can make personality disorders even more pronounced.

Patients with paranoid personality disorder interpret the motives of others as malevolent when they may not be. This results from a pattern of suspiciousness and distrust. These patients believe that others are trying to exploit, deceive, or harm them. Because of such mistrust, they may discharge themselves from treatment. Physical therapists should look for behaviors that indicate paranoid thoughts such as hostile reactions, guardedness, argumentation, and stubbornness, and encourage patients to express their thoughts at that moment. If the patient seems paranoid, the physical therapist should help them to better understand the reality of a specific situation. For instance, if the patient complains about being forced to participate in an elaborate intervention so that, in their view, the therapist can make more money, the therapist should review the pros and cons of various treatments and discuss the clinical reasoning involved. Literature can be very convincing since it does not come directly from the therapist.

Patients with antisocial personality frequently engage in deceit and manipulation. In rehabilitation, they may use an alias, lie to the staff, or malinger. They are irresponsible and often fail to comply with self-care procedures such as hygiene and home maintenance. They seek out and take advantage of weaker staff members, often using wit and charm. When they do not receive what they want, they commonly become irritable and violent, especially when staff members attempt to impose restrictions. They frequently cause disruption to others in rehabilitation. These patients require a cohesive team approach with immediate and strong

intercommunication to minimize disruptive behaviors and refocus on rehabilitation goals.

Patients with borderline personality disorder have instability in emotions, relationships, and self-image; are impulsive; use primitive defense mechanisms such as splitting and devaluation; and tend to engage in self-destructive behaviors such as abusing drugs or self-mutilation. On the surface, they may appear critical of others, but these are signs of deep vulnerability and should be treated as such. Therapists should respond with understanding and empathy instead of anger and should emphasize strengths and strategies for ongoing work. Self-mutilating behaviors, such as repetitive cutting with razor blades, pinpricking, or cigarette burning, should be immediately reported to a doctor and referral made to a psychiatrist.

Patients with histrionic personality disorder seek attention via excessive emotionality. Since these patients respond well to audiences, therapists should provide situations in which patients can gain positive attention from doing well in rehabilitation. Physical therapists should set boundaries to help patients achieve a balance between their need to express themselves and their need to focus on therapeutic interventions. A calm and logical approach to rehabilitation helps settle intense emotions. Patients who have difficulty verbalizing their feelings can be referred to a creative arts therapist to facilitate expression through nonverbal means—such as music, dance, or art.

Patients with narcissistic personality disorder are condescending and have a need for admiration and feelings of superiority. If an illness causes a reduction in this image, they will require help from their physical therapists to identify strengths and feel acceptable.

Patients with schizoid personality disorder have a flat affect, or limited range of emotional expression, and are detached from social interactions. The therapist should attend to the patient's rehabilitation without trying to engage them in a great deal of social interaction. If the disorder has been long-standing, the patient will likely feel uncomfortable socializing.

Patients with schizotypal personality disorder have eccentric behavior, perceptual or cognitive distortions, and marked distress in social relationships. The social intimacy and physical restriction of a rehabilitation environment may cause anxiety. Slow, unforced integration into the therapeutic setting may be required. Asking patients whether their views of reality are accurate may help them remain focused on achieving rehabilitation goals.

Patients with avoidant personality disorder suffer from social inhibition, feelings of inadequacy, and hypersensitivity to criticism. Physical therapists should reassure these patients that they are doing well and emphasize their strengths.

Patients with dependent personality disorder exhibit clinging behavior, need others to care for them, and are submissive. They may fail to function independently in their life roles even after physical functioning has returned, continuing the pattern of dependency. They fear abandonment and require constant reassurances that staff members understand their condition and care about them. Some respond to clear explanations and feedback about their progress and treatment plans. The therapist should reinforce independent behavior through attention and positive feedback while extinguishing dependent behavior by ignoring or redirecting it.

Patients with obsessive-compulsive personality disorder have a long-standing preoccupation with control and order and are often perfectionists. Their self-esteem may suffer if they perceive a loss of control, and they may react by becoming more obstinate, demanding, and inflexible. Those who publicly express their anger may become ashamed. These patients require greater predictability in treatment than usual, dislike change, and do well when given an established routine to follow. The therapist should provide rehabilitative activities that promote a sense of control and predictability and consider allowing patients to set treatment goals, then monitor their daily progress.

Coping Styles

Coping styles are ways that people deal with stress and include behavioral, emotional, and cognitive efforts to cope with internal and external challenges that strain ordinary resources.[53] Theories of coping suggest that it is not what happens to people that is important, but rather how they react.[54] Various coping strategies have been identified in the literature and summarized by Livneh and Antonak.[24] They include planning, problem-solving, wishful thinking, avoiding, minimizing, seeking social support, searching for meaning, emoting feelings, blaming, accepting, negotiating, disengaging, and turning to religion. These and other coping styles can be categorized into three different types: (1) seeking versus avoiding control and information; (2) expressing versus repressing emotional reactions; and (3) seeking versus withdrawing from social interactions and networks.

Coping strategies have been found to be of great importance in rehabilitation. Patients with higher-level coping skills can more easily identify and report symptoms, make treatment decisions, comply with intervention, and accept support. Patients with good problem-solving skills and positive attitudes have been found to make more positive adjustments to their disabilities than patients with low self-esteem and poor self-concept.[55] Coping styles often determine whether patients seek medical help and follow advice.[53]

Social influences, psychological characteristics, and health beliefs have been shown to modify the impact of disability and disease on an individual. Social activism, positive self-acceptance, and information seeking have predicted better ability to cope with a disability.[56]

Krause and Rohe[57] studied the relationship between adjustment and personality following SCI and found that positive values, emotions, actions, and warmth correlated with superior outcomes. Adaptive coping styles that result in positive outcomes for people with disabilities utilize positive, direct, and active problem-solving, social support seeking, and information seeking. Maladaptive coping styles that lead to unfavorable adaptation outcomes include self-blame; nondirect, passive, and escape/avoidance modes of coping; and substance use.

Locus of control is a belief about one's ability to control life conditions and events.[58] Patients with an *external locus of control* believe that other people or outside factors determine outcomes. Patients with an *internal locus of control* take responsibility for change because they believe they can affect their own circumstances. The latter leads to goal-directed activity and active coping.

The ability to intentionally change the relative importance of events that occur in one's life requires constant practice.[59] It has been shown that patients with external loci of control experience stress and anxiety in rehabilitation, whereas patients with internal loci of control have quicker recoveries, better motivation, more hope, and more energy.

Coping styles can be examined through interviews, observations, self-report surveys, checklists, and information from the family. Treatment considerations based on these findings should include emphasis on previous ways of successfully coping and expanding the range of coping strategies, such as maintaining a journal to increase self-expression. Taking care of a pet or using animal assistance can lend help, comfort, and companionship, as well as increase motivation. Group treatment can also be used to increase social networks.[60,61]

Many people with disabilities who have risk factors for emotional problems, such as lower education level, less income, and social isolation, still do well in life because of a certain resilience defined as successful adaptation to stressful situations or events.[62] Researchers of resilience[63] identify protective factors that safeguard people from adverse consequences. Protective factors can arise from the individual, family, and society and are concerned with how these strengths and supports provide security, safety, and positive opportunities.

Turning points are important experiences and realizations that enable people to find new direction, purpose, or meaning in life. King et al.[64] reported four protective factors: determination, perseverance, spiritual beliefs, and social support. Seven protective processes were also identified: transcending, self-understanding, accommodating, receiving a diagnosis that helps explain a patient's experiences, believing in oneself, using anger as motivation, and setting goals. These protective factors and processes help people with disabilities during turning points in their lives. Analysis of turning points revealed three major ways that patients maintained meaning in their lives: through doing, belonging, and understanding themselves in relation to the world. Doing involves participating in activities that are fulfilling and facilitate competency. Belonging involves perceived acceptance by others or membership in a valued group. Understanding oneself in relationship to the larger world provides a sense of identity and sometimes purpose.

■ COMMON DEFENSE REACTIONS TO DISABILITY

Defense mechanisms are coping styles that people use to defend against internal and external stressors. They happen automatically and unconsciously. Some individuals use many different defense mechanisms throughout their lives, but most tend to utilize only one or two. The goal is not to change or modify these defense mechanisms, but to identify them to understand the patient's psychological processes that underlie certain behaviors and resistance. Understanding these behaviors can help physical therapists to motivate or redirect patients during difficult times in their rehabilitation. The defense mechanisms described in Box 26.2 are common reactions to disability and can be further explored in the *Diagnostic and Statistical Manual of Mental Disorders.*[11]

Box 26.2   Common Defense Mechanisms

Acting Out

Instead of expressing feelings verbally, the patient uses actions to release stress. For example, a patient is angry with the insurance company for not funding an athletic wheelchair, so refuses to use the standard wheelchair. Acting out occurs because certain feelings such as anger and hurt are too difficult to express verbally. Unexpressed feelings build anxiety until they are released through action.

The therapist should identify the feeling behind the acting out behavior by asking the patient why they behaved in that way. For instance, the therapist would ask the patient above about using the wheelchair. The patient's responses will eventually trace back to the original unexpressed feeling. Through questioning, the therapist brings to the patient's awareness the link between the feeling and the action. The patient can now verbalize and discuss the feeling. In the case above, the patient may be more willing to use the wheelchair. A patient who does not have difficulty verbalizing feelings tends not to act out.

Altruism

The patient becomes dedicated to helping others to manage their own stress. An altruistic patient may stop treatment to help everyone else in the treatment room, including the therapist. Such a patient receives gratification through these actions, and hence decreases their stress.

Autistic Fantasy

The patient engages in excessive daydreaming instead of pursuing human relationships to decrease stress. The patient may have difficulty following directions, may appear to be in another world, but happily so, and may become emotional and tense when returned to reality. If asked what they were thinking about, the patient may describe their fantasies, which can be a rich source of wishes and desires that can be used by the therapist to motivate the patient to work on short-term goals. For instance, a male patient relates a fantasy of dating his favorite teen idol. However, to engage in dating, he must first develop interpersonal skills and practice them in simulated and real-life settings.

Denial

Denial protects the ego from being overwhelmed by pain through an unrelenting process of disbelief. In the case of disability, denial may be used to protect the patient from reminders of an altered external reality and the resultant sense of loss. Therefore, the patient may refuse to acknowledge an emotionally painful condition or situation that is apparent to others. The patient often denies the severity of a new disability, believing they can return to previous jobs or roles, despite reality testing from the therapist. The patient may refuse rehabilitation, claiming that they just want to leave the hospital to care for their children.

It is important to help the patient work through denial slowly to avoid depression, which may occur if the patient becomes aware of their reality before psychologically ready to accept it. If the patient's denial is so great that treatment cannot proceed, the patient should be referred to a psychologist to explore what disability means to their future.

Devaluation

The patient is overly critical of others and of themself and may insult therapists and other personnel. The therapist should not take such insults personally, but should offer empathy and kindness, which usually decrease devaluation and build rapport. Once a patient trusts the therapist, they may discuss insecurities and fears instead of defending against them through criticism. If the therapist becomes angry with the patient, the insults usually become worse, and a power struggle may ensue.

Box 26.2   Common Defense Mechanisms—cont'd

Displacement

The patient transfers a response to, or feeling about, one object onto a less threatening object to minimize stress. For example, a patient may be angry with a spouse for driving the car recklessly and having an accident but takes the anger out on the physical therapist. In this situation, it may not be safe or helpful for the patient to express anger directly to the spouse, who may be the patient's only emotional support.

   The therapist should help the patient transfer the misplaced feeling back to the object for which it was originally intended. The therapist might accomplish this by asking the patient a series of questions concerning the origin of the anger.

Dissociation

The patient deals with stress through a breakdown in memory, perception, consciousness, or sensorimotor behavior. The patient becomes detached from what is happening in the moment because it is too painful. The patient may stop speaking or participating in therapy and stare blankly into space for up to several minutes without responding to the environment. Afterward, patients may not be aware of their dissociated state, or if they are, patients may state that they "just spaced out." The patient who uses dissociation usually relies on it often; a physical therapist may note its occurrence several times during a session. It is important to notice what happened just before the dissociation to identify the painful thoughts, feelings, or actions that upset the patient.

Help-Rejecting

The patient deals with the stress of having covert hostile feelings toward caregivers by frequently asking for help and then rejecting every suggestion. Working with a patient who uses help-rejecting as a defense mechanism can be very frustrating. Such patients seem to sincerely seek help but reject all advice as ineffectual. In these cases, it may be helpful to point out to the patient that efforts to help have been thwarted. The patient is usually not aware that they have rejected all solutions and may then come up with a solution or be more open to one that has already been proposed.

Humor

Humor can be used to minimize stress by highlighting the ironic or amusing aspects of a stressful situation. For instance, a patient states that he is going to open a hardware store since he has so much hardware (meaning surgically placed pins and plates) in his leg. A patient who uses humor as a defense mechanism usually feels better if the physical therapist laughs at their jokes and participates in joking behavior. It is a safe way for the patient to recognize the difficulty of their situation.

Idealization

A patient endows another individual with overly positive attributes to enhance an otherwise negative situation. This other individual may be the therapist, in which case the therapeutic relationship is often strengthened. Or it could be a spouse, in which case problems could arise if the spouse is not a positive support to the patient. It is important to uncover the reality of the situation so necessary treatment and discharge plans can be made.

Intellectualization

A patient uses intellectual reasoning rather than expressing emotions to avoid painful feelings. For example, the patient describes neurotransmitters and synapses when asked about a head injury. Therapists can relate to such patients by intellectualizing with them. For example, the therapist may speak about the patient's head injury in terms of science and facts instead of emotions.

Isolation of Affect

A patient separates feelings from ideas when thinking about and discussing an upsetting event to minimize negative feelings associated with it. The patient may speak of the details regarding the recent accident that caused a disability without mentioning any feelings associated with the event to avoid reexperiencing them. Therapists should help the patient integrate feelings about an event into their memory of it. This can be achieved by asking patients how they feel about certain aspects of the event while talking about it.

Omnipotence

Patients feel or act as if they are better than others to guard against feelings of inadequacy. For instance, a patient looks down on other patients with disabilities because he does not want to see himself as disabled. A therapist might observe criticism and devaluation of external objects, bragging about accomplishments or skills, conceit, and grandiosity. The therapist could use this defense mechanism to motivate the patient to get better to avoid feeling inferior.

(Continued)

Box 26.2   Common Defense Mechanisms—cont'd

Projection

A patient transfers their own unacceptable feelings, thoughts, and beliefs onto another person and becomes certain that the other person really feels, thinks, and believes that way. A patient cannot tolerate the idea of having unacceptable feelings such as anger, but expresses them by projecting them onto another person, remaining relatively guilt free. For example, a patient says that his therapist is annoyed with him when in fact the patient is annoyed with his therapist.

Rationalization

Patients use elaborate explanations to reassure themselves that personal actions are driven by sound motives when in fact they may truly be unsure. A family member caring for a relative with congestive heart failure asks for a do not resuscitate (DNR) status, citing extensive research studies. The family member states that the relative will die soon anyway, thereby concealing the real and less acceptable reason for seeking the DNR status—to relieve themselves from caregiving responsibilities.

Repression

A patient unconsciously erases negative experiences, wishes, or thoughts from consciousness to decrease stress. For example, a patient finds an endearing letter to a spouse from a student and forgets to mention it because the possibility of the spouse having an affair is painful. Repressed material can be dangerous because it remains in the unconscious. Encouraging the patient to express their feelings, both good and bad, helps free them of these feelings and any possible negative urges to act on them.

Splitting

A patient views a person or event through a positive or negative lens at any given point in time. Later, the patient may flip their feelings to the opposite end of the spectrum regarding the same person or situation, acting in this manner because they have difficulty integrating ambivalent feelings. Some patients will often attempt to split staff, identifying one staff member with unrealistic positive attributes, while identifying another staff member with unrealistic negative qualities. The staff member who has been identified as negative has usually denied some desire the patient requested. The patient may approach the positively identified therapist and complain that the first therapist is insensitive and does not understand their needs. The patient may express that only the positively identified therapist understands their problems. However, when the positively identified therapist also denies the patient's request, the patient then vilifies that therapist as well. The therapist may help the patient to integrate the opposite poles of their emotions by bringing both positive and negative emotions into consciousness. The patient then may be able to see the reality of their situation.

Sublimation

Sublimation occurs when patients transform unacceptable emotions or desires into socially acceptable actions. For example, a patient who is angry about a recent divorce may be unable to consciously express those feelings for fear of losing the affection of their children. Instead of expressing anger, the patient may sublimate those emotions into a more socially acceptable action, such as working out in the gym and eventually training for marathons. By participating in an activity that is valued and admired in society, the patient gains the positive support of others.

Suppression

A patient intentionally avoids thoughts of disturbing feelings, situations, experiences, or problems to reduce stress. When refusing to talk to the therapist about the accident that brought them to rehabilitation, the patient suppresses disturbing thoughts. Therapists can refer patients to creative arts therapists (e.g., dance, music, art, drama, or poetry therapists) to facilitate the expression of disturbing thoughts because such emotions accrue over time if not expressed.

Undoing

A patient uses behavior or words to negate unacceptable actions, thoughts, or feelings. For example, a patient who is frequently bullied by another patient during rehabilitation feels rage against the aggressor but invites them to lunch.

Note: In both undoing and suppression, disturbing feelings are intentionally avoided. In suppression, the feelings are avoided and nothing else happens. Feelings are avoided and concealed through opposing words or actions. Both undoing and suppression differ from repression in that repression is an unconscious act.

■ COMMON PSYCHOSOCIAL ISSUES

Anxiety

Anxiety is the apprehensive anticipation of future danger or misfortune accompanied by feelings of tension and agitation. The anticipated danger may be real or imagined, but it is experienced both psychologically and physiologically.[65] The experience of anxiety varies in different patients. When people are nervous (indicating a moderate level of anxiety), they may experience an upset stomach or headache. When experiencing a panic attack (indicating a high level of anxiety), people may feel impending doom and terror. A symptom of anxiety in one patient may be heart palpitations, while in another it may be shortness of breath. What is anxiety producing to one patient may cause little to no anxiety in another. Given these variables, the following definitions may facilitate physical therapists' understanding of their patients' conditions.

A panic attack is a sudden onset of intense, overwhelming fear that may include feelings of imminent danger or impending doom. These attacks are marked by symptoms of palpitations, chest pain, smothering or choking sensations, shortness of breath, and fear of losing control, dying, or going crazy. Panic attacks may be unexpected (occurring without an internal or external trigger) or situational. It is unclear what kind of physiological change in the brain may trigger such a severe response. A phobia is an anxiety disorder characterized by intense anxiety resulting from thoughts of, or exposure to, a specific feared situation or object (such as heights, spiders, or elevators) leading to avoidance of that object or situation. Generalized anxiety disorder is defined as excessive worry and anxiety without an apparent source persisting for at least 6 months.[11]

Causes of Anxiety

Twenty to 30 million Americans experience anxiety.[28] Some signs and symptoms of anxiety are listed in Table 26.2, and behaviors that may result from anxiety are provided in Table 26.3. Much of the literature on stress and coping has identified major life events as stressors. Life events refer to major changes in lifestyle, status, role, or situation. This view is consistent with the notion that stress, though individually mediated, is to some degree environmentally based and/or exacerbated by environmental and social conditions. Various life event measures have been developed and are used in examining potential environmental stress. One of the more well-known and used instruments is the Holmes-Rahe Social Readjustment Rating Scale (http://www.simplypsychology.org/SRRS.html), which quantifies the effects of life changes on stress and health.[66] Such measures of life events assume a relatively global impact and consider only those items listed. Although there is justified validity in such an approach, there exist potentially more sensitive and valid measures, one of which is the Hassles Scale.

The Hassles Scale, developed by Kanner et al.,[67] requires subjects to identify the irritating and frustrating demands of everyday transactions with the environment.

Table 26.2   Signs and Symptoms Associated With Low, Moderate, and High Levels of Anxiety

Low-Level Anxiety	Moderate-Level Anxiety	High-Level Anxiety
Agitation	Abdominal distress	Chest pains
Apprehension	Aches	Depersonalization
Distress	Chills	De-realization (feeling unreal)
Irritability	Decreased concentration	Difficulty sleeping
Motor restlessness	Diarrhea	Dizziness
Muscle tension	Fear	Dread
Nervousness	Feeling light-headed, unsteady, or faint	Helplessness
Worry	Fever	Horror
	Heart palpitations	Hypervigilance
	Hot flashes	Increased sensitivity to pain
	Increased heart rate	Nausea
	Misperception	Paresthesia
	Shaking or trembling	
	Shortness of breath	
	Sweating	

Table 26.3	Behaviors Associated With Low, Moderate, and High Levels of Anxiety	
Low-Level Anxiety	**Moderate-Level Anxiety**	**High-Level Anxiety**
Avoiding stressful situations	Going to the bathroom frequently	Holding hand over heart
Biting lips	Incessant talking	Reacting to irrelevant cues
Drumming fingers on a tabletop	Mumbling	Throwing up
Fidgeting	Overactivity	
Nail biting	Staring blankly	
Pacing	Verbalizing somatic preoccupations	
Pulling or twirling hair		
Rubbing an object such as worry beads		
Shaking legs		
Sighing heavily		
Tapping feet		

This approach considers the individual's perception of events believed to pose a threat. It is consistent with the theoretical assumption that chronic struggle may tax coping abilities and lead to greater difficulty in the management of daily life events. Considering the enormous changes in a person's function when disability occurs, patients are more likely to expect an increase in daily hassles and stressors. Dealing with life becomes more taxing when disabling circumstances block one's coping style, causing a gap between the person and their fit within the world. Repeat occurrences of stress and the continual need to adjust to new situations can result in repetition of the fight-or-flight response, which can, over time, result in high blood pressure leading to heart attack or stroke.[23]

Anxiety and Rehabilitation

Different levels of anxiety have different effects on patients. If anxiety is completely absent, patients may not be motivated to achieve treatment goals. Mild anxiety can be motivating if directed toward rehabilitation. Severe anxiety can escalate quickly and impair all aspects of the patient's life, including rehabilitation outcomes, by intensifying the perception of pain, inhibiting immunosuppression, and prolonging recovery time.[68,69] Patients who had difficulty managing anxiety before physical illness will probably have more difficulty managing stress brought on by disability.

When a patient is anxious, thought and energy often become focused on the anxiety instead of physical therapy, resulting in decreased concentration. Decreased learning may be observed when a patient is unable to concentrate on the therapist's instructions. The patient may be unable to perform motor tasks that require multiple-step directions. Poor concentration can also result in safety risks as the patient's attention may be alternating between the anxiety and the demands of rehabilitation. To appear functional, the patient may try to perform a task having heard only part of the therapist's instructions. Such a patient may fail to understand directions given by the therapist and may not realize that they have missed important information. Steps may be skipped, and a patient may jump ahead too quickly, resulting in injuries to the patient or others.

If patients become fearful because of anxiety, they may avoid certain behaviors in an attempt to decrease their fear. Fearful, anxious patients are reluctant to try new things. They may refuse treatment, remain in their rooms, request a bedpan when they are capable of using the commode, or be reluctant to progress to the next step in therapy. Such patients will commonly make statements such as, "I can't. I don't feel well. I'm too tired. Leave me alone. Not now, I'll do it later. I'm afraid. You can't help me. You don't look strong enough. I'm going to fall."

Patients who express anxiety through overactivity may attempt to progress too quickly through rehabilitation. They often want to achieve everything at once and appear impatient. They tend to rush through a treatment activity without mastering each step. Such patients frequently talk of discharge before it is an option. They may make rash decisions regarding major life changes, such as purchasing new cars or planning vacations when neither would be in their best interest. Such behaviors may provide immediate relief from anxiety for both patients and their families yet cause more distress in the long run.

When anxiety causes misperception, patients may perceive their level of dysfunction and improvement differently than do their therapists. They often leave therapy sessions with an unrealistic opinion concerning any progress or gains made. Such patients may believe they performed at a higher level than they actually did.

Watching a patient experience a panic attack for the first time can be frightening. It may not be immediately evident to either the patient or physical therapist if the patient has never experienced a panic attack previously. Patients experiencing a panic attack usually report fear of immediate death. They may start to hyperventilate, then experience shortness of breath. Sometimes they believe they are having a heart attack as a result of chest pain, heart palpitations, and increased heart rate. Terror and panic ensue, and the therapist may call a code or, if in an outpatient setting, initiate emergency transport of the patient to the hospital.

How to Address Anxiety

Physical therapists need to help patients control anxiety so they can proceed with treatment. Some patients may find it beneficial to discuss their fears and concerns with their physical therapists. In such cases the therapist should initiate a dialogue with the patient, asking, "How are you feeling?" "What is your greatest concern?" "What is the worst thing you believe may happen?" and so forth. Physical therapists can work with patients to help defuse anxiety by using cognitive restructuring— or the reshaping of the patient's thoughts and beliefs regarding the feared event. For example, a therapist might help the patient to engage in reality testing by assisting the patient to understand that the occurrence of the feared event is unlikely.

Patients with real and imminent crises may benefit from assistance with problem-solving, should their worst-case scenario occur. Such problem-solving can help patients to believe that they can survive and live meaningful lives despite the occurrence of feared events. After patients have expressed their feelings, therapists can help them segue into treatment and redirect their emotion into physical activity.

It should be noted that patients who are verbose and cannot stop talking about their fears should not be encouraged to dwell on them during physical therapy sessions. Encouraging patients to verbalize their anxieties is also contraindicated with patients whose psychosomatic complaints are fueled by conversation regarding their anxieties. For patients who are very anxious, it may help to conduct treatment in a setting that is familiar, calm, and comfortable. An unfamiliar setting, too much stimulation in the environment, too many people, or too much noise can increase anxiety levels. It may be helpful to reorient patients to the therapy room and to treatment expectations—each session—to allow them to feel a greater sense of control.

Physical therapists should choose a purposeful activity with the patient's anxiety in mind. Some anxious patients have been known to respond to activities that consist of one repetitive motor action, as rhythmic motion helps to calm them.[70] Gross motor movements help decrease the physical symptoms of anxiety such as muscle aches, agitation, and restlessness. Therapists should begin by involving patients in a therapeutic activity that is easily performed and then increase the complexity of the task once the patient has gained confidence.

Anxious patients who may interrupt the physical therapist while working with other patients may be reassured that they will be seen on a certain date and time. Physical therapists should ignore, without anger, all subsequent intrusions. Setting limits in this fashion helps patients improve their frustration tolerance. Very anxious people often welcome clear boundaries set by therapists because they have difficulty setting limits for themselves.

Stress management techniques are useful before and after a session. Techniques such as meditation, imagery,[41] relaxation, stretching, stress management diaries, identifying stressors, biofeedback, nutrition, prioritizing, problem-solving, decision-making, anger management, Reiki (a Japanese technique for decreasing stress that involves the transfer of healing energy from the practitioner to the patient), music therapy, therapeutic massage, and prayer have been shown to improve both physical and emotional well-being.[48,71,72] Some of these techniques work more effectively for some patients than others. Choosing one depends on the patient's preference, amount of time available, and materials required.

Relaxation Response

Whichever stress management technique is selected, the overall goal is to teach patients how to experience the relaxation response and replicate it independently during stressful situations.[73] After studying the relaxation response for 20 years, Dr. Herbert Benson identified two essential components that elicit the response: (1) repeating a sound, word, phrase, prayer, or muscular activity and (2) disregarding distracting thoughts and returning to the repetition. Benson[23] suggests that patients use the following techniques:

1. Choose a phrase, word, or prayer that is part of your belief system.
2. Sit comfortably and quietly.
3. Close your eyes.
4. Relax your muscles beginning with your feet and working your way up your body.
5. Breathe naturally and slowly. Say your phrase, word, or prayer silently as you exhale.
6. Rid yourself of all distracting thoughts by letting them flow in and out of your mind like waves on the ocean, always returning to your phrase, word, or prayer.
7. Continue for up to 20 minutes.
8. Sit quietly for a minute, allowing your thoughts to return before opening your eyes. Sit for another minute before standing.
9. Practice this technique daily on an empty stomach if possible.

The relaxation response has proven to be effective in treating headaches, hypertension, anxiety, cardiac rhythm irregularities, mild and moderate depression, and premenstrual syndrome. The relaxation response works by decreasing heart rate, rate of breathing, metabolism rate, oxygen consumption, and carbon dioxide elimination, and returning the body to a healthier balance.[24,73,74] When within-subject comparisons were made between blood pressure before and after meditation using the nine aforementioned steps for several weeks, the average systolic blood pressure for the 36 subjects dropped from 146 to 137 mm Hg, and diastolic pressure dropped from 93.5 to 88.9 mm Hg; both are statistically significant changes.[23] The relaxation response seems to decrease blood pressure through counteracting the activity of the sympathetic nervous system—the same mechanism underlying the action of antihypertensive drugs. Lower blood pressure leads to lower risk for atherosclerosis and related diseases.

Guided Imagery

Another intervention is guided imagery, frequently used as a standard of care to improve rehabilitation through relaxation. Guided imagery is said to work by decreasing the levels of cortisol that can inhibit the immune system and slow tissue repair.[75] As in eliciting the relaxation response, the patient should be guided to a state in which the mind is silent and calm. Through use of a podcast, audiotape, videotape, or therapy guide, the patient is asked to imagine a special place (e.g., the ocean, a forest, a sunset) and focus on vivid details using the five senses. By focusing on this location for increasing lengths of time, patients learn to gain relief from constant worry by releasing concerns for a period of time and returning to a place of relaxation and peace. Guided imagery enhances the mind–body–spirit connection through the induction of an altered state in which the mind communicates more effectively with the body.[68]

The use of guided imagery has achieved improved outcomes of care through significant reductions in pain, blood pressure, stress, side effects of treatments, headaches, uncertainty, depression, insomnia, blood glucose levels, and histamine response to allergies. Significant enhancement of the immune system and wound and bone healing has also been noted.[76] Because music may trigger emotional responses by influencing the limbic system when used with imagery, music used with guided imagery has been shown to decrease pain through increasing endorphin release.[77,78] Guided imagery with music has also been found to reduce the need for large doses of medication and reduce recovery time.[68]

Desensitization

Phobias severe enough to interfere with daily functioning have been reported by one out of every eight American adults.[28] Patients suffering from phobias that interfere with treatment may require desensitization techniques, also called situational exposure exercises.

For example, wheelchair users with a fear of elevators who had always used the stairs before injury now require help in coping with their fears. In a comfortable, calm treatment environment far from an elevator, the physical therapist can have the patient begin to talk about benign aspects of elevators (e.g., what they look like, where they are located, and how many floors are in the building). While the patient is answering these questions, the physical therapist should determine the patient's level of anxiety. What specific issue regarding the elevator is the patient discussing when their anxiety increases? If the patient has not yet become too anxious, the therapist may ask more anxiety-producing questions, such as, "How high is the elevator's ceiling?" "Is there an emergency phone?" "Are you more fearful of taking an elevator by yourself or with a crowd of people and why?" "Have you ever taken an elevator and if so, what happened?" The therapist should continue to examine the patient's level of anxiety during questioning, stopping just before the patient's anxiety reaches a point at which the patient cannot easily be calmed.

The desensitization process allows patients to discuss their fear in a safe environment where they do not feel overwhelmingly anxious. The physical therapist slowly increases the level of anxiety by asking more difficult questions, but only to a tolerable degree. The patient is then asked to imagine visually being in an elevator while practicing relaxation techniques. The patient continues to practice this visualization, over time, until they can do so without experiencing fear. When the patient can visualize themselves in an elevator without experiencing fear, therapy progresses to the real-life experience of riding in an elevator with the therapist. Relaxation techniques continue to be used during such real-life practice. The activity of riding in an elevator with the therapist using relaxation techniques continues until the patient can do so without fear. The final step would be for the patient to practice riding in an elevator alone while using self-induced relaxation techniques. Desensitization therapy has a high rate of effectiveness in the treatment of phobias.

Cognitive-Behavioral Therapy

Cognitive-behavioral therapy (CBT, or cognitive restructuring) can help decrease anxiety by changing maladaptive thought patterns and modifying unhealthy behaviors.[79] Before unhealthy behaviors can be modified, they must first be identified and classified. Because many patients are not conscious of their anxiety, an initial step when using CBT is to help patients recognize anxiety. Determine what the patient's first signs of stress tend to be. Many will reply that they react severely to stress, stating, "I throw up" or "I cannot breathe." In these cases, therapists should ask about the existence of less severe signs, such as nail biting or leg shaking.

Next, patients should count how many times a day they experience stress, recording these in a journal.

Physical therapists should help patients look for patterns in their anxiety. Are patients more anxious in the morning or evening, when they attend therapy, or when family members visit? The more patients can identify patterns of anxiety, the more they can anticipate it and prepare for anxiety before it occurs. Therapists should encourage patients to use stress management techniques as soon as they experience the first sign of stress so that their anxiety does not escalate. Keeping a stress management journal can give patients insight into how their thoughts affect their behavior. Research has shown that CBT can be as effective as medication.[80–84]

Treatment for Panic Attacks

If the therapist knows that a patient has a history of panic attacks, the following techniques can be helpful: Have the patient describe the first signs of discomfort during the attack. Immediately help the patient to breathe long, deep, and slow breaths. This may require the use of a brown paper bag held over the mouth by the patient while breathing into it to slow the inhalation rate. It is beneficial to acknowledge that a panic attack is occurring and that the patient will be all right if they continue to focus on breathing slowly and deeply. The panic attack can become severe within minutes and pass just as quickly. The patient most likely will be seated or lying down throughout the panic attack, as it may render them incapable of doing anything else.

Patients are usually embarrassed after an attack and may avoid all situations in which they believe one may occur. They may sit on the end of the aisle while watching a movie, may avoid crowds, or, in extreme cases, stop leaving their homes entirely (referred to as agoraphobia). Therapists can help patients who experience panic attacks to achieve a more productive life by teaching them techniques to control the attacks before they become severe. Families and patients should be educated to understand that panic attacks involve a real physiological reaction, tend to last only several minutes, and often recur without further intervention. Patients with severe, continuous panic attacks should be referred to a psychiatrist for possible medication management.

When to Make a Referral for Anxiety

Multiple referrals may be necessary. Patients who have panic attacks should be referred to a psychiatrist for a medication consultation. Generalized anxiety can be treated with medication; hence, a referral to a psychiatrist would be appropriate if the anxiety lasts more than a week and interferes with the patient's performance in rehabilitation. Those who continue to experience anxiety from phobias despite desensitization therapy and medication should be referred to a psychologist for a more in-depth exploration of their fears. A referral to a psychologist is indicated if the anxiety seems to be a deeply rooted characteristic of the patient's personality. A social work referral can be helpful if the patient's anxiety results from a lack of necessary resources or involves family members.

In many cases, medication does not fully alleviate patients' anxiety. However, it may decrease it sufficiently enough for patients to begin expressing their fears and implementing strategies to decrease stress. Sometimes a patient may not be forthcoming about their anxiety, and a formal diagnosis may not be present in the chart. If this is the case, the physical therapist may become aware of an anxiety disorder through the type of medication prescribed. By becoming familiar with the names of different antianxiety medications, physical therapists can identify patients suffering from anxiety. The names, effects, and adverse side effects of commonly prescribed antianxiety medications are presented in Box 26.3.

Acute Stress Disorder and Post-Traumatic Stress Disorder

People who were disabled as a result of a traumatic event (e.g., a violent crime, abuse, an accident, a natural disaster, or war)[85,86] or individuals who have witnessed such are at risk for post-traumatic stress disorder (PTSD) or acute stress disorder (ASD). Both are specific forms or subsets of anxiety disorders. The *Diagnostic and Statistical Manual of Mental Disorders* differentiates between both disorders in terms of the duration of the disorder and its symptoms.[11] ASD involves symptoms that must range in duration between 2 days to a maximum of 4 weeks. If symptoms of ASD persist longer than 4 weeks, the diagnosis of ASD is discontinued and changed to PTSD. PTSD is differentiated as *acute* PTSD if symptoms last more than 4 weeks but less than 3 months and as *chronic* PTSD if symptoms last 3 months or longer. Both ASD and PTSD, however, must result from exposure to a traumatic event, and PTSD can be qualified with the term "with delayed onset" if symptoms first occur at least half a year after the traumatic event. Research notes that PTSD is an expected outcome for a certain percentage of patients experiencing even mild traumas.[87,88]

Among the symptoms exhibited are one or more of the following: reexperiencing the traumatic event; numbing of responsiveness to, or reduced involvement with, the external world; and/or a variety of autonomic, dysphoric, or cognitive symptoms. The reexperiencing of the event is described as recurrent, painful, and consisting of intrusive recollections, dreams and nightmares, and on rare occasions, dissociative states during which the individual may act as if reliving the actual traumatic event. This may last only several minutes or occur for hours or even days. The numbing of responsiveness, also called *psychic numbing* or *emotional anesthesia,* is expressed by complaints of feeling detached or estranged from others, a loss of ability or interest in previously enjoyable activities, or the lack of any emotions or feelings. Cognitive symptoms may include impairment of memory, concentration, and task completion

Box 26.3   Effects and Adverse Side Effects of Commonly Prescribed Antianxiety Medications

Alprazolam (Xanax)

- *Summary of effects:* decrease anxiety, seizures, sleep disorders, alcohol abuse, catatonic schizophrenia.
- *Adverse side effects:* sedation, potential for abuse, difficult to taper (gradual dose reduction).

Buspirone hydrochloride (BuSpar)

- *Summary of effects:* decrease depression, anxiety, addictions, and ADHD.
- *Adverse side effects:* tremors, decreased appetite, insomnia, restlessness.

Chlordiazepoxide (Librium, Mitran, Reposans-10)

- *Summary of effects:* decrease anxiety, seizures, sleep disorders, alcohol abuse, catatonic schizophrenia.
- *Adverse side effects:* sedation, potential for abuse, difficult to taper (gradual dose reduction).

Clorazepate dipotassium (Tranxene, Gen-Xene)

- *Summary of effects:* decrease anxiety, seizures, sleep disorders, alcohol abuse, catatonic schizophrenia.
- *Adverse side effects:* sedation, potential for abuse, difficult to taper (gradual dose reduction).

Diazepam (Diastat, Valium)

- *Summary of effects:* decrease anxiety, seizures, sleep disorders, alcohol abuse, catatonic schizophrenia.
- *Adverse side effects:* sedation, potential for abuse, difficult to taper (gradual dose reduction).

Estazolam (Prosom)

- *Summary of effects:* decrease insomnia.
- *Adverse side effects:* cognitive impairments, dizziness, daytime sleepiness, anxiety, uncoordinated motor movements, intoxication, drug accumulation.

Flurazepam hydrochloride (Dalmane)

- *Summary of effects:* decrease insomnia.
- *Adverse side effects:* cognitive impairments, dizziness, daytime sleepiness, anxiety, uncoordinated motor movements, intoxication, drug accumulation.

Hydroxyzine hydrochloride (Vistaril)

- *Summary of effects*: decrease insomnia, tremors, weight gain, anxiety.
- *Adverse side effects:* dizziness, sedation, constipation, cotton mouth, weight gain, urinary retention, blurred vision, hypotension, confusion.

Lithium carbonate (Eskalith, Lithobid)

- *Summary of effects:* decrease mania and suicidal ideation, stabilizes mood.
- *Adverse side effects:* toxicity can be lethal, weight gain, nausea, acne, sedation, psoriasis, diarrhea, polydipsia, tremors, edema, uncoordinated motor movements.

Lorazepam (Ativan)

- *Summary of effects:* decrease anxiety, seizures, sleep disorders, alcohol abuse, catatonic schizophrenia.
- *Adverse side effects:* sedation, potential for abuse, difficult to taper (gradual dose reduction).

Oxazepam (Serax)

- *Summary of effects:* decrease anxiety, seizures, sleep disorders, alcohol abuse, catatonic schizophrenia.
- *Adverse side effects:* sedation, potential for abuse, difficult to taper (gradual dose reduction).

Temazepam (Restoril)

- *Summary of effects:* decrease insomnia.
- *Adverse side effects:* cognitive impairments, dizziness, daytime sleepiness, anxiety, uncoordinated motor movements, intoxication, drug accumulation.

Triazolam (Halcion)

- *Summary of effects:* decrease insomnia.
- *Adverse side effects:* cognitive impairments, dizziness, daytime sleepiness, anxiety, uncoordinated motor movements, intoxication, drug accumulation.

Box 26.3 Effects and Adverse Side Effects of Commonly Prescribed Antianxiety Medications—cont'd

Paroxetine (Paxil)

- *Summary of effects:* decrease depression and anxiety.
- *Adverse side effects:* nervousness, nausea, headache, diarrhea, sexual dysfunction, insomnia, apathy, sweating, hyponatremia, fatigue, and may cause suicidal ideation in children and teens.

Zaleplon (Sonata)

- *Summary of effects:* decrease insomnia.
- *Adverse side effects:* dizziness, drowsiness.

Zolpidem (Ambien)

- *Summary of effects:* decrease insomnia.
- *Adverse side effects:* dizziness, drowsiness.

Note: Brand names are shown in parentheses.
ADHD = attention deficit-hyperactivity disorder

ability. Patients may experience excessive autonomic arousal resulting in hyperalertness, anticipatory anxiety, an exaggerated startle response, constant scanning of the environment, the perception of people and objects that are not real (i.e., hallucinations), or difficulty falling and remaining asleep.[89] Following this state of hypervigilance, the patient may experience a denial reaction marked by a diminution of responsiveness to the environment. Survival guilt may be present in those cases in which others were harmed or killed during a catastrophic event.

Additional associated features that should alert the physical therapist to the presence of PTSD are increased irritability, hostile behavior, constant tension, chronic free-floating anxiety, muscle tension, sexual and social difficulties, and somatic stress symptoms. Box 26.4 summarizes some of the prominent behavioral features of PTSD.

Not everyone who experiences trauma develops PTSD. The triple vulnerability model postulates that three vulnerabilities need to be present to develop an anxiety disorder: (1) a biological vulnerability; (2) a generalized psychological vulnerability (existing from past experiences of lost control over unpredictable events); and (3) a specific psychological vulnerability that links anxiety to specific situations.[90] Keane and Barlow[91] have proposed an explanation for how PTSD develops based on the triple vulnerability model. They suggest that during a traumatic event, a person experiences alarm and other intense emotions. The person is more likely to develop PTSD if the event and resultant emotions are perceived to be unpredictable and beyond the person's control. If the event is perceived to be predictable and within the person's control, it is less likely that PTSD will occur.

Chronic pain frequently occurs concurrently with PTSD, and the occurrence of both disorders tends to negatively affect the treatment outcome for each.[92] Similar processes, such as avoidance, fear, anxiety, oversensitivity,

Box 26.4 Behavioral Features (Warning Signs) of Possible PTSD

Any one of the following behaviors:

- Recurrent, intrusive recollection of traumatic event
- Intrusive and distressing dreams of event
- Dissociative states (behaving as if reliving event; can last for several seconds or minutes)
- Amnesia of events

More than one of the following behaviors:

- Psychic numbing (lack of interest in social or physical environment or activities; significantly lowered participation in social or physical environment)
- Unable to feel emotions (e.g., intimacy, love, sexuality, anger)
- Disturbed sleep patterns
- Hypervigilance
- Exaggerated startle response
- Ongoing level of irritability
- Heightened difficulty with concentration

PTSD = post-traumatic stress disorder.

and catastrophizing (i.e., interpreting an experience as overly threatening), may act to maintain both conditions. Given the high comorbidity of PTSD and chronic pain, physical therapists should examine patients with PTSD for the existence of chronic pain. The Yale Multidimensional Pain Inventory or the McGill Pain Questionnaire can be administered.[93,94] PTSD may be examined using the Clinician Administered PTSD Scale Revised or the PTSD Checklist.[95,96] Examination should also include the patient's beliefs, self-efficacy, level of anxiety, sensitivity, coping style, expectations, and degree of behavioral and cognitive avoidance to understand the mechanisms that may maintain these conditions. See Chapter 25,

Chronic Pain, for a more detailed discussion of instruments designed to measure pain.

The main desired outcome of treatment for PTSD should be engagement in healthy, satisfying, necessary activities. The physical therapist can help patients to build positive self-efficacy through cognitive restructuring, development of healthy coping skills, and learning to use the relaxation response—all in a predictable, safe environment. Techniques used to help decrease catastrophizing and avoidance include situational exposure exercises (mentioned earlier) and interoceptive exposure exercises (such as running in place or spinning in a chair).[97] Interoceptive exposure exercises help patients cope with uncomfortable physiological sensations that may prevent participation in activities. Finally, the therapist should provide the patient with education regarding how PTSD and pain can facilitate each other and result in avoidance. As participation in healthy activities increases, co-occurring disorders—such as depression, anxiety, panic, and substance use—may decrease, and a higher quality of life may ensue for the patient with PTSD.[42]

Depression

Depression refers to feelings of despair and hopelessness, negative shifts in perception, and decreased interest in activities that once provided pleasure. A person may have a depressed personality (referred to as *dysthymia*) and therefore experience sadness throughout their entire life. As in most cases of depression, a person may have one or more episodes of depression, before and after which a normal mood exists. A certain degree of depression is normal in response to life's events, but when depression lasts 2 or more weeks and affects occupational and social functioning, it is considered major depression. Depression may occur as a biochemical imbalance in the brain, which may be triggered by stress, or in response to internal conflicts or life events. For example, the rate of depression in people with SCI is five times higher than that of the general population.[98]

Women with disabilities are more prone to depression (30%)[99] than women without disabilities (10% to 25%),[11] men with disabilities (26%),[99] and the general population (10%).[11] Other researchers support the finding that women with disabilities tend to experience depression more commonly than their male counterparts. In their analysis of 443 women with disabilities, Hughes et al.[100] found depression to be a frequently occurring secondary condition (51% of the sample scored in the mildly depressed range or higher on the Beck Depression Inventory–II). Fifty-nine percent of women with SCI were found to be clinically depressed, compared with a rate of 4.5% to 9.3% of women in the United States at any given time.[101] This high rate of depression among disabled women may be due to the combination of being a woman and having a disability, since both are risk factors for depression. Women are more than twice as likely to have a depressive episode than men due to economic, social, psychological, and biological factors.[102] Female socialization experiences and gender-based roles may also increase their vulnerability to depression. Depression in women has been linked to experiences of abuse and poverty, lack of social support, reduced mobility, chronic pain, lower educational levels, and lower levels of perceived control.[103]

According to *Healthy People 2030*, only 66.3% of people who have depression get treatment.[20] If untreated, depression can spiral into greater severity and may result in suicide. Depression may begin with loss, such as the onset of a physical disability, divorce, death, or the departure of a close friend. Because of such losses, patients may become appropriately sad and mournful. If patients reach out to friends and express their feelings, they can alleviate feelings of loneliness and isolation that commonly occur in response to loss. However, if patients do not take steps to express their feelings, the downward spiral of depression may continue. Over time, patients may lose interest in activities and remain at home. They may lack the energy or motivation to attend to their responsibilities, and feelings of guilt may ensue. A decrease in role participation usually leads to diminished self-esteem and feelings of worthlessness. Eventually, people stop caring about their hygiene. They may avoid social contact and become increasingly lonely. At this point, staying in bed becomes a welcome alternative to dealing with the outside world and the painful feelings it may incur.

Depression and Rehabilitation

Given the signs and symptoms of depression (Table 26.4) and its associated behaviors (Table 26.5), depression may negatively affect the outcome of treatment. Depressed patients may have difficulty getting out of bed and may not be motivated to attend therapy. If they do attend treatment, they may display psychomotor retardation and lack energy and interest; they may also verbalize self-deprecating remarks, feel criticized, and believe that they are progressing inadequately. It may be difficult for physical therapists to leave depressed patients unattended while working with others because the depressed patient may not engage in the prescribed exercises. Patients may feel guilty that they are in the hospital instead of taking care of their children, working to earn money for their family, or engaging in other life roles.

Depression usually affects performance negatively. Depressed patients may not want to make gains in rehabilitation because of decreased motivation and lack of pleasure in life. They may believe that they are unable to progress in rehabilitation as a result of low self-esteem or feelings of hopelessness. Such patients may also have difficulty asserting themselves because of feelings of worthlessness and an inability to express anger. When people feel worthless or have low self-esteem, they may feel unworthy of having or voicing an opinion. Depression may result from anger turned inward. Instead of expressing anger in the moment, depressed patients

Table 26.4	Signs and Symptoms Associated With Mild, Moderate, and Severe Depression	
Mild Depression	**Moderate Depression**	**Severe Depression**
Anger	Decreased self-esteem	Anguish
Anxiety	Despair	Change in appetite and weight
Decreased concentration	Despondence	Decreased sex drive
Depressed mood	Excessive guilt	Desperation
Indecisiveness	Fearfulness	Feeling overwhelmed
Intrusive thoughts	Inadequacy	Helplessness
Irritability	Sensitivity	Hopelessness
Lethargy		Insomnia or excessive sleep
Loneliness		Recurrent thoughts of suicide
Neediness		Worthlessness
Sadness		

Table 26.5	Behaviors Associated With Mild, Moderate, and Severe Depression	
Mild Depression	**Moderate Depression**	**Severe Depression**
Being easily frustrated	Crying	Decreased interest in all activities
Difficulty planning ahead	Feeling pessimistic about the future	Lack of personal hygiene
Obsessing about tasks	Having difficulty making decisions	Staying in bed all day
Sitting alone	Making frequent self-deprecating remarks	Suicide (or suicide attempt)
	Overdependence	
	Reacting strongly to criticism	
	Reporting psychosomatic symptoms	
	Ruminating about problems	
	Ruminating about the past	

may turn their anger against themselves or repress it. People who experience this type of depression may not have been allowed to express hostility in the past.

Depressed patients often become immobilized because they have difficulty making decisions. They may weigh the pros and cons of each choice and become overwhelmed. They may be unable to concentrate on one thought long enough to make decisions. Sometimes depressed patients experience the opposite; when they attempt to execute a decision they may have no thoughts at all (referred to as thought blocking). Consequently, they may need 1 to 2 minutes to think about and answer questions.

Treating Patients With Depression

Depressed patients require assistance with motivation. Physical therapists can facilitate motivation by providing encouragement, emphasizing strengths, offering positive feedback, addressing values, and mobilizing guilt into goal acquisition. Empowering patients by providing activities that offer opportunities for self-control and success has been shown to decrease depression.[104,105]

Depressed patients experience a narrowing of perception. They have difficulty seeing alternate solutions to problems or simple tasks and often feel there is no solution to obstacles. They may perceive their condition as terminal when there is no justification for such a belief. Because of these distortions, it is important to offer reality checks—such as pointing out their strengths when they feel worthless. Cognitive therapy can be used to correct ongoing pessimism by challenging negative thought patterns.

If given choices about their treatment, depressed patients may become ambivalent and unable to decide on a course of action. As a result, they may do nothing. Physical therapists should choose treatment that provides the patient with opportunities for progressive success experiences, avoiding feelings of failure. When reluctant patients perceive that they can succeed in therapy instead of giving up, their chances of continuing treatment increase. Progress made in physical rehabilitation can alleviate depression, as patients report feeling better after having succeeded in an activity they believed they could not accomplish.

Perhaps the most valuable information that a physical therapist can offer depressed patients is that depression will not last forever. Patients will eventually become better through the combination of therapy and possible medication management. Depression can cause an activity or life role that once seemed effortless—such as being a partner in a relationship—to become arduous. It is important for the patient to understand that this does not mean that the relationship caused the depression; more likely, the role of partner has become more difficult to carry out because of depression.

Families often experience a depressed family member as lazy, obstinate, or uncaring, and may not recognize that they are suffering from an illness. Depression can be just as disabling as a physical illness. Families need to be educated that depression, like physical disability, causes decreased functioning and requires treatment. Recovery from depression does not have a specific timeline. Each patient's situation is unique, as is the recovery period. Most patients cannot "snap out of it," as many family members desire.

When to Make a Referral for Depression

If depression is suspected, the physical therapist should determine if the patient is currently being treated for depression or has received treatment in the past. If the patient has never been treated for depression and is experiencing suicidal ideation (see the following section on Suicide) or symptoms of depression that markedly impair life roles, the therapist should refer the patient to a psychiatrist for possible medication management. Medication can enable patients to attend therapy, more readily discuss problems, and express repressed feelings. However, some patients are reluctant to inform their physical therapist of their depression out of stoicism or shame. There is often a negative stigma attached to being depressed because, to the uninformed, it may imply weakness or feeling sorry for one's self. A diagnosis of depression may not be in the chart, and the symptoms may be misinterpreted as fatigue. In these cases, knowledge of the names of medications used to treat depression may help therapists identify patients with depression. The names, effects, and adverse side effects of frequently prescribed antidepressant medications are presented in Box 26.5.

Patients with less severe symptoms who are not suicidal can be referred to a psychologist for verbal therapy. If a patient's depression seems to be caused by family turmoil, a referral to a social worker for family intervention can be made. Patients who have difficulty verbalizing their feelings can be referred to a creative arts therapist to facilitate expression through nonverbal means such as

music, dance, or art. A referral to an occupational therapist can be made to help patients regain function in daily life roles that have been disrupted by depression.

Suicide

There were 45,979 reported suicides in the United States during 2021, according to the Centers for Disease Control and Prevention.[28] More people lose their lives to suicide than to any other cause apart from cancer and cardiovascular disease. Suicide is often a result of poor social support, low self-esteem, ineffective coping skills, and the inability to see a solution to difficult situations. Risk factors include serious illness, previous suicide attempts, family history of suicide, alcohol and substance use/dependence, loss of a loved one through rejection or death, prolonged depression, and financial difficulties.

Recognizing the warning signs of possible suicide risk is important for its prevention. The most frequent signs of suicide risk include the following:

- Direct comments about suicide, such as, "I just want to die"
- Indirect comments about suicide, such as, "My mother will not have to worry about me anymore"
- A plan to commit suicide
- Writing a suicide note
- Preoccupation with death
- A sudden flight into happiness or relief after a long depression
- Excessive risk taking (e.g., driving while inebriated) and a careless attitude
- Final preparations (e.g., composing a will, giving away personal possessions, repairing broken relationships, or writing revealing letters)
- Self-hatred
- Changes in personal appearance, eating habits, sexual drive, sleep patterns, menstrual cycle, behavior (e.g., inability to concentrate or disinterest in activities), or personality (e.g., withdrawal, anxiousness, sadness, irritability, apathy, indecisiveness, or fatigue)
- A recent loss accompanied by an inability to stop grieving

The most important thing for a physical therapist to do when suspecting that a patient is suicidal is to prevent them from carrying out the act. This usually involves obtaining help from a mental health professional, preferably a physician with the knowledge and ability to admit the person to a hospital if needed. It is important not to leave the patient alone while waiting for help. During this period, the following should take place:

- Ask patients whether they are thinking of hurting or killing themselves.
- Listen to patients without expressing shock, without discrediting what they say, and without devaluing their feelings; take all suicide threats seriously even if you do not believe them at the time.

Box 26.5 Effects and Adverse Side Effects of Commonly Prescribed Antidepressant Medications

Amitriptyline hydrochloride (Elavil)

- *Summary of effects:* decrease depression, manage anxiety, insomnia, migraines, and chronic pain.
- *Adverse side effects:* dry mouth, urinary retention, constipation, hypotension, dizziness, tachycardia, blurred vision, impaired memory, and weight gain.

Amoxapine (Asendin)

- *Summary of effects:* decrease depression, manage anxiety, insomnia, migraines, and chronic pain.
- *Adverse side effects:* dry mouth, urinary retention, constipation, hypotension, dizziness, tachycardia, blurred vision, impaired memory, and weight gain.

Bupropion (Wellbutrin)

- *Summary of effects:* decrease depression, anxiety, addictions, and ADHD.
- *Adverse side effects:* tremors, decreased appetite, insomnia, and restlessness.

Celexa (Lexapro)

- *Summary of effects:* decrease depression and anxiety.
- *Adverse side effects:* nervousness, nausea, headache, diarrhea, sexual dysfunction, insomnia, apathy, sweating, hyponatremia, fatigue, and may cause suicidal ideation in children and teens.

Desipramine hydrochloride (Norpramin)

- *Summary of effects:* decrease depression, manage anxiety, insomnia, migraines, and chronic pain.
- *Adverse side effects:* dry mouth, urinary retention, constipation, hypotension, dizziness, tachycardia, blurred vision, impaired memory, and weight gain.

Doxepin hydrochloride (Sinequan, Zonalon)

- *Summary of effects:* decrease depression, manage anxiety, insomnia, migraines, and chronic pain.
- *Adverse side effects:* dry mouth, urinary retention, constipation, hypotension, dizziness, tachycardia, blurred vision, impaired memory, and weight gain.

Fluoxetine (Prozac, Sarafem)

- *Summary of effects:* decrease depression and anxiety.
- *Adverse side effects:* nervousness, nausea, headache, diarrhea, sexual dysfunction, insomnia, apathy, sweating, hyponatremia, fatigue, and may cause suicidal ideation in children and teens.

Fluvoxamine (Luvox)

- *Summary of effects:* decrease depression and anxiety.
- *Adverse side effects:* nervousness, nausea, headache, diarrhea, sexual dysfunction, insomnia, apathy, sweating, hyponatremia, fatigue, and may cause suicidal ideation in children and teens.

Imipramine hydrochloride (Tofranil)

- *Summary of effects:* decrease depression, manage anxiety, insomnia, migraines, and chronic pain.
- *Adverse side effects:* dry mouth, urinary retention, constipation, hypotension, dizziness, tachycardia, blurred vision, impaired memory, weight gain.

Isocurboxazid (Marplan)

- *Summary of effects:* decrease depression and anxiety and used to treat bipolar depression and treatment-resistant depression.
- *Adverse side effects:* dizziness, hypotension, weight gain, sedation, cotton mouth, insomnia, and sexual dysfunction.

Maprotiline (Ludiomil)

- *Summary of effects:* decrease depression and manage anxiety, insomnia, migraines, and chronic pain.
- *Adverse side effects:* dry mouth, urinary retention, constipation, hypotension, dizziness, tachycardia, blurred vision, impaired memory, and weight gain.

(Continued)

Box 26.5 Effects and Adverse Side Effects of Commonly Prescribed Antidepressant Medications—cont'd

Nefazodone (Serzone)
- *Summary of effects:* decrease depression, anxiety, addictions, and ADHD.
- *Adverse side effects:* tremors, decreased appetite, insomnia, and restlessness.

Nortriptyline hydrochloride (Aventyl, Pamelor)
- *Summary of effects:* decrease depression, manage anxiety, insomnia, migraines, and chronic pain.
- *Adverse side effects:* dry mouth, urinary retention, constipation, hypotension, dizziness, tachycardia, blurred vision, impaired memory, and weight gain.

Paroxetine (Paxil)
- *Summary of effects:* decrease depression and anxiety.
- *Adverse side effects:* nervousness, nausea, headache, diarrhea, sexual dysfunction, insomnia, apathy, sweating, hyponatremia, fatigue, and may cause suicidal ideation in children and teens.

Sertraline (Zoloft)
- *Summary of effects:* decrease depression and anxiety.
- *Adverse side effects:* nervousness, nausea, headache, diarrhea, sexual dysfunction, insomnia, apathy, sweating, hyponatremia, fatigue, and may cause suicidal ideation in children and teens.

Phenelzine (Nardil)
- *Summary of effects:* decrease depression and anxiety and used for bipolar depression and treatment-resistant depression.
- *Adverse side effects:* dizziness, hypotension, weight gain, sedation, cotton mouth, insomnia, and sexual dysfunction.

Protriptyline (Vivactil)
- *Summary of effects:* decrease depression, manage anxiety, insomnia, migraines, and chronic pain.
- *Adverse side effects:* dry mouth, urinary retention, constipation, hypotension, dizziness, tachycardia, blurred vision, impaired memory, and weight gain.

Tranylcypromine (Parnate)
- *Summary of effects:* decrease depression and anxiety and used to treat bipolar depression and treatment-resistant depression.
- *Adverse side effects:* dizziness, hypotension, weight gain, sedation, cotton mouth, insomnia, and sexual dysfunction.

Trazodone (Desyrel)
- *Summary of effects:* decrease depression, anxiety, addictions, and ADHD.
- *Adverse side effects:* tremors, decreased appetite, insomnia, and restlessness.

Trimipramine maleate (Surmontil)
- *Summary of effects:* decrease depression, manage anxiety, insomnia, migraines, and chronic pain.
- *Adverse side effects:* dry mouth, urinary retention, constipation, hypotension, dizziness, tachycardia, blurred vision, impaired memory, and weight gain.

Venlafaxine (Effexor)
- *Summary of effects:* decrease depression, anxiety, panic disorder, SAD, addictions, and chronic pain.
- *Adverse side effects:* cotton mouth, sexual dysfunction, nausea, sweating, headache, constipation, dizziness, fatigue, decreased appetite, insomnia, and nervousness.

Note: Brand names are shown in parentheses. ADHD = attention deficit-hyperactivity disorder; SAD = seasonal affective disorder.

- Respond to patients with empathy and understanding; tell them how much you care about them and that you will be available to help them.
- Help patients think of alternatives; offer choices based on your knowledge about the patient's life, rather than generic answers that are easy to offer when under pressure.
- Alert family members, friends, and significant others to the patient's suicide risk; all of these individuals may help prevent the patient from trying to commit suicide; suicidal ideation does not go away in a day; additional help is required from all possible sources over time.

Substance Use

Substance use occurs when an individual demonstrates a dysfunctional pattern of drug and/or alcohol use characterized by recurrent and significant adverse consequences. Substances may include, but are not limited to, alcohol, amphetamines, caffeine, marijuana, cocaine, hallucinogens, inhalants, opioids, or sedatives.[11]

Substance Use and Rehabilitation

If clients come to the clinic under the influence of drugs or alcohol, they may be inappropriate, argumentative, irritable, disinhibited, stubborn, illogical, or angry and will have difficulty following treatment plans. They may also disturb other clients, some of whom may be in their own substance use recovery. For these reasons, intoxicated clients should be escorted out of the treatment area and referred to their substance use programs, with a call to their substance use program provider describing the incident that occurred. If they are not currently engaged in a substance use program, a referral should be made. Many drugs have unique and specific consequences. Table 26.6 presents an overview of common physiological, psychological, and behavioral manifestations associated with substance use.

Table 26.6 Common Physiological, Psychological, and Behavioral Manifestations Associated With Substance Use

Physiological

• Abnormal blood pressure	• Hallucinations	• Reduced perception of pain
• Abnormal pupillary response	• Impaired liver function	• Sensory impairments
• Altered appetite	• Irregular or increased heartbeat	• Shiny ears
• Constipation	• Loss of consciousness	• Sleep disturbances
• Cravings	• Malnutrition	• Tremors (shakiness)
• Dizziness	• Peripheral neuropathy	• Unexplained weight loss or gain
• Drowsiness	• Perspiration	• Visible needle marks (if injecting)
• Enlarged heart	• Psychomotor disturbances	
• Gastrointestinal bleeding	• Red nose or eyes	

Psychological

• Confusion	• Disturbances of perception	• Low self-esteem
• Delusions	• Easily frustrated	• Paranoia
• Denial	• Emotional lability	• Poor concentration
• Depression	• Grandiosity	• Poor memory
• Disturbances in interpersonal behavior	• Intense emotions	• Reduced inhibitions
	• Loneliness	• Thought disturbances

Behavioral

• Anger	• Falling	• Lying
• Associating only with other substance users	• Financial irresponsibility	• Mood swings
• Belligerence	• Hyperactivity (restlessness)	• Nervousness
• Cheating	• Impaired judgment	• Poor hygiene
• Compulsive use of drugs	• Impaired or inability to fulfill major life roles	• Possession of drug paraphernalia
• Decreased ability to manage stress	• Impulsivity	• Spending money on drugs
• Decreased ability to manage time	• Inability to control drug use	• Staying up all night (insomnia)
• Difficulty holding a job	• Irritability	• Stealing
• Discontinuation of usual activities	• Isolation	• Violence
• Drug-seeking and drug-using behaviors	• Lack of interest in favorite sport or activity	• Withdrawal

If patients are not under the influence during treatment but are using drugs or alcohol at home, they may miss treatment sessions or may come to rehabilitation tired, hungry, or late. They may have poor concentration and irritable moods resulting from hangovers. They may experience recurring injuries from falls. Often, patients will not comply with treatment and fail to complete their home exercises or forget to take their prescribed medications. When prescribed medications are ingested along with illegal substances, adverse drug reactions can occur. Patients may lack insight about the extent of their abuse and the trouble that it produces in their lives. They may mask feelings such as anger, guilt, anxiety, or depression through the numbing effect of the substance, but try to present themselves as though they are fine.

Patients in denial commonly do not perceive their need for physical rehabilitation, often neglect to follow precautions, and frequently attempt to obtain discharge before completing rehabilitation goals. Their low frustration tolerance causes them to quit treatment easily. Whether they are actively using substances or not, patients who have abused substances may have cognitive deficits that inhibit their ability to follow or remember instructions. They may experience family discord and lose family support, thus finding themselves homeless. Patients with a history of chronic alcohol abuse tend to have poor balance resulting from changes in the cerebellum and peripheral nerves.[106] To maintain balance, they develop a stereotypic, wide-based gait. Such factors should be considered during gait examination and training. Despite their gruff demeanor, patients who abuse substances can be overly sensitive, easily hurt, suffer from low self-esteem, and easily stressed once they are no longer abusing substances. These patients tend to have poor boundaries. They can be intrusive, flirtatious, or deal-seeking to obtain what they want, such as alcohol, cigarettes, or extra medication.

Treating Patients Who Abuse Substances

Physical therapists can help patients in recovery by providing opportunities that allow them to gain control over their lives again. Such assistance may include opportunities to practice setting boundaries, regulating emotions, and tolerating frustration. Physical therapists can emphasize healthy activities that provide pleasure and decrease cravings. Stress management, time management, ADL, and social skills are usually necessary skills to promote recovery.

Education on Substance Use

Physical therapists, patients, and patients' family members should be aware that substance use is an illness. Like physical or mental illness, it causes a decrease in function, requires skilled intervention for recovery, results in decreased role performance, and can affect anyone. Patients with a diagnosis of substance use

usually cannot stop using drugs and alcohol on their own. They need help, and recovery is a lifelong process that includes developing skills to manage cravings, dealing with stress in healthy ways, expressing feelings, participating in 12-step programs, and engaging in drug-free activities.

When to Make a Referral for Substance Use

For patients going through withdrawal, the physical therapist should immediately refer them to a physician. Signs of withdrawal can include sweating, impaired sleep, seizures, impaired motor coordination, faulty judgment, anxiety, shaking, slurred speech, fluctuating levels of consciousness, and visual and tactile hallucinations. After stabilizing the patient in withdrawal, the physician may transfer them to a detoxification unit. If the patient is not experiencing withdrawal and is not already in a substance use treatment program, physical therapists can make a referral to an appropriate treatment center. Such treatment centers include 28-day inpatient rehabilitation programs, long-term (1 to 1.5 years) inpatient therapeutic communities, 12-step programs for community-dwelling outpatients, and dual diagnosis programs[48] for patients who have also been diagnosed with mental illness.

Patients who have been abusing substances for long periods of time should be referred to a nutritionist for proper dietary regulation. Physical therapy patients who have been abusing substances can be referred to occupational therapists to address regulating emotions, setting and maintaining appropriate boundaries, tolerating frustration, managing time, obtaining social skills, and regaining necessary ADL. Occupational therapists also can help patients learn that healthy activities can be pleasurable through task groups in which patients choose, engage in, and discuss healthy activities. A social work referral can be made if the patient requires community integration, family intervention, or social supports. A referral to a psychiatrist can be made for an evaluation for medication (see Box 26.6 for a list of commonly administered medications for the treatment of substance use and their side effects).

Agitation and Violence

Physical therapists may not expect patients to demonstrate sexual, aggressive, or violent behaviors, yet most have witnessed such behaviors at least once. Therapists should learn how to predict violence, identify signs of escalation, manage aggressive patients, and verbally respond to threats. Violence is not always predictable, but the more therapists understand its signs, the better equipped they will be to handle a dangerous situation.

An initial step involves recognizing the early signs of agitation. Agitation usually does not diminish by itself. Instead, it may build to a verbal altercation or physical act. Some signs of agitation may include clenching fists,

Box 26.6   Medications Commonly Used to Treat Substance Use Disorders

Buprenorphine (Subutex)

- *Summary of effects:* opioid withdrawal, opioid maintenance; stops opioid cravings without euphoria, sedation, or an analgesic effect; pain management related to withdrawal.
- *Adverse side effects:* runny nose and eyes, vomiting, abdominal cramps, diarrhea, nervousness, body aches for up to 7 days, nausea, severe anxiety, dizziness, insomnia, fatigue, headaches.

Buprenorphine and Naloxone (Suboxone)

- *Summary of effects:* opioid withdrawal, opioid maintenance; stops opioid cravings without euphoria, sedation, or an analgesic effect; pain management related to withdrawal.
- *Adverse side effects:* runny nose and eyes, vomiting, abdominal cramps, diarrhea, nervousness, body aches for up to 7 days, nausea, sever anxiety, dizziness, insomnia, fatigue, headaches.

Bupropion (Wellbutrin)

- *Summary of effects:* decrease depression, anxiety, addictions, and ADHD.
- *Adverse side effects:* tremors, decreased appetite, insomnia, and restlessness.

Clonidine (Catapres)

- *Summary of effects:* mild opioid withdrawal; tobacco smoking cessation.
- *Adverse side effects:* runny nose and eyes, vomiting, abdominal cramps, diarrhea, nervousness, body aches for up to 7 days, nausea, sever anxiety, dizziness, insomnia, fatigue, headaches.

Disulfiram (Antabuse)

- *Summary of effects:* prevents alcohol relapse by blocking alcohol breakdown leading to increased levels of toxic acetaldehyde causing violent vomiting; decreases impulsive alcohol consumption.
- *Adverse side effects:* tingling in legs and arms, dark urine, itchy skin or skin rashes, drowsiness, psychosis, eye pain, decreased vision, decreased energy, inflammation of the liver, impotence, white stool, indigestion, jaundice, optic nerve damage.

Imipramine hydrochloride (Tofranil)

- *Summary of effects:* decrease depression, manage anxiety, insomnia, migraines, and chronic pain.
- *Adverse side effects:* dry mouth, urinary retention, constipation, hypotension, dizziness, tachycardia, blurred vision, impaired memory, weight gain.

Methadone Hydrochloride (Methadone)

- *Summary of effects:* heroin detoxification and maintenance; stops heroin cravings without euphoria, sedation, or an analgesic effect; pain management related to withdrawal.
- *Adverse side effects:* must be tapered slowly when discontinuing use to avoid withdrawal symptoms of methadone; dangerous in overdose; at high doses and/or if used in combination with other drugs, can produce an experience of intoxication.

Naltrexone Hydrochloride (ReVia)

- *Summary of effects:* opioid withdrawal; blocks pleasure centers stimulated by opioids; alcohol relapse prevention.
- *Adverse side effects:* Runny nose and eyes, vomiting, abdominal cramps, diarrhea, nervousness, body aches for up to 7 days, nausea, sever anxiety, dizziness, insomnia, fatigue, headaches.

Nalmedfene Hydrochloride (Revex)

- *Summary of effects:* opioid withdrawal; blocks pleasure centers stimulated by opioids; alcohol relapse prevention; used as an injection after anaesthesia to stop the effect of opioids; used orally for alcohol craving reduction; gambling and nicotine addictions.
- *Adverse side effects:* Runny nose and eyes, vomiting, abdominal cramps, diarrhea, nervousness, body aches for up to 7 days, nausea, sever anxiety, dizziness, insomnia, fatigue, headaches.

Nortriptyline hydrochloride (Aventyl, Pamelor)

- *Summary of effects:* decrease depression, manage anxiety, insomnia, migraines, and chronic pain.
- *Adverse side effects:* dry mouth, urinary retention, constipation, hypotension, dizziness, tachycardia, blurred vision, impaired memory, and weight gain.

(Continued)

Box 26.6 Medications Commonly Used to Treat Substance Use Disorders—cont'd

Varenicline tartrate (Chantix)
- *Summary of effects:* tobacco smoking cessation; decreases symptoms of withdrawal and makes smoking a less satisfying experience by binding to brain nicotine receptors.
- *Adverse side effects:* vivid, abnormal, or strange dreams; insomnia; nausea.

Note: Brand names are shown in parentheses.
ADHD = attention deficit-hyperactivity disorder.

pacing back and forth, making angry facial expressions, grunting, groaning, swearing, tapping a foot, spitting, refusing to engage in therapy, throwing objects, and banging weights or other therapeutic equipment.

After observing signs of agitation, physical therapists should identify the source of the agitation to better control it. While many situations can cause agitation, it is important to remember that events that agitate one person may have no effect on another; levels of frustration vary from person to person. People with Alzheimer disease may become agitated because they cannot recall the names of familiar objects or remember familiar motor plans. They may believe that family members are lying to them, deceiving them, or attempting to place them in a nursing home. People can become agitated because of physical pain, memory failure, hunger, fatigue, and dependency on others. Temporal lobe injury, psychosis, and the side effects of certain medications can cause agitation. People with personality disorders who have difficulty managing anger and who have experienced an upsetting event can become easily agitated.

Addressing the underlying circumstance causing the agitation may help to defuse it. If the source of agitation is unknown, the physical therapist should acknowledge to the patient, in a nonaccusatory manner, that they seem upset. Many people are unaware of their agitation and calm down once it is brought to their attention. The therapist can then encourage the patient to verbally express why they feel upset. Therapists can also attempt to redirect patient anger into more productive channels and help alter their perspective regarding the disturbing issue.

Violence also can happen without warning. Many therapists working on inpatient units for patients with TBI have been bitten, kicked, punched, or scratched. Patients may feel that they are being forced to participate in therapy they do not need or that they are being treated like children. They may believe that staff members have assumed control over their lives. To avoid humiliating the patient, therapists can use a client-centered therapy approach in which patients are offered respect and are included in goal setting and treatment planning.

If efforts to defuse the patient's agitation do not work and they become violent, the physical therapist should remove all other patients from the area, then leave and call for help. After an act of violence, members of the rehabilitation team should examine what occurred to learn from the incident, prevent a future recurrence, and provide support and education to those involved. In reviewing the incident, the physical therapist should address the following questions:

- What was the patient's potential for aggression?
- What were the signs of escalating anger?
- Did the patient have a history of violence? If yes, under what circumstances did it occur?
- How did therapists and patients respond to the aggressor before, during, and after the act?
- What could have been done differently during the incident?

In addition to managing an agitated or violent patient, physical therapists need to recognize when a patient is undergoing abuse. It is estimated that 10% of women with disabilities experience sexual, physical, or disability-related violence.[107] Abuse has been related to decreased social support, increased social isolation, and elevated levels of depression and stress.[106] Women with disabilities may be even more susceptible to abuse, due to their dual minority status as people with disabilities and as women. As compared with women without disabilities, women having disabilities experienced longer periods of abuse and abuse from a greater number of perpetrators.[108] Nosek et al.[109] have identified several factors that predict with 80% accuracy whether a woman has experienced abuse within the past year. These include decreased mobility, social isolation, depression, and a lack of education. Examination for abuse should be considered for women with disabilities.[109] Nosek et al. developed a four-item screening tool, the Abuse Assessment Screen—Disability (AAS-D), that examines sexual, physical, and disability-related abuse in the past year.

Hypersexuality

Hypersexuality is a state of heightened sexual arousal that may be accompanied by verbal or physical aggression. These behaviors can be caused by mania, childhood sexual abuse, or brain damage. Patients may desire attention or want to provoke or exert power over others, to impress others, or to show off. Verbal signs of hypersexuality can include whistling; verbalizing sexual desires; or asking for physical closeness, phone numbers, or dates. Physical behaviors include staring, pinching, brushing up against another's body, touching, kissing, exposing genitalia, masturbating, and blocking another's exit from a room.

There are several ways to proceed when a patient exhibits hypersexual behavior. If the therapist feels threatened, they should leave the area and obtain assistance. If the patient's hypersexual behavior is a newly observed behavior, the therapist can describe the behavior to the patient and firmly state that it is inappropriate and will not be tolerated. If the therapist believes that the patient is exhibiting symptoms of mania or hypomania, referral should be immediately made to a psychiatrist. Holding a multidisciplinary team conference may help the patient understand that hypersexual behaviors are not tolerated in the clinic.

■ PSYCHOSOCIAL WELLNESS

According to Jacobs and Jacobs[110] and Donatelle and Davis,[28] wellness is a dynamic process in which people attempt to fully develop their emotional, social, environmental, physical, spiritual, and intellectual health. Donatelle and Davis describe a well individual as someone who can forgive themself and others, learn from mistakes, appreciate all things both grand and small, develop a realistic sense of self and the environment, achieve a balance in life roles and daily activities, respect others and maintain healthy relationships, feel a sense of life satisfaction, understand their needs and express emotions appropriately, and function in their community. Achieving this definition of wellness may require substantial effort for someone with a disability who may experience multiple barriers to wellness.

Barriers to Wellness for People With Disabilities

Healthy People 2030 has identified gaps and disparities in the health and wellness of Americans with disabilities.[99] Authors reported that people with disabilities exhibited more symptoms of psychological distress and tended to not engage in as many physical activities as people without disabilities. Objectives to overcome these barriers included to decrease the number of individuals with disabilities who also suffer from psychosocial issues and decrease depression and anxiety in caregivers of those with disabilities.

More specifically, research has found that women with disabilities experience higher levels of stress than do males with disabilities, possibly owing to higher incidences of poverty, violence, abuse, chronic health problems, and social isolation.[102] Economic disadvantage may be due to stress-inducing factors such as earning a lower income, having less access to disability benefits from public programs, having less education than their male counterparts with disabilities, and having a higher likelihood of being unemployed or unmarried.[111]

People with SCI report a higher level of perceived stress than the general population, and women with SCI tend to have a higher level of perceived stress than men with SCI.[112]

Social Support

Social support is critical in maintaining or achieving psychosocial wellness. Social support is defined as the availability of other persons in the environment who can offer emotional support, financial or material help, a listening ear, guidance, or encouragement. Social support has been associated with increased self-esteem, coping, and adjustment for individuals with disabilities. Evidence suggests that social support plays a strong preventive and palliative role in a wide range of physical and medical conditions. Rintala et al.[113] found that the amount of social support was directly related to a sense of life satisfaction and well-being in patients with SCI. Hardy et al.[114] and Kaplan[115] found that high social support was predictive of a return to vocational functioning after rehabilitation.

Researchers have suggested that failure to recover from depression stemming from disability may correlate to a lack of adequate social support. Social isolation is a frequently encountered condition associated with disability. Physical restrictions such as pain and mobility limitations may discourage connections with others. The combination of diminished social opportunities, negative societal perceptions, and multiple environmental barriers may result in isolation and a lack of emotional intimacy.

Social support can be used to enhance treatment and promote patient adherence. The physical therapist plays an important role in guiding patient education, including access to resources and instruction in use of adaptive equipment and environmental devices designed to improve a patient's access to social networks and socialization. Appendix 26.A (online) provides Web-based resources for patients, families, and caregivers. It provides resources for improving community accessibility (independent living centers), depression, substance use, anxiety, and PTSD.

■ WELLNESS IN REHABILITATION

Psychosocial wellness requires that patients experience success in both rehabilitation activities and long-term relationships and roles. Rehabilitation activities focus on improving functional outcomes, involvement in meaningful events that foster socialization (e.g., playing wheelchair basketball with other patients), and community reintegration. Long-term relationships and roles include being a spouse, parent, worker, and friend. Psychologists, social workers, and occupational therapists can facilitate readjustment to these long-term roles. Both rehabilitation activities and long-term relationships and roles should provide a sense of contentment, happiness, and well-being. Physical therapists can promote and provide opportunities for patients to choose and engage in meaningful activities that promote psychosocial wellness.

Patients who spend a great deal of time dwelling on the past and worrying about the future are unable to be fully cognizant of the present moment.[116] The ability to become absorbed in the present moment can decrease anxiety concerning the past or future—the patient's emotional energy is focused on their immediate activities. Each instance in which a patient can focus on the present offers them the power to change, to break through old habits, to view circumstances differently, and to recognize available choices. Physical therapists can help patients remain focused on the present moment by selecting activities that are both meaningful to and congruent with the patient's goals for rehabilitation.

Having a daily balance of work, leisure, and social activities is important to sustain psychosocial wellness. Any psychological or physical impairment can disrupt this balance. In a study of the relationship between depression and leisure participation in people with SCI, Loy et al.[117] found that patients without depression had wider repertoires and higher levels of leisure activity than patients with depression. Therapists can help patients engage in leisure activities through activity interest surveys and schedules. Activity interest surveys are used to gather information about the types of leisure pursuits patients previously engaged in, which leisure pursuits they currently hold interest in, and which leisure activities they would like to pursue in the future.

A negative outlook inhibits psychosocial wellness. Physical therapists can help patients with negative perspectives to positively alter their expectations through goal setting, identifying optimistic options, using cognitive-behavioral techniques that challenge the validity of negative perceptions, or referring the patient to a psychologist for longer-term intervention.

■ INTEGRATING PSYCHOSOCIAL FACTORS INTO REHABILITATION: CASE EXAMPLE

Chacuka, a 19-year-old who was training to be an Olympic gymnast, sustained an SCI in a motorcycle accident. Chacuka had developed a strong social support system and participated in a variety of extracurricular activities. He was engaged and planning to be married, participated on his college's gymnastics team, and worked as an athletic counselor in the summer camp he had attended since age 7. The SCI he sustained caused a loss of function from his chest down.

All of Chacuka's energy is now focused on getting through each day. He does not view himself as able to work or attend school. The accident has changed his expectations for the future, his outlook on life, his environmental challenges, and his social support system. His depression was compounded by his broken marriage engagement, and Chacuka no longer meets his friends for social events; in fact, he rarely leaves his home other than to attend rehabilitation. Just when he was becoming independent of his parents, Chacuka has now become dependent on them again. He observes his younger sisters and brothers progressing in their lives and feels stagnant, angry, depressed, and ashamed. His self-esteem, which was once high, is now severely diminished, and he has lost his familiar identity.

As part of his rehabilitation, the therapist should provide a safe way for Chacuka to express his anger; a referral to a psychologist is also warranted. The therapist can help him to better understand his physical limitations and capabilities. Based on Chacuka's strengths and limitations, the therapist should help him to redefine interests that could emerge into new roles and a new identity. For instance, it might be helpful if Chacuka could identify a meaningful activity that could take the place of his athletic training (such as coaching a children's gymnastic team). Information about college and distance learning could also be beneficial. The therapist also can assist Chacuka and his family in their understanding of SCI and reasonable expectations for the future.

■ SUGGESTIONS FOR REHABILITATIVE INTERVENTION

Table 26.7 offers a list of behaviors that suggest inappropriate and pathological response patterns to disability. This list is not meant to be fully inclusive, but rather indicates areas requiring further consideration. It is important to understand that even mild expressions of pathological response patterns can become chronic and worsen in severity over time. Table 26.8 identifies patient behaviors that warrant a mental health consultation.

Box 26.7[118] gives examples of general goals and outcomes for patients with psychosocial issues, and Table 26.9 provides instruments typically used to measure these outcomes organized by the International Classification of Functioning, Disability, and Health (ICF) categories.[119] Table 26.10 gives evidence for the effectiveness of psychosocial interventions poststroke. However, human reactions, response patterns, and the adaptation process are variable and individualistic. Each patient must be approached uniquely, and treatment goals should incorporate the patient's individual personality characteristics, responses, and needs. An important component of rehabilitation is the patient–practitioner relationship. Physical therapists can establish a therapeutic atmosphere of communication, understanding, and cooperation with patients, which can serve as the foundation necessary to produce positive rehabilitation outcomes. Therapists can sometimes forget the powerful influence they have in setting the tone of this interaction. The very structure and atmosphere of service delivery and the personality and type

Table 26.7   Behaviors Suggesting Pathological Response Patterns

Grieving	Depression	Damaged Self-Esteem	Heightened Possibility for Suicide	Heightened Possibility for Violence
Grieving for actual or perceived impairment of functioning or actual loss is normal and expected, but the following might serve as clues to a more severe reaction: Denial of problem or its severity Exaggeration or idealizing the loss Obsession with the past or the pre-loss state Obsession with guilt related to loss Regression Difficulty with concentration Loss of interest in activities and events Lability of mood Inability to discuss loss Fear of being left alone Acting out behaviors (tantrums, suicidal gestures, promiscuity) Angry stance	Flat affect (showing little emotion) Very low energy levels Manic energy and behavior Psychomotor retardation (slowing down of movement and action) Ruminating about negative thoughts Change in eating and sleeping patterns (insomnia or hypersomnia) Regression Social withdrawal Self-destructive behaviors Loss of interest in environment, people, and events Self-blame and self-criticism	Isolation from social sphere Self-destructive behavior Inability to sustain eye contact Inability to accept praise Judgmental attitude Self-deprecating and self-critical Unwarranted pessimism Unconcern for appearance Unconcern for personal safety	Depression Giving away possessions Hoarding/hiding medications or potential weapons Writing suicide note Updating will Verbalizing loneliness or hopelessness Statements regarding benefit of release of pain, absence, and so forth Intrusiveness of such thoughts	Low threshold for anger Depression High-anxiety state Motoric agitation Self-mutilation Oversensitive Argumentative Inability to express feelings Fears of abandonment Highly dependent Dissociative states

of communication provided by the practitioner exert a strong influence on patient participation and response to rehabilitation efforts.

Patient Education

Patients should be involved as fully as possible in their own treatment. This includes involvement in goal setting and treatment planning, as well as in the ongoing evaluation of progress. Patient cooperation is also dependent on the therapist's clear explanation of the patient's situation, anticipated goals and expected outcomes, and interventions. Relating to the patient as a partner in therapy can engender cooperation and trust in the therapeutic relationship. When patients feel a heightened sense of control and ability (i.e., locus of control), feelings of despair and helplessness can be mitigated.

Therapists should also maintain a receptive ear to patient concerns and encourage communication. Listening carefully to patients in a nonjudgmental manner will allow them to reveal concerns and issues they may otherwise feel uncomfortable discussing. Clear and articulate communication, however, can be disrupted by emotion, uncertainty, or power discrepancies that exist when patients become passive recipients of service. Although it may sometimes appear easier to do for patients than to witness their struggle—particularly when patients assume a passive role in rehabilitation—promoting self-reliance and independence fosters patients' engagement and responsibility in their recovery. Allowing patients to maintain a passive role fosters helplessness, encourages dependency, and slows progress in the long term.

Patients can also be involved in providing the treatment team with feedback about their treatment and rehabilitation experience. Feedback regarding their care can be used in continuing quality improvement projects for the physical therapy and rehabilitation departments. Continuing quality improvement projects are performed on regularly to provide the best care at the lowest cost.[139,140]

Table 26.8	Patient Behaviors Warranting a Mental Health Consultation
Regression	Regression involves reverting to earlier, more immature patterns of functioning. This may be more commonly observed in children but might be observed in adults as well. For example, children may revert to sucking their thumb or may appear to have lost their toilet training skills. Regression in adults may generally be seen in lost skills and abilities and/or even in the extreme behavior of reverting to taking a fetal position.
Disorientation	Disorientation is confusion as to time, place, activity, self-identity, or identity of others. Occasional, transient disorientation is not wholly uncommon in the average person, yet persistence in frequency or duration of occurrence is cause for examination and intervention. Any more extreme confused behaviors and thought processes need to be carefully examined.
Delusional thinking	Delusional thinking refers to faulty and mistaken beliefs and, although related to inaccurate interpretation of environment, is distinguished by the persistence of this belief system. This can run the gamut from delusions of grandeur or of persecution, to delusions about the nature and scope of a disability. These delusions hold up and persist in the face of contrary information.
Inaccurate interpretation of environment	This is the broadest category in this list, but fortunately is also the most readily understood category. Clearly, when a patient significantly misinterprets and misunderstands the objective situation and reality about them, it is probably most readily noted by non–mental health practitioners in its many expressions. This should draw attention and intervention, not only in its extreme form of a psychotic break, but also in its minor form of small, repeated episodes of misinterpretations.
Inappropriate affect	Affect refers to the mood state displayed by the patient, where feelings such as joy, sadness, fear, and so forth are reflected in body language, facial expression, and verbalizations. Inappropriate affect can be seen in an affective expression alien to the situation; for example, demonstrating and expressing joy on hearing bad news. It also refers to a split between displayed affect and verbalization; for example, the verbal expression of mourning and condolence offered while smiling brightly and jumping for joy.
Hypovigilance or hypervigilance	Hypovigilance can be noted in a patient being oblivious to their surroundings and the events around the patient, socially, as well as physically. Hypervigilance refers to an intense focus and alertness to social and physical surrounds. Each of these has different ramifications and meaning to the mental health team. A consultation is suggested as either extreme is approached.
Mood swings	We all experience changes in mood, yet most of the time these changes are relatively appropriate reactions to external determinants, such as the receipt of news and information or to changing occurrences and circumstances in our environment. Although changeable, moods are generally persistent and stable. When mood shifts either to extremes and/or with some frequency, it suggests either instability or that mood is being driven predominantly by internal rather than external factors.
Self-destructive behaviors	Any self-destructive behavior, particularly that the behavior persists, are cause for serious concern. Self-destructive behaviors can run the gamut from subtle, difficult to detect signs to very clear and frightening overt signs. Subtle signs can include non-adherence with treatment regimen, poor self-maintenance activities such as not eating, overeating, diminishment of personal care and hygiene, or carelessness in negotiating the environment. Clearer signs can include self-inflicted wounds and suicidal ideation and expressions.
Normal behaviors taken to extremes	Normal human behavior enjoys a wide latitude of response repertoire before drawing attention as being out of expected bounds. This latitude must usually be extended further when dealing with someone undergoing a more extreme, traumatic, or stressful experience. Individuals confronted with a disability would be expected to naturally focus their attention, concerns, and anxiety around this issue. The level of focus on a left leg given by someone preparing to have that leg amputated would be considered obsessive in a healthy ambulatory person, yet normal here. Care in judgment is required by the clinician when determining behavior expressions. That said, issues such as obsessiveness, extreme distractibility, immobilization in the face of routine decisions, and unexpected egocentricity or self-denigration may require a consultation. An overly adherent patient, an extremely calm patient, as well as an overly contentious, argumentative, or extremely anxious or hysterical patient also promotes concern. Any response (verbal or behavioral) that appears unwarranted to the stimuli should draw attention. Overreactions in opposite directions or any behavior that appears to be at an extreme, using reasonable judgment, deserves attention.

Box 26.7 Examples of General Goals and Outcomes for Patients With Psychosocial Issues

Impact of pathology is reduced.

- Patient/client, family, and caregiver knowledge and awareness of the disease, prognosis, and plan of care is enhanced.
- Symptom management is enhanced.
- Changes associated with recovery are monitored.
- Risk of secondary impairments and reoccurrence of condition is reduced.
- Intensity of care is decreased.

Impact of impairments is reduced.

- Cognitive function is improved.
- Communication is improved.
- Ability to participate in rehabilitation is improved.

Ability to perform physical actions, tasks, or activities is improved.

- Independence in ADL is increased.
- Problem-solving and decision-making skills are improved.
- Safety of client, family, and caregivers is intact.
- Disability associated with chronic illness is reduced.
- Ability to assume/resume self-care and home management is improved.
- Ability to assume roles such as participation in work activities (job/school/play) and community leisure roles is improved.
- Awareness and use of community resources are improved.

Health status and quality of life are improved.

- Sense of well-being is enhanced.
- Stressors are reduced and/or the ability to manage them is improved.
- Insight, self-confidence, and self-management skills are improved.
- Health and wellness are improved.

Client satisfaction is enhanced.

- Access to and availability of services are acceptable to client and family.
- Quality of rehabilitation services is acceptable to client and family.
- Care is coordinated with client, family, caregivers, and other professionals.
- Discharge placement needs are determined.

Adapted from the *Guide to Physical Therapist Practice*.[118]
ADL = activities of daily living.

Use of Jargon and Labels

Patient–therapist communication should be characterized by simple and easy-to-understand language that matches the cognitive level of the patient. The use of scientific jargon and labels should be avoided when speaking with patients, because it impedes patient understanding and emotionally distances patients from therapists. Similarly, when patients hear therapists referring to fellow patients by their diagnosis, they receive the message that patients are nothing more than disabilities. Such practice should be avoided and, instead, therapists should use language that reflects respect for the patient's dignity and unique life circumstances.[141]

Trauma-Informed Care

"Trauma-informed care is a strengths-based framework that is grounded in an understanding of and responsiveness to the impact of trauma, that emphasizes physical, psychological, and emotional safety for both providers and survivors, and that creates opportunities for survivors to rebuild a sense of control and empowerment."[142] Trauma-informed clinicians understand how pervasive trauma is and how it can influence psychosocial development, lifelong coping strategies, rehabilitation, and adaptation. Staff members within trauma-informed care programs seek to establish and maintain safe environments for clients that enable choice, collaboration, empowerment, and trust throughout all intervention modalities so clients can form healthy relationships with others. They focus on client strengths instead of emphasizing dysfunction and build skills instead of merely addressing symptoms. A trauma-informed care delivery team provides services in a manner that is sensitive to the emotional vulnerability of trauma survivors while avoiding re-traumatization.[143]

There are many trauma-informed care best practice models and frames of references, three of which

Table 26.9 Outcome Measures: Psychosocial Issues[119]

Outcome Measure	ICF Category	Description	Scoring	MCID/MDC
Holmes-Rahe Social Readjustment Scale[66]	Body functions and structures	Paper-and-pencil self-report assessment that measures adaptability, social adjustment, psychosocial adaptation, stress, and life changes	Patients rate 43 life events in the amount of readjustment necessary to cope with each.	NA
The Hassles Scale[67]	Body functions and structures	Measures adult daily life stresses over the past month in areas pertaining to family, work, and leisure	Utilizes a 4-point Likert scale ranging from 1 ("not at all part of my life") to 4 ("very much part of my life"). The higher the score, the higher the level of stress currently being experienced.	NA
Contextual Memory Test[120]	Body functions and structures	Assesses recall, use of strategies, and metacognition of memory ability in adults	Subscores based on the number of correct answers include: recall, recall with cues, strategy use, awareness, and recognition and can be compared to norms to indicate within normal limits, and suspect, mild, moderate, or severe impairment.	NA
Beck Depression Inventory[121]	Body functions and structures	21-question self-report measure of depression over the past week in adults. Also screens for suicidal ideation.	Multiple choice/Likert scale scores range from 0–3, with a score of 0 being "normal." Total score is compared to ranges that indicate the following categories of depression in order of severity: normal, mild, borderline clinical, moderate, severe, and extreme.	NA
Stroop Color and Word Test[122]	Body functions and structures	A timed neuropsychological test of the ability to cognitively sort environmental information and react selectively. It can be used to explore different psychological processes in normal and cognitively impaired adults and children.	Scores measure the ability to inhibit cognitive interference and are compared to age and education matched norms using t-scores. Result patterns are given for various psychiatric diagnoses for comparison.	NA
Neurobehavioral Cognitive Status Examination[123]	Body functions and structures	Cognitive impairment screening tool of 62 items measuring attention, orientation, reasoning, memory, calculations, language, and constructional ability	Each of the subscores are plotted on a graph allowing patients a visual representation of their level of cognitive functioning, which can be either severe, moderate, mild, or average when compared to norms. Results can also be compared to different psychiatric diagnoses.	NA
Generalized Expectancy for Success Scale[124]	Body functions and structures	Self-report 30 item questionnaire utilizing a 5-point Likert scale from 1 (highly improbable) to 5 (highly probable) to measure optimism		NA

Table 26.9   Outcome Measures: Psychosocial Issues[119]—cont'd

Outcome Measure	ICF Category	Description	Scoring	MCID/MDC
Beck Hopelessness Scale[125]	Body functions and structures	21-question self-report measure of three different areas of hopelessness in adults ages 17–80 over the past week: loss of motivation, feelings about the future, and expectations. Also screens for suicidal ideation.	Total scores are compared to normative groups that include suicidal, depressed, and drug abusing patients.	NA
Internal-External Scale[126]	Body functions and structures	Measures the degree to which individuals believe that they can affect their behavior (internal locus of control) versus believing that external events cause them to behave in a certain fashion (external locus of control)	Scores range from 0–23 with 0 being the most internal locus of control and 23 being the most external locus of control. Internal locus of control is correlated with better rehabilitation outcomes.	NA
Self-Efficacy Scale[127]	Body functions and structures	10-item self-report measure of self-efficacy utilizing a 4-point Likert scale from 1 (not at all true) to 4 (exactly true)	Scores are totaled to produce an overall score between 10 and 40, with 40 indicating the highest degree of self-efficacy.	NA
Sentence Completion Attitude Survey[128]	Body functions and structures	Objective and projective sentence completion attitude survey with 40 sentence completions used to identify positive, negative, and neutral attitudes towards eight factors: education, irritants, self-directedness, accomplishment, physical self, psychological self, age-mates/people, and family. Can be used with children (student version) as well as adults.	Total score is compared to mean and standard deviation norms for students and adults yielding "average," "above the mean," or "below the mean." Results can be used to measure individual change over time (within subjects) or between comparison groups (between subjects).	NA
Mini-Mental State Examination[129]	Body functions and structures	11-question quantitative measure of cognition (memory, orientation, recall, calculation, attention, and language) administered by professionals to people with psychiatric or neurological issues	Normative sample mean score was 27.6 with a range of 23–30 (30 being the most cognitively intact).	NA
Occupational Questionnaire[130]	Activity	Measures how individuals spend their time in daily activities and how satisfied individuals are with their use of time	Number of hours spent in each stated activity are totaled to form a visual activity configuration pie chart indicating percentages of time spent in each activity: work, leisure, sleep, etc.	NA

(Continued)

Table 26.9	Outcome Measures: Psychosocial Issues[119]—cont'd			
Outcome Measure	ICF Category	Description	Scoring	MCID/ MDC
Interest Checklist[131]	Activity	Self-report checklist of activities that measures patient's perceived participation in specific activities in the past and present and identifies which activities they would like to do in the future	Results include self-identified activates and motivation for participation in each	NA
Role Checklist[132]	Participation	Self-report checklist that measures patient's perceived participation in 10 specific roles in the past and present and identifies which roles they would like to assume in the future and how they value each	Results include self-identified roles and motivation and the value of each.	NA
Community Adaptation Schedule[133]	Participation	Self-report paper-and- pencil questionnaire with item-analyzed questions on cognition, affect, and behavior	Scores are obtained using a 6-point Likert scale to measure patients' relationship to different community aspects: work, family, social, outer community, commercial, professional, affect, behavior, and cognition. Norms have been established for inpatient psychiatric patients and "average" adults.	NA

**ICF = International Classification of Functioning, Disability, and Health; NA = Not available; MCID/MDC = The smallest amount of change in a domain/minimal detectable change.

are Trauma-Focused Cognitive Behavioural Therapy (TF-CBT); the Attachment, Self-regulation, and Competency Model (ARC); and the Advancing Trauma-Informed Care initiative. Trauma-Focused Cognitive Behavioural Therapy intervention includes reframing distorted beliefs related to trauma, providing a supportive environment, stress management, and parenting skills for parents. By minimizing nonproductive emotions and behaviors, TF-CBT can be used to increase behaviors that promote occupational/social participation and performance skills.[144] It has been used with adults but has also been successful for individuals ages 3 to 21 and their families who have experienced trauma.[145] TF-CBT has been endorsed by The Substance Abuse and Mental Health Services Administration (SAMHSA) and has been shown to be just as affective when delivered through telehealth versus in-person.[146]

The ARC Model emphasizes self-regulation, attachment, competency, and integration and supports the child, family, and organization's ability to engage in the present moment. Grounded in attachment theory and early childhood development, the ARC Model addresses how a child's entire system of care can become trauma

informed.[147–149] The ARC Model has been successful for individuals ages 2 to 21 years and their families who have experienced multiple traumas, chronic traumatic stress, and/or ongoing exposure to adverse life experiences. This intervention resulted in increases in coping and social skills and decreases in children's mental health symptoms including symptoms of posttraumatic stress.[149] The ARC Model is a flexible framework that has been used with different populations (including urban high-risk, pre-/post-adoptive, Native Alaskan, internationally adopted, child welfare involved, juvenile justice-involved, and war refugee youth), in a range of settings (including domestic violence shelters, secure facilities, outpatient, residential treatment, community mental health, and hospital).[149]

Advancing Trauma-Informed Care was a multi-site demonstration project supported by the Robert Wood Johnson Foundation and led by the Center for Health Care Strategies. The Center conducted interviews with nationally recognized experts in the field, including primary care physicians, behavioral health clinicians, academic researchers, program administrators, and trauma-informed care trainers, as well as with state and

Table 26.10	Evidence Summary Studies Addressing the Question: What Is the Need for and Effectiveness of Psychosocial Interventions in Recovery Poststroke?

Cheong et al. (2021)[134]

Design	Scoping review (51 articles) and meta-analysis (42 of the 51 articles in the scoping review) examining correlations between psychosocial factors and motivation for stroke rehabilitation.
Level of Evidence	I
Subjects	All studies were published between January 2011 and February 2021 and were related to client motivation for stroke rehabilitation. The population of interest was South Korea.
Intervention	All studies in the meta-analysis were correlation studies without interventions.
Results	Eighteen psychosocial factors correlated with rehabilitation motivation poststroke: volition, self-esteem, communication, cognition, depression, self-efficacy, sleep pattern, social support, acceptance of disability, resilience, quality of life, empowerment, uncertainty, ADL, rehabilitation environment, financial burden, physical function, and disease-related characteristics.
Comments	Findings in this scoping review and meta-analysis support the need to create psychosocial models of intervention that address the 18 factors above to improve stroke rehabilitation.

Do et al. (2019)[135]

Design	Within subjects pre- and post-test study
Level of Evidence	II
Subjects	N = 12 aged 50–60
Intervention	Four weeks of 4×/week cognitive processing treatment by physical and occupational therapists. Sessions included reality orientation, cognitive exercises, tasks, and reminiscence activities.
Results	There were statistically significant differences between pre- and post-test scores in depression, social cognition, and health-related quality of life.
Comments	Cognitive-processing treatment improved psychosocial factors in stroke survivors within this small sample.

Haynes et al. (2019)[136]

Design	Scoping review of 17 articles that identified psychosocial issues that were barriers to return to work poststroke and interventions aimed at overcoming these barriers in order to sustain gainful employment.
Level of Evidence	I
Subjects	Fifteen (88%) papers identified psychosocial issues that were barriers to return to work and/or sustaining work poststroke. Four (24%) papers identified interventions to treat psychosocial issues that posed work barriers. Psychosocial issues included poor social supports, depression (33%), and inability to accept disability (27%).
Intervention	Work interventions included The Brain Integration Program, awareness and metacognitive training, and contextual workplace interventions.
Results	There are few effectiveness studies measuring psychosocial interventions that address barriers to work among people who have had a stroke even though there are many studies that have identified specific psychosocial factors affecting work poststroke. The effectiveness studies in this paper all showed that overcoming psychosocial barriers to work enhanced positive work outcomes.
Comments	This research supports the need to address psychosocial issues poststroke in order to foster return to work and work sustainability.

(Continued)

Table 26.10	Evidence Summary Studies Addressing the Question: What Is the Need for and Effectiveness of Psychosocial Interventions in Recovery Poststroke?—cont'd
Lund et al. (2018)[137]	
Design	Qualitative study utilizing semi-structured interviews to investigate the effect of a lifestyle group intervention with older adults with stroke
Level of Evidence	III
Subjects	Six older adults with mild to moderate stroke residing in Norway.
Intervention	Person-centered lifestyles groups consisting of group activities administered over a 9-month period.
Results	Participants reported that this group activity intervention allowed them the opportunity to socialize with one another around the topics of their stroke experiences, knowledge, and interests. They believed that group members inspired one another to move forward with their goals, gain self-worth, increase autonomy, and adapt to life poststroke.
Comments	This study is not rigorous enough to generalize to other settings, but by using various activities in life-style groups, it emphasizes the importance of using a long-term, person-centered approach to engaging older adults who have suffered a stroke.
Nott et al. (2021)[138]	
Design	Mixed method pre- and post-intervention study used to examine self-efficacy, satisfaction, and occupational performance.
Level of Evidence	1I
Subjects	Forty patients admitted to a hospital after experiencing a stroke.
Intervention	Twelve-week stroke self-management program tailored to stroke survivors consisting of participation in meaningful occupations, goal setting, self-reflection, problem-solving, sharing experiences, increasing self-confidence and self-efficacy, occupational competence, occupational coaching, performance evaluation, and building local support.
Results	Significant improvements were noted in occupational satisfaction ($p=0.001$) and occupational performance ($p=0.001$). Self-efficacy was a mediator to improvements in occupational performance ($p<0.01$) and satisfaction ($p=0.02$). Thematic analysis revealed three facilitators/barriers: "Reflecting on shared experiences," "Getting back to normal," and "Support in making the transition home."
Comments	This 12-week stroke self-management intervention was effective in improving self-efficacy, satisfaction, and perceived occupational performance. An additional longitudinal data collection would have added information regarding the appropriateness of the length of the intervention.

ICF = International Classification of Functioning, Disability, and Health; ADL = activities of daily living.

federal policymakers. Information from the interviews was used to develop a multifaceted, comprehensive, holistic, evidence-based practice model outlining key steps and skill sets for successful trauma-informed interprofessional care implementation. The model is used to address necessary changes at both organizational and clinical levels. Organizational interventions include: "leading and communicating about the transformation process, engaging patients in organizational planning, training clinical as well as non-clinical staff members, creating a safe environment, preventing secondary traumatic stress in staff, and hiring a trauma-informed workforce." Clinical interventions include: "involving patients in the treatment process, screening for trauma, training staff in trauma-specific treatment approaches, engaging referral sources, and partnering organizations."[150]

It is important to note that many people will have experienced the COVID-19 pandemic as a traumatic event: one which will affect lives for many years to come. Thus, physical therapists may wish to treat everyone that comes to them for help as if they have suffered psychological trauma and use trauma-informed therapy with all of their clients.

Rehabilitation Team Members' Self-Awareness

Finally, and perhaps most important, therapists need to be aware of their own feelings, motivations, and responses. Such self-awareness is critical for therapists to understand their own reactions to patients. It is normal for people to respond to others based on conscious or unconscious memories. Sometimes patients can remind therapists of significant others, such as siblings, parents, spouses, or employers. However, when therapists react to patients based on unconscious associations to others, they can misperceive patient needs and respond inappropriately. For example, unconscious reactions to patients can cause therapists to become overprotective or, at the other extreme, become frustrated with patients without recognizing that their own reactions have more to do with other relationships than with the patient at hand.

Generally, when therapists feel a heightened sense of emotion in response to a particular patient, it may often serve as a cue that such emotions stem from unconscious associations to others. When this occurs, it is important for therapists to step back and evaluate their own feelings to discern the connection between their reactions to the patient and how the patient may be triggering unconscious emotions.

The converse is also true; patients will respond to therapists based on their own unconscious associations with significant others who have similar personality characteristics to those of the therapist. Therapists must be aware of this normal phenomenon and refrain from responding emotionally to the patient's unconscious associations. Rather, the therapist should continue to build a respectful relationship with the patient that, in time, will demonstrate to the patient that their first impressions were misperceptions.

SUMMARY

It is important for physical therapists to identify and understand the individual psychosocial factors that enhance or inhibit the rehabilitation of their patients and intervene accordingly. Successful intervention depends on the following:

- Understanding the psychosocial aspects of each patient, including personality styles and coping skills
- Recognizing and interpreting the common defense mechanisms that patients use in rehabilitation
- Distinguishing the stages of psychosocial adaptation to disability and helping patients' progress in their own adjustment
- Understanding how to identify anxiety, depression, and substance use; determining how to address these problems; and recognizing when referral to other team members is warranted
- Integrating a patient/client-centered approach that emphasizes respect, empathy, and compassion
- Empowering patients and families through psychosocial education and wellness and prevention strategies
- Working together with patients to develop anticipated goals and expected outcomes congruent with their needs, values, and level of functioning
- Collaborating with patients and team members to establish and implement appropriate interventions
- Developing a team approach and providing referrals as necessary

Questions for Review

1. Identify five psychosocial factors and state how each factor may influence rehabilitation.

2. Give examples of interventions for each psychosocial factor identified in question 1.

3. Differentiate between the different mental health professionals who can treat patients with psychosocial issues by describing their roles.

4. What should therapists do to calm an agitated patient?

5. Describe an approach for managing a violent patient and how to analyze an act of violence after it has occurred.

6. What are the manifestations of hypersexuality and how should it be addressed?

7. Identify and describe the phases of psychosocial adaptation to disability.

8. Discuss three coping strategies that have been found to be effective in the psychosocial adaptation to chronic disability and illness.

9. Describe five common defense mechanisms that patients use in response to disability.

10. What are the signs and symptoms of PTSD?

11. Differentiate between typical reactions to grieving and pathological reactions.

12. Explain several ways to optimize patient involvement in the rehabilitation process and promote self-reliance.

13. Why is patient/client-centered intervention important? What strategies can be used to achieve this type of interaction?

14. Describe the GAS.

CASE STUDY

The patient is a 68-year-old female, admitted to an inpatient unit 2 days after sustaining a right femoral neck fracture from falling down her basement stairs. Hip replacement surgery (arthroplasty) was performed on the same day as the fall. The referring documentation indicates "weight-bearing as tolerated." The patient complains that she "can't do anything" for herself owing to the fall.

Before her fall, she was in fair health but was experiencing declining eyesight, poor short-term memory, and osteoporosis. Her hip fracture has placed her at high risk for further deconditioning and loss of function. The patient's wife had suffered a prolonged illness; the patient cared for her during the past 5 years until he passed away. She has a son whom she rarely sees because he is married with children and living in another part of the country. A close friend lives several miles from her, and the rest of her friends have died. The patient is embarrassed to be seen in public in a wheelchair.

Given the deaths of her wife and friends, and given her recent accident, the patient is now very anxious about her own mortality for the first time in her life. She is preoccupied with her wife's death since she was so much a part of her life. She feels that she has no future and nothing to look forward to. She no longer knows who she is and longs to "be reunited with" her wife.

GUIDING QUESTIONS

1. Identify the psychosocial factors apparent in this case study.

2. What relevant questions about the patient remain unanswered (i.e., what relevant information is missing)?

3. How might the patient's emotional condition affect rehabilitation?

4. Develop a problem list for the patient.

5. Identify the patient's assets.

6. Identify the general goals of physical therapy intervention on which specific anticipated goals and expected outcomes will be based.

7. Identify the general categories of procedural interventions appropriate for this patient.

8. Identify referrals to other professionals or resources.

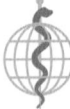 For additional resources, including answers to the questions for review, new immersive cases, case study guiding questions, references and more, please visit **https://www.fadavis.com/product/physical -rehabilitation-fulk-8**. You may also quickly find the resources by entering this title's four-digit ISBN, 4691, in the search field at **http://fadavis.com** and logging in at the prompt.

Supplemental Readings

American Psychiatric Association. *Diagnostic and Statistical Manual of Mental Disorders*, 5th ed. American Psychiatric Publishing; 2013.

Boersma K, Linton SJ. Screening to identify patients at risk: profiles of psychological risk factors for early intervention. *Clin J Pain.* 2005;21(1):38–43. doi:10.1097/00002508-200501000-00005.

Bonder B. *Psychopathology and Function*, 4th ed. Slack; 2010.

Brenes GA, et al. The influence of anxiety on the progression of disability. *J Am Geriatr Soc.* 2005;53(1):34–39. doi:10.1111/j.1532 -5415.2005.53007.x.

Brown C, Stoffel VC, Munoz J. *Occupational Therapy in Mental Health: A Vision for Participation.* FA Davis; 2011.

Drench ED, et al. *Psychosocial Aspects of Health Care*, 3rd ed. Prentice Hall (Pearson Education, Inc.); 2011.

Elfstrom M, et al. Relations between coping strategies and health-related quality of life in patients with spinal cord lesion. *J Rehabil Med.* 2005;37(1):9–16. doi:10.1080/ 1650197041034414.

Falvo D. *Medical and Psychosocial Aspects of Chronic Illness and Disability*, 3rd ed. Jones & Bartlett; 2005.

Hughes RB, et al. Stress and women with physical disabilities: identifying correlates. *Women Health Issue.* 2005;15(1):14–20. doi:10.1016/j.whi.2004.09.00.1.

Kolt GS, Anderson MB, eds. *Psychology in Physical and Manual Therapies*. Churchill Livingstone; 2004.

Miller JF. *Coping with Chronic Illness: Overcoming Powerlessness*. 3rd ed. FA Davis; 2000.

Moldover JE, et al. Depression after traumatic brain injury: a review of evidence for clinical heterogeneity. *Neuropsychol Rev*. 2004;14(3): 143–154. doi:10.1023/B:NERV.0000048181.46159.61.

Precin P, ed. Healing 9/11. Haworth Press; 2006.

Precin P, ed. Posttraumatic Stress Disorder and Work. *WORK*. 2011;38(1). doi:10.3233/wor-2011-1098.

Precin P, ed. Surviving 9/11. Haworth Press; 2003.

Precin P. *Client-Centered Reasoning: Narratives of People with Mental Illness*. Echo Point Books & Media; 2015.

Precin P. *Living Skills Recovery Workbook*. Echo Point Books & Media; 2015.

Rytsala HJ, et al. Functional and work disability in major depressive disorder. *J Nerv Ment Dis*. 2005;193(3):189–195. doi:10.1097/01 .nmd.0000154837.49247.96.

Solet JM. Optimizing personal and social adaptation. In: Trombly CA, Vining Radomski M, eds. *Occupational Therapy for Physical Dysfunction*, 5th ed. Lippincott Williams & Wilkins; 2002:761.

Yerxa EJ. The social and psychological experience of having a disability: implications for occupational therapists. In: Pedretti LW, Early MB, eds. *Occupational Therapy: Practice Skills for Physical Dysfunction*, 5th ed. Mosby, St. Louis; 2001:470.

Cognitive and Perceptual Dysfunction

Carolyn A. Unsworth, BAppSci (OccTher), GCTE, OTR, MRCOT, FOTARA

Chapter 27

LEARNING OBJECTIVES

1. Identify the signs of cognitive and perceptual deficits.
2. Describe how cognitive and perceptual deficits affect a patient's ability to participate in rehabilitation.
3. Explain how a patient can be assisted to compensate for body scheme and/or body image disorders.
4. Describe how spatial relations impairments can affect the patient's ability to follow directions.
5. Compare and contrast the effect of the various agnosias on the patient's ability to recognize stimuli in the environment.
6. Differentiate between ideomotor and ideational apraxia. Describe how a patient with apraxia might behave in response to different instructional sets commonly employed in rehabilitation.
7. Identify how the psychological and emotional status of a patient with cognitive and perceptual deficits may affect participation in rehabilitation.
8. Analyze and interpret patient data, formulate realistic anticipated goals and expected outcomes, and identify appropriate interventions when presented with a clinical case study.

CHAPTER OUTLINE

COGNITION AND PERCEPTION 1055
  Cognition and Higher-Order Cognition 1055
  Perception 1055
RESPONSIBILITIES OF THE PHYSICAL THERAPIST AND THE OCCUPATIONAL THERAPIST 1056
CLINICAL INDICATORS 1056
HOSPITALIZATION FOLLOWING BRAIN DAMAGE 1057
THEORETICAL FRAMEWORKS 1057
  The Retraining Approach 1057
  The Sensory Integrative Approach 1058
  The Neurofunctional Approach 1058
  The Rehabilitative/Compensatory (Functional) Approach 1058
  Cognitive Rehabilitation and the Quadraphonic Approach 1059
EXAMINATION OF COGNITIVE AND PERCEPTUAL DEFICITS 1061
  Purpose of the Examination 1061
  Factors Influencing Patient Examination 1062
  Distinguishing Between Sensory and Cognitive and Perceptual Deficits 1063

Standardized Cognitive and Perceptual Tests 1065
INTERVENTION 1070
  Treatment Approaches 1070
  Patient, Family, and Caregiver Education 1070
  Refocusing Intervention 1071
  The Impact of Managed Care 1071
DISCHARGE PLANNING 1072
OVERVIEW OF COGNITIVE AND PERCEPTUAL DEFICITS 1072
  Attention Deficits 1073
  Memory Impairments 1074
  Impairments of Executive Functions 1075
  Body Scheme and Body Image Impairments 1077
  Spatial Relations Disorders (Complex Perception) 1086
  Agnosias (Simple Perception) 1090
  Apraxia 1092
SUMMARY 1094

Cognitive and perceptual deficits are among the chief causes of poor rehabilitation progress for patients who have sustained brain damage, even among those whose motor skills have returned. Cognitive and perceptual deficits are some of the most puzzling and disabling difficulties that a person can experience. Thinking, remembering, reasoning, and making sense of the world around us is fundamental to carrying out activities of daily living (ADL). When individuals experience problems with these capacities, it can have a devastating effect on their lives and the lives of their families. These people may not be able to live alone, fulfill the responsibilities of paid employment, or sustain a family life and relationships.[1] Thus, effective treatment of many patients with brain damage depends on understanding perception and cognition.

The brain may be damaged through several mechanisms, including infections such as encephalitis; anoxia, as may occur following near-drowning, cardiopulmonary arrest, or carbon monoxide poisoning; tumors that are benign or malignant; trauma resulting from motor vehicle crashes, falls, or violent incidents (e.g., traumatic sports-related injury, gunshot wound); toxins such as alcohol or substance abuse; and vascular disease, which may produce an infarct or hemorrhagic stroke. The largest two groups of people who acquire cognitive and perceptual impairments following brain damage are persons who experienced stroke and traumatic brain injury (TBI).[1] The physical rehabilitation of these patient groups is addressed in Chapter 15, Stroke, and Chapter 19, Traumatic Brain Injury.

The patient who sustained an initial cerebral vascular accident (CVA) is thought to have focal or localized damage to discrete areas of the brain, often resulting in discrete cognitive or perceptual deficits. In contrast, patients who have sustained a TBI are presumed to have generalized brain damage resulting in cognitive impairment with generalized deficits in attention, memory, learning, and so forth, rather than specific difficulties in discrete cognitive or perceptual functions. However, elements of both perceptual and cognitive dysfunction may occur in brain damage owing to either CVA or trauma. The distinctions between the two groups of patients become particularly blurred when one considers the patient who experienced multiple strokes; this patient may in fact present with combined elements of both focal and generalized brain damage. This chapter focuses on the patient with hemiplegia whose brain damage has occurred as a result of a stroke. The overriding goal of this chapter is to introduce the reader to concepts relating to cognitive and perceptual dysfunction following brain damage.

An important focus for the physical therapist should be understanding how a particular cognitive or perceptual impairment might be manifested clinically and how examination and treatment of movement disorders might be adjusted to capitalize on the abilities and minimize the cognitive or perceptual limitations of the patient. Deficits in the cognitive or perceptual domain must be considered to accurately determine the patient's true residual abilities. Using sets of directions that would confuse a patient with apraxia during a specific examination procedure may paint a picture of a greater or different motor disability than that which actually exists. Often the first clue to a cognitive or perceptual problem appears during initial sensorimotor testing. Awareness of the possibility and nature of cognitive or perceptual deficits will signal the therapist to redirect the method of testing, particularly the instructional sets and cues.

■ COGNITION AND PERCEPTION

The perceptual-motor process is a chain of events through which the individual selects, integrates, and interprets stimuli from the body and the surrounding environment. Cognition can be conceived of as the method used by the central nervous system (CNS) to process information. Cognitive processes include knowing, understanding, awareness, judgment, and decision-making.[2] The difficulty of separating perceptual and cognitive deficits is readily apparent, both in patient behavior and in contradictory conceptualizations of these two domains of function. In a review of the literature, Katz and colleagues[3] found that to some authors, cognition is conceived of as a general term that includes perception, attention, thinking, and memory; to other authors, perception is an umbrella term that encompasses both cognition and visual perception as subcomponents. At this time, there is insufficient evidence to suggest which approach most accurately reflects the way we think about and perceive information. What is clear is that normally functioning perceptual and cognitive systems are key to successful interaction with the environment. Because the majority of work in this field does distinguish between cognition and perception[1] and because it is probably easier to learn about these processes individually, they are defined and addressed separately in this chapter.

Cognitive and perceptual capacities are clearly prerequisites for learning,[4] and rehabilitation is largely a learning process.[2] Thus, it is not surprising that patients with cognitive and perceptual disorders are limited in their ability to learn self-care and ADL skills; hence, as a group, they are more restricted in their potential to fully participate in family, work, and other societal roles.[5] In any rehabilitation program geared toward achievement of maximum independence, there is a compelling need for therapists to learn to recognize behavior related to perceptual deficits. The therapist's modification of examination and treatment approaches in light of these deficits will ensure that patients receive the full benefit of these services.

Cognition and Higher-Order Cognition

Cognition is the act or process of knowing, including awareness, reasoning, judgment, intuition, and memory. *Executive functions* are sometimes included under this heading as well. These include the capacity to plan, manipulate information, initiate and terminate activities, recognize errors, solve problems, and think abstractly. Commonly, executive functions are categorized as *higher-order cognitive functions* or *metacognitive functions*.[6–8]

Perception

Lezak[4] defines *perception* as the integration of sensory impressions into information that is psychologically meaningful. Thus, perception is the ability to select those stimuli that require attention and action, to integrate those stimuli with each other and with prior information, and finally to interpret them. The resulting awareness of objects and experiences within the environment enables the individual to make sense out of a complex and constantly changing internal and external sensory environment.[9]

The terms *perception* and *sensation* are often confused with each other. Sensation may be defined as the appreciation (awareness) of stimuli through the organs of special sense (e.g., eyes, ears, nose), the peripheral cutaneous sensory system (e.g., temperature, taste, touch), or internal receptors (e.g., deep receptors in muscles and joints).[9] Perception cannot be viewed as independent of sensation. However, the quality of perception is far more complex than the recognition of the individual sensation.[9] Perceptual deficits do not lie in the sensory ability itself but rather with the individual's ability to interpret the sensation accurately and therefore respond appropriately.[1]

■ RESPONSIBILITIES OF THE PHYSICAL THERAPIST AND THE OCCUPATIONAL THERAPIST

Occupational therapists are the members of the rehabilitation team who are specially trained to examine and treat cognitive and perceptual deficits in relation to functional adaptation. They are responsible for the selection and administration of an appropriate constellation of tests and measures, accurate interpretation of results, and formulation of an overall plan of care for cognitive and perceptual rehabilitation. If appropriate, the occupational therapist may refer a patient to a neuropsychologist for specific intellectual testing.

In the hospital setting, the physical therapist is often the first member of the rehabilitation team to see a patient with brain injury. The physical therapist must understand the nature of cognitive and perceptual dysfunction and recognize that individuals in certain diagnostic categories, such as those with stroke or TBI, are likely to behave in ways that indicate the presence of particular cognitive or perceptual deficits.[10] When this occurs, the physical therapist should refer the patient to occupational therapy for evaluation and treatment.

The tests and measures described in this chapter are included to assist the reader in understanding the nature of the different cognitive and perceptual disabilities and to guide decision-making about referral to another practitioner. They are not a substitute for an intensive evaluation by a trained occupational therapist when referral is deemed necessary.

An understanding of cognitive and perceptual dysfunction may go a long way toward alleviating much of the potential frustration that often accompanies treatment of a patient with brain damage, most of which is the result of inappropriate expectations on the part of team members, the patient, and the family. By collaborating with the occupational therapist, other members of the rehabilitation team, and the family, consistent treatment strategies may be developed and carried out, with obvious benefits to the patient.

■ CLINICAL INDICATORS

Cognitive and perceptual deficits ought to be ruled out as a cause of diminished functioning in all patients who have experienced brain damage. Such problems are particularly likely culprits in cases in which the patient seems unable to participate fully in self-care tasks and has difficulty participating in physical therapy for reasons that cannot be accounted for by lack of motor ability, sensation, comprehension, or motivation. Cognitive and perceptual dysfunction resulting from acquired brain damage must be differentiated from premorbid cognitive perceptual deficits (from previous trauma, illness, congenital abnormality, or dementia and from the general confusion and emotional sequelae that often accompany stroke and brain injury).[4]

Often, patients with cognitive and perceptual difficulties may display an inability to do simple tasks independently or safely, difficulty in initiating or completing a task, difficulty in switching from one task to the next, and a diminished capacity to locate visually or to identify objects that seem obviously necessary for task completion. In addition, they may be unable to follow simple one-step commands, despite apparently good comprehension. They may make the same mistakes over and over. Activities may take an inordinately long time to complete, or they may be done impulsively. Patients may hesitate many times, appear distracted and frustrated, and exhibit poor planning. They are frequently inattentive to one side of the body and extrapersonal space and may deny the presence or extent of their disability. These characteristics, all or some of which may be present, often make participation in ADL and therapy seem an insurmountable problem. These clinical features are explained and expanded on throughout this chapter.

Two typical scenarios are presented to give the reader an idea of when to suspect perceptual dysfunction. The first case involves a patient with a right-hemisphere stroke who presents clinically with a left hemiparesis and good speech. Upon observation in the nursing unit, the patient appears to have functional strength in the unaffected right extremities and fair return on the affected left side. Yet the patient seems to have difficulty with simple range of motion (ROM) activities, even in the intact extremities, appearing confused and unable to move the affected arm up or down on command. The patient cannot seem to follow instructions for walking with a quad cane, constantly confuses the proper step sequence, and is unable to maneuver a wheelchair around the corner without crashing into the wall.

This patient should not be dismissed as uncooperative, intellectually inferior, or confused. In this instance, the patient is likely experiencing difficulty in spatial relations, right–left discrimination, and vertical disorientation, or perhaps left-sided unilateral neglect. Further observation and examination should reveal the precise cause of the difficulties.

The second case involves a patient with left-hemisphere damage and a resulting right hemiparesis and mild expressive and receptive aphasia. The patient can respond reliably to "yes/no" questions and is able to follow simple one-step commands such as, "Put the pencil on the table," or "Give me the cup." However, if asked to point to their arm or to imitate the therapist's movements during an active ROM test even with the unaffected limbs, the patient does not respond and appears totally uncooperative. During therapy, the same patient is on a mat table. The therapist explains and then demonstrates the proper techniques for rolling to one side. The patient does not move. However, a moment later when his wife arrives, the patient quickly initiates rolling in an attempt to sit up to greet his wife.

The astute therapist will realize that this patient may not be confused, stubborn, or uncooperative, as indeed he may appear. Rather, he may be experiencing a lack of awareness of body structure and relationship of body parts (somatoagnosia), as evidenced by the ROM test incident and an inability to perform a task on command or to imitate gestures (ideomotor apraxia), as demonstrated in the rolling episode.

■ HOSPITALIZATION FOLLOWING BRAIN DAMAGE

The brain that has been damaged functions as a whole, just as it does in individuals without brain damage. When one part is damaged, the behavior observed is not merely the result of the brain operating precisely as in the intact individual minus the function of the area that was subject to anoxia. Rather, it is an outward manifestation of the reorganization of the entire CNS, at multiple levels, working to compensate for the loss.[11]

Because of the brain damage, the patient must cope with a nervous system operating without normal sensory input at all levels, both cortical and subcortical.[11] Normal responses to environmental stimuli are difficult to obtain when the input on which they have to act is impaired or incomplete. Recovery of function can be attributed to structural reorganization of the CNS into a new dynamic system widely dispersed within the cerebral cortex and lower segments.[12,13]

A significant contributor to the clinical picture of a patient after a CVA is the response to hospitalization. From a cognitive and perceptual perspective, when a patient is hospitalized (with or without brain damage), the inputs imposed on that patient's nervous system are radically different from the ones normally received. On the one hand, the environment is sensorially impoverished. There is no variation in temperature and lighting, and familiar background noises (e.g., telephones, airplanes, dogs, buses) are missing. On the other hand, an enormous array of unfamiliar noise is present: nurses talking, loudspeakers, and the whir and beeping of machines. Strange and different smells, and unfamiliar, unavoidable, and unpleasant sights abound. Often, because of motor impairment, the patient cannot move around to seek or to escape inputs; therefore, a multiplicity of sensory inputs bombards the nervous system. Even if orienting responses are preserved, there is a profound sense of loss of control. This sensory derangement compounds the problems faced by the patient with brain damage, because those very abilities that enable the individual to select, filter out, and integrate incoming sensations to organize the self for appropriate action often fail in this sensorially bizarre environment.

To gain insight into the experience of the patient under such circumstances, it is enlightening to browse through the biographical and autographical reports of some noted neurologists and neuropsychologists who have experienced CVAs themselves or have close relatives who have experienced a stroke. Particularly instructive are the reports of Bach-y-Rita,[14] Brodal,[15] and Doig.[16]

■ THEORETICAL FRAMEWORKS

The theoretical bases of five approaches to therapy are examined in this section, together with the examination procedures and treatment approaches consistent with the theoretical model. It is important to note that treatment approaches are not mutually exclusive. Many therapists use a combination of approaches, guiding selection by their clinical expertise and the patient's response to the interventions. Specific applications of these approaches are presented following the description of individual cognitive and perceptual deficits in the final section of this chapter. Further information on a variety of theoretical approaches used by occupational therapists when working with patients who have cognitive and perceptual problems can be found in Katz and Toglia[17] and Unsworth.[1]

The Retraining Approach

Katz and Toglia[17] describe the retraining approach that focuses on the remediation of underlying skills the patient has lost. Sometimes this approach is referred to as the *transfer-of-training approach*. The approach is based on the assumption that a disruption in one brain region can have a negative impact on brain functioning as a whole. An underlying assumption is that skills learned for one task can generalize to others. In other words, transfer of training is assumed. The premise is that practice in one task with particular cognitive or perceptual requirements will enhance performance in other tasks with similar perceptual demands.[1,18,19] Thus, doing specifically selected perceptual exercises, such as pegboard (a board with a regular pattern of small holes for pegs) activities or parquetry blocks (inlaid blocks of different woods arranged in a geometric pattern) and puzzles, will result in improving the perceptual skills required to perform those functional tasks. For example, Young et al.[20] demonstrated that training patients with left hemiplegia in block design (constructing shapes using blocks to match a two-dimensional pattern), in addition to *visual scanning* (using the eyes to follow a target) and *visual cancellation tasks* (placing a line through a specific number, letter, or word embedded randomly among other numbers, letters, or words), resulted in improvements in reading and writing, although no specific training in these areas was offered. Because all tasks require the use of multiple perceptual skills, it is difficult to ascertain precisely which perceptual skills are being trained during any one session.[21]

To date, research has not unequivocally demonstrated a generalization from perceptual-motor training to functional skills.[18,21] Neistadt[19] suggests that the patient's capacity to learn must be evaluated and that learning capacity is the key to a patient's ability to generalize material learned in one situation to others. If transfer of training does occur, then strategies to enhance this can be incorporated into other components of the treatment program, such as those aimed at maintaining sitting or standing balance, weight-bearing exercises, or functional use of the more involved extremities.

The Sensory Integrative Approach

Ayres developed the theory of sensory integration in an effort to explain the relationship between neural functioning and the behavior of children with sensorimotor or learning problems.[22] The theory, strongly influenced by the neurobehavioral literature, describes normal sensory integrative development and functioning, defines patterns of sensory integrative dysfunction, and suggests treatment techniques.[22] *Sensory integration* can be defined as the organization of sensation for use.[23,24]

Integration of basic sensorimotor functions (tactile, proprioceptive, and vestibular) proceeds in a developmental sequence in the normal child within the context of goal-directed, meaningful activity. It is assumed that the production of an adaptive response (desired motor response) facilitates sensory integration, which in turn enhances the ability to produce higher level adaptive behaviors. Sensory integration is thought to occur at all levels of the nervous system.

The underlying assumption for treatment is that by offering opportunities for controlled sensory input, the therapist can promote normal CNS processing of sensory information and thus elicit specific desired motor responses.[25] The performance of these adaptive responses, in turn, influences the way in which the brain organizes and processes sensation, thus enhancing the ability to learn.

Some of the treatment modalities employed include rubbing or icing to provide sensory input, resistance and weight-bearing to impart proprioceptive input, and the use of spinning or rocking to provide vestibular input. Following the controlled sensory input, an adaptive motor response is required by the patient to integrate the sensations provided by the therapist. In young children, the use of compensatory or splinter skills (skills acquired in a manner inconsistent with, or incapable of being integrated with, those already present) is avoided in favor of remediating underlying deficits. For more detailed information, the reader is referred to the work of Ayres.[23,24]

Zoltan[2] argues that older adults, who comprise the majority of the stroke population, experience sensory integrative dysfunction similar to that of children with learning disabilities because of age-related physiological changes together with environmentally induced sensory deprivation. The limitations in mobility caused by a stroke further prevent the patient from receiving and thus processing adequate sensory input.

The application of this theory to the adult poststroke population, however, is open to serious debate. Bundy et al.[22] argue that the theory explains mild to moderate learning and behavioral problems resulting from a central deficit in processing sensations but not specifically associated with frank brain damage. Further, there are several problems with the application of this approach to adult populations, even if it is theoretically tenable.

The treatment process is ordinarily quite lengthy. In addition, specific tests and measures and treatment approaches have been developed for and standardized on children, who presumably have sufficiently plastic nervous systems to be influenced by this form of therapy. The neurophysiological literature is replete with examples of skills that children can gain using this approach that would not be possible with mature individuals with similar lesions.[26–28] Furthermore, a mature adult with diffuse cerebral damage may have other complicating medical concerns and deficits in mobility that actually contraindicate the use of the equipment that is essential to the treatment process.[22] It is likely that many of the treatment regimens described as sensory integration are best described as a sensorimotor approach, which utilizes handling or directed sensory stimulation to elicit a specific motor response.[22]

The Neurofunctional Approach

The *neurofunctional approach* was first described by Giles and Wilson in 1992[29] and is based on learning theory. In contrast to the retraining approach, which assumes that transfer of training can occur, the authors of the neurofunctional approach assume that patients with acquired brain injury must practice every activity in its true context in order to recover function. Hence, the focus of this approach is on retraining real-world skills rather than on retraining specific cognitive and perceptual processes.[30] Giles[30] argues that remediation approaches (which include the idea of transfer of training) are largely unproven, and thus may result in little functional improvement for the patient. He also suggests that compensatory skills or techniques are taught to a patient without considering if the gains made in terms of quality of life justify the considerable effort required.

The Rehabilitative/Compensatory (Functional) Approach

Probably the most widely used approach in treating perceptual deficits is the *rehabilitative/compensatory approach*[31–33] (also referred to as the *functional approach*), which offers a great deal of practical support for the physical therapist. The basic assumptions underlying this approach are that adults with brain trauma will have difficulty generalizing and learning from dissimilar tasks.[34] Direct repetitive practice of specific functional skills that are impaired is an efficient means of enhancing the patient's independence in those specific tasks. More recently, Fisher[35] extended the work of Trombly[33] and those who followed[31] by (a) more explicitly articulating assumptions made about people within the rehabilitative/compensatory model; (b) generalizing this model beyond persons with physical disabilities to those with developmental, cognitive, or psychosocial disabilities; and (c) adding collaborative consultation to education and adaptation as strategies used to effect change.

The proponents of this approach favor addressing the functional problem over and above the treatment of its underlying cause when working with an adult poststroke population. For example, a patient with difficulty in depth and distance perception, who is therefore unable to navigate a flight of stairs, would be made aware of the deficit, would be provided with external cues to compensate for the perceptual disorder, and would repetitively practice adapted techniques for safe stair climbing. The more closely the therapeutic practice situation resembles the home and community situation in terms of stair depth and height, amount of traffic, lighting, and so forth, the less generalizing is required, and the more success patients are likely to have when they return home. However, problems might still be displayed in depth and distance perception in other areas of daily function.

In this functional approach, therapy is viewed as learning that takes into consideration the unique strengths and limitations of the individual patient. It is composed of two complementary components: compensation and adaptation.[1] *Compensation* refers to the changes that need to be made in the patient's approach to tasks. *Adaptation* refers to the alterations that need to be made in the human/social and physical environment in order to facilitate relearning of skills. In relation to the human/social environment, the therapist is concerned with altering the actions of others' functioning in the environment to enhance the patient's performance.

To compensate for the disability, the patient first has to be made aware of deficiencies (cognitive awareness) and must then be taught how to circumvent them using intact sensations and perceptual skills. The patient should be instructed in specific techniques and assisted in developing successful functional habits. The patient will need to be taught to attend to cues from the environment to enhance skill performance. The therapist helps the patient identify and then call on these new cues. For example, if the patient has a visual field cut, the therapist should explain that because of a visual problem, the patient is seeing only one half of the environment. The patient should then be shown how to turn the head to compensate for the deficit. Environmental scanning (moving head, and therefore eyes, from side to side to view surroundings) could be incorporated into general therapy sessions as well.

General suggestions when teaching compensatory techniques include (a) using simple directions, (b) establishing and carrying out a routine, (c) doing each activity in a consistent manner, and (d) employing repetition as much as necessary.

Adaptation refers to the alteration not of the patient's strategy but of the environment. For example, if the patient cannot differentiate between right and left or tends to neglect the left side of the body, a piece of red tape on the left shoe during gait training will allow the patient to attend more easily to the left side and thus follow the therapist's instructions more accurately. The therapist can use this functional approach to assist patients in improving specific motor skills related to treatment goals.

There are several inherent benefits to the rehabilitation/compensatory (functional) approach. First, in the current managed care environment, there is a limited amount of time for inpatient rehabilitation.[36] Therefore, therapists need to concentrate on outcome-directed, real-life functional activities, because independent performance of these activities at home is the ultimate goal of therapeutic intervention. Interventions directed toward specific functional outcomes are typically reimbursable.[31] In addition, the activities are age appropriate, specific, and clearly relevant to the patient's concerns. For this reason, they tend to be the most motivating. The tasks can also be incorporated into a daily hospital routine. Dressing can be reinforced at bedside by the nursing staff, and eating skills can be reinforced at each mealtime.

The major limitation of this approach is that the methods learned in one task are not typically generalized to the performance of another task. The functional approach has been criticized as the teaching of splinter skills, in which the causes of the dysfunction are not addressed.

Cognitive Rehabilitation and the Quadraphonic Approach

Cognitive rehabilitation focuses on training individuals with brain injury to structure and organize information.[37] It addresses memory, high language disorders, and perceptual dysfunction under one umbrella.[38] Information processing, problem-solving, awareness, judgment, and decision-making are among the areas included. The therapist using a cognitive remediation approach might be concerned with the patient's perceptual style, including perceptual strategy, response to different types of cues, and rate and consistency of task performance.[39] Cicerone and colleagues[40] provide an evidence-based review of the literature pertaining to rehabilitation strategies for cognitive deficits.

Research has demonstrated that even in a non-brain-injured population, skills learned in one task do not automatically transfer to other tasks.[41] Hence, cognitive strategies can be used to facilitate the carryover of skills learned in therapy to functional activities. In her multi-context treatment approach to cognition, Toglia[41] proposes that learning can be conceptualized as a dynamic interplay between characteristics of the patient, characteristics of the task, and the environment in which it is performed. This has also been termed a *dynamic interactional approach.*[42] Characteristics of the individual patient that might affect learning include information processing strategies, metacognition (including awareness of one's own performance), and prior experience, attitudes, and emotions. Task-related variables that are proposed to affect learning include the nature of the task itself (familiarity with the task, spatial arrangements, instruction set, and movement and postural requirements) and the criteria that are used to determine the learner's abilities. Environmental variables include the social and cultural environment in which treatment occurs, as well as the physical context.

The *cognitive rehabilitation approach* to treatment proposes a number of strategies relevant to physical therapist practice. These treatment strategies include the following:[41]

- Analyzing the characteristics of the task to establish criteria to determine if transfer of learning in fact took place
- Providing interventions to increase patient awareness of abilities, increase the level of difficulty of the task, and promote self-examination of performance
- Relating new information or skills to previously learned ones
- Using multiple environments in which to carry out the training activity to enhance transfer of learning

Although these treatment strategies are well known within the field of cognitive perceptual rehabilitation, the efficacy of the techniques remains to be established with the poststroke population. For a comprehensive understanding and practical guidelines to the evaluation and treatment of patients with cognitive impairments from a dynamic perspective, see Toglia[42] and Abreu.[43]

Abreu and Peloquin[44] have further developed these treatment strategies as the *quadraphonic approach.* The quadraphonic approach is an interactive rehabilitation approach that provides a holistic perspective for the management of stroke, TBI, brain tumors, cerebral palsy, and other neurological conditions. The quadraphonic approach is based on the idea that the therapist can apply both micro (reductionistic) and macro (holistic) perspectives for evaluation and treatment, which is an assumption shared by many occupational therapists who work in this field. Diagrammatic presentations of the components of the four key areas of the macro and four key areas of the micro perspectives (hence the term *quadraphonic*) are provided in Figures 27.1 and 27.2, respectively, and are explained in the text. The *macro* perspective is holistic or humanistic and provides guidelines for the management of functional performance and real-life occupations. In other words, this component of the quadraphonic approach is functional or top-down in focus. In Figure 27.1, the outer square is composed of four characteristics of a client (*lifestyle status, life stage status, health status,* and *disadvantage status*) that the therapist can explore through interviews and by asking clients to tell their stories. The therapist can use this information to explain and predict the client's behavior and performance. An evaluation then needs to be made of the client's will (volition) and goals, as well as the opportunity and capacity for action as depicted in the triangle. From there the therapist can develop an individualized therapy plan with the client (and significant others such as family).

In contrast, the *micro* perspective is more remedial in focus and provides guidelines for the management of performance components or subskills that include

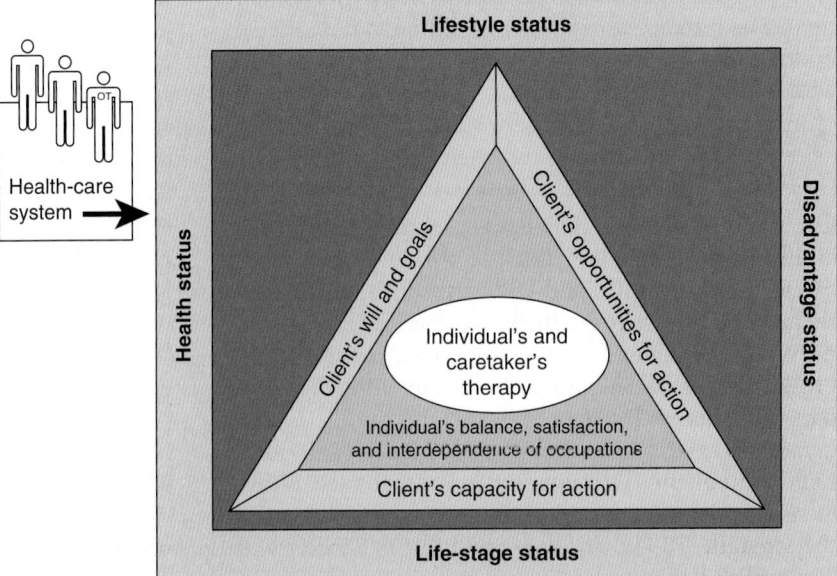

Figure 27.1 The quadraphonic approach—macro perspective. *(From Abreu,[43(p187)] with permission.)*

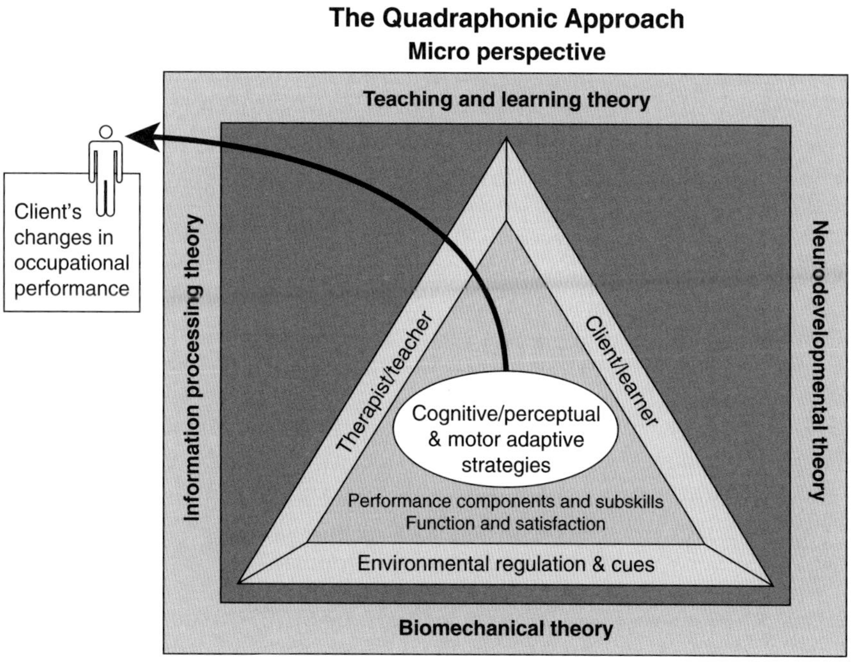

The Quadraphonic Approach
Micro perspective

Figure 27.2 The quadraphonic approach—micro perspective. *(From Abreu,[43(p185)] with permission.)*

attention, visual perception, memory, motor planning, postural control, and problem-solving. Evaluation and treatment of these performance components are based on a frame of reference that incorporates four theories: (a) information processing, (b) teaching and learning, (c) neurodevelopmental, and (d) biomechanical. These theories are listed in the outer square of Figure 27.2. This figure then presents an inner triangle that depicts how changes in the client's condition are further influenced by three dominant factors, which are the therapist (teacher), the environment in which therapy takes place, and what the client brings to therapy. The therapist and client work together to develop cognitive, perceptual, and motor strategies to enhance the client's performance and improve life satisfaction (as shown in the central circle of Fig. 27.1). Hence, the micro perspective is bottom-up, or remedial, in its focus. See Abreu[43] for an example of a therapist using this approach when working with a patient who has memory and learning problems.

■ EXAMINATION OF COGNITIVE AND PERCEPTUAL DEFICITS

The use of systematic data collection provides the scientific basis for guiding intervention. Its importance cannot be overemphasized with respect to all facets of therapeutic intervention, including remediation of cognitive and perceptual dysfunction. Task analysis is the breakdown of an activity or task into its component parts together with a delineation of the specific motor, perceptual, and cognitive abilities necessary to perform each component. Task analysis is another tool critical to appropriate therapeutic intervention. For example, the strength, ROM, and balance abilities necessary to accomplish bed mobility and ambulation activities can

be clearly defined by the physical therapist. However, the specific perceptual and cognitive requirements of each step needed to perform these two tasks may not be known. Without knowledge of the perceptual and cognitive requirements for successful completion of a task, the therapist cannot simplify the task for the patient and progressively upgrade it.

Purpose of the Examination

The presence of cognitive and perceptual dysfunction must be confirmed if it is suspected to be interfering with the patient's ability to carry out functional activities.[1] Perceptual performance is positively correlated with ability to perform ADL; however, it is often difficult to correlate specific perceptual deficits gleaned from testing with specific elements of functional ability and loss.[1,45] Thus, formal testing is indicated when there is a functional loss unexplained by motor or sensory impairments, or deficient comprehension. It should be noted that not all areas of functional loss are typically detected within the hospital setting. It is not uncommon for the patient to perform adequately in self-care skills after therapy in the hospital but to fail on the same tasks in other environmental contexts, such as the home. Higher level tasks, such as driving, banking, or planning a meal, may only emerge as areas of difficulty once the patient is discharged home. When appropriate, the patient's competence in these areas should be considered within the context of an examination of instrumental activities of daily living (IADL) with the occupational therapist while the patient is still hospitalized.

The purpose of patient examination is to determine which cognitive and perceptual abilities are intact and which are impaired. Understanding the manner in which a particular deficit influences task performance will foster the application of a therapeutic strategy in which intact capabilities may be used to compensate for or to overcome deficits.[1]

Failure in the performance of a task may result from any number of processes underlying cognition and perception. For example, a patient's inability to complete a jigsaw puzzle may result from an inability to organize the pieces or problem-solve where they go (disorder of executive function) or difficulty in attending to one half of the picture (unilateral neglect). The patient may be incapable of concentrating on the instructions (attention deficit), unable to know what the pieces are for (ideational apraxia), or unable to manipulate them (ideomotor apraxia). Although it is often difficult to implicate reliably one or another of these problem areas, the therapist must be aware of the different deficits that may produce similar patterns of behavior.[1,5]

A study conducted by Unsworth et al.[46] concerning the prediction of driving ability following stroke in 148 patients underscores the critical nature of carefully selected perceptual and cognitive tests. In this study, 87.5% of actual behind-the-wheel driving performances for people who were fit to drive and 72.2% of actual behind-the-wheel driving performances for people who were not fit to drive were predicted by performance on a selection of tests on the Occupational Therapy Driver Off Road Assessment Battery. Examination of individual test results uncovered the cognitive subtests of the battery where participants had the greatest difficulty, enabling instructors to focus on remediating these specific deficits in preparation for safe driving.

Patient examination is not an end in itself. Careful examination paves the way for realistic and cost-effective intervention.[47] Continuous monitoring of the patient's cognitive and perceptual status will ensure the use of appropriate treatment strategies and their modification when necessary.

Factors Influencing Patient Examination

Psychological and emotional status plays an important role in the patient's ability to cope with disability and with the testing situation. The therapist needs to be aware of behaviors that reflect a patient's psychological response to illness rather than particular cognitive or perceptual abilities. Psychological adjustment to disability depends on many factors, including age, vocational status, education, economic situation, attitude toward the reactions of others, family support, and feelings of competence before the onset of disease[45,48,49] (see Chapter 26, Psychosocial Issues in Physical Rehabilitation).

When examining psychological and emotional status, the following should be noted: whether the patient is confused, the level of comprehension for verbal instructions (written and spoken), whether communication is enhanced through the use of visual cues and demonstration, the ability to recognize errors, the level

of cooperation and initiative (whether the patient is realistic about capabilities and goals), and emotional stability.[50] Disturbances of emotional response are evidenced by rapid and frequent mood changes and low frustration tolerance. Difficult tasks may cause a catastrophic reaction.[45,49]

The patient's ability to detect relevant cues from the environment or to discriminate between relevant and irrelevant stimuli (necessary for cognitive and perceptual competence) may be adversely influenced by poor judgment, fatigue, and prior expectations. Poor judgment is a major contributor to accidents in patients with hemiplegia. This is related in part to the diminished awareness by these patients as to their altered capabilities. The ambiguity of having one set of functional limbs and one set that is not functional may lead the patient to rely on solutions to the problems of daily living that are familiar but now inappropriate.[49]

Anxiety over capabilities may inhibit optimal performance during examination and treatment. The patient's capacity to perform optimally on testing and to learn is enhanced if anxiety can be reduced.[45] Motivation is influenced by many factors, among them premorbid personality. It is of utmost importance for the therapist to structure the therapeutic environment so that the patient will be positively motivated to learn to their maximum ability.[49] To this end, therapeutic tasks should be structured to ensure success, thereby diminishing frustration.

Other factors that may limit a patient's performance on cognitive and perceptual tests include reduced receptive and expressive communication skills, depression, and fatigue. Before a formal examination, the therapist should consider the patient's language skills and confirm these observations with the speech-language pathologist. The therapist should also be aware of any medications the patient is taking and how these may affect performance. For example, many medications produce drowsiness as a side effect, which would impact patient performance during testing.[1] Following stroke, 30% to 70% of people are said to experience depression,[51] the symptoms of which can easily be mistaken for cognitive or perceptual problems. Finally, a determination should be made of the patient's level of fatigue before any examination procedure.

The patient's behavior should not be misinterpreted because of a cultural bias, such as a lack of experience in taking tests. Premorbid intellectual ability should be ascertained from an interview with family or friends, because intellectual abilities may affect performance on some of the tests and measurements and may affect behavior in general. Premorbid memory should also be determined.

Finally, it is very important to conduct a sensory examination *before* cognitive or perceptual testing to establish whether the patient has sufficient sensory abilities to proceed with testing (this includes visual screening). Distinguishing between sensory and cognitive or perceptual problems is explored in more detail in the next section of this chapter. Each of these problems may adversely influence performance and may also reduce the patient's performance in treatment and capacity to learn from treatment. The therapist should be aware of the potential for these problems arising and seek to minimize their impact.

Distinguishing Between Sensory and Cognitive and Perceptual Deficits

Cognitive and perceptual dysfunction must be differentiated from sensory loss, language impairment, hearing loss, motor loss (weakness, spasticity, incoordination), visual disturbances (poor eyesight, homonymous hemianopia), disorientation, and lack of comprehension. The therapist must rule out pure sensory impairments before testing for cognitive and perceptual deficits; otherwise, the therapist may incorrectly attribute poor performance to perceptual problems and design treatment accordingly when in fact the problem has a sensory base and should be treated quite differently. The therapist should conduct tests of deep (proprioceptive) sensations (kinesthesia, position sense, vibration), superficial sensations (pain, temperature, light touch, and pressure), and combined cortical sensations (stereognosis, tactile localization two-point discrimination, barognosis, graphesthesia, and recognition of texture) using methods described in Chapter 3, Examination of Sensory Function. The patient's hearing also requires testing. For example, if the patient does not seem to understand what the therapist is saying, hearing problems should be ruled out before more extensive language and cognitive tests are conducted. The therapist may need to confirm with the family if the patient wears a hearing aid and ensure its availability during therapy. If in doubt, the therapist may need to request testing by the speech-language pathologist or audiologist.

The therapist must also determine if the patient has visual impairments because they can easily be mistaken for perceptual problems. Given the prevalence of sensory-based visual problems, the following section focuses on identification of these impairments and the importance of distinguishing between visual and perceptual origins for treatment purposes.

Visual Impairments

Visual impairments are one of the most common forms of sensory loss affecting the patient with hemiplegia.[52] The lesion resulting from a stroke may affect the eye, optic radiation, or visual cortex and subsequently the reception, transmission, and appreciation of any visual array. Visual impairments commonly encountered by patients with hemiplegia include poor eyesight, diplopia, homonymous hemianopia, and damage to the visual cortex or retina. Awareness of the presence of these deficits is important so as not to confuse them with visual

perceptual deficiencies and to ensure their consideration during treatment planning and therapeutic intervention.

The critical nature of the basic visual skills (i.e., acuity, oculomotor control, and intact visual fields) in forming a basis for higher level visual perception is highlighted by Warren[53,54] in a hierarchical model for the evaluation and treatment of visual perceptual dysfunction. In this developmental model, the basic visual skills enumerated earlier form the foundation for the next level of visual skills, which include *visual attention* (focusing on one aspect of the environment while ignoring others), *visual scanning* (using eyes to follow a target), and *pattern recognition* (recognition of structures that make a recognizable whole). These skills, along with memory, are required to facilitate the highest-level visual skill, termed *visual cognition*.[53,54] This model has implications for the evaluation and treatment of visual perceptual disorders in a bottom-up sequence[54] (i.e., working from the "bottom," initially focusing on underlying skills that will then promote recovery of the next level of skills).

Impairments of oculomotor control (control of eye movements) are a common occurrence following a CVA. Poor visual acuity is another frequent finding following stroke or brain injury, even in the absence of other visual problems.[55] Therefore, it is recommended that the patient receive a comprehensive eye examination and have their eyeglass prescription checked.

Diplopia, or double vision, is often present following brain damage. The patient sees two of the entire environment (horizontally, vertically, or diagonally). Diplopia is usually the result of defective function of extraocular muscles in which both eyes are used but not in conjunction with the other. Treatment usually consists of exercises for the eye muscles. In addition, the patient usually is instructed to wear a patch on alternate eyes until the condition clears. If the condition does not clear, the optometrist may recommend prisms (described later).

Visual field deficit is probably the most common visual deficit affecting patients with hemiplegia[56] and occurs most frequently following damage to the middle cerebral artery near the internal capsule.[49] The diagnostic term for this deficit is homonymous hemianopia. The frequency of homonymous hemianopia in patients with suspected visual deficits following stroke is around 52%.[56] In addition, there is a significant correlation between the presence of visual field deficits and visual neglect.[57] Importantly, the presence of a visual field deficit is a significant prognostic sign, predicting poorer functional outcomes, even following rehabilitation.[56,58]

Figure 27.3 demonstrates the normal functioning of the visual fields, in which the left side of the environment (the tree) is perceived by the nasal retina of the left eye and the temporal retina of the right eye, and the right side of the environment (the car) is perceived by the nasal retina of the right eye and the temporal retina of the left eye.

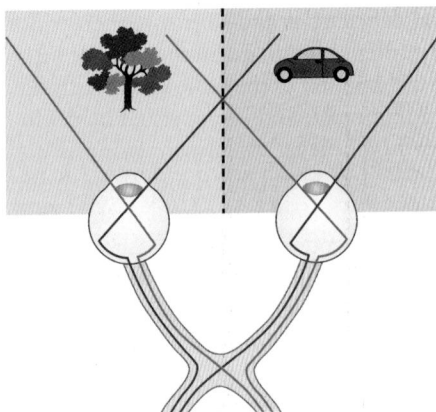

Figure 27.3 Normally functioning visual system; right and left visual fields. See text for explanation.

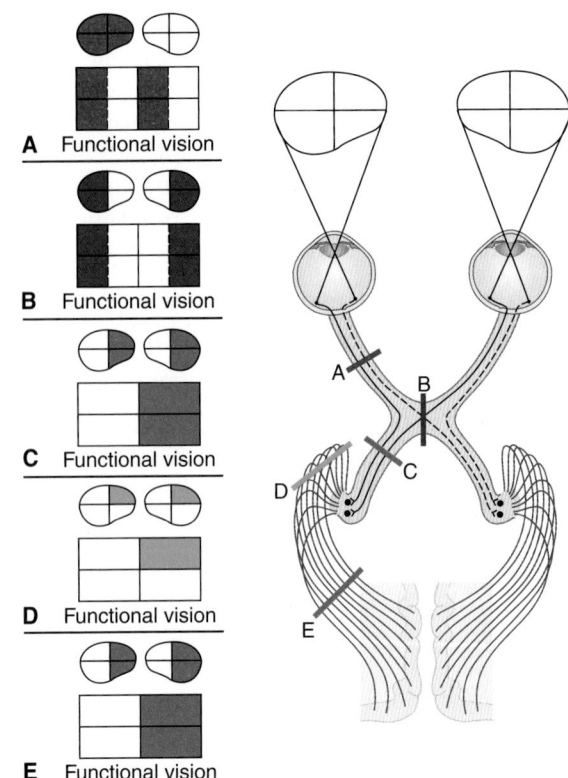

A Functional vision

B Functional vision

C Functional vision

D Functional vision

E Functional vision

Figure 27.4 Visual field deficits (with functional loss) and associated lesions. Vision is shown as clear, and visual loss is colored in examples A–E, which denote (A) blindness in one eye, (B) bitemporal hemianopia (tunnel vision), (C) homonymous hemianopia, (D) quadrantanopia, and (E) homonymous hemianopia.

The lesion producing homonymous hemianopia interrupts inflow to the optic pathways on one side of the brain. This produces a loss of the outer half of the visual field from one eye and the inner half of the visual field of the other eye. The result is a loss of incoming information from half of the visual environment (left or right) contralateral to the side of the lesion. Thus, the loss of the left half of the visual field accompanies left hemiplegia, and loss of the right visual field accompanies right hemiplegia. Zhang et al.[59] suggested that this is a common condition following stroke and noted a spontaneous recovery rate in less than 40% of cases. Figure 27.4 illustrates visual field deficits associated with a number of lesions to the visual system.

The presence of a visual field cut may inhibit performance in many daily activities. The patient is usually unaware of the condition and does not automatically compensate by turning the head unless specifically instructed. One of the dangers in this condition is street crossing (Fig. 27.5). Another example of the effects of a visual field cut is illustrated in Figure 27.6. When presented with a newspaper, a patient with right homonymous hemianopia may attend to only one half of the newspaper page, either to or from the midline.

Because of homonymous hemianopia's prevalence, it is essential for the therapist to determine whether this condition is present or not. A number of testing procedures are currently employed. In the confrontation method, the patient sits opposite the therapist and is instructed to maintain their gaze on the therapist's nose (Fig. 27.7). The therapist slowly brings a target, such as the therapist's finger or a pen, into the patient's field of view simultaneously or alternately from the right or left. Patients are instructed to indicate when and where they see the targets.

To help the patient compensate for the visual field deficit, the patient can first be made aware of the deficit and then be instructed to turn the head to the affected side. Patients usually require constant reminders at

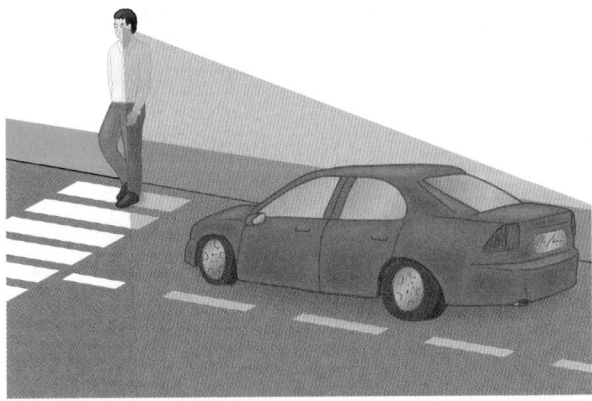

Figure 27.5 The functional significance of hemianopia— it may lead to accidents.

first, which may be tapered off with time and practice. Early in therapy, items such as eating utensils and writing implements should be placed where the patient is most apt to see them (on the less affected side). They can be moved progressively to the midline and then to the more affected side, when appropriate. The nursing staff should be made aware of the condition and be requested to place the patient's essential bedside

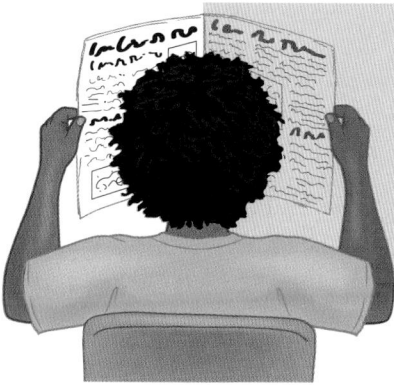

Figure 27.6 A newspaper as it might appear to a patient with right homonymous hemianopia following a stroke. The shading indicates that the patient may be unable to read the right side of the page.

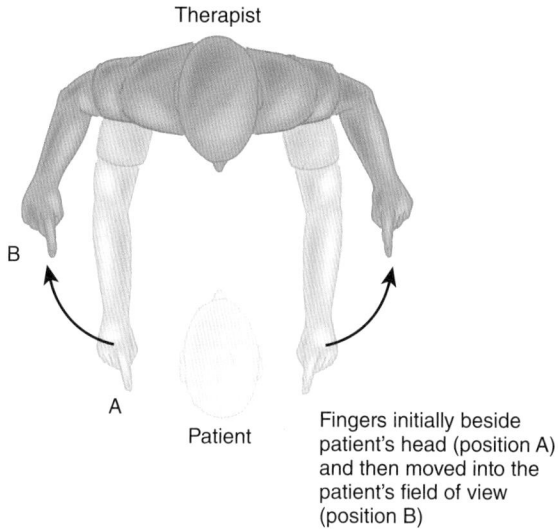

Therapist

B

A

Patient

Fingers initially beside patient's head (position A) and then moved into the patient's field of view (position B)

Figure 27.7 Method for testing hemianopia.

needs such as telephone, tissues, and so forth, within the intact visual field. The therapist initially should sit on the patient's less involved side when instructing or giving demonstrations and should alternate this with the more affected side so that the patient receives maximum stimulation. Of course, the patient will have to be reminded to turn the head at first. External cues can be employed as well. For reading, a red line can be drawn on the side of the page that is not seen. Red tape can be placed on the floor, mat, or parallel bars to attract the patient to scan to the side of the environment that is not seen. The patient should be taught to look for these cues. These external cues can be slowly tapered off over time. Patients can be instructed and encouraged to devise their own cues to clue them in to the unseen side of the environment in situations that have not been addressed per se in therapy. Exercises that require motor crossing of the midline can be used to reinforce visual crossing of the midline and turning of the head.[60,61]

Oculomotor impairment is another area of deficit in basic visual skills that is common in patients who have had a stroke. Eye movements, which are controlled by the extraocular muscles, are used to detect, identify, and derive meaning from objects and the environment. They allow a person to become oriented to and explore the critical visual aspects of the environment.[11] Two types of eye movements are important to examine: (a) visual fixation, which allows the patient to maintain focus on an object as it is brought nearer or farther away, and (b) ocular pursuits, which enable the eyes to follow a moving object and visually scan the environment. Often the eyes will not follow a moving object visually, although the patient seems aware of the presence of that object and can locate it if asked; such patients are visually hypoactive. Oculomotor dysfunction often accompanies visual perceptual dysfunction[62] and may be related to attention deficits.

Visual scanning can be tested as follows. Sit opposite the patient. Hold up a pencil with a colorful pencil topper 18 in. (45.7 cm) in front of the patient's eyes. Slowly move the pencil horizontally, then vertically, then diagonally. Repeat each direction two to three times. Note the smoothness of eye movements, the presence of a midline jerk or jump, and whether the eyes move together.[62,63]

Aside from the visual sensory impairments outlined earlier, many patients experience visual perceptual impairment. Damage to areas of the cortex on which visual information converges with information from other senses may interfere with the recognition and interpretation of visual information, even though the visual stimuli may have arrived at the visual cortex uninterrupted. A total failure to appreciate incoming visual sensory information owing to a lesion in the cortex is referred to as *cortical blindness*.[62] There is no statistical correspondence between the presence of visual field cuts and the presence of visual perceptual disorders.[64] Similarly, there is no correspondence between aphasia, age, and time since infarct and measures of visual perceptual dysfunction.[64] However, within the realm of visual perceptual impairments, there is a significant difference between the performances of patients with right hemiplegia and those with left hemiplegia. Patients with left hemiplegia have frequently been found to perform more poorly on measures of visual perceptual dysfunction than patients with right hemiplegia. Thus, therapists should be aware of the possibility of visual perceptual deficits, particularly in the population with left hemiplegia.

Standardized Cognitive and Perceptual Tests

A standardized test is one that has a uniform procedure to administer and score, provides operational definitions for all terms, is norm-referenced,[65] and has information available concerning its reliability and validity, which is essential for correct interpretation of results.[66] Results from standardized tests of cognition and perception can be communicated to other therapists who will share an understanding of the patient's capacities or abilities. Standardized tests can be administered at both admission and discharge to provide the therapist with a reliable and valid measure of the outcome of therapy.

When conducting a standardized test, the patient should be sitting comfortably and wearing glasses and/or a hearing aid if needed. Ideally, the room should be quiet and free of distraction. The therapist should be positioned opposite or next to the patient. Since the performance of a patient who has had a stroke may vary from day to day, a single testing session may be unreliable.[67] A number of short sessions scheduled on successive days may be preferable. To enhance its practical value, perceptual testing must be done in conjunction with observation in self-care and ADL skills, where the patient's judgment and discriminative abilities with regard to real-life tasks can be determined. It is not uncommon for patients to test poorly for visual perceptual skills but to perform adequately in ADL with minimal effort or assistance.[63]

The quality of the patient's response to the test media (e.g., how the task is approached, how and why the error is made) is as important to note as the success or failure in completing the selected task. Some aspects of response in the testing situation or during ADL can be referred to as the patient's individual *perceptual style*. Included under this rubric are the patient's perceptual strategy, response to various cues (such as auditory, visual, and tactile), rate of performance, and consistency of performance.[37]

Occupational therapists use a variety of standardized tests to determine the presence of cognitive and perceptual impairments and resulting disabilities. When selecting a standardized test, the therapist must consider many factors. The selection depends on what the therapist wants to learn about the patient and what the test can potentially reveal.[1] In many cases, a single test will not provide all the information required by a therapist to plan treatment, so several tests may be administered[5,68-88] (Table 27.1). In addition to those presented in Table 27.1,

Table 27.1   Table of Outcome Measures

Outcome Measure and ICF Category	Description	Scoring	MDC and MCID
A-ONE[5] ICF: 1, 2	This test was developed to measure a patient's neurobehavior through daily living tasks (dressing, grooming, hygiene, transfer and mobility, feeding, and communication). Occupational therapists must undertake a 5-day training and certification course to qualify to administer this test. A wide variety of cognitive and perceptual impairments can be detected with this instrument.	The A-ONE can be administered in 30–40 minutes. The 22 ADL tasks on the FIS and 46 items on the NSIS are rated on a 5-point scale. FIS item scores range from 0 (unable to perform and totally dependent on assistance) to 4 (functionally independent). The FIS total score is derived from the sum of item scores.	MDC: NA MCID: NA
AMPS[68] ICF: 1, 2	The AMPS is a structured, observational assessment of performance in daily living activities. Performance is observed on a choice of two or three familiar instrumental or personal ADLs. Quality of performance is rated on 16 motor and 20 process skills relating to independence, efficiency, effortlessness, and adoption of safe practices in the context of the task undertaken (dynamic interaction of the person with the environment). Training is required before the assessment can be administered.	The AMPS can be completed in 30–60 minutes.[69] Scores range from 1 (deficit) to 4 (competent) for each of the 16 motor and 20 process skills associated with each ADL performed. Higher scores are indicative of more skill competence.	MDC: NA MCID: NA

Table 27.1	Table of Outcome Measures—cont'd			
Outcome Measure and ICF Category	Description	Scoring	MDC and MCID
AusTOMS-OT[70] *ICF: 1, 2, 3*	The AusTOMs-OT is a measure of global functional outcomes for clients of all ages and all diagnoses. The AusTOMS comprises 12 scales that are rated across four domains (Impairment, Activity Limitation, Participation Restriction, and Distress/Well-being). A client's cognitive and perceptual skills are included, but not targeted, as part of this assessment. Training is required before the assessment can be administered.	The AusTOMs-OT outcome measures can be scored in under 5 min. The scores across the four domains range from 0–5, with lower scores indicative of more severe functioning.	MDC: The MDC (90% CI) has been calculated for two scales, from the data from Fristedt.[71] Scale 7 Self-Care-Impairment: MDC = 0.95 Self-Care-Activity/Limitation: MDC = 1.24 Self-Care-Participation/Restriction: MDC = 1.14 Self-Care-Distress/Well-being: MDC = 1.33 Scale 5 Transfers-Impairment: MDC = 1.30 Transfers-Activity/Limitation: MDC = 0.99 Transfers-Participation/Restriction: MDC = 1.13 Transfers-Distress/Well-being: MDC = 1.23 MCID: A change of 0.5 to 1 point on any of the four domains of the AusTOMs-OT scale is considered clinically important.
Behavioural Assessment of the Dysexecutive (BADS)[72] *ICF: 1*	The BADS assesses an individual's executive function skills. The assessment includes six subtests and a 20-item questionnaire that measure everyday executive function and higher level cognitive functions.	The BADS can be completed in 30–45 minutes.[69] Each subtest score ranges from 0–4. An overall profile score is obtained from summing the individual subtest scores. This score can be converted to a standard score with a mean of 100 and a standard deviation of 15.	MDC: NA MCID: NA
Behavioral Inattention Test (BIT)[73] *ICF: 1*	The BIT was developed to examine clients for the presence of unilateral visual neglect and to provide the therapist with information concerning how the neglect affects the client's ability to perform everyday occupations.[74] The BIT is composed of two subtests:	The test can be completed in approximately 1 hr. Total and subscores are obtained by adding the subtests scores together. Max scores: BIT = 227 BITC = 146 BITB = 81	MDC: NA MCID: NA

(Continued)

Table 27.1	Table of Outcome Measures—cont'd		
Outcome Measure and ICF Category	**Description**	**Scoring**	**MDC and MCID**
	BITB subtest consists of nine activity-based subtests such as card sorting and phone dialing. The BITC subtest consists of six pen-and-paper subtests such as representational drawing, line crossing, and figure shape copying. Many of these test items have been used in the past in a nonstandardized way to examine for the presence of neglect.	Higher scores are indicative of more severe visual impairment.	
COGNISTAT The Neurobehavioral Cognitive Status Examination[75] ICF: 1	This cognitive screening assessment comprises 62 items that measure memory, language, attention, calculations, level of consciousness and orientation, and reasoning. Training is required before the assessment can be administered.	The COGNISTAT can be completed in 15–30 minutes.[69] Min score = 0; Max score = 12. Sum score for each domain using the domain raw score to determine the presence and severity of deficits.	MDC: NA MCID: NA
EFPT[76] ICF: 1, 2	The EFPT examines performance on five ADL tasks that involve five executive function constructs as follows: initiation, organization, sequencing, judgment and safety, and completion.	This test can be completed in 30–45 minutes.[77] For each of the five ADL tasks, the five executive function constructs are scored across a range from 0 (independent) to 5 (totally dependent on assistance). A total score for each of the ADL tasks is derived from the sum of the five executive function constructs.	MDC: NA MCID: NA
LOTCA[78] ICF: 1	The LOTCA is a battery-style test lasting 35–40 minutes and composed of 20 subtests that examine four areas: orientation, visual and spatial perception, visuomotor organization, and thinking operations. The instrument was developed for use with people who have experienced stroke, TBI, or tumor.[78] The LOTCA has recently been validated with a Chinese population of patients with stroke.[79] There are several different versions of the LOTCA, including the LOTCA-G,[80] the FLOTCA,[81] the DLOTCA,[82] the DLOTCA-G,[80] and the DOTCA-Ch.[83]	The LOTCA can be completed in 30–45 minutes. Subtests are scored from 1 (low) to 4 (high), except for three subtests, which are scored from 1–5.	MDC: NA MCID: NA

Table 27.1 Table of Outcome Measures—cont'd

Outcome Measure and ICF Category	Description	Scoring	MDC and MCID
MoCA[84] ICF: 1	The MoCA is a comprehensive cognitive screening assessment of memory, language, attention, visuospatial skills, orientation, and abstraction. The MoCA comprises 16 items and 11 categories to assess cognitive abilities in order to detect mild cognitive dysfunction.	This test can be completed in approximately 10 minutes.[77] Max total score = 30.	MDC: NA MCID: NA
RPAB[85] ICF: 1	This instrument was designed to examine visual perceptual impairments in patients following head injury or stroke. The RPAB is a battery consisting of 16 performance tasks that examine form discrimination, color constancy, sequencing, object completion, figure–ground discrimination, body image, inattention, and spatial awareness. For further information on the RPAB, the reader is referred to Jesshope et al.[86]	The RPAB can be completed in approximately 1 hr. Scoring is based on the accuracy of task completion and time to complete task (max time limit range: 3–5 minutes). Max task score range: 4–72. A total score is not recorded.	MDC: NA MCID: NA
RBMT-3[87] ICF: 1	This battery was designed to examine everyday memory abilities. It offers the therapist an initial determination of the client's memory function, provides an indication of appropriate areas for treatment, and enables the therapist to monitor memory skills throughout the treatment program. The RBMT-3 comprises 14 subtests that examine immediate and delayed everyday memory, recall, and recognition. The RBMT-3 also includes a new subtest "Novel Task," which assesses new learning. For further information on the development and validation of the RBMT, the reader is referred to Wilson et al.[87,88]	The RBMT-3 can be administered in approximately 30 minutes by occupational therapists, speech-language pathologists, and psychologists. The RBMIT-3 offers two scoring options: screening and profile score to detect change over time. Subtest raw scores can be converted to scaled scores (based on client age) with a mean of 10 and a standard deviation of 3. An overall General Memory Index can be derived with a mean of 100 and a standard deviation of 15.	MDC: NA MCID: NA

ADL = activities of daily living; AMPS = Assessment of Motor and Process Skills; A-ONE = Arnadottir OT-ADL Neurobehavioral Evaluation; AusTOMS-OT = Australian Therapy Outcome Measures for Occupational Therapy; BADS = Behavioural Assessment of the Dysexecutive; BIT = Behavioral Inattention Test; BITB = Behavioural Inattention Test Behavioral subtest; BITC = Behavioural Inattention Test Conventional; DOTCA-Ch = Dynamic Occupational Therapy Cognitive Assessment for Children; DLOTCA = Dynamic LOTCA; DLOTCA-G = DLOTCA-Geriatric; EFPT = Executive Function Performance Test; FIS = Functional Independence Scale; FLOTCA = Functional LOTCA; ICF = International Classification of Functioning, Disability, and Health; LOTCA = Loewenstein Occupational Therapy Cognitive Assessment; LOTCA-G = LOTCA-Geriatric; MCID = minimal clinically important difference; MDC = minimal detectable change; MoCA = Montreal Cognitive Assessment; NSIS = Neurobehavioral Specific Impairments Subscale; RBMT-3 = Rivermead Behavioural Memory Test; RPAB = Rivermead Perceptual Assessment Battery; TBI = traumatic brain injury.
ICF Category: 1 = Body Structure/Function; 2 = Activity; 3 = Participation.

other instruments used to measure more global outcomes of rehabilitation include the following:

- *Medical Outcomes Study (MOS), Short Form Health Survey (SF-36)*[89]
- *Australian Therapy Outcomes (AusTOMs) (www.austoms.com)*[70]
- *Canadian Occupational Performance Measure (COPM)*[90]
- *Rivermead Rehabilitation Centre Life Goals Questionnaire*[91]
- *Reintegration to Normal Living Index (RNL)*[92]
- *Functional Independence Measure (FIM$_{MR}$)*[93]

Some of these instruments also incorporate items that measure cognition and perception. For example, the FIM$_{MR}$ includes three cognition-related items (social interaction, problem-solving, and memory). The tests described in the section on specific cognitive and perceptual deficits are used widely in the clinic. Although some of the instruments presented are not standardized, they are still useful, particularly for examining the quality of response to the test stimuli.

■ INTERVENTION

Treatment Approaches

Five major approaches to cognitive and perceptual rehabilitation are commonly employed by occupational therapists. They are the *retraining approach,* the *sensory integrative approach,* the *neurofunctional approach,* the *rehabilitation/compensatory approach,* and the *cognitive rehabilitation/quadraphonic approach.* These approaches were described earlier in the chapter. Although research directly comparing the efficacy of the various approaches has been sparse, attempts have been made recently to empirically define and test the methodologies.[21,25,34,94] Issues to consider in examining the approaches are the availability of standardized measures of change in functional status and ADL, group versus individual treatment, specific stimulus properties, format, length and frequency of feedback, and individual information processing styles.[21]

Historically, Neistadt[21,25] described these treatments dichotomously as either remedial or adaptive/compensatory. The remedial approach encompasses the retraining approach, the sensory integrative approach, and the cognitive approach.[1] The neurofunctional approach and the rehabilitation/compensatory approach are described as adaptive or compensatory. The quadraphonic approach brings together aspects of both the remedial and compensatory approaches. A description of the key components of these two main approaches is presented in the following sections. A discussion on education is also provided because no intervention program would be complete without the provision of education to both the patient and the caregivers. Finally, a discussion is provided on integrating these three elements within a rehabilitation program.

The Remedial Approach

Remedial approaches focus on the patient's deficits and attempt to improve functional ability by retraining specific perceptual components of behavior.[25] The assumption uniting this set of tactics is that facilitation of, or training in, underlying skills will enhance the recovery or reorganization of deficient CNS functioning.[21,25] This, in turn, will automatically translate into improvement in functional skills. Remedial approaches are also referred to as *bottom-up approaches.* These approaches work from the bottom, which is the recovery of underlying skills, and assume that the patient will be able to generalize skills to occupational performance, which is at a higher level.[1,47]

The Adaptive/Compensatory Approach

The adaptive or compensatory approach mandates direct training in the functional skills that are deficient. It does not assume automatic carryover from tasks that are not obviously similar to the functional task to be learned and thus minimizes the need for generalization. In an adaptive, or "top-down" approach, the therapist works with the patient on specific tasks that are required, or those that the patient wants to achieve. In other words, the therapist starts at the top, which is the desired functional outcome, rather than working with the patient on the underlying performance components.[35] Table 27.2 presents a comparison of the assumptions underlying the remedial and adaptive approaches.

Patient, Family, and Caregiver Education

Education for the patient, family, and caregivers is essential for continuity of care. Appendix 27.A (online) includes Web-based resources for clinicians, families, and patients with cognitive and perceptual deficits. The patient and caregivers should understand why it is inadvisable or impossible for the patient to do some things safely or independently, and why other things must be done in a specific way. Explaining the reasons why such patients behave in a particular way reduces the likelihood of inappropriate expectations from those without the background to know that brain damage affects not only how patients move but also how they experience and thus respond to the world.

Feedback is essential to the patient's learning. The patient's own feedback may be inaccurate owing to perceptual and cognitive dysfunctions. Thus, the individual may be unaware that a task has not been accomplished or that it has not been performed in the safest or most efficient manner. Feedback should be provided in the form of knowledge of results (KR; information regarding whether or not the patient attained the correct outcome) and knowledge of performance (KP; information regarding the manner in which the task was accomplished).[95]

The form in which this feedback is delivered depends on the specific limitations and strengths of the patient. For example, the physical therapy goal for a patient

Table 27.2 Common Assumptions of Adaptive and Remedial Approaches	
Adaptive Approach	**Remedial Approach**
The adult brain has limited potential to repair and reorganize itself after injury.	The adult brain can repair and reorganize itself after injury.
Intact behaviors can be used to compensate for ones that are impaired.	Repair and reorganization are influenced by environmental stimuli.
Adaptive retraining can facilitate the substitution of intact behaviors for impaired ones.	Cognitive, perceptual, and sensorimotor exercises can promote brain recovery and reorganization.
Adaptive activities of daily living provide training in functional behaviors.	Cognitive, perceptual, and sensorimotor exercises provide training in the cognitive and perceptual skills needed for those exercises.
Training in specific, essential activities of daily living tasks is necessary because adults with brain injury have difficulty generalizing learning.	Remedial training in cognitive and perceptual skills will be generalized across all activities requiring those skills.
Functional activities require cognitive and perceptual skills.	Functional activities require cognitive and perceptual skills.
Adaptation and compensation will lead to improved functional performance.	Cognitive and perceptual remediation will lead to improved functional performance.

with left hemiplegia and visual perceptual involvement might be to walk to the end of the parallel bars. KR would consist of a verbal confirmation by the therapist as to whether the patient reached the end of the parallel bars. KP might include comments by the therapist concerning the adequacy of the patient's visual scanning, positioning of the lower extremities (LEs), correct posture, and appropriate use of the upper limbs. For the patient with communication impairments, feedback would need to be visual. Tactile input also can be used effectively to cue patients with either right or left hemiplegia. A combination of inputs, using a number of sensory modalities, often facilitates patient success at a given task.

When involving the patient in education sessions, the patient must be addressed as a competent adult and not patronized. Patients must be regarded as the principal participants in the rehabilitation process. In situations in which the perceptual deficit does not interfere with assimilation of information, patients should have the major role in the decision-making process regarding the goals of therapy.

Refocusing Intervention

Many clinicians begin an intervention program by adopting remedial strategies. In these circumstances, therapists are aiming to maximize recovery of function and educate their patients about the problems experienced and ways that can improve their function. However, some patients may not make much progress. In some cases, the patient may have inadequate language skills to be able to work with the therapist or may have limited insight to their problems and therefore will not

work with the therapist. In other cases, improvements simply do not seem to occur for a variety of reasons that the therapist may not be able to pinpoint. Finally, in the current climate of managed care, the therapist may not have very much time allocated to work with the patient using remedial techniques. The patient's discharge may be imminent, and yet they may not be independent or safe enough to be discharged. In such cases, the therapist may switch from a remedial approach to a compensatory one.

When using an adaptive compensatory approach, the therapist will address education of the caregivers as well as the patient. Intervention strategies will focus on changing the environment or the strategy for task completion so that the patient can be safe and independent as quickly as possible. In many instances, therapists use a three-point approach to intervention where they educate patients and caregivers, begin the program using remedial techniques, and then switch to compensation techniques when the patient's improvements have plateaued and/or discharge is imminent.

The Impact of Managed Care

Managed care in the U.S. health-care system has many implications for treatment of patients with cognitive and perceptual deficits. The most striking of these is the reduction in time allocated for inpatient evaluation and treatment.[36] Cognitive and perceptual problems are not readily visible and are therefore more easily overlooked than physical problems. Hence, pressure to discharge patients quickly, possibly before the full extent of cognitive and perceptual deficits has been revealed, means that patients may be discharged to potentially hazardous situations at home. Therapists need to do an initial screening of all patients with brain damage to determine potential problems as early as possible and ensure that patients are discharged to a safe environment. Although inpatient rehabilitation time is reduced, there is opportunity for outpatient services conducted in the clinic or in the patient's home.[96] The advantage of home care is that therapists have an opportunity to work with the patient in their own environment and tailor therapy to the patient's current circumstances. Patients with cognitive and perceptual deficits often perform better in their own familiar environments.

The major disadvantage of reduced inpatient treatment time for many patients, including those with cognitive and perceptual deficits, is that a home discharge may not be safe after only limited inpatient rehabilitation. The situation is complicated by having to discharge a patient who does not have family support to another type of institutional care (possibly a nursing home or skilled nursing facility) when in the long term this level of care may not be necessary. It is distressing for patients who are confused, owing to cognitive and perceptual problems, to be moved, particularly when they may believe the move is permanent.

■ DISCHARGE PLANNING

Discharge planning begins as soon as the patient is admitted for rehabilitation, and it draws on a person-centered model of rehabilitation.[97,98] The most important question to be answered during this stage is where the patient will live after discharge. There are two major types of housing available to persons with disabilities: community-based accommodation and residential-care accommodation. Community-based accommodation includes private homes, retirement villages, and hotels or rooming houses. Residential care may be defined as any accommodation that provides personal care and medical services on a consistent, continual, or per-need basis; this includes nursing homes, skilled nursing facilities, assisted living centers, and sheltered or group housing.[98,99]

The key to discharge planning is to consider the match between the patient's skills and the demands of the environment, and then factor in the support systems available from a spouse, friends, or family to assist with tasks that the patient cannot manage.[99,100] This approach works well when patients and their families have insight and an understanding of the patient's problems. However, cognitive and perceptual deficits are often not very visible, and it may be difficult for the family and the patient to understand the functional impact of these deficits. For example, a patient may regain full motor function following a stroke but experience ongoing difficulties with unilateral neglect. This problem is not readily apparent to the untrained onlooker. However, this patient cannot drive and may be in danger when simply crossing the road. These problems have major lifestyle implications for the patient.

Interventions that facilitate a patient's return to community-based housing usually center on enabling the patient to carry out ADL skills in an acceptable and safe manner. If this cannot be achieved and the patient does not have a live-in caregiver, supported housing such as a nursing home may be the only alternative. Research examining the discharge process for a sample of 62 patients following stroke revealed that the majority were reluctant to consider alternatives to returning home despite having significant self-care deficits.[100] Our housing is central to who we are as individuals, and it is very difficult for patients, particularly those with limited insight, to understand and accept that they can no longer live in the community.

■ OVERVIEW OF COGNITIVE AND PERCEPTUAL DEFICITS

This section is divided into seven parts: *attention deficits, memory impairments, impairments of executive function, body scheme and body image impairments, spatial relations impairments, agnosia,* and *apraxia* (Table 27.3). Each category encompasses a constellation of deficits, which are grouped together for ease of understanding. Information pertaining to each deficit will be organized identically as follows:

1. Definition(s)
2. Clinical Examples
3. Lesion Area
4. Testing
5. Treatment Suggestions

The value of dwelling on probable areas of cortical damage is controversial. The indication of cortical loci is an attempt to relate the study of neuroanatomy to actual patient behavior involving cognitive and perceptual dysfunction. An examination of cortical loci will give the reader a sense of which cognitive and perceptual deficits are likely to be seen together.

As therapists, we are required to assist the patient to bridge the gap between maladaptive behavior and independent function in ADL skills. Whether or not the area of the brain purported to produce a particular dysfunction appears damaged on a computed tomography (CT) scan or other neurological or radiological test is not a key determinant of the rehabilitative approach to therapy. The patient's approach to task performance and the relative strengths or weaknesses of the patient (motor, cognitive, and perceptual), which the therapist ascertains through thorough observation and testing, are much more pertinent to the selection of appropriate therapeutic strategies than the locus of the lesion.

Testing tools are described for each cognitive or perceptual deficit to enhance the reader's awareness of the complexity of behavior ascribed to perceptual deficiencies. Familiarity with the tools used to examine cognitive or perceptual deficits can aid in communication

Table 27.3	Summary of Cognitive and Perceptual Impairments
Area of Deficit	**Specific Impairments**
Cognition	
Attention deficits	Sustained attention
	Selective attention
	Divided attention
	Alternating attention
Memory impairments	Immediate recall
	Short-term memory
	Long-term memory
Higher-Order Cognition	
Impairment of executive functions	Volition
	Planning
	Purposive action
	Effective performance
Perception	
Body scheme/body image impairments	Unilateral neglect
	Anosognosia
	Somatoagnosia
	Right–left discrimination
	Finger agnosia
Spatial relation impairments (complex perception)	Figure–ground discrimination
	Form discrimination
	Spatial relations
	Position in space
	Topographical disorientation
	Depth and distance perception
	Vertical disorientation
Agnosias	Visual object agnosia
	Auditory agnosia
	Tactile agnosia
Apraxia	Ideomotor apraxia
	Ideational apraxia
	Buccofacial apraxia

between physical and occupational therapists engaged in the treatment of the same patient.

The following section also includes specific treatment suggestions from the sensorimotor, transfer-of-training, and functional approaches described. The intervention strategies most relevant to physical therapist practice are those dealing with the functional approach and adaptation of the environment. In these sections, examples are given of how to facilitate the patient's success within a treatment session. Information is provided on how the therapist might gear language, demonstrations, feedback, and the use of media and the environment to the individual needs of the cognitively or perceptually impaired patient. The evidence base for treatment is not strong for many of these treatment techniques, and further research is required to support their efficacy.

Attention Deficits

1. *Definitions.* The inability of many patients with hemiplegia to maintain attention during therapy is a frequent complaint of therapists. *Attention* is the ability to select and attend to a specific stimulus while simultaneously suppressing extraneous stimuli.[101] A patient who is inattentive or distractible will have difficulty processing and assimilating new information or techniques.[102] Often, patients who have experienced a CVA will have low arousal levels and require a great deal of sensory input to be alerted to the environment. Low arousal thus must be considered as a cause for seeming inattention.

   Four different kinds of attention are generally discussed in the literature: sustained attention, focused or selective attention, alternating attention, and divided attention. *Sustained attention* is a capacity to attend to relevant information during activity. This implies that a person can maintain a consistent response during a continuous activity. *Focused* or *selective attention* is the capacity to attend to a task despite environmental visual or auditory stimuli. *Alternating attention* is the capacity to move flexibly between tasks and respond appropriately to the demands of each task. *Divided attention* is the capacity to respond simultaneously to two or more tasks or stimuli when all stimuli are relevant.[1]

2. *Clinical Examples.* Patients with a disorder of sustained attention may report that they start to watch a TV program and then "just drift off." A patient who has to stop a dressing activity to talk to the therapist may be demonstrating difficulties with focused attention. Patients who are easily disturbed by music or other forms of background noise may also be experiencing problems with focused attention.

   A problem with focused attention is often referred to as *distractibility*. Divided attention is required when more than one response is needed or more than one stimulus needs to be monitored.[103] Selective attention is required when certain stimuli need to be ignored.[104] Patients who have difficulty with divided and alternating attention may have great difficulties with more complex ADL such as cooking a meal or driving.

3. *Lesion Areas.* Multiple brain regions are thought to be responsible for producing attention. These include the reticular formation (which regulates arousal), the various sensory systems that deliver and code relevant sensory information, and the limbic and frontal regions that underlie the drive and affective components of concentration.[104]

4. *Testing.* General screening tests such as the *Loewenstein Occupational Therapy Cognitive Assessment*[78] or

the *Chessington Occupational Therapy Neurological Assessment Battery*[105] include subtests that examine attentional abilities. To investigate problems of attention, neuropsychologists generally administer the *Stroop Test,*[106] the *Paced Auditory Serial Attention Test,*[107] and the *Trail Making Test.*[108]

5. *Treatment Suggestions.* The purpose of therapy is to increase the patient's attention to appropriate stimuli and disregard inappropriate stimuli.

   a. *Remedial Approach.* Clinically, the ability to attend to a task has implications for the therapeutic process. Patients should be instructed to scan the visual environment in a slow and systematic manner. In the presence of right hemiplegia, the patient should be spoken to more slowly to afford an opportunity to process verbal information and be taught to use visualization techniques to facilitate attendance to verbal tasks. In addition, patients with left hemiplegia should be encouraged to use verbalization to improve performance in visual tasks. A randomized clinical trial (RCT) with 12 patients investigating the effect of training on divided attention skills reported positive outcomes as measured on a rating scale of attentional behavior.[109] Patients were trained to do two computer-based or pen-and-paper tasks simultaneously. However, there was no generalization from this training to nontarget tasks. In other words, the benefits of this training were not transferred to patient ADL. This finding is supported more generally across six RCTs included in a Cochrane Review of treatment effectiveness which concluded that the effectiveness of cognitive rehabilitation for attention deficits following stroke remain unconfimed.[110]

   Some additional tools that may be used for the remediation of attentional deficits and distractibility are setting time or speed limits, amplifying critical stimuli, and making the crucial stimuli salient (noticeable) to the patient.[63] The environment can be graded by having the patient initially perform some aspects of therapy in a nondistracting setting (closed environment) and then slowly increasing potentially distracting elements, both visual and auditory, as patient tolerance improves (progressing to a more open environment).[1]

   b. *Compensatory Approach.* For many patients, the inability to attend to significant stimuli is compounded by distraction due to extraneous stimuli in the environment. Often noise is the most distracting stimulus, causing irritability and diminished concentration. Therefore, a compensatory approach may include providing a quiet, distraction-free environment for therapy activities. Ponsford et al.[111] provide further ideas for working with patients who have limited attention.

A Cochrane Review titled "Cognitive Rehabilitation for Attention Deficits Following Stroke"[110] revealed a small number of controlled trials of attention training in patients with stroke. The results of these six studies suggested that training may improve some aspects of attention (e.g., divided attention), but no evidence of sustained long-term benefits was demonstrated. There was also no evidence to support or refute the use of cognitive rehabilitation for attention deficits to improve functional independence.

Memory Impairments

Memory can be defined as the mental process that enables the storage of perceptions and experiences for recall at a later time. All memory is not localized in one particular place in the nervous system; rather, many and perhaps all regions of the brain may contain neurons with adequate plasticity for memory storage.[112] Memory comprises acquisition or learning, storage or retention, and retrieval or recall.[113] Learning is a crucial element of rehabilitation. If the patient is unable to learn, time in rehabilitation may not be well spent. Hence, it is very important for the therapist to take steps to evaluate the patient's memory before beginning physical rehabilitation programs. Three levels of memory will be examined: immediate recall, short-term memory, and long-term memory.

Immediate Recall and Short-Term Memory

1. *Definitions.* Immediate recall involves retention of information that has been stored for a few seconds. Short-term memory mediates retention of events or learning that has taken place within a few minutes, hours, or days.[4]

2. *Clinical Examples.* A patient with immediate recall difficulties may not be able to remember the instructions given only seconds before by the therapist for what the patient is to do. A patient with a short-term memory problem may not come back to the physical therapy department, even though the therapist asked the patient to return in an hour. Alternatively, the therapist may teach the patient a new transfer technique and on the following day find that the patient has not retained any of the steps involved. Patients with severe short-term memory problems may not even be able to hold a simple conversation.[1]

3. *Lesion Areas.* Memory is a complex capacity involving many brain regions, including four of the major structures of the cerebral cortex (the frontal, parietal, temporal, and occipital lobes) and the limbic system.[4]

4. *Testing.* The *Rivermead Behavioural Memory Test (RBMT)*[87] can be used to examine memory function. Alternatively, the adequacy of memory functions can be ascertained by having the patient recall lists or

collections of objects that have just been presented (immediate recall) or by teaching the patient a new verbal or visual task and asking the patient to recall it a few hours or a day later (short-term memory). Frequently, there is a loss of short-term memory following stroke, and this particularly interferes with the patient's ability to benefit from rehabilitation, especially from those activities involving the use of new and heretofore unfamiliar techniques.[45]

5. *Treatment Suggestions.* The purpose of memory retraining is to enable the patient to effectively encode and recall information so that learning can occur.

   a. *Remedial Approach.* Because good attention skills are vital for memory, the therapist must ensure that attention problems are addressed and improvements are noted before initiating work on memory retraining.[1,43] A primary focus of this approach is working with the patient to effectively encode information so it can be more easily retrieved when appropriate. This may include organizing material to be remembered and making logical associations. A determination should be made of how the patient used to remember information and then build on these past strategies. There is very little evidence to suggest that drills, computer games, or memory tests such as recalling a list of items that have been covered have any effect on retraining memory. On the other hand, if the therapist assists the patient to develop memory strategies when playing these games, then these strategies may be generalized to everyday activities. In a Cochrane Review,[114] the authors drew on findings from 13 studies involving 415 patients following stroke and reported benefits from cognitive rehabilitation on subjective measures in the short term; however, these were not maintained in the longer term. The authors called for more robust and well-designed trials of memory rehabilitation using common standardized outcome measures.

   b. *Compensatory Approach.* The use of a diary or notebook system (memory log) can help many patients to manage their ADL. However, the patient needs to have sufficient memory to use this system. Environmental prompts such as a beeper or a wall calendar can be useful to assist patients to remember their routine or to look at their diary. When external aids are used, the patient needs to be taught how to use them. Guidelines for the use of such devices may be found in Sohlberg and Mateer[115] and Gopi et al.[116]

Long-Term Memory

1. *Definition.* Long-term memory consists of early experiences and information acquired over a period of years. Patients who do not have long-term memory are often described as having amnesia.[112]

2. *Clinical Examples.* Patients who experience long-term memory problems may have difficulty recalling events from many years ago such as a child's birth or their own work experiences. Long-term memory problems are common following brain injury and in Alzheimer disease but are not commonly seen following stroke.[113]

3. *Lesion Areas.* As described, memory is a complex capacity involving many brain regions. For a detailed discussion, see Fuster[117] and Lezak.[4]

4. *Testing.* The adequacy of memory functions can be determined by having the patient recall personal historical events. The RBMT[87] can be used to test memory in a standardized way. It is advisable to question the patient's family as to premorbid memory, because many patients in the stroke-prone age group have already begun to experience declining memory as part of the aging process.

5. *Treatment Suggestions.* Treatments for assisting patients to overcome long-term memory impairments are similar to those outlined earlier for immediate recall and short-term memory impairments. Further information on the management of memory impairments may be found in Baddeley.[118]

Although the literature contains many studies exploring a variety of memory treatments, few of these were designed as RCTs. A Cochrane Review titled "Cognitive Rehabilitation for Memory Deficits After Stroke"[114] included 13 controlled trials of memory training where at least 75% of patients had a stroke. The results of these studies suggested that training improved subjective reports of short-term memory, but no evidence of sustained long-term benefits was demonstrated. There was no evidence to support or refute the use of cognitive rehabilitation for memory deficits to improve functional independence.

Impairments of Executive Functions

1. *Definition.* People with executive function disorder have difficulty taking initiative, being in control, changing strategy, and planning, leading to difficulties across all ADL.[119] According to Lezak, executive functions are capacities for formulating goals, planning, and carrying out plans that enable a person to successfully engage in independent, purposive, and socially constructive behavior.[4] Lezak goes on to describe executive functions as consisting of four overlapping components: volition, planning, purposive action, and effective performance:

   • *Volition* is the capacity to determine what one needs and wants to do. It also encompasses a future realization of one's needs and wants. This encompasses goal planning and task initiation, self-awareness, awareness of the environment, and social awareness.

   • *Planning* is "the identification and organization of the steps and elements (e.g., skills, material, other persons) needed to carry out an intention or achieve a goal."[4(p653)] Planning involves weighing alternatives and making choices.

- *Purposive action* includes productivity and self-regulation. It encompasses the ability to initiate, maintain, switch, and stop complex action sequences in an orderly manner to realize a goal.
- *Effective performance* is the capacity for quality control, including the ability to self-monitor and self-correct one's behavior. Problems with effective performance are associated with ineffective self-monitoring and difficulty with self-correction; for example, patients may not even perceive their mistakes, whereas others may identify them but take no action to correct them.[120]

2. *Clinical Examples.* Although some patients with executive function disorders are unable to formulate realistic goals or intentions (volition) or plan, others may be able to formulate goals and initiate goal-directed task performance, but owing to defective planning, they are not able to realize their goals. Patients with planning problems may say or intend one thing but do another.[4] Family and hospital staff may complain of the patient's apparent apathy, poor or unreliable judgment, inappropriate behavior, difficulty adapting to new situations, and/or lack of attention to the needs and feelings of others.[120]

3. *Lesion Area.* Executive functions have traditionally been associated with the frontal and prefrontal cortex,[6] but the current view is that these capacities are mediated by reciprocal connections with other cortical and subcortical regions via the dorsolateral prefrontal–subcortical circuit.[121]

4. *Testing.* Tests of executive functions include the *Behavioral Assessment of the Dysexecutive Syndrome*[72] and the *Executive Functions Performance Test.*[122] Tests used to assess executive performance were reviewed by Chan et al.[123] and related back to underlying models of executive function.

5. *Treatment Suggestions.* The combination of impulsiveness, poor judgment, poor planning ability, and lack of foresight, does not bode well for independent functioning. The severity of these impairments may diminish somewhat over time.[9] Although some general remedial and adaptive treatment suggestions are described here, for more specific details refer to Ponsford et al.,[110] Duran and Fisher,[120] and Poulin et al.[124]

   a. *Remedial Approach.* By providing structure, feedback, and routine, a person's performance can be enhanced (e.g., providing structure by giving the patient steps to follow, assisting the task to become routine by repeated practice, or providing immediate feedback about the patient's behavior and the effect it has on others). The therapist initially acts as the patient's frontal lobes and gradually transfers these responsibilities to the patient. Unless the patient has

some awareness of the problems, a remedial approach will not be particularly successful.[110] Honda[121] reported a study with three patients over a 6-month period who were provided with self-instructional training, a problem-solving procedure, and physical-set-changing exercises described as moving the four extremities and trunk in time to a metronome. In this study,

> Patients were instructed to follow a videotape for 20 minutes. In the tape, a physical therapist moves four extremities and his trunk in time to a metronome. He changes activities every 2 or 3 minutes. The patients were trained with these methods for a total of 6 months. In the self-instructional procedure and problem-solving training phase, psychologists guided and trained patients 1 hour per day twice a week. In the physical-set-changing exercise phase, patients were advised to practice twice a day watching the instruction videotape. Each training phase lasted 6 weeks.[121(p18)]

While two of the subjects revealed improvements on the neuropsychological test used as an outcome measure, all subjects improved in basic and IADL. Of course, a limitation of this study is the small sample size and lack of control subjects, since it could be expected that these patients would make spontaneous recovery over the 6-month study period.

Hewitt et al.[125] proposed that people with TBI have difficulty with planning because they are not spontaneously using autobiographic memories. The authors asked a control and experimental group of 15 subjects to describe how they would plan common activities. The experimental group underwent a 30-minute training session aimed at prompting retrieval of specific memories to support planning. This intervention was found to be effective in increasing specific memories that could aid planning.

   b. *Compensatory Approach.* The therapist can assist the patient to compensate for poor abilities by utilizing other intact cognitive functions and/or modifying the environment. For example, the therapist might ask the patient to perform a task in a room with minimal distractions or change the demands of the patient's work, home, or community to diminish the need to employ executive functions. A beeper or alarm clock may be used to help a patient overcome poor initiation.

   A Cochrane Review titled "Cognitive Rehabilitation for Executive Dysfunction in Adults With Stroke or Other Adult Non-Progressive Acquired Brain Damage"[126] revealed 13 controlled trials of cognitive rehabilitation to reduce executive dysfunction in adults with TBI, stroke, or other nonprogressive acquired brain injury. No evidence was found to support the use of cognitive rehabilitation to improve the functional independence of people with executive dysfunction.

Body Scheme and Body Image Impairments

Body image is defined as a visual and mental image of one's body that includes feelings about one's body, especially in relation to health and disease.[127] The term *body scheme* refers to a postural model of the body, including the relationship of body parts to each other and the relationship of the body to the environment. Commonly, body scheme and body image problems are termed *difficulties with body awareness*. Body awareness is derived from the integration of tactile, proprioceptive, and interoceptive (visceral) sensations, in addition to the individual's subjective feelings about the body.[127] An awareness of body scheme is considered one of the essential foundations for the performance of all purposeful motor behavior.[127] The terms *body awareness, body image,* and *body scheme* are often used interchangeably; therefore, when researching this topic, close attention should be paid to the particular definition put forth by each author. Specific impairments of body image and body scheme are unilateral neglect, somatoagnosia, right–left discrimination, finger agnosia, and anosognosia.

Unilateral Neglect

1. *Definition. Unilateral neglect* is the inability to register and integrate stimuli and perceptions from one side of the body (*body neglect*) and the environment or hemispace (*spatial neglect* of the area surrounding one side of the body), which is not due to a sensory loss. Unilateral neglect is also referred to as *unilateral spatial neglect, hemi-inattention, hemineglect,* and *unilateral visual inattention*.[128] It is important for the therapist to be familiar with this disorder because it is a frequent clinical finding. In the acute stage, neglect is frequently reported, with visual neglect being reported in 83% of patients following right-sided lesions and in 65% of patients with left-sided lesions.[129] However, reporting rates vary enormously due to differences in time selected for reporting and techniques used to detect the neglect. Although neglect spontaneously resolves in most patients, this disorder is commonly seen as having a functional impact on about 20% of patients. Unilateral neglect usually, although not always, affects the left side of the body or hemispace. For purposes of this discussion, assume that it is the left. If a patient has unilateral neglect, they will seem to ignore the left side of the body and stimuli occurring in the left personal space. This may occur despite intact visual fields, or concomitantly with right or left homonymous hemianopia; however, it is not caused by homonymous hemianopia.[130]

When working with a patient who has unilateral neglect, the therapist should also determine which sensory modalities are affected, including visual, tactile, and auditory. Input from one or all of these modalities may be neglected. Neglect can also be understood in terms of the area of space that is neglected. For example, unilateral neglect may express itself as a disorder of attention and goal-directed behavior in the following:

- Contralesional personal space (defined as pertaining to the body) such as shaving only the right half of the face or failing to wash the left side of the body
- Contralesional peripersonal space (that area of space within arm distance); for example, failing to use objects on the contralesional side of the meal tray
- Contralesional extrapersonal space (that area of space beyond arm length), such as failing to negotiate obstacles, doorways, and so forth, during locomotion[50,128]

Unilateral neglect is also demonstrated by an impaired ability to attend to either the object or the environment as a whole. It is possible that while some patients may neglect half of the environment, others may neglect half of objects in the total environment. In the first case, the patient may neglect most elements of the left side of the entire visual scene (Fig. 27.8). In the second case, a patient may neglect the left side of an object, regardless of its absolute position in the visual display. For example, the patient may neglect the left side of a cup even though it is on their right side or omit the left side of objects when drawing items such as an umbrella, picnic basket, and bucket and spade as depicted in Figure 27.9.

Frequently, a patient with unilateral neglect has sensory loss on the more affected side, which compounds the problem. Although patients with left-sided hemianopia have actual loss of vision from the left visual field of both eyes, they may be aware of the problem and compensate automatically or learn

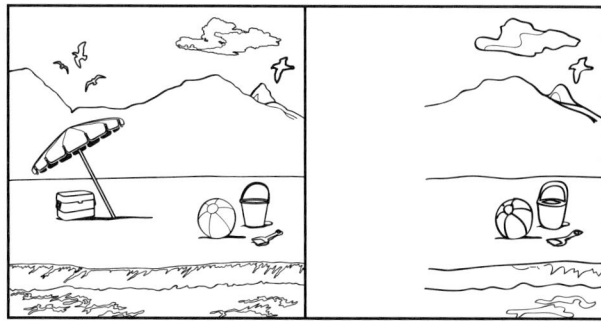

Figure 27.8 Example of a drawing by a patient with unilateral neglect. Therapist's drawing of a beach scene (left). Impaired copying by a patient with unilateral neglect—environment neglect following a stroke (right).

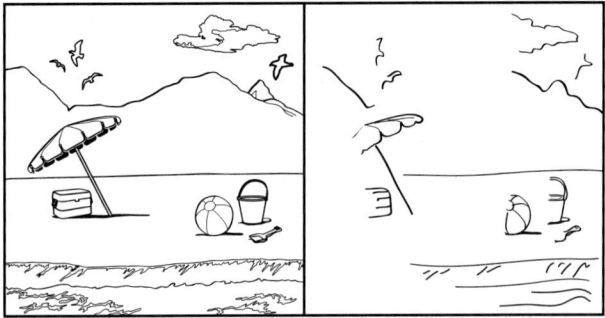

Figure 27.9 Example of a drawing by a patient with unilateral neglect. Therapist's drawing of a beach scene (left). Impaired copying by a patient with unilateral neglect—object neglect following a stroke (right).

to compensate by turning the head. A patient with visual neglect has intact vision but seems unaware of the problem and does not attempt to compensate spontaneously by turning the head. In extreme cases the patient appears totally indifferent to the left side of the body and environment and may deny that the left extremities belong to them.[131] More time seems to be required to learn to compensate for this impairment than for hemianopia. There is great difficulty in integrating all stimuli from the left half of the body and personal space for use in ADL skills. As with hemianopia, the patient with visual unilateral neglect often avoids crossing the midline visually or motorically.[61]

2. *Clinical Examples.* The patient may ignore the left half of the body when dressing and forget to put on the left sleeve or left pants leg, a male patient may forget to shave the left half of his face, and a woman may neglect to put makeup on the left side of her face. The patient may neglect to eat from the left half of a plate and will start reading a newspaper from the middle of the line. Typically, the patient bumps into objects on the left side or tends to veer toward the right when walking or propelling a wheelchair.[129,132]

3. *Lesion Area.* It has been suggested that lesions involving the inferior–posterior regions of the right parietal lobe are significant determinants of neglect.[130,133]

4. *Testing.* A variety of techniques are useful. No single test is adequate to identify unilateral neglect in all patients because the impairment may be manifested differently in each patient.

The *Behavioral Inattention Test*[73] can be used to examine unilateral neglect (see Table 27.1). The patient may also be observed during basic ADL such as dressing or IADL such as preparing a meal. The therapist observes performance and changes in the patient's behavior in response to cueing.

5. *Treatment Suggestions.*
   a. *Remedial Approach.* The purpose of therapy is to increase awareness of the left side of the body and space. Current beliefs concerning the mechanisms underlying unilateral neglect guide the majority of treatment approaches. Rizzolatti and Berti[134] combine the popular attentional and representational models in their premotor theory of neglect. The basis of this theory is that spatial attention is dependent on several independent neural circuits. Attention, and therefore perception of stimuli, is enhanced as a direct result of activation of motor circuits, as occurs when a person moves. Hence, activating motor circuits of the ipsilesional hemisphere (via voluntary movements of the left upper or lower limbs) may facilitate associated sensory circuits. Such movement may in turn lead to improvements in the processing of stimuli from the contralesional (left) side.[128]

   Capitalizing on the rationale of the premotor theory of neglect, the following suggestions are proposed. Stimuli that are specialized for the right side of the brain, such as shapes and blocks, should be used to enhance right brain activation. At the same time, the presence of stimuli that are known to activate the left side of the brain, such as letters and numbers, should be minimized. Use of verbal instructions should be minimized. Simple verbal instructions should be used to encourage the patient to turn the head to the left to anchor their attention to that side of space.[131] In addition, research suggests that conducting motor activities with the left body side, such as simply clenching and unclenching the fist, can improve attention to the left body side and hemispace. Robertson et al.[135] conducted a study with six individuals with hemiplegia who were asked to walk through a doorway. Each of the subject's walking trajectory (pathway) was measured, and it was found that all trajectories were significantly deviated to the right of center. The subjects were then asked to clench and unclench their left hands before and during walking through the doorway. The researchers found that this procedure significantly assisted subjects with centering their walking trajectories.

   Another version of this technique was used by Grattan et al.[136] when they examined the effectiveness of left upper-limb specific training to reduce the effects of unilateral spatial neglect. Their study found small, but statistically significant, improvements in upper-limb function and use can be attained via repetitive task-specific practice, suggesting that this intervention may be promising for people with unilateral neglect. However, the authors note that these findings may not be generalizable to all clients with unilateral neglect and that further evaluation is necessary to determine efficacy. Other techniques that have been used to treat patients with unilateral neglect include mirror therapy, eye patching, optokinetic stimulation and prism adaptation, neck vibration,[137] and trunk rotation.[138] A review of these treatment techniques may be found in Luauté et al.[139]

Pandian et al.[140] conducted an RCT using mirror therapy for unilateral neglect 48 hr after stroke. During mirror therapy, a mirror box was placed vertically on a table in front of subjects to reflect their unaffected hand while their affected hand was inside the mirror box, out of view. Subjects were instructed to flex and extend both hands (limb activation as described by Robertson[135] and Grattan et al.)[136] while they saw the reflection of the unaffected hand movements in the mirror. Subjects received mirror therapy treatment for 1 to 2 hr a day, 5 days a week, for 4 weeks. Results indicated that mirror therapy is a simple intervention that can improve unilateral neglect in stroke patients. Eye patching is another treatment approach, whereby the right visual field of each eye is covered in order to encourage the patient to focus their attention to the left visual space.[141] However, an RCT of 12 subjects conducted by Aparicio-López et al.[142] found that eye patching does not improve functional performance over and above cognitive rehabilitation alone. Prism adaptation involves the use of prism lenses, glasses, or goggles (Fig. 27.10) worn by the patient to shift the left visual field into the right so that there is partial recovery of the left workspace. This provides patients with a representation of the left field of view, facilitating the recall and relearning of previously learned behaviors.[143] An evidence review of studies from 2011 to 2021 investigating the effectiveness of prism adaptation as an intervention to increase visual spatial awareness in patients with unilateral neglect following stroke is included in Table 27.4.[144-152] This review excludes studies that

included patients with neglect following TBI and studies investigating anatomical predictors of the success of prism adaptation.

b. *Compensatory Approach.* The patient is initially educated about the condition, and then strategies to assist managing everyday activities are devised. For example, when reading a book or newspaper, a red ribbon may be placed on the left margin, and the patient is taught to scan back to this point after completing each line. The environment may also be adapted within this approach. The patient is addressed and given demonstrations from the less affected side. The nursing staff should place the patient's call button, telephone, and other essential items on the less affected side. A bold red line may be drawn on the side of the page that is neglected.[128] A mirror may be placed in front of patients while they are dressing or ambulating to draw attention to the neglected side.

An extensive Cochrane Review[153] was conducted concerning the effectiveness of a variety of interventions for unilateral neglect. Longley et al.[153] reviewed 65 controlled trials and concluded that the effectiveness of interventions such as visual interventions, prism adaptation, body awareness, electrical stimulation, and acupuncture remain unproven. Additional, well-designed RCTs of interventions as well as more research including people with experience with the condition to design and run the trials are required.

Anosognosia

1. *Definition.* Anosognosia is defined as a lack of awareness, or denial, of a paretic extremity as belonging to the person, or a lack of insight concerning, or denial of, paralysis and disability.[131] Presence of this condition may greatly compromise rehabilitation potential, because it limits the patient's ability to recognize the need for, and thus to use, compensatory techniques.

2. *Clinical Examples.* Typically, the patient maintains that there is nothing wrong and may disown the paralyzed limbs and refuse to accept responsibility for them. The patient may claim that the limb has a mind of its own or that it was left at home or in a closet.

3. *Lesion Area.* The pathogenesis of anosognosia remains unclear, although the regions of the retrosplenial cortex, left parahippocampal gyrus, thalamus, and left medial superior frontal gyrus have been implicated.[154,155]

4. *Testing.* Anosognosia is identified by talking to the patient. The patient is asked what happened to the arm or leg, whether it is paralyzed, how the limb feels, and why it cannot be moved. A patient with anosognosia may deny the paralysis and disability, say that it is of no concern, and fabricate reasons why a limb does not move the way it should.

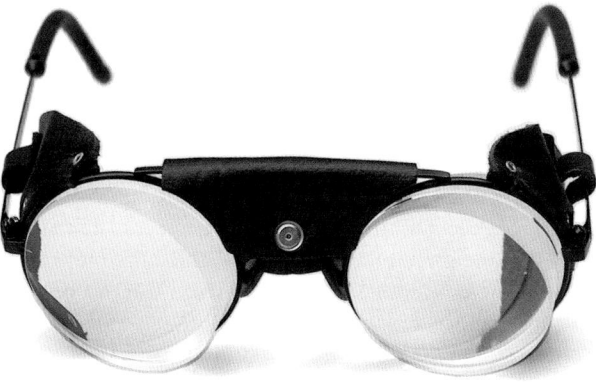

Figure 27.10 An example of prism goggles. *(From Optique Peter, https://optiquepeter.com/en/index.php. Used with permission.)*

Table 27.4	Evidence Summary Evidence Addressing the Use of Prism Adaptation as an Intervention to Increase Visual Function in Patients With Unilateral Neglect Following Stroke

Fortis et al. (2020)[144]

Design	Prospective cohort design
Level of Evidence	II B Moderate evidence
Subjects	Six Ss with L UN completed the study. IC = right-handed, normal or corrected to normal vision, no history of previous neurological or psychiatric disorders. EC = dementia or any other cognitive disorder, not being able to complete the 2 weeks of PA treatment.
Intervention	A home-based carer-assisted PA treatment consisted of Ss wearing neutral goggles (C treatment) during week 1 of treatment and wedge prism goggles (PA) in following 2–4 weeks for 30 minutes, two times per day. The wedge prisms (Bernell Deluxe Prism Training Glasses, 20-diopter) displaced the visual field horizontally rightward 12.4°. In each C and PA session, Ss performed "scheduled activities" for 20 minutes followed by "free activities" for 10 minutes. Scheduled activities included (a) collecting coins into money boxes; (b) dressing rings, bracelets, watch; (c) opening and closing jars; (d) assembling jigsaw puzzles; (e) box and block; (f) sorting and playing cards; (g) serving cup of tea, etc. Caregivers were trained in how to assist these activities. Ss were assessed at baseline, at the end of 2 weeks' PA treatment, and 1, 3, and 6 months follow-up.
Results	PA was assessed by comparing pointing errors in the initial (1–3), middle (28–30), and last (58–60) trials of the exposure period. The main effect of pointing error was significant (F [2, 12] = 72.62, p < 0.001). Significant differences were found between the trials, with participants showing a reduction in rightward error between the initial (M = 7.48°), the middle (M = 2.98°), and the last three exposure trials (M = 0.93°). Aftereffects were also significant, highlighting a leftward deviation. Additionally, the size of the prism-induced deviation diminished during the postexposure phase with a reduction in leftward error.
Comments	The authors concluded that improvement was recorded in chronic stroke survivors with spatial neglect who were treated at home with an ecological PA treatment program.

Goedert et al. (2014)[145]

Design	Prospective cohort design
Level of Evidence	II B Moderate evidence
Subjects	24 Ss with L UN (BIT ≤ 129 or CBS > 1) were divided into groups based on their spatial neglect profile: (1) perceptual-attentional "Where" spatial processing deficit, (2) motor-intentional "Aiming" spatial processing deficit, or (3) both. IC = R-handed within 6–47 days poststroke, exhibiting rightward error on a computerized line bisection task. EC = Ss more than 60 days poststroke with L hemisphere lesions, prior history of neurological or psychiatric conditions, uncorrected ocular disorders, or leftward line bisection error.
Intervention	All Ss wore prism glasses that shifted the field of view 12.4° to the R during PAT on a line bisection task once a day, for 15–20 min, for 10 days. Two pointing tasks were also administered to test for Ss ability to adapt to prisms with and without visual input. Ss assessed on the CBS before, during, and after PAT to examine functional improvement.
Results	Ss with only "Aiming" deficits improved on the CBS, whereas Ss with both deficits showed moderate improvement, and Ss with only "Where" deficits did not improve. Improvement following PA was predicted by spatial neglect profile, whereby Ss with only "Aiming" deficits demonstrated greater improvement compared with Ss with only "Where" deficits or both deficits, respectively.
Comments	The authors suggest that future stroke treatment trials consider classification of Ss based on spatial processing deficits.

Table 27.4 Evidence Summary Evidence Addressing the Use of Prism Adaptation as an Intervention to Increase Visual Function in Patients With Unilateral Neglect Following Stroke—cont'd

Mizuno et al. (2011)[146]

Design	Multicenter, double-blind, RCT
Level of Evidence	I A Strong evidence
Subjects	Thirty-eight Ss with UN were divided into groups based on neglect severity (mild ≥ 55 and severe < 55). IC = first hemiparetic stroke, admission within 3 months of onset, no severe mental deterioration using MMSE, RH damage, and scores on the BIT. EC = unable to sit on wheelchair, unable to understand task due to mental deterioration or aphasia, unable to understand Japanese, extremely impaired eyesight, severe hearing loss, unable to reach with the R upper extremity due to restricted ROM, R UEamputation more proximal to half of the forearm, severe position sense deficits of R fingers due to peripheral neuropathy, and past medical history of head trauma or ventriculoperitoneal shunt. E = 18, C = 20 Gender (M/F): E = 12/6, C = 15/5. No differences between mean days from onset to intervention, mean hospital stay, MMSE score, and SIAS motor score.
Intervention	E = repeated pointing with the index finger of the R nonparetic hand to three targets through the bottom of a table while wearing prism glasses that shifted the field of view 12° to the R twice daily, 5 days per week, for 2 weeks. C = same task while wearing neutral glasses. Data collected: baseline (study entry), post-treatment (after 2-week intervention), and at follow-up (discharge). Measures: BIT, CBS, FIM, and SIAS.
Results	PA found to significantly improve scores on the FIM. In Ss with mild UN, prism adaptation found to significantly improve scores on BIT and FIM, suggesting reduction of neglect symptoms and improvement in ADL, is therefore effective for reducing neglect symptoms and improvement of ADL.
Comments	PA can significantly improve ADL, as measured on FIM, only in patients with mild stroke. This finding suggests that PA could improve rehabilitation outcome for early poststroke patients in a conventional rehabilitation program. There was more than a 3-month delay, on average, postintervention of this study, demonstrating a marked long-term effect of PA compared with previous research. Among studies on prism adaptation, this sample size is the largest reported to date.

Priftis et al. (2013)[147]

Design	Quasi-randomized clinical trial
Level of Evidence	II B Moderate evidence
Subjects	Thirty-one Ss with L UN were divided (quasi-randomly) into three treatment groups (VST, LAT, or PA). VST = 10, LAT = 10, PA = 11. IC = unilateral lesions due to first stroke confirmed by CT or MRI scan, no previous UN treatment received, absence of dementia confirmed by neuropsychological history and interview. EC = medical history of substance abuse and psychiatric disorders.
Intervention	Ss in the VST group were verbally instructed to "look at the pink-colored stripe" placed along the left edge of a A4 landscape sheet of paper as they were required to fill out only parts of drawings that had a little black point inside. Ss in the LAT group were required to fill out the same drawings as the VST group; however, they were instructed to use their L arm to turn off the buzzer on a LAT device that was set to emit a tone at fixed intervals of 240 sec (first week) and 120 sec (second week). Ss in the PA group were required to point toward 90 targets (a pen) presented in random order (90 center, 90 right, 90 left) wearing prism glasses that shifted the field of view 10° to the R. All Ss received treatment for 2 weeks. Data collected over time period of 6 weeks; everyday life task performance was assessed with the CBS four times; baseline (A1), 2 weeks after the end of A1 (A2), immediately after 2-week-long intervention (A3), and 2 weeks after the end of A3 (A4).

(Continued)

Table 27.4	Evidence Summary Evidence Addressing the Use of Prism Adaptation as an Intervention to Increase Visual Function in Patients With Unilateral Neglect Following Stroke—cont'd

Priftis et al. (2013)[147]

Results	All three treatment groups produced improvements, suggesting that they can be considered valid rehabilitation interventions for UN.
Comments	

Rode et al. (2015)[148]

Design	Double-blinded, monocentric RCT
Level of Evidence	II B Moderate evidence
Subjects	Eighteen R-handed Ss with L UN were divided into groups based on neglect severity (mild > 55 and severe ≤ 55). IC = 18–90 years, single stroke, confirmed L UN, and time lapse of at least 1 month after the stroke. EC = multiple lesions, temporospatial disorientation, psychiatric disorders, and associated nonstabilized pathology. Block randomization based on two levels of neglect severity; E = 9 (mild = 6, severe = 3), C = 9 (mild = 6, severe = 3). Gender (M/F): E = 5/4, C = 5/4.
Intervention	E = pointing toward pseudo-randomly alternating targets 10° to the L or R of the middle of Ss body while wearing prism glasses that shifted the field of view 10° to the R; C = same task while wearing neutral glasses. Data collected: baseline (pretest), and 1, 3, and 6 months after each PA session. Measures: FIM, BIT.
Results	At 6-month follow-up, no difference was found between groups. 4 weeks of PA did not provide additional long-term functional benefits in comparison to spontaneous recovery.
Comments	Although benefits produced by PA are maintained at conclusion of treatment, more intensive PAT is suggested to provide additional long-term gains above and beyond spontaneous recovery.

Sarri et al. (2011)[149]

Design	Prospective cohort design
Level of Evidence	II B Moderate evidence
Subjects	11 Ss with L UN.
Intervention	Ss were administered three tasks before and immediately after PA (chimeric face task lateral preference task, gradients lateral preference task, and chimeric/nonchimeric face discrimination task). The chimeric face task was composed of 20 pairs of photographed faces. Each pair of faces consisted of a mirror-reversed image of the same person's photograph divided along the vertical midline with a smiling facial expression on one half or side of the face and a neutral expression on the other side. Ss were asked to choose the face they thought "looked happier." The gradients lateral preference task comprised 20 pairs of grayscale gradient rectangles of a continuous scale ranging from absolute black at one end to absolute white at the other end. Each pair was the mirror-reversed image of the other and separated by 2 cm, one strip placed above the other. Ss were asked to report whether the upper or lower strip of each pair appeared darker. The chimeric/nonchimeric face discrimination task consisted of 40 face stimuli: 20 nonchimeric "real" faces and 20 chimeric faces (as described in the chimeric face task). Ss were asked to indicate whether each face stimulus was "real" or "chimeric." Ss also completed two line bisections and five subjective straight-ahead pointing (with R hand and eyes closed) to measure neglect.

Table 27.4	Evidence Summary Evidence Addressing the Use of Prism Adaptation as an Intervention to Increase Visual Function in Patients With Unilateral Neglect Following Stroke—cont'd

Sarri et al. (2011)[149]

	During PA, Ss pointed toward targets placed in randomly intermingled sequence, 10° to the L or R of the middle of Ss body, while wearing prism glasses that shifted the field of view 10° to the R.
Results	PA did not benefit Ss performance on spatial preference tasks (e.g., chimeric face task lateral preference task, gradients lateral preference task) compared to standard measures of neglect (line bisection, subjective straight-ahead). Results indicated that three out of six Ss benefited from PA on the chimeric/nonchimeric face discrimination task, suggesting that PA may improve awareness for the L side of face stimuli in some cases of UN.
Comments	The authors suggest that further research could provide better understanding of the benefits of PA for certain patients or tasks but not others. This would potentially optimize PA as a tool for rehabilitation for UN.

Scheffels et al. (2021)[150]

Design	Double-blinded, monocentric, crossover design RCT
Level of Evidence	II B Moderate evidence
Subjects	Twenty-four Ss diagnosed with visuospatial neglect were randomly allocated to either a continuous (PA-c) and then an intermittent (PA-i) PA procedure or the reversed order. IC = presence of L visual neglect with >2 omissions on the L side of the page than on R side of the page on Apples Cancellation Test, able to sit in a wheelchair for >45 min, participate in 10 of 15 planned therapy sessions. EC = presence of secondary normal pressure hydrocephalus or premorbid dementia.
Intervention	Ss wore prisms glasses that shifted the field of view 10° to the R; the R visual field was restricted with a cloth (30 × 30 cm) attached laterally to the prism glasses. PA-c = consisted of Ss wearing prisms for the entire session; PA-I = consisted of Ss wearing prisms for two (first series) or three times (second series) within the same session. Sessions lasted for 30-40 min, with a minimum of 50 reaching movement tasks were completed. Ss were evaluated on days 1, 4, 25, and 46. Primary measures = Apples Cancellation Test, ERBI, FIM.
Results	Ss in both conditions improved significantly on all primary measures; however, neither the higher number of opportunities for recalibration (intermittent PA) nor the duration of uninterrupted wearing of the glasses (continuous PA) significantly impacted the recovery from neglect as measured through visual tasks or ADL scores. Spontaneous body orientation was the only domain to demonstrate a beneficial effect following intermittent PA.
Comments	In conclusion, further recalibrations during intermittent PA may have a beneficial impact on body orientation but not on other aspects of neglect or ADL performance.

Ten Brink et al. (2017)[151]

Design	Single center, double-blinded, parallel-group RCT
Level of Evidence	II B Moderate evidence
Subjects	Seventy neglect Ss admitted for inpatient rehabilitation either received PA (34) or SA (35). IC = 18–85 years, stroke (first or recurrent, ischemic or intracerebral hemorrhagic lesion) and sufficient comprehension and communication skills. EC = Interfering psychiatric disorders or substance use, physically or mentally unable to participate, or expected discharge was <3 weeks. All Ss were screened for neglect and were eligible to enroll if neglect present on shape cancellation, line bisection, or CBS.

(Continued)

Table 27.4	Evidence Summary Evidence Addressing the Use of Prism Adaptation as an Intervention to Increase Visual Function in Patients With Unilateral Neglect Following Stroke—cont'd

Ten Brink et al. (2017)[151]

Intervention	E = goggles inducing an ipsilesional optical shift of 10° (PA); C = goggles with plain lenses (SA). Exposure consisted of >100 fast pointing movements to three horizontal axis stimuli (65 cm away). Both left and right stimuli were 10° away from the midline. Treatment was performed daily for 2 weeks in addition to usual care. Primary measure: CBS, 0 (no neglect) to 3 (severe neglect) in ADLs. Measures were taken at baseline and after 1, 2, 3, 4, 6, and 14 weeks.
Results	CBS scores improved over time; however, there was no main difference between groups indicating that the effects of PA and SA were comparable on CBS scores.
Comments	No evidence to support PA as an effective treatment for neglect in subacute stroke; however, results may have been impacted by the heterogeneity of neglect, neurobiological recovery, or standard treatment interventions.

Vaes et al. (2018)[152]

Design	Multicenter, blinded, RCT
Level of Evidence	I A Strong evidence
Subjects	Forty-three Ss with SN were randomly allocated into groups. IC = right-hemisphere stroke, at least four more left-sided omissions than right-sided omissions on star cancellation test or a mean of 10% rightward line bisection deviation. EC = cerebral tumors, TBI, dementia, premorbid mental deterioration or significant oculomotor problems, not demonstrating a PA aftereffect of at least 3°, medical complications or neurological deterioration after inclusion. E = 21, C = 22. Gender (M/F): E = 14/7, C = 14/8. No differences between mean days from stroke onset to intervention, head and gaze deviation, FIM scores, and median line bisection deviation.
Intervention	The PA procedure consisted of three steps; the preexposure baseline measurement of pointing (10 pointing movements), the exposure to prismatic displacement to elicit sensorimotor adaptation (80 pointing movements), and the postexposure aftereffect measurement (1 pointing movement). Seven PA sessions were completed between 7 and 12 days. E = Wedge prisms inducing a rightward optical shift (10° shift) were worn while Ss pointed to dots positioned at 10° from the body midline as fast as possible, which took 5–8 minutes. C = same task while wearing placebo prisms (0° shift). Data collected: baseline and within 2–24 hr (short time interval) after the PA session. Ss who were still in hospital were also followed up at 3 months (long time interval). Measures: consisted of 12 variables from 9 tests inclusive of SLBT, Bells test, Diamond Cancellation, Coloured Rectangle Bisection, Search Time Test, Drawing Test A and B, Extinction Test, Spatial Memory Test, and Visuospatial Navigation Test.
Results	PA found significant differences in six visuospatial variables including the rectangle bisection, drawing test B, extinction tests, spatial memory test, and visuospatial navigation test. Additionally, four variables inclusive of the drawing test B, extinction tests, and the visuospatial navigation test demonstrated a trend toward remaining significantly different in the longer term (3 months post).
Comments	Short-term repetitive PA can improve certain visuospatial deficits in Ss with SN poststroke; however, further research is recommended to confirm these results.

ADL = activities of daily living; BIT = Behavioural Inattention Test; C = control group; CBS – Catherine Bergego Scale; CT = computed tomography; E = experimental group; EC = exclusion criteria; ERBI = Early Rehabilitation Barthel Index; F = female; FIM = Functional Independence Measure; IC = inclusion criteria; L = left; LAT = limbic activation treatment; M = male; MMSE = Mini-Mental State Examination; MRI = magnetic resonance imaging; PA = prism adaptation; PAT = prism adaptation treatment; R = right; RCT = randomized controlled trial; RH = right hemisphere; ROM = range of motion; SA = shape adaptation; Ss = subject, subjects; SIAS = Stroke Impairment Assessment Set; SLBT = Schenkenberg Line Bisection Test; SN = spatial neglect; TBI = traumatic brain injury; UE = upper extremity; UN = unilateral neglect; VST = visual scanning training.

5. *Treatment Suggestions.* Anosognosia may resolve spontaneously in the first 3 months following stroke, however, until the condition resolves, it seriously hampers rehabilitation.[155] It is extremely difficult to compensate for the condition if it persists long term. Safety is of paramount importance in the treatment and discharge planning for patients experiencing anosognosia, because they typically do not acknowledge their disability and will therefore be unaware of potential dangers.

Somatoagnosia

1. *Definition.* Somatoagnosia, or impairment in body scheme, is a lack of awareness of the body structure and the relationship of body parts to oneself or to others. Some authors consider subtypes of somatoagnosia as *autotopagnosia* (referring to the inability to recognize simple and complex body features), *anosognosia* (as previously discussed), and *body agnosia*.[156] Patients with this deficit may display difficulty following instructions that require distinguishing body parts and may be unable to imitate movements of the therapist. Often patients report that the more affected arm or leg feels unduly heavy.

2. *Clinical Examples.* Patient may have difficulty performing transfer activities because they do not perceive the meaning of terms related to body parts; for example, "Pivot on your leg and reach for the armrest with your hand." In addition, a patient with a body scheme disorder will have difficulty dressing. Patients may have a hard time participating in exercises that require some body parts to be moved in relation to other body parts, for example, "Bring your arm across your chest and touch your shoulder."

3. *Lesion Area.* The lesion site is often the dominant parietal lobe.[157] Therefore, this disorder is seen primarily with right hemiplegia. However, impairment in body scheme may also occur with left hemiplegia.

4. *Testing.*
   a. The patient is requested to point to their own body parts when named by the therapist, to the therapist's body parts, and on a picture or puzzle of a human figure. Zoltan[2] provides details of these testing procedures. An example of verbal directives from these tests is, "Show me your feet. Show me your chin. Point to your back." The words *right* and *left* should not be used because they may lead to an inaccurate diagnosis in patients who have difficulty with right–left discrimination. Aphasia should be ruled out as a cause of poor performance.
   b. The patient is asked to imitate movements of the therapist. For example, the therapist touches their own cheek, arm, leg, and so forth. A mirror-image response is acceptable.[2]
   c. The patient is requested to answer questions about the relationship of body parts. For example, "Are

your knees below your head? Which is on top of your head, your hair or your feet?" For patients with aphasia, questions should be phrased to require a yes or no, or true or false response. Patients with intact function in this area should respond correctly most of the time and within a reasonable period of time. Those patients with receptive aphasia are particularly likely to do poorly on tests for somatoagnosia.[156]

5. *Treatment Suggestions.* Using a remedial approach, the therapist aims for the patient to associate sensory input with an adaptive motor response.[2] Facilitation of body awareness is accomplished through sensory stimulation to the body part affected. For example, the patient is asked to rub the appropriate body part with a rough cloth as the therapist names it or points to it. Alternatively, the patient verbally identifies body parts, or points to pictures of them as the therapist touches them.

Right–Left Discrimination

1. *Definition.* A right–left discrimination disorder is the inability to identify the right and left sides of one's own body or those of the examiner.[130] This includes the inability to execute movements in response to verbal commands that include the terms *right* and *left*. Patients are often unable to imitate movements.[130]

2. *Clinical Examples.* The patient cannot tell the therapist which is the right arm and which is the left. The right shoe cannot be discerned from the left shoe, and the patient is unable to follow instructions using the concept of right–left, such as "turn right at the corner." The patient cannot distinguish the right from the left side of the therapist.

3. *Lesion Area.* The lesion site is the parietal lobe of either hemisphere.[130] A close relationship between aphasia (usually owing to left-hemisphere damage) and deficits in right–left discrimination has been reported.[156] In patients without aphasia (usually those with right-hemisphere damage), a relationship has been reported between general mental impairment and right–left discrimination disorder.

4. *Testing.* The patient is asked to point to body parts on command, such as right ear, left foot, right arm, and so forth. Six responses should be elicited on either the patient's own body, on that of the therapist, or on a model or picture of the human body. To rule out somatoagnosia, the patient should be tested first without using the words *right* and *left*.

5. *Treatment Suggestions.* If using a compensatory approach, when giving instructions to the patient, the words *right* and *left* should be avoided. Instead, pointing or providing cues using distinguishing features of the limb may be more effective (e.g., "the arm with the watch"). These guidelines are particularly salient for the therapist teaching locomotion or transfers, where confusing instructions may have dangerous consequences. The right side of all common objects such as shoes and clothing should be marked with red tape or seam binding.

Finger Agnosia

1. *Definition.* Finger agnosia can be defined as the inability to identify the fingers of one's own hands or of the hands of the examiner.[130,156]
2. *Clinical Examples.* The disorder is characterized by difficulty in naming the fingers on command, identifying which finger was touched, and, by some definitions, mimicking finger movements. This deficit usually occurs bilaterally and is more common in the middle three fingers.[158] Finger agnosia correlates highly with poor dexterity in tasks that require movements of individual fingers in relation to each other,[1] such as buttoning, tying laces, and typing.
3. *Lesion Area.* Finger agnosia may be the result of a lesion located in either parietal lobe,[159] often in the region of the angular gyrus of the left hemisphere. It is often found in conjunction with an aphasic disorder, or with general mental impairment.[156] Bilateral finger agnosia along with right–left discrimination problems, agraphia, and *acalculia* is termed *Gerstmann syndrome.*[130] Gerstmann syndrome usually is associated with a focal lesion of the dominant hemisphere in the region of the angular gyrus.[154,156]
4. *Testing.* A portion of *Sauguet's test*[2,158] is recommended. Sauguet's test includes asking the patient to move or point to their finger when named by the therapist to determine if finger agnosia is present. Between five and ten commands from the therapist is adequate. The test is not standardized.
   a. The patient is asked to name the fingers touched by the therapist, with the eyes open (five times) and if successful, with vision occluded (five times).
   b. The patient is asked to point to the fingers named by the therapist on the patient's own hands (10 times), on the therapist's hands (10 times), and on a schematic model (10 times).
   c. The patient is asked to point to the equivalent finger on a life-sized picture when the therapist touches each finger.
   d. The patient is asked to imitate finger movements; for example, curl the index finger, touch the thumb to the middle finger.
5. *Treatment Suggestions.* There is very limited evidence to support the efficacy of treatment techniques for finger agnosia. When using a remedial approach, the patient's discriminative tactile systems (touch and pressure) are stimulated. A rough cloth can be used to rub the dorsal surface of the more affected arm, hand, and fingers, and the ventral surface of the more affected fingers. Pressure can be applied to the ventral surface of the hand. For additional details the reader is referred to Zoltan.[2]

Spatial Relations Disorders (Complex Perception)

Spatial relations disorders encompass a constellation of impairments that have in common a difficulty in perceiving the relationship between the self and two or more objects.[159] Research suggests that the right parietal lobe plays a primary role in space perception. Thus, a spatial relations impairment most frequently occurs in patients with right-sided lesions with resulting left hemiparesis.[159,160]

Spatial relations disorders include impairments of figure–ground discrimination, form discrimination, spatial relations, position in space, and topographical disorientation.[1,160] Additional visuospatial impairments, such as depth and distance perception and vertical disorientation, will also be discussed in this section. In a study comparing the effectiveness of the cognitive remediation (sometimes referred to as the *transfer-of-training technique*) versus the functional approach, Edmans et al.[161] found that both approaches were equally successful in treating perceptual impairments. However, since this study did not control for the effects of spontaneous recovery in both groups, further research is required.

Figure–Ground Discrimination

1. *Definition.* An impairment in visual figure–ground discrimination is the inability to visually distinguish a figure from the background in which it is embedded.[5] Functionally, it interferes with the patient's ability to locate important objects that are not prominent in a visual array. The patient has difficulty ignoring irrelevant visual stimuli and cannot select the appropriate cue to which to respond.[5] This may lead to distractibility, resulting in a shortened attention span,[162] frustration, and decreased independent and safe functioning.[67]
2. *Clinical Examples.* The patient cannot locate items in a pocketbook or drawer, locate buttons on a shirt, or distinguish the armhole from the remainder of a solid-colored shirt. The patient may not be able to tell when one step ends and another begins on a flight of stairs, especially when descending.
3. *Lesion Area.* Parieto-occipital lesions of the right hemisphere and less frequently the left hemisphere commonly produce this disorder.[163]
4. *Testing.*
   a. The *Ayres Figure–Ground Test* (subtest of the *Southern California Sensory Integration Tests*)[164] requires the subject to distinguish the three objects in an embedded test picture, from a possible selection of six items. This test was standardized on children but may be useful as a clinical tool in identifying perceptual disorders in adults with brain damage.[4] Normative data have been generated for normal adult males.[165] Many other tests

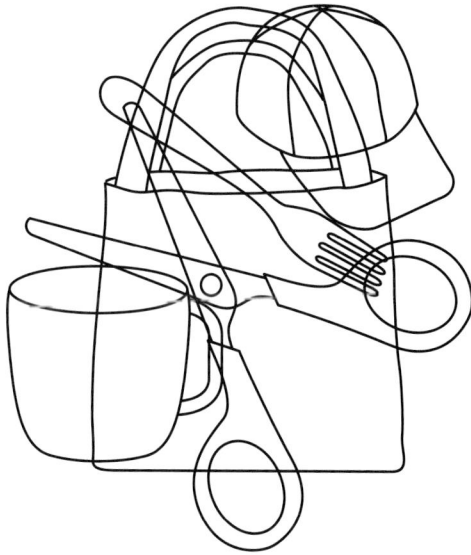

Figure 27.11 An example of a figure–ground perception test.

have since used a similar approach to test figure–ground perception by showing the patient overlapping line drawings of everyday objects and asking clients to name these as illustrated in Figure 27.11.

    b. *Function-Based Tests.* A white towel can be placed on a white sheet, and the patient is asked to find the towel. The patient can be asked to point out the sleeve, buttons, and collar of a white shirt or to pick out a spoon from an unsorted array of eating utensils. It is necessary to rule out poor eyesight, hemianopia, visual agnosia, and poor comprehension to improve the validity of these testing techniques.

5. *Treatment Suggestions.*

    a. *Remedial Approach.* The therapist should arrange for practice in visually locating objects in a simple array (such as three very different objects) and progress to more difficult ones (four or five dissimilar objects and three similar ones).

    b. *Compensatory Approach.* The patient is taught to become aware of the existence and nature of the deficit. The patient should be cautioned to examine groups of objects slowly and systematically and should be instructed to use other, intact senses (e.g., touch) when searching for items such as clothing or silverware. When learning to lock a wheelchair, the patient should be advised to locate the brake levers by touch rather than by searching for them visually. Red tape may be placed over the hook-and-loop closure of the shoe or orthosis to aid the patient in locating it. Few items should be placed in the patient's drawers or nightstand, and they should be replaced in the same location each time. Brightly colored tape can be used to mark the edges on stairs.

Repetition is a key element of this approach, and repeated practice is used in each specific area of difficulty. The same procedure should be employed during each practice session, incorporating verbal cues and touch as adjuncts to vision.

Form Discrimination

1. *Definition.* Impairment in form discrimination is the inability to perceive or attend to subtle differences in form and shape. The patient is likely to confuse objects of similar shape or not to recognize an object placed in an unusual position.

2. *Clinical Examples.* The patient may confuse a pen with a toothbrush, a vase with a water pitcher, a cane with a crutch, and so forth.

3. *Lesion Area.* The lesion site is the parieto-temporo-occipital region (posterior association areas) of the nondominant lobe.[4]

4. *Testing.* A number of items similar in shape and different in size are gathered. The patient is asked to identify them. One set of items might be a pencil, pen, straw, toothbrush, and watch, and the other might be a key, paper clip, coins, and ring. Each object is presented several times in different positions (e.g., upside down). Visual object agnosia must be ruled out as a cause for poor performance by first presenting objects separately and asking the patient to identify them or to demonstrate how they are used (see "Visual Agnosias" later in this chapter).

5. *Treatment Suggestions.*

    a. *Remedial Approach.* The patient should practice describing, identifying, and demonstrating the use of similarly shaped and sized objects. The patient should sort like objects and should be assisted to focus on differentiating object cues.

    b. *Compensatory Approach.* The patient must be made aware of the specific deficit. If the patient can read, frequently used and confused objects can be labeled. The patient should be encouraged to use vision, touch, and self-verbalization in combination when objects are confused.

Spatial Relations

1. *Definition.* A spatial relations disorder, or spatial disorientation, is the inability to perceive the relationship of one object in space to another object, or to oneself. This may lead to, or compound, problems in constructional tasks and dressing.[5] Crossing the midline may be a problem for patients with spatial relations deficits.[160] Spatial relations skills are required to manage most ADL.

2. *Clinical Examples.* The patient might find it difficult to place the cutlery, plate, and spoon in the proper position when setting the table. The patient may be unable to tell the time from an analog clock because of difficulty in perceiving the relative positions of the hands.[2,29] The patient may have difficulty learning to position their arms, legs, and trunk in relation to the wheelchair to prepare for transferring.

3. *Lesion Area.* The lesion site is predominantly the inferior parietal lobe or parieto-occipital-temporal junction, usually of the right side.[5] Arnadottir[160] explains how a patient with perceptual deficits may have difficulty putting on a shirt. This is illustrated in Figure 27.12. Since the CNS works in a holistic way, the task of putting on a shirt requires visual, tactile, and auditory information as well as attentional and memory capacities and motor output. Figure 27.12 suggests that while damage in a variety of brain areas may affect visuospatial processing, the most common lesion site is the right inferior parietal lobe.

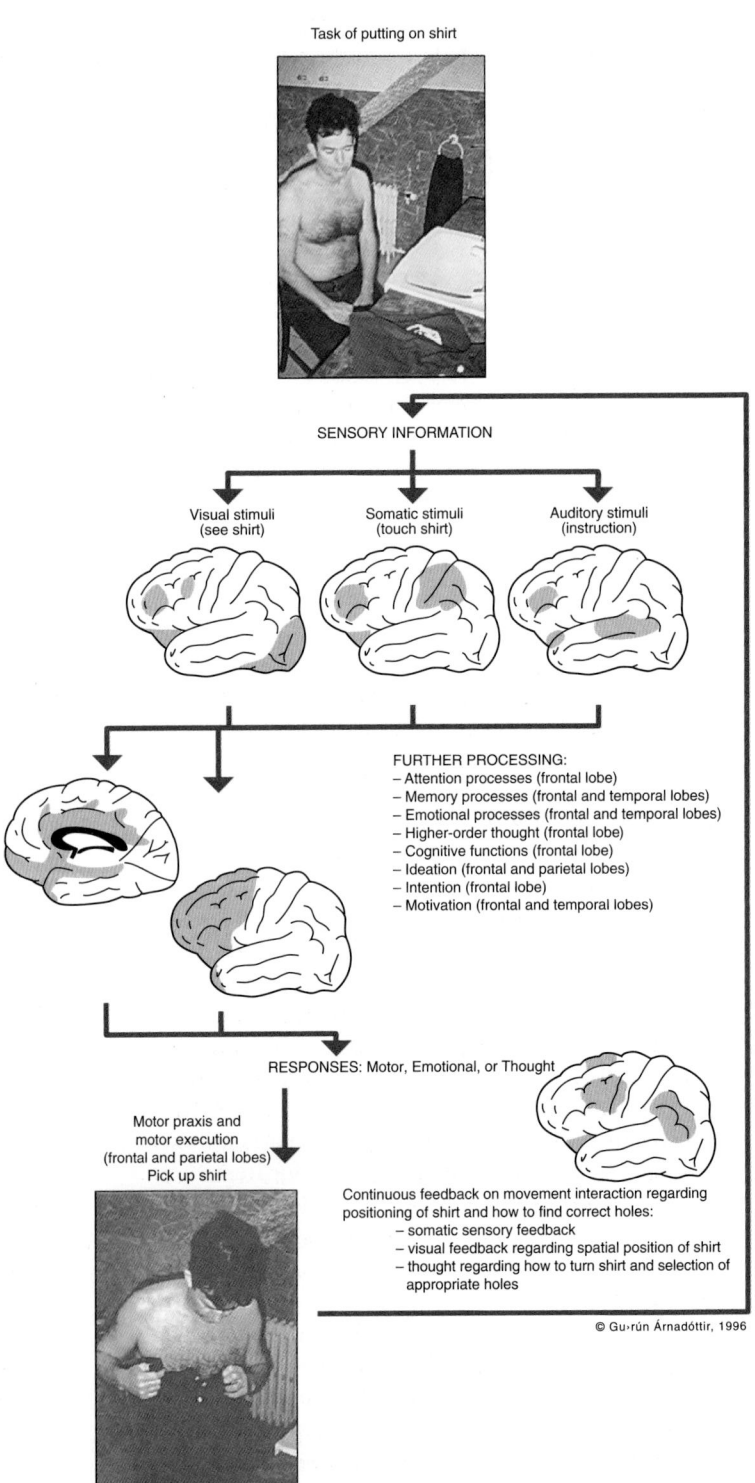

Figure 27.12 Spatial relation processing as a man puts on a shirt. *(From Arnadottir and Gudrun,[160(p405)] with permission.)*

4. *Testing.* Recommended tests include the *Rivermead Perceptual Assessment Battery*[85] and the *Arnadottir OT-ADL Neurobehavioral Evaluation (A-ONE).*[5] To improve the validity of these tests, unilateral neglect and hemianopia should be ruled out as the causes of poor performance. If these impairments are present, the stimulus array should be positioned appropriately.

5. *Treatment Suggestions.* When using a remedial approach, patient ability to orient to other objects can be improved by giving the patient instructions to position themself in relation to the therapist or another object. The therapist might say, "Sit next to me," "Go behind the table," or "Step over the line." In addition, the therapist can set up a maze of furniture (obstacle course). Having the patient copy block or matchstick designs of increasing difficulty will increase awareness of the relationship between one object (block or matchstick) and the next. If the patient avoids crossing the midline, activities that require crossing the midline both motorically and visually can be incorporated into other therapeutic activities (e.g., proprioceptive neuromuscular facilitation chop patterns). One specific activity is to have the patient hold a dowel in front with both hands. The therapist guides it from the less involved side to the more involved side. Later, the patient can progress to manipulating the dowel with only verbal or visual cues, and finally to guiding it independently.[166]

Position in Space

1. *Definition.* Position in space impairment is the inability to perceive and to interpret spatial concepts such as up, down, under, over, in, out, in front of, and behind.

2. *Clinical Examples.* If a patient is asked to raise the arm "above" the head during ROM activities or is asked to place the feet "on" the foot rests, the patient may behave as if they do not know what to do.

3. *Lesion Area.* The lesion is usually located in the nondominant parietal lobe.[163]

4. *Testing.* To test function, two objects are used, such as a shoe and a shoebox. The patient is asked to place the shoe in different positions in relation to the shoebox, for example, in the box, on top of the box, or next to the box. Alternatively, the patient is presented with two objects and asked to describe their relationship. For example, a toothbrush can be placed in a cup, under a cup, and so forth, and the patient is then asked to indicate the location of the toothbrush.

Another mode of testing is to have the patient copy the therapist's manipulations with an identical set of objects. For example, the therapist hands the patient a comb and a brush. The therapist then takes an identical set and places them in a particular relationship to each other, such as the comb on top of the brush. The patient is requested to arrange their comb and brush in the same way. Success in this task may represent sufficient ability to use position in space functionally.

Figure–ground difficulty, apraxia, incoordination, and lack of comprehension should be ruled out when performing these tests. Objects should be positioned to avoid compounding of results with hemianopia and unilateral spatial neglect.

5. *Treatment Suggestions.* If using a retraining approach, three or four identical objects are placed in the same orientation (wrist weights, combs, mugs, etc.). An additional object is placed in a different orientation. The patient is asked to identify the odd one and then to place it in the same orientation as the other objects.

Topographical Disorientation

1. *Definition. Topographical disorientation* refers to difficulty in understanding and remembering the relationship of one location to another.[167] As a result, the patient is unable to get from one place to another, with or without a map. This disorder is frequently seen in conjunction with other difficulties in spatial relations.

2. *Clinical Examples.* The patient cannot find the way from their room to the physical therapy clinic, despite being shown repeatedly. The patient cannot describe the spatial characteristics of familiar surroundings, such as the layout of their bedroom at home.[163]

3. *Lesion Areas.* The majority of cases involve damage to the right retrosplenial cortex, with Brodmann area 30 compromised in most patients.[167] Bilateral parietal lesions, and, more rarely, left-side parietal lesions can produce this problem.[163]

4. *Testing.* The patient is asked to describe or to draw a familiar route, such as the block on where they live, the layout of their house, or a major neighborhood intersection. A patient with topographical disorientation will be unable to succeed in this task. However, the therapist must differentiate between memory problems and topographical orientation difficulties.

5. *Treatment Suggestions.* This deficit usually resolves 8 weeks after onset.[167] However, several treatment techniques can be used to hasten recovery or to assist long term if the condition persists.

   a. *Remedial Approach.* The patient practices going from one place to another, following verbal instructions. Initially, simple routes should be used, and then more complicated ones.[2]

   b. *Compensatory Approach.* Frequently traveled routes can be marked with colored dots. The spaces between the dots are gradually increased and eventually eliminated as improvement takes place.[2] This is an example of taking a normally right-hemisphere task and (because there is right-sided damage) converting it into a left-hemisphere task. In this instance, we take the spatial task of remembering routes (right-hemisphere task) and substitute sequential landmarks (sequencing is typically a left-hemisphere strength) to accomplish the goal of getting from place to place. The patient should be reminded not to leave the clinic, room, or home unattended, because they may get lost.

Depth and Distance Perception

1. *Definition.* The patient with a disorder of depth and distance perception experiences inaccurate judgment of direction, distance, and depth. Spatial disorientation may be a contributing factor in faulty distance perception.
2. *Clinical Examples.* The patient may have difficulty navigating stairs, may miss the chair when attempting to sit, or may continue pouring juice once a glass is filled.[162]
3. *Lesion Areas.* This impairment may occur with a lesion in the posterior right hemisphere in the superior visual association cortices; it may be evident with right-sided or bilateral lesions.[163]
4. *Testing.*
   a. For a functional test of distance perception, the patient is asked to take or to grasp an object that has been placed on a table. The object may also be held in front of the patient or in the air, and the patient is again asked to grasp it. The patient with impaired distance perception will overshoot or undershoot.[2] However, the movements look purposeful and smooth, which distinguishes this problem from a coordination deficit.
   b. To determine depth perception functionally, the patient can be asked to fill a glass of water.[2] A patient with a depth perception deficit may continue pouring once the glass is filled.
5. *Treatment Suggestions.* The patient should be assisted in becoming aware of the deficit (education to increase cognitive awareness). Emphasis should be placed on the importance of walking carefully on uneven surfaces, particularly on stairs.
   a. *Remedial Approach.* The patient is requested to place the feet on designated spots during gait training. Also, blocks can be arranged in piles 2 to 8 in. (5 to 8 cm) high. The patient is asked to touch the top of the piles with the foot. This is done to reestablish a sense of depth and distance.[166]
   b. *Compensatory Approach.* Practice in compensating for disturbances in depth and distance perception occurs intrinsically in many ADL skills, both those that involve moving through space and those that involve manipulation. For example, the patient can hold the armrests of a chair to assist with sitting squarely.

Vertical Disorientation

1. *Definition. Vertical disorientation* refers to a distorted perception of what is vertical. Displacement of the vertical position can contribute to disturbance of motor performance, both in posture and in gait. Early in recovery, most patients post-CVA demonstrate some impairment in the sense of verticality.[168] This is not associated with or affected by the presence of homonymous hemianopia.
2. *Clinical Example.* A person with distorted verticality views the world differently, and this may affect upright posture, as depicted in Figure 27.13.
3. *Lesion Area.* The lesion site is in the nondominant parietal lobe.
4. *Testing.* The therapist holds a cane vertically and then turns it sideways to a horizontal plane. Researchers use a luminous rod with patients seated in a darkened room.[168] The patient is handed the cane and asked to turn it back to the original position. If the patient's perception of the vertical position is distorted, the cane will most likely be placed at an angle, representing the patient's conception of the world around them.
5. *Treatment Suggestions.* Patients must be made aware of the deficit. They should be instructed to compensate by using touch (tactile cues) for proper self-orientation, especially when going through doorways, in and out of elevators, and on the stairs.

Agnosias (Simple Perception)

Agnosia is the inability to recognize or make sense of incoming information despite intact sensory capacities. Although this condition is relatively rare (as listed by the National Institutes of Health Office of Rare Diseases), it

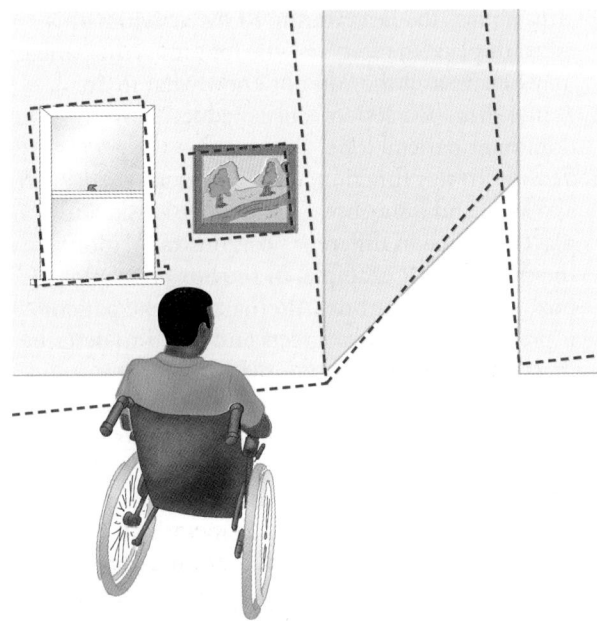

Figure 27.13 Vertical disorientation may contribute to disturbances of posture and gait.

can affect any sensory modality (e.g., vision, audition, touch, taste) and anything (e.g., faces, sounds, colors, familiar or less familiar objects). Although there is an inability to recognize familiar objects using one or two of the sensory modalities, the ability to recognize the same object using other sensory modalities is usually present.[154,169]

Visual Agnosias

1. *Definition.* Visual object agnosia is the most common form of agnosia.[4] It is defined as the inability to recognize familiar objects despite normal function of the eyes and optic tracts.[169]

2. *Clinical Examples.* One remarkable aspect of this disorder is the readiness with which the patient can identify an object once it is handled (i.e., information is received from another sensory modality).[170] The patient may not recognize people, possessions, and common objects. Specific types of visual agnosia include simultanagnosia, prosopagnosia, and color agnosia.

   a. *Simultanagnosia,* also known as Balint syndrome,[4] is the inability to perceive a visual stimulus as a whole. The patient perceives an entire array one part at a time. The lesion is usually in the dominant occipital lobe.

   b. *Prosopagnosia* was traditionally considered to be the inability to recognize familiar faces. Current thought suggests this phenomenon is related to any visually ambiguous stimulus, the recognition of which depends on evoking a memory context, such as different species of birds or different makes of cars. Prosopagnosia is usually accompanied by visual field impairments. Bilaterally symmetrical occipital lesions are thought to be responsible for this impairment.[15,50,171]

   c. *Color agnosia* is the inability to recognize colors; it is not color blindness. The patient is unable to identify or name colors on command, although color chips can be correctly paired.[50] However, the meaning of color is lost so that the patient no longer associates a duckling as yellow or the sea as blue.[169] Color agnosia is frequently associated with facial or other visual object agnosias.[4,163] It is usually the result of a dominant hemisphere lesion.[4] The simultaneous occurrence of left-sided hemianopia, alexia (inability to read; word blindness), and color agnosia is a classic occipital lobe syndrome.[4]

3. *Lesion Area.* The lesions associated with visual object agnosias are thought to occur in the occipito-temporo-parietal association areas of either hemisphere. These areas are responsible for the integration of visual stimuli with respect to memory.[154] Recent evidence suggests visual object agnosias may result from damage in the medial structures of the ventral occipito-temporal cortex.[172]

4. *Testing.* To test for this deficit, several common objects are placed in front of the patient. The

patient is asked to name the objects, point to an object named by the therapist, or demonstrate its use. It is important to rule out aphasia and apraxia, although this is not easily done. Details of other nonstandardized and standardized testing procedures are provided in Laver and Unsworth.[169]

5. *Treatment Suggestions.*

   a. *Remedial Approach.* Drills can be used to practice discrimination between faces that are important to the patient (using photographs) and discrimination between colors and common objects. The therapist should assist the patient in picking out salient visual cues for relating names to faces.

   Note: Another tool for treating visual agnosia, as well as many other cognitive and perceptual deficits, is the Easy Street Environment. These environments have been incorporated into rehabilitation centers in the United States for almost 20 years. The Easy Street Environment is a modular "world" of life-size streets (with a variety of ambulation surfaces, stairs, curbs, etc.), vehicles, shops, and offices, which are constructed in a dedicated area within the rehabilitation setting. The Easy Street Environment has many advantages since it allows occupational therapists, physical therapists, and speech-language pathologists to work with a patient in a safe, private, and comfortable environment where the patient can try out relearned or new skills. The therapist can also save considerable time by taking the patient down the corridor to the Easy Street Environment rather than to their own local community, although ultimately such an outing to the local community may be undertaken. Figure 27.14 shows a patient with a visual object agnosia learning to use the Easy Street Environment automatic teller machine

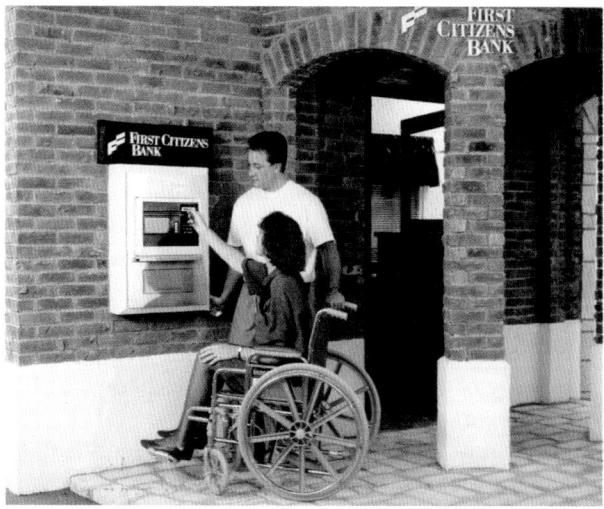

Figure 27.14 A client with an agnosia learns to use an ATM with help from a therapist in the Easy Street Environment. *(Courtesy of Easy Street Environments, Scottsdale, AZ 85260.)*

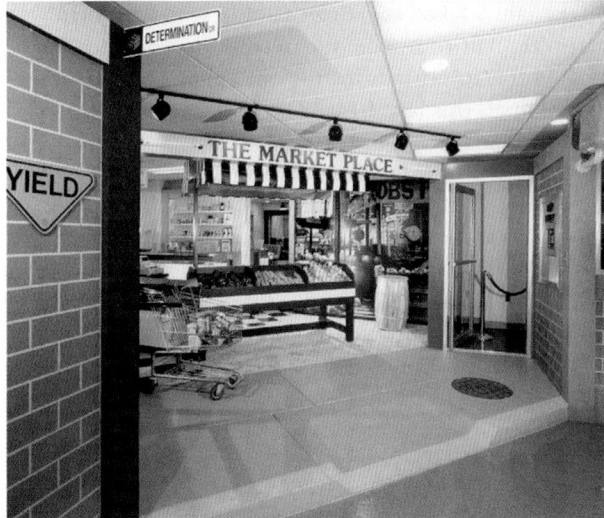

Figure 27.15 Clients with agnosias and many other cognitive and perceptual deficits can practice daily living skills in the controlled Easy Street Environment such as provided in the Market Store. *(Courtesy of Easy Street Environments, Scottsdale, AZ 85260.)*

(ATM). This patient may also learn new strategies to identify groceries and therefore be able to practice shopping in the Easy Street Environment Market Place (Fig. 27.15). Where Easy Street Environments are not available, the therapist can take clients into their own community to practice desired skills. The client's own environment also provides the most ecologically valid environment for rehabilitation. Behrmann et al.[173] have also presented a case study of a 24-year-old male and reported that the patient improved in identifying novel and common objects through recognition training. Positive results were not found for face identification.

b. *Compensatory Approach.* The patient is instructed to use intact sensory modalities, such as touch or audition, to distinguish people and objects.

Auditory Agnosia

1. *Definition.* Auditory agnosia refers to the inability to recognize nonspeech sounds or to discriminate between them. This rarely occurs in the absence of other communication disorders.[4]

2. *Clinical Examples.* The patient with auditory agnosia cannot tell, for example, the difference between the ring of a doorbell and that of a telephone, or between a dog barking and thunder.

3. *Lesion Area.* The lesion is located in the dominant temporal lobe.[4]

4. *Testing.* Testing is usually carried out by a speech-language pathologist. The patient is asked to close the eyes and to identify the source of various sounds. The therapist rings a bell, honks a horn,

rings a telephone, and so forth, and asks the patient to identify the sound (verbally or by pointing to a picture).

5. *Treatment Suggestions.* Treatment generally consists of drilling the patient on sounds, but this has not been found to be particularly effective.[1,2]

Tactile Agnosia or Astereognosis

1. *Definition.* Tactile agnosia, or astereognosis, is the inability to recognize forms by handling them, although tactile, proprioceptive, and thermal sensations may be intact. This impairment commonly causes difficulties in ADL skills, inasmuch as many self-care activities that are normally done in the absence of constant visual monitoring require the manipulation of objects. If tactile agnosia is present in combination with unilateral neglect or other sensory loss, performance in ADL skills may be severely hampered.[67]

2. *Clinical Examples.* If a patient is handed a familiar object (key, comb, safety pin) with vision occluded, they will fail to recognize it.

3. *Lesion Area.* The lesion is in the parieto-temporo-occipital lobe (posterior association areas) of either hemisphere.[4]

4. *Testing.* The patient is asked to identify objects placed in the hand by examining them manually without visual cues.

5. *Treatment Suggestions.*
   a. *Remedial Approach.* The patient practices feeling various common objects, shapes, and textures with vision occluded. The patient is instructed to immediately look at the object for visual feedback and note special characteristics of the object.
   b. *Compensatory Approach.* To improve cognitive awareness, the patient is educated concerning the nature of the deficit and is instructed in visual compensation.

Apraxia

Apraxia is an impairment of voluntary skilled learned movement. It is characterized by an inability to perform purposeful movements, which cannot be accounted for by inadequate strength, loss of coordination, impaired sensation, attentional difficulties, abnormal tone, movement disorders, intellectual deterioration, poor comprehension, or uncooperativeness.[174–176] Many patients with apraxia also present with aphasia, and the two deficits are sometimes difficult to distinguish from each other.[4] Donkervoot et al.[177] report the prevalence of apraxia among patients with first left-hemisphere stroke in rehabilitation as around 28%. The two main forms of apraxia discussed in the literature are *ideomotor* and *ideational apraxia*. Ideomotor and ideational apraxias are generally thought to be the result of dominant hemisphere lesions and may be particularly difficult to test in the patient with aphasia. Although aphasia and apraxia often occur together, there is not a strong correlation between the severity of the aphasia and the severity of the apraxia. A third form of apraxia, *buccofacial apraxia,* is actually a type of ideomotor apraxia and is characterized by difficulties with performing the purposeful movements that involve facial muscles related to the mouth. This may include responding to the command "pretend to blow out a candle" or producing an orderly sequence of phonemes to produce speech. Hence, apraxia is a disorder of skilled movement and not a language disorder.[50] Some rehabilitation texts also describe constructional and dressing apraxias. However, it is generally believed that these are not true apraxias but rather are difficulties in the application of cognitive and perceptual skill to these tasks. In other words, they are terms used to describe specific difficulties with a construction or drawing task or dressing. Both these problems are more frequently associated with right-hemisphere lesions.[178]

In a recent study conducted by Wu et al.,[179] patients with apraxia were found to improve on clinical measures, from admission to discharge from an inpatient rehabilitation facility. However, upon discharge, participants' level of independence was comparable to patients without apraxia at admission, reinforcing the disabling nature of this disorder.

Ideomotor Apraxia

1. *Definition. Ideomotor apraxia* refers to a breakdown between concept and performance. There is a disconnection between the idea of a movement and its motor execution. It appears that the information cannot be transferred from the areas of the brain that conceptualize to the centers for motor execution. Thus, patients with ideomotor apraxia can carry out habitual tasks automatically and describe how they are done but are unable to imitate gestures or perform on command.[180,181] Patients with this form of apraxia often perseverate;[154] that is, they repeat an activity or a segment of a task over and over, even if it is no longer necessary or appropriate. This makes it difficult for them to finish one task and go on to the next. Patients with ideomotor apraxia appear most impaired when requested to perform tasks that require use of many implements and that have many steps. This form of apraxia can be demonstrated separately in the facial areas, upper extremities (UEs), LEs, and total body movements.[182] Patients with apraxia are often observed to be clumsy in their actual handling of objects. Impairment is typically suspected when observing the patient during ADL or during a routine motor examination.

2. *Clinical Examples.* Several examples of ideomotor apraxia follow. The patient is unable to "blow" on command. However, if presented with a bubble wand, the patient will spontaneously blow bubbles. The patient may fail to walk if requested to in a traditional manner. However, if a cup of coffee is placed on a table at the other end of the room and the patient is told, "Please have coffee," the patient is likely to traverse the room to get it.[157] A male patient is asked to comb his hair. He may be able to identify the comb and even tell you what it is used for; however, he will not actually use the comb appropriately when it is handed to him. Despite this observation in the clinic, his wife reports that he combs his hair spontaneously every morning. A female patient is asked to squeeze a dynamometer. She appears not to know what to do with it, although her comprehension is adequate, the task has just been demonstrated, and it is clear that she has adequate strength.

3. *Lesion Area.* Apraxia results most frequently from lesions in the left, dominant hemisphere. There is evidence that both frontal lesions and posterior parietal lesions can result in apraxia.[183]

4. *Testing.* The *Goodglass and Kaplan*[182] test for apraxia is composed of universally known movements, such as blowing, brushing teeth, hammering, shaving, and so forth. It is based on what the authors consider a hierarchy of difficulty for patients with apraxia. First the patient is asked, "Show me how you would bang a nail with a hammer." If the patient fails to do this or uses their fist as if it were a hammer, the patient is told, "Pretend to hold the hammer." If the patient fails following this instruction, the therapist demonstrates the act and asks the patient to imitate it. The patient with apraxia typically will not improve after demonstration but will improve with use of the actual implements.[4] The ability to correct oneself on following verbal cueing is considered not indicative of apraxia. Additional apraxia tests may be found in Butler[178] and the work of van Heugten et al.,[184] who have adapted the A-ONE[5] as an observational method of testing for apraxia.

5. *Treatment Suggestions.*
   a. *Remedial Approach.* In the remediation of apraxias, it is advised that the therapist speak slowly and use the shortest possible sentences. One command should be given at a time, and the second command should not be given until the first task is completed. When teaching a new task, it should be broken down into its component parts. Components are taught one at a time, with the therapist physically guiding the patient through the task if necessary. It should be completed in precisely the same manner each time.[178] When all the individual units are mastered, an attempt to combine them should be made. A great deal of repetition may be necessary.[67] Family members must be advised to use the exact approach found to be successful in the clinic. Performing activities in as normal an environment as possible is also helpful. Butler[178] provides a case example of a young woman relearning how to

drink from a cup using this technique. Using the sensorimotor approach, multiple sensory inputs are used on the affected body parts to enhance the production of appropriate motor responses. See Okoye[185] for additional details on this approach. More recently, researchers in Italy have had some success using mirror box therapy to promote recovery following apraxia,[180] using similar techniques to those described for the treatment of unilateral neglect.

b. *Compensatory Approach.* Donkervoot et al.[186] report an RCT that showed the effectiveness of an occupational therapy treatment program, including "strategy training," over regular occupational therapy. Strategy training involves teaching the patient compensatory techniques to overcome the apraxia, such as use of pictures in the correct sequence to support ADL skills. This approach has been developed further and is now widely used to help patients overcome apraxia. Further studies to support this approach have also come from a group of occupational therapists in the Netherlands and include trials by Donkervoort et al.[187] and Geusgens and colleagues.[188,189]

Ideational Apraxia

1. *Definition.* Ideational apraxia is a failure in the conceptualization of the task. It is an inability to perform a purposeful motor act, either automatically or on command, because the patient no longer understands the overall concept of the act, cannot retain the idea of the task, or cannot formulate the motor patterns required. Often the patient can perform isolated components of a task but cannot combine them into a complete act. Furthermore, the patient cannot verbally describe the process of performing an activity, describe the function of objects, or use them appropriately.[190,191]
2. *Clinical Examples.* When presented in the clinic with a toothbrush and toothpaste and told to brush the teeth, the patient may put the tube of toothpaste in the mouth or try to put toothpaste on the toothbrush without removing the cap. Further, the patient may be unable to describe verbally how toothbrushing is done. Similar phenomena may be evident in all aspects of ADL (washing, meal preparation, etc.) and so may limit the safety and potential independence of the patient.[5] It has been shown that patients with

ideational apraxia who test poorly in the clinical situation appear more able to perform ADL skills at the appropriate time and in a familiar setting.[185]

3. *Lesion Area.* The lesion causing ideational apraxia is thought to be in the dominant parietal lobe. This deficit also may be seen in conjunction with diffuse brain damage, such as cerebral arteriosclerosis.[154]
4. *Testing.* The tests for ideational apraxia are similar to those for ideomotor apraxia. The major expected response difference is that the patient with ideomotor apraxia can perform a motor act spontaneously and automatically at the appropriate time, but the patient with ideational apraxia is unable to do so. Refer to Butler[178] for full testing protocols.
5. *Treatment Suggestions.* The treatment techniques are the same as those for ideomotor apraxia.

Buccofacial Apraxia

1. *Definition.* Buccofacial or oral apraxia involves difficulties with performing purposeful movements with the lips, tongue, cheeks, larynx, and pharynx on command. Pedersen et al.[192] report the prevalence rate of this unusual condition in patients with acute stroke as around 6%.
2. *Clinical Examples.* A patient may have difficulty responding to the command "pretend to blow out a candle" or "blow a kiss." However, in a normal context where the patient may perform these actions automatically, performance is not impaired. In addition, while patients may be able to produce the individual phonemes required for speech, they may have difficulty in producing an orderly sequence of phonemes. Formulaic speech (common, routine phrases) or automatic expressions such as "have a nice day" may be preserved.[193]
3. *Lesion Area.* Difficulties with buccofacial apraxia seem associated with lesions in the frontal and central opercula, anterior insula, and a small area of the first temporal gyrus (adjacent to the frontal and central opercula). Although buccofacial apraxia often coexists with Broca aphasia, the two may be seen independently.[193]
4. *Testing.* The patient should be examined by a speech-language pathologist.
5. *Treatment Suggestions.* The speech-language pathologist can advise the health-care team on strategies to communicate with patients who have buccofacial apraxia.

SUMMARY

Cognition and perception, the processes by which an individual thinks and selects, integrates, and interprets stimuli from the body and surrounding environment, are critical to the normal functioning of each human being. The patient with brain damage may be lacking in those abilities that allow one to make sense of and respond appropriately to the outside world. It is essential for the therapy team to work together to recognize when a patient is experiencing some type of cognitive or perceptual dysfunction and to have the requisite tools to understand the causes of the behavior. The team can then determine the best interventions and consistently deliver these. Although it is often the occupational therapist, neuropsychologist, and speech-language pathologist who will guide the selection and implementation of evaluations and interventions for patients with cognitive and perceptual problems, it is essential that the physical therapist understands how these cognitive and perceptual impairments affect the patient's performance and the strategies that improve performance.

This chapter provided an overview of cognitive and perceptual deficits that may occur following brain damage, particularly those resulting from a stroke, and how such deficits can affect the functioning of the patient, especially within the context of the rehabilitation setting. The importance of differentiating cognitive and perceptual deficits from problems related to lack of motor ability, inadequate sensation, poor language skills, and simple uncooperativeness has been emphasized. Although alluded to in a very abbreviated fashion, activity analysis and systematic data collection remain two of the most powerful tools at the disposal of the therapist attempting to develop a firm rationale for, and to empirically justify the efficacy of, any treatment selected. Treatment in the form of adaptation of the physical environment and instructional sets and the teaching of compensatory techniques has been singled out as one of the most effective avenues for intervention.

Questions for Review

1. Patients with cognitive and perceptual deficits display what general characteristics during execution of a task?

2. Identify the underlying premise of the *transfer-of-training approach* to treatment.

3. What is the underlying assumption of the *sensory integrative approach* to treatment? Provide examples of the treatment modalities employed with this approach.

4. How is the performance of specific functional skills enhanced using the *functional approach* to treatment? What are the inherent benefits of using the functional approach?

5. Describe general suggestions for optimizing teaching/learning strategies when using compensatory techniques.

6. Identify the four treatment strategies included in the *cognitive approach* to treatment.

7. What potential influencing factors must be considered when examining a patient with cognitive and perceptual deficits?

8. What examination procedures will assist the therapist in distinguishing between sensory and cognitive or perceptual problems?

9. Differentiate between feedback provided in the form of KR versus KP.

10. Identify and define the four different types of attention.

11. What is the purpose of memory retraining? Compare and contrast the focus of the *remedial approach* and the *compensatory approach* to memory retraining.

12. Define the following terms: *unilateral neglect, anosognosia, somatoagnosia, finger agnosia,* and *right–left discrimination.*

13. Identify five spatial relations deficits. What general clinical manifestation do these disorders have in common? Define each of the deficits identified and provide an example of how each would influence patient performance of a task.

14. Provide examples of the functional implications of a visual *figure–ground discrimination deficit*. What is the most common lesion site producing this disorder?

15. What is the characteristic feature of apraxia? Define the three types of apraxias and provide examples of task performance characteristics associated with each type of apraxia.

CASE STUDY

The patient is a 72-year-old woman named Shoshana who has just been admitted to a rehabilitation facility following a stroke. Shoshanna experienced a right parietal hemorrhagic stroke. A CT scan revealed a 1.5-in. (4 cm) hemorrhage that was subsequently drained. She will be able to stay in the rehabilitation facility for 20 days. Although the patient has some physical problems, the emphasis of

(Continued)

this case study is on cognitive and perceptual tests and interventions. The occupational therapist and the physical therapist are collaboratively using a combination of cognitive retraining and the functional approach in therapy.

PAST MEDICAL HISTORY

The patient's past medical history includes insulin-dependent diabetes and mild osteoarthritis in both shoulders that causes some morning pain and stiffness.

SOCIAL

The patient lives alone in her own home. Supportive friends and family, her two children, and their families live nearby. A local health maintenance organization provides her insurance. She is retired from the police force and enjoys gardening, reading, and watching television. She previously drove an automobile with an automatic transmission.

PHYSICAL THERAPY EXAMINATION

When the patient was approached from the left, she seemed to ignore the physical therapist and did not respond to greetings. However, when the therapist sat in the chair on the patient's right side, she seemed to have no problems talking to the therapist.

Range of Motion, Muscle Tone, and Balance

Examination revealed functional passive ROM, reduced strength in the left UE with strength generally within the Fair (3/5) range; difficulty manipulating small objects with the left hand; and some reduced dynamic standing balance reactions, with a score of 47/56 on the Berg Balance Scale. She scored 48/66 on the UE component of the Fugl-Meyer Assessment of the Upper Extremity.[194]

Sensation

The physical therapist tested sensation and noted normal sensation in all areas (sharp/dull, light touch, temperature, proprioceptive sensations, cortical sensations) on the right side. However, the patient seemed to have difficulties on the left side, and her performance in detecting stimuli seemed inconsistent. Because the physical therapist suspected cognitive and perceptual deficits, a complete sensory test was deferred until the occupational therapist could fully examine the patient.

Functional Status

The physical therapist examined the patient's transfer abilities and instructed her in a safer way to get in and out of bed. The therapist scored the patient on the *Functional Independence Measure (FIM)*[93] and found the following:

Self-Care
   • Eating: FIM level = 4
   • Grooming: FIM level = 5
   • Bathing: FIM level = 3
   • Dressing—upper body: FIM level = 5
   • Dressing—lower body: FIM level = 4
   • Toileting: FIM level = 6

Transfers
   • Bed, chair, wheelchair: FIM level = 5
   • Toilet: FIM level = 5
   • Tub: FIM level = 4

Locomotion:
   • Walk: FIM level = 5

The physical therapist asked about her family, and she was able to provide many details. However, she seemed puzzled about where she was and expressed concern that she was not looking her best and needed to do her hair. The therapist suggested that she might like to brush her hair. The brush was on the table on the patient's left side, and she said she did not have one. The physical therapist cued her to check her bedside table, but on checking she maintained she did not have a brush. At the end of the session (which lasted about 40 min), the therapist asked her to demonstrate the bed transfer technique again that she had been taught at the beginning of the session. She seemed confused and could not do what the physical therapist had taught her.

CASE STUDY—cont'd

OCCUPATIONAL THERAPY EXAMINATION: COGNITION AND PERCEPTION

The occupational therapist conducted two standardized tests: the *RBMT*[87] (because the patient demonstrates memory impairments) and the *A-ONE*[5] (to examine the impact of the patient's problems on her daily living activities). She received a scaled score of 54 on the RBMT, suggesting the need for ongoing therapy, particularly to support her strength in verbal memory. For the A-ONE, her independence scores for the subtests were Dressing (11/20), Grooming and Hygiene (12/24), Transfer and Mobility (13/20), Feeding (9/16), and Communication (3/8). The occupational therapist also reasoned that further tests of the patient's IADL, including home and driving abilities, would need to be conducted closer to her discharge. The patient's FIM scores for the Social Cognition items were as follows:

Social Cognition FIM
- Social interaction: FIM level = 6
- Problem-solving: FIM level = 6
- Memory: FIM level = 3

GUIDING QUESTIONS

1. What are some of the functional difficulties the patient is having and what cognitive and perceptual deficits might be causing these? Note that there may be more than one deficit impacting the functional problems noted.

2. Develop a clinical asset and problem list across the categories of the ICF.

3. Identify anticipated goals and expected outcomes appropriate for this patient.

4. Identify two treatment strategies to improve spontaneous use of left UE and decrease unilateral neglect.

5. Identify two treatment strategies to improve the patient's memory.

6. How can the success of the patient's rehabilitation program be measured?

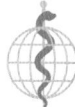 For additional resources, including answers to the questions for review, new immersive cases, case study guiding questions, references, and more, please visit **https://www.fadavis.com/product/physical -rehabilitation-fulk-8**. You may also quickly find the resources by entering this title's four-digit ISBN, 4691, in the search field at **http://fadavis.com** and logging in at the prompt.

Neurogenic Disorders of Speech and Language

Martha Taylor Sarno, CCC-SLP; MA, Fellow ASHA; Honors of the Association, MD (hon)
Jessica Galgano, PhD, CCC-SLP

Chapter 28

LEARNING OBJECTIVES

1. Differentiate the organization of language with respect to the role of phonological, lexical, syntactic, and semantic systems.
2. Understand the role of the motor speech system in the speech production process.
3. Discuss and characterize the classic aphasic syndromes.
4. Identify and explain the critical factors in the evaluation of recovery and rehabilitation of aphasia.
5. Identify and describe general approaches to aphasia rehabilitation and some specific treatment methods.
6. Identify etiologies of cognitive-communication disorders.
7. Compare and contrast deficits in executive function, pragmatic language, and motor speech in persons with cognitive-communication disorders.
8. Describe the primary types of dysarthria and rationales for dysarthria treatment.
9. Describe apraxia of speech and its treatment.
10. Gain an understanding of swallowing disorders.
11. Describe the goals and rationales for the use of augmentative communication systems.

CHAPTER OUTLINE

THE ORGANIZATION OF LANGUAGE *1100*
SPEECH PRODUCTION *1101*
APHASIA *1104*
  Classification and Nomenclature *1104*
  Historical Perspective *1106*
  Aphasia Measures *1107*
  Aphasia Recovery *1108*
  Efficacy of Treatment in Poststroke Aphasia *1108*
  Psychological and Related Factors *1109*
  Treatment of Aphasia *1109*
  Management of the Patient With Aphasia *1110*
COGNITIVE-COMMUNICATION DISORDERS *1111*
  Examination of Cognitive-Communication Disorders *1111*

Treatment of Cognitive-Communication Disorders *1111*
DYSARTHRIA *1112*
  Classification and Nomenclature *1112*
  Treatment of Dysarthria *1113*
APRAXIA OF SPEECH *1114*
  Treatment of Apraxia of Speech *1114*
DYSPHAGIA *1114*
  Treatment of Dysphagia *1115*
COMMUNICATION DISORDERS: IMPLICATIONS FOR THE PHYSICAL THERAPIST *1115*
SUMMARY *1116*

Most people take the ability to produce and understand speech for granted and pay little attention to the nature and function of the processes involved in communication. To develop and engage in oral communication, humans must have a functioning auditory or hearing system. Yet speech, like toolmaking, sets us apart from animals and is one of our most human behaviors. Even in primitive societies, humans have used the oral–motor speech code to share experiences, ideas, and feelings. Not all communities have developed writing and reading systems.

The use of speech for communication contributes to our identity as human beings and to the perception of "self." As a result, disruptions in the ability to communicate, whether caused by structural abnormalities (e.g., cleft palate), neurological conditions (e.g., stroke, Parkinson disease), or nonorganic conditions (e.g., nonorganic articulatory disorders) may affect a person's daily life in important ways. For some, the acquisition of a communication disorder may have sufficient impact to cause an individual to leave the workforce and limit social contact. For those whose communication disorders have persisted since childhood, the disorder may represent a significant vocational handicap. In others, a disorder that does not impede the individual's vocational life may interfere with everyday socialization. Communication disorders are complex, multifaceted behavioral impairments often associated so closely with people's self-image as to threaten the quality of their lives.

The term *communication* encompasses all the behaviors that human beings use to perceive and transmit information and interact with others. The term *language* refers to the quasi-automatic behavior of selecting vocabulary and sentence structures before communicating a message. Understanding what is said requires adequate hearing and the ability to perceive, discriminate, and conceptualize the speaker's thoughts as conveyed through spoken messages.

Speech comprises a delicate and rapid sequence of sensory and motor events requiring the coordinated activity of several parts of the body. The use of speech for communication involves many levels of human activity, ranging from the fine motor coordination of components of the oral–motor system to the subtle shades of meaning that occur at the cognitive/semantic level. Gestures, pantomime, and other nonverbal *pragmatic language* behaviors, such as turn taking, are also essential elements of communication.

Among unimpaired speakers, speech behavior varies greatly, yet the auditory and speech systems are efficient for the exchange of both simple and complicated information. The range of variability is so wide that individuals generally produce different sound waves with different characteristics even when producing the same word. But listeners do not rely solely on information derived from speech waves. We also depend on cues, which are components of what is referred to as *context.* Context includes aspects of a communicative exchange such as the purpose of the activity, location of the exchange, knowledge of the participants, roles of each participant, and level of formality required by the situation.

This chapter addresses *neurogenic disorders of communication,* a category of communication disorders represented by the majority of patients receiving speech-language pathology services in rehabilitation programs. The most common of these disorders are aphasia, a language disorder; dysarthria, a motor–speech disorder; apraxia of speech; cognitive-communication disorders; and dysphagia. The information contained in this chapter does not address neurogenic speech and language disorders in the pediatric population.

The field of SLP began in 1925 with the establishment of the American Speech-Language-Hearing Association (ASHA), an organization of professionals dedicated to the diagnosis and treatment of individuals with congenital or acquired communication disorders. Communication disorders in children and adults are estimated to have prevalence in the United States of 5% to 10% and a cost to the economy of $154 billion to $186 billion per year. The number of persons in the United States with communication disorders is estimated at 14 million.[1,2] These statistics have increased by the addition of a significant number of military personnel returning from active duty who may manifest a host of communication disorders, including hearing loss, speech-language disorders, and/or cognitive-communication disorders. A significant number of returning military personnel and individuals participating in sports have cognitive-communication disorders secondary to traumatic brain injury (TBI), which include deficits in discourse, pragmatic language, and social communication.[3–6]

The National Institute on Deafness and Other Communication Disorders reports that 6 to 8 million people in the United States have an acquired or developmental language disorder. It is estimated that about 180,000 persons acquire aphasia annually, and approximately 1 million people currently have aphasia.[2,7,8] Contemporary data from Aphasia Access suggest that the estimate of people living with aphasia in the United States is closer to 2.4 million, and even that number is conservative.[8] In addition, approximately 7.5 million people in the United States have voice disorders.[2]

Approximately 37.5 million American adults have a hearing loss. Age is the strongest predictor of hearing loss among adults aged 20 to 69, and the degree of loss is significantly greater in those older than age 69.[9,10] It is well known that hearing aids can improve communication function among older adults who suffer from a loss of hearing. Hearing aid technology can be considered either advanced or basic; however, today's basic digital hearing aids offer far more benefit than the best hearing aids of previous generations.

The SLP and audiology professions have grown rapidly. Affiliates (members and certificate holders) in ASHA at year-end 2020 included 188,143 speech-language pathologists (SLPs) and 13,727 audiologists. The abbreviation *SLP* is the official designation of professionals in the field who hold the Certificate of Clinical Competence in speech-pathology (CCC-SLP). The term *speech therapist,* although no longer considered professionally appropriate, is a term that is often used informally. Speech-language pathology and audiology are master's degree entry fields. As of 2009, 50 states require a license for SLPs and audiologists to practice. ASHA awards the CCC-SLP to SLPs who meet specified academic and clinical experience requirements, including a Clinical Fellowship Year, a 9-month period of supervision and mentoring by a speech and language pathologist holding ASHA certification. In 2020, 51.0% of SLPs worked in educational organizations, 39.9% in health-care settings, and 21.7% in private practice.[11] Avenues of service delivery include in-person sessions in a variety of settings.

In 2005, ASHA considered telepractice an appropriate model of service delivery and authorized its use in a wide range of health and educational facilities. This made it possible to deliver SLP services from a distance. Telepractice services must adhere to state and federal laws, the ASHA Code of Ethics, and the ASHA Scope of Practice.

Telepractice has been used in the rehabilitation of a wide range of disorders, including aphasia, motor speech disorders, dysphagia, and cognitive-communication disorders. The effectiveness of employing telepractice in schools as a service delivery model is well documented. SLPs who provide telepractice services must have specialized knowledge and skills in selecting assessments and interventions appropriate to the technology while also considering patient and disorder variables. It is required that the selection of patients for telepractice must consider the unique needs of each individual. A range of factors contribute to a person's ability to benefit from telepractice, including hearing acuity, visual ability, manual dexterity, cognitive status, and physical endurance.

Almost a decade ago, ASHA provided the possibility for many communication-impaired persons to receive treatment that had otherwise been inaccessible as the result of the unavailability of speech-language pathology services and/or travel limitations. The COVID-19 global pandemic further increased inaccessibility to services. ASHA's foresight facilitated access to speech-language pathology intervention during the pandemic. This option for service delivery, which has been effective, suggests that telepractice will be available going forward.

To identify the presence and/or degree of speech or language pathology in a given person, their performance must be compared with a standard of "normal." There are two options for determining what is standard:

1. The language common to the cultural community of unimpaired persons in which the person lives, in which case an individual's verbal function would be compared with that of others in the same community of similar age, gender, education, and achievement.
2. The person's verbal behavior before the onset of illness or trauma. The latter will vary from individual to individual and is based on educational achievement, specific cultural characteristics, personality, and factors such as cognitive function.

Individuals are considered verbally impaired when they deviate in any parameter of language and/or speech processing from the "normal" communication behavior of the community in which they expect to function.

A "normal" standard is implied in the terms *impairment, disability,* and *handicap.* This chapter uses the current World Health Organization (WHO) classification schema, in which the term *disability* is defined as the nature and extent of functioning, and the term *handicap* is defined as a person's involvement in life situations.[12,13]

■ THE ORGANIZATION OF LANGUAGE

When individuals generate an idea they wish to express, it is transformed into words and sentences by calling into play certain physiological and acoustic events. The message is converted into linguistic form. The listener, in turn, fits the auditory information into a sequence of words and sentences that are ultimately understood.

We refer to the system of symbols that are strung together into sentences expressing our thoughts and the understanding of those messages as *language.* In the first few years of life, infants and children gain a great deal of practice and experience in the use of language, until it becomes habitual and is used with different levels of conscious awareness.

Phonology refers to the study of the sound system of language. Words are made up of speech sounds or *phonemes,* which are generally classified as either *vowels* or *consonants.* Phonemes in and of themselves do not symbolize ideas or objects, but when put together they are the basic linguistic units that make words. Words make up the *lexicon,* or vocabulary, of a language. English is composed of 16 vowels and 22 consonants, which are combined into larger units called *syllables.*

A syllable usually consists of a vowel as a central phoneme surrounded by one or more consonants. There are between 1,000 and 2,000 syllables in English. Most languages have their own rules about how phonemes may be combined into larger units. For example, in English, syllables never start with the *ng* phoneme. The most frequently used words in English are sequences of two to five phonemes. Some have as many as 10 phonemes or as few as one. In general, the most frequently used words have few phonemes. Even though only a small number of phoneme combinations are possible, new words are added to the English language every day. Although there are several hundred thousand English words, we use a repertoire of only about 5,000 to 10,000 words 95% of the time.

The grammar, or *syntax,* of a language determines the sequence of words that are acceptable in the formation of sentences. In English, for example, it is possible to say, "The black box is on the table," but the sequence "Box black table on the" is unacceptable. Another example is "The old radio played well," which is syntactically correct, but "Old the well-played radio" is not. The sentence "The boy walked to the store" is meaningful, but the sentence "The book walked to the store" is not. The language system that refers to the meanings of words is called *semantics.*

In addition to the phonological (sounds), lexical (vocabulary), syntactical (grammar), and semantic (meaning) language systems, we also utilize *prosody* (stress and intonation) to help make distinctions among questions, statements, and expressions of emotion.

■ SPEECH PRODUCTION

The speech organs consist of the lungs, trachea, larynx (which contains the vocal cords), pharynx, nose, and mouth. When considered together, these organs comprise a "tube" referred to as the *vocal tract,* which extends from the lungs to the lips. Moving the tongue, lips, and other parts of the vocal tract varies its configuration. The shape of the vocal tract acts to modify the aerodynamic qualities of the air stream during speech (Fig. 28.1).

The primary function of the vocal organs relates to basic life-sustaining functions such as breathing and swallowing. These organs not only take on different roles for speech, but also function differently when engaged in speech production. For example, breathing for life-sustaining purposes is far more rapid than breathing for speech production. A full cycle of inhalation/exhalation takes approximately 5 seconds. When speaking, we control the breathing rate according to the demands of the words and sentences we are producing, sometimes reducing the rate of breathing to as little as 15% of that devoted to inhalation. This is dictated in part by the fact that, when speaking, we generally take in enough air to speak a complete thought and exhale the air gradually during its production.

The steady stream of air exhaled from the lungs is the source of energy for speech production, which is made audible by the rapid vibration of the vocal cords. During speech we alter the shape of the vocal tract continuously by moving the tongue, lips, and other parts of the system. By moving parts of the vocal tract, thereby modifying its acoustic properties, we are able to produce different sounds. By altering the shape of the vocal tract during *phonation*, we transform the air stream into a resonance chamber (Figs. 28.2 and 28.3).

The *larynx* acts as a barrier to prevent food from entering the trachea and lungs by closing the vocal cords automatically during the act of swallowing, which is also helped by the action of the epiglottis. By opening and closing the flow of air from the lungs, the larynx acts as a valve between the lungs and the mouth. The laryngeal valve also acts to lock air into the lungs, which we do automatically when we perform heavy work using our upper extremities. The larynx is not a fixed, rigid organ, but because of its cartilaginous construction and corresponding connecting muscles and ligaments, it moves up and down during both swallowing and speaking.

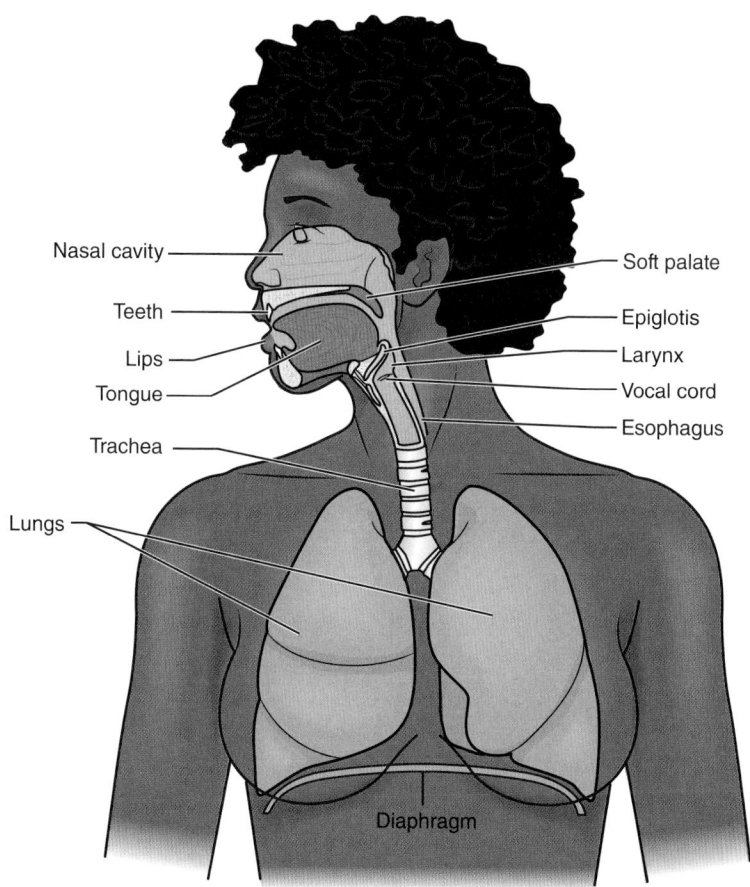

Figure 28.1 The human vocal tract.

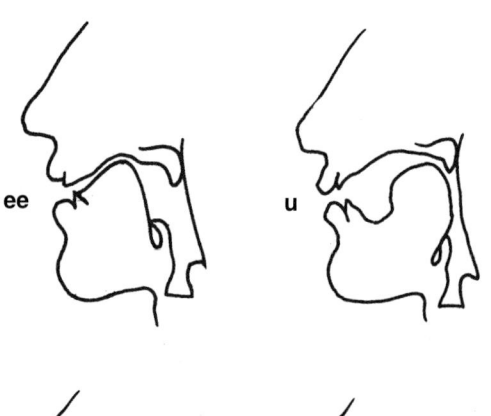

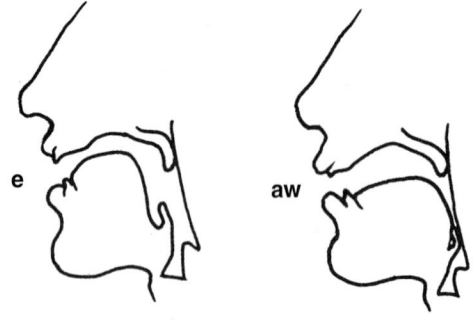

Figure 28.2 Outlines of the vocal tract during articulation of various vowels.

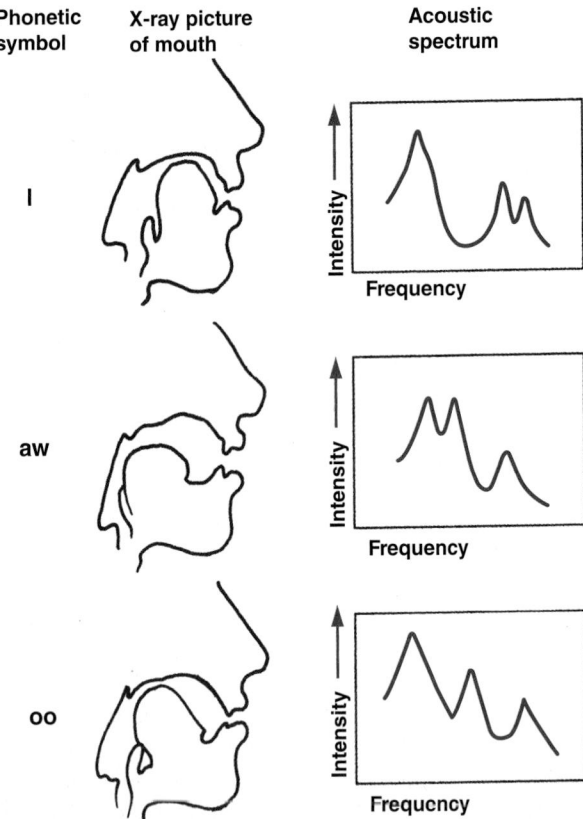

Figure 28.3 Vocal tract configuration and corresponding spectra for three different vowels. The peaks of the spectra represent vocal tract resonances. The vertical lines for individual harmonics are not shown.

The *vocal cords*, which create the sounds of speech, are located on either side of the larynx from the Adam's apple at the front to the arytenoid cartilages at the back. Neuroimaging research has reported findings that reflect the complexity of motor planning and control of vocal cord movement for voice production, showing that subcortical and cortical interactions control the movement of the vocal cords.[14] We refer to the space between the vocal cords as the *glottis*. When the cords are pressed together, the passage of air is sealed off and the valve is shut. Because the cords are held together at the front where they articulate with the Adam's apple, the open glottis is V-shaped, opening only at the back. When we speak, we vibrate the vocal cords in a rhythmic fashion, opening and closing the air passage from the lungs to the oral/nasal cavities.

The frequency of sound produced by the vocal cords is directly related to their mass, tension, and length. The tension and length of the vocal cords are continuously altered while speaking. In normal speech, the range of vocal cord frequencies is from about 60 to 350 cycles per second. Most people use a vocal cord frequency range that covers about one and a half octaves.

The *pharynx* is the area of the vocal tract connecting the larynx with the nose and mouth. We isolate the nasal cavity from the pharynx and back of the mouth by raising the soft palate. The most adjustable component of the vocal tract is the mouth, whose shape and size can be modified more than any other organ of the oral–motor system by changing the relative position of the palate, tongue, lips, and teeth. The lips are rounded, spread, or closed to alter the shape and length of the vocal tract or to stop airflow. The teeth and their relationship to the lips or tongue tip change the airflow, and an important component of this is the *alveolar ridge*, which is a small area covered by the gums just behind the upper front teeth.

The term *articulation* refers to the articulating, or "meeting," of the various organs of the oral–pharyngeal cavity to produce the sounds of speech. Speech *intelligibility* refers to the degree to which speech can be correctly identified by the listener, a significant factor in understanding a speaker. The noise level of the environment is also an important factor influencing speech intelligibility. A number of factors can influence judgments of intelligibility, such as the presence or absence of visual cues or of extraneous movements (i.e., tremor). The precision of the production of consonant sounds is one of the primary factors that contribute to speech intelligibility. Consonants are described by specifying their place and manner of articulation (Table 28.1). The "places" of articulation are the lips (labial), teeth, gums (alveolar), palate, and glottis. The *manner of articulation* refers to the plosive, fricative, nasal, liquid, and semi-vowel categories.

Plosive sounds, sometimes referred to as "stop" sounds, are those produced by building up air pressure

Table 28.1	Classification of English Consonants by Place and Manner of Articulation					
Place of Articulation	Manner of Articulation					
	Plosive	Fricative	Semivowel	Liquids (including laterals)	Nasal
Labial	p b	—	w	—	m
Labiodental	—	f v	—	—	—
Dental	—	_ th	—	—	—
Alveolar	t d	s z	y	l r	n
Palatal	—	sh zh	—	—	—
Velar	k g	—	—	—	ng
Glottal	—	h	—	—	—

in the oral cavity and suddenly releasing it (e.g., *p, t*). The blockage can occur by pressing the lips together or by pressing the tongue against either the gums or soft palate. There are plosive consonants that are labial, alveolar, or velar (consonants articulated with the back part of the tongue).

Fricatives are produced by making the air turbulent (e.g., *f, v*). Most consonants are produced with the soft palate raised, thereby closing off the flow of air to the nasal cavity, except for *nasal sounds* (i.e., *m, n, ng*), which are produced by lowering the soft palate and blocking the oral cavity somewhere along its length. *Liquids* are sounds that are made with the soft palate raised (i.e., *r, l*). *Semivowels* refer to those sounds produced by maintaining the vocal tract in a vowel-like position, then changing the position rapidly for the vowel that follows (e.g., *w, y*).

Speech sounds are affected by their *context*, that is, the sounds that immediately precede or follow. A speech sound wave is a continuous event rather than a sequence of discrete segments. The identification of a speech sound depends on relating acoustic features of the sound wave at different points in time.

A standard reference for the quality of vowels is the eight cardinal vowels (Fig. 28.4). This schema of the positions of the tongue to produce the vowels of the language helps us visualize the tongue's movements during speech. It is, in a sense, a map of the tongue positions for vowel production. Tongue placement is described by specifying the location of the main body of the tongue at its highest point. For example, for the production of vowel "ee," as in the word *beat,* the tongue is high and forward in the mouth, whereas for the production of the vowel "ah," as in the word *father,* the tongue is low and posterior in the oral cavity.

All vowel sounds and some consonant sounds are *voiced.* That is, the vocal cords vibrate during their production. When a sound is produced without vocal cord vibration, we say that it is *unvoiced* or voiceless (e.g., *p, s*).

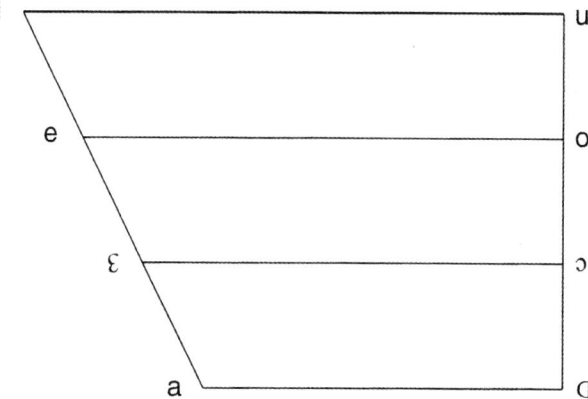

Figure 28.4 The cardinal vowels represented as a vowel quadrilateral. The cardinal vowels are extremely placed reference points for vowel articulation. Vowels on the same horizontal line are believed to have an equally high tongue height while vowels in the left–right position are assumed to be equally backed and fronted. (Adapted from Ladefoged, P: *A Course in Phonetics.* Harcourt Brace Jovanovich, New York, 1975, with permission.)

Speech behavior comprises a complex motor event that goes well beyond the skilled movements required of the oral–motor system. Yet we produce speech without thinking about it, even while we are simultaneously involved in other activities. Transforming thought into speech takes some voluntary, conscious behavior that allows us to take information stored in memory and translate it into a coherent production of words and utterances that follow certain grammatical rules.

In addition to linguistic aspects, neurogenic communication disorders sometimes involve coexisting mild to severe cognitive deficits that may not only aggravate the communication disorder but also make it difficult to differentiate cognitive from communication deficits. The communication disorder manifest in persons with right brain damage, which is addressed in this chapter, is an example of a disorder in which the cognitive component is a major issue.

The importance of the communication process and its underlying systems becomes apparent when we consider the two most common neurogenic communication disorders: *aphasia* and *dysarthria*. This chapter focuses primarily on aphasia and dysarthria but also considers verbal apraxia, dysphagia, cognitive-communication disorders, and the use of augmentative/alternative systems of communication.

Several parameters must be considered when thinking about treatment to address communication, as this behavior calls upon so many complex skills and behaviors in humans. An accurate treatment target(s), intensity of treatment, and factors that facilitate or limit functional generalization comprise the foundation for treatment management in persons with neurogenic communication disorders.

■ APHASIA

The population of persons in the United States increased by over a third (34.2% or 13,787,044) during the past decade and by 3.2% (1,688,924) from 2018 to 2019. Thus, we can anticipate an increase in the population of individuals with aphasia.[15] It is estimated that about 180,000 persons acquire aphasia annually, and approximately 1 million people currently have aphasia.[2,7,8] The actual number may be as high as 4.1 million people.[8] One of the major variables to consider when evaluating the difference in reported numbers is the wide range of potential incidence of aphasia from TBI, which could be between 1% percent (nearly 65,000 people) and 19% (1.2 million).[8] This is a result of the wide range of potential incidence of aphasia from TBI versus stroke.[2,7,8,16–18]

In a study that examined data from the Tulane Stroke Registry from July 2008 to December 2014, 866 of 1,847 patients had aphasia on admission.[19] A smaller number acquired aphasia as the result of head trauma and neoplasms. There are also reports of close, but not always obligatory, relationships between primary progressive aphasia and Alzheimer disease.[20]

Classification and Nomenclature

In this chapter, the term *aphasia* refers to the acquired communication disorder that is manifest in individuals who were previously capable of using language appropriately. It does not refer to developmental language disorders that may be present in individuals who never developed normal language and for whom the ability to use language may never reach age-appropriate performance levels.

In acquired aphasia, central nervous system (CNS) disease or trauma compromises certain structures in a focal rather than generalized fashion. The study of the neuroanatomical correlates of the aphasias has engaged neurologists since the late 19th century, and the correlation between aphasic syndromes and cerebral localization is relatively consistent. Recent advances in neuroradiological technology have provided many new methods for studying the neural substrates of language and language impairment.[21–23]

Aphasiologists generally agree that there are distinct major aphasic syndromes that adhere to specific profiles of impairment. This is not surprising because the lesions that produce aphasia, particularly in the patient with cerebrovascular disease, tend to be in brain loci that are especially vulnerable. It is not always possible, however, to classify patients according to these syndromes.

The characteristics of an individual's speech production provide the basis for determining aphasia classification. Speech output, characterized as hesitant, awkward, interrupted, inaccurate, and/or produced with effort, is referred to as *nonfluent aphasia*. This contrasts with *fluent aphasia*, which is characterized by speech that is easily articulated and is produced at a normal rate with preserved flow and melody.

Fluent Aphasia

Fluent aphasia is characterized by impaired auditory comprehension and fluent speech that is of normal rate and melody. When fluent aphasia is severe, word and sound substitutions may be of such magnitude and frequency that speech may be rendered meaningless. Patients with fluent aphasia tend to have greatest difficulty in retrieving those words that are substantive (nouns and verbs). Since their lesions are in the posterior portion of the brain, distant from motor areas, they also tend to have some degree of impaired awareness and are rarely physically disabled. There are several types of syndromes subsumed under the fluent aphasia classification (Table 28.2).

The most common type of fluent aphasia is *Wernicke aphasia* (also referred to as *sensory aphasia* or *receptive aphasia*) and is correlated with damage to Wernicke area (Fig. 28.5). It is characterized by impaired auditory comprehension and fluent articulated speech marked by word substitutions. Reading and writing are usually severely impaired as well. Although patients with Wernicke aphasia may produce what appear to be complete utterances and use complex verb tenses, they often add words or phrases and ineffectively "augment" speech production. Speech is often produced at a rate faster than normal. Although the production of speech is generally intelligible, patients with Wernicke aphasia may reverse phonemes and/or syllables (e.g., hopspipal/trevilision) and may produce *neologisms* (i.e., nonsense words).

Speech output may also be well articulated yet surprisingly vague or irrelevant and may be characterized by talking around a topic using well-articulated words without being clear or direct.

Nonfluent Aphasia

Nonfluent aphasia is characterized by limited vocabulary; slow, hesitant speech; some awkward articulation; and restricted use of grammar in the presence of

Table 28.2   Classification by Aphasia Syndromes

	Wernicke Aphasia	Broca Aphasia	Global Aphasia	Conduction Aphasia	Anomic Aphasia	Transcortical Motor Aphasia	Pure Word Deafness
Area of infarction	Posterior portion of temporal gyrus	Third frontal convolution	Third frontal convolution and posterior portion of superior temporal gyrus	Parietal operculum or posterior superior temporal gyrus	Angular gyrus	Supplementary motor areas	Both Heschl gyri or connection between Heschl gyrus and posterior superior temporal gyrus
Spontaneous speech	Fluent	Nonfluent	Nonfluent	Fluent or nonfluent	Fluent	Nonfluent	Fluent
Comprehension	Poor	Good	Poor	Good	Good	Good	Poor
Repetition	Poor	Poor (but may be better than spontaneous speech)	Poor	Very poor	Good	Excellent	Poor
Naming	Poor	Poor (but may be better than spontaneous speech)	Poor	Poor	Very poor	Poor	Good
Reading comprehension	Poor	Good	Poor	Good to poor	Good to poor	Good	Good
Writing	Poor	Poor	Poor	Poor	Good to poor	Poor	Good

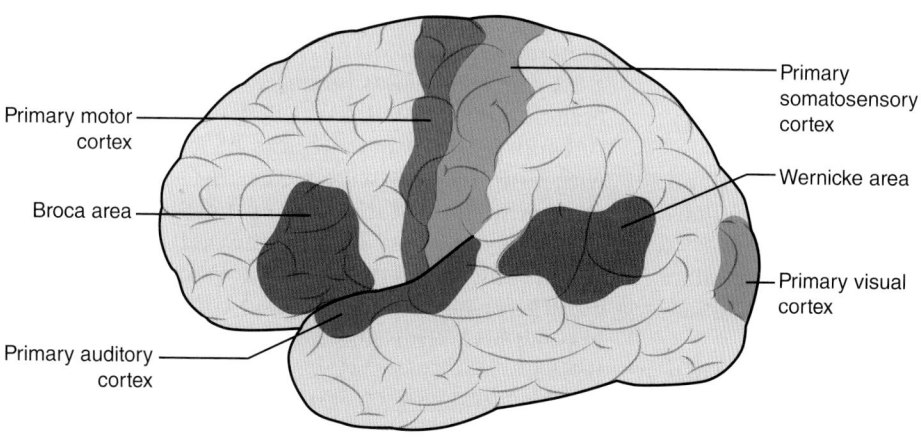

Primary motor cortex
Broca area
Primary auditory cortex
Primary somatosensory cortex
Wernicke area
Primary visual cortex

Figure 28.5 Wernicke and Broca areas. Damage to Wernicke area is associated with fluent aphasia, and damage to Broca area is associated with nonfluent aphasia.

relatively preserved auditory comprehension. Patients with nonfluent aphasia tend to express themselves in vocabulary that is substantive (nouns, verbs) and lack the ability to retrieve fewer substantive parts of speech (prepositions, conjunctions, pronouns). Patients with nonfluent aphasia tend to have awareness of their deficit and usually have impaired motor function on the right side (right hemiplegia-paresis).

Broca aphasia is a nonfluent type of aphasia also sometimes referred to as *expressive aphasia, motor aphasia,* and/or *verbal aphasia* and is correlated with damage to Broca area (Fig. 28.5). It is characterized by awkward articulation, restricted vocabulary, and restriction to simple grammatical forms in the presence of a relative preservation of auditory comprehension. Writing skills generally mirror the pattern of speech, and reading may be less impaired than speech and writing. The patient may be limited to one- and two-word productions for expression and find it impossible to combine words into sentences. Articulation may be awkward and effortful (see the section "Apraxia of Speech"). Nonfluent Broca aphasia is less common after TBI. Anomic disturbances predominate in aphasia secondary to TBI.

Global Aphasia

A severe aphasia with marked dysfunction across all language modalities and with severely limited residual use of all communication modes for oral–aural interactions is referred to as *global aphasia*. Global aphasia is not a type of aphasia but rather a designation of severity. The patient with global aphasia generally has extensive damage, which may be anywhere in the left hemisphere and is sometimes bilateral.[24] As a result, the extensive damage precludes the possibility of spoken or written language use; however, alternative communication methods that are not dependent on speaking or writing may be effective for select patients with global aphasia.[25,26]

Primary Progressive Aphasia

Primary progressive aphasia (PPA) is a condition first described in 1982, which is now a recognized diagnostic category.[27,28] PPA is a slowly progressive isolated aphasia not due to stroke, trauma, tumor, or infection, which does not fit neatly into current aphasia classification schemes. PPA usually begins with difficulties with word retrieval and may progress to an impairment of semantics (i.e., word meaning), syntax (i.e., grammar), and/or phonology (i.e., sounds).[29] Activities of daily living, visuospatial cognition, judgment, insight, memory, personality, and behavior are usually preserved for 1 to 2 years and may remain unimpaired and isolated from the language impairment for a longer period of time.[29–31] A large subset of those with PPA eventually develop symptoms of a more pervasive dementia.[29,32] Spontaneous recovery does not occur.

PPA has been categorized into several subtypes that are usually characterized by the language domain with the greatest impairment.[29] PPA progresses at different rates and in its most severe form can result in the inability to speak.[33] Neuroimaging techniques used for assessment purposes have the potential of being useful biomarkers of clinical decline.[34] It is common practice for individuals with PPA to be referred to or to seek speech pathology services for assessment and treatment. SLP assessment and treatment play an important part within the overall management of individuals who present with PPA symptoms and help to inform the differential diagnosis and monitoring of cognitive-communication status over time.[35]

Historical Perspective

Language disturbances were recorded as early as 3500 BC, and attempts to "retrain" individuals with aphasia have been recorded throughout history.[36] Some of the first documented cases of both natural recovery and intervention were the patients of Nicolo Massa and Francisco Arceo in 1558.[37]

In a landmark paper published in the late 19th century, "Du siège de la faculté du langage articulé," Paul Broca was one of the first to discuss the possibility of retraining in aphasia.[38] Dr. Charles K. Mills was the first to address recovery and rehabilitation in aphasia in an English-language publication. He reported the training of a patient with poststroke aphasia whom he and Donald Broadbent treated, using methods largely determined by the patient, who began by systematically repeating letters, words, and phrases.[39,40] Mills's observations and approach to aphasia rehabilitation, published over a century ago, are remarkably similar to much present-day practice and thought. Mills noted that not all patients benefit from retraining to the same degree and acknowledged that spontaneous recovery might have an influence on the course and extent of recovery.

World War I and its brain-injured combat survivors led to the establishment of treatment centers where patients with post-traumatic aphasia were treated, especially in Europe. Reports of aphasia rehabilitation experiences during and after the war in England and the United States were also published.[41,42] One of the most comprehensive descriptions of the systematic treatment of a large number of patients with aphasia secondary to head trauma, of whom 90 to 100 were followed for a 10-year period, was produced by Kurt Goldstein in Frankfurt during World War II.[43]

Until World War II, reports of retraining civilians with poststroke aphasia were rare. The aphasia literature was based almost exclusively on post-traumatic aphasia. In 1933, Singer[44] reported the case of a 39-year-old woman who suffered an apparent vascular infarct after a full-term delivery and showed continuous language improvement with consistent training over a 10-year period.

In a landmark 5-year study supported by the Commonwealth Fund, Weisenberg and McBride[45] addressed the general topic of aphasia and commented on the effectiveness of reeducation. The study concerned 60 patients who were younger than 60 years of age, a majority of whom had suffered strokes, and concluded that reeducation increased the rate of recovery, assisted in facilitating the use of compensatory means of communication, and improved morale. Their work also documented the psychotherapeutic benefits of treatment.

Before World War II, aphasia and its concomitant neurological deficits in the patient with stroke were generally viewed as natural and necessary components of the aging process. The treatment of aphasia in the civilian population was not an option.

Many variables had an influence on making the treatment of aphasia the common practice that it is today. The advent of SLP as a health profession, the emergence of rehabilitation medicine as a medical specialty, the mass media explosion, a larger and more affluent middle class, an increase in the life span, the number of stroke and brain injury survivors, and public expectations of medicine in the age of technology are among them. The last has been particularly true in the industrialized world, where it is widely believed that there is a treatment for every human ill.[46]

Journals devoted to brain/language issues have become indispensable information sources for aphasiologists (e.g., *Aphasiology, Brain, Brain and Language,* and *Cortex*). Over the years, several scholarly societies and professional organizations have dedicated themselves to aphasia for the purpose of providing information to the public about aphasia, advocating for the aphasia community, providing professional support to aphasiologists (e.g., Academy of Aphasia, Aphasia Access, Connect UK, Aphasia Institute, National Aphasia Association) and encouraging the establishment of a network of support groups, referred to as aphasia community groups.[47] The Academy of Neurologic Communication Disorders and Sciences (ANCDS), founded in 1988, is a nonprofit professional association that supports practitioners who serve individuals with neurologic communication disorders by providing education, training, and certification opportunities to promote high-quality professional service. Several informational publications designed for use by the families and friends of patients with aphasia also appeared in the period following World War II, which paved the way for the development of these professional organizations with a focus on the welfare of people with aphasia and were a testament to the social needs of people with aphasia in the speaking community.[48–53] One of these, *Understanding Aphasia: A Guide for Family and Friends,* has been published in 12 languages.[53]

Aphasia Measures

Many measures of aphasia and related disorders have been developed for use in both clinical and research settings. In an acute care setting, patients with aphasia are generally screened at bedside. The purpose of a bedside screening is to obtain a general idea of a patient's profile of deficits and preserved areas of language function as a basis for recommendations for more comprehensive testing and possible rehabilitation. However, a comprehensive examination is required to provide a baseline measure against which to gauge progress in the course of spontaneous recovery and rehabilitation.

Comprehensive language tests designed to measure aphasic impairment generally contain specific domains of performance. In addition to the general requirements for the construction of tests, such as reliability, standardization, and demonstrated validity, certain factors are important in the design of tests intended to identify and measure aphasia. These include range of item difficulty, efficacy in measuring recovery, and ability to contribute to diagnostic classification.[2,54] Aphasia tests are generally based on examinations of linguistic task performance and at a minimum include tasks of visual confrontation *naming*; a spontaneous or conversational *speech sample* that is analyzed for fluency of output, effort, articulation, phrase length, prosody, word substitutions, and omissions; *repetition* of digits, single words, multisyllable words, and sentences of increasing length and complexity; *comprehension of spoken language* of single words, of sentences that require only "yes" or "no" responses, and pointing on command; *word retrieval* (word finding) measuring the ability to generate words beginning with a particular letter of the alphabet or in a particular semantic category (animals); *reading*; and *writing* from dictation and spontaneously. Some aphasia measures include the *Boston Diagnostic Aphasia Examination (BDAE),*[23] the *Western Aphasia Battery-Revised,*[55] and the *Aphasia Communication Outcome Measure,* which is a patient-reported outcome measure of communicative functioning for persons with aphasia.[56]

In addition to measuring performance on specific linguistic tasks, an aphasia evaluation also requires an examination of *functional communication.* This is necessary because an individual's actual use of language in everyday life may not correspond to the degree of pathology measured by specific language task performance.[57,58] The *Functional Communication Profile (FCP),*[59,60] *Communicative Activities of Daily Living-3rd Edition (CADL-3),*[61] *Communicative Effectiveness Index,*[62] *Functional Life Scale [FLS],*[63] and ASHA's *Functional Assessment of Communication Skills (ASHA FACS)*[64] are measures used for this purpose.

In addition to measures of language and functional communication, new tools have been developed to determine the impact of impaired communication skills on quality of life. The scope of SLP practice now encompasses all of the components and factors specified in the WHO framework.[65–67] Specifically, concern for the effect of aphasia on a person's ability to participate in family, social, and community life is the basis for measures which focus on various aspects which affect quality of life (e.g., *Burden of Stroke Scale [BOSS], Stroke Social Network Scale, Aphasic Depression Rating Scale [ADRS], Frenchay Activities Index, the Barthel Index,* and *Stroke and Aphasia Quality of Life Scale–39 [SAQOL-39]*).[68–75]

Aphasia Recovery

Once aphasia has persisted for years, a complete return to a premorbid state is usually the exception. Language gains in aphasia take place earlier as well as later.[76-81]

Most patients do not consider themselves recovered unless they have fully recovered to previous levels of language performance.[82] When unrecovered patients are satisfied with their level of competence and consider themselves recovered, this is a psychological perception and should not be confused with an objective evaluation of communication abilities. For individuals with aphasia, the true test of rehabilitation outcome is their perception of the quality of their lives. Measures of life function that include activity levels, socialization, mobility, and community reintegration can be used for this purpose.[83,84]

It is useful to distinguish between two separate recovery dimensions in aphasia: one that is objective and attempts to quantify the extent to which a person has regained language abilities and another, which measures the recovery of functional communication.

The concept of a functional dimension of communication behavior emerged logically from the experience of treating patients with aphasia in rehabilitation medicine settings. Historically, rehabilitation medicine has acknowledged that the ability of patients to function in daily life, referred to as activities of daily living (ADL), does not necessarily correlate with the degree of physical disability. Similarly, improvement in quantitative measures of language performance does not necessarily correlate with improvement in functional communication.[46]

Many patients experience a degree of natural recovery with or without intervention in the period immediately following onset. The duration of the *spontaneous recovery* period, however, is unclear.[85-88] The extent of individual variability within the acute, subacute, and chronic stages of poststroke aphasia makes it difficult to reliably predict recovery. Age, gender, educational level, bilingualism, employment status, handedness, health status, and severity and location of lesion have been reported as possible predictors. However, these factors are highly variable, making it difficult to generate a prognosis for individual patients.[89-117] These discrepancies regarding the influence of certain variables may, in part, relate to differences in pathology, methodology, and sampling.

It is generally agreed that posttraumatic aphasia has a better prognosis than aphasia secondary to vascular lesions.[89,94] In fact, some cases of aphasia secondary to TBI have been reported to recover completely.[118] The finding that traumatic aphasia carries a better prognosis than vascular aphasia may be influenced by the fact that patients involved in traumatic events are generally neurologically healthy whereas patients who have had strokes may have widespread vascular involvement.[104]

Both type and severity of aphasia appear to carry predictive value, with global aphasia having the poorest prognosis.[76,119-121] Basso reported that when patients with fluent and nonfluent aphasia of the same severity were compared, there were no differences in degree of recovery. In 881 consecutive acute stroke admissions to a community-based hospital, it was possible to make valid prognoses within 1 to 4 weeks after stroke depending on the initial severity of aphasia.[104]

Not surprisingly, most studies report that patients with severe aphasia do not recover as much as those with mild aphasia.[122] Sarno and Levita found that global aphasia sometimes evolves to Broca aphasia when there is significantly improved comprehension.[76,123] Broca aphasia may become *anomic aphasia,* and Wernicke aphasia may evolve to anomic or *conduction aphasia.*[76,124] When persons with aphasia recover a great deal of language function they are usually left with residual *anomia.*

Functional imaging studies of aphasia secondary to stroke have suggested that language recovery is dependent on several factors. Patients whose computed tomography (CT) scans show large dominant hemisphere lesions, many small lesions, or bilateral lesions are less likely to recover than those with smaller or fewer lesions.[82] Lesions in Wernicke area or those that extend more posteriorly tend to lead to severe and persistent aphasia. The neuroradiological correlates of aphasia recovery have been addressed by some investigators.[125] The neuroplastic changes that are needed during recovery are thought to depend more heavily on left hemispheric changes in activity that slowly manifest over time.[22] Following damage to the left hemisphere, rapid changes have been observed in temporal and frontal areas within the right hemisphere but may reflect maladaptive compensatory activity versus functional reorganization or recovery.[126-135] As technology advances and research continues, new insights into the mechanisms of recovery and treatment will emerge.

The presence of fatigue, stress, and mental health issues, such as depression and anxiety, have been cited as negative factors in recovery, and premorbid personality traits have been identified as important prognostic factors.[136-143] Eisenson and Herrmann felt that patients with outgoing personalities had a better prognosis than those with introverted, dependent, or rigid personalities.[144-146]

Efficacy of Treatment in Poststroke Aphasia

Many methodological problems have limited the number of studies which examine the efficacy of aphasia rehabilitation.[147-153] Nevertheless, treatment accountability issues are compelling and a focus of professional concern.

Studies that investigate treatment effects, specific techniques, and approaches have been reported since the late 1950s.[154] Vignolo,[89] Hagen,[155] and Basso et al.[90]

utilized untreated control and treated groups and showed a positive treatment effect. Edmonds et al.,[156] and Poeck et al.[157] also yielded positive treatment effects with treated and untreated groups. In addition, several reviews and examinations have revealed significant treatment effects (i.e., improvements in communicative ability) with intense intervention provided over a short period of time.[158–160] Variables such as spontaneous recovery,[161,162] age,[163] duration, treatment intensity,[158–160] timing of treatment,[164] and specific treatment techniques[165–167] have been studied.

Although group and single case studies have varied in method and research focus, there have been strong indications for positive treatment effects. Some have maintained that single case studies rather than randomized, controlled trials are the most appropriate method for addressing treatment efficacy.[153,168,169] Negative views of the group study model are based primarily on the view that individuals are unique, especially with respect to communication behavior.

The ANCDS has issued evidence-based practice guidelines for neurogenic communication disorders.[170,171] Until now, SLPs have depended on meta-analyses of efficacy studies reported for 45 studies published between 1946 and 1988 and for 55 studies that support better clinical outcome for patients who receive early, intensive treatment.[152,172]

Psychological and Related Factors

It has been observed that the variability of patients' psychological reactions is rarely determined by lesion type or location but is an expression of the whole life experience of the person who has had a stroke.[104,138,140–143,173,174]

Depression, anxiety, premorbid personality, fatigue, and paranoia are often cited as deterrents to recovery and communication. The social isolation experienced by people with aphasia and their families has a profound impact on quality of life.[175] The effect of aphasia on an individual's sense of "self" can be extremely negative, leading to a loss of self-esteem, feelings of helplessness, and other signs of depression as well as anxiety.[137,139,141] Also, the opportunity for "healing conversation," so essential to individuals who have suffered losses, is often unavailable to those with aphasia, which may be the result of inadequate social support.

In a study of patients participating in an aphasia community group program, Lanyon et al. investigated the experiences and reflections of a group of persons with severe, chronic aphasia.[176] Participants demonstrated a need for increased structure and use of physical materials to facilitate successful interactions and integration with the group when compared to persons with mild to moderate aphasia. Despite the need for increased structure, people with severe aphasia valued groups that offered authentic interactions and arenas to demonstrate their abilities, most notably as active listeners. This study highlights risks, such as exclusion, that

people with severe aphasia experience in group settings if the group is not adequately structured or resourced to support authentic interactions.[176]

Treatment of Aphasia

Aphasia treatment is rarely the same in any two settings. Hundreds of specific speech and language treatment techniques are cited in the aphasia literature. The lack of therapeutic uniformity has undoubtedly impeded an adequate number of carefully controlled studies on the effects of language retraining.[177]

In general, treatment methods can be categorized as those that are largely *indirect stimulation-facilitation* and those that are essentially *direct structured-pedagogic*.[78,80,118,141,178–180] The two principles that underlie most treatment methods reflect contrasting views of aphasia as either impaired access to language or a "loss" of language. The primary assumption that drives the treatment of aphasia is that language is not "erased," but that retrieval of its individual units has been impaired. The stimulation methods generally follow an impaired access model and pedagogic approaches are based on a theory of aphasia as a language loss.

In practice, however, much of aphasia treatment addresses the *performance* aspect of language in which repeated practice and "teaching" strategies are assumed to help restore impaired skills through a "task-oriented" approach (i.e., naming practice). One of the commonly used techniques involves self-cueing and repetition exercises that manipulate components of grammar and vocabulary. Another approach involves "stimulating" the patient to use residual language by encouraging conversation in a permissive setting where a patient's responses are unconditionally accepted and topics are of personal interest.[179]

Significant progress and improvements of language and communication performance have been reported in those with aphasia who have received intensive and/or extended periods of language therapy.[157,181,182] More recent reports of intensive treatment programs have shown significant improvement of communication abilities several years poststroke, when aphasia is in the chronic stage.[182–184] Some benefits may also be received from pharmacological treatment with and without speech therapy.[185–192] In addition, improvements have also been documented with the use of transcranial magnetic stimulation[193] and transcranial direct current stimulation.[194,195]

In recent years, a form of language therapy that has shown promise is contextualized, constraint-induced language therapy (CILT) or constraint-induced aphasia therapy (CIAT), which can be delivered in both intensive and distributed doses. In this treatment method, therapists restrain compensatory communication. Persons with aphasia are required to use and practice only those verbal skills that are difficult or impaired. In this method, forms of communication that may facilitate total communication and are easier for the person with aphasia to use but are not verbal, such as gesturing, drawing, or writing, are constrained.[196,197]

Some investigators have reported the use of writing[198] or drawing as a potential means of communication.[199,201] Others have developed interactive approaches to aphasia treatment. Examples include the *communication partners* approach of Lyon et al.,[202] a treatment plan designed to enhance communication and well-being in settings where the person with aphasia and the caregiver live; the *supported conversation* approach introduced by Kagan and colleagues,[203–207] in which volunteers are trained as conversation partners to facilitate conversation by using all available modalities, thereby revealing the individual's competence and permitting a communicative interaction; and the *social model of aphasia* approach introduced by Simmons-Mackie,[208–216] which focuses on the fulfillment of social needs and the encouragement of a greater conversational burden on the part of communication partners. Partners are trained to facilitate interaction by modifying some of their interactive behavior.

If individuals are unable to make themselves understood, aids can provide a means of communication using manual or electronic devices (e.g., smart device). Use of telecommunications, virtual clinicians and environments, and computer-assisted and Web- or application-based treatments may lead to improvements in language and communication, especially when utilized as an adjunct to clinical therapy. Data suggest that these types of therapies may be effective for patients in various stages of recovery.[217–222]

Management of the Patient With Aphasia

Aphasia rehabilitation should be viewed as a process of patient management in the broadest sense of the term. That is, the task is primarily one of helping patients and their significant others adjust to the alterations and limitations imposed by the disability. Effective aphasia rehabilitation management may often require the participation of a rehabilitation team, including medicine, psychology, physical therapy, occupational therapy, social work, vocational counseling, and, most critically, aphasia therapy.

Speech and language therapy which stimulates and supports the patient through the various stages of recovery is an effective management tool.[223,224] Experienced aphasia therapists recognize that while working on aphasic deficits, they are simultaneously dealing psychotherapeutically with a readjusting personality and a recovery of identity.[143] Speech-language therapy, therefore, serves different purposes at different points along the way. Sometimes it allows patients to "borrow time," as Baerts and Stephenson[225] have aptly stated. Occasionally depression lifts after speech-language therapy has been initiated, which may reflect the significance of the supportive and nurturing nature of the therapeutic

relationship in addition to whatever objective improvement has occurred in communication.

Aphasia recovery can be viewed as a dynamic process consisting of a series of stages, such as the stages of mourning described by Kübler-Ross,[226] through which many patients evolve. Some, of course, never emerge from a state of severe depression.[227,228] Kübler-Ross[226] and other authors have suggested that the stages through which someone with aphasia passes—including denial, rage, bargaining, and acceptance—could be characterized as attempts to overcome the sense of loss.

By directly addressing a patient's linguistic deficits and channeling attention and energies toward constructive goals, speech-language therapy may produce a noticeable reduction in depression. Therapy tasks in this instance act as an equivalent for work, which has long been recognized as an antidote for depression.

Premature attempts to return to work can have a negative psychological impact. There is a tendency to overestimate the capacity of individuals with aphasia to return to work too soon, even if the verbal deficits are mild. Decision-making which addresses a person with aphasia returning to work is complicated and requires the combined efforts and expertise of the aphasia therapist and rehabilitation team.

Experienced aphasia clinicians stress the importance of the patient's family in the rehabilitation process. Some potentially negative reactions on the part of the family include overprotectiveness, hostility, anger, unrealistic expectations, overzealousness, lack of knowledge of the dimensions of the disorder, and inability to cope with practical difficulties. The apparently natural tendency of family members to minimize the patient's communication impairment, particularly in the early stages of recovery, requires understanding and tactful management.[143]

The quality of premorbid relationships generally tends to be intensified after a catastrophic event; those that were problematic may deteriorate further, whereas the bond between a loving couple may become stronger. The reversal of roles, changes in levels of dependency, and a changed economic situation, so often a consequence of chronic disability, can have a critical negative impact on the patient and his or her family.[174]

In a positive family milieu, patients are encouraged to develop regular daily routines as close to premorbid patterns and should, whenever possible, be treated as contributing members of the family. Patients need to be allowed some sense of control. Including the patient in rehabilitation planning promotes the restoration of feelings of self-worth. In this regard, the emphasis on function rather than complete recovery, pointing out success rather than performance failure, adds to a patient's sense of self. It is essential to listen to patients, particularly to their expressions of loss. Commiseration is often more comforting than optimistic prognostic statements.

Aphasia Centers, Intensive Comprehensive Aphasia Programs (ICAPs), group speech therapy, stroke clubs, and other social and support groups are resources that can be effective tools in the management of some patients with aphasia. Other resources include support and social organizations, such as the National Aphasia Association (NAA), which was founded in the United States in 1987, following the lead of existing advocacy organizations established in Finland (1971), Germany (1978), the United Kingdom (1980), and Sweden (1981). These organizations served as models for the NAA, which provides an extensive array of educational and resource information appropriate for patients, families, and professionals on its website (www.aphasia.org).

Group therapy with peers may provide a comfortable atmosphere in which patients can meet new friends and share feelings, although not all individuals with aphasia seek out groups or find them beneficial. Positive effects seem to be related to level of comprehension, time since onset, and personality factors. Although group therapy provides a social context in aphasia rehabilitation, it should be noted that much of its effectiveness depends on the skill and experience of the group facilitator.[229,230]

Aphasia rehabilitation remains eclectic and specifically tailored to the individual patient. Fundamental to this therapeutic philosophy is the acknowledgment and appreciation of the uniqueness of the individual. No two persons with aphasia are exactly alike in pathology, personality, linguistic deficits, reactions to catastrophic illness, life experience, spiritual values, or a host of other factors. The influence of these factors carries different weight and strength at different stages of recovery, and they are all related to recovery outcome.

■ COGNITIVE-COMMUNICATION DISORDERS

When the neural regions responsible for the cognitive processes that support communicative function are damaged, a broad spectrum of deficits can result. Many conditions can cause cognitive-communication disorders, including TBI/concussion, stroke (particularly right hemisphere damage), dementia, brain tumors, aging, degenerative neurological disease, alcohol/drug abuse, and medications. Impairments of executive function, including difficulties with attention and memory, may interfere with a person's ability to transform thoughts and ideas into spoken and/or written language. Impaired memory can also affect word retrieval, topic maintenance, a person's ability to recall and integrate information, and the speed of processing information. In addition, organizing information, interpreting visual stimuli, deficits in abstract reasoning, and decreased orientation to person, place, and time are common symptoms. Impairments in speech production, including reduced fluency and changes in prosodic speech features (i.e., rate and rhythm of speech, stress within words to indicate meaning and within sentences

to express variations of intent or meaning) are also common. Given the nature of these deficits, participating in social situations can be especially difficult.[231] These difficulties may affect all modes of communication, including understanding, nonverbal and verbal expression, reading, and writing. These impairments can be debilitating and socially isolating, because they impair a person's ability to establish and maintain relationships with others.[232,233]

Impairments of certain aspects of pragmatic language (i.e., language use) and nonverbal communication (including difficulty in initiating, maintaining, and ending conversations) may result in difficulties maintaining a topic and taking turns in discourse; being concise; understanding and expressing feeling through facial expressions; comprehending nonverbal methods of communication (i.e., gesturing); maintaining eye contact; engaging in conversation or narrative production that is self-focused; interpreting and expressing emotions appropriately; and reduced ability in understanding humor.

Examination of Cognitive-Communication Disorders

Many factors, including the heterogeneity of individuals, limitations of available standardized testing measures, performance differences in structured versus unstructured contexts, and environmental and personal factors, have made the examination of cognitive-communication disorders a challenging area in need of further study.[234] There have been recent attempts to try to identify what these cognitive communication deficits are and how they relate to an individual's overall communication. The knowledge, experience, and expertise of the examiner continues to play a significant role when evaluating communication disorders coupled by changes in cognition.

Treatment of Cognitive-Communication Disorders

Intervention depends on the type and severity of the cognitive-communication disorder and is usually based on a combination of behavioral, meta-cognitive, and counseling approaches. Patients with cognitive-communication disorders often have reduced insight and/or awareness.[235,236] The importance of providing speech-language pathology treatment using a team approach has been highlighted as an important element in the rehabilitation process. Such collaborative methods consider each person's social network (e.g., family, friends, caregivers).[237]

The management of patients with cognitive-communication disorders begins with determining what environmental factors, if any, can be modified to provide the least visual or auditory distraction. Steps also need to be taken to establish a structured routine or daily schedule. These efforts help to reduce communication

> **Box 28.1** Strategies for Improving Communication in the Presence of Cognitive-Communication Disorder
>
> - Use visual materials/aids to help orient the person to time (e.g., clocks and calendars).
> - Break long, complicated tasks into shorter tasks that are easier to follow.
> - Establish eye contact to initiate and maintain conversation.
> - When giving verbal directions, use simple sentences and repetitions as necessary.
> - Accommodate the presence of visual field deficits by helping the person find compensatory means for reading and writing.
> - Gently state when the topic in a conversation changes prematurely.

breakdowns and facilitate communicative success.[235,236] Cognitive-communication and motor functions can deteriorate under different levels of cognitive-motor interference (e.g., during dual tasking), especially in people with neurological deficits. The simultaneous effects of dual tasking on cognitive communication are especially important to consider in functional environments. Box 28.1 provides several suggested strategies to improve communication for patients with cognitive-communication disorders.

■ DYSARTHRIA

The term *dysarthria* (sometimes called a *motor speech disorder*) refers to an impairment of speech production resulting from damage to the central or peripheral nervous system, which causes weakness, paralysis, and/or incoordination of the motor–speech system. Any one or all of the components of the motor–speech system (respiration, phonation, articulation, resonance) may by compromised by neural damage. The type and degree of dysarthria depend on the underlying etiology, degree of neuropathology, coexistence of other disabilities, and the individual response of the patient to the condition. It is not unusual for dysarthria to coexist with aphasia in patients who have suffered cerebrovascular accident (CVA) or TBI. The severity of dysarthria may range from the production of occasionally imprecise consonant sounds to speech that is rendered totally unintelligible by the degree of impairment to the underlying systems. When patients are unintelligible as the result of severe motor-speech system impairment, they exhibit *anarthria*.

The incidence of dysarthria in the population of individuals with neurogenic disorders is approximately 46%, representing a significant proportion of the patients with communication impairments seen in medical settings.[238] It is difficult to estimate the total number of people affected by dysarthria, because the condition results from a wide range of etiologies (e.g., progressive neurological diseases, TBI, stroke). Dysarthria is generally reflected in deficits occurring in multiple motor-speech systems but may sometimes occur in a single system (e.g., an impairment of soft palate movement resulting in hypernasality). It is most notably prevalent in cerebral palsy, TBI, CVA, demyelinating diseases (e.g., multiple sclerosis), neoplasm, and progressive neurodegenerative diseases, such as Parkinson disease, Huntington disease, and amyotrophic lateral sclerosis (ALS).

There are five primary types of dysarthria: *spastic, flaccid, ataxic, hypokinetic,* and *hyperkinetic.* When two or more types coexist, the term *mixed dysarthria* is used. Coexisting physical disabilities are present in many patients who manifest dysarthria.

Classification and Nomenclature

Spastic Dysarthria

Spastic dysarthria is characterized by one or more of the following: imprecise, slow, and labored articulation, hypernasality, harsh to strained phonation, and monotonous pitch. Syllables may be given equal stress and inflection. There is often reduced control of exhalation, with shallow inhalations and slow breaths. Spastic dysarthria is the result of bilateral pyramidal system damage involving the corticobulbar tracts (upper motor neurons) and can be acquired or congenital. There is a high incidence of spastic dysarthria among those with cerebral palsy.[238]

Flaccid Dysarthria

Flaccid dysarthria is characterized by slow/labored articulation, hypernasality, and hoarse, breathy phonation. Flaccid dysarthria is the result of lower motor neuron weakness and can be acquired or congenital. Phrases may be short, inhalation is shallow, and the control of exhalation may be reduced. There is often a reduction in the variation of pitch and loudness with audible inspirations. Most of these abnormal speech characteristics are related to muscular weakness and reduced muscle tone, which affects speech accuracy.

Ataxic Dysarthria

Ataxic dysarthria is characterized by disturbances of timing, movement, range, control, and coordination of the muscles of speech and respiration. Speech is imprecise, slow, and irregular. There may be intermittent periods of explosive inflection, syllable stress, and loudness patterns. Phonemes may be prolonged; pitch and loudness are monotonous. The lesions producing ataxic dysarthria involve the deep midline nuclei and pathways of the cerebellum. Patients with multiple sclerosis and TBI with cerebellar damage often manifest ataxic dysarthria.

Hypokinetic Dysarthria

Hypokinetic dysarthria is characterized by reduced breath support, variable articulatory precision, impaired rate of speech, voice quality changes, hesitations, prolonged syllables, reduced loudness, and reduced pitch and loudness ranges. Patients with Parkinson disease, atypical Parkinsonisms, or Parkinsonian-like symptoms often manifest hypokinetic dysarthria, usually caused by impairment of the basal ganglia control circuit.

Hyperkinetic Dysarthria

Hyperkinetic dysarthria is characterized by variable articulatory precision, vocal harshness, prolonged sounds and intervals between words, monotonous pitch, and loudness. It is manifest in patients with Huntington disease, also caused by impairment of the basal ganglia control circuit.

Treatment of Dysarthria

Treatment must be individually designed to account for the specific profile of impairment, as well as the variability of its disabling effects. Intensive and other types of treatments have been examined, some of which have been proven to be effective.[239] The focus of treatment is at times based on an approach that emphasizes strengthening and coordinating weakened subsystems, while other approaches emphasize developing and using compensatory strategies. Some of these compensatory techniques tend to encourage the patient to minimize the overall disability by using strategies that may deviate from normal (i.e., slowing down the rate of speech production to increase intelligibility of consonant production). Patients and communication partners must also be trained to facilitate the most optimal situations for communication interactions.

One type of treatment approach is to focus on strengthening residual oral-motor skills (e.g., strength, speed, ROM); however, focusing on strengthening oral-motor movements to address speech clarity is not typically advised because oral-motor (vs. speech-motor) function does not always reflect the intelligibility or comprehensibility of speech.[240] However, an approach that focuses on strengthening and compensating for reduced function of one of the subsystems of speech production, velopharyngeal function, has shown promise in its ability to improve speech in individuals with dysarthria.[241] Other approaches include utilizing loudness as a strategy that results in a spreading of effects and is centered around improving coordination of the subsystems of respiration, phonation, articulation, and resonance.[239,242] Increasing loudness, increasing/decreasing speaking rate, improving clarity, and modifying prosodic features of speech (e.g., stress, intonation, speech rate) have also been investigated for their effectiveness in treating dysarthria.[239]

Increasing amplitude of movement (loudness in the speech motor system and bigger movements in the limb motor system) and addressing changes in sensory processing that may affect a person's ability to speak and move normally are common targets in the treatment of some types of dysarthria, especially those due to Parkinson disease. A significant number of studies have focused on increasing loudness with an intensive mode of delivery and have examined the short- and long-term efficacy of LSVT LOUD for individuals with dysarthria due to Parkinson disease and other neurological disorders. Treatment delivery is intensive and focused on high-effort speech and respiratory-voice exercises to increase vocal loudness to normal levels, as well as a readjustment of the patient's perception of his or her own loudness levels when speaking. The program is based on several exercise physiology principles that drive activity-dependent neuroplastic changes, including intensive practice, movement complexity, emotional saliency of tasks, timing of treatment, accuracy of productions, and continuous/daily exercise to slow symptom progression.[243] Studies that have examined this treatment method have also reported improvement in respiratory kinematics, articulation, intelligibility, swallowing, and facial expression[244–247] and have demonstrated its success in individuals with dysarthria due to stroke,[248,249] TBI,[249] multiple sclerosis,[248] ataxic dysarthria,[248,250] cerebral palsy,[251] and Down syndrome.[252]

In addition to focusing on improving loudness, a variety of strategies are used to manipulate speech rate. Speakers tend to be more intelligible when they speak slowly. The ANCDS' review of studies that investigated the effectiveness of rate control techniques concluded that they are dependent on the type and severity of dysarthria and the specific intervention strategies employed.[239] Further study is still needed to delineate an individual's candidacy for this type of technique, as well as what the carryover can be to the natural communication environment.

A third focus of dysarthria treatment is the improvement of the prosodic aspects of speech (i.e., stress patterns within words and sentences, intonation to express meaning, and rate-rhythm interactions). A variety of strategies that target prosody have been implemented, including those using biofeedback and behavioral instruction. Few conclusions can be drawn about the effectiveness of prosody training because of the small number of examinations and wide range of subject characteristics and techniques used.[239]

Many persons with motor speech impairments have been able to increase their communicative effectiveness using augmentative and alternative communication (AAC). Low- and high-tech aids include specially designed software applications that are available on mobile devices, such as laptops, tablets, and a variety of smartphones. Recommendations of AAC for persons with dysarthria depend on the severity of the communication disorder and the projected course of the disease and must be carefully selected and managed by an experienced, professional speech-language pathologist. Physical and occupational therapists may also play a significant role in managing the patient in need of AAC.

■ APRAXIA OF SPEECH

Apraxia of speech (AOS) is a diagnostic term that refers to symptoms, including speech sound errors (e.g., distortions), slow speech rate, and irregularities, such as slow transitions between sounds, syllables, and words, syllable segregation and equalized stress within words and sentences, reflecting disruptions in motor planning and/or programming with no evidence of impaired strength of the motor speech system.[253–257] Additional behaviors that may be present in persons with AOS include difficulty initiating speech, articulatory struggling, periods of error-free speech production, and a greater number of sound production errors as utterance length and complexity increase. These characteristics may be so severe that the patient is barely intelligible despite having no difficulty in processing the meaning of words. Unlike dysarthric speakers, individuals with AOS do not generally have deficits in performing nonspeech movements of the oral musculature (e.g., chewing and swallowing).

Due to its common co-occurrence with aphasia, AOS is challenging to diagnose.[258] The speech dyspraxia component of this multifaceted communication disorder appears to be especially amenable to direct therapeutic intervention. AOS can be caused by stroke or neurodegenerative disease. The progressive variant of AOS is termed primary progressive apraxia of speech.

Treatment of Apraxia of Speech

A variety of approaches, designed to improve phonetic placement accuracy, typically depend on imitation, stress, and gradually shaping sounds until a desired sound is approximated, which is then drilled using temporal, tactile, kinesthetic, visual, and auditory cues. Treatment guidelines have been published by the ANCDS.[259–261]

The most commonly used approaches are referred to as *articulatory kinematic*. These techniques aim to improve articulatory movements and include modeling, imitation, repetition, shaping, electromagnetic articulography, and multimodal and articulatory placement cueing.[262–270]

Integral stimulation, a method originally introduced by Milisen,[271] was a commonly used articulatory kinematic technique that involved imitation and emphasized the importance of helping the patient focus his or her attention on the auditory and visual models of speech. Rosenbek et al.[264] further developed an eight-step continuum based on this approach that employs a hierarchy of cues in which the timing between the stimulus provided by the clinician and the response produced by the patient is varied.[264]

Wambaugh and colleagues later developed *Sound Production Treatment,* a program that also incorporates principles of motor learning, such as modeling, repetition, integral stimulation, articulatory placement cueing, and verbal feedback. This more commonly used approach has been systematically investigated.[270–274]

AOS treatment methods have focused primarily on these types of articulatory-kinematic approaches. A growing interest in rhythmic/musical approaches and treatments that combine intervention for aphasia and AOS (i.e., speech and language intervention) are being examined. There also has been attention paid to the basic mechanisms of change underlying aspects of treatment that may affect outcomes, such as treatment intensity. Advances in technology also continue to be utilized in AOS treatment.[275–286]

Alternative and augmentative communication approaches are often recommended for persons with AOS. In most cases, the use of multiple communication modalities, such as writing, drawing, gesturing, and signing, with or without communication aids, is suggested as a facilitatory technique to enhance or substitute for impaired speech.[287–291] These approaches employ and combine strategies that can be included in more than one category, such as iconic or rhythmic gestures, rate and rhythm techniques, vibrotactile stimulation, imitation, and modeling.[287–295]

■ DYSPHAGIA

The act of swallowing is composed of a number of complex neuromuscular events. Normal swallowing requires that an individual be able to move food or liquid from the mouth (*oral phase*), through the pharynx (*pharyngeal phase*), and into the esophagus (*esophageal phase*). In the oral phase, food is moistened and collected in the oral cavity in a single mass, or bolus, which is chewed, if necessary, and then propelled into the pharynx and into the esophagus. During the oral phase, the bolus is first held between the tongue and palate and then propelled by the tongue from the front to the back of the oral cavity. The bolus moves over the back of the tongue into the pharynx, triggering the pharyngeal swallow reflex and the neuromuscular events that propel the bolus into the esophagus. Velopharyngeal closure, tongue base posterior motion, pharyngeal contraction, laryngeal elevation and closure, and upper esophageal opening occur to allow bolus passage into the esophagus. Airway protection involves closure of the airway entrance and airway. The true vocal folds and ventricular folds close, and the epiglottis moves downward as the larynx moves upward and forward to prevent food from entering the trachea during this process.

Dysphagia is defined as a condition in which an individual has had an interruption in either swallowing function or the maintenance of nutrition and hydration.[296] Many patients with neurogenic communication disorders and/or individuals who have suffered neuropathology may have mild to severe swallowing disorders.[297-304] In some cases dysphagia is present only in the acute phase, with rapid recovery of swallowing function taking place in the first 3 weeks poststroke.[305] Swallowing deficits in patients poststroke are often due to a combination of weakness and incoordination of the oral, pharyngeal, and laryngeal musculature, resulting in inefficient propulsion of a food bolus or liquid through the oral cavity, pharynx, and into the esophagus. Delayed triggering of swallowing is not uncommon after stroke. Oral or pharyngeal transit times may be slow. Reduced elevation or closure of the larynx may result in material being misdirected into the airway (penetration; aspiration). Dysphagia is also often present in patients with other neurological disorders, such as, but not limited to, Parkinson disease,[300,301,306] Huntington disease,[307] the dystonias and dyskinesias,[308,309] ALS,[310] multiple sclerosis,[304,311] head and neck cancer,[312] dementia,[313,314] cerebral palsy,[315] and TBI.[299,316]

A dysphagia examination begins at bedside, and if a pharyngeal phase swallowing disorder is suspected, is followed by more objective, instrumental techniques. Several examinations may be utilized in the evaluation of swallowing, including a modified barium radiographic study and a flexible fiberoptic endoscopic study, with or without sensory testing. These procedures permit viewing of many components of the oropharyngeal swallow, including structural movement, bolus flow, and penetration and/or aspiration. Physiological swallowing disorders can be precisely identified and described using these measures. In addition, the effects of therapeutic strategies on swallow physiology, safety, and efficiency can be examined. In most settings, the swallowing evaluation is carried out by the speech-language pathologist.

Treatment of Dysphagia

Dysphagia treatment is designed to increase swallowing safety and improve swallowing efficiency for nutritional purposes. This can be accomplished by compensatory strategies and/or techniques designed to change swallowing physiology and reduce the risk of aspiration. Compensatory strategies include postural changes that affect the way food passes through the mouth and pharynx, dietary management, and placing food in the mouth in optimal positions. Specific techniques, exercises, and maneuvers are used to increase the coordination, range of motion, strength, and sensory input of the muscles and structures involved in the oral and pharyngeal phases of swallowing, which includes exercises intended to strengthen muscles involved in airway protection, such as the cough reflex. These exercises are designed to improve initiation of tongue movement, lingual propulsion, laryngeal elevation, closure, and tongue base approximation to the posterior pharyngeal wall.[317-325]

The physical therapist can play an important role by positioning the patient for optimum swallowing and providing treatment to reduce muscle spasticity, improve muscle strength and coordination, and prevent primitive reflex patterns from interfering with swallowing. Additional implications for the physical therapist when treating patients with communication disorders follow. Appendix 28.A (online) presents Web-based resources for patients, families, and caregivers.

■ COMMUNICATION DISORDERS: IMPLICATIONS FOR THE PHYSICAL THERAPIST

Physical therapists often work in settings where they may be the first to become aware of a patient's communication disorder and often refer such patients to an SLP for evaluation. The physical therapist can contribute to the patient's improvement in communication function in two important ways: (1) by providing physiological support for speech, voice, and swallow function and (2) by stimulating and facilitating communication through successful, fulfilling patient-clinician interaction. In either case, the physical therapist will want to work closely with the SLP to ensure that treatment goals and interventions are compatible.

The provision of interdisciplinary support for communication and swallowing function is especially relevant to the patient with neuropathology. Proper posture, for example, can help inhibit reflexes that may trigger primitive movements and facilitate respiratory kinematics. Control of respiration is essential to the improvement of vocalization and speaking. The muscles of respiration can be strengthened, and exercises designed to increase head control, stability, and sitting balance. Proper posture can also enhance the possibility that speech will be audible and clear.

When a patient with a communication impairment is prescribed a communication board, the physical therapist contributes by determining a patient's sitting balance and tolerance, upper extremity motor control, and the best method for responding (e.g., pointing).

Strengthening exercises to increase the speed and range of motion of the tongue, lips, and general facial musculature and improve coordination of the oral–motor system also facilitate the probability of intelligible speech. Postural considerations are especially important for patients with dysphagia, who require individually tailored treatment programs designed to facilitate swallowing and prevent aspiration.

The physical therapy setting is a natural context for communication. The setting can be supportive by providing an atmosphere that is conducive to conversation and allows the patient to engage in successful verbal interactions.

Patients who are neurologically compromised often have difficulty processing information in a distracting setting. Excessive noise, competing voices, and the presence of other stimuli can make communication particularly difficult. When possible, the physical therapist should initially strive to work with communication-impaired patients in a closed environment that is free of distractions. Patients with communication impairments do best when they are positioned in such a way that face-to-face communication is possible, including the visualization of gestures and facial expressions. For this reason, room lighting needs to be sufficient.

Patients who manifest neurogenic speech-language disorders, especially those with aphasia, pose a considerable challenge to effective communication. The nature of aphasia argues for a close working relationship with the SLP to ensure the most effective communication strategies are used with each patient.

One of the greatest difficulties in addressing the needs of patients with acquired aphasia has to do with determining and accounting for the patient's level of auditory comprehension. Virtually all patients with aphasia have some degree of difficulty comprehending spoken language. Physical therapists need to become skilled at recognizing and dealing with auditory comprehension deficits because they can be a major deterrent to successful rehabilitation.

Misconceptions of the auditory comprehension level of a patient with aphasia can range from an assumption that the patient understands everything to the patient comprehends nothing. A guiding principle is that auditory comprehension can vary greatly, depending on the context and complexity of the task at hand. Quickly switching topics, speaking too quickly, background noise, talking while a patient is engaged in physical activity, and conversing with more than one person at a time can impede the individual's ability to process auditory information. Sentences should be short and simple, and the patient should be given sufficient time to process the information and formulate a response. Questions that require elaborate answers, such as "Tell me about your vacation" or "What do you think about the latest news?" are often difficult for patients with aphasia to answer. It is best to ask questions that can be answered with "yes," "no," or a word, phrase, or gesture. Physical cues that aid comprehension, such as gestures, facial expression, and voice inflection, can facilitate and enhance a patient's understanding. Patients with aphasia often find it easier to respond to whole body or axial commands (e.g., "Stand up," "Sit down") rather than distal commands (e.g., "Point," "Pick up").

It can be tempting to try to remedy a laborious communication situation by "talking down" to a patient with aphasia as if speaking to a child or raising one's voice as if speaking to someone with impaired hearing. The best strategy is to speak more slowly, using language that is not too complex. This can be particularly important in the physical therapy setting, where verbal commands are a fundamental element in the patient–therapist interaction. At times, it may be necessary to repeat a sentence to be understood.

Rehabilitation team members almost universally overestimate the degree to which a person with aphasia understands spoken language. Physical therapists, when possible, should consult with the SLP for an indication of the patient's preserved auditory comprehension. It may be necessary to rephrase questions and supplement with body language to ensure comprehension.

The use of accompanying visual cues, such as gestures and facial expressions, can be extremely helpful for some patients. Others may understand best if a message is supplemented by written cues. Sometimes one can assist by asking questions that can be answered by "yes" or "no" in a 20-questions format. When someone with aphasia is having trouble expressing themselves, it usually helps to allow them extra time to speak. If the patient becomes frustrated, it is desirable to remain calm and suggest that the patient wait and try again later.

During physical therapy interventions, patients with aphasia can be encouraged to produce single-word, repetitive speech that coincides with physical movements as a means of providing supplemental speech practice. Activities such as counting movements in a series and using words like *up*, *down*, *left*, and *right* while performing physical movements are examples of such techniques. The physical therapist, however, should always remain sensitive to the possibility of making speech demands that are beyond a patient's level of preserved communicative skill.

SUMMARY

Ever since World War II, SLPs have played an important role on the rehabilitation team in the management of patients with neurogenic speech-language disorders. For the physical therapist, an understanding of normal and pathological communication behaviors can not only make this population of patients more interesting to work with but can also enhance the quality of treatment he or she provides.

Communication using speech is a complex, species-specific behavior that consists of the coordinated interaction of cognitive, motor, sensory, psychological, and social skills. The neurogenic disorders of speech and language dominate the population of patients with communication impairments in the rehabilitation setting. Viewed as a group, patients with neurogenic communication disorders comprise a relatively severely impaired segment of the disabled population.

The impact of neurogenic speech-language disorders on the self, family, community life, and vocational options makes these disorders especially challenging. The close relationship of one's verbal characteristics to personality and identity may cause even the mildest neurogenic communication disorder to affect the psychosocial domain. Current research is addressing the interaction of linguistic, cognitive, sensorimotor, and psychosocial variables and their influence on the outcome of recovery and rehabilitation.

Questions for Review

1. Define aphasia.

2. Describe the distinction between nonfluent and fluent aphasia and give examples.

3. Discuss the components of a comprehensive language test designed to measure aphasic impairment.

4. Describe some critical factors that influence recovery from aphasia.

5. Describe the psychological sequelae that may have a negative effect on the outcome of aphasia rehabilitation.

6. List several causes of cognitive-communication impairments.

7. Define dysarthria.

8. What neurological conditions are generally associated with dysphagia?

9. Describe augmentative communication systems and some specific techniques/devices that may enhance the treatment of aphasia.

10. How can the physical therapist contribute to the physiological support for speech?

CASE STUDY

The patient is a 62-year-old man who teaches high school. He sustained a right hemiplegia and difficulty communicating as the result of a hemorrhagic stroke which occurred 8 months ago. At this time, except for dressing, he is ADL independent and ambulates with a cane.

At 1-month poststroke, the patient was limited to "yes" or "no" responses and a vocabulary ranging from 30 to 50 nouns and verbs as well as everyday greetings ("hello," "goodbye"). During a communicative interaction, he often resorted to writing a letter or word or gesturing to help in his communication efforts. He appeared to understand most of what was said, especially when the topic was familiar. He received rehabilitation services during the acute poststroke phase while hospitalized and received 20 sessions of speech-language pathology services as an outpatient.

At 8 months poststroke, the patient's communication disorder is marked by a slow, hesitant production of one- and two-word utterances; easily produced automatic speech (i.e., everyday greetings); difficulty expressing complex information; awkward and labored articulation, which causes occasional articulatory imprecision; impaired writing; and some difficulty reading lengthy or complex material. Although the majority of his speaking vocabulary consists of nouns and verbs, adverbs and adjectives are now used with greater frequency. There is a persistent lack of conjunctions, articles, and prepositions when speaking, which causes him to have impaired grammar. The patient has no apparent difficulty understanding spoken language except when it is rapid, complex, and/or unfamiliar.

Both the patient and his caregiver report that the frequency of social interactions in his current life has been curtailed dramatically. He continues to see close family members on a regular basis but rarely sees friends or work companions. The family reports that he is frustrated and depressed and feels isolated from the community much of the time. They also indicate that there has been a gradual but noticeable increase in his speaking vocabulary, ability to write, and reading skill. He has recently joined a local stroke group where he hopes to meet others with similar communication difficulties.

GUIDING QUESTIONS

1. A team conference is scheduled the day after you assume treatment responsibilities for the patient. What types of information would you obtain in consultation with the speech-language pathologist?

2. What communication strategies are generally useful with patients who have sustained a stroke?

(Continued)

CASE STUDY—cont'd

3. What approach might you use if a patient became frustrated trying to express themself during a physical therapy treatment?

4. In what ways can physical therapy treatment sessions serve to reinforce communication behavior?

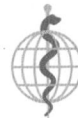

For additional resources, including answers to the questions for review, new immersive cases, case study guiding questions, references, and more, please visit **https://www.fadavis.com/product/physical -rehabilitation-fulk-8**. You may also quickly find the resources by entering this title's four-digit ISBN, 4691, in the search field at **http://fadavis.com** and logging in at the prompt.

Promoting Health and Wellness

Janet R. Bezner, PT, DPT, PhD, NBC-HWC, FAPTA
Jessica Maxwell, PT, DPT, PhD
Beth Black, PT, DSc

Chapter 29

LEARNING OBJECTIVES

1. Explain the importance of health promotion and wellness initiatives.
2. Describe the role of physical therapists in health promotion.
3. Differentiate among the terms *health* and *wellness; illness* and *disease; quality of life, primary, secondary,* and *tertiary prevention; population health management; health promotion; health education; physical activity;* and *exercise.*
4. Discuss the evolution of models of health from the biomedical model to the current International Classification of Functioning, Disability, and Health (ICF) biopsychosocial model of human functioning.
5. Identify measures of health and wellness, health behaviors, and quality of life.
6. Describe key modifiable personal health behaviors.
7. Identify and discuss key theories of behavior change.
8. Explain health coaching and motivational interviewing.
9. Explain how physical therapists can incorporate health promotion and wellness concepts into the plan of care for individuals with impairments and disabilities.
10. Explain how physical therapists can develop and lead health promotion and wellness programs in the community and in institutions and organizations.

CHAPTER OUTLINE

THE IMPORTANCE OF HEALTH PROMOTION AND WELLNESS INITIATIVES *1119*
THE ROLE OF PHYSICAL THERAPISTS IN HEALTH PROMOTION *1122*
KEY TERMS IN HEALTH PROMOTION *1123*
  Health and Disease *1123*
  Wellness and Illness *1123*
  Quality of Life *1124*
  Health Promotion Models *1124*
HEALTH PROMOTION AND HEALTH EDUCATION *1125*
PHYSICAL ACTIVITY AND EXERCISE *1126*
THE INTERNATIONAL CLASSIFICATION OF FUNCTIONING, DISABILITY, AND HEALTH AND HEALTH PROMOTION *1126*
MEASURES OF HEALTH, WELLNESS, QUALITY OF LIFE, AND HEALTH BEHAVIORS *1127*
  Clinical Measures of Health *1127*
  Self-Perceived Health, Wellness, and Quality-of-Life Measures *1127*
  Disease-Specific Measures of Self-Perceived Health, Wellness, and Quality of Life *1128*
KEY MODIFIABLE PERSONAL HEALTH BEHAVIORS *1128*
  Assessing Health Behaviors *1128*

THEORIES OF BEHAVIOR CHANGE *1131*
  Health Belief Model *1131*
  Theory of Reasoned Action and Theory of Planned Behavior *1132*
  Transtheoretical Model (Stages of Change) *1132*
  Self-Determination Theory *1134*
  Social Cognitive Theory *1134*
  Physical Activity Model for People With a Disability *1138*
  Social Ecological Model *1139*
  Community Models *1140*
HEALTH AND WELLNESS COACHING *1140*
  Motivational Interviewing *1140*
HEALTH PROMOTION AND WELLNESS FOR INDIVIDUALS WITH IMPAIRMENTS AND DISABILITIES *1141*
  Examination and Evaluation *1141*
  Interventions *1143*
HEALTH PROMOTION AND WELLNESS AT THE PROGRAM LEVEL *1145*
PHYSICAL THERAPISTS AS ADVOCATES *1145*
SUMMARY *1146*

■ THE IMPORTANCE OF HEALTH PROMOTION AND WELLNESS INITIATIVES

An individual's health is determined by the interaction of numerous factors, including biology and genetics, social and physical environments, health service availability and utilization, and individual behaviors.[1] Unhealthy behaviors are contributing to an increase in chronic disease and disability in the United States and other countries, affecting both the health of individuals and their quality of life.[2,3] It is estimated that over a third of premature deaths in the United States are caused by lack of exercise, poor diet, and cigarette smoking,[4] and these rates are considerably higher in low- or middle-income countries.[2] Obesity rates in the United States continue to climb, contributing to the development of associated chronic diseases such as heart disease, stroke, type 2 diabetes, and certain types of cancer.[5] According to the 2020 Behavioral Risk Factor Surveillance System (BRFSS), the

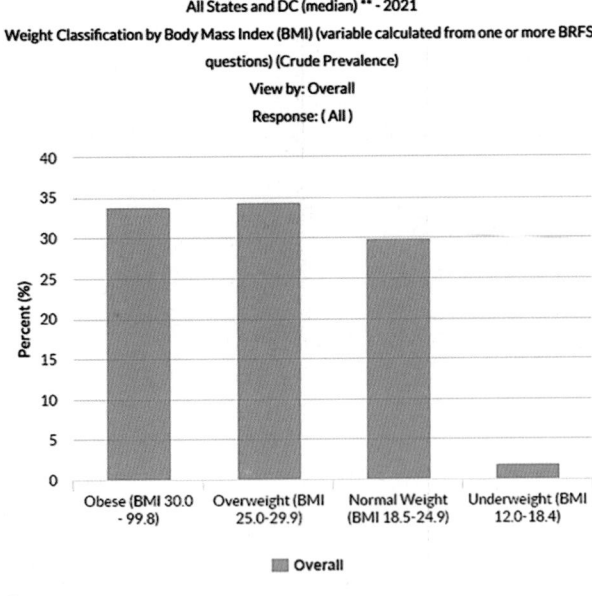

All States and DC (median) ** - 2021

Weight Classification by Body Mass Index (BMI) (variable calculated from one or more BRFSS questions) (Crude Prevalence)

View by: Overall

Response: (All)

Footnote

**   ** Median value reported with no confidence intervals.

Data Source: Behavioral Risk Factor Surveillance System (BRFSS)

Figure 29.1 Weight Classification by Body Mass Index. *(From Centers for Disease Control and Prevention, National Center for Chronic Disease Prevention and Health Promotion, Division of Population Health. BRFSS Prevalence & Trends Data [online]. 2021. Accessed July 15, 2021.* https://www.cdc.gov/brfss/brfssprevalence/index.html*).*

annual telephone survey of more than 400,000 adults in the United States, 67% of the adult population is overweight or obese[6] (Fig. 29.1). In the same survey, when asked if they participated in any exercise during the past month, 22.7% of respondents answered no, and 15.5% of respondents indicated they currently smoke.[6] Fruit and vegetable consumption continues to be low among adults in the United States, with only 23.4% reporting consuming fruits and vegetables five or more times per day in 2009.[7] There is also mounting evidence of the importance of sleep to an individual's health. Sleep insufficiency has been linked to increased risk of motor vehicle and industrial accidents and an increased risk for developing chronic diseases such as hypertension, diabetes, depression, obesity, and cancer.[8] Data from 444,306 adult respondents in all 50 states and the District of Columbia on the 2014 BRFSS indicated that more than one-third of adults in the United States are getting less than the recommended 7 hours of sleep each night.[9]

Not only are adults' health-related behaviors of concern, but there is also growing consensus that the high levels of obesity of children in the United States are related to their health behaviors. Between 2017 and 2020, the prevalence of obesity in children was reported to be 19.7%, affecting 14.7 million children and adolescents aged 2 to 19 years.[10] Behaviors such as consuming high-calorie, low-nutrient foods and beverages, not engaging in sufficient physical activity, spending

too much time on sedentary activities such as watching television or other screen devices, and not getting enough sleep have been identified as contributing to excess weight gain in children and adolescents.[11]

Given the strong relationship between health behaviors and health status, it is clear that the current health-related behaviors of adults and children in the United States are adversely affecting healthy life expectancy, and efforts to support healthier behaviors are essential.

In 1980, the U.S. Department of Health and Human Services began the nation's current health promotion and disease prevention agenda with *Healthy People 1990. Healthy People 2020* was recently concluded, and its final progress status can be found at https://www.cdc.gov/nchs/healthy_people/hp2020/progress-tables.htm.[12] The current set of national health objectives are articulated in *Healthy People 2030.* They have been developed through a wide-reaching collaborative consensus process and published by the U.S. Department of Health and Human Services.[13] Public health experts, government agencies, professional organizations such as the American Physical Therapy Association (APTA), and members of the public all provided input into this important document. The overall framework for *Healthy People 2030* is outlined in Table 29.1.

Given the broad range of factors that contribute to the health of the population, the *Healthy People 2030* goals and objectives address social determinants of health, including economic stability, education access and quality, health-care access and quality, neighborhood and built environment, and social and community context[14] (Fig. 29.2).

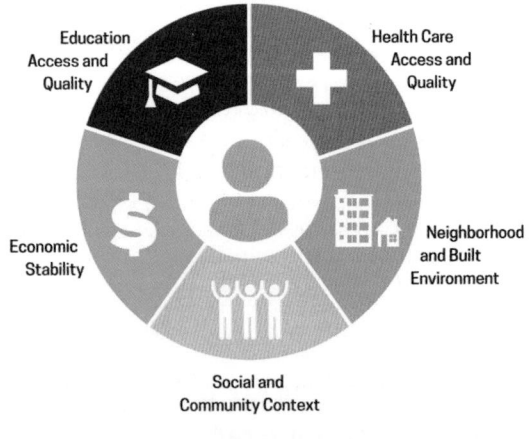

Figure 29.2 Social Determinants of Health. *(From Healthy People 2030, U.S. Department of Health and Human Services, Office of Disease Prevention and Health Promotion.* https://health.gov/healthypeople/objectives-and-data/social-determinants-health*).*

Table 29.1	*Healthy People 2030* Framework
Vision	A society in which all people can achieve their full potential for health and well-being across the lifespan.
Mission	To promote, strengthen, and evaluate the nation's efforts to improve the health and well-being of all people.
Foundational Principles	Foundational principles explain the thinking that guides decisions about *Healthy People 2030*. • Health and well-being of all people and communities are essential to a thriving, equitable society. • Promoting health and well-being and preventing disease are linked efforts that encompass physical, mental, and social health dimensions. • Investing to achieve the full potential for health and well-being for all provides valuable benefits to society. • Achieving health and well-being requires eliminating health disparities, achieving health equity, and attaining health literacy. • Healthy physical, social, and economic environments strengthen the potential to achieve health and well-being. • Promoting and achieving the nation's health and well-being is a shared responsibility that is distributed across the national, state, tribal, and community levels, including the public, private, and not-for-profit sectors. • Working to attain the full potential for health and well-being of the population is a component of decision-making and policy formulation across all sectors.
Overarching Goals	• Attain healthy, thriving lives and well-being, free of preventable disease, disability, injury, and premature death. • Eliminate health disparities, achieve health equity, and attain health literacy to improve the health and well-being of all. • Create social, physical, and economic environments that promote attaining full potential for health and well-being for all. • Promote healthy development, healthy behaviors and well-being across all life stages. • Engage leadership, key constituents, and the public across multiple sectors to take action and design policies that improve the health and well-being of all.
Plan of Action	• Set national goals and measurable objectives to guide evidence-based policies, programs, and other actions to improve health and well-being. • Provide data that is accurate, timely, accessible, and can drive targeted actions to address regions and populations with poor health or at high risk for poor health in the future. • Foster impact through public and private efforts to improve health and well-being for people of all ages and the communities in which they live. • Provide tools for the public, programs, policy makers, and others to evaluate progress toward improving health and well-being. • Share and support the implementation of evidence-based programs and policies that are replicable, scalable, and sustainable. • Report biennially on progress throughout the decade from 2020 to 2030. • Stimulate research and innovation toward meeting *Healthy People 2030* goals and highlight critical research, data, and evaluation needs. • Facilitate development and availability of affordable means of health promotion, disease prevention, and treatment.

From: https://www.healthypeople.gov/2020/About-Healthy-People/Development-Healthy-People-2030/Framework.

Healthy People 2030 identifies 62 topic areas requiring particular attention, organized into the five broad categories of health conditions, health behaviors, populations, settings and systems, and social determinants of health. Under these categories, there are 355 specific objectives, or goals, related to one or more of the topics. For example, within the topic area of physical activity, there are 27 objectives (Table 29.2) accompanied by specific targets to be achieved within the next 10 years. The ecological approach to addressing the topic areas is clear from the breadth of the objectives established for each of these topic areas. For example, in the area of physical activity, Physical Activity Objective–PA1 speaks to increasing individuals' levels of leisure-time physical

Table 29.2 *Healthy People 2030* Physical Activity Objectives	
Healthy People 2030 Physical Activity (PA) Objectives	Topic Area (Objective Short Title)
PA-01	Reduce the proportion of adults who engage in no leisure-time physical activity.
PA-02	Increase the proportion of adults who meet current Federal physical activity guidelines for aerobic physical activity and for muscle-strengthening activity.
PA-03	Increase the proportion of adolescents who meet current Federal physical activity guidelines for aerobic physical activity and for muscle-strengthening activity.
PA-04	Increase the proportion of the Nation's public and private schools that require daily physical education for all students.
PA-05	Increase the proportion of adolescents who participate in daily school physical education.
PA-06	Increase regularly scheduled elementary school recess in the United States.
PA-07	Increase the proportion of school districts that require or recommend elementary school recess for an appropriate period of time.
PA-08	Increase the proportion of children and adolescents who do not exceed recommended limits for screen time.
PA-9	Increase the number of States with licensing regulations for physical activity provided in child care.
PA-10	Increase the proportion of the Nation's public and private schools that provide access to their physical activity spaces and facilities for all persons outside of normal school hours (i.e., before and after the school day, on weekends, and during summer and other vacations).
PA-11	Increase the proportion of physician office visits that include counseling or education related to physical activity.
PA-12	(Developmental) Increase the proportion of employed adults who have access to and participate in employer-based exercise facilities and exercise programs.
PA-13	Increase the proportion of trips made by walking.
PA-14	Increase the proportion of trips made by bicycling.
PA-15	(Developmental) Increase legislative policies for the built environment that enhance access to and availability of physical activity opportunities.

From https://health.gov/healthypeople/objectives-and-data/browse-objectives/physical-activity.

activity, whereas Physical Activity Objective–PA13 identifies the need for parents to limit screen time for their children. Progress toward the objectives and specific targets established for *Healthy People 2030* is tracked by measuring general health status, health behaviors, health-related quality of life and well-being, determinants of health, and measures of health disparities.

■ THE ROLE OF PHYSICAL THERAPISTS IN HEALTH PROMOTION

Interventions aimed at individual, community, state, and national levels by a broad coalition of public health organizations, health professionals, educators, and government agencies will be required to achieve the objectives outlined in *Healthy People 2030*. All health professionals, regardless of their area of practice, have a key role to play in health promotion, either as individual practitioners or as members of an interprofessional health-care team.[15] Physical therapists are participating in health promotion initiatives in a variety of ways, from providing individual interventions and programs to community- and population-level interventions and programs.[16–19] A number of professional publications describe the important role for physical therapists in the area of health promotion and wellness.[20–24]

The APTA's *Guide to Physical Therapist Practice* clearly identifies health promotion and prevention as being within the scope of physical therapist practice:

Physical therapists are involved in prevention and in promoting health, wellness, and fitness in a wide range of populations. Their roles range from helping individuals with chronic conditions engage in physical activity programs to advising elite athletes on sports performance enhancement. These initiatives decrease costs by helping individuals (1) achieve and restore optimal functional capacity; (2) minimize impairments, functional limitations, and disabilities related to congenital and acquired conditions; (3) maintain health (thereby preventing further deterioration or future illness); and (4) create appropriate environmental adaptations to enhance independent function.[25]

The patient history portion of a physical therapy examination should include information about the client's health status and health habits, a systems review, and tests and measures as indicated to screen for potential problems that could affect current or future health status, such as hypertension, obesity, impaired balance, or poor fitness levels. Interventions that physical therapists can utilize to promote health and prevent or minimize impairments, activity limitations, and disabilities are extensive and can include such diverse activities as educational techniques regarding healthy lifestyle choices and healthy behaviors, physical activity and aerobic conditioning programs, fall prevention programs, or consultation in workplace redesign. Referrals to other professionals or special programs (e.g., smoking cessation or nutritional counseling) may also be indicated. As physical therapists expand their practices to include not only rehabilitation, but also health promotion, the principles of evidence-based practice should be considered. Decisions regarding appropriate programs to institute should be based on evidence of effectiveness of the intervention, the knowledge and skill level of the physical therapist, and the appropriateness of that particular intervention for the individual client given his or her unique needs, preferences, and circumstances.

In the document *Professionalism in Physical Therapy: Core Values*, physical therapist behaviors believed to represent the behaviors of a doctoring profession include the following:[23(pp1–3)]

- Participating in the achievement of health goals of patients/clients and society
- Focusing on achieving the greatest well-being and the highest potential for a patient/client
- Facilitating each individual's achievement of goals for function, health, and wellness
- Participating in achievement of societal health goals

These behaviors indicate a broad role and responsibility for physical therapists in health promotion and underscore the need for physical therapists to participate not only at the individual client level but also at a societal level. Physical therapists are participating in discussions at a national level regarding public policy, healthcare reform, and major health initiatives, and are also involved in advocacy efforts to support the objectives articulated in *Healthy People 2030*.[13]

At the Physical Therapy and Society Summit (PASS) meeting held in 2010, future roles for physical therapists were discussed relative to the evolving health-care needs of society.[26] At this conference, the opportunity for physical therapists to take a leadership role in the areas of prevention, health, and wellness were emphasized. There has also been a suggestion that physical therapists should be "birth to death" health practitioners, providing regular consultations on exercise and physical activity using a practice model similar to the dental model and geared toward prevention and health promotion.[27] At the Physical Therapy Summits on Global Health, there was consensus that physical therapists can and should incorporate health promotion and wellness into their practices. Action plans were developed for clinicians, educators, researchers, and professional associations to help move the profession in this direction.[28,29]

Given the tremendous need for health promotion, and the unique knowledge base and skill set of physical therapists, it is the professional responsibility of all physical therapists to engage in health-promotion practice regardless of their practice setting. As physical therapists begin to integrate health promotion interventions into their clinical practice, they should become familiar with the various terms and definitions used in the field of health promotion.

■ KEY TERMS IN HEALTH PROMOTION

Health and Disease

Different terms are used in the field of health promotion to define *health*, and most current definitions of health conceptualize and describe health as a multidimensional construct involving more than the physical domain. In 1948, the World Health Organization (WHO) defined health as "a state of complete physical, mental and social well-being and not merely the absence of disease or infirmity."[30] This definition of health is still used by the WHO today. Health has also been described as "a dynamic balance of physical, emotional, social, spiritual, and intellectual health."[31(piv)] *Health condition* is an umbrella term for acute or chronic disease, disorder, injury, or trauma.[19] *Disease,* often considered the opposite of health, is defined as a pathological condition affecting the body.[20]

Wellness and Illness

The term *wellness* is also frequently used in the field of health promotion. In 1959, Dunn discussed the relationship between body, mind, and spirit, and defined wellness as "a complex state made up of overlapping levels of wellness."[32(p786)] Adams et al.[33] defined wellness as an individual's sense of growth and balance across the physical, spiritual, emotional, intellectual, social, and psychological domains (Fig. 29.3). These two wellness definitions are worded in such a way that individuals with chronic disease could still be considered "well."

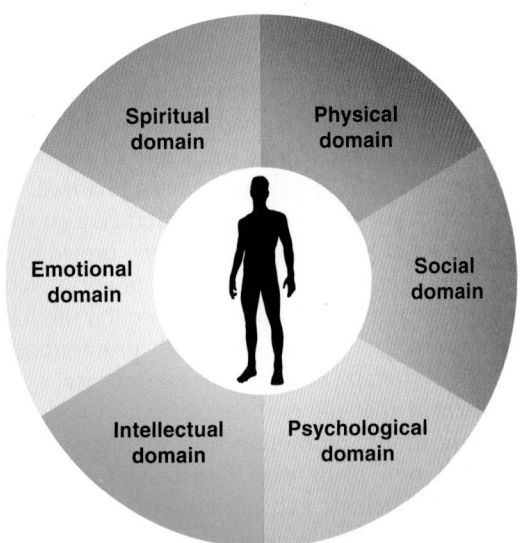

Figure 29.3 Domains of wellness.

The National Wellness Institute defines wellness as "an active process through which people become aware of, and make choices toward, a more successful existence," recognizing that wellness is a process versus a state.[34] Taken together, these various definitions of wellness indicate that wellness is multidimensional; that *salutogenic* or "health-causing" variables are the focus, indicating that wellness is positive or affirming; and that the concept of wellness is specific to each individual. *Illness* is the opposite of wellness, and it has been defined as a social construct where individuals are not achieving balance in their lives and are unable to create a higher quality of life.[35]

Quality of Life

Quality of life (QOL) is a construct with a number of different definitions. The Centers for Disease Control and Prevention (CDC) describes health-related quality of life as an individual's or group's perceived physical and mental health over time.[36] Health-related QOL is influenced by multiple factors (energy level, mood, health risks and conditions, functional status, social support, socioeconomic status, etc.) and is subjective to the individual. The construct of QOL goes beyond direct measures of population health, life expectancy, and causes of death, and focuses on the impact health status has, in addition to other domains, on QOL.[36] The terms *QOL* and *wellness* are similar, both reflecting a person's experience or perception of their life in a general sense.

Health Promotion Models
Primary, Secondary, and Tertiary Prevention

Various health promotion models are used to identify needs and plan health promotion interventions. One such model is the health protection/disease prevention model. Within this model, health is conceptualized as

the absence of disease/pathology, and health promotion is therefore aimed at preventing disease. Interventions in this model are categorized as primary, secondary, or tertiary prevention (see Fig. 29.4).[37(p6)] Physical therapists have traditionally participated primarily in secondary or tertiary prevention, but as they begin to join their fellow health professionals in health promotion practice, they will increasingly add interventions that fall under the category of primary prevention.

Primary prevention includes activities designed to prevent injury or the onset of illness or disease. The use of bicycle helmets and seat belts, water fluoridation, and immunizations are all examples of primary prevention. Physical therapists practice primary prevention when they conduct preseason evaluation and conditioning programs for high school athletes, teach back injury prevention programs at orientation programs for workers in a factory, and support their sedentary patients to adopt regular physical activity habits.

Secondary prevention interventions take place following the development of pathology and are intended to identify and provide treatment for individuals in the early stages of disease in order to minimize the severity of the disease. Screening programs for breast cancer, high blood pressure, and osteoporosis are designed to identify and treat pathology in its earliest stages. Physical therapists engage in secondary prevention when they treat a patient/client with a recent injury or who recently has been diagnosed to be in the early stages of a chronic condition or disease. For example, medically oriented gyms may provide a space for people with prediabetes or prehypertension to exercise in a supervised environment.

Tertiary prevention activities are designed to slow progression of a disease and improve QOL. Physical therapists engage in tertiary prevention when they work with patients/clients who have chronic disease or have sustained an irreversible injury—for example, with patients/clients who have long-standing rheumatoid arthritis.

Population Health Management Model

A similar model to the health protection/disease prevention model is the population health management model (Fig. 29.5). The population health management model examines the health needs of a defined population and provides targeted services for individuals within the group that are appropriate to their level of risk for developing a disease or to their current health status following the development of disease. The goal of the population health management model is to improve the health outcomes of a group by monitoring and providing appropriate interventions to individual members of that group. Interventions are provided across a continuum of care and can include prevention, lifestyle management, disease management, catastrophic care management, and disability management.[38] Magnusson et al. describe

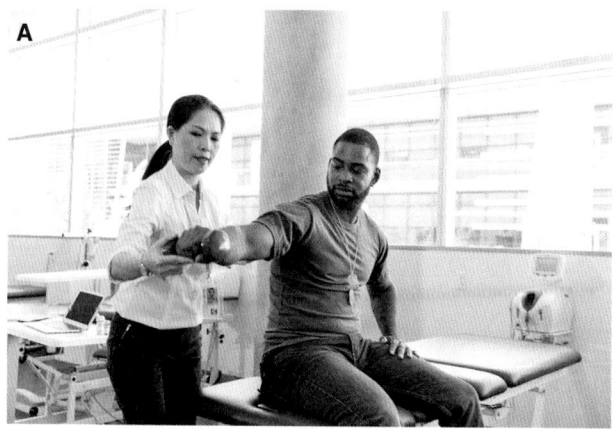
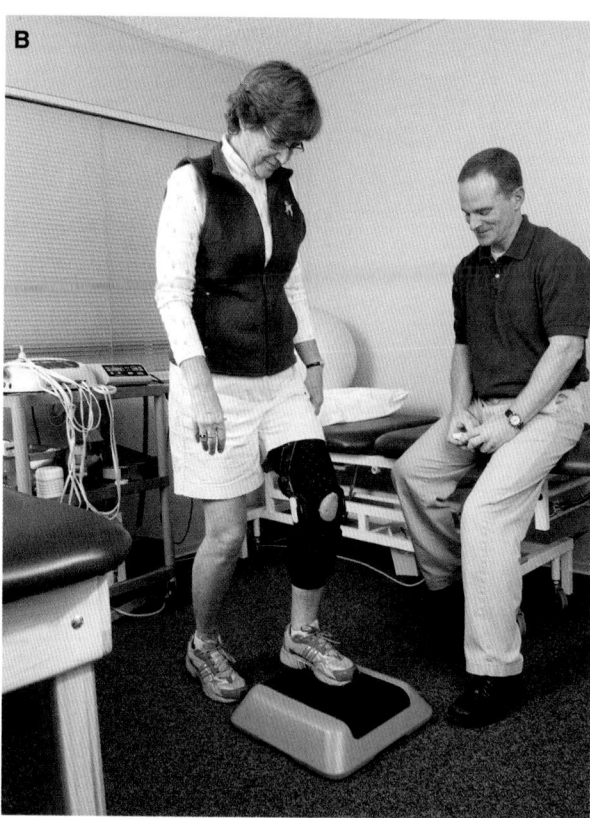
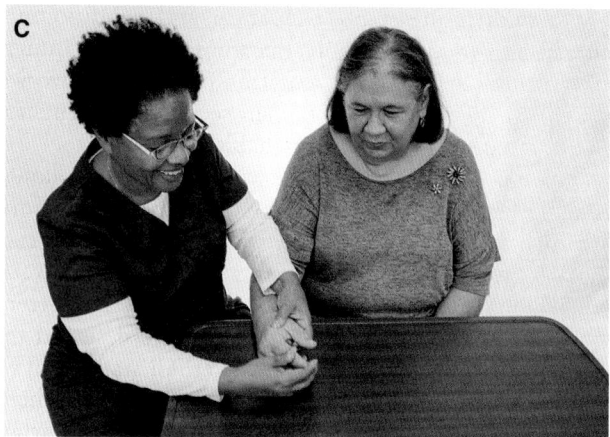

Figure 29.4 Primary, secondary, and tertiary prevention. **A.** Physical therapists practice primary prevention when they help patients to remain healthy and uninjured. **B.** They practice secondary prevention when they provide treatment to minimize the severity of an injury or disease. **C.** Physical therapists practice tertiary prevention when they work with patients who have a chronic disease or irreversible injury to slow the progression of the disorder and improve QOL.

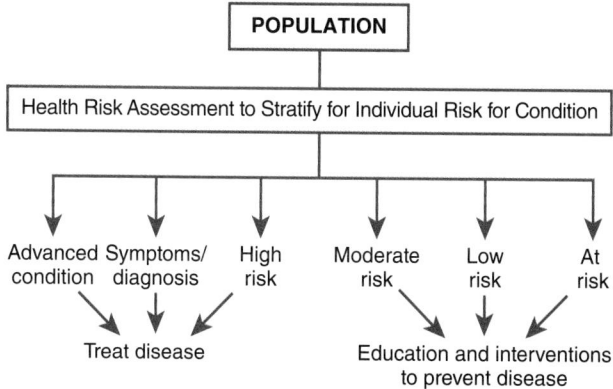

Figure 29.5 Population health management.

approaches physical therapists can use in their practice to incorporate population health frameworks into clinical practice, research, and education, including monitoring of clinical populations using community demographics and health disparities and guiding relevant community-based programming (see Table 29.3).[39]

■ HEALTH PROMOTION AND HEALTH EDUCATION

Green and Kreuter describe *health promotion* as "any planned combination of educational, political, regulatory, and organizational supports for actions and conditions of living conducive to the health of individuals, groups, or communities."[40(pG–4)] WHO defines health promotion as "the process of enabling people to increase control over, and to improve, their health. It moves beyond a focus on individual behavior towards a wide range of social and environmental interventions."[41] Gorin and Arnold[42] describe health promotion as activities undertaken to encourage well-being that are directed toward actualizing an individual's potential. According to Gorin and Arnold, a health promotion model has a more positive orientation and connotation than the prevention models described above that focus on simply preventing disease. *Health education* is one component of health promotion. Green and Kreuter define health education as "any planned combination of learning experiences designed to predispose, enable, and reinforce voluntary

Table 29.3   Population Health Frameworks in Physical Therapy[40]

Application of Population Health Frameworks in Physical Therapist Practice, Research, and Education

Activity	Application
Practice	Enhance monitoring and surveillance of clinical populations
	Identify systematic variations in clinical processes and disparities in health-related outcomes
	Draw attention to the limitations of individual-level interventions as a means of addressing chronic noncommunicable disease and disability
	Facilitate the identification of potential collaborators within and outside the health sector
	Inform the design, implementation, and evaluation of integrated services, programs, and policies
Research	Guide the development of conceptual models that can be systematically tested to establish the nature, strength, and directionality of relationships
	Inform the development of a holistic set of health indicators and the creation of informative data linkages
	Guide the development of quality improvement initiatives or community-based programs as a means of reducing health disparities
	Inform the development of robust prediction models that serve as the foundation for "precision physical therapy"
Education	Serve as a foundation for entry-level physical therapist competencies and curricular guidelines in the areas of prevention and health promotion
	Strengthen the effectiveness of pro bono services by informing the identification of root causes of health inequities, and guiding the development of community and intersectoral partnerships

behavior conducive to health in individuals, groups, or communities."[40] Health education interventions aim to provide information to individuals and groups about health-causing actions and the impact of negative health behaviors in order to make a connection between voluntary behaviors and health. The first step toward positive health behavior change is awareness about the relationship between behavior and disease and injury.

■ PHYSICAL ACTIVITY AND EXERCISE

The definitions for *physical activity* and *exercise* are not synonymous. *Physical activity* is defined as any body movement produced by skeletal muscle contraction that increases energy expenditure above resting level.[43] It includes body movement carried out not only within formal exercise programs but also in occupational activities, leisure activities, and transportation activities such as walking and bicycling. *Exercise* is defined as a subcategory of physical activity and is planned, structured activity that is intended to improve or maintain one or more components of physical fitness.[44] This distinction is important for physical therapists to consider when they work with patients/clients to help them increase their overall levels of physical activity.

■ THE INTERNATIONAL CLASSIFICATION OF FUNCTIONING, DISABILITY, AND HEALTH AND HEALTH PROMOTION

Consistent with the newer multidimensional definitions of health and wellness, there has been a change in the overall framework used to guide evaluation, planning, and interventions to support and promote health. The prevailing model used in 20th century medicine was the *biomedical model*.[45] This model was based on the biological sciences, and health was conceptualized as the absence of disease. The locus of control in the biomedical model was with the health-care providers and the patient was provided with the medical care deemed necessary by health professionals. It was an effective model for managing acute and infectious diseases and illnesses but proved less effective for managing chronic disease[5] or in addressing the psychological, social, or behavioral dimensions of illness.[46] With its primarily biological focus and external locus of control, it was also less useful in the field of health promotion where patients' decisions, behaviors, and environments are considered important elements in understanding and addressing the multiple determinants of health.[47] As the limitations of using a purely biomedical framework to understand the concept of health became apparent, the *biopsychosocial* model evolved. The various biopsychosocial models used today to explain health and illness incorporate those domains missing from the biomedical model, namely the psychological and social domains. The Nagi disablement model[48] is an example of a biopsychosocial model and was the model used to describe practice in the *Guide to Physical Therapist Practice.*[20]

In 2001, WHO endorsed the International Classification of Functioning, Disability, and Health (ICF) biopsychosocial model.[49] The ICF is intended to provide a common language to describe health, function, and disability to facilitate scientific communication within and across health professions. The APTA has endorsed the use of this model as a framework for physical therapists to use in classifying and describing health, function, and disability. In this model, the complex interrelationships of biological, environmental, and personal factors and the impact of these variables on health, activity, and function are recognized. See discussion of the ICF model in Chapter 1, Clinical Decision Making.

Physical therapists have been applying the ICF model to practice in rehabilitation for years.[50-52] However, a number of health professionals, including physical therapists, have also started to demonstrate how the ICF can be used in the field of health promotion research and practice.[53,54] Howard et al.[55] argue that the ICF, with its acknowledgment of the important contribution of the social and physical environment to an individual's health, supports the ecological approach (i.e., the interaction of an individual with others and their environment) used in the field of health promotion. The ICF provides both a rationale for physical therapists to look beyond purely biological and physiological factors when examining and evaluating their clients and a framework to guide their plans of care and interventions. Furthermore, the ICF model is consistent with many of the behavior change theories described later in this chapter that are used to plan and implement behavior change interventions with the goal of promoting health.

■ MEASURES OF HEALTH, WELLNESS, QUALITY OF LIFE, AND HEALTH BEHAVIORS

There is no one standard tool for measuring health, wellness, health behaviors, or QOL. Some tools have been specifically designed to measure the health or health behaviors of a population, whereas other tools are used to measure health and personal health behaviors at the level of the individual patient. A variety of measures of perceived health and QOL have been developed and can be used at the level of a population, as well as at the level of the individual patient.

Clinical Measures of Health

Clinical measures of health include biometric and physiological measures such as body mass index (BMI), aerobic capacity, or blood pressure. Health risk appraisals (HRAs) are increasingly being used in workforce wellness programs to help assess the level and nature of an individual's current health risks based on history, personal behaviors, and clinical variables. HRAs are used to collect information to create risk profiles of individuals and populations, to estimate risk of future adverse health outcomes, and to provide persons with feedback about how to reduce health risk.[56]

The *Guide to Physical Therapist Practice* recommends that an evaluation of a patient/client's general health status, social and health habits (past and current) and potential health risks be included in the initial examination through a thorough history and a systems review.[20] Numerous tests and measures can be used by physical therapists during initial examinations to measure general health status and risk factors.[20]

Self-Perceived Health, Wellness, and Quality-of-Life Measures

The importance of adding a measure of an individual's perception of their general health to the patient/client examination was demonstrated in a landmark study by Mossey and Shapiro in 1982.[57] In this study of 3,128 noninstitutionalized adults over age 64, self-rated health was the strongest predictor of mortality after age 65 and was found to be a better predictor of mortality than a number of morbidity and health-care utilization measures such as medical diagnosis, number of physician visits, number of hospital admissions, and surgical history. The CDC includes a 14-item perceptual measure of health, the *Healthy Days Measure,* in the annual national BRFSS survey and in the National Health and Nutrition Examination Survey.[58]

There are many self-report measures of perceived health, wellness, and QOL that can be completed by clients with a variety of conditions. One of the most commonly used measures of self-perceived health and QOL is the *Medical Outcomes Study 36-Item Short-Form Health Survey (SF-36).*[59] The SF-36 measures self-perceived health and function across eight scales that include physical, psychological, social, and emotional domains. It has been used in general populations and in specific populations, and normative scores for various groups and populations have been documented. WHO has developed the *World Health Organization Quality of Life Questionnaire (WHOQOL-100)*[60] and a shorter version, the *WHOQOL-BREF.* Both versions measure self-perceived physical health, psychological health, social relationships, and the individual's perceptions about his or her environment. WHO tools can be used for the measurement of health at either the population level or the level of the individual patient/client.

Additional measures of self-perceived health used in clinical practice include the *Nottingham Health Profile,*[61] the *Sickness Impact Profile (SIP),*[62] the *Dartmouth Cooperative Functional Assessment Charts (Dartmouth CO-OP charts),*[63] and the *Duke Health Profile.*[64] The *Perceived Wellness Survey (PWS)* measures self-perceived wellness across psychological, physical, emotional, spiritual, social, and intellectual domains.[33] The survey consists of 36 statements with six items for each of the six domains. A composite score, a magnitude score, and a balance score can be computed (Appendix 29.A [online]). This tool has been tested and found to be valid and reliable for use with different populations.[33,65]

Disease-Specific Measures of Self-Perceived Health, Wellness, and Quality of Life

Other measures of health are specific to special populations or people with certain chronic conditions. For example, The National Institutes of Health developed a *Patient-Reported Outcomes Measurement Information System (PROMIS)* that captures important health-related QOL information about patients who have chronic diseases and conditions.[66] The goal of the PROMIS initiative is to be able to develop profiles of PROMIS scores across health domains for various chronic conditions that can then be used in clinical research studies.

Many other disease-specific health and wellness measures have been developed for use with specific clinical populations. The items included in these measures may more specifically address issues related to the health and well-being of a particular population than the general measures described above. The *Arthritis Impact Measurement Scale (AIMS)*[67] and *AIMS2*[68] were developed to measure the physical, mental, and social domains of health in persons with rheumatic diseases. The *Child Health Questionnaire (CHQ)* measures the physical and psychosocial well-being of children and has been found to be a valid and reliable measure of health status across a variety of conditions and disorders.[69] The *Cystic Fibrosis Questionnaire*[70] is a health-related quality-of-life questionnaire that has both parent and child versions to measure the physical, emotional, and social impact of cystic fibrosis on children and their families. Additional disease or condition-specific quality-of-life measures that have been developed include a health and QOL measure for individuals who have had a stroke, such as the *Stroke Adapted Sickness Impact Profile (SA-SIP30)* and the *Stroke Impact Scale,*[71,72] suffer from acute and chronic facial disorders,[73] and have chronic respiratory disease.[74] The *European Organisation for Research and Treatment of Cancer (EORTC)* has developed a series of questionnaires designed to assess the QOL of individuals with cancer. The 30-item EORTC quality-of-life measure has been translated and validated into 81 languages and has disease-specific modules that can be added to it.[75]

■ KEY MODIFIABLE PERSONAL HEALTH BEHAVIORS

The CDC's Healthy Living website provides information about numerous behaviors that contribute to a healthy lifestyle.[76] Some of the health behaviors have the support of organizations, agencies, and schools (e.g., healthy menus in school cafeterias), while others are enforced by local, state, or federal laws, such as seat belt use or nonsmoking environments. Others, though significantly influenced by social, environmental, and economic factors, are primarily the personal responsibility of the individual, such as maintaining a healthy weight, eating a healthy diet, and engaging in physical activity. Some personal health behaviors are considered to be more modifiable than others based on clinical research. Behaviors that are more challenging to change are those with an addictive component, those with compulsive elements, and those strongly associated with cultural or family routines, such as diet.[40] The key behaviors of increasing physical activity, increasing fruit and vegetable consumption, and quitting smoking, all included in the objectives of *Healthy People 2030,* have been shown to be modifiable behaviors if behavior change interventions are appropriately designed and delivered.

Assessing Health Behaviors

Bezner recommends physical therapists include questions about health-related behaviors in initial examinations, including physical activity, nutrition and weight management, sleep, smoking, and stress management.[77] The *Guide to Physical Therapist Practice* also recommends that physical therapists include questions regarding health-related behaviors in initial examinations.[25] The health behaviors of engaging in regular physical activity, eating a healthy diet, abstaining from smoking, and engaging in healthy sleep behaviors and stress management techniques can be determined through patient interview or through a questionnaire. If the anthropometric measures of height and weight are taken, the client's BMI may be calculated, and the physical therapist can determine whether the patient/client is overweight or obese (Box 29.1).

The *International Physical Activity Questionnaire,*[78] originally developed to track levels of physical activity in populations, has also been used in clinical practice

Box 29.1	Body Mass Index
BMI	**Weight Status**
Below 18.5	Underweight
18.5 to 24.9	Normal
25 to 29.9	Overweight
30 or higher	Obese

BMI = body mass index.

to assess individual patient/client's levels of physical activity.[78] The 11-item scale has been used in several studies investigating the impact of employee wellness programs, assessing multiple health behaviors, including physical activity, nutrition habits, healthy living, stress, sleep, QOL, and overall health.[79–82] Table 29.4 contains outcome measures that can be used to document impact of health, wellness, and fitness interventions.

The U.S. Preventive Services Task Force (USPSTF) publishes recommendations for various preventive screening measures and health behavior change interventions based on the most current evidence of the effectiveness of interventions in changing or modifying behavior.[83] For example, there is a recommendation statement for "Healthy Diet and Physical Activity for Cardiovascular Disease Prevention in Adults With

Table 29.4 Outcome Measures of Health, Wellness, and Fitness

Name and Type of Measure	ICF Category	Description	Scoring
6WT[a] *Fitness*	Activity	Submaximal test of aerobic capacity/endurance	Distance walked; person walks as far as possible in 6 minutes without physical assistance; assistive device(s) can be used. Greater distance indicates higher aerobic capacity.
Maximal oxygen uptake (Vo_2 max)[b] *Fitness*	Body Structures and Function	Graded exercise test, typically performed on a treadmill or ergometer; the subject exercises to exhaustion; open-circuit spirometry collects and assesses expired gases from the lungs.	Computerized systems collect and analyze data and directly compute Vo_2 max; submaximal test data can be used to estimate Vo_2 max if collected from at least 2 levels of intensity; norms are available.[b]
International Physical Activity Questionnaire (Short Self-Administered)[77] *Health-Related Physical Activity*	Activity	4-item scale assessing vigorous and moderate PA performed in the last 7 days and time spent sitting; aimed at young and middle-aged adults. Responses gathered for days per week and hours/minutes spent in both vigorous and moderate activity.	For moderate activity, an average MET level of 4.0 is used to calculate MET-minutes/week. For vigorous activity, an average of 8.0 METs is used in the calculation of MET-minutes/week. Sitting is assessed by the time per weekday spent sitting, resulting in a mean per day score.
Self-Efficacy for Physical Activity[c] *Perceptions of Exercise/ Physical Activity*	Personal and Environmental Factors	18-item scale assessing confidence from 0 = cannot do at all to 100 = highly certain can do (10 response options)	Total of all items (range of scores = 0 to 1,800); higher scores = greater self-efficacy.
Life Satisfaction Questionnaire 9[d,e] *Wellness*	Participation	9-item survey to assess various aspects of life satisfaction; items measured on a 6-point Likert scale from 1 = very dissatisfied to 6 = very satisfied	Mean score can be calculated, or individual items can be examined and categorized as dissatisfied (score of 1, 2, 3, or 4) or satisfied (score of 5 or 6); higher scores indicate greater life satisfaction.
Perceived Wellness Survey (see Appendix 29.A [online])[31] *Wellness*	Personal and Environmental Factors	36-item mind–body measure to assess wellness perceptions in six dimensions	Higher scores indicate greater wellness; see http://www.perceivedwellness.com/
SIP-68[f,g]	Body Structures and Function, Activity, Participation	68-question survey to assess QOL and changes in behavior resulting from disability or illness. Items are scored yes/no.	Scores range from 0 = best health to 68 = worst health. Norms established for wheelchair-dependent individuals, acute traumatic brain injury, and acute stroke.

(Continued)

Table 29.4 Outcome Measures of Health, Wellness, and Fitness—cont'd

Name and Type of Measure	ICF Category	Description	Scoring
Quality of Well-Being Scale[h] *Wellness*	Participation	71-item measure of health status and overall well-being over the previous 3 days in four domains.	Scores range from 0 = death to 1 = full function.
WHOQOL—BREF[59] *QOL*	Activity, Participation, Environment Factors	26-item scale, including four domains; items are rated using a 5-point Likert scale from 1 = low to 5 = high	Mean scores can be computed for each domain, ranging from 4–20; higher scores indicate higher QOL; norms exist for individuals with acute stroke, chronic stroke, community-dwelling elderly, and traumatic brain injury.
CDC Measuring Healthy Days[i] *Health-Related QOL*	Body Structures and Function, Participation, Activity	14-item survey used by the BRFSS to assess perceptions of health and their impact on participation in life and work.	Answers to each question are independent. A summary unhealthy days index can be computed by adding the answers to questions 2 and 3 in the healthy days module for a maximum score of 30 unhealthy days due to physical and/or mental health issues.
SF-36[j] *Health-Related QOL*	Body Structures and Function, Activity, Participation	36-item questionnaire measuring physical and mental health constructs of health status using eight subscales.	Likert scale; scores range from 0–100, with a higher score indicating better health status. Norms established for community dwelling and older adults, adults with depression, and people with migraines, arthritis, and epilepsy.
WHO-5[k] *Subjective Well-Being*	Personal Factors	Short, generic global rating scale of subjective well-being using five items, all positively worded.	Scores range from 0 = absence of well-being to 25 = maximal well-being. Raw scores can be multiplied by four to convert to a 100-point scale.

BRFSS = Behavioral Risk Factor Surveillance System; MET = metabolic equivalent; PA = physical activity; QOL = quality of life; SF-36 = Medical Outcomes Short Form Health Survey; SIP-68 = Sickness Impact Profile; WHO-5 = World Health Organization Well-Being Index; WHOQOL = World Health Organization Quality of Life.

[a]Fulk GD, et al. Clinometric properties of the six-minute walk test in individuals undergoing rehabilitation poststroke. *Physiother Theory Pract.* 2008;24(3):195.

[b]America College of Sports Medicine. *ACSM's Guidelines for Exercise Testing and Prescription.* 10th ed. Wolters Kluwer; 2018.

[c]Pajares F, Urdan T. *Self-Efficacy Beliefs of Adolescents.* Information Age Publishing;2006.

[d]Boonstra AM, et al. Reliability of the Life Satisfaction Questionnaire to assess patients with chronic musculoskeletal pain. *Int J Rehabil Res.* 2008;31(2):181.

[e]Borg T, et al. Health-related quality of life and life satisfaction in patients following surgically treated pelvic ring fractures: a prospective observational study with two years follow-up. *Injury.* 2010;41(4):400.

[f]de Bruin AF, et al. The development of a short generic version of the Sickness Impact Profile. *J Clin Epidemiol.* 1994;47(4):407.

[g]Post MW, et al. The SIP68: a measure of health-related functional status in rehabilitation medicine. *Arch Phys Med Rehabil.* 1996;77(5):440.

[h]Anderson JP, et al. Interday reliability of function assessment for a health status measure. The Quality of Well-Being Scale. *Med Care.* 1989;27(11):1076.

[i]Centers for Disease Control and Prevention. Measuring Healthy Days. Atlanta, Georgia: CDC, November 2000. https://www .cdc.gov/emotional-wellbeing/pdfs/mhd.pdf.

[j]McHorney CA, et al. The MOS 36-Item Short-Form Health Survey (SF-36): III. Tests of data quality, scaling assumptions, and reliability across diverse patient groups. *Med Care.* 1994;32(1):40.

[k]Topp CW, et al. The WHO-5 Well-Being Index: a systematic review of the literature. *Psychother Psychosom.* 2015;84(3):167.

Cardiovascular Risk Factors: Behavioral Counseling Interventions."[84] Clinicians can access these guidelines online to quickly obtain this information within the clinical setting. Although more research is needed to support the best counseling approaches, current recommendations support the use of behavioral counseling in the areas of healthful diet, physical activity, and smoking cessation.[83]

A systematic review of the effectiveness of counseling to improve diet and increase physical activity found that behavioral counseling can change these behaviors if the counseling is provided at a sufficient intensity.[85] Given the empirical evidence to support the efficacy of smoking cessation programs, the USPSTF currently recommends that all health-care practitioners ask their patients about tobacco use and make appropriate referrals to cessation programs when indicated.[86] There is also evidence to support the relationship between intensive physical activity interventions and decreased risk of falls in older adults.[87] There are, therefore, clinical research studies that support the value of clinicians addressing the modifiable behaviors of tobacco use, unhealthy eating, and inadequate physical activity with their patients/clients. Research has shown that some physical therapists have already started to address health behaviors with their clients,[16–19,88] but all therapists should be encouraged to engage in these discussions with their patients/clients. Recent studies have shown that many physical therapy educators lack the knowledge to train physical therapy students in the area of health promotion and behavior change techniques, yet most believe that students should learn these skills in entry-level programs.[89] In addition, it may be necessary to ensure that practicing physical therapists receive more training in how to counsel patients/clients in behavior change.[28,29]

■ THEORIES OF BEHAVIOR CHANGE

The decision to engage in or change a health-related behavior is the result of a complex interaction of numerous factors. Just as physical therapists must understand theories of motor control when planning interventions to improve motor function, an understanding of key theories of health behavior change is necessary to be effective in helping clients change their behaviors. Various theoretical models of human behavior have been developed and can be categorized as individual models, interpersonal models, and community and group models.[1] Behavior change interventions based on these theories have been carried out in clinical research trials and have been found to be effective in different situations with different populations.[1]

Health Belief Model

One of the earliest theoretical models developed to explain health behaviors was the *Health Belief Model* (HBM).[90] This individual model of health behavior was initially developed and articulated in the 1950s, when social psychologists in the U.S. Public Health Service found that despite public education about the merits of various screening programs (e.g., tuberculosis screening), large numbers of adults did not participate in the programs. Over the years, the HBM has been developed and extended to incorporate additional concepts and to explain a variety of health-related behaviors beyond screening. In the HBM, it is hypothesized that people's perceptions about their susceptibility to and the severity of the disease, along with beliefs about the benefits and barriers of taking the recommended action, will influence the decision to act (Fig. 29.6). Demographic variables, sociopsychological variables, cues to action (internal and/or external factors promoting the behavior change), and *self-efficacy*, defined as the confidence one has that one can successfully execute the action, will also influence the individual's decision to engage in the behavior. Results from numerous research studies conducted with different populations have provided support for this theoretical model,[1] and interventions based on this model have been found to be effective in supporting behavior change.[91–93] When using this model in the clinical setting to promote healthy behaviors, the clinician would first assess the individual's beliefs and perceptions relative to his or her health condition and the recommended health actions. Based on this assessment, the clinician would then provide appropriate interventions—for example, educating individuals about their risk factors for disease.[94,95]

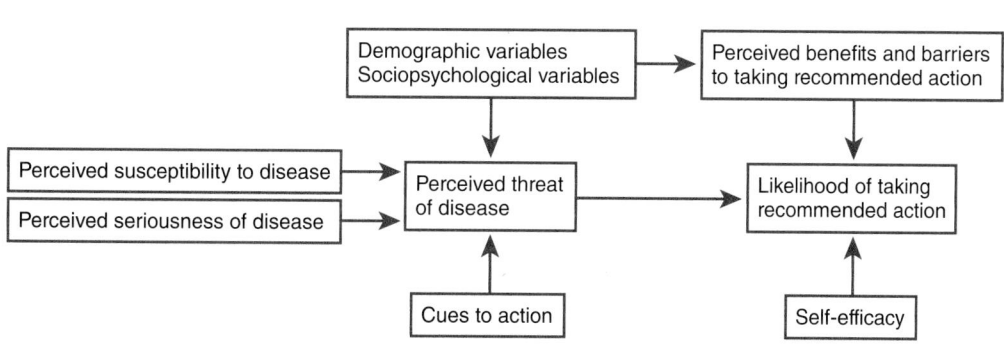

Figure 29.6 Health belief model.

Theory of Reasoned Action and Theory of Planned Behavior

The *Theory of Planned Behavior*, along with its predecessor, the *Theory of Reasoned Action*, is an individual model of health behavior that emphasizes the importance of and relationship between cognitions (thought processes) and behavioral intention. Fishbein proposed the *theory of reasoned action* (Fig. 29.7), in which he hypothesized that an individual's attitudes and beliefs about a particular behavior directly influence the intention to engage in that behavior, which then leads to the actual behavior.[96] The theory was later expanded to include the construct of perceived behavioral control and renamed the theory of planned behavior.[97]

The key constructs in this theoretical model are attitude toward the behavior, subjective norm, perceived behavioral control, and behavioral intention (Table 29.5). Clinical studies that have examined

a variety of health-related behaviors have provided empirical support for the constructs and the relationships articulated in this theory.[1,98–100] A clinician using this theoretical model to design a clinical intervention to change a behavior should begin by assessing the individual's attitude toward the behavior and the individual's perceptions regarding what significant others think about the behavior. The individual's perceived behavioral control can be ascertained by inquiring about any personal, social, or environmental barriers that might limit the ability to successfully engage in the behavior. The clinician can then tailor the intervention to the individual by addressing any areas that were identified. For example, the clinician may need to help the individual problem-solve to address a perceived barrier to engaging in the recommended behavior.

Transtheoretical Model (Stages of Change)

The *Transtheoretical Model* (TTM), first articulated by Prochaska, is categorized as an individual model of health behavior.[101] Key constructs within the TTM include stages of change, decisional balance, self-efficacy, and processes of change (Table 29.6).

Prochaska[101] hypothesized that there are five stages of change: *precontemplation, contemplation, preparation, action,* and *maintenance* (Box 29.2). A sixth stage called *termination* is occasionally included as the final stage of change and is defined as the stage when an individual has engaged in the behavior for more than 6 months, is no longer susceptible to temptation, and has high levels of self-efficacy for maintaining the behavior. An individual progresses through the first five stages as changes are made in a particular behavior. The model

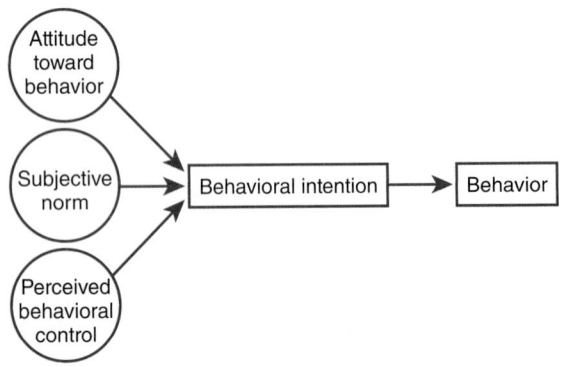

Figure 29.7 Theory of reasoned action.

Table 29.5	Key Constructs in the Theory of Planned Behavior[98]
Construct	**Definition**
Attitude toward behavior	Individual's overall attitude toward the behavior
Subjective norm	Individual's beliefs about whether others approve or disapprove of the behavior
Perceived behavioral control	Individual's perception about the level of control he or she has over the behavior
Behavioral intention	Individual's intention to engage in the behavior, the direct precursor to engaging in the behavior

Table 29.6	Key Constructs in the Transtheoretical Model[100]
Construct	**Definition**
Stages of Change	The stages an individual moves through when changing a behavior
Decisional Balance	The process of weighing the pros and cons of changing a behavior
Self-efficacy	The confidence the individual has that he or she can successfully engage in the behavior
Processes of Change	Activities used to support progress through stages

Box 29.2   Transtheoretical Model: Stages of Change[1]

Precontemplation

- Individual does not intend to take action within the next 6 months.

Contemplation

- Individual intends to take action within the next 6 months.

Preparation

- Individual intends to take action within the next 30 days and has taken some preliminary steps.

Action

- Individual has engaged in the behavior for less than 6 months.

Maintenance

- Individual has engaged in the behavior for more than 6 months.

Termination

- Individual engages in the behavior, has high self-efficacy for the behavior, and is no longer tempted to return to the unhealthy behavior.

is not meant to be linear, meaning individuals can skip stages (e.g., move from contemplation to action in one step). Decisional balance, or considering both pros and cons to a decision and its outcomes, and self-efficacy influence an individual's decision to move from one stage to another.

Different strategies (processes of change) are employed at different stages to support the behavior change (described in Table 29.7). Consciousness raising, dramatic relief, and environmental reevaluation are most useful in the earlier stages of change, whereas counterconditioning, helping relationships, reinforcement management, and stimulus control are most useful in the later stages of change.

Clinical interventions based on this theoretical model have been successful in changing behaviors, particularly in the areas of smoking, diet, and physical activity.[1] The TTM has also been examined in a study looking specifically at the exercise behaviors of adults with physical disabilities, and the key constructs and relationships hypothesized in this theoretical model of behavior were supported by the researchers' findings.[102] A clinician using this theoretical model to support behavior change should begin with an evaluation of the individual's stage of change for the behavior, as well as an evaluation of the individual's level of self-efficacy for the behavior. Box 29.3 provides a sample stage of

Table 29.7   Transtheoretical Model: Processes of Change[1]

Process of Change	Description	Stage in Which Process of Change Is Used
Consciousness raising	Individual increases level of awareness and acquires information about the behavior.	Precontemplation Contemplation
Dramatic relief	Individual experiences negative emotions regarding health risks associated with not changing unhealthy behavior.	Precontemplation Contemplation
Environmental reevaluation	Individual evaluates the negative impact on others of continuing the unhealthy behavior.	Precontemplation Contemplation
Self-evaluation	Individual considers self-image and examines personal values.	Contemplation
Self-liberation	Individual makes a commitment to change behavior.	Preparation
Counterconditioning	Individual substitutes healthy behavior for unhealthy behavior.	Action Maintenance
Helping relationships	Individual seeks social support for behavior change.	Action Maintenance
Reinforcement management	Individual increases rewards for healthy behavior.	Action Maintenance
Stimulus control	Individual removes cues for unhealthy behavior, adds cues for healthy behavior.	Action Maintenance

Box 29.3 Sample Stage of Change Questionnaire

Circle the number before the statement that best describes your current intentions related to walking 150 minutes a week.

1. I currently do not walk 150 minutes a week and have no intentions to start walking 150 minutes a week. (Precontemplation)
2. I currently do not walk 150 minutes a week but plan to start walking 150 minutes a week sometime within the next 6 months. (Contemplation)
3. I currently do not walk 150 minutes a week, but I plan to start walking 150 minutes a week sometime within the next month. (Preparation)
4. I walk 150 minutes a week but have been doing so for less than 6 months. (Action)
5. I walk 150 minutes a week and have been doing so for 6 months or more. (Maintenance)

change questionnaire, and Table 29.8 presents a sample self-efficacy for physical activity questionnaire. Appropriate processes of change can then be selected and implemented by the clinician to match the individual's stage of change and self-efficacy for the behavior (see Table 29.7), while also paying attention to the barriers identified by the individual and assisting to develop strategies to overcome them. Low self-efficacy for the behavior can be addressed by discussing how to maintain the behavior, even under challenging conditions.

Self-Determination Theory

In developing the *self-determination theory* (SDT), Deci and Ryan married two psychological approaches: (1) that humans are growth-oriented beings seeking to actualize their potential and (2) that social environments either support or block this human attempt at growth.[103] According to SDT, humans possess three basic psychological needs that are the constructs of the theory.[104] The construct of *competence* is the degree to

which people feel able to achieve their goals and desired outcomes. *Autonomy,* the second construct, is the degree to which people feel responsible for the initiation and maintenance of their behavior. The third construct, *relatedness,* is the extent to which people feel connected to others in a warm, positive, interpersonal manner. Deci and Ryan suggest that people thrive when environments support these three basic human needs.[103]

SDT can be used to understand and facilitate the development of motivation for a specific behavior, maintaining that when behaviors are based on personal values (intrinsic), they are sustainable, whereas when motivation is extrinsic (e.g., to please another person), they are less likely to be sustainable. Clinical interventions based on this theory have demonstrated positive outcomes for a myriad of behaviors, including exercise and physical activity, smoking cessation, eating, obesity and weight management, and low back pain management.[105–114]

Using the SDT to assist adoption of a behavior involves identifying the type of motivation the patient has, implementing strategies to develop intrinsic motivation (by providing relevant information and meaningful rationales for change), not applying external controls and pressures that detract from choice, and by supporting the individual as he or she explores resistances and barriers to change.[103,104] To build competence, the clinician provides relevant input and feedback, the tools and skills needed for change, support to overcome competence or control-related barriers, and assistance with achieving mastery in the behavior.[103,104] In addition, the clinician should create and maintain an environment in which the patient feels respected, understood, and cared for at all times.[103,104]

Social Cognitive Theory

The previous models, with their emphasis on the cognitions and behaviors of the individual, can be categorized as *individual* models of health behavior.[1] *Social cognitive theory,* with its additional emphasis on the individual's physical and social environment, is an example of a model of *interpersonal* health behavior. In an early article on social learning through observation,

Table 29.8 Sample Self-Efficacy Questionnaire

Place a check mark (✓) in the box that corresponds to how confident you are that you could keep up your walking program in the following situations.

Situation	Not at All Confident	Slightly Confident	Moderately Confident	Very Confident	Extremely Confident
When there is bad weather					
When I am tired					
When I am having pain					
When I am away from home					
When I have too much work to do					

Bandura[115] hypothesized that individuals could learn through watching others' behaviors and rewards. Bandura[116] then further developed the theory, added additional constructs, and changed the name of the theory from social learning theory to social cognitive theory. According to Bandura, an individual's behavior is the result of the constant interaction among the environment, personal factors (including cognitions), and behavior through a process called *reciprocal determinism* (Fig. 29.8).

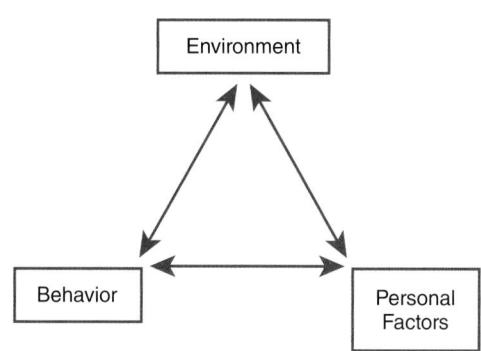

Figure 29.8 Social cognitive theory.

Key constructs within the theory include environment, situation, behavioral capability, expectations, expectancies, self-control, observational learning, reinforcement, self-efficacy, and emotional coping responses (Table 29.9). According to Bandura, self-efficacy, the confidence that one can successfully engage in the behavior across different challenging situations, is the single most important prerequisite for behavior change: It affects the individual's level of effort and persistence in engaging in the behavior in the face of difficulty.[117]

A number of clinical trials support the constructs and relationships proposed by this theory.[1,118–124] Interventions incorporating social cognitive theory constructs have been effective in changing health behaviors (see Table 29.10, Evidence Summary). Clinical application of this theoretical model requires attention to the key constructs as they apply for a given behavior and client. For example, the clinician may want to evaluate the individual's physical and social environment to determine what elements in the environment must be changed in order to support the particular health behavior being promoted. If the individual does not have the behavioral capability to carry out a particular behavior, education and training in the skills needed to perform

Table 29.9 Key Constructs in Social Cognitive Theory[1]	
Construct and Definition	How to Address Construct in Behavioral Change Program
Reciprocal determinism: continuous interaction of individual, behavior, and environment	Consider individual's environment, personal skills, and attitudes when developing strategies to support behavior change.
Environment: factors external to the individual that influences behavior	Consider how to incorporate physical and social support for the behavior.
Situation: the individual's perception of his or her environment	Correct misperceptions about the environment and the behaviors of others.
Behavioral capability: the individual has the knowledge and skills to successfully engage in the behavior	Provide education and skills training.
Expectations: the outcomes the individual anticipates from engaging in the behavior	Provide education regarding positive outcomes of the behavior.
Expectancies: value the individual places on the outcomes of the behavior	Relate the outcomes to the individual's personal values.
Self-control: personal control of the behavior	Incorporate goal-setting and self-monitoring of progress.
Observational learning: learning that occurs through watching others successfully engage in the behavior	Consider the use of peers as role models for the behavior.
Reinforcement: the positive or negative reinforcement the individual receives after engaging in the behavior	Incorporate self-initiated rewards for meeting goals, and support/encouragement from significant others.
Self-efficacy: confidence in ability to successfully perform a specific behavior	Build individual's self-efficacy by breaking the behavior into small achievable steps to ensure success.
Emotional coping responses: how the individual copes with emotions	Teach problem-solving skills and stress management.

Table 29.10	Evidence Summary Evidence Supporting the Use of Theory-Based Coaching to Increase Levels of Physical Activity

Annesi et al (2011)[118]

Design	Randomized Controlled Trial
Level of Evidence	Level II
Subjects	162 women age 21–60 years, BMI of 30–45 kg/m^2, no regular exercise within previous year
Intervention	IG: Exercise prescription for three sessions per week at wellness center over 6 months, nutritional and weight loss information, six 1-hour one-on-one meetings with wellness specialist trained in using "coach approach" based on social cognitive theory (cognitive restructuring, goal setting, behavioral contracting, tailored feedback, instruction in self-regulation). CG: Exercise prescription for 3 sessions per week at wellness center over 6 months, nutritional and weight loss information, six 1-hour one-on-one meetings with study staff focused on the processes of exercise and physiological concerns.
Results	IG had greater exercise session attendance and greater improvements in physical self-concept, exercise barriers self-efficacy, and body areas satisfaction than the CG.
Comments	Participants in the CG received similar amount of personal contact time with exercise specialist as participants in the IG to control for the Hawthorne effect. Separate wellness centers used for the IG and CG to avoid cross-contamination.

Focht et al (2017)[198]

Design	Randomized Controlled Trial
Level of Evidence	Level II
Subjects	80 participants (67 women, 13 men) age 55+ years, with knee pain on most days of the month, less than 20 minutes/week of structured exercise during the prior 6 months, self-reported difficulty with basic daily functional tasks due to knee pain, and radiographic evidence of grade II or III tibio-femoral osteoarthritis on Kellgren-Lawrence Scale.
Intervention	IG: 36 contact hours with study staff over 9 months of the 12-month study. Received exercise prescription and group-mediated cognitive behavioral counseling based on social cognitive theory to facilitate the mastery of key activity-related self-regulatory skills. CG: 36 contact hours with study staff for 3 months performing individualized moderate intensity walking and lower body strengthening in three center-based group exercise sessions per week. Participants in the CG given educational pamphlets with standard osteoarthritis self-management advice.
Results	At the 1-year follow-up, the IG had greater increases in physical activity as measured by accelerometer, increased mobility as measured by the 400-meter walk test, and higher self-regulatory self-efficacy and satisfaction with physical function.
Comments	Outcome assessments carried out by study staff blinded to group assignment to decrease potential for bias. Although total contact hours were equal for both groups, the sequencing of the contact hours was different between groups. The IG had contact with study staff up until month 9, whereas the CG had no contact after month 3, allowing for the potential for a Hawthorne effect.

Froehlich-Grobe et al (2014)[199]

Design	Randomized Controlled Trial
Level of Evidence	Level II
Subjects	128 inactive wheelchair users (64 women, 64 men) with an impairment for >6 months necessitating manual or powered wheelchair use for mobility outside the home, age 18–65, not currently physically active, with sufficient upper arm mobility for aerobic exercise.

Table 29.10	Evidence Summary Evidence Supporting the Use of Theory-Based Coaching to Increase Levels of Physical Activity—cont'd

Froehlich-Grobe et al (2014)[199]

Intervention	IG: Over the 6-month intervention period, participants received exercise prescription, resistance bands, educational information, a 1-day workshop based on social cognitive theory with interventions designed to increase self-efficacy and self-management skills. Over the next 6 months, participants carried out exercises independently and received 15 phone calls, during which study staff provided information tailored to the individual's experiences and needs. CG: Participants received exercise prescription, resistance bands, and educational information. Over the next 6 months, participants in the CG carried out exercises independently and received 15 phone calls during which study staff thanked them for returning (or requested the return of) exercise logs and inquired about any exercise-related injuries.
Results	At the 1-year follow-up, the IG reported more minutes of weekly aerobic exercise than the CG ($p < 0.05$). There was no difference between groups in aerobic capacity or strength.
Comments	Outcome assessments carried out by study staff blinded to group assignment to decrease potential for bias. One third of the participants did not complete the study, although there was no statistically significant difference in number of dropouts by group allocation. Cannot rule out Type II error due to low power.

Knittle et al (2015)[142]

Design	Randomized Controlled Trial
Level of Evidence	Level II
Subjects	78 participants over the age of 18, diagnosed with rheumatoid arthritis according to the American College of Rheumatology criteria, and not currently meeting the physical activity recommendation of 30 minutes of moderate-intensity 5 days per week.
Intervention	IG: Intervention based on social cognitive theory and self-determination theory: one group-based education session in week 1, an individual motivational interview from a physical therapist in week 2, two self-regulation individual coaching sessions from a nurse in weeks 4 and 5, follow-up phone calls by nurse in weeks 6, 12, and 18. CG: one group-based education session in week 1.
Results	At 32 weeks (end of the study), the IG reported increased leisure time activity, more days per week with 30 minutes of physical activity, increased self-efficacy for physical activity, and higher scores for autonomous motivation for physical activity.
Comments	Not clear if participants were blind to group allocation. Contact time for IG higher than CG allowing for possibility of Hawthorne effect. Despite randomization, the CG had significantly more males and higher disease activity scores at baseline.

Motl et al (2011)[122]

Design	Randomized Controlled Trial
Level of Evidence	Level II
Subjects	54 participants with diagnosis of relapsing-remitting multiple sclerosis, independently ambulatory or ambulatory with single-point assistance (i.e., cane), relapse free in past 30 days, not engaging in 30 minutes per day of physical activity on more than 2 days per week over the last 6 months.
Intervention	IG: Over 3 months, participants accessed four multimedia Internet modules that included key elements of social cognitive theory, engaged in twice-weekly online chat sessions, and participated in an online discussion forum. CG: participants received no intervention and were wait-listed to receive the intervention following completion of the study.

(Continued)

Table 29.10	Evidence Summary Evidence Supporting the Use of Theory-Based Coaching to Increase Levels of Physical Activity—cont'd
Motl et al (2011)[122]	
Results	IG had increased physical activity compared to the CG at the end of study as measured by the Godin Leisure-Time Exercise Questionnaire.
Comments	Participants paired at baseline for physical activity level and disability level prior to randomization process to ensure group comparability. Cannot rule out Hawthorne effect as CG did not receive any intervention.
O'Halloran et al (2104)[200]	
Design	Systematic review and meta-analysis
Level of Evidence	Level I
Subjects	10 peer-reviewed RCTs rated as moderate or high quality were included in the review, and eight were included in the meta-analysis. In all selected trials, participants were over the age of 18 and had a chronic health condition.
Intervention	Trials were eligible if the motivational interviewing intervention included (1) a clear focus on changing physical activity, (2) use of reflective listening in a collaborative relationship, and (3) emphasis on evoking the person's motivation for change.
Results	Moderate level of evidence that motivational interviewing had a small effect on increasing self-reported physical activity levels in people with chronic health conditions.
Comments	Authors followed the PRISMA statement and presented a clear search strategy and transparent process for inclusion and exclusion of studies. Variations in treatment fidelity and dose of intervention across studies may have contributed to the modest effect size.
Stacey et al (2015)[201]	
Design	Systematic Review and Meta-Analysis
Level of Evidence	Level I
Subjects	18 RCTs included in full review; seven studies examined effect of intervention on physical activity and diet, 10 studies examined effect of intervention on physical activity only, one study examined effect of intervention on diet only. Meta-analysis was carried out on 12 of the studies that examined effect of intervention on physical activity. All participants in selected studies were age 18 or older, diagnosed with any cancer.
Intervention	Intervention based on SCT or explicitly described and referenced any SCT component such as self-efficacy.
Results	A small to medium effect size found for the effectiveness of the intervention in improving levels of physical activity.
Comments	Authors followed the PRISMA statement. Provided clear search strategy and transparent process for inclusion and exclusion of studies. Studies screened for eligibility by only one reviewer despite Cochrane recommendation that two reviewers carry out this process. Variations in treatment fidelity and dose of intervention across studies may have contributed to the modest effect size.

the behavior may be required. The clinician should also use a tool to measure the client's self-efficacy for the behavior, and if low levels of self-efficacy are found, then specific strategies can be incorporated to build confidence (Box 29.4). The role-modeling construct can be incorporated into a behavioral change program by using peer mentors or group leaders.

Physical Activity Model for People With a Disability

The preceding conceptual models can be applied to a variety of health behaviors with diverse populations. The *Physical Activity for People With a Disability* model was developed to explain the behavior of physical activity in

Box 29.4   Strategies for Enhancing Self-Efficacy[1,115,116]

1. Break the behavior into small achievable steps.
2. Set goals, establish a contract.
3. Problem-solve potential challenges individual might face.
4. Mental practice and imagery.
5. Log progress, document achievement of goals.
6. Use peer role-modeling.
7. Ensure positive reinforcement received from others.
8. Ensure the correct interpretation of internal physiological states produced by the behavior.

a population of people with a disability (Table 29.11).[125] This model is based on the *Attitude, Social Influence, and Self-Efficacy* (ASE) model.[126] It integrates behavioral theoretical models with disability models and uses the ICF framework and terminology. In this model, environmental factors and personal factors interact to influence an individual's intention to engage in physical activity. Environmental factors include such variables as transportation, availability and accessibility of facilities, and assistance from others. Environmental factors also encompass social influence variables such as the opinion of family, friends, or health professionals. Personal factors include attitude, self-efficacy, health condition, and facilitators or barriers such as energy level, time, motivation, and skills. The authors of this model suggest that clinical application can include use

of the TTM's stages of change. The model has been useful in identifying barriers to physical activity in adults and children with disabilities, allowing better design of intervention programs to increase physical activity in these populations.[127,128]

Social Ecological Model

The basic premise of an ecological approach to behavior change is the recognition that there are multiple levels of influence on behavior[1] (see Fig. 29.2). Social ecological models are informed by four principles:

1. There are multiple influences on specific health behaviors, including intrapersonal, interpersonal, organizational, community, and public policy levels.
2. There is interaction of influences across levels.
3. Ecological models should be behavior specific and include identification of the most important influences at each level.
4. Multilevel approaches to behavior change are the most effective.[1]

Numerous researchers have demonstrated that successful behavior change occurs when interventions are planned in a social ecological framework, intervening at multiple levels to support the individual and populations.[129–133] A clinician taking a social ecological approach to facilitating behavior change would select at least two levels of the model and identify interventions that would be appropriate at each level. For example, to facilitate the adoption of a more physically active lifestyle in a patient being seen for low back pain, the

Table 29.11	Physical Activity Guidelines[44]
Age Range	Guidelines
Adults	Aerobic activity every week: 150–300 minutes of moderate-intensity aerobic activity (e.g., brisk walking) **OR** 75–150 minutes of vigorous-intensity aerobic activity (e.g., jogging or running) **OR** an equivalent mix of moderate- and vigorous-intensity aerobic activity. **AND** Muscle-strengthening activities on 2 or more days a week that work all major muscle groups (legs, hips, back, abdomen, chest, shoulders, and arms).
Older Adults	Should include a combination of balance, aerobic, and muscle strengthening activity. If older adults cannot meet the 150-minute guidelines, they should do as much physical activity as their medical status will allow.
Children and Adolescents	Should do at least 60 minutes of physical activity each day. Aerobic activity should make up most of the recommended 60 or more minutes of daily physical activity. Can include moderate-intensity aerobic activity, such as brisk walking, or vigorous activity, such as running, but should include vigorous-intensity aerobic activity on at least 3 days per week. **AND** Muscle-strengthening activities, such as gymnastics or push-ups, at least 3 days a week. **AND** Bone-strengthening activities, such as jumping rope or running, at least 3 days per week.

Source: https://health.gov/sites/default/files/2019-09/Physical_Activity_Guidelines_2nd_edition.pdf.
CG = control group; IG = intervention group; PRISMA = Preferred Reporting Items for Systematic Reviews and Meta Analysis;
  RCT = randomized control trial; SCT = social cognitive theory.

clinician might identify a recreation center (community) the patient could access to swim and a neighbor to take walks with (interpersonal) as two resources that could be woven into an intervention.

Community Models

Several behavior change theoretical models have been developed to explain behavior change at a community level. Although a thorough discussion of community models is beyond the scope of this chapter, physical therapists who are interested in changing the health behaviors of a group or community may want to familiarize themselves with community and group models of health behavior change and intervention planning models such as the *PRECEDE-PROCEED planning model.*[1]

■ HEALTH AND WELLNESS COACHING

In recent years, increased efforts have been made to provide psychological and emotional support for individuals seeking to change health behaviors, in recognition of the challenges to making sustainable behavior change. *Health coaches* are individuals with health-care backgrounds, knowledge of behavior change theories, and skill in building autonomy and self-efficacy in behavior change efforts. A variety of certification programs exist that train health-care providers, such as physical therapists and others, to provide health and wellness coaching services. In an effort to raise the standard of health coaching and create consistency across certification programs, an international set of standards has been developed and was launched in 2017, to which existing certification programs are trying to align.[134]

Health coaching is most commonly delivered face-to-face or virtually, and there is evidence to support the effectiveness of both delivery mechanisms.[135-137] A recent systematic review and meta-analysis on the effect of health coaching on physical activity participation in people over the age of 60 found that while both face-to-face and telephone delivery mechanisms resulted in increased physical activity participation, health coaching delivered face-to-face produced greater effects.[136] Future research on current virtual delivery methods is needed. Experts believe that developing a helping relationship between the client and coach is one key to the effectiveness of health coaching. The competencies the coach should demonstrate include the ability to:[138]

- Apply a patient-centered approach.
- Assist clients to identify their own goals and motivation for change.
- Use a self-discovery process in which clients take an exploratory approach to identifying useful strategies and participate in an active learning process.
- Help clients be accountable to themselves and learn how to monitor their own progress.
- Have relevant content knowledge to assist the client to change a wide variety of behaviors.

A typical approach to health coaching involves the identification of a vision for health and/or wellness, which is a future desired state; identification of health behaviors in which the client can partake that would move the client closer to the vision; identification of previous successful experiences with the behavior and environmental and social supports for behavior change; and establishment of weekly SMART (Specific, Measurable, Attainable, Relevant, Timely) goals and the assessment of self-efficacy for achieving goals.[138] Coaches encourage clients to adopt a "trial and learn" approach, treating goals as experiments to determine what works best to make wellness and health habits sustainable.[139]

Although health coaching is a relatively new intervention, significant evidence exists that generally supports its use as an effective approach to promoting sustainable behavior change. The U.S. Preventive Services Task Force has awarded a grade of B for behavioral counseling to improve diet and increase physical activity in adults who are overweight or obese and at risk for increase cardiovascular disease.[140] A "B" grade indicates that the intervention is recommended and has more potential benefits than potential harms. A systematic review by Frerichs et al.[141] revealed that physical therapists can effectively provide coaching services related to lifestyle behavior change, at least in the short term. These authors identified studies in which physical therapists were involved in smoking cessation, nutrition, weight reduction, and increasing physical activity, acting either independently or as a part of a team of health-care providers. In another study examining the effects of a 5-week intervention on physical activity in patients with rheumatoid arthritis, physical therapists provided group education sessions and a one-on-one motivational interviewing session to all patients in the treatment group and a nurse provided two one-on-one sessions focusing on autonomous motivation. The control group received a group-based education session. The treatment group experienced significant increases in physical activity, self-efficacy, and autonomous motivation, and the increase in physical activity was still present at the 6-month follow-up.[142] The amount of time required to provide health coaching has been shown to vary widely in the literature, but authors indicate that effective change can be promoted with relatively minimal investment of time.[141,142] Thus, physical therapists are well suited to deliver health-coaching interventions given the generous amount of time spent with patients, including within typical physical therapy sessions,[143,144] especially compared to other providers.[78]

Motivational Interviewing

Motivational interviewing is a client-centered counseling method designed to facilitate an internal motivation to change by identifying dissonance between behaviors and values as well as resolving ambivalence.[145] Such interviewing is a valuable tool within the context of health coaching because it generates autonomous motivation, which is a goal of health coaching.[139] This counseling technique, initially developed to support behavior change in the treatment of addiction, is now used with a variety of populations where existing behaviors have adversely affected health or QOL. It has been effectively used to encourage adherence to medical recommendations in general practice populations, to resolve behavioral issues with criminal justice populations, and to assist couples undergoing marital counseling.[145] Physical therapists have used motivational interviewing to improve adherence with rehabilitation programs[146] and to increase physical activity in individuals with chronic disease.[142]

The hallmark of this technique is the emphasis on exploring values and having the client recognize discordance between current behaviors and life goals. The clinician begins by asking probing questions to encourage the client to discuss his or her priorities in life and how current behaviors support or do not support those priorities. Encouraging the client to consider the pros and cons of continuing with current unhealthy behaviors versus changing to healthier behaviors may help resolve ambivalence by tipping the balance in favor of behavior change (identification of more pros than cons). Reflective listening by the clinician will allow a better understanding of the client's point of view and key contextual information related to potential challenges with behavior change. A clinician who is skilled in the motivational interviewing technique is respectful of personal choice and autonomy, is empathetic, avoids arguments, and provides encouragement to support self-efficacy for behavior change[145] (Box 29.5).

Motivational interviewing has been used in the field of health promotion to encourage change in lifestyle behaviors. Regardless of the underlying theoretical behavior change model being used to structure a health behavior change intervention, motivational interviewing can be incorporated as a technique to engage the client in important collaborative discussions about his or her behaviors. There is some empirical evidence of the effectiveness of this technique in supporting behavior change across a number of health-related behaviors, although more research is needed.[147] It has been shown to be effective in encouraging weight loss,[148] physical activity,[149–152] smoking cessation,[153,154] and fruit and vegetable consumption.[152]

■ HEALTH PROMOTION AND WELLNESS FOR INDIVIDUALS WITH IMPAIRMENTS AND DISABILITIES

There is evidence that physical therapists in the United States are moving beyond their traditional roles in secondary and tertiary prevention and engaging in primary prevention and health promotion practice in the general population.[16-19,88] Physical therapists are engaging in screening programs,[155,156] ergonomic consultations,[157] and sports injury prevention and conditioning programs.[158]

There is, however, a great need for physical therapists to engage in more health promotion activities with individuals with disabilities and chronic diseases. One of the specific goals stated in *Healthy People 2030* is to increase the number of health promotion programs for people with disabilities.[13] Research has shown that this population has lower levels of physical activity,[159–162] higher rates of smoking,[163] and higher levels of overweight and obesity than the age-matched general population.[164,165] Physical therapists have a unique knowledge and skill set that positions them well to be leaders in health promotion and wellness initiatives for individuals with disabilities. Unlike other health professionals, therapists also interact with patients over extended periods of time. This extended period of interaction and level of accessibility allows time to develop a rapport with patients and provides the therapist an opportunity to be influential in advocating for healthy behaviors.[166]

Examination and Evaluation

The patient management model in the *Guide to Physical Therapist Practice* provides a framework for therapists to carry out an examination (Box 29.6) and evaluation that will identify potential opportunities for prevention and health promotion interventions.[20] Examples of general prevention and health promotion goals and outcomes are presented in Box 29.7. During the history taking, the therapist should look beyond questions related to a specific impairment and inquire about perceived health or use a self-perceived health, wellness, or QOL questionnaire as described earlier. The therapist should also inquire about health-related behaviors, including physical activity, nutrition and/or weight management, current smoking status, sleep, and stress management.[78]

Box 29.5   Key Principles of Motivational Interviewing[142]

1. Express empathy.
   - Listen respectfully.
   - Do not judge.
   - Build therapeutic alliance.
   - Accept ambivalence.
2. Develop discrepancy.
   - Help client identify discrepancy between present behavior and personal goals and values.
   - Have client present reasons for change.
3. Roll with resistance.
   - Avoid arguing.
   - Accept reluctance to change as natural.
   - Turn problem back to client and encourage client to suggest solutions.
4. Support self-efficacy.
   - Enhance client's confidence in his or her ability to successfully change behavior.

Box 29.6   Elements of the Examination[18]

Patient/Client History

- Demographic information
- Social history
- Employment and work information
- Living arrangements
- General health status
- Perceived health and perceived wellness
- Family history
- Medical and surgical history
- Medications
- Clinical test results
- Functional status and activity level
- Past and current health behaviors: physical activity, smoking, diet, sleep, stress management, substance abuse

Systems Review

- Cardiovascular
- Pulmonary
- Integumentary
- Musculoskeletal
- Neuromuscular
- Communication ability/cognition/learning style

Tests and Measures

- Aerobic capacity/endurance (e.g., fitness level)
- Anthropometric characteristics (e.g., BMI)
- Assistive technology (e.g., appropriate assistive devices to ensure safety and allow participation in activities meaningful to patient)
- Balance (e.g., dynamic balance to safely engage in physical activity)
- Circulation (e.g., claudication or ischemia during activity)
- Community, social, and civic life (e.g., ability to engage in activities meaningful to patient)
- Cranial and peripheral nerve integrity (e.g., peripheral neuropathy creating risk for injury during physical activity)
- Education life: Ability to participate in activities and roles in educational setting
- Environmental factors: Barriers to engaging in physical activity, accessing fitness programs, and safe places to exercise
- Gait (e.g., ability to safely engage in walking and running programs to increase fitness level)
- Integumentary integrity (e.g., assess risk for pressure injuries, examine moles)
- Joint integrity and mobility (e.g., impairments that may affect ability to engage in physical activities)
- Mental functions (e.g., perceived wellness, attitude, and beliefs about physical activity, ability to understand link between health behaviors and health, motivation to change, ability to problem-solve around barriers)
- Mobility (e.g., impairments that could impact activities)
- Muscle performance: Capacity of muscles to generate forces to produce, maintain, sustain, and modify postures and movements required for functional activities
- Pain: Assess pain and impact of pain on levels of physical activity, emotional health, and participation in activities meaningful to patient
- Posture (e.g., body mechanics, ergonomics)
- Range of motion (e.g., impairments that impact ability to engage in physical activities)
- Self-care and domestic life: Assess ability to carry out daily activities and roles
- Sensory integrity: Assess sensory integrity to ensure ability to safely engage in physical activity
- Ventilation and respiration (e.g., assess fitness level)
- Work life (e.g., assess ability to carry out roles and participate in activities related to work life)

Box 29.7   General Prevention and Health Promotion Goals and Outcomes

Impact of pathology/pathophysiology is reduced.

- Fitness levels are improved.
- Health status is improved.
- Self-management of chronic disease is improved.
- Risk factors for development of injury and/or secondary conditions reduced.

Impact of impairments is reduced.

- Aerobic capacity is increased.
- Muscle endurance is increased.
- Gait, locomotion, and balance are improved.
- Motor function is improved.
- Muscle performance is increased.
- Postural control is improved.
- Relaxation is increased.

Activity limitations are reduced.

- Ability to perform physical actions, tasks, or activities related to self-care, home management, work (job/school/play), community, and leisure is improved.
- Tolerance of positions and activities is increased.
- Safety is improved.
- Problem-solving and decision-making skills are enhanced.

Participation restrictions are reduced.

- Ability to assume or resume required self-care, home management is improved.
- Ability to assume work (job/school/play), community, and leisure roles is improved.

Health, wellness, and fitness are improved.

- Self-perceived health and wellness of patient/client is improved.
- Patient/client understanding of health and wellness and health behaviors is increased.
- Self-efficacy is increased.
- Behaviors that support health and wellness are adopted.
- Self-management skills are improved.
- Intrinsic motivation is developed or increased.

Societal resources are utilized.

- Awareness and use of community resources to support health and wellness are improved.
- Patient/client satisfaction is enhanced.
- Therapeutic relationship with physical therapist is valued by patient/client.
- Health coaching skills of physical therapist are valued by patient/client.

Adapted from *Guide to Physical Therapist Practice*, with permission of the American Physical Therapy Association. 2014 American Physical Therapy Association. APTA is not responsible for the translation from English.

A systems review should be carried out to screen for risk factors for disease or injury, and appropriate follow-up by the physical therapist or referral to other health professionals as indicated should occur. For example, physical therapists should routinely take a blood pressure reading before having the patient/client engage in physical activity not only as a component of safe practice but also to be able to identify and report hypertension. Therapists who notice a mole should ask the client if they have discussed this predisposing factor for skin cancer with a physician. Fall risk assessments should be conducted with at-risk populations.

Based on their examination and evaluation, physical therapists may identify the need to engage patients in discussions about healthy behaviors and discuss the impact unhealthy behaviors may have on recovery. For example, discussion can focus on the impact of nicotine on tissue healing, or high BMI on joint health and overall health and wellness. Assessing the patient's stage of change (see Box 29.2) for relevant health behaviors will inform the physical therapist in identifying appropriate interventions. For example, if a patient is in the contemplation stage for becoming regularly physically active, health coaching that includes motivational interviewing may be appropriate in assisting the patient to identify a strong intrinsic motivator and to identify the benefits of regular physical activity so that decisional balance tips toward the benefits side of the benefits/barriers equation and the patient becomes readier to act. Referrals should be made to appropriate programs and health professionals when health issues that fall outside the scope of practice and qualifications of the physical therapist are identified during the examination.

Interventions

Physical Activity/Exercise

The APTA encourages physical therapists and physical therapist assistants to be promoters and advocates for physical activity/exercise.[167] Individuals with chronic disease and disability report lower levels of physical activity and exercise than does the general population.[158–162] The lower levels of physical activity/exercise reported by this population may be due to a host of factors including limited mobility, chronic pain, fatigue, fear of aggravating their condition, or limited access to fitness facilities that have the necessary equipment and personnel to enable safe and effective physical activity.[168–171] Physical therapists are uniquely qualified to evaluate fitness levels and prescribe fitness programs for individuals with medical conditions. The APTA has identified two priority populations requiring the knowledge and skills of physical therapists in physical fitness prescription.[172] The first-priority population consists of individuals with acute and chronic impairments, activity limitations, and disabilities related to movement, function, and health; the second priority population consists of individuals with identified risk for impairments, activity limitations, and disabilities related to movement, function, and health.

A physical therapy exercise program developed for a patient/client to prevent or remediate impairments falls under the category of secondary or tertiary prevention. However, if therapists are truly engaging in primary prevention and health promotion, a physical activity and exercise program to improve overall fitness to the maximal level possible for that patient should also be considered. Participation in physical activity may reduce secondary health problems, improve levels of function, and improve subjective well-being in individuals with chronic medical conditions.[173] There is evidence that exercise can improve QOL in stroke survivors.[174] The CDC recommends that adults participate in 150 to 300 minutes of moderate-intensity or 75 to 150 minutes of vigorous-intensity aerobic activity every week and muscle-strengthening activities on 2 or more days a week.[45] Children should engage in at least 60 minutes of physical activity every day and muscle strengthening activity at least three times a week.[45]

However, these physical activity recommendations were developed for the general population and may not be appropriate for patients/clients with disabilities and medical conditions. For example, people with type 2 diabetes mellitus should engage in 150 minutes of moderate intensity physical activity and strengthening 2 days a week.[45] Physical activity recommendations should be tailored to ensure safety and effectiveness for the patient's unique medical condition. When prescribing a physical activity program, physical therapists must consider not only the patient's condition but also any comorbidities and potential side effects or limitations associated with medical treatments. There are excellent research-based resources to help physical therapists safely test fitness and prescribe exercise for patients with medical conditions.[17,175,176] Beyond appropriate content of a physical activity program, physical therapists should consider the previously mentioned theories of behavior change and motivational interviewing to support patients/clients and optimize their chance for successful behavior change as they begin to increase their level of physical activity. Patients/clients can also be informed about physical activity programs in the community that are geared to specific populations. Physical therapists and patients/clients should refer to the consumer website of the National Center on Health, Physical Activity and Disability (see Appendix 29.B [online]) for education and specific information about exercise, as well as sports and recreational activities recommended for those with disabilities.[177] The benefits of engaging in sports should be discussed with patients/clients; people with disabilities who engage in sports have reported enhanced function, social benefits, and an increased sense of optimism.[178]

Smoking Cessation Counseling

There is strong evidence that even brief counseling of patients can be effective to support smoking cessation.[179,180] Given the strong evidence of the health risks associated with smoking and clinical evidence of the effectiveness of even brief counseling sessions, Bodner and Dean[180] effectively argue that counseling patients about smoking behaviors falls within the role of physical therapists and, given their prolonged contact with patients over the course of treatment, have the opportunity and the rapport necessary to be effective in smoking cessation counseling. As smoking delays tissue healing, physical therapists should feel comfortable engaging in a discussion of smoking behaviors with their patients and clients in all settings. In a systematic review, they found that intervention models based on the motivational interviewing technique are effective. The Agency for Healthcare Research and Quality recommends that clinicians include a question about smoking as part of their examination and evaluation and has designed a specific evidence-based program to assist clinicians in helping their clients address smoking behaviors.[181] The 5 A's tobacco cessation approach recommends that clinicians *Ask* their patients about tobacco use, *Advise* tobacco users to quit, *Assess* the client's readiness to quit, *Assist* the client with a quit plan, and *Arrange* follow-up to review progress toward quitting (Box 29.8). Physical therapists should also be familiar with smoking cessation programs in the local area and refer patients/clients as appropriate to these specialized programs.

Healthy Weight and Healthy Eating Counseling

Overweight and obesity are associated with development of numerous risks, conditions, and diseases[182] (Box 29.9). The *Guide to Physical Therapist Practice* recommends that anthropometric measurements be included in initial examinations. The measurement of height and weight will allow physical therapists to calculate the patient's BMI. Calculators and charts are available on the CDC website (see Appendix 29.C [online]) to assist therapists in calculating the patient/client's BMI.[183]

Patients should be educated about the impact that excessive weight and unhealthy eating have on current condition and future health.[183,184] The APTA encourages physical therapists to speak with their patients about the importance of eating a healthy diet.[185] Physical therapists can screen for unhealthy eating behaviors and make basic recommendations for improving nutrition.[186,187] As nutritional education may be outside the scope of physical therapist practice in some states, it is recommended that therapists review their state practice acts and refer patients to qualified health professionals as appropriate.[188]

Healthy Sleep Counseling

Insufficient sleep or poor sleep quality can adversely affect a patient's overall health and QOL. Current CDC guidelines recommend at least 7 hours of sleep a night for adults, and more for teens and children, increasing hours needed with decreasing age.[189] Health problems found to be associated with insufficient sleep

Box 29.8   Helping Smokers Quit: A Guide for Clinicians

1. Ask about tobacco use.
Implement a system in your clinic that ensures that tobacco-use status is obtained and recorded.

2. Advise all tobacco users to quit.
Use clear, strong, and personalized language. For example, "Quitting tobacco is the most important thing you can do to protect your health."

3. Assess readiness to quit.
Ask every tobacco user if he or she is willing to quit at this time.
- If willing to quit, provide resources and assistance.
- If unwilling to quit at this time, help motivate the patient:
  - Identify reasons to quit in a supportive manner.
  - Build patient's confidence about quitting.

4. Assist tobacco users with a quit plan.
Assist the smoker to:
- Set a quit date, ideally within 2 weeks.
- Remove tobacco products from the smoker's environment.
- Get support from family, friends, and coworkers.
- Review past quit attempts—what helped, what led to relapse?
- Anticipate challenges, particularly during the critical first few weeks, including nicotine withdrawal.
- Identify reasons for quitting and benefits of quitting.

Give advice on successful quitting.
- Total abstinence is essential—not even a single puff.
- Drinking alcohol is strongly associated with relapse.
- Allowing others to smoke in the household hinders successful quitting.

Encourage use of prescribed medications.

Provide resources:
- Recommend toll-free number: 1-800-QUIT NOW (784-8669), the national access number to state-based quit line services.
- Refer to www.smokefree.gov website for free materials.

5. Arrange follow-up.
Schedule follow-up:
- If a relapse occurs, encourage quit attempt.
- Review circumstances that caused relapse. Use relapse as a learning experience.
- Make appropriate referrals.

Adapted from www.ahrq.gov/clinic/tobacco/clinhlpsmksqt.htm.

include hypertension, diabetes, depression, obesity, and cancer.[189] Physical therapists are being encouraged to discuss healthy sleep behaviors with their patients.[27,28,76] A sleep inventory questionnaire can be used to evaluate sleep behaviors, and physical therapists can provide basic recommendations for healthy sleep habits.[190]

Box 29.9   Risks and Health Consequences of Obesity

All-causes of death (mortality)
Hypertension
Dyslipidemia
Type 2 diabetes
Coronary heart disease
Stroke
Gallbladder disease
Osteoarthritis
Sleep apnea and respiratory problems
Some cancers (endometrial, breast, colon, kidney, gallbladder, liver)
Low QOL
Mental illness such as clinical depression, anxiety, and other mental disorders
Body pain and difficulty with physical functioning

From https://www.cdc.gov/obesity/basics/causes.html.

■ HEALTH PROMOTION AND WELLNESS AT THE PROGRAM LEVEL

Patients who are discharged from physical therapy to continue their exercise programs independently often find it challenging to locate a facility with the necessary equipment or personnel who are sufficiently trained to address their unique medical challenges. Physical therapists have begun to recognize and address the need for physical activity programming that is specifically tailored to address the needs of patients with chronic conditions or disabilities. Fitness and health promotion programs geared to this population and offered in rehabilitation settings are growing in popularity. For example, physical therapists are providing fitness classes and health and wellness programs to youths with disabilities,[191] adults poststroke,[192] and individuals with cancer.[193] It is important to remember that these programs should comply with state licensing requirements for physical therapists and that the same standards for physical therapist practice be maintained whether the physical therapist is providing rehabilitation or health promotion interventions.

■ PHYSICAL THERAPISTS AS ADVOCATES

One of the goals stated in *Healthy People 2030* is the need for increased health promotion programming for individuals with disabilities.[13] Physical therapists can make a meaningful contribution to the health of the nation by providing health and wellness to this population within their own practices as described above. In addition, physical therapists should recognize their broader social responsibility, as articulated in the *Core Values* document of the professional association, to advocate for the health and wellness needs of all.[23] The APTA has numerous position statements highlighting the role of physical therapists in health promotion and wellness, including a position titled *Physical Therapists' Role in Prevention, Wellness, Fitness, Health Promotion, and Management of Disease and Disability* (HOD P06-19-27-12) that highlights the role of physical therapists in supporting scientific, educational, legislative, and other policy initiatives that promote regular physical activity and exercise to enhance health and prevent disease; advocating for physical education, physical conditioning, and wellness instruction at all levels of education; and advocating for community design that promotes opportunities for safe physical activity and active forms of transportation for individuals and populations of all ages and abilities.[24] The role of the APTA in advocacy for prevention, wellness, fitness, health promotion, and management of disease and disability is outlined in the position statement, *The Association's Role in Advocacy for Prevention, Wellness, Fitness, Health Promotion, and Management of Disease and Disability* (HOD P06-19-26-11).[194] It discusses advocacy in such areas as appropriate physical activity and exercise goals and priorities as recommended by government or other recognized organizations, appropriate efforts to enhance community design to promote safe physical activity and active forms of transportation,

the inclusion of physical education in schools, and physical therapists making healthy personal lifestyle choices related to active transportation and physical activity as priorities for the association.[194] Clearly, physical therapists have an important role at all levels of government, community, public education, and workplaces to advocate for health promoting policies and practices.

There are several national organizations and efforts in which physical therapists can engage to improve the health of society, including Exercise is Medicine (EIM), a global health initiative managed by the American College of Sports Medicine, whose vision is to make physical activity assessment and promotion a standard in clinical care, connecting health care with evidence-based physical activity resources for people everywhere and of all abilities.[195] EIM makes available free resources on their website to assist health-care providers in this role.

Physical therapists, with their unique knowledge base and clinical experience, are extremely cognizant of the needs and challenges faced by individuals with chronic disease and disability, as well as those of the general population across the life span, and they should participate at both the community and national levels to provide or ensure that all members of society are provided access to health promotion and wellness programming.

SUMMARY

Physical therapists have the knowledge, the skill set, and the opportunity to engage in health promotion practice across the continuum of care. People with medical conditions and disabilities who face unique challenges when trying to incorporate healthy behaviors into their lives may be in special need of the guidance and support of physical therapists. The APTA's 2021-2022 "Scientific Research Priorities for the Physical Therapy Profession"[196] cites population health as one of the three top action items, including investigating health disparities, social determinants of health, and physical therapy interventions related to health promotion and population health.

As the profession continues to define and develop its role in health promotion and wellness, physical therapists should identify and explore opportunities within their current practice environments to promote optimal levels of health and wellness of their patients/clients.

Questions for Review

1. What factors contribute to the health of an individual?
2. What is *Healthy People 2030*?
3. How does the World Health Organization define *health*?
4. Identify the different domains of wellness.
5. Define *primary*, *secondary*, and *tertiary* prevention.
6. Where in the continuum of primary, secondary, and tertiary prevention have physical therapists traditionally practiced?
7. Differentiate between the terms *health promotion* and *health education*.
8. What is the difference between the terms *exercise* and *physical activity*?

9. What tools could a physical therapist use to measure a patient/client's self-perceived health, wellness, or QOL?

10. What health-related behaviors should physical therapists inquire about during initial examination of patients/clients?

11. Describe the following theories of behavior change: health belief model, transtheoretical model and stages of change, theory of planned behavior, SDT, and social cognitive theory.

12. What is health coaching and how can it be used in the context of physical therapist practice?

13. What is the purpose of motivational interviewing?

14. What are the five steps of the 5 A's tobacco cessation approach?

15. What professional documents support the role of physical therapists in health promotion?

16. What are the current physical activity guidelines for children and adults?

CASE STUDY

Mary Boyd is a 53-year-old woman with multiple sclerosis referred to physical therapy by her family physician who reports she is complaining of decreased walking endurance and increased incidence of falls at home.

PATIENT HISTORY

Mrs. Boyd reports she was diagnosed with relapsing/remitting multiple sclerosis 15 years ago. She is being followed by a neurologist and her family physician and currently takes 20 mg of Copaxone and 20 mg of Provigil to help manage the symptoms of her multiple sclerosis. She becomes upset during the initial visit as she describes her growing inability to participate in many family activities outside the home owing to her concerns about falling and increasing levels of fatigue. She is fearful about her deteriorating ability to walk functional distances and worries about what the future holds for her.

SOCIAL HISTORY

Mrs. Boyd lives at home with her husband and three teenage daughters who she describes as very supportive. She does not go out alone, as she cannot drive. During the day, her husband is at work and her daughters are at school. Her primary social circle is her family and her large extended family in town.

PHYSICAL THERAPY EXAMINATION FINDINGS

Mental Status: Alert, oriented
Anthropometric: Height: 5 ft, 8 in, Weight 150 lb
Cardiopulmonary: Resting heart rate: 58, Resting blood pressure: 135/85
ROM: Full ROM all extremities
Strength: Decreased strength in right quadriceps (grade 3), right hamstrings (grade 3), right dorsiflexors (grade 4)
Balance: Difficulty shifting weight in standing
Endurance/Fatigue: Walking tolerance 5 minutes
Gait: Walked 100 ft with no assistive device, was unsteady, demonstrated a slight right foot drop, and used a wide base of support

HEALTH-RELATED BEHAVIORS

- Smoking: Smokes two to three cigarettes/day; she has smoked for 30 years.
- Diet and Nutrition: Has late breakfast due to fatigue first thing every morning. Reports she eats a healthy diet.
- Physical Activity: She does light housework throughout the day, but she spends most of her day sitting on the sofa reading books, working on her computer, or watching TV.

GUIDING QUESTIONS

1. Identify additional tests and/or measures that could be used to assess her level of health.

2. Identify additional tests and/or measures that could be used to assess her level of wellness.

3. What domains of wellness may be at lower levels?

(Continued)

CASE STUDY—cont'd

4. Which health-related behaviors might be adversely affecting her health and wellness?

5. How should a conversation about her health and wellness be initiated?

6. If Mrs. Boyd asked for help in changing her behaviors, select a theory of behavior change to guide the intervention. Which behaviors should be targeted?

7. What level of physical activity should Mrs. Boyd strive to achieve for health-related benefits?

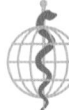 For additional resources, including answers to the questions for review, new immersive cases, case study guiding questions, references, and more, please visit **https://www.fadavis.com/product/physical -rehabilitation-fulk-8**. You may also quickly find the resources by entering this title's four-digit ISBN, 4691, in the search field at **http://fadavis.com** and logging in at the prompt.

Orthotics, Prosthetics, and Seating and Wheeled Mobility

Orthotics

Christopher Kevin Wong, PT, PhD, OCS
Daniel J. Lee, PT, DPT, PhD, GCS, OCS, COMT

Chapter 30

LEARNING OBJECTIVES

1. Relate the major parts of the shoe to the requirements of individuals fitted with lower-limb orthoses.
2. Compare the characteristics, advantages, and disadvantages of plastics, metals, and other materials used in orthoses.
3. Describe the components of contemporary foot, ankle-foot, knee-ankle-foot, hip-knee-ankle-foot, trunk-hip-knee-ankle-foot, and trunk orthoses.
4. Describe common scenarios for upper-limb orthosis use.
5. Explain the orthotic options available for patients with paraplegia.
6. Identify the features of lower-limb and trunk orthoses that are considered during the examination process.
7. Outline the physical therapist's role in management of patients fitted with lower-limb and trunk orthoses.
8. Analyze and interpret patient data, formulate realistic goals and outcomes, and develop a plan of care when presented with a clinical case study.

CHAPTER OUTLINE

TERMINOLOGY AND TYPES OF ORTHOSES *1150*
BIOMECHANICAL INFLUENCES OF ORTHOSES *1150*
LOWER-LIMB ORTHOSES *1150*
  Shoes *1151*
  Foot Orthoses *1152*
  Ankle-Foot Orthoses *1154*
  Knee-Ankle-Foot Orthoses *1160*
  Hip-Knee-Ankle-Foot Orthoses *1162*
  Trunk-Hip-Knee-Ankle-Foot Orthoses *1163*
  Alternative Lower-Limb Orthoses *1163*
SPINAL ORTHOSES *1165*
  Trunk Orthoses *1165*

Cervical Orthoses *1167*
Scoliosis Orthoses *1168*
UPPER-LIMB ORTHOSES *1169*
PHYSICAL THERAPY MANAGEMENT *1169*
  Care Before Orthotic Prescription *1169*
  Care After Orthotic Delivery *1171*
  Orthotic Examination and Evaluation *1172*
  Orthotic Instruction and Training *1173*
CLINICAL CONSIDERATIONS *1175*
  Energy Considerations *1175*
  Psychosocial Considerations *1176*
SUMMARY *1176*

An orthosis is a device worn to restrict or assist motion or to transfer stress from one area of the body to another. Alternate terms include *brace* and *splint*. An orthotist is a health-care professional who designs, fabricates, and fits orthoses for the limbs and trunk; a pedorthist is a health-care professional who designs, fabricates, and fits shoes and foot orthoses. The term *orthosis* is a noun, the term *orthotic* is an adjective.

Archaeological evidence confirms that orthoses have been used for at least four thousand years.[1]

This chapter presents frequently prescribed orthoses for the lower and upper limbs and trunk, as well as new developments in the field. Essentials for teaching patients to use orthoses are considered. Focus is on orthotic designs, materials, biomechanical rationale, and criteria for evaluating orthotic fit, function, and construction. While every attempt is made to use evidence-based research to guide clinical practice, paucity of research and heterogeneity within the population of orthotic users and within orthotic designs confound this effort.[2]

■ TERMINOLOGY AND TYPES OF ORTHOSES

Orthoses are named by the joints they encompass, the motions they control, or the city where they were developed. *Foot orthoses* (FOs) are applied to the foot and placed inside or outside a shoe. *Ankle-foot orthoses* (AFOs) encompass the foot and terminate below the knee. The *knee-ankle-foot orthosis* (KAFO) extends from the shoe to the thigh, while the *hip-knee-ankle-foot orthosis* (HKAFO) extends beyond the hip to the pelvis. A *trunk-hip-knee-ankle-foot orthosis* (THKAFO) covers part of the torso and the lower limbs. *Knee orthoses* (KOs) and *hip orthoses* cover their respective joints. *Cervical orthoses* encircle the neck. Most *trunk orthoses* are named by the motions controlled, although orthoses that manage scoliosis usually are named for the city where they were designed. Upper-limb orthoses, such

as a wrist orthosis, are named after the body segment(s) that they influence.

■ BIOMECHANICAL INFLUENCES OF ORTHOSES

Through the targeted application of force vectors, some orthotic devices can influence postural abnormalities like genu valgum or scoliosis. Abnormal postures are influenced by systematically applying opposing forces to the body segments around the joints that require control in a three-point control system. In the three-point control system, the fulcrum is located along the joint axis and applies a force opposite of two stabilizing forces located equidistant from the fulcrum. The three-point control provides resistance to joint-bending torque, which increases with longer lever length—the distance from the farthest contact point to the joint axis. The force upon the body segment is maintained via attachment to the orthosis by straps, with pressure under the straps dissipated by cushioned padding and/or expanded contact surface area. The amount of force and padding needs to be balanced to allow a comfortable fit while correcting the postural abnormality. Figure 30.1 demonstrates the application of a three-point control system on different joints and in different planes.

■ LOWER-LIMB ORTHOSES

Lower-limb orthoses range from shoes used for clinical purposes to THKAFOs. Characteristics and functions of the principal FOs, AFOs, KAFOs, HKAFOs,

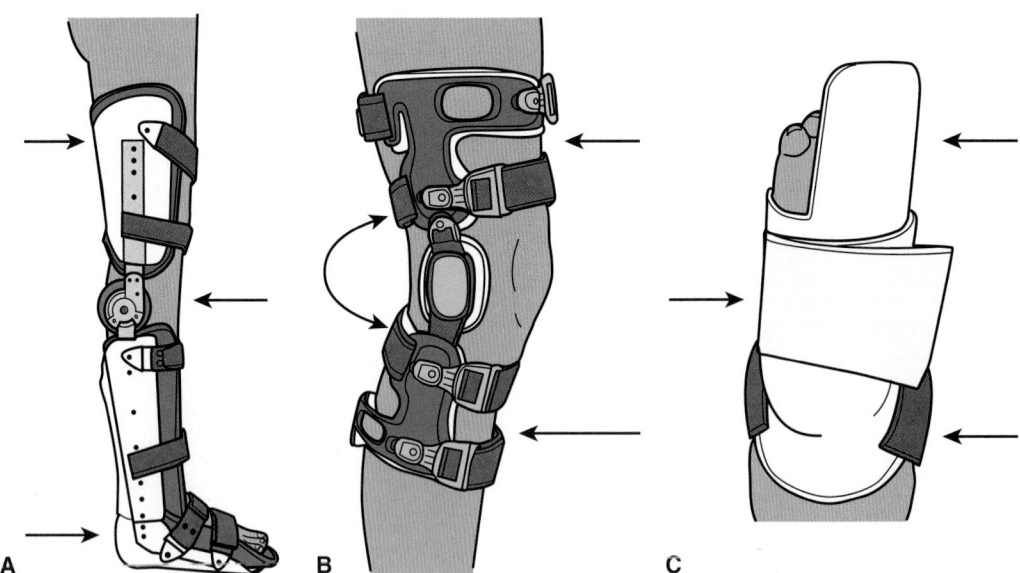

Figure 30.1 Examples of three-point force couples. (A) Sagittal plane: a knee-ankle-foot orthosis promoting extension of the knee joint. Note the long lever arm from the fulcrum decreases the amount of pressure felt on the thigh. (B) Frontal plane: a right knee orthosis limiting genu varum. Note the shorter lever length. (C) Transverse plane: a foot orthosis applying lateral forces to the medial forefoot and hindfoot to normalize the adducted curvature of the foot.

and THKAFOs are described along with a few select orthoses for single joints.

Shoes

The shoe is an orthosis and the foundation for most lower-limb orthoses. Shoes transfer body weight to the ground and protect the foot from the terrain and the weather. The ideal shoe distributes weight-bearing forces to provide optimum comfort and function of the foot. For the patient with an orthopedic disorder, footwear has two additional purposes: (a) reducing pressure on sensitive structures by redistributing force toward pain-free areas, and (b) serving as the foundation for AFOs and more extensive bracing. Unless the shoe is correctly fitted and appropriately modified, the alignment of the orthosis will not provide the designed pattern of weight-bearing. Major parts of a shoe found in dress shoes and athletic footwear are the upper, sole, heel, and reinforcements (Fig. 30.2).

Upper

The *upper* covers the foot dorsum. The anterior component of the upper is the *vamp;* the posterior part is the *quarter.* The vamp of a shoe used with an AFO that includes a footplate insert should cover the proximal portion of the dorsum to secure the shoe and the orthosis onto the foot. In a laced shoe, the vamp contains the *lace stays,* which may have eyelets for the shoelaces (Fig. 30.3). Laces provide more precise adjustment than strap closures. The latter, however, enable individuals with limited manual dexterity to manage the shoe more easily. A *Blucher* lace stay (Fig. 30.3A) is distinguished by the separation between the anterior margins of the lace stays and the vamp. The *Bal,* or *Balmoral,* design lace stay (Fig. 30.3B) is continuous with the vamp. The Blucher design is preferable for orthotic applications because the opening permits greater adjustability and ease of donning, especially important for the patient with edema. An *extra-depth shoe* has an elevated upper to provide more vertical space that accommodates a custom insert, thick surgical dressing, or hammertoes. The shoe *quarter* can also be of various heights. A low quarter

terminates below the malleoli to avoid restricting ankle motion and is satisfactory for most clinical purposes. A high-quarter shoe covers the malleoli to augment ankle stability. If an orthosis molded about the ankle will be worn, a high-quarter vamp is superfluous.

Sole

The *sole* is the bottom portion of the shoe. The sole may have both outer and inner soles with reinforcing material between. The foot rests on the *insole.* The *outsole* contacts the floor. Leather outsoles absorb little impact shock and provide minimal traction as compared to natural or synthetic rubber ones. To absorb shock, the shoe may have resilient material in the outsole, insole, an insert placed over the insole, or any combination of these. Older people should wear shoes with firm, slip-resistant outsoles to reduce the risk of falling.[3] Regardless of material, the anterior outsole should not contact the floor to allow easier toe clearance in swing; the slight rise of the sole is known as the *toe spring* (see Fig. 30.2).

Heel

The *heel* is the shoe portion below the outsole and under the anatomical heel. A broad, low heel provides greatest stability and distributes force between the back and front of the foot most evenly. For adults, a 2-cm heel

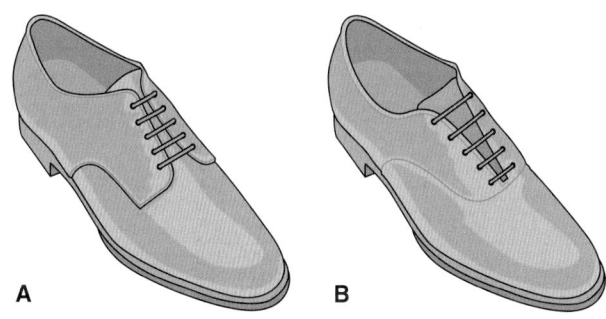

Figure 30.3 Low-quarter shoes: (A) Blucher (open lace) and (B) Bal (Balmoral) (closed lace). The Blucher lace stay is generally preferred for orthotic use owing to ease in donning and adjustability.

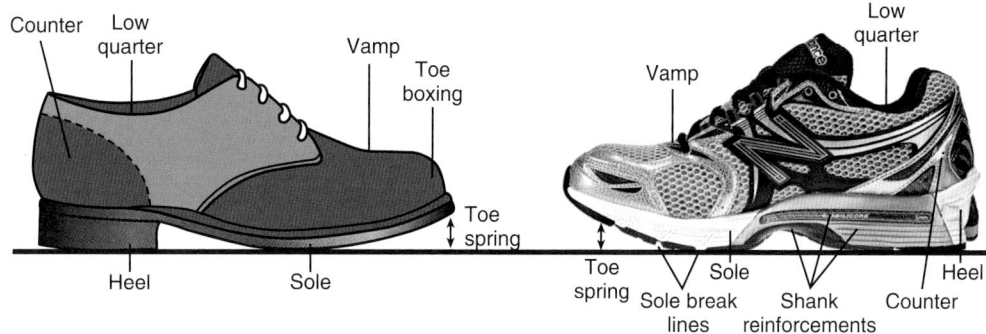

Figure 30.2 (A) Parts of a low quarter with Blucher lace stay. Note that the counter and toe boxing are internal reinforcing structures of the shoe. (B) Parts of a lower quarter athletic shoe.

or heel drop tilts the center of gravity slightly forward to aid transition through stance phase but does not significantly disturb normal knee and hip alignment. A higher heel places the ankle in greater plantarflexion, transfers more weight to the forefoot, and can require more quadriceps activation.[4] Transferring load anteriorly, however, may be desirable if the patient has heel pain. The higher heel accommodates rigid pes equinus and may,[5] or may not,[6,7] reduce tension on the Achilles tendon and other posterior structures. Most heels are made of firm material with a rubber plantar surface to prevent slipping.

Reinforcements

Reinforcements at strategic points preserve the shape of the shoe. *Toe boxing* in the vamp protects the toes from distal and vertical trauma. The *shank* reinforces the sole between the anterior border of the heel and the widest part of the sole at the metatarsal heads to support the midfoot (see Fig. 30.2). The *counter* stiffens the quarter and generally terminates at the anterior border of the heel. A shoe with a long stiff medial counter provides reinforcement along the medial border of the foot that resists medial hindfoot collapse.

Foot Orthoses

An FO may be an *insert* placed in the shoe, an *internal modification* affixed within the shoe, or an *external modification* attached to the sole or heel. FOs apply forces to the foot, which may enhance function and reduce pain by transferring weight-bearing stresses from painful areas to pressure-tolerant sites, correcting biomechanical alignment of bony segments, or accommodating a fixed deformity. Modifications can also improve the wearer's function by altering the rollover point in late stance or by equalizing foot and leg lengths. Many particular therapeutic aims can be achieved by various modifications.

Internal Modifications

An internal modification is an orthosis inside the shoe. Biomechanically, inserts and internal modifications are identical. Both distribute force on the foot more comfortably. An insert is removable, permitting the patient to transfer it from one shoe to another if the shoes have similar heel heights. Most inserts terminate just posterior to the metatarsal heads, a length referred to as three-quarters length, to avoid crowding the toes. Some inserts extend under the metatarsal heads to influence the forefoot, called sulcus length; full-length inserts extend the whole length of the sole. Internal modifications are fixed to the shoe insole to maintain the desired placement, but this limits the patient to the modified shoe. Because inserts and internal modifications reduce shoe volume, proper shoe fit must be judged with these components in place.

Internal modifications made of soft materials, such as rubber or viscoelastic plastics, reduce impact shock and shear, thus protecting painful or insensitive feet.[8,9] Inserts can be constructed of flexible, semirigid, or rigid plastics or carbon composite materials. A flexible heel-spur insert orthosis (Fig. 30.4) absorbs shock and slopes anteriorly to reduce load on the painful heel. Full-length insoles or inserts of semirigid or rigid material limit toe dorsiflexion, thus restricting the windlass mechanism, but can relieve metatarsal head pain.[10–12] FOs may alleviate plantar heel pain[13,14] and improve balance among older adults.[15]

Arch supports are intended to prevent eversion of the subtalar joint with flattening of the arch (pes planovalgus, pes planus). To provide medial arch support, a resilient *scaphoid pad* (Fig. 30.5) may be positioned or integrated into the medial insole with the apex between the sustentaculum tali and the navicular tuberosity. Early use of supportive shoes when children begin to walk, however, may inhibit normal foot development and is associated with higher incidence of pes planus.[16,17]

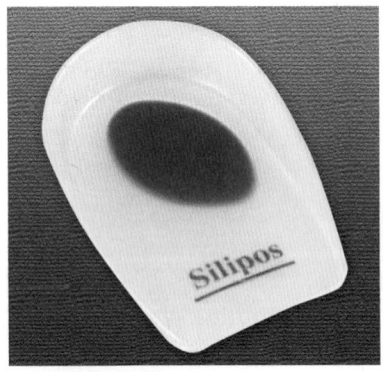
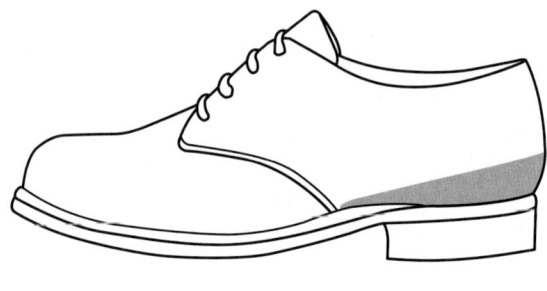

Figure 30.4 (Left) Plastic tapered heel-spur cushion with concave relief to reduce pressure. (Right) The shaded area of the shoe on the far right indicates the relative position of the heel spur when placed in a shoe.

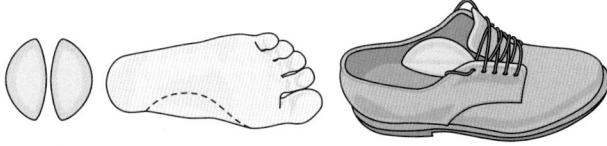

Figure 30.5 Scaphoid pads (left) are available with self-adhesive backing. They are positioned (middle) medial and plantar to the longitudinal arch. Scaphoid pad (right) glued to the inside of the shoe.

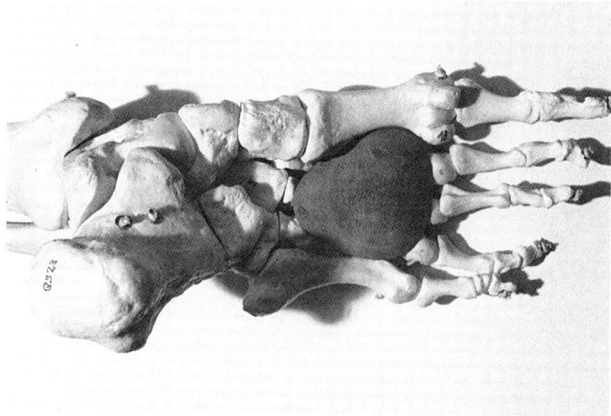

Figure 30.6 Rubber metatarsal pad. Whether used as an internal modification or as part of an insert, the pad should be oriented as shown on the skeletal model.

Older children with pes planus may benefit from wearing longitudinal arch supports.[18]

The *metatarsal pad* (Fig. 30.6) is a convex resilient padded component that may be incorporated in an insert or glued to the inner sole so that its apex is under the metatarsal shafts. The pad transfers stress from the metatarsal heads to the metatarsal shafts and thereby reduces plantar pressure.[19–22]

Some reinforcing modifications are sandwiched between the inner and outer soles to strengthen the sole and eliminate motion at painful metatarsal-phalangeal joints although at the cost of reduced windlass mechanism function.

External Modifications

An external modification involves material added to the exterior of the shoe, such as a heel lift. An external modification allows the patient to wear a shoe of appropriate design and size but may erode as the individual walks and is somewhat conspicuous. In addition, the patient is limited to wearing the modified shoe, rather than being able to wear a wider selection of shoes.

A *heel lift* made of noncompressible lightweight material provides slight plantarflexion and corrects for a leg length discrepancy of more than 1 cm; up to 1 cm can be accommodated inside a low-quarter shoe. A lift applied to both sole and heel can compensate for

greater leg length discrepancy without placing the ankle in plantarflexion.

A *rocker sole* has a marked plantar convexity with the apex posterior to the metatarsophalangeal joints. A *rocker bar* (see Fig. 30.7) is a convex transverse band affixed to the sole proximal to the metatarsal heads. A *metatarsal bar* (see Fig. 30.7) is a flat strip of firm material placed posterior to the metatarsal heads. The rocker sole, rocker bar, and metatarsal bar reduce the distance the wearer must travel during stance phase, allowing transition to forefoot weight-bearing while shifting load from the metatarsal-phalangeal (MTP) joints to the metatarsal shafts.[23,24]

Patients with diabetic neuropathy benefit from extra-depth shoes with spacious toe boxing (see Figure 30.2) to accommodate toe deformities, such as hammertoe, claw toe, and overlapping toes, and to prevent dorsal lesions. A rocker sole or rocker or metatarsal bar can also accommodate for decreased MTP joint motion impact stress on the foot as the wearer walks.[25,26]

A *heel wedge* (Fig. 30.8) alters frontal plane alignment of the rearfoot. A medial heel wedge, by applying laterally directed force, can aid in realigning flexible pes valgus or can accommodate rigid pes varus by filling the void between the sole and the floor on the medial side. A medial wedge is incorporated in a *Thomas heel,* which extends forward on the medial side to augment support for the longitudinal arch in flexible pes valgus (see Fig. 30.7).

Sole wedges alter medial–lateral forefoot alignment. A lateral wedge shifts weight-bearing to the medial side of the front of the foot. Sole wedges also influence forces on the entire lower limb.[22,27]

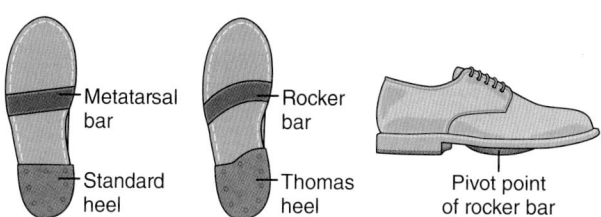

Figure 30.7 (Left) Metatarsal bar and standard heel. (Middle) Rocker bar with a Thomas heel (note the medial extension) and (right) pivot point of rocker bar.

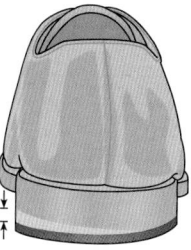

Figure 30.8 Medial heel wedge.

Foot Inserts

An FO is a footplate insert that is placed into the shoe. An FO may include a *wedge* (also called a *post*) to alter foot alignment and forces of the lower limb. For example, medial posting decreases subtalar eversion and increases knee adduction moment or varum.[28] Laterally wedged inserts may benefit some individuals with medial knee osteoarthritis;[29-35] FOs may alleviate patellofemoral pain.[36-40] Flexible flat foot can be realigned with inserts similar in design with varying depths to the semirigid plastic *University of California Biomechanics Laboratory (UCBL) insert* (Fig. 30.9).[41] The insert encompasses the heel and midfoot, applying a medial force to the calcaneus, and lateral and upward force to the medial portion of the midfoot. Table 30.1 presents evidence for the efficacy of lateral wedge insoles.

An FO insert may accommodate pes cavus[42,43] with a convexity that conforms to the contour of the plantar surface of the foot to increase the weight-bearing force area and reduce pressure on sensitive areas.

Ankle-Foot Orthoses

An AFO is composed of a foundation, an ankle control, a foot control, and a superstructure.

Structure

The foundation of an AFO consists of a shoe and a plastic or metal component. An AFO with a footplate foundation, whether thermoplastic or carbon fiber (Fig. 30.10), contacts the plantar surface of the patient's foot. The patient's shoe should close high on the foot dorsum to retain the orthosis. This AFO design can incorporate internal modifications such as a wedge into the footplate to provide good control of the foot. This foundation facilitates donning the orthosis because the

wearer can place the footplate into the shoe before donning the orthosis or strap the orthosis to the foot and leg before sliding the braced limb into the shoe.

Superstructure refers to the portion of the AFO above the ankle and foot components. Plastic AFOs usually

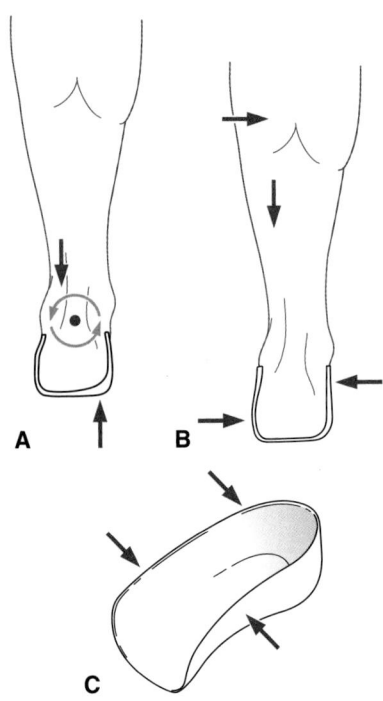

Figure 30.9 University of California Biomechanics Laboratory (UCBL) foot orthosis exerts control at the subtalar joint via a force couple (A) and three-point counterforces to control calcaneal eversion (B). A second counterforce system (C) restricts forefoot abduction. *(From May BJ, Lockard MA. In: Prosthetics and Orthotics in Clinical Practice. F.A. Davis; 2011:12. With permission.)*

Table 30.1	Evidence for the Efficacy of Foot Orthoses for Knee Arthritis
	Zhang et al. (2018)[168]
Design	Systematic Review and Meta-Analysis
Level of Evidence	1
Subjects	Inclusion: 1. Diagnosed knee osteoarthritis 2. Intervention: lateral wedge insoles 3. Outcomes: WOMAC, pain (FTA, Lequesne index)
Intervention	Evaluation of studies examining the effect of laterally wedged versus flat insoles on knee osteoarthritis–related outcomes
Results	Lateral wedge insoles can improve femorotibial angle but are of no benefit for pain and function in knee osteoarthritis.
Comments	Limitations: Limited the analysis to studies that examined lateral wedge insole compared with neutral insole but placed no restrictions on disease severity.

Table 30.1   Evidence for the Efficacy of Foot Orthoses for Knee Arthritis—cont'd

Ferreira et al. (2019)[169]

Design	Systematic Review and Meta-Analysis
Level of Evidence	1
Subjects	Inclusion: 1. Diagnosed medial knee osteoarthritis 2. Intervention: laterally wedged insoles 3. Outcomes: knee adduction angular impulse and moment
Intervention	Evaluation of studies examining the effect of varying degrees of laterally wedged insoles on knee biomechanics
Results	The overall effect suggests that lateral wedge insoles reduce the first peak and knee adduction angular impulse in individuals with medial knee osteoarthritis.
Comments	Limitations: Heterogeneity between study designs and participants makes comparisons difficult between studies.

Zhang et al. (2018)[170]

Design	Meta-Analysis
Level of Evidence	1
Subjects	Inclusion: 1. Diagnosed medial knee osteoarthritis 2. Intervention: laterally wedged insoles 3. Outcomes: WOMAC, pain, Lequesne index
Intervention	This study evaluated the mean difference from the first time point at baseline to the follow-up (12 months) within two groups, the lateral wedge therapy and control treatment.
Results	No significant differences in outcomes were found in groups that received laterally wedged insoles treatment.

Hsieh and Lee (2016)[171]

Design	Randomized Control Trial
Level of Evidence	2
Subjects	Inclusion: 1. Kellgren–Lawrence scores of two or higher in the medial compartment 2. 40–85 years old 3. No prior knee surgery Outcomes: 1. Knee Injury and Osteoarthritis Outcome Score (KOOS) 2. Hospital Anxiety and Depression Scale 3. Pain–pressure threshold 4. Physical activity level 5. Balance 6. Chronic pain grade
Intervention	Participants randomized to two different groups: rigid or soft laterally wedged insoles. Outcomes evaluated at three time points: 1 month, 2 months, and 3 months.
Results	Short-term therapy with soft laterally wedged insoles had improvements in physical activity, activities of daily living, quality of life, and pain.
Comments	Limitations 1. Long-term follow-up not performed 2. Comparison to physical therapy interventions not examined

(Continued)

Table 30.1	Evidence for the Efficacy of Foot Orthoses for Knee Arthritis—cont'd
	Felson et al. (2019)[172]
Design	Randomized Controlled Trial
Level of Evidence	2
Subjects	Inclusion: 1. Kellgren–Lawrence grade of 2–4 or higher in the medial compartment 2. 40–85 years old 3. Knee pain of greater than 4/10 4. Patellofemoral osteoarthritis must have a Kellgren–Lawrence grade of less than three. 5. No prior knee surgery. Outcomes: 1. Knee Injury and Osteoarthritis Outcome Score (KOOS) 2. Pain 3. Bone marrow lesions
Intervention	Participants were randomized with a crossover design between either neutral or laterally wedged insoles.
Results	Lateral wedge insoles produced a greater reduction in knee pain than neutral insoles. However, the treatment effect was small, and most patients did not achieve the minimally clinical important difference.

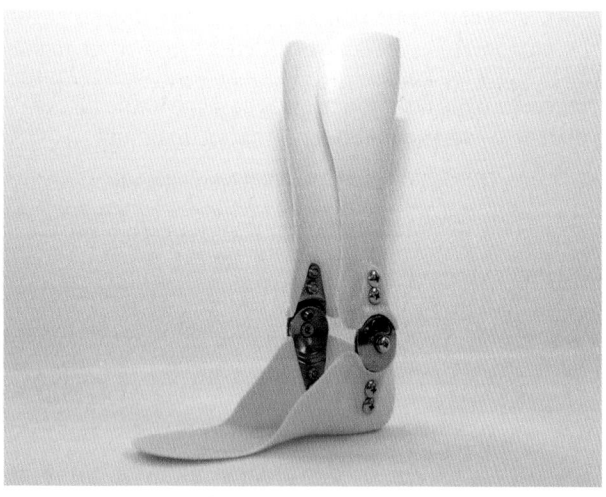

Figure 30.10 Plastic footplate included in a hinged ankle-foot orthosis.

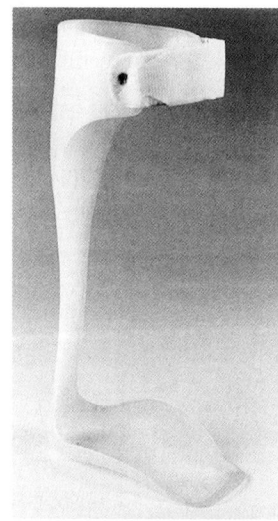

Figure 30.11 Posterior leaf spring ankle-foot orthosis.

have a single upright or shell. The posterior leaf spring AFO (see Fig. 30.11) has a posterior upright that provides leverage for dorsiflexion assistance but does not contribute to frontal or transverse plane control. An AFO with a rigid anterior upright stabilizes the knee. Both the solid ankle and the hinged solid ankle AFOs usually have a posterior shell extending from the anteromedial to the anterolateral midlines of the leg, thus providing excellent medial–lateral control and a broad surface to minimize pressure.

The proximal portion of the plastic AFO consists of a posterior or anterior band, shell, or brim with a strap fastener. The posterior band has an anterior buckled

(Fig. 30.12) or pressure closure strap. The farther the band is from the ankle joint, the more effective the leverage of the orthosis; however, the band must not compress the fibular nerve. An anterior shell that is part of a solid ankle AFO imposes posteriorly directed force near the knee (extension moment), enabling the AFO to resist knee flexion. Such an orthosis is sometimes known as a *floor (ground) reaction orthosis* (Fig. 30.13), although all lower-limb orthoses are influenced by the floor reaction when the wearer stands or is in the stance phase of gait.

Metal orthoses usually have bilateral uprights ending in a posterior leather-covered calf band with an

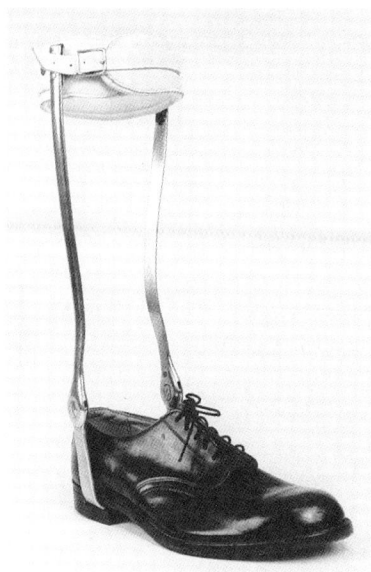

Figure 30.12 Conventional ankle-foot orthosis with stirrup attachment, limited motion ankle joints, bilateral uprights, and upholstered metal calf band.

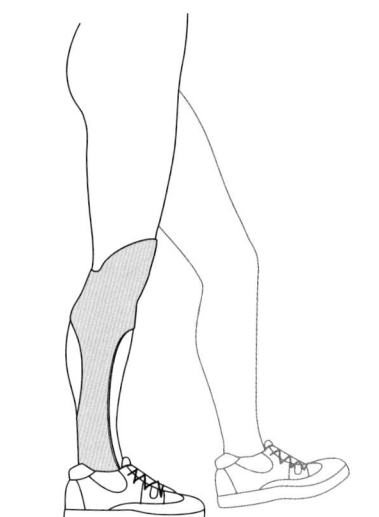

Figure 30.13 Floor reaction ankle-foot with anterior band provides knee extension moment in stance without preventing flexion during swing. *(From May BJ, Lockard MA. In: Prosthetics and Orthotics in Clinical Practice. F.A. Davis; 2011:276. With permission.)*

anterior strap. Carbon graphite and titanium uprights weigh appreciably less than aluminium; however, these materials are more expensive and difficult to modify. The AFO may have a single upright, either medial or lateral, which reduces the weight of the orthosis and is less conspicuous; however, an AFO with one upright is somewhat less stable.

Ankle Control

Most AFOs are worn to control ankle motion by limiting plantarflexion and/or dorsiflexion, or by assisting

motion. Without an orthosis, the patient with dorsiflexor weakness or paralysis risks dragging the forefoot during the swing phase.

A common orthotic solution to control toe drag is the *posterior leaf spring AFO* that arises from a plastic insert (Fig. 30.12). This orthosis can be prefabricated or custom made and is streamlined and lightweight. During early stance, the posterior upright acts as a leaf spring, bending backward slightly. When the patient progresses into swing phase, the upright recoils, "springing" forward to lift the foot. The posterior leaf spring AFO can be adjusted by the orthotist who can remove material to weaken the spring.

Adjustable motion assistance can be achieved with a steel dorsiflexion spring assist (Klenzak joint) (Fig. 30.14) near the ankle. The coiled spring compresses in stance and rebounds during swing. Tightness of the spring can be adjusted by turning a screw on top of the spring. An orthosis with a dorsiflexion spring assist is noticeably bulkier than the posterior leaf spring model. Both the dorsiflexion spring assist and posterior leaf spring orthoses yield into plantarflexion at heel contact, affording the wearer protection against inadvertent knee flexion. Other AFO designs that control toe drag are presented in Figures 30.15 and 30.16.

An alternate approach to prevent toe drag is using plantarflexion resistance provided by a *hinged ankle-foot orthosis*. The hinge may have a plastic overlap joint, a flexible plastic rod, or a metal joint. A hinged AFO permits sagittal motion but can be outfitted with a *posterior stop* (Fig. 30.17). The posterior stop prevents toe drag in swing phase and imposes a flexion force at the knee during early stance, preventing the knee from hyperextending.

During the stance phase, an *anterior stop* at the ankle can limit dorsiflexion and thus resist inadvertent knee

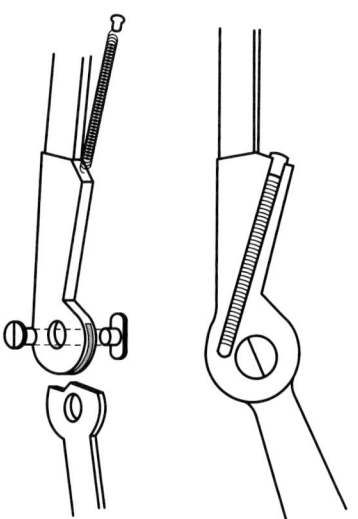

Figure 30.14 Hinged joint with dorsiflexion spring assist.

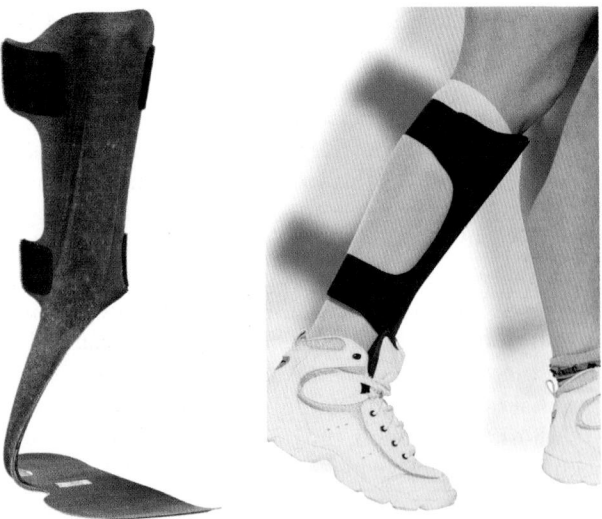

Figure 30.15 ToeOFF ankle-foot orthosis. This fiberglass, carbon fiber, and Kevlar orthosis is designed to provide dorsiflexion assistance in the presence of mild to severe footdrop accompanied by mild to moderate ankle instability. This orthosis is contraindicated in the presence of moderate to severe spasticity or edema. *(Courtesy of CAMP Scandinavia AB. SE 25467 Helsingborg, Sweden.)*

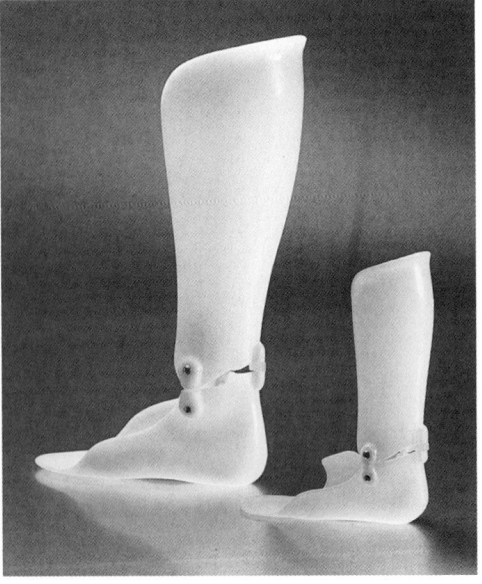

Figure 30.17 Plastic hinged ankle-foot orthoses with plantarflexion stops. *(Courtesy of Otto Bock, Minneapolis, MN 55447.)*

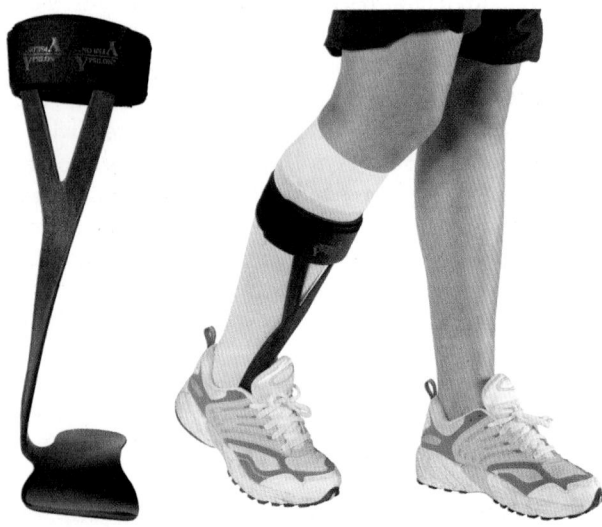

Figure 30.16 Ypsilon ankle-foot orthosis. This carbon composite ankle-foot orthosis is designed to provide dorsiflexion assistance in the presence of mild to moderate isolated drop foot. It promotes free ankle movements (medial, lateral, and rotational). The proximal Y-shape provides tibia crest clearance. This orthosis is contraindicated for an unstable ankle joint or in the presence of moderate to severe spasticity or edema. *(Courtesy of CAMP Scandinavia AB. SE 25467 Helsingborg Sweden.)*

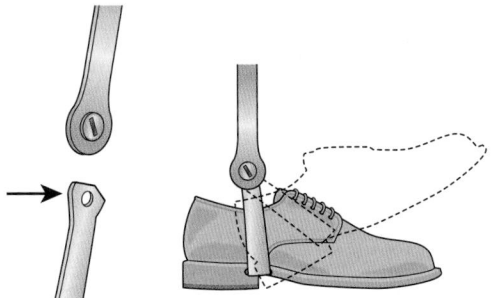

Figure 30.18 Steel stirrup (left) with posterior stop at its distal end (arrow). Posterior stop (right) incorporated into a stirrup. A posterior stop is designed to allow dorsiflexion and prevent or stop plantarflexion.

bending before late stance. Adjustable stops for both dorsiflexion and plantarflexion can be incorporated into the ankle joint of a plastic or metal hinged AFO (Fig. 30.18). Limiting all foot and ankle motion can be achieved with a plastic *solid AFO* (Fig. 30.19); its trimlines (edges) are anterior to the malleoli.

An alternative to the plastic solid ankle AFO is a metal joint called the *limited motion joint*, which resists both plantarflexion and dorsiflexion. One type of limited motion joint is a pair of *bichannel adjustable ankle locks (BiCAALs)* (Fig. 30.20), each of which has an anterior and a posterior spring. The springs can be replaced with metal pins that can be adjusted to allow limited range of motion (ROM). To compensate for lack of plantarflexion in early stance, the shoe worn with the solid AFO or the orthosis with a limited motion stop should have a resilient heel. Similarly, to facilitate rollover in late stance, the shoe sole should have a rocker bar.

Eversion and inversion are restricted by any orthotic design that covers the malleoli including a solid AFO, a hinged AFO, or medial–lateral plastic shells. The posterior leaf spring orthosis does not cover the malleoli

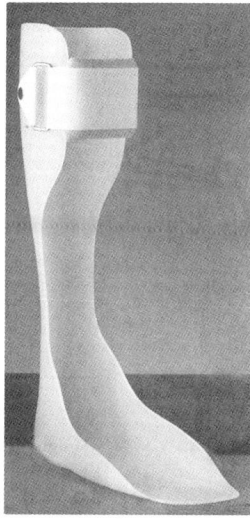

Figure 30.19 Plastic solid ankle-foot orthosis. *(Courtesy of Otto Bock, Minneapolis, MN 55447.)*

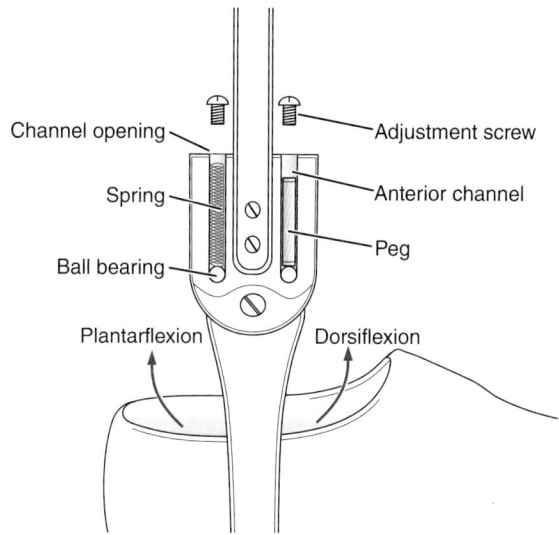

Figure 30.20 Bichannel adjustable ankle locks. Note this ankle joint includes two channels. A spring placed in the posterior channel (shown) provides dorsiflexion assist. A pin placed in the posterior channel creates plantarflexion stop. *(From May BJ, Lockard MA. In: Prosthetics and Orthotics in Clinical Practice. F.A. Davis; 2011:254. With permission.)*

and thus provides no frontal plane control. The solid AFO trimlines are anterior to the malleoli. The hinged AFO is divided transversely at the ankle to form the two portions by overlapping plastic or metal joints (see Fig. 30.10) to permit dorsiflexion and plantarflexion ROM that facilitates foot-flat position in early stance unless motion is limited by a mechanical stop. A plantarflexion stop restricts ankle plantarflexion ROM, thereby preventing footdrop in swing phase but also restricting foot flat in early stance. Regardless, the uprights containing the hinge joints will restrict frontal plane motion. Plastic shells over both medial and lateral malleoli, encircled with straps, provide some frontal plane control depending on the stiffness of the plastic material. Without a foot plate, plastic shells do not interfere significantly with sagittal plane motion, making such a device adequate for use during sports.

Clinical Considerations

Adults with hemiplegia realize several benefits when wearing AFOs.[44] Orthoses can prevent or reduce plantarflexion and inversion contractures,[45,46] improve balance,[47,48] and enhance gait by restoring heel contact, absorbing shock on the paretic limb, increasing midstance stability, improving forward progression in late stance, and enabling the paretic limb to clear the floor during swing phase.[21,49–54] The AFO with posterior ankle stop reduces genu recurvatum.[45] Orthoses with an anterior ankle stop or anterior upright facilitate weight shift to the paretic limb and can prevent knee instability.[50] Patients wearing AFOs increased their velocity[54] and reduced the energy cost of walking.[55,56] They expressed satisfaction with their orthoses, deeming comfort and function more important than the appearance of the device.[57]

Functional electrical stimulation (FES) is an alternative to an AFO for some adults with stroke.[44] Commercially available systems incorporate a cuff worn around the proximal leg; the interior of the cuff contains a skin electrode placed over the fibular nerve. A self-contained electrical unit stimulates the electrode. The systems, such as Bioness L300 (Valencia, CA)[58,59] and Walkaide (Reno NV),[60] enable dorsiflexion in swing phase, thereby reducing the risk of footdrop and tripping. Comparison of performance of those fitted with FES with others who wore AFOs demonstrated that both groups improved gait speed, although the FES users expressed higher satisfaction.[59,61–63] Additionally, preliminary experience with implantable peroneal electrode augmenting an AFO is favorable.[64]

Children with cerebral palsy (CP) improved stride length[65] and gait velocity while wearing AFOs.[66] AFOs also increase dorsiflexion during swing phase and overall function.[67] The most favorable results were achieved with hinged AFOs.[68] Youngsters who exhibited marked knee flexion when walking performed better when wearing AFOs with a solid ankle with an anterior band (floor reaction orthosis).[69] Orthoses also can reduce abnormal hip rotation.[70] Hinged AFOs lessened energy expenditure more than other AFO designs.[71–73] FES may benefit some children with spastic hemiplegia as an alternative to an AFO.[74,75] Orthoses also improved the kinematic and kinetic properties of the gait of children with spina bifida[76] with reduced oxygen cost.[77]

When maximal combined control of the ankle and foot joints is required, the AFO can be incorporated into a boot. A Charcot restraint orthotic walker is a custom device encasing the entire lower leg, ankle, and foot within a two-part clamshell orthosis designed to prevent

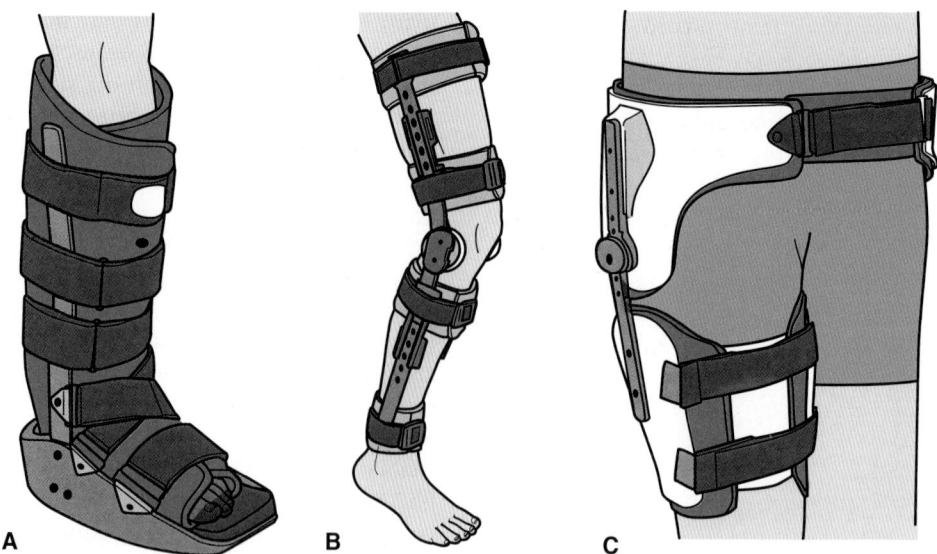

Figure 30.21 Rehab orthoses: (Left) Walking boot. (Middle) Knee orthosis with adjustable lock. (Right) Hip orthosis.

progression of diabetic foot deformity while protecting vulnerable skin.[77] A walking boot is a similar over-the-counter orthosis used after injuries such as ankle sprain, Achilles rupture, or foot fracture to immobilize the entire foot and ankle during healing (Fig. 30.21).[78–80] A plastic shell AO that does not include the foot is often used after ankle sprain to support the lateral ligaments while allowing normal sagittal plane motion as the individual returns to their prior activities.[81]

Knee-Ankle-Foot Orthoses

Individuals with more extensive paralysis/paresis or limb deformity may benefit from KAFOs, which consist of a shoe, foundation, ankle control, foot control, knee control, and superstructure. The shoe, foundation, ankle control, and foot control are selected from components that were already described. Most KAFOs have medial and lateral uprights terminating in one or two thigh bands, which provide structural stability to the orthosis. An alternative to bilateral proximal uprights is a single posterior upright, which is less restrictive.

Knee Control

Most KAFOs include a medial and a lateral upright plus hinges that provide medial–lateral and hyperextension restriction while permitting knee flexion. The *offset joint* (Fig. 30.22) is a hinge placed posterior to the midline of the leg. When the wearer stands and walks on a level surface, the individual's weight line passes in front of the offset joint, stabilizing the knee in extension during the early stance phase of gait. The offset joint does not hamper knee flexion during swing or sitting. The joint may, however, flex inadvertently when the wearer stands on a ramp due to the ground reaction forces traveling posterior to the knee joint.

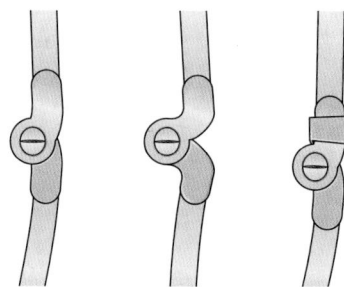

Figure 30.22 Two examples of offset knee joints (left and middle) and a drop ring lock (right).

Knee locks provide security regardless of the terrain. The most common type is the *drop ring lock* (Fig. 30.22). A spring-loaded retention button ensures that the lock will not drop into place while the patient rises from a chair; the user pushes the ring past the button to lock the orthotic knee. For maximum stability, both the medial and lateral knee joints should be locked. A design that provides bilateral locking is the *pawl lock with bail release* (Fig. 30.23). The pawl lock with bail release is bulkier than drop ring locks but allows the wearer to unlock the knee to sit down without using their hands.

Sagittal stability is augmented by an anterior band that completes the three-point pressure system necessary for stability. A rigid anterior band provides posteriorly directed force but does not interfere with sitting. The prepatellar band rests over the proximal portion of the leg; the suprapatellar band fits over the anterodistal thigh (see Fig. 30.1).

Genu valgum or varum is best controlled with a KAFO that incorporates a plastic calf shell shaped to apply corrective force. To reduce genu valgum, the medial portion of the shell extends proximally to apply laterally directed force at the knee. Extending the lateral portion of the shell controls genu varum. The shell does not require extra time in donning and applies force over a broad area without impinging on the popliteal fossa (Fig. 30.24).

A stance control KAFO (SC-KAFO) prevents knee flexion during stance phase yet permits knee flexion during swing phase, thus preventing instability in those with weak knee extensors and allowing for a natural gait.[82,83] While the design of the SC-KAFO appears similar to that of the KAFO, the key design difference is a weight-activated knee joint mechanism that will engage and effectively "lock" the orthotic in a particular ROM to prevent the knee from collapsing into flexion. This safety measure benefits those with neuromuscular disease like polio/postpolio syndrome, spinal cord injury (SCI), and isolate knee extensor weakness. As compared with walking with a KAFO with locked knee, wearing an orthosis with stance control permits faster, more symmetrical gait with less gait deviations, although energy consumption remains unchanged.[84,85] However, recent technological advancements have introduced a microprocessor-controlled KAFO that utilizes hydraulic dampening to provide dynamic control of the orthotic during gait. The microprocessor can detect the phase of gait and provide less or more stability based on the user's specific needs. While the microprocessor-controlled KAFO weighs more than a SC-KAFO, it provides significantly better outcomes on gait, balance, and functional mobility measures.[86]

Mechanical Knee-Ankle-Foot Orthoses for Paraplegia

KAFOs are often prescribed for adults with paraplegia (Fig. 30.25). Each orthosis includes either a plastic solid ankle section or BiCAAL ankle joints set in slight dorsiflexion, a pretibial band, a pawl knee lock with bail release, and a single thigh band. The orthoses enable the patient to stand without crutches by leaning backward; the iliofemoral ligaments restrain excessive lean. Gait requires forearm crutches or a walker. The pattern usually is swing-to or swing-through, with the aid of crutches or a walker. Although the orthoses do not restrict hip motion, the patient with thoracic spinal injury cannot flex the hips voluntarily. Some individuals perform a two- or four-point gait by shifting the trunk enough to allow each leg to swing forward in a pendular manner.

The Walkabout (Polymedic, Sydney, New South Wales, Australia) consists of a pair of KAFOs with a hinge joining the proximal medial uprights of the two

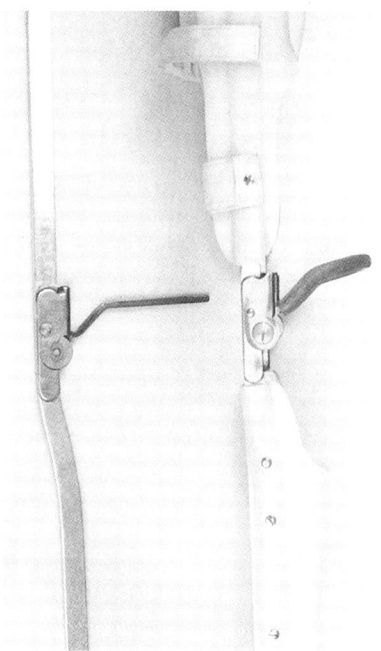

Figure 30.23 Knee joint hinge with pawl lock: (A) basic component and (B) pawl lock installed in knee-ankle-foot orthosis with bail shaped to curve posteriorly.

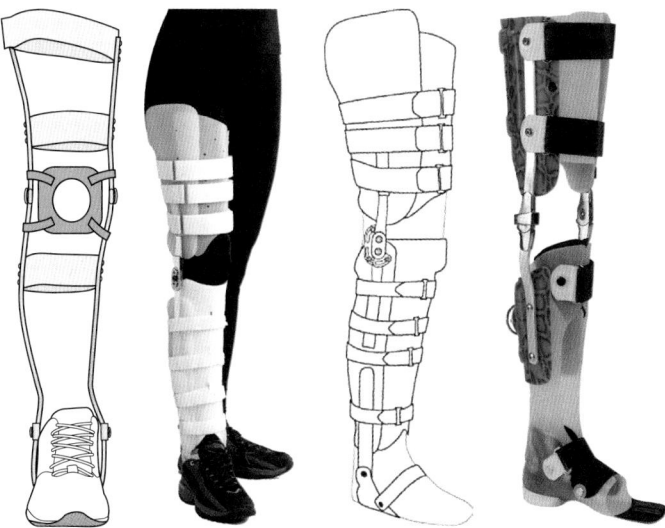

Figure 30.24 (A) Conventional knee-ankle-foot orthosis (KAFO) with knee cap. (B) Plastic KAFO pictured on a subject together with schematic of same orthosis. (C) This orthosis allows conversion between an ankle-foot orthosis and KAFO based on patient requirements. The knee component is detachable. *(Courtesy of Orthomerica Products, Orlando, FL 32810.)*

orthoses (see Fig. 30.26). The mechanism permits hip flexion and extension but restricts hip abduction, adduction, and rotation. The wearer uses crutches or other aids to permit a two- or four-point gait, which is more stable than swinging gait patterns.

Clinical Considerations

Some patients with SCI are fitted with a pair of KAFOs, primarily to obtain the benefits of standing, which assists skeletal,[87] renal, respiratory, circulatory, and

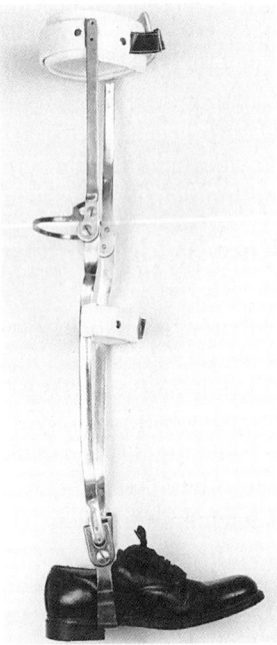

Figure 30.25 Craig-Scott knee-ankle-foot orthoses for paraplegia.

gastrointestinal function and affords the individual psychological advantages. Few children with CP who were fitted with bilateral KAFOs tolerated KAFOs.[88]

After surgery or injury, such as a knee sprain or quadricep rupture, a knee immobilizer may be used to prevent knee motion during healing. The knee is immobilized without interfering with ankle motion using a KO supported by posterior uprights or medial–lateral uprights with adjustable locking hinge joints (see Fig. 30.21). If ongoing support is required during rehabilitation, a functional KO with multiaxial knee joints and plastic shells or fabric straps can be used to mimic anatomical knee kinematics during activity. Evidence suggests that functional bracing after anterior cruciate ligament reconstruction may protect the implanted graft and benefit knee kinematics without sacrificing function, but limited evidence supports routine bracing for prevention or reinjury.[89]

Hip-Knee-Ankle-Foot Orthoses

The addition of a pelvic band and hip joints converts a KAFO to an HKAFO. The orthotic hip joint is a hinge (Fig. 30.27) that connects the lateral upright of the KAFO to a pelvic band. The joint prevents hip abduction, adduction, and rotation. If flexion control is required, a drop ring lock is added to the hip joint (Fig. 30.27).

A solid nylon- or leather-upholstered metal band (Fig. 30.28) anchors the HKAFO to the trunk. HKAFOs are not used very often because they are much more cumbersome to don than KAFOs, and if the hip joints are locked, they restrict gait to the swing-to or swing-through pattern. The pelvic band fitted when the patient is standing may be uncomfortable when the wearer rotates the pelvis when sitting.

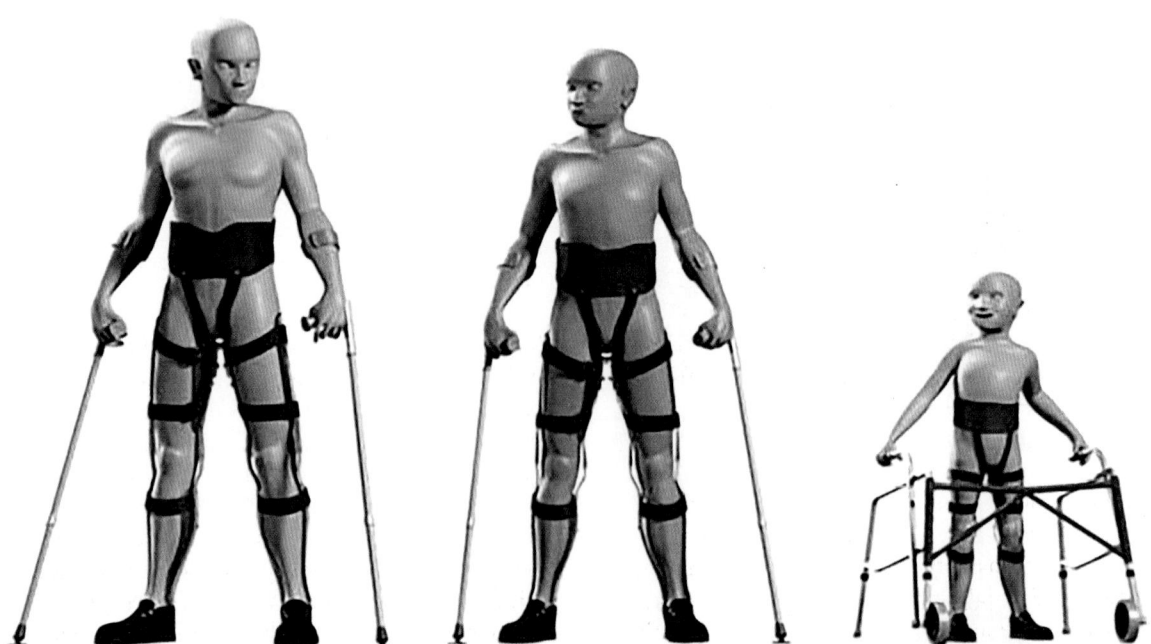

Figure 30.26 Walkabout orthoses. *(Courtesy of Polymedic.)*

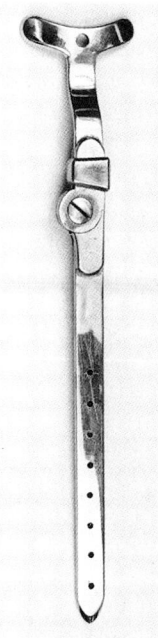

Figure 30.27 Hip joint with drop ring lock.

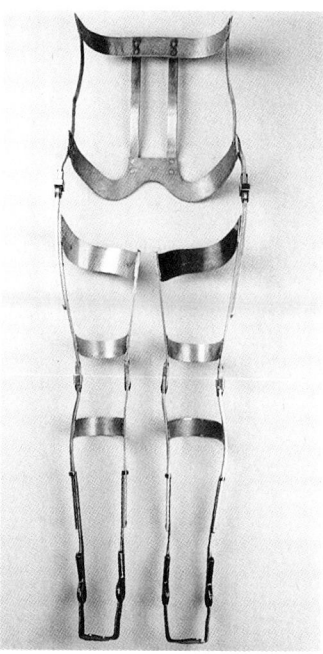

Figure 30.29 Conventional trunk-hip-knee-ankle-foot orthosis without upholstery. This is the foundational structure of these cumbersome orthoses. To this large heavy metal frame, the additional weight of the upholstery, needed straps and pads, and shoes will be added. Patients once leaving the rehabilitation setting often discard such extensive bracing.

Trunk-Hip-Knee-Ankle-Foot Orthoses

Patients who require more stability than provided by HKAFOs may be fitted with THKAFOs (Fig. 30.29), which incorporate a lumbosacral orthosis attached to HKAFOs. The THKAFO is typically prescribed for those with SCI who require trunk control. Because the THKAFO is very difficult to don and is heavy, it is seldom worn after the client is discharged from the rehabilitation facility. Alternative orthoses provide standing stability, with or without provision for walking.

Alternative Lower-Limb Orthoses
Standing Frame

Standing frames consist of a broad base that supports medial and lateral uprights that end at the anterior chest band. A posterior thoracolumbar band and anterior leg bands contribute to stability. The standing frame is used primarily by young children to foster weight-bearing on the skeleton, enable use of the hands to play, promote respiratory and urinary health, and avoid contractures (see Fig. 30.30). Standing frames are also used for the rehabilitation of those with SCI or cerebral vascular accident (CVA) to provide the ability to stand upright, improving blood circulation and trunk stability (see Fig. 30.31).

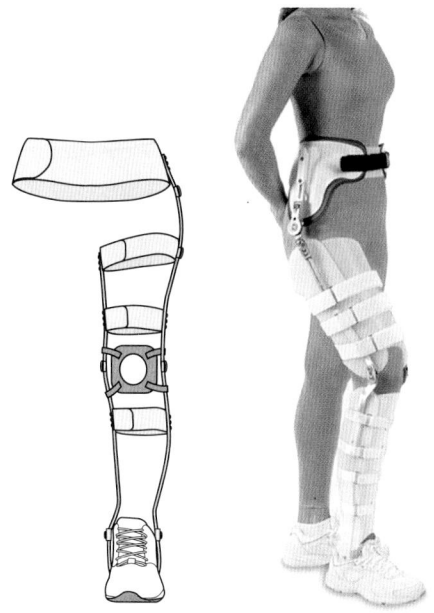

Figure 30.28 Conventional hip-knee-ankle-foot orthosis with stirrup; uprights; hinged ankle, knee, and hip joints; drop ring locks at the knee and hip; and pelvic band.

After injury or surgery, such as a total hip replacement, a hip rehabilitation orthosis can be used to minimize hip motions during healing,[90] although preventing dislocation is not assured.[91,92] Consisting of a plastic pelvic shell and thigh cuff joined by a single lateral upright with single axis locking hip joint, hip motions in all planes including flexion, adduction, and internal rotation are restricted (see Fig. 30.21).

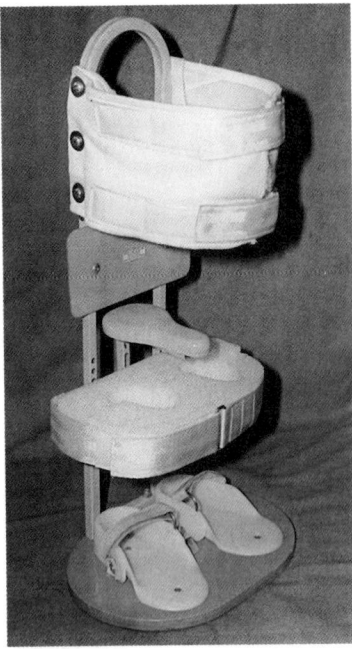

Figure 30.30 Pediatric standing frame. *(Courtesy of Variety Village, Electro Limb Production Centre, Scarborough [Toronto], Ontario, Canada.)*

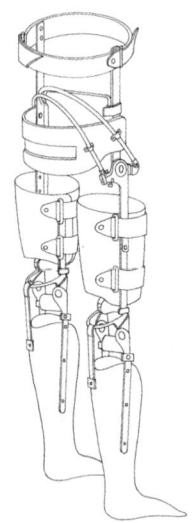

Figure 30.32 Reciprocating gait orthosis. *(Courtesy of Fillauer Companies, Chattanooga, TN 37406.)*

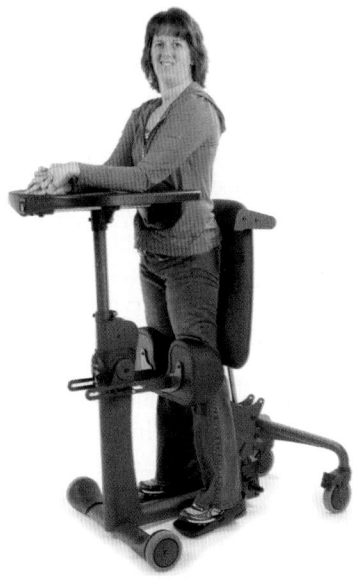

Figure 30.31 Adult standing frame. *(Courtesy of Altimate Medical, Morton, MN 56270.)*

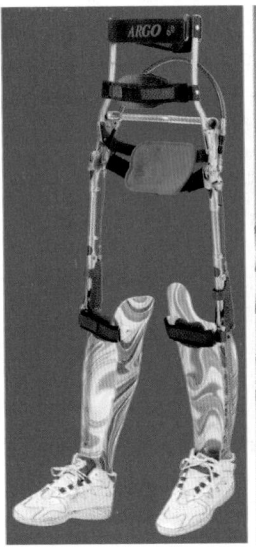
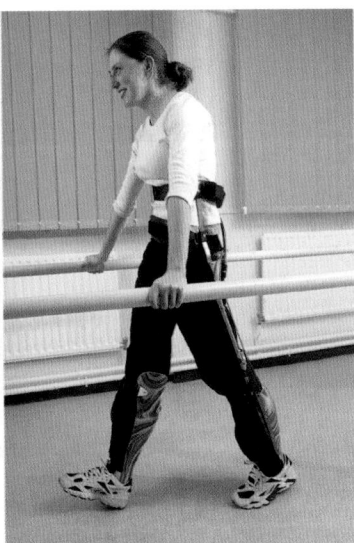

Figure 30.33 A reciprocating gait orthosis. This system includes pneumatic struts at the knee that extend the knees and ensure locks are engaged on standing. *(Courtesy of RSL Steeper, Rochester Kent ME2 4DP, United Kingdom.)*

Reciprocating Gait Orthoses

Children and adults can be fitted with a *reciprocating gait orthosis (RGO)* (Figs. 30.32 and 30.33). The RGO is a HKAFO with a chest strap. The orthotic hip joints are unlocked and are connected posteriorly by one or two metal cables or a bar. Knees are stabilized with locks, and the feet are encased in solid ankle orthoses. To walk, the wearer follows a four-stage procedure: (a) shift weight to the right, (b) tuck the pelvis by extending the upper trunk, (c) press on the crutches to unweight the left leg, and (d) swing the left leg forward. For the next step, one shifts to the left side, tucks, presses, and then swings the right leg. The cable(s) or bar prevents inadvertent hip flexion on the supporting leg. Reciprocal four- or two-point gait is stable, because one foot is always on the floor. For sitting, the wearer releases the cable(s) to enable both hips to flex. The pace is slow,[93–95] and energy is inefficient. Slight improvement in gait velocity is achieved with rocker soles.[96] Training improved patients' performance to a modest extent.[97]

Powered Orthoses

The quest to restore functional ambulation for adults with paraplegia and other ambulatory disorders currently focuses on orthoses with electronic, computer-controlled components. The Parastep (Sigmedics, Wheeling, IL) combines a pair of AFOs with skin electrodes over the quadriceps and glutei maximus to enable wearers to walk short distances[98] with somewhat higher metabolic cost and greater cardiovascular strain than with nonelectronic components.[87,99]

The C-Brace is a microprocessor-controlled KAFO (Otto Bock North America, Austin, TX), suitable for unilateral or bilateral wear and provides the wearer both stance control and variable gait speed abilities.[100,101] However, these benefits may be offset by the weight and bulk of the device for some wearers.

An exoskeleton is a type of orthotic device that aids the wearer in the performance of a functional task. Typically powered by an external battery, an exoskeleton can be used by those with lower thoracic or below SCIs to participate in gait training. Utilizing a system of microprocessors, hydraulics, or motors, an exoskeleton can generate the necessary torque to assist or completely move the user's limbs during gait. Sensors in the suit can detect the phase of gait, stabilizing the suit when needed, but allowing for a reciprocal walking. Commercially available examples include Ekso (Ekso Bionics Holdings, Richmond, CA);[102] Indego (Parker Hannifin, Mayfield Heights, OH);[103] ReWalk (ReWalk Robotics, Marlborough, MA);[104] and Lokomat (Hocoma, Norwell, MA).[105]

Preliminary reports indicate that adults with paraplegia walked slightly faster when using powered orthoses than when wearing other orthoses,[106,107] although speed remained very modest and lacks functionality in real-world scenarios (e.g., crossing a busy street).[108] Exertion was comparable to light to moderate exercise.[109,110] Some robotic orthoses are intended to be worn by patients who are supported by body-weight support apparatus, walking either on a treadmill or overground.[103] These orthoses are a potential resource for physical and psychological fitness, enabling the benefits of upright weight-bearing and the logistical advantage of maneuvering to places inaccessible to a person in a wheelchair.[111] While current technological limitations make the use of exoskeletons for those with SCI impractical, studies have shown that the use of exoskeletons as part of the rehabilitation regimen benefits the cardiovascular and neuromuscular systems.[112]

Clinical Considerations

Although most experience with powered exoskeletons has been with adults with SCI, a few children have been fitted successfully.[113] Those with multiple sclerosis experienced improved balance, reduced pain and fatigue, and a better quality of life.[114]

Current research consists primarily of short-term studies of patients using powered exoskeletons under laboratory conditions. Although these orthoses show promise, much improvement is required before they become a widespread option for people with SCI. Velocity is like that of a manually powered wheelchair.[115]

Candidates for electronic orthoses are those with ankle, knee, and hip mobility within normal limits. Other requirements include access to a rehabilitation facility for specialized gait training and financial resources to cover the increased expense of these devices. For community ambulation, sufficient upper-limb control and overall stamina to manage crutches or a walker are essential. The weight and bulk of powered exoskeletons may not be acceptable to some individuals. Instruction in the care of the orthosis is mandatory. The patient needs a means of obtaining periodic and emergency maintenance of the electronic and mechanical components. Most important, the potential wearer should demonstrate a keen desire to augment wheelchair use with independent ambulation. Consequently, clinicians must assess the degree to which a prospective device will enable the patient to accomplish the desired goals and activities, while fitting with the person's lifestyle.[116]

■ SPINAL ORTHOSES
Trunk Orthoses

Trunk orthoses provide support to thoracic spine, lumbar spine, sacrum, or a combination of multiple segments. They can be combined both with lower-limb and cervical orthoses. The function of a thoracolumbosacral orthoses is to reduce disabilities caused by low back pain, scoliosis, or other skeletal or neuromuscular disorders. Thoracolumbosacral or lumbosacral orthoses are frequently prescribed following vertebral compression fractures to promote healing by restricting motion of the spine. By supporting the trunk, the orthosis assists in controlling spinal motion; however, forces that the orthosis exerts are modified by the skin, subcutaneous tissue, and musculature that surround the vertebral column, and, in the case of higher orthoses, by the thoracic cage.

Corsets

Corsets provide support to the trunk by increasing intra-abdominal pressure and providing proprioceptive feedback (Fig. 30.34). This fabric orthosis has no horizontal rigid structures, although many have vertical reinforcements. The corset may cover only the lumbar and sacral regions, or it may extend superiorly as a thoracolumbosacral corset to also inhibit trunk movement.

Some individuals with low back disorders find that corsets relieve pain.[117,118] The efficacy of orthotic intervention to reduce or prevent low back pain remains controversial.[119,120] The increase in intra-abdominal pressure reduces stress on posterior spinal musculature, thus diminishing the load on the lumbar intervertebral disks. Although temporary reduction of abdominal and erector spinae muscular activity is therapeutic, long-term reliance on a corset may promote muscular atrophy and contracture, as well as psychological dependence on the appliance.

Lumbosacral and Thoracolumbosacral Orthoses

Rigid orthoses are distinguished by the presence of horizontal and vertical rigid plastic or metal components. Motion limitation is accomplished by a series of three-point pressure systems, in which force in one direction is bracketed by two counteracting forces in the opposite direction.

Lumbosacral Flexion, Extension, Lateral Control Orthoses

A typical example of a rigid trunk orthosis is the *lumbosacral flexion, extension, lateral control (LS FEL) orthosis* (Fig. 30.35), also known as a *Knight spinal orthosis*.

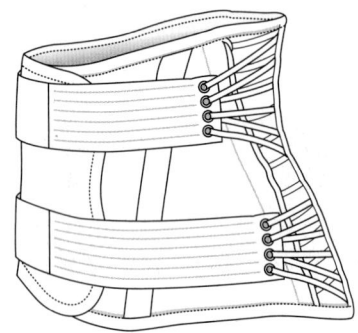

Figure 30.34 Lumbosacral corset (cotton/elastic polymer) with front hook and loop closure.

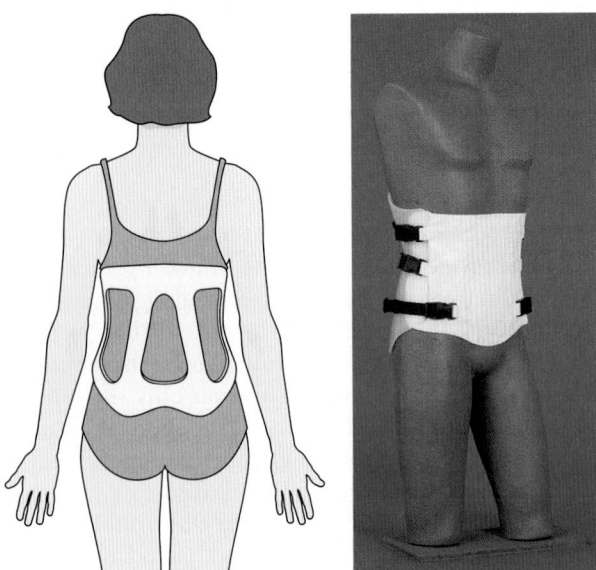

Figure 30.35 (Left) Conventional lumbosacral flexion, extension, lateral (LS FEL) control orthosis. (Right) Custom fabricated plastic LS FEL control orthosis with corset front. *(Courtesy of Orthomerica Products, Orlando, FL 32810.)*

This appliance includes a pelvic band, which should provide firm anchorage over the midsection of the buttocks, and a thoracic band that lies over the lower thorax without impinging the scapulae. The bands, which may be foam-lined rigid plastic or leather-upholstered metal, are joined by a pair of posterior uprights on either side of the vertebral spines, and a pair of lateral uprights placed at the right and left lateral midlines of the torso. A corset or abdominal front completes the LS FEL orthosis. The orthosis restrains flexion by a three-point system consisting of posteriorly directed force from the top and bottom of the abdominal front or corset and an anteriorly directed force from the midportion of the posterior uprights. Extension is controlled by posteriorly directed force from the midsection of the abdominal front or corset and anteriorly directed force from the thoracic and pelvic bands. The lateral uprights resist lateral flexion. Other rigid lumbosacral (LS) orthoses are made entirely of polyethylene with removable, replaceable liners (Fig. 30.36). A plastic LS jacket restricts motion in all directions.

Lumbosacral orthoses limit trunk motion,[121,122] which may alleviate low back pain. Corsets and rigid orthoses appear to produce similar results in treatment of compression fractures.[123]

Orthoses appear to be a primary treatment for athletes and active children.[124,125] The principal effect may be that orthoses act as proprioceptive reminders to the wearer to limit motion.[126] Lumbosacral orthoses do not appear to cause muscle weakness.[127,128]

Thoracolumbosacral Flexion, Extension Control Orthoses

Also called a *Taylor brace*, the *thoracolumbosacral flexion, extension control (TLS FE) orthosis* consists of a pelvic band, posterior uprights terminating at midscapular level, an abdominal front or corset, and axillary straps

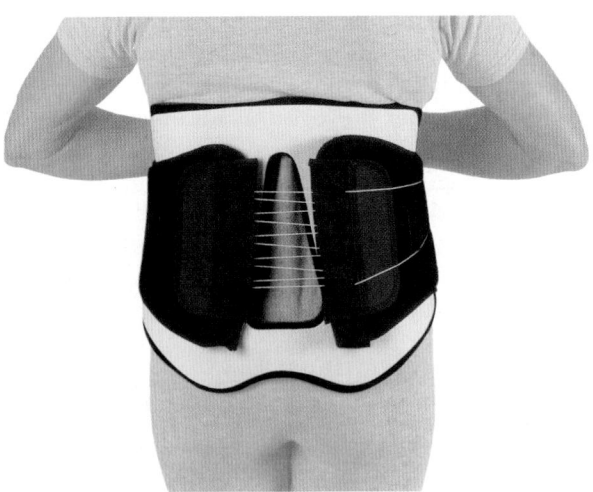

Figure 30.36 Prefabricated adjustable lumbosacral flexion, extension, lateral control orthosis. *(Courtesy of Orthomerica Products, Orlando, FL 32810.)*

attached to an interscapular band. This orthosis reduces flexion by a three-point system consisting of posteriorly directed force from the axillary straps and the bottom of the abdominal front or corset, and anteriorly directed force from the midportion of the posterior uprights. Extension resistance is provided by posteriorly directed force from the midsection of the abdominal front or corset and anteriorly directed force from the pelvic and interscapular bands. The addition of lateral uprights converts the orthosis to a TLS FEL *Knight Taylor* orthosis (Fig. 30.37). A plastic *thoracolumbosacral jacket* limits trunk motion in the frontal, sagittal, and transverse planes providing maximum support. The *thoracolumbosacral flexion control (TLS F) orthosis* is a rigid frame that has sternal and suprapubic plates in front and a dorsolumbar plate; the orthosis limits flexion but permits other trunk motions.

Long-term follow-up of patients with thoracolumbar burst fractures indicates that those who were fitted with an orthosis had at least as good outcomes as patients treated surgically.[129,130] Other case reviews suggest that patients with stable fractures had similar results whether they wore braces.[131,132]

Cervical Orthoses

Cervical orthoses are classified according to design characteristics that provide varying degrees of control. Cervical orthoses can also be joined with thoracic and lumbar braces as needed. Minimal motion control is provided by soft cervical collars (Fig. 30.38) that encircle the neck with fabric and resilient foam. Soft collars

provide minor limitations to motion control, but similar to a knee sleeve brace, the collar can be used to reduce pain, likely resulting from the proprioceptive effect.[133,134] Some patients with cervical radiculopathy benefited from short-term management with a soft collar,[135] while others had comparable results without orthotic use.[136]

Providing more stability are rigid cervical orthotics (e.g., Aspen, Philadelphia, Miami J; see Fig. 30.39). The rigid orthoses have mandibular and occipital extensions and a rigid anterior strut which effectively limit the amount of available ROM.[137] The inside of the brace

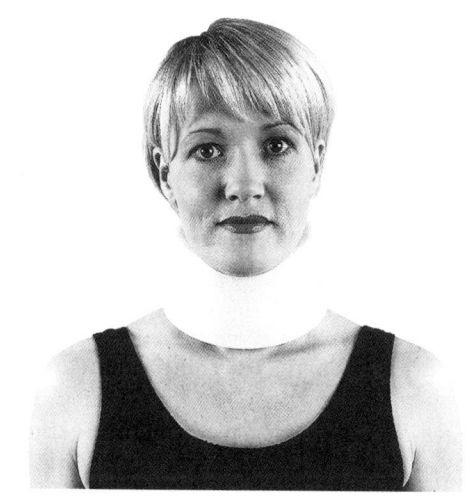

Figure 30.38 Soft foam rubber collar. *(Courtesy of Camp Healthcare Corporation, Jackson, MI 49204.)*

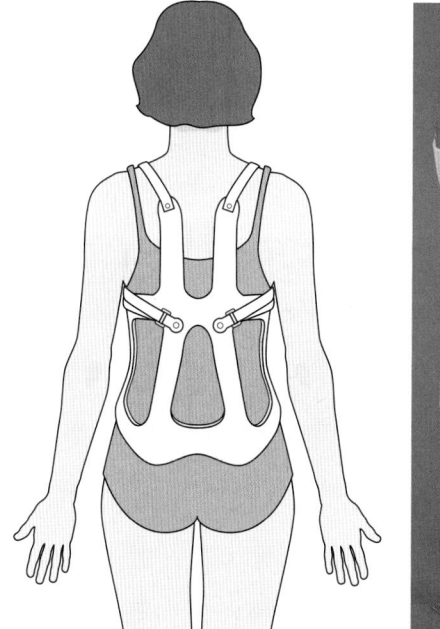 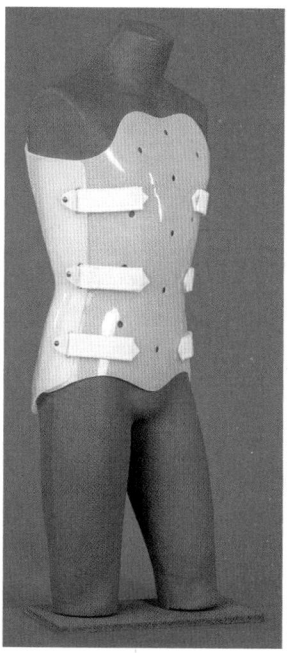 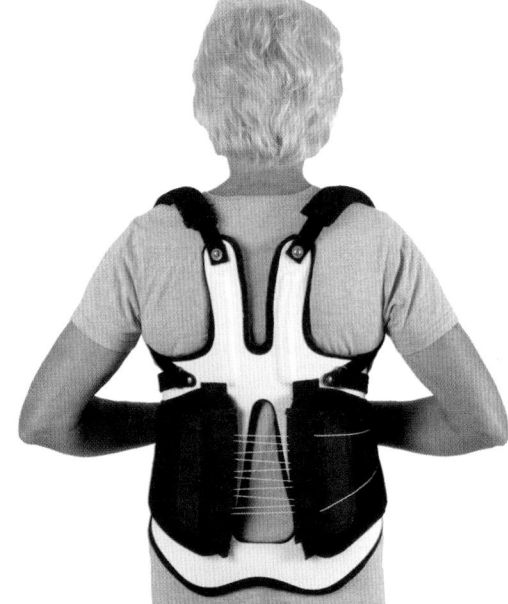

Figure 30.37 (Left) Conventional thoracolumbar flexion, extension, lateral control orthosis (TLS FEL). (Middle) Custom fabricated plastic TLS FEL. (Right) Prefabricated, adjustable TLS FEL. *(Courtesy of Orthomerica Products, Orlando, FL 32810.)*

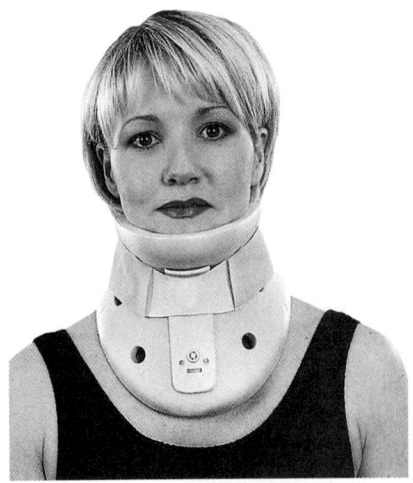

Figure 30.39 Philadelphia collar. *(Courtesy of Camp Healthcare Corporation, Jackson, MI 49204.)*

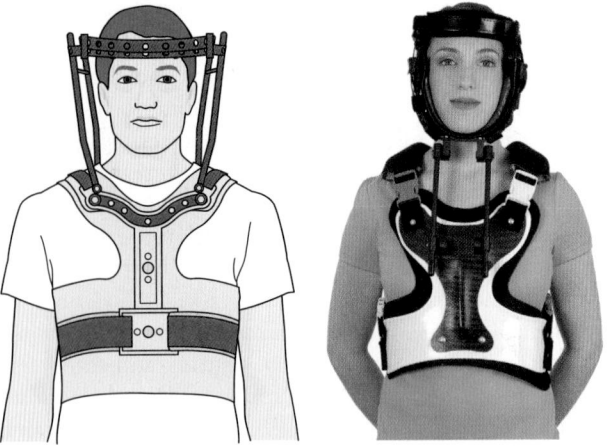

Figure 30.40 (Left) The halo cervical orthosis provides maximum stabilization of the head and cervical spine. The graphite ring (halo) allows placement of titanium pins into the outer skull. (Right) Noninvasive halo devices are also available. They can be used as transitional bracing after removal of the invasive halo cervical orthosis. *(Courtesy of Trulife USA, Jackson, MI 49203.)*

has a removable padded lining that requires cleaning to prevent skin irritation on the patient's neck.

For moderate control, a *post orthosis* is used. A two-post orthosis has an anterior adjustable post joining the sternal and mandibular plates and a posterior upright connecting the thoracic and occipital plates. Straps to join the sternal and thoracic plates and the occipital and mandibular plates complete the orthosis. This orthosis limits cervical flexion and extension. A four-post orthosis has two anterior and two posterior posts to control motion. Maximum orthotic neck control can be achieved with either a *Minerva* or a *halo orthosis* (Fig. 30.40). The Minerva orthosis is a noninvasive appliance with a rigid plastic posterior section extending from head to midtrunk; the superior portion is held in place by a forehead band. The halo orthosis has a circular metal band fixed to the skull by four screws, making it more invasive, with uprights that connect the halo to a thoracic vest. The halo orthosis provides the most restriction to cervical motion.[138] When the wearer walks, the minimal bony stress may foster fracture healing.[139] The most restrictive braces are typically applied following SCIs, cervical spine fractures, and severe segmental instability.

Scoliosis Orthoses

Children and adolescents with idiopathic scoliosis or hyperkyphosis may be fitted with a thoracolumbosacral orthosis (TLSO) that applies distraction, derotation, and bending forces to realign the vertebral column and thoracic cage (see Fig. 30.41) Numerous orthotic designs are in current use. Most are intended to be worn for 18 to 23 hr per day for several years until the patient reaches skeletal maturity. The Milwaukee brace (Fig. 30.42), introduced in 1946, is still prescribed. Its frame is composed of a pelvic girdle, two posterior uprights, an anterior upright, and a superior ring that lies on the upper chest and can be hidden by most clothing. Pads are strapped to the interior of the frame to

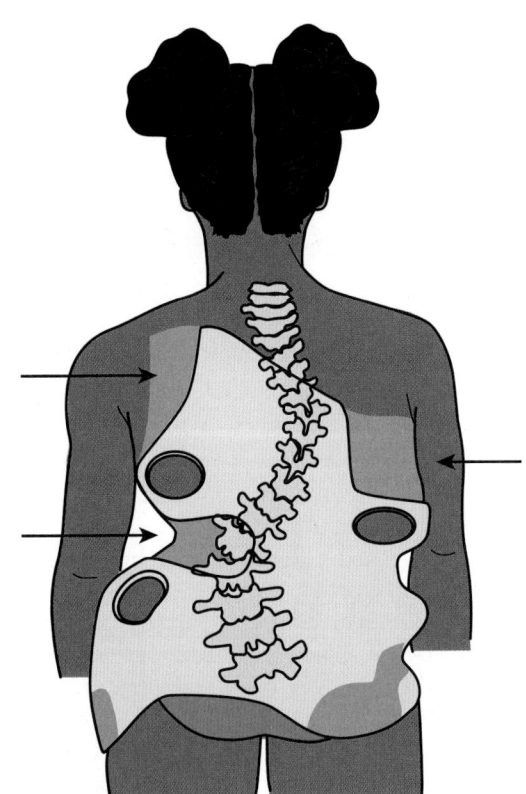

Figure 30.41 Orthotic application of corrective forces for the scoliotic spine.

apply corrective forces.[140] The Boston orthosis, dating from 1972 (Fig. 30.43), usually does not extend as high as the Milwaukee orthosis; its foundation is a mass-produced plastic module that the orthotist alters to fit the individual patient. The effectiveness of the orthosis

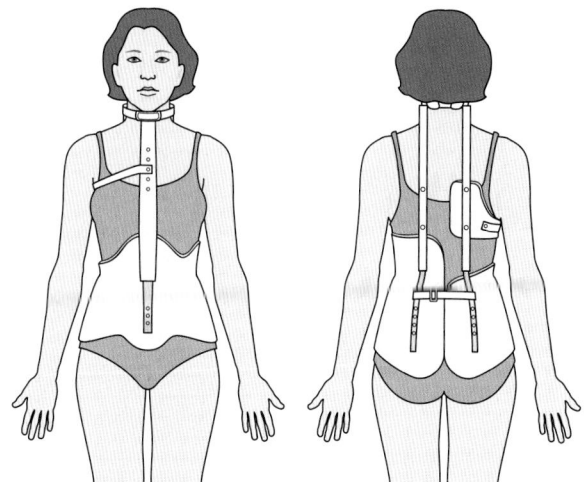

Figure 30.42 Milwaukee plastic and metal orthosis.

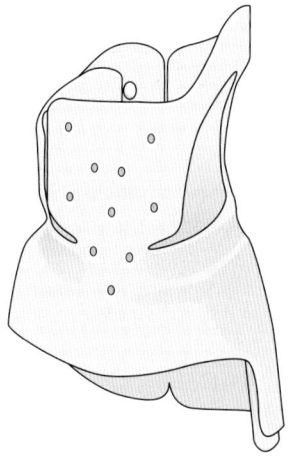

Figure 30.43 Boston thoracolumbosacral orthosis.

is enhanced by interior pads.[141] Another option is the Rigo Cheneau brace, a custom molded plastic TLSO. Its selective openings over the concavities of the curves reduce the bulk of the orthosis.[142,143]

Night bracing is an alternate approach to scoliosis management. When the patient is recumbent, the effect of gravity is minimized, allowing substantial corrective forces to be applied. Both the Charleston bending brace (patented in 1987) and the Providence brace (developed in 1992)[144,145] provide overcorrection of the spinal curve.

Brace effectiveness depends on skeletal immaturity, trunk flexibility, curve less than 35°,[146] snug contact between orthosis and torso, and compliance with the wearing protocol.[147] Long-term follow-up indicates that a variety of braces retard curve progression, although patients with larger curves usually proceed to surgical correction.[148,149]

■ UPPER-LIMB ORTHOSES

Commonly known as splints or braces, upper-limb orthotic devices can accommodate an existing deformity or improve the function of a particular body segment.

While upper-limb orthotics may be prescribed for a variety of reasons, they are commonly used for post-surgical stabilization, accommodating a contracture, or improving the functional grasp of the hand.

Table 30.2 describes common scenarios in which an upper-limb orthosis may be utilized.

■ PHYSICAL THERAPY MANAGEMENT

Physical therapists evaluate and intervene in multiple physiological systems that impact the physical performance of people who use orthoses, including cognitive/communication, cardiopulmonary, neurological, integumentary, and musculoskeletal function. Physical therapists contribute to the care of people using orthoses both before and after orthotic prescription, ideally working as a team with the physician and orthotist to match the person's needs to the best orthotic prescriptive choices and to ensure safe and effective orthotic use to optimize function.

Care Before Orthotic Prescription

Before orthotic prescription, the physical therapist evaluates the individual's potential for function, intervenes to minimize impairments and optimize function, and determines the need for orthotic consultation or intervention. All physiological systems play a role in overall function and can be organized within the larger framework of the International Classification of Functioning, Disability, and Health: (a) body structure/function including passive restraints to movement such as joints, activation of muscle and strength, neuromotor planning, sensory and cardiopulmonary function; (b) activity limitations such as balance and walking; and (c) participation restrictions due to cognitive capacity, environmental barriers, and psychosocial factors. Maximizing physiological ability lessens impairment, activity limitation, and participation restrictions while also minimizing the need for restrictive orthotic designs that can inhibit use and acceptance.

Joint Mobility and Range of Motion

A thorough goniometric examination, including both active and passive ROM, is a prerequisite before orthotic prescription as per the following examples. If passive ankle dorsiflexion remains impaired after joint mobilization and heel cord stretching, then the orthosis and/or shoe may have to be modified to accommodate the plantarflexion contracture and maintain the plantar surface on the ground. Similarly, if knee flexion contracture persists despite joint mobilization and stretching, then the resulting knee flexion moment may have to be counteracted by additional orthotic restraints. Likewise, if hip flexion contracture persists despite joint and hip flexor muscle soft tissue mobilization, then the orthotic designs may require stabilization above the hip.

Table 30.2   Common Upper-Limb Orthoses

	Name of Brace	Purpose
	Shoulder-elbow-wrist orthosis	Used after shoulder surgery (e.g., rotator cuff repair) to limit ROM, stabilize the glenohumeral joint, and prevent external torques from influencing joint motion.
	Wrist-hand orthosis (also known as a cock-up splint)	Used to prevent hand contractures or accommodate existing contractures. May be used after a CVA, for those with spasticity, or those with a non-casted orthopedic injury that requires stabilization. Can have a full-length hand plate or partial (allows for use of fingers).
	Safe position wrist-hand orthosis	This type of splint is prescribed for an individual with burns to their hand and wrist. The POSI is 10°–45° of wrist extension, metacarpophalangeal flexion to 80°–90°, and interphalangeal extension to neutral.
	Radial nerve dynamic wrist-hand orthosis	The purpose of this orthotic device is to prevent contractures caused by the unopposed median nerve muscle actions as well as provide functional grasp. The functional grasp is accomplished through springs or flexible straps that maintain the fingers and wrist in extension so that the tenodesis mechanism of the finger flexors can be used for grasping.

CVA = cerebrovascular accident; FTA = femorotibial angle; POSI = position of safe immobilization; ROM = range of motion; WOMAC = Western Ontario and McMasters Universities Osteoarthritis Index.

Limb length can affect the need for ROM. A difference of more than 1/2 in. (1 cm) should be compensated by a shoe elevation assuming otherwise normal musculoskeletal function. For the patient with chronic weakness or limited active ankle dorsiflexion in one limb, a 1/2-in. (1-cm) lift on the contralateral shoe will aid swing phase clearance of the involved LE.

Muscle Function

Complete manual muscle tests (MMTs) should be augmented by an examination of functional activities such as balance and transfers to determine what substitutions the person uses to accomplish standing and walking. Although the MMT may reveal marked weakness, if the patient can manage without an orthosis, they are unlikely to accept an orthosis. For example, the person with dorsiflexor weakness who can ambulate by exaggerating hip flexion during swing phase may not agree to use an AFO. In the presence of central nervous system dysfunction particularly marked by spasticity, functional tests of motor performance are essential to assess both strength and neuromotor planning.

Even if the patient is being considered as a candidate for a lower limb or trunk orthoses, the therapist must also determine the mobility and muscle power of the upper limbs. Significant weakness, stiffness, or poor coordination will interfere with donning the orthosis or ambulation with assistive devices. If the upper limbs are too weak to use an ambulatory assistive device effectively, the choice of orthoses for walking may be impacted. Standing frames or a standing wheelchair may be indicated to facilitate upright weight-bearing.

Sensation

The presence of any sensory loss (see Chapter 3, Examination of Sensory Function) can determine the orthotic materials chosen. Intimately fitted plastic orthoses are satisfactory for individuals with sensory loss if the edges (trimlines) of the orthosis are smooth and the orthosis does not pinch the patient's flesh. However, particularly vulnerable skin, such as in people with diabetes, may require materials like foam or cork. People using orthoses should be taught to inspect the skin regularly and instructed to alert the physical therapist and orthotist to any changes. Proprioceptive loss may indicate the need for orthotic stabilization, such as an ankle orthosis for chronic ankle instability.[81]

Cardiopulmonary Capacity

Deconditioning occurs quickly after a period of immobility and can have a lasting impact on endurance for walking and activities of daily living. For the person who requires orthotic intervention, the weight of the orthosis combined with loss of limb function contributes to increased energy expenditure. The more controlling the orthosis needs to be, the greater the weight and cardiac demand. Including aerobic exercise to increase or maintain cardiopulmonary capacity can be an important part of preparing people to use their orthoses, particularly those spanning multiple joint segments.

Care After Orthotic Delivery

Orthoses benefit individuals with a wide variety of musculoskeletal and neurological disorders. The particular diagnosis is less important in formulating the prescription than consideration of the patient's impairments and activity limitations. Prognosis also influences prescription: the person who is likely to recover partial or full function should have an orthosis that can be adjusted to accommodate the changing status. An individual with recent hemiplegia, for example, may exhibit marked spasticity and weakness, indicating a need for limiting motion at the ankle. As the person regains voluntary control and strength improves, the orthotic ankle joint can be adjusted to permit more movement.

Lifestyle has a bearing on orthotic selection. A very active patient requires an orthosis made of exceptionally sturdy and lightweight materials, like carbon fiber. The patient's concern with appearance is another practical consideration; it may dictate use of a shoe insert so that reasonably fashionable shoes may be worn. Similarly, plastic shells are less bulky than metal uprights and calf bands and can come in bright colors, using various plastics, or be embossed with decorative designs.

Inspection

Prior to applying an orthosis, an inspection of the patient's skin must be performed. If there are areas of skin breakdown that are not accommodated by the orthosis, the device should not be applied and the orthotist or medical practitioner contacted. An orthotic should first be examined for integrity and cleanliness prior to being applied to the patient. It is imperative that there are no cracks or irregularities in the orthotic

superstructure or foundation as this could prevent the orthosis from performing its function correctly and may cause skin injury. Examine any straps, clasps, or securing elements, including padding that contacts the skin. Clean the device according to the manufacturers or orthotist's recommendation. If there are concerns about either the integrity or cleanliness of the device, referral to the orthotist is indicated. The patient should be educated on how to inspect the orthosis regularly and care for it promptly. Written instructions reinforce the recommendations of the orthotist and therapist.

Shoes and Socks

Whether or not the shoe is attached directly to the orthosis, footwear should be kept in good condition, with replacement as soon as moderate wear is evident. Shoes that are outgrown or distorted will not afford the wearer optimal function from the orthosis. Absorbent socks protect the skin from uprights, shells, and any pads on the interior of the orthosis. Long socks are essential for AFOs and higher lower-limb orthoses. Soft fabric, such as a T-shirt or fabric sheath, is needed when the patient wears a trunk or upper-limb orthosis.

Ankle-Foot Orthoses

The primary candidates for AFOs are patients with ankle-foot weakness, typically occurring with peripheral neuropathy or central nervous dysfunction such as after stroke. Primary gait dysfunctions affected by various AFO designs are footdrop in swing phase that can lead to tripping, frontal plane ankle instability in stance that can lead to sprains and loss of balance, and uncontrolled knee flexion in stance phase that can lead to knee collapse. For footdrop, a variety of AFO designs can be utilized including the posterior leaf spring or solid AFO, and the hinged AFO with dorsiflexion spring assist or plantar flexion stop. Of these four AFO designs, three provide frontal plane support to prevent lateral ankle instability—only the posterior leaf spring does not provide frontal plane support. Two of the AFO options—posterior leaf spring or a metal dorsiflexion spring assist—allow plantarflexion and thus knee extension at foot flat during initial loading in early stance to reduce demand for quadriceps strength for those with moderate weakness or hemiplegia. Only one option, the solid AFO, prevents tibial forward translation past upright and thus knee flexion in stance for people with more severe weakness who cannot maintain knee extension to prevent falling. Prescription, therefore, depends on the plane of dysfunction, the degree of weakness, and combination of gait dysfunctions.

CASE EXAMPLE 30.1

An adult with hemiplegia after a stroke 2 months ago walks slowly, with uncertain balance biased toward the unaffected limb, and hemiplegic side knee instability during gait, requiring assistance to continue. Knee extensor strength on the affected limb is 3+/5 (fair plus), knee flexors are 4/5 (good), dorsiflexors are 2−/5 (poor minus), and plantar flexors are 3/5 (fair). They present with footdrop in swing phase, lateral foot weight-bearing throughout initial loading, and poorly controlled knee flexion in midstance leading to decreased stance time, step length, and balance on the hemiplegic side.

Orthotic prescription: While a locked-knee KAFO would certainly prevent knee collapse, neurological return anticipated at the ankle, knee, and hip would be inhibited by immobilization. A solid AFO would prevent footdrop in swing, stop knee collapse, and provide frontal plane stability to enhance balance without disrupting as much knee and hip function. In addition, as strength improves with recovery, the solid AFO can be modified by cutting back the shell to allow some ankle movement.

Knee-Ankle-Foot and Other Lower-Limb Orthoses

A KAFO may compensate for dysfunction of the entire lower limb. A KAFO with locking knee, for instance, will prevent knee collapse and also confer some stability to the hip via control of the femur. When full control of the hip is needed to prevent jackknifing, a common danger in people with paraplegia or spina bifida, an HKAFO with hips and knees locked in extension can be used to facilitate upright standing and walking. Walking is achieved with bilateral arm support with walking aids. Sitting, however, requires unlocking both the joints and arm support. Core weakness further complicates the scenario and may require a conventional or exoskeletal THKAFO to provide adequate trunk stability.

CASE EXAMPLE 30.2

A 4-year-old child with spina bifida has poor trunk control and paraplegia below L2 and cannot stand or walk without assistance due to ankle and hip weakness. Using their arms for support on a walker and moderate assistance to maintain balance, they are able to walk slowly for a short distance. Hip and ankle control in all planes is poor in both swing and stance phase, however, risking falls and subsequent injury.

ORTHOTIC PRESCRIPTION

While a locked-knee KAFO would prevent knee collapse and HKAFO joined with a pelvic band would stabilize the ankles and hips in all planes, the pelvic band may not provide sufficient trunk stability, and gait would require full upper-extremity weight-bearing for swing-through gait. An RGO would allow reciprocal gait with less upper-extremity weight-bearing while providing support for all lower limb joints in all planes. The RGO would provide the child the opportunity to walk more and develop as normally as possible.

Trunk Orthoses

Isolated trunk weakness or pain can be reduced with a corset to increase intra-abdominal pressure and thereby may reduce the vertical compressive forces through the spine. Where greater motion restriction is indicated, such as for the individual with trunk paralysis, a rigid lumbosacral or thoracolumbosacral orthosis is appropriate. Selection of cervical orthosis depends on the extent of motion control needed.

CASE EXAMPLE 30.3

A 12-year-old female with idiopathic thoracolumbar scoliosis reports worsening pain in her thoracolumbar junction and difficulty turning her trunk to the right. Postural assessment reveals an elevation of the left thoracic cage when viewed posteriorly during the forward bend test. Joint assessment of the spine reveals left rotation and right sidebending of the vertebral segments between T7 and L3, further supported by reduced trunk sidebending left and rotation right. There is evidence that the spinal curvature angle is increasing over time when compared to her prior assessment.

ORTHOTIC PRESCRIPTION

To counteract further development of the scoliotic curvature as she enters a period of growth, a Boston brace could be used. Through the three-point force system, the sidebending to the right and rotation to the left can be reduced progressively over time.

Orthotic Examination and Evaluation

Orthotic examination and evaluation are essential elements of management. The therapist should examine the orthosis through analysis of (a) effects and benefits in terms of improved function, (b) movement while the patient wears the device, (c) fit and alignment, and (d) safety during use of the device. See Appendix 30.A (online), Lower-Limb Orthotic Examination Guiding Questions, and Appendix 30.B (online), Trunk Orthotic Examination Guiding Questions, for more information.

Orthotic Static and Dynamic Examination

Static examination is conducted before donning the orthosis and while the patient wears the orthosis while standing and sitting. *Dynamic examination* is performed during movement, specifically during gait and sit-to-stand transitions.

Static Examination

The patient's skin and the construction of the orthosis are checked with the orthosis off the patient. Prior to use, the fit, function, and appearance should be acceptable for safe application. The orthosis is inspected as the wearer stands and sits.

The patient should stand in parallel bars or another secure environment and be encouraged to bear equal weight on both feet. The sole and heel should rest flat on the floor. Any orthotic ankle joint should be at the distal tip of the medial malleolus to be congruent with the anatomical ankle during gait.

Any calf band should terminate below the fibular head (to avoid pressure on the fibular nerve) and below the popliteal fossa (to allow unobstructed knee flexion when sitting).

Any mechanical knee joints should be congruent with the anatomical knee; for the adult, the usual placement is approximately 3/4 in. (2 cm) above the medial tibial plateau. Knee locks should function properly. Medial uprights should terminate approximately 1.5 in. (4 cm) below the perineum to ensure comfort.

The pelvic joint is set slightly above and anterior to the greater trochanter to compensate for the usual angulation of the femoral neck; setting the joint anterior to the trochanter makes sitting more comfortable. The pelvic band should conform to the contours of the wearer's torso, without undo pressure.

Any thoracic bands should fit flat against the trunk without edge pressure. Uprights should not press against bony prominences, particularly when the patient sits. The abdominal front should extend from just below the xiphoid process to just above the pubic symphysis. The cervical orthosis should hold the head in the best-tolerated position. Rigid components should be shaped to apply maximum area to the body segment.

When the orthosis is taken off after wear, the therapist should inspect the patient's skin to detect any irritations attributable to the orthosis. The cause of any skin breakdown should be analyzed and referral to the orthotist may be required for orthotic adjustments beyond correction of donning method and wear.

Dynamic Examination

The gait pattern exhibited by the person who wears an orthosis reflects both the contribution of the wearer's general health status and the orthotic motion control and assistance. During early stance, the patient may exhibit *foot slap*, striking with toes first, or *flat-foot* contact, indicating inability to restrain plantarflexion tone or failure of the orthosis to support the foot and ankle due to dorsiflexion weakness. Excessive medial or lateral contact may indicate that the orthosis does not track the way the patient's limb does. Knee hyperextension or excessive flexion indicates that the orthosis is not applying adequate control. A posterior stop on the AFO should prevent the lax knee from hyperextending. If the patient wears a KAFO and has knee hyperextension, the stops in the knee joint are set improperly or have eroded, or the calf and thigh shells or bands are too deep. Anterior and posterior trunk bending are seen at early stance when the patient attempts to control a weak knee or hip. If the quadriceps are weak, the patient will bend forward. The person whose knee may collapse may benefit from an AFO with a solid ankle and an anterior band, or a KAFO with a knee lock. If the gluteus maximus is weak, the individual is apt to lean backward. Lordosis indicates hip flexion contracture or a KAFO that does not fit properly.

Lateral trunk bending in early stance phase may result from hip abductor weakness or hip instability; however, uncompensated shortness of the limb will also give rise to this problem, as will a medial upright on a KAFO that is too high, or an abducted pelvic joint on an HKAFO. A wide walking base may be the patient's compensation for a long medial upright or shell that impinges into the perineum.

During late stance, the person may have difficulty maintaining weight-bearing and experience early knee flexion or heel rise. This problem can be mitigated with a rigid full-length foot insert. Conversely, if the person has difficulty transferring weight to the lead limb, a full-length foot insert can be thinned over the toes or cut back to 3/4 length, or a rocker bar or rocker bottom sole can be used.

During swing phase, the patient must be able to clear the floor with the braced LE. *Hip hiking* (swing leg pelvic elevation) occurs when the hip flexors are weak, as well as when the limb is functionally longer than the contralateral limb. Increased length may be produced by a faulty posterior stop that no longer limits plantarflexion or by a locked knee joint. For the unilateral KAFO wearer, foot clearance can be facilitated by adding a 1-cm lift to the contralateral shoe. Excessive medial or lateral foot contact may indicate that the orthosis does not track the way the patient's limb does. A limb that is longer than that on the opposite side can cause a walking base that is abnormally wide. *Vaulting* refers to exaggerated plantarflexion on the contralateral limb during affected side swing phase. Vaulting occurs because the braced leg is functionally too long, possibly because the posterior ankle stop has eroded or a knee lock is used.

Orthotic Instruction and Training

Orthoses are designed to provide the individual with a maximum of function with a minimum of discomfort and effort. Periodic appointments at regular intervals ensure safety by monitoring the integrity of the orthosis, any skin breakdown or other signs of poor fit or disrepair, and the person's functional orthotic use. No single instruction and training program suits every orthosis wearer because of the wide range of disorders for which orthotic management is indicated. To the extent possible, however, the physical therapist should instruct the patient in (a) the correct manner of donning the orthosis, (b) developing standing balance, (c) walking safely, and (d) performing other ambulatory activities. Follow-up visits enable the physical therapist to reinforce skills taught and address new problems that arise.

Donning Orthoses

Orthotic devices may be applied directly to the skin or over clothing. The AFO with shoe insert is most easily donned by applying the orthosis to the foot and leg, prior to placing the braced limb in the shoe.

The same general procedures are useful with KAFOs. The patient may find donning easier if the brace is applied while lying on a bed or a mat table. If the KAFO is donned while the patient sits, the therapist should check the tightness of the orthotic anterior strap or band. Donning HKAFOs and THKAFOs is much more arduous. The beginner should lie on a mat table alongside the orthosis. By rolling to one side, the patient should be able to pull the brace under the legs so as to permit lying in it. Then the patient sits with knees extended to don shoes and fasten straps.

Lumbosacral and TLS corsets and rigid orthoses should be donned while the patient is supine to achieve maximum compression of the abdomen. The orthosis should be fastened from the bottom upward. Note that many trunk orthosis are worn when "out of bed," meaning that when in bed the orthosis can be removed. It is imperative that the physical therapist verify the orders from the managing physician to prevent improper adherence to prescribed wearing requirements.

Wearing Time

In certain circumstances it will be necessary for the patient to immediately start wearing their orthosis with only limited times for its removal. This is typically due to the role of the orthotic in protecting the body segment, as in the case of a cervical fracture and a halo orthosis. In the case of a TLSO for a vertebral compression fracture, the prescription may allow for the removal of the brace when the patient is in bed only. For these scenarios and others warranting immediate and protective bracing, there is no allowance made for slowly accommodating to the brace to the emergent nature of the patient's condition.

However, there are many circumstances where the orthotic should be accommodated through gradual exposure over a period of days to weeks. For example, foot orthotics, lower limb orthotics, and certain spinal bracing solutions can be worn for an hour a day initially.

Each day afterward, an hour is added until the desired wearing time is achieved. This allows for the wearer to observe how their skin reacts to the brace, giving an opportunity to prevent unwanted skin breakdown due to overuse. The decision regarding wearing schedule should be made by the physician and orthotist if the brace is protective in nature. If in doubt, always request clarification on an orthotic order to prevent injury to a patient.

Standing Balance

The problem of standing safely is most difficult for the individual who wears bilateral KAFOs or more extensive bracing.

The person who wears bilateral KAFOs will need crutches or other aids for independent gait. A prerequisite for crutch ambulation is the ability to shift weight. Shifting weight to the heels takes pressure off the hands so they can be moved. Using parallel bars, the beginner shifts all weight to the feet and raises and lowers one hand, then the other hand. The goal is to be able to lift both hands simultaneously, as may be done with crutches when performing a swing-to or similar gait. Once the patient is able to shift weight from the feet to the hands and back to the feet confidently, the same exercise should be done with crutches. Advanced skills, such as moving the hands and eventually the crutches, behind the body, should be practiced. Those who will walk in reciprocal fashion, alternating footsteps, need to practice diagonal weight shifting.

Gait Training

The various crutch gaits differ in the sequence of crutch and footsteps. Patterns vary in speed, safety, and amount of energy required. The patient should learn as many gaits as possible, so as to modify walking in crowds, over long distances, and in situations in which speed is desired. In addition to walking forward, the client needs to be able to walk sideward, turn corners, and maneuver on different surfaces, such as rugs, gravel, grass, and through doors. A repertoire of gaits permits the client to adjust to environmental requirements. Gait selection depends on the individual's functional ability, including the following:

- *Weight-bearing and balance ability:* Can the patient bear weight and remain balanced on one or both LEs?
- *Step ability:* Can the patient take steps with either one or both LEs?
- *Upper-extremity power:* Can the patient push the body off the floor by pressing down on the hands?

Reciprocal Gaits

The four- and two-point gaits require that one move the legs alternately by hip flexion or pelvic elevation. The patient shifts weight as each leg is moved. The four-point sequence is (a) right hand, (b) left foot, (c) left hand, and

(d) right foot. The two-point sequence requires greater balance and coordination but is a faster mode of walking: (a) right hand and left leg and (b) left hand and right leg. The patterns also are useful when one is confronted with crowds or slippery surfaces. These gaits are suited to persons who lack the coordination and balance needed for simultaneous gaits.

Simultaneous Gaits

If both legs are moved simultaneously, the patient places considerable stress on the upper limbs. The series includes the swing-to and swing-through patterns. Although the swing-through gait can be performed rapidly, simultaneous gaits generally are slow and fatiguing. The weight of the orthoses and, in the case of a patient with spinal cord lesion, absence of peripheral sensation, aggravate the problem of using a simultaneous gait pattern.

The swing-to pattern involves the patient swinging the lower extremities. Swinging is accomplished by extending the elbows and depressing the shoulder girdle to elevate the trunk and legs. The swing-through gait is a more advanced pattern, requiring much balance, strength, and coordination of the upper limbs, because the patient swings the legs beyond the hands or crutch tips. The sequence is (a) advance both hands, (b) swing both legs to a point in front of the hands to reverse the basic tripod position, and (c) advance both hands to the starting position. The swing-through gait requires extensive preliminary training, including push-ups to strengthen the arms. Gait is rapid but requires more floor space than the other patterns, to permit alternate swinging of legs and crutches. Detailed instructions in gait training are provided in the appendix of Chapter 11, Strategies to Improve Locomotor Function (online).

The ultimate test of walking proficiency is the ability to conduct a conversation while ambulating (dual tasking), an activity pattern that indicates some degree of automatic functioning. Practice in the clinical setting should be extended to walking on varied terrain, indoors and outdoors.

Related Activities

The patient should learn as many activities as physical condition permits. Daily life often involves negotiating stairs, curbs, and ramps, as well as transferring from the chair to the upright position, and into an automobile. Instruction in driving a suitably equipped car is an important part of rehabilitation. Not all individuals who wear orthoses achieve the full range of ambulatory activities, yet they benefit from partial independence in accomplishing tasks, at least from the psychological and physiological values attendant to ambulation.

Optimal performance depends on the favorable interaction of many factors. Foremost is the extent of skeletal and neuromuscular involvement. The mobility, strength, and coordination of all body segments, especially in the lower extremities and trunk, are important,

as are the individual's muscle tone, cardiovascular and pulmonary health, body weight, psychological status, and chronological age. The quality of the orthosis also influences the client's achievements.

Most orthosis wearers have chronic conditions, such as arthritis, or permanent sequelae from trauma, such as paraplegia following SCI. Orthotic management enhances function without necessarily influencing the underlying pathology. Training people with chronic disorders prepares the patient for lifelong activity with an orthosis. Persons with reversible disorders, such as fibular nerve injury, often benefit from temporary use of an orthosis. Such individuals should learn proper use of the orthosis to prevent secondary disorders and should receive reexamination so that the orthosis may be altered as the condition changes. Patients with progressive disorders, such as muscular dystrophy and multiple sclerosis, require vigilant reexamination so that the extent of physical deterioration may be reflected in orthotic changes, as well as continual training to cope with altered functional abilities. For all situations, an individually devised exercise and activity program should enable the patient to manage efficiently for maximum independence.

Facilitating Acceptance

Interprofessional collaboration is valuable in fostering patient acceptance of the orthosis and achieving maximum rehabilitation benefit. Peer support groups related to disabilities for patients and families are helpful for sharing concerns and workable solutions to common problems. The physical therapist can identify individuals whose response to disability is difficult and refer for psychological attention when needed.

■ CLINICAL CONSIDERATIONS
Energy Considerations

A purpose of rehabilitation is to improve the patient's functional capacity by reducing the amount of energy the individual uses to accomplish meaningful tasks, such as ambulation. However, in the case of orthotic devices, the energy expenditure may either increase or decrease based on the device. The patient's ambulatory ability and capacity for other physical activities reflect both orthotic and anatomical factors. Energy cost is calculated from the amount of oxygen consumed as the subject performs an activity.

If the energy cost is too high, the patient will realize that ambulation is not practical. Sometimes, high-energy cost is tolerable for short distances, as in household ambulation. Community ambulation, however, demands sustained effort for longer distances, plus the ability to maneuver over curbs and other irregularities in the walking surface and cross the street within the time allowed by the traffic light. Following are some scenarios where energy efficiency should be considered.

Hemiplegia

Adults with stroke consume more oxygen than able-bodied people when walking; the difference increases when subjects walk slowly.[150] Shoes with rocker soles worn with an AFO enable the wearer to reduce the energy cost significantly while increasing the preferred walking speed.[151] Handrail support also diminishes the energy cost of walking, primarily by reducing gait velocity.[152] The simplest way to reduce the oxygen demand during walking is by using a cane, which requires less oxygen at a given speed or permits greater speed for the same oxygen consumption. The single-point cane is more efficient than a quad cane or a hemiwalker.[153]

However, the balance between footwear, assisted device, and speed of ambulation must be considered against the need for stability, motion restriction, and safety.

Cerebral Palsy

Children with CP use more energy when walking than other children,[154] consuming as much as 1.3 times more oxygen than able-bodied peers. The higher cost can be attributed to segmental impairments, such as spastic equinus, which increases the mechanical work performed by muscles.[155,156] As compared with barefoot walking, the hinged AFO reduced the children's energy expenditure.[71] Other investigators report that an AFO with a solid ankle reduced energy demand more than hinged AFOs or other orthoses.[72,157]

Paraplegia

The level and extent of spinal cord damage are critical determinants of functional capacity in people with SCI. The trade-off between energy consumption and the ability to ambulate must be balanced. Restraining both plantarflexion and dorsiflexion, as provided by Craig-Scott KAFOs, reduces energy demand very slightly given that degrees of freedom are not restricted. Performance is somewhat more efficient with molded plastic KAFOs, which weigh slightly less than traditional metal and leather braces; however, the user must have adequate trunk and leg strength to ambulate safely. Those with thoracic-level paraplegia use three times their basal oxygen rate ambulating with Craig-Scott KAFOs, and thus must ambulate slowly.[158] Those fitted with KAFOs with dorsiflexion stops performed more poorly during ambulation than patients wearing Craig-Scott orthoses.[159] Ambulation with an RGO facilitated more normal gait movements and stability and less energy expenditure than with traditional orthoses,[93,160] KAFOs, or bilateral KAFOs with a Walkabout medial hinge.[161] RGO use, however, was more arduous than wheelchair use and therefore would not supplant the wheelchair as the primary mode of locomotion.[162,163] Modifications of RGO use, such as FES of thigh muscles[164] or addition of electronic power to the RGO[165] as with powered exoskeletons, appear to improve energy consumption when patients walk.

Physiologically, upright posture stresses the skeleton, improving bone density; otherwise, the patient is vulnerable to fractures. Standing also facilitates respiratory, digestive, and urinary function. The logistical advantage of erect posture enables the patient to reach higher shelves than possible when sitting, improving ability to perform activities of daily living.

Psychosocial Considerations

Orthotic devices can provide the support needed for an individual to participate in community activities; however, the degree of participation is dependent on numerous factors, including the patient's prior level of function, comorbidities, and the activity being pursued. Thus, integration into society may be limited by the orthotic, the patient, the environment, or a combination. When collaborating on treatment goals with the patient, ensure that both restrictions and enabling factors of the orthotic are considered. Examples of restrictions would be movement limitations, orthosis weight, and energy expenditure. Enabling factors would include increased support, decreased pain, and improved biomechanics (e.g., drop foot correction).

Body image and device satisfaction may also impact the wearer's ability to participate meaningfully, as bulkier and more visible orthotic devices are less desirable.[166] The level of satisfaction can be assessed with self-report measures like the Orthotics and Prosthetics User Survey (OPUS) Satisfaction module.[167] If the patient describes low satisfaction on the module, it may increase the likelihood of non-use of the device, prompting the therapist to engage both the patient and the orthotist in a discussion to mitigate the undesirable outcome. Some individuals will be comfortable with clothing obscuring the device; however, when in less-concealing garments (e.g., shorts), they may not want to use the device. Making sure to align the goals of the device with the patient's lifestyle is crucial for acceptance.

SUMMARY

This chapter has focused on lower-limb, upper, and trunk orthoses. The most frequently prescribed orthoses and orthotic components have been presented. In addition, the responsibilities of the physical therapist in orthotic management have been emphasized.

Ideally, an orthotic clinic team composed of a physician, physical therapist, and orthotist aids in the prescription of the orthosis. The prescription should be based on a thorough examination, with particular attention to the specific factors discussed in this chapter. Input from the patient and all team members during the decision-making process is critical. This approach will ensure an optimum match between the patient's biomechanical and psychological requirements and an appropriate orthosis capable of performing its intended function. Once the orthosis has been prescribed, it should be evaluated to ensure satisfactory fit, function, and construction, and the patient should have the benefit of a suitable instruction and training program for donning the orthosis and using it effectively.

Questions for Review

1. Discuss the purpose of a correctly fitted shoe in orthotic management.

2. Describe the purpose (function) of the following external shoe modifications: heel wedge, sole wedge, metatarsal bar, and rocker bar.

3. What are the advantages of a plastic orthotic shoe insert as compared with a shoe?

4. For the patient with dorsiflexor weakness or paralysis, explain how a posterior leaf spring AFO imparts its function during early stance and swing phases of gait.

5. What is the function of the proximal anterior band on a floor reaction AFO?

6. How do tone-inhibiting AFOs improve the patient's function?

7. Indicate the clinical use of an AFO with a patellar-tendon-bearing brim.

8. What strategies can be used to increase the rigidity of plastic orthoses?

9. What is the function of an offset knee joint on a KAFO?

10. Describe the three-point system in a lumbosacral flexion–extension control orthosis.

11. What data should be gathered prior to formulating an orthotic prescription?

12. Compare and contrast the orthotic options for a patient with hemiplegia.

13. What are the purposes of the preorthotic examination?

14. What features of the AFO are considered during the static evaluation?

15. What are the anatomical and orthotic causes of vaulting?

CASE STUDY

PATIENT HISTORY AND CURRENT PROBLEM

The patient is a 60-year-old woman who suffered a left middle cerebral artery stroke 6 months ago and presents to the clinic with persistent mild fluent aphasia, right hemiparesis marked by obligatory upper-limb synergy with some active isolated movements, and right lower limb weakness marked by footdrop in swing phase (associated with both decreased ankle dorsiflexion ROM and decreased ankle dorsiflexion strength) and knee extension throughout stance phase with an occasional buckling into knee flexion, causing instability but not falls (associated with weak hip and knee extensors). She was given an off-the-shelf solid ankle-foot orthosis (SAFO) during inpatient rehabilitation at a skilled nursing facility and has used it ever since. She uses a straight cane and walks with asymmetric weight-bearing (shorter nonparetic step length) and halting pace (0.6 m/sec), minimizing stance time on her right leg. She complains of difficulty rising to stand from the sofa or a chair, which requires her to lean left and backward to use her left hand. She cannot ascend or descend stairs or curbs in step-over-step pattern without assistance for safety and typically uses the "up with the good, down with the bad" approach. In total, impaired transfer, gait, and barrier negotiation ability limits her ability to access the community for social events, which had included a book club, knitting group, and visits to her two sons' homes to see her young grandchildren. She has been referred for outpatient physical therapy to improve her mobility.

PHYSICAL THERAPY EXAMINATION FINDINGS
Body Structure and Function (Impairments)

• Cognition: Alert, oriented, memory intact; flat affect and slow processing; Mini-Mental State Examination 22/30 with difficulty selecting and ordering words and numbers after verbal cues suggests mild cognitive impairment.

• Vision: No visual perceptual deficit noted.

• Cardiopulmonary: Vital signs seated at rest: Blood pressure 130/86, heart rate 84, respiration normal

(Continued)

- Medication: Aspirin 100 mg/day
- Endurance: Exercise capacity 6 min before needing rest
- Integumentary: Intact over foot, ankles, and lower leg areas contacting the SAFO
- Neuromuscular: R-sided impaired sensation
- Musculoskeletal: Passive ROM: hip extension R 10 from neutral (hip flexion contracture), L 10; hip external rotation R 25, L 60; knees normal; ankle DF R 0 L 15
  - Joint mobility: R hip hypomobile
  - Flexibility: SLR R 50 L 70
  - MMT: Difficulty fractionating movement; R ankle DF and R hip extension 3–/5, unable to complete available PROM against gravity; knee extension R 3+/5, L 4+/5
- Orthosis: Polypropylene SAFO with 3/4 footplate

Activity (Limitations)
- Balance: Postural Assessment Scale for Stroke 28/36, with extended time or a little help required for a number of transitional movements, and 43/56 Berg Balance Scale score, with difficulty on small base of support or hemiparetic limb weight-bearing tasks, indicating a risk for falls.
- Gait: 0.6 m/sec with cane over 2 min, putting her in the category of an independent household and limited community walker. Rarely walks longer than 2 min without stopping at any one time. Decreased R-side stance time, increased R-side swing time, and shorter L-side step length with lack of R hip extension past neutral contribute to gait asymmetry. Uses cane in left hand.

Participation (Restrictions)
- Home living: Unsafe for living alone. Needs assistance for most activities of daily living, including all household chores and some self-care activities, such as positioning the shower bench for bathing. Modified independent mobility within the home using a cane and the SAFO. Outside the home, needs assistance to navigate stairs/slopes/curbs/terrain. A home care attendant who comes to her home three times/week assists her in bathing and performs light housework.
- Vocational: Has not returned to work at her office.
- Social: Walks outdoors only for doctor visits; rarely leaves home to shop or socialize.

Individual and Environmental Contextual Factors
She lives with her 70-year-old retired husband in a two-story home with six steps to enter and upstairs bedrooms. She is currently staying in the first-floor guest room. Her two adult sons live with their families within a 1-hr drive, but they are busy working and visit about once or twice per month. She used to enjoy babysitting her young grandchildren and getting together with friends for their book club and knitting group.

PERSON-DESIRED OUTCOME AND GOALS
Improve mobility to allow her to safely leave home to visit grandchildren and friends.

PHYSICAL THERAPY ASSESSMENT AND PLAN FOR CARE
Rehabilitation outcomes are enhanced when the person identifies goals for themselves that implicitly take into account the context of their social life. Reduced pain and improved functional outcomes such as safe and independent community walking and enhanced social participation are common patient goals. The individual seeking physical therapy may not fully understand how those goals are intertwined and that reaching these goals by attaining short and intermediate impairment and activity-level goals will support the desired functional outcome. For instance, short-term goals such as normalized ankle joint dorsiflexion ROM may affect balance reactions and contribute to sit-to-stand or stair-negotiation ability, thus enhancing her ability to leave home and accessing her community for meaningful social activity. Person-specific goals can measure progress with Specific, Measurable, Achievable, Relevant, and Time-bound goals combined with the person's subjective assessment like a Patient-Specific Functional Scale, in which patients list activities that are difficult for them and rate their ability on a 0- (cannot perform at all) to 10-point (can perform fully) scale.

What follows is an example of a long-term participation goal (I), with the underlying activity goals (A) in the context of the individual and environment (B), body structure/function goals (1–3), followed by bulleted suggestions for interventions to address the underlying goals (with guiding notes):

I. Leave the house to see grandchildren once per week by next month.

A. Gait: Ascend and descend stairs step-over-step with upper-limb assist

1. ROM: Ankle dorsiflexion to 10°

CASE STUDY—cont'd

  • Joint mobilization for R ankle (e.g., mobilization with movement in weight-bearing lunge position, supported by wall)
  • Soft tissue mobilization for R ankle plantar flexors, long toe flexors, and hip flexors—particularly rectus femoris
  • Self-stretching for plantar flexors in weight-bearing lunge position, supported by wall
2. MMT: Weight-bearing ankle plantar flexor, knee and hip extension strength

  • R leg forward and lateral step up to blocks of increasing height
  • Prolonged R leg stance time (e.g., in step standing position L leg up)
3. Orthosis: consider a new orthosis
  a. Hinged AFO with plantarflexion stop
   i. (+) will prevent toe drag in swing phase while allowing ankle dorsiflexion for sit-to-stand or stair negotiation
   ii. (–) will prevent plantar flexion upon initial contact, thus requiring ready knee extension strength upon contact
  b. Hinged AFO with dorsiflexion assist
   i. (+) will prevent toe drag while allowing ankle dorsiflexion for sit-stand and stair negotiation while allowing plantarflexion then enhances knee stability upon contact
   ii. (–) additional weight of some metal spring mechanisms adds to metabolic demands during walking
  c. Posterior Leaf Spring Orthosis
   i. (+) will prevent toe drag while allowing ankle dorsiflexion for sit-stand and stair negotiation while allowing plantarflexion then enhances knee stability upon contact
   ii. (–) provides no frontal plane support (which any hinged AFO provides); gives little resistance to ankle motion in either direction
4. Cardiopulmonary (exercise capacity): Walk for 6 min without rest with vital signs in safe range
  • Treadmill walking provides external cue to maintain speed
  • Count steps/day for a week, then increase by 10% per week
  • Walk around block, keeping track of the time, then aim to decrease time by 10%[57]
B. Individual and Environmental Context
  • Stairs/curbs/obstacles: Negotiate safely to facilitate leaving home and entering other people's homes.
  • Dual-task training: Integrate upper-limb carrying/manipulation tasks and cognitive/visual distraction with walking

GUIDING QUESTIONS
1. Formulate a list of other patient-focused participation goals.
2. For a specific participation goal, establish related activity goals and expected outcomes.
3. For a specific activity goal, identify underlying body structure/function impairments and goals.
4. Formulate a physical therapy plan of care to minimize body structure/function impairments and optimize activity outcomes.

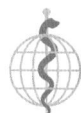
For additional resources, including answers to the questions for review, new immersive cases, case study guiding questions, references, and more, please visit **https://www.fadavis.com/product/physical -rehabilitation-fulk-8**. You may also quickly find the resources by entering this title's four-digit ISBN, 4691, in the search field at **http://fadavis.com** and logging in at the prompt.

Prosthetics

Chapter 31

Christopher Kevin Wong, PT, PhD, OCS
Daniel J. Lee, PT, DPT, PhD, GCS, OCS, COMT

LEARNING OBJECTIVES

1. Describe the components of transtibial and transfemoral prostheses, including advantages and disadvantages of alternative components and materials.
2. Explain the distinctive features of partial foot, ankle disarticulation, knee and hip disarticulation prostheses, and bilateral prostheses.
3. Describe the form and function of upper limb prosthetic devices.
4. Outline the maintenance program for prosthetic components.
5. Conduct static and dynamic evaluation of transtibial and transfemoral prostheses.
6. Summarize the physical therapist's role in management of individuals with lower limb amputation.
7. Analyze and interpret patient data, formulate realistic goals and outcomes, and develop a plan of care when presented with a clinical case study.

CHAPTER OUTLINE

LOWER LIMB PROSTHESES 1181
PARTIAL FOOT AND ANKLE PROSTHESES 1181
TRANSTIBIAL PROSTHESES 1182
  Foot-Ankle Assemblies 1182
  Shanks 1185
  Sockets 1186
  Liners 1187
  Socks 1188
  Suspension 1188
TRANSFEMORAL PROSTHESES 1191
  Foot-Ankle Assemblies and Shanks 1191
  Knee Units 1191
  Sockets 1194
  Suspensions 1195
DISARTICULATION PROSTHESES 1197
  Knee Disarticulation Prostheses 1197
  Hip Disarticulation Prostheses 1197
BILATERAL PROSTHESES 1198
  Bilateral Ankle Disarticulation and Transtibial Prostheses 1198
  Bilateral Transfemoral Prostheses 1198
UPPER LIMB PROSTHESES 1198
  Passive 1198
  Body Powered 1199

  Myoelectric 1199
  Hybrid 1200
  Activity Specific 1200
PROSTHESIS MAINTENANCE 1200
  Foot-Ankle Assemblies 1200
  Shanks 1200
  Joints 1201
  Sockets and Suspensions 1201
PROSTHETIC FIT AND ALIGNMENT 1201
  Prosthetic Fit 1201
  Prosthetic Alignment 1202
PHYSICAL THERAPY MANAGEMENT 1203
  Prescription Considerations 1203
  Physical Examination 1203
  Cognition and Psychosocial Conditions 1204
  Temporary Prostheses 1205
  Prosthetic Prescription 1205
  Prosthetic Examination 1208
  Prosthetic Training 1212
  Community Integration: Work, Sports, and Other Activities 1219
SUMMARY 1220

Physical therapists play an important role in the care of individuals with lower- and upper-limb amputations. To replace the absent part of the leg or arm, patients are often fitted with a *prosthesis*. In the broadest sense, prostheses also include dentures, titanium femoral heads, and plastic heart valves. A *prosthetist* designs, fabricates, and fits limb prostheses.

The major causes of amputation are peripheral vascular disease, trauma, malignancy, and congenital deficiency. In the United States, vascular disease accounts for most leg amputations, particularly among patients with diabetes.[1] Individuals older than 60 years constitute the largest group of people with amputation. Men are more likely to sustain amputation because of vascular disease and trauma. Among younger adults and adolescents, trauma is responsible for most amputations.

Bone and soft tissue tumors are sometimes treated by amputation, with adolescence the period of peak incidence. *Congenital deficiency* refers to the absence or abnormality of a limb evident at birth.

Physical therapists are key members of the rehabilitation team, working with prosthetists, physicians, occupational therapists, and others to foster the patient's welfare. For individuals with lower limb amputation, physical therapists have the major role in assisting the person to regain function. Lower limb and upper limb prostheses will be described, together with a program for training patients in their use. Read Chapter 22, Amputation, of this text for more information about amputations and postoperative rehabilitation.

A *prosthesis* is the artificial device that replaces an anatomical structure, while the term *prosthetic* is an adjective used to describe the device (e.g., prosthetic limb). Therefore, when instructing a patient to walk with their artificial limb, you would say "Please walk with your prosthesis" or "Please walk with your prosthetic leg" and not "Please walk with your prosthetic." Additionally, since not all individuals underwent amputation, the term *individual with limb loss* is preferred to amputee. For those born with congenital deficiency, the term *limb difference* should be used.

■ LOWER LIMB PROSTHESES

The principal lower limb prostheses are partial foot, ankle disarticulation (Syme), transtibial, and transfemoral as well as knee and hip disarticulations. The purposes of lower limb prostheses are to (a) restore as much function as possible, particularly in walking, and (b) simulate the shape of the missing segment(s). The physical therapist should be familiar with their characteristics and maintenance as well as the rehabilitation of patients fitted with these devices.

■ PARTIAL FOOT AND ANKLE PROSTHESES

Phalangeal amputation or disarticulations can be accommodated with a functional passive prosthesis that allows for improved gait mechanics during terminal stance and midstance (see Fig. 31.1). An additional foot orthotic helps to maintain alignment of the amputated foot, especially if one or more proximal phalanges have been amputated.[2] Prostheses for ankle disarticulations include a foot-ankle assembly and socket for the residual lower limb.

Transmetatarsal amputation disturbs foot appearance and function more noticeably. A prosthesis consisting of a plastic socket affixed to a rigid plate extending the full length of the inner sole of the shoe restores form and function of the foot (see Fig. 31.2). *Socket* refers to a shell that conforms to the residual limb, allowing for the transfer of forces between the anatomical and

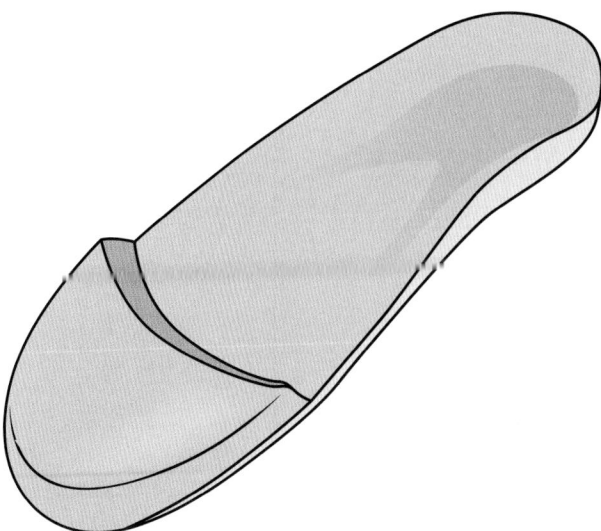

Figure 31.2 Foot plate to accommodate transmetatarsal amputation. *(Courtesy of Infinite Technologies Orthotics & Prosthetics, Fairfax, VA 22030.)*

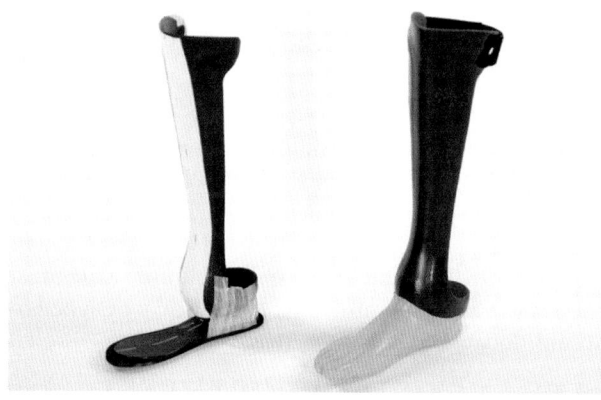

Figure 31.3 Prosthesis for Chopart tarsal disarticulation amputation. *(Courtesy of Otto Bock, Minneapolis, MN 55447.)*

prosthetic segment. To aid late stance, the bottom of the prosthesis or the sole of the shoe may have a convex rocker bar.[3]

Disarticulation through the tarsals, such as Lisfranc (tarsometatarsal disarticulation) and Chopart disarticulations,[4] poses the additional problem of retaining the small foot segment in the shoe during swing phase. Foot length is apt to be diminished further by an equinus deformity of the amputated limb, resulting from unbalanced contraction of the triceps surae. For a tarsometatarsal disarticulation, a prosthesis described for transmetatarsal amputation may be augmented with a plastic calf shell, similar to that of an ankle-foot orthosis (AFO), which is discussed in Chapter 30, Orthotics.[5,6] For a Chopart disarticulation (see Fig. 31.3), a prosthetic socket is designed to accommodate the remaining tarsal bones (calcaneus and talus) and attaches to a foot plate (similar to that of an AFO).

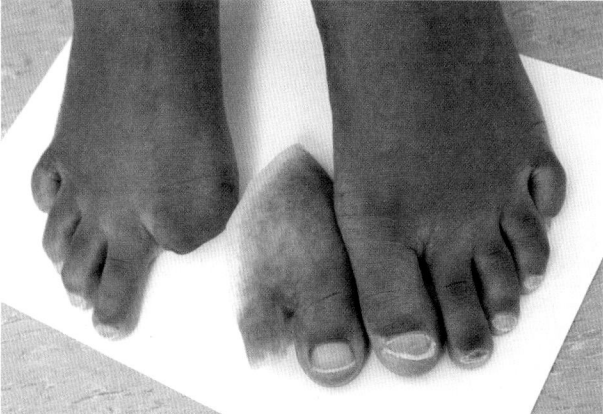

Figure 31.1 Passive prosthesis for great toe amputation. *(Courtesy of Medical Art Resources, Inc, Milwaukee, WI 53227.)*

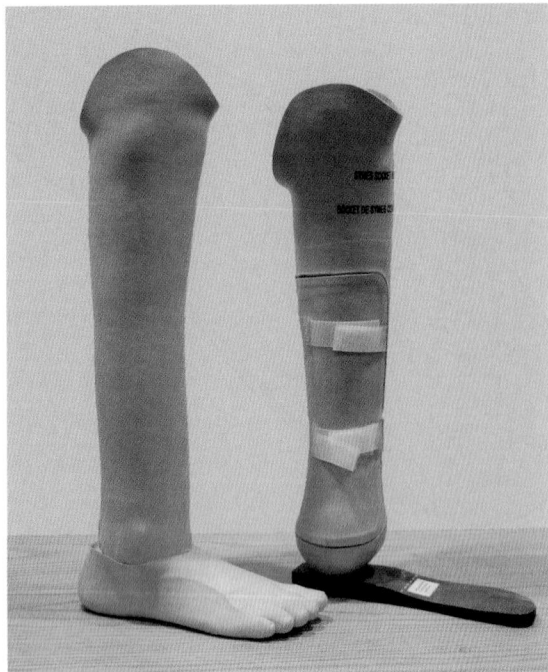

Figure 31.4 Ankle disarticulation prostheses. (Left) Socket with medial opening. (Right) Socket with continuous walls and flexible liner.

Ankle disarticulation involves surgical sectioning through the distal tibia and fibula to leave a flat distal weight-bearing surface, which can be the preserved heel fat pad. The patient can usually bear significant weight through the distal end of the residual limb.[7,8] The prosthesis includes a low-profile foot specifically designed to accommodate the long socket (Fig. 31.4).

■ TRANSTIBIAL PROSTHESES

The *transtibial level,* also known as *below-knee,* refers to an amputation in which the tibia and fibula are transected. The patient retains the anatomical knee with its motor and sensory functions. This is the predominant site of amputation, particularly for individuals with vascular disease.[9] Prostheses for transtibial amputations include a foot-ankle assembly, a shank (lower leg), a socket, and a suspension component.

Foot-Ankle Assemblies

A foot-ankle assembly restores the general contour of the patient's foot, absorbs shock at initial contact, plantar flexes in loading response, and simulates metatarsophalangeal extension (toe-off action) in terminal stance. A balance between rigidity and flexibility must be maintained for efficient gait, with preference for a foot with a relatively rigid forefoot.[10] The foot maintains neutral positioning during swing phase allowing for toe clearance.

In response to ground reaction forces, many assemblies provide slight motion in the frontal and/or transverse planes to approximate physiological foot motion.[11,12] Rubber encases the stiff inner portion called the *keel,*

made of wood, high-temperature plastic, metal, or carbon fiber.

Nonarticulated Foot-Ankle Assemblies
Solid Ankle Cushion Heel Foot

The nonarticulated *solid ankle cushion heel (SACH)* assembly is commonly available around the world (Fig. 31.5) due to its simplicity and low manufacturing costs. The keel, which provides stability, is wooden or metal and terminates at a point corresponding to the metatarsophalangeal joints. The keel is encased in rubber; the posterior portion is resilient to absorb shock and permit plantarflexion at initial contact. Terminal stance is facilitated by the junction of the rubber toe section and the keel. The SACH foot is manufactured in a wide range of sizes to accommodate infants, adolescents, and adults. The SACH foot is available with heel cushions of varying degrees of compressibility for people who place different amounts of force through the heel.

A patient's weight must be considered when prescribing a SACH foot as the heel will fail to perform weight acceptance correctly during initial contact if it is too soft or firm. A very firm heel will result in uncontrolled plantarflexion and foot slap, while a soft heel will delay plantarflexion and prolong the loading response. SACH feet can be ordered in several plantarflexion angles to fit shoes with diverse heel heights. Most nonarticulated foot designs also have rigid ankle blocks and stiff keels of different materials surrounded by rubber, though newer materials may provide more flexibility (Fig. 31.6)

Feet made with materials that bend slightly under the force of weight-bearing as the wearer moves over the foot during midstance before recoiling in late stance as the wearer transfers loading to the opposite foot are described as *energy-storing* or *dynamic feet.* The *Flex-Foot* (Fig. 31.7) and feet of similar manufacture include a long length of carbon fiber, extending from the toe to the proximal shank. The long carbon fiber length acts as a leaf spring, enabling the foot to store considerable energy in early and midstance, and then to release

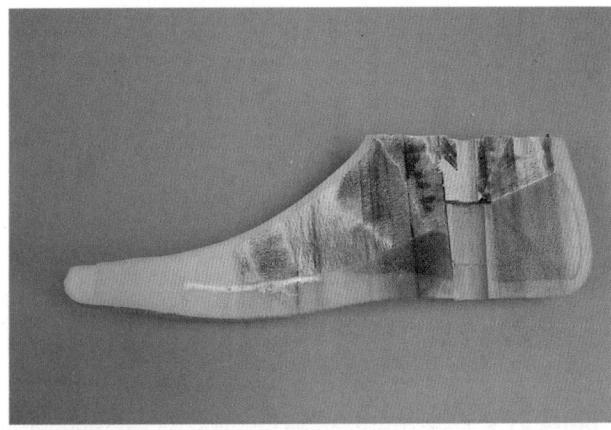

Figure 31.5 Cross section of a solid ankle cushion heel nonarticulated foot-ankle assembly.

energy in the late stance phase of gait. A posterior heel length is optional.

Active wearers, such as those who play basketball, run, or engage in other high-impact activities, can best utilize the energy-storing/energy-releasing capacity of these feet (Fig. 31.8A, D). Other energy-storing prosthetic feet, all more expensive than SACH feet, are shown in Figure 31.8. The anterior keel can be split into two to allow different degrees of bending on the medial or lateral keel and thus provide some frontal plane motion (Fig. 31.8A, C, D, F). Many of these feet can be sheathed in a cosmetic cover (Fig. 31.9). Athletes may opt to interchange the basic prosthetic foot for one designed for sprinting (Fig. 31.10).

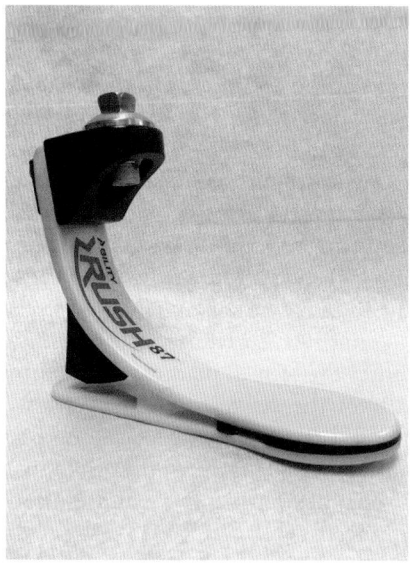

Figure 31.6 The Rush foot made of glass composite.

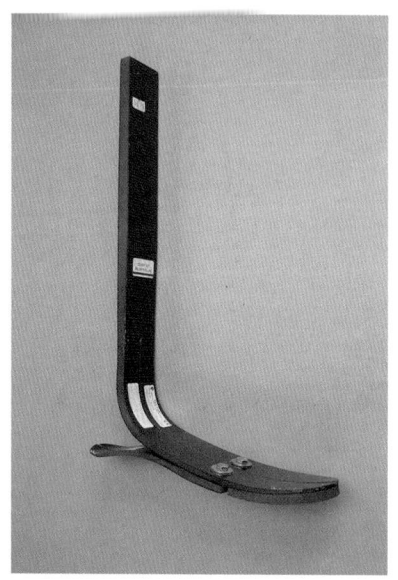

Figure 31.7 Flex-Foot posterior leaf spring.

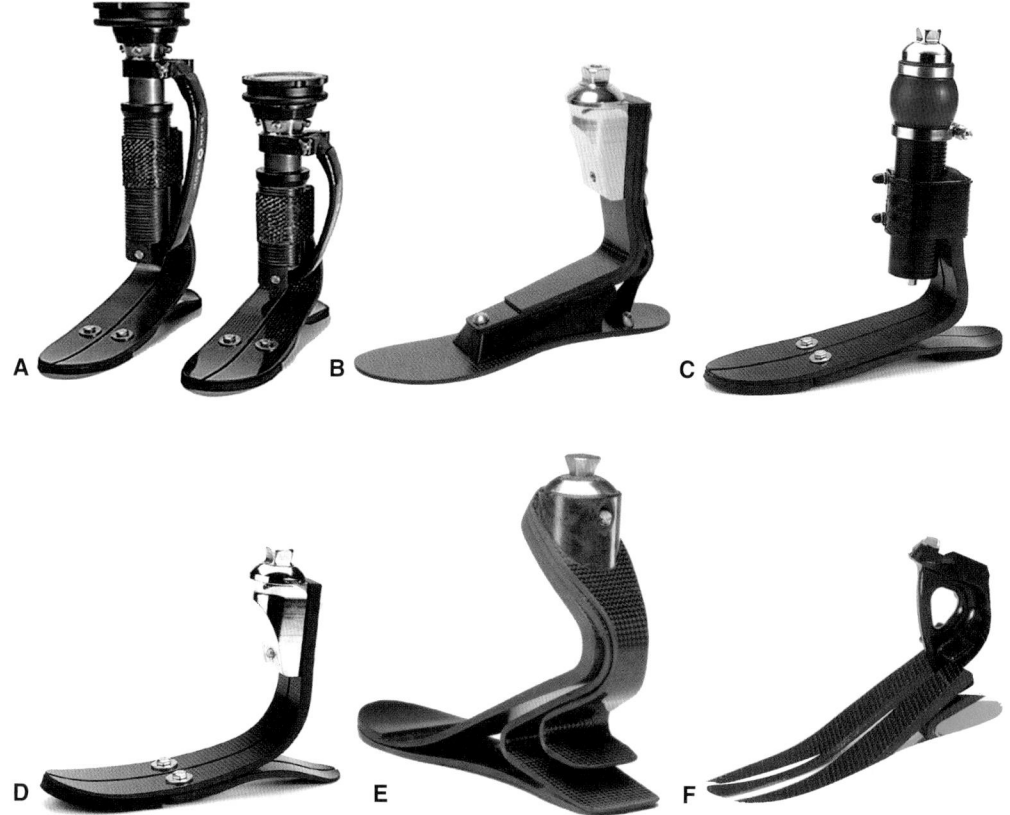

Figure 31.8 Nonarticulated energy-storing prosthetic feet. (A) Re-Flex VSP and Re-Flex VSP Low Profile. (B) Talux. (C) Ceterus. (D) Vari-Flex. *(Courtesy of Össur, Aliso Viejo, CA, 92656.)* (E) Renegade. (F) ELITE 2. *(Courtesy of Endolite, Miamisburg, OH 45342.)*

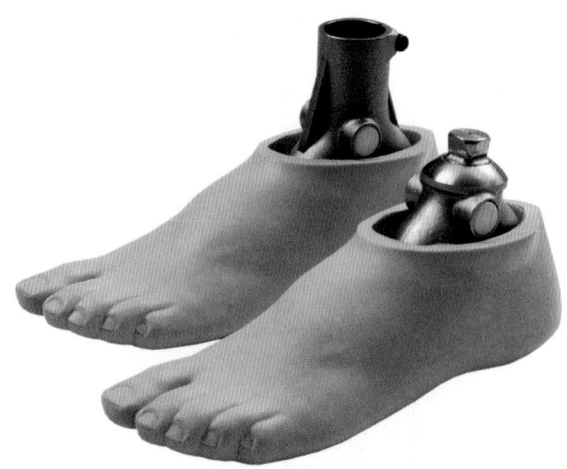

Figure 31.9 Cosmetic foot covers. *(Courtesy of Össur, Aliso Viejo, CA 92656.)*

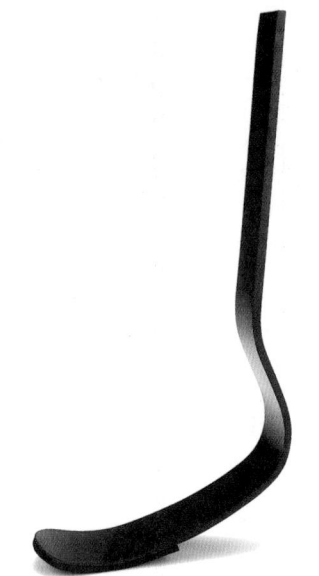

Figure 31.10 Flex-Foot Cheetah. *(Courtesy of Össur, Aliso Viejo, CA 92656.)*

Articulated Foot-Ankle Assemblies

Articulated foot-ankle assemblies can offer enhanced mobility when compared to nonarticulating foot-ankle assemblies. This is due to the inclusion of mechanical joints, potential spaces, and purposeful leverage. Rubber bumpers or hydraulics may be used to improve the timing and magnitude of the motion but require regular maintenance to preserve normal function.

Single-Axis Foot-Ankle Assemblies

The most common example of an articulated foot is the *single-axis foot* (Fig. 31.11). A posterior bumper absorbs shock and controls plantarflexion excursion; it is easy for the prosthetist to substitute a firmer or softer bumper, depending on the force that the patient applies in early stance. A heavy or very active client requires a firm bumper, whereas a frail individual needs a bumper that is soft enough to permit the foot to plantarflex with minimal loading. At initial contact, bearing weight on the heel causes the foot to plantarflex, ensuring that the wearer achieves the stable foot-flat position. An anterior bumper resists dorsiflexion and absorbs force as the wearer transfers weight forward over the foot. The total amount of dorsiflexion-plantarflexion motion provided by an articulated ankle (20° to 25°) is roughly double that provided by a nonarticulated ankle (11° to 14°) but does not approach the anatomical movement.[13] The single-axis foot does not allow medial–lateral or transverse motion.

Multiaxial Foot-Ankle Assemblies

These components move slightly in all planes to aid the wearer in maintaining maximum contact with the walking surface, even if the surface slopes or has slight irregularities (Fig. 31.12). Multiaxial foot-ankle assemblies are heavier and less durable than single-axis or nonarticulated feet. A recent version of a multiaxial foot-ankle assembly is the ProprioFoot (Fig. 31.13),

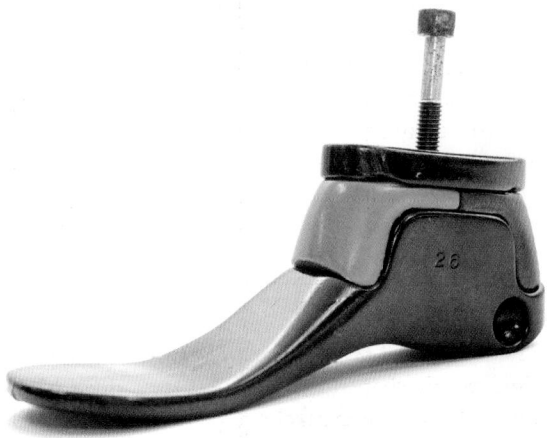
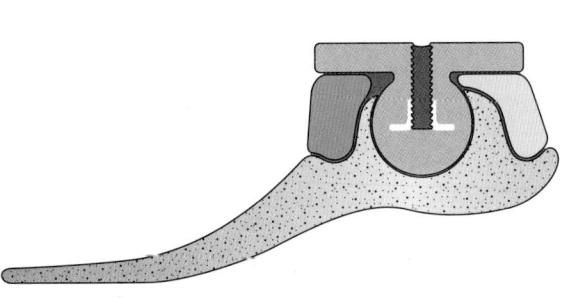

Figure 31.11 Single-axis foot with cross-sectional view; anterior bumper controls dorsiflexion, posterior bumper controls plantarflexion.

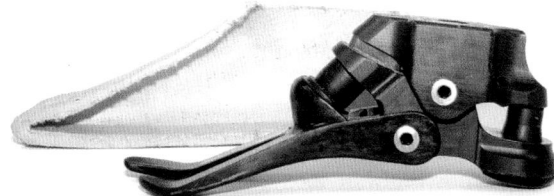

Figure 31.12 Multiaxial foot with cosmetic cover cross section

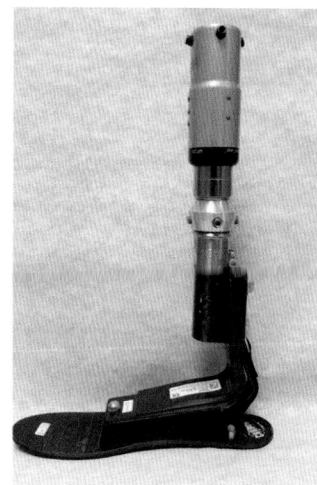

Figure 31.14 Delta Twist torsion adapting.

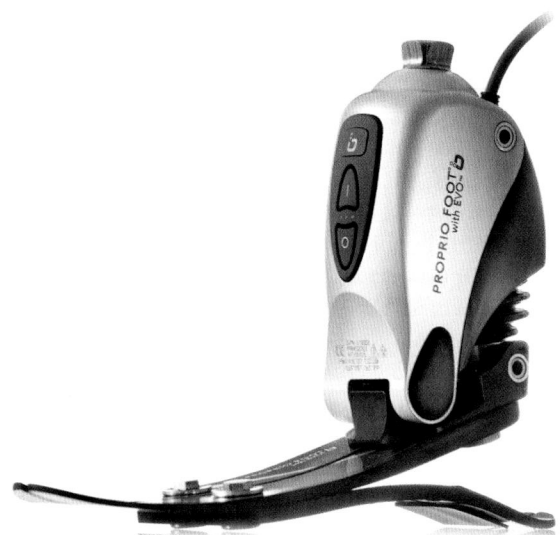

Figure 31.13 ProprioFoot. *(Courtesy of Össur, Aliso Viejo, CA 92656.)*

which includes electronic sensors to detect when the wearer needs dorsiflexion; it also provides greater ankle excursion than other foot-ankle assemblies and reduces pressure on the residual limb.[14,15]

Selection of the appropriate foot is based on the needs of the individual, considering the wearer's activity level, weight, level of amputation, environment, and length and shape of the residual limb.

Rotators and Shock Absorbers

A rotator is a component placed above the prosthetic foot-ankle assembly to promote rotational motion in the transverse plane during weight-bearing. A shock absorber reduces vertical impact, such as from jumping. These components protect the user from skin chafing, which would otherwise occur if the socket were permitted to slide against the skin.[16,17] Rotators and shock absorbers are most often used with single-axis feet and by very active individuals, especially those with transfemoral amputations. A rotator with or without a shock absorber may be contained within a prosthetic foot, such as Ceterus (see Fig. 31.8C), or may be installed in

the shank, such as the Delta Twist (Otto Bock, Minneapolis, MN 55447) (Fig. 31.14) to provide transverse plane motion. Though motion is minimal, enhanced comfort during gait can result from the reduced joint stress.[18]

Shanks

The shank is the substitute for the human leg, restoring leg length and transmitting body weight from the socket to the prosthetic foot. The shank is located between the foot-ankle assembly (or rotator) and the socket in a transtibial prosthesis. The two types of shanks are *endoskeletal* (most common) and *exoskeletal.*

Endoskeletal Shank

The *endoskeletal* (Fig. 31.15), or *modular shank,* consists of a central aluminum or rigid plastic tube (called a *pylon*) usually covered with foam rubber made to resemble the leg. With its cover, the endoskeletal shank is more natural in appearance than the exoskeletal shank, which is made from a hard material unlike skin. The pylon permits adjustment to the prosthesis alignment, which is described in greater detail in the section on Prosthetic Alignment later in this chapter. A variety of prosthetic foot-ankle assemblies, such as the Flex-Foot, incorporate an endoskeletal shank. Some patients wear prostheses without a cover over the pylon as it is not necessary for the device to function.

Exoskeletal Shank

The *exoskeletal shank* (Fig. 31.16) is typically made of rigid plastic shaped to simulate the contour of the anatomical leg. The exoskeletal shank is very durable and impervious to liquids. Because they are less lifelike, heavier, and do not permit alignment changes, exoskeletal shanks are less frequently prescribed.

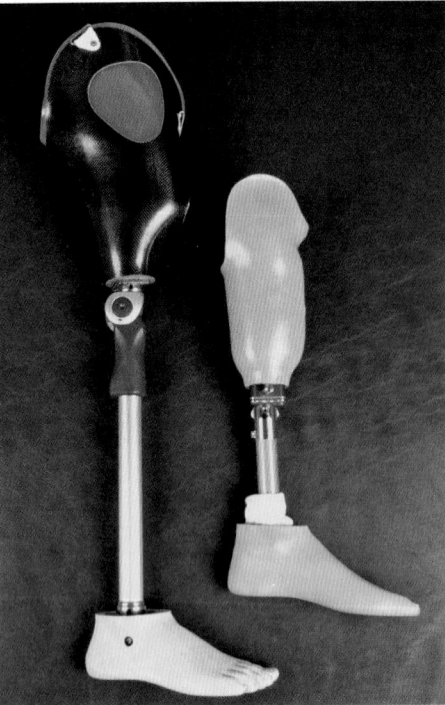

Figure 31.15 Endoskeletal (modular) shank on (left) trans-femoral prosthesis and on (right) transtibial prosthesis. *(From Roy SH, Wolf SL, Scalzitti DA. The Rehabilitation Specialist's Handbook. 4th ed. F.A. Davis; 2013:953. With permission.)*

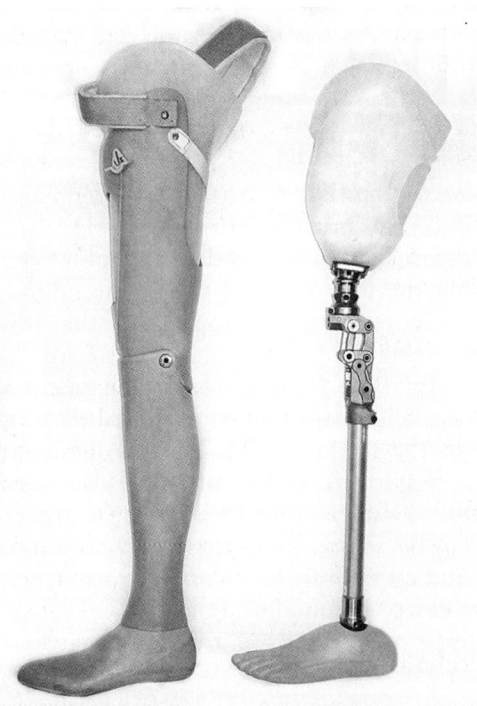

Figure 31.16 (Left) Exoskeletal transfemoral prosthesis. (Right) Endoskeletal transfemoral prosthesis with cosmetic foam cover removed.

Sockets

The residual limb fits into a receptacle called the *socket* (Fig. 31.17). The socket serves at the attachment point of the residual limb to that of the shank and as such is the primary weight-bearing point of contact. There are numerous types of sockets, each serving a different purpose based on the prosthetic user's particular needs. For example, a *patellar-tendon-bearing* socket uses an indentation in the socket wall to increase weight-bearing through the patellar tendon. More commonly prescribed is a *total surface bearing* socket, which has a shallower anterior indentation and allows for a greater distribution of forces over the entirety of the residual limb.[19]

Sockets are custom-made to intimately fit the patient's residual limb. The socket may be produced from a plaster cast of the amputation limb or by *computer-aided design/computer-aided manufacture*. The latter involves an electronic scanner that transmits a detailed map of the limb to a computerized program consisting of socket-shape variations; the prosthetist selects the appropriate shape, which is transmitted to an electronic carver that creates the model over which the socket is shaped.

Whether the socket is made by hand or by computer, a series of pressure-relieving *reliefs* are integrated into the socket over sensitive structures, such as bony prominences (Fig. 31.18). Reliefs are typically located over the fibular head, tibial crest, tibial condyles, and anterior-distal tibia. The posterior socket trimline or *brim* is shaped to provide adequate room and thus comfort for the medial and lateral hamstring tendons when the person bends the knee to, for instance, sit. *Buildups* are convexities in the socket over areas contacting pressure-tolerant tissues, such as the belly of the gastrocnemius; patellar ligament; proximal medial tibia, corresponding to the pes anserinus; and the tibial and fibular shafts. The combination of pressure reliefs and buildups allow for maximal skin contact, weight distribution, and comfort for the wearer, while also reducing the prevalence of pressure-related skin breakdown.

When viewed from above, the socket resembles a triangle, with the apex forming the relief for the tibial tubercle and crest, and the base angles forming the hamstring reliefs. The anterior wall terminates at the mid-patella or above. The medial and lateral walls extend at least to the femoral epicondyles. The posterior wall lies across the popliteal fossa.

The socket is aligned on the shank in slight flexion to enhance loading on the patellar ligament, prevent genu recurvatum, and resist the tendency of the amputation limb to slide too deeply into the socket. Flexion also facilitates contraction of the quadriceps muscle. The socket is also aligned with a slight lateral tilt to reduce loading on the fibular head.[20,21] See the section on Prosthetic Alignment for more details.

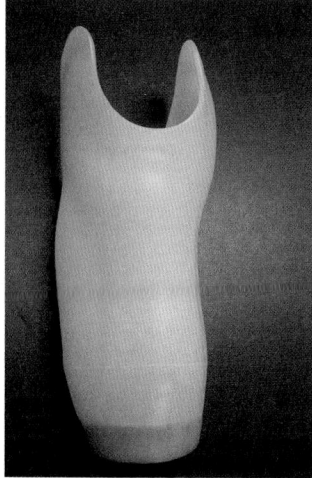

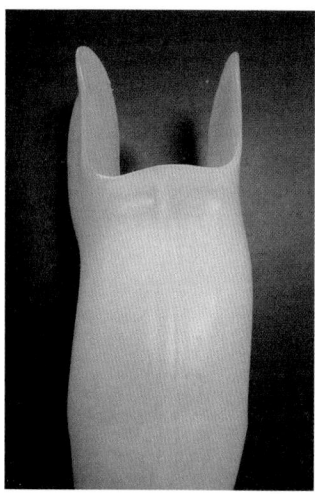

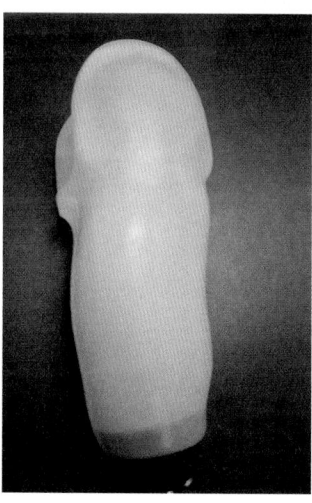

Figure 31.17 Transtibial patellar tendon-bearing socket from three directions.

Liners

The transtibial socket may include a resilient liner made of polyethylene foam,[22] polyurethane,[23] silicone,[24] or similar materials. In addition to cushioning the residual

limb, the removable liner facilitates alteration of socket size; the prosthetist can add material to the inside of the liner, reducing the volume of the socket while preserving smooth interior contours. The liner, however, adds to the bulk of the prosthesis and is a heat insulator, which the wearer may find uncomfortable in hot weather.

Silicone gel liners cushion the residual limb and function as a primary or secondary suspension system. The liner is applied directly to the skin, providing a barrier to friction and compressive forces. The primary types of silicon liners are locking and nonlocking liners. Locking liners (Fig. 31.19) have a pin, strap, or other mechanism that physically engages with the socket to suspend the prosthesis. Nonlocking liners may only provide cushioning or in some cases have a seal that creates a vacuum inside of the socket in order to suspend the prostheses.

Socks

Fabric socks are woven in various thicknesses referred to as *ply*, designating the number of threads knitted together. The purpose of the socks is to ensure that a congruent fit is maintained as the residual limb volume fluctuates throughout the day. Socks are worn over the silicon liner in order of the smallest ply to the largest ply. Cotton socks are the least allergenic; they are made in two, three, and five ply, the last being the thickest. Wool socks provide good cushioning, woven in three and five ply; they are expensive and must be laundered carefully. Orlon/Lycra socks are manufactured in two- and three-ply thicknesses. They can be washed easily without shrinking.

It is common practice to add more socks as the amputation limb volume reduces. When the patient requires socks equaling 15 ply to achieve a snug fit, the socket should be altered or replaced by the prosthetist. Excessive sock padding distorts the weight-bearing characteristics of the socket, losing the effect of strategically placed buildups and reliefs.

Suspension

During the swing phase of walking, or whenever the wearer is not standing on the prosthesis, such as when climbing stairs or jumping, the prosthesis requires some form of suspension to hold it in place. There are a myriad of suspension solutions available, many region or prosthetist specific. Sometimes the prosthetist will design the suspension to combine multiple types, as in the case of a pin suspension with a vacuum component. Presented next are common suspension systems found clinically.

Cuff Variants

The modern transtibial prosthesis originated with a supracondylar cuff (Fig. 31.20). The cuff may be a leather, flexible plastic, or fabric-webbing strap. It encircles the

Transtibial Limb   **Transfemoral Limb**

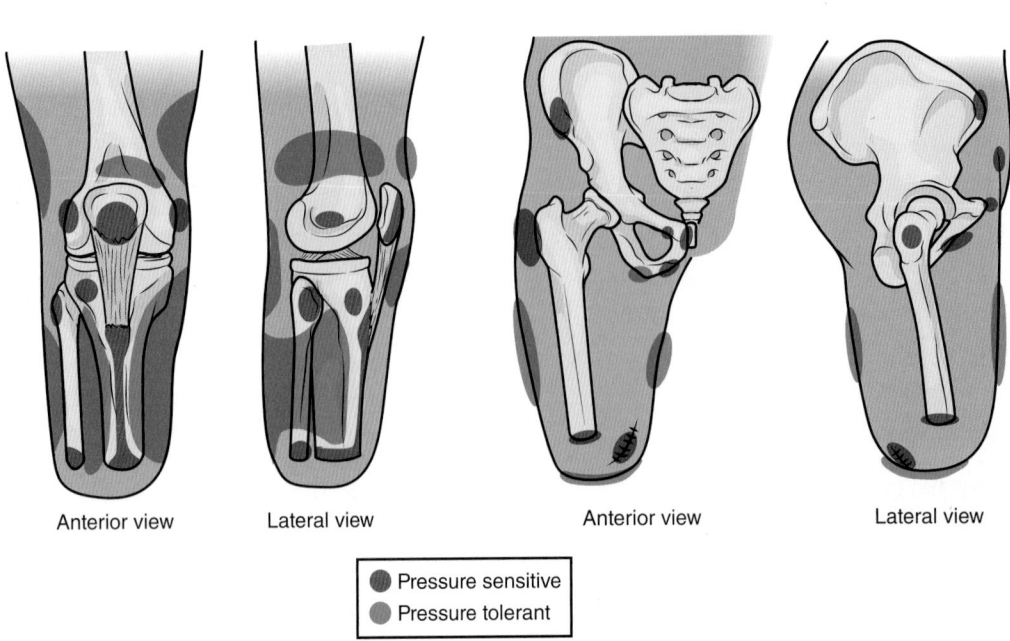

Anterior view   Lateral view   Anterior view   Lateral view

● Pressure sensitive
● Pressure tolerant

Figure 31.18 Transtibial and transfemoral limb–socket interfaces with pressure-tolerant (green) and pressure-sensitive (red) areas demarcated. Areas of relief (also called *channels*) reduce pressure over sensitive tissues. Buildups (also called *bulges*) contact pressure-tolerant tissues.

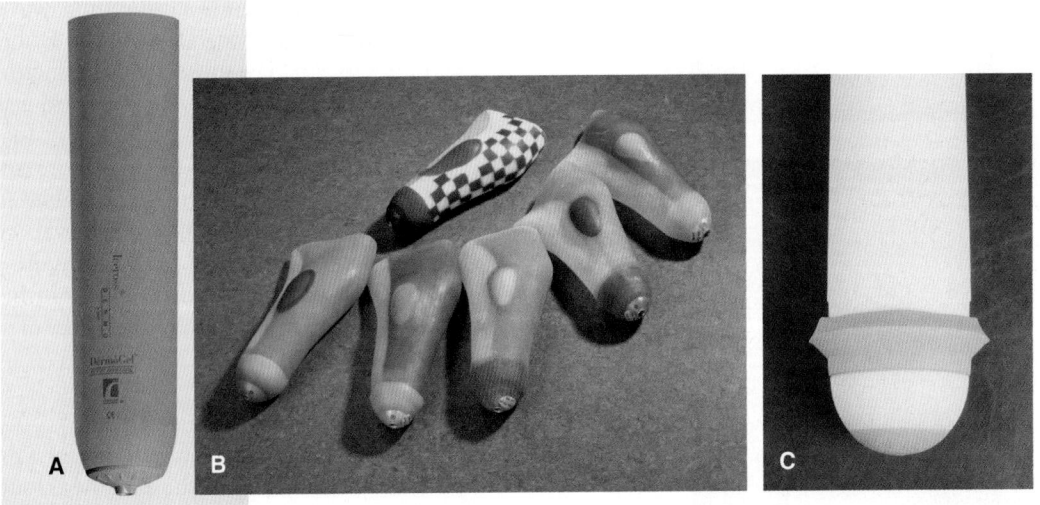

Figure 31.19 Silicone liners: (A) Iceross Dermo locking silicone gel liner. *(Courtesy of Össur, Aliso Viejo, CA 92656.)* (B) Custom liners with fibular head padding. *(Courtesy of Otto Bock, Minneapolis, MN 55447.)* (C) Seal-in designs. *(From Roy SH, Wolf SL, Scalzitti DA. The Rehabilitation Specialist's Handbook. 4th ed. F.A. Davis; 2013:977. With permission.)*

thigh immediately above the femoral epicondyles and permits the user to easily adjust the snugness of suspension. Some individuals, however, object to the profile of the distal thigh created by the cuff. Others who have severely arthritic hands or limited vision have difficulty engaging the buckle or pressure hook-and-loop closure on the cuff (see Fig. 31.20).

A fork strap and waist belt may be used to augment the cuff. The elastic fork strap extends from the outside of the anterior portion of the socket to a waist belt. The fork strap and waist belt may be indicated for individuals who climb ladders or engage in other activities during which the prosthesis is unsupported by the ground for long periods. An alternative to the cuff is a rubber

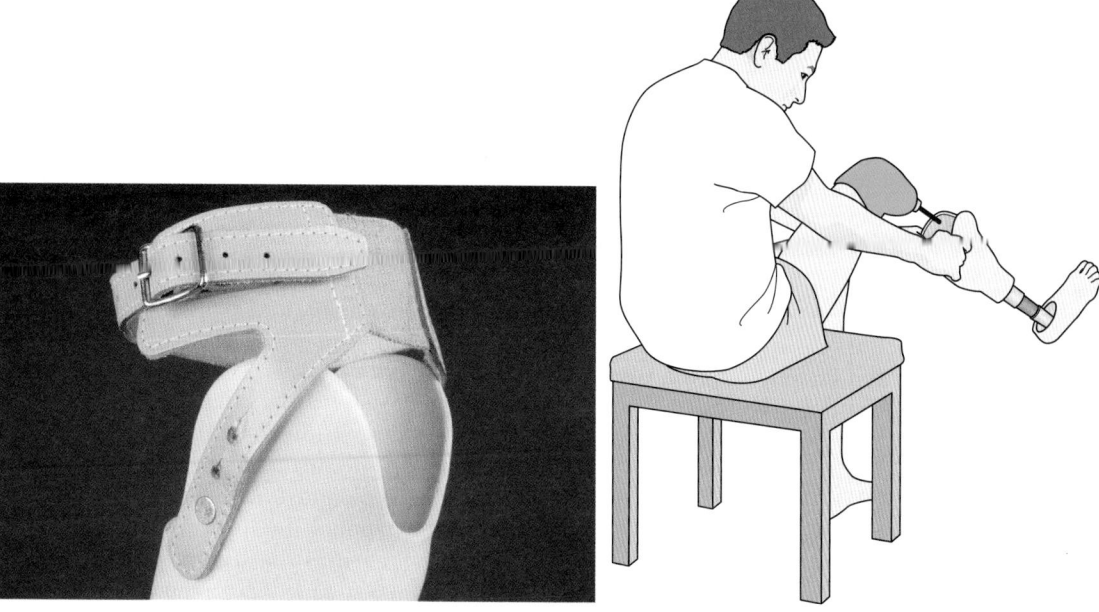

Figure 31.20 (Left) Supracondylar cuff suspension for transtibial prostheses. *(From Roy SH, Wolf SL, Scalzitti DA. The Rehabilitation Specialist's Handbook. 4th ed. F.A. Davis; 2013:977. With permission.)* (Right) Patient donning a transtibial prosthesis using a roll-on sleeve that includes a pin and shuttle lock assembly.

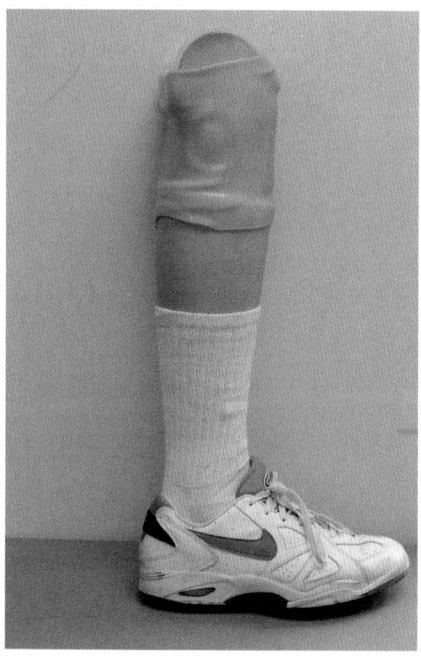

Figure 31.21 Transtibial suspension sleeve. Note round relief for fibular head.

sleeve, a tubular component that covers the proximal socket and the distal thigh (Fig. 31.21). The sleeve provides excellent suspension and a streamlined silhouette when the wearer sits. Donning the sleeve, however, requires two strong hands and a thigh that does not have excessive subcutaneous tissue.

Shuttle Lock and Pin

Secure suspension is achieved with the use of a silicone gel liner with a distal metal pin (Fig. 31.22). The user inserts the residual limb into the prosthesis, guiding the attached pin into the shuttle lock located at the bottom of the socket (see Fig. 31.20, Right). The resultant interface between the pin and shuttle lock creates a strong bond between the silicon liner and the socket, preventing the prosthesis from falling off during mobility. An alternative to the pin system is a lanyard or cord suspension, in which instead of a metal pin protruding

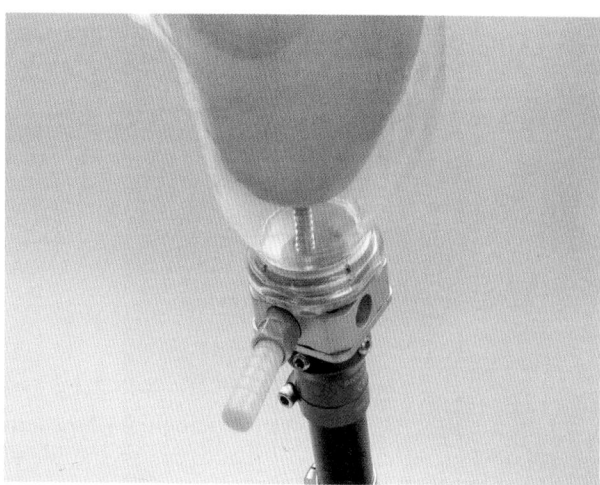

Figure 31.22 Transtibial distal pin attachment. The pin fits into a receptacle in the socket bottom and is then tightened into place.

from the liner, a cord extends through a receptacle and is anchored externally on the prosthesis.

Suction

Suction suspensions come in a variety of forms, but all serve the same function: suspend the residual limb in the socket through the creation of negative pressure. This is accomplished by expelling air distally from the socket when donning the socket, and sealing the socket to the skin proximally with a neoprene sleeve. The expulsion of the air occurs at a valve incorporated into the distal aspect of the socket, and may be a one or two-way valve. To release the suction, a button on the valve is pressed, allowing air to flow into the socket and releasing the negative pressure.

Vacuum-Assisted Suspension

Vacuum-assisted suspension is another alternative mode of suspension (Fig. 31.23). There are two primary types of vacuum suspension: mechanical and electric. An electric system actively creates a vacuum inside of the socket once loss of suction occurs. A mechanical type is typically integrated into the prosthetic foot, drawing air out of the socket with each step to maintain negative pressure. The system combines a pump, liner, and sleeve to achieve negative pressure in an airtight environment. Vacuum promotes fluid exchange, reduces moisture buildup, regulates volume fluctuations, and increases proprioceptive awareness of the limb's position in space. While similar to suction suspension, a vacuum is more efficient at maintaining the negative pressure, albeit at a greater weight of the suspension system.

A surgical approach to distal attachment is known as *osseointegration*,[25] in which the surgeon implants a metal post in the distal bone. The post protrudes through the skin and locks into a mechanism in the prosthesis. Osseointegration eliminates the need for other suspension apparatus; however, fluid drainage and infection at the skin–post interface are sometimes troublesome. The procedure was developed in Europe and was approved in the United States in 2016.

Brim Variants

The socket walls may be extended proximally to suspend the prosthesis. With *supracondylar (SC) suspension* (see Fig. 31.20), the medial and lateral walls extend above the femoral epicondyles. When donning the prosthesis, the patient applies the liner and then inserts the limb with the liner into the socket. Supracondylar suspension may increase medial–lateral stability of the knee.

Presenting a contour of medial and lateral walls similar to the supracondylar suspension, the supracondylar/suprapatellar (SC/SP) suspension (Fig. 31.24) also features an anterior wall that terminates above the patella.

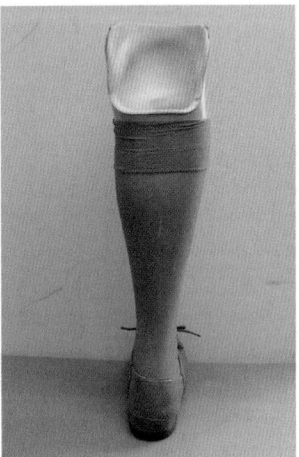

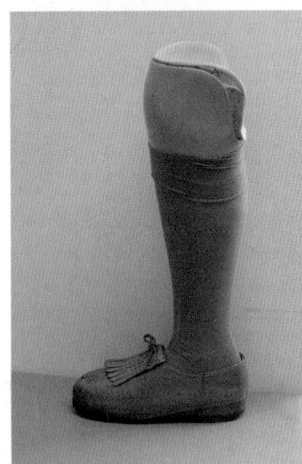

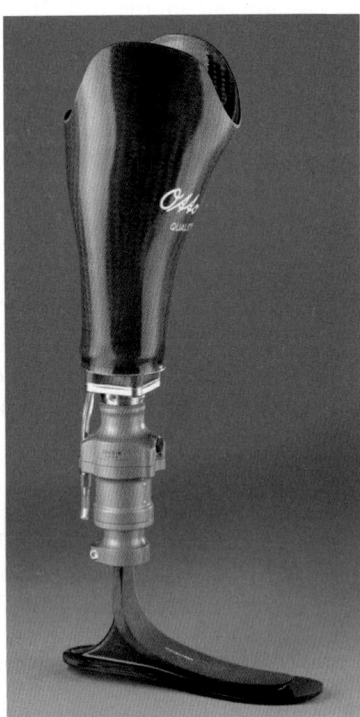

Figure 31.23 Vacuum-assisted suspension: Harmony Volume Management System. *(Courtesy of Otto Bock, Minneapolis, MN 55447.)*

Figure 31.24 Brim variant: Transtibial prosthesis with supracondylar/suprapatellar suspension with posterior and lateral views.

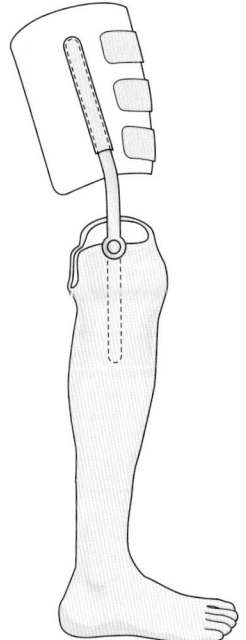

Figure 31.25 Transtibial prosthesis with thigh corset suspension.

A short amputated limb is well accommodated by SC/SP suspension. The high anterior wall may interfere with kneeling and presents a conspicuous contour when the wearer sits.

Thigh Corset

Some individuals with unusual limb contours or very short limb length, such as after rotationplasty surgery, may benefit from thigh corset suspension (Fig. 31.25). Metal hinges within medial and lateral uprights connect the socket to a flexible plastic corset. The hinges enhance frontal plane knee stability which is important post-rotationplasty because the ankle joint lacks the inherent frontal plane stability of the anatomical knee joint. The resulting prosthesis, however, is heavy and allows limb pistoning. To don a prosthesis with corset suspension, the wearer must fasten the corset laces or pressure-closure straps.

■ TRANSFEMORAL PROSTHESES

Individuals with amputation between the femoral epicondyles and greater trochanter are fitted with transfemoral (above-knee) prostheses. Those whose limbs retain the distal part of the femur can wear a knee disarticulation prosthesis, which differs from the transfemoral prosthesis in the type of knee unit and socket (described later). If the amputation is proximal to the greater trochanter, the patient cannot retain or control a transfemoral prosthesis and is therefore a candidate for a hip disarticulation prosthesis (described later). The transfemoral prosthesis consists of (a) foot-ankle assembly, (b) shank with rotation and shock-absorbing modification if needed, (c) knee unit, (d) socket, and (e) suspension device.

Foot-Ankle Assemblies and Shanks

Although the SACH foot is often prescribed for transtibial prostheses, the single-axis foot is more frequently used for transfemoral than for transtibial prostheses. The single-axis foot reaches the foot-flat position with minimal application of weight-bearing load. Nevertheless, almost any foot, including the energy-storing/energy-releasing designs, can be incorporated in a transfemoral prosthesis. Either the sturdy exoskeletal shank or the more lifelike endoskeletal shank may be used (see Fig. 31.16). The latter creates a more pleasing appearance, allows adjustable alignment, and is lighter than an exoskeletal shank. While greater prosthetic weight may increase metabolic energy cost, the weight may provide added sensory feedback that can lead to longer step lengths and improved gait symmetry.[26] Problems of durability remain, particularly at the knee, where constant bending of the joint, especially when the wearer is kneeling, accelerates deterioration of the rubber cover. A rotator (see Fig. 31.8C and Fig. 31.14) incorporated in the shank allows rotational motion that can diminish shear stress on the amputation limb.[27]

Knee Units

The prosthetic knee enables the user to bend the knee when sitting or kneeling and, in most instances, permits knee flexion during the latter portion of the stance phase and throughout the swing phase of walking. Commercial knee units may be described according to four features: (a) axis, (b) friction mechanism, (c) extension aid, and (d) mechanical stabilizer. Many combinations of features are available; not every knee unit has all four components.

Axis System

The thigh piece can be connected to the shank either by a *single-axis hinge,* which is the usual arrangement, or by *polycentric linkage.* Polycentric systems (Fig. 31.26) have four or more pivoting bars that provide greater stability to the knee, inasmuch as the momentary center of knee rotation is posterior to the wearer's weight line during most of the stance phase, resulting in a more fluid gait cycle.[28] The trade-off of stability and fluidity comes at a longer length and heavier weight of the knee component, which may make it impractical for some prosthesis users.

Friction Mechanism

In the simplest sense, the leg of the transfemoral prosthesis is a pendulum swinging about the knee hinge. For the individual who walks slowly for short distances, a basic pendulum is adequate. More energetic walkers, however, benefit from adjustable friction mechanisms that modify the pendulum action of the leg to reduce the asymmetry between the motions of the sound and prosthetic limbs. If the prosthetic knee does not have sufficient friction to control its natural pendulum action, the person who walks rapidly experiences

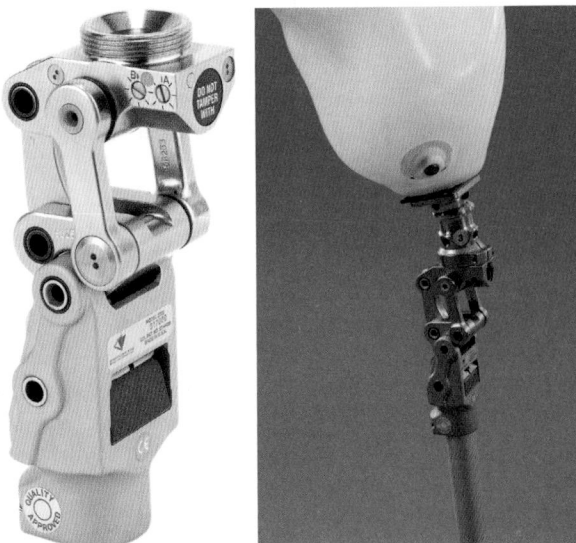

Figure 31.26 (Left) Polycentric knee unit designed to provide stability during stance. *(Courtesy of Össur, Aliso Viejo, CA 92656.)* (Right) Polycentric knee in place on a transfemoral prosthesis.

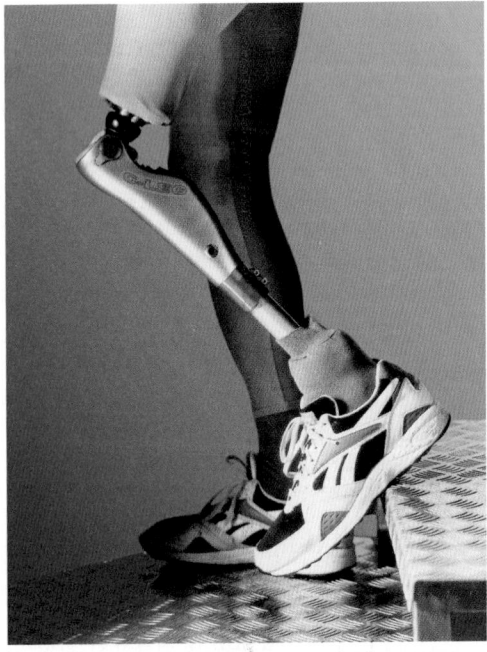

Figure 31.27 Friction mechanism: C-Leg. *(Courtesy of Otto Bock, Minneapolis, MN 55447.)*

abrupt transitions at terminal stance and initial contact. Friction mechanisms can resist knee flexion in the stance phase to enable stair descent (Fig. 31.27), which is activated by the ground reaction forces transferring from the foot through the prosthetic knee.

Constant and Variable

The most commonly prescribed knee unit has *constant friction* within the joint. A more-sophisticated device applies *variable friction,* in which the amount of friction

changes during a given portion of gait. At initial swing, high friction is applied to control excessive knee flexion; during midswing, friction diminishes to permit the knee to swing easily; at terminal swing, friction increases to dampen impact and to stabilize for initial contact.

Friction Brake

A more elaborate stabilizing system, the *friction brake,* provides very high friction during early stance as the wearer bears weight on the prosthesis, resisting the tendency of the knee to flex.[29] One design, the load-dependent friction unit, applies resistance to knee flexion during the initiation of prosthetic limb weight-bearing during initial contact to prevent collapse (see Fig. 31.28). Another version of friction brake is found in some hydraulic units; during early stance, additional fluid resistance markedly controls piston descent within the fluid cylinder and thus stabilizes the knee. From midstance through initial contact, friction brakes do not interfere with knee motion. In addition, they do not impede the patient who transfers from sitting to standing. Such devices may not protect the patient from falling when the knee is flexed beyond 20° or if insufficient weight-bearing is applied.

Medium

The medium through which friction is applied influences performance. A load-dependent friction unit applies a mechanical brake to knee flexion when weight-bearing is borne through the limb. A more complex approach is *fluid friction,* either oil (*hydraulic friction*) (Fig. 31.29) or air (*pneumatic friction*). Unlike a load-dependent friction unit, fluid friction varies directly with velocity. Thus, with a hydraulic or pneumatic unit, if the wearer walks faster, the knee increases friction instantly to prevent excessive knee flexion and abrupt extension. Consequently, the movements of the prosthetic and sound limbs are less asymmetrical than would be the case with load-dependent friction. Oil or air is contained in

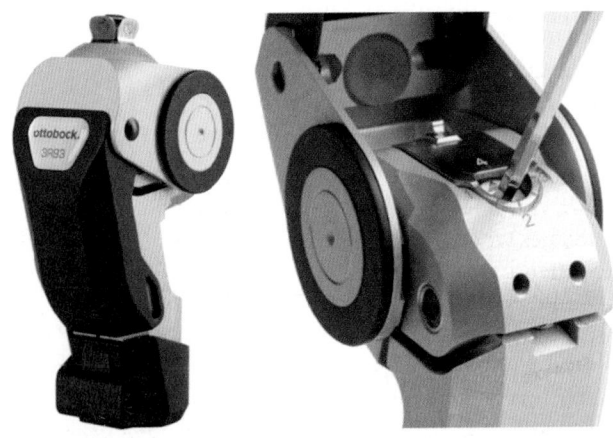

Figure 31.28 The SR93 load-dependent friction knee. *(Courtesy of Otto Bock, Minneapolis, MN 55447.)*

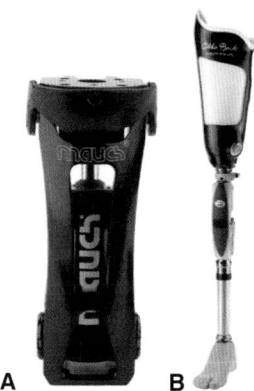

A   **B**

Figure 31.29 (A) Mauch (SNS) single-axis hydraulic knee unit with swing and stance control. *(Courtesy of Össur, Aliso Viejo, CA 92656.)* (B) The SR60 Ergonomically Balance Stride (EBS) hydraulic system controls the knee during swing, allowing greater ease in initiating swing and a greater range of walking speeds. Note that this prosthesis includes a flexible socket supported within a rigid frame. *(Courtesy of Otto Bock, Minneapolis, MN 55447.)*

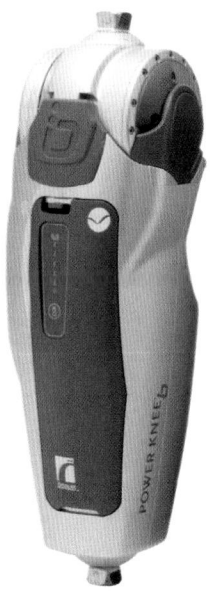

Figure 31.30 Power Knee. *(Courtesy of Össur, Aliso Viejo, CA 92656.)*

a cylinder in the knee unit. A piston descends in the cylinder during early swing, causing the knee to flex. The speed of piston descent depends on the type of fluid and the walking speed. Later, the piston ascends, extending the knee. Hydraulic units provide more friction than do pneumatic devices. Both types are more expensive than the simpler load-dependent friction designs.

Microprocessor-controlled hydraulic units such as the C-Leg (see Fig. 31.27) utilize electronic sensors, which detect the rate and range of movement 50 or more times per second, providing almost instant friction adjustment to changes in the gait pattern.[30,31] Units are programmed with a computer and may provide stumble recovery, locking option, and accommodation to walking on various terrain and bicycle riding. An alternative to oil-filled hydraulic units is the Rheo knee (Össur, Aliso Viejo, CA 92656), which has magnetized fluid and sensors that detect knee action in much smaller time units.[32]

Extension Aid

Many knee units include a mechanism to assist knee extension during the latter part of swing phase. The simplest type is an *external extension aid,* consisting of an elastic strap in front of the knee axis. The elastic stretches when the knee flexes in early swing and recoils to extend the knee in late swing. Strap tension is easily adjusted but tends to pull the knee into extension when the wearer sits. The *internal extension aid* is an elastic strap or coiled spring within the knee unit. It functions identically to the external aid during walking, but unlike the external aid, the internal type keeps the knee flexed when the individual sits. Fluid-controlled knee units incorporate an internal extension aid.

Although most extension aids affect the wearer's performance during late swing and early stance phases, the Power Knee (Össur, Aliso Viejo, CA 92656) (Fig. 31.30) also assists the user to ascend stairs step-over-step and to rise from a chair. The unit incorporates accelerometers, gyroscopes, a torque sensor, an on-board computer, and a motor. The motor makes a noise when engaged that will be noticeable to the wearer.

Mechanical Stabilizer

Most knee units do not have a special device to increase stability. The patient controls prosthetic knee action by hip motion, aided by the alignment of the knee in relation to other components of the prosthesis. The knee axis is usually aligned posterior to a line extending from the greater trochanter to the ankle (trochanter-knee-ankle [TKA] line) in order to promote stability at midstance and allow for knee flexion at terminal stance.

Manual Lock

The simplest mechanical stabilizer is a manual lock (Fig. 31.31), in which a rod lodges in a receptacle and is released only when the wearer manipulates an unlocking lever by pulling on the cable. Other U-shaped manual locks are located at the posterior aspect of the knee unit (Fig. 31.32). When engaged, the manual lock prevents knee flexion. The user is secure not only during early stance when stability is desired but also throughout the entire gait cycle. To compensate for difficulty in advancing the locked prosthesis, the shank should be shortened approximately 1/2 in. (1 cm). The manual lock must be manually disengaged when the wearer sits. Nevertheless, some people with impaired balance prefer the stability of the locked knee.[33]

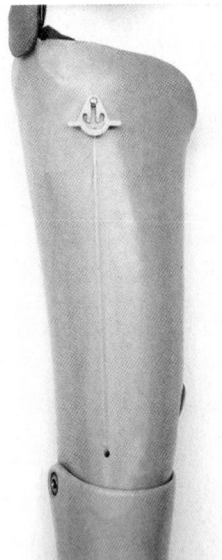

Figure 31.31 Single-axis knee unit with manual lock. Note that this configuration has a proximal release cable attached to the knee. For patients with impaired balance, the proximal release eliminates the need to flex forward and reach down to the knee to unlock the unit.

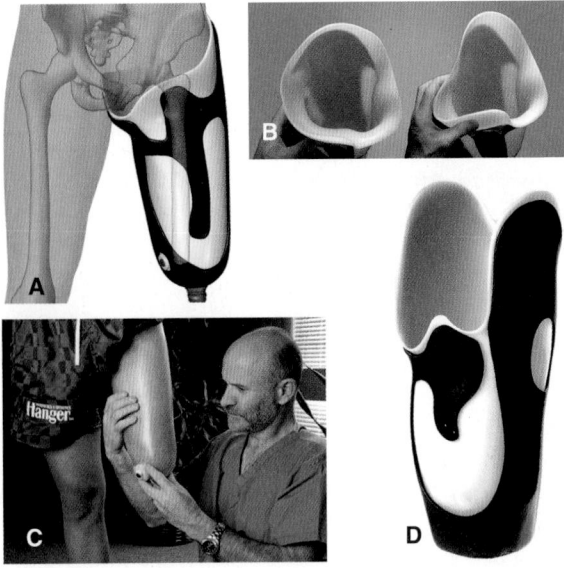

Figure 31.33 ComfortFlex socket design. (A) Anatomical orientation of transfemoral socket. (B) Overhead view of transfemoral socket (thumb and finger pressure illustrating socket flexibility). (C) Socket without carbon frame. (D) Transtibial socket design. *(Courtesy of Hanger, Inc., Oklahoma City, OK 73118.)*

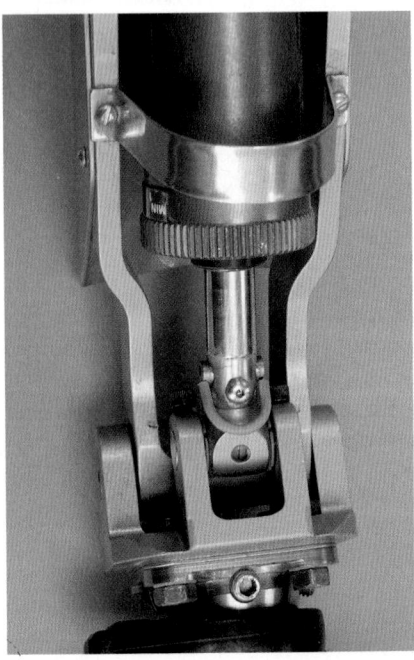

Figure 31.32 Manual lock (blue) on a hydraulic prosthetic knee unit.

Sockets

As with all prosthetic sockets, the transfemoral one should be a total-contact receptacle to distribute load over the maximum area, thereby reducing pressure. Total-contact fitting also provides counterpressure to assist venous return and prevent distal edema, and it enhances sensory feedback to foster better control of the

prosthesis. Most transfemoral sockets are made of a flexible thermoplastic socket (Fig. 31.33), similar to that of a transtibial socket.

Transfemoral sockets are designed to emphasize loading on pressure-tolerant structures, such as the gluteal musculature, sides of the thigh, and, to a lesser extent, the distal end of the amputated limb. The socket must avoid excessive pressure on the pubic symphysis and perineum.

Quadrilateral Socket

One transfemoral socket shape is quadrilateral when viewed from above (Fig. 31.34). The socket features a horizontal posterior shelf for the ischial tuberosity and gluteal musculature, a medial brim at the same level as the posterior shelf, an anterior wall 2.5 to 3 in. (6 to 8 cm) higher to apply a posteriorly directed force to the thigh to retain the ischial tuberosity on its shelf, and a lateral wall the same height as the anterior wall to aid in medial–lateral stabilization. Concave reliefs are (a) anteromedial, for the pressure-sensitive adductor longus tendon and obturator nerve; (b) posteromedial, for the sensitive hamstring tendons and sciatic nerve; (c) posterolateral, to permit the gluteus maximus to contract and bulge without being crowded; and (d) anterolateral, to allow adequate room for the rectus femoris. The anterior wall has a convexity to maximize pressure distribution in the vicinity of the femoral triangle. The lateral wall may have reliefs for the greater trochanter and the distal end of the femur.

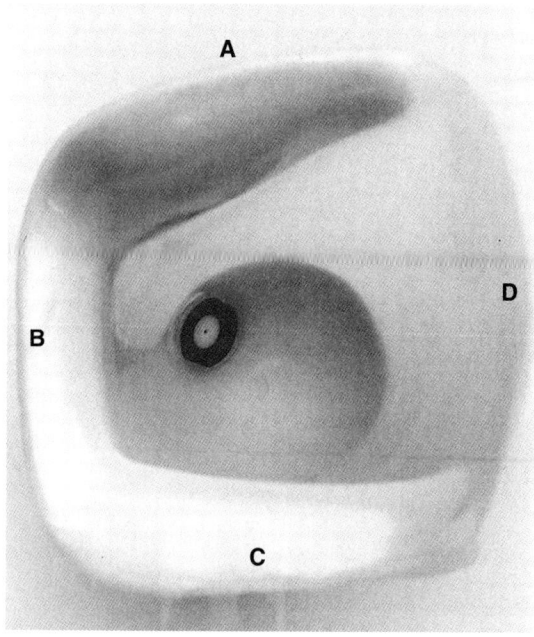

Figure 31.34 Quadrilateral socket viewed from above.
(A) Anterior wall. (B) Medial wall. (C) Posterior wall.
(D) Lateral wall.

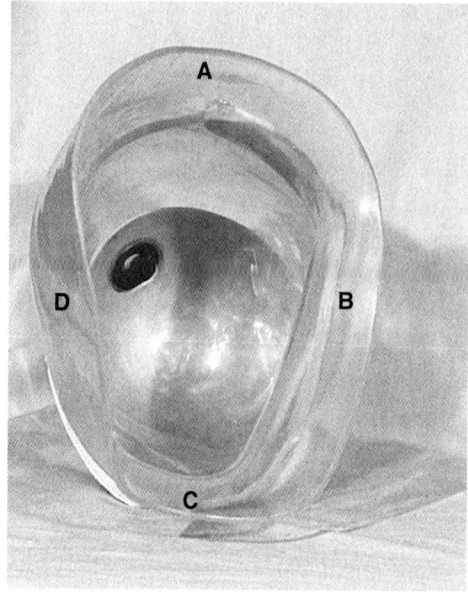

Figure 31.35 Ischial containment flexible transfemoral
socket. (A) Anterior brim. (B) Medial brim. (C) Posterior
brim. (D) Lateral brim.

Ischial Containment Socket

An alternate design type is the ischial containment
socket (Fig. 31.35). This socket is commonly encountered clinically with walls that cover the ischial tuberosity and part of the ischiopubic ramus to augment socket
stability. To increase frontal plane stability and minimize bulk between the thighs, the mediolateral width
of the socket is narrower than that of the quadrilateral
socket. The anterior wall is lower than in the quadrilateral socket, whereas the lateral wall covers the greater
trochanter. Alternating vertical reliefs and buildups can
reduce rotation of the limb in the socket.[34] Weight-
bearing occurs on the sides and bottom of the amputated limb.

Slight socket flexion is desirable to (a) facilitate
contraction of the hip extensors, (b) reduce lumbar
lordosis, (c) emphasize posterior thigh weight-bearing,
and (d) provide a zone through which the thigh may be
extended to permit the wearer to take steps of approximately equal length. For wearers of quadrilateral sockets,
socket flexion also enhances positioning of the ischial
tuberosity on the posterior brim. Socket adduction
allows lateral thigh weight-bearing (Fig. 31.36). More
information can be found in the section on Prosthetic
Alignment.

Suspensions

Similar to the transtibial suspension systems, there are
many possibilities. Depending on the level of activity
and user's needs, an elastic waist belt can be added to

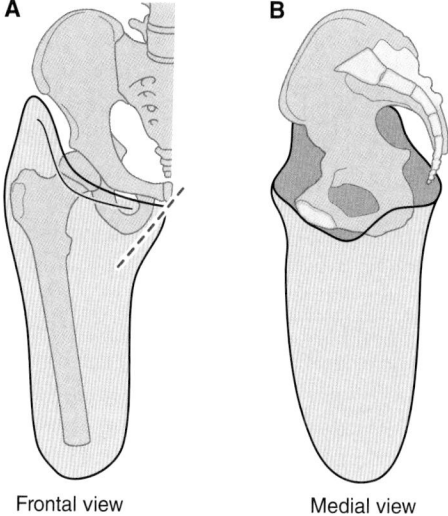

Figure 31.36 (A) Frontal view of the femur and pelvis
in the ischial containment socket. (B) Medial view of the
pelvis in the ischial containment socket. *(From May BJ,
Lackard MA. Prosthetics and Orthotics in Clinical Practice.
F.A. Davis; 2011:95.)*

the suspension system to add more proximal stability.
Common suspension types encountered clinically are
presented in the following sections.

Suction Suspension

Much like its transtibial counterpart, suction suspension results from creating a closed system where the
air is expelled distally and the socket sealed proximally.
Unlike the transtibial counterpart, a neoprene sleeve is

not typically used, but rather a unique silicone liner with gaskets circumferentially wrapping around the midportion is used. The gaskets create a tight seal to the socket, preventing the entry of air into the socket that would reduce the suction effect.

Another form of suction involves placing the limb directly into the socket without any liner, sometimes called a "skin fit." The suction occurs between the intimate fit of the prosthesis on the residuum, creating a seal. Distally, a valve still expresses air to create the negative-pressure environment.

Locking Liners

Either a pin or lanyard system can be used to suspend the residuum in the prosthesis. The pin system mimics what is used in the transtibial counterpart but is less frequently prescribed. Alternatively, the lanyard is prescribed more frequently at the transfemoral than the transtibial level. The Keep It Simple System is a popular option, which uses a broad strap that must be directed internally to externally through the inferior aspect of the socket in order to don. Once the strap is external, it is anchored on the surface of the socket through an anchoring mechanism (usually a ring) before being attached to itself via Velcro. An example of this system can be visualized in Figure 31.37.

Vacuum

A vacuum system can also be utilized for transfemoral prostheses. There is no difference in the mechanism of suspension when compared to a transtibial. Depending on the system used, a neoprene sleeve may be used between the proximal socket brim and the thigh to create a tight seal.

Osseointegration is the newest alternative suspension method that has the advantage of obviating the need for a socket.[25] A metal implant is inserted and integrated into existing bone with an attachment that permanently extrudes through the skin at the distal residual limb to attach to the prosthetic components.[35]

Osseous integration raises concern among some regarding the potential for perioperative site infection[36] or osseous failure or fracture,[25] though incidents have been rare.[37] Over time, proximal bony remodeling occurs in response to biomechanical loading[38] (Fig. 31.38).

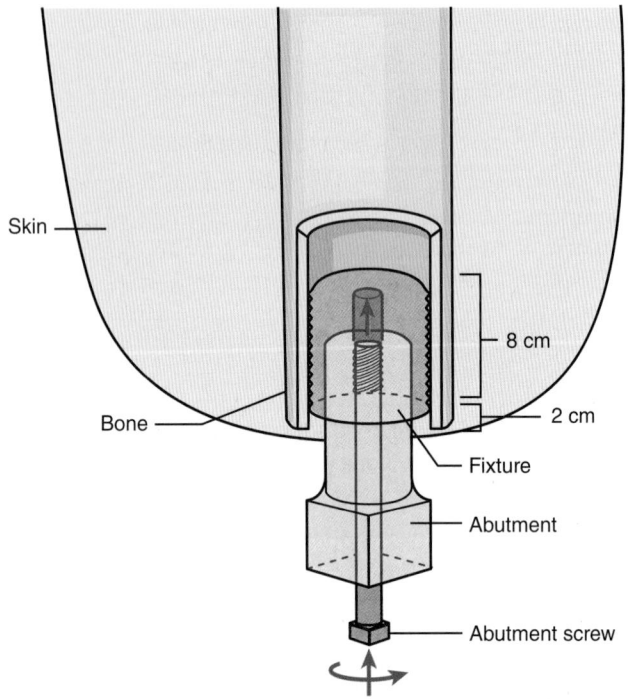

Figure 31.38 (Left) Osseous integration hardware. *(Reproduced from Figure 1 in Tillander et al., Clin Orthop Rel Res., 2017, as originally published from Cecilia Berlin, PhD, Chalmers University of Technology, Gothenburg, Sweden, and used under Creative Commons Attribution 4.0 International License [http://creativecommons.org/licenses/by/4.0].)* (Right) Osseous integration in place visualized by x-ray. *(Originally published as Figure 3-C in Hoellwarth JS et al., JBJS, 2020, and used under the terms of the Creative Commons Attribution-Non Commercial-No Derivatives License 4.0 [CCBY-NC-ND].)*

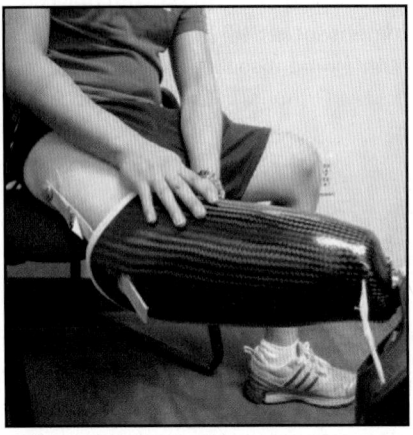
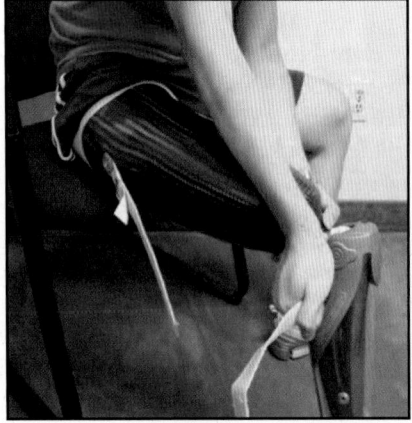
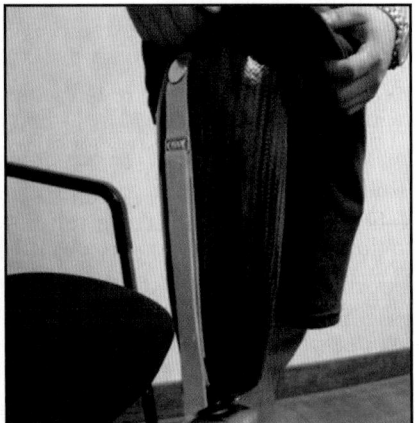

Figure 31.37 Locking liner system with external lanyard.

■ DISARTICULATION PROSTHESES

Individuals with knee or hip disarticulation wear prostheses that include the same distal components as prostheses for lower levels. Any prosthetic foot can be used with either an endoskeletal or exoskeletal shank. The user, however, is less likely to produce sufficient weight-bearing force to benefit from an energy-storing/energy-releasing foot. The major distinction, therefore, is in the proximal portion of the prostheses.

Knee Disarticulation Prostheses

When amputation is at or distal to the femoral epicondyles, the patient should have excellent prosthetic control because (a) thigh leverage is maximum, (b) most of the body weight can be borne through the distal end of the femur, and (c) the broad epicondyles provide rotational stability.[39,40]

Knee Units

Several units are specifically manufactured for knee disarticulation. All have a thin proximal attachment plate to minimize added thigh length. One may choose among hydraulic, pneumatic, and weight-activated friction units, with or without polycentric linkage. Even with a special knee unit, the thigh will be slightly longer. Consequently, the shank is shortened equivalently, so that when the person stands, the pelvis is level. When the individual sits, the thigh on the prosthetic side will project farther by several centimeters.[41]

Sockets

Two types of sockets are currently in use. Both are made of plastic and usually terminate below the ischial tuberosity. Generally, no additional suspension aids are needed. One version features an anterior opening to accommodate a bulbous amputation limb. After the limb is inserted, the wearer closes the socket with lacing or hook-and-loop closure. The other design has no anterior opening and is suitable for limbs that are not bulbous.

Hip Disarticulation Prostheses

A hip disarticulation prosthesis[42] is fitted to a person with amputation above the greater trochanter (very short transfemoral), removal of the femoral head from the acetabulum (hip disarticulation), or removal of the femur and any portion of the pelvis (transpelvic amputation, also known as *hemipelvectomy*) (Fig. 31.39). The modern prosthesis was developed in Toronto and is sometimes called the *Canadian hip disarticulation prosthesis*. Prostheses for proximal levels share common hip, knee, and foot assemblies but differ with regard to socket design. The endoskeletal thigh and shank predominate because they save appreciable weight in these massive prostheses. The prosthesis may be shortened

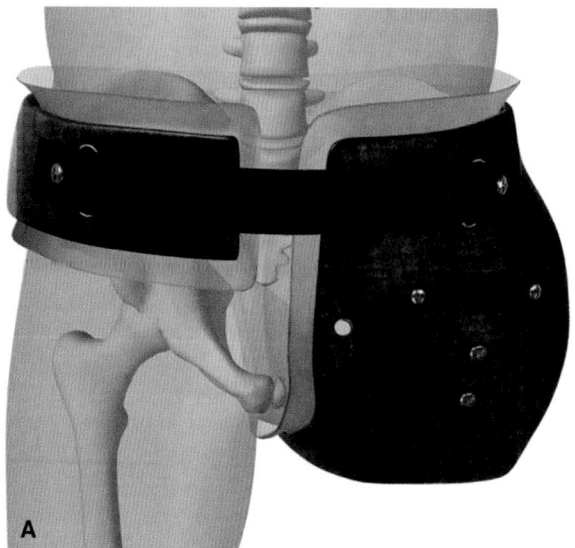

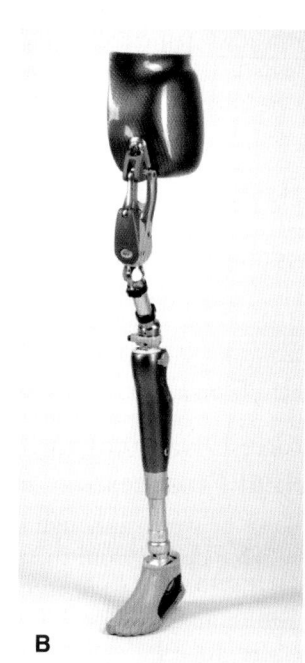

Figure 31.39 (A) Anatomical orientation of the Comfort-Flex hip disarticulation socket. *(Courtesy of Hanger, Oklahoma City, OK 73118.)* (B) Additional components of the completed prosthesis include a Helix 3D hip joint, rotator, knee unit, endoskeletal pylon, and foot. *(Courtesy of Otto Bock, Minneapolis, MN 55447.)*

slightly to aid clearance during swing phase, encourage the wearer to apply maximum weight to the prosthesis, and increase stability.

Sockets

The basic socket is plastic molded to provide weight-bearing on the ipsilateral ischial tuberosity and buttock (gluteal musculature). The person with transpelvic amputation who does not retain the ipsilateral tuberosity or iliac crest has a socket with a higher proximal trimline, sometimes encompassing the lower thorax. The individual supports weight on the remainder of the pelvis, on the abdomen, and perhaps on the lower ribs.

Hip Units

The prosthetic hip joint has an extension aid to bias the prosthesis toward the stable neutral position. Positioning the mechanical hip anterior to a point corresponding to the anatomical hip also contributes to hip stability. The joint is set below the normal hip so that when the wearer sits, the prosthetic thigh will not protrude unattractively. All hip joints provide hip flexion; some also allow transverse rotation[43,44] (see Fig. 31.39).

Knee Units

Although virtually any knee unit can be incorporated in a hip disarticulation prosthesis, an extension aid can be used to assist limb advancement during the swing phase of gait. The prosthetic knee should resist knee flexion in stance phase or be aligned posteriorly to contribute to stability.

■ BILATERAL PROSTHESES

Bilateral amputations occur either simultaneously, as in the case of trauma or congenital limb deficiency, or sequentially, as is seen with peripheral vascular disease. In the latter instance, previous experience with a unilateral prosthesis is invaluable in determining whether the patient will benefit from a pair of prostheses.

Bilateral Ankle Disarticulation and Transtibial Prostheses

Any foot design can be worn, although both prosthetic feet must be the same design from the same manufacturer to reduce the likelihood of gait asymmetry. Ideally, foot and shoe size should be shorter than the person's preamputation size to facilitate transition through stance phase; wider feet contribute to stability. Shanks, sockets, and suspensions need not match; each component should suit the characteristics of the individual amputation limb.[45]

Bilateral Transfemoral Prostheses

Other than matching prosthetic foot design and size, each amputation limb is fitted on an individual basis. The patient will perform activities in a manner similar to someone with unilateral transfemoral amputation.

The patient can be fitted with short, nonarticulated prostheses, sometimes referred to as foreshortened or "stubbies" (see Fig. 31.40). The lower center of gravity provides the individual with more stability and can serve as transition between early gait training and full-length prostheses. Gait is awkward, with exaggerated trunk rotation; crutches or canes need to be adjusted to suit the person's short stature. Transferring into an adult-size chair, as well as climbing stairs, is more difficult

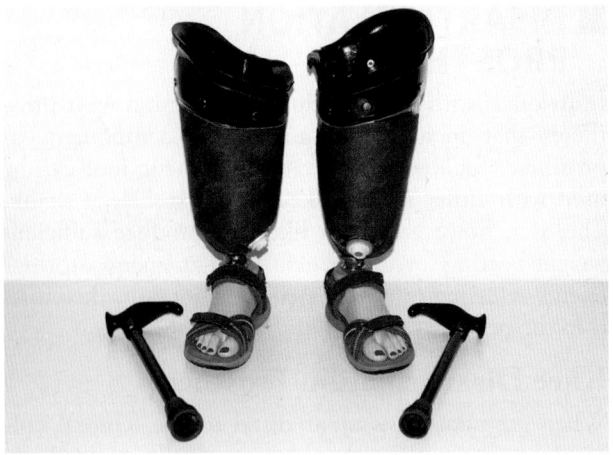

Figure 31.40 Foreshortened prostheses or "stubbies."

than with longer prostheses. Patients who object to the markedly altered appearance created by these short prostheses may refuse to wear them but may utilize the prostheses as part of their training.

Longer prostheses should include a matched pair of feet. Endoskeletal shanks are highly desirable to reduce prosthetic weight and enable minute changes in alignment; typically, the shanks are shortened by several inches to reduce the effort required to walk with the prostheses. Any type of knee unit may be worn. Sockets do not have to match; however, a pair of ischial containment sockets will minimize the walking base because the sockets have a relatively narrow mediolateral dimension, as compared with quadrilateral sockets. Any type of suspension may be worn.[46,47]

■ UPPER LIMB PROTHESES

The primary etiology of acquired upper limb loss is trauma associated with occupational hazards, such as power tools or industrial equipment.[48] Limb difference, typically occurring during fetal development, is the most common cause of upper limb prosthesis use.[49] Unlike those with lower limb loss, individuals with upper limb loss or difference have adherence rates of 10% to 80% depending on amputation level.[50] Those with more proximal amputations levels have lower adherence rates compared to people with more distal levels (e.g., transhumeral versus transradial),[51] similar to those with a lower limb prosthesis.

Many individuals choose not to utilize a prosthesis at all. For those who are able or choose to utilize an upper limb prosthesis, five primary types are commonly available: (a) passive, (b) body powered, (c) myoelectric, (d) hybrid, and (e) activity specific.

Passive

Passive prostheses (Fig. 31.41), sometimes known as passive functional prostheses, are designed to replicate the missing limb segment and provide limited terminal

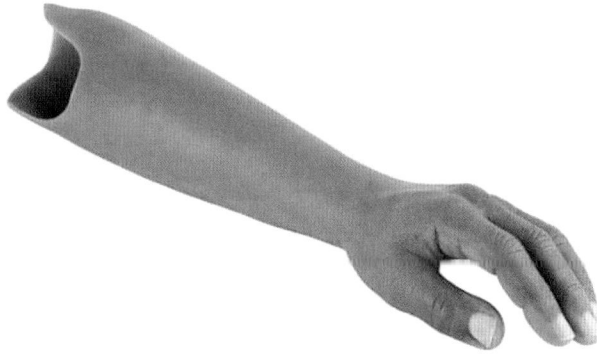

Figure 31.41 Passive hand prosthesis. *(Courtesy of Otto Bock, Minneapolis, MN 55447.)*

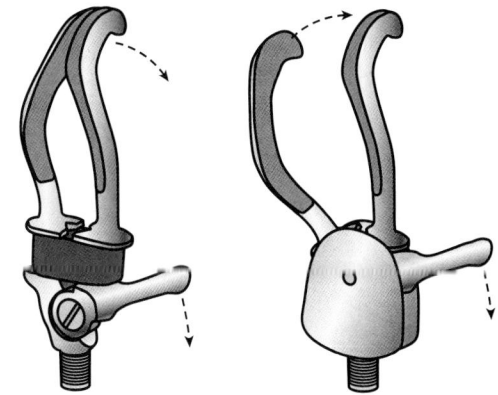

A Voluntary opening device   **B** Voluntary closing device

Figure 31.42 Terminal devices with voluntary opening and voluntary closing controls. *(Courtesy of Jon Sensinger, https://www.ece.unb.ca/jsensing/.)*

functionality. Passive prosthetic devices are manually positioned to provide support and function during grasping tasks, though the degrees of freedom are limited with the prosthesis maintaining only one position at a time. Passive prostheses typically have a silicone cover to cosmetically match the individual's anthropomorphic characteristics.

Body Powered

Body-powered prostheses are manipulated by performing a predetermined pattern of movements of the user's intact body segments to articulate each joint and control the terminal device via a series of cables. The terminal device is the hand, hook, or operating device. The prosthesis allows for movement with degrees of freedom based on amputation level and terminal device capabilities. Depending on the amputation level, a combination of shoulder, elbow, and wrist prosthetic components will be needed, in addition to the terminal device. For instance, when the shoulder is intact, shoulder flexion is commonly used to operate the terminal device.

Terminal devices can be categorized as voluntary opening (VO) or voluntary closing (VC) (see Fig. 31.42). As the name implies, the device can either be opened or closed based on volitional movement patterns elicited by the prosthesis user. While in a small study the VC was found to be faster to operate than the VO,[52] it remains the preference of the prosthesis user and designing prosthetist to determine which device type they will receive. Adults typically use a VO device, while children often receive VC.

Transhumeral prosthetic users wear a figure-eight harness secured around the back and controlled through a series of scapular and shoulder movements that work the elbow and terminal device. The harness also serves to aid suspension. Depending on harness design and prosthesis, cables extending between the harness and device cause elbow or terminal device movement, sometimes simultaneously. To control both elbow and terminal device, a two-cable system is used: ipsilateral shoulder locking or elbow motion are controlled with one

cable, while bilateral scapular abduction manipulates the terminal device with the other cable. Thus, natural shoulder and scapular movements manipulate the prosthesis, such as shoulder flexion to cause the elbow joint to bend, or protracting the scapula to open or close the terminal device. A limitation of body-powered prostheses is that the elbow joint usually needs to be locked, typically through quick shoulder extension and scapular depression, before the terminal device can be manipulated. Transradial body-powered prosthetic devices use a similar harness as a transhumeral device; however, the anatomical elbow joint simplifies the process. The same shoulder and scapular movements manipulate the terminal device.

Myoelectric

Myoelectric prostheses utilize a combination of sensors and externally powered actuators to influence movement. The sensors are placed at specific intervals along the residual limb in areas that can sense muscle contractions and are integrated into the socket liner. The sensors interpret contraction magnitude from the muscle sensors and activate powered actuators that transform the muscle signal into controlled terminal device movement. For example, an individual with a transradial amputation can still utilize their flexor and extensor musculature; thus sensors placed over these muscles allow for natural grasping and releasing, respectively. For a transhumeral prosthesis, the wearer will have additional control over the powered elbow unit but can typically only control one joint at a time. A microprocessor unit employing pattern recognition technology may be used to act as an intermediary between the sensation of the signal and the desired output, increasing the natural manipulation of the device while minimizing the amount of effort required to create the desired motions. Figure 31.43 illustrates a typical transradial myoelectric prosthesis.

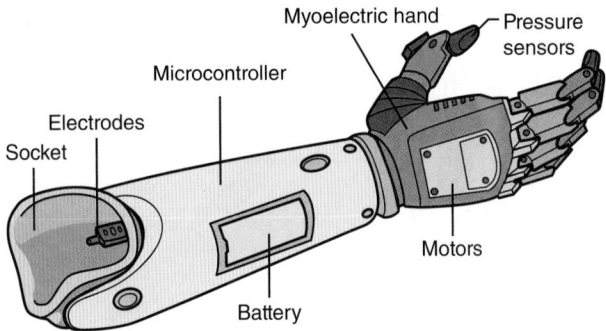

Figure 31.43 Hybrid myoelectric and body-powered prosthesis.

Hybrid

Hybrid prostheses are a combination of the aforementioned prosthesis types. An example of a hybrid with advantages over single systems is a transhumeral prosthesis. A body-powered elbow and a myoelectric hand allow for simultaneous reaching and grasping, rather than the segmented approach afforded by a singular system. The benefits of hybrid systems can make for a more functional prosthesis, improving the natural look and feel of the device.

Activity Specific

Activity-specific devices come in a variety of types, forms, and functions. Much like their lower limb counterparts, activity-specific devices can be used to perform a purposeful singular role but are cumbersome and complex to use daily. For the mountain climber, a specifically engineered terminal device is manufactured to allow for the rigorous and particular needs of the activity (Fig. 31.44). There are devices for fishing, bowling, and every other activity one can think of, increasing the benefit of an upper limb prosthesis for those who are able or choose to use one.

■ PROSTHESIS MAINTENANCE

Optimal function depends on proper care of socks or liners, prosthesis, residual limb, intact limb, as well as general health maintenance. As with any medical device, the prosthesis benefits from regular maintenance, which generally avoids costly, time-consuming repairs. Timely referral to the prosthetist can improve the user's function and avoid unnecessary discomfort. In addition to ensuring cleanliness, the individual should wear a well-fitting sock and shoe on the sound foot. Guidelines for personal hygiene are presented in Chapter 22, Amputation.

Foot-Ankle Assemblies

Most prosthetic foot-ankle assemblies are vulnerable to water, dirt, and sand. Dampness or direct or excessive heat can degrade the foot material; sand or similar substances can restrict or damage prosthetic joints.

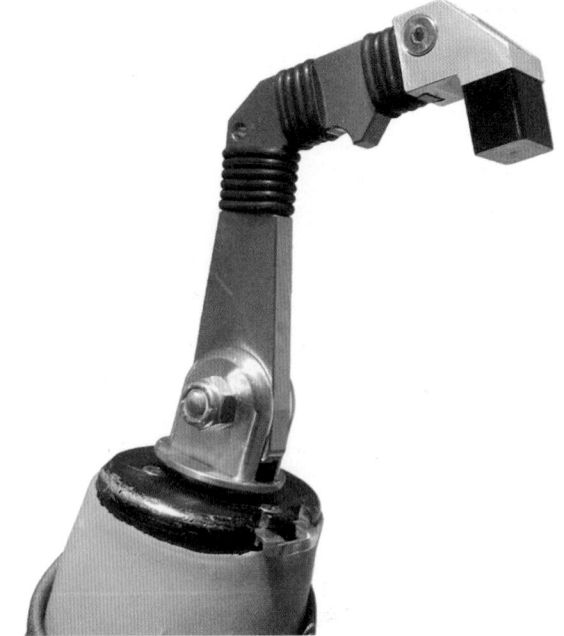

Figure 31.44 Mountain climber sport-specific prosthesis (Raptor Sky Hook). *(Courtesy of Fillauer TRS, Inc., Boulder, CO, 80301.)*

Prosthetist intervention may be required to disassemble and clean the foot-ankle assembly. It is imperative that the user of the prosthesis follow the manufacturer's guidelines for the prosthetic device as certain models are capable of exposure to environmental elements, while others are not. The physical therapist must also be aware of these restrictions for appropriate goal setting and patient education.

Most prosthetic foot-ankle assemblies are not designed to be walked on without a shoe. Prosthetic alignment typically factors in shoe heel height; thus, standing on a prosthesis without a shoe causes an unplanned-for leg length discrepancy as well as knee extension moment pushing the wearer backward. Wearing shoes of the same heel height as the prosthesis had when initially aligned allows consistent biomechanical effects (Fig. 31.45). Too low a heel interrupts late stance; an unduly high heel makes the knee less stable. A small internal heel lift up to 1 cm can be placed inside both shoes at the heel for minor differences in heel height. High-heeled shoes require a different foot or an adjustable heel height foot as in certain models of feet (e.g., Runway [Freedom Innovations, Fayette, UT 84630] or Elation [Össur, Aliso Viejo, CA 92656]). Boots will restrict the dorsiflexion and plantarflexion action of any articulated foot and can be difficult to don. A shoehorn can aid with prosthetic donning.

Shanks

The soft foam cover of the endoskeletal prosthesis requires reasonable caution against exposure to direct

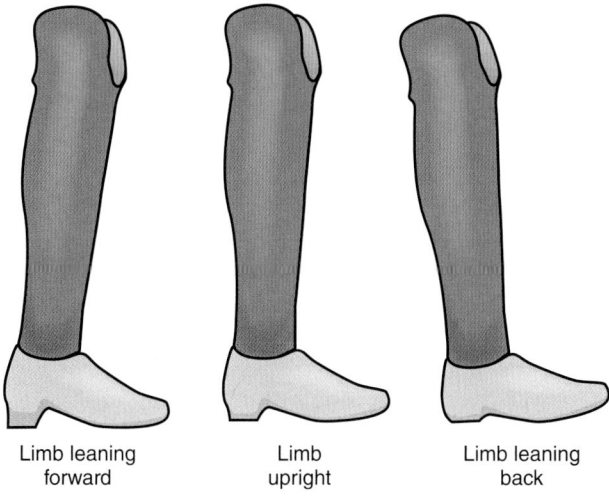

Limb leaning forward   Limb upright   Limb leaning back

Figure 31.45 Influence of heel height on knee stability.

heat, penetrating objects, and solvents. The outer covering will need replacement whenever it becomes unacceptably soiled or torn. Transfemoral foam covers deteriorate, particularly at the knee. Exoskeletal shanks are impervious to most liquids and can be cleaned with a dampened cloth and gentle detergent.

Joints

Squeaking or unusual noise at any joint indicates the need for maintenance by the prosthetist. Springs and joints can squeak and can need adjustment or replacement. Bumpers erode after prolonged or vigorous use, and the wearer will notice an impact noise with full joint motion such as knee hyperextension. A joint that becomes difficult to move may not make a sound but may need maintenance to ensure that pneumatic, hydraulic, and electrical components work correctly. Hydraulic or pneumatic microprocessor joints should be plugged in to recharge the battery at night. Prosthetist intervention is required for joint maintenance and should never be attempted by the user or physical therapist.

Sockets and Suspensions

The inside of sockets should be washed with a cloth dampened in warm water that has a very small amount of mild soap dissolved in it. The socket is then wiped with a damp, soap-free cloth and dried with a fresh towel. Socket sheaths and liners should be maintained according to the manufacturer's instructions. This typically involves turning the liner inside out so the gel is facing outward, washing with a damp lint-free cloth, then rinsing under warm water. The liner is then placed inside out on a liner tree designed to dry liners. Avoid contact with environmental contaminants as these can embed into the gel of the liner and cause skin breakdown. Suspension locks and components including the suction valve should be brushed daily to remove talcum

and lint, which might interfere with the mechanisms. Inability to maintain suspension or residual limb discomfort related to socket fit can require prosthetic consultation or intervention.

■ PROSTHETIC FIT AND ALIGNMENT

Prosthetic Fit

Prosthetic fit plays a vital role in the prosthesis user's comfort when wearing the prosthesis.[53] The interface between prosthetic socket and residual limb influences limb comfort and impacts walking pattern and quality of life.[23,24] Pressure is reduced over the whole limb by maintaining total contact with the limb, thereby maximizing surface area to reduce pressure according to the formula for pressure, $P = F/A$. Maximizing skin contact area also reduces movement and shear forces within the socket. The prosthetist can further optimize comfort by minimizing pressure on pressure-sensitive areas such as bony prominences, nerves, and blood vessels. Socket reliefs or indentations over the sensitive areas are balanced with socket buildups or bulges that press into nearby pressure-tolerant areas of the residual limb. In this way, pressure-tolerant areas receive more pressure than the sensitive areas (see Fig. 31.18).

Prosthetic fit is assessed with specifically designed outcome measures. The Comprehensive Lower-Limb Amputee Socket Survey (CLASS) is a valid and reliable self-assessment of the fit of the prosthesis.[54] The assessment consists of 16 items that address stability, suspension, comfort, and appearance. An alternative to the CLASS is the Socket Comfort Score (SCS) that asks a single question of the prosthesis user: "Rate the comfort of your socket on a scale from 0–10, with 0 being the most uncomfortable and 10 being the most comfortable."[55] While the SCS is the fastest way to assess socket comfort, the CLASS should be used if a more comprehensive understanding of fit is needed.

Transtibial Socket Fit

Due to the presence of superficial bones and nerves, the fit of a transtibial socket is more difficult than that of a transfemoral.[56] Pressure-sensitive areas of the transtibial residual limb include the distal ends of the tibia and fibula, tibial crest and lateral condyle, fibular head and adjacent nerves, patella, and medial and lateral femoral condyles. Pressure-tolerant areas include the tibial medial and lateral flares, lateral fibula, patella ligament, and posterior calf.

Transfemoral Socket Fit

Pressure-sensitive areas of the transfemoral residual limb include the distal-lateral end of the femur, ischial-pubic rami, greater trochanter, and adductor longus tendon. Pressure-tolerant areas include the ischial tuberosity, lateral residual femur, and posterior thigh.

Prosthetic Alignment

The prosthetic alignment affects the forces applied to the limb via ground reaction forces and thus influences the kinetic chain during walking. Assessment of prosthetic alignment begins with bench alignment—alignment of the prosthetic components when not being worn. When the prosthesis is worn, the static alignment is assessed to ensure optimal adjustment for all body segments in weight-bearing. Dynamic alignment is performed during walking to account for the impact of individual movement variations above the prosthesis, such as trunk rotation, as well as step length or width. When issues arise with prosthetic alignment during rehabilitation, timely referral to the prosthetist should be made.

Transtibial Alignment

The standard bench alignment for a transtibial prosthesis is based on the relationship of the socket and foot, accounting for the intended heel height. In the sagittal plane, a vertical line from the proximal socket center falls between the foot center and the anterior ankle. In the frontal plane, a vertical line from the proximal socket center falls ~1 cm lateral of the heel center indicating foot inset. In the transverse plane, the foot should be externally rotated 5° (Fig. 31.46).

Typically, the transtibial socket is flexed forward 5° in the sagittal plane. Socket flexion creates a flexion moment at the knee and of the prosthesis forward over the foot that must be matched by the quadricep muscle to maintain stability. Note that the term *socket flexion* denotes the whole socket is rotated over the pylon.

Any prosthetic alignment that decreases the toe lever—the distance from the vertical line from the socket center to the end of the keel within the prosthetic foot—will further increase this knee flexion moment and destabilize the knee. Examples include excess socket flexion, anterior socket shift, excess foot external rotation, or a short foot (Fig. 31.47).

Typical bench alignment in the frontal plane includes an inset foot 1 cm from the vertical socket center line. The inset foot allows a normal walking base of support and minimizes horizontal motion during gait. Any prosthetic alignment that creates a larger base of support will create more side-to-side motion and greater demand on the hip abductors. Examples include lateral socket shift and lateral socket tilt, also called socket adduction (see Fig. 31.47).

Transfemoral Alignment

The standard bench alignment for a transfemoral prosthesis must take into account the relationship of the socket and foot, accounting for the intended heel height, and the TKA line. In the sagittal plane, a vertical line from the proximal socket center falls just anterior to the ankle and knee, producing a knee extension moment for weight-bearing stability. In the frontal plane, a vertical line from the proximal socket center falls 1 cm lateral of the heel center to minimize horizontal motion in gait (see Fig. 31.46).

Typically, the transfemoral socket is flexed backward 5° in the sagittal plane such that the anatomical hip is in slight flexion. Socket flexion in a transfemoral socket faces the opposite direction of the transtibial socket

Transtibial Prosthesis

Sagittal plane   Frontal plane

Transfemoral Prosthesis

Sagittal plane   Frontal plane

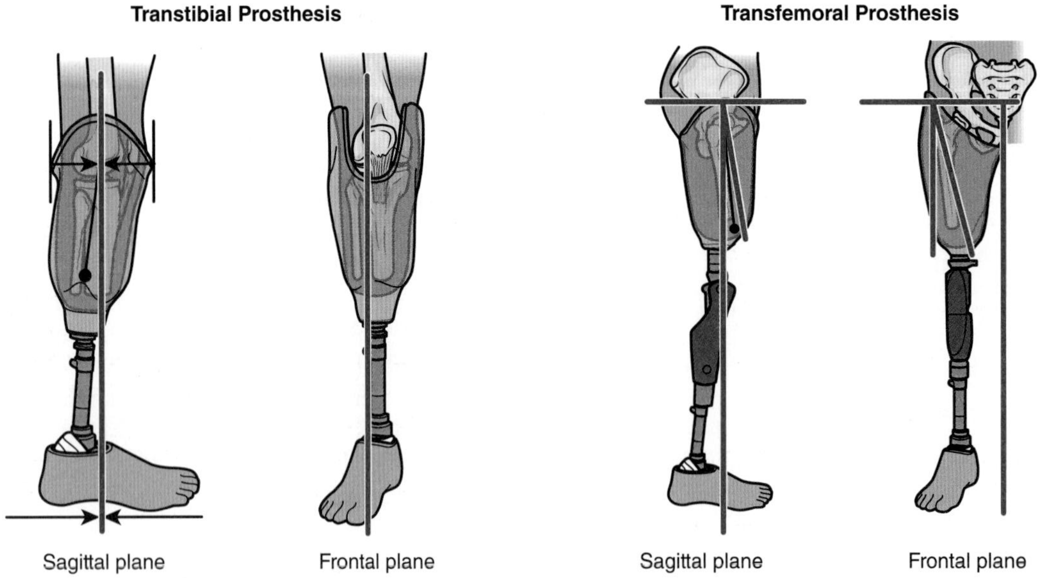

Figure 31.46 Socket alignment for transtibial and transfemoral prostheses. Typical transtibial bench alignment includes 5° of socket flexion to shift some weight from the distal to the anterior limb. Typical transfemoral alignment includes 7° of socket adduction to shift some weight to the lateral thigh.

Right Lateral View-Sagittal Plane Alignment

Right Posterior View-Frontal Plane Alignment

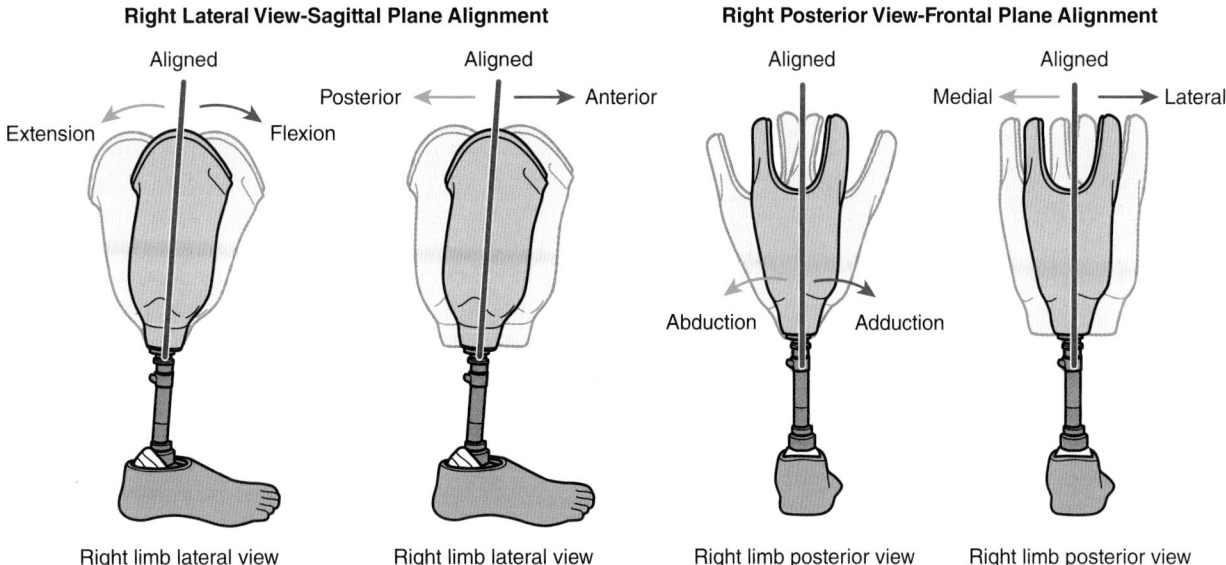

Figure 31.47 Adjustments for transtibial prosthesis socket alignments. Sagittal plane abnormalities include persistent knee flexion contractures that may have to be accommodated with increased socket flexion. Posterior socket shift lengthens the toe lever to create an extension moment and stabilizes the knee. Frontal plane abnormalities of the anatomical knee require socket alignment accommodation with frontal plane tilt. For example, lateral socket tilt accommodates for the knee adduction seen in genu varum common with knee osteoarthritis.

to shift weight from the distal femur to the pressure-tolerant posterior thigh. However, positioning the hip in flexion can inhibit full hip extension after midstance and limit contralateral limb advancement. A persistent hip flexion contracture may have to be accommodated with increased socket flexion.

Typical transfemoral bench alignment in the frontal plane includes 7° of lateral tilt or socket adduction, such that the anatomical hip maintains its normal relationship with the pelvis. Socket adduction shifts some weight from the distal femur to the pressure-tolerant lateral limb. Because pelvic width can vary among individuals, particularly of different sexes, the degree of socket adduction also varies. A persistent hip abduction contracture unresponsive to manual therapy and stretching may have to be accommodated with reduced socket adduction and corresponding increased inset foot to maintain the normal base of support.

■ PHYSICAL THERAPY MANAGEMENT

Physical therapists participate in the management of people with limb loss at several key stages: (a) perioperative, (b) preprosthetic, (c) prosthetic training, and (d) lifelong care.

The first three stages are described in Chapter 22, Amputation. The following section emphasizes the role of the physical therapist in helping people manage their prosthesis. The physical therapist coordinates their work with the physician and prosthetist, as well as other professionals such as social workers, occupational therapists, vocational counselors, and psychologists as needed. An interprofessional team provides the most comprehensive and efficient lifelong care.[57] The physical therapist has an integral part to play in all stages of rehabilitation including encouraging lifelong physical activity and participation in wellness activities.

Prescription Considerations

Successful prosthetic rehabilitation depends on matching the individual's physical and psychosocial characteristics to a prosthesis composed of carefully selected components. Not everyone with limb loss or difference will receive or choose to utilize a prosthesis. For some, significant comorbidities such as severe dementia, loss of neuromotor control, or cardiopulmonary disease may preclude safe prosthesis use. Some people with hip disarticulation or high-level amputations find prosthesis use unduly cumbersome and prefer to ambulate with crutches without a prosthesis or use a wheelchair for mobility. Several competitive sports, particularly swimming and soccer, are performed without prostheses to eliminate the influence of device inequality among athletes.

Physical Examination

The physical therapist should perform a complete examination, described in Chapter 22, Amputation. Physical examination components with direct impact on prosthetic prescription and use described here include anthropometrics, integument, and sensation of the residual and sound limbs; joint mobility, muscle flexibility, and strength; functional ability; and cardiovascular capacity. Cognition and psychosocial factors including satisfaction and motivation follow.

Anthropometric dimensions of the residual and sound limbs require careful scrutiny because limb length, limb shape, and surface area impact the choice of prosthetic components. Residual limb length impacts joint and suspension systems selections. Circumferential residual limb measurements provide insight into limb volume and shape that impact socket fit. Limb volume changes due to edema or atrophy can alter socket fit; temporary adjustment can be made by adding or subtracting sock ply thickness. A loose socket causes increased pistoning in the socket, distal residual limb weight-bearing, and pain; additional sock ply increases total volume and improves fit. A too-tight socket makes it difficult to don completely, preventing full distal contact and complete suspension; removing sock ply decreases total volume and improves fit. Obesity may influence limb volume stability but has not been shown to impact prosthetic function.[58]

Integument inspection of skin and any lesions, using a mirror to visualize difficult-to-see surfaces, is an important indicator of socket fit. Identifying skin lesions, abrasions, or bruises can indicate prosthetic fit and alignment issues and facilitate referral to the prosthetist for corrective measures before ulceration ensues. Most minor wounds and incompletely healed incisions, in the absence of major comorbidities, will continue to resolve with prosthetic weight-bearing.[59] Early identification of potential infections and keeping the sound foot clean and dry with clean socks/stockings and well-fitting shoes are vital in preventing subsequent amputations in people with vascular disease (see Chapter 14, Vascular, Lymphatic, and Integumentary Disorders).

Sensory assessment to identify impaired sensation to touch or pressure may require prosthetic accommodation to protect vulnerable skin. Someone with impaired knee proprioception may need extra prosthetic stability. Painful neuromas can persist and may require surgical or medical intervention if prosthetic accommodation is insufficient.

Joint mobility, muscle flexibility, and active and passive range of motion (ROM) of all lower limb joints is important for optimal prosthetic use. Knee and hip flexion contractures compromise prosthetic alignment and function; thus, reducing contractures and maintaining joint mobility is an important physical therapy goal. Joint contractures can be caused by both joint hypomobility and limited muscle flexibility, and both the joint and musculature should be addressed to improve passive ROM. Severe contractures may prevent prosthesis provision. Older people with chronic vascular disease may have diminished ROM and strength, from reduced physical activity prior to amputation, that need to be addressed to optimize their ability.

Strength of all limb and trunk muscles is important for preventing contractures, maintaining ROM, and performing functional activities. Muscle strength, particularly gluteal muscle hip extension and abduction and quadricep strength for people with intact knee joints, is essential for prosthetic use. A locked-knee transfemoral prosthesis may be needed initially until the patient develops confidence and stability in standing. Prosthetic limb weight-bearing serves the multiple purposes of facilitating wound healing, promoting sensory adaptation, strengthening muscle, and increasing confidence wearing the prosthesis.

Functional examination is essential in physical therapy management (see Chapter 8, Examination of Function). The person's ability to transfer from sit-to-stand or bed-to-wheelchair provides insight into their strength, coordination, balance, and cardiovascular status. Just prolonged standing can challenge the patient's aerobic capacity and endurance. Monitoring walking and overall exercise tolerance can indicate the level of deconditioning and demonstrate improving aerobic capacity. A lightweight prosthesis with locked joints may be indicated for severely deconditioned individuals. People able to walk both slowly and rapidly with endurance to navigate community distances and obstacles are more likely candidates for energy-storing foot/ankle assemblies and/or fluid-controlled knee units. Chapter 22, Amputation, describes functional outcome measures specific to prosthetic use, including the Amputee Mobility Predictor (AMPpro) and Comprehensive High-Level Activity Mobility Predictor.

Cognition and Psychosocial Conditions

Assessment of the person's ability to learn and retain new information, including short- and long-term memory, provides insight into cognitive function that can impact the use and prescription of a prosthesis in older adults.[60] Neurological conditions such as cerebrovascular accidents complicate fitting and training. Ipsilateral hemiplegia is not as detrimental to prosthetic rehabilitation as contralateral paralysis. In both instances, the prosthesis should be designed for maximum stability. Patients with mild neurological impairments often respond favorably to altered training strategies, which the therapist designs on an individualized basis.

The physical therapist works closely with the patient and may be most attuned to changes in the individual's psychosocial status. Many people after amputation confront psychosocial issues that should be recognized and addressed.[61-64] The Trinity Amputation and Prosthesis Experience Scales-Revised (TAPES-R) can be used to assess limb loss–specific psychosocial disposition.[65] Expression of suicidal ideation is not uncommon and should prompt referral for appropriate support and psychological care.[66] Ample evidence supports the psychological and physical benefits of clinic team management.[57]

Patient satisfaction with their prosthetic device and care, assessed with the Orthotics Prosthetics User Survey (OPUS), Satisfaction with Device and Service modules, can also influence outcomes. Since low satisfaction is linked with undesirable outcomes like prosthetic non-use, individual satisfaction should not be overlooked.[67]

Motivation is a cardinal determinant of prosthetic outcome. Strong motivation demonstrated by prosthesis use and adherence with the rehabilitation program can predict successful prosthetic rehabilitation. However, one should guard against unrealistic expectations. Involving the person and family in groups of people with amputation during rehabilitation or in community settings fosters supportive and social constructive lifelong wellness attitudes.

Temporary Prostheses

Immediate Postoperative Prostheses

Persons undergoing amputation without comorbidities anticipated to delay wound healing may receive a prosthetic fitting immediately after surgery by the prosthetist. Such prostheses are plaster casts with attached pylon and simple prosthetic foot for temporary use. The immediate postoperative prosthesis provides total contact to the residual limb to improve wound healing, a rigid protective barrier to prevent physical trauma, potential for early weight-bearing to facilitate transfers, and a motivational boost. It is not meant for ambulation.[68]

Prosthetic Prescription

No prosthesis is ideal for all clients; selected components should meet each individual's needs. Alternatives to every element of the prosthesis have advantages and disadvantages. The physical therapist, in consultation with the prosthetist and physician, judges the relative merits of various prosthetic foot/ankle and knee units, suspensions, and other components in light of their evaluation findings and knowledge of the individual's goals, environment, and personal factors. Ultimately, the medical doctor prescribes the prosthetic components after a comprehensive examination by the physical therapist and prosthetist.

In 1995, Medicare listed functional levels applicable to individuals with unilateral transtibial and transfemoral amputations that determine the medical necessity, and thus reimbursement, of prosthetic knee and ankle-foot units.[69] There are five functional levels with corresponding suggested componentry classes. See Table 31.1 for details. Medicare K-level classifications parallel walking speed.[70]

Medicare requires consideration of the following information in determining K-level: prior, current, and perceived future level of function. Therefore, the physical therapist includes a complete history to define current and past functional levels with the thorough examination as part of the rehabilitation team. Depending on the level of the amputation, prior level of function, and available prosthetic options, goals may meet or exceed the prior functional level. For example, an individual who had

Table 31.1	Medicare Functional K Levels		
K-Level	Description	Knee (for Transfemoral only)	Foot/Ankle System
0	• Prosthesis will not enhance quality of life or mobility potential.	N/A	N/A
1	• Transfers • Ambulate on level surfaces • Fixed cadence • Limited or unlimited household ambulator	• Single axis	• SACH • Single axis
2	• Traverse low-level barriers: curbs, stairs, uneven surfaces • Limited community ambulator	• Polycentric	• Flexible-keel • Multiaxial
3	• Variable cadence ambulator • Unlimited community ambulator • Traverse most environmental barriers • Prosthetic use beyond simple locomotion	• Hydraulic/pneumatic • Microprocessor	• Dynamic response • Multiaxial microprocessor
4	• Exceeds basic ambulation skills • Exhibits high-impact, stress, or energy levels • Typical of child, athlete, or active adult	• Any system	• Any system "blades"

SACH = solid ankle cushion heel.

limited mobility prior to amputation due to nonhealing plantar ulcers may be free to move without restriction after amputation. Alternatively, an individual who underwent bilateral transfemoral amputations will likely be less mobile than before amputation. Goal setting to justify the perceived future level of function is critical.

A critical factor in determining K-level is ability to walk with variable cadence. Variable cadence is the ability of prosthesis users to change the step rate per time while walking, an important aspect of safe community ambulation and prosthetic function. For instance, an individual may have to speed up their cadence to cross the street at a busy intersection and also slow down to navigate the curb. For an individual to be a candidate for hydraulic/pneumatic knee units, variable cadence is necessary.

Some people can be expected to function best with a sophisticated prosthesis that enhances the wearer's ability to engage in vigorous walking and athletics. Others are well served by simple, inexpensive devices. The most accurate predictor of future function is the patient's performance with a previous prosthesis. For people who seek a replacement prosthesis, use of the previous limb, health status, and lifestyle changes are relevant factors. For example, a person using a simple transfemoral prosthesis who now plans to become more active and participate in sports may need a prosthesis with hydraulic knee unit and energy-storing foot configuration. Some prosthetic components can also have functional benefits (see Table 31.2).

Prescription for the new patient is more difficult. Depending on the interval between amputation surgery

Table 31.2	Table of Evidence: Prosthetic Interventions for Gait Speed
	Gardiner et al. (2016)[125]
Design	Systematic Review
Level of Evidence	1
Subjects	Inclusion: Studies that 1. Included people with unilateral transtibial amputation 2. Included SACH feet and energy-storing feet 3. Reported metabolic cost of walking data, either per minute or per meter Exclusion: Studies that 1. Involved people with vascular amputation.
Intervention	A systematic review to assess whether use of energy-storing feet improved energy cost compared to SACH feet.
Results	Energy-storing feet reduced the cost of walking (per meter) in subjects with transtibial amputation versus conventional SACH feet. The reduction is very small: mean energy cost of walking for all energy-storing feet was 97.3% of that with a SACH foot.
Comments	Energy-storing feet marginally improve energy cost of walking for people with traumatic transtibial amputation using SACH feet. The limited push-off power provided by energy-storing feet likely makes the difference. The statistically significant difference may not translate into a clinically significant improvement in function.
	Kannenberg et al. (2014)[126]
Design	Systematic Review
Level of Evidence	1
Subjects	Inclusion: Studies that have 1. Randomized or nonrandomized comparative studies that included comparison of results of a microprocessor knee with those of one or more non-microprocessor knees 2. People with a unilateral transfemoral or knee disarticulation amputation classified as MFCL-2 mobility grade 3. Quantifiable results of performance objective and/or self-reported outcome measures in the areas of safety, function and mobility, and prosthetic function and satisfaction Exclusion: Studies that 1. Investigate implantable knee joints 2. Include people with bilateral amputations or an amputation level higher than transfemoral or lower than knee disarticulation 3. Report no data for independent appraisal

Table 31.2	Table of Evidence: Prosthetic Interventions for Gait Speed—cont'd

Kannenberg et al. (2014)[126]

Intervention	A systematic review to assess whether individuals with a unilateral TFA and MFCL-2 mobility grade benefit from using microprocessor prosthetic knees compared to non-microprocessor knees
Results	• One study (Kahle et al.) found a decrease in stumbles and uncontrolled fall frequency and improved confidence while walking with microprocessor knee use • For abilities necessary for community ambulation, improvements were demonstrated in all MFCL-2 subgroups in slow to medium walking velocity. • No one article demonstrated that NMPK use is superior.
Comments	The use of microprocessor prosthetic knees for hydraulic stance only or both stance and swing control may improve safety, function, and mobility in people with unilateral transfemoral amputations.

Sawers and Hafner (2013)[127]

Design	Systematic Review
Level of Evidence	1
Subjects	Inclusion: Studies that 1. Compared microprocessor and non-microprocessor prosthetic knees 2. Included subjects with transfemoral or knee disarticulation amputations Exclusion: Studies that included 1. People with bilateral amputations 2. People who required walking aids, such as crutches, canes, or walkers
Intervention	A systematic review to assess whether the prescription, fit, and use of microprocessor knees change outcomes for individuals with unilateral transfemoral amputations compared with non-microprocessor knees
Results	• Moderate evidence exists to suggest that swing and stance microprocessor knees are associated with increased confidence during ambulation, increased self-reported mobility, reduced self-reported cognitive demand while walking, improved self-reported well-being, and equivalent overall societal costs when compared with NMPKs. • Microprocessor knees appear to have similar total prosthetic rehabilitation costs compared with non-microprocessor knees. • Microprocessor knees do not appear to influence O_2 consumption, physiological measures of cognitive demand, or the amount of daily activity performed.
Comments	The provision of a microprocessor knee is likely to improve safety and ability to descend stairs and/or negotiate uneven terrain as well as increase patient satisfaction and perception of mobility. However, the limited literature reflects a small subset of commercially available prosthetic knees and is mostly derived from outcomes of two specific models (Compact C-Leg and SmartIP).

Samitier et al. (2016)[128]

Design	Quasi-experimental
Level of Evidence	2
Subjects	Inclusion: 1. Older than 50 years of age 2. Unilateral amputation 3. Six months or longer prosthesis use 4. Independent or modified independent indoor ambulation Exclusion: 1. Cognitive impairments

Table 31.2   Table of Evidence: Prosthetic Interventions for Gait Speed—cont'd

Samitier et al. (2016)[128]

Intervention	Participants were evaluated at baseline and after 4 weeks of using a vacuum-assisted socket system on the following outcomes of interest: Medicare Functional Classification Level, BBS, Four Square Step Test, Timed Up and Go Test, the 6MWT, the LCI, SAT-PRO questionnaire, and Houghton Scale.
Results	Those classified as having a K-level 2 (*n* = 6) had significant improvements in Four Square Step Test and Houghton Scale scores. For those with K-level 3 classifications (*n* = 10), significant differences were found in all outcomes of interest except the Houghton Scale and SAT-PRO.
Comments	A small sample size (*n* = 16) and nonexperimental design limits its generalizability. Approximately 50% of participants in the K-level 2 subgroup experienced blisters with the vacuum suspension.

Paradisi et al. (2015)[129]

Design	Quasi-experimental
Level of Evidence	2
Subjects	Inclusion: **1.** Body mass less than 125 kg **2.** K-level 1 or 2 **3.** Uses a SACH foot for 6 months or longer **4.** Is ambulatory 4 hr/day or more Exclusion: **1.** Residual limb or medical complications
Intervention	Participants (*n* = 20) performed a battery of physical performance and self-report measures wearing a SACH foot, then after 4 weeks, with a multiaxial foot-ankle system. Outcomes of interest were LCI-5, 6MWT, HAI, SAI, BBS, upper-body accelerations, and PEQ.
Results	Significant differences favoring the multiaxial foot demonstrated significant improvements in the overall 6MWT, HAI, SAI, LCI-5, BBS, and specific PEQ scales.
Comments	Long-term follow-up needed to determine influence on ADLs, community ambulation, and societal participation.

ADL = activities of daily living; BBS = Berg Balance Scale; HAI = Hill Assessment Index; LCI-5 = Locomotor Capability Index-5;
MFCL-2 = Medicare Functional Classification Level-2; NMPK = non-microprocessor-controlled prosthetic knee;
PEQ = Prosthesis Evaluation Questionnaire; SACH = solid ankle cushion heel; SAI = Stairs Assessment Index;
SAT-PRO = Satisfaction With Prosthesis; 6MWT = 6-minute Walk Test; TFA = transfemoral amputation.

---

and prescription, the amputation limb may not have stabilized in volume; the patient may not have achieved maximum benefit from preprosthetic rehabilitation. The best criterion for prosthetic prescription in such an instance is performance with a temporary prosthesis complete with a well-fitting socket, suitable suspension, pylon, foot/ankle unit, and a knee unit for transfemoral prostheses. The temporary prosthesis is designed for easy alteration in case of limb volume changes and allows assessment of preliminary gait and activities training. The major difference between the temporary and definitive (permanent) prosthesis is appearance. Ordinarily, little attention is paid to the color and exterior shape of temporary prostheses.

Prosthetic Examination

The prosthesis should be examined to determine the adequacy of prosthetic fit and function, as well as the wearer's overall satisfaction. This process typically includes examination of prosthetic and skin analysis, static standing analysis, and dynamic gait analysis. A full evaluation may include negotiation of stairs and a ramp. Appendix 31.A, Transtibial Prosthetic Evaluation (online), and Appendix 31.B, Transfemoral Prosthetic Evaluation (online), contain the checklists referred to in the following sections.

Transtibial Examination

Most items on the checklist in Appendix 31.A (online) are self-explanatory. Each contributes to forming an accurate judgment of the adequacy of the prosthesis.

Prosthetic and Skin Analysis With Prosthesis Off the Patient

The residual limb and prosthesis are examined. The prosthesis should be compared with the prescription, with any deviation noted and communicated to the prosthetist and physician. The socket size and brim should be appropriate for the individual, any straps should be secured, and vacuum or suspension components should be operational. The skin should be inspected to allow for comparison after prosthetic gait. Skin discomfort, redness, or abrasion after dynamic gait analysis can inform the therapist regarding potential relationships with observed gait deviations.

Static Analysis

The prosthesis is examined while the wearer stands and sits. With the wearer standing in parallel bars or another secure environment, ability to bear equal weight on both feet is assessed, and subjective comments about comfort are solicited. Estimates of anteroposterior and mediolateral weight-bearing can be gleaned by slipping a sheet of paper under various parts of the shoe. Ideally, the patient should stand with both heels and soles flat on the floor. Misalignment, indicated by excessive weight-bearing on one portion of the shoe, may be confirmed during dynamic gait analysis.

Most prostheses are constructed so that when the individual stands, the pelvis is level.[30] A residual limb that sinks too far into the socket will make the prosthetic side appear short, and the wearer may complain of discomfort. This can be rectified through the addition of sock ply to account for the diminished residuum volume. If an excessive leg length discrepancy still exists despite obtaining a proper socket fit, referral to the prosthetist is required.

Pistoning is vertical residual limb motion in the socket. Movement can be determined in standing by marking the sock at the socket brim and then having the patient elevate the ipsilateral pelvis. The socket should slip less than 1/4 in. (0.5 cm). Loose or inadequate suspension causes socket pistoning; the socket should fit snugly.

Comfortable sitting is a primary need for all people. The posterior transtibial brim should not press into the popliteal fossa, and hamstring reliefs especially for the medial semitendinosus and semimembranosus tendons should be adequate.

Dynamic Analysis

Analysis of the gait pattern and performance of other ambulatory activities is an essential part of rehabilitation. No prosthesis completely eradicates the anatomical and physiological changes produced by amputation, such as sensation, musculoskeletal continuity, or full body weight. Anatomical differences are accentuated in the presence of pain, contracture, weakness, instability, or incoordination. When walking, the person who wears a prosthesis compensates for anatomical and prosthetic deficiencies.[71-74] Because virtually all people walk with a prosthesis in a manner different from the normal walking pattern, prosthetic gait represents compensation for the altered locomotor apparatus. The term *gait compensation* may be more accurate than the more commonly used *gait deviation* inasmuch as the patient with limb loss is unlikely to walk exactly like a person without limb loss.

Some gait deviations common after amputation can be attributed to factors related to the prosthesis or person. Prosthetic components do not replace every function of the missing limb. For example, prosthetic feet do not include dorsiflexion that occurs at the anatomical toes. As a result, the prosthetic limb is relatively longer in swing phase and thus is typically designed to be up to 1 cm shorter than the anatomical limb to aid swing phase toe clearance. The lack of toe dorsiflexion also restricts normal progression from heel-off to toe-off, though this is mitigated by flexible designs that allow slight forefoot dorsiflexion. Prosthetic problems such as poorly fitted sockets, prosthetic misalignments, malfunctioning components, and improper length compel the wearer to adopt gait compensations that should be minimized to promote efficient and pain-free functional mobility. Factors related to the person such as incorrect prosthetic donning and inappropriate shoes also cause compensations. The physical therapist determines potential gait compensation causes so that corrective action may be taken; otherwise the patient will expend excess energy walking and exhibit more conspicuously abnormal gait. The new wearer is unlikely to have a smooth gait initially, but prosthetic- or person-related causes of observed gait compensations usual for those with similar prostheses should be assessed. Ultimately, gait with a transtibial prosthesis should closely resemble gait without a prosthesis in the absence of musculoskeletal and neuromuscular impairments.

Transtibial gait analysis focuses on step length and stance duration, which are both affected by prosthetic-side knee function during stance phase. Knee stability while flexing during early and late stance phases is best observed from the side. At initial contact, uncontrolled prosthetic-side knee flexion leads to instability and potential collapse; thus the wearer may shorten prosthetic-side stance duration. After midstance, excessive prosthetic-side knee flexion, referred to as early heel-off, leads to short sound limb step length. Person causes of excessive and uncontrolled knee flexion include residual limb pain, quadricep and gluteal weakness, or fear or low confidence with prosthetic weight-bearing. Prosthetic causes of excessive or uncontrolled knee flexion include socket alignment too far anterior to the foot and or dorsiflexed foot alignment, both of which cause a short toe lever and limit resistance to anterior translation over the foot. If the knee flexes excessively only during initial contact, the cause may be a too firm heel cushion. Conversely, insufficient knee flexion results from posterior socket displacement, inadequate socket flexion, or plantarflexed foot alignment, all causes of a long toe lever that resists the body's translation over the foot. Table 31.3 summarizes the prosthetic and anatomical causes of transtibial gait compensations/deviations.

Transfemoral Examination

A similar checklist is used to evaluate the transfemoral prosthesis (Appendix 31.B [online]). It is important to

Table 31.3   Prosthetic Gait Analysis: Typical Gait Deviations

Deviation	Phase of Gait	Level	Prosthetic Cause	Person Cause
			Viewed From Behind	
Abducted hip	Stance	TF/TT	• Long prosthesis • Poor suspension • Improper socket fit or alignment	• Hip abduction contracture • Hip weakness • Residual limb pain • Poor balance or confidence
Circumduction and/or hip hiking	Swing	TF/TT	• Long prosthesis • Excessive (TF) knee resistance • Poor suspension • Improper socket fit or alignment • Long toe lever	• Limited (TT) knee flexion • Hip flexion weakness • Limited terminal stance loading • Poor motor control
Whips	Swing	TF	• Loose socket fit • Loose componentry	• Limited hip rotation motion • Hip weakness
			Viewed From the Side	
Forward trunk shifting	Stance	TF/TT	• Unstable prosthesis • Improper socket fit or alignment	• Hip flexion contracture • Gluteal weakness • Pain, fear avoidance
Short sound limb step length	Stance	TF	• Long toe lever • Improper socket fit • Improper socket alignment: excess TF socket flexion, insufficient TT socket flexion	• Hip flexion contracture • Gluteal weakness • Residual limb pain • Fear avoidance of loading prosthesis • Poor balance or confidence
Long step on prosthetic side	Swing	TF	• Excessive friction in knee component	• Fear avoidance of loading prosthesis • Lack of terminal stance loading • Lack of pelvic initiation
Insufficient knee flexion	Swing	TF/TT	• Excessive TF knee friction • Loose socket fit • Loose componentry	• Limited TT knee flexion • Hip flexion weakness • Poor motor control
Excess knee flexion	Stance	TF/TT	• Short toe lever (TT) • Insufficient TF knee friction	• Gluteal (TF/TT) or quadricep (TT) weakness • Residual limb pain • Poor balance or confidence

TF = transfemoral; TT = transtibial.

recognize that seldom is one item of major significance. For example, misalignment detected in static analysis should be confirmed during gait.

Prosthetic and Skin Analysis With Prosthesis Off the Patient

As with the transtibial prosthesis, the prosthesis should be compared with the prescription, with deviations noted and communicated to the prosthetist and physician. Socket size and brim should match the individual, and all straps and suspension components should be operational. The residual limb skin should be inspected to allow for comparison after prosthetic gait.

Static Analysis

The patient who has a flesh roll above the socket either did not don the socket properly or has a socket that is too small for the thigh. Perineal pressure results from sharpness of the medial brim or insufficiency of the adductor longus relief in a quadrilateral socket. If the socket is opaque, the only way to judge its snugness is by palpating tissue protruding through the valve hole when the valve is removed.

The knee unit should be stable enough to maintain extension after a firm push by the therapist to the posterior aspect of the unit when the patient stands. Stability is influenced by knee *alignment* in relation to the hip and prosthetic ankle, the trochanteric-knee-ankle line. The farther posterior the knee bolt, the more stable the knee is, but the more difficult it is for the knee to bend smoothly into terminal stance. Polycentric knee joints also contribute to stability.

The checklist is designed to help the clinician determine the fit of the socket, regardless of shape or material. For a quadrilateral socket, proper adductor longus tendon and ischial tuberosity location indicates correct socket donning and alignment. A horizontal posterior brim allows gluteal musculature and ischial tuberosity weight-bearing. The ischial containment socket is intended to provide stability via three-point contact with the ischial tuberosity, pubic ramus, and greater trochanter that minimizes motion in the frontal and transverse planes. The wearer can still move the hip in all directions comfortably, without socket gapping. Some sockets allow adjustment for fit (Fig. 31.48).

A transfemoral suspension sleeve can be used to aid suspension (Fig. 31.49). A Silesian belt for additional stability should have the lateral attachment superior and posterior to the greater trochanter to best control prosthetic rotation (Fig. 31.50). Anteriorly, the attachment should be at the ischial tuberosity level, or slightly below, to aid in adducting the prosthesis.

The patient should be able to sit comfortably with the prosthesis. Socket alterations that allow for more

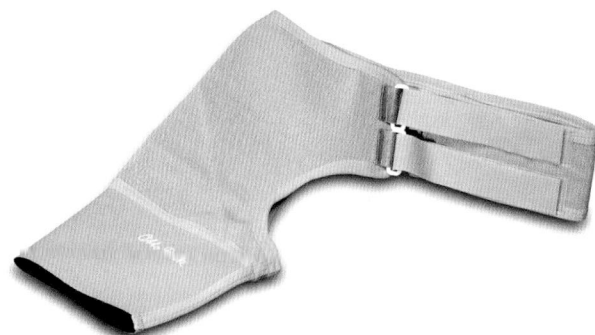

Figure 31.49 Transfemoral suspension sleeve. *(Courtesy of Otto Bock, Minneapolis, MN 55447.)*

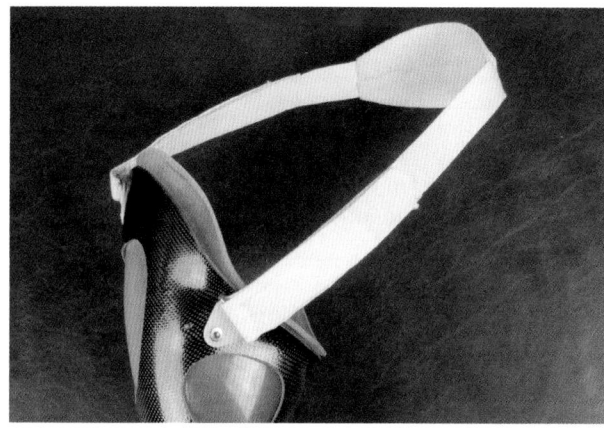

Figure 31.50 Silesian belt. *(From Roy SH, Wolf SL, Scalzitti DA. The Rehabilitation Specialist's Handbook. 4th ed. F.A. Davis; 2013:977. With permission.)*

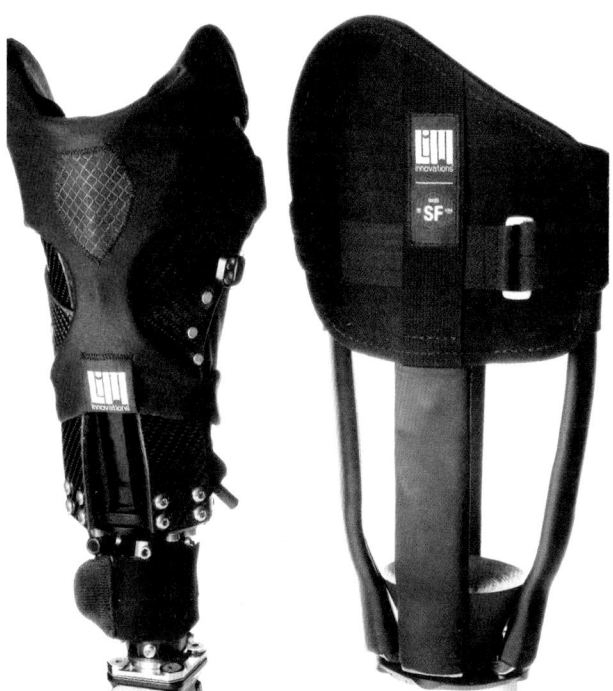

Figure 31.48 LIM Innovations adjustable sockets for transtibial (left) and transfemoral (right) amputations.

comfortable sitting may be made by the prosthetist (see Fig. 31.51).

Dynamic Analysis

The goal of walking with a transfemoral prosthesis is a comfortable, safe, efficient gait, rather than duplicating the gait of someone who does not have an amputation.[75] Both prosthetic factors such as socket fit and alignment and personal factors such as the presence of joint contractures and muscular contraction influence gait. Table 31.3 summarizes the prosthetic and anatomical causes of transfemoral gait compensations/deviations. The primary difference in transfemoral gait, compared to transtibial gait, is dependence on prosthetic knee function which affects base of support, step length, and stance duration.

COMPENSATIONS/DEVIATIONS BEST VIEWED FROM BEHIND

For many individuals with transfemoral amputation, a wide base of support that enhances frontal plane balance may be apparent when viewed from behind.

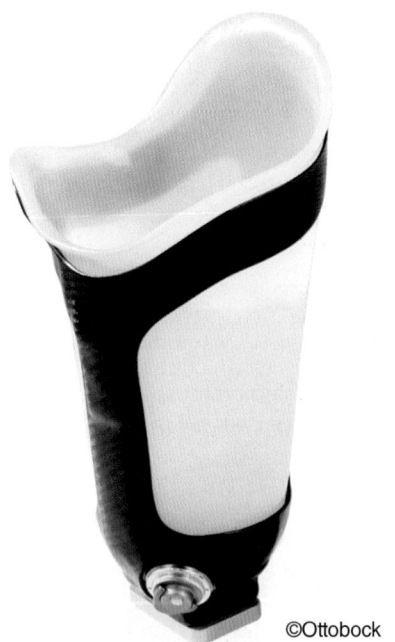

©Ottobock

Figure 31.51 Socket alterations including large fenestrations. *(Courtesy of Otto Bock, Minneapolis, MN 55447.)*

Hip abduction contracture predisposes patients to *abducted gait* and may occur with a wide stance phase base of support or swing phase circumduction. *Circumduction* can occur due to inadequate socket adduction, socket looseness, medial socket brim discomfort, or when the prosthesis is too long. The prosthetic limb is effectively too long in the swing phase when the prosthetic knee flexes inadequately, whether the resistance to knee flexion is excessive or the person has yet to learn to control the knee. *Lateral trunk bending* toward the prosthetic side during stance phase can accompany abducted gait due to lateral momentum generated by weight shifting onto the shorter prosthetic limb. Even when the anatomical hip and gluteus medius are in good condition, shorter prosthetic stance duration can limit lateral weight shifts and lead to a wide base of support.

Whips refer to medial or lateral rotation of the heel at early swing. If the socket does not fit well, contraction with bulging of the thigh musculature will cause the prosthesis to rotate abruptly as it is being unloaded at the end of stance phase. Although less likely, malrotation of the knee unit or foot-ankle assembly may contribute to whipping. *Rotation of the foot on heel contact* indicating inadequate compression of the heel cushion or hip weakness is a much more serious deviation that can lead to a fall.

COMPENSATIONS/DEVIATIONS BEST VIEWED FROM THE SIDE

Prosthetic knee function and asymmetric step length and stance time may be apparent when gait is viewed from the side. *Forward trunk shifting* in stance phase is a compensation used to cope with knee instability and is accentuated by walker or assistive device use. Lumbar *lordosis* results from inadequate socket flexion and is aggravated by a hip flexion contracture and weakness of the gluteal muscles important for knee stability in the absence of the quadriceps.

Improper adjustment of the knee unit gives rise to *uneven heel rise* (excessive knee flexion) and *terminal swing impact* (abrupt knee extension). If both deviations are present, the probable cause is insufficient knee unit resistance. Excessive knee resistance causes inadequate flexion in swing phase. Referral to the prosthesis is appropriate for adjustment of resistance settings.

To compensate for reduced knee motion, the vigorous walker may demonstrate *vaulting* by excessively plantarflexing the sound ankle to afford extra room to clear the prosthesis during prosthetic swing phase. A less strenuous compensation for excessive actual or functional prosthesis length is *hip hiking*, when the patient elevates the pelvis on the prosthetic side.

Unequal step length will be evident if the patient has a hip flexion contracture, fear of the knee collapsing in initial loading, or inadequate balance. A longer step taken with the prosthesis gives the person more time on the sound limb and reduces prosthetic stance duration. A flexion contracture or insufficient socket flexion limiting hip extension range prevents the sound limb from passing the prosthetic side during swing phase on the sound limb.

Prosthetic Training

Learning to use a prosthesis effectively involves donning it correctly, problem-solving the residual limb–socket interface, developing good balance and coordination, walking in a safe and reasonably symmetrical manner, and performing other ambulatory and self-care activities. Anticipated goals and expected outcomes depend on the patient's physical and psychological status, preprosthetic experience, and quality of prosthesis. Using the prosthesis only for transfers from the wheelchair to toilet or bed may be an appropriate outcome for individuals with multiple comorbidities limiting function prior to the amputation, whereas the program for the individual with traumatic amputation might extend to a full range of sports.

Donning

Correct application of the prosthesis is very important in preventing discomfort or skin breakdown. Patients with partial foot, ankle disarticulation, and transtibial amputations can don the prosthesis while seated. The individual simply inserts the residual limb into the socket, applying the correct number and sequence of socks and/or liners, and secures the suspension component. The correct use of socks and liners for the prosthetic suspension system is imperative.

Those with transfemoral amputation also can begin the donning process while seated. Total suction wearers may use either a pulling or pushing method. To pull oneself into the socket, the patient applies a light dusting of talcum powder to the thigh to reduce friction. Then one applies a pull sock, a tubular cotton stockinette, or length of elastic bandage to the residual limb up to the groin to capture proximal thigh tissues. After placing the sock-encased thigh into the socket, the distal end is drawn out of the valve hole to pull the limb completely into the socket. Most prefer to stand while pulling the pull sock through the valve hole after which the valve is inserted and tightened. Another approach to donning is to coat the thigh with light lubricating lotion and push the limb into the socket until all air is expelled, after which the valve is closed.

Self-Management

Self-management for persons with limb loss is the process of caring for the residual limb and prosthesis, problem-solving the interface between the residuum and the socket, making decisions regarding self-care, and recognizing red-flag scenarios that may require the assistance of a clinician.[76] Failure to properly self-manage can result in injury to the residual limb, falls, or secondary complications like musculoskeletal pain. Thus, self-management is critical for the physical therapist to teach. The main self-management topics are (a) residual limb care, (b) decision-making regarding assistance, and (c) problem-solving the fit of the prosthesis.

Residual Limb Care

Residual limb care primarily involves skin hygiene and red-flag recognition. Proper skin hygiene requires that the individual regularly wash their residual limb, ensuring that any skin folds are cleansed. After drying the residual limb, lotion should be applied to keep the skin hydrated. During this hygiene ritual, the individual should use a mirror to inspect their skin for breakdown, irritation, or rash formation. Since mundane conditions like folliculitis or contact dermatitis can lead to infection, the individual must be vigilant in examining their integument.

Decision-Making Regarding Assistance

Red-flag recognition is the process of identifying residual limb issues that could become problematic if not attended to in a timely manner. Examples of red flags that require emergent care are signs and symptoms of infection, wound formation in an individual with vascular or metabolic disease, or significant residuum volume fluctuation. If the individual identifies an area of concern, they should be instructed to contact their medical provider for care. Generally, red flags also indicate discontinuing prosthetic wear until the residual limb is evaluated.

Problem-Solving the Fit

Problem-solving the fit of the prosthesis is one of the most difficult tasks a wearer may experience, yet one of the most common issues.[77] Part of the education process entails teaching the individual to adjust sock ply, adjust suspension components, and respond to volume fluctuations throughout the day. Complicating matters further is the myriad suspension options, each requiring a different approach to effectively problem-solve the fit. While clinical experience and working together with the prosthetist can help the clinician properly educate the patient, certain clinical tools can assist the problem-solving process. An example is a decision tree, which illustrates a step-by-step process to problem-solve prosthetic fit issues. While paper versions may be complex to follow, displaying the decision trees in a digital format improves the usability and acceptability.[78] An example of a paper-based decision tree is presented in Fig. 31.52.[79]

The ability to independently problem-solve depends on the individual's physical and cognitive function. Physically, the individual must be able to manipulate suspension components to achieve a congruent and comfortable fit. Hand deformities, visual impairments, or generalized weakness create a barrier to effective problem-solving. Additionally, cognitive impairments make it less likely the individual can functionally utilize the prosthesis and more likely that complications develop.[80] Therefore, both cognitive and physical impairments should be considered in the educational plan.

Decision-making entails recognizing an issue that the individual with limb loss can either solve themselves (e.g., modifying sock ply) or should seek professional help for (e.g., sounds emitted from the prosthesis during gait). The decision-making component of self-management depends on vigilance, education, and the external support structures available to the individual. Since not everyone will live within a relatively short distance to seek assistance, patients should be educated on what issues require external help and how to connect with the right professional. When the prosthesis or residual limb has developed a new issue, not utilizing the prosthesis until a professional can evaluate the situation is recommended.

Exercises to Stretch and Strengthen

Exercises are similar for most individuals with limb loss, although the individual with a transfemoral or hip disarticulation prosthesis may be expected to encounter more difficulty controlling the mechanical knee, as compared to those with two anatomical knees. Because flexibility and strength depend on the underlying joint mobility, joint mobility of the lumbo-pelvic-hip complex is an important starting place.[81] Hip flexor flexibility is often limited but important to allow advance of the body over the pelvis (Fig. 31.53). Hip strength can be developed prior to and after prosthetic fitting without wearing the prosthesis by pressing the residual limb against a bolster or towel roll (Fig. 31.54). With the prosthesis, an elastic band can be used to apply resistance at the level

Trans-femoral (Above Knee): Suction Suspension With Liner

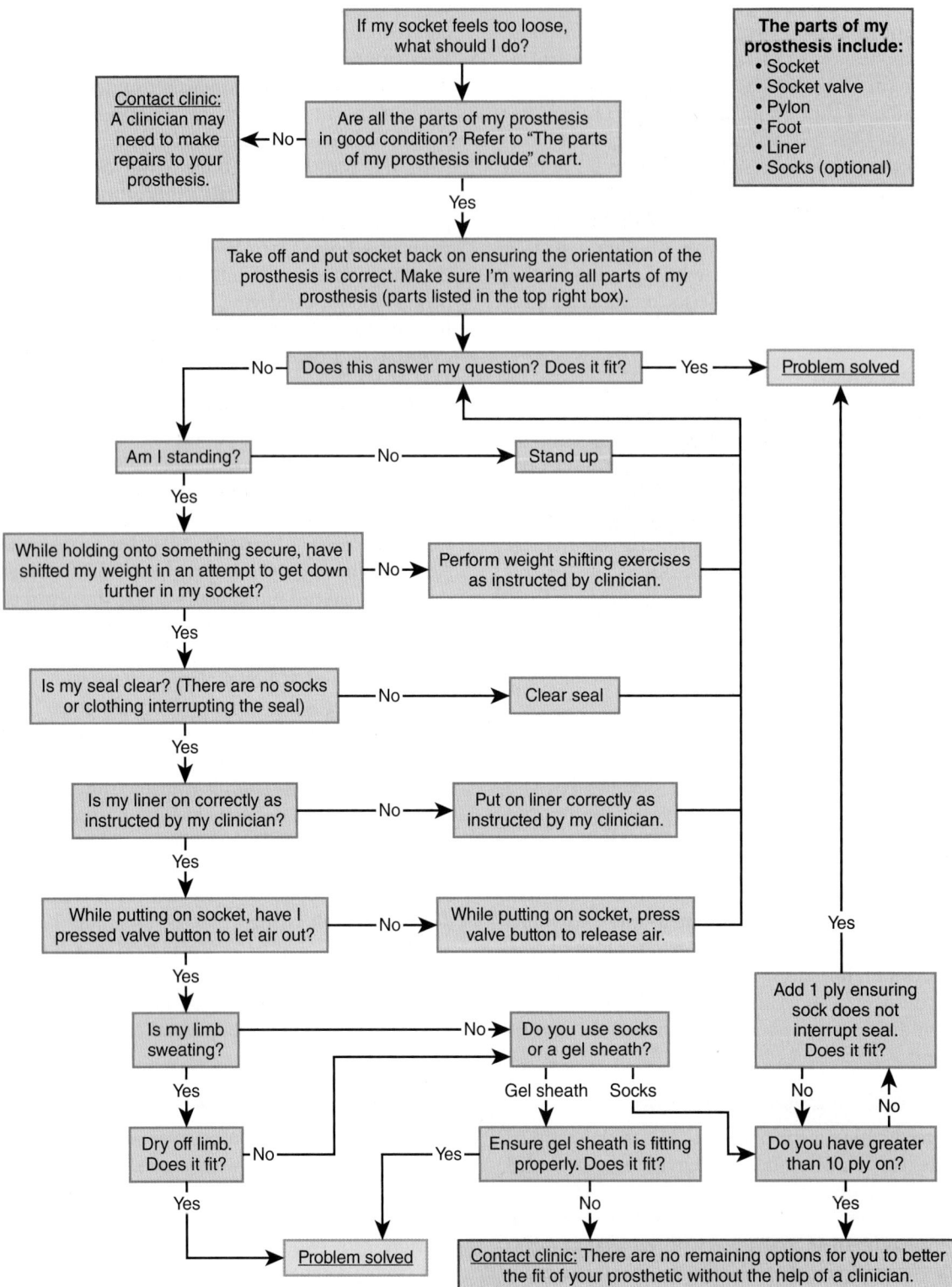

Figure 31.52 An example of a paper-based decision tree. *(Courtesy Dr. Daniel J. Lee, with permission.)*

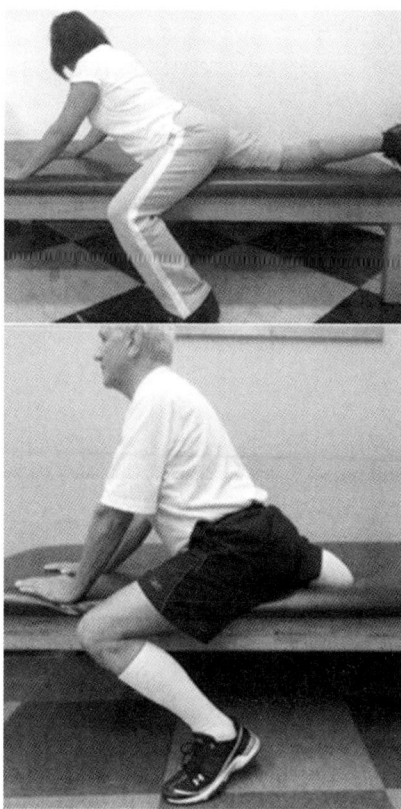

Figure 31.53 Hip flexor muscle stretching can be performed with or without the prosthesis for transtibial and transfemoral amputation levels.

of the residual limb to accentuate the forceful sensation against the prosthetic socket needed to control the prosthetic limb (Fig. 31.55). See Chapter 22, Amputation, for more information on exercise prescription for people with lower limb amputations.

Transfers

Rising from different chairs, the toilet, and the car are primary skills that need to be relearned after amputation. Most patients enter the physical therapy department in a wheelchair. Initially, the patient can park the chair at the parallel bars or at a plinth. After locking the wheelchair and raising the footrests, the patient should sit forward and transfer weight to the intact leg, then push down on the armrests. The individual will find that placing the sound foot close to the chair enables rising by extending the knee and hip on the sound side. Sitting is accomplished by placing the sound foot close to the chair and lowering oneself by controlling hip and knee flexion on the sound side with eccentric strength or assist of the arms.

For both standing and sitting, the beginner should have the advantage of a chair with armrests that enables use of the hands to control and assist trunk movement. This is particularly true for the person with bilateral amputations. Later the person should practice sitting in deep upholstered sofas and low chairs, as well as benches, the toilet, and other seats that do not have armrests. Transfer into an automobile should be an integral part

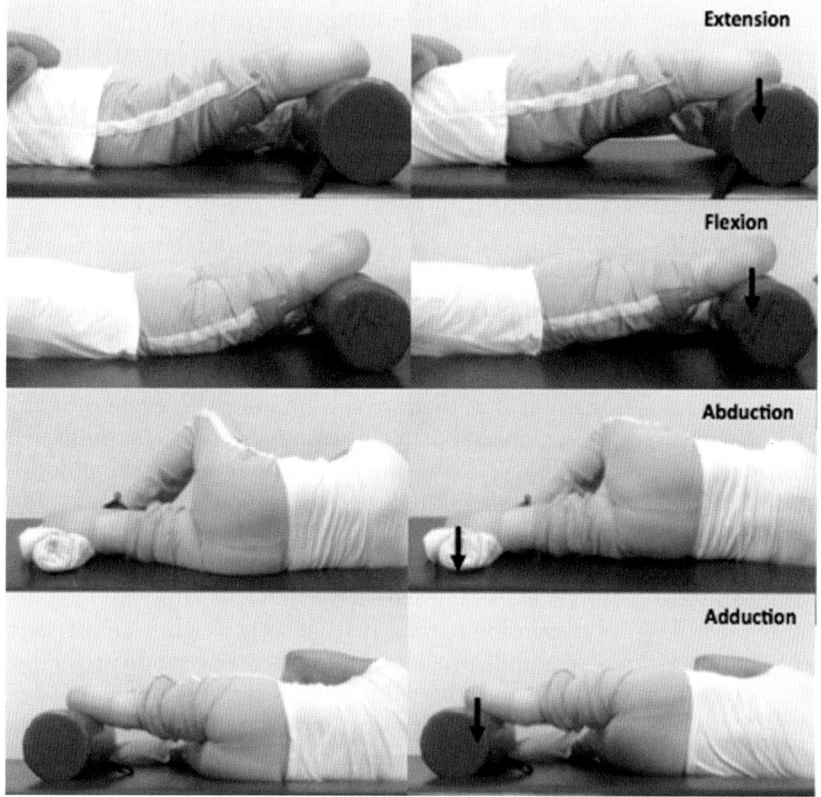

Figure 31.54 Hip-strengthening exercises can be performed without the prosthesis by pressing down against a bolster with the residual limb to lift the pelvis off the table. *(Courtesy of Dr. Christopher Kevin Wong, with permission.)*

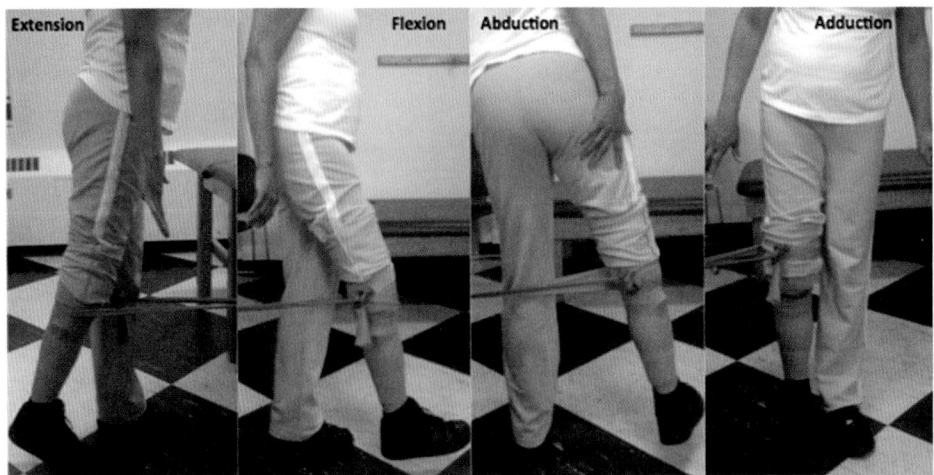

Figure 31.55 Elastic band resistance can be used for hip strengthening with the prosthesis. *(Courtesy of Dr. Christopher Kevin Wong, with permission.)*

of the training activities; otherwise, the patient faces a gloomy future, confined to home or dependent on special transportation systems.

To enter the right (passenger) side of an automobile, the prosthesis wearer faces the front of the car. The person with a right prosthesis puts the right hand on the door post and the left hand on the back of the front seat, then swings the left leg into the car, slides onto the car seat, and finally places the prosthesis in the car. The individual with a left prosthesis may find that sitting sideways with both feet out the car door is easiest. The person pivots on the seat while swinging the prosthesis into the car, then puts the intact right foot inside the car.

Balance and Coordination

All people with lower limb amputations must learn to balance on the amputated side.[82,83] For people with lower limb amputations, use of the Berg Balance Scale provides a reliable and valid assessment across the range of ability levels.[84,85] A graduated program for increasing prosthetic tolerance minimizes the danger of skin abrasion, particularly if the residual limb presents skin grafts, poor circulation, or diminished sensation. The patient should alternately exercise and rest, with cardiopulmonary monitoring a routine part of the program, especially for high-risk individuals.

Some clinicians eschew parallel bars because the fearful patient pulls on them, which will be fruitless when progressing to a cane. When bars are used, the therapist should encourage the patient to rest the open hand on the bar for support, rather than using a tight grip. A plinth or sturdy table offers the dual advantages of providing good support on only one side, and unidirectional control, because the patient can only push, never pull, for balance.

Static erect balance reintroduces the novice to bipedal posture. The patient should strive for level pelvis and shoulders, vertical trunk without excessive lordosis, and equal weight-bearing. The therapist should guard and assist the patient as necessary. When the physical therapist stands near the prosthesis, this encourages the patient to shift their weight onto it. The client must learn to utilize proximal sensory receptors to maintain balance and perceive the position of the prosthesis without looking at the floor. Some patients respond well to increased use of visual feedback (e.g., using a mirror) or dual task training.[86–88]

Static exercises to improve medial–lateral, sagittal, and rotary control can later be progressed to dynamic exercises (Fig. 31.56). The patient learns that hip flexion causes the knee to bend, and hip extension stabilizes the knee during stance phase. Placing the sound foot ahead of the prosthesis makes the prosthetic knee more stable. Patients should be instructed in weight shifting in both symmetrical and stride positions and in stepping movements. Stepping on a low stool or step platform with the sound foot obliges the patient to shift weight onto the prosthesis and increases stance phase duration on the prosthesis. Having all exercises performed rhythmically with both the right and left lower limbs fosters symmetrical performance.

Gait Training

Walking is a natural progression from dynamic balance exercises as the patient takes successive steps. Patients tend to place greater load and exert more propulsive force on the intact side; consequently, gait training should emphasize symmetrical performance.[74,81,82,87] Inasmuch as hamstrings become the main muscles of propulsion, strengthening exercises are indicated (Fig. 31.57). Some people respond well to proprioceptive neuromuscular facilitation[89,90] (Fig. 31.58). Rhythmic counting and walking in time with music in 2/4 time also improves gait symmetry and speed. In the physical therapy department, an apparatus that includes a suspension harness (partial body weight support) over a treadmill provides a protected environment for the patient to learn gradual weight-bearing on the prosthesis. A balance apparatus providing electronic feedback with or without emphasis on psychological awareness of bodily position is another training option.[91]

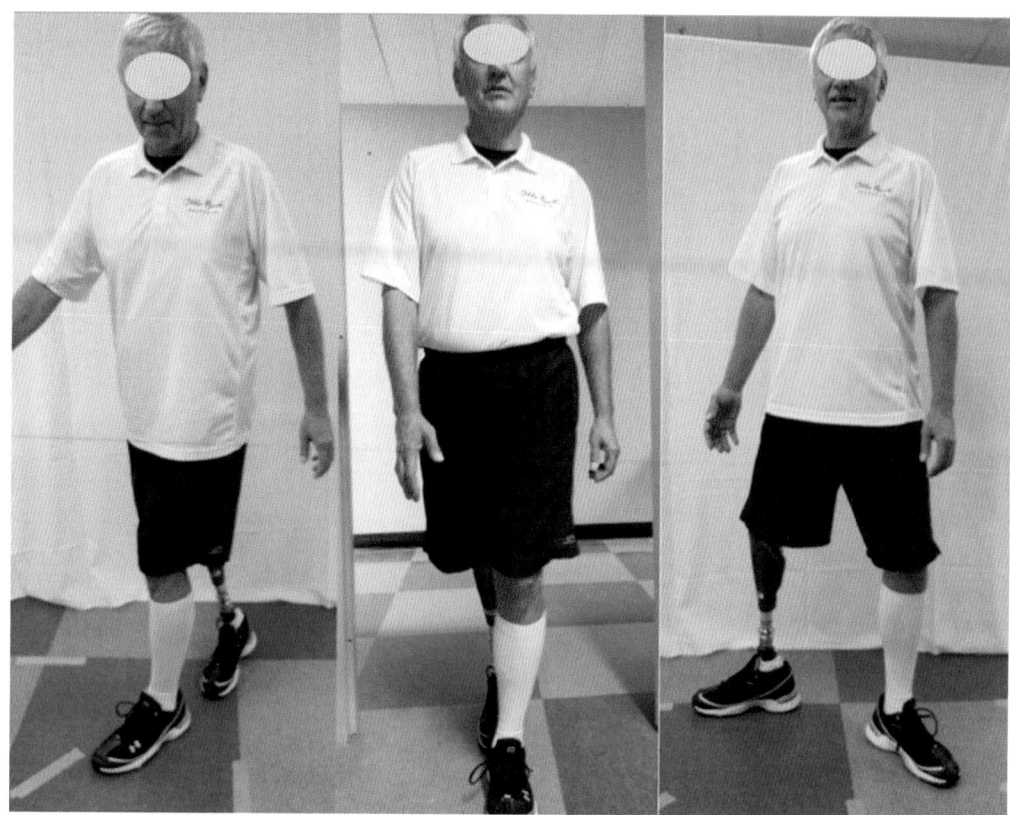

Figure 31.56 Static balance exercises incorporating hip rotation and a narrow base of support. *(Courtesy of Dr. Christopher Kevin Wong, with permission.)*

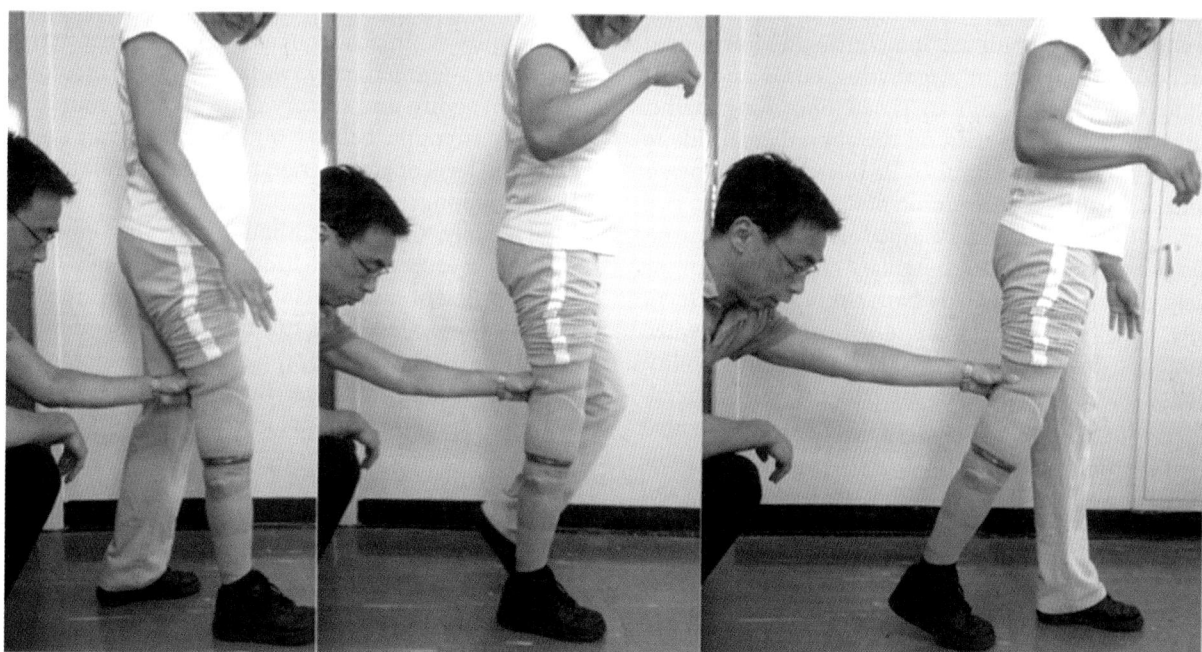

Figure 31.57 Resistance applied to the prosthetic-side limb to develop hip extension strength throughout the gait cycle. *(Courtesy of Dr. Christopher Kevin Wong, with permission.)*

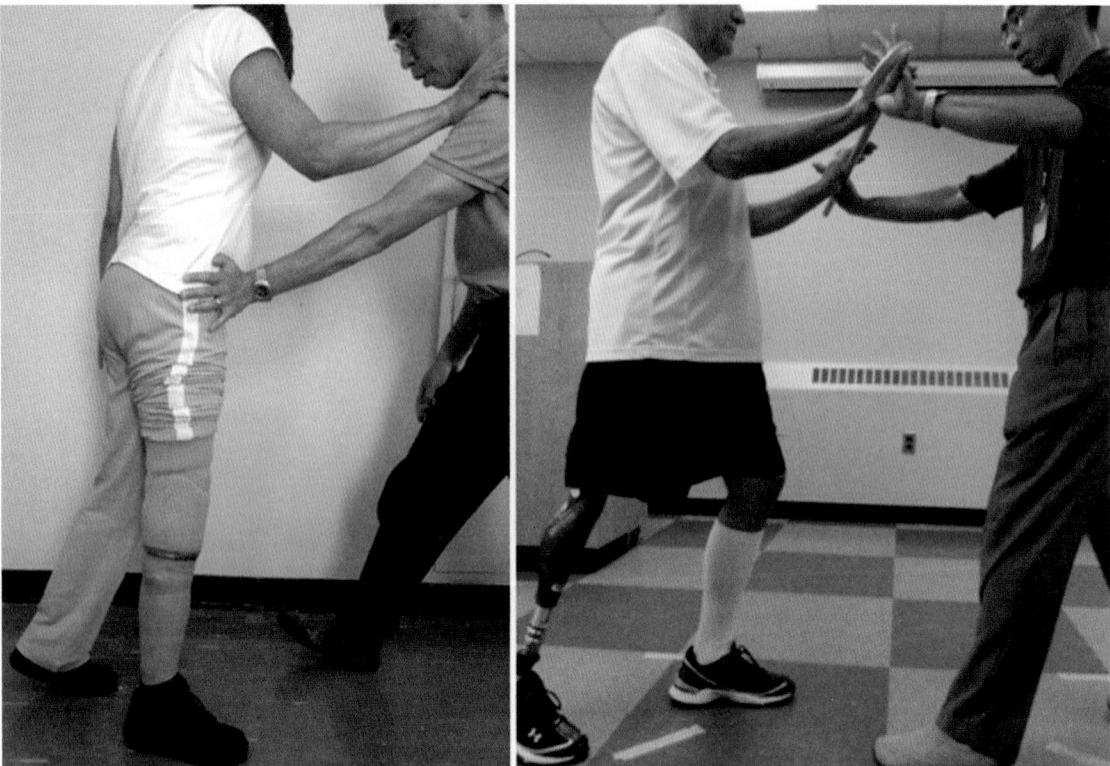

Figure 31.58 Resistance applied through the pelvis or trunk via the arms to develop hip extension strength during gait. *(Courtesy of Dr. Christopher Kevin Wong, with permission.)*

Either a cane or pair of forearm crutches is an appropriate aid for the client who is unable to achieve a safe gait without undue fatigue. Sometimes the cane is used only outdoors to aid in negotiating curbs and other ground irregularities and to signal oncoming traffic. Ordinarily the cane is used on the contralateral side to enhance frontal plane balance. If bilateral assistance is required, a pair of forearm crutches is preferable to two canes. The crutches remain clasped around the forearms when the user opens a door. Axillary crutches tempt the patient to lean on the axillary bars, risking impingement of the radial nerves; they are also inconvenient when climbing stairs. A walker provides maximum stability, which is particularly useful for patients with generalized weakness. The walker should be adjusted so that the user does not lean too far forward. Ultimately, some people will need walking aids to maintain balance[92] and have confidence to maximize prosthetic function and participate in community social activities.[93,94]

Functional Training

The prosthesis wearer who is learning to walk also should gain experience in performing a wide variety of functional mobility skills both indoors and outdoors. The training program for vigorous individuals includes stair climbing, negotiating ramps, retrieving objects from the floor, kneeling, sitting on the floor, running, multiple terrains, driving a car, and engaging in sports.[95]

The fundamental difference between these activities and walking is the way each lower limb is used. Walking implies symmetrical usage, but the other activities are done asymmetrically, with greater reliance on the strength, agility, and sensory control of the sound limb. Overall, strength, balance ability, etiology of amputation, and level of amputation predict the extent of activity restriction.[96]

Generally, the patient should have the opportunity to analyze each new situation and arrive at a solution to the problem rather than depend on directions from the therapist. Most tasks can be accomplished safely in several ways. The learner profits from practice in clinical decision-making and observing other prosthesis wearers as well as from professional instruction.

Community Mobility: Climbing Stairs, Ramps, and Curbs

Patients with ankle disarticulations and transtibial amputations generally ascend and descend stairs and inclines with steps of equal length in step-over-step progression.[97,98] Those with unilateral transfemoral amputation, in contrast, usually ascend by leading with the sound foot and learn to descend by first placing the prosthesis on the lower step. Some individuals with transfemoral amputation using a hydraulic prosthetic knee component can learn to control the knee and descend step-over-step, however, must still ascend step-to. Some may be able to use a handrail to ascend step-over-step, particularly if the prosthetic knee such as the Genium locks in weight-bearing even at large angles of knee flexion; others fitted with a knee that provides a knee extension assist such as the PowerKnee may be able to ascend stairs step-over-step (see Fig. 31.30).

Curbs present a slightly different problem because there is no handrail. The techniques are basically the same, however.

Ramps may be difficult if the prosthetic foot and ankle do not have sufficient dorsiflexion and plantarflexion.[99–101] With steep stairs, ramps, and curbs, the individual may climb diagonally or sidestep with the prosthesis kept on the downhill side. Patients should also learn how to maneuver over obstacles on the walking surface.[102]

Community mobility can be limited by cardiovascular capacity for physical activity. People with limb loss on average demonstrate markedly lower levels of physical activity measured by steps per day than able-bodied people, even those with diabetes or peripheral artery disease.[103] Physical activity and overall function may be influenced by increased energy cost for people with limb loss.[104,105] A unilateral transtibial prosthesis requires slightly more oxygen when walking at a comfortable speed,[106] but a transfemoral prosthesis requires nearly 50% more oxygen than normal.[107] The lower the amputation level, the less is the metabolic disadvantage. The absence of the knee is critical; people with bilateral transtibial amputations expend less energy than those with unilateral transfemoral amputations. Use of a hip disarticulation prosthesis demands even greater energy expenditure.[108] People wearing bilateral prostheses consume even more oxygen and walk more slowly than those with unilateral amputation at a given level.[109] While selection of prosthetic feet and knee units can modify energy demand somewhat,[110–112] the biggest factor may be the health of the individual.

The increased metabolic expenditure results in part from the socket, which surrounds semifluid tissue, giving imperfect anchorage. The foot-ankle assembly transmits no plantar tactile or proprioceptive sensation, does not move through as large an excursion as the anatomical foot, and does not initiate the dynamic propulsion characteristic of normal gait. The prosthesis is operated by remotely located muscles that contract longer and more forcefully than in normal gait, the resulting motion alterations reflected in gait asymmetry and energy expenditure.

Community Integration: Work, Sports, and Other Activities

Initial prosthetic training can sometimes be brief, with many people not receiving formal physical therapy after prosthetic provision and initial training. Thus, exercise, balance, and gait training progressing to advanced functional activities apply during prosthetic

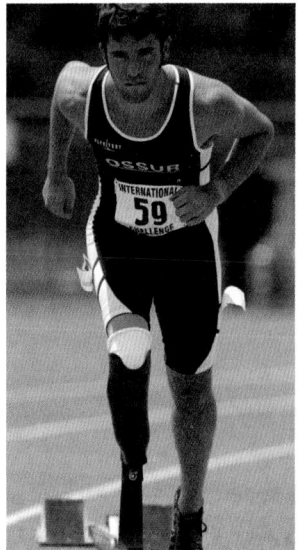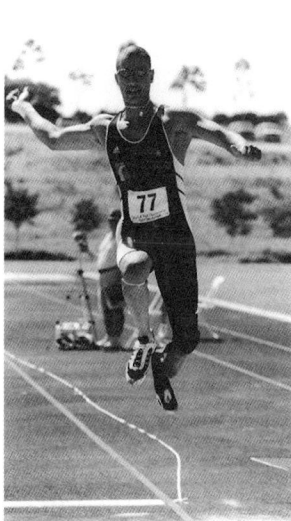

Figure 31.59 Participants in a distance run (left) and long jump (right) event. *(Courtesy of Össur, Aliso Viejo, CA 92656.)*

training, community reintegration, and lifelong care. Full community integration can mean a return to work or school and participation in leisure activities such as sports (Appendix 31.C [online]). Sports participation (Fig. 31.59) is an excellent extension of rehabilitation for patients of all ages.[113–120] Nearly any sport can be performed with accommodation, and most sports do not require any adaptive or special prosthesis.

For activities that involve vigorous walking or running, an energy-storing/energy-releasing foot is most suitable. The socket should fit snugly with very secure suspension paired with a shock-absorbing liner to minimize abrasion and bruising of the residual limb. Those with a transfemoral prosthesis typically use hydraulic knee units to take advantage of variable stance and swing phase control. Activities that involve jumping, as in basketball, require substantial vertical power generation and absorption primarily achieved with the sound leg which can be assisted by energy-storing foot/ankle assemblies such as J-spring–type prostheses which provide some power (Appendix 31.D [online]).

Activities such as dancing do not require prosthetic adaptation, though torque converters may be useful. Other activities such as kite surfing benefit from specialized prostheses that are saltwater tolerant.[121] Some activities such as horseback riding or bicycling are facilitated by minor modification of the equipment, such as a toe loop on an adapted bicycle pedal prosthesis.

Other activities are generally performed without a prosthesis, such as swimming and skiing. The skier will probably use ski poles equipped with small rudders, in a "three-track" manner. Soccer is usually played without a prosthesis, with the player using a pair of crutches. Many competitive activities such as tennis and field events are performed in a wheelchair. Equipment and techniques developed for individuals with paraplegia usually can be adapted for people with amputations.

Recreational programs designed for adults with limb loss help the participants to return to active lifestyles.

The physical therapist should refer patients to convenient recreational clubs, adaptive sports groups, or competitive sporting events. The desired outcome is to maximize each person's functional capacity and quality of life.

SUMMARY

This chapter has focused on the prosthetic management of adults with limb loss and limb difference. Characteristics and function of the principal prostheses and prosthetic components have been discussed. In addition, the responsibilities of the physical therapist in prosthetic management have been emphasized. Successful prosthetic rehabilitation depends on close collaboration among the patient, physical therapist, physician, prosthetist, and other team members. This will provide an environment for information exchange and foster coordinated management. The result will be an optimum match between the patient's physical and psychosocial characteristics and a prosthesis capable of fulfilling its intended purposes.

Questions for Review

1. What are the principal causes of amputation based on demographics?

2. Describe appropriate prostheses for individuals with various partial foot amputations.

3. Distinguish between the ankle disarticulation and the transtibial residual limbs and prostheses.

4. What prosthetic feet are especially suitable for older adults? Why?

5. What is the purpose of the reliefs and buildups in the transtibial socket.

6. Contrast the modes of suspension for the transtibial prosthesis. Which suspension is indicated for an individual with a very short residual limb?

7. Classify knee units according to friction mechanisms.

8. Compare the quadrilateral and the ischial containment transfemoral sockets.

9. Describe the modes of suspension of the transfemoral prosthesis. In which type(s) does the client wear a sock?

10. How is the wearer of a hip disarticulation prosthesis prevented from inadvertently flexing the prosthetic hip and knee?

11. Outline a maintenance program for a transfemoral prosthesis with hydraulic knee unit and endoskeletal shank.

12. What factors should be considered prior to formulating a prosthetic prescription?

13. How can the physical therapist determine and improve the patient's psychological status?

14. What features of the transtibial prosthesis are considered in static evaluation? In dynamic evaluation?

15. Delineate the training program for a patient with a transfemoral prosthesis.

CASE STUDY

The patient is a 55-year-old man and former college athlete who has peripheral artery disease and lost his right leg at the transfemoral level a year ago. Delayed wound healing prolonged his hospital stay and delayed prosthetic fitting for 6 months, during which time he received a short episode of home-based physical therapy. The therapist had reinforced consistent care, and inspection of the left foot and right residuum prepared him for his prosthesis with weight-bearing residual limb exercises and general mobility with forearm crutches. He received a K2-rated prosthetic limb at the prosthetic clinic, at which time he "learned to walk" in the parallel bars before going home using one crutch. Over the next 6 months, he began walking on his own with a cane indoors and outdoors, though mostly just to his car to commute to work from his suburban home. He does not like slowing people down or getting so exhausted that he has to rest while people wait for him, so he limits his social activities to avoid having to walk too much. He has been referred to physical therapy because of a

CASE STUDY—cont'd

recent fall on his sloping driveway that resulted in low back pain (NRPS 3/10) aggravated by walking a few minutes. Although the low back pain has diminished over time, he presents with notable limitations in all domains of the International Classification of Functioning, Disability, and Health.

PHYSICAL THERAPY EXAMINATION FINDINGS

Body Structure and Function
- Cognition: Alert, oriented, memory intact
- Vision: Intact with corrective lens
- Cardiopulmonary:
  - Vital signs seated at rest: Blood pressure 140/86, heart rate 84, respiration normal
  - Endurance: Exercise capacity less than 10 min before needing rest
- Integumentary: Incision well healed without adherent scar
- Neuromuscular: Sensation and reflexes normal bilateral
- Musculoskeletal:
  - ROM: Hip extension R –15, L –5; hip adduction R –15, L –5
  - Joint mobility: Hip and sacrum hypomobile bilateral
  - Flexibility: L SLR 50, PKB 90
  - MMT: Hip extension, abduction, and flexion R 3+/5, L 4+/5
  - Prosthesis related:
    - Residual limb: ~50% of femur length
    - Prosthesis:
      - Silicone liner for suspension with pin-lock
      - Endoskeletal shank with flexible inner and fenestrated outer sockets
      - Weight-activated knee (Ottobock 3R93)
      - Non-energy-storing multiaxial foot/ankle (Greissinger foot + multiaxial ankle)

Activity
- Balance: Berg Balance Scale (BBS) score performed with his prosthesis 46/56, placing him in the second lowest of the four balance ability strata[85] with the following items not receiving maximum scores:
  - Turning 360° in a circle
  - Retrieve object from floor
  - Stand in tandem
  - Alternate steps
  - Stand on one leg (either)
  - Stand from sitting without hands
- Gait: 0.7 m/sec with cane over 2 min, putting him in category of independent household and limited community walker.[70] Rarely walks longer than 5 min at one time. Decreased prosthetic-side stance time with lateral trunk lean and shorter sound-side step length with lack of prosthetic-side hip extension past neutral contributes to asymmetric gait appearance.
- AMP(PRO): Total score 30, placing him within the range of AMP scores for K1, K2, and K3 prosthetic users.[122,123]

Participation
- Home living: Independent but limited from some household chores such as laundry and shopping that involve carrying while walking or navigating stairs/slopes/curbs.
- Vocational: Goes to work in an office independently.[124]
- Social: Walks outdoors only to commute; rarely leaves home to go shopping or socialize.

Individual and Environmental Contextual Factors
He lives with his wife in a split-level home with a sloping yard. He works in an office near home, his wife works full-time in the nearby city, and his adult daughter lives in an apartment in the same city. He used to enjoy nature walks with his wife, dining out with his family, and jogging and golfing but has not returned to any of these activities. In fact, the back pain combined with distal residual limb pain after walking and phantom limb pain at night have contributed to decreasing activity in the past year and some anxiety about his future.

PERSON-DESIRED OUTCOME AND GOALS
Reduce back pain, improve walking ability, and prevent future falls are his stated goals.

(Continued)

CASE STUDY—cont'd

GUIDING QUESTIONS

The primary outcome around which rehabilitation efforts may focus will be the patient-centered goal of participating more fully in life by leaving the home for social and community activities. However, addressing impairment-based goals at the level of the body structure and function are critical supporting blocks upon which to build future abilities. In addition, maximizing body structure and functions to optimize ability in functional activities such as walking speed can also help an individual qualify for more advanced prosthetic components that can in turn benefit social-community integration. For instance, K3-level prosthetic users can qualify for hydraulic knees that make descending stairs and slopes safer, which was his recent mechanism of injury. Consideration of a person's limitations in all domains of the International Classification of Functioning, Disability, and Health as well as broad examination across systems and treatment for all relevant body structures and function with the overall goal of achieving a SMART patient-identified participation goal may well provide the best results for any individual case.

1. Identify the impairments, activity limitations, and participation restrictions you will address in developing the plan of care.
   a. Body structure and function impairments
      i. Impaired ROM, particularly at the hip
      ii. Impaired muscular strength, particularly of the hip
      iii. Impaired cardiovascular endurance
   b. Activity limitations
      i. Reduced balance ability
      ii. Reduced walking ability as measured by speed, distance, or endurance
   c. Participation restrictions
      i. Restricted social interaction
      ii. Restricted community integration

2. Establish reasonable expected outcomes (long-term participation goal) and anticipated goals (short-term).
   • For each long-term participation goal, identify activity limitations that should be ameliorated to facilitate participation.
   • For each activity limitation, identify body structure/function impairments that, if reduced, can minimize the activity limitation.
   • Plan interventions to address body structure/function impairment and functional activity limitations.
   • Note safety precautions that should be observed during treatment of this patient.
   • Note strategies to develop self-management and self-efficacy in achieving goals and outcomes.

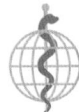 The reader is referred to Immersive Case G: A Patient With Limb Loss Following Amputation, an interactive case that guides users through the interview, examination, diagnosis, and writing of goals and the plan of care for a patient with limb loss following amputation, available online at **fadavis.com**.

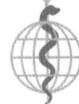 For additional resources, including answers to the questions for review, new immersive cases, case study guiding questions, references, and more, please visit **https://www.fadavis.com/product/physical -rehabilitation-fulk-8**. You may also quickly find the resources by entering this title's four-digit ISBN, 4691, in the search field at **http://fadavis.com** and logging in at the prompt.

Seating and Wheeled Mobility

Laura J. Cohen, PhD, PT, ATP/SMS, RESNA Fellow
Faith Saftler Savage, PT, ATP

"Mobility devices enable persons with disabilities to achieve personal mobility, and access to these devices is a precondition for achieving equal opportunities, enjoying human rights and living in dignity."[1]

LEARNING OBJECTIVES

1. Identify when a wheelchair user has basic, intermediate, or complex needs.
2. List the eight basic steps of the wheelchair seating and mobility service delivery process.
3. Explain the difference between a reference neutral sitting posture and a person's *optimal* sitting posture.
4. Describe the components of the examination process for determining the most appropriate wheelchair seating and mobility device (WSMD).
5. Discuss the relationship between elements of the assessment interview and the wheelchair prescription/selection.
6. Explain the different methods of seating simulation and the expected outcomes.
7. Describe factors that affect determination of seat and back support features.
8. Discuss the benefits and contraindications of various seating system features.
9. Apply the components of a problem-solving model when presented with a clinical case study.
10. Describe at least five basic elements that should be included in the clinician documentation for a WSMD.

CHAPTER OUTLINE

INTRODUCTION 1223
  The Wheelchair User 1224
  Mobility-Related Assistive Technology Defined 1225
  The Person-Technology Match 1226
WHEELCHAIR SEATING AND MOBILITY SERVICE DELIVERY TEAM 1227
WHEELCHAIR SEATING AND MOBILITY SERVICE DELIVERY PROCESS 1227
  Wheelchair Service Delivery Steps 1227
PRINCIPLES OF WHEELCHAIR SEATING AND MOBILITY 1230
  Principles of Sitting Posture 1230
  Pressure Injuries 1233
  Principles of Mobility 1234

WHEELCHAIR SEATING AND MOBILITY EXAMINATION AND SPECIALTY EVALUATION 1235
  Communication Tips 1235
  Examination 1235
  Specialty Evaluation 1242
  Intervention 1249
WHEELCHAIR SEATING AND MOBILITY TECHNOLOGIES 1250
  Seating Support System 1251
  Wheeled Mobility Devices 1258
FUNDING 1280
DEFENSIBLE DOCUMENTATION 1280
OUTCOME MEASUREMENT 1280
SUMMARY 1282
ACKNOWLEDGMENTS 1282

■ INTRODUCTION

According to estimates from the Centers for Disease Control and Prevention, approximately 61 million, or one in four adult Americans has a disability of some type, and the number is increasing daily.[2,3] Roughly 2.7 million people in the United States depend on a wheelchair for day-to-day tasks and mobility.[4,5] Wheelchair users are limited in their ability to walk. This may include people who are unable to walk at all and who will need a wheelchair full-time for mobility in all environments; others may need a wheelchair only for longer distances or in certain environments.

In 2001, the International Classification of Functioning, Disability and Health (ICF) introduced language and a framework for describing disability.[6–8] The ICF carefully defines key concepts, including functioning, disability, activity, participation, and personal and environmental factors. Wheelchair seating and mobility (WSM) technologies are, from an ICF perspective, considered an *environmental factor* that has an impact on a person's functioning and can facilitate *activity and participation*.[9]

A functional mobility limitation such as an inability to walk does not always equate to a functional limitation.

For example, the function of walking may cease to be disabling if accommodations are made to compensate for the limitation, such as with the use of equipment (e.g., wheelchair, walker, cane) and/or accommodations to the environment, such as a ramp or elevator, to enable access to buildings and the community.

The Wheelchair User

People of any age may need a wheelchair—children, adults, and older adults. The need for a wheelchair can be permanent, or it can be temporary. People with a variety of diagnoses, such as multiple sclerosis (MS), cerebral palsy (CP), or cerebrovascular accident (CVA), may need a wheelchair because their walking ability is limited. Other people need wheelchairs because they have no ability to walk, including individuals with spinal cord injury (SCI), amyotrophic lateral sclerosis (ALS), traumatic brain injury (TBI), CP, or severe

rheumatoid arthritis. The needs of each wheelchair user will vary, depending on lifestyle, life roles, type of mobility impairment, and the environments routinely encountered.

Hierarchy of Wheelchair User Seating and Positioning Need

Providing wheelchairs and seating systems for people with mobility limitations is both a science and an art that, for people with more complex needs, requires more training than that which is covered in this chapter. Adapted from the World Health Organization's (WHO's) Wheelchair Service Training Program, a service delivery model based on a hierarchy of wheelchair users' seating and positioning needs is used to distinguish among three levels: *basic, intermediate,* and *complex*[10-13] (Table 32.1). Three variables considered are (1) balance and postural control in sitting, (2) the ability to achieve a neutral sitting posture,

Table 32.1 Hierarchy of Wheelchair User Seating and Positioning Needs

Sitting and Positioning Needs	Basic	Intermediate	Complex
Balance and postural control in sitting	Good sitting balance, hands-free sitter	Fair sitting balance and trunk control	Poor sitting balance
Ability to achieve neutral sitting posture	Achieves neutral posture without support	Achieves close to neutral posture	Unable to achieve neutral posture
Degree of postural support required	No additional postural supports needed	Needs postural supports	Needs custom supports

and (3) the degree of postural support needed to achieve a neutral posture.

A wheelchair user with a *basic* level of seating and positioning needs has good sitting balance and can sit with their hands free to function (also known as a "hands-free" sitter). Additionally, this person can sit in a neutral upright sitting posture without any additional postural supports in the wheelchair. An example of a user with basic needs is an older adult who has lower extremity (LE) weakness but can sit with good balance in a neutral or upright posture. Another example is a person with a T12 complete SCI who does not require additional postural support around the trunk or pelvis to sit upright but requires a seat cushion and back support to help minimize risk of pressure injuries and to provide a stable base to support a neutral trunk alignment.

A wheelchair user with an *intermediate* level of seating and positioning need has only fair sitting balance and trunk control and needs to use their hands to help them balance in sitting (also known as a "hands-dependent" sitter). They may be able to sit close to a neutral posture but will require additional postural supports (such as hip and trunk supports) to sit symmetrically as well as to help balance to free up their hands for function. Some examples of users with intermediate needs include people with mild CP (e.g., Gross Motor Function Classification System [GMFCS] Level III) or with TBI without joint contractures, significant spasticity, or other abnormal muscle tone problems. Even if the person has pelvic or spinal asymmetries, the asymmetries are flexible enough to allow the individual to achieve a neutral sitting posture. These wheelchair users will require appropriate seating and postural supports such as special seat cushions and lateral hip and lateral trunk supports.

Wheelchair users with *complex* seating and positioning needs have poor trunk control and cannot sit upright without a lot of postural support (e.g., maximal). They are unable to achieve a neutral sitting posture and may require custom postural supports to accommodate significant abnormalities in muscle tone, joint contractures, and spinal deformities. Examples of users with complex needs include people with progressive diseases such as secondary progressive MS and people with severe tone, weakness, or contractures such as people with CP with spastic quadriplegia (GMFCS Levels IV and V), TBI, or tetraplegia.

This categorization is useful because a more complex level of need requires that the therapist and wheelchair service delivery team have a more advanced level of knowledge and skill. This chapter introduces the knowledge and skills to assess and provide wheeled mobility and seating for users with basic needs and some users with intermediate needs. Wheelchair users with complex needs should be referred to a wheelchair seating specialist who regularly practices with individuals who have these higher levels of need. Those interested in developing their expertise to serve wheelchair users with complex needs will require additional advanced training.

Wheelchair User Rights

Wheelchair users come from all walks of life and have mobility limitations for many different reasons. They rely on their wheelchairs to provide them with optimal support, mobility, and function to perform their jobs, care for their families, attend school, and actively participate in many different life roles and activities. Statistics show that less than 5% of those in the world who need a properly fitted wheelchair actually have one.[14] Notice the emphasis is not only on having a wheelchair, but also on having a properly fitting wheelchair, which is essential for supporting the lives and livelihoods for those who need them.

In 2006, the United Nations Convention on the Rights of Persons with Disabilities (UNCRPD) was signed. In 2008, the UNCRPD became international law. While the United States signed the UNCRPD on July 30, 2009, Congress has yet to ratify or confirm it into law. There are 50 different articles in the Convention, and article number 20 is about the right to "personal mobility," stating that all people have a right to personal mobility.[15] The Convention also defines personal mobility as "the ability to move in a manner and at the time of one's own choice."[14] For many people with a mobility impairment, having an appropriate wheelchair is the only way that they can have personal mobility and is therefore supported by this very important international convention.

Mobility-Related Assistive Technology Defined

The *Technology-Related Assistance for Individuals with Disabilities Act (Tech Act)* was first passed in 1988 and again in 1998, increasing access to, availability of, and funding for assistive technology through state and national initiatives.[16] This legislation defines *assistive technologies (AT)* as any item, piece of equipment, or product system—acquired commercially off the shelf (prefabricated), modified, or customized—that is used to increase, maintain, or improve an individual's functioning and independence to facilitate participation and to enhance overall well-being.[16] Assistive technology can also help reduce impairments and decrease risk for secondary health conditions. The purpose of this chapter is to focus on mobility-related assistive technology.

Consistent with the *APTA Guide to Physical Therapist Practice,* wheeled mobility technology is an *aid to locomotion* used to assist a person to move from one location to another when walking is not safe or functional.[17] *Seating and positioning technology* is individually selected, configured and/or custom-designed for one or more of the following purposes: "(1) to provide support to a person's body in a desired sitting position, (2) to provide support in positions other than a sitting position (e.g., standing, side-lying, supine), (3) to provide support in a way that will assist in maintaining or restoring skin integrity, or (4) to provide a mechanical method to change position relative to gravity (e.g., tilt, recline, elevate, stand)."[16] An implied purpose, although not specifically stated, includes facilitating the use of a wheeled mobility device. This chapter is specific to and limited to seating support systems for use in wheeled mobility devices.

The Person-Technology Match

Achieving a good match between the person and the technology requires attention to the environments in which the technology will be used, the needs and preferences of the user, and the functions and features of the technology. If the match is not a quality one from the standpoint of the person, the technology may not be used or will not be used optimally. The Matching Person and Technology (MPT) model was developed to support the AT assessment and service delivery process.[18,19] It is goal directed, person-centered, and designed to facilitate the identification and selection of AT that is most likely to be used by the individual.[18,19] Several wheelchair-specific and general assistive technology outcome measures suitable for use in evaluating the person–technology match are presented later in the chapter.

Appropriate versus Inappropriate Wheelchair Seating and Mobility Device

Personal mobility for people who use wheelchairs largely depends on access to an appropriate wheelchair seating and mobility device (WSMD), which includes devices such as strollers, manual and powered wheelchairs, and scooters. A combination of the seating support system and a wheeled mobility device when integrated together is considered a WSMD. There are several characteristics that make a WSMD more, or less, appropriate for any individual wheelchair user. Most WSMDs have multiple features that can be selected (added or omitted), depending on an individual's specific needs. Most WSMDs require some sort of individual configuration to fit the person to the technology and address environmental considerations.

An appropriate WSMD meets the user's mobility needs, positioning needs, and environmental conditions. For example, an appropriate WSMD must provide proper fit and postural support, be safe and durable, be readily available in the person's geographic region, be obtained and maintained at an affordable cost, and be accessible to local skilled service and repair by a qualified durable medical equipment (DME) supplier ("supplier") or rehab technology professional (RTP). In addition to meeting the mobility and positioning needs of a wheelchair user, it must be usable where the person typically goes. For example, if a user

resides in a rural environment, the tires must be able to manage rocks, dirt, and mud versus a more urban environment, in which the wheels must allow the user to manage uneven pavement, curbs, and side slopes.

A WSMD can be inappropriate for many different reasons. An inappropriate WSMD has characteristics that do not meet one or more of the needs of a wheelchair user. A few examples of these characteristics include ill-fitting; too large or small, impacting ability to self-propel; inadequate skin protection; insufficient postural support; does not meet functional needs (e.g., seat height too low impeding independent transfers or ability to access standard table or desk). Any WSMD that is inappropriate for the environments in which it will be used will either limit mobility or will fail prematurely, requiring frequent repairs or early replacement.

While there are many benefits of an appropriate wheelchair, they can be organized into four primary categories: (1) mobility, (2) access to community life, (3) health, and (4) self-esteem (or confidence), as described in Box 32.1. Appropriate wheelchairs optimize a wheelchair user's abilities in all four of these categories, and the categories frequently influence each other as well. For example, independence in mobility usually helps a person to optimize their health and access to the community. The primary benefit of a wheelchair is mobility. Wheelchairs provide personal mobility to individuals, allowing them to engage in typical life activities in multiple environments. However, it is not enough to have just any wheelchair. If the wheelchair fits properly, a person has greater potential to be independent in their personal mobility, allowing them to access their community, including going to school or work. A properly fitting wheelchair may also improve the person's overall health by increasing the person's activity level; improving posture, breathing, and circulation; and potentially minimizing risk for impairments such as pressure injuries. All these benefits can also improve self-esteem and self-confidence, leading to improved overall quality of life for the wheelchair user.

Box 32.1 Benefits of a Wheelchair

Mobility: Allowing people to get around with the greatest independence and engage in typical life activities, including functional ADL/IADLs in multiple environments.
Access to community life: A wheelchair allows people to go to work, school, visit friends, attend places of worship, or other community activities.
Health: A well-fitting wheelchair can increase the person's physical activity, improve posture, and prevent pressure injuries.
Self-esteem and confidence: With a well-fitting wheelchair, people can feel better about themselves.

ADLs = activities of daily living; IADLs = instrumental activities of daily living.

WHEELCHAIR SEATING AND MOBILITY SERVICE DELIVERY TEAM

The first part of understanding the wheelchair seating and mobility (WSM) service delivery process is to understand the participants, referred to as the *WSM service delivery team* (WSM team). This team is configured with specific team members, depending on the circumstances related to the referral and the complexity of the person to be evaluated. Regardless of the team size and members, it is commonly accepted as best practice that in order to provide the wheelchair user with the most appropriate WSMD, an interdisciplinary team approach is necessary. Key participants typically involved in the team process at a minimum include:

- The wheelchair user.
- Family members and caregivers.
- A physician or nonphysician practitioner (e.g., nurse practitioner, physician assistant, clinical nurse specialist), recognized by policymakers and payers as the *prescriber*.
- A physical therapist and/or occupational therapist, recognized by policymakers as the *licensed or certified medical professional (LCMP)*.
- A *supplier* or *rehabilitation technology professional (RTP)*, recognized by policymakers as the *certified, registered,* or *otherwise credentialed RTP*.

The team collectively provides *clinical-related services* and *technology-related services*. An individual's medical and functional needs are identified by the clinical team, who are responsible for assessing the person's body structures and functions and identifying the medically necessary and appropriate features needed in a WSMD. The supplier/RTP brings equipment and technology knowledge that matches features identified by the clinical team, with specific make/model products that are then configured into custom-designed systems with input from the clinical team.

Each member of the WSM service delivery team has specific roles and responsibilities relative to obtaining an appropriate WSMD. It is very important to keep in mind the principle that the wheelchair user is an equal partner and is frequently the key player on the service delivery team. Experienced wheelchair users know what they like and what they don't like, what works and what does not work for them. The experienced wheelchair user often helps guide the assessment and delivery process. In this instance it is often the role of the clinician(s) and supplier to provide education and discuss new and emerging technologies, trade-offs between function and equipment choice, and recommendations that are needed to address health, activity, and participation. Even if the disability is not progressive in nature, as a wheelchair user ages, their needs may change, and their technology needs may as well. New wheelchair users will need more information and guidance, as this will likely be their first exposure to the WSM service delivery process and the range of WSM technologies available to address their personal mobility issues. It is essential to really listen to the wheelchair user and help guide them to an appropriate WSMD that will match their needs and goals.

WHEELCHAIR SEATING AND MOBILITY SERVICE DELIVERY PROCESS

Evaluating a person and then recommending and prescribing a WSMD is a complex therapy intervention. Providing an appropriate wheelchair to a person is not a singular event; it is a process that does not end when the user receives the WSMD. The provision of WSM services consists of two interrelated components:

- The *clinical-related component* done by the therapist: the physical and functional evaluation, treatment plan, goal setting, preliminary device feature determination, trials/simulations, documentation and justification, fittings, function-related training, determination of outcomes, and follow-up.[20]
- The *technology-related component* done by the supplier/RTP: the technology assessment; the accessibility survey of the home environment; transportation assessment; equipment demonstration/trial/simulation; product feature matching to identified medical, physical, and functional needs; system configuration; fitting; adjustments; programming; determination of outcomes; and product-related training and follow-up.[20]

The service delivery process can be time-consuming and may require several visits to complete, depending on complexity. Additional time spent up front to be thorough often decreases errors and future costs associated with mistakes created by incomplete information, examination, and trials.

Wheelchair Service Delivery Steps

Each step in the wheelchair service delivery process is important to the overall outcome for the individual.[10,11,21–23] Summarized here are the crucial components of the *wheelchair service delivery process,* as outlined by the World Health Organization.[10,11,24] These steps as performed in a *wheelchair examination* and *specialty evaluation* are explored in greater detail later in the chapter.

Step 1: Identification of Need and Referral

People are referred for WSM services by a range of different sources: hospital or health-care providers (e.g., physician/NP/PA, case manager, discharge planner), community resources (vocational counselors, educators), family and friends, disability organizations, or other wheelchair users. It is important to identify the reason(s) for referral and the complexity of the person's mobility impairment. This information will assist in routing the person to an appropriate clinic, therapist, complex rehabilitation technology (CRT) supplier, or DME supplier. Preliminary questions may include the following: Is this the person's first wheelchair? Is the person being seen for problems with their existing wheelchair? Are there problems with skin integrity or sitting posture, or are the needs solely related to mobility, or both? Answers to these questions (and more) will help determine whether the person's WSM needs are at a basic, intermediate, or complex level. The identification of these needs and the referral into the service delivery process is the first step in obtaining an appropriate WSMD.

Step 2: Assessment

The assessment is divided into two primary components: the *assessment interview* and the *physical assessment* (also known as the *Wheelchair Examination & Specialty Evaluation*) (Table 32.2). The interview is used to gather information about the wheelchair user's physical condition (medical diagnoses), lifestyle and environment (including home, school, work, and community issues), and existing equipment. The physical assessment begins with the assessment of the person as they arrive to the clinic in their present wheelchair (if they have one) and includes a description of the person's current seated posture and mobility function. A *mat examination* is performed to assess the person out of the wheelchair in both a supine (gravity eliminated) and a sitting position (with the effects of gravity). Presence, risk, or history of pressure injury is assessed and pressure under bony prominences is considered and often measured at this time, particularly if the person is at risk for a pressure injury. Finally, body measurements are taken of the person while seated in an optimal sitting posture. The purpose of the assessment is to begin to identify the person's problems and potentials and determine the amount, type, and location of needed postural supports, and WSMD features and functions.[21,22]

Step 3: Prescription/Selection

A *prescription* means selecting the best available wheelchair (WSMD) for the wheelchair user. This entails matching a person's identified physical and functional needs, goals, and environments identified in the assessment to necessary equipment features (*person/feature match*).[24] After the equipment features are identified, the wheelchair base, seating system, and wheelchair accessories and options are specified (*feature/product match*).[21,22] As stated previously, the prescription and selection decisions made by the clinician(s) should include involvement of the wheelchair user, his or her family members or caregivers (if appropriate), and a qualified RTP or DME supplier.

Step 4: Funding and Ordering

The next step in the process involves securing funding and ordering the appropriate WSMD and all parts and accessories that go with it. It is essential to know the payer source for the WSMD if a third-party payer is involved, or alternately, to determine if it is being donated, purchased self-pay, or being provided from a facility-owned fleet of available equipment. Documentation is a professional responsibility, a legal requirement, and the most important factor to successful coverage and payment for a WSMD. The person's medical records are expected to reflect clear rationale and justification of the medical need for the care you provide and WSM equipment you recommend. The supplier/RTP typically takes the lead for understanding the coverage and payment policies for the WSMD, compiling required documentation, and submitting it to the payer (e.g., health insurance company), obtaining *prior authorization,* ordering, and billing for the equipment.

Step 5: Product Preparation (WSMD)

This step is normally completed by the supplier/RTP and/or rehab technician. The WSMD that was selected and ordered, once delivered by the manufacturer to the supplier, is prepared for fitting and delivery to the user. It is important to make sure that the wheelchair base, seating, and accessories that were ordered are the ones that were received. For CRT devices, it is not uncommon for a WSMD to have upward of three or more different manufacturer's products included. During the assembly process, the WSMD is configured by the supplier/RTP as specified and inspected for safety and function. It is helpful for all members of the WSM team to have some familiarity with how to assemble some of the basic components of the wheelchair, as they may be needed to assist with this process to some extent.

Step 6: Fitting

If everything has gone as planned, accurate information was obtained during the assessment and the equipment was ordered properly and met the ordering specifications on delivery, then this step should be straightforward; however, it is no less important! During the fitting, the wheelchair user, the therapist, and the supplier together check that the wheelchair is the correct size and that all the necessary modifications and adjustments have been made to ensure proper fit. Next, they check that the wheelchair and seating system (seat, back, head support, etc.) supports the wheelchair user in their optimal sitting posture. Finally, if a pressure-relieving cushion has been prescribed, they check that the cushion relieves pressure adequately for the user. Wheelchair fitting is essential to the success of an appropriate wheelchair, as there are many adjustments that need to be made to ensure the proper support of the wheelchair user in an optimal position. Without this fitting process, a perfectly appropriate wheelchair may become inappropriate!

Table 32.2   Wheelchair Examination and Specialty Evaluation

Examination					Specialty Examination		Intervention
Assessment interview	Equipment assessment	Functional assessment	Screening of body function	Physical assessment	Wheelchair assessment	Evaluation and plan of care	Wheelchair fitting, delivery, and training
Demographic information	Existing equipment	ADL/IADL status:	Status of:	Supine and sitting mat assessment	Measurement	Diagnosis related to positioning and mobility limitation	Function from WC
Reason for referral	Prior equipment	• Toileting	• Cardiovascular system	Sensation	Simulation	Problem list	WC mobility
Diagnosis	Current seating and mobility equipment	• Dressing	• Pulmonary system	Pain	Technology trial	Goals for interventions:	WC skills and training
Medical and surgical history	Sitting posture in existing equipment	• Eating	• Circulatory system	Skin integrity	Person and technology match	• Treatment	Maintenance and repairs
History of WSM problems		Mobility status:	• Gastrointestinal system	Postural alignment		• WSMD	Follow-up
Goals of user, family, caregiver		• Bed mobility	• Vision and hearing	Balance		Equipment prescription and justification	
Social determinants of health		• Transfers	• Bowel and bladder function	Strength, endurance, and muscle power			
Environmental accessibility (home and community)		• Weight shift	• Communication ability	ROM and flexibility (supine and sitting)			
Employment/work status (job/school)		Ambulation	Cognitive and behavioral status:	Neuromuscular status:			
General health status		Propulsion method	• Attention	• Muscle tone			
Functional status and activity level			• Judgment	• Reflexes			
Transportation			• Motor planning	• Motor control and impact on function			
			• Memory				

ADL/IADL = activities of daily living/instrumental activities of daily living; ROM = range of motion; WC = wheelchair; WSM = wheelchair seating and mobility; WSMD = wheelchair seating and mobility device.

Step 7: User Training

An essential step in the service delivery process is education and training for the wheelchair user and, if appropriate, for family/caregivers, in the care and proper use of the new WSMD. It is critically important that the wheelchair user knows how to safely and effectively use their wheelchair. The therapist is responsible for teaching the wheelchair user how to function from the wheelchair, how to get in and out of it, and techniques to minimize risk for pressure injuries. The user will need to know how to propel a manual wheelchair, as well as how to navigate stairs, ramps, and environmental obstacles. Or, if the recommended equipment is a power wheelchair, the user will need to know how to turn the wheelchair on/off, adjust the speed settings, and access any seat functions, as well as operate the wheelchair safely indoors and outdoors. The supplier/RTP is responsible for providing user training on handling the wheelchair (such as folding, taking parts on/off the wheelchair, charging the wheelchair), safe use, care, and maintenance of the WSMD, and what to do in the event of a mechanical problem.

Step 8: Maintenance, Repairs, and Follow-Up

All wheelchairs will require ongoing maintenance, intermittent repairs, and general follow-up to be sure they still fit the users properly and still meet the users' needs. Therefore, follow-up appointments are an important step in a wheelchair service delivery program. During a follow-up appointment, the therapist or supplier/RTP checks the WSMD fit and function and provides further training and support if needed. If the wheelchair is found to no longer be appropriate, the process should start again with an appropriate referral for an assessment for a new wheelchair or a substantial modification of the existing wheelchair. This process should be systematic and is often iterative, but it leads to the greatest possibility of success.

■ PRINCIPLES OF WHEELCHAIR SEATING AND MOBILITY

Most wheelchair users spend many hours sitting each day, so the way in which the person sits in the wheelchair can have a profound effect on health, function, and comfort. For that reason, the wheelchair is not just a mobility aid; it also helps to support the wheelchair user in a comfortable upright sitting posture. Therefore, it is important to understand some basic concepts related to sitting posture and mobility.

Principles of Sitting Posture

The term *posture* refers to the way a person's body segments are arranged, and *sitting posture* is the way a person's body segments are arranged in the sitting position. When providing a wheelchair, it is important to consider the supports in the wheelchair that are needed to help wheelchair users sit in a posture that is comfortable, healthy, and functional.

Reference Neutral Sitting Posture

It is imperative to have a good understanding of the *reference neutral sitting posture* to understand when good posture can be achieved and to assist in determining the amount of support needed. It will also help to understand when an individual's needs are complex and requires services from a seating specialist to obtain the most appropriate system. The objective of the seating system is to allow the person to sit with good pelvic and trunk alignment, neutral LE alignment, and neutral head positioning.

Pelvic Position

The pelvis is the base for sitting upright. Just like a building needs a strong, stable foundation, the pelvis is the foundation for a stable, neutral sitting posture. The pelvis can move and be oriented in different ways. Changes in the orientation of the pelvis affect the posture of the spine and other body segments both above and below the pelvis. The movement and/or position of the pelvis in sitting can be seen from the sagittal, frontal, and transverse views, as shown in Table 32.3.

A reference neutral pelvic position is characterized by a neutral pelvic tilt where a line between the anterior superior iliac spine (ASIS) and posterior superior iliac spine (PSIS) is horizontal or parallel to the seat plane (sagittal view) and the ASIS is level and straight when viewed from the front and top (frontal and transverse views).

The position of the pelvis is critical in creating an optimal foundation for the sitting position. By supporting a neutral to slightly anteriorly tilted pelvis that is level (not oblique or rotated), the pelvis assists with the following:

- Maintains the normal spinal curves (lumbar, thoracic, and cervical)
- Provides symmetrical weight-bearing on bilateral ischial tuberosities (ITs) and pressure distribution over the surface area of the ITs (rather than weight-bearing on the bony prominences of the sacrum or coccyx, which increases pressure risks)
- Promotes symmetry and provides a more stable upright position for active trunk movement and co-contraction of trunk muscles
- Supports flexion at the hips and extension in the lumbar spine; often effective in decreasing abnormal tonal patterns
- Improves alignment in body segments above and below the pelvis
- Provides proximal stability, improving distal mobility and function

Table 32.3   Reference Neutral Sitting Posture

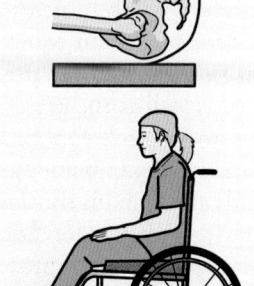 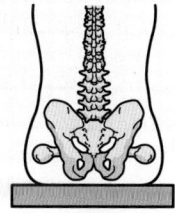 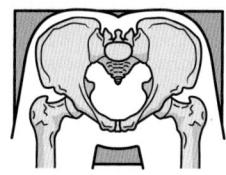

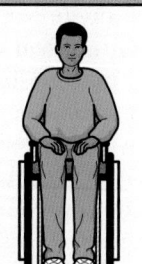 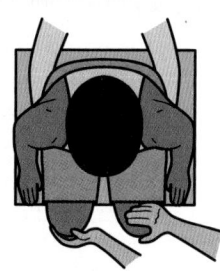

Sagittal View	Frontal View	Transverse View
• Pelvis is neutral to slight anterior tilt • Shoulders are aligned above or slightly behind hips • Spine maintains natural lumbar, thoracic, and cervical curves • Head is vertical and balanced over trunk with neutral horizontal visual gaze • Hips are flexed 80°–90° • Knees and ankles are flexed near 90° • Heels directly below the knees or slightly forward or back • Feet flat on the footrests	• Pelvis (ASIS) is level • Trunk is in midline • Head is in midline, balanced over body • Shoulders are level, relaxed and arms are free to move • Thighs are in slight abduction • Lower legs are vertical with neutral hip rotation • Feet are under the knees	• Pelvis (ASIS) and trunk (shoulders) are not rotated • Head is forward facing and free to rotate • Knees are pointing forward with mild symmetrical abduction • Feet are pointing forward or slightly outward

ASIS = anterior superior iliac spine.

Optimal Postural Alignment

The *neutral reference posture* is used as a reference point for determining optimal postural alignment. Not everyone can achieve a symmetrical "neutral" resting posture. Each person's *optimal sitting posture* will be unique to them due to limitations in joint range of motion (ROM), muscle shortening, spasticity, or scoliosis, as seen with individuals with complex WSM needs. Also it is important to note that optimal sitting posture will be influenced by health needs, personal preferences, and functional requirements.

A person's optimal sitting posture is as symmetrical and balanced as possible, enabling the person to relax comfortably, while also being ready to move. The person's optimal posture is also their "home base" or resting posture, a place to come back from between extremes of movement, but it is not a place of collapse. To achieve optimal postural alignment, fixed ROM limitations and deformities must be accommodated. Additionally, flexible deformities must be corrected and/or supported.

Factors Influencing Postural Alignment

It must be determined whether a person can maintain optimal postural alignment using their own muscular effort or if external supports are required. First it must be determined if improved alignment can be achieved passively (flexible), with the effects of gravity eliminated, supine and/or side-lying on a mat table and in the seated position with the effects of gravity.

Attention is first directed toward alignment of the pelvis and then other body segments. If good alignment can be achieved (corrected), it must be determined whether the person can maintain alignment using muscular effort or if external supports are required.

For joints and/or body segments that are not flexible (*fixed*) to passive alignment, *accommodation* is needed. For example, accommodation would be needed for a person who presents with long-standing fixed hip ROM limitations from hip subluxation and prolonged sitting in a *"windswept lower extremity (LE) posture"* (Fig. 32.1), where one hip is positioned in abduction and external rotation and the opposite hip is in either a neutral sitting position (flexion/adduction) or in adduction and internal rotation. Given a fixed deformity, attempts at aligning the LEs will cause pelvic and/or trunk rotation. The LEs therefore must be accommodated by supporting positioning in the windswept posture (see Fig. 32.1). Alignment of the pelvis takes priority over alignment of other body segments. Providing optimal pelvic and trunk alignment is most important and sometimes trade-offs are needed to maintain or improve function.

Time must be allocated to practice motor skills and movement within the context of improved postural alignment, especially if dramatic alignment changes have resulted. A person's posture is affected by tone, strength, gravity, habitual patterns of movement, and activities. New skill acquisition should be promoted to foster independence rather than dependence on equipment. This is especially important to the younger person who is growing and changing, as well as the person who has not had the opportunity to improve function due to poor positioning and excessive equipment use. Supports can be used intermittently throughout the day to provide learning opportunities (acquisition of new skills) over time. Using minimum supports can improve cosmetic appearance and self-esteem. Other equipment may need to be used for specific activities or for opportunities to improve strength and skills.

Frequently, it is necessary to encourage wheelchair users to sit with "optimal sitting posture," especially if

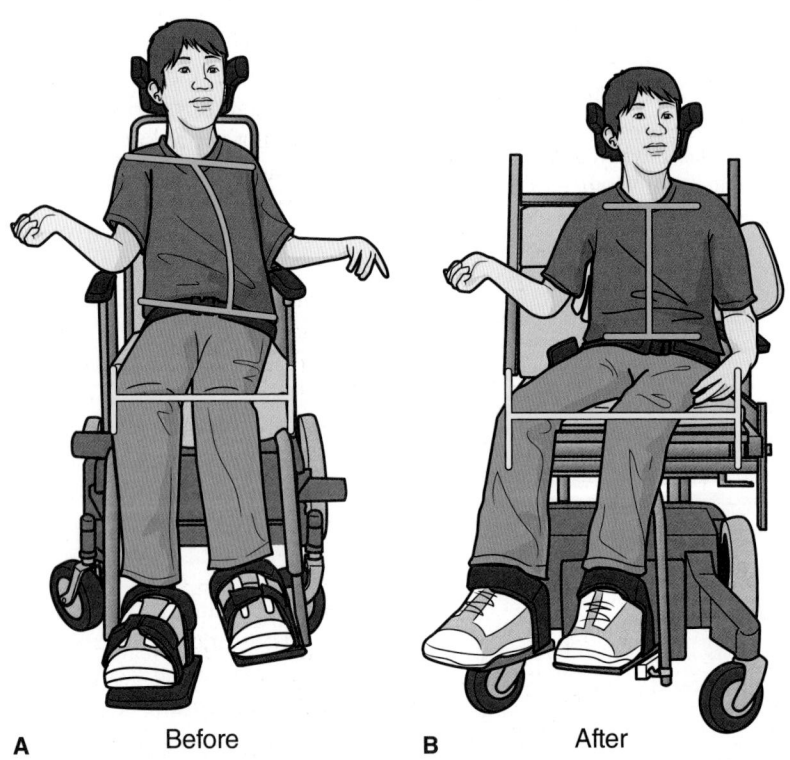

A   Before   **B**   After

Figure 32.1 Person with a right windswept deformity due to fixed right hip extension/abduction contractures on right and scoliosis. (A) Postural presentation in standard wheelchair seating prioritizing a LE forward-aligned position instead of accommodating for hip ROM limitations. The result is causing a compensatory left pelvic obliquity (left ASIS lower than the right by 2 in.), left thoracic scoliosis, and right forward rotation of shoulder/trunk/pelvis to open hip angle. (B) "Accommodating" right hip flexion and adduction range limitations (through seating system) allows a neutral pelvic position without obliquity or rotation. The spine is straight with neutral curves, neutral trunk rotation, and forward head position. The right LE is abducted and slightly extended to accommodate ROM limitations. The left LE and hip is in a neutral sitting posture with neutral adduction and flexion. The lower body lines show the overall sitting width. To accommodate a windswept position often it is necessary to allow the lower body to rotate to achieve a more functional upper body and face forward position.

they are accustomed to sitting and functioning from a suboptimal posture. It is recommended that the therapist spend time discussing the rationale for pursuing the optimal sitting posture to gain the person's understanding and agreement. Ultimately it is the decision of the wheelchair user, but at the same time it is the therapists' responsibility to provide the education and document their professional opinion and recommendation.

Benefits of Optimal Sitting Posture

Optimal sitting posture has benefits for an individual's overall health, comfort, and functioning from the wheelchair. In the optimal sitting posture, the person's muscles do not have to work hard to maintain their posture, yet they are not collapsed and inactive. The individual is ready for action.

Sitting with optimal body alignment supports health benefits, including facilitating healthy body functioning such as safe swallowing, optimal breathing, and digesting food. Sitting with an optimal posture can also help to reduce the risk of pressure injuries. This is because the person's body weight is evenly distributed across their buttocks and thighs when they are sitting in a symmetrical, neutral posture, and this helps prevent skin breakdown from asymmetrical loading of the person's body weight onto their buttocks. Finally, sitting with an optimal posture can help reduce the chance of developing deformities of the spine or joint contractures from sitting asymmetrically for long periods of time.

There are also many potential *functional benefits* of an optimal sitting posture. When the core of the body is balanced and stable, this can help improve motor control of the head, trunk, arms, and hands. This can translate to increased ability to reach with arms, propel a wheelchair, grasp and manipulate objects, control eye gaze, communicate and project voice, or operate switches that can control other devices in the environment. Imagine having to sit on an exercise ball without your feet planted on the floor. You would have to work your core muscles to maintain your balance. Now imagine threading a needle while balancing on the ball. This is what it is like for some wheelchair users who have poor trunk control or who experience abnormal movement patterns from muscle spasticity. If they cannot stabilize their core on their own, it is difficult to have optimal control of their head or arms to do functional tasks from their wheelchair. If the wheelchair is designed to fit appropriately, it can help to align and stabilize the body core, resulting in improved ability to engage in functional tasks. Proximal stability facilitates distal mobility and function.

Finally, sitting in an optimal posture provides *comfort benefits* for the wheelchair user. When the body is symmetrical, and weight is distributed evenly on weight-bearing surfaces, the person is usually more comfortable and uses less energy. They feel balanced and stable. When a person is comfortable, they can more effectively participate in work, learning, or play. Comfort leads to improved endurance, attentiveness, concentration, and use and adoption of the equipment. Sitting in an optimal posture can also help wheelchair users feel better about themselves, increasing self-esteem and self-confidence. Critical to the provision of equipment is involvement of the user, who should participate in the process and be allowed an opportunity to express likes and dislikes of the system.

Pressure Injuries

In April 2016, the National Pressure Ulcer Advisory Panel redefined the term *pressure injuries,* previously referred to as *pressure ulcers, pressure sores,* or *decubitus ulcers.* Pressure injuries are a major health concern for wheelchair users, especially for those who lack sensation or are unable to reposition themselves. Pressure injuries develop quickly and can lead to serious and costly health issues. It is estimated that hospital costs for pressure injuries in the United States are approaching $26.8 billion annually, with a cost for a stage 3, 4, or unstageable pressure injury between $75,000 and $150,000 per individual.[25] Pressure injuries are preventable, and physical therapists can assist people with maintaining good skin integrity by providing appropriate seating, training, and education.

A pressure injury is an area of damaged skin, usually over a bony prominence, that results from excessive prolonged pressure, friction, shear, heat and/or moisture. It may also be related to use of a medical or other device. The skin may be intact or open, and the area may be painful. The tolerance of soft tissue for pressure and shear may also be affected by microclimate (meaning heat and moisture), nutrition, perfusion, and comorbidities affecting the condition of the soft tissue.[26,27] A pressure injury can develop in a few hours but can take months to heal or be seen. If the injury becomes infected, the infection can spread to the blood, heart, or bone and can lead to serious illness and/or death.

The majority of all pressure injuries develop over primary bony areas, including the sacrum, coccyx, greater trochanter, IT, calcaneus, and lateral malleolus. In sitting, the seat cushion and pelvic posture affect weight-bearing and pressure on the sacrum, coccyx, greater trochanters, and ITs. Foot positioning in the wheelchair may result in injuries to the lower leg and feet.

There are six categories of pressure injuries as defined by the National Pressure Injury Advisory Panel:[27]

- *Stage 1 Pressure Injury:* Nonblanchable erythema of intact skin—a red or dark mark on the skin that doesn't blanche within 30 minutes after pressure is removed.
- *Stage 2 Pressure Injury:* Partial-thickness skin loss with exposed dermis—a shallow wound with the top layer of skin beginning to peel away or blister; involvement of the dermis.

- *Stage 3 Pressure Injury:* Full-thickness skin loss—a deep wound with full thickness loss of skin. Adipose tissue is visible, and there may be rolled wound edges, slough, and/or eschar visible.
- *Stage 4 Pressure Injury:* Full-thickness skin and tissue loss—a very deep wound extending through the muscle and possibly down to the bone. Tunneling and undermining often occur, making this wound more difficult to heal with greater possibility for systemic infection.
- *Unstageable Pressure Injury:* Obscured full-thickness skin and tissue loss—cannot be confirmed because it is obscured by slough or eschar.
- *Deep Tissue Pressure Injury:* Persistent nonblanchable deep red, maroon, or purple discoloration—results from intense and/or prolonged pressure and shear forces at the bone-muscle interface and may evolve rapidly to reveal the actual extent of tissue injury or may resolve without tissue loss.

Factors Influencing Pressure Injuries

Therapists play an important role in educating wheelchair users in the prevention of pressure injuries. Risk factors in developing pressure injuries include decreased sensation, decreased ability to move, excessive heat and/or moisture, poor sitting posture, previous or current pressure injury, poor diet and inadequate fluid intake, aging, and being underweight or overweight.[28–32] In examining risk for pressure injuries, the therapist should consider all situations that place the person at risk, including but not limited to bed positioning, shower commode chair positioning, car seat positioning, and the transfer technique used between different surfaces. Risks for pressure injuries can be minimized by improving posture, nutrition, transfer skills, and pressure relief techniques.[33]

Pressure injuries are typically caused by prolonged pressure over bony prominences from sitting or lying in the same position for too long without moving. This often occurs when an individual has decreased sensation in these areas, so the person is not cued to shift weight or change positions due to pain or discomfort.

The two primary factors causing pressure injuries are friction and shear. *Friction* is defined as the force that resists the relative motion of two objects sliding against each other.[34] This is a contributing factor to shear. *Shear* is a distortion of the body tissues resulting from two opposing forces parallel to the surface.[34] This occurs when the pressure of the body or gravity is now added to friction. Shear happens when the skin stays still and is stretched as the bones move over the skin. The bottom line is this: It is not possible to have shear without friction, but it *is* possible to have friction without shear. For example, an arm rubbing on a wheel as a wheelchair moves will create friction. When a person slides down in the bed or slides forward on a wheelchair cushion, this also creates friction and can contribute to the development of shear stresses within underlying tissues by tending to keep the skin in place against the support surface while the person's body, or more specifically their bony structure, continues to move.

A combination of good sitting posture and an appropriate seat cushion can minimize risk for pressure injury and assist with healing. Sitting in a neutral, upright posture distributes pressure over the greatest surface area (the buttocks and thighs) and decreases pressure over bony areas. An appropriate seat cushion can assist in both supporting a neutral upright posture and distributing pressure more evenly. Ensuring the wheelchair fits the user correctly and allows the person to transfer and reposition themselves with minimal friction and shear (e.g., scraping or rubbing against wheelchair parts) will also decrease risk.

Some wheelchair cushion properties and materials can assist with dissipating heat and moisture and can be a factor to consider during selection. Avoiding moisture such as wet or soiled clothing or seat cushion can improve skin integrity. Oftentimes a bowel and bladder management program may be needed to address these issues and require a referral from the therapist.

Changing position regularly, utilizing effective pressure relief techniques (e.g., forward bending, side leaning, press-ups) or positioning features (e.g., tilt, recline, and stand) are crucial for reducing pressure injury risk. Also transferring out of the wheelchair to other surfaces (e.g., bed, sofa, chair) is another strategy that can be used for breaks throughout the day.

Drinking water will help keep the skin and body tissues healthy. Increasing protein and eating a well-balanced diet also assists with wound healing and decreasing risk for pressure injuries. Smoking can have a negative effect on circulation and should be avoided. See Chapter 14, Vascular, Lymphatic, and Integumentary Disorders for a more detailed discussion of pressure injuries.

Principles of Mobility

The term *mobility* refers to the way a person moves by changing body positions or locations (locomotion) or by transferring from one place to another.[35] This includes ambulation and wheeled mobility. The determination that a wheeled mobility device is reasonable and necessary for a person is based on the clinical assessment and judgment of the WSM team. Factors include the person's:

- Past history, including prior level of functioning and assistive device use, if applicable.
- Current condition, including present functional mobility status, temporary or permanent nature of the condition, static or progressive nature of condition, nature of other medical problems.
- Ability to functionally ambulate safely and sufficiently to perform mobility needs during typical daily activities in a timely manner.

When providing a wheelchair, it is important to think about the person's daily mobility needs, environments and terrains typically encountered, and distances necessary to accomplish typical daily tasks without pain or excessive signs of fatigue (i.e., dyspnea, discoloration, rapid respirations, diaphoresis, and so forth).[36] Decisions about the wheeled mobility device (intervention) selected are based on the goals identified, such as improving independence and function, optimizing safety, decreasing risk of falls, reducing risk for pressure injuries, and improving physical capacity, health status, activity, and participation.

WHEELCHAIR SEATING AND MOBILITY EXAMINATION AND SPECIALTY EVALUATION

A wheelchair seating and mobility examination and specialty evaluation involves different components based on key information and methods used for collecting the data. An outline of the components of the WSM Examination and Specialty Evaluation are found in Table 32.2. For the purposes of this chapter, the examination process, which is part of Steps 2, 3, and 4 of WHO's Wheelchair Service Delivery Steps described above, is divided into three major sections: examination, specialty evaluation, and intervention. These components may be completed in one or more therapy visits. Each component described is essential to the process. A problem-solving model is used to match the person to the technology and the environments typically encountered, known as the *person/technology/environmental match*. The result is a plan of care (POC) that includes a prescription, justification, and recommendations for specific WSM equipment and additional clinical interventions such as fitting, training, and follow-up.

Communication Tips

It is important to take time at the beginning of the examination process to explain to the user, family, and caregivers the overall process, the type of information that will be gathered, and why it is important. Time should be allocated during data collection for comments or questions from the wheelchair user, caregivers, and other team members. Each team members' input is necessary and valuable to the process. While questions may be personal, remind everyone that information discussed is confidential and necessary to help the team identify and select the most appropriate WSMD. Remember to directly address the wheelchair user (not the caregiver/family member) unless he or she is a small child or unable to understand your questions or communicate answers. Box 32.2 lists effective communication tips and considerations to use during the assessment process.

The APTA Mobility Device Documentation Guide (link provided in Appendix 32.A: Internet Resources [online]) details the elements of the wheelchair

| **Box 32.2** | Effective Interview and Communication Tips |

- Always address the wheelchair user (not the caregiver/family member).
- Speak clearly.
- Make good eye contact (when appropriate).
- Be respectful.
- Use straightforward terms.
- Explain what is going to happen before it happens.
- After explaining something, check that the wheelchair user understands.
- Listen carefully and check to make sure you have understood the wheelchair user correctly.
- Show you are interested.
- Don't assume you know best

evaluation to consider and document and is a valuable tool to keep handy and reference.[35,37] Although time-consuming, it is absolutely critical that documentation of the examination and specialty evaluation is complete and accurate because changes to the WSMD prescription may be difficult to make once equipment is ordered. Accurate and detailed notes provide a permanent record of why certain decisions were made. During the ordering or manufacturing process, additional decisions concerning configuration may be needed. If accurate measurements are on file, decisions can often be made without recalling the person to the clinic.

Examination

The examination is individually tailored by the therapist to the person's condition and needs. While not all examination components may be relevant for a particular individual, all components should be considered and relevant details documented, even if it is merely to indicate a component is not applicable. Remember, the majority of the time, your examination findings will be reviewed by another professional responsible for deciding to approve or disapprove the equipment request. Include as much objective quantitative and qualitative information as possible to paint a clinical picture of the person on paper and communicate clearly to an unfamiliar reader.

Assessment Interview

The purpose of the assessment interview is to describe the person's environments, functions, and activities/participation on a typical day, including limitations and restrictions. The assessment interview components follow.

Demographic Information

General demographics about the person such as name, contact information, age, gender, height, weight, and so on.

Reason for Referral

The reasons a person is referred for the WSM examination will be different for each person. It may be due to a new or progressive mobility impairment, a first-time device, or modifications or replacement for an existing device.

Diagnosis

The diagnosis(es) relevant to the positioning and/or mobility impairment is specified, including the corresponding ICD-10 diagnostic code. In particular, specify any pertinent diagnoses related to positioning such as scoliosis, hip subluxation or dislocation, pressure injuries past or present, contractures, and so on. Unlike mobility devices where eligibility is based on functional criteria, eligibility for positioning devices is frequently diagnostic specific, requiring particular ICD-10 codes.

Medical/Surgical History

Document pertinent history related to the positioning and/or mobility impairment. Include the onset date, prognosis, course, and rate of progression. Include past and planned surgeries if known.

History of WSM Problems

Describe the progression of the positioning/mobility limitation, technology used or tried in the past, medical/surgical/treatment interventions to improve the impairment, and the results of the interventions.

Goals (User, Family/Caregiver)

Specify the goals for the recommended WSM equipment and any recommended clinical related services (e.g., wheelchair skills training, transfer training, person/family teaching).

Social Status

Describe the person's living situation (e.g., lives alone; lives with family; receives attendant care, including hours/week and assistance provided).

Environmental Accessibility (Home and Community)

Describe the person's home (e.g., ranch, split-level house, apartment, mobile home, assisted living). Discuss the home environment and accessibility, such as entrance (steps, ramp, elevator), floor surfaces (low-pile carpet, tile, wood), and measurements (narrowest doorway, heights of table, sink, bed, and so forth). Home adaptations, assistive equipment, and sometimes entire modifications may be needed for safety and improved wheelchair access (see Chapter 9, Examination and Modification of the Environment). Discuss the environments the person typically encounters in the course of their daily activities. Describe terrain encountered (e.g., grass, gravel, hills, side slopes, inclement weather, environmental obstacles), and describe environmental facilitators and barriers that will affect safe access to the community.

Employment/Work Status (Job/School)

Describe the person's occupation (typical job duties), school/work tasks, functions, workstation accessibility needs, distances traveled, and so on.

General Health Status

Provide a general description of the person's overall social/health habits (past/current). A change in health status can impact a person's weight and therefore impact the size and capacity of the WSMD. Relevant information about weight gain or loss, planned surgical interventions (e.g., gastrointestinal tube placement), medications, and other risk factors that might contribute to pressure injuries, infections, aspiration, changes in weight, safety concerns, and so on, should be included.

Functional Status and Activity Level (Roles/Responsibilities)

Describe the person's primary roles, responsibilities (e.g., parent, primary caregiver for spouse or elderly parent, student), activity level, and prior level of functioning. Have the person describe a typical day, including self-care and routine daily activities (e.g., medical appointments, cooking/cleaning, shopping, recreation) to get a sense of functional status and activity level. Include time spent in wheelchair daily (hours/day) and distances traveled.

Transportation

Discussing the transportation plan for the person and the wheelchair is critical to the decision-making process. Specific wheelchair features will determine how the wheelchair can be transported and how it can be secured and stowed. Describe how the person and the wheelchair will be transported. Note if the person will be a driver or passenger in a vehicle seat or in the wheelchair, transfer type, transportation and/or vehicle type (make/model car, van, bus, public transportation); wheelchair storage location, method, and dimensions (passenger seat, trunk, exterior or interior lift, ramp); wheelchair securement (tie down, docking system, other); and occupant restraint.

Understanding whether the person will load/unload the wheelchair alone or have assistance may factor into decisions about overall wheelchair weight and how the wheelchair collapses or folds. If the person rides in a van in their wheelchair, measurements of the door opening and height will be necessary to ensure sufficient head clearance and wheelchair access into the van. If the person drives from the wheelchair, the measurements of the van will be necessary to ensure the person will be able to safely maneuver in/out of the van and fit in the driving station.

Equipment Assessment
Existing Equipment

Detail existing equipment the person owns or uses (e.g., cane, walker, manual/power wheelchair, scooter); bathroom equipment; lifts; bed equipment; other devices, including but not limited to home, vehicle modifications, prosthetics/orthotics, and so on. Include problems or concerns about existing equipment and plans for future changes or modifications.

Current WSM Equipment

List the make/model, serial number, condition, size, age, supplier, payer, and reason for new equipment. Explain what worked/didn't work about current equipment (e.g., no longer meets the person's needs because . . . , or the cost to repair exceeds the cost of new technology).

Sitting Posture in Existing Equipment

Observing the person in their existing wheelchair provides a great deal of information. The person should be in the best or most commonly assumed position, with supports and straps in place as they arrive to the clinic. Questions should include how the person and/or caregiver perceives current posture, if person has any new pain and location of pain, any new pressure injuries and location of injuries, any weight loss or weight gain since receiving equipment. For questions about the WSMD, ask the person what works well and what doesn't work well related to mobility, positioning, and function. Ask if they are having any difficulty using the equipment.

Functional Assessment

The next part of the examination involves subjective and objective evaluations of performance and functional abilities to establish activity level, positioning needed for function, and extent of mobility impairment. It is important that the persons' prognosis (potential for restoration or enhancement) for function is established.

Activities of Daily Living/Instrumental Activities of Daily Living Status

Describe the person's typical activities of daily living (ADLs) and instrumental activities of daily living (IADLs). A critical part of the functional assessment is identifying functional activities performed from the wheelchair such as dressing, self-catheterization, cooking, laundry, and so on. When seated in a wheelchair, accessing kitchen appliances, cabinets, the sink, bathtub, shower, laundry, and shelves is frequently more difficult. Specify adaptive equipment or assistive technology used, accessibility considerations, efficiency (timeliness), and safety concerns. Describe assistance needed to perform typical daily activities.

Explore the person's usual community activities. Information from the assessment interview may prompt further discussion about distances traveled, terrain, climate/weather, transportation, and accessibility

barriers. These details will drive decisions about product features needed such as product durability, robustness, range, power, speed, and maneuverability. Important ADL/IADL topics that significantly contribute to the decision-making process for WSMD selection follow.

TOILETING

Toilet transfers are probably the most difficult transfer performed and often are required multiple times per day. Discussion about toilet height, transfer technique, transfer equipment, and toilet seat pressure management are critical factors. Power wheelchair seat lifts can facilitate transfers to toilets of differing heights. If the person uses a urinal, the wheelchair seat style needs to be discussed to prevent accidental tipping of the urinal. If the person will be self-catheterizing from the wheelchair, positioning in the wheelchair needs to be considered. If the person has an indwelling catheter and independently empties the collection bag, maneuvering close to the toilet is necessary. If the person experiences episodes of incontinence or accidents, cushion properties and materials must be considered, such as a waterproof cover, closed cell foam, and antimicrobial seat cushion materials.

DRESSING

Some individuals find it easier to don/doff clothing when in their wheelchair; others prefer a bed. Depending on the person's technique, footrest and armrest style and durability, or back cane type and height are discussed to ensure the system will accommodate the extra force placed on these components during dressing and other functional activities. Use of tilt seating or a reclining back system to unweight the lower body may be useful for the person who dresses in the wheelchair.

EATING

The wheelchair seat and armrest height may prevent positioning the wheelchair close to some tables or desks. The style of table or desk may interfere with wheelchair access (e.g., number and arrangement of legs, height of working surface, presence of drawers). If a person needs assistance during mealtime, caregivers need to have ease of access to ensure safety during mealtime. Positioning of head/neck and trunk are important considerations while eating to optimize swallowing and minimize risk for aspiration or choking.

Mobility Status
BED MOBILITY, TRANSFERS, WEIGHT SHIFT

Current mobility status, prior level of functioning, and potential anticipated functioning are documented. The person's bed mobility, transfer status, and ability to weight shift are examined. Equipment and assistance needed for mobility are noted (e.g., slide board, mechanical lift, mattress overlay, electric hospital bed). For weight shift, the method (e.g., press-up, leaning, bridging, tilt, recline, stand), frequency, duration, and effectiveness are discussed and observed (throughout the duration of the examination).

AMBULATION

Documenting the quantitative and qualitative ambulation status of the person is an essential part of the examination and often the key factor in qualifying a person for a wheeled mobility device. Describe how the person arrived at your clinic, distance they can typically walk, speed, duration of walking or standing prior to needing a rest, balance, and incidences of falls or close calls (detail injuries, frequency, and factors attributing to incident).

Keep in mind that assessing ambulation is done to determine if the person requires a WSMD temporarily, permanently, or would benefit from physical therapy or another intervention to achieve independent, safe, functional, and timely ambulation. Consider if a lower-level device or intervention will meet the person's mobility needs and justify your decision-making process clearly in your written report. For instance, make clear your professional opinion about whether the person's mobility impairment could be ameliorated with the use of a mobility device such as a cane, walker, orthotic, and so on, with or without a therapy intervention.

Although a person may require a wheelchair to accomplish daily mobility needs, the person may still be able to ambulate short distances (e.g., "wall walk"), albeit not functionally for the purposes of meeting all daily mobility needs. Documentation to paint a clinical picture of the person's mobility status is critical. For example, if a person with MS is able to take a few steps in the morning with a walker, but symptoms fluctuate day to day and morning to afternoon, be sure to present these details in your report. Remember, if the person does utilize an assistive device (e.g., cane, walker, crutches) for transfers or taking a few steps, a means to mount the device on the wheelchair needs to be determined to ensure availability and access.

PROPULSION METHOD

The next aspect of the functional assessment is considering the person's wheelchair skills and potential. Is the person a first-time wheelchair user, or have they previously used a wheelchair (manual or power)? If the person uses a manual wheelchair, how do they propel the wheelchair (both UEs, hemi-propel) (one arm/one leg, both LEs, all four extremities)? Does the person have adequate motor control to self-propel? Do they have sufficient strength and muscular endurance to self-propel for the demands of typical daily activities? Note any functional limitations using quantitative and qualitative objective data to include decreased strength, motor control, pain, and endurance.

If the person operates a scooter (power-operated vehicle [POV]) or power wheelchair, describe the access method (tiller, switch, joystick, head array) and controls (multidrive controls, proportional, latched). Specify if the person is independent and safe or indicate if a different access method or controller is needed.

Propulsion method is a primary factor in the decision-making process for a person/feature match. For users of manual wheelchairs, the propulsion method establishes wheelchair configuration needs. For example, if the person uses their feet to self-propel, a seat-to-floor height that allows the feet to easily contact the floor is critical and often a deciding factor in narrowing available products. For another person, the controller (e.g., joystick) position alone might determine if they can independently operate the power wheelchair. If the person is unable to use a standard joystick controller with their hand, alternative drive controls exist (e.g., chin control, sip and puff, track pad, head array). Identifying a consistent, nonfatigable access site will lead to options for controllers and access site to optimize independent power wheelchair control. If the person is dependent for mobility, caregivers will be moving the wheelchair. Considerations to discuss include style and height of push handles, wheel lock styles, and/or attendant controls.

Screening of Body Functions and Structures

During the assessment interview, the wheelchair user describes medical issues that may influence wheelchair selection. This section addresses further screening of essential body functions and structures that impact the person's positioning and mobility. If indicated, a more detailed evaluation is conducted, or the person may be referred to another professional.

Cardiovascular/Pulmonary/Circulatory Status

In terms of cardiovascular/pulmonary and circulatory issues, it may be relevant to take the heart and respiratory rates, blood pressure, and/or oxygen saturation level at rest and with activity. It will be important to note how the person responds to activity (e.g., endurance tolerance for self-propulsion). Does the person require supplemental oxygen, ventilator, or suction? It is also a good practice to examine the person's body for edema and/or lymphedema, especially in the lower extremities.

Gastrointestinal System Review

For the gastrointestinal system, note if the person has any digestive issues, such as reflux or elimination issues, that may affect seating and positioning. If the person receives nourishment via tube, note the method (e.g., nasogastric tube, gastrostomy tube, and so forth); the location may affect type and mounting position for postural supports and straps. Also, it is important to determine if the person requires specific positioning for digestion, swallowing, or following meals, particularly if they will be eating while in the wheelchair.

Communication

Communication is assessed from the beginning of the examination. Expressive and receptive communication abilities are noted. For wheelchair purposes, if the person is unable to speak, do they use an augmentative communication device? If so, considerations for how and where a device will need to be mounted and accessed are discussed. Even if the person is unable to speak, discuss with the caregiver how to discern yes/no, comfort/pain issues so that you do not miss any needs of the individual.

Cognitive Status

When assessing the person's cognitive status, determine their ability to safely utilize the wheelchair, taking the environments they routinely encounter into consideration. Focus on the person's memory, pathfinding, problem-solving, judgment, motor planning, attention, behavior, and learning skills.

Vision and Hearing

The person's vision and hearing must be functional in order to operate the wheelchair safely and independently. Vision affects a person's ability to operate a power or manual wheelchair. Consider spatial awareness, visual fields, and depth perception. It is important to determine if visual problems exist, how they affect mobility, and if the person can learn compensatory techniques to be independent and safe (otherwise known as *minimizing or ameliorating impairments*). Full or partial vision loss may affect the person's ability to see curb cuts, potholes, drop-offs, and other environmental barriers. Hearing deficits, too, can pose safety concerns. For example, when driving outdoors, a person with a hearing impairment may not hear a car horn or someone calling to them to stop. Note use of hearing aids.

Bowel/Bladder Functions

The management of bowel and bladder function is critical to the person's wheelchair/seating choices. Note if the person is continent or incontinent, uses a catheter, if it is indwelling or intermittent, and if the person will be self-catheterizing from the wheelchair. Oftentimes, issues of incontinence can require referrals to other professionals such as urologist, neurologist, physiatrist, or enterostomal nurse for bowel and bladder interventions and management.

Physical Assessment

Information gathering was initiated during the interview and functional assessment. If further detail is needed, this is the time to collect it. In this section, first the supine and sitting mat assessment is described; then the components of the physical assessment and how the various physical findings interact and influence selection of WSMD features are discussed.

As you proceed with the physical assessment, communicate with the person about what you are doing and why. Be mindful that some people are sensitive to loud speech or quick movements, which may trigger reflexes, increase muscle tone, or cause anxiety. As you go, a "think aloud" approach, explaining what is being observed or measured, allows team members, including the person and their family/caregivers, an opportunity to ask questions and contribute information.[37] This practice allows all stakeholders to hear the findings and contribute to the clinical problem-solving process that results in the WSM recommendations.

Mat Assessment

The physical assessment is typically performed during a mat assessment in both sitting and supine positions. To start, if not already completed, document the person's baseline position and function when they are sitting in their current WSMD. When done, have the person transfer onto a mat table, noting observations and/or inconsistencies that may not have been identified during the functional assessment.

Supine Mat Assessment

The person is examined in a gravity-minimized position to learn about his or her strength, range of available movement, and how movement of one body part affects tone, comfort, position, control, and performance in other body segments. This is typically performed supine on a firm surface. A mat table or floor works well. A bed is often too soft. If modification for supine positioning is needed, try using a wedge or side-lying position.

It is important that the maximum range of available pelvic and hip movement as it relates to spinal and pelvic alignment is determined. The goal is to preserve spinal alignment whenever possible, maintaining the natural lumbar curve and determining the presence of any flexible and/or fixed deformities. Postural tendencies should be noted when the person is supine on the mat. Range of motion and muscle length are assessed to determine muscle limitations that will affect a person in the seated position. For example, since the hamstring muscle is a two-joint muscle, it affects the range at both the hip and knee. If the hip is extended, the knee can be extended even if there is hamstring tightness. But if the hip is flexed, knee extension will be limited if hamstring tightness is present. The gastrocnemius is also a two-joint muscle with tightness affecting the knee and ankle ROM. In the supine position, preliminary linear measurements may be obtained, including buttock/thigh length, lower leg length, chest width, and hip width (Fig. 32.2).

Sitting Mat Assessment

While seated on a mat table or firm surface, with thighs and lower legs fully supported, the person is assessed upright with the effects of gravity (Fig. 32.3). If the

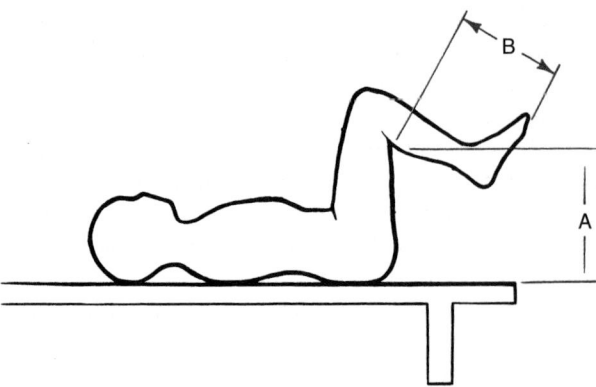

Figure 32.2 (A) With the person in the supine position with the hips and knees flexed, the examiner can measure the under surface of the thigh from the popliteal fossa to a firm support surface. (B) Note that this position can also be used to measure lower leg length from the popliteal fossa to the heel.

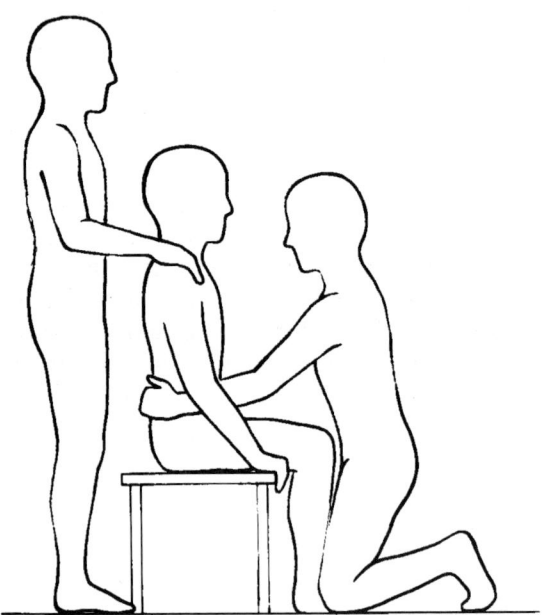

Figure 32.3 The sitting position can be used to determine the amount and location of required support.

person has significant physical involvement, oftentimes more than one person is needed to provide support while the therapist completes the assessment. Assess the person in all three reference planes (i.e., frontal, sagittal, transverse) and record all positional issues and postural anomalies. Compare the current posture with the reference neutral posture discussed earlier in the chapter.

Assess the pelvis, hips, knees, ankles, feet, trunk, head, and upper extremities, palpating as needed and measuring linear and angular asymmetries. Record specific postural alignment findings, noting fixed and/or flexible deformities and postural tendencies of the pelvis, spine, lower and upper extremities, and head/neck in the

sitting position. See detailed description in the "Postural Alignment" section.

Components of Physical Assessment

The components of the physical assessment include sensation, pain, skin integrity, postural alignment, balance, strength and endurance, ROM and flexibility, and neuromuscular status.

SENSATION

Sensory impairment is a very important risk factor for pressure injuries. Assess whether the person has intact, impaired, or absent sensation and describe level of involvement and location. Pay particular attention to skin that is in contact with the seating surface (buttocks, thighs, coccyx, sacrum, pelvis). Note if there are any other sensory concerns such as deep pressure, proprioception, kinesthesia, phantom sensation, pain, and so on.

PAIN

Document location and severity of pain. Indicate what exacerbates and relieves the pain. It is critically important to understand any pain that is potentially related to sitting and/or the wheelchair seating environment. If the person is nonverbal, body movements or facial expressions may help you determine areas and extent of pain.

SKIN INTEGRITY

Individuals who use a wheelchair for locomotion have an increased chance of developing pressure injuries from prolonged sitting, making an in-depth assessment of current and past skin integrity issues an important consideration. Location, size, and stage of current or previous healed pressure injuries, surgeries, or treatments related to skin integrity are noted. Existing pressure injuries are examined and investigated to determine what the injury is attributed to—shear, friction, maceration, injury/trauma (e.g., hitting wheelchair wheel during transfer), bed mattress with no cushion or overlay, prolonged sitting on shower/toilet commode with no cushion, and so on. Pressure under bony prominences is assessed, especially for users at risk or with a history of a pressure injury. Measurement tools such as pressure mapping are available to quantitively assess pressure, offering a visual graphic showing areas of high pressure and pressure distribution.

Remember, once a pressure injury occurs, there is permanent change to the tissue affected. Therefore, even if there is a healed pressure injury, inspect the skin and document the details, including scars; for example, "Healed Stage 3 pressure injury R IT with healed flap incision noted—June 2022."

POSTURAL ALIGNMENT

Postural alignment is assessed by looking at the orientation of body segments in relation to each other in three reference planes (frontal, sagittal, transverse). In the sagittal plane, the amount of anterior or posterior pelvic tilt and curves of the spine are assessed, noting any abnormal curves or spinal postures. For example, a posterior pelvic tilt is frequently associated with a decreased (or absent) lumbar lordosis and an increased thoracic kyphosis.

In the frontal plane (from the front and rear), the spine is observed for scoliosis. The lateral curve of the spine is named based on the convex side of the curve. For example, in Figure 32.4, lateral flexion would be named *right thoracic lateral flexion* or *C curve*. A lateral curvature with two curves is frequently referred to as an *S curve*. In this example, there is also a left cervical compensatory curve.

In the transverse plane, looking at the person from above, rotation of the pelvis or trunk is observed. The posture is typically determined based on the pelvis relative to shoulders or lower trunk relative to upper trunk.

Often, lateral flexion in the frontal plane and rotation occur simultaneously. In the right column of Figure 32.4 the pelvis is rotated forward on the right and the upper trunk is counter-rotated posteriorly (or backward) on the right.

BALANCE

Sitting balance status is assessed to determine (1) the type of postural support the wheelchair user will require (size, location, force) and (2) the hierarchy of user need (basic, intermediate, complex). Remember that hierarchy of user need is dependent on the user's sitting balance and postural control (see Table 32.1). As described

in the "Hierarchy of Wheelchair User Seating and Positioning Need" section, note if the person is a hands-free sitter, hands-dependent or prop sitter, or dependent sitter who requires a lot of external support.

Users with fair to poor sitting balance and trunk control require additional postural supports to sit symmetrically to free up their hands for function and are considered users with intermediate to complex needs. These individuals require a therapist and RTP with advanced level knowledge and skills for their wheelchair service provision. Referral may be needed.

STRENGTH AND ENDURANCE

Physical assessment of strength includes muscle power and muscle endurance utilizing objective measures as much as possible. Standard manual muscle testing alone may or may not be appropriate, depending on the person's neuromuscular function. If strength is found to be within 3 to 5/5, it is critical to objectively measure, describe, and document if muscular endurance and power are sufficient to meet the individual's daily mobility needs. Keep in mind that the reason for this important objective assessment is to demonstrate the capacity for strength and muscular endurance to safely and effectively self-propel and/or operate a wheeled mobility device.

Upper and lower extremity strength impacts a person's ability to transfer and self-propel a manual wheelchair with their UEs, LEs, or combination of both. A consistent, nonfatiguable movement (e.g., hand, finger, head, foot) is identified as a potential access site to operate a power wheelchair user interface (input device), such

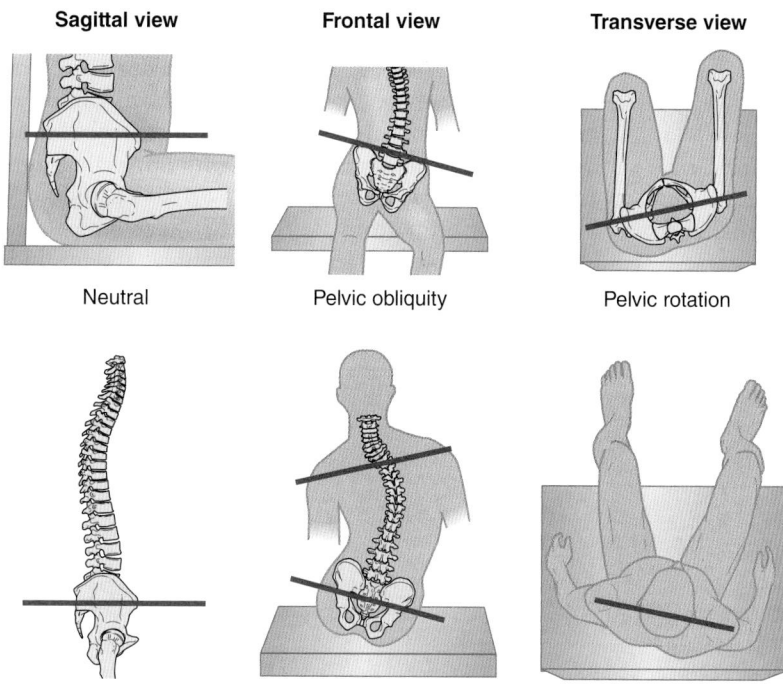

Figure 32.4 Trunk and pelvis postures in the sagittal, frontal, and transverse planes.

as a joystick, head array, chin microcontroller, or foot switch. Trunk strength and endurance will impact the amount of external postural support needed and the person's endurance for sitting upright in the wheelchair.

Findings from the comprehensive strength assessment are critical to qualifying a person for a specific wheeled mobility device. As a result, it is important to connect the dots, paint a clinical picture of the person's function in the context of daily mobility needs, and note their ability to perform functional activities throughout the day. As an example, a person might function well for 1 hour initially in the morning and need no assistance during that time with mobility but may need moderate assistance with mobility in the afternoon due to waxing and waning symptoms, medication schedule, and/or poor endurance and fatigue.

RANGE OF MOTION AND FLEXIBILITY

Joint ROM and flexibility of the pelvis, spine, and extremities determine if a person can achieve a neutral, or upright, sitting posture. Pelvic mobility is assessed with the person supine and their hips and knees flexed. Placing thumbs on the person's ASIS and fingers on the PSIS, the pelvis is shifted in all three planes, assessing anterior/posterior tilt, pelvic obliquity, and pelvic rotation to achieve a neutral position in all planes. Flexible, partially flexible, and fixed deformities are noted.

Hip flexion is measured with the person in the supine position (Fig. 32.5). Knees are flexed to decrease the influence of the hamstring muscles. The pelvis is positioned in a neutral to slight anterior tilted position (or as neutral as possible). Both hips are flexed slowly, keeping one hand flat under the person's lumbosacral spine until posterior movement of the pelvis is palpated. The hip joints must be able to achieve true hip joint movement of at least 90° of flexion, meaning that there is no compensatory movement of the pelvis or lower spine in order to sit in a standard wheelchair with a 90° seat to back angle. The hips also need approximately 5 to 8° of hip abduction, typical of a neutral sitting posture, and 0° of internal and external rotation. Goniometric values for hip abduction, adduction, and internal and external rotation are obtained.

Knee popliteal angle (thigh to lower leg angle) is measured with the person in the supine position with both hips flexed to 90° (or their maximum amount of true flexion) and the knees initially flexed (see Fig. 32.5).[38,39] While maintaining the hip angle and keeping one hand under the lumbosacral spine, the knees are slowly extended until the pelvis begins to move posteriorly or excessive tightness/tension is felt in the hamstring muscles. It is especially important to maintain the appropriate hip position while extending the knees since the hamstring muscles are a two-joint muscle and the amount of range achieved is dependent on the position of the hips.[39] When the hips are extended, knee extension range tends to be increased, and when the hips are flexed, knee extension range tends to be decreased due to hamstring muscle tightness. If the knees are extended greater than the available ROM, the pelvis will rotate posteriorly due to the pull on the hamstring muscles.

Ankle dorsiflexion ROM is also measured in the supine position. Hips and knees are positioned in available hip flexion and knee extension alignment (as described previously). The ankle is maintained in a neutral inversion/eversion position, and an attempt is made to achieve neutral dorsiflexion/plantarflexion position at the ankle. The gastrocnemius muscle is a two-joint muscle, and ROM at the ankle is affected by the position at the knee. If the knee is extended and muscle tightness is present, decreased dorsiflexion is noted. With the knee flexed, increased dorsiflexion is achieved. Although it is important to measure ROM with knee extended (bed positioning, standing, and ambulation), this is an assessment for seating, and muscle tightness limitations must be addressed in a simulated position on the mat to better understand posture achieved in sitting.

A complete ROM examination of both UEs and LEs, head/neck, trunk, and pelvis is needed since limitations in these areas will affect a person's ability to propel the wheelchair, position the head for safe eating and functional vision, and sit with optimal upright alignment.

Postural limitations are noted, specifying if it is fixed, flexible, or partially flexible. If significant

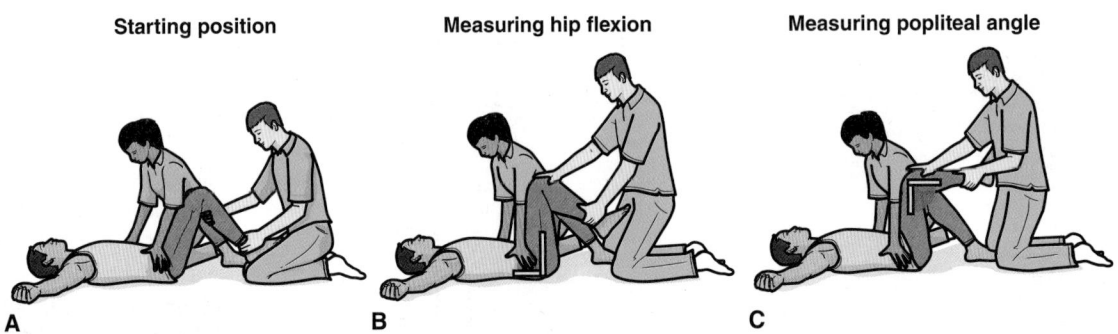

Starting position   **Measuring hip flexion**   **Measuring popliteal angle**

A   B   C

Figure 32.5 Measuring hip and knee ROM: (A) Starting, neutral pelvic/lumbar posture. (B) Measuring hip flexion. (C) Measuring popliteal angle.

deformities are identified, decisions will need to be made regarding the amount and method to correct, support, or accommodate the deformity while optimizing function. In the instance of a moderate fixed scoliosis with pelvic obliquity, decisions are made about accommodating the pelvic obliquity and supporting the trunk above and below the apex of the primary spinal curve.

Contractures in the neck region affect head and eye position impacting vision. In the instance of a fixed or partially fixed cervical lateral flexion contracture, attempts to align the head to support and accommodate a midline horizontal gaze can instead result in the trunk shifting laterally to the opposite side, affecting the shoulders, spine, pelvis, hips, knees, and ankles. To support the person in a position with improved functional vision, additional postural supports will need to be considered to accommodate and support the impact on downstream postural changes. When done intentionally this is an example of a "trade-off" to improve functional vision. The team weighs the trade-offs for achieving full midline horizontal gaze versus the extent of downstream changes. Simulation, described below, is a process used to inform the decision-making process. Often a compromise is needed, prioritizing function over optimal posture.

Remember that UE position and function, once proximal trunk stability is established, becomes critical when determining ability to self-propel the wheelchair or operate a power wheelchair controller. If specific UE positioning (e.g., arm trough, UE support tray, angle adjustable forearm support) is required to maintain current ROM, enable optimal wheel access for self-propulsion or UE position for reliable controller access, and be sure to describe it.

NEUROMUSCULAR STATUS

Neuromuscular status includes muscle tone, reflexes, coordination, and motor control in the context of function. Each of these elements may potentially impact the person's ability to operate a mobility device and factors into the equipment selection process. Note if the person has hyper/hypotonia, ataxia, athetosis, clonus, or tremor. Consider abnormal reflexes such as asymmetric tonic neck reflex and symmetric tonic neck reflex, as these will affect decisions related to head position and orientation in space. Motor control and coordination will impact operation of both manual and power mobility devices.

Specialty Evaluation
Wheelchair Assessment

The wheelchair assessment includes measurements, simulation, technology trial, and the person/technology match.[10,24,38–41]

Measurements

Following the physical assessment and simulation process, measurements of the person's body are taken and recorded to help determine the dimensions of the wheelchair and seating equipment that will be required (Fig. 32.6).[10] Some considerations that need to be made when taking measurements to ensure they are accurate are as follows:

- Initial thigh length and calf length measurements should be taken in supine position to increase accuracy (see Fig. 32.2).
- The person is measured when sitting as upright as possible or in an optimal sitting posture (sometimes a second or third person may be needed to provide external support, depending on the complexity of the individual's need) (see Fig. 32.3).

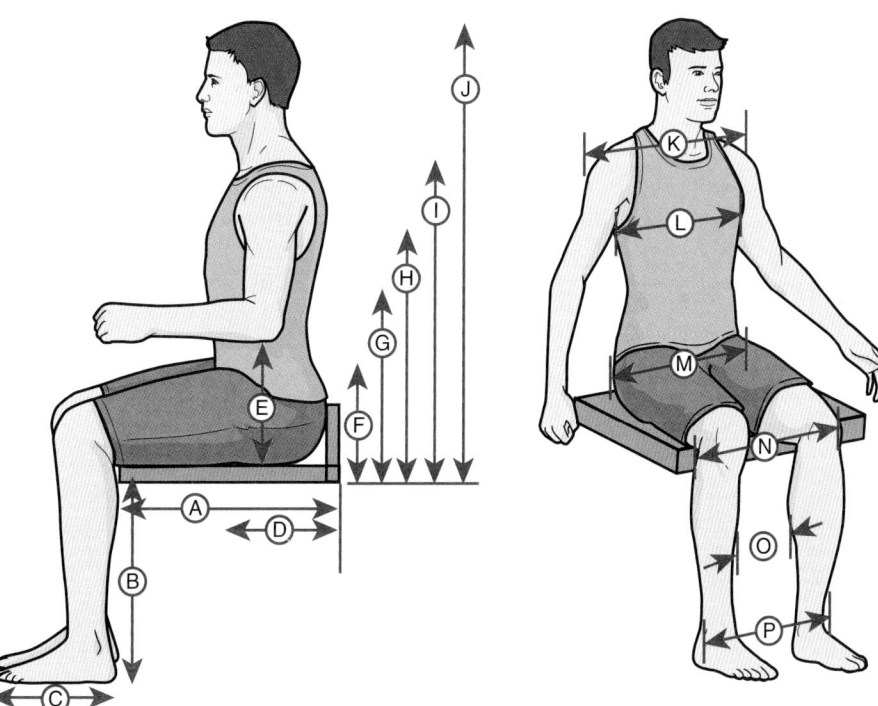

Figure 32.6 Body measurements: (A) buttock/thigh depth. (B) Lower leg length. (C) Foot depth. (D) Ischial depth. (E) Elbow height. (F) PSIS height. (G) Inferior angle of scapula height. (H) Axilla height. (I) Shoulder height. (J) Maximum sitting height. (K) Shoulder width. (L) Chest width. (M) Hip width. (N) External knee width. (O) Internal knee width. (P) External foot width.

- Provide as much thigh support as possible for postural stability.
- Use foot blocks to position and support the feet.
- Use a metal retractable tape measure, preferably 1-in. width, and calipers to minimize error (flexible/bendable tape measures increase errors).
- Consider using clipboards to define outer limits of curved body surfaces when calipers aren't available.
- Align your line of sight with the tape measure at the correct angle.

As you can see from Figure 32.6, there are many body measures that can be taken during the evaluation and used to determine the features of the wheelchair and postural supports. It is critical to note that we are measuring and recording the person and not the equipment. The information about the person is used to make final decisions about the measurements of the equipment.

The specific measurements needed for an individual assessment will depend on the body supports that will be necessary in the wheelchair. Hip width and buttock/thigh depth will be required to determine basic wheelchair seat width and depth and will be required for all wheelchair users. Additionally, to determine back support height, it is useful to know the height of the PSIS, the inferior angle of the scapula, axilla height, and the top of the shoulder. Lower leg length is also necessary to determine the height of the foot supports that will be needed; however, these are typically adjustable items, so this measurement is used to determine the needed range. Additional measures may be needed, depending on the complexity of the body support system that will be used. *A Clinical Application Guide to Standardized Wheelchair Seating Measures of the Body and Seating Support Surfaces, Revised Edition,* is a downloadable practical reference and guide for linear and angular measurements in sitting.[38] (See https://www.ucdenver.edu/centers/center-for-inclusive-design-and-engineering/clinical-services/wheelchair-seating-measures-guide.)

LINEAR BODY MEASUREMENTS

A. Buttock/thigh depth: Hold a rigid flat surface, such as a hardcover book or clipboard, against the back of the buttocks, parallel to the seat surface. Measure from the book to the back of the knees. If a hamstring tendon is prominent, measure to the edge of the hamstring tendon (see Fig. 32.6A).

B. Lower leg length: Measure from the back of the knee to heel (or weight-bearing area) (see Fig. 32.6B).

C. Foot depth: Measure from the back of the heel to the front of the toes (or shoes) (see Fig. 32.6C).

D. Ischial depth: Measure from the back of the buttocks (the book) to the front of the IT. This measurement will be important for an antithrust seat cushion and any pressure-relieving cushions (see Fig. 32.6D).

E. Elbow height: Measure from the seat surface to the bottom of the elbow. This is helpful for arm supports and lap trays (see Fig. 32.6E).

F. PSIS height: Measure from the seat surface (contact point of the buttocks) to PSIS. If you cannot find the PSIS, measure from the seat surface to 1 in. below the iliac crest. This will be helpful if the person needs a lower back support at the PSIS (see Fig. 32.6F).

G. Inferior angle of the scapula height: Measure from the seat surface to the inferior angle of the scapula. This measurement is good for shorter back supports, unencumbered scapular motion for self-propulsion, or to make reliefs for the scapula (see Fig. 32.6G).

H. Axilla height: Measure from the seat surface to under the axilla. This is necessary if the person needs lateral trunk supports (see Fig. 32.6H).

I. Shoulder height: Measure from the seat surface to the top of shoulders for higher back supports. This measurement is also needed to ensure proper line of pull for certain shoulder straps (see Fig. 32.6I).

J. Maximum sitting height: Measure from the seat surface to the top of the head. This measurement will assist in determining head clearance needs (see Fig. 32.6J).

K. Shoulder width: Measure from the outside of the upper arms. This measurement will assist in specifying the width of the back support and determine wheelchair frame size (see Fig. 32.6K).

L. Chest width: Your hands should simulate the support the person requires. Measure between your hands (or the flat supports). The supports should be at least 1 in. below the armpit so as not to press on brachial nerves in the axilla. Calipers can also be used (see Fig. 32.6L).

M. Hip width: Place a rigid flat surface such as a hardcover book or clipboard along each hip. Make sure the books are held at 90° to the seat surface. Measure the width between the books at the widest point. This is easier to do with two people or with calipers (see Fig. 32.6M).

N. External knee width: Measure the width between the outside of the knees. This measurement will assist with determining the width of the seat cushion and wheelchair (see Fig. 32.6N).

O. Internal knee width: Measure the distance between the inside of the knees. This measurement will assist with specifying the dimensions of a medial knee support (see Fig. 32.6O).

P. External foot width: Measure the distance between the outermost borders of the feet. This measurement will assist with determining placement of foot supports and frame dimensions (see Fig. 32.6P).

If the person sits asymmetrically, it will be necessary to measure across the widest span of the person's seated body (e.g., outside hip on the adducted side to outside knee of the abducted leg) to determine the maximum sitting width (see Fig. 32.1). To ensure accurate recommendations, it is important to consider orthoses, clothing, and recent weight loss or gain, as well as the person's potential for growth, and make notations as appropriate. If it takes more than a few months between the evaluation and the ordering of the equipment (e.g., delay in prior authorization process), it may be necessary to remeasure the person prior to placing the order to determine if they have changed (e.g., grown or experienced weight loss or gain).

BODY SEGMENT ANGLES

Thigh to Trunk Angle

Measuring hip flexion assists in determining the thigh to trunk angle and ultimately the seat to back support angle.[41–43] As seen in Figure 32.7, if hip flexion is 75°, the thigh to trunk angle is 105°. Identifying the optimal alignment of the head and trunk over the center of mass (COM), or seat base, considers factors, including but not limited to, tone, reflexes, motor control, endurance, body shape or contour, function, and comfort. These factors taken together guide selection of the final seat to back support angle. As shown in Figure 32.8A, hip flexion is 95° and the thigh to trunk angle is 85°. This

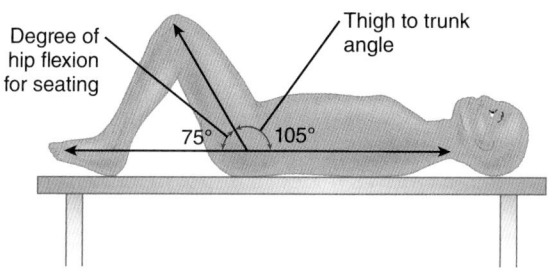

Figure 32.7 The amount of hip flexion determines the trunk angle. If the degree of hip flexion for seating is 75°, the thigh to trunk angle is 105°.

position, however, may not provide the person sufficient postural stability, promoting instead trunk flexion or difficulty maintaining an upright sitting posture (Fig. 32.8B). In this example, the person may benefit from a final seat to back support angle of 100° to allow the shoulders to move posterior to the hips. Shifting the COM posterior to the center of gravity is known as *gravity-assisted positioning*, as illustrated in Figure 32.8C.

Thigh to Lower Leg Angle

The thigh to lower leg angle (popliteal angle) is documented (Fig. 32.9). The final seat to lower leg support angle is determined by considering factors such as the thigh to lower leg angle, hamstring flexibility, abnormal tone, movement patterns, and comfort.[38,41–43] Hamstring muscle tightness must be accommodated to prevent the pelvis from being pulled into a posterior pelvic tilt. Some people will require a seat to lower leg support angle less than 90° to accommodate tight hamstrings or fixed knee flexion contractures in order to maintain a neutral pelvic tilt position.

Lower Leg to Foot Angle

Available ankle dorsiflexion ROM, deformities, abnormal tone, and movement patterns factor in to determining lower leg support to foot support angle (Fig. 32.10 and 32.11).[38,41–43] The use of ankle–foot orthoses (AFOs) will also affect the final lower leg support to foot support angle.

Simulation

Often it is difficult to determine the specific features and configuration of the equipment through the physical assessment process alone. *Simulation* is a process using your hands and/or equipment to determine the

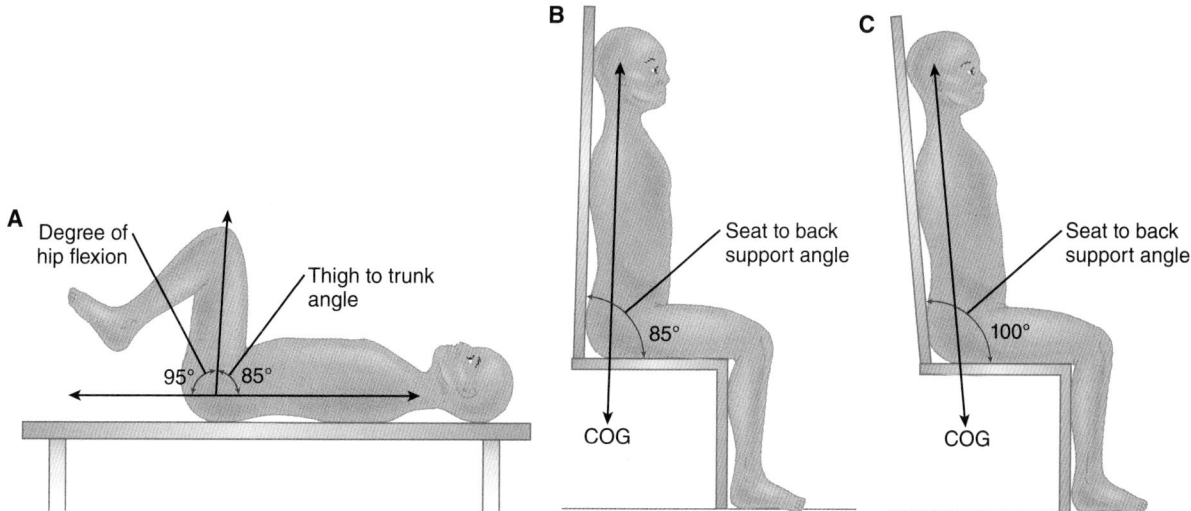

Figure 32.8 (A) If the degree of hip flexion for seating is to 95°, the thigh to trunk angle is 85°. (B) Seat to back support angle does not always correlate with thigh to trunk angle. In this example, if the seat to back support angle is set at 85°, tolerance to sitting in this position may be poor and cause the person to fall forward or constantly be working to hold themselves upright. Body shape, COM, and sitting tolerance must be addressed. (C) Opening the seat to back support angle to 100° better accommodates body shape and COM, and tolerance to sitting upright improves.

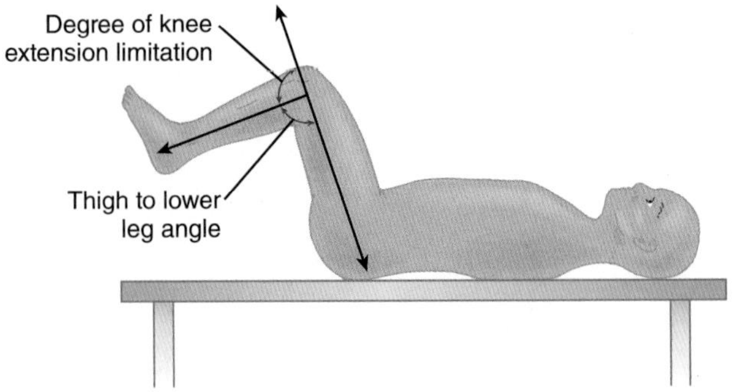

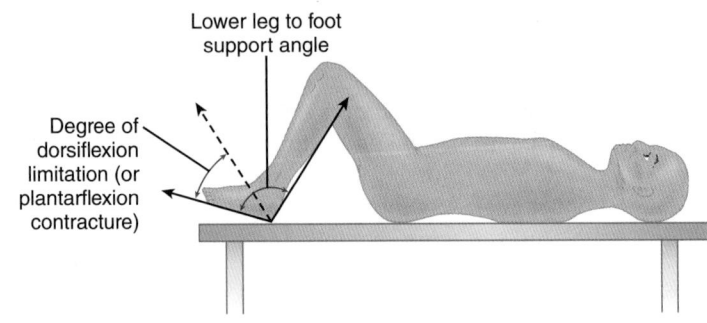

Figure 32.9 Thigh to lower leg angle is determined during the mat examination and is based on the popliteal angle (degree of knee extension limitation) when the hip is flexed to identified optimal position.

Figure 32.10 Lower leg support to foot support angle is determined during mat examination and is based on ankle ROM.

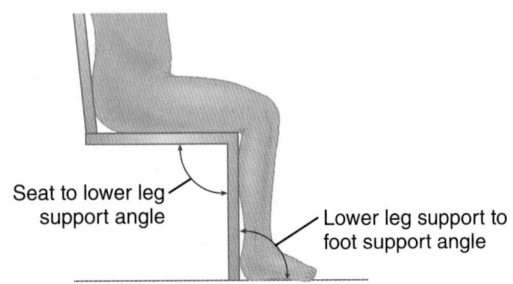

Figure 32.11 Seat to lower leg support angle and lower leg support to foot support angle are the final seating angles determined during seating simulation accommodating ROM, tone, and comfort at the knees and ankles.

person's tolerance to the recommended angles and linear measurements identified in the physical assessment. Simulation provides an opportunity to observe tone, movement, postural alignment, and function, and to assess equipment features and the effectiveness of postural supports in achieving the desired goals. In this way, hypotheses can be tested regarding position; orientation to gravity; and location, dimensions, angles, and sizes of postural supports needed. Seating simulation provides the opportunity to add and subtract supports to determine the amount of postural support a person tolerates (correction or accommodation) and the influence of gravity on a person's ability to function. If significant changes are being made to a seating system, simulation provides the person an opportunity to "test" and provide feedback about the seating recommendations.

Hand simulation is one form of simulation frequently performed during or immediately after the sitting mat assessment described previously. Placing one's hands (or other body parts) on the wheelchair user's body and providing corrective forces helps us to understand the optimal location of the forces needed, the magnitude and direction of the forces, and the size of the support structures (see Fig. 32.3). When needed, towel rolls, foam, or other available materials in the clinic can be used to assist with simulation, especially under the pelvis. Having this understanding assists with the feature matching process, another critical element of the wheelchair assessment.

A *seating simulator*, as seen in Figure 32.12, is a commercially available assessment chair. It provides the therapist with the ability to assess an individual's optimal sitting posture and can be used with a variety of people. Unfortunately, seating simulators are generally available only in specialty wheelchair clinics. The ideal seating simulator is adjustable for linear and angular measurements, and orientation in space. Additionally, some simulators are capable of using generic and commercial postural supports and power wheelchair input devices to simulate access and driving.[44]

If unable to access a seating simulator, a tilt-in-space and/or a recliner wheelchair may be used for simulation purposes instead. Try to obtain the necessary seat to back support angle, buttock/thigh depth, and wheelchair width if using trial equipment to *mock up* a system for seating simulation.

As with the assessment of the sitting posture, it is helpful to be systematic with simulation. First, provide support at the pelvis and move distally from there. Make only one change at a time. Observe carefully how changes in one part of the body affect other parts.

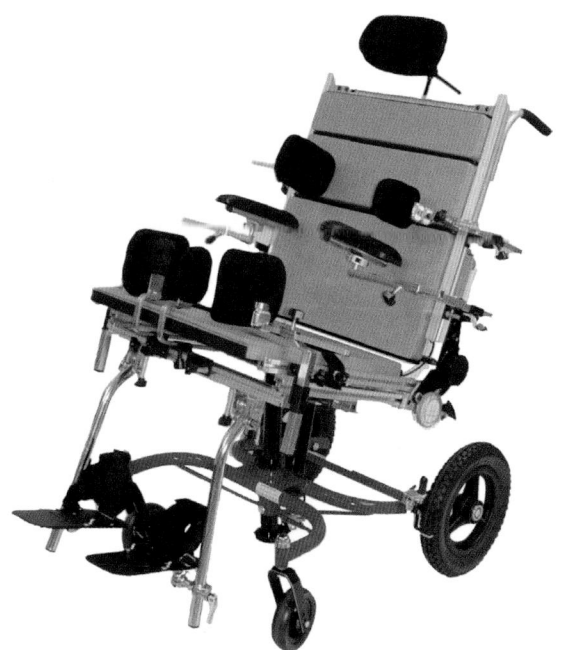

Figure 32.12 Planar seating simulator. *(Courtesy of Permobil Corp. Lebanon, TN 37090.)*

Technology Trial

Another very important part of the evaluation process is to provide a variety of equipment for the wheelchair user to compare and try out. If there is any uncertainty about the type of mobility device or seating equipment that will optimize function, trials of this equipment will help determine which features work best for the person. Allowing the person to compare and contrast features is beneficial in making educated decisions.

Trials of different wheelchairs (manual wheelchairs, power mobility devices) and seating equipment add to the evidence of what does and does not work well for the person. Documentation should describe mobility trials specifying the basic features and configuration of the mobility bases tried and ruled out. Also discuss seating and postural support trials and pressure management considerations. Describe the results of the trials and effectiveness of attaining identified goals with different equipment. Documentation of the trial results is a critical component of the evidence used by third-party payers in making decisions for coverage and payment.

Person/Technology Match (Prescription)

The person/technology match is matching the person with necessary and appropriate equipment features. Oftentimes it is necessary to make trade-offs between ideal positioning, function, and environmental access.

On occasion, new strategies for function or modifications to the environment are needed. Other times trade-offs are made in equipment features to retain function and/or access. The important message here is providing information and opportunity for trial equipment helps the person and team make educated decisions to maximize the opportunity for a positive outcome and minimize surprises at the fitting and delivery.

Evaluation and Plan of Care

The evaluation and POC is the synthesis of all information gathered so far. This portion of the specialty wheelchair evaluation is called the *prescription* step in WHO's eight steps of wheelchair service delivery process. The MPT problem-solving model is a four-step process that is specific to the Assistive Technology Assessment and provides a framework that considers the characteristics and interaction of the person, environment, and technology when selecting assistive technology for a particular person's use.[45,46] The process is person-centered rather than product-centered. This problem-solving approach provides a foundation for critical thinking, communication, and specification of products during the assessment process. It guides selection of appropriate and necessary WSM products by using a sequence of (1) identifying equipment-related clinical problems, (2) establishing objectives for the equipment intervention, (3) making equipment feature recommendations, and (4) deciding product specifications. The process structures the decision-making process and ensures that all issues are addressed. When documented, the systematic approach communicates rationale for selecting each specific WSM feature and product. Readers unfamiliar with the client (e.g., reviewers, auditors) will be able to follow the clinical rationale for choosing specific WSM products.

The first step in the decision-making process is to develop a list of *problems* and *potentials*. Information obtained during the WSM examination and specialty evaluation is used to generate a list of the person's unique characteristics, problems, and potentials related to their mobility and seating needs. Next, for each listed problem or potential, a specific *objective* is written individualized to the person and related to positioning, alignment, motor control, health, function, environmental access, activity, and participation. Objectives should be specific and relate to the equipment features needed. For example, "Reduce risk for pressure injury under left ischial tuberosity by providing accommodation for a fixed pelvic obliquity." The third step in the MPT problem-solving model is to consider the different WSM *equipment features* required for the person to achieve the stated objectives, the *person/feature match*. Attention is given to product properties, materials, configuration, and specific details of the final product. In the final step (*feature/technology match*), the list of identified equipment features is reviewed by the therapist and RTP. Specific make/model of *product specifications* are identified. The RTP ensures that multiple products from different manufacturers will interface and be configured as intended. If no commercial option is available with the necessary properties, custom fabrication is explored. Box 32.3 provides an example of this strategy illustrating the rationale for justifying the WSMD.

Box 32.3   Example of Matching Person and Technology Problem-Solving Model Grid

Problems and Potentials	Objectives	Equipment Features	Product Specifications
Diagnosis of CP diplegia, currently uses a MWD power wheelchair for outdoor mobility for work and complains of back pain and buttock discomfort when driving the wheelchair over uneven terrain. Able to use a standard joystick for driving the power wheelchair.	Increase sitting tolerance and comfort to ensure ability to drive power wheelchair outdoors on varied terrain with decreased stress on body.	MWD wheelchair with frame suspension system to decrease stress on body. Tilt seating system to assist with pressure and pain management, comfort, and sitting tolerance.	Compare a variety of MWD power wheelchairs with tilt seating to determine most optimal device for suspension, accessibility, and outdoor mobility.
Presents with poor sitting posture with posterior pelvic tilt and kyphotic spine (10° forward for upper trunk and 20° posterior tilt) in current power wheelchair with planar seat and back supports (current seat depth = 19 in., seat to back support angle = 90°.	Support trunk in upright midline posture with slight anterior pelvic tilt, no obliquity and no rotation. Support trunk extension to decrease kyphotic tendencies. Provide seat depth and seat-to-back support angles that match body measurements.	Planar seat and back supports with 2 in. of dense foam set at 100° seat-to-back angle and seat depth adjusted to 16 in. to accommodate body measurements. Compared materials and shapes for a variety of planar and precontoured seats and backs. It was determined that a simple planar back and a gel seat cushion will achieve stated objectives.	Planar with 2 in. of dense foam back support and seat cushion with gel in buttock region with set up of 100° seat to back support angle (see ROM information) and seat depth of 16 in.
B Hip flexion = 80°, B abduction = 0°, B knee extension with hip flexed = 90°, B ankle DF with knee flexed = 0°. Able to achieve neutral pelvic position and straight trunk alignment in supine position. No UE or head/neck limitations.	Accommodate BLE ROM limitation to assist in optimal pelvic position and neutral positioning of lower extremities in the seated position.	Seat to back seat support angle = 100°, seat to lower leg support angle = 90° and lower leg support to foot support angle = 90°.	Angle adjustable back post to support 100° seat to back angle. Center mount footrest system to accommodate LE contractures with a seat to lower leg support angle = 90° and lower leg to foot support angle = 90°.
Performs stand pivot transfers independently	Ensure ability to move footplates out of way and use armrests to perform a stand pivot transfer independently.	Center mount flip-up footrest system. Height-adjustable armrests.	Height-adjustable full-length armrests. Center mount flip-up footplate.
Uses desk computer daily	Maintain independence in computer, desk, counter, and table access.	Ensure optimal seat height for table access. Provide easy access release mechanism to move joystick out of the way independently due to impaired UE dexterity.	Swing away retractable joystick mount with easy access release mechanism due to impaired UE dexterity.

CP = cerebral palsy; DF = dorsiflexion; LE = lower extremity; MWD = mid-wheel drive; ROM = range of motion; UE = upper extremity.

Intervention

Wheelchair Fitting, Delivery, and Training

The wheelchair fitting, delivery, and training are done to ensure that the equipment is configured, fits and functions as anticipated, and that the wheelchair user and caregivers know how to use the wheelchair safely and effectively. Documenting this process and providing instructions is an important safeguard to reduce risk for liability. Training is required for first-time users as well as users who are making dramatic equipment switches (e.g., moving from a folding frame wheelchair to a rigid frame wheelchair or moving from a manual wheelchair to a power wheelchair).

All equipment is set up prior to the delivery process to ensure the fitting/delivery is completed in an efficient manner. At the delivery, the person is positioned in the new equipment and all components are adjusted to meet their needs. Check that the seat depth, back height, arm height, and foot position fit appropriately. Compare positioning angles (seat to back support angle, seat to lower leg support angle, lower leg support to foot support angle, pelvic support angle of attachment, and so forth) to specifications. Verify fixed and/or variable position in space (e.g., tilt, recline, procline) is as planned. Ensure all primary and secondary supports are adjusted and final posture is compared to the expected results determined during the evaluation.

Function From Wheelchair

The user is instructed in how to use all moving parts. This includes functions such as operating the wheel locks on a manual wheelchair, operating the motor releases on a power wheelchair to enable moving the wheelchair manually, moving the foot supports, adjusting the armrests, and adjusting the seat cushion and back cushions. Care is taken to instruct the user in how to function from the wheelchair while minimizing the risk of tipping or falling during use.

The person and their family/caregivers, if appropriate, are instructed in methods to reduce the risk of pressure injuries. This includes instruction and education on safety, pressure management (weight relief, frequency, and duration), skin inspection, and positioning. If additional training is needed beyond the initial wheelchair fitting, it is incorporated into the POC for follow-up.

Transfer training is critical for safety and independence. An important part of the fitting and training is to ensure the person can safely transfer in and out of the wheelchair as independently as possible. Therefore, transfers (e.g., stand pivot transfers, sliding board transfers, lift transfers, and modified transfers) are practiced. Care is taken to ensure the seat height is optimal for safe transfers and components can be moved out of the way as needed (swing away footrests and removable armrests) or adjusted (e.g., adjustable height armrest), depending on the specific type of transfer.

Car and van transfers are also practiced if needed. The therapist's role is to teach the wheelchair user how to manage the WSMD (such as folding or disassembling for transportation) and how to transfer in and out of the vehicle.[47,48] If the person drives the car, they may need to lift the wheelchair into the car either by placing it behind the front seat or lifting it across their body into the passenger seat. The weight of the wheelchair, method of folding, and ability to remove components (wheels, footrests, armrests, back support) are important considerations when lifting a wheelchair into the car, and the person may need training and practice to master new skills.

Wheelchair Mobility

Wheelchair mobility involves ensuring that the WSMD is configured for optimal propulsion and driving. For individuals receiving a manual wheelchair, the system is assessed for the person's position relative to the drive wheel and wheelchair responsiveness (center of gravity adjustment/tippyness). Adjustment of the seat and axle position will impact the person's UE position (extremes of movement) and contact with the drive wheel. Adjustments are made to the wheelchair configuration to optimize UE contact with the drive wheel and avoid extremes of movement if propelling with the UEs. If propelling with the LEs or hemi-propelling, care is taken to ensure the person has firm foot contact with the floor. Techniques for efficient and effective wheelchair propulsion are demonstrated. The center of gravity position is configured for more or less stability or tippyness, dependent on the person's wheelchair skills and functional needs. If additional training is needed, follow-up is included in the POC.

For an individual receiving a power wheelchair, the user input device (joystick, switch, and so forth) is adjusted for access. The person is instructed in how to turn the wheelchair on/off, change speeds or drive programs, and use all features. Electronic programming is individualized to ensure the person can drive the wheelchair safely indoors and outdoors and at an appropriate speed to minimize risk for injury to themselves or to others.

It is also important for wheelchair users and caregivers to understand how the wheelchair works and how much assistance the user needs either to move the wheelchair, transfer in and out of the wheelchair, or transport the wheelchair. Finally, it is important that the wheelchair user learn how to instruct others to help them with their wheelchair should assistance be needed.

Wheelchair Skills Training

Wheelchair skills training includes, but is not limited to, how to propel and turn the wheelchair, how to go up and down ramps and curbs or instruct a caregiver to assist, and if appropriate how to perform higher level wheelchair skills, such as rear wheel balancing (wheelie)[47-52] (Fig. 32.13).

User Training

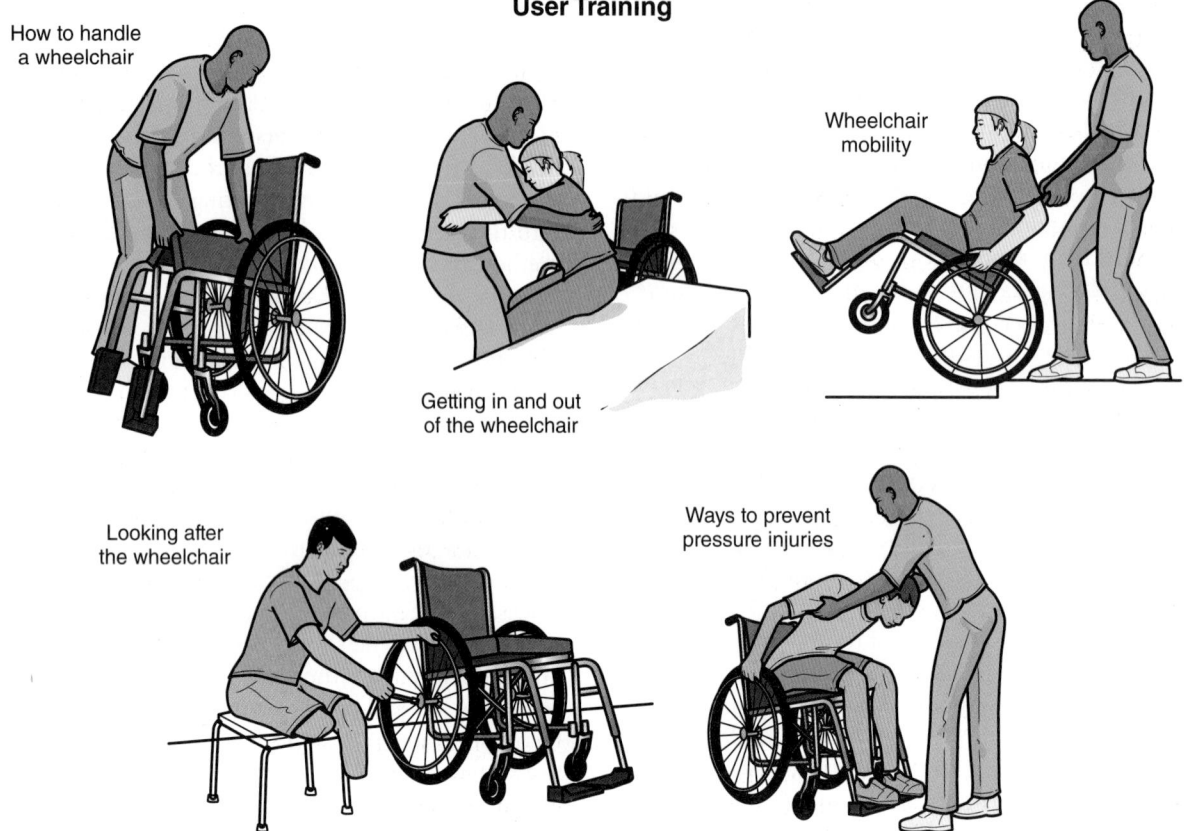

How to handle
a wheelchair

Getting in and out
of the wheelchair

Wheelchair
mobility

Looking after
the wheelchair

Ways to prevent
pressure injuries

Figure 32.13 Important skills for wheelchair users and caregivers.

Wheelchair mobility also includes operating the wheelchair on a variety of surfaces and terrains, including indoor flooring, outdoor sidewalks, driveways, and maneuvering down narrow hallways and turning into rooms, making three-point turns, and pulling up to counters or tables. The objective is to ensure that the person can safely operate and maneuver the wheelchair in a variety of situations that they will typically encounter.

Wheelchair management and skills training is considered a skilled therapeutic service. It is very important to document what was taught to the wheelchair user and what instructions were provided (written and verbal). Written instructions and resources are useful for the person to refer to later.

Maintenance/Repairs/Follow-Up

Individuals receiving new equipment or modifications to existing equipment should make a follow-up appointment with the clinician and equipment supplier after they have had time to practice with the wheelchair if adjustments or further training is needed. All wheelchairs require maintenance and/or repairs if used on a regular basis. The person should be provided with instructions on how to care for their WSM equipment and what they can do to keep the wheelchair clean and in good working order. The person should understand

when the equipment supplier needs to be notified to assist with repairs, such as new upholstery, new wheels, casters and bearings, and new arm pads. If it is a power wheelchair, new replacement batteries will be needed periodically depending on usage.

If the person's condition changes and feels the equipment is no longer working for them to maintain optimal posture, function, or optimal mobility, they should contact the clinician who assisted them in obtaining the equipment to set up an appointment for a reassessment of needs.

■ WHEELCHAIR SEATING AND MOBILITY TECHNOLOGIES

Thus far we have discussed the wheelchair examination and specialty evaluation, identified the person/feature match, and initiated the prescription process. At this time, in collaboration with the RTP, the therapist determines the feature/product match identifying the wheelchair and specific frame components and seating supports for the final WSM prescription. This section presents an organizational framework and foundational knowledge about *seating support systems* and *wheeled mobility devices*. This framework can be used for categorizing equipment, identifying unique features and functions, and making comparisons between manufacturers' products and models. The *Glossary of Wheelchair Terms and Definitions* provides the framework for the terminology used for seating support systems and wheeled mobility devices.[53] For more information and to download the e-book go to https://www.ucdenver.edu/centers/center-for-inclusive-design-and-engineering/clinical-services/wheelchair-seating-measures-guide.

A combination of the seating support system and a wheeled mobility device when integrated together is a WSMD (Fig. 32.14). The *seating support system* is considered the surfaces that directly contact, support, or contain the user's body.[53] *Primary seating supports* are primary weight-bearing components, including the seat, back support, foot support, arm support, and head support.[53] The contact surfaces that provide support to maintain postural alignment are considered *secondary support surfaces*.[53] These components are selected based on the persons' need for external supports to achieve their optimal sitting posture. Secondary supports may include components such as lateral supports for the trunk, hips, and knees, and medial supports for the knees and UE support surfaces.

A *wheeled mobility device* consists of the *wheelchair frame or base,* arm support assembly, foot support assembly, and wheels, and may also include additional *wheelchair options/accessories.* Wheeled mobility devices may be either manual or power operated. Wheel bases come in various wheel configurations (e.g., front, mid, or rear-wheel drive) and wheelbase lengths that impact the maneuverability of the device. The person/feature/product match (MPT problem-solving model) details the decision-making process linking the person's problems/potentials, objectives, equipment features, and recommended products to clinical rationale to justify the necessity and appropriateness of the items prescribed.

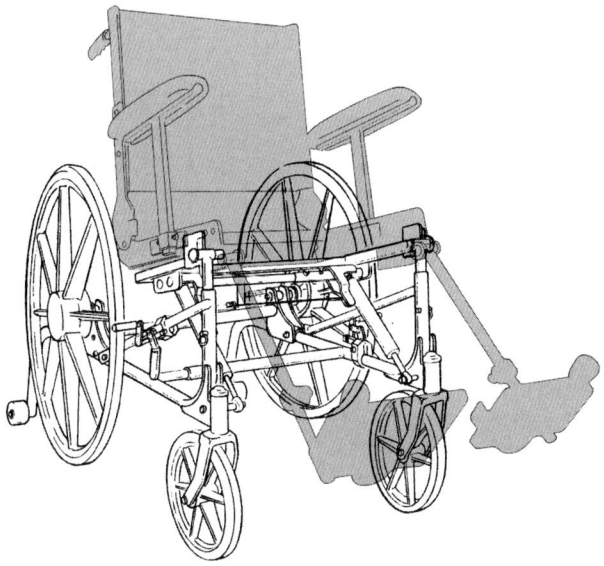

Figure 32.14 A WSMD consists of the seating support system and the wheeled mobility device.

While users with basic level seating and positioning needs can sit *hands-free* to function and will unlikely require much of the seating support equipment discussed below, it is important that therapists understand the range of WSM equipment available to people with basic, intermediate, and complex mobility limitations. In particular, it is important for therapists to recognize the limits of their WSM knowledge and skills, especially with regard to people with intermediate to complex needs, and to know when it is necessary to refer a person to a clinician with advanced WSM knowledge and skills.

Policymakers and payers have identified, and in many cases require therapists, professionals with no financial ties, to manage the evaluation and recommendation process. Consequently, it is our ethical and professional responsibility to ensure users receive skilled services and appropriate and necessary recommendations, and that fiscally responsible decisions are made with their valuable (and often limited) resources.

Seating Support System

Specifying the primary and secondary seating support system means detailing the size, location, shape, and attachment method of the supports. The size and location of the supports are dependent on the linear and angular measurements established during the wheelchair assessment. Critical dimensions to specify include, at a minimum, seat width, seat depth, back height, and lower leg length. Similarly, critical angular measurements to consider and document include (1) seat to back support angle, (2) seat to lower leg support angle, and (3) lower leg support to foot support angle.

The size and location of the secondary supports are specified to provide optimal body alignment without interfering with function. The shape and size of the supports are dependent on the amount of support and pressure distribution required. Dimensions are specified for all primary and secondary support surfaces.

Seating supports, including the seat, back, and postural supports, come in different shapes: *planar, precontoured, and custom contoured.* A planar seating support surface is flat (Fig. 32.15). Pre-contoured is a generically shaped seating support surface (Figs. 32.16 and 32.17). Custom contoured (carved or molded) is a seating support surface that is uniquely shaped to match the body contours of the person (Fig. 32.18). Matching the shape of the person with the support is critical to maximizing contact between the user and the seating support system. A properly shaped support distributes pressure over bony prominences and body surface area, increases comfort, and results in improved postural control.[54-57]

Once the postural support is selected, a method to mount or attach the support and the location of the support are identified and specified. Mounting hardware can be fixed (requires tools), removable, or swingaway. The type and size of the mounting hardware

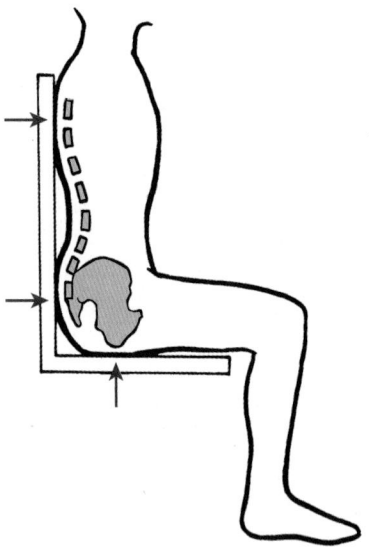

Figure 32.15 Persons seated on planar surfaces may show increased pressure over bony prominences.

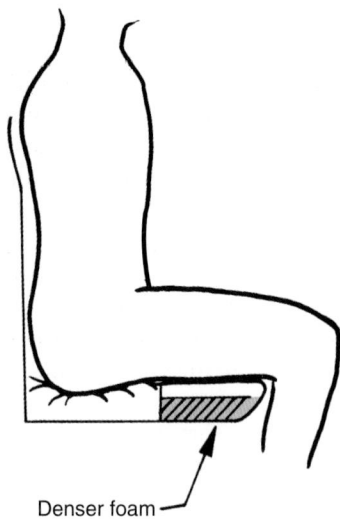

Figure 32.17 An option for creating contoured seats is use of varying density (firmness) foam.

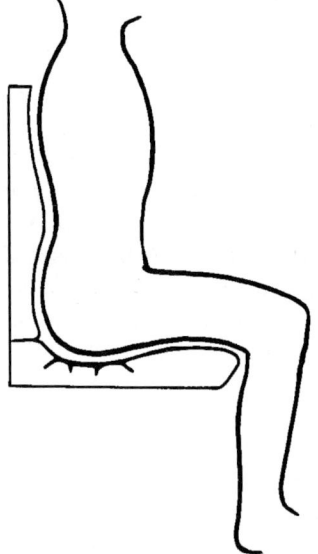

Figure 32.16 Some types of foam will contour as a response to body weight.

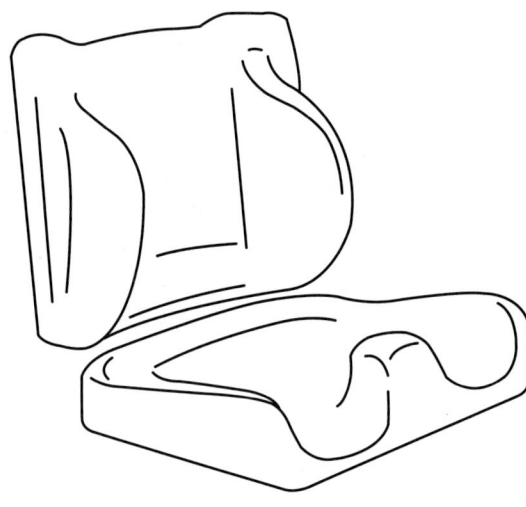

Figure 32.18 Custom-contoured cushions match the person's body contours.

selected often are dictated by the space available on the WMD to mount the support in the desired location. The rationale for the type of hardware selected is dependent on the objectives identified. For instance, if the wheelchair needs to be folded, removeable hardware may be necessary. If the person has multiple caregivers and there is a risk the supports may be misplaced or incorrectly positioned, fixed hardware may be desirable. If the person is able to transfer alone or with the assistance of another, swing-away hardware that remains mounted to the wheelchair may be the best option.

Primary Support Surfaces

Seat

The seat is the postural support device intended to contact the buttocks and thighs. Seat options include sling upholstery, solid base, or van seat that come included as part of the WMD. Alternately, a seat cushion can be added to a WMD when specified and purchased separately. The most critical dimensions to accurately specify are seat depth, seat width, and seat or cushion height (thickness). If the seat depth is too long, it promotes a posterior pelvic tilt and kyphotic posture. If the seat width is too wide, it will make wheel access and self-propelling the wheelchair more difficult and result in poor shoulder alignment and biomechanics (Figs. 32.19 and 32.20). If the wheelchair is too narrow it can cause increased pressure on the hips from the armrests and leg rest system, placing the person at risk for a pressure injury. If the cushion is too thin, the person could "bottom out" on the solid seat below, resulting in pressure injury.

A firm seat support is critical to providing a solid base to support neutral LE alignment, promote pressure distribution, and improve comfort. Basic manual wheelchairs typically are standardly equipped with sling

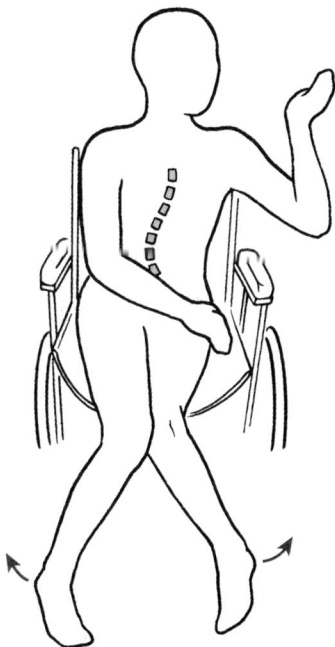

Figure 32.21 Overall poor sitting posture and asymmetries created by a sling seat and sling back.

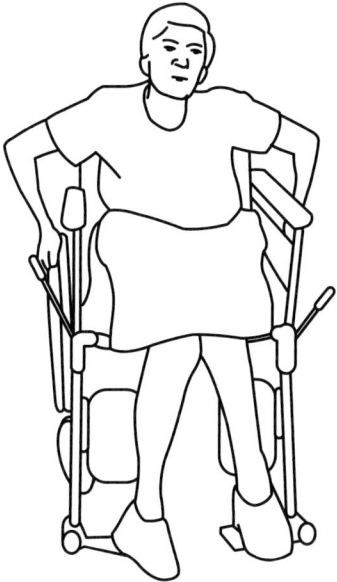

Figure 32.19 A wheelchair that is too wide will make wheel access and propulsion more difficult for the person.

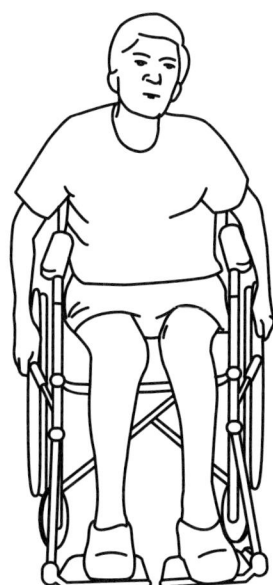

Figure 32.20 A narrower wheelchair allows easier wheel access and propulsion.

upholstery. Over time, the sling material stretches, creating hammocking and poor pelvic positioning—posterior pelvic tilt, hip adduction, and internal rotation (Fig. 32.21). Sling upholstery is generally provided to facilitate ease of folding and storing of the wheelchair. However, if the WSMD is used daily for more than 2 hours at a time, and not just for intermittent mobility, then a firm seat support should be added to the wheelchair. A solid seat insert can be placed under the cover of a seat cushion to provide a firm base of support and used on top of the seat upholstery and seat frame. Alternatively, a solid seat pan (metal or plastic) can be mounted directly to the seat frame (with upholstery removed) and a seat support (e.g., cushion) placed on top of the pan (Fig. 32.22).

Cushion shape (planar, precontoured, custom contoured) and material properties are selected based on the person's needs. Goals of a seating support (cushion) might include promoting improved positioning, maximizing postural stability for UE activities and function, distributing pressure to minimize risk of pressure injury, and improving sitting tolerance time (e.g., comfort).[58]

Once the shape of the seat cushion is established, the properties of the cushion materials are determined. Cushion properties affect sitting stability, pressure relief, ability to transfer, and comfort. Different materials ensure these objectives are met. Cushions are made of different materials, including foam (open or closed cell, foam elastomer), air, fluid (gel, water, viscoelastic fluid), or a combination of materials. Foam cushions come in different densities. Firm foams provide increased stability. Different densities of foam can also be used to achieve

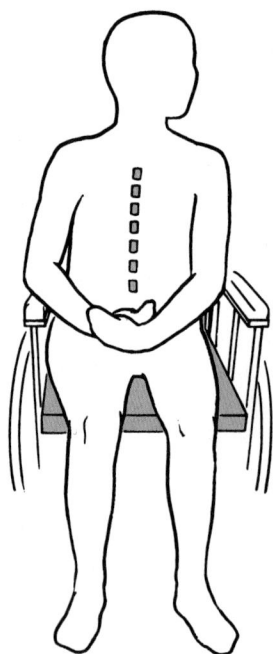

Figure 32.22 A firm sitting surface enhances sitting posture and provides a stable base of support.

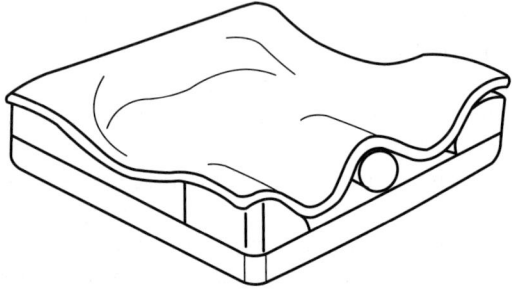

Figure 32.23 Firmer foam shapes can be placed under a more flexible foam to create a contoured cushion.

shaping and pressure redistribution (Fig. 32.23). Different materials allow for varying degrees of envelopment of the person (immersion) in the cushion, distributing pressure over a greater surface area. In general, the continuum of immersion properties for different materials from lesser to greater is foam, gel, air.

Cushion maintenance is another consideration during the selection process. Foam cushions require little maintenance other than keeping dry and clean. Air cushions need to be monitored for proper inflation for optimal pressure redistribution. Over- or underinflation can result in a pressure injury. Changes in temperature and altitude can affect cushion inflation, requiring reinflation or deflation. Air cushions are also subject to puncture. Gel cushions settle with use and require kneading to redistribute gel to prevent "bottoming out" on the cushion base or solid seat below.

Some cushions are made with a combination of materials to benefit from the different material properties.

For instance, a combination foam and gel cushion will allow for envelopment of the gel around the bony prominences of the ITs and the firm support of the foam base to support the trochanters and femurs for stability. Specialty off-loading cushions are custom shaped, may be made from one or more different materials, and generally require little maintenance once fabricated. Off-loading cushions can reduce interface pressure and compression at ITs and sacral/coccygeal regions by loading and containing surrounding tissues and managing tissue deformation.

Cushion covers are made with materials with different properties that also factor into the selection process. If the cover is loose and stretchy, it will allow the person to be immersed in the cushion. However, if the fabric is tight or taut, the full effects of the cushion material underneath will be diminished. Cover(s) can be *waterproof* or *water resistant*. If a person is incontinent, a waterproof cover is necessary, especially if the person is using a foam cushion. If a person is prone to incontinence, a second cushion cover is useful to prevent exposure of the cushion material to urine or feces during cleaning of the cover. Cushions that are not permanently mounted to the wheelchair frame are typically attached to the seat pan with hook and loop fastener (e.g., Velcro) to secure the cushion in place, prevent slippage, and make removal for cleaning easier. Care is needed when placing the cushion cover back on the cushion to make sure that the cushion is in the proper orientation and positioned in the wheelchair as intended. Inappropriately placed cushions (upside down or backward) may result in a pressure injury and should be part of your instructions and markings on the cushion.

If permanently mounting a seating system, decisions are needed for selecting mounting hardware. If using a solid seat pan, the original seat upholstery is removed. Fixed or removeable hardware can be used, depending on the needs of the person. Adjustable hardware allows for height and angle adjustment, ensuring the linear and angular dimensions are appropriate for the person. If the person needs a seat incline angle of 10°, the front seat pan hardware can be set higher than the rear to achieve this angle. If the wheelchair needs to be folded for transportation, removable hardware is appropriate. If the weight of the wheelchair is an issue, fixed hardware may be lighter.

Whenever possible, the person should try different seat cushions (shapes and materials) to compare products and determine the best person/product match for their specific needs. Box 32.4 provides a list of questions that should be considered when finalizing the seat support.

Back Support

The back support is the surface behind the sacrum, lumbar, and/or thoracic segments of the trunk. A firm back support is critical to support a neutral trunk posture.

Box 32.4 Questions to Consider When Finalizing the Seat Support

- Does the seat provide adequate support and stability to promote good sitting posture?
- Will the pressure distribution on the seat prevent pressure injuries?
- Is the shape of the seat cushion appropriate for the person's body contours?
- Does the person need a custom shape to accommodate deformities and maximize support?
- Is pressure relief provided if the person is unable to complete weight shifts independently using UEs or through a tilt or recline option?
- Are special combinations of foam, air, or gel seat cushions needed to maximize comfort and pressure relief?
- Is the seat depth an appropriate length?
- Is the seat width appropriate for propelling the wheelchair and for comfortable positioning?
- Is the seat surface appropriate for safe transfers into and out of the wheelchair?
- Does the seat cushion provide optimal comfort?
- Is the seat cushion able to dissipate heat and moisture? Does the cushion function effectively in different climates?

Some people require back support plus additional secondary supports such as lateral trunk supports to maintain their optimal sitting posture.

Basic manual wheelchairs typically come equipped with sling-back upholstery. Like seat upholstery, back upholstery stretches over time, promoting one or more of the following: a kyphotic posture, scoliotic spine, posterior pelvic tilt, or hyperextended neck. Tension adjustable back upholstery is one available option that uses strapping to accommodate mild pelvic and trunk positioning needs and provide support and stability, and it can be retightened over time. If the person uses the wheelchair for longer than 2 hours at a time and not merely for intermittent mobility, firm back support should be provided. Most back supports require hardware (fixed or removeable) or Velcro loops to attach the back support to the wheelchair.

The same properties considered for the seat are considered for the back support, including the dimensions, surface shape, stability (firmness), and mounting or attachment method.

Back supports come in a range of dimensions (heights and widths). The shape selected is dependent on the needs of the individual.[38,56] Back support height is determined based on the person's trunk control, functional abilities, and comfort. A shorter back support may be appropriate for a person with good trunk control and hands-free sitting balance who self-propels. A shorter

back height, below the inferior angle of the scapula, allows for unobstructed movement of the scapula and shoulder girdle. A taller back support may be needed for a person who is unable to sit without support or uses a tilt-in-space feature and requires full back support. Back width is generally dictated by the width of the wheelchair frame or the location needed for mounting trunk supports that may be required.

The shape of the back support is assessed and selected to ensure contact is provided behind the buttocks, sacrum, lumbar, and thoracic segments of the trunk. When considering a precontoured back support, the person's shape must be considered. For instance, if a person has a narrower upper trunk and wider hips, the precontoured lateral supports may interfere with the hips, making it impossible for full lower back contact. In this instance, a precontoured back with built-in lateral supports may not be an appropriate option for optimal pelvic/low back support; instead, mounted lateral supports may be the better option.

Back supports frequently are made with foam of different densities determined by comfort and pressure relief needs. Back supports frequently are designed with insets or reliefs made with different materials: air, gel, or a combination (discussed in seat section). Inset material is selected based on the properties desired, including the need for pressure relief, shape, and location. The person should be given an opportunity to trial various back cushions to determine which works best to attain the identified goals.

Mounting hardware is an important consideration, especially when attaching the back support to the wheelchair. The type of hardware is chosen based on the type of wheelchair, the angular dimensions required, the need to fold the wheelchair, the need to keep the wheelchair as light as possible, or the need to increase durability. Mounting hardware may be heavy and affect a person's ability to self-propel the wheelchair or lift/load the wheelchair into the car. Box 32.5 presents questions that should be considered when finalizing the back support.

Foot Support

The foot support is the postural support device used to support or position the foot and lower leg and is considered a primary support surface. Placement of the foot support directly affects the position of the entire lower body, tone, and posture (trunk, head, arms). To achieve appropriate positioning of the foot on the foot support, one needs to match the linear and angular dimensions determined during the mat assessment and seating simulation, including (1) lower leg length, (2) seat to lower leg support angle, and (3) lower leg to foot support angle.

Adequate lower leg length is required to maintain good pelvic position and distribute the weight of the thighs on the seat. Foot supports that are too low will

---

Box 32.5   Questions to Consider When Finalizing the Back Support

- Is the back support in an appropriate position for upright trunk posture (seat to back support angle, orientation in space)?
- Is the back support an appropriate shape to fit the person's body contours? (If using a commercially available back support with contour, it should be examined to ensure the support will fit the person. At times, the person's hips may be too wide to fit between the fixed lateral supports of a commercial back.)
- Does the person require a custom shape to provide full contact and support?
- Does the back support provide adequate control for muscle weakness and trunk asymmetries?
- Is the back comfortable when used in a tilted or reclined position?
- Does the back support allow performance of functional activities (propelling, reaching, transfers)?
- Is pressure distribution/relief adequate for a person with a bony spine or protruding sacrum, or to prevent pressure sores?
- Are special combinations of foam, air, or gel needed to maximize comfort and pressure relief?

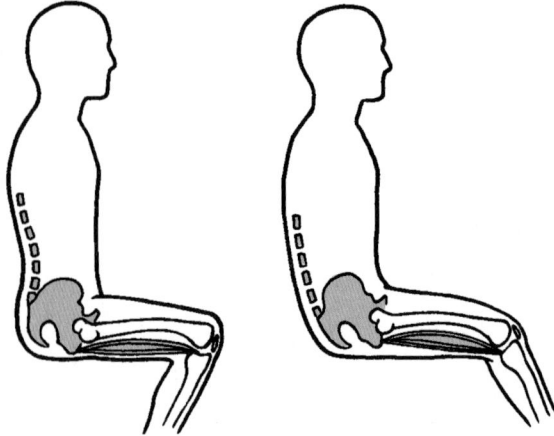

Figure 32.24 Sitting alignment with the hamstrings on slack and the knees flexed (*left*) and positioning assumed with feet resting on elevating leg rests (*right*), causing tension on the hamstring that pulls the pelvis into a posterior tilt.

result in the knees being lower than the hips, placing the hips in a more open angle and encouraging forward sliding of the pelvis. Also, foot supports that are too low, with inadequate ground clearance, can cause the wheelchair to tip should the foot support interfere with the ground or an obstacle (e.g., ramp, doorjamb). Two inches of ground clearance is a target to keep in mind. Foot supports that are too high may unload the thighs, placing increased weight on the ITs, coccyx, and sacrum and increasing the risk for developing pressure injuries.

The seat to lower leg support angle and the lower leg support to foot support angle guide the selection of the foot support assembly. Foot supports that are mounted too far forward when hamstring muscles are tight will pull the pelvis into a posterior tilt and promote forward sliding of the pelvis (Fig. 32.24). This is an important consideration, especially when using elevating leg rests, one type of foot support assembly. Foot support devices that are mounted close to or below the seat may cause interference with the casters. This is important to avoid, as caster interference can cause wheelchair tips, falls, or injury to the lower leg or foot.

Any limitation of motion imposed by the hamstring muscle and gastrocnemius muscle will directly influence the choice of foot support. With tight hamstrings, to achieve the person's optimal sitting posture and maximum available hip flexion, it may be necessary to flex the knees more than 90° to place the hamstrings

on slack. This approach may require special positioning of the foot supports.

Arm Support

Arm supports are the postural support device intended to contact the inferior surface of the forearms. This surface provides support to the UE and trunk, off-loading weight from the spine. The height, length, and width of the arm supports are the critical measurements needed for decision-making. Correct armrest height generally allows for 30° shoulder flexion and 90° of elbow flexion. If arm support placement is too high, shoulders become elevated, placing stress on the shoulders and neck. If armrest placement is too low or too wide, inadequate support can lead to leaning or slumping to reach the supports.

The arm pad directly contacts the forearm or hand and, in addition to providing upper trunk support, is used for function, such as pushing up to standing, making clothing adjustments, and performing weight reliefs (forward bending, side leaning, and press-ups). If the arm pad support is too wide, it may interfere with lifting or flipping back the armrests or grasping the armrests for transfers or interfere with propulsion. If the arm pad support is too narrow, it may cause concentrated pressure on the forearms or elbows, or the upper extremities may slip off the pads, providing ineffective support. Arm pads come in different materials such as plastic, foam, or gel and are selected based on the person's needs.

For some individuals, arm supports will be used to mount a *UE support surface* such as a UE support tray or wedge. A tray surface provides several important functions. It can promote symmetrical positioning of the UEs or accommodate alignment of the glenohumeral joint and scapula, support the weight of the upper limbs, decrease shoulder subluxation, and provide trunk support. Importantly, UE support trays are used for function: for meals, work or school, or supporting a communication device, computer, book, and so on.

Head Support

A posterior head support is a support intended to contact the posterior aspect of the head. This is beneficial for a person who is unable to hold their head upright and needs a resting support surface or for a person who needs support when the wheelchair is tilted rearward or when the back is reclined. Important issues to consider include the size, shape, and material of the support; the adjustability/durability of the attaching hardware; and the final placement of the support. For example, a curved shape will support the person's head in the center of the headrest while a flat support will not provide any cues for positioning of the head, and the head may tend to slide on the flat surface. Adjustable hardware will allow accommodation for a forward head position or a laterally flexed position. Swing-away hardware may be needed when transferring from behind so that the caregiver can get close for lifting and repositioning. Proper support and positioning of the head affect posture, visual gaze, swallowing, and communication. Depending on a person's needs, head supports sometimes may also incorporate secondary support surfaces such as lateral support pads, facial pads, forehead head straps, chin supports, and so on.

Secondary Support Surfaces

Secondary supports include lateral and medial trunk, hip, knee, foot, UE, anterior chest, and pelvic supports.[53] Secondary supports may or may not be necessary for positioning, stability, pressure relief, and comfort. When determining the need for the support, consideration should be given to surface shape, stability or support (firmness/flexibility), size, placement, and attachment method. The supports are named according to their location and the terms used are standard medical terms to increase the ease of understanding the location of the supports. Using the MPT problem-solving model, document the objective and rationale to justify each recommended support.

Anterior Supports

Anterior supports are positioned on the anterior aspect of the body. Common anterior supports include anterior pelvic support, anterior trunk supports, and anterior shoulder supports. Anterior trunk supports and shoulder supports tend to be made of flexible materials such as neoprene or fabric. Measurements and placement of the supports are critical to ensure the support is secure and does not slide or ride up, creating a hazard (e.g., choking).

ANTERIOR PELVIC SUPPORT

An anterior pelvic support is a device intended to contact the anterior aspect of the pelvis, just inferior to the ASIS. This device can be a flexible strap or seat belt or a rigid pelvic positioner (padded bar). The decision about the necessary pelvic support features is dependent on the support or accommodation needed to (1) control pelvic position (tilt, obliquity, or rotation), (2) maintain the person's optimal pelvic position, and (3) ensure safety.[59] In specifying an anterior pelvic support, decisions about the direction of pull, angle of pull, number of securement or anchor points, attachment hardware, location, and release mechanism are made.[60] For example, if the person has a tendency, secondary to tone, for the left hip to consistently rotate forward, it may be useful to have the belt tighten by pulling toward the left hip, creating a counterpressure. The angle of pull of the pelvic support in relation to the seating surface is a critical decision for safety and effectiveness. It is important for safety to prevent the pelvic support from lifting up into the abdomen or for the pelvis to slide underneath the support. Therefore, specifying the angle of pull is necessary. Attachment points are generally 30° to 45° to the seat to control for anterior pelvic tilt, 60° to 90° for posterior pelvic tilt, and around 60° for obliquity and rotation (Fig. 32.25).[59] Some users respond well to supports that have a 90° attachment angle with the sitting surface. This angle of pull secures the thighs against the seat support and inhibits hypertonia in persons who tend to extend in their wheelchairs as a result of increased tone. A 90° placement also leaves the pelvis free for forward trunk inclination, often necessary for reaching and function (Fig. 32.26). Some users can benefit from pelvic supports with more than one angle of pull from two securement points. A four-point belt

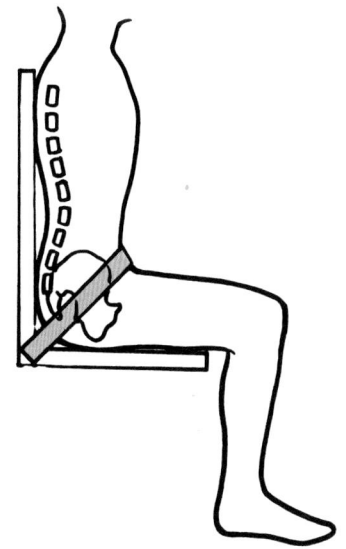

Figure 32.25 The pelvic belt should cross the pelvic-femoral junction at approximately a 45° to 60° angle to the seating surface.

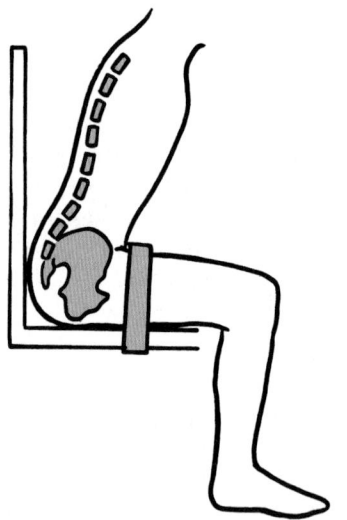

Figure 32.26 A belt placed over the upper thigh (at a 90° angle to the sitting surface) will free the pelvis for natural anterior tilting.

provides four places to anchor it. The top two anchors assist in securing the pelvis against the back support and the bottom two anchors assist in securing the femurs against the seat support, limiting the pelvis from shifting forward. Setting specific objectives for the pelvic position will drive the decision-making process for determining the optimal anterior pelvic support and securement parameters.

LATERAL SUPPORTS

Lateral supports are postural support devices contacting the lateral sides of the body. Lateral supports (pelvis, trunk, hip, knee, foot, and so forth) assist a person in maintaining optimal alignment. Each support requires a corresponding objective and rationale to support medical necessity.

If a person has poor trunk control and leans to the left side, lateral trunk supports can be used to support an upright midline position and decrease leaning to the left.[60] To correct a flexible or accommodate a fixed scoliosis, *three points of control* are needed. This is done by placing a pad at the apex of the curve on one side and on the opposite side a pad above and below the apex. In this example, for right (convex) scoliosis, a lateral trunk support would be placed on the right at the apex of the curve and on the left side above the apex, with a third pad below the apex at the pelvis or hip.

If both LEs abduct and the person doesn't have the muscle strength in their lower extremities to maintain neutral alignment, then lateral thigh/knee supports will help maintain LE position and limit excessive abduction.

Properties to consider include the surface size, shape, firmness, location, and method of attachment. The dimensions are necessary to ensure the supports aren't too large or too small. The location ensures the support provides the forces needed to attain the person's identified optimal sitting alignment. As an example, if the person's trunk width measures 12 in. but the width between the lateral trunk supports is 16 in., then the person will not benefit from contact of the lateral trunk support and will therefore continue to lean to the left side until they reach it. Be sure to consider adjustability and adjust the position of the supports to optimize postural control and comfort, taking into consideration factors such as future growth needs, weight gain, and seasonal clothing (e.g., winter coat, sweaters).

The attachment method can facilitate or impede transfers and mobility. The supports might need to be moved out of the way in order to perform sit pivot transfers, mechanical lift transfers, or stand pivot transfers. The style of the support attachment will determine if the person is able to move the support out of the way independently or require assistance. Defining objectives for posture and transfers will guide you in selecting the most effective equipment features. Other less common lateral supports include forearm, elbow, head, lower leg, and foot support, but the same concepts apply for shape, firmness, dimensions, placement, and attachment method.

MEDIAL SUPPORTS

Medial supports are postural support devices contacting the medial side of the body. The most common supports are medial knee and thigh supports. Other medial supports include forearm and foot supports.

POSTERIOR SUPPORTS

Posterior supports are postural support devices contacting the posterior aspect of the body. The most common include posterior foot, lower leg (calf), and arm support (elbow). A head support, although included in the primary support surface section, is considered a posterior head support. Objectives and equipment features are determined.

Wheeled Mobility Devices

A wheelchair can be divided into two parts: the seating support system that provides support to the person's body (discussed above) and the mobility base that provides movement within the environment (discussed below). Wheeled mobility devices may provide mobility in different positions such as sitting, lying, or standing and allow a person to be out of bed or out of a stationary chair and mobile in their environment. This chapter is devoted to seated wheeled mobility. A person may be able to operate the wheeled mobility device independently such as self-propelling a manual wheelchair or independently driving a power wheelchair, or he or she may be dependent in wheeled mobility, reliant on a caregiver to move in the environment. The wheeled mobility device provides a person with the ability to move to different rooms in their home and leave their home and participate in community activities. The wheeled mobility device framework is shown in Figure 32.27 and can be used for a reference for categorizing equipment.[53]

Wheelchair Frame/Base Considerations

In this section, adjustable frame considerations are discussed, including but not limited to linear, angular, and other configurable frame features. Figure 32.28 provides an overview of configurable wheelchair components that can be selected to individualize the wheelchair frame for the person's needs. These concepts and product considerations are factored into the decision-making process when matching equipment features to product specification (feature/model match).

Frame Linear Adjustments

Wheelchairs are available in different widths and depths. Sizing for optimal propulsion and posture was discussed in the primary support section above. Some manual wheelchair frames have built-in adjustability of the frame to accommodate for changes in width or depth without needing to purchase a new wheelchair and if

available is noted in the manufacturer literature. The growth option is most often used to accommodate for growth, as this can be a concern for children; however, it can also be used to accommodate for weight gain or loss. Care should be taken to select the most appropriate range, considering the person's immediate and future anticipated needs. For instance, if a frame width of 20 in. (50.8 cm) is needed, a frame may be selected that can be adjusted from 16 to 20 in. (40.6 to 50.8 cm), or 20 to 24 in. (50.8 to 60.9 cm). If the person has the potential to gain weight, the larger size should be considered.

Wheelchair seating dimensions (width and depth) are specific to the person's body size and posture needs. The overall wheelchair frame dimensions, however, dictate overall size, maneuverability, and accessibility. It results in extra width and length based on the style of the wheels, footrests, and other wheelchair features (e.g., anti-tip tubes).

The overall width is considered to ensure ability to move safely through doorways. This may be more difficult in a manual wheelchair since the wheels and handrims add 8 to 10 in. to the overall wheelchair width. In addition, hand clearance needs to be factored

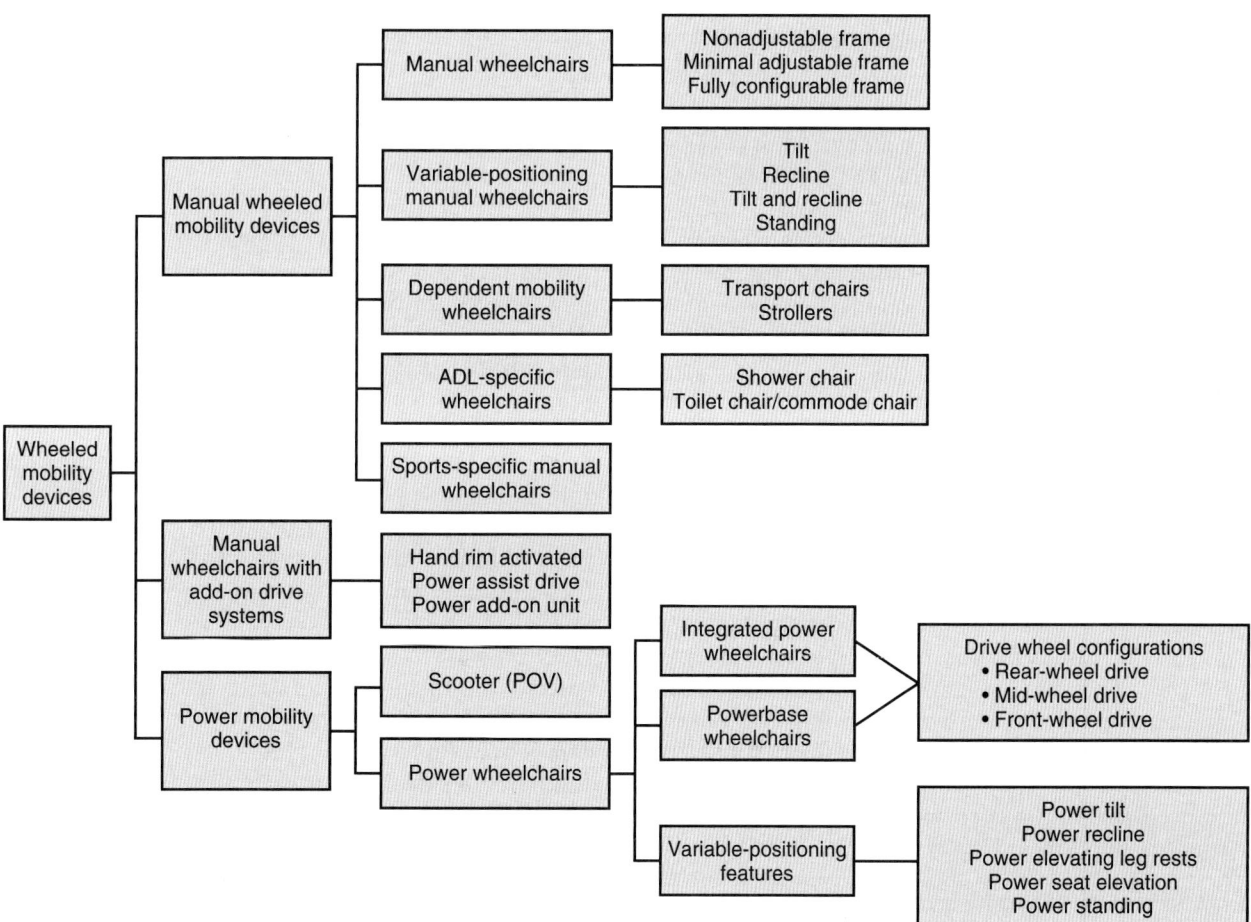

Figure 32.27 Wheeled mobility device framework.

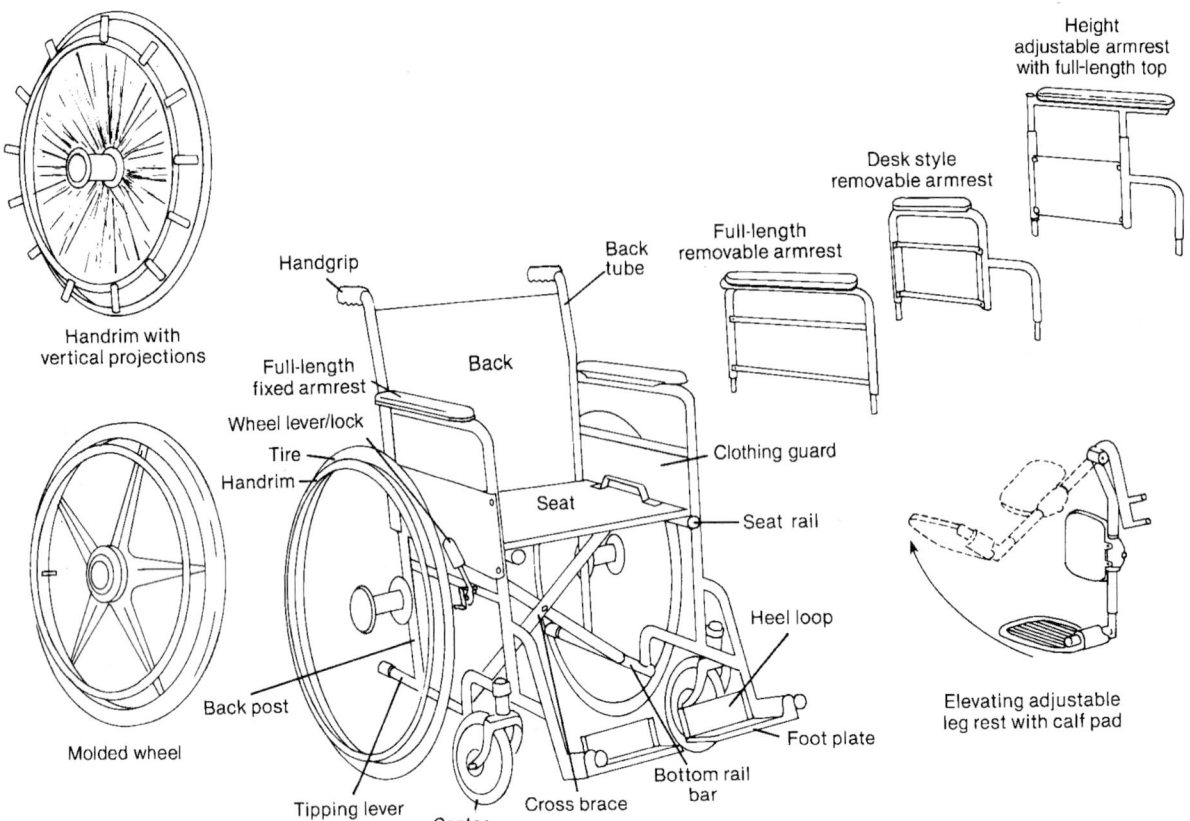

Figure 32.28 Overview of wheelchair components.

to enable the person to use their hands to propel while also allowing doorway clearance. Some people, however, prefer to use a compensatory strategy, such as using the doorjamb to pull through the opening instead of pushing on the wheel rim to decrease the risk of hand injuries. Regardless, doorway clearance is a critical consideration and sometimes requires environment adaptation (e.g., offset door hinges).

Wheelchair overall length determines turning radius and the ability to maneuver the wheelchair safely in confined spaces. The addition of tilt, recline, and elevating leg rests increases the overall frame length and turning radius, often making 90° turns from a hallway into a room difficult or impossible.

The overall wheelchair height (floor to the top of person's head) is a critical measurement when considering van access to ensure the van door height and interior space (floor to ceiling height) provide adequate head clearance. For van access, overall turning radius and maneuverability are important considerations for a person riding in their wheelchair to ensure the person and the wheelchair can be safely loaded and positioned for transportation.

Angular Frame Adjustments

Angular frame adjustments such as seat to back support angle, seat to lower leg support angle, and seat sagittal angle (seat incline or tilt) are used to narrow down make/model wheelchair frame options and determine the position of different frame components.

Manufacturers of manual wheelchairs preset seat frame angles and configurations based on the specifications detailed during the ordering process. Some manual wheelchairs are *made to order* (manufactured for the individual and nonadjustable) and others are *made to measure* (configured for the individual as specified). Even made to order manual wheelchairs typically have minimal adjustability or limited options of some features such as axle position or seat to back angle.

Some manual wheelchairs have axle plates and caster forks that have one or more adjustment options. These features provide the ability to specify a rear wheel size, caster size, front and rear frame heights, wheel placement, and wheel axle position (horizontal/vertical adjustment) (Fig. 32.29). By design, selection and configuration (e.g., frame height, seat angles, person's relation to rear wheel, wheelchair tippyness) are dependent on the objectives and features identified in the wheelchair assessment. For example, by selecting a small caster and caster fork size and raising the rear axle vertical position, a low seat to floor height can be accomplished so the person can reach the floor for foot propulsion. For a person with tight hamstrings requiring the feet to flex back under the seat, raising the front

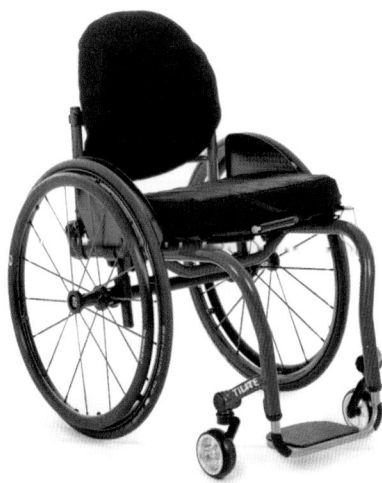

Figure 32.29 Wheelchair frame with adjustable axle plates, adjustable forks, and adjustable back posts to achieve specific heights and frame angles. *(Courtesy of Permobil, Lebanon, TN 37090.)*

frame height in relation to the rear frame can increase foot and caster clearance. Similarly, this configuration can provide a person with difficulty sitting upright in a fixed tilt position for gravity-assisted positioning.

Some power wheelchairs also have adjustable seat frames that can be adjusted for seat height and fixed tilt, depending on the style of the wheelchair. Power wheelchairs that have a base and separate seating system come preconfigured for seat height and angle if specified when ordering the wheelchair. Most power wheelchairs have limited adjustability after delivery. Configuration considerations are an important part of the selection process, as decisions can affect the person's ability for function (e.g., transfers, reaching, sitting balance, sitting endurance).

Many manual and power wheelchairs and most tilt-in-space wheelchairs have the capacity for one or more back post angle adjustments allowing configuration to meet the person's identified seat to back angle needs. The identified seat to back angle may determine which frame options are available. Some wheelchairs only have 10° of adjustment while others have 30° or more of adjustment.

For a person who can tolerate a fixed tilt or fixed recline position, an adjustable seat to back angle feature may be all that is needed to accommodate a person with a mild hip flexion limitation or a person who is unable to tolerate sitting upright but who does not need a variable tilt-in-space system. Opening the seat to back angle 5° to 15° alone (fixed recline) or in combination with adjusting the seat position (fixed tilt) can help position the person for better balance, sitting tolerance, and comfort. Specifying the configuration of the wheelchair frame is as important as verifying it has accomplished the intended objective, which is assessed at the fitting and delivery and fine-tuned as necessary.

Wheelchair Frame Options

There are many wheelchair accessories, a few of which are highlighted here. *Anti-tippers* are used to prevent a wheelchair from tipping rearward. *Wheel lock extensions* are used on a manual wheelchair to increase the lever and ease of applying or removing the wheel lock. Various wheel lock styles are available (e.g., push to lock, pull to lock, scissor, low mount, high mount). Wheelchair *push handles* are available in a variety of shapes and configurations (fixed, flip down, removeable), depending on the person's needs. If a person uses the push handles to hook for balance during weight shift or clothing adjustments, a particular height and durable style may be required. If a person is lifted while in their wheelchair by the push handles, removable handles are not advised. If a person is dependent for mobility, the push handle height or the addition of an *adjustable stroller handle* may be needed for the caregiver, especially when there is a height difference between caregivers or when used on a pediatric or tilt-in-space wheelchair.

Wheelchair securement sites (transportation securement brackets or *transport option*) are an important feature to consider for individuals transported while riding in their wheelchair. Many transport options meet voluntary safety standards for vehicle crash testing and are important to discuss during the ordering process.

These are only a few of the multitude of available wheelchair options and accessories. Manufacturers offer a variety of accessories available with their wheelchair bases. There also exist numerous manufacturers that offer accessories that are not product specific (aftermarket manufacturers). Importantly, review the identified objectives and determine if additional wheelchair accessories or options are required prior to completing the final recommendation.

Attachment Mechanisms

Options and accessories are attached to the wheelchair frame in different ways. Decisions about options include, but are not limited to, attachment style (fixed, removeable, swing-away), release (push button, lever, cam lock, and so forth), durability (heavy duty, shock absorbing), and functionality (swing out, swing in, lift off, and so forth). These important decisions can be the difference between independence and the need for assistance. Specifying the objective, feature, and rationale in your documentation will support the medical necessity for the items requested. Examples related to foot and arm supports follow.

FOOT SUPPORT ASSEMBLY

The foot support assembly (footrest) includes the components that mount the foot support surface to the frame of the wheelchair. Most foot support assemblies are mounted from the side rails of the frame while some systems are center mounted on the wheelchair. The foot support assembly may be fixed, lift off, or swing in or out. In the case of rigid manual wheelchairs, the foot support assembly is most often not removeable but may flip up and may include a swing-away option.

Transfer style and final foot position placement (determined during the wheelchair assessment) will affect decision-making and selection. If a person transfers independently, retaining independence and the ability to manage foot support are essential. Each wheelchair manufacturer provides different release mechanisms for moving the foot support assembly out of the way, and dexterity will dictate which option will work best. A footplate or foot platform are components of the foot support assembly that are also an important part of the technology selection. These may include dual-sided, standard size, non-adjustable, large, or angle adjustable, as well as a single platform. If using a flip-up style foot plate, it is important to verify that the person can lift the foot plate out of the way. If the person transfers independently and the footplate position interferes, they must be able to move the foot support assembly out of the way but still be close enough to transfer safely to a toilet, bed, or chair. In this example, a swing-in foot support may be desirable.

ARM SUPPORT ASSEMBLY

The arm support assembly is the components of the wheelchair that attach the arm support surface to the frame of the wheelchair. Different styles may include single post, dual post, tubular swing-away, and flip-up mounted to back cane.

The arm support assembly is chosen when finalizing the wheelchair. The method to release and remove the arm support is discussed, and functional issues such as transfer type, pressure relief technique, and durability are considered. The style of transfer, access to tables, and ability to move the arm support out of the way independently will determine which arm support assembly is optimal. In addition, the armrest pad style, length (full versus desk), and width are also important options that must be determined.

Manual Wheeled Mobility Devices

Manual wheeled mobility devices are used by a person with a mobility limitation and require the occupant or an attendant to move it. There are five types of devices in this category: manual wheelchairs, variable positioning manual wheelchairs, dependent mobility wheelchairs, ADL-specific manual wheelchairs, and sports-specific manual wheelchairs (refer to Fig. 32.27). Each are presented below and classified or grouped by features and functions.

Manual Wheelchairs

NONADJUSTABLE FRAME

The most basic type of manual wheelchair has no frame adjustability (wheel axle position, caster position, seat to back angle, armrest height, leg rest or footplate

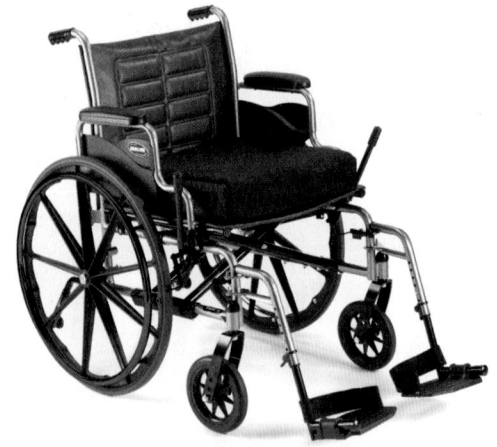

Figure 32.30 Upright manual wheelchair with nonadjustable frame. *(Courtesy of Invacare Corporation, Elyria, OH 44035.)*

position). It is typically available in limited sizes (e.g., 16 in., 18 in. seat width and depth) (Fig. 32.30). Sling seat and back upholstery is the standard option on this style wheelchair. Standard armrests are fixed height (non/removeable), with desk length or full length arm pads. Leg rests are frequently nonremoveable and fixed (not swing away) with flip-up footrests that are only length adjustable in a limited range. Removeable height adjustable armrests and elevating swing away leg rests may be available and ordered separately depending on the manufacturer.

A basic nonadjustable wheelchair allows the user to be moved from place to place to safely perform or participate in daily tasks. A basic manual wheelchair is typically used as a rental or for temporary/intermittent use. Few options are available to properly fit this wheelchair to the user's size or positioning needs. This type of basic wheelchair is primarily for individuals who cannot independently self-propel, require a wheelchair intermittently for short durations (<2 hours), and transfer to other sitting surfaces frequently throughout the day.

MINIMALLY ADJUSTABLE FRAME

Wheelchairs that meet this frame description generally provide more limited adjustability (e.g., limited vertical and/or horizontal wheel axle options, limited caster positions and options). These wheelchairs may have additional seat widths, depths, and seat to floor heights than the non-adjustable frame.

This type of wheelchair will allow the user to move or be moved from place to place to perform daily tasks, typically in accommodated environments. Minimally adjustable configurations may allow a fixed hemi height (lower seat to floor height) or standard seat to floor height for self-propulsion (e.g., hemi-propulsion, LE propulsion) or to facilitate independence with transfers. Sling seat and back upholstery are standard options on these wheelchairs. However, the seat and back upholstery can be removed and replaced with a firm support with bracket hardware or adjustable tension upholstery to imitate a slightly opened seat to back angle. Although the seat upholstery can be removed, for the seat it is more common to insert a solid seat surface under the cover of a cushioned seat that is then Velcroed to the wheelchair seat upholstery. Changes to the configuration of the wheelchair are only functional if the wheelchair has the capacity to adjust caster alignment perpendicular to the floor to optimize rolling ability; otherwise, this adjustment will make self-propulsion more difficult.

FULLY CONFIGURABLE FRAME

Fully configurable frames are the most complex type of manual wheelchairs and are categorized as CRT. This category includes wheelchairs with modular and non-modular frames.

Modular wheelchair frames have a seat frame, side frame, front rigging(s), and rear frame. Modular frames can either fold (side to side, front to back) or are rigid. These frames can be modified after delivery, for a cost, by ordering replacement frame parts to reconfigure the frame to meet the changing needs of the person (e.g., weight, height, function). This wheelchair can accommodate a more complex seating system and is indicated for an individual with a changing condition or disorder that requires a more supportive seating system. Configurable frame adjustments (i.e., seat to back angle, seat depth, back height, rear wheel axle position, camber, seat inclination angle, seat to floor height, caster alignment) (Fig. 32.31) provide a means to adequately configure the wheelchair to meet an individual's moderate and/or

changing postural support and functional needs at the time of order, at the time of delivery, and to meet anticipated future needs. Configuring the wheelchair to the individual is necessary to enhance wheelchair propulsion, improve maneuverability, and minimize rolling resistance. Also, configurable frame adjustments can improve sitting posture by accommodating hip and knee contractures, improve sitting balance, and improve transfer and access to tables for function. These wheelchairs often have folding back canes and removeable rear wheels, allowing for disassembly for transportation and stowage.

Rigid frame (nonmodular) wheelchairs are welded solid frames, designed, and built to provide an intimate fit based on individual measurements. As a result, there is limited adjustability after delivery (e.g., wheel axle position, camber, seat to back angle, back height) (Fig. 32.32). Changes to the frame base requires a new wheelchair frame. Consequently, it is rare for a nonmodular rigid wheelchair to be recommended as a first wheelchair for new manual wheelchair users and are instead more often recommended for people with stable conditions.

Rigid frame wheelchairs (nonmodular and modular) by design have less hardware and moving parts because they have less adjustability; therefore, these wheelchairs are often lighter in weight than folding frame wheelchairs. The rigid frame also reduces frame flex or movement, making them more durable and efficient for propulsion. By design, these wheelchairs have a smaller front rigging profile, shortening the overall length and optimizing maneuverability.

Rigid frame wheelchairs are typically used by an active person who puts great demands on the wheelchair frame and parts. Usually, this individual is independent

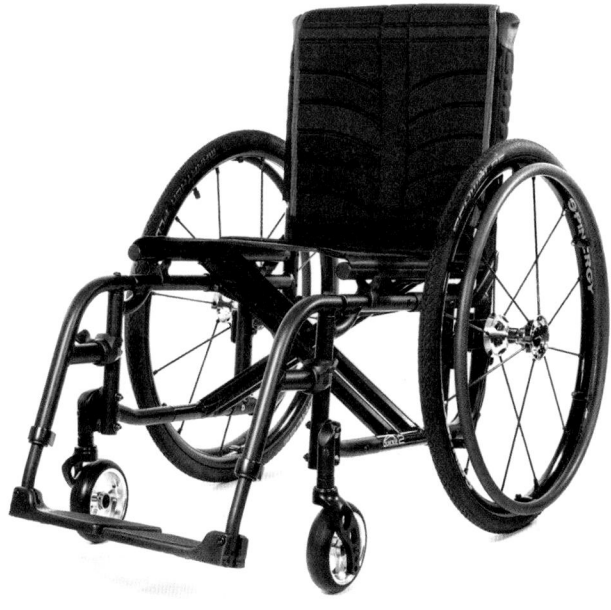

Figure 32.31 Fully configurable manual wheelchair. *(Courtesy of Sunrise Medical, Fresno, CA 93727.)*

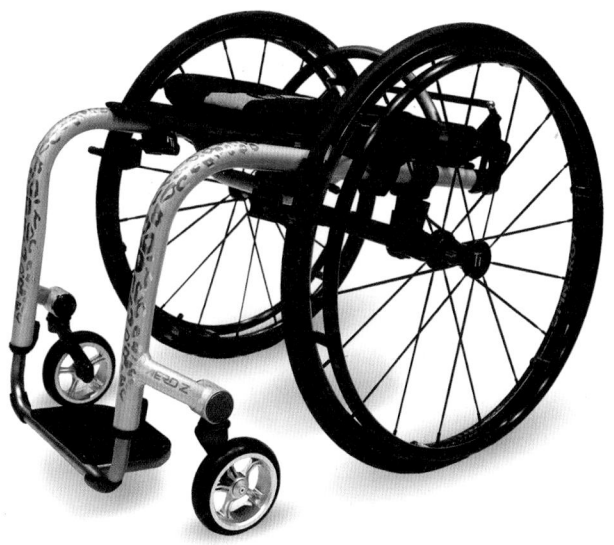

Figure 32.32 Fully configurable rigid frame manual wheelchair showing back support in fold-down position. Rear wheels are removable for transportation and stowage. *(Courtesy of Permobil, Lebanon, TN 37090.)*

and safe negotiating ordinary environmental obstacles (e.g., door thresholds), can achieve and maintain a rear wheel balancing position (wheelie), maneuvers in and around doors, safely negotiates ramps, and requires a specially configured wheelchair for maximum independent functioning. The majority of rigid frames have a fixed front end (leg angle, foot supports and caster position); as a result, LE management during transfers need to be considered.

PROPULSION CONFIGURATION

There are four typical methods of manual wheelchair self-propulsion: (1) both UE, (2) both LE, (3) hemi-propulsion, and (4) all four extremities.

Both UE (BUE) propulsion is the most common method used, requiring good UE function, strength, and muscular endurance. The location of the drive wheel in relation to the user is critical for efficiency and proper UE body mechanics.

Most manual wheelchairs are configured with rear drive wheels. However, drive wheels can also be positioned in the center or front of the base, as primarily seen and used with children (Fig. 32.33). Positioning the drive wheels in different configurations can improve the ability to access and propel the wheelchair. This is especially critical when considering the possible implications for long-term function of the shoulder girdle and to minimize risk for *repetitive strain injuries* (RSIs).

RSIs can result in damage to soft tissue (tendons, ligaments, nerves) or bony structures secondary to frequent repeated motions such as wheelchair push strokes. The damage can include inflammation, compression, and/or tears in the shoulder joint and surrounding structures, resulting in pain and decreased function.[61,62]

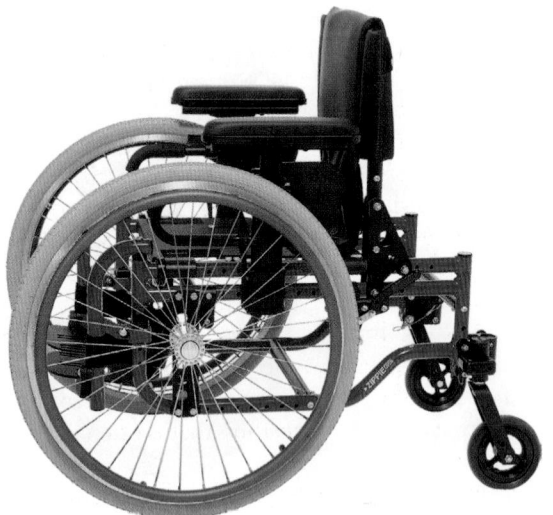

Figure 32.33 Wheelchairs with large front wheels and small rear casters may be easier for some people to push but are more difficult to use outdoors. *(Courtesy of Sunrise Medical, Fresno, CA 93727.)*

RSIs are often seen in the shoulders, wrists, and hands of wheelchair users. Even persons without documented RSIs report increased pain in these joints with prolonged wheelchair use.[61,63] Small muscles are required to produce large forces repeatedly to move the wheelchair through space. These same muscles are typically required for a variety of ADL tasks such as transfers and reaching, thus increasing the demands placed on the same muscles and the potential of causing injury. Prolonged wheelchair use and/or improper wheelchair configuration can result in muscle imbalances, pain, and injury. Stress on the muscles and joints increases with wheelchair rolling resistance, overall wheelchair weight (frame, seating, user, accessories, backpacks, and so forth), and environmental factors (terrain, surface type, and so forth). RSI symptoms may not be felt until the condition is well advanced. Common conditions include rotator cuff injuries, medial epicondylitis, and carpal tunnel syndrome.

When prescribing wheelchairs and features for people who are able to self-propel, consideration must be given to minimizing risk for RSIs by carefully evaluating the position of the person in relation to the drive wheel to decrease stress and strain on the shoulders, elbows, wrists, and hands. Importantly, UE positioning must allow for an efficient stroke, reducing the force needed per stroke and the frequency of strokes required to move the wheelchair. Attention to shoulder biomechanics and alignment is critical.

For efficient pushing, the elbows should be bent at an angle of about 120° when the hands are resting atop the push rims. The wheelchair user should be able to comfortably reach the front and back of the push rim at the height of the wheel axle. To attain this position, the wheels need to be adjusted horizontally (fore and aft), and the wheels or seat need to be adjusted vertically. The back height and camber of the wheels are adjusted so that the arms and shoulder girdle are unrestricted over the entire propulsion phase.[64-66] Frequently, there are trade-offs between optimal position for propulsion and configuration needed for function or environmental access that need to be discussed and decided.

Some people with functional use of one UE (e.g., hemiplegia) use a one-arm drive mechanism for self-propulsion. The one-arm drive mechanism has two concentric handrims of different sizes mounted on one wheel, on the side being used to propel the wheelchair. The outer rim controls one wheel, enabling the wheelchair to turn in one direction; the inner rim controls the other wheel, enabling the wheelchair to turn in the other direction. Propelling both rims simultaneously enables the wheelchair to move forward and backward (Fig. 32.34). A one-arm drive mechanism is useful for maneuvering/aligning the wheelchair and moving short distances; however, it is seldom effective for efficient independent self-propulsion in a range of environments.

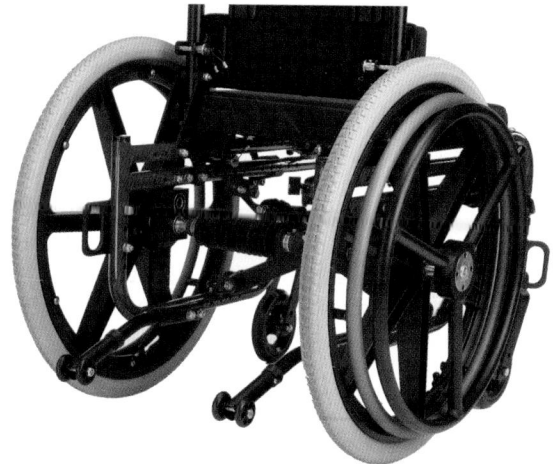

Figure 32.34 A double handrim on one side allows the user to propel a one-arm drive wheelchair with one hand. *(Courtesy of Sunrise Medical, Fresno, CA 93727.)*

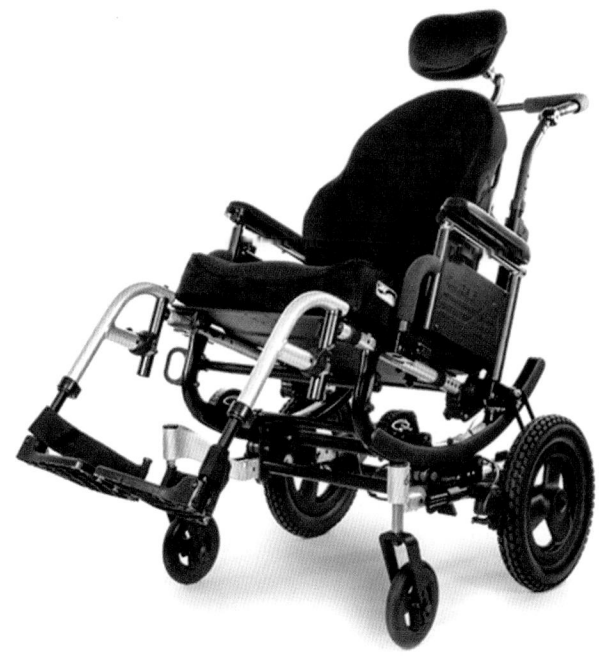

Figure 32.35 A manual wheelchair with tilt to assist with positioning, pressure relief, and posture. *(Courtesy of Sunrise Medical, Fresno, CA 93727.)*

Self-propulsion with both LEs requires a low seat to floor height so the person can firmly plant their foot on the floor without sliding forward in the wheelchair.

The hemi-propulsion method of self-propulsion uses a combination of one arm and one leg. Care is taken to configure the wheelchair with a seat to floor height to enable LE propulsion, positioning of the person in relation to the drive wheel, and drive wheel placement for maximal UE contact with the wheel. In this configuration, the person uses their hand and foot together to propel the wheel and steer.

For people who use all four extremities to self-propel, the same wheelchair setup needs are considered as described above.

Variable Positioning Manual Wheelchairs

Variable positioning manual wheelchairs are available in a range of pediatric and adult sizes and may include tilt, recline, tilt and recline, and standing features.

Tilt

A manual wheelchair with a variable tilt system allows for frequent angular repositioning of the seat and back, within a predefined range, relative to upright, whereby the seat orientation in space (relative to gravity) changes to assist with positioning, pressure relief, and posture (Fig. 32.35). Manual tilt systems are mostly operated by a caregiver; however, there exist a few manual tilt systems that can be self-operated by the user, and a few power tilt systems that can be configured on a manual wheelchair operated by the user. There exist *positioning tilt systems* (usually ~ 0° to 25°) and *full tilt systems* (>45°). In order to be considered a *full tilt system*, for purposes of effective weight shifting (moving body weight from the seat to the back) the wheelchair needs to tilt at least 45°. Both types of tilt systems can be

moved through the available ROM, incrementally, and as often as needed for repositioning.

A positioning tilt system (usually ~ 0° to 25°) is typically used to accommodate for muscle weakness, paralysis, or fatigue of neck and trunk muscles; to provide a neutral head/neck position for safe swallowing and saliva control; and to provide gravity-assisted positioning for rest and when traversing challenging terrain. A few manufacturers offer a positional tilt system that can be operated by the user to change their position independently; however, most products require caregiver operation of the tilt system. Table 32.4 presents evidence for the use of positional tilt systems.[67-79]

A primary benefit of a full tilt system (>45°) is pressure relief/pressure redistribution, which is accomplished by shifting weight and pressure away from the bony prominences under the pelvis to the posterior pelvis and back. Increasing the amount of tilt exponentially increases the amount of pressure redistributed away from the pelvis. Beyond 45°, the body weight starts to load through the back surface, providing pressure relief/pressure redistribution, minimizing the shear forces and the potential loss of user position that is often associated with recline.[80]

The location of the tilt pivot will determine various aspects of tilt. Two of the most common tilt pivot types are center of gravity (COG) pivot (curvilinear or adjustable pivot) and front (knee) pivot (Fig. 32.36). A front pivot tilt keeps knee height constant as the tilt system lowers the rear of the frame so the feet can be

Table 32.4   Evidence Summary Studies Addressing the Impact of Positional Tilt Less Than 45°

Aissaoui et al. (2002)[106]

Design	Experimental design with randomized repeated measures
Level of Evidence	IIB: Moderate Evidence
Subjects	14 older (range 64–77 yrs) experienced wheelchair users living independently. Eligibility criteria: (1) able to propel WC on a daily basis with two-hand synchronous pattern, (2) no pressure sores >1 year, (3) able to give informed consent, (4) able to propel for a period of 10 minutes during a 1-hr experiment
Intervention	Three seat-to-back rest angles (95°, 100°, and 105°) and three system tilt angles (0°, 5°, and 10°) were selected. The nine conditions were randomized for each subject. Rear wheel camber was set at 0° and handrim and rear wheel radii were 0.267 meters and 0.305 meters, respectively. The horizontal distance between the wheel axle and the acromion marker in the sagittal plane was set to 4 centimeters independent of tilt and backrest positioning. Subjects were asked to propel on a friction roller cylinder ergometer between 0.96 and 1.01 m/sec.
Results	The kinetics of wheelchair propulsion can be affected by seat and backrest adjustments. System tilt angle but not back recline significantly affects biomechanical efficiency.
Comments	Tilting the system by 10° and reclining the back by 10° increase the biomechanical efficiency of the subject by 10%. This is a very important finding for older adults, many of whom benefit from positional tilt system for enhancement in mobility, postural support, and pain management.

Desroches et al. (2006)[107]

Design	Experimental design
Level of Evidence	IIB: Moderate Evidence
Design	14 elderly MWC users, seven women and seven men, mean age 68.2 +/– 5.2 yr; use BUE for self-propulsion daily, no pressure ulcers for >1 yr able to propel MWC 6 meters < 30 seconds, informed consent, 1 yr minimum MWC use
Level of Evidence	Friction roller cylinder to control resistance—all subjects used the same wheelchair, and the seat and backrest had independent movement. STA 0°, 5°, 10° and SBA 95°, 100°, and 105° (configurations were randomly tested twice)
Subjects	No significant difference for the various STA and SBA combinations were revealed. Changing the seat angle while keeping the wheel-axle position constant in both vertical and horizontal locations maintained the shoulder load at the same level.
Intervention	Seat angle can be determined with goals of user comfort and decreasing risk for pressure ulcers without increasing risk of overuse shoulder injuries. Positional tilt systems may be used for comfort, posture management, or pressure management without interfering with independent propulsion.

Dewey et al. (2004)[108]

Design	Qualitative research design. Phenomenology aims to reveal the different experiences of a phenomenon by talking about it.
Level of Evidence	IVC: Weak evidence
Subjects	Inclusion criteria: were severely disabled, full-time wheelchair users requiring hoisting, had significant spasticity. Exclusion criteria: low tone, posture problems unrelated to spasticity. Where possible, caregivers were invited to participate; 23 participants— tilt in space WC *n* = 7 (manual *n* = 2, power *n* = 5) and conventional WC users *n* = 16 (manual *n* = 8, power *n* = 8).

Table 32.4 Evidence Summary Studies Addressing the Impact of Positional Tilt Less Than 45°—cont'd

Dewey et al. (2004)[108]

Intervention	Participants were asked the following questions: What were the experiences of conventional/tilt-in-space WCs and the benefits and disadvantages of their present wheelchair? What other factors influenced the quality of life of people with MS who had significant spasticity and were full-time wheelchair users?
Results	Tilt-in-space WCs offer acceptable levels of comfort and enable severely disabled people with MS to sit out of bed for many hours, requiring fewer transfers throughout the day, which is important to them. Tilt-in-space wheelchairs are described as comfortable, and clients can rest for many hours in them without the need to return to bed. Overall benefits included increased comfort, improved postural support and control through gravity-assisted positioning, enhanced sitting stability, and improved pressure management. Difficulties reported were bulkiness or reduced maneuverability of the device and difficulty transporting the device in the community. Use of a tilt-in-space WC usually involves buying a rear access adapted vehicle. Overall, participants reported higher satisfaction with positional tilt systems (six out of seven) compared to a control group using conventional wheelchairs (eight out of 16).
Comments	The study showed that medical professionals are often most focused on physical health while clients are more concerned with vitality, general health, and mental health rather than physical disability.

Stavness (2006)[109]

Design	Evidence Review
Level of Evidence	IIB: Moderate evidence
Subjects	Sixteen journal articles published after 1980 were used. Specific key terms were searched: positioning, wheelchair, postural control, posture, adaptive seating devices, patient positioning, CP, movement disorders, UE, reaching, grasping, and occupational therapy. Articles were excluded if they were purely descriptive, did not involve children with CP, included surgery as part of the intervention, explored only one individual case, did not study UE function, or were published before 1980.
Intervention	This review focuses on determining the most appropriate sitting positioning for children with CP to promote energy conservation and optimal functional abilities.
Results	Neutral pelvic positioning does improve functional abilities. Children with CP benefit most from the entire functional sitting positioning package rather than some components (i.e., minus tray and/or abduction orthoses). Neutral or forward positioning show the greatest long-term UE functional improvements (whole wheelchair tilted).
Comments	Evidence supports that an upright position improves a child with CP's UE function such as reaching and pressing to use a communication device. Children with CP should be fitted with a wheelchair that places them in a functional sitting position. The exact seat tilt should be determined on an individual basis. One should ensure that the line of gravity from the child's trunk, shoulders, and head are anterior to his/her ischial tuberosities. A more upright position would force the child to waste energy to fight against his/her trunk. This energy can be used for functional tasks. Individuals with neuromuscular conditions may benefit from positional tilt system to optimize postural control, maximize comfort, and facilitate control of their UE depending on position of the tilt.

BUE = both upper extremities; CP = cerebral palsy; MS = multiple sclerosis; MWC = manual wheelchair; SBA = seat to backrest angle; STA = system tilt angle; UE = upper extremity; WC = wheelchair.

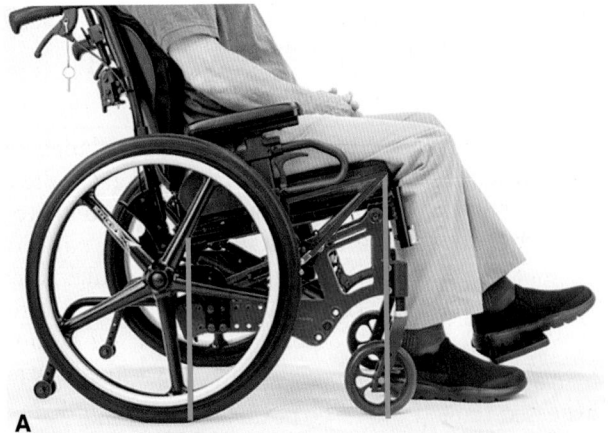

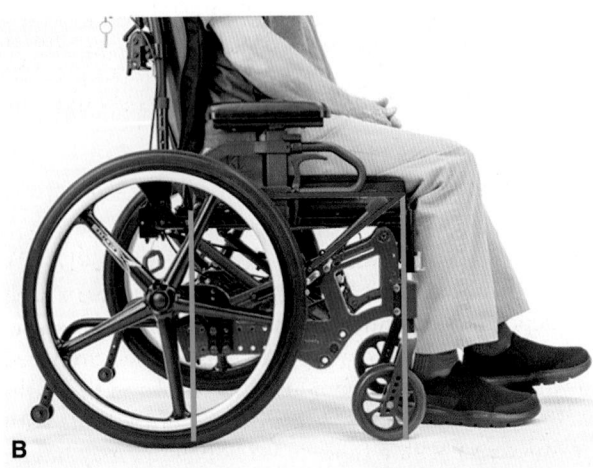

Figure 32.36 A manual wheelchair with front (knee pivot) tilt system. Please note that the foot is flat on the ground in both the upright and tilted positions to improve foot propulsion. *(Courtesy of Ki Mobility, Stevens Point, WI 54481)*

maintained on the floor even when tilted 20°. This feature therefore may allow for self-propulsion with arms and/or foot propulsion. Also, the user may be rolled up to a table even while in tilt. If manual propulsion is a goal, the individual should trial the various systems to determine if the rear wheels can be configured for effective propulsion of the wheelchair. With a COG tilt, the person's COG aligns with the center of rotation of the tilt mechanism, there is no displacement of the person's COG, the tilt system shifts the seating system through an arc of movement to maintain or improve the stability of the wheelchair and prevent tipping rearward. With increasing tilt, the knee height rises and the back height lowers. This may compromise surface access (e.g., table/desk), and should be considered if needed while in a tilted position. An individual with good UE function may be able to effectively self-propel a COG style tilt wheelchair but it is rarely effective for functional daily mobility, dependent on wheel position and the amount of tilt needed during propulsion. Different wheelchair

frames with tilt need to be tested to determine which wheelchair is optimal for self-propulsion.

RECLINE

A reclining wheelchair has a manually adjustable seat to back angle to allow for a change in position (Fig. 32.37). The recline feature is operated by a caregiver and may be used to accommodate a hip extension contracture or cast; change of position to minimize an individual's risk of contracture or pain; weight relief/pressure redistribution; rest, gravity-assisted positioning and to perform functional tasks without transferring out of the wheelchair (e.g., catheterizing, clothing change).

A reclining wheelchair is typically used as a rental item for a temporary need (such as status post-surgery, spica cast, halo, and so forth) or may be used with an individual who requires changes in position due to medical condition(s) such as autonomic dysreflexia or hypotension.

This wheelchair is available in a very limited number of seat widths and depths. Although a reclining wheelchair is not designed for self-propulsion, a user may have the ability to maneuver the wheelchair if they have functional UE ROM and strength to adjust their alignment at a table for eating, a sink for hygiene, or a desk for writing or computer use. The rear wheel axles are set at or behind the wheelchair back canes to increase the base of support and stability needed for safety as the back support is reclined. By design, this increases

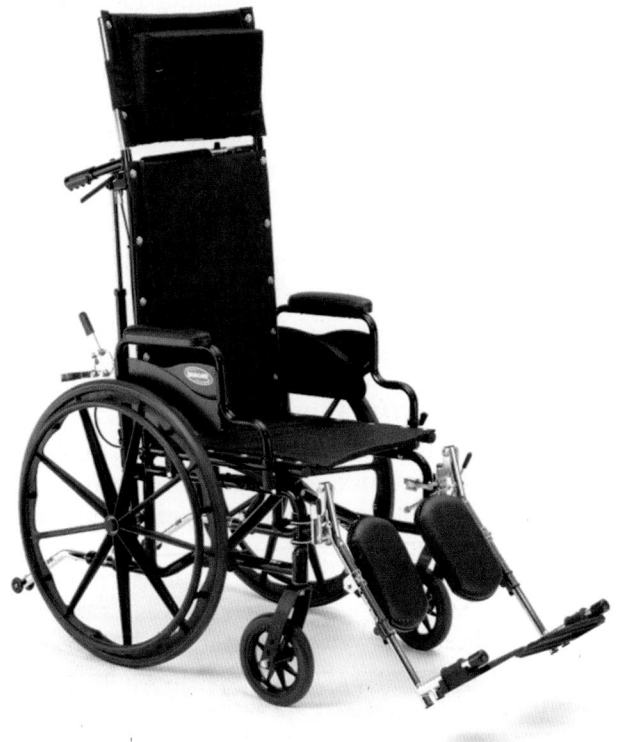

Figure 32.37 A manual wheelchair with adjustable back recline. *(Courtesy of Invacare Corporation, Elyria, OH 44035.)*

the length of the wheelchair and makes UE access to the wheels problematic. Reclining wheelchairs have the largest overall turning radius of manual wheelchairs making accessibility and maneuverability challenging or impossible in most homes. Most individuals who require this type of wheelchair for support require maximum assistance, are dependent in mobility, and do not have the potential to independently self-propel. Reclining manual wheelchairs do not allow for individual configuration for full time wheelchair users with moderate and/or changing postural support needs but instead are frequently used as a rental item for a temporary or changing need until stabilized.

TILT AND RECLINE

Few manual wheelchairs have a combination of tilt and recline for positioning, pressure relief, personal care, and posture. In most cases, the person who uses a combination manual tilt/recline wheelchair has a fixed recline (e.g., open seat to back angle to accommodate a postural deformity) with a variable full tilt system. Not many manufacturers offer a combination of variable tilt and variable recline. Most models have limitations on the amount of recline and/or tilt offered due to safety and wheelchair frame stability.

STANDING

A standing manual wheelchair offers a means for independent mobility plus enables the person to move from a sitting to standing position for weight-bearing and pressure redistribution (relief) in a single device (Fig. 32.38A, B, C). The wheelchair standing mechanism requires the person to use their own arm strength with a hydraulic assist mechanism to move from a sitting to a standing position. Therefore, the person must be able to independently self-propel and have sufficient UE strength to operate this feature. The standing mechanism does increase the overall weight of the wheelchair but enables the person to independently and frequently change their position throughout the day as needed to stand, stretch, reach, and work without needing to transfer to a dedicated standing device.

Dependent Mobility Wheelchairs

Depending on the person's positioning and mobility needs, they may require a manual wheelchair frame (discussed previously) even though the person may not be able to self-propel.

TRANSPORT CHAIRS

Transport wheelchairs have four small wheels with sling seat and back upholstery (Fig. 32.39). These wheelchairs tend to be lightweight and are easily folded and lifted by a caregiver and transported by car. Due to limited postural support, this type of wheelchair is intended for short-term use and is primarily used to assist moving a person from point A to point B. People who have

the ability or potential to self-propel should consider a manual wheelchair base instead.

STROLLERS

Pediatric and adult adaptive strollers are included in this category (Fig. 32.40). Like transport chairs, these devices are lightweight, offer minimal support, and provide for folding and ease of transport. Some strollers are available with added positioning features, including tilt, recline, and combination tilt/recline. Many adaptive strollers have been voluntarily tested by manufacturers to meet transportation safety standards (e.g. crash test). If needed, an integrated transit option can be purchased. This is an important consideration if a person is transported while riding in the device. Many children use adaptive strollers with transit options to ride the adapted school bus. Once again, people who have the ability or potential to self-propel should consider a manual wheelchair base instead.

ADL-Specific Wheelchairs

ADL-specific manual wheelchairs include shower wheelchairs and toilet/commode wheelchairs (Fig. 32.41A, B). These wheelchairs have either small or large drive wheels for dependent or independent propulsion. These specialty wheelchairs allow a person to transfer from bed to wheelchair in one room and then move to the bathroom to perform ADLs. These devices often come with a padded seat with a front or side opening, may have a commode pail, and are usually made of materials that will endure water (e.g., aluminum, stainless steel, plastic). There are a variety of adjustable systems available in this category, but most devices offer limited positioning options. For people with more complex postural needs, specialty rehab commode chairs are available with tilt, recline, and a range of primary and secondary postural supports.

Sports-Specific Manual Wheelchair

Many wheelchair users are active in recreational and competitive sports. As a result, the person may use more than one wheelchair: a daily-use wheelchair and a specially designed *competition* or *recreational wheelchair* to meet the demands of the activity or sport.

Wheelchair features to consider when aiming for wheelchair performance include the ability to camber the wheels (move top of the wheel closer to the user and the bottom farther away) to provide a more stable wheelchair. A durable wheelchair frame built to endure high impact, such as a rigid frame with large-diameter tubing, made with high-strength, lightweight materials, will increase the strength, durability, and lifetime of the wheelchair.

When properly configured for the individual, wheel and caster placement, tire type, axle position, and bearings make a significant difference in wheelchair performance. Users who participate in more than one activity

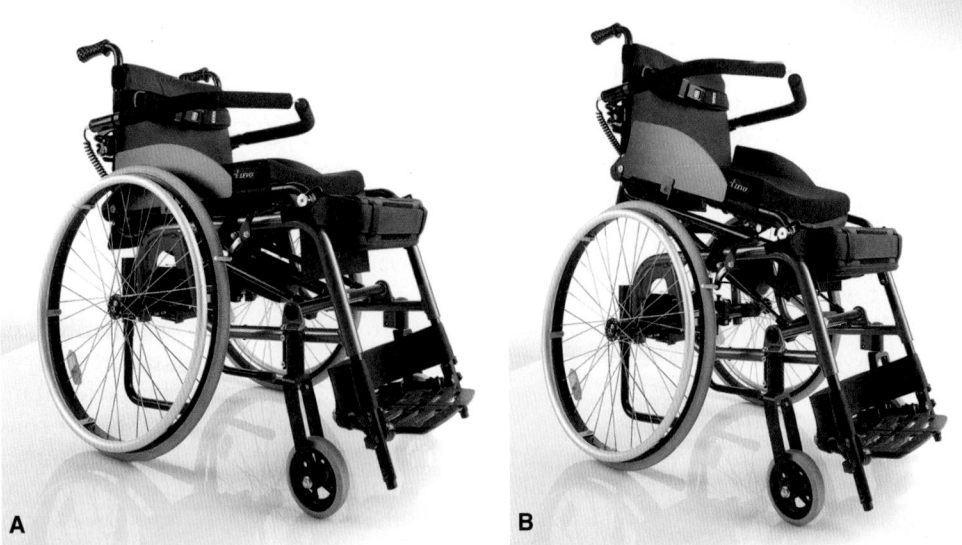

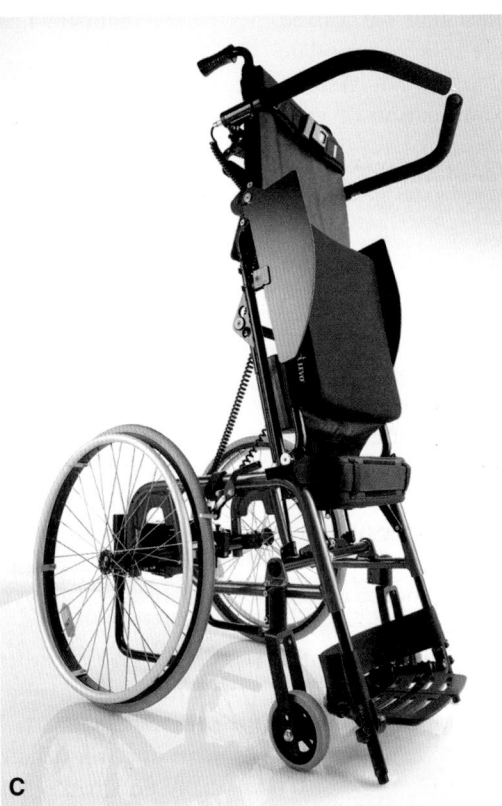

Figure 32.38 A manual wheelchair with a standing feature. (A) Sitting position. (B) Semi-standing position. (C) Full standing position. *(Courtesy of Levo USA Inc., Brooklyn Park, MN 55443.)*

may prefer a sports wheelchair with a great deal of adjustability (with or without tools) to allow changes to the wheelchair configuration for various activities (e.g., changing shoes) versus requiring multiple sports wheelchairs.

Specialty wheelchairs are designed for a specific category of sports. For example, a tennis wheelchair (Fig. 32.42) is designed with a low COM with built-in camber for responsiveness, stability, and control. The

functionality of this type of wheelchair also meets the demands needed for dancing. A basketball wheelchair (Fig. 32.43) and other contact-sport wheelchairs (e.g., rugby and soccer) (Fig. 32.44) are designed for maneuverability, durability, and stability. All-terrain wheelchairs have wide wheelbases for stability and large casters and rear wheel tires with knobby tread to optimize traction and maneuverability for self-propulsion on uneven ground and terrain (Fig. 32.45). Road racing

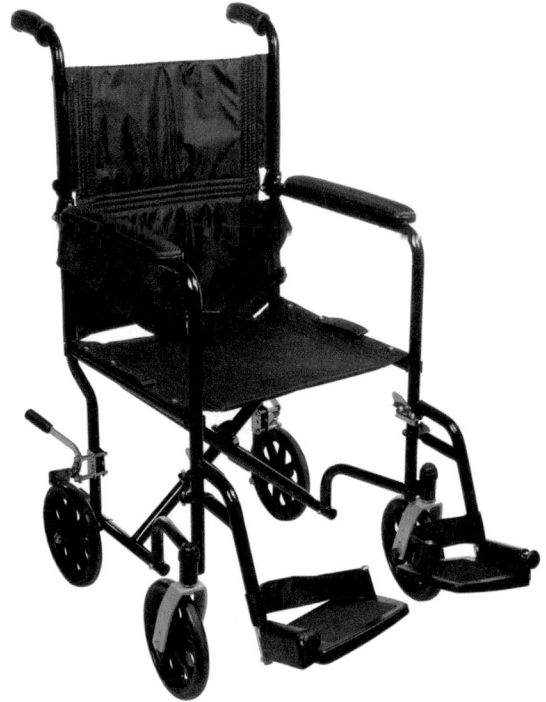

Figure 32.39 A transport wheelchair with sling back and seat upholstery. *(Courtesy of Sunrise Medical, Fresno, CA 93727.)*

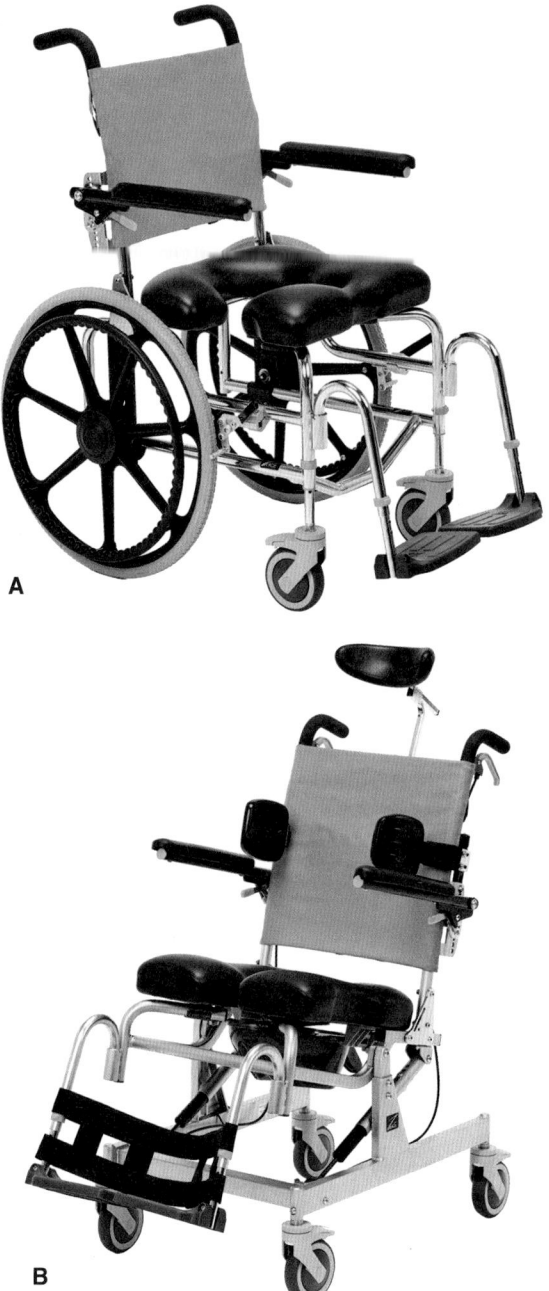

A

B

Figure 32.41 (A) A basic upright toilet/commode chair. (B) A shower chair with the tilt feature that can be used as a commode chair as well. *(Courtesy of Raz Designs, Niagara Falls, NY 14305.)*

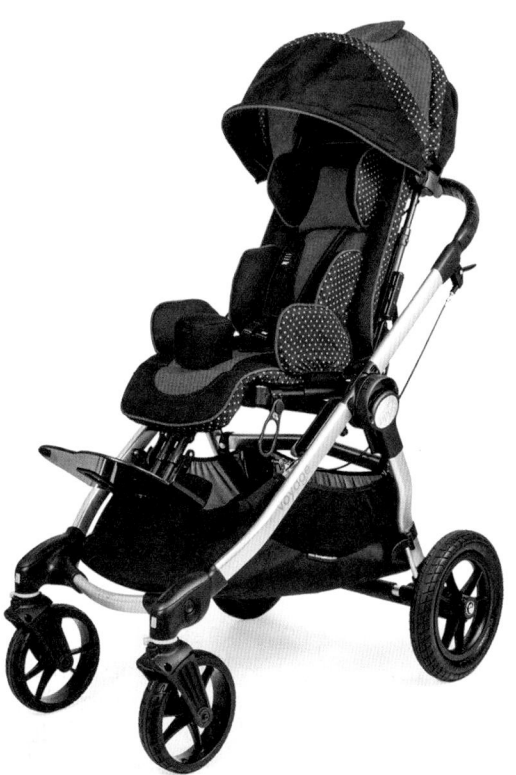

Figure 32.40 A pediatric adaptive stroller with moderate seating support. *(Courtesy of Sunrise Medical, Fresno, CA 93727.)*

wheelchairs support the person in a tucked position. By design, these wheelchairs are built low to the ground to minimize wind resistance and increase propulsion efficiency (Fig. 32.46). Specialty beach wheelchairs are available for people for attendant-assisted access on sand and for beach swimming (Fig. 32.47).

A competition/recreational wheelchair is not traditionally covered by most medical insurance plans; however, it is often covered for veterans through their benefits. Various philanthropic organizations and

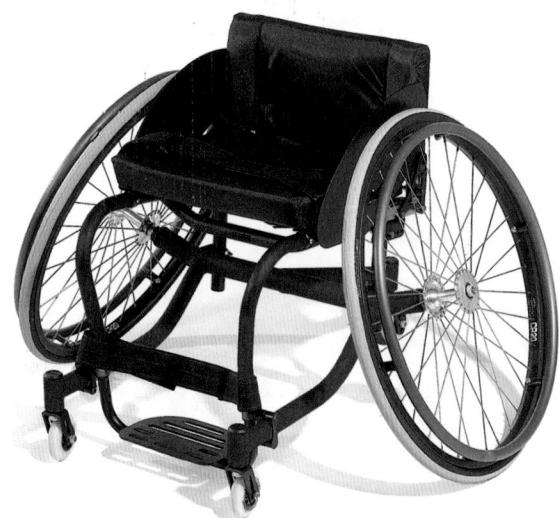

Figure 32.42 A sports wheelchair designed for tennis. Note the low back and cambered wheels. *(Courtesy of Sunrise Medical, Fresno, CA 93727.)*

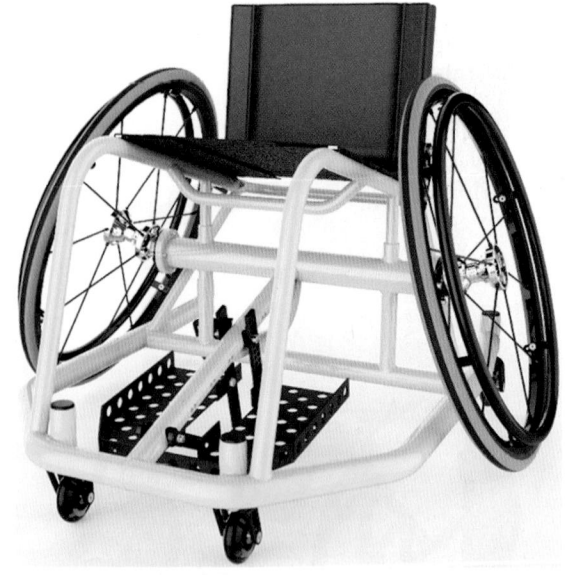

Figure 32.44 A contact sports wheelchair designed for rigidity and strength. *(Courtesy of Colours, Corona, CA 92879.)*

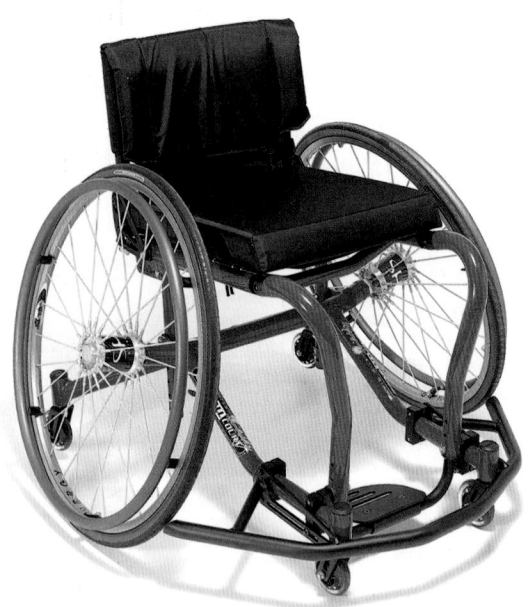

Figure 32.43 A basketball wheelchair designed for maneuverability and power that can be used for other court sports. *(Courtesy of Sunrise Medical, Fresno, CA 93727.)*

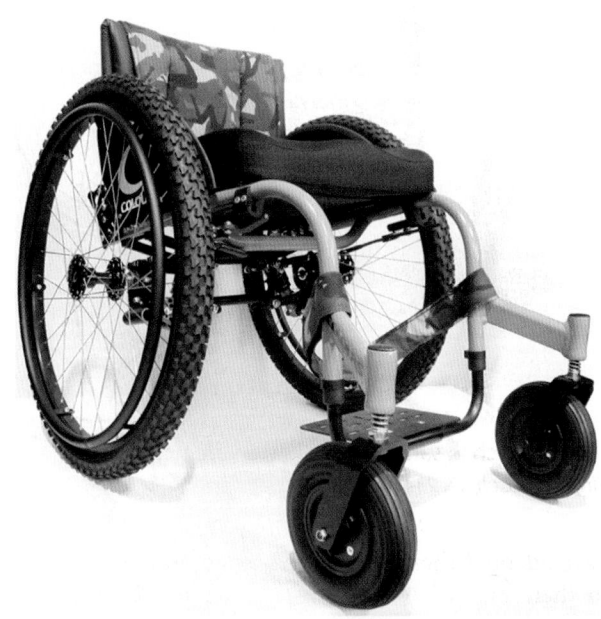

Figure 32.45 An all-terrain wheelchair with wide knobby tires, wide front casters, and casters attached farther forward for wheelchair stability. *(Courtesy of Colours, Corona, CA 92879.)*

nonprofit groups assist with fundraising to obtain equipment for individuals who are unable to pay privately (see "Funding" section). The ability to participate in competition and recreational activities can improve health, self-esteem, and confidence and provides a positive social network.

Manual Wheelchair With Add-on Drive Systems

Manual wheelchairs can become difficult for a person to self-propel due to a change in condition, injury, or aging. Power add-on drive systems enable a user to continue using their manual wheelchair while benefiting from the addition of a power assist system to reduce risk of injury or impairment secondary to self-propulsion.

While there are numerous power wheelchairs available on the market, a person's transition from a manual wheelchair to a power wheelchair is often challenging. Although appropriate seating can be provided in either a manual or power wheelchair, many other factors must be considered when making the transition. Many experienced users with fully configurable manual wheelchairs

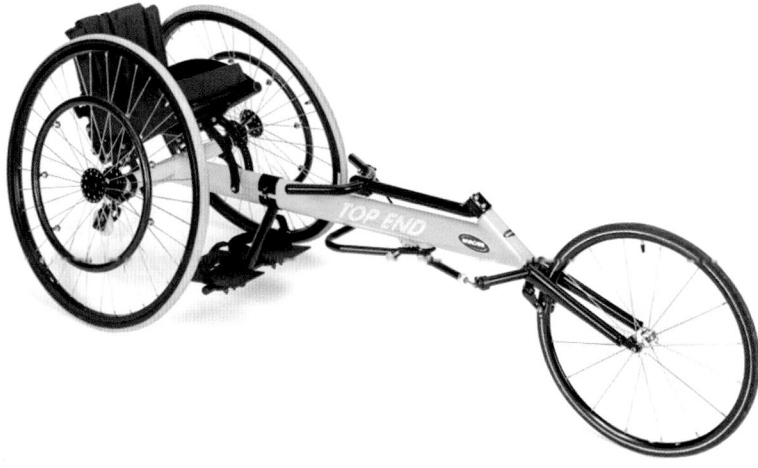

Figure 32.46 A sports wheelchair used for road racing. *(Courtesy of Invacare Corporation, Elyria, OH 44035.)*

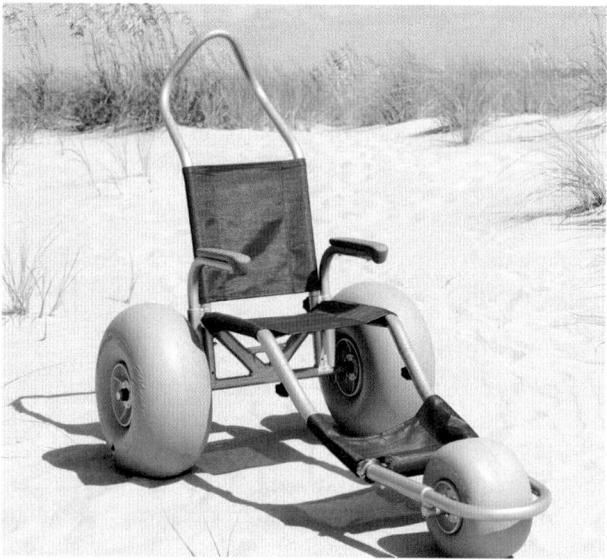

Figure 32.47 A special wheelchair designed for use on the beach in sand and water. *(Courtesy of Sand Rider, Virginia Beach, VA 23455.)*

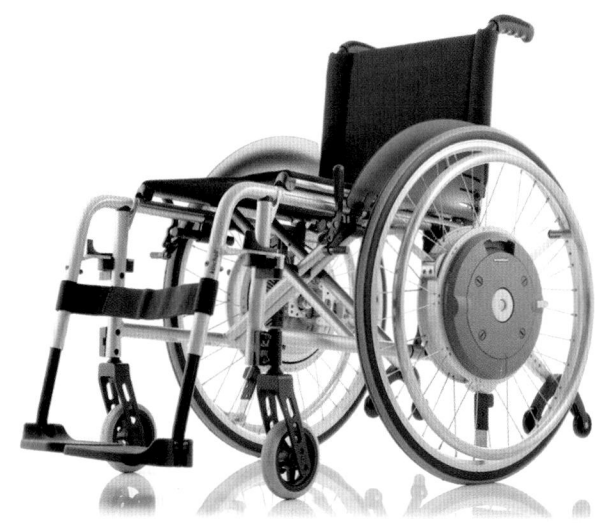

Figure 32.48 Handrim activated power assist wheels provides person with an assist on each propulsion. *(Courtesy of Alber [Germany], Albstadt-Tailfingen 72461.)*

have adapted their lifestyle, environment, and vehicles to their manual wheelchair and are not equipped to make the transition to power mobility. For example, some users are faced with insurmountable environmental barriers (e.g., inaccessible house or mobile home) that preclude the use of power mobility. Some of the challenges of using power wheelchairs include size, maneuverability, accessibility, transportation, and even stigma. Because power add-on drive systems are used as an option with a manual wheelchair, the combination of the manual wheelchair and add-on drive system is costly and may exceed the cost of a dedicated power wheelchair. Therefore, rationale is needed to justify why a dedicated power wheelchair will not work instead.

Handrim-Activated System

Handrim activated power assist systems come as a modular add-on option for the manual wheelchair. The wheels are equipped with motors and batteries in

the hubs (Fig. 32.48). These wheels replace the standard rear wheels on the manual wheelchair and can be interchanged as needed for use in the home and out in the community. This option allows the motorized wheels to be removed from the wheelchair frame for folding and stowage in a vehicle. The handrim-activated power assist system provides the person with supplemental power augmented assist with each push, increasing a person' travel distance and propulsion efficiency while reducing overall fatigue, effort, and stress on shoulders.[81–84] Newer systems can be programmed with different amounts (percent) of assist per wheel to accommodate differences in strengths of each UE.

Power Assist Drive System

A modular power add-on unit can be mounted to most adjustable manual wheelchair frames and used without changing the wheelchair wheels (Fig. 32.49). The person uses the wheels to steer the wheelchair

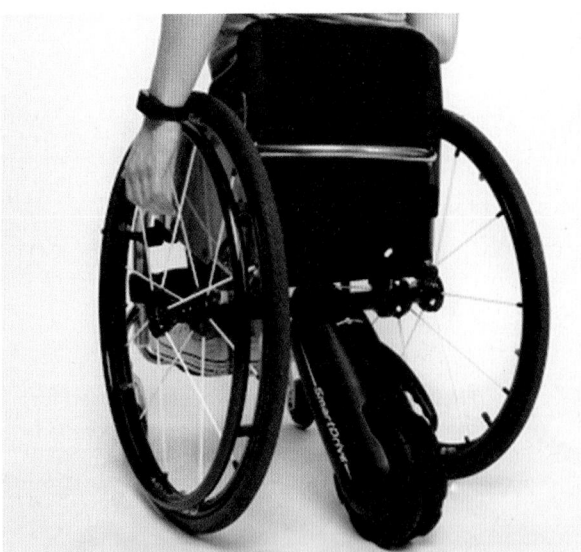

Figure 32.49 A power add-on unit attached to the back of the wheelchair. *(Courtesy of Max Mobility, Antioch, TN 37013.)*

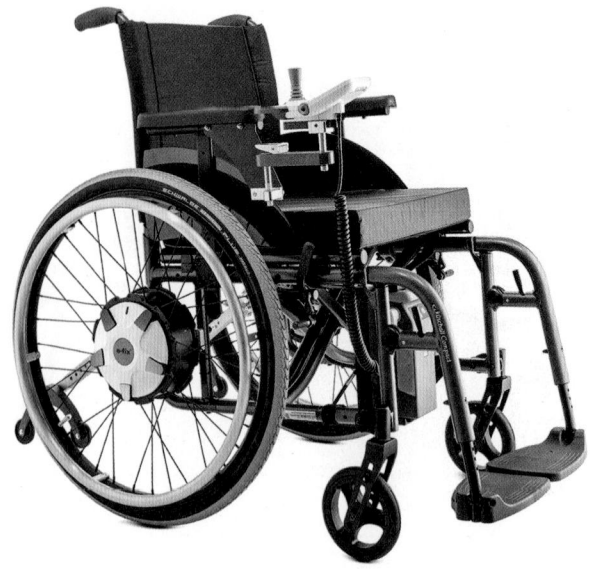

Figure 32.50 A manual wheelchair converted to a power wheelchair by replacing the wheels and adding a battery and joystick. *(Courtesy of Alber [Germany], Albstadt-Tailfingen 72461.)*

and the motor attached to the back of the wheelchair provides the power assist to go up steep hills, uneven terrain, and over long distances. The person controls the speed of the wheelchair using an application (e.g., watch, phone), control unit, or switch depending on the chosen manufacturer and model. This type of power assist system also increases a person' travel distance and reduces overall fatigue, effort, and stress on the shoulders. Once the motor is activated, the person is assisted going up steep hills, through thick carpet and over long distances by adjusting directions using the handrims to steer the wheelchair. This can be a smart solution for someone with an intermittent need for power mobility as it is beneficial indoors, outdoors, and for long distances.[81,82,84] The module is easily removed for transport and charging.

Power Add-on Unit

A power add-on unit converts a manual wheelchair to a portable lightweight power mobility device. These units are added to a manual wheelchair system (usually with tools) and include batteries, motors, and an alternative input method such as a joystick, tiller, handlebars, etc. (Fig. 32.50). This solution may be appropriate for a person who requires power mobility for long distances but does not have a method to transport a power wheelchair. It can be disassembled for loading into a vehicle with the heaviest component other than the wheelchair, weighing approximately 20 pounds. It is important to be mindful that the manual wheelchair frame by design is not intended to be used as a power wheelchair; thus, it is not as durable and not designed for the same terrain, distance, and conditions. Therefore, an active heavy-duty user may benefit instead from a dedicated

power wheelchair. Trade-offs and considerations should be discussed.

Power Mobility Devices

If a person is unable to independently and functionally use a manual wheelchair for all of their mobility needs and is cognitively aware of their surroundings, power mobility should be considered.[85–88] For example, a person may be able to move around in a manual wheelchair indoors and on flat outdoor surfaces (*accommodated environments*), yet be unable to functionally self-propel in all environments regularly encountered. For instance, the person may be unable to traverse door thresholds, thick carpet, uneven sidewalks, side slopes, steep ramps, and hills (*nonaccommodated environments*) encountered in the home and community due to pain, weakness, diminished muscular endurance, and cardiovascular strain. The therapist should discuss with the person risks involved with long-term UE overuse and RSI and strategies to mitigate risk. As part of the decision-making process, it is important to educate the person about implications of acute and chronic injury and impact on long-term function for activities such as transfers, mobility, and ADLs/IADLs.[61–66,85–89]

Scooter (Power-Operated Vehicle)

Scooters, or power-operated vehicles (POVs), come in three- or four-wheeled configurations operated with a tiller that controls speed and steering (Fig. 32.51). A tiller controller functions similarly to manual steering in a car, thereby requiring sufficient UE strength and endurance to operate. The scooter base has a platform and long wheelbase that serves as both the foot support and structural support for the wheels, seating

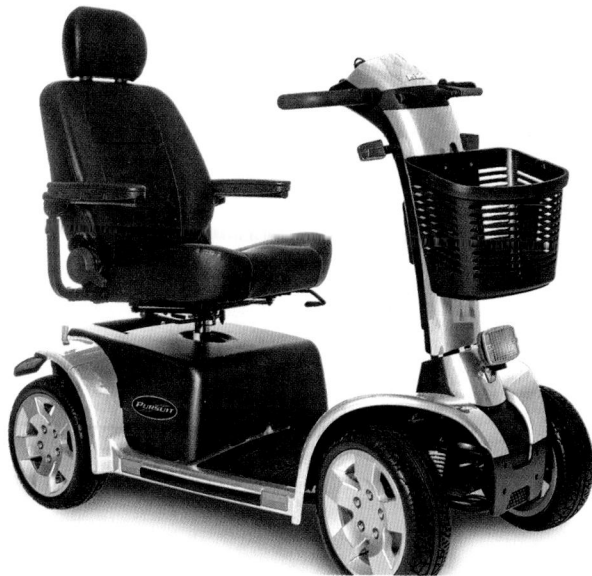

Figure 32.51 A scooter with four wheels for a more stable drive. *(Courtesy of Pride, Exeter, PA 18643.)*

system, and steering mechanism. The scooter seat and back support generally provided is either a captain-style van seat or a plastic flip-down boat seat type, available in limited widths and depths. Depending on the seat to floor height required, scooters can have a high COM, making them more tippy than a power wheelchair. The person must have adequate hands-free sitting posture and balance and adequate UE strength and endurance for a scooter to be a functional WMSD.

Due to the long wheelbase and overall length of scooters, the turning radius is larger than a power wheelchair, making maneuverability in small spaces difficult or impossible. Turning requires an arcing turn, three-point turn, or backing out of a tight space. Because of the tiller controller and scooter platform, a person is unable to pull straight forward up to a table or counter and instead must pull alongside the desired surface (e.g., parallel park) and rotate the scooter seat for access.

Some scooters can be disassembled for transport, yet the components can be heavy or awkward to lift for loading into the vehicle. Scooters are designed to be used on accommodated surfaces. Scooter electronics and motors have limited speed and range capabilities that need to be considered in the decision-making process. Although scooters tend to be less costly, consideration of a person's disability, changing needs, and environmental issues need to be discussed when deciding between pursuing a scooter versus a power wheelchair.

Power Wheelchairs

Power wheelchairs are categorized based on criteria such as frame style and seating system, drive-wheel configuration, performance, power seat options, electronic capability, and input options. Power wheelchairs are designed for use in particular environments (indoor,

outdoor, combination) and categorized based on performance criteria such as weight capacity, stability (tippyness), durability (life cycle), obstacle climbing, range, and speed. The person's clinical and postural needs, preferences, and environmental demands are matched with the performance capabilities of the power wheelchair considered. Significant power wheelchair features include frame type (integrated system or power base), wheelbase configuration (front, mid, rear drive), power positioning features, electronics, motors, controller, and input device.[53]

INTEGRATED POWER WHEELCHAIR

An integrated power wheelchair system combines the seating system and drive system as one unit that cannot be separated Fig. 32.52. This type of wheelchair is available in limited sizes and cannot be retrofitted with different seat frame systems once ordered.

POWERBASE WHEELCHAIR

A powerbase frame is a modular system with a separate base that contains the drive control system, batteries, motors, and wheels. It can be separated from the seating system and modified or replaced in the future if needed (Fig. 32.53).

DRIVE WHEEL CONFIGURATIONS

Power wheelchairs are available in three drive wheel configurations: rear, mid-, and front wheel drive (Fig. 32.54). Specific parameters to consider when comparing performance of different drive wheel configurations include stability, incline transition, transfers, control, obstacle

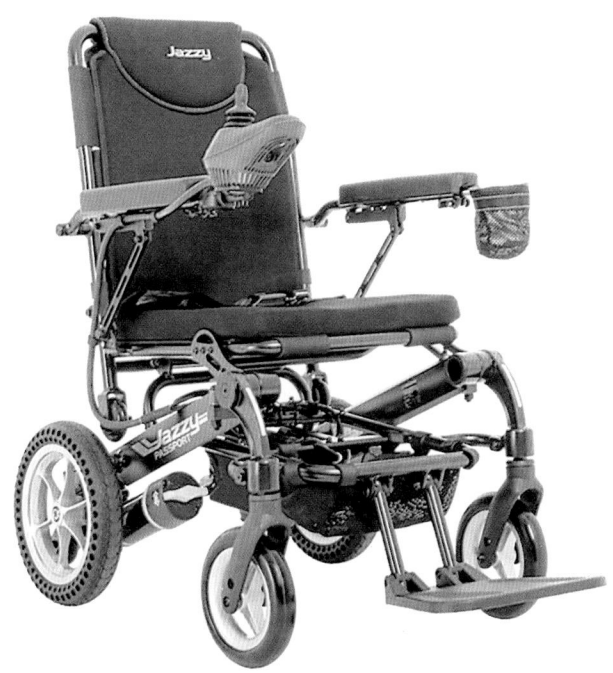

Figure 32.52 An integrated power wheelchair. *(Courtesy of Pride, Exeter, PA 18643.)*

handling, maneuverability, and positioning. Each drive wheel configuration has benefits and drawbacks, and no one configuration is clearly better than another in all circumstances. Center of gravity greatly affects the performance of all drive wheel configurations and therefore must be set for optimal wheelchair performance. Whenever possible, new and experienced users should have an opportunity to try different drive wheel configurations for comparison prior to committing to a final decision. Power wheelchair drivers will experience a learning curve when changing from one configuration to another.

Rear Wheel Drive Bases

A rear wheel drive (RWD) wheelchair has the fixed drive wheels in the rear and small front casters (see Fig. 32.54C). RWD chairs have good control, drive in a predictable manner in response to joystick input, and accurately maneuver in different situations and environments. A RWD wheelchair has a wider turning radius that might make it more difficult to maneuver in small spaces. Because of the front caster position, RWD chairs can be challenging to achieve optimal foot positioning to accommodate for a persons' knee and ankle contracture(s) or long lower leg length and it may be difficult to get close to objects from the front (e.g., sink, counter, etc.).

Mid-Wheel Drive Bases

Mid-wheel drive (MWD) wheelchairs have the fixed drive wheels in the middle of the wheelchair and small casters both in front and in the rear of the wheelchair (see Fig. 32.54B). Center-wheel drive power wheelchairs are a "type of MWD in which the drive wheels are located in the center and equidistant from the front and rear caster wheels."[53]

MWD chairs turn from the center and have the smallest turning radius (same length of wheelchair in front and behind the drive wheel). MWD chairs are intuitive to operate because the person's COM is closest to the COM of the wheelchair. The lower extremities can be positioned closer to the body due to decreased caster interference compared to RWD.

Front Wheel Drive Bases

A front wheel drive (FWD) wheelchair has the fixed drive wheels in the front of the wheelchair and swiveling caster wheels in the rear (see Fig. 32.54A). FWD

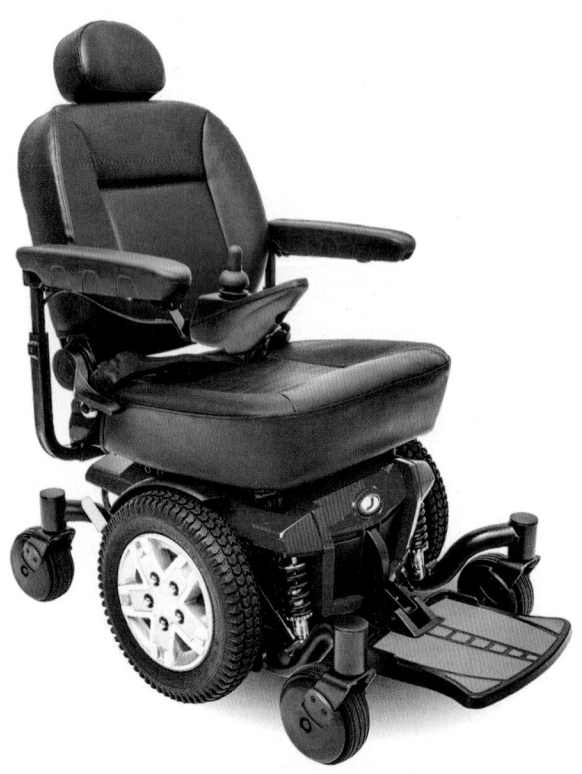

Figure 32.53 A power base that contains the drive control system, motors, and wheels and can be separated from the seating system. *(Courtesy of Pride, Exeter, PA 18643.)*

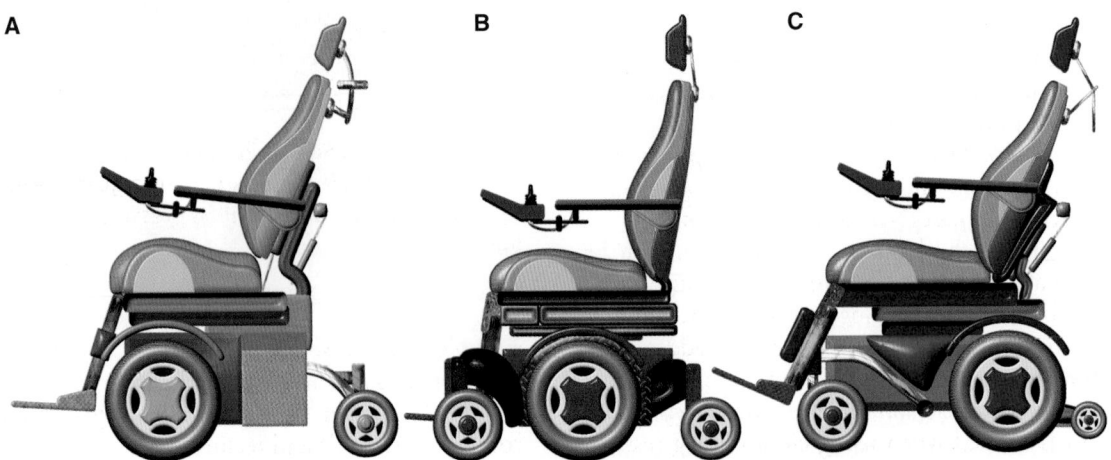

Figure 32.54 The wheel configurations for power base wheelchairs. (A) Front-wheel drive base. (B) Center- and mid-wheel drive base. (C) Rear-wheel drive base. *(Courtesy of Mobility Management, Irvine, CA 92618.)*

chairs have excellent stability, incline transition, obstacle handling, maneuverability, and positioning, allowing the feet to be positioned close to the body with no caster clearance issues. The turning radius is wider than the MWD and this may be a consideration in the user' living environment. There is a learning curve with this base configuration, as the back end moves first, and care must be taken to ensure sufficient posterior clearance. This configuration allows closer access to tables and sinks.

VARIABLE POSITIONING FEATURES FOR POWER WHEELCHAIRS

Just as manual mobility wheelchairs have variable positioning features (tilt, recline, elevating leg rests), so do power wheelchairs. Variable positioning power features can be operated independently by the user unlike most manual wheelchair positioning options. Power seat functions can be operated by a separate switch at any other access site or integrated into the drive system of the power wheelchair and operated by the same system used to drive the power wheelchair (e.g., joystick, track pad, or head control). Even the most physically involved person can be set up to independently control their own position and make changes as frequently as needed throughout the day without requiring caregiver assistance.

Power Tilt

Certain power wheelchairs can be equipped with a variable power tilt system and be mounted on an integrated or modular frame. For power wheelchairs, the tilt system is comprised of the seat and back frame and leg supports that move with the seat as it tilts (Fig. 32.55). The range of rearward and forward tilt available is dictated by the product selected. Just like the manual tilt system, power tilt provides the person with a resting position, assists with gravity-assisted repositioning in the wheelchair after transfers or a weight shift, improves sitting balance and trunk and head position, and improves comfort.[90,91]

Power Recline and Power Elevating Leg Rest System

A power recline system is typically paired with a power elevating leg rest system to allow the person to recline supine in their wheelchair (Fig. 32.56). These features can be operated simultaneously or independently. Some power wheelchairs have an option for manually elevating leg rests; however, in this instance the person is usually dependent on a caregiver for leg positioning.

Power recline with elevating leg rest system can be beneficial to assist with pressure relief or redistribution, change in joint ROM, stretching, rest, comfort, management of orthostatic hypertension, bowel/bladder care, and clothing management.[91] These features are available on certain power wheelchairs and are ordered separately.

Caution is needed when using elevating leg rests to ensure the person has sufficient hamstring length. If the person has hypertonia affected by change in hip or knee position, power recline may induce spasms, pulling the person out of position. Rarely do elevating leg

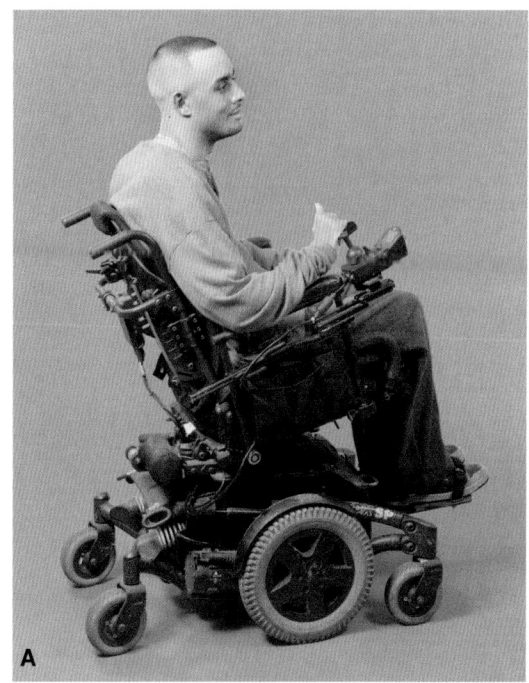

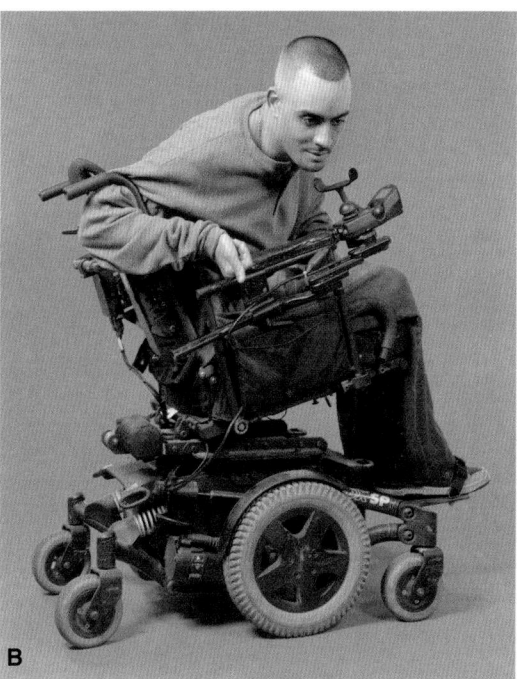

Figure 32.55 (A) Power tilt seating system on center-wheel drive base. System is infinitely adjustable in a preset range. (B) Person performing pressure-relief maneuver in tilt wheelchair.

rests alone decrease edema. For effective edema management, legs must be elevated above the level of the heart.[92,93] This can be accomplished by tilt alone or a combination of tilt and recline.[94]

Power Seat Elevation

Power seat elevation (seat lift) allows the wheelchair seat system to be raised or lowered. The distance of travel

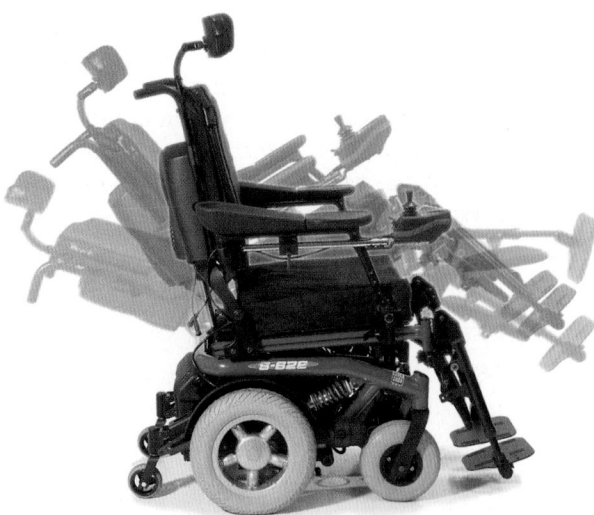

Figure 32.56 This wheelchair is equipped with power recline and power elevating leg rests. *(Courtesy of Sunrise Medical, Fresno, CA 93727.)*

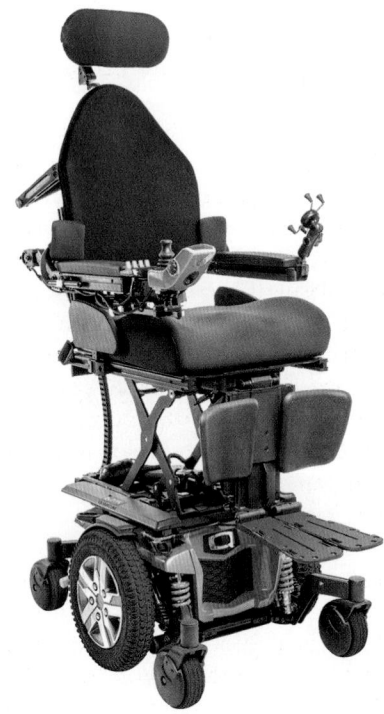

Figure 32.57 Power wheelchair with power seat elevation. Seat is in the raised position. *(Courtesy of Pride, Exeter, PA 18643.)*

(range) is dependent on the product selected (Fig. 32.57). Power seat elevation can improve reach, function, and safety; improve the person's access to tables, sinks, cabinets, and so on; and improve transfers by providing a level or downhill transfer—for example, on and off the toilet, bed, and so on.

When in the elevated position, the person may safely access the burners on the stove and the controls on the washing machine, reach items in the closet, and have improved eye to eye (social) interactions. Most power wheelchairs can be driven while the seat is in the elevated position. A built-in electronic safety mechanism will automatically slow the wheelchair speed or shut it off completely to prevent driving when the COM reaches an unsafe height for movement.

Power Standing

A power standing wheelchair allows the person who ordinarily would not be able to stand to independently move from a seated to a standing position. A combination power wheelchair and standing device allows the person to frequently change position throughout the day without transferring to another device and has the same benefits as described with a manual standing wheelchair system. Carefully explain the rationale to justify an integrated power standing feature and be sure to document why a separate dedicated standing device will not meet the person's needs.

Other Custom Seat Functions

Custom power seat functions are available to a limited extent by manufacturers to assist with improving a person's transfers, posture, and function, and are described here. *Power anterior tilt* moves the front of the seat lower than the rear of the seat, moving the feet toward the floor and the knees lower than the hips to facilitate weight-bearing or standing. An *adjustable height foot plate* allows the user to lower the footplate to the floor and actually stand on the footplate for transfers rather than moving the footplate out of the way. A *power seat to floor feature* is a pediatric feature that lowers to the ground for floor to seat transfers. *Power lateral tilt* is the ability to tilt the seat system to the side. This feature is seldom needed and only for the person with severe fixed scoliosis. When available, this feature is often paired with tilt to manage pressure, to facilitate digestion and gastric emptying, and to optimize function and comfort.

Power Wheelchair Input Devices

An input device is the method used by the person to operate the power wheelchair and to control the direction, speed, and functions of the wheelchair. Input devices are either proportional or nonproportional and are configured and programmed to meet the individual needs of the user.

A *proportional controller* is like a gas pedal. The farther you push it, the faster it goes. There exists a variety of specialty proportional controllers that can be mounted in different locations, depending on the person's most reliable and nonfatigable movement and identified access location.

A *nonproportional controller* is more like a light switch; it is either on or off. Speed is controlled with either a rheostat dial controller that allows the person to increase the speed only within the predefined available range, or via a separate input method (e.g., separate switch to toggle to a different mode and adjust speed). A nonproportional input device does not offer the fine adjustment that can be performed with a proportional input device and require additional steps to accomplish the same result. People who use nonproportional input devices typically have less control of their bodies and therefore fewer reliable access site options.

PROPORTIONAL DRIVE CONTROLS

A *conventional joystick* operated with the hand is the most common input device used by most power wheelchair users and is typically a standard option. It provides the user the ability to incrementally speed up, slow down, and change direction dependent on the extent and direction of joystick displacement. The final placement of the joystick is important to ensure that the person can reach the control without difficulty and without putting excessive stress on the wrist, elbow, or shoulder. Access to the on/off switch, mode switch, and/or speed dial must be assessed to ensure independent control and prevent accidental activation when driving. These features are incorporated into the conventional proportional joystick and may include power indicator lights or program indicators.

A *compact joystick* is mounted and positioned where needed. When controlled by the hand the joystick can be mounted in the center (midline) of the wheelchair using specialty swing-away mounting hardware. When controlled by the chin, it is mounted on a swing-away bracket and positioned slightly below and forward of the chin. When controlled by the foot, the compact joystick is mounted on a foot control mounting platform that allows for wheelchair control through plantar and dorsiflexion combined with right and left foot movements. Compact joysticks work much the same as a conventional joystick. Depending on the person's needs, the knob on the joystick can be replaced with a small cup or other shaped piece.

Finger and touchpad drive control systems can be mounted just about anywhere the user can comfortably reach it. The person places one finger on the device and moves the finger in the direction they want the wheelchair to move. This system is basically the same principle as a proportional drive joystick, but the person uses the movement of a finger for activation.

NONPROPORTIONAL DRIVE CONTROLS

Proximity switch drive controls do not require any pressure to be activated. The person only needs to move some part of their body (e.g., finger, head, elbow) near the switch to activate it. Proximity switches can be purchased unattached and mounted virtually anywhere on the wheelchair the person can reach. Typically, these switches are mounted on the underside of a tray.

Head controls can be proportional, nonproportional or a combination. The majority of *head controls* are nonproportional. Proximity switches are imbedded in a head support, mechanical switches can be attached to the head support, or a combination of proximity and mechanical switches can be used in the head support. A simple system consists of three switches. The switch behind the head allows the wheelchair to move forward, the one to the left side of the head turns the wheelchair left, and the one to the right side of the head turns the wheelchair to the right. Activating a combination of the switches allows the user to move diagonally or make small corrections to control direction with increased ease. A fourth switch can be used for reverse or to toggle the system so the rear pad on the head array becomes reverse. This fourth switch can also be used to change the speeds and operate other wheelchair functions such as seat functions or drive modes. If needed, a fifth switch may be used with the fourth switch for reverse, and the fifth switch can be designated for mode changes. Good head control is needed to operate this type of system. Programming is extremely important to ensure the person can rest their head against the rear head pad without accidentally operating the wheelchair (e.g., driving the wheelchair forward).

Single switch scanning array systems are available for a person who has only one switch placement site available. This is a nonproportional, digital input device. A light scan systematically around a display highlighting different directions. When the light hits the direction of travel desired, activation of the switch moves the wheelchair in that direction. Once the contact is removed from the switch, the scanner light continues to move around the display in a preset fashion. Although this rare type of system can be slow and tedious, the ability to drive independently makes it useful and valuable to the person with few access sites for reliable and nonfatiguable input.

Sip-n-puff drive control are for those users who are unable to use any other part of their body to operate a control device on their power wheelchair. These systems are nonproportional controls and require practice to learn. A straw is used in the mouth. A hard puff allows the wheelchair to move forward, a hard sip for reverse, a soft puff is right, and a soft sip is left. Systems can be calibrated through electronic programming for easier or harder puffs and sips. The system can be set up in latch mode (forward is locked after a hard puff) so the person is not required to constantly be puffing into the straw to keep the wheelchair moving forward. Once in latch mode, small puffs or sips provide steer correction. A hard sip stops the wheelchair. When using this type of system, it is important to have good lip closure without leakage through the mouth or nose for optimal efficiency. A combination of sip-n-puff and switches can be used for driving a wheelchair if a person has difficulty differentiating the hard and soft sips and puffs.

■ FUNDING

Fiscal awareness and responsibility are particularly important given today's environment of shrinking funding and limited resources for WSMD. Errors can have deleterious effects, wasting valuable medical benefits and personal resources. In the United States, most medically necessary WSM technologies used to enhance physical functioning and mobility are covered and paid in part or in full by third-party insurance, including Medicare, Medicaid, the Veterans Administration, and private payers.[95] The Medicare program is widely accepted as the model that other payers use as a basis to establish their own coverage, coding, and pricing policies; therefore, Medicare is used here as an example.

Therapists are often called on by physicians, nonphysician practitioners (e.g., physician assistants, nurse practitioners), and third-party payers to evaluate an individual and recommend appropriate WSM technologies. Because therapists have no financial interest in prescribing or selling WSM technologies, payers have identified therapists as the LCMP responsible for performing the WSM examination and specialty evaluation to qualify individuals for certain medically necessary and appropriate WSM equipment. Medicare, Medicaid, and many private payers require a physical therapist or occupational therapist to perform a wheelchair and seating specialty evaluation as a condition for coverage and payment.[96,97]

DME/CRT suppliers are typically paid by third-party payers for the provision of the equipment only. The supplier's DME-related services are considered by most payers in the price of the equipment and, therefore, for the most part, are not billable separately.

Medicare considers medical equipment needed at home to treat or ameliorate a beneficiary's illness or injury under the DME benefit. WSM technologies are classified as DME for which CRT is a subset. To qualify as DME, the equipment must (1) withstand repeated use, (2) primarily serve a medical purpose, (3) generally not be useful to a person without an illness or injury, and (4) be appropriate for use in the home.[98]

WSM products and services can be described as "standard" DME or CRT. Because Medicare defines DME as an item that can withstand repeated use and could normally be rented and used by successive patients, it includes commodity-type mobility devices such as canes, walkers, crutches, and standard wheelchairs.[96] Unlike DME, CRT products include medically necessary, individually configured devices that require evaluation, configuration, fitting, adjustment, or programming. CRT products and services are designed to meet the specific and unique medical, physical, and functional needs of an individual. CRT is used primarily by people with complex needs with a primary diagnosis typically resulting from a congenital disorder, progressive or degenerative neuromuscular disease, or certain types of injury or trauma, referred to here as *CRT diagnoses*.[20] People using CRT typically have more functional and medical needs that require more advanced interventions beyond standard DME. At present, Medicare does not recognize CRT as a separate benefit category but groups these technologies together in one DME benefit category. Legislation has been introduced in Congress and in multiple states to establish a separate Medicare benefit category and separate benefit recognition for CRT (www.access2crt.org). Appendix 32.A, Internet Resources (online), provides helpful links to information about Medicare policies and funding DME through state Medicaid programs.

■ DEFENSIBLE DOCUMENTATION

Funding agencies require letters of justification or specific documentation from the therapist to support recommended equipment. Most third-party payers have a prior authorization process. Once all decisions are made, including equipment specification and justification, documentation is generated that explains why each component of the WSM system is needed. Justification and rationale for the wheeled mobility base, positioning features, seating technologies, and wheelchair accessories and options are specified. The justification should follow the problem-solving process detailing the individual's problems/potentials, goals of the WSM intervention, equipment features recommended, make/model equipment, and justification/ rationale to support necessity. The DME or CRT supplier is responsible for compiling all the required documentation and submitting to the payer for prior authorization, claims processing, and payment. The company gathers the documentation from the referring physician, including the referral, written order/ prescription, and medical documentation (face-to-face evaluation, pertinent tests and measures, history/ physical). As part of the interdisciplinary team, the supplier/RTP is also required to prepare and submit supplier documentation, including the technology assessment, home accessibility survey, detailed product description, and delivery ticket. All paperwork is prepared and submitted to the funding agency. Appendix 32.A, Internet Resources (online), includes links to a documentation guide and an example electronic fillable seating/mobility evaluation form and more.

■ OUTCOME MEASUREMENT

Every aspect of the WSM service provision process impacts the overall outcome for the user. Without a doubt, the process is complex, evaluated by the success of the services and utilization of the WSMD by the user. Understanding and measuring outcomes is not straightforward. The provision of WSMD reflects the diverse contexts of the user's health needs, goals, social roles, and environment. In addition, outcomes can be confounded by the users' satisfaction with service provision and device availability.[99] Outcomes can be measured

Table 32.5   Wheelchair Seating and Mobility Outcome Measures

Name	Domain of Measurement	Description	Mode of Administration	Administrative Time
WHOM	Activity and participation		Administered by clinician	30 minutes
FEW	Activity. Evaluation of participation from both the user's and clinician's perspective.	Measures performance in 10 environment- and activity-based situations	Self-administered or by evaluator	<15 minutes
WST	Evaluation of wheelchair mobility skills (activity)	Assesses 30 manual wheelchair skills for safety and performance	Administered by clinician	~30 minutes
TAWC	Wheelchair comfort	20 items assess factors affecting discomfort, discomfort location, and intensity	Administered by clinician	Not stated
PIDA	Indoor driving skills (mobility)	30 items designed to describe a user's mobility status at a single point in time	Administered by clinician	Not stated
QUEST	User satisfaction with device and services	12 items (eight device and four services)	Self-administered or by evaluator	6–30 minutes
PIADS	Measures the impact of assistive technology on quality of life	26-item questionnaire: adaptability, competence, self-esteem	Self-report	5–10 minutes
OTFACT	Functional performance	Measures five domains (role integration, activities, integrated skills, components of performance, and environment)	Administered by clinician	15 minutes
ATOM	Assesses assistive technology usability and service	Demographics and 18 items	Administered by clinician	Not stated
GAS	Attainment of client-identified goals.	User sets personally relevant goals and self-rates achievement to measure change over time.	Collaborative goal setting between user and clinician	60 minutes

ATOM = Assistive Technology Outcome Measure; FEW = Functioning Every Day with a Wheelchair; GAS = Goal Attainment Scale; OTFACT = Occupational Therapy Functional Assessment Compilation Tool; PIADS = Psychosocial Impact of Assistive Technology; PIDA = Power Mobility Community Driving Assessment; QUEST = Quebec User Evaluation of Satisfaction with Assistive Technology Version 2.0; TAWC = Tool for Assessing Wheelchair Discomfort; WHOM = Wheelchair Outcome Measure; WST = Wheelchair Skills Test 4.1.

in clinical, functional, psychosocial, and cost terms. Regardless of intent, all outcome measurements seek information designed to capture change.

While measuring outcomes is regarded as an essential component of practice, it is not regularly incorporated in practice for many reasons, including limited time, lack of available information, and an undervaluing or lack of prioritization for program and service evaluation.[73] Yet the demand for outcome measurement continues to grow. With the high cost of WSM services and technology, policymakers increasingly are relying on outcomes evidence to determine eligibility, coverage, and payment policy.

Table 32.5 presents a select sample and description of five wheelchair outcome measures and five assistive technology outcome measures suitable for use in evaluating WSM provision.

Because there are multiple aspects of a WSMD intervention (the services and the technology), and because numerous constructs can be measured, an instrument must be selected to match the goals of the research or purpose of the program evaluation.[100–105]

SUMMARY ▮▮▮▮▮▮▮▮▮▮▮

This chapter discussed the basics of seating and wheeled mobility with an emphasis on the eight steps of the wheelchair service delivery process. The three most critical steps are identification of need, assessment, and prescription/selection. Using the problem-solving model approach, attention to evaluation details will ensure that the person will be provided with the most appropriate WSMD. The person–technology match is essential to ensure positive outcomes. An overview of mobility equipment and seating equipment has been provided, and while a good start, there are many more products and features that are not covered here. This chapter focused on a user with basic to intermediate needs and provides the entry-level clinician with foundational knowledge about WSM examination and wheelchair evaluation and a base for organizing and understanding the range of equipment and features available. Specialized training in WSM technology to develop expertise is needed for the clinician interested in providing seating and mobility services to people with intermediate to complex needs.

■ ACKNOWLEDGMENTS

We would like to acknowledge Jean Anne Zollars MA PT, Physical Therapy, Inc.; Kelly Waugh MA PT, ATP, Assistive Technology Partners; and Barbara Crane PhD, PT, ATP/SMS, Plymouth State University, for their expertise, contribution, and effort in developing entry-level curriculum materials for WSM education as part of a Craig H. Neilsen Foundation funded project and a corresponding curriculum. We would also like to thank the Academy of Neurologic Physical Therapy for their leadership and support in developing and hosting the quality supportive web-based training materials entitled *An Introduction to Practice in Wheelchair Seating & Mobility* for professionals wishing to develop expertise in the area of WSM practice and to supplement their learning beyond this chapter.[39]

Questions for Review

1. Describe the differences between a wheelchair user with basic, intermediate, or complex needs.

2. List four factors that play a role in determining an optimal wheelchair system for a wheelchair user.

3. Explain what information or data are gathered during each of the following portions of the examination process:
   a. Assessment interview
   b. Functional assessment in existing equipment
   c. Supine mat assessment
   d. Seated simulation

4. Discuss the importance of using principles of sitting posture when performing seating assessments.

5. Explain optimal sitting posture in the sagittal plane, frontal plane, and transverse plane.

6. How do you achieve optimal posture for a person with ROM limitations?

7. Explain the difference between ROM for a seating assessment and ROM for a standard physical therapy examination.

8. When determining seat-to-back support angle, what parameters are used to finalize this angle?

9. What techniques should be used when measuring seat depth?

10. Why should recommended equipment be tested by the intended user? What specific issues need to be tested?

11. When would you recommend a wheelchair with sling seat and back upholstery?

12. When would you recommend the following types of cushions?
    a. Firm seat cushion
    b. Contoured seat cushion
    c. Air seat cushion
    d. Custom-molded seat cushion

13. Why is a pelvic positioner important, and what methods can be used to make it more effective?

14. Describe the following wheelchair components; compare and contrast their functional benefits:
    a. Detachable swing-away footrests versus elevating leg rests
    b. Fixed-height armrests versus adjustable-height armrests
    c. Single-axle placement versus multiple-axle placement

15. Identify four methods of self-propulsion in manual mobility and the benefits of each method.

16. Explain the benefits and contraindications of power mobility.

17. Describe the various power wheelchair bases available and the benefits of each system.

18. Discuss the pros and cons of a tilt system versus a recline system with elevating leg rests.

CASE STUDY

Ms. Black is a 70-year-old woman with a primary diagnosis of MS who resides at home independently. She currently has no other medical issues. She has been experiencing increased right LE weakness this past year. Her ambulation abilities have decreased, and she is no longer able to ambulate functionally or safely in her home with any assistive device and currently depends on a manual wheelchair for full-time mobility. She continues to be able to perform a stand pivot transfer and wears an AFO on her right foot for stability. She uses a basic manual wheelchair with sling seat and back upholstery, fixed-height full-length armrests, and swing-away footrests. She propels the wheelchair with both UEs. Ms. Black prefers not to use her footrests in her home due to the difficulty of maneuvering the wheelchair around corners and through doorways with the extra length. Instead, she holds her feet off the floor when propelling and rests her feet on the floor once she reaches her destination.

Ms. Black is independent in dressing, eating, and using the bathroom. She uses her wheelchair to move around her home for her various activities. She is in the wheelchair 15 hrs a day with breaks throughout the day. Skin integrity is intact. She works out at the gym, goes food shopping, and performs home activities. She depends on friends to take her to the various activities using their cars for transportation.

Ms. Black's posture is poor in her current manual wheelchair. She sits with a right pelvic obliquity of 15° (right side lower by 2 in.), neutral pelvic tilt, and no pelvic rotation noted. She has a mild right thoracic C-curve scoliosis, and both LEs are adducted with feet resting on the floor. Although she does have footrests, she usually doesn't use them since it is difficult to move around her home and get close to the sink and stove.

Ms. Black was assessed on the mat in the supine position to determine passive ROM limitations that affect her seating position.

	Right	Left
Hip Flexion	85°	85°
Hip Abduction	10°	0°
Hip Internal Rotation	40°	0°
Knee Extension With Hips Flexed	−90°	−90°
Ankle Dorsiflexion With Knee Flexed	0°	0°
Ankle Dorsiflexion With Knee Extended	−10°	−5°

Mobility is within functional limits in the pelvis and trunk, but due to weakness, Ms. Black tends to position herself in a right pelvic obliquity and right thoracic scoliosis. The range of head/neck and both UEs is within functional limits. Thigh length is 17 in., calf length is 17 in., and hip/thigh width is 17 in., measured in supine position. Ms. Black has 4/5 strength for both UEs. Right LE is 3 to /5 and left LE is 3+/5. Trunk strength is 2+/5.

Ms. Black was assessed in the sitting position on the mat table. She demonstrated improved pelvic and LE position but was unable to maintain her trunk posture independently. She used her arms to prevent herself from falling and continued to collapse into a right thoracic scoliosis but was able to maintain a neutral pelvic position when sitting on a firm surface.

Ms. Black was assessed in a seating simulation chair with a firm back, firm seat, arm support, and foot support. Posture continued to improve but she continued to assume a scoliotic position. A right lateral trunk support was tested, and she maintained straight trunk alignment. Although three points of control are usually needed when working with someone with a scoliosis, the support that she received from the seat surface and arm surface was adequate to achieve straight trunk alignment, and she can reposition herself as needed to maintain neutral pelvic alignment.

(Continued)

CASE STUDY—cont'd

Ms. Black currently uses a standard 18 in. wide by 16 in. deep wheelchair with 24 in. rear wheels and 8 in. casters. A firm back with a right lateral trunk support and a firm seat were attached to this manual wheelchair. Overall posture improved, and Ms. Black stated she was much more comfortable. However, function decreased. The seat was too high, and she needed to use the footrests for support. Maneuvering the wheelchair in her home was more difficult and she was constantly hitting door-jambs and walls when attempting to turn the wheelchair. It was more difficult to reach her sink and stove. She is unable to get her legs under her table for meals or under her computer desk with this higher seat height. Due to the addition of the firm back, the seat depth was too short, and she was unable to position her hips far enough back in the wheelchair, decreasing her access to the wheels.

Ms. Black tested various other wheelchair styles and noted a difference in propelling a lighter weight wheelchair with less stress on her shoulders and improved mobility and access.

CASE STUDY GUIDING QUESTIONS

1. What type of manual wheelchairs would you have Ms. Black test?
2. Based on ROM limitations, what areas need to be addressed on the seating system?
3. What features would you recommend for a manual wheelchair?
4. What type of seat cushion would you recommend?
5. What type of back cushion would you recommend?
6. Fill out a problem-solving grid and address issues of posture, skin integrity, health/medical issues, functional tasks and abilities, environmental issues, caregiver needs, social and emotional issues, and mobility issues. Use the following four column headings in developing the grid: Clinical Problems and Potential Problems, Objectives for Equipment Intervention, Equipment Properties and Recommendations, and Product Specifications.

Clinical Problems and Potential Problems	Objectives for Equipment Intervention	Equipment Properties and Recommendations	Product Specifications

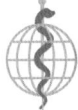

For additional resources, including answers to the questions for review, new immersive cases, case study guiding questions, references, and more, please visit **https://www.fadavis.com/product/physical-rehabilitation-fulk-8**. You may also quickly find the resources by entering this title's four-digit ISBN, 4691, in the search field at **http://fadavis.com** and logging in at the prompt.

■ INDEX

Note: Page numbers followed by *(b)* indicate box; *(f)*, figure; and *(t)*, table.

A

Abarognosis, 89(t)
Abbreviated MFIS (MFIS-5), 609
ABCD assessment tool, 385, 386(f)
ABCDE model, 457, 461, 465
Abdominal binder, 790
Abdominal reflex, 150, 150(t)
Abducens nerve (CN VI), 98(t), 151, 153(t)
Abducted gait, 1210(t), 1212
Ability
  defined, 127(b)
  to perform, in measures of function, 277
Abnormal central vestibular function, 838
Abnormal synergies, 144–145
Abrasive strips, 302, 302(f)
Absent pulse, 489
Academy of Acute Care, 26, 105
Academy of Cardiovascular and Pulmonary
        Physical Therapy, 26
Academy of Geriatric Physical Therapy, 26
Academy of Neurologic Communication Disorders
        and Sciences (ANCDS), 1107, 1109,
        1113, 1114
Academy of Neurologic Physical Therapy (ANPT)
  CPGs published by, 26
  EDGE Taskforce Outcome Measures, 133
  Framework, 12(f)
  Jimmo settlements and implementation
        resources, 697
  Movement System Task Force, 16, 137
  online resources guide for locomotor function,
        372, 373
  PDEDGE, 707
  spinal cord injury resources, 807
  StrokEDGE workgroup, 547
  stroke examination resources, 547
  traumatic brain injury resources, 746
Academy of Neurologic Physical Therapy Outcome
        Measures Recommendations, 742
Academy of Orthopedic Physical Therapy, 26
Acalculia, 76, 1086
Acapella, 408, 411, 411(f)
Acceleration, 218, 219(t), 246(t), 248, 249, 261,
        262, 335
Accelerometers, 248–249, 249(f)
Accessibility, 294
Accessible design, 294–295
Accessory joint motions, 116–118, 116(t), 117(f),
        118(f)
Accessory nerve (CN XI), 151, 154(t)
Accuzyme, 951
Acetic acid solution, 501
Acetylcholine (ACh), 129, 130(f), 167, 682
Acetylcholinesterase inhibitors, 602
Achilles, 149(t)
Acknowledgment, psychosocial adaptation and,
        1018
Acting out, 1022(b)
Action observation training (AOT), 716
Action potentials, 129, 130(f), 165, 167, 170, 173
Action Research Arm Test (ARAT), 145, 197(t),
        551, 552, 558
Action stage of change, 1132, 1133(b)
Action tremor/kinetic tremor, 684
Active cycle of breathing techniques (ACBT),
        410(f), 410–411
Active engagement, 355
Active exercise, 959, 960–961

Active markers for tracking motion, 256, 257
Active range of motion (AROM), 113–114, 698,
        699, 709
Active restraint, 141
Activities Balance Confidence Scale, 610, 702(t)
Activities of daily living (ADLs), 6, 136
  amyotrophic lateral sclerosis, 669, 669(t)
  eye-hand coordination, 182
  Falls Efficacy Scale, 211
  multidimensional functional assessment
        instruments, 287(t)
  OASIS-D, 288(t)
  spinal cord injury, expectations for patients with,
        784–787(t)
  WSM examination and specialty evaluation, 1237
Activities-Specific Balance Confidence (ABC)
        scale, 212, 298, 608(t), 754, 754(t)
Activity, 6, 7(b), 273. *See also* Activities of daily
        living (ADLs); Activity limitations;
        Physical activity (PA)
Activity Balance Confidence (ABC), 348(t)
Activity diary, 621
Activity limitations, 6, 7(b), 273
  osteoarthritis, 909
  rheumatoid arthritis, 901
  spinal cord injury, 772–773, 781–782
    assistive technology, 782
    community, social, and civic life, 782
    functional balance and, 781
    locomotion and, 781
    self-care and domestic life, 782
    upper extremity function, 781–782
  traumatic brain injury, 730
Activity Measure for Post-Acute Care (AM-PAC),
        286, 289, 456(t)
Activity pacing, 412, 621
Activity-Specific Balance Confidence Scale (ABC),
        989
Activity specific upper limb prostheses, 1200,
        1200(f)
Activity/step-count monitors, 249
Acute care, 3(b)
Acute cerebral ischemia, 540
Acute confusional state, 536
Acute coronary syndrome (ACS), 428–438
  angina, 432–433, 452(t), 454(b), 457(t), 462
  cardiac enzymes, 436
  clinical manifestations, 428, 432
  electrocardiographic changes, 434–436, 435(f),
        436(f)
  evaluation of patients with (evaluation triad),
        433–436, 434(f)
  injury and infarction, 433, 433(f)
  medical management, 436–438
    coronary artery bypass graft, 436–437
    percutaneous transluminal coronary
        angioplasty, 436
    physical therapy clinical implications,
        437–438
  pathophysiology, 428
  referral pattern for chest pain, 434, 434(f)
  reported symptoms, 434
  risk factors for endothelial dysfunction and
        atherosclerosis, 428, 432(t)
  See also Myocardial infarction (MI)
Acute cyanosis, 35(b)
Acute disseminating encephalomyelitis (ADEM),
        596
Acute exercise overdose, 353

Acute inflammation stage, 122
Acute pain, 970
Acute phase of stroke recovery, 543–544
Acute PT3D, 1029
Acute relapse, of multiple sclerosis, 596
Acute stage, 122
Acute stress disorder, 1029, 1030–1032
ADA Accessibility Guidelines (ADAAG), 322
Adaptation, 158, 344, 346
  cognitive and perceptual dysfunction, 1070,
        1071(t)
  defined, 158, 159(b)
  motor learning, 129, 132(b), 158, 159(b)
  rehabilitative/compensatory approach, 1059
Adaptive approach, 1070, 1071(t)
Adaptive DBS (aDBS), 695
Adaptive equipment and devices, 317
  amyotrophic lateral sclerosis, 669, 669(t)
  Parkinson disease, 720–721
  vascular, lymphatic, or integumentary disorders,
        488
Adaptive postural control, 199
*ADA Regulations and Technical Assistance
        Materials*, 322
Adenosine triphosphate (ATP), 527
Adhesive capsulitis, 577
Adjustable height foot plate, 1278
Adjustable stroller handle, 1261
Adjustment, psychosocial adaptation and, 1018
Adjuvant medications, 1007
Adrenocorticotropic hormone (ACTH), 1016
Adult Support Groups, 964
Advanced cardiac life support (ACLS), 447
Advanced Mechanical Technology, Inc. (AMTI),
        262, 262(f)
Advanced performers, 341, 342(t)
Advance of movement, 68
Advancing Trauma-Informed Care, 1048, 1050
Adventitious breath sounds, 53–54, 397
Advisory Council on Clinical Trials in Multiple
        Sclerosis, NMSS, 590
Aerobic capacity/endurance
  amyotrophic lateral sclerosis, 659
  measurement of, in pulmonary disease, 398
  motor function, 353
  multiple sclerosis, 606(b), 610
  Parkinson disease, 698(b)
  physical assessment for WSM, 1241, 1242
  prosthetics, 1204
  spinal cord injury, 780, 792(f), 792–793
  stroke, 581–583
  vascular, lymphatic, and integumentary
        disorders, 486
Aerobic conditioning
  amyotrophic lateral sclerosis, 659
  arthritis, 932
  health and wellness, 1123
  heart disease, 423–426, 425(f) (*See also under*
        Exercise)
  mild TBI, 755
  motor function, 353–354
  multiple sclerosis, 619–620
  Parkinson disease, 719
  pulmonary rehabilitation, 401
  stroke, 582
  traumatic brain injury, 747
Aerobic Exercise Recommendations to Optimize
        Best Practices in Care After Stroke
        (AEROBICS), 353

Aesthesiometer, 85, 85(f)

Affect, inappropriate, 1044(t)

Affective function
    multidimensional functional assessment
        instruments, 287(t)
    multiple sclerosis, 592(b), 595, 608
    stroke, 536

Affective pain, 971

Affordances, 349(t), 350(t), 363

Afterload, 419

Afterload reducers, 438, 443

Age-adjusted HR formula, 45

Agency for Healthcare Research and Quality
    (AHRQ), 462, 491, 500, 1144

Age-related changes
    blood pressure, 57, 57(t)
    cell senescence, 432(t)
    coordination impairments, 191–192
    heart rate, 44
    microglia, 73
    multiple sclerosis, 588
    myelin, 73
    respiration, 52–53
    sensory function, 72–73, 74–75(t)
    temperature, 39
    training-induced plasticity, 339(t)
    See also Older adults

Agility, 181–182

Aging-in-place design, 294–295

Agitated Behavior Scale, 740, 743(t)

Agitation, 1038, 1040

Agnosias, 134, 201, 538, 1090–1092
    auditory, 1092
    summary, 1073(t)
    tactile (astereognosis), 1092
    visual, 1091–1092, 1091–1092(f)

Agoraphobia, 689

Agraphia, 1086

Aids for daily living, 319(b)

Air conduction hearing, 77

Air plethysmography (APG), 490

Airsplints, 575–576

Airway clearance, 410

Airway obstruction, 689

Airway oscillation devices, 408

Akathisia, 687, 694

Akinesia, 188, 190(t), 684, 699

Alarm system, 143

Alemtuzumab (Lemtrada), 598(t)

Alert, defined, 75

Alert flags
    arthritis, 914, 915(t)
    chronic pain, 979, 979(t), 982(f), 984–985, 992
    musculoskeletal, 105, 108, 109

Alertness, 535

Algometer, 988

Algorithm for selecting upper extremity
    interventions, 568, 569(f)

Alginates, 510–511, 511(f)

Alignment, prosthetic, 1202–1203
    transfemoral, 1202–1203, 1202–1203(f)
    transtibial, 1202, 1202–1203(f)

Allergic asthma, 389

Allergic sensitivity, 389

Allesthesia, 89(t)

Allodynia, 89(t), 972, 988

Allogenic skin substitute, 952

Allograft, 952

Allostasis model of pain, 972

Aloe vera-loaded gelatin (OP-Gel), 511

Alpha-adrenergic blocking agents, 602

Alpha-synuclein, 682

Alprazolam (Xanax), 1030(b)

ALS Association Recognized Treatment Centers,
    646

ALS CNTF Treatment Study Group, 660

ALS Cognitive Behavioral Screen (ALS-CBS), 660

ALS Functional Rating Scale (ALSFRS), 660, 664

ALS Functional Rating Scale-Revised
    (ALSFRS-R), 646, 660–661, 662

ALS Severity Scale (ALSSS), 660

ALS Specific Quality of Life-Short Form
    (ALSSQOL-SF), 662

Altered consciousness, 134–135, 532

Alternate heel-to-knee; heel-to-toe test, 194(t)

Alternate nose-to-finger test, 193(t)

Alternating attention, 1073

Alternating pulse, 44

Alternative therapies
    arthritis pain relief, 926–927
    chronic pain relief, 1008

Altruism, 1022(b)

Alveolar ridge, 1102

Alveoli, 51, 51(f)

Alzheimer disease, gait analysis and, 234(t), 235(t)

Amantadine (Symmetrel), 602, 693(t), 694

Ambient vision, 201

Ambulation
    burns, 961
    classification of, stroke, 551, 551(t)
    postsurgical phase of amputation, 860
    profiles and scales, 233–241
        Emory Functional Ambulation Profile, 240
        Functional Ambulation Profile, 240
        Functional Independence Measure (FIM),
            241, 241(t)
        Iowa Level of Assistance Scale, 240–241
        outcome measures, 234–240(t)

Ambulation Index (AI), 610

Ambulatory Blood Pressure Monitoring (ABPM),
    58

American Academy of Neurology (AAN)
    Quality Measurement and Reporting
        Subcommittee, 647, 648

American Association of Cardiovascular and
    Pulmonary Rehabilitation, 402

American Burn Association (ABA), 939, 940, 963

American Chronic Pain Association, 993

American College of Cardiology (ACC), 57, 416,
    426, 439, 441, 443

American College of Chest Physicians, 399, 402

American College of Sports Medicine (ACSM),
    351–352, 352(t), 353, 456(t), 573, 792,
    1146

American Foundation for the Blind, 612

American Heart Association (AHA), 57, 416, 426,
    439, 440, 441, 443, 465, 525

American Lung Association, 408

American National Standards Institute, 294

American Physical Therapy Association (APTA)
    Academy of Orthopedics, 14
    aerobic exercise for Parkinson disease, 719
    biopsychosocial model endorsed by, 1127
    Clinical Research Agenda, 24
    documents available from, 23
    EDGE, 133, 207
    evidence-based practices, in motor function
        examination, 133
    evidence-based resources, 14, 24, 25(t)
    on exercise, 517
    Guide to Physical Therapist Practice, 2, 8, 16, 19,
        20(f), 265, 941
    health promotion and prevention, 1123
    ICD-10 codes, 24
    Mobility Device Documentation Guide, 1235
    movement system defined by, 8
    Movement System Task Force, 16
    MS-EDGE, 610
    Musculoskeletal Preferred Practice Patterns, 122
    OPTIMAL, 278
    performance-based measures, 298
    Physical Therapy journal, 26
    position statements on role of physical
        therapists, 1146
    priority populations requiring physical
        therapists, 1143
    process for establishing CPGs, 25–26
    on sharp débridement, 499
    Standards of Measurement, 282
    Telehealth and, position statement on, 297
    See also Academy of Neurologic Physical
        Therapy

American Speech-Language-Hearing Association
    (ASHA), 1099–1100, 1107

American Spinal Injury Association (ASIA), 762

Americans with Disabilities Act (ADA), 326–327
    curb cuts, 321
    disability access symbols, 295
    disability defined in, 326
    publications, 322, 327
    public transportation systems, 327
    Standards for Accessible Design, 294
    workplace guides, 322

American Thoracic Society, 397, 399

Amitriptyline (Elavil), 501, 602, 648, 650, 1035(b)

Amnesia, 531

Amorphous, 510

Amount of movement (AOM), 552

Amoxapine (Asendin), 1035(b)

Amplitude-scaling strategies, 709

Amputation, 849–888
    case study, 886–888
    causes, 850–851
    functional outcome measurements, 803–805,
        804–805(t)
    gait analysis
        footswitches and footswitch systems, 256
        heart rate data, 267
        measuring kinetic variables, 262, 264
        outcome measures, 234(t), 236(t), 237(t),
            238(t), 239(t)
        physiological energy cost measures, 266
    healing process, 854–855
    levels, 851(t), 851–852
    older adult with, 865
    phases of care, 857(b), 857–874
        bilateral amputation, 874
        education, 874
        postsurgical phase, 857–861, 858(b), 859(f)
        preoperative phase, 857
        preparatory and definitive prostheses,
            873–874
        preprosthetic phase, 861–873
        prosthetic training, 876–885, 877–880(t)
    surgery, 852–854, 853(f), 854(f)

Amputee Mobility Predictor (AMPpro), 369, 1204

Amygdala, 337

Amyotrophic lateral sclerosis (ALS), 635–678,
    636(t)
    aerobic capacity, 659
    apoptosis, 638
    balance, 661–662
    behavioral impairments (ALSbi), 641(t),
        642–643
    bulbar, 636, 640, 641(f), 641(t)
    bulbar function, 659
    case study, 675–678
    classifications, 643–644, 644(f)
    clinically definite, 643–644, 644(f)
    clinically possible, 643, 644, 644(f)
    clinically probable, 643, 644, 644(f)
    clinically probable, laboratory-supported, 643,
        644, 644(f)
    clinical manifestations, 640–643
        bulbar pathology impairments, 641(t), 642
        cognitive impairments, 641(t), 642–643
        LMN pathology impairments, 640–641,
            641(t)

other impairments, 641(t), 643
  rare impairments, 643, 643(t)
  respiratory impairments, 641(t), 642
  UMN pathology impairments, 641(t), 642
cognition, 660
cognitive and behavioral impairment, 641(t),
  643
cognitive impairment, 641(t), 642–643
composite impairment, 658
control, 661–662
cranial nerve integrity, 659–660
diagnosis, 643–644, 644(f)
direct impairment, 658
disease course, 644–645, 645(t)
environmental barriers, 660
environmental factors, 638
epidemiology, 636–637
etiology, 637–638
exercise, 671–672
  disuse atrophy, 671
  overuse damage, 671, 672(f)
  prescription, 671–672, 673(b)
familial, 636–637, 638, 639, 644
fasciculations, 170
fatigue, 143, 660
with frontotemporal dementia, 638, 641(t), 660
functional status, 660
gait, 660–661
genetics, 636–638
glutamate, 638
immune response, 638
indirect impairment, 658
instruction, 672, 673–674
integument, 661
intraneuronal protein aggregates, 638
joint integrity, 661
management, 645–650
  anxiety, 650
  communication impairments, 649
  depression, 650
  disease-modifying agents, 646
  dysphagia, 648–649
  evidence summary, 651–656(t)
  fasciculations, 649–650
  fatigue, 650
  multidisciplinary approach, 646, 646(f),
    647(t)
  muscle cramps, 649–650
  pain, 649–650
  performance measurement set, 647(t)
  pseudobulbar affect, 648
  respiratory impairments, 649
  sialorrhea affect, 648
  spasticity, 649–650
  symptomatic management, 647–648
motor function, 661
muscle length, 661
muscle performance, 661
neuroinflammation, 638
neurotrophic factors, 638
non-familial, 636
pain, 661
pathophysiology, 638–640, 639(f), 640(f)
physical therapy examination, 658–663, 659(b)
  aerobic capacity, 659
  balance, 661–662
  bulbar function, 659
  cognition, 660
  control, 661–662
  cranial nerve integrity, 659–660
  elements, 659(b)
  environmental barriers, 660
  fatigue, 660
  functional status, 660
  gait, 660–661
  integument, 661

joint integrity, 661
motor function, 661
muscle length, 661
muscle performance, 661
pain, 661
postural alignment, 661–662
psychosocial function, 662
quality-of-life measures, 662
range of motion, 661
reflexes, 663
respiratory function, 662–663
sensation, 663
tone, 663
physical therapy interventions, 663–671
  activities of daily living, 669, 669(t)
  cervical muscle weakness, 664, 666(f), 667(t)
  decreased mobility, 669, 670
  disease stages and general intervention
    strategies, 665(t)
  dysarthria, 664
  dysphagia, 664
  lower extremity muscle weakness and gait
    impairments, 669
  muscle cramps, 670
  pain, 667–668
  psychosocial issues, 670–671
  respiratory muscle weakness, 668
  role of physical therapist, 663
  spasticity, 670
  upper extremity muscle weakness, 668
postural alignment, 661–662
prognosis, 645
psychosocial function, 662
quality-of-life measures, 662
range of motion, 661
reflexes, 663
rehabilitation, 650, 656–658, 657(b), 658(f)
  framework, 650, 658(f)
  goals and outcomes, 657(b)
respiratory function, 662–663
risk factors, 637(f)
sensation, 663
staging, 644–645, 645(t), 650, 656, 665(t)
tone, 663
viral infections, 638
Amyotrophic Lateral Sclerosis Assessment
  Questionnaire (ALSAQ-40), 662
Amyotrophic Lateral Sclerosis Association
  (ALSA), 646, 673–674
Amyotrophic Lateral Sclerosis Depression
  Inventory (ADI-12), 662
Analgesia, 89(t)
Analgesics, 500, 501, 772
Analytical/objective learning style, 160
Anarthria, 1112
Anarthric, 642
Anatomical dead space, 383
Aneroid manometer, 59
Aneroid sphygmomanometer, 59, 60(b)
Angina, 432–433
  outcome measures, 457(t)
  presentation, 452(t)
  scale, 454(b)
  as symptom of coronary heart disease, 462
  types, 432–433
Angina pectoris, 434
Angina Scale, 454(b)
Angiogenesis, 353, 472, 476, 509, 527
Angiotensin-converting enzyme (ACE) inhibitors,
  428, 429(t), 438, 443
Angiotensin II receptor antagonists, 543(b)
Angiotensin receptor blockers (ARBs), 428, 430(t),
  438, 443
Angiotensin receptor neprilysin inhibitor (ARNI),
  430(t), 443
Angle of Louis, 416, 453(t)

Angular acceleration, 246(t)
Angular velocity, 245(t), 249, 261, 267
Ankle-brachial index (ABI), 479, 480, 489, 489(f),
  489(t), 505(t), 512, 513, 516
Ankle disarticulation (Syme's), 851(t), 852
Ankle disarticulation, bilateral, 1198
Ankle-foot orthoses (AFO), 1150, 1154,
  1156–1160
  amyotrophic lateral sclerosis, 669
  ankle control, 1157–1159, 1157–1159(f)
  care after delivery, 1171
  clinical considerations, 1159–1160, 1160(f)
  functional electrical stimulation, 565, 566,
    566(b), 567
  gait examination, 255–256
  multiple sclerosis, 626, 627(f)
  structure, 1154, 1156(f), 1156–1157
Ankle plantar flexors, strengthening of, 374, 375(f)
Ankle prostheses, partial, 1181(f), 1181–1182,
  1182(f)
Ankle(s)
  clonus, 150
  gait deviations, 227–228(t)
  rheumatoid arthritis, 898
  spasticity in UMN syndrome, 146(t)
  strategies, 204, 204(f), 359
Anomia, 1108
Anomic aphasia, 1105(t), 1108
Anorgasmia, 689
Anosmia, 687
Anosognosia, 134, 529, 538, 1079, 1085
Anoxia, 63
Anterior cerebral artery (ACA), 528, 529(f)
Anterior cerebral artery (ACA) syndrome, 528,
  529(t)
Anterior cord syndrome, 764
Anterior pelvic support, for WSM, 1257–1258,
  1257–1258(f)
Anterior stop, 1157, 1158, 1158(f)
Anterior view, in postural alignment, 110
Anterolateral spinothalamic system, 78, 81, 82(f),
  83(t)
Anteropulsive gait, 686
Anthropometric characteristics, 486–487
  bioelectrical impedance, 487
  girth measurement, 486–487, 487(f)
  height and weight, 486
  tonometry, 487
  volumetric measurement, 486, 486(f)
Antianxiety medications, 1030–1031(b)
Antiarrhythmics, 429(t)
Antibacterials, 501
Antibiotics,
  burns, 946
  chronic pulmonary dysfunction, 395
  topical, 500, 951(t)
Anticholesterol agents/statins, 543(b)
Anticholinergics, 393, 394(t), 602, 692(t), 694
Anticipation timing (time to contact), 138, 139(b)
Anticipatory balance, 359
Anticipatory motor control, 126, 127(b)
Anticipatory postural adjustments (APAs), 685,
  686
Anticipatory postural control, 199, 206, 550
Anticoagulants, 104, 429(t), 539, 543(b)
Anticonvulsants, 538, 543(b), 649, 772
Antidepressants, 543(b), 602, 772, 1035–1036(b)
Anti-dopaminergics, 681
Antiepileptics, 602, 681
Antihypertensives, 58, 543(b)
Antimicrobials, 500
Antiplatelet therapy, 429(t), 543(b)
Antipsychotics, 693(t), 694
Anti-scald valves, 313, 315
Antiseizure agents, 53
Antiseptics, 500–501

Antisocial personality disorder, 1020
Antispasmodics, 543(b)
Antispastics, 543(b), 602, 622
Anti-tippers, 1261
Anxiety, 1013, 1014, 1025–1029
　addressing, 1027–1029
　　cognitive-behavioral therapy, 1028–1029
　　desensitization, 1028
　　guided imagery, 1028
　　panic attacks, 1029
　　relaxation response, 1027–1028
　amyotrophic lateral sclerosis, 650
　antianxiety medications, 1030–1031(b)
　behaviors associated with, 1026(t)
　causes, 1025, 1026
　Parkinson disease, 689
　psychosocial adaptation, 1016–1017
　referral, 1029
　rehabilitation, 1026–1027
　signs and symptoms, 1025(t)
Aortic area, 417
Aortic bodies, 56
Aortic sinuses, 56
Apathy, 536, 689
Aphasia, 532, 1104–1111
　classification and nomenclature, 1104–1106,
　　1105(t)
　　fluent aphasia, 1104, 1105(f)
　　global aphasia, 1106
　　nonfluent aphasia, 1104, 1105–1106
　　primary progressive aphasia, 1106
　historical perspective, 1106–1107
　management, 1110–1111
　measures, 1107
　post-stroke aphasia, efficacy of treatment,
　　1108–1109
　psychological and related factors, 1109
　recovery, 1108
　treatment, 1109–1110
Aphasia Centers, 1111
Aphasia Communication Outcome Measure, 1107
Aphasic Depression Rating Scale (ADRS), 1107
Apical pulse, 43, 46, 48(f), 48–49
Apical-radial pulse, 49
Apligraf, 511
Apnea, 54(f), 55
Apoptosis, 638
Appel ALS Scale (AALS), 660
Appliance
　environmental control units, 318
　kitchen, 316
Appraisal of Guidelines for Research and
　　Evaluation Enterprise (AGREE), 26
Apraxia, 529, 557, 1073(t), 1092–1094, 1114
　buccofacial apraxia, 1094
　deficits, 134
　ideational apraxia, 1094
　ideomotor apraxia, 1093–1094
　treatment, 1114
Aquacel, 511
Architectural Barrier Act of 1968, 327
Architectural Transportation Barriers and
　　Compliance Board, 327
Areflexic bladder, 770
Areflexive bowel, 771
Arm coordination, outcome measures of,
　　196–197(t)
Arm cradling, 575
Arm ergometry, 423, 426
Arm support, for WSM, 1256–1257
Arnadottir OT-ADL Neurobehavioral Evaluation
　　(A-ONE), 1089, 1093
Arousal
　altered level of, in motor function examination,
　　134–135
　examination, 488

preliminary tests, 75
　traumatic brain injury, 735
Arrhythmias, 416, 444, 445(f), 451(t)
Arterial insufficiency and ulceration, 478–479
　brief overview of disorders, 478
　clinical presentation, 478, 479(f)
　defined, 478
　history, 478–479
　intervention, 479
　tests and measurements, 479
Arterial perfusion, 488–489, 489(f), 489(t)
Arterial system, 470
Arterial wounds, compression treatment and, 515
Arteries, 56–57, 470
Arteriography, 541
Arterioles, 470
Arteriosclerosis, 478, 489
Arteriosclerosis obliterans, 478
Arteriovenous malformation (AVM), 525, 542
Arthritis, 889–938
　balance, 922
　cardiovascular status, 916–917
　case study, 936–938
　education and self-management, 935
　environmental factors, 923
　gait, 922
　history, 914
　joint stability, 916
　joint tenderness, 914, 915
　medical management, 910–914
　mobility, 922
　observation, 914
　outcome measures, 917–921(t), 917–922
　physical activity, 932–934
　　balance training, 932, 933
　　functional training, 932
　　gait training, 932, 933, 934(t)
　　mobile and internet applications, 933(t)
　physical therapy examination, 914–923
　　balance, 922
　　cardiovascular status, 916–917
　　environmental factors, 923
　　gait, 922
　　history, 914
　　joint stability, 916
　　joint tenderness, 914, 915
　　mobility, 922
　　observation, 914
　　outcome measures, 917–921(t), 917–922
　　psychosocial status, 922–923
　　range of motion, 915–916
　　red flag signs and symptoms, 914, 915(t)
　　sensory integrity, 915
　　socioeconomic factors, 923
　　strength, 916
　　yellow flag signs and symptoms, 914, 915(t)
　physical therapy interventions, 923–932
　　cardiovascular training, 930, 932
　　evidence summary of therapeutic exercise,
　　　929(t), 930–931(t)
　　flexibility exercise, 927
　　goals and outcomes, 923(b), 923–924
　　pain relief, 924–927
　　range of motion exercise, 927
　　strengthening exercise, 927–928, 930
　psychosocial status, 922–923
　range of motion, 915–916
　red flag signs and symptoms, 914, 915(t)
　rehabilitative management, 914–935
　sensory integrity, 915
　socioeconomic factors, 923
　strength, 916
　telehealth/telerehabilitation, 935
　yellow flag signs and symptoms, 914, 915(t)
　See also Osteoarthritis; Rheumatoid arthritis
Arthritis Foundation, 322

Arthritis Impact Measurement Scale (AIMS),
　1128
Arthrokinematics, 116, 117, 117(f)
Articulated foot-ankle assemblies, 1184–1185,
　1184–1185(f)
Articulated foot assemblies, 1184–1185,
　1184–1185(f)
Articulation, 135, 1102
Articulatory kinematic approach, 1114
Artificial dermal template (partially temporary),
　953
Ascending reticular activating system, 134
Ashworth Scale (AS), 148
Ashworth Spasticity Scale. See Modified Ashworth
　Scale
ASIA Impairment Scale, 763(b), 763–764
Aspen collar, 774
Aspiration, 535
Aspiration pneumonia, 594
Assessment interview, for WSM, 1235–1236
　demographic information, 1235
　diagnosis, 1236
　employment/work status, 1236
　environmental accessibility, 1236
　functional status and activity level, 1236
　general health status, 1236
　goals, 1236
　history of WSM problems, 1236
　medical/surgical history, 1236
　referral, 1236
　social status, 1236
　transportation, 1236
Assessment of Life Habits, 348(t)
Assisted cough, 790, 790(f)
Assistive devices
　chronic pain, 1006
　gait training with, 379
　multiple sclerosis, 626–628, 627(f), 628(f)
　vascular, lymphatic, and integumentary
　　disorders, 488
Assistive listening devices (ALDs), 99
Assistive technology (AT), 300, 317–318, 319(b),
　782, 1225
Assistive Technology Act of 2004, 317
Assistive technology device, defined, 317
Assistive Technology Outcome Measure (ATOM),
　1281(t)
Assistive technology professional (ATP), 318
Assistive Technology Society of North America,
　318
Associated motor learning, 341, 342(t)
Associated reactions reflex, 145, 152(t), 556
Association for Palliative Medicine of Great Britain
　and Ireland, 649
Associative learning, 340
Associative stage of motor learning, 155, 158(b)
Astereognosis, 89(t), 538, 1092
Asthenia, 187, 190(t), 195(t)
Asthma, 389–390
　clinical course, 390
　clinical presentation, 389–390
　diagnosis, 389
　etiology, 389
　pathophysiology, 389, 389(f)
　pharmacological management, 393, 395(t)
Astrocytoma, 186, 186(f)
Asymmetric tonic neck reflex (ATNR), 144, 152(t)
Asynchronization, 685
Asynergia, 187, 190(t)
Ataxia, 354, 593–594
　cerebellar, 242, 253(t)
　cerebellar impairments, 186–187
　Friedreich, 186, 252–253(t)
　gait, 187–188
　optic, 201
　sensory, 202

Ataxic dysarthria, 1112
Ataxic hemiparesis, 531
Atelectasis, 390
Atherosclerosis, 415, 428, 432, 432(t), 433, 436,
    450, 478, 524, 525, 527
Atherothrombotic brain infarction (ABI), 524, 525
Athetoid movements, 188–189
Athetosis, 188–189, 190(t)
Atopognosia, 89(t)
Atopy, 389
Atrial fibrillation (A-fib), 416, 444, 445(f),
    447–448, 525
Atrial gallop, 453(t)
Atrial kick, 419, 447
Atrioventricular (AV) valves, 418
Atrophy, 142
Atropine, 648
Attachment, Self-regulation, and Competency
    Model (ARC), 1048
Attention
    deficits, 1073–1074
    defined, 535, 1073
    examination, 488
    preliminary tests, 76
    stroke, 535
    traumatic brain injury, 735, 740
Attitude, Social Influence, and Self-Efficacy (ASE)
    model, 1139
Atypical antipsychotics, 693(t), 694
Atypical neuroleptics, 681
Auditory agnosias, 134, 538, 1092
Augmentative/alternative communication, 319(b)
Augmentative and alternative communication
    (AAC), 649, 1113–1114
Augmentative sensory devices, 99
Augmented feedback, 97
Aurix System, 502
Auscultation
    chest, 387
    heart, 440, 452–453(t)
    lungs, 397–398, 398(f), 440, 453(t), 455(f)
Auscultatory gap, 59
Australian Therapy Outcome Measures for
    Occupational Therapy (AusTOMs-OT),
    1067(t)
Australian Therapy Outcomes (AusTOMs), 1070
Authoritative personality, 1019
Autistic fantasy, 1022(b)
Autogenic drainage (AD), 408, 411
Autograft, 952
Autologous skin cell spray, 952
Autolytic débridement, 473, 500
Automated sphygmomanometers, 59, 60(b)
Automated thermometers, 40, 42
Automatic implantable cardiac defibrillator
    (AICD), 447
Automatic movements, motor control and, 336
Autonomic dysreflexia (AD), 765–767
Autonomic function/dysfunction
    mild TBI, 753
    neuromuscular impairments, 143–144
    Parkinson disease, 689, 704–705
Autonomic nervous system (ANS)
    actions of, 143
    chronic pain, 973
    divisions, 143
    stimulation, 144(t)
Autonomous motor learning, 155–156, 158(b),
    341, 342(t)
Autonomy, 1134
Autoregulatory mechanisms, 527
Autosomal recessive trait (Mendelian), 390(f)
Autotopagnosia, 1085
AVERT (A Very Early Rehabilitation Trial),
    362(t), 363
Avoidant personality disorder, 1020

Awakenings (Sacks), 680
Aware in Care kit, 691
Axis system, 1191, 1192(f)
Axonal degeneration, 165
Axonal regeneration, 128, 130, 132(f), 166
Axons, 128–129, 129(f)
Ayres Figure-Ground Test, 1086

B
Babinski sign, 145, 150, 150(t)
Baciguent, 501
Bacitracin, 501, 951
Back Range of Motion II (BROM II), 699
Back support, for WSM, 1254–1255, 1256(b)
Backward walking, 372
Baclofen (Lioresal), 601, 649–650
Bacteria, in wounds, 474
Balance
    amyotrophic lateral sclerosis, 661–662
    arthritis, 922
    chronic pain, 989–990
    confidence measures, 211–212
        Activities-Specific Balance Confidence scale,
        212
        Falls Efficacy Scale, 211
        Falls Efficacy Scale International, 211–212
    gait combination tests, 209–211, 210(f), 211(f)
        Dynamic Gait Index, 210
        Four-Square Step Test, 210, 211(f)
        Get Up and Go Test, 209–210
        Performance-Oriented Mobility Assessment,
        210
        Timed Up and Go Test, 209–210, 210(f)
        Walking While Talking Test, 211
    multiple sclerosis, 593–594
        physical therapy examination, 610
        physical therapy interventions, 623(f),
        623–625, 624(f), 625(f)
    during overground walking, 375–377, 376(b),
    376(f)
    Parkinson disease, 700–701, 704
    performance-based tests, 207–209, 209(t)
        Balance Evaluation Systems Test, 209, 209(t)
        Berg Balance Scale, 208
        Fullerton Advanced Balance Scale, 208
        Functional Reach Test, 207–208, 208(t)
        Function in Sitting Test, 207
        modified Functional Reach Test, 208
        Multidirectional Reach Test, 208, 208(t)
    physical assessment for WSM, 1241
    preprosthetic phase of amputation, 870–872,
    871(f)
    prosthetic training, 1216, 1217(f)
    safe, strategies to promote, 100
    strategies, 201–206
        motor, 204(f), 204–206, 206(t)
        sensory, 201–204, 203(f), 203(t), 204(f)
    stroke
        examination, 548–550
        interventions, 561–563
    training
        arthritis and, 932, 933
        Parkinson disease, 712–715, 713(f), 714(f)
        postsurgical phase of amputation, 860
    traumatic brain injury, 747
    unilateral vestibular hypofunction, 836(t)
    vascular, lymphatic, and integumentary
    disorders, 490
    vestibular disorders, 827, 827(t)
    See also Postural control and balance
Balance Error Scoring System (BESS), 754, 754(t)
Balance Evaluation Systems Test (BESTest), 209,
    209(t), 610, 700–701, 754
Balance point, 802
Balint syndrome, 1091

Balmoral lace stay, 1151, 1151(f)
Bandages, for compression
    four-layer bandage system, 513
    long-stretch and short-stretch, 513, 513(f)
    lymphedema bandaging, 513–514, 514(f)
Bandages, for wounds. See Dressings
Barbiturates, 53
Barefoot walking, 263
Bariatric equipment, 306(b)
Bariatric patients
    classification, 304, 305(t)
    environmental needs, 304, 306(b)
    exterior accessibility to home, 304
    risks and health consequences of obesity, 1144,
    1145(b)
Barognosis (recognition of weight) test, 93, 93(f)
Baroreceptors, 56
Barrier, contextual factors as, 273
Barriers, 7, 7(b), 294
Barthel Index, 552, 1107
Basal ganglia
    motor control, 337, 337(f), 354
    overview, 185, 185(f)
    Parkinson disease, 681(f), 681–682, 685–686
    pathology, 188–189, 190(t)
Basal ganglia-thalamocortical loops, 681
Baseline Dyspnea Index (BDI), 398, 399(t)
Baseline hemodynamic instability, 452(t)
Baseline hemodynamic stability, 451(t)
Base of support (BOS)
    balance training, 562
    closed chain movements, 351
    coordination and balance, 187, 199, 202, 205
    gait, 247
    locomotor function, 375
    motor function, 137, 138, 140, 145
Basic activities of daily living (BADL), 6, 136, 552,
    706, 733
Basilar artery, 532
Bathroom accessibility, 310, 311–315
    additional considerations, 313
    bariatric considerations, 306(b)
    door frames, 310, 311
    grab bars, 311(f), 311–312, 312(f)
    minimum space requirements, 314, 315(f)
    mirrors, 314, 314(f)
    roll-in shower water containment strategies, 314,
    314(f)
    shower entries, 314, 314(f)
    shower stalls, 313, 313(f)
    sinks, 314, 314(f)
    toilets, 311, 311(f)
    tub transfer bench, 312–313, 313(f)
B-cell activation, 589
Beau lines, 34
Becaplermin gel, 502
Beck Depression Inventory, 538, 608, 662,
    1046(t)
Beck Hopelessness Scale, 1047(t)
Bed, 310
Bed mobility
    descriptive terminology, 279(b)
    spinal cord injury, 793–797
        coming straight to long-sitting position from
        supine, 796–797, 797(f)
        prone-on-elbows, 794–795, 795(f)
        rolling, 793–794, 794(f)
        supine-on-elbows, 795, 796(f)
        transitioning supine to/from sitting, 794
        walking on elbows to assume long-sitting
        position, 795, 796, 796(f)
    stroke, 579, 579(f)
Bedroom accessibility, 306(b), 310, 310(f), 311(f)
Bedside nightstand, 310
Behavioral Assessment of the Dysexecutive
    Syndrome, 1076

Behavioral capability, in social cognitive theory, 1135, 1135(t)
Behavioral deficits, stroke and, 536–538, 537(t)
Behavioral Inattention Test (BIT), 1067–1068(t), 1078
Behavioral interventions
   locomotor function, 378–379
   motor control, 349(t)
   multiple sclerosis, 613
   smoking cessation, 393
Behavioral Risk Factor Surveillance System (BRFSS), 1119–1120, 1127
Behavior change, theories of, 1131–1140
   community models, 1140
   Health Belief Model, 1131, 1131(f)
   Physical Activity for People with a Disability model, 1138–1139, 1139(t)
   self-determination theory, 1134
   social cognitive theory, 1134, 1135(f), 1135(t), 1135–1138, 1136–1138(t), 1139(b)
   social ecological model, 1139, 1140
   Theory of Planned Behavior, 1132, 1132(t)
   Theory of Reasoned Action, 1132, 1132(f)
   Transtheoretical Model (stages of change), 1132(t), 1132–1134, 1133(b), 1133(t), 1134(b), 1134(t)
Behavior(s)
   anxiety, 1026(t)
   chronic pain, 979–980, 980(t)
   depression, 1033(t)
   modifiable personal health, 1128–1131
   PTSD, 1031(b)
   substance use, 1037(t)
   suggesting pathological response patterns, 1043(t)
   traumatic brain injury, 740, 749, 750(t)
   warranting mental health consultation, 1044(t)
Behavioural Assessment of the Dysexecutive (BADS), 1067(t)
Beighton Score, 987
Bell shape diaphragm, 59
Bendopnea, 441
Benign arrhythmias, 416, 444
Benign paroxysmal positional vertigo (BPPV), 831, 832–833
   Brandt-Daroff exercises, 833
   canalith repositioning maneuver, 832(f), 832–833, 833(f)
   liberatory (Semont) maneuver, 833
   nystagmus, 831, 832(t)
   traumatic brain injury, 747, 753, 754–755
   treatment techniques, 834(t)
Benzodiazepines, 53, 649, 650
Benztropine (Cogentin), 648
Berg Balance Scale (BBS), 208, 286, 298, 345, 348(t), 549, 558, 562, 563, 608(t), 610, 661, 700–701, 703(t), 740, 743(t), 777(t), 781, 989
Berg Balance Test, 456(t)
Beta-2 agonists, 393, 394(t)
Beta-adrenergic blockers, 428, 430(t), 438
Better Breathing Club, 408
Biceps, 149(t)
Bichannel adjustable ankle locks (BiCAALs), 1158, 1159(f), 1161
Bicuspid valve, 418
Bigeminal pulse, 44
Bigeminy, 444, 445(f)
Bilateral amputation, 874
Bilateral prostheses, 1198
   bilateral ankle disarticulation and transtibial prostheses, 1198
   bilateral transfemoral prostheses, 1198, 1198(f)
Bilateral stance time, 240, 246(t)
Bilateral vestibular hypofunction, 837, 838, 838(t), 839–843(t)

Binaurals, 59
Biobag, 500
Biobrane, 511
Bioburden, 474, 476
Bioelectrical impedance, 487
Biological dressings, 511
Biomarkers, 540
Biomechanical influences of orthotics, 1150, 1150(f)
Biomechanics Framework, 12(f)
Biomedical model, 971, 1126–1127
Bioness L300, 1159
Biopsy, 474
Biopsychosocial model, 971, 1127
Biopsychosocial-spiritual model, 971
Biosurgery, 499–500, 500(f)
Bio-Thesiometer, 96, 97(f)
Biot's respirations, 54(f)
Biventricular failure, 438
Black flags, 979(t)
Bladder function
   Functional Independence Measure (FIM), 287(t), 288
   multiple sclerosis, 592(b), 595, 602–603, 620–621
   screening for WSM, 1239
   spinal cord injury, 770
   stroke, 538–539
Blanch, 943
Blanchable erythema, 483
Blocked practice, 343–344, 345(t), 356–357, 370, 560, 708
Blood flow, 419–420, 488
Blood oxygen level dependent (BOLD) signal, 162
Blood pressure (BP), 55–63
   with activity, 452(t)
   brachial, measuring, 61–62, 62(f)
   cardiovascular health, 526(t)
   defined, 55
   equipment requirements, 586–59, 60(b)
   factors influencing, 56–58
      age, 57, 57(t)
      arm position, 58
      blood volume, 56
      cardiac output, 57
      diameter and elasticity of arteries, 56–57
      exercise, 57
      medications, 58
      orthostatic hypotension, 58
      Valsalva maneuver, 57–58
   invasive or direct measures, 58
   Korotkoff sounds, 59, 61
   noninvasive or indirect measure, 58
   normal, 426–427
   popliteal, measuring, 62–63
   regulation, 56
   stroke risk, 525
Blood pressure cuff, 58–59, 62(f)
Blood stasis, 479
Blood urea nitrogen (BUN), 423
Blood volume, 56
Blucher lace stay, 1151, 1151(f)
Blue flags, 979, 979(t)
Bluetooth capabilities of heart rate monitors, 49
BODE index, 389
Body agnosia, 1085
Body diagram, 490, 982
Body function and structure (BFS)
   ICF framework, 6, 6(f), 7(b), 272–273, 273(f), 274(t)
   musculoskeletal impairments, 140–143
   neuromuscular impairments, 144(t), 143–155, 146(t)
   spinal cord injury, 765–772, 779–781
      aerobic capacity/endurance, 780
      autonomic dysreflexia, 765–766

      bladder dysfunction/management, 770
      bowel dysfunction/management, 770–771
      cardiovascular impairment, 767–768
      initiating stimuli, 766, 766(t)
      integument, 779–780, 780(t)
      intervention, 766, 767
      mental function, 780
      motor and sensory function, 765, 776, 779
      pain, 772, 780–781
      pulmonary impairment, 768–769, 769(t)
      range of motion, 780
      reflex integrity, 781
      respiratory function, 779
      secondary and other impairment, 772
      sexual dysfunction, 771–772
      signs and symptoms, 766
      spastic hypertonia, 767
      thermoregulation impairment, 768
   stroke
      examination, 552–557, 555(t)
      goals, 558(b)
      interventions, 581
   traumatic brain injury, 728–730, 740
      cognitive impairments, 729
      communication impairments, 729–730
      disordered sleep, 730
      neurobehavioral impairments, 729
      neuromuscular impairments, 728–729
      paroxysmal sympathetic hyperactivity, 730
      posttraumatic seizures, 730
      secondary impairments and medical complications, 730, 730(b)
   wheelchair seating/mobility, 1238–1239
      bowel/bladder functions, 1239
      cardiovascular/pulmonary/circulatory status, 1238
      cognitive status, 1239
      communication, 1239
      gastrointestinal system review, 1238
      vision and hearing, 1239
Body heat
   conservation and production, 37–38
   heart rate, 46
   loss, 38
Body image, defined, 1077, 1146
Body mass index (BMI), 304, 305(t), 384, 427, 1120(f), 1127, 1128(b)
Body neglect, 1077
Body odor, 34
Body powered upper limb prostheses, 1199
Body scheme, defined, 1077
Body scheme/body image impairments, 134
   cognitive and perceptual dysfunction and, 1073(t), 1077–1086
      anosognosia, 1079, 1085
      finger agnosia, 1086
      right-left discrimination, 1085–1086
      somatoagnosia, 1085
      unilateral neglect, 1077–1078(f), 1077–1079, 1079(f), 1080–1084(t)
   stroke, 538
Body segment angle measurements, 1245, 1245(f)
Body size/stature, respiration and, 53
Body structures, 6, 6(f), 7(b), 272, 273, 273(f), 274(t)
Body weight support (BWS)
   motor function, 345(t), 360
   multiple sclerosis, 626
   spinal cord injury, 787
   stroke, 564–565, 565(f)
Body weight support treadmill training (BWSTT), 361–362(t), 363, 626, 787
Bone conduction hearing, 77
Bony prominences, pressure points of, 483, 483(f)
Borderline personality disorders, 1020

Borg Rating of Perceived Exertion (RPE), 143, 353, 401(t), 401–402, 462, 462(t), 610, 706
Boston Diagnostic Aphasia Examination (BDAE), 1107
Boston orthosis, 1168–1169, 1169(f)
Botox injections, 351, 355
Bottom-up approaches, 1070
Botulinum toxin (BT) injections, 601–602
Bounding pulse, 44, 45(f), 489
Bowel function
    bowel training, 603
    Functional Independence Measure (FIM), 287(t), 288
    multiple sclerosis, 592(b), 595, 602–603
    screening for WSM, 1239
    spinal cord injury, 770–771
    stroke, 538–539
Box and Blocks Test (BBT), 197(t)
Brachial blood pressure, measuring, 61–62, 62(f)
Brachial pulse, 46(f), 47(b)
Brachioradialis, 149(t)
Braden Scale for Predicting Pressure Sore Risk, 493, 780
Bradycardia, 43
Bradykinesia, 189, 190(t), 195(t), 354, 684
Bradyphrenia, 684
Bradypnea, 54(f), 55
Brain attack, 526
Brain damage. See Traumatic brain injury (TBI)
Brain-derived neurotrophic factor (BDNF), 338, 339, 353–354
Brain Injury Specialist Training, 749
Brain/language journals, 1107
Brain MRI with gadolinium (GAD), 596
Brain pathology, Parkinson disease and, 683, 683(t)
Brain regions that change with chronic pain, 974, 974(f)
Brain stem herniation, 527
Brandt-Daroff exercises, 833
Breakthrough symptoms of bronchoconstriction, 394–395
Breathing
    adventitious breath sounds, 53–54, 397
    bronchial breath sounds, 397
    decreased breath sounds, 397
    exercises, 411–412
    patterns, assessment of, 452(t)
    vesicular breath sounds, 53, 397
Brief International Cognitive Assessment for MS (BICAMS), 608
Brief Pain Inventory (BPI), 609, 661, 981
Brief Symptom Inventory-18, 348(t)
Brim, socket, 1186
Brim variants, 1190(f), 1190–1191
Broca aphasia, 532, 1105(t), 1105–1106, 1108
Brodmann areas, 82, 183
Bronchi, 51, 51(f)
Bronchial breath sounds, 397
Bronchodilators, 53, 393
Brown-Séquard syndrome, 764, 764(f)
Bruce protocol, 458(f)
Bruit, 489
B-type natriuretic peptide (BNP), 442
Buccofacial apraxia, 134, 1093, 1094
Bucket Model, 977, 977(f), 978(b), 992
Buerger disease, 478
Buffalo Concussion Bike Test (BCBT), 753, 754(t)
Buffalo Concussion Treadmill Test (BCTT), 753, 754(t), 755
Buildups, socket, 1186
Bulbar function, 641(t), 642, 659
Bulbar-onset ALS, 636
Bundle of His, 420, 448
Buprenorphine (Subutex), 1039(b)
Buprenorphine and naloxone (Suboxone), 1039(b)

Bupropion (Wellbutrin), 602, 1035(b), 1039(b)
Burden of Stroke Scale (BOSS), 1107
Burn Camps, 964
Burn Rehabilitation Therapist Competency Tool (BRTCT), 958
Burn(s), 939–965
    case study, 965
    classifications, 941–946
        burn wound zone, 945(f), 945–946
        deep partial-thickness burn, 943(f), 943–944
        differential diagnosis, 942(f)
        electrical burn, 945
        epidermal burn, 942, 942(f)
        extent of burned area, 946, 946(f), 947(f)
        full-thickness burn, 944(f), 944–945
        subdermal burn, 945, 945(f)
        superficial partial-thickness burn, 942–943, 943(f)
    community programs, 963–964
    complications, 946–948
        cardiovascular complications, 948
        heterotopic ossification, 948
        infection, 946
        metabolic complications, 946, 947–948
        neuropathy, 948
        pathological scars, 948
        pulmonary complications, 946
    cutaneous functional units, 960(f), 960–961
    dressings, 950, 951
    epidemiology, 939–940
    medical management, 950–953
        initial treatment, 950–951, 951(t)
        surgical management, 951–953, 952–953(f)
    physical therapy management, 953–964
        assessment of burn scars, 954, 955–957(t)
        examination, 954
        goals and outcomes, 954
        intervention, 954, 958(t), 958–964, 959(f), 960(f), 962(f)
    Rule of Nines, 946, 946(f)
    scars
        assessment, 954, 955–957(t)
        contracture, 953
        management, 961–962, 962(f)
        pathological, 948
    skin anatomy, 940(f), 940–941, 941(t)
    wound healing, 948–950
        dermal healing, 949–950
        epidermal healing, 948–949
    wound pathology, 940–941, 941(t)
Burn scar contracture (BSC), 961
Burn wound zone, 945(f), 945–946
Buspirone (BuSpar), 650, 1030(b)

C

C9orf72, 636, 637, 638, 642, 645
Cabinets, kitchen, 315, 316(f)
Cadence, 245(t), 247, 248, 249, 250, 250(f), 256, 262, 264, 265
Calcaneus, 483, 483(f)
Calcium alginate, 510
Calcium channel blockers, 428, 430(t), 438, 681
Calcium influx, stroke and, 527
Calculation ability, preliminary tests of, 76
Call bells, 313
Calluses, 110
Camouflage makeup, 963
Camptocormia, 685
Canadian hip disarticulation prosthesis, 1197
Canadian Occupational Performance Measure (COPM), 1070
Canadian Stroke Guidelines, 574, 576
Canalith repositioning maneuver (CRM), 832(f), 832–833, 833(f)

Capabilities of Upper Extremity Instrument (CUEI), 777(t), 781
Capacity, 6, 6(f), 7(b)
    improved motor performance, 350
    lung, 383(f), 383–384
    measures of function, 276, 277
    performance vs. capacity vs. patient-reported outcomes, 379
    qualifiers, 6–7
    selective, stroke and, 555–556
    tests as functional performance measures, 277
Capsular end-feel, 116
Capsular patterns, 116
Carbamazepine (Atretol, Tegretol), 601, 602, 649
Carbidopa/levodopa, 691, 692(t), 693–694
Carbon dioxide (CO$_2$), 384
Carbon monoxide alarms, 309
Cardiac anatomy and physiology, 416(f), 416–423
    blood flow and hemodynamic values, 419–420, 420(t)
    cardiac cycle, 419, 420(f)
    cardiac index, 419
    cardiac output, 418–419
    coronary arteries, 417–418, 418(f)
    electrical conduction of the heart, 420–421, 421(f)
    heart tissue, 417, 417(f)
    heart valves, 418
    laboratory values, 422(t), 422–423
    myocardial oxygen supply and demand, 422
    neurohormonal influences on cardiovascular system, 421–422
    stroke volume, 419, 419(f)
    surface anatomy of the heart, 416(f), 416–417
Cardiac cycle, 419, 420(f)
Cardiac enzymes, 436
Cardiac index (CI), 419
Cardiac muscle dysfunction, 438, 439(b)
Cardiac output (CO), 57, 418–419
Cardiac rehabilitation
    coronary artery disease, 454
    inpatient, 459–460(t)
    outpatient, exercise prescription parameters utilized in, 461(t)
    phase I, 454, 459(t)
    phase II, 457, 461(t)
    research on effectiveness, 459(t)
Cardiac tamponade, 417
Cardinal signs. See Vital signs
Cardinal vowels, 1103, 1103(f)
Cardiomyopathies, 417
Cardiopulmonary interventions
    amputation, 872
    motor control, 349(t)
Cardiopulmonary resuscitation (CPR), 447
Cardiovascular deconditioning, 456(t)
Cardiovascular disease (CVD)
    clinical presentations, 426
    epidemiology, 415, 416
    hypertension, 416, 426–428
Cardiovascular function
    arthritis, 916–917
    burns, 948
    Parkinson disease, 705–706
    rheumatoid arthritis, 900
    screening for WSM, 1238
    spinal cord injury, 767–768
    stroke, 526(t), 539
Cardiovascular system
    anatomy and physiology, 416(f), 416–423 (See also Cardiac anatomy and physiology)
    cardiac pathologies and physical therapy implications, 426–450 (See also Heart disease)
    responses to exercise, 423–426 (See also under Exercise)

Cardiovascular training
  arthritis, 930, 932
  spinal cord injury, 792(f), 792–793
Care paths and delivery, Parkinson disease and, 696–697, 697(t)
Carina, 51
Carotid bodies, 56
Carotid Doppler ultrasound, 541
Carotid endarterectomy, 542
Carotid pulse, 43, 46(f), 47(b)
Carotid sinuses, 56
Carpeting, home accessibility and, 306–307
Carpometacarpal (CMC) joints
  capsular patterns, 116(t)
  rheumatoid arthritis, 898
Cartilage, osteoarthritis and, 902–903
Case manager, traumatic brain injury and, 733
Cast shoes, 518
Catechol-O-methyltransferase (COMT), 692(t), 694, 978
Catheterization, heart, 420, 420(t)
Cauda equina, 765
Cauda equina injuries, 764–765
Caudate, 338
Caudate nucleus, 185, 185(f), 681
Causalgia, 89(t), 973
C-Brace, 1165
Ceiling effects, 156
Celexa (Lexapro), 1035(b)
Cell phone apps, 305
Cellulitis, 482, 488
Center for Health Care Strategies, 1048
Center for International Rehabilitation Research Information and Exchange, 25(t)
Center for Neurologic Study Bulbar Function Scale (CNS-BFS), 659
Center for Outcome Measurement in Brain Injury (COMBI), 742
Center for Universal Design, 295
Center of Epidemiologic Study Depression Scale, 662
Center of force (COF), 200
Center of gravity (COG), 145
Center of mass (COM)
  alignment, 200, 201, 375
  coordination and balance, 199–200, 202, 205, 561–562
  gait, 261, 261(t), 262, 267
  locomotor function, 375–376
  motor function, 138, 140
Center of pressure (COP), 200, 261, 261(t), 262, 264
Centers for Disease Control and Prevention (CDC), 33, 209–210, 485, 1034, 1124, 1127, 1128, 1144
Centers for Medicare and Medicaid Services (CMS), 23, 24, 136, 288, 552, 604, 697, 741, 782
Centigrade scale, 35, 36(f)
Central chemoreceptors, 52
Central cord syndrome, 764
Central cyanosis, 35(b)
Central elements of motor system, 183
Central nervous system (CNS)
  depressant agents, 53
  differential diagnosis of major types of CNS disorders, 175–177(t)
  electrophysiologic neuromuscular assessment, 163, 172(t), 173
  magnetic resonance imaging, 161
  motor coordination, 138
  motor learning, 126
  motor structure/function, 127
  muscle tone, 147, 148
  nerve conduction studies, 165
  neural plasticity, 130

neuromuscular control factors, 140–141
  PET/SPECT, 163
  reflexes, 149, 151
  task systems, 126
  vestibular system dysfunction, 830
Central neuropathic pain (CNP), 969(t), 970, 975
Central pattern generators, 126
Central poststroke pain (CPSP), 531, 553–554
Central Sensitivity Index (CSI), 984, 985(t)
Central sensitization (CS), 967, 974(f), 974–975
Central vestibular system, 817, 817(f)
Cerebellar ataxia, 242, 253(t)
Cerebellar pathology, 186–188, 187(f), 190(t)
Cerebellum, 184–185, 187(f), 338, 338(f)
Cerebral blood flow, stroke and, 524, 526–528, 528–529(f)
Cerebral cortex, 185, 185(f)
Cerebral edema, 527
Cerebral embolus (CE), 524
Cerebral hemorrhage, 525, 528, 538, 540, 541(f)
Cerebral infarction, 524, 527, 529, 540
Cerebral palsy (CP)
  coordination impairments, 182
  gait analysis
    observational gait scale scores, 226
    outcome measures, 234(t), 236(t)
    6-minute Walk Test, 247
    walkway systems, 251(t)
  orthotics
    ankle-foot orthotics for children, 1159
    energy considerations, 1176
Cerebral perfusion pressure (CPP), 734
Cerebral shock, 147
Cerebral thrombosis, 524
Cerebrospinal fluid (CSF) analysis, 596
Cerebrovascular accident (CVA). See Stroke
Cerebrovascular imaging, 540–541, 541(f)
  arteriography, 541
  computed tomography, 540, 541(f)
  digital subtraction angiography, 541
  Doppler ultrasound, 541
  magnetic resonance angiography, 541
  magnetic resonance imaging, 540–541, 541(f)
Certificate of Clinical Competence in speech-pathology (CCC-SLP), 1099
Cervical collars, 664, 666(f)
Cervical Range of Motion instruments, 699
Cervical spine
  mild TBI, 753–754
  muscle weakness, ALS and, 664, 666(f), 667(t)
  orthoses, 774, 774(f), 1167(f), 1167–1168, 1168(f)
  rheumatoid arthritis, 893, 895(f)
Cervicogenic dizziness, 846
Chaddock sign, 150, 150(t)
Chair glides, 670
Challenge point theory, 342–343, 343(f), 356
Challenge pressure, 350(t)
Change, stages of, 1132(t), 1132–1134, 1133(b), 1133(t), 1134(b), 1134(t)
Change-in-support strategies, 205, 359
Charcot joint, 488
Charcot triad, 588
Charleston bending brace, 1169
Chemical débridement, 499
Chemical thermogenesis, 37
Chemoreceptors, 56, 78, 79(b)
Chessington Occupational Therapy Neurological Assessment Battery, 1074
Chest pain referral pattern, 434, 434(f)
Cheyne-Stokes respirations, 54(f), 55, 527
Child Health Questionnaire (CHQ), 1128
Chlamydia pneumoniae, 589
Chlordiazepoxide (Librium, Mitran, Reposans-10), 650, 1030(b)
Chlorpromazine, 681

Cholesterol, 525, 526(t)
Cholinesterase inhibitors, 693(t), 694
Chopart disarticulations, 1181, 1181(f)
Chorea, 189, 190(t)
Choreiform movements, 189
Choreoathetosis, 189, 190(t), 531
Chronic care, 2, 3(b)
Chronic illness, psychosocial adaptation to, 1018
Chronic inflammation, 122, 472
Chronic inflammatory demyelinating polyradiculoneuropathy, 235(t)
Chronic kidney disease, 525
Chronic low back pain (CLBP), 989
Chronic lung diseases, 384–393
  asthma, 389–390
  COPD, 384–389
  COVID-19, 392–393
  cystic fibrosis, 390–391
  restrictive lung diseases, 391–392
Chronic obstructive pulmonary disease (COPD), 384–389
  ABCD assessment tool, 385, 386(f)
  clinical presentation, 387(f), 387–389, 388(f)
  course and prognosis, 389
  gait analysis, 235(t), 242
  pathophysiology, 385, 386–387
  pharmacological management, 384(t), 393
  risk factors, 385
  supplemental oxygen, 395
Chronic pain, 966–1011
  alert flags, 979, 979(t)
  basic concepts, 867–971
  biopsychosocial model of pain, 971
  brain regions that change in patients with, 974, 974(f)
  Bucket Model, 977, 977(f), 978(b)
  case study, 1009–1011
  chronification of neuropathic pain, 976–977
  complementary and alternative approaches, 1008
  defined, 970
  diagnosis, 990–992, 991(f)
  examination of patients with, 980, 981–990
    general flow, 981, 982(f)
    impact of pain on physical and psychosocial function, 981, 982
    mnemonics for assessing, 982, 984(b)
    pain characteristics, 982, 984, 984(b)
    pain classification tools, 985(t)
    pain severity and functional assessment tools, 983(t)
    physical therapy tests and measures, 987–990, 989(t)
    PSCEBSM model for taking a biopsychosocial history, 986(b)
    psychosocial factors impacting pain, 984, 986, 986(b)
    review of systems, 987
    subjective examination, 986–987
    systems review, 987
  Fear-Avoidance Model, 980, 981(f)
  IASP definition, 967(b)
  ICD-11 classification, 970(b)
  medically unexplained pain, 971
  medical management, 1007
    medical diagnostic testing, 1007
    other, 1007
    pharmacological management, 1007
  neural processing changes, 972–976, 974(f), 976(f)
  pain behavior clusters, 980(t)
  pathophysiology, 971–977
  physical therapy evaluation, 990–992, 991(f)
  physical therapy management, 993–1007
    assistive devices, 1006
    biophysical and other modalities, 1006–1007

chronic pain interventions by mechanism, 996–997(t)
cognitive behavioral therapy, 999, 1000, 1001(b)
cognitive functional therapy, 1000
CPGs for chronic pain, 993, 994–995(t), 1007
exercise, 1004–1005, 1006(t)
instruction, 995, 997, 999
manual therapy, 1005, 1006
multidisciplinary pain management team, 993, 995
neuromuscular reeducation, 1003–1004
pain coping skills, 999–1002, 1001(b)
physical self-care strategies, 1002–1003
therapeutic alliance, 995
prognosis, 992993
risk factors, 977(f), 977–980, 978(b)
genetic, 978
pain beliefs and behaviors, 979–980, 980(t)
psychosocial, 978–979
subjective and objective characteristics, 969(t)
terminology, 967(b), 968(b)
types, 967, 969–971
Chronic phase of stroke recovery, 544–545
Chronic primary pain, 970
Chronic PTSD, 1029
Chronic pulmonary dysfunction, 382–414
case study, 413–414
chronic lung diseases, 384–393
asthma, 389–390
COPD, 384–389
COVID-19, 392–393
cystic fibrosis, 390–391
restrictive lung diseases, 391–392
exercise intensity, 401–402
interval vs. continuous exercise, 403–405(t)
as a percentage of peak workload, 402
as a percent of heart rate, 401
as a percent of VO$_{2peak}$, 401
by rating of perceived exertion/perceived dyspnea, 401(t), 401–402
interventional management, 396
medical management, 393–395
pharmacological management, 393–395, 394–395(t)
smoking cessation, 393–396
supplemental oxygen, 395
physical therapy management, 396–412
education, 408, 408(b)
examination, 397–400
exercise prescription, 400, 401–402
goals and outcomes, 396, 396(b)
home exercise programs, 407, 407(f)
multispecialty team, 407–408
pulmonary rehabilitation, 402, 405–406
secretion removal techniques, 408–412
respiratory physiology, 383(f), 383–384, 384(f)
surgical management, 396
Chronic Respiratory Questionnaire, 398, 399(t)
Chronic stage, 122
Chronic venous insufficiency (CVI), 471, 479–481, 515. See also Venous insufficiency
Chronic wound, 477(f), 477–478
Chronification of neuropathic pain, 976–977
Chronotropic competence, 44
Chronotropy, 421
Circadian rhythm, 39
Circle of Willis, 528
Circuit class training (CCT), 582
Circuit-training physical therapy (CTPT), 351, 352(t), 377, 377(b), 378(f), 582–583
Circuit-training workstations, 573
Circulation, 488–490
arterial perfusion, 488–489, 489(f), 489(t)
lymph vessel integrity, 490

pain, 489–490
special tests, 490
status, in screening for WSM, 1238
temperature, 488
trophic changes, 489
venous patency, 490
Circumduction, 227, 230(t), 1210(t), 1212
Civic life, 782
Cladribine (Mavenclad), 598(t)
Clasp-knife response, 145, 146
Classical conditioning, 340
Classification of Walking Handicap After Stroke, 551
Classification System for Chronic Pain in SCI, 781
Claudication, intermittent, 236(t)
Claudication Scale, 490
C-Leg, 1192(f), 1193
C-Leg prostheses, 266
Clinical Application Guide to Standardized Wheelchair Seating Measures of the Body and Seating Support Surfaces, Revised Edition, 1244
Clinical Assessment Scale for Contraversive Pushing, 550
Clinical COPD Questionnaire, 399(t)
Clinical decisions, 2, 3(f), 5, 14, 23
feedback in motor learning, 345
motor learning, 342
orthotics, 1175–1176
energy considerations, 1175–1176
psychosocial considerations, 1176
stroke, 545
vital signs, 32
See also Clinical reasoning; Integrated framework
Clinical exercise testing, 619–620
Clinical Fellowship Year, 1099
Clinically definite ALS, 643–644, 644(f)
Clinically established PD, 691
Clinically isolated syndrome (CIS), 590, 590(b)
Clinically possible ALS, 643, 644, 644(f)
Clinically probable, laboratory-supported ALS, 643, 644, 644(f)
Clinically probable ALS, 643, 644, 644(f)
Clinically probable PD, 691
Clinical pain, 971
Clinical practice environments, 2, 4(b)
Clinical Practice Guideline for Locomotor Training, 2020, 360
Clinical practice guidelines (CPGs), 14, 24, 26
chronic pain, 993, 994–995(t), 1007
locomotor training, 360, 372, 373
stroke, 547, 559
traumatic brain injury, 752
Clinical Practice Guideline to Improve Locomotor Function Following Chronic Stroke, Incomplete Spinal Cord Injury, and Brain Injury, 372, 373
Clinical practice terminology, 3–4(b)
Clinical reasoning, 2
elements, 5–8
HOAC, 5
ICF, 5–8, 6 (f), 7(b)
movement science and movement system, 8
shared decision-making, 5
Clinical Sensory Test, 988, 989(t), 990
Clinical Stride Analyzer, 250
Clinical stroke rehabilitation specialist (CSRS), 542
Clinical syndromes, spinal cord injury and, 764(f), 764–765
anterior cord syndrome, 764
Brown-Séquard syndrome, 764
cauda equina injuries, 764–765
central cord syndrome, 764
conus medullaris syndrome, 765

Clinical Test of Sensory Interaction on Balance (CTSIB), 202–204, 203(t), 348(t), 610
Clinical Trials Registry, National Institutes of Health (NIH), 25(t)
Clinician Administered PTSD Scale Revised, 1031
Clonazepam (Klonopin), 649
Clonidine (Catapres), 1039(b)
Clonus, 148, 149, 150
Clorazepate, 650
Clorazepate dipotassium (Tranxene, Gen-Xene), 1030(b)
Closed chain movements, 351, 352(t)
Closed-ended questions, 9
Closed environment, 158, 560, 562
Closed-loop system, 126, 184–185, 336, 349(t), 350(t)
Closed-loop theory, 341
Closed skills, 138, 139(b)
Closed technique, 950
Close guarding, defined, 279(b)
Closet clothes bar, 310, 310(f)
Closets, 295, 308, 310, 310(f)
Clot-dissolving enzymes, 526
Clothing, donning/doffing from wheelchair, 1237
Clubbing, 34, 35(f), 110
Cluster analysis, 266
C-Mill, 262
Coaching, health and wellness, 1140–1141
Coccyx, 483, 483(f)
Cochrane Central Register of Controlled Trials (CCTR), 25(t)
Cochrane Database of Systematic Reviews, 24, 25(t), 352, 353, 357, 360, 377, 393, 459(t), 545, 565, 566, 571, 572–573, 576, 580, 582–583, 616(t), 651(t), 652(t), 670, 839(t), 842(t), 1005, 1074, 1075, 1076, 1079, 1138(t)
Cock-up splint, 1170(t)
Co-contraction, 354
Codamotion, 256
Code of Ethics, ASHA, 1100
COGNISTAT, 1068(t)
Cognition
amyotrophic lateral sclerosis, 660
decision-making, 335
defined, 76
examination, 488
higher-order, 1055
mild TBI, 752–753
motor learning, 341, 342(t)
multiple sclerosis, 608
preliminary tests, 76
prosthetics, 1204–1205
rehabilitation, 630, 1059–1061
tests, 1065–1070
traumatic brain injury, 735, 740, 753
vision, 201
Cognitive behavioral therapy (CBT)
anxiety, 1028–1029
chronic pain, 999, 1000, 1001(b)
multiple sclerosis, 602, 603, 630, 631
Cognitive-communication disorders, 1111–1112
examination, 1111
treatment, 1111–1112, 1112(b)
Cognitive dysfunction, 1054–1097
amyotrophic lateral sclerosis, 641(t), 642–643
case study, 1095–1097
chronic pain, 1000
clinical indicators, 1056–1057
cognition and higher-order cognition, 1055
discharge planning, 1072
examination, 1061–1070
differentiating sensory loss from cognitive/perceptual deficits, 1063–1065, 1064–1065(f)
factors influencing, 1062–1063

Cognitive dysfunction (*continued*)
  outcome measures, 1066–1069(*t*)
  purpose, 1061–1062
  standardized cognitive and perceptual tests, 1065–1070
hospitalization following brain damage, 1057
intervention, 1070–1072
  education, 1070, 1071
  impact of managed care, 1071–1072
  motor control, 349(*t*)
  refocusing, 1071
  treatment approaches, 1070, 1071(*t*)
motor function examination, 135
motor learning stage, 155, 158(*b*)
multiple sclerosis, 591–592(*b*), 594, 602, 630
overview, 1072–1094
  agnosias (simple perception), 1090–1092, 1091–1092(*f*)
  apraxia, 1092–1094
  attention deficits, 1073–1074
  body scheme and body image impairments, 1077–1078(*f*), 1077–1086, 1079(*f*), 1080–1084(*t*)
  executive function impairments, 1075–1077
  memory impairments, 1074–1075
  spatial relations disorders (complex perception), 1086–1090, 1087(*f*), 1088(*f*), 1090(*f*)
Parkinson disease, 705
perception, 1055
physical/occupational therapist's responsibilities, 1056
screening for WSM, 1239
stroke, 535–536
summary, 1073(*t*)
theoretical frameworks, 1057–1061
  cognitive rehabilitation, 1059–1061
  neurofunctional approach, 1058
  quadraphonic approach, 1059–1061, 1060–1061(*f*)
  rehabilitative/compensatory (functional) approach, 1058–1059
  retraining approach, 1057–1058
  sensory integrative approach, 1058
traumatic brain injury, 729
Cognitive-evaluative dimension, 972
Cognitive mapping, 155
Cognitive-motor interference (CMI), 594
Cognitive rehabilitation approach, 1060
Cognitive rehabilitation/quadraphonic approach, 1070
Cognitive Timed Up-and- Go (CTUG), 700
Cogwheel rigidity, 146, 189, 190(*t*), 684
Cold laser therapy, 508
Cold therapy, 924
Collagenase, 951
Collagen synthesis, 472, 476
Collateral sprouting, 130, 132(*f*), 170
Collectors, 470
College of Chest Physicians, 397
Color agnosia, 1091
Coloration
  integumentary integrity, 490–491
  wound drainage by, 491, 491(*t*)
Coma, 75, 532, 729
Coma Recovery Scale-Revised (CRC-R), 735, 743(*t*)
Combined cortical sensations, 78, 91–93
  barognosis (recognition of weight), 93, 93(*f*)
  double simultaneous stimulation, 92–93
  graphesthesia (traced figure identification), 93
  recognition of texture, 93
  stereognosis perception, 91
  tactile localization, 91–92
  two-point discrimination, 92
ComfortFlex socket design, 1194(*f*), 1197(*f*)

Commercial building requirements, 294
Commercial skin and wound cleansers, 498
Communication
  augmentative and alternative, 649, 1113–1114
  defined, 1099
  functional, 1107
Communication impairments
  amyotrophic lateral sclerosis, 649
  augmentative and alternative communication, 319(*b*)
  Functional Independence Measure (FIM), 287(*t*)
  integumentary system disorders, 495
  interventions, 19
  lymphatic system disorders, 495
  motor function examination, 135
  screening for WSM, 1239
  traumatic brain injury, 729–730
  vascular system disorders, 495
  See also Neurogenic disorders of communication
Communication partners approach, 1110
Communicative Activities of Daily Living-3rd Edition (CADL-3), 1107
Communicative Effectiveness Index, 1107
Community Adaptation Schedule, 1048(*t*)
Community Balance and Mobility Scale (CB&M), 233, 242, 369, 740, 743(*t*)
Community-dwelling older adults, 26, 204, 211
Community environment
  access, 322–324
    facilities, 324
    transportation, 323(*f*), 323–324, 324(*f*), 325(*f*)
  burn programs, 963–964
  models of behavior change, 1140
  prosthetic training and mobility, 1218–1219
  reentry/reintegration
    prosthetics and, 1219–1220
    traumatic brain injury, 742, 749, 751(*t*)
  spinal cord injury, 782
Community Integration Questionnaire (CIQ), 742
Community walker, 551, 551(*t*)
Compact joystick, 1279
Compendium of Physical Activities, 423
Compensated HF, 440
Compensation, 347
  motor, 129, 132(*b*)
  permanent loss, 347
  rehabilitative/compensatory approach, 775, 1059
Compensatory-based interventions, 19–20
  cognitive and perceptual dysfunction, 1070, 1071(*t*), 1074
  multiple sclerosis, 604
  sensory function, 97
  spinal cord injury, 804–806, 805–806(*f*)
  stroke, 545
  traumatic brain injury, 742, 744, 744(*t*), 745(*t*)
Compensatory intervention, 663
Compensatory training approach, 317
Competence, 1134
Complementary therapies, for arthritis pain relief, 926–927
Complete basilar artery syndrome, 533(*t*)
Complete decongestive therapy (CDT), 482, 512, 514
Complete injury, 763
Complete spinal cord injury, 763
Complex motor skill, 138, 139(*b*)
Complex regional pain syndrome (CRPS), 578, 1003
Complex rehabilitation technology (CRT), 1228, 1263, 1280
Complex repetitive discharges (CRDs), 168
Complicated MI, 433
Composite dressings, 511

Compound motor action potential (CMAP), 165(*f*), 165–166, 166(*f*), 167
Comprehensive High-Level Activity Mobility Predictor, 1204
Comprehensive Lower-Limb Amputee Socket Survey (CLASS), 1201
Comprehensive Rehabilitation Services Amendments of 1978, 327
Comprehensive stroke center (CSC), 526
Compression (accessory motion), 117
Compression garments, 514(*f*), 514–515
Compression therapy, 480, 512–516
  compression garments, 514(*f*), 514–515
  compression guidelines, 515–516
  elevation, 512–516
  four-layer bandage system, 513
  guidelines, 515–516
  intermittent pneumatic compression, 516, 516(*f*)
  limb containment systems, 515, 515(*f*)
  long-stretch and short-stretch bandages, 513, 513(*f*)
  lymphedema bandaging, 513–514, 514(*f*)
  sequential pneumatic compression with truncal component, 516, 516(*f*)
  Unna boot, 512–513
Computed tomography (CT), 160–161, 161(*f*), 164(*t*), 525, 526, 540, 541(*f*)
Computer-aided design/computer-aided manufacture, 1186
Computer applications, 319(*b*)
Computerized adaptive test (CAT), 289
Computer workstations, 321–322, 322(*f*)
Concave-convex rule, 117, 118(*f*)
Concentric contractions, 351
Concurrent validity, 283
Conditioned pain modulation (CPM), 988, 1004
Conditioning
  burns, 961
  multiple sclerosis, 614, 619
Condition of Participation, 288
Conducting zone, 51, 52(*f*)
Conduction, 38
Conduction aphasia, 1105(*t*), 1108
Conduction delays and blocks, 165, 448
Confabulation, 535
Confrontation method, 201
Confusion, stroke and, 535
Congestive heart failure (CHF), 415–416, 440–441
  biventricular pacer, 444
  chest x-ray to confirm, 442, 442(*f*)
  clinical presentation, 440–441
  edema, 453(*t*)
  education, 464(*b*)
  epidemiology, 415–416, 438
  nutrition, 462
  self-monitoring, 461–462
  stroke risk, 525
  See also Heart failure (HF)
Consciousness, levels of, 134–135, 532
Consciousness raising (change process), 1133, 1133(*f*)
Consecutive task training (CTT), 719
Consensus-based standards for the selection of health measurement instruments (COSMIN), 282, 283
Consensus Statement from the Concussion in Sport Group, 752
Consonants, 1100, 1102–1103, 1103(*t*)
Consortium for Spinal Cord Medicine, 517
Consortium of Multiple Sclerosis Centers, 596, 608
Constant error, 157(*t*)
Constant fever, 38(*b*)
Constant friction, 1193

Constant practice, 344, 345(*t*), 356–357, 370
Constipation, 539, 603, 689
Constraint-induced aphasia therapy (CIAT), 1109–1110
Constraint-induced language therapy (CILT), 1109–1110
Constraint-induced movement therapy (CIMT), 544, 570–571, 571(*f*), 747
Construct validity, 204
Contact guarding, 279(*b*)
Contact inhibition, 475, 476
Contemplation stage of change, 1132, 1133(*b*)
Content validity, 283
Context, 1099, 1103
Contextual factors, 5, 6(*f*), 7, 7(*b*), 783
Contextual interference, 343–344, 560, 686
Contextual Memory Test, 1046(*t*)
Continuity Assessment Record and Evaluation (CARE), 136, 288, 608(*t*), 610, 706, 741, 782
Continuous fever, 38(*b*)
Continuous gait control problems, 686
Continuous moderate aerobic exercise, 463(*t*)
Continuous motor skill, 138, 139(*b*), 340
Continuous shortwave diathermy (CSWD), 506
Continuum of care, traumatic brain injury and, 732
Contractility, 419
Contraction
    muscle, 140–142
    wound healing, 474–475
Contracture
    burn scars, 953
    lower extremities, 685
Contralateral hemiplegia, 531
Contralateral loss of proprioception, 764
Contralesional extrapersonal space, 1077
Contralesional peripersonal space, 1077
Contralesional personal space, 1077
Contrast CT, 160, 164(*t*)
Contrast sensitivity, 335
Contraversive pushing, 550, 563
Control. *See* Postural control and balance
Control unit, 318
Conus medullaris syndrome, 765
Convection, 38
Conventional double upright/dual channel AFO, 567
Conventional joystick, 1279
Conversion disorder, 1013
Cool-down period of exercise, 351, 352(*t*)
Coordination
    age-related impairments, 191–192
        changes in skilled motor performance, 191–192
        decreased ROM, 191
        decreased strength, 191
        postural changes, 191
        slowed reaction time, 191
    basal ganglia pathology, 188–189, 190(*t*)
    cerebellar pathology, 186–188, 187(*f*), 190(*t*)
    defined, 126, 127(*b*), 138, 181, 354
    dorsal (posterior) column-medial lemniscal pathology, 189
    examination
        administering, 192–193, 194–196
        arm, hand, and finger coordination, 196–197(*t*)
        case study, 214–215
        coordination tests, 192, 193–194(*t*), 195(*t*)
        documentation, 195–196
        examples, 198(*b*)
        outcome measures of upper extremity coordination, 196–198, 196–197(*t*), 198(*b*)
        patient considerations, 192
        preliminary observation, 192–193

    preparation, 192–193
    purposes of performing, 182(*f*), 182–183
    testing environment/equipment, 192
integumentary system disorders, 495
interventions, 19, 354–355
lymphatic system disorders, 495
motor, 138, 139
multiple sclerosis, 593–594, 623(*f*), 623–625, 624(*f*), 625(*f*)
prosthetic training, 1216, 1217(*f*)
stroke, 556–557
terms associated with, 181–182
tests, 192, 193–194(*t*), 195(*t*)
types, 182
vascular system disorders, 495
Coordinative structures (synergies), 126, 127(*b*), 144–145
Copaxone, 601
COPD assessment test (CAT), 398, 399(*t*)
COPD Control Questionnaire (CCQ), 398
Coping styles, 1021–1022
Core Sets, 8
Coriolis acceleration, 249
Corium, 941
Coronary arteries, 417–418, 418(*f*)
Coronary artery bypass graft (CABG), 436–437
Coronary artery disease (CAD)
    angina, 432–433, 452(*t*), 454(*b*), 457(*t*), 462
    cardiac muscle dysfunction, 439(*b*)
    cardiac rehabilitation, 454
    clinical manifestations, 428, 432
    epidemiology, 415–416, 438
    heart tissue, 417
    pharmacological management, 438
    primary prevention, 465
    See also Acute coronary syndrome (ACS)
Coronary blood flow, 422
Coronary computed tomography angiography (CCTA), 443
Coronary heart disease (CHD). *See* Coronary artery disease (CAD)
Coronavirus disease 2019. *See* COVID-19 pandemic
Cor pulmonale, 386
Corrigan's (water-hammer) pulse, 45(*f*)
Corsets, 1165–1166, 1166(*f*)
Cortex, 127, 127(*f*)
Cortical-basal ganglionic degeneration (CBGD), 681
Cortical blindness, 531, 1065
Cortically controlled movement, 336
Corticobulbar tract, 184
Corticospinal impairments, 355
Corticospinal tract (CST), 558
Corticosteroids, 104, 393, 394(*t*)
Corticotropin-releasing factor (CRF), 1016
Cougar Home Safety Assessment, 300(*t*)
Cough assist device, 668
Cough/coughing, 34, 50, 51, 410
Counter, 1151(*f*), 1152
Counterconditioning (change process), 1133, 1133(*t*)
Countertops, kitchen, 315, 315(*f*)
Couplets, 444, 445(*f*), 447
COVID-19 pandemic, 392–393, 601, 990, 1005, 1050, 1100
COVID-19-related postencephalitic parkinsonism, 680
Crackles (rales), 54, 387, 390, 397, 440, 453(*t*)
Craig Handicap Assessment and Reporting Technique (CHART), 299(*t*), 773, 778(*t*), 782
Craig Hospital Inventory of Environmental Factors (CHIEF), 299(*t*)
Cranial nerves (CNs)
    function
        abnormal, 151, 153–155
        components, 98(*t*)

documentation, 151
sensory examination, 97
tests, 99(*b*)
integrity, 58, 68
    amyotrophic lateral sclerosis and, 639, 659(*b*), 659–660
    chronic pain and, 988
    examination of, 151, 153–155(*t*)
    multiple sclerosis, 609
    traumatic brain injury, 739(*b*)
stroke
    dysphagia, 535
    motor control, 557
    visual field defects, 553
CRASH (corticosteroid randomization after significant head injury), 731
Creams, antibacterial, 501
Creatine kinase (CK), 436
Creatine kinase MB (CK-MB), 436
Creatinine, 423
Credé maneuver, 602
Cremasteric reflex, 150
Creutzfeldt-Jakob disease, 681
Criterion-related validity, 283
Crossed extension reflex, 152(*t*)
Crosstalk, 977
CRT diagnoses, 1280
Cryotherapy, 622
Cuff variants, 1187–1189, 1189(*f*)
Cuing strategies, 708–709
Cultural competence, 33
Culture
    defined, 33
    vital signs, 33
Cultured autologous composite grafts, 951
Cultured dermis, temporary/definitive, 953
Cultured epidermal autografts (CEAs), 951
Cumulative Index to Nursing and Allied Health Literature (CINAHL), 25(*t*)
Curb cuts, 321
Curbs, prosthetic training and, 1218–1219
Cusps, 418
Cutaneous functional units (CFUs), 960(*f*), 960–961
Cutaneous inputs, 335
Cutaneous reflexes, 150, 150(*t*)
Cutaneous sensory receptors, 78–80, 79(*b*), 80(*f*)
Cutis anserina, 37
Cyanosis, 35(*b*), 110
Cycle ergometry, 557, 581, 706
Cycle time, 217, 246(*t*), 255
Cystic fibrosis (CF), 390–391
    clinical presentation, 391
    course and prognosis, 391
    diagnosis, 391
    etiology, 390, 390(*f*)
    pathophysiology, 390–391
Cystic Fibrosis Questionnaire, 1128
Cystic fibrosis transmembrane conductance regulator (CFTR), 390, 391
Cysts, 482
Cytosolic copper-zinc superoxide dismutase (CuZnSOD), 637

D

Daclizumab (Zinbryta), 598(*t*)
Dakin solution (bleach and boric acid), 501
Dance therapy, 428
Dantrolene sodium (Dantrium), 601
Dartfish, 226
Dartmouth Cooperative Functional Assessment Charts (Dartmouth CO-OP charts), 132
DASH diet, 427–428
Database of Abstracts of Reviews of Effects (DARE), 25(*t*)

Data gathering tools, 295, 296, 297(t), 320(t)
Dawson fingers, 596
Débridement, 498–500
　autolytic, 473
　burns, 950
　defined, 498
　nonselective, 498
　selective, 499–500, 499(f), 500(f)
Deceleration, 218, 219(t), 262
Decerebrate rigidity, 147
Decerebration experiments, 204
Decision flowchart, 990, 991(f)
Decision-making
　clinical reasoning, shared, 5
　cognition, 335
　motor control and motor learning, 159(b),
　　159–160
Decision aids, 5
Declarative memory, 340
Decompensated HF, 440
Deconditioning, 900
Decorticate rigidity, 146–147
Decreased breath sounds, 397
Decreased resistance (vasodilation), 56
Deep brain stimulation (DBS), 695
Deep partial-thickness burn, 943(f), 943–944
Deep sensations, 78, 90–91
　kinesthesia awareness, 90
　proprioceptive awareness, 90–91
　vibration perception, 91
Deep sensory receptors, 78, 79(b), 80
　joint receptors, 79(b), 80
　muscle receptors, 79(b), 80, 81(f)
Deep somatic pain, 969(t), 982
Deep tendon reflexes (DTRs), 142, 149(t),
　149–150
Deep tissue pressure injury, 1234
Deep vein thrombosis (DVT), 479, 490, 491, 539
Defense mechanisms, 1022, 1022–1024(b)
Degrees of freedom (DOF), 127(b), 138, 341
Dehiscence, 474, 474(f)
Delayed onset muscle soreness, 143
Delayed primary wound closure, 475
Delayed reaction time, 188, 190(t)
Delirium, 536
Delphi process, 776
Delta Twist, 1185, 1185(f)
Delusional thinking, 1044(t)
Dementia
　frontotemporal, 681
　multi-infarct, 535–536
　PD, 688
Dementia syndromes, 681
Denervation, 639, 640(f), 671
Denial, 1017, 1022(b)
DePaul Symptom Questionnaire-Post-Exertional
　　Malaise short form (DSQ-PEM), 982
Dependence, defined, 278
Dependent mobility wheelchairs, 1269
　strollers, 1269, 1271(f)
　transport chairs, 1269, 1271(f)
Dependent personality disorder, 1020–1021
Depressant agents, 53
Depression, 1032–1037
　amyotrophic lateral sclerosis, 650
　antidepressant medications, 1035–1036(b)
　behaviors associated with, 1033(t)
　Geriatric Depression Scale, 348(t)
　motor function, 338
　multiple sclerosis, 592(b), 594–595, 602
　Parkinson disease, 688
　pathological response patterns, 1043(t)
　Patient Health Questionnaire for Depression
　　and Anxiety, 109
　psychosocial adaptation, 1017
　referral, 1034

　rehabilitation, 1013, 1014, 1032, 1033
　signs and symptoms, 1033(t)
　stroke, 536
　suicide, 1034, 1037
　treating, 1033–1034
Depression Anxiety Stress Scales, 780
Depth and distance perception, 77, 134, 335
Depth of respiration, 53
Dermagraft, 511
Dermal healing, in burns, 949–950
　inflammatory phase, 949
　maturation phase, 949–950
　proliferative phase, 949
Dermatome, 953
Dermatome map, 70–71(f), 71–72, 87, 88(f)
Dermatomes, 70–72, 86, 111, 112(f)
Dermis, 471, 477, 940–941, 941(t). See also
　　Dermal healing, in burns
Descending corticospinal tract (CST), 336
Descending motor pathways, 184
Descriptive parameters, 278
Desensitization, 1028
Desipramine (Norpramin), 602, 1035(b)
Desquamate, 942
Destabilizing functional activities, 562
Deteriorating stroke, 527
Devaluation, 1022(b)
Dexterity, 181
Dexterity Questionnaire 24 (DextQ-24), 706
Dextromethorphan hydrobromide, 648
Diabetes mellitus (DM), 525
Diabetic neuropathy, 484(f), 484–485
Diabetic polyneuropathy, 162, 176(t)
Diagnosis, 15–16
　motor function examination, 174, 175–177(t)
　physical therapy, 15–16, 174, 175–177(t)
　See also Differential diagnosis
Diagnosis-specific organizations, 326
Diagnostic and Statistical Manual of Mental
　　Disorders, 1022, 1029
Diaphoresis, 34
Diaphragm, 51, 51(f)
Diaphragm pacing (DP), 789
Diastole, 419
Diastolic blood pressure (DBP), 423, 426
Diastolic dysfunction, 439
Diastolic murmur, 453(t)
Diastolic pressure, 55–56, 57, 57(t), 58, 59, 61, 62
Diazepam (Diastat, Valium), 601, 602, 649, 650,
　　1030(b)
Diet. See Nutrition
Dietary Approaches to Stop Hypertension
　　(DASH), 427–428
Difference score, 156
Differential diagnosis, 15–16
　burns, 942(f)
　CNS disorders, 175(t)
　hemorrhagic vs. ischemic cerebral strokes, 160
　lymphedema, 482
　neuromuscular degenerative diseases,
　　176–177(t)
　sensory function examination, 68, 72
　traumatic brain injury, 160
　UMN and LMN syndromes, 174(t)
Differential Diagnosis for Physical Therapists
　　(Goodman and Snyder), 992
Different skills practice, 343–344, 345(t)
Difficulty, defined, 2778
Diffuse axonal injury (DAI), 727
Diffuse Lewy body disease (DLBD), 681
Diffusion tensor imaging (DTI), 161–162, 162(f),
　　164(f)
Digital subtraction angiography, 541
Digital video recorder (DVR), 225–226
Dilated cardiomyopathy, 417
Diltiazem, 681

Dimethyl fumarate (Tecfidera), 598(t)
Dimmer switches, 305
Diphasic dyskinesia, 694
Diplopia, 592, 1063
Direct intervention, 19–20, 22
Direct motor loop, 681–682, 682(f)
Direct structured-pedagogic treatment, 1109
Diroximel fumarate (Vumerity), 598(t)
Disabilities of the Arm, Shoulder, and Hand
　　(DASH), 289
Disabilities of the Arm, Shoulder and Hand
　　questionnaire (DASH), 107
Disability, 6(f), 7, 7(b)
　access symbols, 295, 296(f)
　barriers to wellness for people with, 1041
　defense reactions, 1022, 1022–1024(b)
　defined, 272, 326
　gait analysis
　　accelerometer data, 249
　　Dynamic Gait Index, 243
　　heart rate data, 267, 268
　　outcome measures, 236(t), 238(t)
　　walkway systems, 250, 251(t), 252(t), 253(t),
　　　254(t)
　health promotion and wellness, 1141–1145
　　examination and evaluation, 1141–1143,
　　　1142(b), 1143(b)
　　interventions, 1143–1145, 1145(b)
　psychosocial adaptation, 1018
　specific measures, 145
Disability Status Scale (DSS), 610–611
Disarticulation prostheses, 1197–1198
　hip, 1197(f), 1197–1198
　knee, 1197
Discharge planning, 22, 22(b)
　cognitive and perceptual dysfunction, 1072
　postsurgical phase of amputation, 860–861
　stroke, 583
Discrete motor skill, 138, 139(b)
Discrete skills, 340
Discriminant analysis, 266
Discriminative sensory receptors, 82(f)
Disease
　characteristics, 272
　defined, 1123
　health promotion and wellness, 1123
Disease-modifying therapies (DMTs), 597–601,
　　598–600(t), 646, 647, 647(t)
Disease-specific measures
　health and wellness, 1128
　multiple sclerosis, 610–611
　Parkinson disease, 707
Dishwashers, 316, 317(f)
Disinfectants, 500
Disordered sleep
　stroke, 539–540
　traumatic brain injury, 730
Disorders of Consciousness Scale (DOCS), 735
Disorientation, 535, 1044(t)
Displacement, 220, 1023(b)
Dissemination in space (DIS), 596
Dissemination in time (DIT), 596
Dissociation, 1023(b)
Distal interphalangeal (DIP) joints, 897
Distal sensing microphones, 59
Distractibility, 1073
Distraction (accessory motion), 117
Distributed practice, 343, 345(t), 560
Disulfiram (Antabuse), 1039(b)
Disuse atrophy, 142, 671
Diuretics, 428, 431(t), 443
Divided attention, 1073
Division of Vocational Rehabilitation, 326
Dix-Hallpike test, 753, 754(t)
Dizziness Handicap Inventory (DHI), 348(t), 354,
　　753, 754(t), 821, 821(t)

Documentation, 23–24
  coordination examination, 195–196
  defensible, in WSM, 1280
  electronic documentation software, 87
  examination and modification of environment,
    324, 326
    community access, 326
    examples, 297(t)
    workplace, 320(t)
  integumentary system disorders, 495
  lymphatic system disorders, 495
  lymphedema using body diagram, 490
  motor function examination
    motor coordination, 138, 139
    motor learning, 158, 159
    musculoskeletal impairments, 141–143
    neuromuscular impairments, 145, 148, 151
    tests and measures, 133
  sensory examination, 87
  vascular system disorders, 495
  vital signs, 32, 64–65
  wound closure, 475
Domains of disorientation, 76
Domestic life, spinal cord injury and, 782
Donning
  orthotics, 1174
  prosthetics, 1212–1213
Donor site, 953
Door handles, 304, 308, 308(f)
Doorknob lever adapter, 308, 308(f)
Door locks, 304
Door openers, automatic, 304
Doorways
  exterior, 304
  interior, 307–308, 308(f)310–311
Dopamine, 682, 693
Dopamine agonists, 692(t), 694
Dopamine replacement therapy, 693–694
Doppler effect, 50
Doppler ultrasound (DUS), 50, 489, 489(f)
  heart rate, 50
  stroke, 541
Dorsal (posterior) column-medial lemniscal
    (DCML)
  pathology, 189
  pathway, 186
Dorsal column-medial lemniscal system, 78, 81,
    82(f), 83(t)
Dorsalis pedis pulse, 46(f), 48(b)
Dorsal root reflex, 973
Dorsiflexion, 145, 148, 149(t), 150, 150(t)
Dorsiflexors, 141, 227, 261
Double limb stance, 217, 218(f), 219
Double simultaneous stimulation test, 92–93
Double vision, 592, 1063
Down Syndrome, gait analysis and, 234(t)
Doxepin (Sinequan, Zonalon), 1035(b)
Dramatic relief (change process), 1133, 1133(t)
Drawing a circle test, 194(t)
Dressing, wheelchairs and, 1237
Dressings
  amputation, postsurgical, 855(t), 855–857
    rigid dressings, 855, 856
    semirigid dressings, 856
    soft dressings, 856(f), 856–857
  burns, 950–951, 962, 962(f)
  wounds, 508–512
    alginates, 510–511, 511(f)
    biological/skin substitutes, 511
    composite, 511
    foam, 507(f), 507–508, 509(f), 509–510
    gauze/fiber, 508(f), 508–509
    hydrocolloids, 510, 510(f)
    hydrofibers, 511, 511(f)
    hydrogels, 510, 510(f)
    impregnated gauze, 509

innovative, 512
    medical-grade honey, 500
    moisture-retentive, 473
    primary, 508
    secondary, 508
    transparent films, 509, 509(f)
    wet-to-dry, 498
Drills, 343–344, 345(t)
Drive wheel configurations, 1275–1276, 1276(f)
  mid-wheel drive bases, 1276, 1276(f)
  rear wheel drive bases, 1276, 1276(f)
Drop ring lock, 1160, 1160(f), 1162, 1163(f)
Drug-eluting stents, 436
Drug-induced parkinsonism, 681
Drugs. See Pharmacological management
Dual-task (DT), 686, 716
Dual-task control, 206, 686
Dual-task interference, 704, 716
Dual-task interventions
  motor function, 342(t), 349(t), 350(t), 354,
    357
  motor learning, 156
  motor skills, 139(b)
  stroke, 562
  traumatic brain injury, 747–748, 748(f)
Dual-task performance, 741
Dual-task training (DTT)
  Parkinson disease and motor-cognitive,
    716–719, 717–718(t)
  stroke, 562
  traumatic brain injury, 748, 755
Duke Health Profile, 1128
Duloxetine (Cymbalta), 602
Durable medical equipment (DME), 1226, 1280
Dying-back hypothesis, 638, 640(f)
Dying-forward hypothesis, 638, 640(f)
Dynamical systems stages, 341, 342(t)
Dynamic balance, 349(t), 360
Dynamic examination, 1173
  transfemoral, 1211–1212
    compensations/deviations best viewed from
      behind, 1211–1212
    compensations/deviations best viewed from
      the side, 1212
  transtibial, 1209
Dynamic Exertion Test, 753
Dynamic Gait Index (DGI), 209, 210, 233, 237(t),
    242–243, 348(t), 354, 551, 608(t), 610,
    700, 703(t), 704, 754, 754(t)
Dynamic interactional approach, 1059–1060
Dynamic level of demand, 343
Dynamic mechanical allodynia, 988
Dynamic neural representation of pain, 972
Dynamic postural control, 137, 138(t)
  multiple sclerosis, 610, 623, 623(f)
  overground walking, 372–373(f), 375–377,
    376(b), 376(f)
Dynamic posturography, 200, 202, 203, 205, 610
Dynamic systems, 336–337
Dynamic visual acuity (DVA), 826, 827
Dynamic weight transfer rate, 246(t)
Dynamometers, 609
Dysarthria, 135, 187, 190(t), 642, 1112–1114
  amyotrophic lateral sclerosis, 642, 664
  ataxic, 1112
  classification and nomenclature, 1112–1113
  flaccid, 1112
  hyperkinetic, 1113
  hypokinetic, 1113
  multiple sclerosis, 594
  spastic, 1112
  stroke, 532
  treatment, 1113–1114
Dysarthria/clumsy hand syndrome, 531
Dysautonomia, 144
Dyscalculia, 76

Dysdiadochokinesia, 187, 190(t), 195(t), 593
Dysequilibrium, 820
Dysesthesias, 89(t), 592, 602, 613
Dyskinesia, 354
Dysmetria, 187, 190(t), 195(t), 593–594
Dysphagia, 1114–1115
  amyotrophic lateral sclerosis, 642, 648–649,
    664
  Parkinson disease, 688
  stroke, 535
Dysphonia, 594
Dyspnea, 54, 55
  on exertion, 452(t)
  high altitudes, 53
  left-sided CHF, 440–441
  oral temperatures contraindicated for, 42
  outcome measures and quality of life, 398,
    399(t)
  Perceived Level of Dyspnea, 452(t)
Dyspnea ALS-15 (DALS-15) scale, 663
Dyspnea Scale, 454(b), 610
Dysrhythmia, 43
Dyssynergia, 187, 190(t), 195(t), 593
Dyssynergic bladder, 595, 602
Dysthymia, 1032
Dysthymic disorder, 688
Dystonia, 145, 147, 189, 190(t), 531, 694
Dystonic posture, 147, 189

E

Early learning, 344
Early mobilization, 736, 737
Early or myopathic recruitment, 171
Easy Pivot, 670
Easy Street Environment, 1091–1092,
    1091–1092(f)
Eating, wheelchair positioning and, 1237
Eccentric contractions, 351
Ecchymosis, 35(b)
Echocardiography, 442
ECRI Guidelines Trust, 25(t)
Ectopic beats, 444–445, 445(f)
Edema
  cerebral, stroke, 527
  compression treatments, 516 (See also
    Compression therapy)
  musculoskeletal examination, 110, 111, 113
  pitting, 440, 453(t)
  residual limb care, 865–866
  weight gain, 440, 453(t)
  See also Lymphedema
EDGE (Evaluation Database to Guide
    Effectiveness), 133
EDGE Taskforce Outcome Measures, 133
Edinburgh Cognitive and Behavioural ALS Screen
    (ECAS), 660
Education. See Patient and family/caregiver
    education
Effective performance, 1076
Effector organs, 36–38
  conservation and production of body heat,
    37–38
  loss of body heat, 38
Ejection fraction (EF), 419
Ekso, 1165
Elastic end-feel, 116
Elastic loads, 351, 352(t)
Elastic shrinkers, 856(f), 856–857, 866
Elastic wraps, 856
Elastomer putty, 519, 519(f)
Elbow complex, 116(t)
Elbow(s)
  rheumatoid arthritis, 894
  spasticity in UMN syndrome, 146(t)
Electrical burn, 945

Electrical conduction of the heart, 420–421, 421(*f*)
abnormalities, 444–450
atrial fibrillation, 416, 444, 445(*f*), 447–448
automatic implantable cardiac defibrillator, 447
calculating heart rate from electrocardiography, 449–450, 450(*f*)
conduction delays and blocks, 448
ectopic beats, 444–445, 445(*f*)
electrocardiogram complex for viewing, 420–421, 421(*f*)
pacemakers, 448–449, 449(*t*)
supraventricular ectopy, 445(*f*), 445–446
ventricular ectopy, 445(*f*), 446–447, 446(*f*)
ventricular fibrillation, 416, 444, 445(*f*), 447
ventricular tachycardia, 416, 444, 445(*f*), 447
Electrical controls, home accessibility and, 305
Electrical stimulation (ES), 502, 506, 506(*f*), 571–572
Electrocardiogram (ECG)
calculating heart rate, 449–450, 450(*f*)
changes in acute coronary syndrome, 434–436, 435(*f*), 436(*f*)
electrical conduction of heart, 420–421, 421(*f*)
following myocardial infarction, 433, 433(*f*)
12-lead, 434–436, 435(*f*)
Electroencephalography (EEG), 172(*t*), 173
Electrogoniometers, 256
Electromagnetic motion analysis system, 259, 260
Electromagnetic (photic) receptors, 78, 79(*b*)
Electromechanically assisted locomotor training, 565
Electromyographic biofeedback (EMG-BFB), 352–353
Electromyography (EMG), 167–171
advantages, disadvantages, and clinical use, 172(*t*)
complex repetitive discharges, 168
fasciculation potentials, 168, 170
fibrillation potentials, 168, 169(*f*)
gait analysis, 233, 255, 256, 257, 257(*f*), 259, 260(*f*), 262, 263
insertional EMG activity, 168, 168(*f*)
kinesiologic, 168
motor unit action potentials, 170(*f*), 170–171
nerve conduction studies, 168
polyphasic potentials, 170, 170(*f*), 171
positive sharp waves, 168, 169(*f*)
resting potentials, 168, 170(*f*)
Electronic databases, 25(*t*)
Electrophysiologic neuromuscular assessment, 163, 165–174
characteristics of techniques, 171–172(*t*)
electroencephalography, 173
electromyography, 167–171, 168(*f*), 169(*f*), 170(*f*)
nerve conduction studies, 165(*f*), 165–167, 166(*f*), 167(*f*)
transmagnetic stimulation, 173–174
Electrotherapy, 924
Elephantiasis, 482
El Escorial criteria, 643
Elevation, 512–516
Elevators, home, 308–309, 309(*f*)
Emed system, 263, 264
Emergency care, for spinal cord injury, 773
EMG-triggered NMES, 571–572
Emory Functional Ambulation Profile (EFAP), 233, 240
Emotional anesthesia, 1029, 1031
Emotional coping responses, in social cognitive theory, 1135, 1135(*t*)
Emotional dysregulation syndrome, 536
Emotional impairments
amputation, 864–865
multiple sclerosis, 595, 602
stroke, 536, 537(*t*), 538

Emotional incontinence, 595
Emotional lability, 536
Emotional Well-Being index of PDQ-39, 705
Emotions/stress
heart rate, 44
respiration, 53
temperature, 39
Empathy fatigue, 987
En bloc turning style, 686
Encephalitis lethargica, 680
End-feels, 116
Endobronchial lung volume reduction interventions, 396
Endocardium, 417
Endocrine system, chronic pain and, 975–976, 976(*f*)
End-of-dose deterioration, 694
End-of-life decision-making, 643, 647(*t*)
Endoneurium, 128, 131(*f*)
Endoskeletal shank, 1185, 1186(*f*)
Endothelial dysfunction, 428, 432(*t*)
Endotypes, 904
End-stage pulmonary disease, 396
End-stage renal disease, 525
Endurance. *See* Aerobic capacity/endurance
Energy conservation
arthritis pain, 924
multiple sclerosis, 621
Energy considerations, for orthotics, 1175–1176
cerebral palsy, 1176
hemiplegia, 1176
paraplegia, 1176
Energy cost analysis during gait, 266–268
heart rate data, 267–268
mechanical energy cost determination, 267
physiological energy cost measures, 266–267
Energy effectiveness strategies (EES), 621–622
Energy expenditure, measures of, 423
Energy-storing prosthetic feet, 1182–1183, 1183(*f*)
Enteroviruses, 638
Entrance wound, 945
Entryways, accessibility of, 302(*f*), 302–304
entrances, 303–304
route of entry, 302(*f*), 302–303, 303(*f*)
Environment, 6(*f*), 7, 7(*b*)
amyotrophic lateral sclerosis, 660
arthritis, 923
body temperature, 39
closed, 158, 560, 562
coordination, 192
data gathering tools, 297(*t*), 320(*t*)
demands, 136
function examination, 273, 275, 275(*t*)
ICF, 294
inaccurate interpretation of, 1044(*t*)
motor examination, 340
motor function, 340, 363–364
motor skills, 138, 139(*b*)
multiple sclerosis, 610
open, 158, 560, 562
respiration, 53
sensory examination, 84
social cognitive theory, 1135, 1135(*t*)
spinal cord injury, 783
stroke, 559–560, 562
temperature, 39
worker-job-environment relationship, 318
See also Environmental accessibility
Environmental accessibility, 293–331
adaptive equipment, 317
assistive technology, 317–318, 319(*b*)
case study, 328–331
community access, 322–324
facilities, 324
transportation, 323(*f*), 323–324, 324(*f*), 325(*f*)

disability access symbols, 295, 296(*f*)
documentation, 297(*t*), 320(*t*), 324, 326
examination strategies, 295–300
data gathering tools, 297(*t*)
description of physical environment, 298
documentation, 297(*t*)
environmental factors outcome measures, 298, 299–300(*t*)
interview, 297–298
on-site visits, 298, 300
performance-based measures of function, 298
self-report measures, 298
tests and measures, 297(*t*)
funding sources, 326
home examination, 300–317, 494 (*See also under* On-site visits)
intervention strategies, 300
legislation, 326–327
objects, modification or altered location of, 300
patient-environment relationship, 295
physical environment, 294
purpose of examination, 295
universal design, 294–295
workplace examination, 318–322
data gathering tools, 320(*t*)
documentation, 320(*t*)
functional capacity evaluation, 320–321, 321(*f*)
job requirements, 318
on-site visit, 321–322
tests and measures, 320(*t*)
Environmental control units (ECUs), 318, 319(*b*)
Environmental reevaluation (change process), 1133, 1133(*t*)
Enzymatic débridement, 499
Ephedrine, 768
Epibole, 476
Epicardium, 417
Epidermal burn, 942, 942(*f*)
Epidermal healing, burns and, 948–949
Epidermis, 471, 940–941, 941(*t*)
Epiglottis, 50, 51(*f*)
Epinephrine, 37
Epineurium, 128, 131(*f*)
Epithelial healing, 948–949
Epithelialization, 474, 475, 476
Equilibrium reactions, 204
Equilibrium Score, 203
Equipment assessment, for WSM, 1237
Equitable use, in universal design, 295
Erectile dysfunction, 689
Ergonomic evaluation, 121
Ergotamine, 768
Error augmentation, 343
Error enhancement, 343
Erythema, 35(*b*)
Eschar, 473, 483, 944
Escharotomy, 944, 944(*f*)
Estazolam (Prosom), 1030(*b*)
Estrogen deficiency, 432(*t*)
Euphoria, 536
Eupnea, 54, 54(*f*)
European Multicenter Study on Human Spinal Cord Injury, 783
European Organisation for Research and Treatment of Cancer (EORTC), 1128
European Pressure Ulcer Advisory Panel (EPUAP), 496
EuroQOL-5D (EQ-5D), 662
Evaluation, 14–15, 15(*t*)
defined, 174
motor function examination, 174, 175–177(*t*)
Evaluation triad, in acute coronary syndrome, 433–436, 434(*f*)
Evaporation, 38
Evidence-based care, for mild TBI, 755

Evidence-based design (EBD), 294
Evidence-based practice (EBP), 24–27, 559
    clinical decisions guided by, 24, 26
    clinical practice guidelines, 24, 26
    clinical question elements, 24
    components, 26(f)
    critical analysis of research findings, 26
    electronic databases, 25(t)
    essential steps, 24
    levels of evidence and grades of
        recommendation, 27(t)
    systematic review, 26
Evidence Database to Guide Effectiveness, 14
Evoked potentials (EPs), 596
Exacerbation
    arthritis, 893, 910, 915(t), 926, 928
    asthma, 389–390, 395(t)
    COPD, 406
    COVID, 392
    heart failure, 438, 440, 442, 454, 462
    lymphedema, 490
    multiple sclerosis, 590–591, 596
    protocol, 408
    pseudoexacerbation, 591, 609
Examination, 12(f), 12–13
    body function structure, 13
    burns, 954
    chronic pain, 980, 981–990
        characteristics, 982, 984, 984(b)
        classification tools, 985(t)
        general flow, 981, 982(f)
        impact on physical and psychosocial function,
            981, 982
        mnemonics for assessing, 984(b)
        physical therapy tests and measures,
            987–990, 989(t)
        PSCEBSM model for taking a
            biopsychosocial history, 986(b)
        psychosocial factors impacting pain, 984, 986,
            986(b)
        review of systems, 987
        severity and functional assessment tools,
            983(t)
        subjective examination, 986–987
        systems review, 987
    chronic pulmonary dysfunction, 397–400
        laboratory tests, 397
        patient history, 397
        tests and measures, 397–400
    cognitive and perceptual dysfunction,
        1061–1070
        differentiating sensory loss from cognitive/
            perceptual deficits, 1063–1065,
            1064–1065(f)
        factors influencing, 1062–1063
        outcome measures, 1066–1069(t)
        purpose, 1061–1062
        standardized cognitive and perceptual tests,
            1065–1070
        visual impairments, 1063–1065, 1064(f),
            1065(f)
    heart disease, 450–454
        medical record review, 450
        patient interview, 450–451
        tests and measures, 451–453(t), 451–454,
            456–457(t)
    movement analysis of tasks, 13
    orthotic, 1172–1173
    participation goal mapping, 12, 13
    prosthetic, 1208–1212, 1210(t), 1211(f), 1212
    purposes, 12
    relevant activities/tasks, 12, 13
    respiration, 55
    stroke, 540, 545–557
        activities, 548–552, 549(t), 551(t)
        ANPT resources, 547

body function and structure, 552–557, 555(t)
    clinical practice guidelines for outcome
        assessment, 547, 548(t)
    elements, 546–547(b)
    interview, 545–546
    order, 547
    participation, 547, 548
    patient/client history, 546(t)
    purposes, 545
    systems review, 546(t)
    tests and measures, 546–547(t), 547
vestibular disorders
    history and systems review, 820
    symptoms, 820(t), 820–821
    tests and measures, 821(t), 821–828,
        822–827(f), 827(t)
wheelchair seating and mobility, 1235–1250
    assessment interview, 1235–1236
    equipment assessment, 1237
    functional assessment, 1237–1238
    physical assessment, 1239–1243
    screening of body functions and structures,
        1238–1239
Excessive daytime somnolence, 689
Excitatory amino acid transporter 2 (EAAT2), 638
EXCITE (Extremity Constraint-Induced Therapy
    Evaluation), 361(t), 363, 571
Execution, motor performance and, 335–337
Executive function
    cognitive and perceptual dysfunction,
        1075–1077
    defined, 535
    motor function examination, 135
    stroke, 535
Executive Function Performance Test (EFPT),
    1068(t)
Executive functions, 1055
Executive Functions Performance Test, 1076
Exercise
    adherence, 1006(t)
    amyotrophic lateral sclerosis
        disuse atrophy, 671
        overuse damage, 671, 672(f)
        prescription, 671–672, 673(b)
    arthritis, 927–928, 929(t), 930–931(t)
    blood pressure, 57
    burns, 959, 960–961
        active and passive exercise, 959, 960–961
        resistive and conditioning exercise, 961
    capacity, 423, 428, 454, 456(t)
    chronic pain, 1004–1005, 1006(t)
    chronic pulmonary dysfunction
        exercise log, 407(f)
        home exercise programs, 407, 407(f)
        intensity, 401–402
        multispecialty team, 407–408
        prescription, 400, 401–402
    defined, 1126
    duration
        chronic pulmonary dysfunction, 402
        pulmonary rehabilitation, 406
        strength training, 351, 352(t)
    frequency
        chronic pulmonary dysfunction, 402
        strength training, 351, 352(t)
    habituation, 340, 836, 837, 837(f)
    health promotion and wellness, 1126
    heart disease, 423–426
        abnormal responses, 426, 426(b)
        blood pressure with activity, 452(t)
        dance therapy, 428
        dyspnea on exertion, 452(t)
        energy expenditure measures, 423
        exercise capacity, 423, 428, 454, 456(t)
        exercise intolerance signs and symptoms, 426,
            426(b)

exercise prescription in outpatient cardiac
    rehabilitation, 461(t)
heart failure, 463(t)
heart rate and rhythm, 451(t)
hemodynamic stability, 451–452(t)
metabolic equivalents, 423, 424(t)
normal responses, 423, 425(f), 426
outcome measures, 456(t)
oxygen requirements, 458(f)
respiratory rate, 451(t), 452(t)
therapeutic exercise, 454
heart rate, 44, 45–46
intensity
    chronic pulmonary dysfunction, 401–402
    determining, 351, 352(t)
    feedback, 346, 347(t)
    locomotor training, 370
    neuroplasticity principle, 339(t)
mode, for chronic pulmonary dysfunction, 401
multiple sclerosis, 614–620, 615–618(t)
Parkinson disease, 709(f), 709–711, 710(f),
    710(t)
    flexibility exercises, 709–711, 710(f), 710(t)
    relaxation exercises, 709, 709(f)
    strength training, 711
prescription
    amyotrophic lateral sclerosis, 671–672,
        673(b)
    chronic pulmonary dysfunction, 400,
        401–402
    Guidelines for Exercise Testing and Prescription
        (ACSM), 456(t)
    multiple sclerosis, 620
    outpatient cardiac rehabilitation, 461(t)
    Parkinson disease, 719–720
    prosthetics, 1203
    pulmonary rehabilitation, 402, 403–405(t),
        405, 406
    respiration, 53
    spinal cord injury, 810–811, 811(f)
    stroke
        endurance, 557
        precautions, 582–583
    temperature, 39
    wound healing, 517–518
    See also Aerobic capacity/endurance; Physical
        activity (PA)
Exercise-induced hypoalgesia (EIH), 1004
Exercise is Medicine (EIM), 1146
Exercise Management for Persons with Chronic
    Diseases and Disabilities (ACSM), 353
Exercise science, 2
Exercise Tolerance Tests (ETTs), 398, 399–400,
    400(b), 456(t)
Exergaming, 373–374
Exertional tolerance, mild TBI and, 753
Exhaustion, defined, 143
Exit wound, 945
Exoskeletal shank, 1185, 1186(f)
Exoskeleton interventions, 379
Expanded Disability Status Scale (EDSS), 604,
    610–611, 614, 623
Expectancies, in social cognitive theory, 1135,
    1135(t)
Expectations, in social cognitive theory, 1135,
    1135(t)
Experimental pain, 971
Expert performers, 341, 342(t)
Expiration, 51
Expiratory reserve volume (ERV), 383
Explain Pain, 971, 998, 999, 1000(t)
Explicit vision, 201
Expressive aphasia, 532, 1105(t), 1105–1106, 1108
Extension aid, 1193, 1193(f)
Extension phase, 580
External extension aid, 1193

Externalized hostility, 1017
External locus of control, 1021
Externally-paced skills, 138, 139(b)
External modifications, 1152, 1153, 1153(f)
External respiration, 50, 385(f)
Exteroceptors, 78
Extracellular superoxide dismutase (ECSOD), 637
Extra-depth shoes, 493, 518–519, 519(f), 1151
Extremity strength training, 405–406
Extrinsic factors, in wound healing, 477
Extrinsic feedback, 370
Exudate, 473, 474, 480
Eye-hand coordination, 182
Eye-hand-head coordination, 182
Eye movement examination, 822–823, 823(f)

F

Face validity, 283
Facial nerve (CN VII), 98(t), 151, 153(t), 639, 659
Facial Pain Scale, 981
Facilitator
    contextual factors as, 273
    defined, 7, 7(b)
Facilitator and Barriers Survey (FABS/M), 299(t)
Faded frequency schedule, 346, 347(t), 357
Fahrenheit scale, 35, 36(f)
Fair Housing Amendment Act of 1988, 294, 327
Falls and fall risk
    fall diary, 704
    fear of falling and balance confidence measures, 211–212
    floor-to-stand examination, 212–213, 213(f)
    at home, 317
    Parkinson disease, 685, 704
    STEADI, 212(f), 212–213
    threshold scores for fall risk, 209–210
Falls Efficacy Scale (FES), 211, 348(t)
Falls Efficacy Scale International (FES-I), 211–212
Familial ALS (FALS), 636–637, 638, 639, 644
Fasciculations, 168, 170, 641, 649–650
Fast Evaluation of Mobility, Balance, and Fear (FEMBAF), 233, 243
Fasting plasma glucose, 526(t)
FASTRAK, 260
FAST signs of stroke, 525
Fast speed, 245(t)
Fatigue
    amyotrophic lateral sclerosis, 143, 643, 650, 660
    defined, 353
    empathy, 987
    interventions, 353
    motor endurance, 142–143
    multiple sclerosis, 143, 156, 593, 602, 609
    muscle endurance, 143
    neuromuscular endurance, 353
    Parkinson disease, 143, 685, 705
Fatigue Assessment Scale, 987
Fatigue Impact Scale (FIS), 348(t)
Fatigue Scale for Motor and Cognitive Functions (FSMC), 353, 607(t), 609
Fatigue Severity Scale (FSS), 143, 660, 705, 987
Faucets
    bathroom, 313, 314
    kitchen, 315
Fear avoidance, 979, 980(t)
Fear-Avoidance Beliefs Questionnaire (FABQ), 107
Fear-Avoidance Model, 980, 981(f)
Feedback
    control, 68
    defined, 126, 127(b)
    motor control, 335, 355–356
    motor learning, 345, 346, 347(t), 357–358, 370–371

clinical decisions about, 345
    initial kinematic, 341
    intensity, 346, 347(t)
    mode, 345, 346, 347(t)
    scheduling, 346, 347(t)
    stroke, 560, 562–563
Feedforward, 126
    control, 68, 184, 336
    responses, 36
Feet. See Foot
Femoral pulse, 46(f), 47(b)
Festination, 686
Fever, 38(b), 38–39
Fiber, for constipation, 603
Fiberoptic endoscopic evaluation of swallowing, 535, 629
Fibrillation potentials, 168, 169(f)
Fibrin, 949
Fibroblasts, 949
Fibrosis, 480, 490
Fight-or-flight responses, 143, 622
Figure-ground discrimination, 134, 538, 1086–1087, 1087(f)
Figure-of-8 Walk Test (F8W), 233, 243–244
Filariasis, 481
FIM Locomotion: Walk/Wheelchair Guide, 241, 241(t)
The FIM System Clinical Guide, Version 5.2, 241
Final common pathway, 127
Fine motor movements, 192
Fine motor skill, 138, 139(b)
Finger agnosia, 538, 1086
Finger and touchpad drive control systems, 1279
Finger Dexterity Test, 198(b)
Finger nails, 34, 35(f)
Finger opposition test, 193(t)
Finger(s)
    coordination, outcome measures, 196–197(t)
    flexors, 149(t)
    osteoarthritis, 906–907, 907(f)
    rheumatoid arthritis, 895–897(f), 895–898
Finger-to-finger test, 193(t)
Finger-to-therapist's finger test, 193(t)
Fingolimod (Gilenya), 598(t)
Fire extinguishers, 316
First-degree heart block, 448
Fistulas, 482
Fit, prosthetic, 1201
    problem-solving, 1213, 1214(f)
    transfemoral socket fit, 1201
    transtibial socket fit, 1201
Fitbit activity monitors, 249
Fitbit Charge, 249
Fitts and Posner 3-stage model, 155–156, 158(b)
5 A's tobacco cessation approach, 1144, 1145(b)
5-meter Walk Test (5MWT), 248, 369
Five Times Sit to Stand Test, 9, 11, 13, 298, 345, 348(t), 398, 453(t), 703(t), 706
Fixation, 192
Fixation test, 194(t)
Fixed support strategies, 204(b), 204–205
Flaccid bladder, 770
Flaccid bowel, 771
Flaccid bulbar palsy, 642
Flaccid dysarthria, 1112
Flaccidity, 145, 147
Flaccid or big bladder, 595
Flat-disk diaphragm, 59
Flat-foot contact, 1173
Flex-Foot, 1182, 1183(f)
Flexibility
    arthritis, 927
    motor function, 350–351
    multiple sclerosis, 620, 621(f)
    Parkinson disease, 709–711, 710(f), 710(t)

physical assessment for WSM, 1242(f), 1242–1243
    stroke, 552–553
    in use, in universal design, 295
Flexion-momentum phase, 580
Flexion-momentum stage, 580
Flexor withdrawal reflex, 151, 152(t)
Floor effects, 156
Floor (ground) reaction orthosis, 1156, 1157(f)
Floors, home accessibility and, 306–307, 307(f)
Floor-to-stand examination, fall risk and, 212–213, 213(f)
Floor-to-wheelchair transfers, 800–801, 800–801(f)
Floor transfers, 712
Flow rates, 384
Fludrocortisone, 768
Fluency, problems of, 135
Fluent aphasia, 135, 532, 1104, 1105(f)
Fluid friction, 1192
Fluoxetine (Prozac, Sarafem), 602, 650, 1035(b)
Flurazepam (Dalmane), 650, 1030(b)
Flushing, 35(b)
Flutter, 408, 411
Fluvoxamine (Luvox), 648, 1035(b)
Foam dressings, 507(f), 507–508, 509(f), 509–510
Foam soft collar, 774
Focal deficits, stroke and, 523–524
Focal dystonia, 147
Focal vision, 201
Focused attention, 1073
Food and Drug Administration (FDA), 448, 499, 501, 502, 597, 646, 660, 662, 663
Foot
    clonus, 150
    gait deviations, 227–228(t)
    orthoses, 1152–1154
        external modifications, 1153, 1153(f)
        foot inserts, 1154, 1154(f)
        internal modifications, 1152–1153, 1152–1153(f)
        knee arthritis, 1154–1156(t)
    osteoarthritis, 908, 908(f)
    prostheses, partial, 1181(f), 1181–1182, 1182(f)
    rheumatoid arthritis, 898, 899(f)
    spasticity in UMN syndrome, 146(t)
    support, for WSM, 1255–1256, 1256(f)
Foot and Ankle Ability Measure (FAAM), 289
Foot-ankle assemblies
    maintenance, 1200, 1201(f)
    transfemoral prostheses, 1191
    transtibial prostheses, 1182–1185, 1182–1185(f)
        articulated, 1184–1185, 1184–1185(f)
        nonarticulated, 1182–1184, 1182–1184(f)
        rotators and shock absorbers, 1185, 1185(f)
Foot-ankle controls, 567
Foot flat, 218, 219(t), 227(t), 260(f)
Foot inserts, 1154, 1154(f)
Foot orthoses (FOs), 1150, 1152–1154
    external modifications, 1153, 1153(f)
    foot inserts, 1154, 1154(f)
    internal modifications, 1152–1153, 1152–1153(f)
    knee arthritis, 1154–1156(t)
Foot slap, 1173
Footswitches/footswitch systems, 250, 255(f), 255–256
Forced expiratory volume in 1 sec (FEV$_1$), 384
Forced vital capacity (FVC), 383
Forceful irrigation, 496(f), 496–497, 498
Force plate technology, 262–263
Force platform biofeedback, 562–563

Forearm
   capsular patterns, 116(*t*)
   spasticity in UMN syndrome, 146(*t*)
Form discrimination, 134, 538, 1087
Forward trunk shifting, 1210(*t*), 1212
Foundation for Peripheral Neuropathy, 98
Four-Item Dynamic Gait Index, 243
Four-layer bandage system, 513
Four-Square Step Test, 210, 211(*f*)
Four-Stage Balance Test, 213
Fractionated (isolated) movement, loss of, 354
Fracture
   risk, stroke and, 539
   stabilization, spinal cord injury and, 773
Free nerve endings, 79, 79(*b*), 80, 941(*t*)
Free speed, 245(*t*)
Freezing of gait (FOG), 354, 684, 686–687,
      702(*t*), 716, 719
Freezing out, 341
Frenchay Activities Index, 1107
Frequency, intensity, time, type (FITT) equation,
      20, 21(*b*), 356, 560, 614, 620
Fricatives, 1103
Friction, defined, 1234
Friction brake, 1193, 1193(*f*)
Friction mechanism, 1191–1193, 1192(*f*)
   constant friction, 1193
   friction brake, 1193, 1193(*f*)
   medium, 1193–1194, 1194(*f*)
   variable friction, 1193
Friedreich ataxia, 186, 252–253(*t*)
Frontotemporal dementia (FTD), 636, 641(*t*),
      660, 681
Front wheel drive (FWD) wheelchair, 1276(*f*),
      1276–1277
F-Scan Bipedal In-Shoe Plantar Pressure/Force
      Measurement System, 264
Fugl-Meyer Assessment (FMA), 145, 554, 555,
      558
Fullerton Advanced Balance (FAB) scale, 208,
      700–701
Full pulse, 44, 45(*f*)
Full-thickness burns, 491, 492(*t*), 944(*f*), 944–945
Full-thickness skin graft, 953
Full tilt systems, 1265
Fully accessible, defined, 327
Function
   balance
      grades, descriptive terminology, 279(*b*)
      spinal cord injury, 781
   defined, 272
   imaging techniques, 162–163, 163(*f*), 164(*t*)
   mobility outcome measures, 400(*t*)
   mobility skills, 136, 552
   movement analysis, 121
   performance
      descriptors used to qualify, 278, 279(*b*)
      measures, 277, 298
   plan to optimize, 321
   spinal cord injury, 784–787(*t*)
Function, examination of, 276–290
   case study, 290–292
   case vignettes, sample, 282(*t*)
   general considerations, 276
   ICF framework, 272–275
   impairment terminology, 279(*b*)
   instrument parameters, 278–280
      descriptive, 278
      quantitative, 279–280
   instrument quality, 282–284
      minimal clinically important difference, 284
      minimally detectable change, 284, 285(*b*),
         285(*t*)
      reliability, 282–283
      responsiveness, 284, 285(*b*), 285(*t*)
      validity, 283–284, 284(*b*)

instrument selection, 284–286, 285(*b*)
   instruments to assess function, 277–278,
      287–290
      Activity Measure for Post-Acute Care, 289
      Functional Independence Measure, 287(*t*),
         287–288
      Medical Outcomes Study Short Form 36,
         286, 287, 289, 289(*t*)
      Outcome and Assessment Information Set,
         288, 288(*t*)
      Patient-Specific Functioning Scale, 289–290
      performance-based tests, 277
      self-reports, 277–278
   multidimensional measures, 286–287, 287(*t*)
   purpose, 276
   response formats, 280–281
      interval/ratio measures, 280–281, 281(*f*)
      nominal measures, 280
      ordinal measures, 280
   results, interpreting, 281–282
   single *vs.* dimensional measures, 286
   testing perspectives, 276–277
Functional activities, examination of, 136
Functional Ambulation Classification Scale, 551
Functional Ambulation Profile (FAP), 233, 240
Functional assessment, WSM, 1237–1238
   ADL and IADL status, 1237
      dressing, 1237
      eating, 1237
      toileting, 1237
   mobility status, 1237–1238
      ambulation, 1238
      bed mobility, transfers, weight shift,
         1237–1238
      propulsion method, 1238
Functional Assessment Measure (FAM), 233, 241,
      242, 741, 743(*t*)
Functional Assessment of Chronic Illness
      Therapy-Fatigue scale, 11
Functional Assessment of Communication Skills
      (ASHA FACS), 1107
Functional capacity evaluation (FCE), 320–321,
      321(*f*)
Functional Classification Scale, 441, 441(*f*)
Functional communication, 1107
Functional Communication Profile (FCP), 1107
Functional cough, 779
Functional electrical stimulation (FES)
   ankle-foot orthoses, 1159
   motor function, 351, 354, 355, 360
   spinal cord injury, 792, 792(*f*)
   stroke, 565, 566(*b*), 575
Functional Examination of MS (FAMS), 611
Functional Gait Assessment (FGA), 210, 233,
      238–239(*t*), 243, 298, 348(*t*), 369, 379,
      700–701, 703(*t*), 704, 754, 754(*t*)
Functional imaging techniques, 162–163, 163(*f*)
Functional Independence Measure (FIM), 18, 660,
      782, 1070
   function assessed by, 286, 287(*t*), 287–288
   gait examination, 233, 241, 241(*t*), 242
   GG codes in place of, 136, 288, 552, 741, 782
   heart disease, 457(*t*)
   interrater reliability, 288
   locomotor function, 369
   multiple sclerosis, 610
   traumatic brain injury, 741
Functional K levels, 1205(*t*), 1205–1206
Functional Life Scale (FLS), 1107
Functional magnetic resonance imaging (fMRI),
      162–163, 163(*f*), 164(*t*), 571
Functional Mobility Assessment, 136
Functional Reach Test (FRT), 207–208, 208(*t*),
      277, 549, 562, 608(*t*), 610, 661, 700, 703(*t*)
Functional residual capacity (FRC), 383
Functional restoration, 993

Functional status, 272
   amputation, 803–805, 804–805(*t*), 864
   amyotrophic lateral sclerosis, 660
   multiple sclerosis, 610
   Parkinson disease, 706–707
   stroke, 552, 578–581, 579(*f*)
      bed mobility, 579, 579(*f*)
      sitting, 579–580
      sit-to-stand transfers, 580
      stand-to-sit transfers, 580–581
      transfers, 581
      upper extremities, 578–581, 579(*f*)
Functional training
   arthritis, 932
   multiple sclerosis, 628–629
   Parkinson disease, 711–712, 712(*f*)
      bed mobility, 711–712, 712(*f*)
      floor transfers, 712
      sit-to-stand, 712, 712(*f*)
   postsurgical phase of amputation, 859–860
   prosthetic training, 1218
Function-induced recovery, 132(*b*)
Functioning, 6, 6(*f*), 7, 7(*b*)
Functioning Every Day with a Wheelchair (FEW),
      1281(*t*)
Function in Sitting Test (FIST), 145, 207
Funding sources, 326
Fund of knowledge, 76
Furniture arrangement and features, 304
Fused in sarcoma (FUS), 636, 637, 638
F-waves, 165, 167, 171(*f*)

G

Gabapentin (Neurontin), 602
GABA (gamma-amino butyric acid) receptor
      antagonists, 543(*b*)
Gadolinium (GAD), brain MRI with, 596
Gait
   amplitude abnormalities, 220
   amyotrophic lateral sclerosis, 660–661
   analysis (*See* Gait analysis)
   arthritis, 922
   balance and gait combination tests, 209–212,
      210(*f*), 211(*f*)
   cycle, 217–220, 218(*f*), 219(*t*) (*See also* Stance;
      Swing)
   defined, 216
   deviations, 227–232
      ankle and foot, 227–228(*t*)
      hip, 230–231(*t*)
      knee, 229(*t*)
      pelvic and trunk, 231–232(*t*)
   freezing, 354, 684, 686–687, 702(*t*), 716, 719
   locomotion differentiated from, 216
   multiple sclerosis, 591(*b*), 594, 610
   normal features, 220–224(*t*)
   observation, 11
   Parkinson disease, 686–687
      freezing of gait, 716
      tests and measures, 704
   pattern classification, 265–266
      cluster analysis, 266
      normalcy index, 266
   phases, 218(*f*), 218–220
      initial contact, 218(*f*), 219, 219(*t*), 220,
         221–223(*t*)
      initial swing, 218(*f*), 219, 219(*t*), 220,
         221–223(*t*)
      loading response, 218(*f*), 219, 219(*t*),
         221–223(*t*), 256, 262
      midstance, 218(*f*), 219, 219(*t*), 221–223(*t*),
         226, 227, 267
      midswing, 218(*f*), 219, 219(*t*), 220,
         221–222(*t*), 224(*t*)
      pre-swing, 218(*f*), 219, 219(*t*), 221–223(*t*)

Gait (continued)
 terminal stance, 218(f), 219, 219(t), 221–223(t), 227
 terminal swing, 218(f), 219, 219(t), 220, 222(t), 224(t), 259
 prosthetic training, 1216–1218, 1217(f), 1218(f)
 speed (See Gait speed)
 spinal cord injury, 804–809, 805–806(f), 807(f)
 stroke
  examination, 550–551
  interventions, 563–567
 task-specific training, 360, 363
 terminology, 217–220, 219(t)
 tests for disturbances, 195(t)
 timing abnormalities, 220
 training (See Gait training)
 variables (See Kinetic gait variables; Spatial and temporal gait variables)
 vestibular disorders, 827
Gait Abnormality Rating Scale (GARS), 233, 242, 244
Gait analysis, 216–270
 approach, 217
 case study, 269–270
 energy cost analysis, 266–268
 gait pattern classification, 265–266
 purposes, 216–217
 types, 220–268 (See also Kinematic gait analysis; Kinetic gait analysis)
 vascular, lymphatic, integumentary disorders, 490
Gait ataxia, 187–188, 190(t)
Gait compensation, 1209
Gait deviation, 1209
GAITRite, 250, 250(f), 251–255(t)
Gait speed
 chronic pulmonary dysfunction, 399–400
 locomotor function, 369, 369(t), 371, 372, 373, 374(f), 379
 prosthetics
  interventions, 1206–1208(t)
  transtibial compensations/deviations, 1210(t)
  typical, 1210(t)
 stroke, 551
Gait training
 amputation, 876, 880
  ESAR prosthetic foot, 880(b)
  evidence summary, 881–882(t)
  postsurgical phase of amputation, 860
  prosthetics for amputation, 876, 880, 880(b), 881–882(t)
  skills required for efficient prosthetic gait, 876(b)
 arthritis, 932, 933, 934(t)
 with assistive devices, 379
 orthotic, 1174–1175
  reciprocal gaits, 1174–1175
  related activities, 1175
  simultaneous gaits, 1175
Gaitway, 262
Galveston Orientation and Amnesia Test (GOAT), 731, 740
Garamycin, 501
Gas exchange, 51
Gastrointestinal (GI) disorders, 689, 987
Gastrointestinal system review, for WSM, 1238
Gauze/fiber dressings, 508(f), 508–509
Gaze stability exercises (GSE), 835, 835(f)
Gelo-Cast, 513
Gender
 heart disease, 416
 multiple sclerosis, 588
 stroke, 524, 525, 526
General adaptation syndrome (GAS), 1016
General Health Questionnaire, 348(t)

Generalizability, 158, 344–345, 345(t)
Generalized Expectancy for Success Scale, 1046(t)
Generalized motor programs (GMPs), 126, 127(b), 336
Genetic risk factors, for chronic pain, 978
Gentamicin, 501
Gentile's taxonomy, 559–560
Geriatric Anxiety Inventory, 705
Geriatric Depression Scales (GDS), 348(t), 705
Gerstmann syndrome, 1086
Get Up and Go (GUG) Test, 209–210, 277
GG codes, 136, 288, 552, 741, 782
GHORT, 224
Girth measurement, 486–487, 487(f)
Glasgow Coma Scale (GCS), 134, 532, 731, 731(f), 731(t)
Glasgow Outcome Scale (GOS), 731
Glass mercury thermometers, 40
Glatiramer acetate (Copaxone), 599(t)
Glatopa, 599(t)
Glenohumeral friction, 577
Glenohumeral joint
 capsular patterns, 116(t)
 rheumatoid arthritis, 898
Glial activation, markers of, 540
Glial neoplasms, 186, 186(f)
Glide (slide) motion, 116, 117, 117(f), 118(f)
Global aphasia, 532, 1105(t), 1106
Global functioning, traumatic brain injury and, 741–742
Global health measures, Parkinson disease and, 707
Global Initiative for Asthma (GINA), 389
Global Initiative for Chronic Obstructive Lung Disease (GOLD), 384
Global Pain Scale, 981
Globus pallidus, 185, 185(f), 681
Globus pallidus internus (GPi), 695
Glossary of Wheelchair Terms and Definitions, 1250–1251
Glossopharyngeal breathing, 790
Glossopharyngeal nerve (CN IX), 98(t), 151, 154(t), 639, 659
Glottis, 1102
Glove and stocking distribution, 72
Glutamate, 638
Glycopyrrolate (Robinul), 648
Goal Attainment Scale (GAS), 348(t), 547, 1281(t)
Goal-oriented training, stroke and, 563–564
Goals and outcomes
 amyotrophic lateral sclerosis, 657(b)
 arthritis, 923(b), 923–924
 burns, 954
 chronic pulmonary dysfunction, 396, 396(b)
 motor function, 348(t)
 multiple sclerosis, 607–608(t), 611, 612(b)
 Parkinson disease, 707, 707(b)
 plan of care, 18, 19(b)
 psychosocial rehabilitative intervention, 1045(b), 1046–1048(t)
 sensory impairment, 100, 100(b)
 SMART, 1140
 spinal cord injury, 783–787
  examples, 787(b)
  functional expectations for spinal cord injury by level of injury, 784–787(t)
 stroke, 558, 558(t), 559, 563–564
 traumatic brain injury, moderate to severe
  during active rehabilitation, 742, 743(t)
  early after injury, 736, 737(b)
 See also Outcome measures
Golgi tendon organs, 79(b), 80, 81(f)
Golgi-type endings, 79(b), 80
Go-No-Go boxing task, 716
"Go/No Go" decision, 335

Good exercise practice, 351
Goodglass and Kaplan test, 1093
Gosnell Scale-Pressure Sore Risk Assessment, 493
Grab bars, 311(f), 311–312
Gracile and cuneate nuclei, 82(f)
Graded and Redefined Assessment of Sensibility Strength and Prehension (GRASSP), 778(t), 782
Gradient of dopaminergic depletion, 693
Grading. See Staging or grading
Grammar of language, 1100
Granulation tissue, 472, 474
Graphesthesia (traced figure identification) test, 93
Grasp reflex, 151, 152(t)
Gravity-assisted positioning, 1245, 1245(f)
Gravity-eliminated position, 354
Greater trochanter, 483, 483(f)
Grief, 1015–1016, 1043(t)
Gross Motor Function Classification System (GMFCS), 1225
Gross Motor Function Measure, 226
Gross motor movements, 192
Gross motor skill, 138, 139(b)
Ground fault circuit interrupter (GFCI), 305
Ground reaction forces (GRFs), 261, 261(t), 262–263
Group speech therapy, 1111
Growth factors, 475, 501–502
Guidance for Patient Reported Outcomes (PRO), 660, 663
Guided imagery, 1028
Guided movement, 357
Guide for a Uniform Data Set for Medical Rehabilitation, 241
Guideline for the Prevention, Detection, Evaluation, and Management of High Blood Pressure in Adults (ACC/AHA), 57
Guidelines for Exercise Testing and Prescription (ACSM), 456(t)
Guidelines for Pulmonary Rehabilitation, 402
Guidelines International Network (GIN), 25(t)
Guide to Physical Therapist Practice (APTA), 2, 8, 16, 19, 20(f), 265, 941
Guillain-Barre syndrome, 128, 141, 143, 144, 167, 353
Guy's Neurological Disability Scale, 609
Gyroscopes, 249

H

Habitual performance, 276
Habituation, 340, 836, 837, 837(f)
Hair follicle endings, 79, 79(b)
Half-and-half nails, 34
Halo orthosis, 774, 774(f), 1168, 1168(f)
Haloperidol, 681
Hamilton Depression Rating Scale (HAMD-17), 705
Hamstrings, 149(t)
Handheld dynamometry (HHD), 118, 119–120, 120(f), 777(t)
Hand hygiene, 42
Handrails, 302, 303(f), 308
Hand rim-activated system, 1273, 1273(f)
Hand(s)
 coordination outcome measures, 196–197(t)
 osteoarthritis, 905(b), 906–907, 907(f)
 rheumatoid arthritis, 895–897(f), 895–898
  distal interphalangeal joints, 897
  metacarpophalangeal joints, 895–896, 896(f)
  mutilans deformity (opera-glass hand), 898
  proximal interphalangeal joints, 896–897, 897(f)
  thumb, 897–898
 spasticity in UMN syndrome, 146(t)

Hand simulation, 1246
Hand-spray faucet attachment, 312, 312(f)
Hand Tool Dexterity Test, 198(b)
Hard end-feel, 116
Hassles Scale, 1025, 1026, 1046(t)
Head controls, 1279
Head-hips movement strategy, 775
Head Impulse Test (HIT), 823–824, 824(f), 825(f)
Headmaster collar, 664, 666(f), 667(t)
Head position relative to gravity and self-motion, 335
Head-shaking induced nystagmus (HSN) test, 824
Head support, for WSM, 1257
Head Up collar, 664, 666(f), 667(t)
Health
    health promotion and wellness, 1123
    ICF description, 5, 7(b)
    measures, 1127–1128
        quality-of-life, 1127–1128
        self-perceived health, 1127–1128
        wellness, 1127–1128
    WHO's definition, 272
Health Belief Model (HBM), 1131, 1131(f)
Health Care Financing Administration, 288
Health condition, 5, 7(b), 1123
Health education, 1125, 1126
Health Information Research Unit, McMaster University, 25(t)
Health Insurance Portability and Accountability Act (HIPAA), 23–24
Health literacy universal precautions, 5
Health promotion, defined, 2, 4(b), 1125
Health promotion and wellness, 1119–1148
    behavior change theories, 1131–1140
        community models, 1140
        Health Belief Model, 1131, 1131(f)
        Physical Activity for People with a Disability model, 1138–1139, 1139(t)
        self-determination theory, 1134
        social cognitive theory, 1134, 1135(f), 1135(t), 1135–1138, 1136–1138(t), 1139(b)
        social ecological model, 1139, 1140
        Theory of Planned Behavior, 1132, 1132(t)
        Theory of Reasoned Action, 1132, 1132(f)
        Transtheoretical Model (stages of change), 1132, 1133(b), 1133(t), 1134(b), 1134(t), –1134 1136(t)
    case study, 1147–1148
    coaching, 1140–1141
    education, 1125, 1126
    Healthy People 2030
        framework, 1121(t)
        Physical Activity Objectives, 1121–1122, 1122(t)
    ICF, 1126–1127
    impairments and disabilities, 1141–1145
        examination and evaluation, 1141–1143, 1142(b), 1143(b)
        interventions, 1143–1145, 1145(b)
    importance, 1119–1122
    key terms, 1123–1125
        health and disease, 1123
        health promotion models, 1124–1125, 1125(f), 1126(t)
        quality of life, 1124
        wellness and illness, 1123–1124, 1124(f)
    measures, 1127–1128
        health, 1127
        quality-of-life, 1127–1128
        self-perceived health, 1127–1128
        wellness, 1127–1128
    modifiable personal health behaviors, 1128–1131
        assessing, 1128(b), 1128–1131
        outcome measures, 1129–1130(t)

motivational interviewing, 1140–1141, 1141(b)
    physical activity and exercise, 1126
    physical therapists
        as advocates, 1145–1146
        role, 1122–1123
    at program level, 1145
    social determinants of health, 1120(f)
    spinal cord injury, 810–811, 811(f)
    weight classification by body mass index, 1120(f)
Health promotion models, 1124–1125
    population health management model, 1124, 1125, 1125(t), 1126(t)
    primary prevention, 1124, 1125(f)
    secondary prevention, 1124, 1125(f)
    tertiary prevention, 1124, 1125(f)
Health-related quality of life, 272
Health risk appraisals (HRAs), 1127
Healthy Days Measure (CDC), 1127, 1130(t)
Healthy eating counseling, 1144, 1145(b)
Healthy People 2020, 1120
Healthy People 2030
    goals, 72–73
    health promotion programs for people with disabilities, 1141, 1145
    modifiable health behaviors, 1128
    national health objectives, 1120–1122, 1121(t)
    Physical Activity Objectives, 1121–1122, 1122(t)
    social determinants of health, 1120, 1120(f)
    treatment for depression, 1032
Hearing
    augmentative sensory devices, 99
    preliminary tests, 77
    screening for WSM, 1239
    technology, 319(b)
Heart auscultation, 440, 452–453(t)
Heart blocks, 448
Heart catheterization, 420, 420(t)
Heart disease (HD), 415–468
    acute coronary syndrome, 428, 432(t), 432–438
    arrhythmias, 416
    cardiac pathologies and physical therapy implications, 426–450
    cardiovascular disease (See Cardiovascular disease (CVD))
    case study, 466–468
    education, 461–464
        activity guidelines, 461
        lifestyle issues, 462
        medications, 462
        nutrition, 462
        self-monitoring, 461, 462
        sexual activity, 462, 464
        suggested topics, 464(b)
        symptom recognition and response, 462, 464(f)
    electrical conduction abnormalities, 444–450
    epidemiology, 415–416
    examination, 450–454
        medical record review, 450
        patient interview, 450–451
        tests and measures, 451–453(t), 451–454, 456–457(t)
    gender, 416
    heart failure (See Heart failure (HF))
    heart transplantation, 450
    hypertension, 416, 426–428, 429–431(t)
    pathophysiology, 415
    physical therapy interventions, 454–461
        cardiac rehabilitation, 454–455, 457, 459–461(t)
        heart failure, 457, 461, 463(t)
        therapeutic exercise, 454
    psychological/social issues, 464–465
    stroke risk, 525

valvular heart disease, 444
    See also Cardiovascular system; Coronary artery disease (CAD)
Heart failure (HF), 438–444
    baseline instability, 452(t)
    classification, 441(t)
    clinical manifestations, 440–441, 441(f)
    echocardiography and nuclear imaging, 442–443
    electrocardiogram changes, 442
    epidemiology, 415–416
    hemodynamic pressures, 430, 439(t)
    interventions, 457, 461, 463(t)
    laboratory findings, 442
    left-sided, 438, 440
    mechanical and surgical support, 443–444
    medical examination and evaluation, 442
    with mild reduction in ejection fraction (HFmrEF), 439
    pathophysiology, 439–440
    pharmacological management, 443
    with preserved ejection fraction, 439
    radiological findings, 442, 442
    with reduced ejection fraction (HFrEF), 438, 439
    right-sided, 438
    shortness of breath, 432, 438, 440–441, 451, 452(t), 454
    See also Congestive heart failure (CHF)
Heart Failure Guidelines, 439
Heart Failure Society of America, 439
Heart murmurs, 440, 453(t)
Heart rate (HR), 43
    bradycardia, 43
    doppler ultrasound, 50
    exercise, 451(t)
    factors influencing, 44–46
        age, 44
        emotions/stress, 44
        exercise, 44, 45–46
        medications, 46
        sex, 44
        systemic or local heat, 46
    gait analysis data, 267–268
    heart rate monitors, 49–50, 50(f)
    palpitations, 43
    tachycardia, 43
Heart rate monitors (HRMs), 49–50, 50(f)
Heart Rate Reserve (HRR), 353
Heart rate variability (HRV), 988, 997(t)
Heart rhythm
    cardiovascular disease, 451(t)
    stroke risk, 525
Heart sounds, abnormal, 452–453(t)
Heart tissue, coronary artery disease and, 417, 417(f)
Heart transplantation, 450
Heart valves, 418
Heat, body. See Body heat
Heat exhaustion, 38
Heating units, home accessibility and, 309
Heat stroke, 39
Heat therapy, 924
Heel lift, 1153
Heel off, 218, 219(t)
Heel-on-shin test, 194(t)
Heel strike, 217–218, 219(t), 242, 247
Heel wedge, 1153, 1153(f)
Height, measurement of, 486
Helper T cells, 589
Helping relationships (change process), 1133, 1133(t)
Help-rejecting, 1023(b)
Hemarthrosis, 104
Hemianopsia, 576–577
Hemiballismus, 189, 190(t)
Hemicorporectomy, 851(t)

Hemi-inattention, 1077
Hemineglect, 1077
Hemiparesis, 524
Hemipelvectomy, 851(t), 1197
Hemiplegia
    defined, 141
    energy considerations for orthotics, 1176
    stroke, 524, 566(b)
Hemispheric behavioral differences, 536–538,
        537(t)
Hemodynamic stability with exercise
    blood pressure with activity, 452(t)
    exercise heart rate and rhythm, 451(t)
    respiratory rate, 451(t)
Hemodynamic values, 419–420, 420(t), 438,
        439(t)
Hemorrhagic stroke, 523, 524, 525, 526, 540, 542
Hemosiderin staining, 480
Hering-Breuer reflex, 52
Heterograft, 952
Heterotopic ossification (HO), 948
Hick's law, 335
Hidden hypoxemia, 64
Hierarchical control model, 355
Higher-order cognition, 1055, 1073(t)
Higher-order cognitive functions, 1055
High-frequency chest compression (HFCC)
        devices, 408, 411, 411(f)
High-frequency chest wall oscillation (HF-CWO),
        668
High-intensity interval training (HIIT), 373,
        463(t), 582
High-Level Mobility Assessment Tool
        (HiMAT), 233, 243–244, 369, 740,
        741(f), 746, 754
High resting pressure, 513
High-temperature stops, 313
High working pressure, 513
Hinged ankle-foot orthosis, 1157, 1157(f),
        1158(f)
Hip disarticulation, 851(t), 852
    prostheses, 1197(f), 1197–1198
Hip extensors, strengthening of, 374, 375(f)
Hip hiking, 227, 1173, 1210(t), 1212
Hip joints
    capsular patterns, 116(t)
    center, determining, 257
    hip-knee-ankle-foot orthoses, 1162–1163,
        1163(f)
    prosthetic, 1198
    seating and wheeled mobility, 1242
Hip-knee-ankle-foot orthoses (HKAFO),
        804–805, 1150, 1162–1163, 1163(f),
        1172
Hippocampal system, 337
Hip(s)
    gait analysis
        fracture, 235(t)
        gait deviations, 230–231(t)
        normative sagittal plane data and impact of
            weakness, 223–224(t)
        osteoarthritis, 236(t), 905(b), 907–908
        rheumatoid arthritis, 898
        spasticity in UMN syndrome, 146(t)
        strategies, 204(f), 204–205, 359
    See also Hip joints
Hip units, hip disarticulation prosthesis, 1197(f),
        1198
Histrionic personality disorder, 1020
Hoehn and Yahr Classification of Disability Scale
        (H&Y), 683, 683(t)
Holmes-Rahe Social Readjustment Rating Scale,
        1025, 1046(t)
Holter monitors, 49–50
Homans sign, 490
Homans Test, 490

Home, on-site visits of, 300–317
    bariatric considerations, 304, 306(b)
    exterior accessibility, 301, 302(f), 302–304
        entrance, 303–304
        route of entry, 302(f), 302–303, 303(f)
    home examination forms, 301
    interior accessibility, 301, 304–309, 310–317
        bathroom, 310, 311(f), 311–315, 312(f),
            313(f), 314(f), 315(f)
        bedroom, 310, 310(f), 311(f)
        doors, 307–308, 308(f)
        electrical controls, 305
        fall risk and, 317
        floors, 306–307, 307(f)
        furniture arrangement and features, 304
        heating units, 309
        kitchen, 315–316(f), 315–317, 317(f)
        stairs, 308–309, 309(f)
        windows, 308
    preparation, 300–301
    smoke and carbon monoxide alarms, 309
Home and Community Environment (HACE),
        299(t)
Home Assessment Profile (HAP), 299(t)
Home exercise program (HEP)
    chronic pulmonary dysfunction, 407, 407(f)
    motor function, 337, 344
    motor learning, 156, 158
    multiple sclerosis, 622
    Parkinson disease, 719–720
Homeostasis, 143
Homograft, 952
Homoiothermic, 35
Homonymous hemianopia, 1064–1065, 1065(f),
        1077
Homonymous hemianopsia, 529, 531
Hook-lying, 622–623
Hormonal regulation, 37–38
Horner syndrome, 533(t), 534(t)
Hospital Anxiety and Depression Scale (HADS),
        662
Household walker, 551, 551(t)
Housing and Urban Development Office, 326
Hoyer Lift, 670
H-reflexes, 165, 167, 171(f)
HTC VIVE headset, 572
Huffing, 410
Human endogenous retroviruses (HERVs), 589
Humor, 1023(b)
Huntington disease, 182, 189
Hybrid upper limb prostheses, 1200
Hydraulic friction, 1192
Hydrocolloids, 510, 510(f)
Hydrofibers, 511, 511(f)
Hydrogels, 510, 510(f)
Hydrogen peroxide solution, 501
Hydronephrosis, 770
Hydrotherapy, 613, 622
Hydroxyzine (Vistaril), 1030(b)
Hypalgesia, 89(t)
Hyperalgesia, 89(t), 687, 972
Hyperbaric oxygen therapy (HBOT), 506–507
Hypercapnea, 386
Hypercholesterolemia, 432(t)
Hyperesthesia, 89(t)
Hyperextensibility of joints, 147
Hyperhidrosis, 34, 689
Hyperinflation, 386, 387, 388(f)
Hyperkeratosis, 482
Hyperkinesis, 189, 190(t)
Hyperkinetic dysarthria, 1112, 1113
Hypermetria, 187, 190(t)
Hypermobile Ehlers-Danlos syndrome (hEDS),
        987, 992, 1006
Hypermobility, 114
Hyperpathia, 592

Hyperpyrexia, 38
Hyperreflexic bladder, 770
Hypersexuality, 1040–1041
Hypertension (HTN), 426–428
    ABPM for diagnosing, 58
    ACC/AHA guidelines, 57, 58, 62
    age-related, 57
    auscultatory gap, 59
    categories, 427
    epidemiology, 416
    isolated systolic, 427
    labile, 427
    management, 427–428
        pharmacological, 46, 428, 429–431(t)
        physical therapy, 427–428
    prevalence, 416, 426
    stroke risk, 525
    Valsalva maneuver, 57
    white coat or nonsustained, 57, 427
Hyperthermia, 768
Hypertonicity, 735, 736, 738
Hypertrophic cardiomyopathy, 417
Hypertrophic scarring, 476
Hypertrophic scars, 944
Hypertrophy, 948
Hyperventilation, 53, 55
Hypocalcemia, 422–423
Hypodermis, 471
Hypoesthesia, 89(t)
Hypoglossal nerve (CN XII), 98(t), 151, 155(t),
        639, 659
Hypokalemia, 422
Hypokinesia, 189, 190(t), 354, 684, 699
Hypokinetic dysarthria, 688, 1112, 1113
Hypomagnesemia, 422–423
Hypometria, 187, 190(t)
Hypomimia, 684
Hypomobility, 114
Hypoplasia, 481
Hypothalamic-pituitary-adrenal (HPA) axis,
        975–976, 976(f)
Hypothermia, 39
Hypothesis-Oriented Algorithm for Clinicians
        (HOAC), 2, 4, 5, 16, 545
Hypotonia, 145, 147, 188, 190(t), 195(t)
Hypovigilance/hypervigilance, 1044(t)
Hypoxemia, 31, 63, 64, 386, 452(t)
Hypoxia, 63

I

Iatrogenic factors, in wound healing, 477
ICARE (Interdisciplinary Comprehensive Arm
        Rehab Evaluation), 361(t), 363
    elliptical trainer, 266
ICD-10, 23–24, 272, 970(b)
ICD-11, 272, 970, 970(b), 971
ICF Core Sets, 286
Idealization, 1023(b)
Ideational apraxia, 134, 557, 1092, 1094
Ideomotor apraxia, 134, 557, 1092, 1093–1094
Idiopathic parkinsonism. See Parkinson
        disease (PD)
Idiopathic pulmonary fibrosis (IPF), 391
Illness
    defined, 272, 1124
    health promotion and wellness, 1123–1124,
        1124(f)
Imaging
    arthritis
        osteoarthritis, 905
        rheumatoid arthritis, 892
    central nervous system, 161
    characteristics of imaging modalities, 164(t)
    computed tomography, 160–161, 161(f)
    diffusion tensor, 161–162, 162(f), 164(t)

functional imaging techniques, 162–163, 163(f)
functional magnetic resonance imaging, 162–163, 163(f), 164(t), 571
magnetic resonance imaging, 161, 162(f), 164(t), 540–541, 541(f), 596, 597(f), 601
molecular imaging techniques, 163, 163(f), 164(t)
multiple sclerosis, 596, 597(f), 601
musculoskeletal examination, 104
nuclear, in heart failure, 443
radiography (x-ray), 160, 161(f)
spinal cord injury, 162
stroke, 540–541, 541(f)
    arteriography, 541
    computed tomography, 540, 541(f)
    digital subtraction angiography, 541
    Doppler ultrasound, 541
    magnetic resonance angiography, 541
    magnetic resonance imaging, 540–541, 541(f)
structural imaging techniques, 160–162, 161(f), 162(f)
traumatic brain injury, 161–162
Imipramine (Tofranil), 602, 650, 1035(b), 1039(b)
Immediate Post-Concussion and Cognitive Testing (ImPACT), 751, 753
Immediate recall, 1074
Immobilization, 774–775
cervical orthoses, 774, 774(f)
thoracolumbosacral orthosis, 774(f), 774–775
Immune response, 638
Immune system, chronic pain and, 973
Immunomodulating agents, 601
Impairment, 5–6, 7(b), 272, 273
Implicit learning, 158(b)
Implicit vision, 201
Impregnated gauze, 509
Improving Functional Outcomes in Physical Rehabilitation, 800–801, 804
Impulse generator (IPG), 695
Inactivity, clinical manifestations of, 603(f)
Inappropriate affect, 1044(t)
Inclusive design, 294–295
Incomplete SCI (iSCI), 763, 765, 781, 792, 793, 804
Incomplete tetraplegia, 760
Incontinence, 538–539, 603, 689
Increased peripheral resistance (vasoconstriction), 56
Incremental cycle ergometry testing, 398, 399
Incremental Shuttle Walk Test (ISWT), 399
Indego, 1165
Independent, defined, 278, 279(b)
Indirect motor loop, 682, 682(f)
Indirect stimulation-facilitation, 1109
Indurated tissues, 483
Inertial loads, 351, 352(t)
Infection
burns, 946, 950
wound healing, 476–477
Inflammation phase
dermal healing, 949
wound healing, 471–472, 476
Inhalation injury, 946
Inhibitory cutoff, 819–820
In-Home Occupational Performance Evaluation (I-HOPE), 300(t)
In-Home Occupational Performance Evaluation for Providing Assistance (I-HOPE Assist), 300(t)
Initial contact, 218(f), 219, 219(t), 220, 221(t), 222(t), 223(t)
Initial double limb stance, 217, 218(f), 219
Initial kinematic feedback, 341
Initial observation, 147
Initial swing, 218(f), 219, 219(t), 220, 221(t), 222(t), 223(t)

Initiating stimuli, 766, 766(t)
Injury, acute coronary syndrome and, 433, 433(f)
Innovative dressings, 512
Inotropes, 431(t), 443
Inotropy, 421
Input device, 318
Insert, foot, 1152, 1152(f)
Inside-out model, 589
Insomnia, 540, 689
Inspection
chronic pulmonary dysfunction, 397
integumentary, 110
musculoskeletal, 110(f), 110–111
Inspiration, 51
Inspiratory capacity, 383
Inspiratory muscle training, 406, 406(f), 463(t)
Instruction. See Patient and family/caregiver education
Instrumental activities of daily living (IADL), 6, 136, 287(t), 288(t), 552, 733, 1237
Instrumentation and technology to assess motor function, 160–174
characteristics of imaging modalities, 164(t)
electrophysiologic neuromuscular assessment, 163, 165(f), 165–174, 166(f), 167(f), 168(f), 169(f), 170(f), 171–172(t)
functional imaging techniques, 162–163, 163(f)
molecular imaging techniques, 163, 163(f)
structural imaging techniques, 160–162, 161(f), 162(f)
Instrumented systems for determining gait parameters, 249–256
footswitches/footswitch systems, 250, 255(f), 255–256
low-cost, 248–249
accelerometers, 248–249, 249(f)
gyroscopes, 249
walkways, 250, 250(f), 251–255(t)
Integral stimulation, 1114
Integrated framework, 2, 4(f)
elements of clinical reasoning, 5–8
patient/client management, 8–13
Integrated power wheelchair, 1275, 1275(f)
Integrating Manual Therapy and Pain Neuroscience: Twelve Principles for Treating the Body and the Brain, 998
Integumentary system
anatomy and physiology, 471
disorders, 482–485
neuropathy, 484–485
pressure injuries, 482–484
resources for patients with, 495
evaluation, 494
examination, 485–490
arousal, attention, and cognition, 488
assistive and adaptive devices, 488
circulation, 488–490
gait, locomotion, and balance, 490
history, 485–486
muscle performance, 493
orthotic, protective, and supportive devices, 493
pain and, 493
posture and, 493
range of motion and, 493–494
risk factor assessment, 493
self-care and home management, 494
sensation and, 494, 494(f)
systems review, 486
tests and measures, 486–488
ventilation and respiration, 494
inspection, 110
integumentary integrity, 490–491
amyotrophic lateral sclerosis, 661
coloration, 490–491
fibrosis, 490

motor control, 349(t)
observation and palpation, 490
Parkinson disease, 706
spinal cord injury, 779–780, 780(t)
stroke, 554
temperature, 491
trophic changes, 490
intervention, 494–496
coordination, communication, and documentation, 495
instruction, 495
procedural, 495–496
Intellectual deficits, stroke and, 536, 537(t)
Intellectualization, 1023(b)
Intelligibility, speech, 1102
Intensive Comprehensive Aphasia Programs (ICAPs), 1111
Intention tremor, 188, 190(t), 195(t)
Intention (action) tremors, 593
Intercom system, 304
Interdisciplinary team, TBI and, 732–734
case manager/team coordinator, 733
neuropsychologist, 733
occupational therapist, 733
other team members, 734
patient and family, 732
physician, 732
rehabilitation nurse, 733
social worker, 733
speech-language pathologist, 732–733
vocational rehabilitation counselor, 733–734
Interest Checklist, 1048(t)
Interference, neuroplasticity principle of, 339(t), 357
Interferon beta-1a (Avonex, Rebif), 599(t)
Interferon beta-1b (Betaseron, Extavia), 599(t)
Interferon drugs, 597, 601
Interleukin-6, 540
Interlimb coordination, 182
Intermittent catheterization, 770
Intermittent claudication (IC), 236(t), 478, 489
Intermittent control hypothesis, 336
Intermittent fever, 38(b)
Intermittent pneumatic compression (IPC), 516, 516(f)
Intermittent self-catheterization (ISC), 602
Internal carotid artery (ICA), 528, 529
Internal carotid artery (ICA) syndrome, 529
Internal extension aid, 1193
Internal-External Scale, 1047(t)
Internalized anger, 1017
Internal locus of control, 1021
Internal modifications, 1152–1153, 1152–1153(f)
Internal respiration, 50, 385(f)
International Advisory Committee on Clinical Trials of MS, 590
International Association for the Study of Pain (IASP), 967, 967(b)
International Classification of Diseases
10th revision (ICD-10), 23–24, 272, 970(b)
11th revision (ICD-11), 272, 970, 970(b), 971
International Classification of Functioning, Disability and Health (ICF), 2, 5–8
burns, 954
community activities, 212
coordination examination, 182–183, 197(t)
enablement language and structure for organizing information, 545
function examination, 272–275
body functions and body structures, 272, 273, 273(f), 274(t)
classification of activities and participation, 274(f)
classification scheme for coding, 275
contextual factors, 273, 275
Core Sets, 286

International Classification of Functioning, Disability and Health (ICF) (continued)
   defined by components, 272–273
   environmental factors, 273, 275, 275(t)
   functioning and disability model, 273(f)
   gait analysis, 234–240(t)
   health promotion and wellness, 1126–1127
   heart disease examination, 451, 451–453(t)
   information on function and disability, describing and organizing, 334, 334(f)
   outcome measures, 14
   pain model, 971, 992
   Parkinson disease, 701–703(t), 707
   physical environment, 294
   psychosocial issues, 1043(t), 1046–1048(t)
   spinal cord injury, 765–773
      activity limitations, 772–773
      body structure/function impairments, 765–772, 766(t), 769(t)
      outcome measures, 777–778(t)
      participation restrictions, 772–773
      quality of life, 772–773
   standardized assessments organized by, 548(t)
   structure, 6(f)
   terminology, 7(b)
   traumatic brain injury, 743(t), 744(t)
International Classification of Impairments, Disabilities, and Handicaps (ICIDH), 2
International Cooperative Ataxia Rating Scale (ICARS), 196
International Parkinson and Movement Disorder Society, 705
International Physical Activity Questionnaire, 1128–1129, 1129(t)
International Society of Lymphology Staging System, 487–488
International Standards for Neurological Classification of Spinal Cord Injury (ISNCSCI), 762–763, 764, 776
Internet applications, 933(t)
Internuclear ophthalmoplegia (INO), 592
Interpersonal health behavior model, 1134
Interphalangeal (IP) joints
   capsular patterns, 116(t)
   osteoarthritis, 908
   rheumatoid arthritis, 896, 897
Interrater reliability, 282, 288
Interstitial lung diseases. See Restrictive lung diseases
Intertrial variability, 344
Interval/ratio measures, 280–281, 281(f)
Interval training, 351, 352(t)
Intervention, 19–22
   behavioral
      locomotor function, 378–379
      motor control, 349(t)
      multiple sclerosis, 613
      smoking cessation, 393
   coordination and communication, 19
   direct intervention, 19–20, 22
   dual-task
      motor function, 342(t), 349(t), 350(t), 354, 357
      motor learning, 156
      motor skills, 139(b)
      stroke, 562
      traumatic brain injury, 747–748, 748(f)
   education, 22
   FITT equation for exercise intervention, 20, 21(b)
   restorative, 20
      amyotrophic lateral sclerosis, 663
      multiple sclerosis, 603
      neural plasticity, 745
      stroke, 545
      traumatic brain injury, 742, 744, 744(t), 745, 745(t)

task-specific training, 20, 21(b)
   See also Physical therapy interventions
Interview
   environmental accessibility, 297–298
   heart disease, 450–451
   musculoskeletal examination, 108–110
   stroke, 545–546
   See also Assessment interview, for WSM; Patient interview
Interviewer report, 277
Intra-aortic balloon pump (IABP), 433
Intracerebral hemorrhage (IH), 525
Intraclass correlation coefficient (ICC), 226, 243, 249, 250, 284
Intracranial pressure (ICP), 527, 734
Intralimb coordination, 182
Intraneuronal protein aggregates, 638
Intrarater reliability, 282
Intrinsic factors, in wound healing, 477
Intrinsic feedback, 97, 370
Intuitive/global learners, 160
Invariant characteristics, 336
Inverted-U principle, 135
Involuntary emotional expression disorder, 595
Involuntary movements. See Dystonia
Involved stance time, 240, 246(t)
Iowa Level of Assistance Scale (ILAS), 233, 240–241
Ipsilateral loss of proprioception, 764
Ipsilateral pushing, 550, 563
Ischemia, vascular, 483
Ischemic cascade, 527
Ischemic stroke, 523, 524–525, 526–527, 540, 543(b)
Ischial containment socket, 1195, 1195(f)
Ischial tuberosity, 483, 483(f)
Isocarboxazid (Marplan), 1035(b)
Isokinetic dynamometer, 142
Isokinetic dynamometry, 118, 120
Isokinetic measurement system, 264
Isokinetic testing, 142
Isolated systolic hypertension (ISH), 427
Isolated writer's cramp, 147
Isolation of affect, 1023(b)
Isometric contractions, 351
Isometric torque measurement system, 264
Isovolumetric contraction, 419

J

Jargon, psychosocial issues and, 1045
Jaundice, 35(b)
Jaw. See Temporomandibular joint (TMJ)
Jebsen-Taylor Hand Function Test, 198(b)
Jendrassik maneuver, 150
JFK Coma Recovery Scale Revised (CRS-R), 75
Jimmo Settlement Agreement webpage, 604
Jimmo v. Sibelius, 604, 697
Job requirements, examination of workplace and, 318
Joint impairments
   amyotrophic lateral sclerosis, 661
   hypomobility/hypermobility, 114
   osteoarthritis, 903, 904(f), 906–908
   rheumatoid arthritis, 893–901, 894(f)
   stroke, 552–553
   See also Arthritis
Joint kinematics (motion), evaluation of, 256–260
   electrogoniometers, 256
   electromagnetic motion analysis system, 259, 260
   optical marker-based motion analysis systems, 256–259, 257(f), 258(f), 259(f), 260(f)
   optical markerless motion analysis system, 260
   video-based motion analysis systems, 256
Joint mobilization, 117

Joint play motions, 116, 117(f)
Joint prosthetics, 1201
Joint receptors, 79(b), 80
Journal of Orthopedic and Sports Physical Therapy, 14
Joystick, 1279
J point, 435
Jugular venous distention, 438, 453(t), 455(f)
Jump response, 989
Juvenile Huntington disease, 681

K

Karvonen formula, 45
Keep It Simple System, 1196
Keloid, 476, 950
Keloid scars, 944
Keratinocytes, 475, 476, 477, 498, 511
Kickplate, 304
Kidney damage, 595
Killer T cells, 589
Kinematic feedback, 341, 357
Kinematic gait analysis
   qualitative, 220, 224–244
      ambulation profiles and scales, 233–241
      Community Balance and Mobility Scale, 242
      displacement examined, 220
      Dynamic Gait Index, 242–243
      Fast Evaluation of Mobility, Balance, and Fear, 243
      Figure-of-8 Walk Test, 243–244
      Functional Assessment Measure, 241, 242
      Functional Gait Assessment, 243
      Gait Abnormality Rating Scale, 242
      High-Level Mobility Assessment Tool, 243–244
      observational gait analysis, 220, 224–233
      summary, 265, 265(f)
      Tinetti Performance Oriented Mobility Assessment, 244
      Walking Index for Spinal Cord Injury II, 244
   quantitative, 244–260
      joint kinematics evaluation, 256–260
      spatial and temporal variables, 245–246(t), 245–256
   summary, 265, 265(f)
   See also Joint kinematics (motion), evaluation of
Kinesiologic EMG, 168
Kinesio Taping (KT), 926
Kinesthesia awareness test, 90
Kinesthetic and Visual Imagery Questionnaire (KVIQ), 566, 572
Kinesthetic imagery, 377
Kinetic feedback, 357
Kinetic gait analysis, 261–264, 265
Kinetic gait variables, 261(t), 261–264
   force plate technology for measuring, 262–263
   isokinetic and isometric torque measurement systems, 264
   plantar pressure measurement systems, 263(f), 263–264, 264(f)
   software for processing, analyzing, and displaying, 264
   See also Spatial and temporal gait variables
Kinetic tremor, 188
King's staging system, 645, 645(t)
Kinovea, 226
Kistler Instrument Corp., 262
Kitchen, 315–316(f), 315–317, 317(f)
Knee-ankle-foot orthoses (KAFO), 567, 1150, 1160–1162
   care after delivery, 1172
   clinical considerations, 1162
   knee control, 1160(f), 1160–1161, 1161(f)
   mechanical, for paraplegia, 1161–1162, 1162(f)
   spinal cord injury, 804–805, 806(f)

Knee controls, 567
Knee disarticulation, 851, 851(t)
  prostheses, 1197
Knee injury and Osteoarthritis Outcome Score,
    107
Knee orthoses (KOs), 1150
Knee(s)
  arthritis
    foot orthoses, 1154–1156(t)
    osteoarthritis, 905(b), 908
    rheumatoid arthritis, 898, 898(f)
  gait analysis, 229(t), 254(t)
    gait deviations
      Iowa Level of Assistance Scale, 241
      knee arthroplasty, 234(t), 237(t), 241, 245,
        254(t)
      normative sagittal plane data and impact of
        weakness, 222(t)
      osteoarthritis and, 236(t), 239(t)
      outcome measures, 234(t), 236(t), 237(t),
        239(t)
  spasticity in UMN syndrome, 146(t)
  tibiofemoral joint, 116(t)
Knee units
  disarticulation prostheses, 1197
  transfemoral prostheses, 1191–1194
    axis system, 1191, 1192(f)
    extension aid, 1193, 1193(f)
    friction mechanism, 1191–1193,
      1192–1194(f)
    mechanical stabilizer, 1193, 1194(f)
Knight Taylor orthosis, 1167, 1167(f)
Knowledge of performance (KP), 126, 159(b),
    560, 561
Knowledge of results (KR), 126, 156, 159(b), 346,
    370–371, 560, 561
Korotkoff sounds, 59, 61
Krause end bulbs, 79, 79(b), 941(t)
Krusen Limb Load Monitor, 250
Kussmaul's respirations, 54(f)

L

Labeled line principle, 78
Labels, psychosocial issues and, 1045
Labile HTN, 427
Laboratory tests/values
  cardiac anatomy and physiology, 422(t),
    422–423
  chronic pulmonary dysfunction, 397
  chronic pulmonary dysfunction examination,
    397
  heart disease, 422
  heart failure, 442
  medical record review of heart disease, 450
  musculoskeletal examination, 105
  normal, online access of, 105
  rheumatoid arthritis, 891, 892
  vital signs, 33
Lacunar strokes, 531
Lambert-Eaton myasthenic syndrome (LEMS),
    167
Language
  deficits, stroke and, 532
  defined, 1099
  journals, 1107
  organization, 1100–1101
  pathology, normal, 1100
  pragmatic language behaviors, 1099
Laryngopharynx, 50
Lateral gaze palsy, 592
Lateral inferior pontine syndrome, 533(t)
Lateral malleolus, 483, 483(f)
Lateral medullary (Wallenburg) syndrome, 533(t)
Lateral midpontine syndrome, 534(t)
Lateral spinal pathways, 127, 128(f)

Lateral spinothalamic tract, 81, 82(f)
Lateral superior pontine syndrome, 534(t)
Lateral supports, for WSM, 1258
Lateral trunk bending, 1212
Lateral view, in postural alignment, 110, 110f
Lead-pipe rigidity, 145, 146, 189, 190(t)
Lead pipe rigidity, 684
Lead-up practice, 344
Leaflets, 418
LEAPS (Locomotor Experience Applied
    Post-Stroke), 360, 362(t), 363
Learned nonuse, 132(b), 544, 553, 576
Learner, in interventions for stroke, 559
Learner specific level of demand, 343
Learning networks, 337–338, 337–338(f)
Leeds Assessment of Neuropathic Symptoms and
    Signs (LANSS), 984, 985(t)
Left anterior descending (LAD), 418, 418(f),
    436
Left bundle branch block (LBBB), 448
Left circumflex (CX), 418, 418(f), 436
Left hemiplegia, 537, 538
Left hemisphere lesions, 537, 537(t)
Left-sided heart catheterization, 420, 420(t)
Left-sided heart failure, 438, 440
Left ventricle (LV)
  failure, 433, 439(t), 440, 453(t)
  function, 415–416, 419(f), 420, 422, 442, 447
Left ventricular assist devices (LVADs), 443
Left ventricular-end diastolic volume (LVEDV),
    419, 420, 443, 453(t)
Leg ergometry, 423, 426
Legislation, in examination and modification of
    environment, 326–327
Length-tension relationship, 354
Lesion level in spinal cord injury, designation of,
    762(f), 762–763
Lethargic, defined, 75
Lethargy, 532
Leukotriene antagonists, 393, 394(t)
Levels of Cognitive Function (LOCF), 134, 735,
    736, 736(b)
Levine sign, 452(t)
Levodopa, 681, 685, 691–695, 692(t), 704, 711,
    719
Levodopa-induced dyskinesias (LIDs), 694
Lewy bodies, 682
Lexicon, 1100
Liberatory (Semont) maneuver, 833
Licensed or certified medical professional (LCMP),
    1227
Lidocaine, 501
Life Satisfaction Questionnaire (LISAT-9), 348(t),
    773, 778(t), 783, 1129(t)
Life span design, 294–295
Lifestyle factors
  heart disease, 462
  stroke, 525
  vital signs, 33
Lifts devices, 670
Light-emitting diodes (LEDs), 256
Light-headedness, 820
Lighting, 302, 305, 308
Likert scale, 143
Limb containment systems, 515, 515(f)
Limb holding, 192
Limbic system, 337
Limb-onset (spinal) ALS, 636
Limited community walker, 551, 551(t)
Limited household walker, 551, 551(t)
Limited motion joint, 1158, 1159(f)
Limits of stability (LOS), 191, 199–201, 205, 375,
    561–562
Lindsay nails, 34
Linear velocity, 245(t)
Line of gravity, 110, 110f, 199

Liners
  locking, 1196, 1196(f)
  transtibial prosthetics, 1187, 1188(f)
Lipodermatosclerosis, 480
Liquids (sounds), 1103
Lisfranc disarticulations, 851(t), 859, 1181
Lithium carbonate (Eskalith, Lithobid), 1030(b)
LMN bladder, 770
Loading response, 218(f), 219, 219(t), 221(t),
    222(t), 223(t), 256, 262
Locked-in syndrome (LIS), 532, 533(t)
Locking liners, 1196, 1196(f)
Locomotion, defined, 216
Locomotor Experience Applied Post-Stroke
    (LEAPS), 360
Locomotor function, 368–381
  case study, 380–381
  examination, 490
  Functional Independence Measure (FIM),
    287(t), 288
  gait speed, 369, 369(t), 371, 372, 373, 374(f), 379
  gait training with assistive devices, 379
  multiple sclerosis, 610
  performance vs. capacity vs. patient-reported
    outcomes, 379
  physical therapy interventions, 370–379
    behavioral change support, 378–379
    circuit training, 377, 377(b), 378(f)
    exoskeleton, 379
    intensity, 370
    motor imagery, 377–378
    motor learning, 370–371
    muscle force production, augmenting,
      374–375, 375(f)
    neuromodulation, 379
    neuroplasticity, 371, 371(b)
    overground walking for balance and postural
      control, 375–377, 376(b), 376(f)
    task-specific walking training/treadmill
      training, 371–373, 372–373(f)
    virtual reality and exergaming, 373–374, 374(f)
  spinal cord injury, 781, 801–809
    gait/walking skills, 804–809, 805–806(f),
      807(f)
    wheelchair skills, 801–803(f), 801–804
  task-specific training, 360, 363
  traumatic brain injury, 740–741, 741(f)
  walking function examination, 368–370
  See also Locomotor training (LT)
Locomotor training (LT)
  multiple sclerosis, 625–628, 626(f), 627(f),
    628(f)
  Parkinson disease, 715(f), 715–716
  stroke
    ambulation classification, 551(t)
    electromechanically assisted locomotor
      training, 565
    examination, 550–551
    functional electrical stimulation and
      ankle-foot orthosis, 565, 566(b)
    interventions, 563–567
    motor imagery, 566–567
    orthotics for lower extremity, 567
    overground locomotor training, 563–564
    task-specific/goal-oriented training and,
      563–564
    treadmill training with/without body weight
      support, 564–565, 565(f)
    virtual reality, 566–567
    wheelchairs, 567
  traumatic brain injury, 745, 746
Locus coeruleus (LC), 682, 975
Loewenstein Occupational Therapy Cognitive
    Assessment (LOTCA), 1068(t), 1073
Lokomat, 807, 1165
Long-acting beta-2 agonist (LABA), 393, 394(t)

Long COVID, 392–393, 990, 1005
Long-stretch and short-stretch bandages, 513, 513(f)
Long-term depression, 338
Long-term (remote) memory, 77
Long-term potentiation (LTP), 338
Long transfemoral (above knee) amputation, 851(t)
Long transtibial (below knee) amputation, 851(t)
Lorazepam (Ativan), 649, 650, 1030(b)
Lordosis, 664, 1212
Lou Gehrig disease. See Amyotrophic lateral sclerosis (ALS)
Lower extremities (LE)
    amyotrophic lateral sclerosis, 669
    range of motion, 114, 115(f)
    stroke
        balance training, 562
        obligatory synergies, 554, 555(t)
        orthotics, 567
Lower Extremity Functional Scale (LEFS), 289
Lower leg to foot angle measurements, 1245, 1246(f)
Lower-limb orthoses, 1150–1165
    alternative, 1163–1165, 1164(f)
        clinical considerations, 1165
        powered orthosis, 1165
        reciprocating gait orthosis, 1164, 1164(f)
        standing frame, 1163, 1164(f)
    ankle-foot orthoses, 1154, 1156–1160
        ankle control, 1157–1159, 1157–1159(f)
        care after delivery, 1171
        clinical considerations, 1159–1160, 1160(f)
        functional electrical stimulation and, 565, 566, 566(b), 567
        gait examination and, 255–256
        multiple sclerosis, 626, 627(f)
        structure, 1154, 1156(f), 1156–1157
    foot orthoses, 1152–1154
        external modifications, 1153, 1153(f)
        foot inserts, 1154, 1154(f)
        internal modifications, 1152–1153, 1152–1153(f)
        knee arthritis, 1154–1156(t)
    hip-knee-ankle-foot orthoses, 1162–1163, 1163(f)
    knee-ankle-foot orthoses, 1160–1162
        care after delivery, 1172
        clinical considerations, 1162
        knee control, 1160(f), 1160–1161, 1161(f)
        mechanical, for paraplegia, 1161–1162, 1162(f)
    shoes, 1151(f), 1151–1152
    trunk-hip-knee-ankle-foot orthoses, 1163
Lower limb prostheses, 1181
Lower motor neuron (LMN) injuries, 765
Lower motor neuron syndrome (LMN), 140, 636, 636(t)
    amyotrophic lateral sclerosis, 640–641, 641(t), 642, 643–644, 644(f)
    deep tendon reflexes, 149
    differential diagnosis, 174(t)
    hypotonia/flaccidity, 147
    impairments, related, 640–641, 641(t)
    motor weakness/muscle atrophy, 141, 142
Lower trunk rotation (LTR), 622–623
Low-level cold laser, 508
Low-level infrared laser, 508
Low physical effort, in universal design, 295
Low-quarter shoes, 1151, 1151(f)
Low resting pressure, 513
Lub-dub, 49
Lumbar puncture (LP), 596
Lumbosacral flexion, extension, lateral control (LS FEL) orthosis, 1166, 1166(f)
Lumbosacral orthoses, 1166
Lung auscultation, 397–398, 398(f), 440, 453(t), 455(f)
Lung capacities, 383(f), 383–384
Lung transplantation, 396

Lung volume recruitment (LVR) technique, 668
Lung volume reduction surgery (LVRS), 396
Lung volumes
    COPD, 387, 388(f)
    pulmonary system, 383, 383(f)
    restrictive lung disease, 392, 392(f)
Lymphangions, 470–471
Lymphatics, 470–471
Lymphatic system
    anatomy and physiology, 470–471
    evaluation, 494
    examination, 485–494
        arousal, attention, and cognition, 488
        assistive and adaptive devices, 488
        circulation, 488–490
        gait, locomotion, and balance, 490
        history, 485–486
        muscle performance, 493
        orthotic, protective, and supportive devices, 493
        pain and, 493
        posture and, 493
        range of motion and, 493–494
        risk factor assessment, 493
        self-care and home management, 494
        sensation and, 494, 494(f)
        systems review, 486
        tests and measures, 486–488
        ventilation and respiration, 494
    intervention, 494–496
        coordination, communication, and documentation, 495
        instruction, 495
        manual lymphatic drainage, 512, 512(f)
        procedural, 495–496
    lymphedema, 481–482
    resources, 495
Lymphedema, 481–482
    bandaging, 513–514, 514(f)
    classifying, 481, 481(f)
    clinical presentation, 481(f), 482
    compression treatments, 516 (See also Compression therapy)
    defined, 481
    history, 482
    intervention, 482
    manual lymphatic drainage, 512, 512(f)
    staging or grading, 487–488
    tests and measures, 482
Lymphedematous limb, 482
Lymph fluid, 470–471
Lymphorrhea, 482
Lymphoscintigraphy, 482, 490
Lymph vessel integrity, 490

M

Maddocks questions, 753
Mafenide acetate, 501, 951
Maggot débridement therapy (MDT), 499–500, 500(f), 510
Magnetic resonance angiography, 541
Magnetic resonance imaging (MRI), 161, 162(f), 164(t)
    multiple sclerosis, 596, 597(f), 601
    stroke, 540–541, 541(f)
Maintenance drugs, for chronic pulmonary dysfunction, 393–395, 394(t), 395(t)
Maintenance stage of change, 1132, 1133(b)
Maintenance therapy, 604, 696–597
Major histocompatibility complex (MHC), 589
Major stroke, 527
Maladaptive pain, 971
Mal de Debarquement, 845
Malignant arrhythmias, 416, 444
Managed care, 1071–1072
Manner of articulation, 1102

Manometer, 59
Manual lock, 1193, 1194(f)
Manual lymphatic drainage (MLD), 471, 482, 512, 512(f), 513, 514, 516
Manual muscle testing (MMT), 13, 118–120, 141, 167, 348(t), 351, 354
    amyotrophic lateral sclerosis, 661
    as break test, 118, 120
    chronic pulmonary dysfunction, 398
    grading system, 118–119, 119(t)
    as make test, 118, 120
    multiple sclerosis, 609
    recording form, 112(f)
    spinal cord injury, 762–763, 776
    stroke, 556
Manual resistance, 351, 352(t)
Manual sphygmomanometer, 59, 60(b)
Manual stretching, spinal cord injury and, 790–791
Manual therapy
    cervicogenic dizziness, 846
    chronic pain, 994(t), 997(t), 998(f), 1005, 1006
    hip and knee osteoarthritis, 927
    manual lymphatic drainage, 512
    traumatic brain injury, 754
Manual wheelchairs, 1262–1265
    with add-on systems, 1272, 1273–1274
        hand rim-activated system, 1273, 1273(f)
        power add-on unit, 1274, 1274(f)
        power assist drive system, 1273–1274, 1274(f)
    ADL-specific, 1269, 1269(f)
    fully configurable frame, 1263(f), 1263–1264
    minimally adjustable frame, 1262–1263
    nonadjustable frame, 1262, 1262(f)
    propulsion configuration, 1264(f), 1264–1265, 1265(f)
    sports-specific, 1269, 1270–1272, 1272(f), 1273(f)
    variable positioning, 1265–1269
        recline, 1268(f), 1268–1269
        standing, 1269, 1270(f)
        tilt, 1265(f), 1265–1268, 1266–1267(b), 1268(f)
        tilt and recline, 1269
Maprotiline (Ludiomil), 1035(b)
Marcus Gunn pupil, 592
Massage
    amputation, 868
    amyotrophic lateral sclerosis, 670
    anxiety, 1027
    arthritis, 924, 926
    chronic pain, 997(t), 1002, 1003
    multiple sclerosis, 613
    Parkinson disease, 711
    scar management
        burns, 954, 962–963
        wounds, 519
    stroke, 575, 581
    supraventricular ectopy, 446
    traumatic spinal cord injury, 767, 771, 772
Massed practice, 343, 345(t), 742
Mass grasp test, 193(t)
Mat assessment, for WSM, 1239–1240
    sitting mat assessment, 1239–1240, 1240(f)
    supine mat assessment, 1239, 1240(f)
Matching Person and Technology (MPT), 1226
Mat examination, 1228
Matrix metalloproteinase (MMP-9), 540
Mat-Scan System, 264
Mattress, 310
Maturation phase
    dermal healing, 949–950
    wound healing, 472, 476
Maximal oxygen consumption (VO₂max), 423
Maximal oxygen uptake (Vo₂ max)ᵇ, 1129(t)
Maximum assistance, defined, 279(b)
Maximum inspiratory pressure (PI_max), 384
Maximum voluntary isometric contraction (MVIC), 661

Mayo-Portland Adaptability Inventory, 742
McDonald Criteria of the International Panel on Diagnosis of MS, 596
McGill Pain Questionnaire (MPQ), 105, 108(f), 609, 984, 985(t), 1031
MDA ALS Research and Clinical Centers, 646
MDS Clinical Diagnostic Criteria for Parkinson Disease, 691
Mean absolute percent errors (MAPEs), 249
Measles, 589
Mechanical energy cost determination, 267
Mechanical insufflation–exsufflation (MI-E) device, 668
Mechanical KAFOs, for paraplegia, 1161–1162, 1162(f)
Mechanical modalities, 502–506
    electrical stimulation, 502, 506, 506(f)
    thermal and nonthermal diathermy, 506
    ultrasound, 502, 502(f), 503–505(t)
    ultraviolet radiation, 506
Mechanical stabilizer, 1193
    manual lock, 1193, 1194(f)
Mechanical thrombectomy, 542
Mechanisms and Management of Pain for the Physical Therapist, 971
Mechanoreceptors, 78, 79(b), 81, 83, 83(t)
Medial inferior pontine syndrome, 533(t)
Medial lemnisci, 81, 82(f), 186
Medial longitudinal fasciculus (MLF), 592
Medial medullary syndrome, 533(t)
Medial midpontine syndrome, 534(t)
Medial supports, for WSM, 1258
Medical complications
    diabetic neuropathy, 485
    spinal cord injury, 760, 770
    stroke, 544
    traumatic brain injury, 730, 730(b)
Medical device-related pressure injury, 492(t)
Medical diagnosis, 16
    Parkinson disease, 691
    stroke, 540
Medical diagnostic testing, chronic pain and, 1007
Medical-grade honey, 500
Medical labeling, 272
Medically unexplained pain, 971
Medical management
    acute coronary syndrome, 436–438
        coronary artery bypass graft, 436–437
        percutaneous transluminal coronary angioplasty, 436
        pharmacological management, 438
        physical therapy clinical implications, 437–438
    amyotrophic lateral sclerosis, 646–650
    arthritis, 910–914
        osteoarthritis, 912–914
        rheumatoid arthritis, 910–912
    burns, 950–953
        initial treatment, 950–951, 951(t)
        surgical management, 951–953, 952–953(f)
        topical medications, 951(t)
    chronic pain, 1007
        medical diagnostic testing, 1007
        other, 1007
        pharmacological management, 1007
    chronic pulmonary dysfunction, 393–395
        pharmacological management, 393–395, 394(t), 395(t)
        smoking cessation, 393–396
        supplemental oxygen, 395
    early traumatic brain injury, 734
    multiple sclerosis, 596–603, 598–601(t)
        acute relapse, 596
        disease-modifying therapeutic agents, 597–601, 598–600(t)
        symptoms, 601–603
    Parkinson disease, 691–695

deep brain stimulation, 695
    nutritional management, 695
    pharmacological management, 691–694, 692–693(t)
    spinal cord injury, 773–774
        emergency care, 773
        fracture stabilization, 773
        immobilization, 774(f), 774–775
    stroke, 541–542
    traumatic brain injury, 734
See also Pharmacological management
Medical Outcomes Study (MOS), 289, 611, 1070
    Short Form 36, 286, 287, 289, 289(t)
Medical record review
    amputation, 858(b)
    heart disease, 450
    traumatic brain injury, 734
    wound healing, 474
Medical Research Council (MRC), 558, 731
Medicare
    Continuity Assessment Record and Evaluation (CARE), 136, 288, 608(t)
    functional classification levels, 875, 875(b)
    functional K levels, 1205(t), 1205–1206
    OASIS as a Condition of Participation, 288
Medications. *See* Pharmacological management
Medicopaste, 513
Medium, friction, 1193–1194, 1194(f)
MEDLINE, 25(t)
Medulloblastoma, 186, 186(f)
Mee lines, 34
Meissner corpuscles, 79(b), 80
Meissner's corpuscle, 941(t)
Memory
    classifying, 340
    defined, 535, 1074
    impairments, 1074–1075
        immediate recall and short-term memory, 1074–1075
        long-term memory, 1075
    loss, stroke and, 535
    preliminary tests, 77
Memory trace, 341
Mendelian trait, 390(f)
Ménière Disease, 843–844
Mental health, 10(f)
    age-related sensory changes, 73
    aphasia, 1108
    arthritis, 909(b), 931(t), 935
    behaviors warranting mental health consultation, 1044(t)
    body functions and body structures, 274(t)
    electrophysiological assessment, 173
    examination, 1014–1015, 1014–1015(b)
    heart disease, 465
    multiple sclerosis, 611
    as predictor of physical health, 1013
    quality of life, 1124
    spinal cord injury, 780
    suicide, 1034
    36-Item Short Form Health Survey, 289, 289(t)
    traumatic brain injury, 739(b), 752
    See also Psychosocial issues
Mental Health Services Administration (SAMHSA), 1048
Mental practice, 344, 345(t)
Mercury manometer, 59
Merkel disks, 79, 79(b), 941(t)
Mesh graft, 953, 953(f)
Metabolic complications
    active range of motion, 114
    amputation, 872, 872(b)
    burns, 946, 947–948
    orthoses, 1165
    Parkinson disease, 681
    stroke, 540

Metabolic Equivalent Chart, 424(t)
Metabolic equivalents (METs), 423, 424(t), 451(t), 459–460(t)
Metacarpophalangeal (MCP) joints
    capsular patterns, 116(t)
    rheumatoid arthritis, 895–896, 896(f)
Metacognitive functions, 1055
Metatarsal bar, 1153, 1153(f)
Metatarsal pad, 1153, 1153(f)
Methadone, 1039(b)
Methicillin-resistant *Staphylococcus aureus* (MRSA), 499–500, 506
Methylxanthines, 393
Metoclopramide, 681
Miami J collar, 774
Miami-J Select collar, 667(t)
Microglia, age-related changes in, 73
Micrographia, 684
Micro perspective, 1060, 1061
Microprocessor-controlled KAFO, 1161, 1165
Microsoft Kinect, 373–374
Microwave ovens, 316
Micturition, 770
Middle cerebral artery (MCA), 528, 529, 530(f)
Middle cerebral artery (MCA) syndrome, 528, 529, 530(t)
Middle East respiratory syndrome, 392
Midodrine, 768
Midstance, 218(f), 219, 219(t), 221(t), 222(t), 223(t), 226, 227, 267
Midswing, 218(f), 219, 219(t), 220, 221(t), 222(t), 224(t)
Midtarsal joint, 116(t)
Mid-wheel drive bases, 1276, 1276(f)
Milano-Torino (MiToS) staging system, 645, 645(t)
Mild cognitive impairment (MCI), 688
Mild TBI
    clinical trajectories, 751–752
    defined, 751
    diagnosis, 751
    evidence-based care, 755
    physical therapy examination, 752–754
        autonomic/exertional tolerance, 753
        cervical musculoskeletal, 753
        cognition, 752–753
        motor function, 754
        symptoms, 752–753
        vestibular-oculomotor, 753
    physical therapy management, 752–755
        physical therapy examination, 752–754
        physical therapy interventions, 754–755
        return to sport/activity, 752
    postconcussion symptoms, 751(t)
Milroy disease, 481
Milwaukee brace, 1168, 1169(f)
Mineralocorticoid receptor antagonists, 431(t)
Minerva orthosis, 774, 1168, 1168(f)
Mini-Balance Evaluation Systems Test (Mini-BESTest), 209, 700–701, 701(t), 781
Minimal assistance, defined, 278, 279(b)
Minimal clinically important difference (MCID)
    amputation, 883
    arm, hand, and finger coordination, 196, 197(t)
    gait analysis, 234–240(t)
    gait speed, 369, 369(t)
    outcome measures to create goals, 347, 348(t)
    Parkinson disease, 701–703(t)
    postural control and balance, 207
    responsiveness of functional status, 284
    spinal cord injury, 778(t), 782
Minimal data set (MDS), 9
Minimal detectible change (MDC)
    amputation, 883
    arm, hand, and finger coordination, 196, 197(t)
    outcome measures to create goals, 347, 348(t)
    Parkinson disease, 701–703(t)

Minimal detectable change (MDC) (*continued*)
respiratory function, 663
responsiveness of functional status, 284
spinal cord injury, 778(*t*), 781–782
Minimal Examination of Cognitive Function in MS (MACFIMS), 608
Minimally conscious state, 729
Minimally detectable change (MDC), 196, 197(*t*), 207
formulas to determine, from reliability coefficient, 285(*b*)
gait analysis, 234–240(*t*)
responsiveness of functional status, 284, 285(*t*)
Minimally invasive direct coronary artery bypass, 437
Mini-Mental State Examination (MMSE), 536, 608, 780, 1047(*t*)
Minimum data set (MDS), 457(*t*)
Minnesota Living With Heart Failure Questionnaire (MLHFQ), 457(*t*)
Minnesota Manual Dexterity Test, 198(*b*)
Miosis, 533(*t*), 534(*t*)
Mirror neuron system, 337, 355
Mirrors, in accessible bathroom, 314, 314(*f*)
Mirror therapy, 572, 576
Mitoxantrone (Novatrone), 599(*t*)
Mitral valve, 418
Mnemonics
FAST, in stroke, 984(*b*)
PQRST and SOCRATES, in chronic pain, 982, 984(*b*)
VITAMINS, in multiple sclerosis, 596
Mobile applications
activity tracking, 932, 933(*t*), 935
cognitive impairment, 630
gait analysis, 226
motor speech impairments, 1113
spinal cord injury, 807
Mobility
amyotrophic lateral sclerosis, 669, 670
arthritis, 922
defined, 1234
post-acute care measures, 457(*t*)
preprosthetic phase of amputation, 870–872, 871(*f*)
spinal cord injury, 793–809
bed mobility, 793–797, 794–795(*f*), 796(*f*), 797(*f*)
functional expectations, 784–787(*t*)
locomotor rehabilitation, 801–803(*f*), 801–809, 805–806(*f*), 807(*f*)
sitting balance, 797–798, 798(*f*)
transfers, 798–801, 799–801(*f*)
technology, 319(*b*)
wheelchair seating, 1234–1235
Mobility-related assistive technology, defined, 1225–1226
Mobitz type I and Mobitz type II heart blocks, 448
Modafinil (Provigil), 602
Modality, defined, 78
Modality of sensation, 78
Mode, feedback, 345, 346, 347(*t*)
Moderate assistance, defined, 278, 279(*b*)
Modifiable personal health behaviors, 1128–1131
assessing, 1128(*b*), 1128–1131
outcome measures, 1129–1130(*t*)
Modified AFO, 567
Modified Ashworth Scale (MAS), 148, 148(*t*), 348(*t*), 553, 609, 663, 670, 735, 736, 779
Modified barium swallow, 535
Modified British Medical Council (mMRC) Dyspnea Scale, 398, 399(*t*)
Modified CIMT (mCIMT), 571
Modified Clinical Test of Sensory Interaction in Balance (mCTSIB), 203–204, 204(*t*), 209
Modified Cumulative Illness Rating, 348(*t*)

Modified Dynamic Gait Index (mDGI), 238(*t*), 242–243
Modified Emory Functional Ambulation Profile (mEFAP), 233, 240
Modified Fatigue Impact Scale (MFIS), 143, 607(*t*), 609, 622
Modified Functional Reach Test (mFRT), 208
Modified GARS (GARS-M), 233, 242, 244
Modified Tardieu Scale, 148
Modified Walking and Remembering Test (WART), 741
Modular shank, 1185, 1186(*f*)
Moisture in wound healing, role of, 472–473
Moisture-retentive dressing, 473
Molecular imaging techniques, 163, 163(*f*), 164(*t*)
Molecular mimicry, 589
Monoamine oxidase-B (MAO-B) inhibitors, 692(*t*), 694
Monochromatic infrared energy (MIRE), 508
Monofilaments, 90, 95, 494, 494(*f*)
Monomethyl fumarate (Bafiertam), 599(*t*)
Montreal Cognitive Assessment (MoCA), 701(*t*), 705, 780, 1069(*t*)
Mood swings, 1044(*t*)
Moro reflex, 152(*t*)
Moss Attention Rating Scale (MARS), 740
Motion, musculoskeletal, 113–118
accessory joint motions, 116, 116(*t*), 117(*f*), 118(*f*)
active range of motion, 113–114
lower extremity, 114, 115(*f*)
passive range of motion, 114, 116
Motion Analysis, 256
Motion Sensitivity Quotient (MSQ), 822, 822(*f*)
Motivation, in stroke interventions, 560–561, 580
Motivational-affective dimension, 972
Motivational interviewing, 5, 108–109, 984, 1140–1141, 1141(*b*)
Motor ability, 127(*b*)
Motor Activity Log (MAL), 551, 552, 571
Motor aphasia, 532, 1105(*t*), 1105–1106, 1108
Motor balance strategies, 204(*f*), 204–206
change-in-support strategies, 205
fixed support strategies, 204(*b*), 204–205
movement strategies, 205–206, 206(*t*)
sitting strategies, 205
Motor circuit, of basal ganglia, 185
Motor-cognitive dual-task training, 716–719, 717–718(*t*)
Motor control, 118, 334–340
chronic pain, 989
defined, 126, 127(*b*), 334
examination, 136–139
documentation, 138, 139
functional activities and movements, 136
motor coordination, 138, 139
motor skills, 137–138, 138(*t*), 139(*b*)
movement observation and analysis, 136–137, 137(*b*)
interventions, 349–350(*t*)
learning networks, 337–338, 337–338(*f*)
multiple sclerosis, 591(*b*), 593
neuroplasticity, 338–339, 339(*t*)
stroke, 554–557, 555(*t*)
coordination, 556–557
cranial nerves, 557
Fugl-Meyer Assessment of Physical Performance, 554, 555
motor planning, 557
motor recovery stages, 554, 555(*t*)
muscle performance, 556
obligatory synergy patterns following stroke, 555(*t*)
selective capacity, 555–556
systems/processes underlying, 334, 335–337
cognition, decision-making and, 335
dynamic systems, 336–337

motor performance, execution and, 335–337
reflexive/automatic movements, 336
sensation/perception, 334, 335
voluntary/cortically controlled movement, 336
terms, 127(*b*)
treatment planning, 355(*f*), 355–356, 356(*b*)
vestibular disorders, 818–820
inhibitory cutoff, 819–820
push-pull mechanism, 819, 819(*f*)
tonic firing rate, 818
velocity storage system, 820
vestibulo-ocular reflex (VOR), 818(*f*), 818(*t*), 818–819, 819(*f*)
See also Sensory function
Motor Control Framework, 12(*f*)
Motor coordination, 138, 139
Motor cortex, 183–184
Motor endurance, 142–143
Motor-evoked potentials (MEPs), 558
Motor function, 333–367
amyotrophic lateral sclerosis, 661
case study, 365–367
constraints on, 339–340
individual, 339–340
Newell's model, 334, 334(*f*), 335(*t*)
task and environment, 340
examination, 125–180
altered consciousness and arousal, 134–135
body structure and function, 140–155
case study, 178–180
cognitive impairments, 135
communication impairments, 135
components, 132–133
constraints, 133–135
decision-making/problem-solving skills, 159(*b*), 159–160
evaluation and diagnosis, 174, 175–177(*t*)
executive functions, 135
functional imaging techniques, 162–163, 163(*f*)
imaging modalities, 164(*t*)
instrumentation and technology, 160–174
(*See also* Electrophysiologic neuromuscular assessment)
molecular imaging techniques, 163, 163(*f*)
motor control, 136–139
patient history, 132–133
perceptual impairments, 134
sensory impairments, 134
structural imaging techniques, 160–162, 161(*f*), 162(*f*)
systems review, 133
tests and measures, 133
foundational concepts/theoretical models, 334, 334(*f*), 335(*t*)
mild TBI, 754
motor control, 334–340
motor learning, 340–347
motor structure, 127(*f*), 127–129, 128(*f*), 129(*f*)
multiple sclerosis, 609
neural plasticity, 129–130, 132(*b*)
Parkinson disease, 685–686, 699–700
physical therapy interventions, 347–364, 349–350(*t*)
aerobic conditioning, 353–354
coordination, 354–355
electromyographic biofeedback, 352–353
environment and, 363–364
flexibility, 350–351
instruction, 364
measuring outcomes and writing objective goals, 348(*t*)
motor control, 349–350(*t*), 355–356
motor learning, 356–358

neuromuscular endurance and fatigue, 353
neuromuscular reeducation, 354
strength training, 351–352, 352(t)
task, 358(f), 358–363
technology, 364
recovery, 129, 132(b)
spinal cord injury, 776, 779, 783
strategies, 333–367
systems theory, 126
See also Motor control; Motor learning
Motor homunculus, 128(f), 173
Motor imagery (MI)
amputation
gait training, 876, 880
phantom limb pain, 873
chronic pain, 1003–1004
locomotor function, 377–378
Parkinson disease, 709
stroke, 566–567, 572
Motor impairments
amyotrophic lateral sclerosis, 644
basal ganglia pathology, 188–189, 190(t)
cerebellar pathology, 186–187, 190(t)
dorsal column-medial lemniscal pathology, 189
Parkinson disease, 716
spinal cord injury, 765, 797, 811
stroke, 536, 571, 573, 584, 1057
Motor interventions
locomotor, 370, 371
traumatic brain injury, 754–755
Motorized scooters, 323(f), 325(f)
Motor learning, 155–159, 340–347
defined, 126, 127(b), 158(b), 340
documentation, 158, 159
feedback, 345, 346, 347(t)
clinical decisions about, 345
intensity, 346
mode, 345, 346
scheduling, 346
treatment planning, 357–358
instruction, 341, 342, 356
knowledge of performance, 126, 159(b)
knowledge of results, 126, 156, 159(b)
locomotor function, 370–371
measures
adaptation, 158, 159(b)
performance measures, 156, 157(t), 159(b)
retention tests, 156, 158, 159(b)
transfer of learning, 158, 159(b)
transfer tests, 158, 159(b)
Parkinson disease, 708–709
amplitude-scaling strategies, 709
cuing strategies, 708–709
patient populations and special considerations, 346
practice considerations, 342–345
blocked *vs.* random practice, 343–344, 345(t)
challenge point theory, 342–343, 343(f)
clinical decisions, 342
constant *vs.* variable practice, 344, 345(t)
massed *vs.* distributed practice, 343, 345(t)
mental practice, 344, 345(t)
part task practice, 344, 345(t)
practice organization and strategies, 345(t)
simplification, 344, 345(t)
summarized, 345(t)
transfer of training/generalizability, 344–345, 345(t)
treatment planning, 356–357
stages, 155–156, 158(b), 341, 342(t)
associative, 155, 158(b)
autonomous, 155–156, 158(b)
cognitive, 155, 158(b)
terms, 158–159(b)
theories, 340–341
traumatic brain injury, 742

treatment planning, 356–358
types, 340
Motor level, 762
Motor memory, 126, 127(b), 340
Motor Neuron Disease Dyspnea Scale (MND-DS), 663
Motor neuron disease-parkinsonism, 681
Motor neuron diseases (MNDs), 636, 636(t).
See also Amyotrophic lateral sclerosis (ALS)
Motor performance
arousal, 135
coordination, 184, 185
age-related changes, 191–192
basal ganglia, 185
cerebellum, 184
execution, 335–337
homeostatic stability, 144
measures, 157(t)
multiple sclerosis, 615(t)
musculoskeletal examination, 122
orthotics, 1170
Parkinson disease, 690(b), 694, 695, 696, 709, 711
sensory function, 68, 83, 97
stroke, 552, 553, 563, 572
traumatic brain injury, 740, 742
vertical disorientation, 1090
Motor planning
apraxia of speech, 1114
chronic pain, 974(f)
cognitive rehabilitation, 1061
defined, 127(b)
functional status, 281
motor control, 337
orthoses, 1169, 1170
Parkinson disease, 686, 690(b), 704
sensory function, 68, 334
speech production, 1102
stroke, 15(t), 547(b), 557
wheelchair seating and mobility, 1229(t), 1239
Motor praxis, 127(b), 557. *See also* Motor planning
Motor priming, 353
Motor program
cognitive mapping, 155
coordination and balance, 183, 185
defined, 126, 127(b)
generalized, 126, 127(b), 336
motor skills, 139(b), 340
Parkinson disease, 686
sensory function, 68
sensory representations, 183
stroke, 557
Motor recovery
defined, 129, 132(b)
neuroplasticity, 129, 132(b), 364
normal function, 347
spinal cord injury, 773, 783, 793
stroke, 542, 543–545, 583–584
acute phase, 543–544
chronic phase, 544–545
prognosis and diagnosis, 557–558
rates, 584
simultaneous bilateral training, 572–573
stages, 554, 555(t)
subacute phase, 544
virtual reality, 567
traumatic brain injury, 744(t), 745(t)
Motor Relearning Programme for Stroke (Carr and Shepherd), 559
Motor skills, 137–138
categorizing, 137–138, 138(t), 139(b)
defined, 126, 127(b), 340
environment, 139(b)
Motor strip, 337
Motor structure, 127(f), 127–129, 128(f), 129(f)

Motor symptoms
multiple sclerosis, 591(b), 605(t)
Parkinson disease, 684–687
bradykinesia, 684
dual-task training, 716
gait, 686–687
motor function, 685–686
muscle performance, 685
postural instability, 684–685
rigidity, 684
tremor, 684
Motor system, 183–186
areas, 183–186
basal ganglia, 185, 185(f)
cerebellum, 184–185
descending motor pathways, 184
dorsal (posterior) column-medial lemniscal pathway, 186
motor cortex, 183–184
divisions, 183
parallel arrangement, 183
sensory input, 183
Motor unit, 127–128, 129(f)
Motor unit action potentials (MUAPs), 170(f), 170–171
Mourning, 1015–1016
Movement
accuracy, 192
analysis of tasks, 13
composition, 192
observation and analysis, 136–137, 137(b)
parameters, 336
science, 2, 4, 4(b), 8, 13
sensation, 68
strategies, 205–206, 206(t)
anticipatory postural control, 206
dual-task control, 206
seated control, 206, 206(t)
standing control, 205–206
system, 4, 4(b), 8, 9
time, 191
Movement Coordination Test, 205
Movement Disorder Society (MDS), 691
Movement Disorders Society Unified Parkinson Disease Rating Scale (MDS-UPDRS), 683, 700, 701(t)
Movement System Task Force, 137
Movement time, 157(t), 188, 191, 556–557, 699, 713
MSA Thermotest, 96, 97(f)
MS Clinical Trials, 610
MS Daily Activity Diary, 621
MS-EDGE, 610
MS Impact Scale (MSIS-29), 611
MS Quality of Life Inventory-54, 607(t), 611
Mucolytics, 393, 394(t)
Mucosal membrane pressure injury, 492(t)
Multiaxial foot-ankle assemblies, 1184–1185, 1185(f)
Multidimensional Fatigue Inventory (MFI), 705
Multidimensional function
assessment instruments, 286–287, 287(t)
measures, 286–287, 287(t)
Multidimensional Pain Inventory, 986
Multidirectional Reach Test (MDRT), 208, 208(t)
Multidisciplinary approach, 646, 646(f), 647(t)
Multidisciplinary pain clinic, 613
Multidisciplinary pain management team, 993, 995
Multi-infarct dementia, 535–536
Multi-infarct vascular disease, 681
Multiple sclerosis (MS), 588–634
active/not active, 590
age, 588
case study, 632–634
cerebellar impairments, 186
clinical subtypes, 590, 590(b)

Multiple sclerosis (MS) (*continued*)
coordination impairments, 182
diagnosis, 595–596, 597(*f*)
diplopia, 134
disease course, 590–591
disease-specific measures, 610–611
expanded Disability Status Scale for MS, 610–611
Functional Examination of MS, 611
MS Impact Scale, 611
MS Quality of Life Inventory, 611
Multiple Sclerosis Functional Composite, 611
Multiple Sclerosis Quality of Life-54, 611
dysautonomia, 144
education, 631
epidemiology, 589
etiology, 589
exacerbating factors, 590–591
fatigue, 143, 156
gait analysis
Dynamic Gait Index, 242
outcome measures, 237(*t*), 238(*t*)
walkway systems, 250
gender, 588
goals and outcomes, 607–608(*t*), 611, 612(*b*)
medical management, 596–603, 598–601(*t*)
acute relapse, 596
disease-modifying therapeutic agents, 597–601, 598–600(*t*)
symptoms, 601–603
onset, 588
outcome measures, 607–608(*t*), 611, 612(*b*)
pathophysiology, 589–590
patient/client history, 604, 606, 606(*b*)
physical therapy examination, 604, 606(*b*), 606–612
elements, 606(*b*)
goals and outcomes, 607–608(*t*), 611, 612(*b*)
patient/client history, 604, 606, 606(*b*)
systems review, 606, 606(*b*)
tests and measures, 606(*b*), 606–611
physical therapy interventions, 612–630
aerobic conditioning, 619–620
assistive devices, 626–628, 627(*f*), 628(*f*)
bladder control management, 620–621
cognitive training, 630
coordination and balance deficits, 623(*f*), 623–625, 624(*f*), 625(*f*)
exercise training, 614–620, 615–618(*t*)
fatigue management, 621–622
flexibility exercises, 620, 621(*f*)
functional training, 628–629
locomotor training, 625–628, 626(*f*), 627(*f*), 628(*f*)
orthotic devices, 626, 627(*f*)
pain management, 613
sensory deficits and skin care management, 612–613
sexual function management, 621
spasticity management, 622–623
speech and swallowing management, 629
strength and conditioning, 614, 619
psychosocial issues, 630–631
race/ethnicity, 588–589
rehabilitation framework, 603(*f*), 603–604
stages, 605(*t*)
symptoms, 591–592(*t*), 591–595
affective, 592(*b*), 595
bladder dysfunction, 592(*b*), 595, 602–603
bowel dysfunction, 592(*b*), 595, 602–603
cognitive impairment, 591–592(*b*), 594, 602
coordination and balance, 593–594
depression, 592(*b*), 594–595
emotional impairments, 595, 602
fatigue and fatigability, 593, 602
gait, 591(*b*), 594

gait and mobility, 591(*b*), 594
medical management, 601–603
motor, 591(*b*), 593
pain, 591, 592, 602
patterns, 592(*b*)
sensory, 591
sexual dysfunction, 595
spasticity, 593, 601–602
speech and swallowing, 594
visual, 591(*b*), 592–593
weakness, 593
systems review, 606, 606(*b*)
tests and measures, 606(*b*), 606–611
transmagnetic stimulation, 173
vestibular disorders, 845
with/without progression, 590
Multiple Sclerosis Coalition, 597
Multiple sclerosis EDGE (MSEDGE), 133
Multiple Sclerosis Functional Composite (MSFC), 610, 611
Multiple Sclerosis Quality of Life-54 (MSQOL-54), 611
Multiple Sclerosis Society, 322
Multiple Sclerosis Walking Scale, 370
Multiple Sclerosis Walking Scale-12 (MSWS-12), 610
Multiple system atrophy, 845–846
Multiple system atrophy syndromes, 681
Multi-Podus boot, 737(*f*)
Multisensory cuing, 708
Multispecialty team, 407–408
Muscarinic antagonists, 393
Muscle relaxants, 53, 1007
Muscle(s)
atrophy, 142
cardiac dysfunction, 438, 439(*b*)
contraction, 140–142
cramps, 649–650, 670
delayed onset muscle soreness, 143
endurance
defined, 118, 351
documenting, 143
health and wellness, 1143(*b*)
Parkinson disease, 699
seating and wheeled mobility, 1241
fatigue, 143
force production, augmenting, 374–375, 375(*f*)
function
amputation, 852, 858(*b*), 869–870, 870(*f*)
arthritis, 927–928
heart failure, 440
orthotics, 1170
respiratory, 406, 662–663
spinal cord injury, 762, 763(*b*), 765, 779
Valsalva maneuver, 57
inspiratory, 406, 406(*f*), 463(*t*)
length
amyotrophic lateral sclerosis, 661
assistive devices, 1006
cardiac cycle, 419
multiple sclerosis, 606(*b*)
muscle spindles to monitor changes, 80, 81(*f*)
Parkinson disease, 698(*b*)
seating and wheeled mobility, 1239
stroke, 547(*b*)
overwork weakness, 143
palpation, 147
performance, 118–120, 120(*f*), 140–143
amyotrophic lateral sclerosis, 661
chronic pain, 989
defined, 118
examination, 493
grading system, 118, 119, 119(*t*)
handheld dynamometry, 118, 119–120, 120(*f*)
isokinetic dynamometry, 118, 120

manual testing (*See* Manual muscle testing (MMT))
multiple sclerosis, 609
Parkinson disease, 685
resisted isometric testing, 118, 119(*t*)
stroke, 556
power, 118, 140, 351, 374, 1170, 1241
receptors, 79(*b*), 80, 81(*f*)
rheumatoid arthritis, 899–900
strength
amputation and, 863–864
defined, 118, 351
inspiratory, 453(*t*)
musculoskeletal impairments, 140–141
peripheral, 440, 453(*t*)
synergies
abnormal, 144–145
defined, 126, 127(*b*), 138
obligatory, 144, 554, 555(*t*)
stereotypic, 354, 355
tone
abnormal, 145–148, 146(*t*), 148(*t*)
amyotrophic lateral sclerosis, 663
decerebrate rigidity, 147
decorticate rigidity, 146–147
defined, 145
documentation, 148
dystonia, 147
examination, 147–148, 148(*t*)
factors influencing, 145
hypotonia, 147
initial observation, 147
Modified Ashworth Scale, 148, 148(*t*)
passive motion testing, 147–148
rigidity, 145, 146
spasticity, 145, 146(*t*)
stroke, 553
Tardieu/Modified Tardieu Scale, 148
Muscle spindles, 79(*b*), 80
Muscular Dystrophy Association (MDA), 646, 673–674
Musculoskeletal examination, 103–124
additional tests and measurements, 121–122
case study, 123–124
evaluation of findings, 122–123
functional movement analysis, 121
impairments, 140–143
documentation, 141–143
limitations in ROM and alignment, 140
motor endurance and fatigue, 142–143
motor weakness and muscle atrophy, 140–142
muscle endurance and fatigue, 143
muscle performance, 142
muscle strength, 141
mild TBI, 753, 754
motion, 113–118 (*See also* Range of motion (ROM))
motor control interventions, 349(*t*)
observation/inspection, 110(*f*), 110–111
palpation, 113
Parkinson disease, 698, 699, 699(*f*)
patient history, 104–110
imaging, 104
medical history, 104–105, 106–107(*f*), 108(*f*)
medications, 104
patient interview, 108–110
patient-reported outcome measures, 105, 107–108
systems review, 105
procedures, 104–122
purposes, 103–104
screening examination, 111(*f*), 111–113
tissue-specific tests, 120–121
See also Muscle(s)

Musculoskeletal Preferred Practice Patterns (APTA), 122
Mutilans deformity (opera-glass hand), 898
Mutism, 688
Myalgic encephalomyelitis/chronic fatigue syndrome (ME/CFS), 990, 1005
Myasthenia gravis (MG), 167
Myelin
  age-related changes, 73
  multiple sclerosis, 589, 590
Myelinopathy, 165
Myocardial infarction (MI)
  anatomical classifications, 435, 436
  angina, 432
  blood work to determine presence of, 436, 450
  complicated, 433
  electrocardiogram following, 433, 433(*f*), 434–436, 436(*f*)
  epidemiology, 415, 416
  injury, 433
  nontransmural, 435
  NSTEMI, 435
  STEMI, 435
  subendocardial, 435
  time frames for healing and convalescence, 451
  transmural, 433(*f*), 435
  See also Acute coronary syndrome (ACS)
Myocardial oxygen demand (MVO₂), 422, 428, 432
Myocardial oxygen supply, 422
Myocardium, 417
Myoelectric upper limb prostheses, 1199, 1200(*f*)
Myofibroblasts, 475, 476
Myopathic recruitment, 171
Myoplasty, 444
Myotome/dermatome tests, 11
Myotomes, 111, 121, 121(*t*)

N

Nagi disablement model48, 1127
Nalmefene (Revex), 1039(*b*)
Naltrexone (ReVia), 1007, 1039(*b*)
Narcissistic personality disorder, 1020
Nasal sounds, 1103
Natalizumab (Tysabri), 599(*t*)
National Aphasia Association (NAA), 1111
National Association for Visually Handicapped, 612
National Center on Health, Physical Activity and Disability, 1144
National civic groups, 326
National Easter Seal Society, 322
National Federation of the Blind, 612
National Health and Nutrition Examination Survey, 304, 1127
National Heart, Lung, and Blood Institute (NHLBI), 384, 389
National Institute for Health and Care Excellence (NICE), 25(*t*)
National Institute of Handicapped Research, 241
National Institute on Deafness and Other Communication Disorders, 1099
National Institutes of Health (NIH), 25(*t*)
  Stroke Scale (NIHSS), 348(*t*), 540, 558
National Lymphedema Network, 482
National Multiple Sclerosis Society (NMSS), 590, 631
National Parkinson Foundation, 691
National Pressure Injury Advisory Panel (NPIAP), 491, 517, 1233–1234
National Pressure Ulcer Advisory Panel (NPUAP), 482–483, 496
National Rehabilitation Information Center (NARIC), 25(*t*)
National Standards for Culturally and Linguistically Appropriate Services in Health Care (HHS OMH), 33

National Stroke Association, 525, 540, 542
National Wellness Institute, 1124
Natriuretic peptide assays, 442
Neck Disability Index (NDI), 107, 289, 753, 754(*t*)
Neck reflexes, tonic, 151
Neck weakness, 664
Necrosis, 471, 476
Needs Assessment Checklist (NAC), 773
Nefazodone (Serzone), 1036(*b*)
Negative affect, 977–978
Negative inspiratory pressure (PI_{max}), 398
Negative predictive value, 283
Negative pressure wound therapy (NPWT), 507(*f*), 507–508
Negative self-talk, 1001
Negative transfer, 158
Neologisms, 1104
Neomycin sulfate, 501
Neosporin, 501
Nerve conduction studies (NCS), 165–167
  compound motor action potential, 165(*f*), 165–166, 166(*f*), 167
  disadvantages, 166
  distal motor and sensory latencies, 165–167, 166(*f*)
  electromyography performed with, 168
  F-waves, 165, 167, 171(*f*)
  H-reflexes, 165, 167, 171(*f*)
  nerve conduction velocity, 165, 166(*f*)
  repetitive nerve stimulation, 167, 167(*f*), 171(*t*)
  sensory nerve action potential, 165, 165(*f*)
  supramaximal stimulus, 167, 171(*t*)
  temporal dispersion, 165
Nerve conduction velocity (NCV), 165, 166(*f*)
Nerve growth factors, 338
Nerve injury, classification of, 128, 131(*f*)
Neural connectome, 682
Neural plasticity. *See* Neuroplasticity
Neural processing, chronic pain and, 972–976
  autonomic system, 973
  central sensitization, 974(*f*), 974–975
  endocrine system, 975–976, 976(*f*)
  immune system, 973
  peripheral sensitization, 972
Neurectomy, 602
Neuritis, 592
Neurobehavioral Cognitive Status Examination, 1046(*t*), 1068(*t*)
Neurobehavioral impairments, 729, 731, 749
Neurobehavioral Rating Scale-Revised (NRS-R), 740
Neurobehavioral Symptom Inventory (NSI), 752, 753, 754(*t*)
Neurocardiogenic syncope, 144
NeuroCom Sensory Organization Test (SOT), 754, 754(*t*)
Neurodevelopmental treatment, 355
Neurofunctional approach, 1058, 1070
Neurogenesis, 353, 997(*t*)
Neurogenic atrophy, 142
Neurogenic disorders of communication, 1098–1118
  aphasia, 1104–1111, 1105(*f*), 1105(*t*)
  apraxia of speech, 1114
  case study, 1117–1118
  cognitive-communication disorders, 1111–1112
  dysarthria, 1112–1114
  dysphagia, 1114–1115
  implications for physical therapist, 1115–1116
  language organization, 1100–1101
  speech production, 1101–1102(*f*), 1101–1104, 1103(*f*), 1103(*t*)
Neurogenic inflammation, 973
Neurogenic pain, 970
Neurogenic shock, 768

Neurohormonal influences, 421–422
Neuroinflammation, 638
Neuroleptics, 53
Neurological complications/conditions
  gait analysis
    Dynamic Gait Index, 243
    energy cost analysis, 266
    footswitches and footswitch systems, 255
    observational gait analysis, 232–233
    outcome measures, 236(*t*)
    walkway systems, 251–252(*t*)
  rheumatoid arthritis, 900
  stroke, 532, 534–540
Neurological level of injury, 762
Neurological pins, 84, 85(*f*)
Neuromatrix model of pain, 971–972
Neuromodulation, 379
Neuromuscular disease (NMD), 143–155
  abnormal synergies, 144–145
  autonomic function, abnormal, 143–144
  autonomic nervous system stimulation, 144(*t*)
  cranial nerve function, abnormal, 151, 153–155(*t*)
  documentation
    abnormal movements, 145
    CN integrity, 151
    reflex abnormalities, 151
    tone abnormalities, 148
  exercise, 671
  muscle tone, abnormal, 145–148, 146(*t*), 148(*t*)
  physical therapy interventions
    endurance, 353
    motor control, 349(*t*)
    reeducation considerations, 354
  postural control, abnormal, 145
  reflex function, abnormal, 149(*t*), 149–151, 150(*t*), 152(*t*)
  respiratory muscle weakness, 668
  traumatic brain injury, 728–729
Neuromuscular electrical stimulation (NMES), 463(*t*), 571–572, 581, 629
Neuromuscular junction (NMJ), 128, 130(*f*), 167
Neuromuscular Recovery Scale (NRS), 782
Neuromuscular reeducation (NMR), 1003–1004
Neuromuscular status, 1243
Neuromuscular transmission, 127–129
Neuromyelitis optica (NMO), 596
Neuropathic Diagnostic Questionnaire (DN4), 984, 985(*t*)
Neuropathic pain, 970
  amputation, 873
  causalgia, 973
  central, 968(*b*), 970, 974, 975, 990
  chronification, 976–977
  desensitization, 1003
  measures to identify or quantify, 981
  multiple sclerosis, 591, 602, 609
  nociceptive, 967, 968(*b*), 969, 969(*t*), 982, 988, 993, 1007
  peripheral, 968(*b*), 969, 976, 977, 992
  peripheral sensitization, 972
  questionnaires, 984
  spinal cord injury, 772
  See also Pain
Neuropathic Pain Scale, 609, 984, 985(*t*)
Neuropathic recruitment, 171
Neuropathic walker, 518, 518(*f*)
Neuropathic wounds, 516
Neuropathy, 484–485
  burns, 948
  clinical presentation, 484(*f*), 485
  defined, 484
  diabetic, 484(*f*), 484–485
  history, 485
  intervention, 485
  tests and measures, 485

Neuroplasticity, 129–130, 338–339
  defined, 130, 132(b), 338, 370
  locomotor function, 371, 371(b)
  motor control, 338–339, 339(t)
  motor learning, 360–363, 361–363(t)
  principles, 339(t), 355, 356, 357, 358, 360, 363
  traumatic brain injury, 745
Neuroprosthetics, 354
Neuroprotection, 353, 773
Neuropsychologist, 733
Neurosurgical management for stroke, 542
Neurothesiometer, 609
Neurotoxins, 543(b)
Neurotrophic factors, 638
Neutral reference posture, 1231
Newell's model of constraints, 334, 334(f), 335(t)
New England Journal of Medicine, 427
New Freezing of Gait Questionnaire (NFOG-Q),
    702(t), 704
New learners, 341, 342, 342(t), 343, 347(t), 349(t),
    350(t), 356, 357
New York Heart Association (NYHA), 441, 443
Ng phoneme, 1100
Night bracing, 1169
Night-lights, 305
Nike+ FuelBand, 249
Nine Hole Peg Test (9HPT), 197(t), 607(t),
    702(t), 706
Nintendo Wii, 373, 713
Nitrates, 431(t), 438
Nitro-L-arginine methyl ester, 768
Nocebo, 974
Nociceptive pain, 772, 967, 968(b), 969, 969(t),
    982, 988, 993, 1007. See also Chronic pain
Nociceptors, 78, 79(b), 81
Nociplastic pain, 592, 969(t), 970
Nominal measures, 280
Nonallergic asthma, 389
Nonarticulated foot assemblies, 1182–1184,
    1182–1184(f)
Nonassociative learning, 340
Noncapsular patterns, 116
Noncompressible vessels, 489
Noncontact infrared thermometers (NCIT), 41,
    41(f)
Noncontact low-frequency ultrasound (MIST),
    502, 502(f), 503–505(t)
Noncontrast CT, 160, 164(t)
Non-familial ALS, 636
Nonfluent aphasia, 135, 532, 1104, 1105–1106
Nonforceful irrigation, 497, 497(f)
Nonfunctional cough, 779
Noninvasive brain stimulation (NIBS), 379
Noninvasive ventilation (NIV), 649
Nonmotor symptoms in Parkinson disease, 687–690
  anxiety, 689
  apathy, 689
  autonomic dysfunction, 689
  depression, 688
  dysphagia, 688
  sensory symptoms, 687–688
    auditory dysfunction, 688
    olfactory dysfunction, 687
    vestibular dysfunction, 687
    visual and visuospatial perception, 687
  sleep disorders, 689
  speech disorders, 688
  tests and measures, 704 705
Nonmotor Symptoms Questionnaire
    (NMSQuest), 701(t), 704
Nonmotor Symptoms Scale (NMSS), 702(t), 704
Nonorganic pain, 971
Nonpatient-identified problems (NPIPs), 5, 14,
    15(t), 16, 18, 20
Nonproportional controller, 1278–1279
Nonproportional drive controls, 1278–1279

Non-Q-wave myocardial infarction (NQMI), 428,
    434, 435
Nonselective débridement, 498
Nonselective phosphodiesterase inhibitors, 393
Nonsteroidal anti-inflammatory drugs (NSAIDs),
    1007, 1010(t)
Non-ST-segment elevation myocardial infarction
    (NSTEMI), 428, 434, 435
Nonsustained clonus, 150
Nonsustained hypertension, 57
Nonsustained V-tach, 447
Nonthermal diathermy, 506
Nontransmural myocardial infarction, 435
Nontraumatic spinal cord injury (SCI), 760
Non-Violent Crisis Intervention Training, 749
Noradrenaline, 682
Norepinephrine, 37, 39, 73, 421, 688, 693(t), 694
Normal behaviors taken to extremes, 1044(t)
Normal consciousness, 532
Normalcy index (NI), 266
Normal pressure hydrocephalus, 681
Normal pulse, 489
Normal sensation, 494
Normal sinus rhythm, 420
Norris Scale, 660
Norton Risk Assessment Scale, 493
Nortriptyline (Aventyl, Pamelor), 1036(b), 1039(b)
Nosings, 302, 302(f)
Nottingham Health Profile, 1128
Nottingham Sensory Assessment, 609
Novantrone, 601
Novel Electronics, 263
Novices, 341, 342(t)
N-terminal pro-BNP (NT-proBNP) assays, 442
Nuclear imaging in heart failure, 442–443
Nucleus basalis of Meynert, 682
Nuedexta (DMQ), 648
Numeric pain rating scale, 780–781
Numeric Rating Scale (NRS), 981
Nutrition
  amyotrophic lateral sclerosis, 648
  cardiovascular health, 526(t)
  chronic pain, 978
  heart disease, 462
  Parkinson disease, 695
  wound healing, 473–474
Nystagmus
  benign paroxysmal positional vertigo, 831, 832(t)
  defined, 188, 190(t)
  head-shaking induced nystagmus test, 824
  multiple sclerosis, 592
  observation, 822–823, 823(f)
  types, 832(t)

O

Obesity. See Bariatric patients
Object manipulation, 337, 350(t)
Obligatory reflexes, 151
Obligatory synergies, 144, 554, 555(t)
Observation
  arthritis, 914
  chronic pulmonary dysfunction, 397, 397(f)
  defined, 34
  integumentary integrity, 490
  musculoskeletal examination, 110(f), 110–111
  vital signs, 34–35, 35(b), 35(f)
Observational gait analysis (OGA), 220, 224–233,
    369, 550
  advantages, 224
  digital video recording, 225–226
  gait deviations and possible causes, 227–232
    ankle and foot deviations, 227–228(t)
    hip deviations, 230–231(t)
    knee deviations, 229(t)
    pelvic and trunk deviations, 231–232(t)

  guidelines for performing, 232
  mobile device software applications, 226
  neuromuscular disorders, 232–233
  podiatrists, 224
  process, 226–227
  Rancho Los Amigos, 220, 224, 225(f)
  training and practice needed for performing, 224
  traumatic brain injury, 740
Observational learning, in social cognitive theory,
    1135, 1135(t)
Obsessive-compulsive disorder, 689
Obsessive-compulsive personality disorder, 1020,
    1021
Obstructive sleep apnea (OSA), 539–540
Obtundation, 532
Obtunded, 75, 729
Occipital infarction, 531
Occult hypoxemia, 64
Occupational Information Network (O*NET),
    321
Occupational Questionnaire, 1047(t)
Occupational therapist (OT)
  responsibilities, 1056
  traumatic brain injury, 733
Occupational Therapy Driver Off Road
    Assessment Battery, 1062
Occupational Therapy Functional Assessment
    Compilation Tool (OTFACT), 1281(t)
O'Connor Tweezer Test, 198(b)
Ocrelizumab (Ocrevus), 599(t), 601
Ocular complications
  mild TBI, 753–755
  rheumatoid arthritis, 900
Oculomotor impairment, 1065
Oculomotor nerve (CN III), 98(t), 151, 153(t)
Ofamtumab (Kesimpta), 600(t)
Office of Minority Health (OMH), 33
Off-pump procedures, 437
Offset hinges, 307
Offset joint, 1160, 1160(f)
Ointments, antibacterial, 501
Olanzapine, 681
Older adults
  amputation, 865
  blood pressure, 57, 57(t)
  cell senescence, 432(t)
  community-dwelling, 26, 204, 211
  coordination impairments, 191–192
  gait analysis
    accelerometer data, 248, 249
    Dynamic Gait Index, 242
    Fast Evaluation of Mobility, Balance, and
        Fear, 243
    Figure-of-8 Walk Test, 243–244
    Modified GARS, 242
    outcome measures, 234(t), 235(t), 236(t),
        237(t), 238(t), 239(t)
    Performance Oriented Mobility Assessment,
        244, 244(f)
    plantar pressures patterns, 263
    walkway systems, 250, 252(t), 254(t), 255(t)
  heart rate, 44
  microglia, 73
  multiple sclerosis, 588
  myelin, 73
  respiration, 52–53
  sensory function, 72–73, 74–75(t)
  temperature, 39
  training-induced plasticity, 339(t)
  See also Falls and fall risk
Olfactory nerve (CN I), 98(t), 151, 153(t)
Oligodendrocytes, 589
Omnipotence, 1023(b)
O*NET Career Exploration Tools, 321
O*NET OnLine, 321
"On-off" phenomenon, 693–694

On-site visits
    examination strategies, 298, 300
    home, 300–317
        exterior accessibility, 301, 302(f), 302–304
        interior accessibility, 301, 304–309, 310–317
        preparation, 300–301
        smoke and carbon monoxide alarms, 309
    workplace, 321–322
        external accessibility, 321
        internal accessibility, 321–322, 322(f)
Onufrowicz nucleus (Onuf nucleus), 639
Onycholysis, 34
Opal sensor-based analysis system, 248
Open chain movements, 351, 352(t)
Open-ended questions, 9
Open environment, 158, 560, 562
Open loop system, 126, 336, 349(t), 350(t)
Open skills, 138, 139(b)
Open technique, 950
Operant conditioning, 340
Ophthalmoplegia, 643
Opioids, 1007
Opisthotonus, 147
Oppenheim sign, 150(t)
Optical marker-based motion analysis systems, 256–259, 257–260(f)
Optical markerless motion analysis system, 260
Optic ataxia, 201
Optic flow, 335
Optic nerve (CN II), 98(t), 151, 153(t)
Optic neuritis, 592
Optimal Screening for Prediction of Referral and Outcome Yellow Flag (OSPRO-YF), 109, 984
Optimal sitting posture, 1231, 1232–1233
Optimal Theory, 559
Optimizing Performance Through Intrinsic Motivation and Attention for Learning (OPTIMAL), 355, 355(f)
Oral airway oscillation devices, 408, 411, 411(f)
Oral apraxia, 1093–1094
Oral temperature, 42
Oral thermometers, 40, 41(f)
Orange flags, 979(t), 982(f)
Ordinal measures, 280
Orientation, preliminary tests of, 76, 76(b)
Orientation Log (O-Log), 731, 740
Orpington Prognostic Scale (OPS), 557
Orthopnea, 55, 441, 452(t)
Orthostatic hypotension (OH), 58, 689, 706, 768
Orthotics, 1149–1179
    arthritis, 925–926
    assessment, 493
    biomechanical influences, 1150, 1150(f)
    case studies, 1171–1172, 1177–1179
    cast shoes, 518
    clinical considerations, 1175–1176
    delivery care after, 1171–1172
        ankle-foot orthoses, 1171
        inspection, 1171
        knee-ankle-foot and other lower-limb orthoses, 1172
        shoes and socks, 1171
    donning, 1174
    energy considerations, 1175–1176
    examination and evaluation, 1172–1173
    extra-depth shoes, 493, 518–519, 519(f)
    instruction and training, 1173–1175
    lower-limb orthoses (See Lower-limb orthoses)
    multiple sclerosis, 626, 627(f)
    neuropathic walker, 518, 518(f)
    physical therapy management, 1169–1175
        care after orthotic delivery, 1171–1172
        care before orthotic prescription, 1169, 1170–1171

    orthotic examination and evaluation, 1172–1173
    orthotic instruction and training, 1173–1175
    prescription, 1169, 1170–1171
        cardiopulmonary capacity, 1171
        joint mobility and range of motion, 1169, 1170
        muscle function, 1170
        sensation, 1170–1171
    psychosocial considerations, 1176
    spinal orthoses, 774–775, 1165–1169
        cervical orthoses, 774, 774(f), 1167(f), 1167–1168, 1168(f)
        four-point pattern, 806
        gait/walking skills, 804–806, 805–806(f)
        push-ups, 806
        putting on and removing, 805
        scoliosis orthoses, 1168(f), 1168–1169, 1169(f)
        sit-to-stand activities, 805
        static standing balance, 805
        swing-through pattern, 806
        thoracolumbosacral orthosis, 774(f), 774–775
        trunk orthoses, 1165–1167, 1166(f), 1167(f)
        weight shifting in standing, 805–806
    splinting, 518
    terminology, 1150
    total contact casting, 518
    types, 1150
    upper-limb orthoses, 1169, 1170(t)
Orthotics and Prosthetics User Survey (OPUS) Satisfaction module, 1176
Orthotics Prosthetics User Survey (OPUS), 1205
Oscillopsia, 820
Osseointegration, 1190, 1196, 1196(f)
Osteoarthritis, 901–910
    activity limitations, 909
    case study, 937–938
    classification, 904–905, 905(b)
    clinical presentation, 905–909, 906–909(f), 909(b)
    consequences, 908–909, 909(b)
    diagnostic criteria, 904–905
    disease onset and course, 904
    epidemiology, 901–902
    etiology, 902, 902(f)
    gait analysis, 236(t), 239(t), 244
    joint impairments, 906–908
        feet and toes, 908, 908(f)
        hands and fingers, 905(b), 906–907, 907(f)
        hips, 905(b), 907–908
        knees, 905(b), 908
        spine, 908, 909(f)
    participation restrictions, 909
    pathophysiology, 902–904
        endotypes, 904
        joint, 903, 904(f)
        normal cartilage, 902–903
        phenotypes, 903–904
    pharmacological management, 912–914
    prognosis, 910
    radiography/diagnostic imaging, 905
    risk factors, 902(b)
    signs and symptoms, 905–908
    See also Arthritis
Osteokinematics, 113
Osteopenia, 104
Osteoporosis, 539, 685
Oswestry Disability Index, 107
Oswestry Low Back Pain Disability Questionnaire, 989
Oswestry Low Back Pain Questionnaire, 289
Otolith organs, 817, 817(f)
Otolith tests, 828
Ottawa Ankle Rules, 111

Ottawa Knee Rules, 111
Outcome and Assessment Information Set (OASIS), 286, 287, 288, 288(t), 457(t)
Outcome measures
    amputation, 803–805, 804–805(t)
    arthritis, 917–921(t), 917–922
    burns, 954
    cardiovascular disease, 457–456(t)
    chronic pain, 981, 982(f)
    chronic pulmonary dysfunction, 396, 396(b), 398, 399(t), 400(t)
    cognitive and perceptual dysfunction, 1066–1069(t)
    environmental examination and modification, 298, 299–300(t)
    gait capability, 234–240(t)
    health promotion and wellness, 1129–1130(t)
    heart disease, 456–457(t)
    locomotion function, 379
    motor function, 347, 348(t)
    motor performance, 157(f)
    multiple sclerosis, 607–608(t), 611, 612(b)
    musculoskeletal examination, 105, 107–108
    neurological disorders, 236(t)
    patient-reported
        function examination, 277
        musculoskeletal examination, 105, 107–108
        performance vs. capacity vs., in locomotor function, 379
    postural control and balance, 206–213
        balance and gait combination tests, 209–212, 210(f), 211(f)
        fall risk and floor-to-stand examination, 212–213, 213(f)
        fear of falling and balance confidence measures, 211–212
        primary balance performance-based tests, 207–209, 209(t)
    psychosocial issues, 1046–1048(t)
    spinal cord injury, 776, 777–778(t)
    stroke, 547, 548(t), 558, 558(t), 583–584
    traumatic brain injury
        during active rehabilitation, 739(b), 740–741, 741(f)
        activity, 740–741
        arousal, 735
        attention, 735, 740
        behavior, 740
        body structure/function, 740
        cognition, 735, 740
        early after injury, 735–736, 736(b)
        hypertonicity, 735, 736
        locomotion, 740–741, 741(f)
        participation, 740–741
        safety, 740
        spasticity, 735, 736
    wheelchair seating and mobility, 1280, 1281(t)
    See also Goals and outcomes
Outpatient Physical Therapy Improvement in Movement Assessment Log (OPTIMAL), 278
Outside-in model, 589
Ovens, 316
Overground locomotor training
    stroke, 563–564
    walking overground, 372–373(f), 375–377, 376(b), 376(f)
Overtraining, 353
Overuse damage, 671, 672(f)
Overuse weakness, 353
Overweight. See Bariatric patients
Overwork weakness (injury), 143
Oxazepam (Serax), 1030(b)
Oxidizing agents, 501

Oxygen
  cost, 266
  demand, myocardial, 422, 428, 432
  levels, determining, 488
  rate, 266
  therapy, 507
  topical, 507
  wound healing role, 472
Oxygen saturation (SaO₂), 63, 395, 397, 399, 405
Ozanimod (Zeposia), 600(t)

P

Paced Auditory Serial Attention Test, 1074
Pacemakers, 448–449, 449(t)
Pacing, 1001
Pacinian corpuscles, 79(b), 80, 941(t)
Paciniform endings, 79(b), 80
Pain
  acute, 970
  amyotrophic lateral sclerosis, 643, 649–650,
    661, 667–668
  arthritis relief, 924–927
    cold, 924
    complementary and alternative therapies,
      926–927
    electrotherapy modalities, 924
    energy conservation, 924
    heat, 924
    joint protection, 925
    Kinesio Taping, 926
    orthoses, 925–926
    rest, 924, 927
  central neuropathic, 969(t), 970
  circulation, 489–490
  clinical, 971
  coping skills, 999–1002, 1001(b)
  deep somatic, 969(t), 982
  defined, 967, 967(b)
  experimental, 971
  inflammatory, 967, 969
  key notes, 967, 967(b)
  medically unexplained, 971
  multiple sclerosis, 591, 592, 602, 609, 613
  neurogenic, 970
  neuropathic, 772, 970
  nociceptive, 772, 967, 968(b), 969, 969(t), 982,
    988, 993, 1007
  nociplastic, 592, 969(t), 970
  numeric pain rating scale, 780–781
  peripheral neuropathic, 969(t), 969–970
  physical assessment for WSM, 1240
  spinal cord injury, 772, 780–781
  visceral, 967, 969(t)
  visual analog scale for measuring, 281, 281(f)
  wounds, 493
  See also Chronic pain; Neuropathic pain
Pain behavior clusters, 980(t)
PainDETECT, 984, 985(t)
Pain Disability Index, 981
Pain neuroscience education (PNE), 998, 999
Pain Neuroscience Education: Teaching People About
  Pain, 971, 998
Pain perception test, 84, 85(f), 87
Pain persistence, 979, 980, 980(t)
Pain Quality Assessment Scale (PQAS), 985(t)
Pain readiness to change, 992
Palatal lift prosthesis, 649
Pallanesthesia, 89(t)
Palliative care, 647, 696
Pallor (pale), 35(b)
Palpation
  chronic pain examination, 988, 989
  chronic pulmonary dysfunction examination,
    397
  integumentary examination, 490

muscle, 147
  musculoskeletal examination, 113
  scale, 487
Palpation/Pitting Scale, 440, 453(t)
Palpitations, 43
Panic attack, 1029
Panic disorder, 689, 1013
Pan Pacific Pressure Injury Alliance (PPPIA), 496
Paper-based decision tree, 1213, 1214(f)
Papillary dermis, 940, 941, 941(t)
Papillomas, 482
Papules, 482
Paradoxical pulse, 44
Parallel bar ambulation, 240, 246(t)
Paralysis, 765
Paranoid personality disorder, 1020
Paraplegia, 760
  defined, 141
  orthotics
    energy considerations, 1176
    mechanical KAFOs, 1161–1162, 1162(f)
Parastep, 1165
Parasympathetic nervous system (PNS), 143,
  144(t)
Paratonia, 147
Paresis, 765
Paresthesias, 89(t), 591
Parietal pericardium, 417
Parking spaces, 321
Parkinson Anxiety Scale (PAS), 705
Parkinson Database to Guide Effectiveness
  (PDEDGE), 707
Parkinson disease (PD), 679–725
  adaptive and supportive devices, 720–721
  bed mobility, 711–712, 712(f)
  care paths and delivery, 696–697, 697(t)
  case study, 722–725
  classification, 680(b)
  coordination impairments, 182
  COVID-19-related postencephalitic
    parkinsonism, 680
  disease course, 683
    Hoehn and Yahr Classification of Disability
      Scale, 683, 683(t)
    Movement Disorders Society Unified Parkin-
      son Disease Rating Scale, 683
  dysautonomia, 144
  education, 721(b), 721–722
  etiology, 680(b), 680–681
    Parkinson disease, 680
    Parkinson-plus syndromes, 681
    secondary parkinsonism, 680–681
  falls and fall risk, 685, 704
  fatigue, 143, 685, 705
  gait analysis
    accelerometers, 248
    Dynamic Gait Index, 242
    Figure-of-8 Walk Test, 244
    Functional Gait Assessment, 243
    outcome measures, 234(t), 235(t), 236(t),
      237(t), 238(t), 239(t)
    Performance Oriented Mobility Assessment,
      244
    6-minute Walk Test, 247
    walkway systems, 250, 250(f)
  global health measures, 707
  goals and outcomes, 707, 707(b)
  incidence, 679–680
  medical diagnosis, 691
  medical management, 691–695
    deep brain stimulation, 695
    nutritional management, 695
    pharmacological management, 691–694,
      692–693(t)
  pathophysiology, 681(f), 681–682, 682(f)
  patient/client history, 697, 698

PET/SPECT, 163
physical therapy examination, 697–707
  global health measures, 707
  goals and outcomes, 707, 707(b)
  patient/client history, 697, 698
  systems review, 698
  tests and measures, 698, 699–707,
    701–703(t)
physical therapy examination and evaluation,
  697–707
physical therapy interventions, 708–720
  aerobic exercise, 719
  balance training, 712–715, 713(f), 714(f)
  community-based exercise prescription and
    home exercise programs, 719–720
  exercise training, 709(f), 709–711, 710(f),
    710(t)
  functional training, 711–712, 712(f)
  locomotor training, 715(f), 715–716
  motor-cognitive dual-task training, 716–719,
    717–718(t)
  motor learning strategies, 708–709
psychosocial issues, 721
rehabilitation, 695–697
rigidity, 145–146
sleep disorders, 687, 689
stages and models of brain pathology, 683,
  683(t), 696
symptoms, 684–690
  cardinal features and clinical manifestations,
    690(b)
  motor, 684–687
  nonmotor, 687–690
systems review, 698
tests and measures, 698, 699–707, 701–703(t)
transmagnetic stimulation, 173
Parkinson disease EDGE (PDEDGE), 133
Parkinson disease-mild cognitive impairment
  (PD-MCI), 688, 701(t)
Parkinson Disease Questionnaire-8 (PDQ-8),
  702(t)
Parkinson Disease Questionnaire-39 (PDQ-39),
  702(t), 705, 707
Parkinson Disease Society UK Brain Bank, 691
Parkinson Disease Summary Index, 707
Parkinson Fatigue Scale-16 (PFS-16), 701(t), 705
Parkinson-plus syndromes, 681, 691
Parkinson's Disease Quotient (PDQ-39), 348(t)
Paroxetine (Paxil), 602, 1031(b), 1036(b)
Paroxysmal atrial tachycardia, 445–446
Paroxysmal nocturnal dyspnea (PND), 441, 452(t)
Paroxysmal pain, 602
Paroxysmal sympathetic hyperactivity, 730
Partial ankle prostheses, 1181(f), 1181–1182,
  1182(f)
Partial foot amputation, 851(t), 852, 859
Partial foot prostheses, 1181(f), 1181–1182,
  1182(f)
Partially immersive systems, 373
Partial neuropraxia, 165
Partial pressure of oxygen (Pao₂), 52
Partial-thickness burns, 491, 492(t)
Partial toe amputation, 851(t)
Participation, 6, 6(f), 7(b)
  chronic pain, 990
  defined, 273
  restrictions, 6, 7(b), 273
    osteoarthritis, 909
    rheumatoid arthritis, 901
    spinal cord injury, 772–773, 781–782
    traumatic brain injury, 730
  stroke, 547, 548
    goals, 558(b)
    physical therapy interventions, 561
    Stroke Impact Scale, 547, 548
  traumatic brain injury, 740–741

Participation Assessment With Recombined Tools-Objective (PART-O), 742
Participation goal mapping, 12, 13
Part task practice, 344, 345(t)
Passive-aggressive personality, 1019
Passive exercise, 959, 960–961
Passive markers for tracking motion, 256–257, 257(f)
Passive motion testing, 147–148
Passive range of motion (PROM), 114, 116, 698, 699, 700, 709
Passive restraint, 141
Passive upper limb prostheses, 1198–1199, 1199(f)
Patellar-tendon-bearing socket, 1186
Pathological pain, 971
Pathological scars, burns and, 948
Pathophysiology
    acute coronary syndrome, 428
    amyotrophic lateral sclerosis, 638–640, 639(f), 640(f)
    arthritis
        osteoarthritis, 902–904, 904(f)
        rheumatoid arthritis, 890–891, 891(f)
    asthma, 389, 389(f)
    chronic pain, 971–977
        changes in neural processing, 972–976, 974(f), 976(f)
        chronification of neuropathic pain, 976–977
    heart disease, 415
    multiple sclerosis, 589–590
    Parkinson disease, 681(f), 681–682, 682(f)
    respiratory, 383(f), 383–384
        anatomy, 383(f)
        external and internal respiration, 384(f)
    restrictive lung diseases, 391
    stroke, 526–532
    traumatic brain injury, 727–728
        primary injury, 727–728
        secondary injury, 728
    vestibular disorders, 818–820
        inhibitory cutoff, 819–820
        push-pull mechanism, 819, 819(f)
        tonic firing rate, 818
        velocity storage system, 820
        vestibulo-ocular reflex (VOR), 818(f), 818(t), 818–819, 819(f)
    wounds, 471–478
Patient and family/caregiver education, 22
    amputation, 860, 874
    amyotrophic lateral sclerosis, 672, 673–674
    arthritis, 935
    chronic pain, 995, 997–999
        Explain Pain, 999, 1000(t)
        pain neuroscience education, 998, 999
    chronic pulmonary dysfunction, 408, 408(b)
    cognitive and perceptual dysfunction, 1070, 1071
    health education defined, 1125, 1126
    heart disease, 461–464
    integumentary system disorders, 495
    lymphatic system disorders, 495
    lymphedema, 482
    mild TBI, 754, 754(b)
    motor function, 364
    motor learning, 341, 342, 356
    multiple sclerosis, 631
    orthotic, 1173–1175
        donning orthoses, 1174
        facilitating acceptance, 1175
        gait training, 1174–1175
        standing balance, 1174
        wearing time, 1174
    Parkinson disease, 721(b), 721–722
    pressure management, 484
    sensory impairment, 97, 98–100, 99(f)

    stroke, 583
    substance use, 1038
    traumatic brain injury, 732, 738, 748–749
    vascular system disorders, 495
    vestibular disorders, 838
Patient autonomy, 355
Patient/client history, 8–9
    chronic pulmonary dysfunction examination, 397
    data generated from, 10(f)
    motor function examination, 132–133
    multiple sclerosis examination, 604, 606, 606(b)
    musculoskeletal examination, 104–110
        imaging, 104
        medical history, 104–105, 106–107(f), 108(f)
        medications, 104
        patient interview, 108–110
        patient-reported outcome measures, 105, 107–108
        systems review, 105
    Parkinson disease examination, 697, 698
Patient/client management, 8–30
    case study, 28–30
    documentation, 23–24
    evidence-based practice, 24–27
    examination, 12(f), 12–13
    history and interview, 8–9, 10(f), 11(b)
    sensory impairment, 99(f)
    steps, 4(f), 8
    systems review, 9, 11–12
    tests and measures, 13–23
Patient Health Questionnaire 9 (PHQ-9), 780
Patient Health Questionnaire for Depression and Anxiety (PHQ-4), 109
Patient-identified problems (PIP), 5, 15(t), 18
Patient interview, 8–9, 10(f), 11(b)
    examination strategies, 297–298
    heart disease, 450–451
    motivational interviewing, 5, 108–109, 1140–1141, 1141(b)
    musculoskeletal examination, 108–110
    representative interview questions, 9, 11(b)
Patient-Reported Outcomes Measurement Information System (PROMIS), 379, 1128
Patient-Specific Functional Scale (PSFS), 107, 289–290, 981, 982
Pattern recognition, 1063
Pawl lock with bail release, 1160, 1161(f)
PD dementia (PDD), 688
PD EDGE Task Force, 703(t)
Peak expiratory flow (PEF), 384
Pedal pulse, 46(f), 48(b)
Pedar system, 263–264, 264(f)
Pediatric Balance Scale, 249
PEDro (Physiotherapy Evidence Database), 25(t)
Pedunculopontine nucleus (PPN), 682, 695
Peginterferon beta-1a (Plegridy), 600(t)
Pelvic girdle pain, pregnancy and, 234(t), 235(t)
Pelvic position, 1230, 1231(t)
Pelvis
    gait deviations, 232(t)
    spasticity in UMN syndrome, 146(t)
Penn Spasm Frequency Scale, 779
Perceived Level of Dyspnea, 452(t)
Perceived Wellness Survey (PWS), 1128, 1129(t)
Perceptible information, in universal design, 295
Perception
    defined, 134, 1055
    motor control, 349(t)
    sensation differentiated from, 1055
Perceptual dysfunction, 1054–1097
    case study, 1095–1097
    clinical indicators, 1056–1057
    cognition and higher-order cognition, 1055

    discharge planning, 1072
    examination, 1061–1070
        differentiating sensory loss from cognitive/perceptual deficits, 1063–1065, 1064–1065(f)
        factors influencing, 1062–1063
        outcome measures, 1066–1069(t)
        purpose, 1061–1062
        standardized cognitive and perceptual tests, 1065–1070
    hospitalization following brain damage, 1057
    intervention, 1070–1072
        education, 1070, 1071
        impact of managed care, 1071–1072
        refocusing, 1071
        treatment approaches, 1070, 1071(t)
    motor control, 334, 335
    motor function, 134
    overview, 1072–1094
        agnosias (simple perception), 1090–1092, 1091–1092(f)
        apraxia, 1092–1094
        attention deficits, 1073–1074
        body scheme and body image impairments, 1073(t), 1077–1078(f), 1077–1086, 1079(f), 1080–1084(t)
        executive function impairments, 1075–1077
        memory impairments, 1074–1075
        spatial relations disorders (complex perception), 1086–1090, 1087(f), 1088(f), 1090(f)
    stroke, 538
Perceptual style, 1066
Perceptual tests, 1065–1070
Perceptual trace, 341
Percussion, 409
Percussion Test, 490
Percutaneous endoscopic gastrostomy (PEG), 648–649
Percutaneous transluminal coronary angioplasty (PTCA), 436
Perfectionistic personality, 1019
Performance, 6, 6(f), 7(b)
    vs. capacity vs. patient-reported outcomes, 379
    errors, 342
    function tests, 277
    measures
        amyotrophic lateral sclerosis, 647(t)
        function, 298
        motor learning, 156, 157(t), 159(b)
    plateaus, 156
    qualifiers, 6, 7, 7(b)
Performance-Oriented Mobility Assessment (POMA), 207, 210, 233, 239(t), 244
Perfusion, 386, 472
Pericardial friction rub, 417, 453(t)
Pericarditis, 417, 453(t)
Pericardium, 417
Perilymphatic fistula, 844
Perineurium, 128, 131(f)
Periodic fever, 38(b)
Peripheral arterial disease (PAD), 525
Peripheral chemoreceptors, 52
Peripheral cyanosis, 35(b)
Peripheral elements of motor system, 183
Peripheral field vision, 77
Peripheral nerve, 131(f)
Peripheral nerve integrity
    chronic pain, 988
    multiple sclerosis, 606(b)
    Parkinson disease, 698(b)
    stroke, 546–547(b)
Peripheral nervous system (PNS) stimulation, 143, 144(t)
Peripheral neuropathic pain, 969(t), 969–970
Peripheral neuropathy, 174(t)

Peripheral pulse, 43, 46, 46(f)
Peripheral sensitization, 972
Peripheral vascular disease (PVD), 415, 427, 478
Peripheral vascular resistance, 421
Peripheral vestibular pathology, 828–830
   decreased receptor input, 829, 830
   mechanical, 828–829, 829(f)
   symptoms associated with, 831(t)
Peripheral vestibular system, 816
Peripheral vision, 201
Periwound area, 474
Persantine thallium test, 443
Perseveration, 535
Persistent reflexes, 151
Personal factors, 6(f), 7, 7(b), 275, 294
Personality disorders, 1020–1021
Personality types, 1019–1020
Person/technology/environmental match, 1226,
   1235, 1247, 1248(b)
Perspiration, 34
Perturbed stance, 202
Petechiae, 35(b)
Phantom limb pain, 864, 872–873
Pharmacological management
   acute coronary syndrome, 438
   amyotrophic lateral sclerosis, 645–650
   anxiety, 1030–1031(b)
   arthritis
      osteoarthritis, 912–914
      rheumatoid arthritis, 910–912
   asthma, 393, 395(t)
   blood pressure, 58
   burns, 950–951, 951(t)
   chronic pain, 1007
   chronic pulmonary dysfunction, 393–395,
      394– 395(t)
      antibiotics, 395
      maintenance drugs, 393–395, 394(t), 395(t)
      rescue drugs, 394, 395
   coronary artery disease, 438
   depression, 1035–1036(b)
   heart disease, 462
   heart rate, 46
   hypertension, 428, 429–431(t)
   multiple sclerosis, 597–601, 598–600(t)
   musculoskeletal examination, 104
   Parkinson disease, 691–694, 692–693(t)
      atypical antipsychotics, 693(t), 694
      carbidopa/levodopa, 691, 692(t), 693–694
      catechol-O-methyl transferase, 692(t), 694
      cholinesterase inhibitors, 693(t), 694
      dopamine agonists, 692(t), 694
      implications for physical therapist, 694
      monoamine oxidase-B inhibitors, 692(t), 694
      norepinephrine precursors, 693(t), 694
   respiration, 53
   smoking cessation, 393
   stroke, 542, 543(b)
      deep vein thrombosis, 539
      exercise precautions, 582
      pulmonary embolus, 539
      seizure, 538
   substance use, 1039–1040(b)
   temperature, 39–40
Pharynx, 50, 51(f), 1102
Phase models of psychosocial adaptation,
   1016–1018
   acknowledgment, 1018
   adjustment, 1018
   anxiety, 1016–1017
   denial, 1017
   depression, 1017
   externalized hostility, 1017
   internalized anger, 1017
   shock, 1016
PhaseSpace, 256

Phenelzine (Nardil), 1036(h)
Phenotypes, 590
Phenytoin (Dilantin), 602, 649
Philadelphia collar, 774
Phoenix Society for Burn Survivors, 964
Phoenix Technologies, 256
Phonation, 50, 1102(f)
Phonemes, 1100
Phonology, 1100
Phosphodiesterase 4 inhibitors, 393, 394(t)
Phosphodiesterase type 5 inhibitors (PDE5i), 771
Photic (electromagnetic) receptors, 78, 79(b)
Physical activity (PA)
   arthritis, 932–934
      balance training, 932, 933
      functional training, 932
      gait training, 932, 933, 934(t)
      mobile and internet applications, 933(t)
   blood pressure with exercise, 452(t)
   chronic pain, 990
   community, 212
   defined, 1126
   demands, in plan of care, 137
   functional examination, 136
   health promotion and wellness, 1126
   heart disease, 452(t), 461
   ICF classification, 274(f)
   limitations (See Activity limitations)
   mild TBI, 752
   pacing, 412
   self-efficacy, 1129(t)
   stroke, 581–583
      cardiovascular health, 526(t)
      examination, 548–552, 549(t), 551(t)
      exercise precautions, 582–583
      gait and locomotion, 563–567
      goals, 558(b)
      ipsilateral pushing, 563
      postural control and balance, 561–563
      training with visual feedback, 562–563
      upper extremity use, 568–581
   task, required for success, 349–350(t)
   traumatic brain injury, 740–741
   See also Activity limitations
Physical Activity for People with a Disability
   model, 1138–1139, 1139(t)
Physical Activity Scale for the Elderly, 348(t)
Physical assessment, for WSM, 1239–1243
   components, 1240–1243
      balance, 1241
      neuromuscular status, 1243
      pain, 1240
      postural alignment, 1240–1241, 1241(f)
      range of motion and flexibility, 1242(f),
         1242–1243
      sensation, 1240
      skin integrity, 1240
      strength and endurance, 1241, 1242
   mat assessment, 1239–1240
      sitting mat assessment, 1239–1240, 1240(f)
      supine mat assessment, 1239, 1240(f)
Physical environment, 294, 298. See also Environmental accessibility
Physical examination, prosthetics and,
   1203–1204
Physical function, pain and, 981, 982
Physical Performance and Mobility Examination,
   277
Physical therapist, responsibilities of, 1056
   amyotrophic lateral sclerosis, 663
   health promotion and wellness, 1122–1123,
      1145–1146
   neurogenic disorders of speech and language,
      1115–1116
   pharmacological management of Parkinson
      disease, 694

Physical Therapists' Role in Prevention, Wellness,
   Fitness, Health Promotion, and Management
   of Disease and Disability (APTA), 1146
Physical therapy diagnosis, 15–16, 174, 175–177(t)
Physical therapy examination
   amyotrophic lateral sclerosis, 658–663
      aerobic capacity, 659
      balance, 661–662
      bulbar function, 659
      cognition, 660
      control, 661–662
      cranial nerve integrity, 659–660
      elements, 659(b)
      environmental barriers, 660
      fatigue, 660
      functional status, 660
      gait, 660–661
      integument, 661
      joint integrity, 661
      motor function, 661
      muscle length, 661
      muscle performance, 661
      pain, 661
      postural alignment, 661–662
      psychosocial function, 662
      quality-of-life measures, 662
      range of motion, 661
      reflexes, 663
      respiratory function, 662–663
      sensation, 663
      tone, 663
   arthritis, 914–923
      balance, 922
      cardiovascular status, 916–917
      environmental factors, 923
      gait, 922
      history, 914
      joint stability, 916
      joint tenderness, 914, 915
      mobility, 922
      observation, 914
      outcome measures, 917–921(t), 917–922
      psychosocial status, 922–923
      range of motion, 915–916
      red flag signs and symptoms, 914, 915(t)
      sensory integrity, 915
      socioeconomic factors, 923
      strength, 916
      yellow flag signs and symptoms, 914, 915(t)
   mild TBI, 752–754
      autonomic/exertional tolerance, 753
      cervical musculoskeletal, 753
      cognition, 752–753
      motor function, 754
      symptoms, 752–753
      vestibular-oculomotor, 753
   multiple sclerosis, 604, 606–612
      elements, 606(b)
      goals and outcomes, 607–608(t), 611, 612(b)
      patient/client history, 604, 606, 606(b)
      systems review, 606, 606(b)
      tests and measures, 606(b), 606–611
   Parkinson disease, 697–707
      global health measures, 707
      goals and outcomes, 707, 707(b)
      patient/client history, 697, 698
      systems review, 698
      tests and measures, 698, 699–707,
         701–703(t)
   spinal cord injury, 776–783
      activity/participation, 781–782
      body structure/function, 776, 779–781,
         780(t)
      contextual factors, 783
      history, 776
      outcome measures, 776, 777–778(t)

Physical Therapy Healthy Lifestyle Appraisal, 986
Physical therapy interventions
  acute coronary syndrome, 437–438
  amyotrophic lateral sclerosis, 663–671
    activities of daily living, 669, 669(t)
    cervical muscle weakness, 664, 666(f), 667(t)
    decreased mobility, 669, 670
    disease stages and general intervention
      strategies, 665(t)
    dysarthria, 664
    dysphagia, 664
    lower extremity muscle weakness and gait
      impairments, 669
    muscle cramps, 670
    pain, 667–668
    psychosocial issues, 670–671
    respiratory muscle weakness, 668
    role of physical therapist, 663
    spasticity, 670
    upper extremity muscle weakness, 668
  arthritis, 923–932
    cardiovascular training, 930, 932
    evidence summary of therapeutic exercise,
      929(t), 930–931(t)
    flexibility exercise, 927
    goals and outcomes, 923(b), 923–924
    pain relief, 924–927
    range of motion exercise, 927
    strengthening exercise, 927–928, 930
  burns, 953–964
    active and passive exercise, 959, 960–961
    ambulation, 961
    assessment of burn scars, 954, 955–957(t)
    camouflage makeup, 963
    community programs, 963–964
    examination, 954
    follow-up care, 963
    goals and outcomes, 954
    massage, 962–963
    physical therapy interventions, 954, 958(t),
      958–964, 959(f), 960(f), 962(f)
    positioning, 958, 958(t), 959(f)
    pressure dressings, 962, 962(f)
    resistive and conditioning exercise, 961
    scar management, 961–962
    silicone gel, 962
    splinting, 958, 958(t), 959, 959(f), 960(f)
  chronic pain, 993–1007
    assistive devices, 1006
    biophysical and other modalities, 1006–1007
    chronic pain interventions by mechanism,
      996–997(t)
    cognitive behavioral therapy, 999, 1000,
      1001(b)
    cognitive functional therapy, 1000
    CPGs for chronic pain, 993, 994–995(t), 1007
    evaluation, 990–992, 991(f)
    exercise, 1004–1005, 1006(t)
    instruction, 995, 997–999
    manual therapy, 1005, 1006
    multidisciplinary pain management team,
      993, 995
    neuromuscular reeducation, 1003–1004
    pain coping skills, 999–1002, 1001(b)
    physical self-care strategies, 1002–1003
    therapeutic alliance, 995
  chronic pulmonary dysfunction, 396–412
  cognitive and perceptual dysfunction,
    1070–1072
    adaptive/compensatory approach, 1070,
      1071(t)
    education, 1070, 1071
    impact of managed care, 1071–1072
    refocusing, 1071
    remedial approach, 1070
    treatment approaches, 1070, 1071(t)

  heart disease, 454–461
    cardiac rehabilitation, 454–455, 457,
      459–461(t)
    heart failure, 457, 461, 463(t)
    therapeutic exercise, 454
  hypertension, 427–428
  impairments and disabilities, 1143–1145
    healthy weight and healthy eating counseling,
      1144, 1145(b)
    physical activity/exercise, 1143–1144
    sleep counseling, 1144, 1145
    smoking cessation counseling, 1144, 1145(b)
  locomotor function, 370–379
    behavioral change support, 378–379
    circuit training, 377, 377(b), 378(f)
    exoskeleton, 379
    intensity, 370
    motor imagery, 377–378
    motor learning, 370–371
    muscle force production, augmenting,
      374–375, 375(f)
    neuromodulation, 379
    neuroplasticity, 371, 371(b)
    overground walking for balance and postural
      control, 375–377, 376(b), 376(f)
    task-specific walking training/treadmill
      training, 371–373, 372–373(f)
    virtual reality and exergaming, 373–374,
      374(f)
  mild TBI, 752–755
    aerobic exercise, 755
    cervical musculoskeletal, 754
    instruction, 754, 754(b)
    motor, 755
    physical therapy examination, 752–754
    return to sport or activity, 752
    vestibular-oculomotor, 754–755
  motor function, 347–364, 349–350(t)
    aerobic conditioning, 353–354
    coordination, 354–355
    electromyographic biofeedback, 352–353
    environment and, 363–364
    flexibility, 350–351
    instruction, 364
    measuring outcomes and writing objective
      goals, 348(t)
    motor control, 349–350(t), 355–356
    motor learning, 356–358
    neuromuscular endurance and fatigue, 353
    neuromuscular reeducation, 354
    strength training, 351–352, 352(t)
    task, 358(f), 358–363
    technology, 364
  multiple sclerosis, 612–630
    aerobic conditioning, 619–620
    assistive devices, 626–628, 627(f), 628(f)
    assistive devices, 626–628, 627(f), 628(f)
    bladder control, 620–621
    bladder control management, 620–621
    cognitive training, 630
    coordination and balance deficits, 623(f),
      623–625, 624(f), 625(f)
    exercise training, 614–620, 615–618(t)
    fatigue, 621–622
    fatigue management, 621–622
    flexibility exercises, 620, 621(f)
    functional training, 628–629
    locomotor training, 625–628, 626(f), 627(f),
      628(f)
    orthotic devices, 626, 627(f)
    pain management, 613
    sensory deficits and skin care, 612–613
    sensory deficits and skin care management,
      612–613
    sexual function, 621
    sexual function management, 621

    spasticity, 622–623
    spasticity management, 622–623
    speech and swallowing, 629
    speech and swallowing management, 629
    strength and conditioning, 614, 619
  orthotics, 1169–1175
    care after orthotic delivery, 1171–1172
    care before orthotic prescription, 1169,
      1170–1171
    orthotic examination and evaluation,
      1172–1173
    orthotic instruction and training, 1173–1175
  Parkinson disease, 708–720
    aerobic exercise, 719
    balance training, 712–715, 713(f), 714(f)
    community-based exercise prescription and
      home exercise programs, 719–720
    evaluation, 697–707
    exercise training, 709(f), 709–711, 710(f),
      710(t)
    functional training, 711–712, 712(f)
    locomotor training, 715(f), 715–716
    motor-cognitive dual-task training, 716–719,
      717–718(t)
    motor learning strategies, 708–709
  prosthetics, 1203–1220
    cognition and psychosocial conditions,
      1204–1205
    community integration: work, sports, and
      other activities, 1219–1220
    physical examination, 1203–1204
    prescription considerations, 1203
    prosthetic examination, 1208–1212, 1210(t),
      1211(f), 1212
    prosthetic prescription, 1205(t), 1205–1208,
      1206–1208(t)
    prosthetic training, 1212–1219, 1214(f),
      1215(f), 1216(f), 1217–1218(f), 1219(f)
    temporary prostheses, 1205
  spinal cord injury, 766, 767, 787–809
    activity-directed upper extremity training,
      809
    cardiovascular/endurance training, 792(f),
      792–793
    head-hips relationship, 788, 788(f)
    mobility skills, 793–809, 794–803(f),
      805–806(f), 807(f)
    momentum, 788
    muscle substitution, 788
    precautions, 788(b)
    respiratory, 789(f), 789–791, 790(f)
    skin care, 791(f), 791–792, 792(f)
    strengthening, 789
    task modification, 788
    working in and out of the task, 788
  stroke, 558, 559–583
    activities, 561–581
    aerobic capacity, 581–583
    body function and structure, 581
    dose and, 560
    environment, structuring, 559–560
    feedback, 560
    motivation, 560–561
    participation, 561
    physical activity, 581–583
    practice schedule, 560
    progression, 560
    self-efficacy, 560–561
    structure, 559–561
    task, goal, learner, 559
  traumatic brain injury, 739–751
    during active rehabilitation, 739–751, 744(t),
      745(t), 748(f)
    aerobic conditioning, 747
    balance, 747
    behavioral factors, 749, 750(t)

Physical therapy interventions (*continued*)
  community reentry/reintegration, 742, 749, 751(*t*)
  dual-task interventions, 747–748, 748(*f*)
  early after injury, 734–738, 737(*f*)
  early mobilization, 736, 737
  education, 738, 748–749
  examination during active rehabilitation, 739(*b*), 739–742, 741(*f*)
  examination early after injury, 734–736, 736(*b*)
  global functioning, 741–742
  goals and outcomes, 736, 737(*b*), 742, 743(*t*)
  hypertonicity, 738
  locomotor training/walking recovery, 745, 746
  motor (re)learning strategies, 742
  outcome measures, 735–736, 736(*b*), 739(*b*), 740–741, 741(*f*)
  quality of life, 742
  resistance training, 747
  restorative interventions and neural plasticity, 745
  restorative *versus* compensatory-based interventions, 742, 744, 744(*t*), 745(*t*)
  secondary impairments, 737–738, 737–738(*f*)
  sensory stimulation, 738
  spasticity, 738
  task-oriented approach, 745
  upper extremity function, 746(*f*), 746–747
  vestibular disorders, 831–843
    abnormal central vestibular function, 838
    benign paroxysmal positional vertigo, 831, 832(*f*), 832(*t*), 832–833, 833(*f*), 834(*f*), 834(*t*)
    bilateral vestibular hypofunction, 837, 838, 838(*t*), 839–843(*t*)
    education, 838
    mild TBI, 754–755
    unilateral vestibular hypofunction, 833, 834–837, 835(*f*), 836(*f*), 836(*t*), 837(*f*)
  wheelchair seating and mobility, 1249–1250
    function from wheelchair, 1249
    maintenance/repairs/follow-up, 1250
    wheelchair delivery, 1249
    wheelchair fitting, 1249
    wheelchair mobility, 1249
    wheelchair skills training, 1249–1250, 1250(*f*)
Physical Therapy Journal, 457
Physical therapy management
  burns, 953–964
    assessment of burn scars, 954, 955–957(*t*)
    examination, 954
    goals and outcomes, 954
    intervention, 954, 958(*t*), 958–964, 959(*f*), 960(*f*), 962(*f*)
  chronic pain, 993–1007
    assistive devices, 1006
    biophysical and other modalities, 1006–1007
    chronic pain interventions by mechanism, 996–997(*t*)
    cognitive behavioral therapy, 999, 1000, 1001(*b*)
    cognitive functional therapy, 1000
    CPGs for chronic pain, 993, 994–995(*t*), 1007
    exercise, 1004–1005, 1006(*t*)
    instruction, 995, 997–999
    manual therapy, 1005, 1006
    multidisciplinary pain management team, 993, 995
    neuromuscular reeducation, 1003–1004
    pain coping skills, 999–1002, 1001(*b*)
    physical self-care strategies, 1002–1003
    therapeutic alliance, 995

chronic pulmonary dysfunction, 396–412
  education, 408, 408(*b*)
  examination, 397–400
  exercise prescription, 400, 401–402
  goals and outcomes, 396, 396(*b*)
  home exercise programs, 407, 407(*f*)
  multispecialty team, 407–408
  pulmonary rehabilitation, 402, 405–406
  secretion removal techniques, 408–412
orthotics, 1169–1175
  care after orthotic delivery, 1171–1172
  care before orthotic prescription, 1169, 1170–1171
  orthotic examination and evaluation, 1172–1173
  orthotic instruction and training, 1173–1175
prosthetics, 1203–1220
  cognition and psychosocial conditions, 1204–1205
  community integration: work, sports, and other activities, 1219–1220
  physical examination, 1203–1204
  prescription considerations, 1203
  prosthetic examination, 1208–1212, 1210(*t*), 1211(*f*), 1212
  prosthetic prescription, 1205(*t*), 1205–1208, 1206–1208(*t*)
  prosthetic training, 1212–1219, 1214(*f*), 1215(*f*), 1216(*f*), 1217–1218(*f*), 1219(*f*)
  temporary prostheses, 1205
traumatic brain injury, 734–755
  during active rehabilitation, 739–751
  aerobic exercise, 755
  behavioral factors, 749, 750(*t*)
  cervical musculoskeletal, 754
  community reentry, 749, 751(*t*)
  community reentry/reintegration, 742, 749, 751(*t*)
  early after injury, 734–738, 737(*f*)
  early mobilization, 736, 737
  education, 738, 754, 754(*b*)
  examination during active rehabilitation, 739(*b*), 739–742, 741(*f*)
  examination early after injury, 734–736, 736(*b*)
  global functioning, 741–742
  goals and outcomes, 736, 737(*b*), 742, 743(*t*)
  hypertonicity, 738
  mild TBI, 752–755
  motor, 755
  outcome measures, 735–736, 736(*b*), 739(*b*), 740–741, 741(*f*)
  quality of life, 742
  secondary impairments, 737–738, 737–738(*f*)
  sensory stimulation, 738
  spasticity, 738
  vestibular-oculomotor, 754–755
Physician, traumatic brain injury and, 732
Physiological Cost Index (PCI), 267
Physiological energy cost measures, 266–267
Physiological manifestations, substance use and, 1037(*t*)
Physiological walker, 551
Physiology. *See* Pathophysiology
Physiotherapy Evidence Database (PEDro), 14
PICO, 24
Piezoelectric technology, 261
Piloerection, 37
Pisa syndrome, 685
Pistoning, 1209
Pitting, 34
Pitting edema, 113, 440, 453(*t*)
Pitting scale, 487
Placebo, 974
Plan for risk reduction, 321

Planning, 1075–1076
Plan of care (POC), 17–23
  cranial nerve function, 97
  discharge planning, 22, 22(*b*)
  elements, 22(*b*)
  goals and outcomes, 18, 19(*b*)
  Guide to Physical Therapist Practice for organizing, 19, 20(*f*)
  implementation, 23
  interventions, 19–22
  motor function examination
    activity demands and, 137
    decision-making and, 159–160
    discharge placement/resources and, 174
    executive functions and, 135
    goals and outcomes, 133
    neural plasticity, 130, 131
  reexamination of patient and evaluation of expected outcomes, 23
  specialty evaluation for WSM, 1247
  stroke, 542, 543–545
Plantarflexion, 146(*t*), 147, 150, 150(*t*)
Plantarflexors, 141, 227, 261
Plantarflexor weakness, 218, 233
Plantar pressure measurement systems, 263(*f*), 263–264, 264(*f*)
Plan to optimize function, 321
Plaques, 589
Plastic footplate, 1154, 1156, 1156(*f*), 1157(*f*)
Plegia, defined, 141
Plosive sounds, 1102, 1103
Plyometrics, 351, 352(*t*)
Pneumatic friction, 1192
Pocket doors, 307
Podiatrists, 224
Poikilothermia, 768
Poikilothermic, 35
Pointing and past pointing test, 194(*b*), 194(*t*)
Point of maximal impulse (PMI), 49, 417, 452(*t*)
Pole-striding groups, 720
Polycentric linkage, 1191
Polycentric systems, 1191, 1192(*f*)
Polycythemia, 386–387
Polyneuropathy, 162, 166, 167, 170, 171(*t*), 176(*t*)
Polyphasic potentials, 170, 170(*f*), 171
Polysporin, 951
Ponesimod (Ponvory), 600(*t*)
Pool therapy, 613
Popliteal blood pressure, measuring, 62–63
Popliteal pulse, 43, 46(*f*), 47(*b*)
Population health management model, 1124, 1125, 1125(*t*), 1126(*t*)
Positional testing, 826, 826(*f*), 827(*f*)
Position holding test, 194(*t*)
Positioning
  burns, 958, 958(*t*), 959(*f*)
  postsurgical phase of amputation, 858–859, 859(*f*)
  pressure injuries, 484
  stroke, 574, 574(*b*)
  wound healing, 517
Positioning tilt systems, 1265
Position in space, 134, 538, 1089
Positive expiratory pressure (PEP), 411, 411(*f*)
Positive expiratory pressure (PEP) devices, 408
Positive inotropes, 443
Positive predictive value, 283
Positive sharp waves (PSWs), 168, 169(*f*)
Positive supporting reflex, 152(*t*)
Positive transfer, 158
Positron emission tomography (PET), 163, 163(*f*), 164(*t*)
Post, 1154
Postcentral gyrus, 82
Postconcussion Scale (revised) (PCS), 753, 754(*t*)
Postconcussion Symptom Inventory (PCSI), 753
Postconcussion symptoms, 751(*t*)

Post-COVID conditions, 392
Postencephalitic parkinsonism, 680
Posterior cerebral artery (PCA), 529, 529(f), 531
Posterior cerebral artery (PCA) syndrome, 529, 531, 531(t)
Posterior column, 82(f)
Posterior descending artery (PDA), 418, 418(f)
Posterior leaf spring (PLS), 567
Posterior leaf spring AFO, 1157, 1157(f)
Posterior leaf spring ankle-foot orthosis, 1156, 1156(f)
Posterior stop, 1157, 1158(f)
Posterior supports, for WSM, 1258
Posterior tibial pulse, 46(f), 48(b)
Posterior view, in postural alignment, 111
Post orthosis, 1168
Post-polio syndrome, 143
Post-stroke aphasia, 1108–1109
Postsurgical phase of amputation, 857–861, 858(b), 859(f)
    ambulation and gait training, 860
    balance training, 860
    care of remaining lower extremity, 860
    discharge planning, 860–861
    functional training, 859–860
    instruction, 860
    positioning, 858–859, 859(f)
    residual limb care, 860
Posttraumatic amnesia (PTA), 729, 730, 731(t), 740, 751
Post-traumatic rehabilitation, 1018–1019
Posttraumatic seizures, 730
Post-traumatic stress disorder (PTSD), 1029, 1031–1032, 1031(b)
Postural alignment
    amyotrophic lateral sclerosis, 661–662
    examination, 200(f), 200–201
    normal, 199(f), 199–201
    observation/inspection, 110f, 110–111
    physical assessment for WSM, 1240–1241, 1241(f)
Postural Assessment Scale for Stroke Patients (PASS), 145, 550
Postural control and balance, 199–213
    abnormal, 145
    amyotrophic lateral sclerosis, 661–662
    balance strategies, 201–206
        motor, 204(f), 204–206, 206(t)
        sensory, 201–204, 203(f), 203(t), 204(f)
    examination, 493
    multiple sclerosis, 610, 623, 623(f)
    outcome measures, 206–213
        balance and gait combination tests, 209–211, 210(f), 211(f)
        fear of falling and balance confidence measures, 211–212
        fall risk and floor-to-stand examination, 212–213, 213(f)
        primary balance performance-based tests, 207–209, 209(t)
    overground walking, 375–377, 376(b), 376(f)
    Parkinson disease, 684–685, 700–701, 704
    postural alignment and weight distribution, 199(f), 199–201, 200(f)
    postural stability exercises, 836, 836(f), 836(t)
    respiratory patterns, 35
    resting posture observation, 147
    stroke
        examination, 548–550
        interventions, 561–563
        postural alignment deviations, 549(t)
    tests for posture disturbances, 195(t)
Postural drainage, 408, 409(f), 410(b)
Postural instability gait disorder (PIGD)
    group, 683
    phenotype, 680

Postural orthostatic tachycardia syndrome (POTS), 144, 987
Postural reflex mechanism, 204
Postural sway, 191, 200(f), 200–201
Postural syncope (postural hypotension), 144
Postural tone, 145
Postural tremor, 188, 190(t), 195(t), 593, 684
Posture, defined, 1230
Posture forward, 116(t)
Posturography, dynamic, 200, 202, 203, 205
Povidone-iodine (PVI), 500–501, 502
Power add-on unit, 1274, 1274(f)
Power anterior tilt, 1278
Power assist drive system, 1273–1274, 1274(f)
Powerbase wheelchair, 1275, 1276(f)
Powered orthosis, 1165
Power elevating leg rest system, 1277, 1278(f)
Power Knee, 1193, 1193(f)
Power lateral tilt, 1278
Power Mobility Community Driving Assessment (PIDA), 1281(t)
Power mobility devices, 1274–1279
    power wheelchairs, 1275(f), 1275–1278
    scooters/power-operated vehicles, 670, 1274–1275, 1275(f)
Power-operated vehicles (POVs), 1274–1275, 1275(f)
Power recline, 1277, 1278(f)
Power seat elevation, 1277–1278
Power seat functions, 1278
Power seat to floor feature, 1278
Power standing, 1278
Power tilt, 1277, 1277(f)
Power wheelchairs, 1275(f), 1275–1278
    amyotrophic lateral sclerosis, 670
    drive wheel configurations, 1275–1276, 1276(f)
        mid-wheel drive bases, 1276, 1276(f)
        rear wheel drive bases, 1276, 1276(f)
    front wheel drive wheelchair, 1276(f), 1276–1277
    input devices, 1278–1279
        nonproportional drive controls, 1278–1279
        proportional drive controls, 1278, 1279
    integrated power wheelchair, 1275, 1275(f)
    positioning features, 1277–1278
        custom power seat functions, 1278
        power recline and power elevating leg rest system, 1277, 1278(f)
        power seat elevation, 1277–1278
        power standing, 1278
        power tilt, 1277, 1277(f)
    powerbase wheelchair, 1275, 1276(f)
    variable positioning features, 1277–1278
        custom power seat functions, 1278
        power recline and power elevating leg rest system, 1277, 1278(f)
        power seat elevation, 1277–1278
        power standing, 1278
        power tilt, 1277, 1277(f)
PQRST mnemonic, 984(b)
Practice
    evidence-based, 24–27, 559
    motor learning, 342–345, 356–357, 370–371
    schedule, for stroke, 560
Pragmatic language behaviors, 1099
PRECEDE-PROCEED planning model, 1140
Precentral gyrus, 183
Preclinical lymphedema, 488
Precollectors, 470
Precontemplation stage of change, 1132, 1133(b)
Predicting reward, 340
Predictive validity, 284
Preference-based health-related quality-of-life (PB HRQL) measure, 662
Prefrontal cortex, 338
Pregabalin (Lyrica), 602

Pregnancy, pelvic girdle pain and, 234(t), 235(t)
Preload, 419
Premature atrial contractions (PACs), 444, 445(f)
Premature junctional contraction (PJC), 444
Premature ventricular contractions (PVCs), 444, 445(f), 447
Premotor area (PMA), 183–184, 185
Premotor reaction time, 191
Preoperative phase of amputation, 857
Preparation stage of change, 1132, 1133(b)
Preprosthetic phase of amputation, 861–873
    examination, 861–864
        guide, 862–863(b)
        muscle strength, 863–864
        range of motion, 861, 863, 863(f)
        residual limb, 861
    goals, 861(b)
    intervention, 865–872
        balance and mobility activities, 870–872, 871(f)
        cardiopulmonary endurance exercise, 872
        muscle function exercises, 869–870, 870(f)
        range of motion, 869
        residual limb care and edema/volume management, 865–866
        residual limb wrapping, 866, 866(b), 867(b), 867(f), 868(f)
        shrinkers, 866
        skin care, 866, 868–869
    phantom limb pain management, 872–873
    status of uninvolved limb, 864–865
        cognition, 865
        emotional and psychological status, 864–865
        functional status, 864
        phantom limb, 864
Pressoreceptors, 56
Pressors, 431(t)
Pressure and light touch, 335
Pressure dressings, 962, 962(f)
Pressure injuries, 482–484
    bariatric patients, 306(b)
    categories, 1233–1234
    clinical presentation, 483, 484(f)
    defined, 482
    history, 483
    hypodermis, 471
    intervention, 484
    medical device-related, 492(t)
    mucosal membrane, 492(t)
    multiple sclerosis, 613
    pressure points of bony prominences, 483, 483(f)
    pressure-redistributing devices, 517, 517(f)
    staging or grading, 491, 492(t), 1233–1234
    tests and measures, 484
    wheelchair seating/mobility, 1233–1234
Pressure mapping, 263(f), 263–264, 264(f), 484
Pressure pain threshold (PPT), 988
Pressure perception test, 90
Pressure points of bony prominences, 483, 483(f)
Pressure-redistributing devices (PRDs), 477, 484, 485, 517, 517(f), 554, 613
Pressure Sore Status Tool, 493
Pressure Ulcer Scale for Healing, 493
Presupplementary motor area, 338
Pre-swing, 218(f), 219, 219(t), 221(t), 222(t), 223(t)
Prevention, 2, 4(b)
Prevention of Falls Network Europe (PROFANE), 211
Preventive interventions, 20, 545, 604, 663
Prilocaine, 501
Primary care, 2, 3(b)
Primary dressings, 508
Primary excision, burns and, 951
Primary (or essential) HTN, 427

Primary injury, traumatic brain injury and, 727–728
Primary intention wound closure, 474
Primary lateral sclerosis, 636(t)
Primary lymphedema, 481, 481(f)
Primary motor cortex, 183
Primary prevention, 4(b), 1124, 1125(f)
Primary progressive aphasia (PPA), 1106
Primary progressive MS (PPMS), 590, 590(b), 596, 614
Primary sensory cortex, 82(f)
Primary support surfaces, for WSM, 1252–1257
    arm support, 1256–1257
    back support, 1254–1255, 1256(b)
    foot support, 1255–1256, 1256(f)
    head support, 1257
    seat, 1252–1254, 1253–1254(f), 1255(b)
Primitive reflexes, 151, 152(t)
Principal components analysis, 266
Prinzmetal angina, 432–433
Prism adaptation, 1079, 1080–1084(t)
Prism goggles, 1079, 1079(f)
Proactive motor control, 126, 127(b)
Proactive postural control, 199, 550
Problem list, 15, 15(t)
Problem-solving skills, 159(b), 159–160, 1001.
    See also Decision-making
Procedural interventions, 495–508
    cold laser therapy, 508
    débridement, 498–500
    hyperbaric oxygen therapy, 506–507
    mechanical modalities, 502(f), 502–506, 503–505(t), 506(f)
    negative pressure wound therapy, 507(f), 507–508
    topical agents, 500–502
    wound cleansing, 496–498
Procedural learning, 158(b)
Procedural memory, 126, 127(b), 340
Prodromal period, 682
Professionalism in Physical Therapy: Core Values, 1123, 1145–1146
Profile of Function and Impairment Level Experience with Parkinson Disease (PROFILE PD), 707
Profore, 513
Program level, of health promotion and wellness, 1145
Progressive bulbar palsy, 636(t)
Progressive multifocal leukoencephalopathy (PML), 601
Progressive muscular atrophy, 636(t)
Progressive overload principle, 711
Progressive Return to Activity Following Mild TBI (PRA), 752
Progressive supranuclear palsy, 681
Projection, 1024(b)
Prolapse, 444
Proliferative phase
    dermal healing, 949
    wound healing, 472, 476
PRO Measures, 662
Pronation/supination test, 193(t)
Prone-on-elbows, 794–795, 795(f)
Proportional controller, 1278
Proportional drive controls, 1278, 1279
Proprioception, 335
Proprioception deficits, 988
Proprioceptive awareness test, 90–91
Proprioceptive feedback, 624
Proprioceptive loading, 612, 624
Proprioceptive losses, 612, 619
Proprioceptive neuromuscular facilitation (PNF), 351
Proprioceptors, 78
Prosody, 1101

Prosopagnosia, 531, 1091
Prospective surveillance model, 481
Prosthetics, 1180–1222
    alignment, 1202(f), 1202–1203, 1203(f)
    amputation
        Medicare functional classification levels, 875, 875(b)
            predicting potential, 874–875, 875(b)
            preparatory and definitive, 873–874
            training, 876(b), 876–883, 877–880(t)
    bilateral, 1198, 1198(f)
    case study, 1220–1222
    cognition, 1204–1205
    community integration, 1219–1220
    disarticulation, 1197–1198
        hip, 1197(f), 1197–1198
        knee, 1197
    examination, 1208–1212, 1210(t), 1211(f), 1212
        transfemoral, 1209, 1210–1212
        transtibial, 1208–1209
    fit, 1201, 1213, 1214(f)
    gait speed, 1206–1208(t), 1210(t)
    immediate postoperative, 1205
    lower limb, 1181
    maintenance, 1200–1201
        foot-ankle assemblies, 1200, 1201(f)
        joints, 1201
        shanks, 1200–1201
        sockets and suspensions, 1201
    Medicare functional K levels, 1205(t)
    partial foot and ankle, 1181(f), 1181–1182, 1182(f)
    physical examination, 1203–1204
    physical therapy management, 1203–1220
        cognition and psychosocial conditions, 1204–1205
        community integration: work, sports, and other activities, 1219–1220
        physical examination, 1203–1204
        prescription considerations, 1203
        prosthetic examination, 1208–1212, 1210(t), 1211(f), 1212
        prosthetic prescription, 1205(t), 1205–1208, 1206–1208(t)
        prosthetic training, 1212–1219, 1214(f), 1215(f), 1216(f), 1217–1218(f), 1219(f)
        temporary prostheses, 1205
    prescription, 1203, 1205(t), 1205–1208, 1206–1208(t)
    psychosocial conditions, 1204–1205
    temporary, 1205
    training, 1212–1219, 1214(f), 1215(f), 1216(f), 1217–1218(f), 1219(f)
    transfemoral, 1191–1196
    transtibial, 1182–1191
    upper limb, 1198–1200
Prosthetic training, 876–883, 1212–1219
    advanced, 880, 882–883
        steps and ramps, 880, 882, 883
        transfemoral activities, 883(t)
    balance and coordination, 1216, 1217(f)
    community mobility, 1218–1219
    decision-making regarding assistance, 1213
    donning, 1212–1213
    elements, 877–880(t)
        knee control, 877
        pelvic control, 879
        proprioception, 878
        prosthetic control, 878
        sidestepping; backward stepping, 880
        stability—both legs, 877
        stability on prosthesis, 877–878
        stepping with prosthesis, 879
        stepping with sound leg, 879
    exercises to stretch and strengthen, 1213, 1215, 1215(f), 1216(f)

functional training, 1218
gait, 876, 880
    evidence summary, 881–882(t)
    patients using ESAR prosthetic foot, 880(b)
    skills required for efficient prosthetic gait, 876(b)
    training, 1216–1218, 1217(f), 1218(f)
    problem-solving the fit, 1213, 1214(f)
    residual limb care, 1213
    self-management, 1213
    transfers, 1215, 1216
Protective devices, 493
Protective sensation, 485, 494, 494(f)
Protective withdrawal reflexes, 150
Protriptyline (Vivactil), 1036(b)
Proverb interpretation, preliminary tests of, 76
Providence brace, 1169
Provisional Best Practices Guidelines for the Evaluation of Bulbar Dysfunction in ALS, 648
Proximal interphalangeal (PIP) joints, 896–897, 897(f)
Proximity switch drive controls, 1279
PSCEBSM model, 984, 986(b)
Pseudobulbar affect (PBA), 536, 595, 643, 648
Pseudoexacerbation, 591, 609
Pseudomonas aeruginosa, 391, 501, 506, 946
Psychic numbing, 1029, 1031
Psychogenic erections, 771
Psychogenic pain, 971
Psychological issues
    amputation, 864–865
    heart disease, 464–465
    substance use, 1037(t)
Psychopath, 1020
Psychopharmacology, 602
Psychosocial adaptation, 1015–1019
    chronic illness/disability, 1018
    grief, mourning, and sorrow, 1015–1016
    phase models, 1016–1018
    post-traumatic rehabilitation, 1018–1019
Psychosocial function, pain and, 981, 982
Psychosocial Impact of Assistive Devices, 782
Psychosocial Impact of Assistive Technology (PIADS), 1281(t)
Psychosocial issues, 1012–1052
    acute stress disorder, 1029, 1030–1032
    agitation, 1038, 1040
    amyotrophic lateral sclerosis, 662, 670–671
    anxiety, 1013, 1014, 1025–1026(t), 1025–1029, 1030–1031(b)
    arthritis, 922–923
    case study, 1052
    chronic pain, 978–979
    conversion disorder, 1013
    coping styles, 1021–1022
    defense reactions to disability, 1022, 1022–1024(b)
    depression, 1013, 1014, 1032–1037, 1033(t), 1035–1036(b)
    hypersexuality, 1040–1041
    integrating into rehabilitation, 1042
    lifetime prevalence, 1013(t)
    mental health examination, 1014–1015, 1014–1015(b)
    motor control, 349(t)
    multiple sclerosis, 608, 630–631
    orthotics, 1176
    pain, 984, 986, 986(b)
    panic disorder, 1013
    Parkinson disease, 705, 721
    personality disorders, 1020–1021
    personality types, 1019–1020
    post-traumatic stress disorder, 1029, 1031–1032, 1031(b)
    prosthetics, 1204–1205
    psychosocial adaptation, 1015–1019

chronic illness/disability and, 1018
grief, mourning, and sorrow, 1015–1016
phase models, 1016–1018
post-traumatic rehabilitation, 1018–1019
psychosocial wellness, 1041
barriers to wellness for people with
disabilities, 1041
social support, 1041
rehabilitative intervention, 1042, 1043(t)
education, 1043
effectiveness of psychosocial interventions
post-stroke, 1049–1050(t)
goals and outcomes, 1045(b), 1046–1048(t)
integrating psychosocial factors, 1042
jargon and labels, 1045
patient behaviors warranting mental health
consultation, 1044(t)
rehabilitation team members' self-awareness,
1051
trauma-informed care, 1045, 1048, 1050
substance use, 1037(t), 1037–1038
education, 1038
medications used to treat, 1039–1040(b)
referral, 1038
rehabilitation and, 1037, 1038
treating patients who abuse substances, 1038
violence, 1038, 1040
wellness in rehabilitation, 1041–1042
Psychosocial wellness, 1041
people with disabilities, 1041
social support, 1041
Psychotherapy, 602
Ptosis, 533(t), 534(t)
PTSD Checklist, 1031
Public building requirements, 294
Public Buildings Act of 1983, 327
Public transportation systems, ADA and, 327
PubMed, 25(t)
Pulmonary artery (PA), 420
Pulmonary artery (PA) catheter, 420
Pulmonary capillary wedge pressure (PCWP), 420,
439(t), 440, 441, 453(t)
Pulmonary complications
burns, 946
rheumatoid arthritis, 900
Pulmonary dysfunction, 539
Pulmonary edema, 53
Pulmonary embolus (PE), 539
Pulmonary impairment, 768–769, 769(t)
Pulmonary rehabilitation, 402, 405–406
exercise progression, 406
exercise training, 402, 405
program duration, 406
strength training, 405–406
Pulmonary status, in screening for WSM, 1238
Pulmonary veins (PVs), 420
Pulmonic area, 417
Pulmonic valve, 418
Pulsatile lavage with suction (PLWS), 496(f),
496–497, 498
Pulse, 43–50
defined, 43
monitoring, 46, 48–49
apical pulse, 48(f), 48–49
apical-radial pulse, 49
radial pulse, 48
normal and abnormal, 45(f)
quality, 44, 44(t)
rate (See Heart rate)
rhythm, 43
sites, 46, 46(f), 47–48(b)
Pulse deficit, 49
Pulsed radiofrequency stimulation (PRFS), 506
Pulsed shortwave diathermy (PSWD), 506
Pulse oximeters, 63, 64(f)
Pulse oximetry, 63–64, 452(t)

Pulse pressure, 56
Pulse quality, 489
Pulsus alternans, 44, 45(f)
Pulsus bigeminus, 45(f)
Pulsus bisferiens, 45(f)
Pulsus paradoxus, 44, 45(f)
Pupillary size and reaction, examination of, 134
Purdue Pegboard Test, 198(b)
Pure motor lacunar stroke, 531
Pure sensory lacunar stroke, 531
Pure word deafness, 1105(t)
Purkinje fibers, 420
Purposive action, 1076
Pus, 472
Pusher syndrome, 550, 563
Push handles, 1261
Push-off, 219, 226
Push-pull mechanism, 819, 819(f)
Putamen, 185, 185(f), 338, 681
Pylon, 1185
Pyrexia, 38(b), 38–39

Q
QRS complex, 421, 446, 447, 448
Quadraphonic approach, 1059–1061, 1060–1061(f)
Quadriceps, 149(t)
Quadrilateral socket, 1194, 1195(f)
Qualifiers, 7
Qualisys Motion Analysis system, 256, 257,
257(f), 258(f)
Qualitative assessment of motor function, 133
Qualitative gait analysis. See under Kinematic gait
analysis
Quality, pulse, 44, 44(t)
Quality of life (QOL), 18, 19(b), 25
amyotrophic lateral sclerosis, 662
defined, 1124
dyspnea, 398, 399(t)
health promotion and wellness, 1124
intermittent claudication, 489–490
measures, 1127–1128
spinal cord injury, 772–773
traumatic brain injury, 742
Quality of Life After Brain Injury tool, 742, 743(t)
Quality of movement (QOM), 552
Quality of Well-Being Scale, 1130(t)
Quantitative assessment of motor function, 133
Quantitative gait analysis. See under Kinematic gait
analysis
Quantitative parameters, 279–280
Quantitative sensory testing (QST), 94–97, 988
Bio-Thesiometer, 96, 97(f)
MSA Thermotest, 96, 97(f)
Rolltemp II, 96, 96(f)
Rydel-Seiffer tuning fork, 96, 96(f)
Touch Test Sensory Evaluator, 95–96, 96(f)
TSA-II NeuroSensory Analyzer + VSA 3000
Vibratory Sensory Analyzer, 94(f), 94–95,
95(f)
von Frey Aesthesiometer II, 95, 95(f)
Quebec User Evaluation of Satisfaction with
Assistive Technology (QUEST), 782
Quebec User Evaluation of Satisfaction with
Assistive Technology Version 2.0
(QUEST), 1281(t)
Questionnaires
examination of environmental factors, 295,
297(f)
musculoskeletal examination, 105, 107, 108(f)
nonmotor symptoms, 691
pain, 981, 984
patient-reported outcome measures, 105, 107
QOL of cancer patients, 1128
self-assessment, 143
Quiet stance, 202

Quinidine sulphate, 648
Q-wave myocardial infarction (QMI), 428, 435

R
Radial nerve dynamic wrist-hand orthosis, 1170(t)
Radial pulse, 43, 46(f), 47(b), 48
Radiation, 38
Radicava/Radicut (edaravone), 646
Radiculopathy, 167, 172(t), 174(t)
Radiography (x-ray), 160, 161(f), 164(t)
heart failure, 442
osteoarthritis, 905
rheumatoid arthritis, 892
Radiometer, 488
Rales (crackles), 54, 440
Ramps, 302, 303(f), 307(f), 325(f), 1218–1219
Rancho Los Amigos (RLA)
Levels of Cognitive Function, 134, 735, 736,
736(b)
National Rehabilitation Center, 219, 224
Observational Gait Analysis, 220, 369
drawback to using, 224
Full Body Gait Analysis Form, 225(f)
spinal cord injury, 781
traumatic brain injury, 740
RAND Health Insurance Study, 289
Randomized controlled trials (RCTs), 24, 26,
27(t), 403–405(t), 559, 1074
Random practice, 343–344, 345(t), 370, 742
Random practice order, 708
Range of motion (ROM)
age-related coordination impairments, 191
amputation, 861, 863, 863(f), 869
amyotrophic lateral sclerosis, 661
arthritis, 915–916, 927
examination, 493–494
goals and outcomes, 18, 19(b)
measurements, 9, 13
multiple sclerosis, 609
musculoskeletal examination, 113–118
accessory joint motions, 116–118, 116(t),
117(f), 118(f)
active range of motion, 113–114
capsular patterns, 116
end-feels, 116
lower extremity, 114, 115(f)
passive range of motion, 114, 116
musculoskeletal impairments, 140, 141–142
neuromuscular impairments, 148
Parkinson disease, 698, 699, 709, 710(t)
physical assessment for WSM, 1242(f),
1242–1243
spinal cord injury, 780
stroke
joint flexibility, 552–553
self-ROM, 575
upper extremities, 574(b), 574–575, 575(f)
systems review, 9
Ranvier, nodes of, 128
Rapid alternating movements (RAM), 700
Rasch analysis, 288
Rasch Overall ALS Disability Scale (ROADS),
660
Rate of perceived dyspnea (RPD), 399
Rate of perceived exertion (RPE), 399
Rate pressure product (RPP), 422
Rating of Perceived Exertion (RPE), 143, 353,
401(b), 401–402, 462, 462(t), 557, 610,
706
Rationalization, 1024(b)
Raynaud disease, 478
Ray resection, 851(t)
Reaching movements, 205
Reaction time, 157(t), 191, 335, 359–360, 556,
684, 699, 716, 753

Reactive balance, 359
Reactive motor control, 127(b)
Reactive postural control, 549
Rear wheel drive bases, 1276, 1276(f)
Rebound phenomenon, 188, 190(t)
Rebound test, 193(t)
Recall schema, 341
Receptive aphasia, 1104, 1105(t), 1106, 1108
Receptor specificity, 77–78
Reciprocal determinism, 1135, 1135(t)
Reciprocal gaits, 1174–1175
Reciprocal motion, 192
Reciprocating gait orthosis (RGO), 1164, 1164(f)
Reclining wheelchair, 1268(f), 1268–1269
Recognition schema, 341
Recovery. See Motor recovery
Recovery of function, 775
Recurrent fever, 38(b)
Red flags
    arthritis, 914, 915(t)
    chronic pain, 979(t), 982(f), 987, 992
    compression therapy, 512
    musculoskeletal examination, 105, 108, 109
    prosthetics, 1213
Reepithelialization, 472, 475
Reference neutral sitting posture, 1230, 1231(f)
Reference of correctness, 341
Referral
    anxiety, 1029
    depression, 1034
    substance use, 1038
Reflex bowel, 770
Reflexes
    abnormal, 149–151
        cutaneous reflexes, 150, 150(t)
        deep tendon reflexes, 149(t), 149–150
        documentation, 151
        primitive and tonic reflexes, 151, 152(t)
        superficial reflexes, 150, 150(t)
    amyotrophic lateral sclerosis, 663
    cutaneous, 150, 150(t)
    defined, 149
    grading, 150, 151
    motor control, 336
    spinal cord injury, 781
    testing, 111
Reflexogenic erections, 771
Refocusing, 1071
Refrigerators, 316
Regression, 1044(t)
Regulatory conditions, 138, 139(b)
Regulatory features for success, 346, 349(t), 355
Regulatory T cells, 589
Regurgitation, 444
Rehabilitation, 2, 3(b)
    amyotrophic lateral sclerosis, 650, 656–658,
        657(b), 658(f)
        framework, 650, 658(f)
        goals and outcomes, 657(b)
    anxiety, 1026–1027
    arthritis, 914–935
        education and self-management, 935
        physical activity, 932–934, 933(t), 934(t)
        physical therapy examination, 914–923,
            915(t), 917–921(t)
        physical therapy interventions, 923(b),
            923–932, 929(t), 930–931(t)
        telehealth/telerehabilitation, 935
    cardiac
        coronary artery disease, 454
        inpatient, 459–460(t)
        outpatient, exercise prescription parameters
            utilized in, 461(t)
        phase I, 452, 454
        phase II, 457, 461(t)
        research on effectiveness, 459(t)

depression, 1032, 1033
locomotor function, 370–379
    circuit training, 377, 377(b), 378(f)
    intensity, 370
    motor imagery, 377–378
    motor learning, 370–371
    muscle force production, augmenting,
        374–375, 375(f)
    neuroplasticity, 371, 371(b)
    overground walking for balance and postural
        control, 375–377, 376(b), 376(f)
    task-specific walking training/treadmill
        training, 371–373, 372–373(f)
    virtual reality and exergaming, 373–374,
        374(f)
multiple sclerosis, 603(f), 603–604
Parkinson disease, 695–697, 697(t)
psychosocial issues, 1042, 1043(t)
    education, 1043
    effectiveness of psychosocial interventions
        post-stroke, 1049–1050(t)
    goals and outcomes, 1045(b), 1046–1048(t)
    integrating psychosocial factors, 1042
    jargon and labels, 1045
    patient behaviors warranting mental health
        consultation, 1044(t)
    rehabilitation team members' self-awareness,
        1051
    trauma-informed care, 1045, 1048, 1050
pulmonary dysfunction, 402, 405–406
    exercise progression, 406
    exercise training, 402, 405
    program duration, 406
    strength training, 405–406
spinal cord injury, 775(f), 775–776
stroke, 542, 543–545
substance use, 1037, 1038
vestibular, 846
wellness, 1041–1042
Rehabilitation Act of 1973, 295, 327
Rehabilitation Measures Database (RMD), 14,
    25(t), 133, 207, 348, 379, 742, 776
Rehabilitation nurse, traumatic brain injury and, 733
Rehabilitation Reference Center, 24
Rehabilitation technology specialist, 318
Rehabilitative/compensatory (functional)
    approach, 1058–1059, 1070
Rehab technology professional (RTP), 1226, 1227
Rehawalk, 262
Reinforcement, in social cognitive theory, 1135,
    1135(t)
Reinforcement management (change process),
    1133, 1133(t)
Reinnervation, 639, 640(f), 671
Reintegration to Normal Living Index (RNL),
    783, 1070
Relapses
    defined, 589
    multiple sclerosis, 590–591
Relapsing fever, 38(b)
Relapsing-remitting MS (RRMS), 590, 590(b),
    596, 614, 630
Relatedness, 1134
Relative overdosing, 694
Relaxation
    anxiety, 1027–1028
    chronic pain, 1001(b), 1001–1002
    Parkinson disease, 709, 709(f)
Reliability
    ambulation profiles and scales, 233
    coefficient values, 283
    instrumented walkways, 250, 251–255(t)
    instrument measures of function, 282–283
    interrater/intrarater reliability, 282
    sensory examination, 93–94
    test-retest reliability, 282

Reliefs, pressure-relieving, 1186
Remedial approach, 1070, 1071(t)
Remission criteria, 901
Remissions, 589
Remittent fever, 38(b)
Remodeling, 433, 472, 476
Remote-controlled features
    curtains, 308
    door openers, 304
    lights, 305
    locks, 304
    smart appliances, 305
REM sleep behavior disorder (RBD), 687, 689
Remyelination, 130, 132(f)
Repetitions, 351, 352(t)
Repetitive nerve stimulation (RNS), 167, 167(f),
    171(t)
Repetitive strain injuries (RSIs), 1264
Repetitive transcranial magnetic stimulation
    (rTMS), 173, 379
Repression, 1024(b)
Rescue drugs, 394, 395
Reserpine, 681
Residual limb care
    edema/volume management, 865–866
    examination, 861
    postsurgical phase of amputation, 860
    preprosthetic phase of amputation, 861
    prosthetic training, 1213
    wrapping, 866, 866(b), 867(f), 868(b), 868(f)
Residual volume (RV), 383
Resistance generation, point of peak, 351
Resistance training, 374, 463(t), 747
Resisted isometric testing, 118, 119(t)
Resistive breathing training program, 629
Resistive exercise, burns and, 961
Resistive strengthening, 351
Respiration, 50–55, 384
    amyotrophic lateral sclerosis, 641(t), 642, 649,
        662–663, 668
    depth, 53
    examination, 55
    factors influencing, 52–53
        age, 52–53
        body position, 53
        body size and stature, 53
        emotions/stress, 53
        environment, 53
        exercise, 53
        pharmacological management, 53
        spinal cord integrity, 53
    monitoring, 55
    parameters, 53–54
    Parkinson disease, 705–706
    patterns, 54(f), 54–55
    regulatory mechanisms, 51–52
    respiratory system, 50–51, 51(f), 52(f)
    rhythm, 53
    sounds, 34, 53–54
    spinal cord injury
        abdominal binder, 790
        assisted cough and, 790, 790(f)
        examination, 779
        glossopharyngeal breathing, 790
        manual stretching, 790–791
        muscle training, 789(f), 789–790
        physical therapy interventions, 789–791
        respiratory muscle training, 789(f), 789–790
    tests and measures, 494
Respiratory rate, 451(t)
Respiratory system
    physiology, 383(f), 383–384
        anatomy, 383(f)
        external and internal respiration, 385(f)
    structures, 50–51, 51(f), 52(f)
Respiratory zone, 51, 52(f)

Response
  formats, 280–281
    interval/ratio measures, 280–281, 281(f)
    nominal measures, 280
    ordinal measures, 280
  instrument measures of function, 284, 285(b), 285(t)
  programming, 335
  selection, 335
  stimulus and, association between, 335
Rest-activity ratios, 621
Rest for arthritis pain, 924, 927
Resting heart rate and rhythm, 451(t)
Resting-state fMRI, 162, 164(t)
Resting tremor, 189, 190(t), 195(t), 684
Restless legs syndrome (RLS), 540
Restorative interventions, 20
  amyotrophic lateral sclerosis, 663
  multiple sclerosis, 603
  neural plasticity, 745
  stroke, 545
  traumatic brain injury, 742, 744, 744(t), 745, 745(t)
Restrictive cardiomyopathy, 417
Restrictive lung diseases, 391–392
  clinical presentation, 391–392, 392(f)
  course and prognosis, 392
  etiology, 391
  pathophysiology, 391
Restrictive lung dysfunction, 689
Retention
  defined, 156
  interval, 156
  tests, 156, 158, 159(b)
Rete peg region, 941
Rete pegs, 477
Reticular dermis, 940, 941, 941(t)
Reticulospinal tract, 184
Retraining approach, 1057–1058, 1070
Retropulsive gait, 686
Return to sport (RTS), 752
Reverse transfer, 339(t), 357
Reverse transfer effect, 345, 356, 360
ReWalk, 1165
Reward, predicting, 340
Rheo knee, 1193
Rheumatoid arthritis, 889–901
  activity limitations, 901
  cardiovascular complications, 900
  case study, 936–937
  classification, 892–893
  clinical presentation, 893–901, 894–899(f)
  diagnostic criteria, 892–893
  disease onset and course, 893
  epidemiology, 890
  etiology, 890
  joint impairments, 893–901, 894(f)
    ankle, 898
    cervical spine, 893, 895(f)
    deconditioning, 900
    elbow, 894
    feet, 898, 899(f)
    hand, 895–897(f), 895–898
    hip, 898
    knee, 898, 898(f)
    muscle involvement, 899–900
    ocular complications, 900
    rheumatoid nodules, 900
    shoulder, 893, 894
    temporomandibular joint, 893
    tendon involvement, 900
    wrist, 894, 895, 895(f)
  laboratory tests, 891, 892
  neurological complications, 900
  ocular complications, 900
  participation restrictions, 901

  pathophysiology, 890–891, 891(f)
  pharmacological management, 910–912
  prognosis, 901
  pulmonary complications, 900
  radiography/diagnostic imaging, 892
  remission criteria, 901
  systemic features, 893
  vascular complications, 900
  See also Arthritis
Rheumatoid nodules, 900
Rhizotomy, 602
Rhythm
  pulse, 43
  respiration, 53
Rhythmic auditory stimulation (RAS), 708
Right bundle branch block (RBBB), 448
Right coronary artery (RCA), 418, 418(f), 435
Right hemiplegia, 537
Right hemisphere lesions, 537, 537(t)
Righting reactions (RRs), 204
Right-left discrimination, 134, 538, 1085–1086
Right-sided heart catheterization, 420, 420(t)
Right-sided heart failure, 438
Right ventricle (RV), 416, 418, 420, 438, 439(t)
Rigid dressings, 855, 856
Rigidity, 145, 146, 189, 190(t), 195(t), 339, 684, 686
Rigo Cheneau brace, 1169
Riluzole (Rilutek), 646
Risk reduction plan, 321
Risperidone, 681
Rivermead Behavioural Memory Test (RBMT), 1069(t), 1074
Rivermead Mobility Index, 145, 608(t)
Rivermead Perceptual Assessment Battery (RPAB), 1069(t), 1089
Rivermead Post-Concussion Symptom Questionnaire (RPQ), 753, 754(t)
Rivermead Rehabilitation Centre Life Goals Questionnaire, 1070
Robert Wood Johnson Foundation, 1048
Robot-assisted gait training (RAGT), 715, 807
Robot-assisted treadmill training (RATT), 626
Robotic-assisted training, 573
Rocker bar, 1153, 1153(f)
Rocker sole, 1153, 1153(f)
Roeder Manipulative Aptitude Test, 198(b)
ROHO Quadtro Select High Profile cushion, 517(f)
Role Checklist, 1048(t)
Rolling, 793–794, 794(f)
Roll-in shower water containment strategies, 314, 314(f)
Roll motion, 116, 117, 117(f)
Rolltemp II, 96, 96(f)
Romberg sign, 189
Romberg test, 11, 202, 989
Rotation of the foot on heel contact, 1212
Rotators, 1185, 1185(f)
Rubella, 589
Rubor of dependency, 490
Rubrospinal tract, 184
Ruffini endings, 79, 79(b), 80
Ruffini's corpuscle, 941(t)
Rugs, 307
Rule of Nines, 946, 946(f)
Rush Dyskinesia Scale, 700
Rush foot, 1182, 1183(f)
Rydel-Seiffer tuning fork, 96, 96(f)

S

Sacrum, 483, 483(f)
Safe position wrist-hand orthosis, 1170(t)
Safety
  devices, 300
  traumatic brain injury, 740

Safety Assessment of Function and the Environment for Rehabilitation (SAFER tool), 299(t)
St. George's Respiratory Questionnaire, 398, 399(t)
Salience, neuroplasticity principle of, 339(t)
Salience network, 972
Saltatory conduction, 589
Salutogenic variables, 1124
Salvos, 447
Same skill practice, 344, 345(t)
Sarcopenia, 191
Sarcoplasmic reticulum, 130(f)
Satisfaction with Life Scale, 348(t), 783
Sauguet's test, 1086
Scald-guard valves, 313, 315
Scale for the Assessment and Rating of Ataxia (SARA), 196
Scanning speech, 187
Scaphoid pad, 1152, 1153(f)
Scapula, 146(t)
Scar management
  burn
    assessment, 954, 955–957(t)
    contracture, 953
    management, 961–962, 962(f)
    pathological, 948
    wounds, 519, 519(f)
SCEBS model, 984
Schedule for Evaluation of Individual Quality of Life-Direct Weighting (SEIQoL-DW), 662
Scheduling, feedback, 346, 347(t)
Schema, 127(b), 336
Schema theory, 341
Schizoid personality disorder, 1020
Schizotypal personality disorder, 1020
School Reentry Programs, 964
Schwab and England Activities of Daily Living Scale (SE), 660
SCI Pressure Ulcer Scale (SCIPUS), 780
SCIPUS-Acute, 780
SCI Research Evidence, 776
SCI Special Interest Group of the Academy of Neurologic Physical Therapy, 776
Scleroderma, 494
Sclerosis in plaques, 588
Scoliosis orthoses, 1168(f), 1168–1169, 1169(f)
Scooters, 670, 1274–1275, 1275(f)
Scope of Practice, ASHA, 1100
Scotoma, 592
Screening examination
  body functions and structures for WSM, 1238–1239
  musculoskeletal, 111(f), 111–113
  sensory function, 705
  systems review, 9, 11–12, 133
Seat, for WSM, 1252–1254, 1253–1254(f), 1255(b)
Seated control, 206, 206(t)
Seating and positioning technology, 319(b), 1225–1226
Seating and wheeled mobility. See Wheelchair seating and mobility (WSM)
Seating simulator, 1246, 1247(f)
Seating support system, for WSM, 1251–1258, 1252(f)
  primary support surfaces, 1252–1257
    arm support, 1256–1257
    back support, 1254–1255, 1256(b)
    foot support, 1255–1256, 1256(f)
    head support, 1257
    seat, 1252–1254, 1253–1254(f), 1255(b)
  secondary support surfaces, 1257–1258
    anterior pelvic support, 1257–1258, 1257–1258(f)
    lateral supports, 1258

Seating support system, for WSM (continued)
    medial supports, 1258
    posterior supports, 1258
Seating system, spinal cord injury and, 809–810
Seattle Angina Questionnaire (SAQ), 457(t)
Seborrhea, 689
Seborrheic dermatitis, 689
Secondary care, 2, 3(b)
Secondary chronic pain, 970
Secondary dressings, 508
Secondary (or nonessential) HTN, 427
Secondary impairments
    spinal cord injury, 772
    traumatic brain injury, 730, 730(b), 737–738,
        737–738(f)
Secondary injury, traumatic brain injury and, 728
Secondary lymphedema, 481, 481(f)
Secondary parkinsonism, 680–681
    drug-induced parkinsonism, 681
    postencephalitic parkinsonism, 680
    toxic parkinsonism, 681
Secondary prevention, 4(b), 604, 1124, 1125(f)
Secondary progressive MS (SPMS), 590, 590(b),
        596
Secondary support surfaces, for WSM, 1257–1258
    anterior pelvic support, 1257–1258, 1257–1258(f)
    lateral supports, 1258
    medial supports, 1258
    posterior supports, 1258
Secondary wound closure, 474–475
Second-degree heart block, 448
Secretion removal techniques, 408–412
    active cycle of breathing techniques, 410(f),
        410–411
    activity pacing, 412
    airway clearance, 410
    breathing exercises, 411–412
    high-frequency chest compression devices, 411,
        411(f)
    manual, 408–410
        percussion, 409
        postural drainage, 408, 409(f), 410(b)
        shaking, 410
    oral airway oscillation devices, 411, 411(f)
    positive expiratory pressure, 411, 411(f)
Section GG Functional Abilities and Goals, 136,
        288, 552, 741, 782
Segmental dystonia, 147
Seizures, stroke and, 538
SelectAir MAX, 517(f)
Selective attention, 1073
Selective capacity, stroke and, 555–556
Selective débridement, 499–500, 499(f), 500(f)
    autolytic débridement, 500
    biosurgery, 499–500, 500(f)
    enzymatic débridement, 499
    medical-grade honey, 500
    sharp débridement, 499, 499(f)
Selective serotonin and norepinephrine reuptake
        inhibitors (SSNRIs), 602, 1007
Selective serotonin reuptake inhibitors (SSRIs),
        648, 650, 1007
Self-administered report, 277
Self-assessment questionnaires, 143
Self-awareness, in psychosocial intervention, 1051
Self-care
    chronic pain, 1002–1003
    Functional Independence Measure (FIM),
        287(t), 287–288
    spinal cord injury, 782
    vascular, lymphatic, and integumentary
        disorders, 494
Self-control, in social cognitive theory, 1135,
        1135(t)
Self-destructive behaviors, 1044(t)
Self-determination theory, 1134

Self-efficacy, 355
    Attitude, Social Influence, and Self-Efficacy
        model, 1139
    defined, 1131
    enhancing, 1139(b)
    health belief model, 1131, 1131(f)
    health coaching, 1140
    motivational interviewing, 1141, 1141(f)
    multiple sclerosis, 631
    physical activity, 1129(t)
    for physical activity questionnaire, 1129(t),
        1134, 1134(t)
    questionnaire, 1134(t)
    social cognitive theory, 1135, 1135(t), 1138
    stroke, 560–561
    Transtheoretical Model, 1132, 1132(t), 1133, 1134
Self-Efficacy Scale, 1047(t)
Self-esteem, damaged, 1043(t)
Self-evaluation (change process), 1133, 1133(t)
Self-liberation (change process), 1133, 1133(t)
Self-management, prosthetic training and, 1213
Self-monitoring, heart disease and, 461, 462
Self-paced skills, 138, 139(b)
Self-perceived health measures, 1127–1128
Self-report Leeds Assessment of Neuropathic
        Symptoms and Signs (S-LANSS), 985(t)
Self-report measures, 136, 277–278, 298
Semantics, 1100
Semicircular canals (SCCs), 201, 816(f), 816–817
    tests, 827, 828
Semilunar valves, 418
Semirigid dressings, 856
Semivowels, 1103
Semmes-Weinstein monofilament, 494, 609, 988
Sensations
    amyotrophic lateral sclerosis, 663
    combined cortical, 78, 91–93
        barognosis (recognition of weight), 93, 93(f)
        double simultaneous stimulation, 92–93
        graphesthesia (traced figure identification), 93
        recognition of texture, 93
        stereognosis perception, 91
        tactile localization, 91–92
        two-point discrimination, 92
    deep, 78, 90–91
    examination, 494, 494(f)
    motor control, 334, 335
    movement, 68
    multiple sclerosis, 609
    normal, 494
    perception differentiated from, 1055
    physical assessment for WSM, 1240
    protective, 485, 494, 494(f)
    stroke, 553–554
    superficial, 78, 87, 89–90
Sensitivity, test, 196, 207, 283, 284(b)
Sensitization, 340
Sensorimotor integrative treatment, 576
Sensorimotor vision, 201
Sensory aphasia, 1104, 1105(t), 1106, 1108
Sensory ataxia, 202
Sensory balance strategies, 201–204, 203(f),
        204(f)
    Romberg test, 202
    Sensory Organization Test, 202–204, 203(t)
Sensory decussation, 82(f)
Sensory-discriminative dimension, 972
Sensory examination
    administering, 84–86
    clinical indications, 69–72
        pattern (distribution) of sensory impairment,
            70–71(f), 70–72
        spinal cord tracts, 72
    combined cortical sensations, 91–93
    cranial nerve function, 97, 98(t), 99(b)
    data generated by, 86

deep sensations, 90–91
documentation, 87
elements, 69(b)
equipment, 84–86, 85(f)
    light touch, 84
    pain, 84, 85(f)
    recognition of texture, 86
    stereognosis (object recognition), 84
    temperature, 84, 85(f)
    two-point discrimination, 85, 85(f)
    vibration, 84
order, 86–87
patient preparation, 86
preliminary tests, 74, 75–77
    arousal, 75
    attention, 76
    calculation ability, 76
    cognition, 76
    elements, 69(b)
    hearing, 77
    memory, 77
    orientation, 76, 76(b)
    proverb interpretation, 76
    visual acuity, 77
quantitative sensory testing, 94–97
reliability, 93–94
sample sensory examination form, 88(f)
superficial sensations, 87, 89–90
testing environment, 84
trial run or demonstration, 86
Sensory function, 67–102
    age-related sensory changes, 72–73, 74–75(t)
    case study, 101–102
    multiple sclerosis, 591, 609, 612–613
    Parkinson disease, 705
    sensation and movement, 68
    sensory integration, 67–68
    sensory integrity, 68, 97 (See also Sensory
        examination; Sensory impairment)
    somatic sensory signals, 81, 82(f)
    somatosensory cortex, 82, 83–84, 84(f)
    spinal cord injury examination, 776, 779
    stroke, 538, 576
Sensory homunculus, 83
Sensory impairment
    augmentative sensory devices, 99
    education, 97, 98–100, 99(f)
    goals and outcomes, 100, 100(b)
    motor function examination, 134
    Parkinson disease, 687–688
    patient management elements, 99(f)
    pattern (distribution), 70–71(f), 70–72
    safe balance, strategies to promote, 100
    self-monitoring, 99
    spinal cord injury, 765
    terminology describing common, 89(t)
Sensory input
    balance training, 562
    motor system role, 183
Sensory integration, 67–68, 97, 1058, 1070
Sensory Integration Model, 97
Sensory integrity, 58, 68, 97
    arthritis, 915
    chronic pain, 988, 989(t)
    See also Sensory examination; Sensory
        impairment
Sensory level, 762–763
Sensory/motor stroke, 531
Sensory nerve action potential (SNAP), 165,
        165(f)
Sensory Organization Test (SOT), 202–204,
        203(t), 562, 754, 754(t)
Sensory receptors, 77–78
    classification, 78, 79(b)
    divisions, 78
    types, 78–80

Sensory retraining programs, 576
Sensory stimulation, 576, 738
Sensory system, 77–78
    sensory receptors, 77–78
    spinal pathways, 78
Sentence Completion Attitude Survey, 1047(t)
Septum, 420
Sequential pneumatic compression with truncal
    component, 516, 516(f)
Serial casting, 737, 738(f)
Serial motor skill, 138, 139(b)
Serial skills, 340, 344
Serotonin syndrome, 987, 1007
Sertraline (Zoloft), 602, 650, 1036(b)
Severe acute respiratory syndrome (SARS), 392
Severe acute respiratory syndrome coronavirus 2
    (SARS-CoV-2), 392–393, 589, 601, 681
Sexual activity, heart disease and, 462, 464
Sexual dysfunction
    multiple sclerosis, 595, 621
    spinal cord injury, 771–772
        female response, 771–772
        male response, 771
SF-12, 289
Shaking, as manual secretion removal technique,
    410
Shank, 1151(f), 1152
Shanks, prosthetic
    maintenance, 1200–1201
    transfemoral, 1191
    transtibial, 1185–1186
        endoskeletal shank, 1185, 1186(f)
        exoskeletal shank, 1185, 1186(f)
Shared decision-making, 5
Sharp debridement, 950
Sharp débridement, 499, 499(f)
Sharp/dull discrimination test. See Pain perception
    test
Shear, 1234
Sheet graft, 953, 953(f)
Sheffield Support Snood, 664
Shirley Ryan Ability Lab, 298, 348, 379, 742, 776
Shivering, 37
Shock, 1016
Shock absorbers, 1185, 1185(f)
Shod walking, 263
Shoes, orthotic, 1151–1152
    heel, 1151–1152
    reinforcements, 1152
    sole, 1151
    upper, 1151, 1151(f)
Short-acting beta-2 agonist (LABA), 393, 394(t)
Short Form 36, 783
Short Form MPQ (SF-MPQ), 984, 985(t)
Shortness of breath (SOB)
    angina, 432, 452(t)
    heart failure, 438, 440–441, 451, 454
    orthopnea, 452(t)
    paroxysmal nocturnal dyspnea, 452(t)
Short Physical Performance Battery (SPPB), 277,
    990
Short-term memory, 77
Short transfemoral (above knee) amputation,
    851(t)
Short transtibial (below knee) amputation, 851(t)
Shoulder-elbow-wrist orthosis, 1170(t)
Shoulder-hand syndrome (SHS), 578
Shoulder impingement syndrome, 577
Shoulder(s)
    amyotrophic lateral sclerosis pain, 667–668
    pain management, 577–578
    rheumatoid arthritis, 893, 894
    spasticity in UMN syndrome, 146(t)
    See also Glenohumeral joint
Shower entries, 314, 314(f)
Shower seat, 313, 313(f)

Shower stalls, 313, 313(f)
Shrinkers, 856(f), 856–857, 866
Shuttle lock and pin, 1189(f), 1189–1190
Shy-Drager syndrome, 681
Sialorrhea, 642, 648, 688
Sialorrhea affect, 648
Sickness Impact Profile (SIP), 662, 707, 1128,
    1129(t)
Sidestepping, 372, 372(f), 373(f), 376(f)
Sigh, 54
Silent myocardial ischemia, 415
Silicone gel/gel sheets, 519, 519(f), 962
Silvadene, 501, 502
Silver sulfadiazine, 501, 502, 951
Simple and intuitive, in universal design, 295
Simple motor skill, 138, 139(b)
Simplification, 344, 345(t)
Simulation, in wheelchair assessment, 1245–1246,
    1247(f)
Simulator II Functional Capacity Evaluation
    System, 321(f)
Simultanagnosia, 1091
Simultaneous bilateral training, 572–573
Simultaneous gaits, 1175
Single-axis foot-ankle assemblies, 1184, 1184(f)
Single-axis hinge, 1191
Single-dimensional measures, of function, 286
Single Leg Stance, 11
Single limb support, 217, 218(f), 219, 220
Single limb support time, 217
Single photon emission computed tomography
    (SPECT), 163, 164(t)
Single pulse TMS (spTMS), 173
Single switch scanning array systems, 1279
Sinks
    bathroom, 314, 314(f)
    kitchen, 315–316
Sinus tracts, 474
Sip-n-puff drive control, 1279
Siponimod (Mayzent), 600(t)
SIRROWS (Stroke Inpatient Rehab with Reinforce-
    ment of Walking Speed), 356, 362(t), 363
Sit-pivot transfers, 798–800, 799(f)
Sitting
    balance, 797–798, 798(f)
    postural alignment, 199–200, 200(f)
    strategies, 205
    stroke, 579–580
Sitting mat assessment, 1239–1240, 1240(f)
Sitting posture, WSM and, 1230–1233
    benefits of optimal sitting posture, 1233
    defined, 1230
    factors influencing postural alignment,
        1231–1233, 1232(f)
    optimal postural alignment, 1231
    pelvic position, 1230, 1231(t)
    reference neutral sitting posture, 1230, 1231(f)
Sit to stand (STS)
    Parkinson disease, 712, 712(f)
    stroke, 580
Situation, in social cognitive theory, 1135, 1135(t)
Situational syncope, 144
6-minute Arm Test (6MAT), 780
6-Minute Pegboard and Ring Test, 398
6-minute Walk Test (6MWT), 9, 143, 157(t),
    235–236(t), 247–248, 277, 285(t), 298,
    348(t), 369, 379, 392, 395, 399, 400,
    456(t), 548(t), 551, 557, 607(t), 610, 661,
    701, 702(t), 706, 739(b), 740–741, 743(t),
    777(t), 781, 875, 922, 990, 1129(t)
Six Spot Step Test, 610
Size and space, in universal design, 295
Skin
    color changes, 34, 35(b)
    observation, 34
    substitutes, 511

Skin anatomy, 940(f), 940–941, 941(t)
Skin care
    amputation, 866, 868–869
    multiple sclerosis, 612–613
    spinal cord injury, 791(f), 791–792, 792(f)
Skin grafts, burns and, 951–953, 952–953(f)
Skin integrity
    multiple sclerosis, 610
    physical assessment for WSM, 1240
Skin perfusion, determining, 488
Skin perfusion pressure (SPP), 490
Skin segment innervation, 70–71(f), 70–72, 86
Skin substitutes, 952–953
Skin surface thermometers, disposable, 40
Sleep counseling, 1144, 1145
Sleep disorders
    amyotrophic lateral sclerosis, 650
    cardiovascular health, 526(t)
    chronic pain, 978
    Parkinson disease, 687, 689
    sleep apnea, 525
    stroke, 539–540
Slide (glide) motion, 116, 117, 117(f), 118(f)
Slings, 577
Slow speed, 245(t)
Small, spastic bladder, 595
Smart appliances, 305
SMART (Specific, Measurable, Attainable,
    Relevant, Timely) goals, 1140
Smartphones, apps for, 226
Smoke alarms, 309
Smoking cessation, 1128
Smoking cessation, 393–396
Smoking cessation counseling, 1144, 1145(b)
Smoking/tobacco use
    cardiovascular health, 526(t)
    stroke risk, 525
    temperature affected by, 35
Snellen chart, 77
SnNOut, 283
Social cognition, 287(t)
Social cognitive theory, 1134, 1135(f), 1135(t),
    1135–1138, 1136–1138(t), 1139(b)
Social determinants of health (SDOHs), 603,
    1120(f)
Social ecological model, 1139, 1140
Social function, 287(t)
Social issues, 464–465
Social life, 782
Social model of aphasia approach, 1110
Social phobia, 689
Social support, 1041
Social worker, 733
Socioeconomic factors, 923
Sociopath, 1020
Socket Comfort Score (SCS), 1201
Socket flexion, 1202
Sockets, prosthetic, 1181
    disarticulation, 1197
    fit, 1201
    hip, 1197(f), 1197–1198
    ischial containment socket, 1195, 1195(f)
    maintenance, 1201
    quadrilateral socket, 1194, 1195(f)
    transfemoral, 1194(f), 1194–1195, 1195(f)
    transtibial, 1186, 1187(f), 1188(f), 1201
Socks, 1187
SOCRATES mnemonic, 984(b)
Sodium hypochlorite (household bleach), 501
Soft dressings, 856(f), 856–857
    elastic shrinkers, 856(f), 856–857
    elastic wraps, 856
Soft end-feel, 116
Software for kinematic/kinetic data, 264
Sole wedges, 1153
Solid AFO, 1158, 1159(f)

Solid ankle AFO, 567
Solid ankle cushion heel (SACH), 1182, 1182(f)
Sollerman Hand Function Test (SHFT), 197(t)
Somatagnosia, 538
Somatic dimensions of pain, 982, 984(b)
Somatic sensory signals, 81, 82(f)
Somatoagnosia, 134, 1085
Somatosensation, 68
Somatosensory cortex, 82, 83–84, 84(f), 184
Somatosensory feedback, 335
Somatosensory inputs, 201
Sorrow, 1015–1016
Sound of respirations, 53–54
Sound Production Treatment, 1114
Southern California Sensory Integration Tests, 1086
Spark Motion, 226
Spasmodic torticollis, 147
Spasmolytics, 543(b)
Spastic bladder, 770
Spastic bowel, 770
Spastic bulbar palsy, 642
Spastic dysarthria, 1112
Spastic hypertonia, 767
Spasticity
    amyotrophic lateral sclerosis, 649–650, 670
    multiple sclerosis, 593, 601–602, 609, 622–623
    strategies, 339, 349(t), 351, 355
    stroke, 553, 575–576
    traumatic brain injury, 735, 736, 738
    upper motor neuron syndrome, 145, 146(t)
Spatial and temporal gait variables, 245–246(t),
        245–256
    description, 245–246(t)
    measurement, 247–256 (See also Instrumented
        systems for determining gait parameters)
        simple methods, 247–248
        timed walked tests, 247–248
Spatial disorganization, 529
Spatial neglect, 1077
Spatial relations disorders, 1086–1090
    clinical examples, 1087–1088
    defined, 1087
    depth and distance perception, 1090
    figure-ground discrimination, 1086–1087, 1087(f)
    form discrimination, 1087
    lesion area, 1088, 1088(f)
    perception, 134, 538
    position in space, 1089
    testing, 1089
    topographical disorientation, 1089–1090
    treatment suggestions, 1089
    vertical disorientation, 1090, 1090(f)
Spatial relations syndrome, 538
Special tests
    arterial and venous function, 490
    lymphoscintigraphy, 482
    synovitis, 898
    tissue-specific tests, 120–121
Specialty evaluation, for WSM, 1243–1248
    evaluation and plan of care, 1247
    wheelchair assessment, 1243–1247, 1248(b)
        measurements, 1243(f), 1243–1245, 1245(f),
            1246(f)
        person/technology match (prescription),
            1226, 1247, 1248(b)
        simulation, 1245–1246, 1247(f)
        technology trial, 1247
Specificity
    neuroplasticity principle, 339(t), 357
    test, 283, 284(b)
Specificity model of pain, 971
Speech deficits
    multiple sclerosis, 629
    Parkinson disease, 688
    stroke, 532
Speech intelligibility, 1102

Speech-language pathologist (SLP), 648, 649,
        732–733, 1099–1100, 1107
Speech pathology, normal, 1100
Speech production, 1101–1102(f), 1101–1104,
        1103(f), 1103(t)
Speech therapist, 1099
Speed, defined, 245(t)
Speed-accuracy trade-off, 156, 686
Sphincter control, 287(t), 288
Sphygmomanometers, 58–59, 60(b)
Spinal accessory nerve, 98(t)
Spinal Cord Independence Measure (SCIM),
        778(t), 782
Spinal cord injury (SCI), 759–814
    activity/participation, 781–782
    body structure/function, 776, 779–781, 780(t)
    case study, 812–814
    classification, 760–765
        ASIA Impairment Scale, 763(b), 763–764
        clinical syndromes, 764(f), 764–765
        complete injuries, 763
        incomplete injuries, 763
        lesion level designation, 762(f), 762–763
        neuroanatomical organization and structure,
            760–762, 761(f)
        zone of partial preservation, 763
    contextual factors, 783
    demographics, 760
    diffusion tensor imaging, 162
    dysautonomia, 144
    etiology, 760
    exercise, 810–811, 811(f)
    gait analysis
        heart rate data, 267
        outcome measures, 234(t), 235(t), 236(t), 240(t)
        Walking Index for Spinal Cord Injury II, 244
    goals and outcomes, 783–787, 784–787(t),
        787(b)
    health, wellness, and prevention, 810–811
    history, 776
    impact, across ICF, 765–773
        activity limitations, 772–773
        body structure/function impairments,
            765–772, 766(t), 769(t)
        participation restrictions, 772–773
        quality of life, 772–773
    isokinetic testing, 142
    medical management, acute, 773–774
        emergency care, 773
        fracture stabilization, 773
        immobilization, 774(f), 774–775
    muscle substitutions, 141–142
    outcome measures, 776, 777–778(t)
    physical rehabilitation, 775(f), 775–776
    physical therapy examination, 776–783
        activity/participation, 781–782
        body structure/function, 776, 779–781, 780(t)
        contextual factors, 783
        history, 776
        outcome measures, 776, 777–778(t)
    physical therapy interventions, 766, 767, 787–809
        activity-directed upper extremity training,
            809
        cardiovascular/endurance training, 792(f),
            792–793
        head-hips relationship, 788, 788(f)
        mobility skills, 793–809, 794–803(f),
            805–806(f), 807(f)
        momentum, 788
        muscle substitution, 788
        precautions, 788(b)
        respiratory, 789(f), 789–791, 790(f)
        skin care, 791(f), 791–792, 792(f)
        strengthening, 789
        task modification, 788
        working in and out of the task, 788

    prognosis for recovery of motor function and
        walking ability, 783
    respiration, 53
    secondary care, 2
    wheelchair and seating system, 809–810
Spinal cord injury EDGE (SCIEDGE), 133
Spinal Cord Injury Functional Ambulation Inven-
        tory (SCI-FAI), 781
Spinal Cord Injury: Functional Rehabilitation,
        801, 804
Spinal Cord Injury Locomotor Trial, 361(t), 363
Spinal cord tracts, 72
Spinal inclinometers, 699
Spinal orthoses, 1165–1169
    cervical, 1167(f), 1167–1168, 1168(f)
    scoliosis, 1168(f), 1168–1169, 1169(f)
    trunk, 1165–1167, 1166(f), 1167(f)
Spinal pathways
    anterolateral spinothalamic system, 78, 81, 82(f)
    dorsal column-medial lemniscal system, 78, 81,
        82(f)
Spinal shock, 147
Spine
    osteoarthritis, 908, 909(f)
    rheumatoid arthritis, 893, 895(f)
Spin motion, 117, 117(f)
Spinoreticular tract, 81
Splinter hemorrhages, 34
Splinting
    burns, 958, 958(t), 959, 959(f), 960(f)
    orthotics, 518
Split-thickness skin graft, 953, 953(f)
Splitting, 1024(b)
Spontaneous recovery, 132(b), 1108
Sporadic ALS, 636
Sporadic olivopontocerebellar atrophy (OPCA),
        681
Sport Concussion Assessment Tool 5 (SCAT5),
        753
Sports prosthetics, 1219–1220
Sports-specific manual wheelchairs, 1269,
        1270–1272, 1272(f), 1273(f)
SpPIn, 283
Sprague Rappaport-type stethoscope, 59
SPRINT-Mind Trial, 427, 428
Sprouting, 639, 640(f), 671
Stability, 137–138, 138(t), 351, 352(t)
Stabilization phase, 580
Stable angina, 432
Staging or grading
    amyotrophic lateral sclerosis, 644–645, 645(t),
        650, 656, 665(t)
    lymphedema, 487–488
    Parkinson disease, 683, 683(t), 696
    pressure injuries, 491, 492(t), 1233–1234
Stairs
    abrasive strips, 302, 302(f)
    exterior, 302, 302(f), 303, 303(f)
    handrails, 302, 303(f), 308
    interior, 308–309, 309(f)
    nosings, 302, 302(f)
    prosthetic training, 1218–1219
    ramps, 302, 303(f)
    stairway lifts, 302–303, 303(f), 308, 309(f)
    tactile warning strips, 308
    vertical platform lifts, 302, 303(f)
Stairway lifts, 302–303, 303(f), 308, 309(f), 670
Stance, 217–219, 218(f), 219(t)
    double limb stance, 217, 218(f), 219
    initial contact, 218(f), 219, 219(t), 221(t),
        222(t), 223(t)
    loading response, 218(f), 219, 219(t), 221(t),
        222(t), 223(t), 256, 262
    midstance, 218(f), 219, 219(t), 221(t), 222(t),
        223(t), 226, 227, 267
    phase of gait cycle, 369

terminal stance, 218(f), 219, 219(t), 221(t), 222(t), 223(t), 227
time, 217, 245, 246(t), 255
Stance control KAFO (SC-KAFO), 1161
Standard deviation (SD), 284
Standard error of measurement (SEM), 284
Standardized Assessment of Concussion, 753
Standards for Accessible Design, ADA and, 294
Standing
control, 205–206
postural alignment, 199, 199(f)
Standing frames, 1163, 1164(f)
Standing wheelchairs, 1269, 1270(f)
Stand/Lean Test, 987
Stand-to-sit transfers, 580–581
Staphylococcus aureus, 391, 946
Start hesitation, 686
Startle reflex, 152(t)
State-Trait Anxiety Inventory, 662
Static allodynia, 988
Static analysis
transfemoral examination, 1210–1211, 1211(f), 1212(f)
transtibial examination, 1209
Static balance, 345, 349(t)
Static examination, 1173
Static postural control, 137–138, 138(t)
Statins, 431(t), 543(b)
Steadiness, 200
Stemmer sign, 482, 490
Stenosis, 444
Stents, drug-eluting, 436
Step length, 217, 218(f), 233, 244, 246(t), 247, 250, 250(f), 262, 265
Stepping over obstacles, 372
Stepping strategy, 204(f), 205
STEPS (Step Training Effectiveness Post Stroke), 345, 360, 361–362(t)
Step time, 218
StepWatch Activity Monitor (SAM), 248, 249, 249(f)
Stereognosis perception, 91
Stereognosis (object recognition) test, 84
Stereotypic synergy, 354, 355
Sternal precautions, 437
Sterno-occipital-mandibular immobilizer (SOMI), 774
Stertor, 54
Stethoscopes, 58, 59, 61(f)
Stimulus
identification, 335
response and, association between, 335
subconscious response, 340
Stimulus control (change process), 1133, 1133(t)
Stool softeners, 603
Stopping Elderly Accidents, Deaths, and Injuries (STEADI), 212(f), 212–213
Stop sounds, 1102, 1103
Stops Walking While Talking Test, 211
Storage areas, kitchen, 316
Stoves, 316, 316(f)
Strain gage technology, 261
Stratum basale, 940–941
Stratum corneum, 940
Stratum granulosum, 940
Stratum spinosum, 940, 941(t)
Strength
arthritis, 916
measurement, in pulmonary disease, 398
multiple sclerosis, 614, 619
physical assessment for WSM, 1241, 1242
Strength training
arthritis, 927–928, 930
motor function, 351–352, 352(t)
Parkinson disease, 711

prosthetic training, 1213, 1215, 1215(f), 1216(f)
pulmonary rehabilitation, 405–406
extremity strength training, 405–406
inspiratory muscle training, 406, 406(f)
spinal cord injury, 789
stroke, 573(f), 573–574
Stress echo, 443
Stretching exercises
prosthetic training, 1213, 1215, 1215(f), 1216(f)
spinal cord injury, 790–791
Striatonigral degeneration (SND), 681
Striatum, 681, 681(f)
Stride, 217–218, 218(f)
Stride Analyzer, 249–250, 251(t), 255, 256
Stride length, 246(t)
Stride time, 218, 246(t)
Strideway Walkway system, 249
Stridor, 54
Stroke, 523–587, 558(t)
activities
examination, 548–552, 549(t), 551(t)
goals, 558(b)
ipsilateral pushing, 563
physical therapy interventions, 561–581
training with visual feedback, 562–563
aerobic capacity, 557
examination, 557
interventions, 581–583
affective status, 536
age, 524
altered consciousness, 532
ambulation classification, 551(t)
balance
examination, 548–550
interventions, 561–563
bladder dysfunction, 538–539
body function and structure
examination, 552–557, 555(t)
goals, 558(b)
interventions, 581
bowel dysfunction, 538–539
cardiovascular dysfunction, 539
cardiovascular health, 526(t)
case study, 585–587
cerebellar impairments, 186
cerebrovascular imaging, 540–541, 541(f)
arteriography, 541
computed tomography, 540, 541(f)
digital subtraction angiography, 541
Doppler ultrasound, 541
magnetic resonance angiography, 541
magnetic resonance imaging, 540–541, 541(f)
children, 527
clinical decision-making, 545
cognitive deficits, 535–536
deep vein thrombosis, 539
defined, 523
diagnosis, 557–558
discharge planning, 583
disordered sleep, 539–540
dysphagia, 535
endurance, 557
epidemiology and etiology, 524–525
examination, 540, 545–557
activities, 548–552, 549(t), 551(t)
ANPT resources, 547
body function and structure, 552–557, 555(t)
clinical practice guidelines for outcome assessment, 547, 548(t)
elements, 546–547(b)
interview, 545–546
order, 547
participation, 547, 548
patient/client history, 546(t)

purposes, 545
systems review, 546(t)
tests and measures, 546–547(t), 547
FAST early warning signs, 525
flexibility, 552–553
focal deficits, 523–524
fracture risk, 539
functional status, 552, 578–581, 579(f)
bed mobility, 579, 579(f)
sitting, 579–580
sit-to-stand transfers, 580
stand-to-sit transfers, 580–581
transfers, 581
gait
examination, 550–551
interventions, 563–567
gait analysis
accelerometer and gyroscope data, 249
cluster analysis, 266
Community Balance and Mobility Scale, 242
Dynamic Gait Index, 242
footswitches and footswitch systems, 255
Functional Ambulation Profile, 240
Functional Assessment Measure, 242
Functional Gait Assessment, 243
heart rate data, 267
Modified Emory Functional Ambulation Profile, 240
normalcy index, 266
observational gait analysis, 226
outcome measures, 234(t), 235(t), 236(t), 237(t), 238(t), 239(t)
Performance Oriented Mobility Assessment, 243
quantitative gait analysis, 244–245
6-minute Walk Test, 247, 248
StepWatch Activity Monitor, 248
2-minute Walk Test, 249
walkway systems, 250, 251(t), 252(t), 253(t), 254(t)
gender, 524, 525, 526
goals and outcomes, 558, 558(t), 583–584
hemispheric behavioral differences, 536–538, 537(t)
hemorrhagic, 523
history, 540
instruction, 583
integumentary integrity, 554
ipsilateral pushing, 550, 563
ischemic, 523
joint integrity, 552–553
language deficits, 532
locomotor training
ambulation, 551(t)
electromechanically assisted locomotor training, 565
examination, 550–551
functional electrical stimulation and ankle-foot orthosis, 565, 566(b)
interventions, 563–567
motor imagery, 566–567
orthotics for lower extremity, 567
task-specific/goal-oriented training, 563–564
training using body weight support and treadmill training, 564–565, 565(f)
virtual reality, 566–567
wheelchairs, 567
management categories, 527
medical diagnosis of stroke health condition, 540–541
medical management, 541–542
modifiable risk factors, 525
motor control, 554–557, 555(t)
coordination, 556–557
cranial nerves, 557

Stroke (*continued*)
Fugl-Meyer Assessment of Physical Performance, 554, 555
motor planning, 557
motor recovery stages, 554, 555(*t*)
muscle performance, 556
obligatory synergy patterns following stroke, 555(*t*)
selective capacity, 555–556
muscle tone, 553
neurological sequelae and associated conditions, 532, 535–540
neurosurgical management, 542
osteoporosis, 539
participation
examination, 547, 548
goals, 558(*b*)
physical therapy interventions, 561
Stroke Impact Scale, 547, 548
pathophysiology, 526–532
perceptual deficits, 538
pharmacological management, 542, 543(*b*)
physical activity
cardiovascular health, 526(*t*)
examination, 548–552, 549(*t*), 551(*t*)
exercise precautions, 582–583
gait and locomotion, 563–567
goals, 558(*b*)
interventions, 581–583
ipsilateral pushing, 563
postural control and balance, 561–563
training with visual feedback, 562–563
upper extremity use, 568–581
physical therapy interventions, 558, 559–583
activities, 561–581
aerobic capacity, 581–583
body function and structure, 581
dose and, 560
environment, structuring, 559–560
feedback, 560
motivation, 560–561
participation, 561
physical activity, 581–583
practice schedule, 560
progression, 560
self-efficacy, 560–561
structure, 559–561
task, goal, learner, 559
plan of care, 542, 543–545
postural control
common postural alignment deviations, 549(*t*)
examination, 548–550
interventions, 561–563
prevention, 525–526
problem list, 15(*t*)
prognosis, 557–558
psychosocial interventions post-stroke, 1049–1050(*t*)
pulmonary dysfunction, 539
pulmonary embolus, 539
race/ethnicity, 524
recovery, 583–584
rehabilitation, 542, 543–545
risk factors, 525
seizures, 538
sensation, 553–554
spasticity, 553
speech deficits, 532
stages of recovery, 542, 543–545
acute phase, 543–544
chronic phase, 544–545
subacute phase, 544
tests and measures, 145, 540, 546–547(*t*), 547
upper extremity use
algorithm for selecting upper extremity interventions, 568, 569(*f*)

constraint-induced movement therapy, 570–571, 571(*f*)
electrical stimulation, 571–572
examination, 551, 552
functional status, 578–581, 579(*f*)
hemianopsia, 576–577
interventions, 568–581
mirror therapy, 572
motor imagery, 572
range of motion management, 574(*b*), 574–575, 575(*f*)
robotic-assisted training, 573
sensory function management, 576
shoulder pain management, 577–578
simultaneous bilateral training, 572–573
spasticity management, 575–576
strengthening, 573(*f*), 573–574
supportive devices, 577
task-specific training, 568–570, 569(*f*), 570(*f*)
unilateral neglect, 576–577
video games, 572
virtual reality, 572
vascular syndromes, 527–532
anterior cerebral artery syndrome, 528, 529(*t*)
cerebral blood flow, 527–528, 528–529(*f*)
internal carotid artery syndrome, 529
lacunar strokes, 531
middle cerebral artery syndrome, 528, 529, 530(*t*)
posterior cerebral artery syndrome, 529, 531, 531(*t*)
vertebrobasilar artery syndrome, 531–532, 533–534(*t*)
vision, 553–554
Stroke Adapted Sickness Impact Profile (SA-SIP30), 1128
Stroke and Aphasia Quality of Life Scale-39 (SAQOL-39), 1107
Stroke Center Network, 526
Stroke clubs, 1111
StrokEDGE, 133, 545, 547
Stroke Impact Scale (SIS), 145, 348(*t*), 547, 548, 1128
Stroke Social Network Scale, 1107
Stroke volume (SV), 43, 419, 419(*f*)
Strollers, 1269, 1271(*f*)
Stroop Test, 716, 1046(*t*), 1074
Structural alterations, 300
Structural imaging techniques, 160–162
characteristics, 164(*t*)
computed tomography, 160–161, 161(*f*)
diffusion tensor imaging, 161–162, 162(*f*)
magnetic resonance imaging, 161, 162(*f*)
radiography (x-ray), 160, 161(*f*)
ST-segment elevation myocardial infarction (STEMI), 428, 433, 435
Stubbies, 1198, 1198(*f*)
Stupor, 75, 532, 729
Subacute phase of stroke recovery, 544
Subacute stage, 122
Subarachnoid hemorrhage (SH), 525, 540
Subconscious response, 340
Subcutaneous layer, 471
Subdermal burn, 945, 945(*f*)
Subendocardial myocardial infarction, 435
Sublimation, 1024(*b*)
Subordinate part, 282
Substance use, 1037–1038
education, 1038
manifestations, 1037(*t*)
medications, 1039–1040(*b*)
patient treatment, 1038
referral, 1038
rehabilitation, 1037, 1038
Substantia nigra, 185, 185(*f*), 681

Substitution, muscle, 129, 132(*b*), 141–142
Subtalar joint
arthritis, 926
capsular patterns, 116(*t*)
foot orthoses, 1152
Subthalamic nucleus (STN), 185, 185(*f*), 681, 695
Suction, 1190
Suction suspension, 1195–1196
Sudden cardiac death, 415, 428
Suicide, 1034, 1037, 1043(*t*)
Sulfamylon, 501
Superficial burns, 491
Superficial partial-thickness burn, 942–943, 943(*f*)
Superficial reflexes, 150, 150(*t*)
Superficial sensations, 78, 87, 89–90
pain perception, 87
pressure perception, 90
temperature awareness, 89, 90(*f*)
touch awareness, 90
Superior canal dehiscence syndrome, 846
Superoxide dismutase 1 (SOD1), 636–638
Superoxide dismutases, 637
Superstructure, 1154, 1156
Supervision, defined, 279(*b*)
Supervision Rating Scale, 740
Supine mat assessment, 1239, 1240(*f*)
Supine-on-elbows, 795, 796(*f*)
Supine roll test, 753, 754(*t*)
Supplemental motor area, 338
Supplemental oxygen, 395
Supplementary motor area (SMA), 183–184, 185, 682
Supported conversation approach, 1110
Supportive devices
Parkinson disease, 720–721
peripheral vascular disease, 493
stroke, 577
Suppression, 1024(*b*)
Supracondylar (SC) suspension, 1189(*f*), 1190, 1190(*f*)
Supramaximal stimulus, 167, 171(*t*)
Suprapubic tapping, 770
Supraventricular ectopy, 445(*f*), 445–446
Supraventricular tachycardia (SVT), 445(*f*), 446
Surface anatomy of the heart, 416(*f*), 416–417
Surgical débridement, 498
Surgical management
amputation, 852–854, 853(*f*), 854(*f*)
postsurgical phase, 857–861, 858(*b*), 859(*f*)
preoperative phase, 857
biosurgery, 499–500, 500(*f*)
burns, 951–953
correction of scar contracture, 953
primary excision, 951
skin grafts, 951–953, 952–953(*f*)
chronic pulmonary dysfunction, 396
joint replacement, 265, 369, 904
Suspension, prosthetic
maintenance, 1201
transfemoral, 1195–1196
locking liners, 1196, 1196(*f*)
suction suspension, 1195–1196
vacuum system, 1196, 1196(*f*)
transtibial, 1187–1191
brim variants, 1190(*f*), 1190–1191
cuff variants, 1187–1189, 1189(*f*)
shuttle lock and pin, 1189(*f*), 1189–1190
suction, 1190
thigh corset, 1191, 1191(*f*)
vacuum-assisted suspension, 1190, 1190(*f*)
Sussman Wound Healing Tool, 493
Sustainable design, 294–295
Sustained attention, 1073
Sustained clonus, 150
Sustained fever, 38(*b*)
Sustained stretching, 575

Sustained V-tach, 447
Swallowing, 629
Swan-Ganz catheter, 420
Sway envelope, 200
Sweat gland activity, 37
Swedish Knee Cage, 567
Swing, 217–219, 220
  initial swing, 218(f), 219, 219(t), 220, 221(t),
    222(t), 223(t)
  midswing, 218(f), 219, 219(t), 220, 221(t),
    222(t), 224(t)
  pre-swing, 218(f), 219, 219(t), 221(t), 222(t),
    223(t)
  terminal swing, 218(f), 219, 219(t), 220, 222(t),
    224(t), 259
Swing-clear hinges, 307
Swing phase of gait cycle, 369
Swing time, 217, 245, 246(t), 255
Sydenham chorea, 182
Syllables, 1100
Symbol Digit Modalities Test (SDMT), 608
Symmetrical tonic neck reflex (STNR), 152(t)
Sympathetic nervous system (SNS), 143, 144(t)
Symptomatic management, 647–648
Synergies
  abnormal, 144–145
  defined, 126, 127(b), 138
  obligatory, 144, 554, 555(t)
  stereotypic, 354, 355
Syntax of language, 1100
Synthetic interferon drugs, 597, 601
Systems models, 355
Systems review (SR), 9, 11–12, 26
  cardiovascular, 9
  chronic pain, 987
  cognition and communication screening, 9
  endocrine, 11
  identification of areas to be examined, 12
  integumentary, 9
  motor function examination, 133
  multiple sclerosis, 606, 606(b)
  musculoskeletal, 9, 105
  neuromuscular, 11
  other major body systems, 12
  Parkinson disease, 698, 698(b)
  pulmonary, 9
  screening for healthy populations, 12
  sensory function, 69(b)
  stroke, 546(t), 559
  vascular, lymphatic, and integumentary
    disorders, 486
  vestibular disorders, 820
Systems theory, 126
Systole, 419
Systolic blood pressure (SBP), 422, 426
Systolic dysfunction, 438, 439
Systolic murmur, 453(t)
Systolic pressure, 55–56, 57, 59, 61, 62, 63

T

Tables, kitchen, 316
Tabletop polishing, 575
Tablets, apps for, 226
Tachycardia, 43, 53, 144
Tachypnea, 54(f), 55
Tactile agnosia, 134, 538, 1092
Tactile localization test, 91–92
Tactile warning strips, 308
Talk test, 451(t)
Talocrural joint, 116(t)
Tampa Scale of Kinesiophobia (TSK), 107
Tamponade, cardiac, 417
Tandem Walking Test, 11
Tapping (foot) test, 193(t)
Tapping (hand) test, 193(t)

Tardieu/Modified Tardieu Scale, 148
Tardieu Scale, 148
TAR DNA-binding protein 43 (TDP-43), 636,
  637, 638, 642
Tarsometatarsal (Lisfranc) amputation, 851(t),
  859, 1181
Task
  activities required for success, 349–350(t)
  analysis, 358
  modification, 300
  motor examination, 340
  motor function, 349(t), 358(f), 358–363
  performance, 129, 156, 158, 535, 537, 537(t)
  stroke, 535, 537, 537(t)
  systems, 126
Tasked-based fMRI, 162, 164(t)
Task-oriented circuit training, 370
Task-specific training, 20, 21(b)
  stroke, 559, 563–564
    upper extremities, 568–570, 569(f), 570(f)
  walking, 371–373, 372–373(f)
Teach back, 5
Team coordinator, 733
Technology
  electronic databases, 25(t)
  motor function assessment, 160–174, 364
  related services, 1227
  wheelchair seating and mobility, 1250–1279,
    1251(f)
    seating support system, 1251–1258, 1252(f)
    technology trial in wheelchair assessment,
      1247
    wheeled mobility devices, 1258–1279,
      1259(f)
Technology-Related Assistance for Individuals
  with Disabilities Act (Tech Act), 1225
Tectospinal tract, 184
Tekscan, 264
Telecommunications Act of 1996, 327
Telecommunications device for the deaf (TDD),
  296(f)
Telehealth/telerehabilitation, 3(b), 296, 297, 646,
  935
Telemetry oximetry, 63
Telephone typewriter (TTY), 295, 296(f)
Telepractice, 1100
Temazepam (Restoril), 1030(b)
Temperature, body, 35–43
  abnormalities, 38(b), 38–39
    decreased body temperature (hypothermia), 39
    increased body temperature (fever), 38(b),
      38–39
  centigrade scale, 35, 36(f)
  circulation, 488
  conversion formula, 36
  factors influencing, 39–40
    age, 39
    emotions/stress, 39
    exercise, 39
    external environment, 39
    measurement site, 40
    medications, 39–40
    time of day, 39
  Fahrenheit scale, 35, 36(f)
  hand hygiene, 42
  integumentary integrity, 491
  measuring, 42–43
  multiple sclerosis, 609
  normal, 36
  temperature-regulating center, 36
  temporal artery temperature, measuring, 42–43
  thermometers, 40–41, 41(f)
  thermoregulatory system, 36–38, 37(f)
Temperature awareness test, 89, 90(f)
  equipment, 84, 85(f)
Temperature-regulating center, 36

Temporal artery temperature
  measuring, 42–43
  thermometers, 40–41, 42–43
Temporal dispersion, 165
Temporal gait variables. See Spatial and temporal
  gait variables
Temporal pulse, 46(f), 47(b)
Temporal summation, 975, 988
Temporary prostheses, 1205
Temporomandibular joint (TMJ), 149(t), 893
10-meter Walk Test (10MWT), 157(t), 234–235(t),
  240, 247, 248, 251(t), 252(t), 276, 286, 298,
  348(t), 369, 379, 456(t), 551, 610, 702(t),
  704, 740, 743(t), 777(t), 990
Tendonotomy, 602
Tendons, 900
Tenodesis grasp, 775, 775(f)
Tensile strength, 472
Teriflunomide (Aubagio), 600(t)
Terminal double limb stance, 217, 218(f), 219
Terminal double limb stance time, 217
Terminal stance, 218(f), 219, 219(t), 221(t),
  222(t), 223(t), 227
Terminal swing, 218(f), 219, 219(t), 220, 222(t),
  224(t), 259
Terminal swing impact, 1212
Termination stage of change, 1132, 1133(b)
Tertiary care, 2, 3(b)
Tertiary intention wound closure, 475
Tertiary prevention, 4(b), 604, 663, 1124, 1125(f)
Test of Everyday Attention, 740
Test-retest reliability, 282
Tests and measures, 13–23
  aerobic capacity/endurance, 486
  anthropometric characteristics, 486–487
    bioelectrical impedance, 487
    girth measurement, 486–487, 487(f)
    height and weight, 486
    tonometry, 487
    volumetric measurement, 486, 486(f)
  arterial insufficiency and ulceration, 479
  chronic pain, 987–990
    activity measures, 990
    balance, 989–990
    cranial nerve integrity, 988
    medical diagnostic testing, 1007
    motor control, 989
    muscle performance, 989
    palpation, 988, 989
    participation measures, 990
    peripheral nerve integrity, 988
    sensory integrity, 988, 989(t)
  chronic pulmonary dysfunction, 397–400
    auscultation of the lungs, 397–398, 398(f)
    dyspnea and quality of life measurement, 398,
      399(t)
    exercise tolerance test, 398, 399–400,
      400(b)
    inspection, 397
    observation, 397, 397(f)
    palpation, 397
    strength and endurance measurement, 398
    vital signs, 397
  diagnosis, 15–16
  discharge planning, 22, 22(b)
  environment
    examples, 297(t)
    workplace, 320(t)
  evaluation, 14–15, 15(t)
  goals and outcomes, 23
  heart disease, 451–454
    angina scale, 454(b)
    body structure and function impairment,
      451–453(t)
    dyspnea scale, 454(b)
    outcome measures, 456–457(t)

Tests and measures (continued)
integumentary system, 486–488
lymphatic system, 486–488
lymphedema, 482
staging or grading, 487–488
motor function, 133
multiple sclerosis, 606(b), 606–611
affective and psychosocial function, 608
balance, gait, and locomotion, 610
cognition, 608
cranial nerve integrity, 609
disease-specific measures, 610–611
environment, 610
fatigue, 609
functional status, 610
general health measures, 610
ICF outcome measures, 607–608(t)
motor function, 609
muscle performance, 609
pain, 609
posture, 610
range of motion, 609
sensation, 609
skin integrity and condition, 610
temperature sensitivity, 609
visual acuity, 609
neuropathy, 485
palpation/pitting scale, 487
Parkinson disease, 698, 699–707, 701–703(t)
autonomic function, 704–705
cardiorespiratory function, 705–706
cognitive function, 705
disease-specific measures, 707
falls and fall risk, 704
fatigue, 705
functional status, 706–707
gait, 704
global health measures, 707
integumentary integrity, 706
motor function, 699–700
musculoskeletal function, 698, 699, 699(f)
nonmotor symptoms, 704–705
orthostatic hypotension, 706
postural control and balance, 700–701, 704
psychosocial function, 705
sensory function, 705
plan of care, 17–22, 23
pressure injuries, 484
problem list, 15, 15(t)
prognosis, 16–17
reexamination of patient, 23
stroke, 540, 546–547(t), 547
vascular system, 486–488
venous insufficiency and ulceration, 480
vestibular disorders, 821(t), 821–828
balance, 827, 827(t)
Dizziness Handicap Inventory, 821, 821(t)
dynamic visual acuity, 826, 827
eye movements, 822–823, 823(f)
gait, 827
Head Impulse Test, 823–824, 824(f), 825(f)
head-shaking induced nystagmus test, 824
Motion Sensitivity Quotient, 822, 822(f)
nystagmus, 822–823, 823(f)
positional testing, 826, 826(f), 827(f)
vestibular function tests, 827, 828
Vestibular Rehabilitation Benefit Questionnaire, 821
visual analogue scale, 821
websites for information, 14
Tetraplegia, 760
Tetraplegia, defined, 141
Texture recognition test, 86, 93
Thalamic syndrome, 89(t)
Theoretical construct, 58

Theoretical frameworks, 1057–1061
cognitive rehabilitation, 1059–1061
neurofunctional approach, 1058
quadraphonic approach, 1059–1061, 1060–1061(f)
rehabilitative/compensatory (functional) approach, 1058–1059
retraining approach, 1057–1058
sensory integrative approach, 1058
Theories, motor learning, 340–341
Theory of Planned Behavior, 1132, 1132(t)
Theory of Reasoned Action, 1132, 1132(f)
TheraPEP PEP Therapy System, 408
Therapeutic alliance, 995
Thermal and nonthermal diathermy, 506
Thermal-tactile stimulation, 629
Thermal testing, 89, 90(f)
Thermanalgesia, 89(t)
Thermanesthesia, 89(t)
Thermhyperesthesia, 89(t)
Thermhypoesthesia, 89(t)
Thermistor, 488
Thermometers, 40–41, 41(f)
automated, 40, 42
glass mercury, 40
noncontact infrared, 41, 41(f)
oral, 40, 41(f)
skin surface, disposable, 40
temporal artery, 40–41, 42–43
tympanic, 41, 41(f), 43
Thermoreceptors, 36, 78, 79(b), 81, 83(t)
Thermoregulation impairment, 768
Thermoregulatory dysfunction, 689
Thermoregulatory system, 36–38, 37(f)
effector organs, 36–38
temperature-regulating center, 36
thermoreceptors, 36
Thigh corset, 1191, 1191(f)
Thigh to lower leg angle measurements, 1245, 1246(f)
Thigh to trunk angle measurements, 1245, 1245(f)
Thigmanesthesia, 89(t)
Thioridazine, 681
Third-degree heart block, 448
30-meter Walk Test, 248
30-second Chair Rise Test, 213, 453(t)
30-second Sit to Stand Test, 990
36-Item Short Form Health Survey (SF-36), 286, 287, 289(t), 610, 662, 707, 1070, 1130(t)
Thomas heel, 1153, 1153(f)
Thoracolumbosacral flexion, extension control (TLS FE) orthosis, 1166–1167, 1167(f)
Thoracolumbosacral flexion control (TLS F) orthosis, 1167
Thoracolumbosacral orthosis (TLSO), 774(f), 774–775, 1166, 1168, 1168(f)
Thready pulse, 44, 45(f), 489
3-minute Walk Test, 248
Three-dimensional (3D) video-based motion analysis systems, 256, 257(f), 258(f), 260
Thresholds, doorway, 304, 307(f)
Thromboangiitis obliterans, 478
Thrombolysis, 526
Thrombolytics, 543(b)
Thumb, 897–898
Thyroxine, 37
Tibiofemoral joint
capsular patterns, 116(t)
osteoarthritis, 926
Tidal volume (TV or V_t), 383
Tilt and recline wheelchairs, 1269
Tilt wheelchairs, 1265(f), 1265–1268, 1266–1267(b), 1268(f)
Timed 25-ft Walk, 608(t), 610
Timed performance, 143, 706

Timed Up and Go (TUG) Test, 11, 209–210, 210(f), 234(t), 249, 277, 284, 285(t), 354, 456(t), 549, 608(t), 610, 661, 662, 700, 703(t), 704, 990
Timed walk tests, 247–248. See also individual walk tests
Time to fatigue, 619
Timing, neuroplasticity principle of, 339(t), 356
Tinetti Balance Test, 661
Tinetti Falls Efficacy Scale (FES), 211
Tinetti Gait Assessment, 701
Tinetti Performance Oriented Mobility Assessment (POMA), 207, 210, 233, 239(t), 244, 610, 661–662
TipSheet, 596
Tip-therm, 84, 85(f)
Tissue plasminogen activator (tPA), 526
Tissue-specific tests (TSTs), 120–121
Title II and Title III of the ADA, 326–327
Titubation, 188, 190(t)
Tizanidine (Zanaflex), 601, 649–650
Toe boxing, 1151(f), 1152
Toe off, 218, 219(t)
Toe(s)
disarticulation, 851(t)
gait deviations, 227(t), 228(t)
osteoarthritis, 908, 908(f)
rheumatoid arthritis, 898, 899(f)
Toe spring, 1151, 1151(f)
Toe-to-examiner's finger test, 194(t)
Toilets
accessible, 311, 311(f)
transfers, 1237
Tolerance for error, in universal design, 295
Tone, muscle
abnormal, 145–148, 146(t), 148(t)
amyotrophic lateral sclerosis, 663
decerebrate rigidity, 147
decorticate rigidity, 146–147
defined, 145
documentation, 148
dystonia, 147
examination, 147–148, 148(t)
factors influencing, 145
hypotonia, 147
initial observation, 147
Modified Ashworth Scale, 148, 148(t)
passive motion testing, 147–148
rigidity, 145, 146
spasticity, 145, 146(t)
stroke, 553
Tardieu/Modified Tardieu Scale, 148
Tonic firing rate, 818
Tonic reflexes, 151, 152(t)
Tonometry, 487
Tool for Assessing Wheelchair Discomfort (TAWC), 1281(t)
Topical agents, 500–502
acute wounds, 502
analgesics, 501
antibacterials, 501
antiseptics, 500–501
burns, 946, 951(t)
growth factors, 501–502
Topical hyperbaric oxygen (THBO), 507
Topical oxygen, 507
Topographical disorientation, 134, 201, 538, 1089–1090
Torque, 120, 261, 261(t)
Total body surface area (TBSA), 940, 946, 947(f), 948, 954, 961
Total contact casting (TCC), 518
Total Heart Beat Index, 268
Total lung capacity (TLC), 383
Total surface bearing socket, 1186
Touch, decreased sensitivity to, 612–613

Touch awareness test, 84, 90
Touch Test Sensory Evaluator, 95–96, 96(f)
Towel racks, 313
Toxic parkinsonism, 681
Trachea, 51, 51(f)
Tracheostomy, 51
Traction injury, 577
Traction reflex, 151, 152(t)
Traffic light approach, 402, 401(f)
Trail Making Test, 1074
Trail Making Test Part B, 740
Transcortical motor aphasia, 1105(t)
Transcranial direct current stimulation (tDCS), 379
Transcranial Doppler ultrasound, 541
Transcranial magnetic stimulation (TMS), 650, 783
Transcutaneous electrical nerve stimulation
    (TENS), 1002, 1006–1007
Transcutaneous oxygen (TcPO₂), 490
Transdermal hyoscine (scopolamine), 648
Transfemoral (above knee) amputation, 851(t)
    balance training, 860
    causes, 850–851
    contracture, 859
    elastic wraps, 856
    exercises for muscle function, 870(f)
    functional status, 864
    muscle strength, 863
    postsurgical dressings, 855(f), 856, 856(f)
    range of motion, 861, 869
    residual limb examination, 861
    residual limb wrapping, 866, 866(b), 868(b),
        868(f)
    shrinkers, 856(f)
    surgery, 852, 853(f), 854
Transfemoral examination, 1209, 1210–1212
    dynamic analysis, 1211–1212
        compensations/deviations, viewed from
            behind, 1211–1212
        compensations/deviations, viewed from the
            side, 1212
    prosthetic and skin analysis with prosthesis off
        the patient, 1210
    static analysis, 1210–1211, 1211(f), 1212(f)
Transfemoral prostheses, 1191–1196
    alignment, 1202(f), 1202–1203, 1203(f)
    bilateral, 1198, 1198(f)
    foot-ankle assemblies and shanks, 1191
    knee units, 1191–1194, 1192(f), 1193(f),
        1194(f)
    sockets, 1194(f), 1194–1195, 1195(f)
    suspensions, 1195–1196, 1196(f)
Transference, neuroplasticity principle of, 339(t),
    360
Transfer of learning, 158
Transfer of training, 344–345, 345(t)
Transfer-of-training approach, 1057, 1086
Transfer(s)
    descriptive terminology, 279(b)
    Functional Independence Measure (FIM),
        287(t), 288
    prosthetic training, 1215, 1216
    spinal cord injury, 798–801, 799–801(f)
        floor-to-wheelchair transfers, 800–801,
            800–801(f)
        sit-pivot transfers, 798–800, 799(f)
    stroke, 581
Transfer tests, 158, 159(b)
Transient ischemic attack (TIA), 527
Transitional mobility, 137, 138(t)
Translatory accessory motions, 117
Transmagnetic stimulation (TMS), 172(t),
    173–174
Transmetatarsal amputation, 851(t), 852, 1181
Transmural MI, 435
Transparent films, 509, 509(f)
Transpelvectomy, 851(t)

Transpelvic amputation, 1197, 1197(f)
Transportation, 323–324
    community access, 323(f), 323–324, 324(f),
        325(f)
    public transportation systems, ADA and, 327
Transport chairs, 1269, 1271(f)
Transtheoretical Model (TTM), 1132–1134
    key constructs, 1132(t)
    processes of change, 1133(t)
    self-efficacy questionnaire, 1134(t)
    stage of change questionnaire, 1134(b)
    stages of change, 1133(b)
Transtheoretical Model of Behavior Change, 992
Transtibial (below knee) amputation, 851(t)
    balance and mobility activities, 871, 871(f)
    causes, 850–851
    contracture, 859
    elastic wraps, 856
    exercises for muscle function, 870(f)
    muscle strength, 863
    positioning strategies, 859, 859(f)
    postsurgical dressings, 855, 855(t), 856, 856(f)
    range of motion, 861, 869
    residual limb care, 860
    residual limb examination, 861
    residual limb wrapping, 866, 866(b), 867(f)
    shrinkers, 856(f), 866
    surgery, 852, 853, 853(f), 854(f), 858(b)
Transtibial examination, 1208–1209
    dynamic analysis, 1209
    gait compensations/deviations, 1210(t)
    prosthetic and skin analysis with prosthesis off
        the patient, 1208–1209
    static analysis, 1209
Transtibial prostheses, 1182–1191
    alignment, 1202, 1202(f), 1203(f)
    bilateral ankle disarticulation, 1198
    foot-ankle assemblies, 1182–1185
        articulated, 1184–1185, 1184–1185(f)
        nonarticulated, 1182–1184, 1182–1184(f)
        rotators and shock absorbers, 1185, 1185(f)
    liners, 1187, 1188(f)
    shanks, 1185–1186
        endoskeletal shank, 1185, 1186(f)
        exoskeletal shank, 1185, 1186(f)
    sockets, 1186, 1187(f), 1188(f)
    socks, 1187
    suspension, 1187–1191
        brim variants, 1190(f), 1190–1191
        cuff variants, 1187–1189, 1189(f)
        shuttle lock and pin, 1189(f), 1189–1190
        suction, 1190
        thigh corset, 1191, 1191(f)
        vacuum-assisted suspension, 1190, 1190(f)
Transverse myelitis, 596
Tranylcypromine (Parnate), 1036(b)
Trauma-Focused Cognitive Behavioural Therapy
    (TF-CBT), 1048
Trauma-informed care, 1045, 1048, 1050
Traumatic axonal injury (TAI), 727–728
Traumatic brain injury (TBI), 726–758
    abnormal autonomic function, 143, 144
    abnormal postural control, 145
    case study, 756–758
    characteristics, 731, 731(t)
    compensatory interventions, 20
    continuum of care, 732
    coordination impairments, 182
    defined, 727
    diagnosis, 731
    electroencephalography, 173
    gait analysis
        Functional Assessment Measure, 242
        outcome measures, 235(t), 238(t)
    Glasgow Coma Scale, 731, 731(f)
    hospitalization, 1057

    imaging, 161–162
    impact, 728(b), 728–731
        activity limitations, 730
        body structure/function impairments,
            728–730, 730(b)
        long-term impact, 730–731
        participation restrictions, 730
    interdisciplinary team, 732–734
    mechanism of injury and pathophysiology,
        727–728
        primary injury, 727–728
        secondary injury, 728
    medical management, early, 734
    mild TBI
        clinical trajectories, 751–752
        defined, 751
        diagnosis, 751
        evidence-based care, 755
        physical therapy management, 752–755
        postconcussion symptoms, 751(t)
    neurobehavioral impairments, 729, 731, 749
    physical therapy interventions
        aerobic exercise, 755
        cervical musculoskeletal, 754
        motor, 755
        vestibular-oculomotor, 754–755
    physical therapy management, 734–755
        during active rehabilitation, 739–751
        behavioral factors, 749, 750(t)
        community reentry, 749, 751(t)
        community reentry/reintegration, 742, 749,
            751(t)
        early after injury, 734–738, 737(f)
        early mobilization, 736, 737
        education, 738, 754, 754(b)
        examination during active rehabilitation,
            739(b), 739–742, 741(f)
        examination early after injury, 734–736,
            736(b)
        global functioning, 741–742
        goals and outcomes, 736, 737(b), 742, 743(t)
        hypertonicity, 738
        mild TBI, 752–755
        outcome measures, 735–736, 736(b), 739(b),
            740–741, 741(f)
        quality of life, 742
        secondary impairments, 737–738,
            737–738(f)
        sensory stimulation, 738
        spasticity, 738
    plan of care, 23
    prevalence, 727
    prognosis, 17, 731
    secondary care, 2
Traumatic brain injury EDGE (TBIEDGE), 133
Traumatic spinal cord injury (SCI), 760
Trazodone (Desyrel), 1036(b)
Treadmills, 262
Treadmill training (TMT)
    locomotor function, 370, 371–373
    multiple sclerosis, 626
    robot-assisted, 626
    spinal cord injury, 787
    stroke, 557, 564–565, 565(f)
Tremor, 188, 189, 190(t), 195(t), 684
Tremor-dominant (TD) phenotype, 680
Trendelenburg Test, 490
Triaxial accelerometers, 248
Triazolam (Halcion), 1030(b)
Triceps, 149(t)
Tricuspid valve, 418
Tricyclic antidepressants (TCAs), 53, 650, 1007
Trigeminal nerve (CN V), 98(t), 151, 153(t), 639,
    659
Trigeminal neuralgia, 592
Trigeminy, 444, 445(f), 447

Trihexyphenidyl (Artane), 648
Trimipramine maleate (Surmontil), 1036(b)
Trinity Amputation and Prosthesis Experience
    Scales-Revised (TAPES-R), 1204
Triple network model of pain, 972
Trochanter-knee-ankle (TKA) line, 1193, 1202
Trochlear nerve (CN IV), 98(t), 151, 153(t)
Trophic changes
    circulation, 489
    integumentary, 490
Trunk
    gait deviations, 232(t)
    spasticity in UMN syndrome, 146(t)
Trunk-hip-knee-ankle-foot orthoses (THKAFO),
    1150, 1163, 1172
Trunk Impairment Scale, 607(t)
Trunk movements, balance training and, 562
Trunk orthoses, 1150, 1165–1167
    corsets, 1165–1166, 1166(f)
    lumbosacral flexion, extension, lateral control
        orthosis, 1166, 1166(f)
    lumbosacral orthoses, 1166
    thoracolumbosacral flexion, extension control
        orthosis, 1166–1167, 1167(f)
    thoracolumbosacral orthoses, 1166
TSA-II NeuroSensory Analyzer + VSA 3000
    Vibratory Sensory Analyzer, 94(f), 94–95,
    95(f)
Tub transfer bench, 312–313, 313(f)
TUG cognitive (TUGcog), 210, 608(t)
TUG manual (TUGman), 210
Tulane Stroke Registry, 1104
Tuning reflexes, 151
Tunneling, 474, 476, 483
Turning schedules, 484
12-item MS Walking Scale, 607(t)
12-lead electrocardiogram (ECG), 434–436,
    435(f)
12-minute Walk Test (12MWT), 157(t), 248,
    557, 706
TWIST prediction tool, 558
2-minute Step Test (2MST), 456(t)
2-minute Walk Test (2MWT), 9, 11, 236–237(t),
    248, 249, 456(t), 557, 610, 655(t), 706,
    882(t), 990
Two-dimensional (2D) video-based motion
    analysis systems, 256
Two-point discrimination test
    combined cortical sensations, 92
    equipment, 85, 85(f)
    variations, 83
2010 ADA Standard for Accessible Design, 322
Tympanic membrane temperature, measuring, 43
Tympanic thermometers, 41, 41(f), 43
Type A personality, 1019
Typical neuroleptic drugs, 681
Tysabri, 601

U

Uhthoff symptom, 591
Ulceration, 479–480
    arterial insufficiency, 478–479
    clinical presentation, 480, 480(f)
    defined, 478, 479
    history, 480
    intervention, 480
    pressure-redistributing devices, 517, 517(f)
    tests and measures, 480
    venous insufficiency, 479–480
Ultrasound (US), 502, 502(f), 503–505(t)
Ultraviolet (UV) radiation, 506
Umbilical deviation, 150, 150(t)
UMN bladder, 770
Underdosing, 353
Undermining, 474, 476, 483

Understanding Aphasia: A Guide for Family and
    Friends, 1107
Undoing, 1024(b)
Unequal step length, 1212
Uneven heel rise, 1212
Unified Dyskinesia Rating Scale (UDysRS), 700
Unified Parkinson's Disease Rating Scale
    (UPDRS), 369, 683, 709
Uniform Data System for Medical Rehabilitation
    (UDSMR), 136, 287. See also Functional
    Independence Measure (FIM)
Uniform Federal Accessibility Standards, 294
Unilateral neglect, 1077–1078(f), 1077–1079,
    1079(f)
    body scheme/body image impairments, 134
    clinical examples, 1078
    defined, 1077–1078
    lesion area, 1078
    stroke, 529, 538, 576–577
    testing, 1078
    treatment suggestions, 1078–1079
        compensatory approach, 1079
        prism adaptation, 1079, 1080–1084(t)
        remedial approach, 1078–1079
Unilateral spatial neglect, 1077
Unilateral vestibular hypofunction, 833, 834–837
    gaze stability exercises, 835, 835(f)
    habituation exercises, 836, 837, 837(f)
    postural stability exercises, 836, 836(f), 836(t)
Unilateral visual inattention, 1077
Uninvolved stance time, 240, 246(t)
United Nations Convention on the Rights of
    Persons with Disabilities (UNCRPD),
    1225
U.S. Department of Defenses (DoD), 752
U.S. Department of Health and Human Services
    (HHS), 33, 72, 465, 517, 1120
U.S. Department of Justice, 322
U.S. Department of Labor, 321
U.S. Department of Veterans Affairs (VA), 752
U.S. Preventive Services Task Force (USPSTF),
    58, 427, 1129, 1131
Universal design (UD), 294–295
University of Buffalo Foundation Activities, 241
University of California Biomechanics Laboratory
    (UCBL) insert, 1154, 1154(f)
Unna boot, 512–513
Unna-FLEX, 513
Unobservable event, 58
Unresponsive wakefulness, 729
Unstable angina, 432
Unstageable pressure injury, 1234
Unvoiced sound, 1103
Upper extremities (UE)
    amyotrophic lateral sclerosis, 668
    spinal cord injury, 781–782, 809
    stroke
        algorithm for selecting interventions, 568,
            569(f)
        balance training, 562
        constraint-induced movement therapy,
            570–571, 571(f)
        electrical stimulation, 571–572
        examination, 551, 552
        functional status, 578–581, 579(f)
        hemianopsia, 576–577
        interventions, 568–581
        mirror therapy, 572
        motor imagery, 572
        obligatory synergies, 554, 555(t)
        range of motion management, 574(b),
            574–575, 575(f)
        robotic-assisted training, 573
        sensory function management, 576
        shoulder pain management, 577–578
        simultaneous bilateral training, 572–573

        spasticity management, 575–576
        strengthening, 573(f), 573–574
        supportive devices, 577
        task-specific training, 568–570, 569(f),
            570(f)
        unilateral neglect, 576–577
        video games, 572
        virtual reality, 572
    traumatic brain injury, 746(f), 746–747
Upper-limb orthoses, 1169, 1170(t)
Upper limb prostheses, 1198–1200
    activity specific, 1200, 1200(f)
    body powered, 1199
    hybrid, 1200
    myoelectric, 1199, 1200(f)
    passive, 1198–1199, 1199(f)
Upper motor neuron (UMN) injuries, 765
Upper motor neurons (UMNs), 336
Upper motor neuron syndrome (UMN), 140, 593,
    636, 636(t)
    abnormal postural control, 145
    abnormal synergies, 144
    amyotrophic lateral sclerosis, 640–641, 641(t),
        642, 643–644, 644(f)
    deep tendon reflexes, 149
    differential diagnosis, 174(t)
    hypotonia, 147
    impairments, 641(t), 642
    motor weakness/muscle atrophy, 141
    positive and negative features, 140(t)
    primitive/tonic reflexes, 151
    rigidity, 145
    spasticity, 145, 146(t)
    superficial reflexes, 150, 150(t)
Urinary incontinence, 529(t), 538, 554, 620–621,
    689, 770
Urinary tract infections (UTIs), 595, 602, 765
Usual interstitial pneumonia, 391

V

Vacuum-assisted closure (VAC), 507
Vacuum-assisted suspension, 1190, 1190(f)
Vacuum system, 1196, 1196(f)
VA/DoD CPG, 752
Vagus nerve (CN X), 98(t), 151, 154(t),
    639, 659
Validity
    ambulation profiles and scales, 233
    instrumented walkways, 250, 251–255(t)
    instrument measures of function, 283–284,
        284(b)
Valproate, 681
Valsalva maneuver, 57–58, 351, 398, 770
Valves
    heart replacements, 444
    vein, 470
Valvular heart disease, 444
Vamp, 1151, 1151(f)
Vancomycin-resistant enterococcus, 506
Varenicline tartrate (Chantix), 1040(b)
Variable error, 157(t)
Variable friction, 1193
Variable Intensity Early Walking Post-Stroke
    (VIEWS), 360
Variable positioning manual wheelchairs,
    1265–1269
    recline, 1268(f), 1268–1269
    standing, 1269, 1270(f)
    tilt, 1265–1268, 1266–1267(b),
        1268(f)
    tilt and recline, 1269
Variable practice, 344, 345(t), 370
Variable practice schedule, 560
Variant or Prinzmetal angina, 432–433
Varicella-zoster viruses, 589

Vascular syndromes, 527–532
  anterior cerebral artery syndrome, 528, 529(t)
  cerebral blood flow, 527–528, 528–529(f)
  internal carotid artery syndrome, 529
  lacunar strokes, 531
  middle cerebral artery syndrome, 528, 529, 530(t)
  posterior cerebral artery syndrome, 529, 531, 531(t)
  vertebrobasilar artery syndrome, 531–532, 533–534(t)
Vascular system
  anatomy and physiology, 470
  arterial system, 470
  disorders, 478–480
    arterial insufficiency and ulceration, 478–479
    instruction, 495
    resources, 495
    rheumatoid arthritis, 900
    venous insufficiency and ulceration, 479–480
  evaluation, 494
  examination, 485–490
    arousal, attention, and cognition, 488
    assistive and adaptive devices, 488
    circulation, 488–490
    gait, locomotion, and balance, 490
    history, 485–486
    muscle performance, 493
    orthotic, protective, and supportive devices, 493
    pain, 493
    posture, 493
    range of motion, 493–494
    risk factor assessment, 493
    self-care and home management, 494
    sensation, 494, 494(f)
    systems review, 486
    tests and measures, 486–488
    ventilation and respiration, 494
  intervention, 494–496
    coordination, communication, and documentation in, 495
    procedural, 495–496
  venous system, 470
Vasoconstriction, 37, 56, 470
Vasodilation, 56, 470
Vasodilators, 428, 431(t), 438
Vasomotor center, 56
Vasomotor tone, 56
Vasovagal syncope, 144
Vaulting, 1173, 1212
Veins, 470
Velocity storage system, 820
Venlafaxine (Effexor), 602, 1036(b)
Venous Filling Time, 490
Venous insufficiency, 479–480
  clinical presentation, 480, 480(f)
  defined, 479
  history, 480
  intervention, 480
  tests and measures, 480
Venous patency, 490
Venous reflux, 470
Venous stasis ulcer, 479
Venous system, 470
Venous thromboembolism (VTE), 670
Venous wounds, 515–516
Ventilation, 383, 384
  accessory muscles, 388(f)
  tests and measures, 494
Ventricular bigeminy, 445(f), 447
Ventricular ectopy, 445(f), 446–447, 446(f)
Ventricular fibrillation (V-fib), 416, 444, 445(f), 447
Ventricular gallop, 453(t)
Ventricular tachycardia (V-tach), 416, 444, 445(f), 447

Ventrolateral (VL) nucleus, 682
Ventromedial pathways, 127, 129(f)
Ventroposterolateral (VPL) nucleus, 81, 82(f)
Verapamil, 681
Verbal aphasia, 532, 1105(t), 1105–1106, 1108
Verbal instructional sets, 715
Verbal Rating Scale, 981
Vertebral arteries, 528, 531–532
Vertebrobasilar arteries, 528(f), 531–532
Vertebrobasilar artery syndrome, 531–532, 533–534(t)
Vertical disorientation, 134, 1090, 1090(f)
Vertical platform lifts, 302, 303(f)
Vertigo, 820
Vesicoureteral reflux, 770
Vesicular breath sounds, 53, 397
Vestibular anatomy, 816–817
  central vestibular system, 817, 817(f)
  otolith organs, 817, 817(f)
  peripheral vestibular system, 816
  semicircular canals, 816(f), 816–817
Vestibular atelectasis, 844
Vestibular disorders, 815–848
  case study, 847–848
  coordination impairments, 182
  diagnoses, 843–846
    cervicogenic dizziness, 846
    Mal de Debarquement, 845
    Ménière Disease, 843–844
    multiple sclerosis, 845
    multiple system atrophy, 845–846
    perilymphatic fistula, 844
    superior canal dehiscence syndrome, 846
    vestibular atelectasis, 844
    vestibular migraine, 845
    vestibular paroxysmia, 845
    vestibular schwannoma, 844
  examination, 820–828
    duration and circumstances of symptoms, 821
    history and systems review, 820
    identification of symptoms, 820, 820(t)
    mild TBI, 753
    tests and measures, 821(t), 821–828, 822–827(f), 827(t)
  gait analysis
    Dynamic Gait Index, 242, 243
    Functional Gait Assessment, 243
    outcome measures, 237(t), 238(t), 239(t)
  pathology, 828–831
    central nervous system pathology, 830
    peripheral/central vestibular pathology, differentiating, 830–831, 831(f), 831(t)
    peripheral pathology, 828–830, 829(f)
  physical therapy interventions, 831–843
    abnormal central vestibular function, 838
    benign paroxysmal positional vertigo, 831, 832(f), 832(t), 832–833, 833(f), 834(f), 834(t)
    bilateral vestibular hypofunction, 837, 838, 838(t), 839–843(t)
    education, 838
    mild TBI, 754–755
    unilateral vestibular hypofunction, 833, 834–837, 835(f), 836(f), 836(t), 837(f)
  physiology and motor control, 818–820
    inhibitory cutoff, 819–820
    push-pull mechanism, 819, 819(f)
    tonic firing rate, 818
    velocity storage system, 820
    vestibulo-ocular reflex (VOR), 818(f), 818(t), 818–819, 819(f)
    VOR gain and phase, 818(f), 818–819
  postural control and balance, 201–202
  rehabilitation contraindications, 846
  vestibular system dysfunction, 828–831

central nervous system pathology, 830
  peripheral/central vestibular pathology, differentiating, 830–831, 831(f), 831(t)
  peripheral pathology, 828–830, 829(f)
Vestibular dysfunction EDGE (VestibularEDGE), 133
Vestibular-evoked myogenic potentials (VEMPS), 687
Vestibular feedback, 335
Vestibular function tests, 827–828
  otolith tests, 828
  semicircular canal tests, 827, 828
Vestibular migraine, 845
Vestibular/Ocular Motor Screening (VOMS), 753, 754(t)
Vestibular paroxysmia, 845
Vestibular positional tests, 753, 754(t)
Vestibular Rehabilitation Benefit Questionnaire (VRBQ), 821
Vestibular schwannoma, 844
Vestibulocochlear nerve (CN VIII), 98(t), 151, 154(t)
Vestibulo-ocular reflex (VOR), 202, 818(f), 818(t), 818–819, 819(f)
Vestibulo-spinal reflexes, 202
Vestibulospinal tracts, 184
Vest System, 408, 411(f)
Veterans Administration, 322, 326
Vibration, decreased sensitivity to, 612–613
Vibration perception test, 84, 91
Vibratron, 609
Vicon, 256
Video-based motion analysis systems, 256
Videofluoroscopic swallowing studies (VFSSs), 535, 629
Video games, 572
Videography, 226
Video-recorded case studies, 139
VIEWS (Variable Intensity Early Walking Post-Stroke), 362–363(t), 363
Violence, 1038, 1040, 1043(t)
Viral infections, 638
Virtual reality (VR)
  locomotor function, 373–374, 374(f)
  multiple sclerosis, 614
  Parkinson disease, 715
  stroke, 563, 566–567, 572
Visceral pain, 967, 969(t)
Visceral pericardium, 417
Viscous loads, 351, 352(t)
Vision, 201
  cognitive and perceptual dysfunction, 1063–1065, 1064(f), 1065(f)
  motor coordination, 182
  multiple sclerosis, 609, 612
  preliminary tests, 77
  role in motor control, 334, 335
  screening for WSM, 1239
  stroke, 537(t), 553–554
  technology, 319(b)
Visual 3D software, 264
Visual agnosias, 201, 531, 1091–1092, 1091–1092(f)
Visual analogue scale (VAS), 281, 281(f), 661, 821, 981
  fatigue, 607(t), 609
Visual attention, 1063
Visual cancellation tasks, 1057
Visual cognition, 1063
Visual cues, 708
Visual feedback, 357, 562–563
Visual field deficit, 1063–1064, 1064(f)
Visual imagery, 377
Visual object agnosia, 134, 538
Visual perceptual impairment, 1065
Visual proprioception, 201

Visual scanning, 1057, 1063, 1065
Vital capacity (VC), 779
Vital signs, 31–66
  alterations in values, 33
  baseline values, 32
  case study, 65–66
  chronic pulmonary dysfunction examination, 397
  clinical decision-making, 32
  culture, 33
  lifestyle patterns, 33
  normative values, 32(t), 32–33
  observation, 34–35, 35(b), 35(f)
  patient characteristics, 33
  recording results, 32, 64–65
  resources, 32(t), 32–33, 65
  See also Blood pressure; Pulse; Respiration;
    Temperature, body
VITAMINS mnemonic, 596
Vocal cords, 50, 51(f), 1102
Vocal tract, 1101(f), 1101–1102, 1102(f)
Vocational rehabilitation counselor (VCR),
  733–734
Voice- and noise-activated (clapping) lighting
  controls, 305
Voiced sound, 1103
Volition, 1075
Volumetric measurement, 486, 486(f)
Voluntary closing (VC) controls, 1199, 1199(f)
Voluntary movement, 336
Voluntary opening (VO) controls, 1199, 1199(f)
Voluntary saccades, 687
Von Frey Aesthesiometer II, 95, 95(f)
VOR gain and phase, 818(f), 818–819
Vowels, 1100, 1103
V/Q matching, 440–441

W

Wagner Ulcer Grade Classification, 493
Walkabout, 1161–1162, 1162(f)
Walkaide, 1159
Walking Impairment Questionnaire, 489
Walking Index for Spinal Cord Injury (WISCI),
  369, 777(t), 781
Walking Index for Spinal Cord Injury II (WISCI
  II), 233, 240(t), 244
Walking skills
  balancing training, 562
  capacity measures, clinic-based, 369
  compensatory-based approach, 804–806,
    805–806(f)
  four-point pattern, 806
  functional, recovery-based approach, 806–807,
    807(f)
  function examination, 368–370
  overground walking, 372–373(f), 375–377,
    376(b), 376(f)
  performed in parallel bars, 805–806
  performed in parallel bars progressed to
    overground, 806
  performed in sitting or supine, 805
  push ups, 806
  putting on and removing orthoses, 805
  sit-to-stand activities, 805, 806(f)
  spinal cord injury, 783, 804–809, 805–806(f),
    807(f)
  static standing balance, 805
  swing-through pattern, 805(f), 806
  technologies to enhance walking recovery,
    808–809
  traumatic brain injury, 745, 746
  walking while carrying objects, 372, 373(f)
  weight shifting in standing, 805, 806
Walking Trail-Making Test, 716
Walking velocity, 244, 245(t), 250(f), 264
Walking While Talking (WWT) Test, 211

Walk tests. See individual walk tests
Walkway systems
  GAITRite, 250, 250(f), 251–255(t)
  Zeno Walkway system, 250, 254(t), 255(f)
Wallerian degeneration, 128, 131(f), 165
Wardrobe lifts, 310, 310(f)
Warm-up decrement, 156
Warm-up period of exercise, 351, 352(t)
Water volume-control mechanisms, 313
Weak functional cough, 779
Weakness, defined, 141
Weak pulse, 44, 45(f), 489
Wearing-off, 694
Wedge, 1154
WeeFIM, 288
Weight
  acceptance, 217, 218(f), 219
  classification by body mass index, 1120(f)
  counseling, healthy, 1144, 1145(b)
  distribution, 199(f), 199–201, 200(f)
  gain from edema, 440, 453(t)
  measurement, 486
  test for recognition (barognosis), 93, 93(f)
Well-being, 272
Well Criteria for DVT, 490
Wellness, 2, 4(b)
  defined, 1123, 1124
  domains, 1124(f)
  health promotion and, 1123–1124
  measures, 1127–1128
  rehabilitation, 1041–1042
Wenckebach, 448
Wernicke aphasia, 1104, 1105(t), 1106, 1108
Wernicke/sensory/receptive aphasia, 532
Western Aphasia Battery-Revised, 1107
Western Ontario and McMaster Universities
  Osteoarthritis Index (WOMAC), 107
Westmead Home Safety Assessment (WeHSA),
  299(t)
Wet-to-dry (WTD) dressing, 498, 509
Wheelchair Examination & Specialty Evaluation,
  1228, 1229(t)
Wheelchair Outcome Measure (WHOM),
  1281(t)
Wheelchair propulsion, 781
Wheelchairs
  amyotrophic lateral sclerosis, 670
  benefits, 1126(b)
  delivery, 1249
  fitting, 1249
  flaccid arm support, 577
  function from, 1249
  joystick control, 627–628, 628(f)
  maintenance/repairs/follow-up, 1250
  measurements, 1243(f), 1243–1245, 1245(f),
    1246(f)
    body segment angles, 1245, 1245(f)
    considerations, 1243(f), 1243–1244
    linear body measurements, 1243(f),
      1244–1245
  mobility, 1249
  multiple sclerosis, 627–628, 628(f)
  person/technology match (prescription), 1226,
    1247, 1248(b)
  shower entries, 314, 314(f)
  simulation, 1245–1246, 1247(f)
  skills
    ascending and descending inclines, 801–802
    power wheelchair driving tasks, 804
    propulsion on even surfaces, 801, 801(f)
    training, 1249–1250, 1250(f)
    wheelies, 802–803(f), 802–804
  spinal cord injury, 801–803(f), 801–804,
    809–810
  stroke, 567, 577
  technology trial, 1247

  training, 1249–1250, 1250(f)
  transfers, 798–801, 799–801(f)
    floor-to-wheelchair transfers, 800–801,
      800–801(f)
    sit-pivot transfers, 798–800, 799(f)
  user rights, 1125
  user seating and positioning needs, 1124(f),
    1224–1225
  wheelchair-accessible bathroom, space
    requirements for, 314, 315(f)
  See also Manual wheelchairs; Power wheelchairs;
    Wheelchair seating and mobility (WSM);
    Wheeled mobility devices
Wheelchair seating and mobility (WSM), 1223–1284
  appropriate vs. inappropriate device, 1226
  case study, 1283–1284
  communication tips, 1235
  defensible documentation, 1280
  examination, 1235–1243
    assessment interview, 1235–1236
    equipment assessment, 1237
    functional assessment, 1237–1238
    physical assessment, 1239–1243
    screening of body functions and structures,
      1238–1239
  funding, 1280
  intervention, 1249–1250
  maintenance/repairs/follow-up, 1250
  mobility principles, 1234–1235
  mobility-related assistive technology, defined,
    1225–1226
  outcome measurement, 1280, 1281(t)
  person-technology match, 1226
  pressure injuries, 1233–1234
  principles, 1230–1235
  service delivery process, 1227–1230
    assessment, 1228, 1229(t)
    fitting, 1228
    funding and ordering, 1228
    identification of need and referral, 1227–1228
    maintenance, repairs, and follow-up, 1230
    prescription/selection, 1228
    product preparation, 1228
    user training, 1230
  service delivery team, 1227
  sitting posture, 1230–1233
    benefits of optimal sitting posture, 1233
    factors influencing postural alignment,
      1231–1233, 1232(f)
    optimal postural alignment, 1231
    pelvic position, 1230, 1231(t)
    reference neutral sitting posture, 1230, 1231(f)
  specialty evaluation, 1243–1248
    evaluation and plan of care, 1247
    wheelchair assessment, 1243–1247, 1248(b)
  technologies, 1250–1279, 1251(f)
    seating support system, 1251–1258
    wheeled mobility devices, 1258–1279
  See also Wheelchairs
Wheelchair seating and mobility device (WSMD),
  1226
Wheelchair Skills Test, 778(t), 781, 804
Wheelchair Skills Test 4.1 (WST), 1281(t)
Wheelchair Skills Training Program, 804
Wheelchair symbol, 295
Wheelchair Users Shoulder Pain Index (WUSPI),
  777(t), 781
Wheeled mobility devices, 1258–1279, 1259(f)
  angular frame adjustments, 1260–1261, 1261(f)
  attachment mechanisms, 1261–1262
    arm support assembly, 1262
    foot support assembly, 1261–1262
  components, 1260(f)
  dependent mobility wheelchairs, 1269
    strollers, 1269, 1271(f)
    transport chairs, 1269, 1271(f)

frame linear adjustments, 1259–1260
framework, 1259(*f*)
manual wheelchairs, 1262–1265
wheelchair frame/base considerations, 1259–1262, 1260(*f*)
wheelchair frame options, 1261
See also Power mobility devices; Wheelchairs; Wheelchair seating and mobility (WSM)
Wheel lock extensions, 1261
Wheeze/wheezing, 53–54, 387, 390, 397–398
Whiplash, 989
Whips, 1210(*t*), 1212
Whirlpool
debridement, 498
wound cleansing, 496
White coat hypertension, 57, 427
Whole task training, 344
Width of the walking base, 246(*t*)
Wilson disease (WD), 681
Windows, 308
Windows Media Player, 226
Windswept lower extremity (LE) posture, 1232, 1232(*f*)
Wind-up summation, 975, 988
Wolf Motor Function Test (WMET), 145, 197(*t*), 571
Wolf Motor Function Test Functional Ability Scale (WMFT-FAS), 197(*t*)
Worker-job-environment relationship, 318
Workers' Compensation Commission, 326
Working pressure, 513
Work life integration or reintegration, 320(*t*)
Workload (WL), 423, 426
Workplace, examination of, 318–322
ADA guides, 322
data gathering tools, 320(*t*)
documentation, 320(*t*)
functional capacity evaluation, 320–321, 321(*f*)
job requirements, 318
on-site visits, 321–322
external accessibility, 321
internal accessibility, 321–322, 322(*f*), 323(*f*)
tests and measures, 320(*t*)
Work prosthetics, 1219–1220
Workstations, 321–322, 322(*f*)
Work-to-rest ratio, 343, 345(*t*), 351
World Federation of Neurology Research Group on Motor Neuron Diseases, 643
World Health Organization (WHO), 334, 384, 389
classification schema, 1100
Core Sets, 8
enablement model, 2
hand washing recommendations, 87
health defined by, 272, 1123
ICF endorsed by, 272, 1127
ICIDH disablement model, 2
motor recovery and compensation across levels of ICF, 744(*t*)
pain in children, 1007
palliative care and QOL, 647
Quality of Life BREF (WHO QOL-BREF), 773, 778(*t*), 783

Quality of Life Questionnaire (WHOQOL-100), 662, 1127, 1130(*t*)
scope of SLP practice, 1107
Well-Being Index, 1130(*t*)
Wheelchair Service Delivery Steps, 1227, 1235
See also International Classification of Functioning, Disability and Health (ICF)
Wound Care: A Collaborative Practice Manual for Health Professionals (Bates-Jensen and Sussman), 502
Wound contraction, 949
Wound healing
abnormal, 476–478
clinical signs, 476
complications of chronicity, 477(*f*), 477–478
extrinsic factors, 477
iatrogenic factors, 477
infection, 476–477
intrinsic factors, 477
burns, 948–950
dermal healing, 949–950
epidermal healing, 948–949
cold laser therapy, 508
compression therapy, 480, 512–516
dressings, 508–512
exercise, 517–518
hyperbaric oxygen therapy, 506–507
manual lymphatic drainage, 512, 512(*f*)
mechanical modalities, 502(*f*), 502–506, 503–505(*t*)
negative pressure wound therapy, 507(*f*), 507–508
normal, 471–475
moisture role, 472–473
nutrition role, 473–474
oxygen role, 472
wound characteristics, 474
orthotics, 518–519, 518–519(*f*)
phases, 471–472
inflammation (phase I), 471–472, 476
maturation/remodeling (phase III), 472, 476
proliferation (phase II), 472, 476
positioning, 517
pressure-redistributing devices, 517, 517(*f*)
scar management, 519, 519(*f*)
tools, 493
topical agents, 500–502
acute wounds, 502
analgesics, 501
antibacterials, 501
antiseptics, 500–501
burns, 946, 951(*t*)
growth factors, 501–502
wound closure, 474–475
primary intention, 474
secondary intention, 474–475
tertiary intention, 475
Wound Healing: Evidence-Based Management (McCulloch and Kloth), 502
Wound(s)
burn pathology, 940–941, 941(*t*)
case study, 520–522
cleansing, 496–498

commercial skin and wound cleansers, 498
nonforceful irrigation, 497, 497(*f*)
pulsatile lavage with suction, 496(*f*), 496–497, 498
whirlpool, 496
closure, 474–475
documentation, 475
primary intention, 474
secondary intention, 474–475
tertiary intention, 475
débridement, 498–500
autolytic, 477
burns, 950
defined, 498
nonselective, 498
selective, 498–500, 499(*f*), 500(*f*)
depth, 491
drainage by color and thickness, 491, 491(*t*)
physiology, 471–478
size, 491
staging, 491, 492(*t*)
text on management, 502
See also Wound healing
Wrist-hand orthosis, 1170(*t*)
Wrist(s)
capsular patterns, 116(*t*)
rheumatoid arthritis, 894, 895, 895(*f*)
spasticity in UMN syndrome, 146(*t*)
WSM service delivery team (WSM team), 1227
WWT-simple, 211

X

Xenograft, 952

Y

Yale Multidimensional Pain Inventory, 1031
Yamax Digi-Walker SW-701, 249
Yellow flags
arthritis, 914, 915(*t*)
chronic pain, 979, 979(*t*), 982(*f*), 984–985, 992
musculoskeletal, 105, 108, 109
Yerkes-Dodson law, 135
Young stroke, 527

Z

Zaleplon (Sonata), 1031(*b*)
Zeno Walkway system, 250, 254(*t*), 255(*f*)
Zolpidem (Ambien), 1031(*b*)
Zone of coagulation, 945, 945(*f*)
Zone of hyperemia, 945–946
Zone of infarction, 433(*t*)
Zone of injury, 433(*t*)
Zone of ischemia, 433(*t*)
Zone of partial preservation, spinal cord injury and, 763
Zone of stasis, 945
Zones of partial preservation (ZPPs), 72, 763
Z-plasty, 953, 953(*f*)